# REESE AND BETTS'

# A PRACTICAL APPROA[illegible] TO INFE[illegible]ES

[illegible]ON



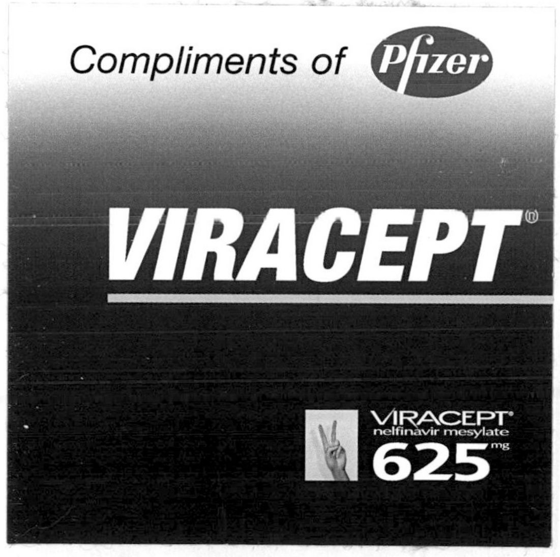

## CONTENTS

## CONTRIBUTING AUTHORS

**Robert F. Betts, M.D.**
*Professor of Medicine, Department of Medicine, Division of Infectious Diseases, University of Rochester School of Medicine and Dentistry, Rochester, New York*

**James R. Burton, Jr., M.D.**
*Hepatology Fellow, Oregon Health Sciences University, Portland, Oregon*

**Stanley W. Chapman, M.D.**
*Professor of Medicine, Associate Professor of Microbiology, Vice Chairman, Department of Medicine, Director, Division of Infectious Diseases, University of Mississippi Medical Center, Jackson, Mississippi*

**Susan E. Cohn, M.D.**
*Associate Professor of Medicine, University of Rochester Medical Center, Rochester, New York*

**J. Thomas Cross, Jr., M.D., M.P.H.**
*Associate Professor, Department of Medicine, Section of Infectious Diseases, Louisiana State University Health Sciences Center–Shreveport, Shreveport, Louisiana*

**Richard D. deShazo, M.D.**
*Professor of Medicine and Pediatrics, Chairman, Department of Medicine, Division of Allergy and Immunology, University of Mississippi Medical Center, Jackson, Mississippi*

**Nancy J. Dorman, M.D., Ph.D.**
*Professor, Department of Medicine, Division of Infectious Diseases, University of Mississippi Medical Center, Jackson, Mississippi*

**Marlene L. Durand, M.D.**
*Assistant Professor, Department of Medicine, Harvard Medical School; Director, Infectious Disease Service, Massachusetts Eye and Ear Infirmary; Assistant Physician, Massachusetts General Hospital, Boston, Massachusetts*

**Paul J. Edelson, M.D.**
*Professor of Pediatrics, Center for the Study of Society and Medicine, College of Physicians and Surgeons, Columbia University, New York, New York*

**Paul S. Graman, M.D.**
*Associate Professor of Medicine, University of Rochester School of Medicine and Dentistry, Rochester, New York*

**Caroline Breese Hall, M.D.**
*Professor of Pediatrics and Medicine, Division of Infectious Diseases, University of Rochester Medical Center, Rochester, New York*

**Rayhan H. Hashmey, M.D.**
*Assistant Professor of Internal Medicine, Division of Infectious Diseases, University of Texas Medical Branch, Galveston, Texas*

**Harold M. Henderson, M.D.**
*Associate Professor, Department of Medicine, Division of Infectious Diseases, University of Mississippi Medical Center, Jackson, Mississippi*

**David R. Hill, M.D., D.T.M.&H.**
*Professor of Medicine, Division of Infectious Diseases, University of Connecticut School of Medicine, Farmington, Connecticut*

**Eric R. Houpt, M.D.**
*Fellow in Infectious Diseases, Department of Internal Medicine, Division of Infectious Diseases, University of Virginia Health System, Charlottesville, Virginia*

**Sally H. Houston, M.D., F.A.C.P**
*Associate Professor of Medicine, University of South Florida College of Medicine, Infectious Diseases Center, Tampa, Florida*

**Stephen R. Jones, M.D.**
*Associate Professor of Medicine, Oregon Health Sciences University; Chief, Department of Medicine, Good Samaritan Hospital and Medical Center, Portland, Oregon*

**Adolf W. Karchmer, M.D.**
*Professor of Medicine, Harvard Medical School; Chief, Division of Infectious Disease, Beth Israel Deaconness Medical Center, Boston, Massachusetts*

**Stephen F. Kemp, M.D.**
*Assistant Professor of Medicine and Pediatrics, Department of Medicine, Division of Allergy and Immunology, University of Mississippi Medical Center, Jackson, Mississippi*

**Fred A. Lopez, M.D.**
*Assistant Professor and Vice Chair, Department of Medicine and Section of Infectious Diseases, Louisiana State University School of Medicine, New Orleans, Louisiana*

**Amneris E. Luque, M.D.**
*Associate Professor of Medicine, University of Rochester School of Medicine and Dentistry, Rochester, New York*

**C. Richard Magnussen, M.D.**
*Associate Professor of Medicine, University of Rochester School of Medicine and Dentistry; Associate Medical Director, Highland Hospital, Rochester, New York*

**Peter R. Mariuz, M.D.**
*Associate Professor of Medicine, University of Rochester School of Medicine and Dentistry, Rochester, New York*

**Marilyn A. Menegus, Ph.D.**
*Professor, Department of Microbiology and Immunology, University of Rochester Medical Center, Rochester, New York*

**Candace L. Mitchell, M.D.**
*Fellow, Department of Medicine, Section of Infectious Diseases, Louisiana State University Health Sciences Center–Shreveport, Shreveport, Louisiana*

**Rathel L. Nolan, M.D.**
*Associate Professor, Department of Medicine, Division of Infectious Diseases, University of Mississippi Medical Center, Jackson, Mississippi*

**Richard D. Pearson, M.D.**
*Professor of Medicine and Pathology, Department of Medicine, Division of Geographic and International Medicine, University of Virginia School of Medicine, Charlottesville, Virginia*

**Robert L. Penn, M.D.**
*Professor of Medicine, Chief Infectious Diseases Section, Department of Medicine, Louisiana State University Health Sciences Center, Shreveport, Louisiana*

**Richard E. Reese, M.D.**
*Clinical Professor, Department of Medicine, University of New England College of Osteopathic Medicine, Beddeford, Maine*

**Michael F. Rein, M.D.**
*Professor of Medicine, Department of Internal Medicine, Division of Infectious Diseases, University of Virginia Health System, Charlottesville, Virginia*

**Norbert J. Roberts, Jr., M.D.**
*Paul R. Stalnaker Distinguished Professor of Internal Medicine, Professor of Microbiology and Immunology, Director, Division of Infectious Diseases, University of Texas Medical Branch, Galveston, Texas*

**Charles V. Sanders, M.D.**
*Edgar Hull Professor and Chairman, Department of Medicine and Section of Infectious Diseases, Louisiana State University School of Medicine, New Orleans, Louisiana*

**W. Michael Scheld, M.D.**
*Professor of Medicine and Neurosurgery, Division of Infectious Diseases, University of Virginia Health Sciences Center, Charlottesville, Virginia*

**Deborah E. Sentochnik, M.D.**
*Bassett Healthcare, Cooperstown, New York*

**Kent A. Sepkowitz, M.D.**
*Head, Clinical Infectious Disease Section, Memorial Sloan Kettering Cancer Center; Associate Professor of Medicine, Weill Medical College of Cornell University, Memorial Sloan Kettering Cancer Center, New York, New York*

**Thomas A. Shaw-Stiffel, M.D.C.M., M.M.M., F.A.C.P**
*Medical Director of Liver Transplantation and Director of Hepatology, University of Rochester; Department of Medicine, Strong Memorial Hospital, Rochester, New York*

**JoAnn Palumbo Shea, A.R.N.P, M.S.N.**
*Clinical Instructor of Internal Medicine, University of South Florida College of Medicine, Tampa, Florida*

**George K. Siberry, M.D., M.P.H.**
*Fellow, Department of Pediatric Infectious Diseases, Johns Hopkins University School of Medicine, Baltimore, Maryland*

**John T. Sinnott, M.D., F.A.C.P**
*Professor of Medicine, Chief, Division of Infectious Diseases and Tropical Medicine, University of South Florida College of Medicine, Tampa General Hospital, Tampa, Florida*

**John W. Sixbey, M.D.**
*Departments of Microbiology, Immunology, and Medicine, Feist-Weiller Cancer Center, Louisiana State University Health Sciences Center, Shreveport, Louisiana*

**Mark C. Steinhoff, M.D.**
*Professor, School of Public Health and School of Medicine, Johns Hopkins University; Department of Pediatrics, Johns Hopkins Hospitals, Baltimore, Maryland*

**Jin S. Suh, M.D.**
*Assistant Clinical Professor of Medicine, Columbia University College of Physicians and Surgeons; Associate Medical Director, The Center for Comprehensive Care, St. Luke's-Roosevelt Hospital, New York, New York*

**John J. Treanor, M.D.**
*Associate Professor of Medicine, University of Rochester School of Medicine and Dentistry, Rochester, New York*

**Allan R. Tunkel, M.D., Ph.D.**
*Professor of Medicine, MCP Hahnemann University, Philadelphia, Pennsylvania*

**Thomas T. Ward, M.D.**
*Associate Professor of Medicine, Oregon Health Sciences University; Chief of Infectious Diseases Section, Veterans Affairs Medical Center, Portland, Oregon*

**Geoffrey A. Weinberg, M.D.**
*Associate Professor of Pediatrics, University of Rochester School of Medicine and Dentistry, Rochester, New York*

# PREFACE

When our chief resident was asked what he thought of *Reese and Betts' A Practical Approach to Infectious Diseases,* he responded, "It is logically organized and thoroughly referenced. It provides a comprehensive, up-to-date guide for diagnosing and managing common and obscure infectious diseases. It is an invaluable resource for any resident or practicing physician."

This book was written to provide helpful information on infectious disease problems for medical students, house officers, community practicing physicians, and other health care practitioners such as hospitalists, nurses, and infection control officers.

*Reese and Betts' A Practical Approach to Infectious Diseases* uses an outline format to make the information readily available and succinct. This approach provides the reader with rapid access to the information that they need to find, while at the same time it leads their thinking in a logical fashion step-by-step through the management of the problem at hand. Up-to-date references are provided for readers to expand their understanding of the specific problem with which they are confronted.

The original intent of this text, when it was conceived by Dr. Richard Reese during his fellowship in infectious diseases in the late 1970's, was to answer the questions most often asked of the infectious disease consultant by the practicing physician. That philosophy is maintained in this edition. The difference between this edition and the earlier ones is that some of the questions have changed, and some quite dramatically.

This new edition provides the reader with up-to-date information in several areas: In-depth discussions of the rapidly emerging resistant gram positive, gram-negative, and mycobacterial infections, and the newest antimicrobial approach to combat these problems of resistance is discussed in detail in the respective chapters; analysis of evolving fungal infections and the new antifungal agents, some of which are not yet fully approved; an in-depth analysis of antivirals available to combat HIV infection is provided, as well as thoughtful analysis of their use in adults, in children, and in pregnant women, and will bring the generalist and the infectious diseases expert up-to-date in this field; investigational new antiretroviral agents are presented; emerging problems in bioterrorism can be found in the pneumonia and skin and soft tissue chapters; and each of the organ system chapters provides new information that has emerged since the last edition.

Whether in the intensive care unit, in the emergency department, or in the office, the practitioner can turn to this compact, yet complete, text to find the answers that he or she needs. The problem may be as complicated as a bone marrow transplant patient with fever and a new pulmonary infiltrate; or an HIV-infected patient who has failed previous regimens; or it may be as straightforward as the office patient with an upper respiratory infection or with cellulitis. The information to help the practitioner think through a logical approach to these and many other problems is provided.

An additional, and unusual, feature of this text is the inclusion of hard-to-find information on the approach to infection in the neonate, infections of the eye, use of vaccines to prevent infectious diseases problems, in-depth information on international travel, infections in transplantation patients, and management of employee health problems.

What prompted us to bring this new edition forward is the excellent response we have had from the house staff and students who have used our book previously. They have urged us to update the information and we have responded with this new edition.

We thank all of our contributors for their outstanding effort to update their contributions and Dr. Geneen Gibson, who provided the important cost information concerning antibiotics. Dr. Richard Reese was most helpful with suggestions along the way. We acknowledge Margaret Aldrich, who helped prepare portions of the text. We extend our sincere appreciation to Hal Pollard and Denise Martin of Lippincott Williams & Wilkins for helping us keep up the momentum that led to the completion of the task. Most of all, we thank our wives Sherrill, Rachel, and Stephanie, without whose patient understanding and support we could not have completed this work.

Robert F. Betts, M.D.
Stanley W. Chapman, M.D.
Robert L. Penn, M.D.

thus, active transport systems have been postulated as a potential entry mechanism [28,29]. It also has been proposed that the cytokines may circumvent the BBB by acting on the **organum vasculosum laminae terminalis** (OVLT), an organ that lacks the BBB. More recently, chemosensitive abdominal vagal afferents have been shown to participate in neural pyrogen signaling to the brain [30–33].

A relatively recent field of investigation has arisen from the recognition that **several endogenous antipyretic systems exist that can modulate the fever response.** Exogenous pyrogens such as viruses induce the concomitant production of both IL-1 and inhibitors of IL-1, or IL-1 receptor antagonists (IL-1ra), by monocytes-macrophages [34,35]. Treatment of rats with anti–IL-1ra at the time of LPS injection significantly prolonged the duration of fever [36]. IL-10 and TNF-$\alpha$ (in subpyrogenic doses) inhibit LPS-induced fever in mice [37,38]. In addition, IL-1 induces the release of stress hormones—including adrenocorticotropic hormone (ACTH), melanocortin, and vasopressin—which possess a broad range of antiinflammatory and cytokine-inhibitory properties [6,22,37–40]. The full breadth of biologic activity of these endogenous cryogens are currently being determined, and it is likely that the febrile and other acute responses to infection or similar pyrogenic challenges are regulated in an integrated fashion by the several mediators that are produced [40,41]. Such observations extend our knowledge well beyond the long-recognized activation of the pituitary–adrenal axis during an infection, and the cortisol-mediated or other glucocorticoid-mediated suppression of the immune response, including production of the proinflammatory cytokines IL-1, TNF, and IL-6.

**B. The sepsis syndrome and septic shock.** (Sepsis is discussed in detail in Chapter 2.) It is important to note here that many of the features of the sepsis syndrome and septic shock have been related to production of the proinflammatory cytokines associated with fever, particularly TNF [24]. Interference with the inflammatory cascade, it was thought, would provide non–etiology-specific intervention that would likely affect the outcome by providing support until specific medical intervention (administration of antimicrobial or other appropriate agents) or specific immune responses become effective. However, blockade of cytokine mediators and their receptors has not proved therapeutically successful, because blockade of mediators alone does not block the direct activation of processes such as coagulation and complement in efforts to reduce the morbidity and mortality of sepsis and septic shock [42–44].

**C. Central nervous system events in the production of fever.** The **preoptic area (POA)** of the anterior hypothalamus appears to be the major thermoregulatory center. Although the POA reacts rapidly to locally injected IL-1, it is unclear whether pyrogenic cytokines cross the BBB in sufficient amounts to induce fever directly, or act by release of secondary mediators, especially prostaglandin-E from the OVLT [30,45–48]. The POA contains temperature-sensitive neurons that respond not only to changes in core temperature by altering firing rates, but also react to afferent sensory input from thermoreceptors throughout the body. Because of the rapidity of onset of fever after injection of LPS and the delay in appearance of cytokines in the blood, neural pathways of pyrogen signaling to the brain have been proposed with evidence emerging especially for the vagus nerve [30–33].

**III. Metabolic and physiologic responses, and the acute-phase reaction.** A variety of physiologic and metabolic alterations begin at the onset of an infection or shortly thereafter [3,24,49–53]. Many of these changes were considered to be the results of the accompanying fever, but they also might ensue from the direct action of the proinflammatory cytokine mediators induced by the invading microorganisms or their products (see section **II.A**). The extent to which physiologic responses are due to, or aggravated by, temperature elevation of a fever as opposed to resulting from direct coordinated effects of proinflammatory cytokines is still being delineated.

**A.** Prominent **metabolic changes** associated with pyrogenic infections and other etiologies of fever include:

1. **Metabolic rate increases** of approximately 10% to 12% with each 1°C elevation in body temperature. If the need for calories and amino acids is not met, body wasting can eventually ensue.

2. **Increased insensible water loss,** which is influenced by the degree of fever, hyperpnea, humidity, and ambient temperature. Generally, there will be an increased loss of 300 to 500 mL/m$^2$/°C/day.
3. **Heart rate increases** of up to 15 beats/min per °C increase in temperature, which could induce heart failure or angina in individuals with significant cardiovascular disease.
4. **Electrolyte depletion** through loss via sweating and, if associated with the infection, via diarrhea or vomiting.

B. **Secondary nutritional consequences** (the "costs") of an acute infection or recurrent mild infections are unlikely to be significant for the well-nourished child or adult but may be substantial for those who are marginally nourished and are severely or frequently challenged by infection [3]. The latter individuals are susceptible to a vicious cycle: malnutrition leading to increased susceptibility to infection leading to increasing malnutrition [3].

C. **Altered hepatocyte functions** in acute generalized infection include the following [24,53,54]: increased uptake of free amino acids from plasma, increased gluconeogenesis with glycogenolysis, increased ureagenesis, increased liponeogenesis, impaired ketogenesis, increased uptake and sequestration of iron (in transferrin and hemosiderin) and zinc (with metallothionein), and synthesis of acute-phase proteins (see section **D**).

Some metabolic changes vary during the course of an infection. For example, hyperglycemia may be a prominent feature early in the infection, whereas hypoglycemia secondary to depletion of carbohydrate stores may be troublesome later in the course of an uncontrolled infection.

D. In the **acute-phase response,** certain proteins, referred to collectively as **acute-phase reactants,** are synthesized by the liver in response to the proinflammatory cytokines IL-1, TNF, and IL-6 [53,55,56]. Changes in these proteins (C-reactive protein, $\alpha_1$-antitrypsin, haptoglobin, serum amyloid P component, serum amyloid A protein, and others) commonly are associated with the temperature elevation of a fever, but their precise roles in host defense are not entirely clear [56]. Despite production of acute-phase proteins, there is an overall negative nitrogen balance. Furthermore, additional changes in other body constituents such as circulating iron or zinc, which decrease in this setting [51,54,57], are commonly associated with infection and the febrile response and may play integrated roles in host defense (see section **V**).

## IV. Fever patterns

A. **Background.** Before the advent of modern diagnostic techniques, the pattern of the febrile response was stressed as an important diagnostic clue. **Generally, a fever pattern (temperature course) cannot be considered pathognomonic for a particular infectious agent in a given patient** [19]. (See section **B.7** and the next major section of this chapter regarding drug fever, which illustrate this important point.) Despite this general concept, in certain circumstances (and especially when combined with other information) the fever curve may provide a clue to the etiology of the fever.

B. **Types of fever** (temperature over time). Because fever patterns often are discussed in the literature and at times provide some clinical clues, they are summarized briefly here. As noted earlier, diurnal variation often is preserved during a febrile episode, with more than 90% of patients with remittent or intermittent fever due to infection showing diurnal variation in one study [19].

1. **Intermittent fevers** are characterized by wide swings in temperature (>0.3°C [0.5°F] and <1.4°C [2.5°F]), with the temperature returning to normal at least once during any 24-hour period. This is the second most common type of fever encountered by an infectious diseases consulting service [19].
   a. **Pyogenic abscesses and irregular use of antipyretics are the most common causes** of the intermittent pattern. This pattern also can be seen in disseminated tuberculosis, acute pyelonephritis with bacteremia, and malaria.
   b. **A double fever spike** occurring daily is said to be suggestive of gonococcal endocarditis and has been noted with miliary tuberculosis. It is also

much more commonly associated with sporadic use of antipyretics in a febrile patient.

c. **Variants of intermittent fevers**

(1) Alternate-day fever may be seen in *Plasmodium vivax* infections and steroid withdrawal fevers (patients on alternate-day dosage schedules).

(2) Fever spikes every third day occur in *Plasmodium malariae* infections.

(3) Any form of malaria in the early stages of infection may present with intermittent or remittent fevers without periodicity.

2. **Remittent fever** is similar to intermittent fever except the fluctuations in temperature are less dramatic and the temperature does not return to normal. This is the most common type of fever encountered by an infectious diseases consulting service [19]. Examples include acute respiratory viral infections, mycoplasmal pneumonia, and *Plasmodium falciparum* malaria.
3. **Hectic ("septic") fever** can be either an intermittent or a remittent fever with a difference of 1.4°C (2.5°F) or more between peak and trough temperatures.
4. **Sustained (continuous) fever** is a moderately persistent elevation in temperature with only minimal fluctuations. Examples include gram-negative bacterial pneumonia, brucellosis, typhoid fever, tularemia, psittacosis, pneumococcal pneumonia, rickettsial infections, and fever in a comatose patient with central nervous system (CNS) damage.
5. **Relapsing (recurrent) fever** is characterized by periods of fever and periods of normal temperature alternating cyclically. During the febrile episodes, the fever may follow any of the previously listed patterns. Examples include lymphomas, rat-bite fever, borreliosis, and dengue.
6. **Temperature-pulse disparity** (i.e., high temperature with a relatively slow pulse) may be seen in factitious fever, brucellosis, typhoid fever, psittacosis and Legionnaires disease. A clue to factitious fever may be the absence of diurnal variation when there is no hypothalamic disease.
7. **Drug fever** may present with any of the patterns described in sections **1 through 6** [18,19]. Hectic fever spikes may simulate sepsis at times. Drug fever is discussed in more detail later in this chapter.

C. **Hyperpyrexia, heatstroke (hyperthermia), and malignant hyperthermia.** Extreme temperature elevation often generates concern in both parents and physicians. However, as noted earlier, temperatures exceeding 41°C (105.8°F) are rare even with infections commonly associated with high fevers [22]. Thermoregulatory failure resulting in hyperpyrexia is more likely to occur at extremes of age and in patients with debilitating illness. Infection appears to be an important trigger. During the 1995 heat wave in Chicago, 57% of heatstroke victims had evidence of infection on admission to the hospital [58]. Patients present with signs of fluctuating consciousness and autonomic nervous system lability. Tachycardia and blood pressure instability are common. Hyperpyrexia also can be triggered in susceptible individuals after severe exercise in hot conditions or exposure to suxamethonium or halogenated anesthetic agents [20]. When precipitated by the effects of neuroleptic drugs (e.g., butyrophenones, loxapine, phenothiazines, thioxanthenes, antidepressants, and antiemetics), it is called **neuroleptic malignant syndrome.** A dangerous hypermetabolic state results, often accompanied by increased muscle tone and rhabdomyolysis. A specific inherited muscle membrane defect related to mutation in the ryanosine receptor (RYR) gene has been detected in 20% of cases [20,59,60]. There is increasing evidence that tissue injury, especially endothelial damage, results from extreme elevations in temperature [21,61]. Immediate action to decrease the core body temperature using external cooling methods is imperative (see section **VII**). **Dantrolene sodium is considered the drug of choice to treat malignant hyperthermia** (2.5 mg/kg intravenously (i.v.) initially, with total doses up to 10.0 mg/kg i.v. to control the event) [20].

D. **Attenuated fever responses.** Although significant infection may exist, fever sometimes may be absent.

1. **Seriously ill newborns** with infection may lack a fever or may even have subnormal temperatures. (In contrast, young children may have exaggerated febrile responses to relatively insignificant infections.)

2. **Elderly patients** occasionally do not exhibit a febrile response [62] or, when febrile, have a limited response compared with a younger patient.
3. Patients with **uremia** may not have a fever or may have a fever with temperatures normally not considered febrile. (Such patients may have a basal temperature somewhat lower than normal, and a temperature in the usual high-normal range might therefore represent a fever for them.)
4. **Significantly malnourished individuals** may show reduced production of the proinflammatory cytokines and a diminished febrile response [3].
5. Patients receiving **corticosteroids** or **continuous treatment with antiinflammatory or antipyretic agents** may not have a febrile response.

V. **Potential reasons for not treating fever.** There seems to be a tendency—almost a reflex—among physicians as well as parents to attempt to lower body temperature in a patient with fever, an attitude that likely stems from a general belief that fever is noxious to the body [63,64]. Although associated with seizures in young children, fever per se has not been shown to be harmful in humans and there is no evidence to suggest that its suppression, at least in the short term, is beneficial. In fact, conservation of the febrile response across the animal kingdom argues strongly that fever is a protective and adaptive response, and the decision to use antipyretic therapy should be weighed carefully.

Experiments using animal models have demonstrated the beneficial effect of fever in enhancing resistance to infection. Elegant experiments using the poikilothermic lizard *Dipsosauras dorsalis* showed a direct correlation between temperature and survival from infection with *Aeromonas hydrophilia* [65]. Increased resistance to a variety of viruses also has been demonstrated using mice, dogs, and ferrets [64,66]. Immunologic pathogen-specific responses are generally enhanced in the setting of temperature elevation within the physiologic range [41]. Temperature elevation appears to affect primarily the phase of recognition and sensitization or activation of mononuclear leukocytes. Evans et al. showed that fever-range temperatures caused a three- to fourfold increase in L-selectin and $\alpha_4\beta_7$ integrin-dependent trafficking of lymphocytes to secondary lymphoid tissues [67,68].

Good clinical data regarding the role of fever in recovery from infection are lacking. Studies based on retrospective analysis and chart reviews support the relationship between a febrile response and favorable outcome [6,64]. Antipyretic therapy has not been shown to protect against recurrence of febrile seizures in children [69]. In addition to the inherent toxicities of antipyretic compounds [70], studies have shown adverse effects of aspirin or acetaminophen therapy on parameters associated with recovery from infection (e.g., prolonged shedding of rhinovirus or varicella virus [during chickenpox] [71]).

Fever remains one of the sentinel indicators of disease and is one of the most frequent causes prompting patients to seek medical attention. Its persistence may aid in the evaluation of a chosen therapeutic regimen, as well as redirect investigation to rule out noninfectious etiologies. **The decision regarding whether to treat a fever per se (and if so, how) should be a considered decision every time,** not merely a routine, predetermined response to detection of a fever.

VI. **Potential reasons to treat fever.** The preceding section discusses reasons why most individuals and the human species overall may benefit from the existence of the febrile response. Nonetheless, individual subjects may be anticipated to have morbidity—derived from the fever—that is unacceptable in the context of current therapeutic capabilities and sound medical judgment regarding relative risks. Specific situations exist where use of antipyresis may be justified. It has been argued that elderly individuals with pulmonary and cardiovascular disease are particularly vulnerable to the additional metabolic and cardiovascular effects of a fever-related temperature elevation, which could lead to greater morbidity or even increased risk of mortality. Additionally, persistence of fever could have detrimental metabolic consequences, exacerbating poor nutrition or dehydration, particularly if the fever is prolonged. Risks considered in the analysis should also include nonmedical factors such as interference with required daily activities due to illness (which might be alleviated by analgesia or antipyresis). It is thus reemphasized that **the decision regarding whether to suppress a fever should be specific for the individual patient.**

**VII. Methods of lowering temperature.** Antipyretic orders commonly are written imprecisely and as a routine for hospitalized patients; acknowledgment of the intervention appears in the progress notes for only a small percentage of patients, with a rationale appearing even less frequently [72].

The most common antipyretic order may be for as-needed administration, often not even prompted by detection of a fever. If aspirin or another antipyretic agent is given intermittently in response to fever spikes, its use may cause precipitous decreases in temperature and produce a hectic fever that is more stressful for the host than maintenance of a continued febrile temperature.

**If the decision is made to suppress a patient's fever, it is usually more appropriate to do so by continuous administration of the antipyretic for a period of time** (24–48 hours) after the fever's characteristics have been noted, followed by withholding of the antipyretic agent to determine whether the fever persists. The withholding of antipyretic therapy allows one to observe the temperature curve for evidence of therapeutic efficacy if antimicrobial or other agents have been administered (i.e., absence of fever with appropriate specific therapy for the infection or illness responsible for inducing the fever) and, in the absence of such evidence, indicates the potential need for further evaluation.

**A. Antipyretics**

1. **Nonsteroidal antiinflammatory drugs (NSAIDs). Aspirin** is the prototypic drug of this class and has been in clinical use for more than 100 years. Examples of other drugs in this class include indomethacin, ibuprofen, naproxen, and diclofenac. NSAIDs act by inhibiting cyclooxygenase (COX), the rate-limiting enzyme in prostaglandin synthesis, thereby producing potent antipyretic, analgesic, and antiinflammatory effects [73]. Inhibition of COX is also responsible for the serious toxicities associated with NSAIDs, which include renal insufficiency, gastrointestinal (GI) tract ulcers, and coagulation abnormalities [70]. More recently, the discovery of two distinct isozymes of COX (COX-1, present constitutively in cells and involved in tissue homeostasis; and COX-2, the inducible, "inflammatory" form) has led to the development of isozyme-specific drugs (COX-2 selective), with safer toxicity profiles [74–76]. Two drugs, celecoxib and rofecoxib, are currently available. However, it appears that these drugs are not completely devoid of GI side effects, with cost-effective benefit demonstrable only in patients at high risk for GI bleeding [77].
2. **Alternatives to NSAIDs** are necessary in allergic or anticoagulated patients, or in patients who have hemostatic or platelet abnormalities or GI tract ulcers, or who are otherwise intolerant of these agents. Additionally, it is **advisable to avoid salicylates to treat fever in children with viral illnesses, particularly chickenpox and influenza-like illnesses, because salicylate use has been associated with Reye syndrome** (see Chapter 10). **Acetaminophen** is often used as an aspirin substitute and is approximately as effective as aspirin in reducing fever in either adults or children [78]; however, it possesses weak antiinflammatory properties. It has been postulated that acetaminophen acts on a yet unidentified isoform of COX (?COX-3), mainly in the central nervous system [73].
3. **Duration.** In patients with infectious causes of fever, specific antibiotic therapy alone usually controls infection and fever within 24 to 72 hours (or, in a viral syndrome, the acute febrile phase may be over in 1–3 days). At this point if not before, it is advantageous to withhold antipyretic therapy as noted previously and to monitor the temperature to determine whether it would be appropriate to discontinue the aspirin (or alternate antipyretic agent).

**B. Sponging the body** with isopropyl alcohol or water may be done. Because water has the highest heat of vaporization, it is the preferred liquid. Tepid (rather than cold) water may decrease the tendency toward peripheral vasoconstriction, a counterproductive reflex.

**C.** The **Turkish massage of Weinstein** [79] is a method of reducing fever by rubbing the patient's skin with a Turkish towel and tepid water. This method takes advantage of the heat of vaporization while encouraging cutaneous vasodilatation. The increased cutaneous blood flow functions as a heat exchanger, and core temperature is lowered.

**D. Cooling blankets** also are popular and may have an appropriate role in temperature reduction. These blankets enhance conductive heat loss and are effective. However, the clinician should not attempt to reduce the temperature to normal, which may result in hypothermia by "overshooting." The body responds with peripheral vasoconstriction and shivering, making the patient feel miserable. **The cooling blanket should be turned off when body temperature reaches approximately 37.7° to 38.3°C (100°–101°F), to minimize overshooting.** When possible, an antipyretic drug should be used in association with the cooling blanket in an attempt to blunt wide swings in temperature.

**E. Combined evaporation and convection.** Sprays of tepid water at an ambient temperature of 20°C have been used effectively to treat heatstroke victims during the annual pilgrimage at Mecca [80]. Water can be atomized under pressure and combined with air blown by a fan.

**F. Ice water immersion.** Although there is no agreement on the most effective way of quickly reducing the core body temperature, one commonly used method is to immerse the patient in an ice-water bath until the temperature is reduced to 39.5°C (103°F) [81]. At this point more moderate measures (see sections A, B, and D) should be continued to control the fever.

## DRUG FEVER

Drugs are a fairly common cause of fever [18,82,83]. **Drug fever should be suspected** whenever a fever occurs (with or without associated findings) in a patient who is taking a drug known to produce fever (Table 1.1). The diagnosis should always be considered, but **especially when the patient either looks or feels well** on current therapy and has no obvious uncontrolled or superimposed infections or is at least hemodynamically stable with no localized infection. Antimicrobial agents, as a group, have been linked to the greatest number of cases [84]. Rigors (43% [corrected calculation]), myalgias (25%), rashes (18%, less than half pruritic), headache (18%), relative bradycardia, leukocytosis (22%), eosinophilia (22%), serum sickness, abnormal liver function tests, and proteinuria may occur [18].

**Onset** occurs typically within 10 days after a patient begins taking a drug [85]. **Discontinuation of the suspect drug** with a decrease in the temperature within 1 or 2 days lends support to the diagnosis. **Rechallenge with the offending agent is not generally recommended** unless done carefully in a controlled setting (i.e., in a hospital). However, one study suggested that rechallenge with agents responsible for drug fever (>45% of cases reported) was associated with a low risk of serious sequelae, although it was not altogether free from risk [18].

Table 1.1. Agents Responsible for Episodes of Drug Fever

| Common | Less Common | Rare |
|---|---|---|
| Atropine | Allopurinol | Salicylates |
| Amphotericin B | Azathioprine | Corticosteroids |
| Asparaginase | Cimetidine | Aminoglycosides |
| Barbiturates | Hydralazine | Macrolides |
| Bleomycin | Iodides | Tetracyclines |
| Methyldopa | Isoniazid | Clindamycin |
| Diuretics | Rifampin | Chloramphenicol |
| Penicillins | Streptokinase | Quinolones |
| Cephalosporins | Imipenem | Linezolid |
| Phenytoin | Vancomycin | |
| Procainamide | Calcium channel blockers | |
| Interferon | Beta blockers | |
| | Nonsteroidal antiinflammatory drugs | |

Adapted from Johnson DH, Cunha BA. Drug fever. *Infect Dis Clin North Am* 1996;10:85–91; with permission.

## FEVER OF UNKNOWN ETIOLOGY

**I. Definitions.** Fever of unknown origin (FUO) was defined by Petersdorf and Beeson [86] in 1961 as a febrile illness of more than 3 weeks' duration. To qualify as FUO, temperatures must exceed 38.3°C (101°F) on several determinations with no diagnosis reached after 1 week of study in the hospital. These criteria are chosen because they tend to eliminate acute, self-limited infectious illnesses such as common viral diseases, postoperative fevers, and febrile illnesses of obvious cause; the criteria exclude patients who defervesce spontaneously, and they also allow time for the completion of the usual initial laboratory studies. Because of the expense of hospitalization and the frequent ability to investigate an FUO as an outpatient, **Petersdorf** [87] **modified this definition** by proposing that, in lieu of 1 week in hospital, 1 week of intelligent and intensive investigation be undertaken, which in most patients is possible on an outpatient basis.

**Durack and Street** [88] **have recommended further modifications. They have proposed subdividing FUO into four groups:**

**A. Classic FUO**

1. Fever of 38.3°C (101°F) or higher on several occasions.
2. Fever of more than 3 weeks' duration.
3. Diagnosis uncertain, despite appropriate investigations, after at least three outpatient visits or at least 3 days in hospital.

**B. Nosocomial FUO**

1. Fever of 38.3°C (101°F) or higher on several occasions in a hospitalized patient receiving acute care.
2. Infection not present or incubating on admission.
3. Diagnosis uncertain after 3 days despite appropriate investigation, including at least 2 days' incubation of microbiologic cultures.

**C. Neutropenic FUO**

1. Fever of 38.3°C (101°F) or higher on several occasions.
2. Fewer than 500 neutrophils/$mm^3$ within 1 to 2 days.
3. Diagnosis uncertain after 3 days despite appropriate investigation, including at least 2 days' incubation of microbiologic cultures.

**D. Human immunodeficiency virus (HIV)-associated FUO** [89–93] (see Chapter 18)

1. Fever of 38.3°C (101°F) or higher on several occasions.
2. Confirmed positive serology for HIV infection.
3. Fever of more than 4 weeks' duration for outpatients or more than 3 days' duration in hospital.
4. Diagnosis uncertain after 3 days despite appropriate investigation, including at least 2 days' incubation of microbiologic cultures.

**II. Causes of FUO** [87,94,95]

**A.** Although **infections are still the most common cause of FUOs,** the incidence of multisystem or collagen vascular diseases remains significant and there is a decrease in the number of tumors presenting as FUOs. However, Barbado et al. [96] found that collagen vascular diseases, especially vasculitides, are more frequent (29%) than infections (11%). Endocarditis, abdominal abscesses, and hepatobiliary diseases have become less important causes of FUOs. Tuberculosis remains an important cause of FUO.

1. **Infections (23%–36%).** Tuberculosis, bacterial endocarditis due to slow-growing organisms, culture-negative endocarditis, localized suppurative process (within the biliary tract, liver, or kidney), intraabdominal abscesses, septic pelvic vein thrombophlebitis, and certain viral infections such as cytomegalovirus (CMV) and Epstein-Barr virus (EBV) should be considered. **In HIV-positive patients, however, opportunistic infections (OIs) account for most FUOs** and fever should not be attributed to HIV-infection itself without extensive investigation to rule out other infections [89–93]. Common OIs in the United States include tuberculosis, atypical mycobacterial infections, *Pneumocystis carinii* infection, disseminated fungal infections (e.g., histoplasmosis), and CMV infection. Infection due to *Coccidioides immitis* (Southwest United States), *Trypanosoma cruzii* (Latin America), and *Penicillium marneffei* (Southeast Asia) are endemic in those regions [91,97,98].

2. **Neoplasms (7%–31%).** Lymphoma, leukemia, renal cell carcinoma, GI tumor, and metastatic ovarian carcinoma are the most common neoplasms associated with FUOs. In more recent studies of FUOs [95], there was a marked decrease in the incidence of neoplasms. This is believed to be due to the widespread use of ultrasonography and computed tomography (CT) scanning. In HIV-positive patients, tumors account for only 10% of FUOs, 90% of which are lymphomas [90–92]. Observational and time-trend data indicate that the incidence of Kaposi sarcoma (KS) and primary brain lymphoma have decreased, but suggest that current therapies have not had a proportionate effect on systemic non-Hodgkin lymphomas [99–101]. It is likely that lymphoma will become proportionately more important as an FUO in these patients.
3. **Collagen vascular diseases (9%–20%).** Systemic lupus erythematosus, rheumatoid arthritis, mixed connective tissue diseases, temporal arteritis, juvenile rheumatoid arthritis of the adult (adult Still disease), and vasculitis can present as an FUO.
4. **Miscellaneous causes (17%–24%)** include drug fever, recurrent pulmonary emboli, inflammatory bowel disease (especially regional enteritis), sarcoidosis, and factitious or fraudulent fever. However, there are numerous unusual causes of FUOs [102,103].
5. **In adults, 10% of FUOs remain undiagnosed.** In Knockaert's study [95], there was a noticeably higher incidence of undiagnosed cases (26%). This is because, in contrast to other reports, Knockaert and co-workers [95] categorized as FUOs fever in patients with diseases of unknown origin, such as granulomatous hepatitis or pericarditis; these were labeled *nondiagnosis* rather than being relegated to the miscellaneous category [87]. It is reassuring, though, that the vast majority of patients that remain undiagnosed do well in follow-up [104–106].
6. **The spectrum of causes** of FUOs among community hospital patients and the elderly (≥65 years old) is similar to the general population, with a few noticeable differences [107–109]. In the community hospital group, infections (abscesses, tuberculosis, endocarditis, acute HIV infection, and CMV) represented approximately 33% of the FUO population; neoplasms, primarily lymphomas, were present in 24% of the population; and 16% had collagen vascular diseases. Alcoholic hepatitis and recurrent pulmonary emboli are relatively common in this group. The most common causes of FUOs in the elderly are leukemias, lymphomas, abscesses, tuberculosis, and temporal arteritis.

B. **Factitious fever** refers to fever produced artificially by the patient.

1. **A diagnosis of factitious fever** [110] should be considered in any FUO, especially in young women or persons with medical training, or if the patient looks clinically well and there is a disparity between temperature and pulse. The advent of digital thermometers has reduced the frequency of this diagnosis.
2. **Absence of the normal diurnal pattern** should alert the physician to this diagnostic possibility.
3. Some practitioners recommend several temperature determinations in the presence of a nurse or physician. Others have suggested the use of a thermocoupling device (electric thermometer) to allow immediate recording of results. Urine temperatures also have been suggested as a means to uncover factitious fever due to manipulation of the glass thermometer.
4. The diagnosis should be considered especially in paramedical personnel.

C. **Fraudulent fever** is akin to factitious fever. In this case, the fever is authentic but is induced by the patient's self-inoculation or ingestion of foreign material.

III. **Approach to the FUO.** Although the clinical investigation of a patient with FUO should be individualized, Knockaert [111] has developed a detailed diagnostic strategy for the patient with an FUO. This report also presents an algorithmic approach to the diagnosis of FUOs.

A. **Rule out common infections or other causes of fever.** Although it may seem obvious, initial assessment of the nonseptic febrile patient must rule out the common infections causing fever, including respiratory and urinary tract infections, wound and pelvic infections, GI infections, and superficial and deep phlebitis, including intravenous-related phlebitis in hospitalized patients.

**B. Determine whether the patient has a true FUO.** Before launching what may be an intensive workup for FUO, the fever should be present, at least by history, for a prolonged period as noted above, and the routine evaluation should be unremarkable. Only then may a case be defined as an FUO.

**C. Workup of the patient with a true FUO.**

1. **A careful history is essential** to discover clues from the patient's travel background, exposure to tuberculosis, animal exposure, drug use, work environment, hobbies, geographic origins, HIV risk factors, and other habits. With the differential diagnosis of FUO in mind, the physician explores each of the diagnostic categories. If the workup is unrewarding initially, **serial follow-up histories** may provide additional clues to a specific diagnosis. Interviews with the immediate family or close relatives may be helpful.
2. **A complete and careful physical examination** should be repeated if the patient is believed to have a true FUO. Again, the differential diagnosis is kept in mind and particular attention is directed to the skin, lymph nodes, hepatosplenomegaly, rectal and pelvic examination, and cardiac examination. **Serial physical examinations are crucial!** While the patient is hospitalized, his or her clinical status might change, and a new lymph node, murmur, or rash could appear and provide an important clue to the diagnosis.
3. **Laboratory examinations and biopsies.** By definition, the routine complete blood count, urine and sputum cultures, chest radiograph, and other determinations have already been unrewarding in the early evaluation of the FUO. Studies of antibodies to EBV and CMV, especially IgM antibodies, may be helpful (see Chapter 9). **Further testing must be individualized,** and a variety of tests are available.

**IV. Laboratory and diagnostic aids in the FUO evaluation**

**A. Blood cultures.** Advances in blood culture methodology have resulted in earlier detection of pathogens causing bloodstream infections [112]. **In continuous bacteremia** (such as endocarditis), three sets of blood cultures will be adequate to recover the organism in more than 95% of cases [113]. However, any oral or parenteral antibiotic therapy given before the initial blood cultures are drawn may inhibit the growth of the organisms (e.g., in partially treated BE). In addition, some fastidious organisms may take several days or weeks (e.g., *Brucella*) to grow or may have special growth requirements [112]. Fungal and mycobacterial blood cultures are of particular importance in HIV-positive patients [89–93]. **Culture-negative endocarditis** is a recognized entity that accounts for 5% to 15% of cases of endocarditis (see Chapter 12) [114]. It can occur even in patients who have had no prior exposure to antibiotics and is well described in the literature of the preantibiotic era. **This diagnosis should be considered in the patient with FUO, negative initial blood cultures, and underlying cardiac disease** (such as rheumatic or congenital heart disease). When possible, infectious disease consultation should be sought for such patients before one commits a patient to a prolonged course of antibiotics.

**B. Sedimentation rate.** The erythrocyte sedimentation rate (ESR) is a nonspecific marker of inflammation and can be elevated in noninfectious conditions, for example, in uremia. In the older patient ($\geq$55 years) with FUO and an ESR in excess of 100 mm/h, the diagnosis of **temporal arteritis** should be considered. The patient's history should be reviewed carefully with respect to headaches, visual problems, and myalgias. **When temporal arteritis is suspected, the patient should undergo bilateral temporal artery biopsies** for definitive diagnosis. Initiation of high-dose steroid therapy (e.g., oral prednisone 60–80 mg/day) may help to prevent blindness, a major complication of temporal arteritis.

**C. Collagen vascular disease screening.** Because up to 15% of adult patients with FUO have a collagen vascular disease, histories must be elicited carefully.

1. **ESR** and **antinuclear antibody studies** generally are used for screening.
2. **Muscle or skin biopsies** (or both) of suspicious rashes may uncover a vasculitis.

**D. Serology.** As a general rule, serologic tests assume importance when a fourfold or greater increase in titer can be demonstrated (see Chapter 25). Serologic studies should only be ordered if potential diagnostic clues to a particular infection exist. In a recent prospective study of 167 patients, serologic tests were never helpful in the absence of diagnostic clues [115].

1. **An acute-phase blood sample** should be drawn; serum should then be frozen and set aside in an FUO evaluation. This will assure an early specimen if careful serologic studies are indicated as the workup proceeds.
2. **Blood for convalescent titer** usually is drawn 2 to 4 weeks after the acute titer.
3. Occasionally only a single serum specimen is available for study. Characteristic titer elevations may be very suggestive, or even diagnostic, in certain clinical settings. For example, an indirect fluorescent antibody titer of 1:1,024 or greater to *Toxoplasma gondii* is suggestive of toxoplasmosis. A specific IgM antibody response is highly suggestive of a recent primary infection, more so than is the presence of IgG antibody.

**E. Skin tests**

1. **The intermediate purified protein derivative (PPD) test** should be performed routinely unless the patient is known to be a reactor. A negative test should be repeated in approximately 1 week to test for a "booster effect" (see Chapter 11) [116]. Anergy testing is not routinely recommended [117].
2. **Fungal skin tests** generally are not helpful (see Chapter 17). For example, skin tests with histoplasmin and blastomycin are not useful diagnostically, especially in an endemic area. In addition, these tests may induce an antibody response that would either lead to a false diagnosis or preclude future serologic studies.

**F. Imaging**

1. **CT and magnetic resonance imaging (MRI).** The advent of modern imaging modalities such as CT and MRI has almost completely supplanted older radiographic techniques such as intravenous pyelograms, nephrotomograms, and barium imaging of the GI tract. Due to their greater resolution, they provide a sensitive tool for identifying and localizing intracranial, intraabdominal, and intrathoracic abscesses. MRI with gadolinium contrast is the study of choice for diagnosing intracranial lesions in patients with HIV infection. Due to their wide availability, CT scan and ultrasonography are often used in a blind fashion for detection of intraabdominal abscesses and lesions; thus, their overall diagnostic yield per test performed has been quite low [118]. CT imaging is also used in the guidance of percutaneous procedures in order to enhance the diagnostic yield.
2. **Ultrasonography. Abdominal or pelvic studies** may help localize an abscess or differentiate a solid from a cystic mass. Ultrasonography is useful in visualizing hepatobiliary and renal abnormalities. **Transesophageal echocardiography** has added a new dimension to the sensitivity of detecting valvular vegetations, especially those on prosthetic valves [119]. **Venous duplex imaging** may be useful in identifying cases of deep venous thrombosis as a cause of FUO [120].
3. **Radionuclide scans.** Of the various radiopharmaceutical-based tests available, gallium-67 and indium 111–labeled leukocyte scanning have the highest yield [121]. Indium 111–labeled polyclonal human immunoglobulin (HIG) has not proved to be superior to $^{111}$In leukocyte scanning [121]. Total-body gallium scanning has occasionally been useful in detecting occult abscesses and lymphoma as well as thyroiditis and unusual tumors, such as leiomyosarcoma and pheochromocytoma. Indium 111 is less likely to accumulate in noninfected foci. Bone scans and $^{111}$In scans appear to be useful in distinguishing osteomyelitis from a cellulitis that is in close proximity to the bone. Three-phase bone scanning frequently is not specific enough to delineate cellulitis clearly from osteomyelitis (see Chapter 5). More recently, [(18)F]fluoro-deoxyglucose positron emission tomography scan was used in 58 consecutive cases of FUO and was helpful in reaching a diagnosis in 35% of abnormal scans as compared with 25% with gallium scintigraphy [122].

**G. Tissue biopsies**

1. **Lymph nodes** that are pathologically enlarged should be examined via biopsy early in the workup, because underlying malignancy or granulomatous disease might be uncovered.
2. **Liver.** In patients with hepatomegaly, abnormal liver function test results, or possible miliary tuberculosis or disseminated fungal disease, a liver biopsy may

provide the diagnosis either by histologic examination or by culturing. **The biopsy should be cultured aerobically and anaerobically and for acid-fast organisms and fungi.** The yield in HIV-related FUO appears to be much higher [123]. Rarely, the organism involved in infective endocarditis may be cultured from the liver biopsy.

3. **Bone marrow biopsy.** The overall yield for bone marrow biopsy in FUO is less than 15% [87,94,95], but, as for liver biopsy, it is useful in diagnosing disseminated mycobacterial and fungal infection in the setting of HIV infection, where its diagnostic yield has been as high as 40% [124].
4. **Skin nodules and rashes** may provide a clue to metastatic disease or an underlying vasculitis.
5. **Temporal artery biopsy** (bilateral) may be diagnostic in the elderly patient with an unexplained elevated ESR.

**H. Indications for exploratory laparotomies in patients with FUO.** Exploratory laparotomy seldom is indicated if scanning procedures, ultrasonographic studies, and percutaneous biopsies are used appropriately. Laparotomy is not considered a routine procedure but is reserved as a concluding step in the workup of selected patients [125–127] and for use when abnormalities apparent on scanning need clarification, biopsy, or possible drainage. However, laparoscopy should be considered first if it is technically feasible [128].

**I. Therapeutic drug trials in patients with FUO.** In general, the use of medication in the absence of a definitive diagnosis is discouraged. However, a therapeutic trial may be justified if, after one has done careful investigation and culturing, the clinical and laboratory data support certain etiologies, but a definitive diagnosis cannot be reached. **Infectious disease consultation should be sought in such situations.** A trial of antibiotics in culture-negative endocarditis, and of antituberculous agents in granulomatous hepatitis and cases suspicious for tuberculosis can be life saving.

**V. Miscellaneous diseases that cause FUOs**

**A. Granulomatous hepatitis** may be documented by a liver biopsy performed as part of the FUO evaluation. This represents a histologic reaction pattern with many etiologies, among which are tuberculosis, histoplasmosis, brucellosis, Q fever, syphilis, sarcoidosis, Hodgkin disease, berylliosis, Wegener granulomatosis, and drug reactions.

**B. Juvenile rheumatoid arthritis** is characterized in children by fever, polyarticular or monoarticular arthritis, salmon-colored maculopapular rash, generalized lymphadenopathy, hepatosplenomegaly, and, occasionally, pericarditis (rarely, myocarditis). Iridocyclitis occurs frequently and should be sought by an ophthalmologist, even if ocular symptoms are minimal. Rheumatoid factor is absent. A similar clinical picture may be seen in young adults.

**C. Familial Mediterranean fever (periodic disease)** is an autosomal-recessive disease characterized by periodic fevers contracted predominantly by men, particularly those of Italian, Sephardic Jewish, or Irish descent. Peritonitis, pleuritis, arthritis, and skin lesions may accompany the fever.

**D. Whipple disease** is seen in middle-aged to older men and is characterized by low-grade fever, progressive weight loss, diarrhea, malabsorption, arthralgias, abdominal pain, increased skin pigmentation, and lymphadenopathy. Jejunal biopsy can establish the diagnosis.

**E. Bacterial hepatitis** is comprised of chronic nonsuppurative bacterial infections of the liver (e.g., *Staphylococcus aureus*) other than those causing a granulomatous reaction. Fever and minimally elevated alkaline phosphatase may be the only evidence of liver involvement. A liver biopsy will be helpful and, as usual, the biopsy specimen should be cultured aerobically and anaerobically.

**F. Hyperimmunoglobulinemia D and periodic fever** is a rare syndrome of fever in children of Dutch ancestry that has been linked to a deficiency of mevalonate kinase [129]. The clinical picture is similar to that of familial Mediterranean fever.

**G. Ehrlichiosis.** The majority of symptomatic patients with ehrlichiosis present with an abrupt onset of fever, chills, and headache, often accompanied by nausea, myalgias, arthralgias, and malaise. Roland et al. [130] reported six patients in whom the principal finding was protracted fever ranging from 17 to 51 days' duration. The diagnosis was delayed due to lack of consideration of the diagnosis, patient's delay in seeking medical care, or both [130]. See Chapter 21.

**H. Other** unusual causes of FUO have been described [102,103].

**VI. Recurrent or episodic FUO.** In some patients with a classic FUO, the fever spontaneously resolves for at least 2 weeks and then recurs. On further workup, approximately 20% of these patients will have demonstrable underlying infection, tumor, or connective tissue diseases [106]. Miscellaneous causes (e.g., Crohn disease, factitious fever) are common. Overall, these patients generally do well [106] and often can simply be followed carefully and assessed serially as outpatients.

## REFERENCES

1. McGowan JE Jr, Rose RC, Jacobs NF, et al. Fever in hospitalized patients. With special reference to the medical service. *Am J Med* 1987;82:580–586.
2. Norman DC. Fever in the elderly. *Clin Infect Dis* 2000;31:148–151.
3. Santos JI. Nutrition, infection, and immunocompetence. *Infect Dis Clin North Am* 1994;8:243–267.
4. Lewin S, Brettman LR, Holzman RS. Infections in hypothermic patients. *Arch Intern Med* 1981;141:920–925.
5. Mackowiak PA, Bartlett JG, Borden EC, et al. Concepts of fever: recent advances and lingering dogma. *Clin Infect Dis* 1997;25:119–138.
6. Mackowiak PA. Concepts of fever. *Arch Intern Med* 1998;158:1870–1881.
7. Kluger MJ, Kozak W, Conn CA, et al. *The adaptive value of fever.* In: Mackowiak PA, ed. *Fever: basic mechanisms and management, 2nd ed.* Philadelphia: Lippincott-Raven, 1997:225–226.
8. Schmitt BD. Fever phobia: misconceptions of parents about fevers. *Am J Dis Child* 1980;134:176–181.
9. May A, Bauchner H. Fever phobia: the pediatrician's contribution. *Pediatrics* 1992;90: 851–854.
10. Mackowiak PA, ed. *Fever: basic mechanisms and management, 2nd ed.* Philadelphia: Lippincott-Raven, 1997.
11. Mackowiak PA, Wasserman SS, Levine MM. A critical appraisal of 98.6 degrees F, the upper limit of the normal body temperature, and other legacies of Carl Reinhold August Wunderlich. *JAMA* 1992;268:1578–1580.
12. Amoateng-Adjepong Y, Del Mundo J, Manthous CA. Accuracy of an infrared tympanic thermometer. *Chest* 1999;115:1002–1005.
13. Giuliano KK, Scott SS, Elliot S, et al. Temperature measurement in critically ill orally intubated adults: a comparison of pulmonary artery core, tympanic, and oral methods [see comments]. *Crit Care Med* 1999;27:2188–2193.
14. Giuliano KK, Giuliano AJ, Scott SS, et al. Temperature measurement in critically ill adults: a comparison of tympanic and oral methods. *Am J Crit Care* 2000;9:254–261.
15. Huang HP, Shih HM. Use of infrared thermometry and effect of otitis externa on external ear canal temperature in dogs. *J Am Vet Med Assoc* 1998;213:76–79.
16. Lanham DM, Walker B, Klocke E, et al. Accuracy of tympanic temperature readings in children under 6 years of age. *Pediatr Nurs* 1999;25:39–42.
17. Modell JG, Katholi CR, Kumaramangalam SM, et al. Unreliability of the infrared tympanic thermometer in clinical practice: a comparative study with oral mercury and oral electronic thermometers [see comments]. *South Med J* 1998;91:649–654.
18. Mackowiak PA, LeMaistre CF. Drug fever: a critical appraisal of conventional concepts. An analysis of 51 episodes in two Dallas hospitals and 97 episodes reported in the English literature. *Ann Intern Med* 1987;106:728–733.
19. Musher DM, Fainstein V, Young EJ, et al. Fever patterns. Their lack of clinical significance. *Arch Intern Med* 1979;139:1225–1228.
20. Denborough M. Malignant hyperthermia. *Lancet* 1998;352:1131–1136.
21. Duthie DJ. Heat-related illness. *Lancet* 1998;352:1329–1330.
22. Mackowiak PA, Boulant JA. Fever's glass ceiling. *Clin Infect Dis* 1996;22:525–536.
23. Roberts NJ Jr, Lu ST, Michaelson SM. Hyperthermia and human leukocyte functions: DNA, RNA, and total protein synthesis after exposure to less than 41 degrees or greater than 42.5 degrees hyperthermia. *Cancer Res* 1985;45:3076–3082.

24. Dinarello CA. Cytokines as endogenous pyrogens. *J Infect Dis* 1999;179(suppl 2):294–304.
25. Dinarello CA. Cytokines as endogenous pyrogens. In: Mackowiak PA, ed. *Fever: basic mechanisms and management, 2nd ed.* Philadelphia: Lippincott-Raven, 1997:87–116.
26. Tavares E, Minano FJ. RANTES: a new prostaglandin dependent endogenous pyrogen in the rat. *Neuropharmacology* 2000;39:2505–2513.
27. Akarsu ES, House RV, Coceani F. Formation of interleukin-6 in the brain of the febrile cat: relationship to interleukin-1. *Brain Res* 1998;803:137–143.
28. Banks WA, Kastin AJ. Relative contributions of peripheral and central sources to levels of IL-1 alpha in the cerebral cortex of mice: assessment with species-specific enzyme immunoassays. *J Neuroimmunol* 1997;79:22–28.
29. Banks WA, Kastin AJ, Broadwell RD. Passage of cytokines across the blood-brain barrier. *Neuroimmunomodulation* 1995;2:241–248.
30. Blatteis CM, Sehic E, Li S. Pyrogen sensing and signaling: old views and new concepts. *Clin Infect Dis* 2000;31(suppl 5):168–177.
31. Maier SF, Goehler LE, Fleshner M, et al. The role of the vagus nerve in cytokine-to-brain communication. *Ann NY Acad Sci* 1998;840:289–300.
32. Romanovsky AA, Ivanov AI, Szekely M. Neural route of pyrogen signaling to the brain. *Clin Infect Dis* 2000;31(suppl 5):162–167.
33. Sehic E, Blatteis CM. Blockade of lipopolysaccharide-induced fever by subdiaphragmatic vagotomy in guinea pigs. *Brain Res* 1996;726:160–166.
34. Dinarello CA. Role of interleukin-1 in infectious diseases. *Immunol Rev* 1992;127:119–146.
35. Roberts NJ Jr, Prill AH, Mann TN. Interleukin 1 and interleukin 1 inhibitor production by human macrophages exposed to influenza virus or respiratory syncytial virus. Respiratory syncytial virus is a potent inducer of inhibitor activity. *J Exp Med* 1986;163:511–519.
36. Cartmell T, Luheshi GN, Hopkins SJ, et al. Role of endogenous interleukin-1 receptor antagonist in regulating fever induced by localised inflammation in the rat. *J Physiol* 2001;531(part 1):171–180.
37. Leon LR, Kozak W, Kluger MJ. Role of IL-10 in inflammation. Studies using cytokine knockout mice. *Ann NY Acad Sci* 1998;856:69–75.
38. Kozak W, Kluger MJ, Tesfaigzi J, et al. Molecular mechanisms of fever and endogenous antipyresis. *Ann NY Acad Sci* 2000;917:121–134.
39. Bicego-Nahas KC, Steiner AA, Carnio EC, et al. Antipyretic effect of arginine vasotocin in toads. *Am J Physiol* 2000;278:1408–1414.
40. Tatro JB. Endogenous antipyretics. *Clin Infect Dis* 2000;31(suppl 5):190–201.
41. Roberts NJ. Impact of temperature elevation on immunologic defenses. *Rev Infect Dis* 1991;13:462–472.
42. Glauser MP. Pathophysiologic basis of sepsis: considerations for future strategies of intervention. *Crit Care Med* 2000;28(suppl):4–8.
43. Hasday JD, Fairchild KD, Shanholtz C. The role of fever in the infected host. *Microbes Infect* 2000;2:1891–1904.
44. Reinhart K, Karzai W. Anti-tumor necrosis factor therapy in sepsis: update on clinical trials and lessons learned. *Crit Care Med* 2001;29(suppl):121–125.
45. Blatteis CM, Sehic E. Prostaglandin $E_2$: a putative fever mediator. In: Mackowiak PA, ed. *Fever: basic mechanisms and management, 2nd ed.* Philadelphia: Lippincott-Raven, 1997:117–145.
46. Netea MG, Kullberg BJ. Van der Meer JW. Circulating cytokines as mediators of fever. *Clin Infect Dis* 2000;31(suppl 5):178–184.
47. Ushikubi F, Segi E, Sugimoto Y. et al. Impaired febrile response in mice lacking the prostaglandin E receptor subtype EP3. *Nature* 1998;395:281–284.
48. Coceani F, Akarsu ES. Prostaglandin $E_2$ in the pathogenesis of fever. An update. *Ann NY Acad Sci* 1998;856:76–82.
49. Dinarello CA. Interleukin-1. *Rev Infect Dis* 1984;6:51–95.
50. Beisel WR. Effects of infection on nutritional status and immunity. *Fed Proc* 1980;39:3105–3108.
51. Beisel WR. Magnitude of the host nutritional responses to infection. *Am J Clin Nutr* 1977;30:1236–1247.

52. Baumann H, Gauldie J. The acute phase response. *Immunol Today* 1994;15:74–80.
53. Ramadori G, Christ B. Cytokines and the hepatic acute-phase response. *Semin Liver Dis* 1999;19:141–155.
54. Rosenzweig PH, Volpe SL. Iron, thermoregulation, and metabolic rate. *Crit Rev Food Sci Nutr* 1999;39:131–148.
55. Gabay C, Kushner I. Acute-phase proteins and other systemic responses to inflammation. *N Engl J Med* 1999;340:448–454.
56. Steel DM, Whitehead AS. The major acute phase reactants: C-reactive protein, serum amyloid P component and serum amyloid A protein. *Immunol Today* 1994;15:81–88.
57. Weinberg ED. Iron and infection. *Microbiol Rev* 1978;42:45–66.
58. Dematte JE, O'Mara K, Buescher J, et al. Near-fatal heat stroke during the 1995 heat wave in Chicago. *Ann Intern Med* 1998;129:173–181.
59. Gencik M, Gencik A, Mortier W, et al. Novel mutation in the RYR1 gene (R2454C) in a patient with malignant hyperthermia. *Hum Mutat* 2000;15:122.
60. Robinson RL, Curran JL, Ellis FR, et al. Multiple interacting gene products may influence susceptibility to malignant hyperthermia. *Ann Hum Genet* 2000;64(part 4):307–320.
61. Bouchama A, Hammami MM, Haq A, et al. Evidence for endothelial cell activation/injury in heatstroke. *Crit Care Med* 1996;24:1173–1178.
62. Bruunsgaard H, Pedersen M, Pedersen BK. Aging and proinflammatory cytokines. *Curr Opin Hematol* 2001;8:131–136.
63. Plaisance KI, Mackowiak PA. Antipyretic therapy: physiologic rationale, diagnostic implications, and clinical consequences. *Arch Intern Med* 2000;160:449–456.
64. Mackowiak PA. Physiological rationale for suppression of fever. *Clin Infect Dis* 2000;31(suppl 5):185–189.
65. Kluger MJ, Ringler DH, Anver MR. Fever and survival. *Science* 1975;188:166–168.
66. Conti C, De Marco A, Mastromarino P, et al. Antiviral effect of hyperthermic treatment in rhinovirus infection. *Antimicrob Agents Chemother* 1999;43:822–829.
67. Evans SS, Bain MD, Wang WC. Fever-range hyperthermia stimulates alpha4beta7 integrin-dependent lymphocyte-endothelial adhesion. *Int J Hyperthermia* 2000;16:45–59.
68. Evans SS, Wang WC, Bain MS, et al. Fever-range hyperthermia dynamically regulates lymphocyte delivery to high endothelial venules. *Blood* 2001;97:2727–2733.
69. Rosman NP. Febrile convulsions. In: Mackowiak PA, ed. *Fever: basic mechanisms and management, 2nd ed.* Philadelphia: Lippincott-Raven, 1997:267–277.
70. Plaisance KI. Toxicities of drugs used in the management of fever. *Clin Infect Dis* 2000;31(suppl 5):219–223.
71. Stanley ED, Jackson GG, Panusarn C, et al. Increased virus shedding with aspirin treatment of rhinovirus infection. *JAMA* 1975;231:1248–1251.
72. Isaacs SN, Axelrod PI, Lorber B. Antipyretic orders in a university hospital. *Am J Med* 1990;88:31–35.
73. Simmons DL, Wagner D, Westover K. Nonsteroidal anti-inflammatory drugs, acetaminophen, cyclooxygenase 2, and fever. *Clin Infect Dis* 2000;31(suppl 5):211–218.
74. Goldstein JL, Silverstein FE, Agrawal NM, et al. Reduced risk of upper gastrointestinal ulcer complications with celecoxib, a novel COX-2 inhibitor. *Am J Gastroenterol* 2000;95:1681–1690.
75. Kurumbail RG, Stevens AM, Gierse JK, et al. Structural basis for selective inhibition of cyclooxygenase-2 by anti-inflammatory agents. *Nature* 1996;384:644–648.
76. Langman MJ, Jensen DM, Watson DJ, et al. Adverse upper gastrointestinal effects of rofecoxib compared with NSAIDs. *JAMA* 1999;282:1929–1933.
77. Silverstein FE, Faich G, Goldstein JL, et al. Gastrointestinal toxicity with celecoxib vs nonsteroidal anti-inflammatory drugs for osteoarthritis and rheumatoid arthritis: the CLASS study: A randomized controlled trial. Celecoxib Long-term Arthritis Safety Study. *JAMA* 2000;284:1247–1255.
78. Koch-Weser J. Drug therapy. Acetaminophen. *N Engl J Med* 1976;295:1297–1300.
79. Keusch GT, Fever. To be or not to be. *NY State J Med* 1976;76:1998–2001.
80. Yaqub BA, Al-Harthi SS, Al-Orainey IO, et al. Heat stroke at the Mekkah pilgrimage: clinical characteristics and course of 30 patients. *Q J Med* 1986;59:523–530.

81. Armstrong LE, Crago AE, Adams B, et al. Whole-body cooling of hyperthermic runners: comparison of two field therapies. *Am J Emerg Med* 1996;14:355–358.
82. Cunha BA. Antibiotic side effects. *Med Clin North Am* 2001;85:149–185.
83. Johnson DH, Cunha BA. Drug fever. *Infect Dis Clin North Am* 1996;10:85–91.
84. Mackowiak PA. Drug fever: mechanisms, maxims and misconceptions. *Am J Med Sci* 1987;294:275–286.
85. Anderson JA. Allergic reactions to drugs and biological agents. *JAMA* 1992;268:2844–2857.
86. Petersdorf RGB, Beeson PB. Fever of unexplained origin. Report on 100 cases. *Medicine* 1961;40:1–30.
87. Petersdorf RG. Fever of unknown origin. An old friend revisited. *Arch Intern Med* 1992;152:21–22.
88. Durack DT, Street AC. Fever of unknown origin—reexamined and redefined. *Curr Clin Top Infect Dis* 1991;11:35–51.
89. Sullivan M, Feinberg J, Bartlett JG. Fever in patients with HIV infection. *Infect Dis Clin North Am* 1996;10:149–165.
90. Sepkowitz KA. FUO and AIDS. *Curr Clin Top Infect Dis* 1999;19:1–15.
91. Armstrong WS, Katz JT, Kazanjian PH. Human immunodeficiency virus-associated fever of unknown origin: a study of 70 patients in the United States and review. *Clin Infect Dis* 1999;28:341–345.
92. Miller RF, Hingorami AD, Foley NM. Pyrexia of undetermined origin in patients with human immunodeficiency virus infection and AIDS. *Int J STD AIDS* 1996;7:170–175.
93. Miralles P, Moreno S, Perez-Tascon M, et al. Fever of uncertain origin in patients infected with the human immunodeficiency virus. *Clin Infect Dis* 1995;20:872–875.
94. Larson EB, Featherstone HJ, Petersdorf RG. Fever of undetermined origin: diagnosis and follow-up of 105 cases, 1970–1980. *Medicine* 1982;61:269–292.
95. Knockaert DC, Vanneste LJ, Vanneste SB, et al. Fever of unknown origin in the 1980s. An update of the diagnostic spectrum. *Arch Intern Med* 1992;152:51–55.
96. Barbado FJ, Vazquez JJ, Pena JM, et al. Pyrexia of unknown origin: changing spectrum of diseases in two consecutive series. *Postgrad Med J* 1992;68:884–887.
97. Supparatpinyo K, Khamwan C, Baosoung V, et al. Disseminated. *Penicillium marneffei* infection in southeast Asia. *Lancet* 1994;344:110–113.
98. Sirisanthana T, Supparatpinyo K. Epidemiology and management of penicilliosis in human immunodeficiency virus-infected patients. *Int J Infect Dis* 1998;3:48–53.
99. International Collaboration on, H.I.V. and Cancer. Highly active antiretroviral therapy and incidence of cancer in human immunodeficiency virus–infected adults. *J Natl Cancer Inst* 2000;92:1823–1830.
100. Matthews GV, Bower M, Mandalia S, et al. Changes in acquired immunodeficiency syndrome–related lymphoma since the introduction of highly active antiretroviral therapy. *Blood* 2000;96:2730–2734.
101. Grulich AE. AIDS-associated non-Hodgkin's lymphoma in the era of highly active antiretroviral therapy. *J AIDS* 1999;21(suppl 1):27–30.
102. Wolff SM, Fauci AS, Dale DC. Unusual etiologies of fever and their evaluation. *Annu Rev Med* 1975;26:277–281.
103. Mackowiak PA, Lipscomb KM, Mills KJ, et al. Dissecting aortic aneurysm manifested as fever of unknown origin. *JAMA* 1976;236:1725–1727.
104. Kerttula Y, Hirvonen P, Pettersson T. Fever of unknown origin: a follow-up investigation of 34 patients. *Scand J Infect Dis* 1983;15:185–187.
105. Weinstein L. Clinically benign fever of unknown origin: a personal retrospective. *Rev Infect Dis* 1985;7:692–699.
106. Knockaert DC, Vanneste LJ, Bobbaers HJ. Recurrent or episodic fever of unknown origin. Review of 45 cases and survey of the literature. *Medicine* 1993;72:184–196.
107. Kazanjian PH. Fever of unknown origin: review of 86 patients treated in community hospitals. *Clin Infect Dis* 1992;15:968–973.
108. Goetz MB. Fever of unknown origin in the elderly. *Infect Dis Clin Pract* 1993;2:377–380.
109. Cunha BA. Commentary: FUO in the elderly. *Infect Dis Clin Pract* 1993;2:380–383.
110. Sarwari AR, Mackowiak PA. Factitious fever: a modern update. *Curr Clin Top Infect Dis* 1997;17:88–94.

111. Knockaert DC. Diagnostic strategy for fever of unknown origin in the ultrasonography and computed tomography era. *Acta Clin Belg* 1992;47:100–116.
112. Brouqui P, Raoult D. Endocarditis due to rare and fastidious bacteria. *Clin Microbiol Rev* 2001;14:177–207.
113. Aronson MD, Bor DH. Blood cultures. *Ann Intern Med* 1987;106:246–253.
114. Tunkel AR, Kaye D. Endocarditis with negative blood cultures. *N Engl J Med* 1992;326:1215–1217.
115. de Kleijn EM, van Lier HJ, van der Meer JW. Fever of unknown origin (FUO). II. Diagnostic procedures in a prospective multicenter study of 167 patients. The Netherlands FUO Study Group. *Medicine* 1997;76:401–414.
116. Thompson NJ, Glassroth JL, Snider DE. The booster phenomenon in serial tuberculin testing. *Am Rev Respir Dis* 1979;119:587–597.
117. Anonymous. Targeted tuberculin testing and treatment of latent tuberculosis infection. American Thoracic Society. *MMWR* 2000;49:1–51.
118. Arnow PM, Flaherty JP. Fever of unknown origin. *Lancet* 1997;350:575–580.
119. Jessurun C, Mesa A, Wilansky S. Utility of transesophageal echocardiography in infective endocarditis. A review. *Tex Heart Inst J* 1996;23:98–107.
120. AbuRahma AF, Saiedy S, Robinson PA, et al. Role of venous duplex imaging of the lower extremities in patients with fever of unknown origin. *Surgery* 1997;121:366–371.
121. Corstens FH, van der Meer JW. Nuclear medicine's role in infection and inflammation. *Lancet* 1999;354:765–770.
122. Blockmans D, Knockaert D, Maes A, et al. Clinical value of [(18)F]fluoro-deoxyglucose positron emission tomography for patients with fever of unknown origin. *Clin Infect Dis* 2001;32:191–196.
123. Garcia-Ordonez MA, Colmenero JD, Jimenez-Onate F, et al. Diagnostic usefulness of percutaneous liver biopsy in HIV-infected patients with fever of unknown origin. *J Infect* 1999;38:94–98.
124. Benito N, Nunez A, de Gorgolas M, et al. Bone marrow biopsy in the diagnosis of fever of unknown origin in patients with acquired immunodeficiency syndrome. *Arch Intern Med* 1997;157:1577–1580.
125. McNeil BJ, Sanders R, Alderson PO, et al. A prospective study of computed tomography, ultrasound, and gallium imaging in patients with fever. *Radiology* 1981;139:647–653.
126. Rothman DL, Schwartz SI, Adams JT. Diagnostic laparotomy for fever or abdominal pain of unknown origin. *Am J Surg* 1977;133:273–275.
127. Greenall MJ, Gough MH, Kettlewell MG. Laparotomy in the investigation of patients with pyrexia of unknown origin. *Br J Surg* 1983;70:356–357.
128. Henning H. Value of laparoscopy in investigating fever of unexplained origin. *Endoscopy* 1992;24:687–688.
129. Frenkel J, Houten SM, Waterham HR, et al. Clinical and molecular variability in childhood periodic fever with hyperimmunoglobulinaemia D. *Rheumatology (Oxford)* 2001;40:579–584.
130. Roland WE, McDonald G, Caldwell CW, et al. Ehrlichiosis—a cause of prolonged fever. *Clin Infect Dis* 1995;20:821–825.

# 2. SEPSIS

Nancy J. Dorman

The development of penicillin during World War II transformed the practice of medicine dramatically. The advent of antimicrobial therapy in the latter half of the 20th century was associated with a precipitous decline in mortality and morbidity from infections. Since that time, however, the incidence of severe sepsis is rising, and associated mortality rates remain high despite an ever-increasing armamentarium of antibiotics and continued advances in critical care medicine.

The leading cause of death in intensive care units, sepsis is one of the most important modifiable causes of death overall in the United States. Lacking uniformly accepted definitions and specific International Classification of Diseases codes for septic shock and other life-threatening complications of infection, typical morbidity and mortality reports probably do not reflect the true magnitude of sepsis-associated disease. Nevertheless, based on discharge codes for bacteremia and septicemia, the Centers for Disease Control and Prevention reported a distressing 139% rise in the incidence of sepsis from 1979 to 1987 [1]. Figures reporting 500,000 septic episodes per annum in the United States underestimate the incidence of sepsis. More recent estimates conclude there are 751,000 new cases of sepsis annually in the United States, leading to nearly a quarter of a million fatalities [2], rivaling myocardial infarction as one of the most important causes of death in the developed world. Furthermore, because most studies focus on short-term outcome (<30 days), reported 30% to 50% mortality rates underestimate the overall impact of sepsis on survival. Independent of underlying disease, sepsis is associated with increased mortality risks for at least 1 year and probably as long as 5 years beyond the acute septic episode [3].

Reporting problems aside, the incidence of sepsis and associated mortality rates are rising despite better understanding of underlying pathophysiology, technologic improvements in critical care, and advances in antimicrobial therapy. In addition to improved reporting, factors that probably contribute to the increasing incidence of sepsis include the expanding use of invasive procedures, emergence of increasingly resistant pathogens, increasing number of patients with compromised immune status, and aging populations. Medical progress, undoubtedly, drives the rising incidence of sepsis. Comorbid illnesses are major outcome determinants, and patients presenting with sepsis today typically have severe underlying conditions not seen a few decades ago. Despite aggressive antimicrobial therapy and intensive medical care, mortality rates for sepsis remain high because we lack specific treatment for the systemic inflammatory response triggered by infection and reliable diagnostic assays to identify those patients at risk for developing severe sepsis.

A practical approach to sepsis requires working knowledge of current terminology, fundamental understanding of etiology or pathophysiology, appropriate utilization of innovative diagnostic technology, clinical application of new therapeutic interventions as these become available, and implementation of advancing strategies for prevention.

## I. Definitions

Sepsis is a syndrome, not a specific clinical entity. Over the past two decades, clinical trials examining new treatment strategies for septic shock generated disappointing failures and occasional surprising toxicities (see section IV). Similar to the difficulties determining accurate incidence and prevalence statistics for sepsis, a lack of uniformly accepted definitions hinders clinical research. Without consistent clinically applicable definitions for sepsis and its major sequelae, appropriate patient enrollment in multicenter clinical trials is unfeasible. Until rapid, sensitive, and specific diagnostic laboratory tests become available, sepsis remains a bedside diagnosis defined in clinical terminology.

In 1992, the Society of Critical Care Medicine (SCCM) and the American College of Chest Physicians (ACCP) published consensus definitions for sepsis and organ failure along with guidelines for the use of innovative therapies in sepsis [4]. These definitions serve as a framework for consistent clinical descriptions of sepsis and its sequelae, providing a common language among clinicians and investigators from center to center. Acknowledging the complexity of the systemic inflammatory response to infection and the importance of timely diagnosis, the definitions are intentionally rather simple in context and broad in scope. Some experts assert that broad nonspecific ACCP/SCCM consensus definitions lack practical applicability, especially in clinical research protocols. ACCP/SCCM Consensus Conference participants recognized these problems with their current definitions, anticipating modifications as our understanding of sepsis evolves [4]. Until future refinements improve the discriminatory value of sepsis terminology, these definitions provide clinicians and researchers with a consistent vocabulary that is currently accepted widely in clinical practice and in research.

**A.** **Infection** describes a microbial phenomenon characterized by an inflammatory response to the presence of microorganisms or the invasion of otherwise sterile host tissues by those organisms.

**B.** **Bacteremia** describes the presence of viable bacteria in the blood. Similarly, the presence of other pathogens in the blood would be described appropriately as viremia, fungemia, or parasitemia. Used previously to describe the presence of microorganisms or their toxins in the blood, the term septicemia was eliminated from the Consensus Conference definitions for sepsis because of ambiguities that cause confusion and difficulties in data interpretation.

**C.** **Systemic inflammatory response syndrome (SIRS)** denotes a generalized inflammatory response to a medley of severe clinical insults. Perhaps the most controversial definition from the Consensus Conference [5,6,22,23], the term SIRS was not developed as a stand-alone entity and should be viewed in combination with other clinical information [7]. As developed, SIRS deliberately presents low threshold clinical evidence for defining systemic inflammatory response regardless of cause. The definition of SIRS may be refined as prospective studies using the consensus definitions identify new variables that will improve prognostic accuracy and clinical applicability [8]. As it stands currently, the new term highlights the systemic inflammatory response as a syndrome, or constellation of signs and symptoms, that warrants early recognition and aggressive search for the underlying cause. SIRS is triggered by a number of noninfectious pathologic processes including, but not limited to, pancreatitis, burns, severe trauma, major tissue injury, ischemia, hemorrhagic shock, immune-mediated organ injury, and exogenous administration of putative mediators (**e.g., certain cytokines such as tumor necrosis factor** [TNF]) (Fig. 2.1). During diagnostic evaluation, only physiologic alterations representing an **acute change from baseline without other known causes (e.g., chemotherapy-induced neutropenia, drug-induced tachycardia, etc.)** should be used as clinical criteria to define SIRS. The term SIRS describes the presence of two or more of the following clinical manifestations, including but not limited to

1. Temperature higher than 38°C or lower than 36°C;
2. Heart rate higher than 90 beats/min;
3. Tachypnea (**respiratory rate >20 per minute**) or hyperventilation (**$P_{CO_2}$ <32 Torr**);
4. White blood cell count alterations more than 12,000/$\mu$L or less than 4,000/$\mu$L or the presence of more than 10% immature neutrophils.

**D.** **Sepsis** is defined as the systemic inflammatory response to infection. In association with infection, the manifestations of sepsis are the same as described above for SIRS. The term sepsis should be reserved for those instances when the clinical manifestations of systemic inflammation are related directly to an infectious process. Recognizing that sepsis and its sequelae represent a continuum of clinical and pathophysiologic severity, the degrees of which may independently affect prognosis, additional definitions are used to describe clinically recognizable stages of sepsis.

**E.** **Severe sepsis** describes sepsis associated with organ dysfunction, hypoperfusion, or sepsis-induced hypotension. Clinically recognizable hypoperfusion and perfusion abnormalities include but are not limited to

1. Lactic acidosis;
2. Oliguria;
3. Acute mental status changes.

**F.** **Sepsis-induced hypotension** is defined by a systolic blood pressure less than 90 mm Hg or a decrease of at least 40 mm Hg from baseline in the absence of other causes (**e.g., cardiogenic shock**).

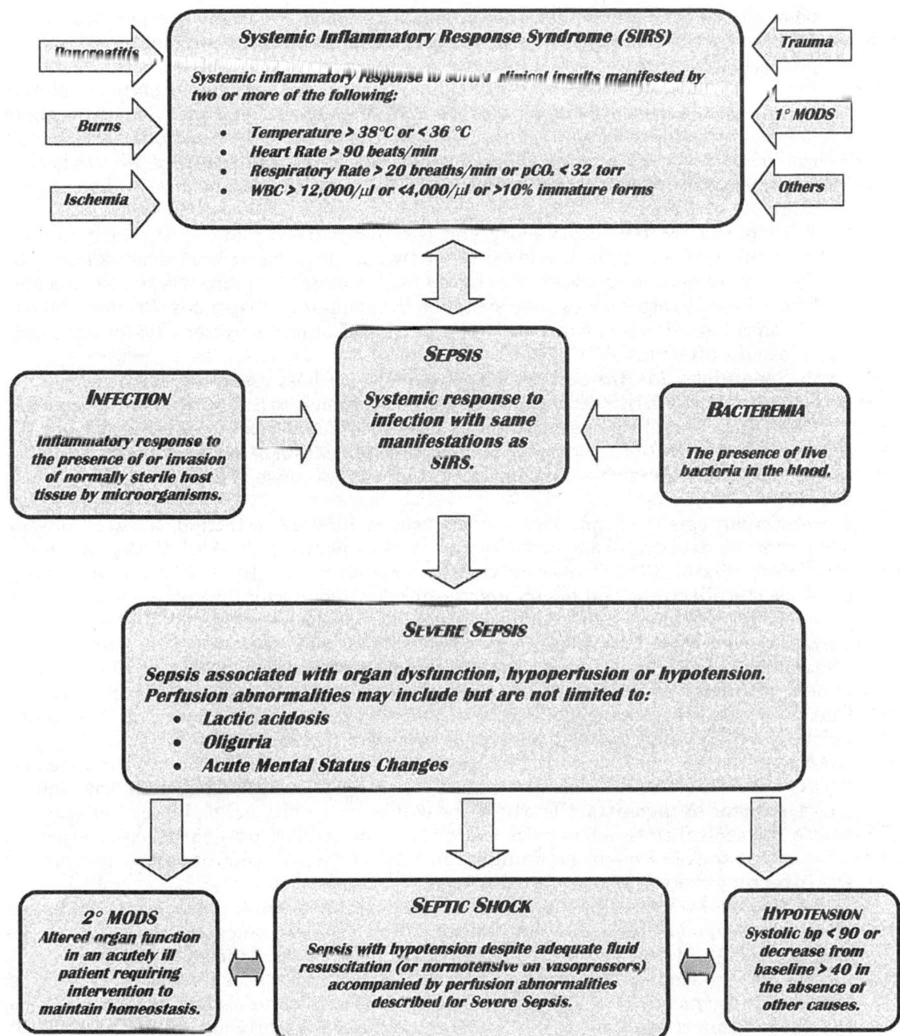


**FIG. 2.1** Sepsis-related definitions and interrelationships. (Based on Bone RC, Balk RA, Cerra FB, et al. American College of Chest Physicians/Society of Critical Care Medicine Consensus Conference. Definitions for sepsis and organ failure and guidelines for the use of innovative therapies in sepsis. *Crit Care Med* 1992;20:864–874).

G. **Septic shock** describes a subset of severe sepsis characterized by sepsis-induced hypotension unresponsive to adequate volume resuscitation, in addition to hypoperfusion abnormalities or organ dysfunction. The term **septic shock** still applies to patients with **severe sepsis** whose systolic blood pressure normalizes on vasopressor or inotropic support before developing hypoperfusion abnormalities or organ dysfunction.

H. **Multiple organ dysfunction syndrome (MODS)** describes a syndrome characterized by a continuum of physiologic derangements in organ function such that homeostasis cannot be maintained. Older terminology referring to organ failure implies that organ function is present or absent, thus excluding the dynamic physiologic process more characteristic of the syndrome encountered clinically. As defined during the Consensus Conference, multiple organ dysfunction may be absolute or relative but is more readily viewed as a continuum of change over time. Currently, there are no universally accepted criteria for quantifying organ dysfunction in MODS, but consensus criteria may evolve from outcomes data in the near future. MODS is classified as **primary** or **secondary** based on two pathogenetic pathways that are not mutually exclusive.

1. **Primary MODS** occurs early and is directly attributable to a clearly defined insult. One example would be chest trauma leading to lung dysfunction. The initiation and progression of primary MODS stem from direct response to a specific insult rather than host systemic inflammatory responses. Primary MODS can trigger SIRS, subsequently instigating other organ system dysfunction (secondary MODS).
2. **Secondary MODS** occurs as a consequence of host responses identified within the context of SIRS rather than as a direct response to a specific insult. Secondary MODS characteristically develops after a latent period separating it from the primary insult and is most commonly a complication of severe sepsis. Secondary MODS is viewed as a consequence rather than a cause of SIRS.

## II. Etiology

Invading pathogens do not cause septic shock directly. Infection triggers physiologic changes evolving from sophisticated and exquisitely complex interplay among multiple mediators. Over the past decade, important scientific advances identifying cytokine cascades provided a solid foundation for understanding the pathophysiology of sepsis. Despite these major advances, medical science has only begun to scratch the surface of comprehension prerequisite to developing reliable therapeutic interventions for treating severe sepsis and septic shock. Early excitement surrounding the discovery of new inflammatory mediators engendered enthusiastic search for therapeutic agents that attenuate adverse physiologic responses to infection. Unfortunately, therapeutic agents used successfully to treat sepsis in animal models typically lack efficacy in clinical trials [14], as seen with multiple earlier studies evaluating cyclooxygenase (COX) inhibitors, antiendotoxin antibodies, anti-TNF antibodies, and interleukin (IL)-1 receptor antagonists. Clearly, there will be no single "magic bullet" for treating sepsis. As medical science has unraveled the complexities of host–pathogen interaction, interest has shifted from intervening at the level of single mediators toward modifying the **interplay** among important pathways.

The view that severe sepsis stems from a predominance of proinflammatory mediators is now challenged as an over-simplification of the complex interplay among intracellular, intercellular, local, and systemic responses to infection. Indeed, recent arguments question the concept that overwhelming systemic inflammation causes severe sepsis, focusing on the notion that although local response to infection is proinflammatory, the clinically manifest systemic response overall is predominantly antiinflammatory [10]. Most likely, the **balance** between **proinflammatory** and **antiinflammatory** processes determines the final outcome during infection, with deleterious sequelae resulting when the scales tip too far in either direction (Fig. 2.2).

Whereas medical science once focused on pathogen virulence factors, current sepsis research has shifted toward exploring genetic variations in host response as outcome determinants [11–13]. Clearly, as biomedical research strives to define better ways to treat severe sepsis, clinicians must come to grips with a growing array of immunologic mediators and, eventually, genetic variations therein if they hope to apply new therapeutic options. Although detailed discussion of all potential pathogen- and host-derived inflammatory mediators is beyond the scope of this text, certain key areas of current interest warrant consideration, recognizing there are still major gaps in our knowledge base and that new horizons in sepsis research are expanding rapidly.

A. **Cytokines** are small pleiotropic proteins that signal cells and orchestrate the immune response by binding to appropriate receptors on multiple tissues [16,19]. The birth of "cytokine biology" dates back to the isolation of "endogenous pyrogen" and

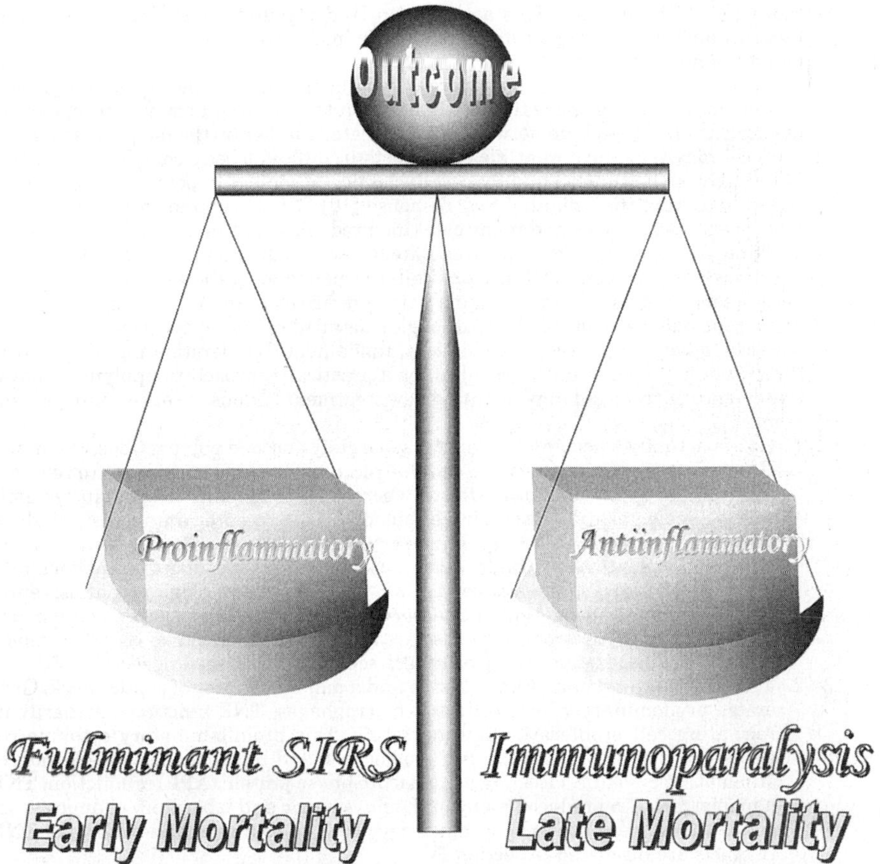


**FIG. 2.2** Balance between proinflammatory and counter-regulatory antiinflammatory events in response to infection determines clinical outcome. Infection triggers several inflammatory cascades, including proinflammatory cytokine, complement, coagulation system, and neutrophil activation. Compensatory antiinflammatory mechanisms, including antiinflammatory cytokine production, natural inhibitor release, stress hormone response, and immune cell inactivation, regulate the inflammatory response to prevent systemic toxicity. Localized proinflammatory response is essential for host defense against microbial invasion. Excessive proinflammatory response causes systemic toxicity clinically manifested as sepsis. Excessive antiinflammatory response causes immunoparalysis associated with increased propensity for overwhelming infection and late mortality.

the subsequent recognition that IL-1 is a potent pyrogen. Since that time, a number of cytokines have demonstrated pyrogenicity, linking the ancient concept of fever to a present-day understanding of inflammation-induced perturbations in cell biochemistry [15]. Historically, different research groups discovered certain cytokines simultaneously, each applying various descriptive names to a single mediator. For example, IL-6 has also been called B-cell stimulating factor and hybridoma growth factor. Cytokine nomenclature remains rather confusing. The term interleukin improved nomenclature somewhat but is still misleading because cells other than leukocytes may produce these factors. Currently, when a cytokine is characterized sufficiently, it is assigned an IL designation (**e.g., IL-1, IL-2, IL-6, etc.**). To date, there are 18 cytokines with the name IL. Despite these more recent designations, certain cytokines still bear descriptive names such as TNF, colony-stimulating factor (CSF), and interferon, even though these names tend to represent only one of many biologic activities. In addition to confusing nomenclature, clinical application of the cytokine network is complicated further by the fact that any given cytokine may have divergent biologic effects in different body compartments; this is highlighted in Munford and Pugin's discussion of context-dependent mediator activity regulating the inflammatory response [10]. Most cytokines are produced by more than one cell type, and many cytokine-producing cells generate more than one cytokine. Any given cytokine may regulate its own production in addition to modifying the release of other cytokines or similar components of the regulatory network. Host defense mediators and cytokine networks are examined in a number of texts and recent publications [15–19]. Although a detailed review of cytokine network intricacies is beyond the scope of this text, fundamental understanding of currently recognized key mediators is essential for a practical approach to applying innovative diagnostic tests and implementing new treatment options in sepsis management plans.

1. **IL-1** is actually a designation for two separately encoded polypeptides, IL-1$\alpha$ and IL-1$\beta$. Both recognize the same cellular receptors, but IL-1$\alpha$ appears to regulate intracellular events and local effects, whereas IL-1$\beta$ is more involved in systemic effects. Their naturally occurring antagonist, IL-1 receptor antagonist, binds to the same receptors. IL-1 is a proinflammatory cytokine produced by many cell types during acute and chronic inflammation, but mononuclear cells, particularly macrophages, are a major source. IL-1 has highly diverse biologic activities, reproducing many physiologic changes observed in septic patients. Fever, acute phase response, and corticotrophin release are major biologic effects of IL-1. Therapies directed against IL-1 for treating severe sepsis are discussed in section IV.
2. **TNF-$\alpha$** is a proinflammatory cytokine and a major mediator of septic shock. Generated predominantly by T cells and macrophages, TNF functions primarily in regulating cell proliferation and apoptosis. This proinflammatory cytokine recruits and activates neutrophils, lymphocytes, and macrophages, in addition to stimulating cytokine, eicosanoid, and acute phase protein (APP) production. TNF administration reproduces many of the physiologic and laboratory changes associated with severe sepsis. Therapies developed to counteract the effects of TNF in sepsis are discussed in section IV.
3. **IL-6** has both proinflammatory and antiinflammatory properties by virtue of diverse biologic activities. IL-1 and TNF stimulate the release of IL-6, which subsequently influences a number of inflammatory responses. IL-6 plays a major role in the APP response, stimulating hepatocytes to produce noncytokine proteins such as C-reactive protein (CRP), fibrinogen, $\alpha_1$-antitrypsin, serum amyloid A, and $\alpha_1$ acid glycoprotein. In contrast to the more toxic effects of TNF and IL-1, exogenous IL-6 administration induces only mild symptoms such as fever and chills. Generally regarded as a proinflammatory cytokine, IL-6 also has antiinflammatory influences by decreasing TNF and IL-1 production and increasing circulating levels of the natural inhibitors, soluble TNF receptors and IL-1 receptor antagonist. IL-6 is present in the serum during sepsis, and levels correlate with the disease severity and outcome in patients with severe sepsis. Serum IL-6 measurement may provide useful diagnostic and prognostic data in patients with sepsis, as discussed in section III.

**B. CSFs** are growth factors produced by a number of cell lines such a monocytes, macrophages, endothelial cells, and fibroblasts. Four CSFs isolated and characterized to date are granulocyte CSF (G-CSF), granulocyte-macrophage CSF (GM-CSF), macrophage CSF (m–CSF), and IL-3 (multi-CSF). G-CSF and GM-CSF are available commercially, and growing clinical experience has prompted studies exploring their potential as adjunct therapy for infections (see section IV). Produced by a number of cell lines, G-CSF specifically targets neutrophil proliferation and activity, whereas GM-CSF has broader hematopoietic effects on multiple cells lines, particularly monocytes, macrophages, and eosinophils. G-CSF stimulates committed stem cell proliferation and differentiation into mature neutrophils, mobilizes mature granulocytes from the marrow, and enhances neutrophil functions such as phagocytosis, oxidative burst, microbicidal activity, and chemotaxis. Unlike the proinflammatory effects on neutrophil function, G-CSF appears to have antiinflammatory effects on mononuclear cells. When exposed to endotoxin or other bacterial stimuli *in vitro*, whole blood from human volunteers treated with G-CSF generated less TNF than pretreatment samples [24]. Furthermore, antiinflammatory mediators IL-1 receptor antagonist and soluble TNF receptors increase after G-CSF treatment. Added to its previously known stimulatory effect on neutrophil antimicrobial function, the discovery that G-CSF attenuates TNF production and enhances antiinflammatory mechanisms fosters continued interest in clinical trials using G-CSF as adjunct therapy for treating infection. In contrast, animal studies suggest that GM-CSF increases circulating TNF levels and is actually associated with increased mortality in some infections. GM-CSF also increases leukotriene (LT) biosynthesis in mature human leukocytes [39]. Currently, recombinant human G-CSF (filgrastim) and GM-CSF (sargramostim) are available commercially for clinical use in the United States. Potential clinical applications for CSF in the management of sepsis are discussed in section IV (Table 2.1).

C. **Chemokines** are small chemotactic cytokines that play a central role in trafficking inflammatory cell migration and extravasation. Chemokines also influence the inflammatory response by altering cytokine profiles and mediating leukocyte migration and degranulation. Chemokine receptors are an attractive target for therapeutic interventions to limit deleterious inflammatory responses [37].

D. **Other mediators** implicated in sepsis include a vast array of substances ranging from acute phase proteins to phospholipase $A_2$ (PLA) with its resultant arachidonic acid (AA) metabolites and associated highly reactive oxygen species.

1. **PLA** plays a pivotal role in cellular metabolism by hydrolyzing the *sn*-2 acyl bond of phospholipids releasing free fatty acid (**commonly AA**) and 2-lysophosphospholipid. Decades ago, PLA was recognized as one of several enzymes comprising pancreatic secretions and snake venoms. More recently discovered diverse intracellular PLAs are now known to generate inflammatory mediator precursors. This association with inflammation prompts further research to characterize these enzymes with an eye toward developing new antiinflammatory agents [25].

   Mechanical trauma, specific cytokines, growth factors, and other stimuli (**e.g., collagen and adenosine diphosphate in platelets, thrombin and bradykinin in endothelial cells**) initiate cell signals that activate PLAs with subsequent AA release. The resultant secondary mediators act in an autocrine fashion, orchestrating PLA activity via exquisitely intricate interplay that is currently only partially understood [26].

   PLA appears to play a vital role in the pathogenesis of acute lung injury associated with infection (**acute respiratory distress syndrome [ARDS]**) [28], a common and potentially lethal consequence of sepsis for which there is no specific treatment beyond supportive measures [31,32]. Increased PLA activity associated with multiple organ failure in severely injured patients has spurred interest in investigating these enzymes as both prognostic markers and clinical targets for inflammatory processes [33]. PLA also appears to play an important role during pathogen invasion in infectious diseases such as bacterial meningitis [29]. Forthcoming advances in phospholipid and eicosanoid biology will likely engender novel therapeutics for treating harmful systemic inflammatory responses associated with sepsis [31].

2. **AA metabolites** are a class of lipid mediators also called **eicosanoids** based on their derivation from the parent 20-carbon polyunsaturated essential fatty acid. In addition to the somewhat better understood role of eicosanoids in inflammation [26], medical science is beginning to define lysophospholipid functions in cell signaling and immunity [27]. Nonsteroidal antiinflammatory drugs (NSAIDs) used commonly as antipyretics to reduce core temperature during infection impact eicosanoid production at many levels. Reducing infection-associated febrile response does not clearly improve outcome [50], and some would argue

Table 2.1. Colony-Stimulating Factors as Potential Adjunct Therapy for Treating Sepsis

| | G-CSF | GM-CSF |
|---|---|---|
| Cellular source | • Endothelial cells<br>• Fibroblasts<br>• Monocytes<br>• Macrophages<br>• Stromal cells | • Endothelial cells<br>• Fibroblasts<br>• Monocytes<br>• Macrophages<br>• T lymphocytes<br>• Smooth muscle cells |
| Receptor cells | • Neutrophils | • Neutrophils<br>• Monocytes<br>• Macrophages<br>• Eosinophils<br>• Endothelial cells |
| Biologic effects | • Neutrophil leukocytosis<br>• ↑ Chemotaxis<br>• ↑ Phagocytosis<br>• ↑ Microbicidal activity<br>• ↑ Ab-dependent cytotoxicity<br>• ↑ Oxidative activity<br>• ↑ sTNFr release<br>• ↑ IL-1ra release<br>• Delayed apoptosis | • Neutrophil leukocytosis<br>• Eosinophil leukocytosis<br>• Chemotaxis<br>• ↑ Phagocytosis<br>• ↑ Microbicidal activity<br>• ↑ Ab-dependent cytotoxicity<br>• ↑ Oxidative activity<br>• Free arachidonic acid<br>• ↑ LTB4 production<br>• ↑ IL-1, TNF, IL-6 |
| Clinical effects | • Antiinflammatory effects | • Proinflammatory effects |
| Pneumonia | • Decreased ARDS, DIC, Mortality | • Possible ↑ ARDS |
| Diabetic foot infections | • Faster response, better outcome | |
| Comparative safety | • Well-tolerated<br>• Mild–moderate bone pain<br>• Rare allergic reactions | • Fever, myalgias flu-like Sx<br>• Flushing, tachycardia<br>• Musculoskeletal pain<br>• Nausea, vomiting<br>• Dyspnea, $O_2$ desaturation<br>• Capillary leak syndrome<br>• Rare autoimmune Sx |

Biologic activities are summarized from *in vitro,* animal, and human studies. Clinical activities are summarized from preliminary clinical trials.
G-CSF, granulocyte colony stimulating factor; GM-CSF, granulocyte-macrophage colony stimulating factor; TNF, tumor necrosis factor; IL-1ra, interleukin-1 receptor antagonist; ARDS, acute respiratory distress syndrome; DIC, disseminated intravascular coagulation.

that fever is potentially beneficial as a natural physiologic response to pathogen invasion [51,52]. Recently reviewing the clinical use of antipyretics in fever suppression, Aronoff and Neilson [53] cautioned against using antipyretics indiscriminately and, like others, advocated reserving NSAID use for clinical situations where infection-associated fever risks may outweigh benefits. Over the last few decades, it has become clear that most antipyretics work by inhibiting COX. Medical science, however, has yet to resolve how inhibiting this pivotal enzyme impacts host defense overall and whether shifting eicosanoid production can affect outcome by altering the balance between proinflammatory and antiinflammatory mediators.

**a. Prostaglandins (PGs)** are synthesized *de novo* by most cells in response to PLA-mediated AA release from membrane phospholipids. Prostaglandin G

(PGG) synthase, known more commonly as COX, converts AA into the initial eicosanoid intermediate endoperoxide $PGG_2$, which is rapidly hydrolyzed into $PGH_2$. COX currently has two recognized isoforms, known as COX-1 and COX-2. COX-1 is constitutively expressed in most tissues, minimally affected by proinflammatory stimuli, and considered responsible for homeostatic PG formation. In contrast, COX-2 activity is absent in most tissues until inflammatory or mechanical stress induces enzyme expression with resultant proinflammatory PG synthesis. Although oversimplified, this classification has found application as selective COX-2 inhibitors are now used clinically as analgesics and NSAIDs. Although $PGH_2$ formation is common to most cell types, its fate is more cell specific. For example, platelets convert $PGH_2$ predominantly to thromboxane, endothelial cells to prostacyclin, uterine cells to $PGF\alpha_2$, and brain and mast cells to $PGD_2$. Extremely potent biologic mediators with very short half-lives, PGs typically exert direct biologic activity at or near their sites of synthesis. However, PG interplay with other mediator cascades should be viewed within the context of a complex milieu, culminating either in systemic inflammation or its control. For example, $PGE_2$ induces biochemical changes that mediate features of inflammation such as edema [46] but can also downregulate host inflammatory responses [47], perhaps by enhancing lipoxin synthesis [45] in addition to feedback on COX-2. The biosynthesis and actions of PGs were reviewed recently [26]. Inhibiting COX-2 (**selectively or nonselectively**) impacts all "downstream" eicosanoid production.

**b. Prostacyclin ($PGI_2$),** synthesized by endothelial cells from COX-derived precursor $PGH_2$, is an extremely potent antiplatelet mediator and vasodilator with a short (**5-minute**) half-life. $PGI_2$ inhibits platelet aggregation, neutrophil attachment to endothelium, and endothelial cytokine production (IL-6, IL-8, TNF). High circulating prostacyclin levels are associated with increased mortality in patients with sepsis [34]. Although not required for the development of systemic hypotension, prostacyclin may mediate sepsis-induced increases in oxygen consumption, arterial hypoxemia, and lactic acidosis [35,36].

**c. Thromboxane $A_2$,** the predominant AA metabolite synthesized by platelets, is an extremely potent vasoconstrictor with a fleeting (**30-second**) half-life. COX inhibitors such as NSAIDS block thromboxane $A_2$ production by decreasing $PGH_2$, the substrate for platelet thromboxane synthetase. Opposed by vascular endothelial cell derived prostacyclin, thromboxane $A_2$ is a powerful platelet aggregation inducer. High circulating thromboxane levels are associated with increased mortality in patients with sepsis [34] and apparently contribute to increased oxygen consumption, arterial hypoxemia, and lactic acidosis [36] exhibited during severe sepsis. Thromboxane production is essential for normal hemostasis and an important outcome determinant during vascular endothelium–platelet interplay.

**d. LTs** are biologically active AA metabolites with potent proinflammatory characteristics. So named because they were discovered in leukocytes and share a characteristic conjugated triene feature, LTs are formed from AA by leukocyte 5-lipoxygenase via pathways unrelated to COX. LT synthesis is diminished by PLA inhibitors such as steroids but unaffected by COX inhibitors such as NSAIDs. Indeed, Samuelsson [38] discovered LTs two decades ago while searching for novel AA metabolites that might account for differences noted between the antiinflammatory effects of NSAIDS and steroids. It took an additional 15 years to develop anti-LT agents for treating human disease (see section IV). Collectively, LTs recruit and activate leukocytes, enhance vascular permeability, and induce vascular and nonvascular smooth muscle contraction. The slow-reacting substance of anaphylaxis, first described in 1938, is now recognized as a mixture of interrelated LTs. Interest in blocking LT synthesis to prevent allergic bronchoconstriction led to developing anti-LT drugs for treating asthma [40]. The cysteinyl-LTs ($LTC_4$, $LTD_4$, and $LTE_4$) cause bronchoconstriction, vasoconstriction, endothelial contraction, and plasma extravasation (**1,000 times more potent than histamine**). The dihydroxy acid $LTB_4$, on the other hand, recruits leukocytes and induces neutrophil degranulation in addition to causing plasma extravasation [41]. Still in its infancy, LT research is evolving beyond asthma therapy and exploring potential intervention in other inflammatory diseases, including sepsis [42,43].

**e. Lipoxins** are AA derivatives that antagonize LT actions such as $LTB_4$-induced chemotaxis, leukocyte-endothelial adhesion, and plasma extravasation. Formed via 15-lipoxygenase pathways, lipoxins constitute a distinct eicosanoid class characterized as antiinflammatory mediators and modulators [44]. Lipoxins are generated at sites of injury or inflammation during cell–cell interactions, limiting the inflammatory response through a complex mediator-modulator network [45]. Although detailed discussion of these complex biochemical pathways is beyond the scope of this text, clinicians should recognize that drugs targeting one pathway (**e.g., COX-2 inhibitors, aspirin**) might impact other pathways with consequences yet unrecognized. For example, low dose aspirin-acetylated COX-2 no longer produces PG but remains catalytically active to generate biologically active endogenous lipoxin mimics, 15-epi-lipoxins, which likely contribute to aspirin's beneficial effects [44,45]. Other NSAIDs can negate this desirable aspirin effect. Medical science has not yet established clearly the temporal relationships among eicosanoid classes. Defining these complex temporal relationships is essential for understanding lipid mediator roles in inflammation and timing therapeutic interventions to control dangerous sequelae without paralyzing appropriate immune function. NSAIDs feasibly have unrecognized effects on sepsis-induced inflammation and its resolution. Presently it is uncertain what impact the pervasive use of NSAIDs as antipyretics might have on clinical outcome in patients with severe sepsis.

**3. Platelet-activating factor (PAF)** is a proinflammatory cell membrane phospholipid metabolite implicated in the sepsis cascade [48,49]. PAF amplifies inflammatory mediator release and produces many physiologic changes associated with septic shock. Many cell types, including neutrophils, monocytes, basophils, eosinophils, lymphocytes, endothelial cells, and platelets, produce PAF from phospholipase-generated lysophospholipids. Proinflammatory cytokines and other factors that activate PLA, *de facto*, also trigger PAF production. Conversely, drugs that inhibit PLA, such a glucocorticoids, decrease PAF production. PAF binds to specific receptors present on numerous inflammatory cells, activates neutrophils, aggregates platelets, and facilitates nitric oxide (NO) production. PAF is implicated in sepsis-associated coagulation abnormalities, pulmonary hypertension, myocardial depression, and gut ischemia. Like other proinflammatory mediators, PAF increases during sepsis. Furthermore, the enzyme responsible for degrading PAF to an inactive metabolite is decreased in patients who die from sepsis [54]. The important role PAF plays in the sepsis cascade prompted research into developing antagonists that prevent associated adverse physiologic events. Encouraging results from experimental studies culminated in clinical trials investigating PAF receptor antagonist use for treating patients with severe sepsis (see section IV).

**4. NO** plays a central role in regulating vascular tone and determining responsiveness to endogenous and exogenous vasopressors [55]. NO is formed from the amino acid L-arginine by the enzyme nitric oxide synthase (NOS). NOS exists in both constitutive (calcium/calmodulin-dependent) and inducible (calcium/calmodulin-independent) isoforms. The constitutive enzymes are found in endothelial (NOS III) and neuronal cells (NOS I), the former responsible for generating NO in response to sheer stresses and vasorelaxing substances such as histamine, bradykinin, or acetylcholine. Normal function of this constitutive enzyme is essential for maintaining normal vasomotor tone. In contrast, inducible NOS (NOS II) is formed by endothelial cells, smooth muscle cells, macrophages, and cardiac myocytes in response to inflammatory mediators such as endotoxin, peptidoglycan, lipoteichoic acid, IL-1, TNF, and PAF. The inducible NOS generates considerably more NO than its constitutive counterpart (**nanomolar vs. picomolar quantities**), accounting for the high levels of circulating NO noted in patients with septic shock [56]. NO activates guanylate cyclase, increasing cGMP levels with subsequent smooth muscle relaxation. As reviewed recently [57], NO is thought to mediate the hypotension and low systemic vascular resistance (SVR) observed in sepsis. NO is also implicated in sepsis-associated myocardial depression. If NO attains cytotoxic concentrations, it might participate in tissue and, ultimately, organ damage during sepsis. On the other hand, NO also has beneficial potential. For example, NO-induced vasodilation promotes microvascular and visceral blood flow, serving as a counter-regulatory mechanism for thromboxane-initiated vasoconstriction. By decreasing platelet aggregation and leukocyte adhesion, NO may help counterbalance mediators that promote microvascular stasis and thrombosis [57]. Given the high circulating levels observed in septic shock, however, NO (**along with its biologically active metabolites**) is considered the penultimate mediator of sepsis-associated cardiovascular dysfunction. As such, controlling NO production to reverse sepsis-induced cardiovascular dysfunction and hypotension is an attractive interventional target. Accordingly, after promising results in animal models of sepsis, NOS inhibitors have entered clinical trials for treating patients with sepsis (see section IV).

5. **APPs** reflect systemic changes, or acute phase response, accompanying inflammation. Defined as a serum proteins whose concentrations increase (**positive APPs**) or decrease (**negative APPs**) by 25% during inflammatory disorders [58], the term APP is somewhat misleading in that altered levels occur in chronic and in acute inflammatory processes. Interest in APPs dates back to 1930 when CRP was identified in patient serum during the acute phase of pneumococcal pneumonia [59]. Numerous APPs are recognized currently. Medical science continues to identify new acute phase response markers and their significance in the sepsis cascade. Conditions that cause sizable changes in APP concentrations include infection, immune-mediated inflammatory conditions, tissue infarction, surgery, burns, trauma, and advanced cancer. Smaller changes can occur with strenuous exercise, childbirth, heatstroke, and even psychological stress. Induced by cytokines, particularly IL-6, individual APP level changes vary both in timing and degree during the acute phase response. More than just reflecting inflammatory syndrome presence and intensity, APPs influence the process [60]. Despite lacking specificity as diagnostic markers in sepsis, APP (**e.g., CRP**) measurements can provide useful prognostic and treatment response information. In contrast to APPs, increased procalcitonin levels observed in sepsis appear more specific for infection-induced inflammation. Pending further study, procalcitonin holds promise as a possible diagnostic marker for sepsis (see section III).
6. **Pathogen factors** responsible for triggering the cytokine cascade are numerous and diverse. In addition to immune cell interaction with intact invading pathogens, microbial components can also induce host inflammatory responses culminating in shock and multiple organ failure [68–70,76].
   a. **Endotoxin,** a glycopeptide comprising a major portion of the outermost membrane in gram-negative bacteria, can induce pathophysiologic changes associated with severe infection. The discovery that endotoxin can cause septic shock generated prolific research investigating antiendotoxin strategies for treating sepsis. Notwithstanding promising data from animal studies, clinical trials using antiendotoxin therapies in patients with sepsis yielded disappointing results (see section IV).
   b. **Other toxins.** Lacking endotoxin, gram-positive pathogens can cause septic shock clinically indistinguishable from gram-negative counterparts. Gram-positive bacterial cell wall components currently known to have proinflammatory activity include **teichoic acid, lipoteichoic acid, and peptidoglycan** [67,69,70]. **Exotoxins,** such as toxic shock syndrome toxin from *Staphylococcus aureus* or pyrogenic exotoxins from *Streptococcus pyogenes* (group A streptococci), and **enterotoxins,** such as staphylococcal enterotoxins A–H,

act as **superantigens** [69]. Superantigens induce excessive proinflammatory cytokine production and are associated with septic shock in humans.

c. **Bacterial DNA** itself is proinflammatory, although approximately 10-fold less potent on a per weight basis than endotoxin [71].

d. **Other bacterial components** also participate in host inflammatory response during infection [67,69]. A century ago, Jarisch [72] and Herxheimer and Krause [73] described a complex clinical reaction that occurred in patients within hours of initiating treatment for secondary syphilis. Now well known as the Jarisch-Herxheimer reaction, the complex systemic reaction to initial treponemal killing is manifested by fever, chills, headache, myalgias, hyperventilation, tachycardia, vasodilation, and hypotension. Although the responsible treponemal components are currently unidentified, recent data demonstrating that anti-TNF antibodies block the Jarisch-Herxheimer reaction suggest bacterial lysis induces cytokine production [74]. In gram-negative bacteria, a Jarisch-Herxheimer–like reaction was first described in patients treated for typhoid fever. Increasing understanding of what bacterial components induce host inflammatory responses and how these substances participate in sepsis-induced injury has renewed interest in studying antimicrobial-induced bacterial lysis. Certain cell-wall active antibiotics (**e.g., $\beta$-lactams**) cause a rapid cell lysis and release of proinflammatory or toxic bacterial components. The resulting sudden increase in proinflammatory bacterial components may sway clinical outcome. Studies to date suggest that bacterial component release varies across and within antibiotic classes. Antibiotic concentration also influences bacterial component release. High antibiotic concentrations are associated with less bacterial component release compared with drug levels closer to the minimum inhibitory concentration. Antibiotics that interfere with bacterial protein synthesis (e.g., **clindamycin, rifampin, macrolides, tetracyclines, quinolones, streptogramins**) inhibit bacterial component release. Combining protein synthesis inhibitor antibiotics with $\beta$-lactams attenuates the release of proinflammatory compounds from bacteria. In a recent review, Nau and Helmut [67] summarized current information from studies investigating antibacterials as inflammatory response modulators and how antibiotic choices may influence outcome in sepsis and meningitis. Although intriguing, pending confirmatory clinical trials, the therapeutic relevance of antibacterial immune modulating effects is currently unclear. However, these concepts are applicable in certain circumstances where antibiotics that inhibit protein synthesis are used for more than their bactericidal activity. For example, in addition to its bactericidal activity, clindamycin also inhibits toxin production providing added therapeutic advantage when included in antimicrobial regimens for treating patients with necrotizing fasciitis caused by group A streptococci (*S. pyogenes*). Despite current limited therapeutic application, choosing antimicrobial therapy based on potential immunomodulatory actions is not currently recommended for clinical routine.

E. **Microbiology.** Sepsis has an extensive microbiologic differential diagnosis. Although, in theory, virtually any microorganism can trigger systemic inflammatory responses, bacteria and fungi are the most common pathogens identified in practice. Unfortunately, cultures are often negative, leaving the microbiologic diagnosis uncertain in approximately 50% of patients with clinically suspected sepsis [61]. Nevertheless, data from documented bloodstream infections provide useful information, because bacteremias reflect the microbiology of sepsis.

1. **Among nosocomial bloodstream pathogens,** gram-positive organisms currently predominate [62]. However, gram-negative bacteremias are more common in patients with septic shock [63]. *Candida* and *Enterococcus* species currently comprise the third and fourth most common bloodstream isolates in hospitalized patients (63–65).
2. **Various factors influence recovery of causal pathogens** from cultures such as prior antimicrobial therapy, source accessibility, specimen collection or handling, and microorganism growth characteristics.

3. **The microbiology of any given infection reflects its clinical source.** Likewise, the clinical source of infection determines its microbiology. For example, bacteremias from urinary tract sources most often involve gram-negative pathogens, whereas intravenous (i.v.) line sources more frequently involve gram-positive pathogens. Intra-abdominal and pelvic infections typically involve polymicrobial mixtures of gram-negative enteric flora, anaerobes, and enterococci.
4. **Identifying the infection source is crucial** for choosing appropriate antimicrobial therapy pending culture results or for treating clinically suspected sepsis in the absence of positive cultures. Sepsis-associated mortality risks increase when diagnostic evaluation fails to identify the causal pathogen(s) and clinical source of infection. Further details regarding the microbiologic etiology of specific infections are detailed in subsequent chapters spotlighting noteworthy infections.

## III. Diagnosis

Timely diagnosis and early intervention are key factors in preventing morbidity and mortality from sepsis. Sepsis is most amenable to treatment when identified early during incipient phases, before irreversible damage occurs. Infection is often accompanied by suggestive clinical and laboratory findings such as fever, tachycardia, and leukocytosis. These signs and symptoms are not present in all patients with impending sepsis, however, and may be manifestations of inflammatory diseases with noninfectious etiologies. The clinical challenge lies in not only recognizing early signs of systemic infection, but also distinguishing between patients with infection and those with noninfectious causes of SIRS. In this era of increasing antimicrobial resistance, clinicians must balance the indiscriminate or unnecessary use of antibiotics against treatment delays that increase risk for infection-associated morbidity and mortality. Definitive microbiologic diagnoses eliminate the need for empiricism. Unfortunately, clinicians must deal frequently with clinical signs of sepsis in patients without evident sources of infection. **Common diagnostic dilemmas** stem from wide variation in clinical signs and symptoms; classic signs of sepsis without clinically apparent source; false-positive cultures due to contamination or colonization; false-negative cultures due to fastidious pathogens, prior antimicrobial therapy, or improper collection techniques; and lack of specific and sensitive clinical or laboratory parameters that distinguish between infection and other causes of systemic inflammatory responses.

In the search for sensitive and specific markers for sepsis, some laboratory parameters have merit in certain clinical circumstances. Because no parameter is 100% sensitive and specific for diagnosing sepsis and its cause, appropriate management remains embedded in clinical judgment based on careful consideration of data from multiple sources.

A. **History** and physical examination are the foundation for all diagnoses. In most cases, a sagacious clinician leaves the bedside with an accurate diagnosis, using diagnostic tests to confirm clinical impressions, obtain baselines for following treatment efficacy, and establish a definitive microbiologic etiology. Once the infection source is established and appropriate cultures obtained, antimicrobial therapy should commence without delay. Pending culture results, the suspected infection source guides antibiotic choice, focusing on the most likely pathogens. However, if an infection source is not readily apparent from routine assessment, a more detailed approach is crucial, including painstaking attention to **clinical history.**
   1. **Underlying diseases.** Underlying diseases predispose patients to certain types of infections or particular pathogens. Certain medical conditions also alter the clinical presentation of common infections or predispose to infection with uncommon pathogens.
      a. **Immunosuppression,** whether due to underlying disease or induced by treatment, increases mortality risks from common infections and predisposes to infections uncommon in immunocompetent individuals. Determining whether the immunodeficiency primarily affects cell-mediated versus humoral immunity alerts clinicians to consider particular pathogens in the microbiologic differential diagnosis.
      b. **Diabetes mellitus** predisposes to pulmonary, urinary tract, and soft tissue infections. Concurrent neuropathy and vascular disease attenuate symptoms and physical signs of infection, increasing tissue damage. Patients with diabetes are prone to malignant otitis externa (*Pseudomonas aeruginosa*)

and its complications. Diabetes-associated infections are discussed further in Chapter 5.

c. **Hormonal abnormalities** or shifts can alter immune function and increase risk for certain infections. For example, hormonal changes in late pregnancy and excessive adrenocorticotrophic hormone production in Cushing disease cause cellular immune dysfunction, increasing risk for serious infections associated with decreased cell-mediated immunity.

d. **Chronic obstructive pulmonary disease** increases risk for bronchitis and pneumonia. Underlying lung disease increases mortality risk from other serious infections as well as pneumonia. Infections due to *Haemophilus, Moraxella, Legionella,* and other gram-negative pathogens are more common in persons with chronic obstructive pulmonary disease [21]. Gram-negative pathogens are more difficult to treat, require broader spectrum antimicrobial therapy, and increase mortality risk.

e. **Valvular and congenital heart diseases** predispose to infective endocarditis [20]. Endocarditis prevention, microbiology, and treatment are discussed in Chapter 12. Preexisting cardiovascular disease increases mortality risk in patients with sepsis.

f. **Hyposplenism or asplenia (functional or surgical)** predisposes to infection with certain pathogens such as *Streptococcus pneumoniae, Haemophilus influenzae, Neisseria meningitidis, Capnocytophagia canimorsus, Salmonella* species, and *Babesia* species. Infections in asplenic patients are frequently fulminant, rapidly progressing to septic shock barring early intervention.

g. **Cirrhosis** increases infection risk at a number of levels. Cirrhosis is associated with neutrophil chemotactic defects, predisposing to infection with *S. pneumoniae* and *H. influenzae*. Concurrent ascites, edema, hypoglobulinemia, hypoalbuminemia, portal hypertension with varices, and other associated abnormalities increase risk for developing infection (e.g., **spontaneous bacterial peritonitis, cellulitis**) and decrease appropriate immune response. Cirrhosis and its associated complications increase mortality risk for infections in other organ systems (e.g., **pneumonia**).

h. **Malignancies** increase risk for infection in a number of ways. Organ dysfunction from primary or metastatic disease can predispose to sepsis by (a) disrupting natural barriers (e.g., **skin, mucous membranes**), (b) obstructing passages (e.g., **ureters, bronchi, bowel**), (c) creating fistulas between sterile sites and contaminated tissues (e.g., **bronchopleural fistulas, esophageal perforation by mediastinal tumors**), (d) causing metabolic derangements that alter host defense and acute phase responses (e.g., **hypoalbuminemia, hypogammaglobulinemia cachexia**), and (e) infiltrating tissues essential to immune function (e.g., **bone marrow, liver, spleen**). Treatment inevitably impairs normal host defenses and often damages healthy tissue, increasing risk for invasive infection. Frequently colonized with multiply resistant pathogens resulting from prior antimicrobial therapy, infections in this patient population require rapid aggressive treatment to prevent sepsis and its high mortality risk.

i. **Malnutrition** compromises host defenses by causing metabolic derangements that decrease, in particular, cellular immune function. Iron deficiency, for example, decreases neutrophil killing capacity and T-lymphocyte function *in vitro*. Certain nutritional abnormalities predispose to infection with particular pathogens, as exemplified in the association between iron overload and increased risk for listeriosis and mucormycosis. Furthermore, malnutrition-associated abnormalities impact clinical outcome as epitomized in the association between hypoalbuminemia and increased mortality in patients with community-acquired pneumonia.

2. **Medication history.** Knowledge regarding a patient's past and present medications provides vital clues to infection type and severity. By modifying host flora, **prior antimicrobial therapy** alters disease epidemiology and warrants broadening microbiologic differential diagnoses to include resistant or unusual pathogens. Resistant or unusual pathogens, in turn, can increase mortality risks

and influence empiric antibiotic choices. Antimicrobial therapy influences diagnostic culture results and affects microbiologic data interpretation. **NSAIDs** and **corticosteroid therapy** attenuate fever and other signs or symptoms of infection, delaying diagnosis. **Corticosteroids** or other **immunosuppressive drugs** increase risk for unusual infections or opportunistic pathogens. **Beta-blockers** may prevent infection-induced tachycardia, mimicking the pulse-temperature disassociation classically linked with certain intracellular pathogens such as *Brucella*. **Drug-related adrenal insufficiency,** as seen with sudden cessation of chronic corticosteroid therapy, mimics septic shock clinically. **Allergic reactions** to medications can also cause distributive shock mimicking sepsis.

3. **Invasive procedures or surgery.** Invasive and surgical procedures increase risk for sepsis from particular pathogens. Although antimicrobial therapy for surgical prophylaxis covers typical flora for the system involved, clinicians should include iatrogenic infections in the differential diagnosis when evaluating septic patients. Even seemingly minor wound infections involving toxin-producing staphylococci or streptococci may cause toxic shock or toxic strep syndromes. Prior antimicrobial therapy alters colonizing flora, resulting in procedure-related infections with unusual or resistant pathogens. Central lines, antibiotics, and hyperalimentation predispose to sepsis from *Candida* species. Procedure-related infections due to difficult pathogens such as vancomycin-resistant enterococci, methicillin-resistant *Staphylococcus aureus*, *Stenotrophomonas*, *Pseudomonas*, *Enterobacter*, *Acinteobacter*, and *Burkholderia* show considerable geographic and demographic variation. It is important for clinicians to check local microbiologic trends and report unusual causes of postprocedure infections.
4. **Obstetric and gynecologic history.** Obstetric and gynecologic histories are important for assessing sepsis in women. Tampon use is associated with toxic shock syndrome caused by exotoxin TSST-1 producing *S. aureus*. Not typically isolated from blood cultures, the causal *S. aureus* is at times recovered from other sites such as vagina, cervix, or nares. Obstetric and gynecologic history is also important to assess risk for infection from a pelvic source. Characteristically polymicrobial, pelvic infections typically involve enteric gram-negative bacteria, anaerobes, and enterococci.
5. **Social history.** A patient's social history often provides vital clues to sepsis etiology. Social history and exposure history are often synonymous. Exposure history identifies infection risks, directs preventive therapy (**postexposure prophylaxis, immunization**), and guides empiric antimicrobial therapy pending culture results.
   a. **Travel** is commonplace. **Foreign travel** raises concern for otherwise uncommon causes of sepsis, such as malaria, plague, and hemorrhagic fevers. **Domestic travel** is associated with exposure to indigenous pathogens such as Rocky Mountain spotted fever, brucellosis, babesiosis, leptospirosis, and endemic mycoses. Even **intrastate travel** is associated with exposure to prevailing local pathogens, influencing the microbiologic differential diagnosis (e.g., **influenza, Legionnaires**).
   b. **Residence** locale may increase exposure to certain pathogens such as tick-borne rickettsia in wooded areas. Local disease outbreaks, such as methicillin-resistant *S. aureus* and Legionnaires, factor into the microbiologic differential diagnosis of sepsis. Infections in the homeless, including the high risk for blood-borne diseases, have been reviewed recently [75].
   c. **Occupation** at times poses certain exposure risks, such as *Salmonella* species, *Vibrio* species, and *Escherichia coli* in poultry, seafood, and beef processing industries, respectively. Veterinarians and others working with animals are at increased risk for various zoonoses. Some occupations involve extensive travel with attendant exposure to endemic infections. Other occupations, such as teaching or health care professions, involve close association with particular populations at risk for certain communicable diseases (e.g., **tuberculosis**).
   d. **Recreational activities** can expose individuals to otherwise unexpected pathogens as seen in leptospirosis, brucellosis, and tularemia. Recreational activities often also involve travel with attendant exposure risks.

e. **Alcoholism,** with or without cirrhosis, increases risk for serious infections with *S. pneumoniae* and *H. influenzae*. Alcohol intoxication can increase risk for aspiration pneumonia involving anaerobes and other oral flora not routinely involved in community-acquired pneumonia. Gastrointestinal disease associated with alcoholism can predispose to infections involving gut flora. Severe pancreatitis at times mimics sepsis and causes distributive shock indistinguishable from septic shock. Alcohol withdrawal, particularly delirium tremens, can obscure symptoms associated with serious infections such as bacterial meningitis or brain abscess.

f. **Smoking** inhibits mucociliary function and diminishes local immune defense, predisposing to respiratory tract infections (e.g., **pneumonia, sinusitis**).

g. **Recreational drug use history** can provide important clues when assessing patients with sepsis. Intravenous drug use increases risk for serious staphylococcal infections, including bacteremia. Marijuana is often contaminated with molds, particularly *Aspergillus*, that may cause serious infection in immunocompromised hosts. Cocaine and other illicit drugs are at times obtained in exchange for sexual favors, increasing risk for sexually transmitted diseases such as gonorrhea and human immunodeficiency virus (HIV).

h. **Sexual history** provides important information regarding potential pathogens that cause sepsis (e.g., **gonococcemia**) or predispose to infections that can alter host response to infection (e.g., **HIV**).

6. **Epidemiology.** Although many characteristics of sepsis are documented, the epidemiologic picture remains incomplete. Hampered by lack of reliable case definitions and the remarkable complexity of the condition, epidemiologic studies continue seeking to clarify risk factors, course, treatment, and outcomes.

   a. **Currently identified mortality risk factors** include antibiotic inadequacy, underlying disease, shock, need for vasopressors, multiple organ failure, neutropenia, infection source, and cause [8,76].

   b. **Gender and genetic predisposition factors** are gaining recognition as important epidemiologic issues in sepsis [77].

   c. **Infection site** can influence outcome, with higher mortality rates reported for intraabdominal or lower respiratory tract infections or when source is unidentified [8,78].

   d. **Microbiology** also influences sepsis outcome as suggested by high attributable mortality rates associated with bloodstream infections caused by *Candida* species and *Enterococcus* species [79]. In addition to affecting antimicrobial therapy, the type of invading pathogen also influences treatment response to sepsis interventions. In a recent review, Opal and Cohen [80] discussed clinical trials with antiinflammatory agents (e.g., **corticosteroids, IL-1 receptor antagonists, PAF antagonists**), noting poorer outcomes in patients with gram-positive versus gram-negative sepsis.

   e. **Changing epidemiology.** In a recent retrospective review spanning 40 years, Friedman et al. [81] noted several important factors in the changing epidemiology of septic shock, most notably the infection site and pathogen type. Infection site shifted from the abdomen before 1990 to chest in subsequent years. Causal pathogen type also shifted over the same time course with gram-positive pathogens becoming proportionately much more important.

   f. **Hospital-acquired infections** require special consideration compared with community-acquired counterparts. Nosocomial infections often involve multiply resistant pathogens, affecting both antimicrobial therapy choice and efficacy. Most hospital microbiology laboratories track antimicrobial susceptibility data to document resistance trends and facilitate appropriate antibiotic prescribing practices. Knowledge regarding these resistance patterns is especially relevant when selecting empiric antimicrobial therapy for treating sepsis. Awareness regarding community outbreaks and resistance patterns is also useful, alerting clinicians to increased risk for less common or resistant pathogens in otherwise common infectious diseases (e.g., **postinfluenzal staphylococcal pneumonia, Legionnaires disease, penicillin (PCN)-resistant pneumococcal disease, vancomycin-resistant enterococci**).

**B. Physical examination.** Meticulous physical examination is central to diagnosing sepsis, its cause, and appropriate treatment. The initial exam must rapidly ascertain overall clinical stability and guide prompt resuscitation to correct physiologic abnormalities such as hypotension, hypoxia, and impaired tissue oxygenation. The presence of shock constitutes a medical emergency. Because early recognition and prompt treatment of sepsis chiefly determine outcome, confirming infection and identifying its source are supremely important. Failure to initiate prompt appropriate empiric antimicrobial therapy increases sepsis mortality rates by 10% to 15% [82]. Because blood cultures are negative in approximately 70% of patients with sepsis, identifying the infection source is essential for guiding empiric antimicrobial therapy and recovering the causal pathogen(s) from infected sites. Typically, the most common infection sites are lung, abdomen/pelvis, and urinary tract [83]. Routine physical examination often identifies the site of infection. However, a definite infection site is not identified in 20% to 30% of patients with sepsis [82,83]. The fact that empiric antimicrobial choices cannot possibly cover every pathogen contingency for all cases underscores the merit in meticulous search for frequently overlooked subtle clinical clues to the site and cause of sepsis. A practical approach to diagnosing and treating sepsis begins at the bedside with heightened perspicacity for subtle findings.

1. **Vital signs.** Routine vital signs often provide the first clues to impending or evolving sepsis. Although "normal" ranges are common knowledge, sagacious clinicians recognize that baselines vary among individuals and interpret vital signs accordingly. **Vital sign trends** are often more informative than actual numbers.
   a. **Temperature. Fever,** often accompanied by **chills** or **rigors,** is a common early sign of infection and should prompt evaluation for impending sepsis. Temperature data should be interpreted along a continuum from the patient's personal baseline. As discussed in Chapter 1, fever pattern occasionally suggests underlying cause. **Fever does not always accompany serious infection,** most notably in neonatal or geriatric age groups and in debilitated patients, age notwithstanding. Steroidal and nonsteroidal **antiinflammatory drugs can attenuate or delay fever.** In some patients, temperature abnormalities are inexplicably delayed or absent. **Hypothermia,** although less common than fever, is also seen in septic patients and portends poor prognosis.
   b. **Pulse. Tachycardia** is common and frequently due to fever or compensatory changes associated with sepsis-induced hypotension. However, tachycardia without fever or hypotension is not rare and can be an early sign of impending sepsis. In febrile patients, a normal or low pulse, commonly termed "temperature-pulse disparity or disassociation," can indicate infection with certain intracellular pathogens (e.g., Legionella, Brucella, Chlamydia). Other common conditions that cause temperature-pulse disparity include beta-blockade, intrinsic conduction abnormalities, and diabetes mellitus.
   c. **Blood pressure. Hypotension,** defined as systolic blood pressure less than 90 mm Hg and mean arterial pressure (MAP) less than 70 mm Hg, or more than a 40 mm Hg decrease from baseline, should prompt immediate volume resuscitation. **Volume depletion** is commonplace in patients with sepsis due to reduced intake and increased losses (**fever, tachypnea, etc.**). In euvolemic febrile patients without underlying cardiac disease, hypotension implies maldistribution of blood flow, heralding severe sepsis. High cardiac output with bounding pulses and wide pulse pressure characterize early sepsis. Low cardiac output with rapid weak pulses typifies late sepsis. **Hypotension unresponsive to adequate volume resuscitation** connotes **shock** and must be regarded as a **medical emergency.**
   d. **Respiratory rate. Hyperventilation,** often overlooked because it precedes the onset of fever and chills, is the **earliest clinical manifestation of bacteremia.** In critical care settings, otherwise unexplained hyperventilation foreshadows bacteremia and warrants blood cultures along with clinical evaluation for signs of impending sepsis.

2. **General findings.** In **early sepsis,** patients frequently appear apprehensive, tachypneic, and toxic or ill. Malaise occurs often but irritability is not uncommon. Typically, extremities are warm and dry. Rigors suggest bacteremia but also are associated with fungemia, viremia, and parasitemia. At times, mental confusion is evident, especially in the elderly. Sepsis-associated capillary leak causes peripheral edema that evolves rapidly with fluid resuscitation, mimicking intravascular volume overload. Peripheral edema alone does not justify fluid restriction. In **late sepsis,** clinical findings reflect progressive organ dysfunction. Depressed respiration, decreased pulses, cyanosis, cold extremities, lethargy, and coma characterize terminal phases.
3. **Skin.** At times subtle and easily overlooked, cutaneous manifestations of infectious diseases are valuable diagnostic opportunities as well as clues to cause (Table 2.2). When evaluating patients with sepsis, otherwise elusive microbiologic diagnoses are at times established simply from Gram stain and culture of material from cutaneous lesions. Direct fluorescent antibody stains performed on specimens collected from suspicious skin or mucosal lesions provide rapid diagnostic data for certain viral infections (e.g., **varicella zoster, herpes simplex**). In addition to intimating primary infection focus and microbiologic etiology, skin findings provide useful staging and prognostic information. In septic patients, certain important skin findings are at times subtle, evanescent, or temporally variant, underscoring the need for meticulous serial inspections. Antimicrobial therapy may alter, trigger (e.g., **ampicillin-induced rash in Epstein-Barr virus infections**), or cause rashes outright. Nevertheless, when analyzed in conjunction with historical, clinical, and epidemiologic clues, it is possible to construct a reasonable differential diagnosis when evaluating the acutely ill patient with fever and cutaneous lesions or rash.
   a. **Petechiae,** although less specific than other cutaneous manifestations of infectious diseases, are associated with several rapidly fatal diseases. These small red or brown spots do not blanch with pressure and may coalesce into larger areas of discoloration or ecchymosis. Formed by bleeding into the skin, petechial rashes comprise purpuric eruptions, including purpuric vesicles. Any bacteremia can cause petechial rash, with or without disseminated intravascular coagulation (DIC). Acutely ill patients with fever and petechial rash typically have bacteremia or rickettsial disease. Petechial rashes are commonly associated with meningococcemia, gonococcemia, and staphylococcemia. Petechiae are the most common skin finding in patients with endocarditis, although Osler nodes, Janeway lesions, splinter hemorrhages, and conjunctival hemorrhages are more readily associated with the disease. Microbiologic etiology notwithstanding, petechial lesions in septic patients connote striking underlying pathology warranting further evaluation, including platelet count, coagulation studies, and DIC panel. Other infectious diseases associated with petechial rashes are listed in Table 2.2. Noninfectious mimics of sepsis, particularly certain rheumatologic diseases, can also present with petechiae or other vasculitic skin lesions associated with SIRS.
   b. ***Ecthyma gangrenosum,*** characteristically oval or round lesions with erythematous indurated borders and necrotic ulcerated centers, implies gram-negative bacteremia, most notably *Pseudomonas aeruginosa*. Gram stain and culture may recover the causal pathogen.
   c. **Purpuric macules, papules, or vesicles,** signaling poor prognosis in patients with meningococcemia, at times accompany bacteremias involving *S. aureus, Neisseria gonorrheae, and P. aeruginosa*. These lesions can also reflect bacterial endocarditis, drug hypersensitivity, allergic vasculitis, enteroviral illness, rickettsial disease, acquired immunodeficiency syndrome (AIDS), systemic lupus erythematosus, and other processes that trigger systemic inflammation. Biopsy with appropriate stains and cultures can often distinguish between infectious and noninfectious causes.
   d. **Diffuse erythroderma** is associated with toxin-producing gram-positive infections such as toxic shock or toxic streptococcal syndromes, with or without

Table 2.2. Rash Etiologies in the Evaluation of Patients with Sepsis

| Rash Type | Bacterial | Other Infectious | Noninfectious |
|---|---|---|---|
| Petechial | • Endocarditis<br>• Staphylococcemia<br>• Pseudomonas bacteremia<br>• Meningococcemia<br>• Gonococcemia<br>• Rocky Mountain spotted fever<br>• Endemic typhus<br>• Rat-bite fever | • Dengue fever<br>• Enterovirus<br>• Hepatitis B<br>• Epstein-Barr virus<br>• Rubella | • Drug allergy<br>• Hypersensitivity vasculitis<br>• Acute rheumatic fever<br>• Henoch-Schönlein purpura<br>• SLE<br>• HIV<br>• Thrombocytopenia<br>• Hyperglobulinemia<br>• Amyloidosis<br>• Scurvy |
| Erythematous | • Streptococci<br>• Staphylococci<br>• Toxic shock syndrome<br>• Erlichiosis<br>• C hemolyticum<br>• Kawasaki disease | • Enterovirus | • Allergy<br>• Vasodilation<br>• Lymphoma<br>• Eczema<br>• Psoriasis<br>• Pityriasis rubra<br>• Sézary syndrome |
| Maculopapular | • Endocarditis<br>• Meningococcemia<br>• Toxic shock syndrome<br>• Scarlet fever<br>• Kawasaki disease<br>• Rickettsial diseases<br>• Typhoid fever<br>• Secondary syphilis<br>• Lyme disease<br>• Mycoplasma<br>• Psitticosis | • Enteroviruses<br>• Adenovirus<br>• Epstein-Barr virus<br>• Rubella<br>• Rubeola<br>• Parvovirus B19<br>• HHV-6<br>• HIV | • Drug allergy<br>• Toxic epidermal necrolysis<br>• Erythema multiforme<br>• Erythema marginatum<br>• Serum sickness<br>• SLE<br>• Dermatomyositis<br>• Sweet syndrome |
| Vesicobullous | • Endocarditis<br>• Staphylococcemia<br>• Meningococcemia<br>• Pseudomonas Bacteremia<br>• Erysipelas<br>• Toxic shock syndrome<br>• Scalded skin syndrome | • Varicella-Zoster virus<br>• Herpes simplex virus<br>• Enterovirus<br>• Parvovirus B19<br>• HIV | • Drug allergy<br>• Toxic epidermal necrolysis<br>• Erythema multiform bullosum<br>• Eczema vaccinatum<br>• Plant dermatitis |
| Urticarial | • Mycoplasma<br>• Lyme disease | • Enteroviruses<br>• Adenovirus<br>• Epstein-Barr virus<br>• Hepatitis<br>• HIV | • Drug allergy<br>• Vasculitis<br>• Malignancy<br>• Idiopathic |

SLE, systemic lupus erythematosus; HIV, human immunodeficiency virus; HHV-6, human herpes virus.

bacteremia. In lieu of positive blood cultures, uncovering the occult site is vital to management as in cases involving drainable abscess or other removable source.

**e. Cellulitis** often suggests both microbiology and source. In addition to primary soft tissue infections (see Chapter 4), occult infections such as infected i.v. lines, drug injection sites, sinusitis, septic arthritis, or osteomyelitis can manifest as focal cellulitis, the source governing empiric antimicrobial therapy pending definitive microbiologic diagnosis.

f. **Furuncles, pustules, or vesicles** offer readily accessible diagnostic opportunity. Properly collected specimens submitted for appropriate stains and cultures can recover otherwise elusive pathogens.

g. **Nodules,** at times more subtle than other cutaneous manifestations of infectious diseases, are often overlooked. Discrete, raised, mildly erythematous skin nodules suggest **candidemia.** In neutropenic patients with candidemia, the erythema associated with these nodules is often subtle or absent. Biopsy specimens readily obtained at bedside yield rapid diagnosis, because Gram stain results showing the budding yeast are available immediately, days earlier than blood culture results.

4. **Head and neck.** Head or neck infection is the primary focus for sepsis in some patients. Sinus or ear infections can lead to meningitis or central nervous system (CNS) abscesses. Rheumatic fever associated with group A streptococcal pharyngitis is associated with clinical manifestations consistent with systemic inflammatory responses. At times, peritonsillar and retropharyngeal abscesses are foci for life-threatening infectious sequelae, including septic shock. Sinusitis involving toxin-producing staphylococci or streptococci can cause toxic shock syndrome without bacteremia or other invasive infection. Sinusitis occasionally leads to septic cavernous sinus thrombosis with attendant morbidity or mortality if not treated appropriately. Odontogenic infections can cause endocarditis and other life-threatening diseases, such as Ludwig angina and Vincent angina/Lemierre disease. Funduscopic examination, often difficult and deferred in the acutely ill patient, provides rapid diagnostic clues in sepsis, such as Roth spots associated with infectious endocarditis or retinal findings connoting disseminated candidiasis. When the differential diagnosis of sepsis includes infectious diseases with characteristic funduscopic findings, timely diagnosis justifies ophthalmology consultation for thorough retinal examination.

5. **Heart murmurs** characterizing valvular abnormalities or septal defects raise suspicion for infective endocarditis. Scrupulous baseline and serial cardiac examinations are important for detecting new or changing murmurs that connote endocarditis. Clinical findings suggesting pericarditis or myocarditis are also helpful diagnostic clues to underlying etiology (see Chapter 12).

6. **Lungs.** Community-acquired and nosocomial pneumonias are common causes of sepsis. Subtle clinical findings such as egophony or whispered pectoriloquy may precede radiographic signs of consolidation. Both clinical and radiographic findings suggesting pneumonia are often minimal during early disease, particularly in dehydrated, elderly, or immunocompromised patients. Chest radiographs are warranted in all patients with sepsis, because roentgenographic studies may reveal infiltrates or other pulmonary pathology imperceptible on clinical exam. Serial clinical examination and chest radiographs often detect abnormal findings because pulmonary disease manifestations evolve with hydration and time. In septic patients, pulmonary infiltrates may represent infectious or noninfectious processes such as noncardiogenic (**ARDS**) or cardiogenic pulmonary edema. In critically ill patients, pulmonary infiltrates are often multifactorial. Microbiologic studies typically distinguish between infectious and noninfectious causes.

7. **Abdominal, rectal, and pelvic examinations** provide important clinical data for determining septic foci and choosing appropriate empiric antimicrobial therapy. If a detailed history is unreliable or unavailable, telltale scars from prior abdominal (e.g., **splenectomy, cholecystectomy, appendectomy**) or pelvic (e.g., **hysterectomy, laparoscopy, prostatectomy**) surgery provide important clues to underlying pathology and risk for certain infections. Localized or early manifestations of intraabdominal or pelvic infections are often subtle in elderly, neurologically compromised, or immunosuppressed patients, especially those taking steroids. Often deferred in acutely ill patients, rectal and pelvic examinations are crucial for identifying rectal abscess (**especially in patients with neutropenia or inflammatory bowel disease**), prostatitic abscess,

attempted abortion, or pelvic inflammatory disease. Splenomegaly is occasionally the only clinical finding in febrile patients with subacute bacterial endocarditis. Duodenal ulcers occasionally perforate into the pancreas, presenting with signs of fulminant pancreatitis, peritonitis, and septic shock.

8. **Extremities.** In septic patients, inflammatory arthritis is both a diagnostic sign and opportunity. In the absence of penetrating joint trauma, septic arthritis points toward systemic infection, most notably staphylococcemia, streptococcemia, meningococcemia, and gonococcemia. Acute joint pain as a presenting complaint warrants assessment for systemic infection, especially if the patient has fever or complete blood count shows neutrophilia and/or increased immature forms. Early diagnosis and timely antimicrobial therapy can prevent sepsis and its sequelae. Arthrocentesis for synovial fluid analysis and culture provides rapid diagnostic data. Synovial fluid Gram stain often discloses the invading pathogen long before blood or joint aspirate cultures yield a microbiologic diagnosis. Septic arthritis and its causes are detailed in Chapter 5. Osteomyelitis also implicates systemic infection, therefore warranting full skeletal evaluation in septic patients, including examination for vertebral point tenderness. When examining extremities, signs of phlebitis implicate pulmonary emboli as cause for fever, tachypnea, and/or hypotension in acutely ill patients, stipulating further diagnostic studies.
9. **Central nervous system.** Fever associated with focal neurologic deficits demands timely evaluation for CNS infection, particularly brain or spinal cord abscess. Meningitis at times causes focal neurologic findings, particularly when the basilar meninges are involved extensively (**notably tuberculosis or fungal meningitis, although bacterial infections may also do so**). (CNS infections are detailed in Chapter 6.) Unless otherwise contraindicated, lumbar puncture for appropriate cerebrospinal fluid analysis is imperative for diagnosing CNS infections. Stroke in the febrile septic-appearing patient warrants evaluation for infectious endocarditis (see Chapter 12). Evaluation for endocarditis (especially subacute bacterial endocarditis [SBE]) is justified in all patients with embolic stroke, even if lacking overt signs of infection.
10. **Wounds and soft tissues.** Skin and soft tissues are important infection foci in sepsis. Although most suppurative wounds are apparent on routine physical examination, certain noteworthy soft tissue infections present with minimal clinical findings and progress so rapidly that septic shock develops before the underlying infection is apparent. Group A streptococcal necrotizing fasciitis often presents with severe localized pain without objective clinical findings to implicate infection, commonly eluding timely diagnosis unless clinical vigilance motivates further evaluation and appropriate laboratory tests. Immature granulocytes, lymphopenia, hypoalbuminemia, and hypocalcemia are diagnostic clues warranting further evaluation with an eye toward rapid surgical intervention and timely antimicrobial therapy. Seemingly minor wound and soft tissue infections, when caused by certain toxin-producing staphylococci or streptococci, can present as a toxic shock syndrome. Soft tissue crepitance identified during physical examination or air visualized in radiographic studies (e.g., **computed tomography** [CT]) suggests infection with gas-producing pathogens such as *Clostridium* or mixed enteric gram-negative bacteria.

**C. Diagnostic microbiology**

1. **Blood cultures** are essential tools for diagnosing sepsis. True positive blood cultures constitute the best criteria for defining sepsis and its cause. Unfortunately, blood cultures are negative in a substantial number of patients with sepsis. Multiple factors obscure blood culture yield. **Transient bacteremias** accompany most serious infections [84] but pass before fever or other clinical manifestations motivate orders for blood cultures. **Intermittent bacteremias,** recognized as recurrent transient bacteremias, are associated with sporadic obstruction or manipulation of infected sites. **Continuous or sustained bacteremias,** defined by multiple positive blood cultures obtained at intervals from several hours to days, typify intravascular infections such as endocarditis, suppurative thrombophlebitis, and intravascular catheter or graft infections. Occasionally,

continuous bacteremia accompanies extravascular infections (e.g., **intraabdominal abscess)** in immunosuppressed hosts. **Persistent bacteremia** despite appropriate antimicrobial therapy portends endovascular infection and warrants rigorous search for an intravascular source. Prior antimicrobial therapy decreases blood culture yield. Using resin-containing media to lower antibiotic concentrations in blood cultures, although attractive theoretically, does not improve sensitivity and may decrease specificity by facilitating recovery of contaminants, most notably coagulase-negative staphylococci [85]. Fastidious or slow-growing blood-borne pathogens, often overlooked by standard blood culture protocols, are recoverable if clinicians inform the microbiology lab that the differential diagnosis includes such pathogens. The single most important factor governing blood culture sensitivity is the volume of blood cultured [86]. False-negative blood cultures are less common than false-positive ones. Blood culture specificity is not absolute, requiring appropriate interpretation to distinguish true pathogens from possible contaminants. False-positive cultures due to contamination or colonization pose diagnostic problems, especially in patients with increased risk for infection caused by otherwise typical skin contaminants (e.g., **coagulase-negative staphylococci or diphtheroids cultured from patients with indwelling i.v. catheters, prosthetic heart valves, or joint prostheses**). Several factors influence the predictive value of positive blood cultures, including pattern (number of positive culture sets), pathogen identity, and clinical context.

a. **Blood volume.** Blood volume is the single most important variable governing blood culture yield or sensitivity [86]. Pathogen concentration is no more than 1 colony-forming unit (CFU) per mL of blood in 50% of bacteremic adults and less than 0.1 CFU/mL in 20% of bacteremic adults [87]. Pediatric bacteremias are often higher grade, with blood pathogen concentrations reaching more than 100 CFU/mL [88], although low-level bacteremias (**1–10 CFU/mL blood**) are also documented [89]. In adults, blood culture yield increases 3% per mL of blood cultured [86]. In adults, culturing at least 10 mL and preferably 20 mL of blood maximizes bloodstream pathogen recovery. Culturing more than 20 mL of blood does not increase yield substantially and is not recommended except, possibly, in cases of suspected viridans streptococcal subacute bacterial endocarditis. In pediatric patients, recommended blood volumes per culture are as follows: 1 to 2 mL for neonates, 2 to 3 mL for infants aged 1 month to 2 years, 3 to 5 mL for older children, and 10 to 20 mL for adolescents [88]. Because low-level bacteremia can occur in pediatric populations, some experts recommend using weight-based determinations, culturing up to 4.5% of a child's estimated total blood volume [89].
b. **Blood culture set number.** Although a single blood culture is inadequate for documenting bacteremia or fungemia, two to three properly collected blood cultures will detect 99% of clinically important bloodstream infections caused by common bacterial and fungal pathogens [90,91]. It is rarely necessary to collect more than two blood culture sets in a 24-hour period, although many clinical microbiology laboratories will process more if notified that the clinician suspects subacute bacterial endocarditis. When treating patients with intravascular infections, daily blood cultures (**until negative**) are warranted to assess antimicrobial efficacy, establish adjunct interventional requirements (e.g., **heart valve replacement**), and determine treatment duration.
c. **Site selection.** Venipuncture site selection is a controllable variable that has significant impact on blood culture results. Blood obtained from femoral vessels is associated with higher contamination rates than specimens collected from antecubital veins or other upper extremity vessels [90]. Blood obtained from sites with overlying cellulitis or dermatologic disease is also associated with higher contamination rates. Culturing arterial blood offers no higher yield than venous blood [92]. The American College of Physicians guidelines [93] and expert opinion [94] discourage culturing blood from intravascular catheters. A recent retrospective analysis comparing 551 paired venipuncture and i.v. catheter specimens from hospitalized cancer patients demonstrated a high negative but low positive predictive value in blood cultures obtained

through indwelling central i.v. catheters [95]. Although negative blood cultures obtained from central i.v. lines may rule out bacteremia, positive cultures require careful clinical interpretation and likely require confirmation to distinguish true bacteremia from line colonization. When clinical circumstance necessitates culturing blood from central i.v. lines, these specimens should be paired with blood cultures obtained by peripheral venipuncture [88,94].

**d. Timing.** The optimal time for obtaining blood culture specimens is immediately before onset of rigors. Because predicting such clinical events is impossible, a practical approach calls for blood cultures as soon as fever or rigors are detected. In acutely ill patients likely requiring immediate antimicrobial therapy, it is reasonable to obtain two sets of blood cultures simultaneously from different sites. In less urgent situations, blood cultures may be spaced at intervals. Spacing blood collection over a 24-hour period does not improve yield [96] but may provide useful clinical information by distinguishing between transient and continuous bacteremia or fungemia.

**e. Incubation duration.** Five-day incubation periods are adequate for detecting most pathogens via the continuous-monitoring blood culture systems used in contemporary U.S. clinical microbiology laboratories. By protocol, blood culture specimens are discarded if negative after 5 to 7 days of incubation. Some fastidious pathogens such as *Legionella, Bartonella, Brucella,* and certain fungi require longer incubation periods. Alerting the clinical microbiology laboratory when fastidious pathogens are suspected averts untimely discard of blood culture specimens. Fungal and mycobacterial blood cultures are incubated for 4 to 6 weeks.

**f. Positive blood culture interpretation.** Blood culture interpretation is straightforward in many cases such as when multiple blood cultures grow *S. aureus* in the clinical context of infective endocarditis. In contrast, recovery of less credible microorganisms such as coagulase-negative staphylococci and diphtheroids is commonplace and complicates blood culture interpretation. Because any microorganism can, given the right circumstance, become a blood-borne pathogen, clinicians must interpret accurately the clinical relevance of positive blood cultures. Several factors improve blood culture predictive values.

**(1) Pattern.** When all or most blood cultures obtained from a series of separate venipunctures yield the same isolate, bloodstream infection is highly probable regardless of microorganism identity.

**(2) Microorganism identity.** Certain blood isolates virtually always (**>90%**) represent true infection such as *Streptococcus pneumoniae, S. aureus, N. meningitidis* and *gonorrhoeae, E. coli* and other *Enterobacteriaceae, Pseudomonas aeruginosa, Candida albicans, Histoplasma capsulatum,* and *Cryptococcus neoformans*. In contrast, *Corynebacterium* species, *Propionibacterium acnes*, and *Bacillus* species rarely (**<5%**) cause true bloodstream infections and, with rare exception (e.g., ***Corynebacterium jekeium* in neutropenic patients with permanent i.v. catheters**), likely represent contaminants when recovered sporadically in blood cultures. Coagulase-negative staphylococci, viridans streptococci, and enterococci are particularly problematic blood culture isolates, representing true bacteremia in 15%, 38%, and 78% of cases, respectively [97]. Because there are no laboratory gold standards for distinguishing between true bloodstream pathogens and contaminants, judging positive blood culture relevance remains embedded in clinical context.

**g. Clinical context.** Blood culture isolates are virtually always relevant when the microorganism identity parallels clinical context. Credible pathogens as related to specific infections are discussed in their respective chapters. Less plausible blood culture isolates gain relevance in certain clinical situations and deserve further consideration.

**(1) Endocarditis or endovascular infections.** *S. aureus* bacteremias are common in patients with high carriage or colonization rates such as individuals with (a) atopic dermatosis, (b) diabetes, (c) chronic renal failure requiring hemodialysis, (d) chronic indwelling catheters, (e) i.v. drug use, (f) recent or chronic corticosteroid therapy, (g) recent hospitalization, and (h) institutional living requirements, such as nursing homes or prisons. ***S. aureus* bacteremia** without an identifiable source or as a community-acquired infection often signifies endocarditis. Coupled with clinical evidence suggesting subacute bacterial endocarditis, especially when temporally related to dental procedures, blood cultures growing **viridans streptococci** signify true bacteremia. **Coagulase-negative staphylococci** occasionally cause native valve endocarditis but assume greater importance as a bloodstream isolate in patients with indwelling central i.v. catheters, prosthetic heart valves or other artificial endovascular devices, joint prostheses, and ventriculoperitoneal (VP) shunts. Community-acquired **enterococcal bacteremia** without an identifiable source in patients with valvular heart disease warrants further evaluation for endocarditis. **Candidemia** may represent serious endovascular infection in certain patients, most notably those with neutropenia or prolonged hospitalization involving central i.v. catheters, broad-spectrum antimicrobial therapy, and total parenteral nutrition. Persistent bacteremia or fungemia, especially in patients receiving appropriate antimicrobial therapy, suggests intravascular infection such endocarditis, suppurative thrombophlebitis, or infected i.v. catheters or grafts. Endocarditis and its causes are discussed further in Chapter 12.

(2) **Pneumonia and respiratory tract infections.** Common pulmonary pathogens such as *S. pneumoniae* or *H. influenza* isolated from blood cultures in patients with pneumonia inarguably represent true bacteremias. Less virulent organisms such as *Stenotrophomonas maltophilia, Burkholderia cepacia,* and *Acinetobacter baumanii* gain relevance as blood culture isolates in patients at increased risk for pneumonia caused by these bacteria (e.g., **ventilator-associated pneumonia, nosocomial pneumonia in patients receiving broad-spectrum antibiotics, patients with cystic fibrosis**). In patients with pneumonia, recovering even unusual organisms from multiple blood cultures and purulent sputum helps distinguish true bacteremia from contaminants. Occasionally, lung abscess is associated with polymicrobial bacteremia.

(3) **Abdominal and pelvic infections.** Positive blood cultures yielding multiple organisms may reflect inappropriate collection technique or central i.v. line contamination, particularly when drawn from femoral sites. However, true **polymicrobial bacteremias (accounting for 6%–18% of all bacteremias)** commonly stem from intraabdominal or pelvic infections. In patients with documented or suspected intraabdominal or pelvic infections, appropriately collected polymicrobial positive blood cultures likely represent true bacteremia, particularly if the isolates include *Enterobacteriaceae*, anaerobes, enterococci, *S. aureus*, *Pseudomonas*, and *Candida*. True polymicrobial bacteremia in the absence of intraabdominal or pelvic sources often represents line-related nosocomial infection. *Streptococcus bovis* identified in blood cultures from patients with colon cancer signifies bacteremia. Conversely, identifying *S. bovis* bacteremia in patients with no known malignancy calls for painstaking evaluation for colon cancer or other occult gastrointestinal pathology.

(4) **Urinary tract.** In patients with clinical findings consistent with urinary tract infection, blood cultures growing typical pathogens (e.g., *E. coli, Klebsiella pneumoniae*) undoubtedly represent true bacteremia. Disparate results from urine and blood cultures raise doubt and justify repeat studies. Indwelling urinary catheter use is a common hospital practice, especially in critical care settings, increasing risk for urinary tract infections caused by atypical pathogens. Polymicrobial urinary tract colonization is common in patients with urinary catheters. If clinical and laboratory data suggest a urinary tract source in patients with sepsis, positive blood cultures yielding isolates matching those from urine likely represent true bacteremia.

*S. aureus* recovered from both blood and urine cultures suggests hematogenous seeding of the urinary tract rather than a primary urinary source and warrants careful evaluation for intravascular infection. A similar approach applies when both urine and serial blood cultures grow *Candida, Enterococcus,* or coagulase-negative staphylococci in patients with indwelling central i.v. lines.

**(5) Soft tissue infections.** Positive blood cultures with what might otherwise represent skin contaminants may represent true bacteremia in patients with serious skin or soft tissue infections. Appropriately collected serial blood cultures usually distinguish between potential contaminants and true bloodstream infection, especially when coagulase-negative staphylococci are isolated. At times, decubitus ulcer sepsis is associated with polymicrobial bacteremia, in which case blood isolates should match those obtained from wound cultures. For obvious reasons, blood cultures must not be collected from venipunctures through infected appearing skin or soft tissues. *N. meningitiditis* or *P. aeruginosa* recovered from vasculitic appearing or ecthyma-like skin lesions and blood cultures reflects systemic infection rather than a primary soft tissue source and warrants careful evaluation for other cause.

**(6) Central nervous system.** Positive blood cultures in patients with meningitis usually yield obvious pathogens such as pneumococcus and reflect true bacteremias. Positive blood cultures with what might otherwise represent contaminants may represent true bacteremia in patients with meningeal signs when associated with extenuating clinical history such as neurosurgical procedures, ventriculostomy or epidural catheter placement, VP shunts, or spina bifida. In these patients, coagulase-negative staphylococci, enterococci, or unusual gram-negative bacteria isolated from blood cultures and cerebrospinal fluid signifies true bloodstream infection.

2. **Gram stain and other stains.** The three main methods for rapid detection of infection in critically ill patients are detecting pus in a normally sterile site, demonstrating microorganisms (**bacteria, fungi, viruses, or parasites**) in a normally sterile site by stains or culture, and detecting pathogen genome in a normally sterile site using molecular biology techniques. For most bacterial pathogens, Gram stain remains the fastest, simplest, and most universally available diagnostic tool for identifying infection. In settings where antimicrobial therapy is initiated before obtaining specimens for microbiologic studies, the Gram stain may be the only way to diagnose infection if cultures prove negative. A positive Gram stain facilitates rapid distinction between infectious and noninfectious causes of inflammatory exudates obtained from normally sterile sites such as the peritoneal cavity and pleural, pericardial, epidural, or articular spaces. Interpreting Gram-stained specimens obtained from normally nonsterile sites (e.g., **lung, sinuses, wounds**) is less straightforward but often valuable nonetheless, especially when visualized organisms corroborate clinical impression. Acid-fast stains (e.g., **Kinyoun**) are rapid diagnostic tools for identifying mycobacteria when differential diagnoses include tuberculosis or nontuberculous mycobacterial disease. In some clinical laboratories, gene probe technology permits rapid identification of *Mycobacterium tuberculosis* and other clinically important mycobacterial species. Modified acid-fast stains are used to detect *Nocardia* in clinical specimens. Direct fluorescent antibody stains permit rapid detection of certain pathogens where cultures are unreliable or require prolonged incubation (e.g., **Legionella, Varicella zoster virus**). Fungal stains often provide rapid diagnostic data where culture results are not available for several weeks.

3. **Cultures.** Although microbiologic stains often provide valuable diagnostic data, definitive microbiologic diagnoses are established by isolating the causative pathogens from appropriate cultures. Cultures also permit *in vitro* susceptibility testing, an important clinical tool for guiding antimicrobial therapy and epidemiologic tool for monitoring resistance trends. Certain clinical situations call for special culture media or techniques. Good communication between the

clinician and microbiology laboratory is imperative when microbiologic differential diagnoses include unusual or fastidious pathogens that may require special handling or unconventional selective media. **Quantitative cultures** defining precise bacterial numbers in clinical specimens are useful for diagnosing infection in certain sites. It is now standard clinical laboratory practice to perform quantitative cultures on urine specimens based on the widely accepted premise that more than $10^5$ CFU/mL correlates with urinary tract infection. For other sites, bacterial colony counts are only semiquantitative (e.g., **colony counts from bronchoalveolar lavage specimens for diagnosing ventilator-associated pneumonia or i.v. catheter tips for diagnosing catheter-associated bloodstream infections**). No unequivocal clinical data show presently that quantitative blood culture results improve diagnostic accuracy or medical management of sepsis [98].

4. **Molecular diagnostics.** Recent advances in automated molecular testing methods are changing clinical microbiology laboratory diagnostic practice for infectious diseases. Previously relegated to detecting slow-growing or uncultivatable pathogens, technological advances now make molecular diagnostic testing adaptable for use in clinical microbiology laboratories and applicable for detecting common pathogens [99]. Molecular (**genotypic**) susceptibility testing is gaining similar practical application in infectious disease treatment and epidemiology [100]. Molecular testing is available presently for diagnosing group A streptococcal pharyngitis, pulmonary tuberculosis, HIV, hepatitis C virus infection, Herpes simplex virus encephalitis, CNS toxoplasmosis, progressive multifocal leukoencephalopathy, and *Chlamydia trachomatis* and *N. gonorrhoeae* urogenital infections. Molecular biology testing methods hold promise for clinical application in the rapid diagnosis of life-threatening infections, especially in situations where prior antimicrobial therapy or pathogen characteristics render standard microbiologic methodology inadequate [101]. Clinicians should check with their clinical microbiology laboratory regarding the applicability and availability of specific molecular diagnostic tests.

D. **Hematology.** Complete blood count with differential is a simple, rapid, readily available test that provides valuable clinical and diagnostic information.

1. **Granulocytosis with increased immature forms** ("left shift") suggests infection. Granulocyte counts can be normal or reduced in severe sepsis, but the differential will still reveal the telltale left shift. Granulocyte count and differential consistent with infection is one of several recommended drug utilization criteria for using human recombinant activated protein C (hrAPC; drotrecogin alpha [activated]) in the treatment of patients with severe sepsis (see section IV.D). Neutropenia (**absolute granulocyte counts $<$1,000**) increases risk for severe infection with both common and opportunistic pathogens, disseminated fungal infections, nosocomial infections, poor response to antimicrobial therapy, and increased mortality.
2. **Thrombocytopenia** portends DIC and justifies further tests to assess for this common complication of sepsis (**fibrinogen, D-dimers, prothrombin time/partial thromboplastin time**). Platelet count is both an inclusion and exclusion criterion for using rhAPC in the treatment of severe sepsis (see section IV.D). Sepsis-associated thrombocytopenia can be severe, requiring platelet transfusions to prevent life-threatening hemorrhage.
3. **Anemia** diminishes oxygen-carrying capacity of the blood and potentially worsens tissue hypoxia in septic patients, especially when hemoglobin concentration drops below 8 g/dL.
4. **Peripheral blood smears** occasionally detect bloodstream pathogens such as *Histoplasma capsulatum*, *Plasmodium* species, *Babesia* species, certain spirochetes, and even bacteria in cases of overwhelming sepsis (**most notably *S. pneumoniae***). Both **thick and thin blood smears** should be ordered and scrutinized for *Plasmodium* parasites when **malaria** is suspected.

E. **Coagulation studies**. Prothrombin time and partial thromboplastin time provide useful information when evaluating septic patients. Prothrombin time/partial thromboplastin time are prolonged in sepsis-associated DIC. Prothrombin time/partial thromboplastin time are also excellent markers for liver function and, when prolonged in the absence of DIC or anticoagulation therapy, herald hepatic dysfunction and secondary MODS in patients with sepsis.

F. **Chemistry.** Routine chemistries are readily available and provide rapid prognostic and diagnostic data when assessing patients with sepsis.

1. **Serum electrolytes** provide important information regarding metabolic status. In septic patients, an elevated anion gap metabolic acidosis implies lactic acidemia from tissue hypoxia and warrants checking serum lactate levels. Serum electrolytes should be monitored closely during volume resuscitation to assess efficacy and detect potentially life-threatening electrolyte abnormalities (**notably hypokalemia and hypophosphatemia**) that can develop rapidly as renal function improves and acidosis resolves.
2. **Baseline and serial renal panels** provide information for guiding and assessing resuscitative measures. Elevated serum creatinine and blood urea nitrogen at presentation may simply reflect volume contraction that should respond rapidly to volume repletion or, more ominously, connote renal failure due to sepsis-induced acute tubular necrosis. Severe pyelonephritis occasionally causes acute renal failure directly, in which case urinalysis will detect white blood cell casts.
3. **Liver panel** abnormalities are common in patients with severe sepsis and can reflect underlying cause or imply end-organ dysfunction.
   a. **Isolated baseline alkaline phosphatase elevation** in the absence of severe sepsis may connote liver abscess.
   b. **Elevated direct bilirubin** levels can signify underlying gallbladder disease as a source of sepsis. Elevated direct bilirubin levels in the absence of gallbladder disease likely reflects sepsis-associated intrahepatic cholestasis and accompanies other liver panel abnormalities due to liver dysfunction in the continuum of secondary MODS.
4. **Amylase and lipase** elevation in the absence of shock suggests pancreatitis as an underlying cause for systemic inflammatory responses mimicking sepsis. Elevated amylase and lipase levels associated with refractory hypotension in patients with septic shock signifies end-organ damage and is a part of the organ dysfunction constellation comprising secondary MODS. Procalcitonin levels offer promise for distinguishing between SIRS caused by pancreatitis versus sepsis (see following).
5. **Procalcitonin,** a calcitonin propeptide normally produced in the C cells of the thyroid gland, has recently drawn attention as a specific marker of systemic inflammatory response to infection. During systemic infection, extrathyroid tissues produce procalcitonin; the exact site of production during sepsis is uncertain. Procalcitonin levels increase dramatically in patients with sepsis, are detectable within 3 hours of induction onset (**at least 20 hours earlier than CRP**), have a much longer half-life than cytokines, and are stable in serum or plasma at room temperature (**>90% in 12 hours**). Various stimuli, other than bacterial infection, may increase procalcitonin levels in certain clinical conditions (e.g., **severe trauma, major surgical procedures, prolonged circulatory failure**). As a rule, however, procalcitonin levels detected under these conditions are substantially lower than those seen in patients with sepsis. Procalcitonin levels, presently, can be measured with a commercially available immunoluminometric assay. Procalcitonin assays, although not widely available in clinical laboratories presently, hold promise for clinical application by rapidly detecting invasive bacterial infection, discriminating between infectious and noninfectious causes of SIRS, and following response to therapy in patients with sepsis. Establishing optimal procalcitonin thresholds for appropriate application in clinical settings is the subject of ongoing investigations. Procalcitonin measurements, in the near future, probably will become a part of routine diagnostic testing for rapid identification of infection in several clinical settings.
   a. **Elevated procalcitonin levels (>0.5 ng/mL)** in emergency department patients with suspected infectious or inflammatory disease **indicate ongoing and potentially severe systemic infection with an increased risk of**

**fatal outcome** [102]. The specificity of procalcitonin threshold more than 0.5 ng/mL approaches 100%, but levels below this threshold do not rule out infection.

b. **Procalcitonin levels correlate strongly with infection severity** and therefore may provide useful objective data for stratifying patients into various sepsis stages [103,104]. There are those, however, who question the value of procalcitonin as a marker for infection [105]. Optimal procalcitonin thresholds for discriminating among the various stages of the sepsis continuum are not defined clearly at present but remain the subject of ongoing clinical investigations.

c. **In critically ill pediatric patients,** procalcitonin concentration appears to be a better diagnostic marker for sepsis than CRP in children but no better than CRP in neonates [106].

d. **Procalcitonin helps discriminate between infectious and noninfectious causes of early ARDS.** Limited clinical data suggest that procalcitonin is a useful diagnostic tool for differentiating between infectious and noninfectious underlying disease in patients with early ARDS [107].

e. **Procalcitonin discriminates between infection and acute graft rejection** in organ transplant patients [108,109].

f. **Procalcitonin discriminates between bacterial and viral infections.** Bacterial meningitis, in neonates and children, is associated with substantially higher procalcitonin levels than viral meningitis.

g. **Procalcitonin predicts infectious complications in patients with necrotizing pancreatitis and abdominal sepsis.** Procalcitonin in patients with necrotizing pancreatitis appears to be a good predictor of infection versus noninfectious pancreatic necrosis [110]. Procalcitonin, similarly, appears to have clinical applicability for identifying septic complications after abdominal surgery [111].

6. **CRP** is used widely to determine inflammatory status but is not specific for infection and does not correlate with severity. In patients with documented sepsis, however, CRP provides useful prognostic information for after treatment efficacy as levels normalize with successful therapy and is readily available presently in most clinical laboratories.

7. **Cytokine levels** rise rapidly during sepsis and are detectable earlier than procalcitonin. The short half-life of cytokines, however, causes rapid fluctuations in plasma levels, making serial assessments difficult and reducing clinical applicability.

   a. **IL-6 and IL-8,** among all cytokines studied to date, show most consistent correlation with outcome in critically ill patients but do not discriminate between infectious and noninfectious causes of systemic inflammation [101].

   b. **IL-6 levels** appear to provide useful prognostic information and may be useful for following therapeutic response in patients with sepsis [101]. Whether IL-6 levels offer an advantage over procalcitonin levels presently is uncertain.

G. **Arterial blood gases**. Arterial blood gases should be checked in all patients with impending or established sepsis.

1. **Respiratory alkalosis,** reflecting hyperventilation, is an early sign of impending sepsis.
2. **Respiratory acidosis** signifies ventilatory failure and calls for careful evaluation of lungs and CNS to identify cause. Arterial blood gases facilitate decisions regarding the need for ventilatory support and timing of intubation.
3. **Metabolic acidosis** cannot be assessed on the basis of serum chemistries alone. Arterial blood gases in patients with sepsis-associated metabolic acidosis provide accurate blood pH measurements useful in formulating management plans (e.g., **dialysis needs**) and following treatment efficacy (e.g., **resolution of lactic acidosis with resuscitative measures**).
4. **Elevated $AaO_2$ gradient,** calculated from arterial blood gas results, often precedes the appearance of infiltrates on chest roentgenogram in patients with ARDS and certain forms of pneumonia (e.g., ***Pneumocystis carinii*** **pneumonia [PCP]**).

**H. Urinalysis**. Urinalysis provides useful data relevant to both cause and effect in patients with sepsis. Urinary tract infections are a leading cause of sepsis, and urinalysis provides rapid diagnostic information in acutely ill patients, especially when white blood cell or fungal casts are detected. Urinalysis results consistent with urinary tract infection justify urine cultures to corroborate infection and identify its cause. In the absence of primary urinary tract infection, abnormal sediment may reflect end organ damage associated with secondary MODS (e.g., **acute tubular necrosis [ATN]**).

**I. Serology.** Serologic tests for detecting microbial antigens and host antibodies can, in limited clinical circumstances, provide diagnostic information in the workup of sepsis.

1. **Legionellosis** presents a diagnostic challenge. Sputum cultures often fail to grow the pathogen, and sputum direct fluorescent antibody stains, in most clinical laboratories, lack adequate specificity and sensitivity. An enzyme immunoassay currently is available for detecting *L. pneumophila* serogroup 1 antigen in urine and may be useful in areas with high prevalence of this serovariant but does not detect the 62 other Legionella serovariants. A test kit for detecting a broad group of Legionella serovariants has recently become available, but performance characteristics must be established to determine widespread clinical applicability [112].
2. **Cryptococcal antigen testing** is available in most clinical laboratories and is useful for rapidly detecting *C. neoformans* in serum and CSF of immunosuppressed patients (e.g., **AIDS, organ transplant recipients**) with cryptococcemia and meningitis.
3. **Acute and convalescent antibody titers,** although useful for confirming diseases such as rickettsiosis, ehrlichiosis, viral encephalitis, and hemorrhagic fevers, do not provide immediate diagnostic data in the acute setting. Treatment, in these settings, must be based on clinical assessment with serologic data providing confirmatory and epidemiologic diagnoses.

**J. Radiology.** A wide variety of imaging techniques is available to facilitate evaluation and intervention in the management of sepsis. Appropriate diagnostic imaging presupposes thorough clinical evaluation and close consultation with the imaging specialist. Diagnostic imaging in sepsis has been reviewed, including the advantages and limitations of imaging studies for specific conditions, and in specific anatomic areas [113].

1. **Plain radiographs** are rapid, inexpensive, and portable; require no special preparation; and carry low risks limited to minimal radiation exposure. Plain radiographs are relatively nonspecific and insensitive in many situations but, in some cases, provide rapid diagnostic data (e.g., **some pneumonias, visceral perforation**).
   a. **Lung.** Chest radiographs are helpful for diagnosing community-acquired pneumonia, and lung abscess but are less reliable for ventilator-associated pneumonia [114] and PCP. Pulmonary effusions, adenopathy, and masses detected on plain radiographs can be detailed further by chest CT, which also provides direct visualization for guiding invasive diagnostic and interventional measures.
   b. **Abdomen and pelvis.** Plain radiographs, at times, provide diagnostic data when images detect free air or demonstrate classic signs of bowel obstruction. Contrast studies are useful for evaluating hollow viscera; soluble contrast should be used when clinical findings suggest perforation. Masses and organomegaly, at times, are discernible with plain radiographs, but ultrasound, CT, and magnetic resonance imaging (MRI) are more reliable and provide better detail.
2. **CT and MRI** offer diagnostic information as well as diagnostic and interventional opportunity.
   a. **Chest CT or MRI** provides detailed images for detecting subtle abnormalities in lung, mediastinum, and bony thorax. Contrasted studies help distinguish between inflammatory and noninflammatory processes. CT or MRI allows image-guided fine-needle aspiration and biopsy that often establish microbiologic and histopathologic diagnoses in lieu of higher risk open

surgical procedures. CT or MRI of chest, abdomen, and pelvis is recommended for disclosing infection foci in septic patients when the source is uncertain despite detailed clinical evaluation.

b. **Abdomen and pelvis CT or MRI** are preferred when clinical circumstance calls for a global view of intraabdominal and pelvic structures [113]. MRI or CT using i.v. and oral contrast can detect (a) abscesses (**including hepatosplenic microabscesses commonly associated with disseminated staphylococcal and fungal infections**); (b) cholecystitis and cholangitis; (c) pancreatitis (**with or without phlegmon**); (d) renal and perinephric abscesses; (e) enteric and peritoneal conditions associated with sepsis (e.g., **bowel wall inflammation, including extension into mesenteric or peritoneal regions, localized phlegmon, pneumatosis intestinalis, obstruction, fistulas, etc.**); (f) neutropenic typhlitis; (g) perirectal abscess (**particularly in septic neutropenic patients**); (h) prostatic, tuboovarian, and other pelvic abscesses; (i) endometritis; and (j) arterial or venous thrombosis. CT or MR image-guided percutaneous fine-needle aspiration and drain placement, in many cases, provide both diagnosis and intervention in patients with focal sources of infection.

c. **Head and neck CT or MRI** is recommended when clinical evaluation suggests meningitis, encephalitis, intracranial abscess, or serious infections of soft tissues not detected by physical examination (e.g., **retropharyngeal abscess**). **Sinus CT or MRI is justified in patients with sepsis of uncertain origin**, particularly in critically ill patients with *in situ* endotracheal or nasogastric tubes. Sinus-associated toxic shock syndrome has been described [115]. MRI with i.v. gadolinium is superior to CT for detecting basilar meningitis and other CNS-related inflammatory processes, including intraspinous, epidural, and paraspinous abscesses.

d. **Extremity and spine CT or MRI** is a valuable diagnostic tool for assessing patients with suspected myositis, necrotizing fasciitis, or osteomyelitis. Vertebral osteomyelitis and discitis, extremely difficult diagnoses to establish clinically, are characterized well using MRI technology. Spinal MRI provides accurate anatomic information and allows diagnostic fine-needle aspiration and biopsy.

3. **Ultrasonography** is a simple and inexpensive means of detecting abnormal fluid collections in the soft tissues and joints. Ultrasound offers advantages over CT and MRI in certain clinical situations by virtue of portability (**particularly in critically ill patients unable to tolerate transport**), safety (**scans do not involve contrast or radiation exposure**), and low cost. Ultrasound is useful for detecting visceral and soft tissue abscesses, cholelithiasis and nephrolithiasis, and obstruction (e.g., **hydronephrosis, biliary ductal dilation**).

4. **Nuclear medicine imaging** provides information on pathophysiologic and pathobiochemical processes not visualized using other imaging procedures. In patients with fever of unknown origin, nuclear medicine techniques provide whole body imaging and can localize inflammatory foci, permitting subsequent CT- or MRI-guided biopsy for definitive diagnosis. Conversely, nuclear medicine imaging can be used after CT or MRI localization to ascertain whether an identified focus represents an inflammatory or noninflammatory process. Decisions to perform specific infection or inflammation nuclear medicine scans must be based on applicability and clinical circumstance. There is no general consensus regarding the appropriate sequencing of imaging technology in septic patients [113]. In critically ill patients, it is reasonable and expedient to begin with cross-sectional scans and, if negative, follow with nuclear medicine imaging when clinical circumstances permit. In patients who are not critically ill, nuclear medicine scanning can be used as the initial diagnostic imaging modality. A detailed review has been published recently discussing the current and future role of nuclear medicine imaging in infection and inflammation [116].

## IV. Treatment

Ideally, prevention is the best "treatment" for sepsis. In reality, there are no absolute methods for anticipating or preventing sepsis. Effective treatment of sepsis requires (a) timely institution of appropriate antimicrobial therapy; (b) aggressive supportive measures, including immediate resuscitative measures in patients with impending or established septic shock; and (c) appropriate adjunct interventions such as surgical drainage of abscesses and debridement of necrotizing soft tissue infections.

A. **Antimicrobial therapy.** Selecting appropriate initial antimicrobial therapy is a high priority for treating sepsis. The life-threatening nature of sepsis justifies empiric broad-spectrum antibiotic coverage administered by parenteral route. **Specific antibiotic choices and dosing regimens are governed by** the presumed **source** of infection, suspected or known **organism**(s), **Gram stain** results, and **resistance patterns** of common pathogens prevalent within the acquisition setting (**community-acquired vs. hospital-acquired**). **Antimicrobial selection** must also account for **host factors** such as **immune status** (**especially patients with neutropenia or receiving immunosuppressive drugs**), **allergies**, **hepatic dysfunction**, and **renal failure**. Most hospitals limit the number of antibiotics on formulary based on availability, recognized hospital resistance patterns, and patient demographics and associated clinical variables. Hospital formulary listings and regional patient demographics aside, general guidelines apply for choosing antimicrobial therapy based on the documented or suspected source of sepsis [117,118]. Efficacy and safety are prime directives when selecting empiric antimicrobial therapy to treat life-threatening infections. Antibiotic selection is governed by target site and tailored to individual patient variables (e.g., **drug allergy or interactions, renal function, hepatic dysfunction**). Detailed discussions of individual antibiotics are included in Chapter 27.

1. **Severe sepsis or septic shock without identifiable source.** Broad-spectrum antimicrobial therapy for treating patients with severe sepsis or septic shock without identifiable source requires combination regimens.
   a. **Antipseudomonal cephalosporin** (e.g., **cefepime, ceftazidime**) or **antipseudomonal penicillin** (e.g., **piperacillin, mezlocillin**) + **aminoglycoside** (e.g., **gentamicin, tobramycin, amikacin**) or **quinolone** (e.g., **ciprofloxacin, levofloxacin**). The $\beta$-lactam/aminoglycoside combination is a synergistic alliance, but in patients at increased risk for nephrotoxicity a quinolone may be preferred. With rare exception, aminoglycoside therapy may be discontinued and another suitable agent substituted in its place when clinical recovery is certain and signs of sepsis have resolved.
      (1) **Clindamycin** or **metronidazole** should be added to these regimens if **anaerobes** are suspected.
   b. **Imipenem, meropenem,** and **piperacillin-tazobactam,** as single agents offer broad coverage (**including anaerobes, methicillin-susceptible staphylococci, and gram-negative aerobes including *Pseudomonas* species**).
      (1) **Aminoglycoside** or an **antipseudomonal quinolone** should be added if *P. aeruginosa* is suspected. None of these regimens covers methicillin-resistant staphylococci, common causes of hospital-acquired wound, or vascular catheter infections (see sections IV.5.b and IV.6).
   c. **Vancomycin** should be added to the antimicrobial regimen if methicillin-resistant staphylococci are suspected. A **streptogramin** (e.g., **dalfopristin/quinupristin**) or an **oxazolidinone** (e.g., **linezolid**) is an acceptable alternative in patients with vancomycin allergy.
   d. **Linezolid** or **dalfopristin-quinupristin** should be added to the antimicrobial regimen in place of vancomycin when vancomycin-resistant *Enterococcus faecium* (VRE) or vancomycin intermediate susceptible *Staphylococcus aureus* (VISA) are highly suspected. Linezolid has a better safety profile, is active against both *E. faecalis* and *E. faecium*, and offers an oral formulation for step-down therapy. Specific details regarding indications, contraindications, and warnings are included in Chapter 27.
2. **Pneumonia.** Sepsis related to community-acquired pneumonia in the immunocompetent host may be treated with antimicrobial regimens appropriate for community-acquired pneumonia as detailed in recent guidelines published by the Infectious Diseases Society of America [119] or the American Thoracic Society [120]. **Pneumonia in immunosuppressed patients,**

**patients with structural lung disease, hospital-acquired pneumonia,** and **ventilator-associated pneumonia** are at risk for multidrug-resistant or unusual pathogens. Appropriate antimicrobial regimens for specific clinical circumstances can be summarized as follows.

a. **Immunocompetent patients with severe sepsis and community-acquired pneumonia**. Suitable antimicrobial regimens include
   (1) **Third-generation cephalosporin** (e.g., ceftriaxone, cefotaxime, cefepime) + **macrolide** (e.g., erythomycin, azithromycin), or **quinolone** (gatifloxacin, levofloxacin, moxifloxacin). Ceftazidime and older fluoroquinolones (**ciprofloxacin, ofloxacin, lomafloxacin**) lack adequate activity against *S. pneumoniae*. When treating community-acquired pneumonia in elderly or critically ill patients, a quinolone may be preferable in place of a macrolide in combination with an appropriate $\beta$-lactam agent.
   (2) **$\beta$-Lactam/$\beta$-lactamase inhibitor** (e.g., ampicillin-sulbactam, piperacillin-tazobactam, ticarcilli-/clavulanate) + **macrolide** or **quinolone** as described above in section IV.1.a.(1).
   (3) **Clindamycin + quinolone** is an alternative regimen in patients with $\beta$-lactam allergy **unless meningitis accompanies pneumococcal disease,** in which case **vancomycin plus rifampin** should be added to the antimicrobial regimen.
   (4) **Vancomycin** or a **quinolone** must be included in the antimicrobial regimen when **penicillin-resistant *S. pneumoniae* is suspected** and adding **rifampin** should be considered. **Linezolid** or **dalfopristin/quinupristin** are appropriate alternatives to vancomycin **unless meningitis is present.**

b. **Immunosuppressed patients with severe sepsis and community-acquired pneumonia.** When community-acquired pneumonia is the source of sepsis in immunocompromised hosts, invasive diagnostic testing (**bronchoscopy or open lung biopsy**) should be considered to detect opportunistic pathogens such as mycobacteria, fungi, parasites, and *Nocardia*. When medical circumstances prevent invasive diagnostic testing, expanded empiric antimicrobial therapy to cover for opportunistic pathogens must be based on clinical judgment.
   (1) **Trimethoprim-sulfamethoxazole** should be added to regimens described section IV.2.a for **patients with HIV**.
   (2) **Trimethoprim-sulfamethoxazole (unless PCP or *Nocardia* are unlikely) + a regimen described in section IV.2.a that includes, specifically, those agents with antipseudomonal activity (e.g., cefepime, piperacillin/tazobactam) for organ transplant recipients and patients receiving chronic or high dose corticosteroid therapy**.
   (3) **Neutropenic patients** should receive antimicrobial therapy as described for sepsis of unknown source (see section IV.1) **provided the regimen selected includes adequate coverage for *S. pneumoniae* (e.g., antipseudomonal $\beta$-lactams, imipenem, or meropenem for PCN-susceptible isolates; levofloxacin, vancomycin, dalfopristin/quinupristin, or linezolid $\pm$ rifampin for PCN-resistant isolates) and *Legionella pneumophila* (a quinolone or a macrolide).** A common contaminant in respiratory secretions, *Aspergillus* detected in sputum from neutropenic hosts justifies including **amphotericin B** empirically in the antimicrobial regimen based on the premise that this patient population is at extremely high risk for invasive aspergillosis.

c. **Patients with severe sepsis, structural lung disease, and community-acquired pneumonia.** Patients with structural lung disease such as cystic fibrosis are at increased risk for infection involving multidrug-resistant pathogens. Suitable regimens include the following.
   (1) **Antimicrobial regimens as detailed in section IV.2.b.(2) for immunosuppressed patients.**

(2) **Vancomycin** or **linezolid** or **dalfopristin-quinupristin** should be included for patients with cystic fibrosis to cover *S. aureus* pending susceptibility testing results or unless staphylococci are unlikely.

**d. Patients with severe sepsis and lung abscess and postobstructive or aspiration pneumonia.** Lung abscesses, postobstructive pneumonia, and aspiration pneumonia typically involve polymicrobial flora, including oral anaerobes. Recommended antimicrobial therapy includes the following.

(1) **Regimens described in section IV.2.a or IV.2.b,** based on the patient's immune status, **provided the selected regimen includes adequate coverage for anaerobes.**

(2) Regimens containing **$\beta$-lacatm/$\beta$-lactamase inhibitor** combinations, **imipenem**, or **meropenem** provide sufficient anaerobic coverage. **Ertapenem** provides anaerobic coverage similar to the other carbapenems but, unlike imipenem and meropenem, lacks adequate activity against certain multidrug-resistant gram-negative aerobes, including *P. aeruginosa*.

(3) **Clindamycin** or **metronidazole** should be added to those regimens lacking sufficient anaerobic coverage.

**e. Patients with severe sepsis and ventilator-associated or nosocomial pneumonia.** Nosocomial pneumonia is the most common infection among patients in intensive care units. Traditional diagnostic methods, including chest radiographs and respiratory secretion cultures, are suboptimal. Up to 50% of cases are polymicrobial; *Enterobacter* species, *Klebsiella* species, *P. aeruginosa*, and *S. aureus* are the major pathogens [121]. Appropriate antimicrobial therapy includes the following.

(1) **Antibiotic regimens described in section IV.1 for sepsis of unknown source.**

**f. Nursing home patients with severe sepsis and pneumonia.** *S. pneumoniae* is the most common bacterial cause of pneumonia in nursing home patients, but aerobic gram-negative pathogens, including *P. aeruginosa*, are commonly encountered. Empiric treatment in these cases includes the following.

(1) **Extended-spectrum cephalosporin (e.g., cefepime) + clindamycin.**

(2) **Piperacillin-tazobactam or carbapenem (e.g., imipenem or meropenem).**

**3. Abdominal and pelvic infections.** Serious abdominal and pelvic infections associated with severe sepsis typically involve polymicrobial flora, most notably enteric gram-negative aerobes, enterococci, and anaerobes. Arguably, in a limited number of clinical situations, when *P. aeruginosa* and enterococci are unlikely, monotherapy using imipenem, meropenem, ampicillin/sulbactam, or piperacillin/tazobactam might be considered adequate; combination therapy, however, is recommended in most cases. Recommended combination therapy includes the following.

**a. Ampicillin + gentamicin** or **tobramycin + metronidazole** or **clindamycin** if multidrug-resistant pathogens are unlikely.

**b. Ampicillin/sulbactam + gentamicin** if multidrug resistant pathogens are unlikely.

**c. Piperacillin/tazobactam** or **imipenem + gentamicin** or **tobramycin** if multidrug-resistant pathogens are suspected. **Neutropenic patients** should receive combination regimens that provide double coverage for *P. aeruginosa*. For patients with serious $\beta$-lactam allergy, treatment options are less clearly defined but might reasonably include the following.

**d. Ciprofloxacin** (or other quinolone if *P. aeruginosa* is unlikely) + **aminoglycoside** or **aztreonam** (if *P. aeruginosa* is likely) + **metronidazole + enterococcal coverage.**

Note: Enterococci, intrinsically resistant to cephalosporins, are particularly relevant in sepsis associated with intraabdominal or pelvic infections. Cell-wall active agents (**penicillins, imipenem, vancomycin**) are only bactericidal in synergistic combination with aminoglycosides. For life-threatening enterococcal infections, bactericidal combinations including an aminoglycoside are recommended despite potential for nephrotoxicity or ototoxicity. Streptomycin may be an alternative for synergy against enterococci that are highly resistant to gentamicin. Serious infections involving enterococci resistant to both gentamicin and streptomycin should be treated aggressively with alternative antibiotics in lieu of aminoglycoside synergy. Ampicillin is the drug of choice for treating penicillin-susceptible strains, but piperacillin or imipenem provide adequate coverage in regimens recommended above. Enterococci are resistant to ticarcillin (**with or without clavulanate**), nafcillin, and oxacillin. Imipenem is the only carbapenem reliably active against ampicillin-susceptible enterococci. Meropenem and ertapenem are not reliably active against enterococci. Vancomycin and linezolid are alternatives for treating ampicillin-resistant enterococci or as alternative agents in patients with β-lactam allergy. Linezolid and dalfopristin/quinupristin are options for treating vancomycin-resistant *Enterococcus faecium*. Linezolid is active against *E. faecalis* and *E. faecium*; dalfopristin/quinupristin is active against *E. faecium* but not *E. faecalis*.

4. **Urinary tract infection.** Urinary tract obstruction (e.g., **calculi, prostatism, congenital abnormalities; functional obstruction associated with neurogenic bladder)** is the major intrinsic risk factor for developing overwhelming sepsis associated with urinary tract infections. Major extrinsic risk factors include urinary tract instrumentation and indwelling Foley catheters. In addition to appropriate antimicrobial therapy, adjunct treatment includes removal of catheter or obstruction and surgical drainage of abscesses (e.g., **prostate**). Urosepsis is usually caused by gram-negative aerobes. Therapeutic options for treating septic patients due to urinary tract infections include the following.
   a. **Third-generation cephalosporin + aminoglycoside.**
   b. **Aztreonam** or **quinolones** are suitable alternatives for patients with β-lactam allergies.
   c. **Antipseudomonal β-lactam, aztreonam, imipenem** or **meropenem + aminoglycoside** or **quinolone** are recommended when *P. aeruginosa* or other multidrug-resistant gram-negative aerobes are suspected (e.g., **nosocomial or catheter-associated urinary tract infection**).
   d. **Enterococcal coverage** should be included when urine Gram stain shows streptococci. Suitable regimens when enterococci are suspected include the following.
      (1) **Regimens, preferably synergistic combinations, as described in section IV.3.**
   e. **Antifungal coverage** should be added if *Candida* species are likely. *Candida* species are being identified with increased frequency in severe hospital-acquired urinary tract infections. Clinical suspicions of systemic candidiasis can be corroborated expediently with urinalysis or urine Gram stain and antifungal treatment implemented pending urine and blood culture results.
      (1) **Amphotericin B** should be used in life-threatening fungal infections pending culture results.
      (2) **Fluconazole** may be appropriate if candidiasis is caused by *Candida albicans* or related species with known susceptibility to azoles.
5. **Skin and soft tissue infections.** Staphylococcal and streptococcal toxic shock syndrome associated with cellulitis, wound, and necrotizing soft tissue infections are well described. Necrotizing soft tissue infections (e.g., **cellulitis, fasciitis, myositis**) caused by *Clostridium perfringens* or *Clostridium septicum* are characterized by rapid development of pain, erythema, swelling, foul-smelling drainage, gas formation, and marked systemic toxicity. Clostridial infections may be difficult to distinguish from mixed synergistic necrotizing infections involving other anaerobes (e.g., **Bacteroides** *species* and **Peptostreptococcus** *species*) in combination with nongroup A streptococci and aerobic gram-negative bacteria (see Chapter 4). Treatment includes emergent surgical debridement and broad-spectrum antibiotics. Antimicrobial therapy may be modified based on intraoperative Gram stain and culture results.

a. **Toxic shock syndrome associated with soft tissue infections** typically involves *S. aureus* or *S. pyogenes*. Appropriate antibiotic regimens include the following.
   (1) **Nafcillin or oxacillin**, appropriate for treating infections caused by methicillin-susceptible *S. aureus*, also covers most nonenterococcal streptococci.
   (2) **Vancomycin** should be used in place of antistaphylococcal penicillins if methicillin-resistant *S. aureus* or coagulase-negative staphylococci are suspected.
   (3) **Clindamycin** should be added, particularly if *Streptococcus* is suspected, based on the premise that, in addition to inhibiting bacterial growth, it suppresses bacterial exotoxin production. Neutralization of toxins using intravenous immunoglobulin (IVIG) appears to provide additional clinical benefit in patients with streptococcal toxic shock syndrome.

b. **Other necrotizing soft tissue infections** typically involve polymicrobial flora as described above. Suitable antibiotic regimens include the following.
   (1) **Ampicillin-sulbactam + aminoglycoside** if multidrug-resistant pathogens are unlikely.
   (2) **Piperacillin-tazobactam** or **imipenem** or **meropenem + aminoglycoside** if multidrug-resistant pathogens are likely.
   (3) **Vancomycin** or **linezolid** or **quinupristin-dalfopristin** should be added if methicillin-resistant *S. aureus* or coagulase-negative staphylococci are suspected.

c. **Unique causes of severe sepsis associated with soft tissue infections** warrant consideration in special circumstances.
   (1) ***Vibrio vulnificus*** and ***Aeromonas hydrophila,*** particularly in patients with underlying liver disease, cause fulminant infections associated with bacteremia, cutaneous lesions, and septic shock. Bacterial invasion occurs via wounds or penetrating injury during salt-water exposure. Vibrio sepsis associated with raw shellfish consumption has been reported in patients with underlying liver disease. Appropriate antimicrobial regimens in these settings include the following.
      (a) **Quinolone** or **third-generation cephalosporin.**
      (b) **Doxycycline** if *V. vulnificus* is documented.
   (2) ***Capnocytophagia canimorsus*** can cause fulminant sepsis after dog bite injuries, most notably in asplenic individuals or those with underlying chronic liver disease. Peripheral blood Gram stain, in such cases, may reveal gram-negative bacilli within neutrophils and is considered diagnostic in the appropriate clinical setting. This gram-negative anaerobe, part of the normal oral flora in canines, is resistant to aminoglycosides and trimethoprim-sulfamethoxazole. **Quinolones** or **$\beta$-lactams** provide suitable antimicrobial therapy for infections caused by this pathogen.

6. **Intravascular catheter infections.** Infected intravascular catheters cause as many as 150,000 bloodstream infections annually with associated mortality rates of 10% to 20%. Risk factors for intravascular catheter-related bloodstream infections include longer duration of line placement, underlying acute leukemia, AIDS, and IL-2 therapy. Staphylococci cause most line-related infections. On the other hand, line-related infections are the most common cause of *S. aureus* bacteremia in hospitalized patients. Gram-negative bacteria (e.g., *Enterobacter, Pseudomonas, Acinetobacter*) and *Candida* species also commonly cause intravascular catheter-associated infections, especially after prior broad-spectrum antimicrobial therapy. Central venous catheters should be removed from patients with severe sepsis who have no obvious source of infection. Persistent fever and bacteremia after intravascular catheter removal warrant evaluation for endocarditis, septic thrombophlebitis, or metastatic foci of infection. Pending blood and catheter-tip cultures, appropriate antibiotic regimens include the following.

   a. **Vancomycin + aminoglycoside** or **extended-spectrum cephalosporin** (e.g., **cefepime, ceftazadime**) or **aztreonam** (**if $\beta$-lactam allergy documented**).

b. **Rifampin** should be considered for patients with intravascular or life-threatening staphylococcal infections, especially when accompanied by persistent bacteremia.
c. **Persistent bacteremia justifies multidrug combinations** for prolonged periods, as described for endocarditis in Chapter 12.

B. **Supportive care.** Effective treatment for patients with sepsis requires resuscitation, supportive care, and monitoring. The first priority in the management of septic patients is to assess airway, respiration, and perfusion, implementing appropriate supportive measures as needed. Unstable acutely ill patients should be monitored closely in an intensive care setting.

1. **Airway.** Intubation, for airway protection, may be required when sepsis is complicated by encephalopathy and depressed level of consciousness.
2. **Oxygenation.** All patients with sepsis should receive supplemental oxygen. Baseline arterial blood gases should be obtained and oxygenation monitored using continuous pulse oximetry.
3. **Perfusion.** Sepsis-associated hypotension results from plasma volume loss into interstitial spaces, decreased vascular tone causing maldistribution of blood flow, and myocardial depression limiting compensatory increases in cardiac output. Intravenous fluids, packed red blood cells, and vasopressors are administered based on intravascular volume, cardiac status, and severity of shock. A detailed discussion of hemodynamic support measures is beyond the scope of this text. The SCCM recently published practice guidelines for hemodynamic support of adult patients with sepsis [122] that can be summarized briefly as follows.
   a. **Fluid resuscitation.** Fluid resuscitation represents the best initial therapy for treatment of hypotension in sepsis. Isotonic crystalloid solutions (e.g., **0.9% sodium chloride [normal saline], lactated Ringer solution**) or iso-oncotic colloid solutions (e.g., **albumin, dextrans, hydroxy ethyl starch, plasma protein fraction, gelatins**) and packed red blood cells can be used for intravascular volume repletion. Crystalloid and colloid solutions are equally effective when titrated to the same hemodynamic end points [122].
   b. **Vasopressor therapy.** Vasopressor therapy should be implemented in patients with clinical signs of septic shock unresponsive to aggressive empiric fluid challenge. Dopamine is considered the first-line agent for increasing blood pressure. Pulmonary artery catheterization is useful to guide therapy. Details regarding specific vasopressor selection, indications, contraindications, monitoring, dosage, and administration are included in the practice guidelines published by the SCCM [122].
   c. **Inotropic therapy.** Patients with sepsis-associated myocardial dysfunction may benefit from inotropic therapy as detailed in guidelines published by the SCCM [122].
   d. **Transfusion therapy.** Hemoglobin concentrations should be maintained above 8 to 10 g/dL. Higher hemoglobin concentrations may be desirable in patients with low cardiac output, mixed venous oxygenation desaturation, lactic acidosis, widened gastric-arterial $P_{CO_2}$ gradients, or coronary artery disease [122].
4. **Nutritional support.** Optimal nutritional support is vital for maintaining immune function and appears beneficial for both preventing and treating sepsis. Early enteral nutrition appears to enhance gut function and deter bacterial translocation. Immunonutritional therapy is discussed in section V.
5. **Control of infection source.** Antimicrobial therapy, at times, may not eradicate infection unless the source is removed. Physical measures to eradicate ongoing infectious sources may include (a) changing or removing intravascular or urinary tract catheters; (b) changing or removing VP shunts or other implanted CNS devices; (c) removing or replacing intravascular grafts; (d) removing prosthetic heart valves, pacemakers, or defibrillator implants; (e) removing prosthetic joints or internal fixation devices; (f) draining abscesses or other infected fluid collections (**percutaneously or surgically**); (g) debriding infected tissues; and (h) removing obstructions that prevent normal drainage or emptying function.

## V. Immunomodulatory Interventions

Immunomodulatory interventions are attractive potential strategies for the treatment of life-threatening inflammatory responses associated with infection. Recent clinical research, focused on reducing sepsis-associated mortality by way of modulating immune response during sepsis, has identified several promising agents or interventions that warrant consideration presently or if clinical trials corroborate efficacy. Immunomodulatory therapies, for convenience, can be roughly grouped into categories [123], recognizing there is overlap that reflects the complex nature of the SIRS called sepsis.

**A. Nonspecific interventions.** A number of potential nonspecific immunomodulatory therapies involve innovative application of conventional treatments used for diseases other than sepsis.

1. **Steroids.** Corticosteroid therapy, proposed as early as 1940 for treating patients with severe sepsis or septic shock [124], has been debated for decades. Despite initial enthusiasm engendered by anecdotal reports and early clinical trials, data from well-designed prospective studies published in 1987 showed no overall outcome benefit from empiric high-dose steroid therapy implemented early in septic shock [125,126]. Subsequent meta-analyses confirmed that brief high-dose corticosteroid treatment were ineffective [127] or possibly harmful [128]. A recent retrospective report examining prognostic factors in 80 critically ill adults with pneumococcal meningitis suggested that corticosteroids, as adjunct to appropriate antimicrobial therapy, might improve clinical outcome in patients with life-threatening meningitis [129]. Current evidence suggests that septic shock causes relative adrenal insufficiency [130]. Recent clinical trials, based on this premise, suggest that lower doses of glucocorticoids administered over longer periods (5–14 days) have beneficial hemodynamic effects and improve survival in patients with septic shock [131–133]. Presently, there are neither speculative nor corroborating guidelines for using corticosteroid therapy in the treatment of septic shock.
2. **Pentoxifylline.** Pentoxifylline, a phosphodiesterase inhibitor, licensed by the U.S. Food and Drug Administration (FDA) for the treatment of intermittent claudication in patients with atherosclerotic peripheral vascular disease, has multiple effects on the inflammatory cascade, including TNF and NO production. There is an increasing number of reports in the medical literature describing beneficial effects from pentoxifylline in a number of clinical syndromes such as cerebral malaria [134], acute alcoholic hepatitis [135], and postoperative organ dysfunction [136]. Small clinical trials investigating pentoxifylline effects in sepsis and ARDS, however, have not produced reliable evidence that its use improves outcome [137,138].
3. **Hemofiltration.** Hemofiltration, the principal underlying continuous renal replacement therapy, is effective at removing molecular weight compounds in ranges that include putative mediators of sepsis. Favorable outcome trends have been reported in limited clinical trials using hemofiltration as adjunct treatment in patients with septic shock [139], but as yet there have been no controlled clinical trials to corroborate efficacy in general. Barring more convincing evidence, it is doubtful that hemofiltration for the nonspecific removal of inflammatory mediators will prove widely applicable for treating septic shock [140]. Polymyxin B effectively binds to lipopolysaccharide and, when bound to polystyrene fibers in dialysis filters, creates a system that removes endotoxin during hemofiltration. Limited clinical reports using such a system in the treatment of patients with septic shock are encouraging [123].

**B. Antimodulator interventions.** Treatment interventions aimed at influencing specific mediators of the systemic inflammatory response include those that effect coagulation, cytokine, and eicosanoid cascades or modulate the production of oxygen free radicals and nitrous oxide. Although a complete review of all antimodulator therapies is beyond the scope of this text, FDA-approved drugs and a select number of other agents merit discussion.

1. **APC**, a natural endogenous anticoagulant, interrupts several pathways in sepsis and decreases morbidity and mortality in some patients with severe sepsis. [141]. APC inhibits thrombin generation by proteolytic inactivation of clotting factors

Va and VIIIa. Although generally not viewed as antiinflammatory agents, recent scrutiny suggests that some anticoagulant strategies affect inflammatory pathways distinct from the coagulation system. Three anticoagulant strategies tested in patients with sepsis that have drawn attention include antithrombin [142], tissue-factor-pathway inhibitor [143], and APC. Presently APC is the only agent in this class licensed by the FDA for use in patients with severe sepsis. A recent large, randomized, placebo-controlled, double-blind, international, multicenter study reported on the safety and efficacy of rhAPC (drotrecogin alpha [activated]) in 1,690 patients with severe sepsis and organ failure [144]. In two decades of failed sepsis treatment trials, this is the first investigation to demonstrate a positive effect on 28-day all-cause mortality. The only safety concern identified in the trial involved an increased incidence of serious bleeding in the rhAPC-treated group, including fatal intracranial hemorrhage in two patients. Differences in the incidence of serious bleeding were limited to the infusion period only, after which the incidence was similar in the rhAPC and placebo groups. In the study by Bernard et al. [144], rhAPC (drotrecogin alpha [activated]) administration was associated with reduced plasma D-dimer and serum IL-6 levels, evidence that the treatment diminishes the procoagulant effects of sepsis and attenuates the inflammatory cascade. In late November 2001, the FDA approved drotrecogin alpha for use in patients with severe sepsis and organ failure. However, physicians should recognize that currently the reported drotrecogin alpha success story is limited to patients meeting very specific inclusion criteria for severe sepsis, including evidence of end-organ dysfunction with shock, acidosis, oliguria, or hypoxemia (see Table 2.3). Furthermore, physicians should note the very important exclusion criteria used in this landmark clinical trial. Most notably, the study excluded patients at increased bleeding risk, including those with chronic renal failure requiring dialysis, chronic liver disease, recent surgery, organ-transplant recipients, thrombocytopenia (<30,000), and aspirin therapy. The study also excluded patients under 18 years of age. Unless further trials show benefit in these other groups, rhAPC (drotrecogin alpha) should not be given to patients with clinical signs of mild to moderate sepsis without evidence of end-organ damage, in those with increased bleeding risk, or individuals younger than 18 years old (Table 2.3) [145,146]. Guidelines for utilization of drotrecogin alpha are summarized in Table 2.4. Currently, there are no published clinical studies evaluating rhAPC efficacy beyond the 28-day mortality figures reported by Bernard et al. The predicted cost for drotrecogin alpha therapy at current recommended doses is $8,000 to $10,000.

2. **Anti-TNF therapy.** Therapies directed aimed at modulating TNF proinflammatory effects offered promise in early studies [147,148]. Subsequent large clinical trials found no beneficial effects on outcome in patients treated with anti-TNF monoclonal antibody or soluble TNF receptor preparations [123]. Infliximab, a humanized monoclonal against TNF-$\alpha$, is licensed for use in the United States and elsewhere for the treatment of rheumatoid arthritis and Crohn disease. Recent reports identifying increased rates of tuberculosis in patients treated with infliximab suggests that TNF may play an important role in protecting against certain infections [149].
3. **PAF antagonist therapy.** Clinical trials involving PAF antagonists have not demonstrated reduced mortality rates in patients with sepsis [123]. Preliminary studies using recombinant PAF acetylhydrolase report promising results; confirmatory clinical data from a large multicenter clinical trial are, presently, not available.
4. **Antioxidant therapy.** Antioxidant therapy using *N*-acetyl cysteine, an agent that restores cellular antioxidant capacity, showed some promise in early studies. However, subsequent clinical trials have yielded conflicting results [123]. Selenium supplementation may be beneficial effects on renal function and outcome in patients with SIRS, but currently data are from pilot studies and require corroboration in larger clinical trials [150].
5. **NO inhibition therapy. NOS blockade** has mixed hemodynamic effects, increasing blood pressure and systemic and pulmonary vascular resistance while lowering the cardiac output. **Methylene blue**, more selective in its modulatory

Table 2.3. Recommended Indications and Contraindications for Treating Severe Sepsis with Recombinant Human-Activated Protein C (Drotrecogin Alpha [Activated])

| | |
|---|---|
| Infection criteria | • Known infection or<br>• Suspected infection (one or more of the following):<br>WBC in normally sterile body fluid<br>Perforated viscus<br>CXR evidence of pneumonia + purulent sputum<br>Syndromes with high risk for infection |
| SIRS criteria (modified) | At least 3/4 of the following:<br>• Core temperature ≥38°C or ≤36°C<br>• Heart rate ≥90<br>• Respiratory rate ≥20 or $Paco_2$ ≤32<br>• Mechanical ventilation for acute respiratory process<br>• WBC ≥12,000 or ≤4,000 or >10% immature neutrophils |
| Organ dysfunction criteria | One or more of the following:<br>• SBP ≤90 or MAP ≤70 (for ≥1 hr despite adequate volume resuscitation or vasopressor support)<br>• Urine output ≤0.5 mL/kg/hr (for ≥1 hr despite adequate volume resuscitation)<br>• $Pao_2/Fio_2$ ≤250 + other organ dysfunction or <200 alone<br>• Platelets <80,000 or 50% decrease over 3 days<br>• Metabolic acidosis: pH ≤7.30 or base deficit ≥5 mmol/L + plasma lactate >1.5 × normal |
| Contraindications | Clinical situations with increased bleeding risk:<br>• Active internal bleeding<br>• Hemorrhagic stroke within 3 mo<br>• Intracranial-intraspinal surgery within 2 mo<br>• Severe head trauma within 2 mo<br>• Trauma with increased risk of life-threatening bleeding<br>• Epidural catheter<br>• Intracranial neoplasm<br>• Intracranial mass lesion<br>• Evidence of cerebral herniation<br>• Known hypersensitivity to drotrecogin or components |

WBC, white blood cell count; CXR, chest x-ray; SBP, systolic blood pressure; MAP, mean arterial pressure.

effects on NO activity, has been used in small uncontrolled studies and appears to have beneficial hemodynamic effects. These effects were transient in earlier studies using short-term infusions of methylene blue. A more recent pilot study found that continuously infused methylene blue, in a small number of patients with septic shock, counteracted myocardial depression, maintained oxygen transport, and reduced adrenergic support requirements when compared with conventional treatment alone [151]. Larger trials are needed to delineate efficacy and safety of this antioxidant therapy.

**C. Immunostimulation therapies.** Immunostimulation therapies include treatment regimens directed toward enhancing immune function and recovery during sepsis.

1. **Immunonutrition** involving specific nutrients such as arginine, glutamine, and omega-3 fatty acids influences nutritional, immunologic, and inflammatory parameters in critically ill patients. It is unclear whether these observed nutritional effects translate into improved clinical outcomes. Treatment effects may vary with patient populations, specific nutritional formulations, and study methodology. In trials to date, immunonutrition has not clearly reduced mortality, and in one published study a certain enteral formulation was associated with increased mortality [152]. However, overall, arginine-enriched formulas may decrease

Table 2.4. Recombinant Human-Activated Protein C (Drotrecogin Alpha [Activated]) Guidelines

| | |
|---|---|
| Administration | • Initiate within 24 h onset of severe sepsis<br>• 24 μg/kg/h × 96 h<br>• No known antidote for overdose<br>• Stop immediately if clinically significant bleeding develops |
| Surgery and invasive procedures | • Stop infusion 2 h before surgery or invasive procedure<br>• Restart 12 h after achieving adequate hemostasis<br>• Restart immediately after uncomplicated less invasive procedures |
| Pregnancy and lactation | • Pregnancy category C—effects on fetus unknown<br>• Effects on reproductive capacity unknown<br>• Concentration in breast milk unknown |
| Pediatric use | • Safety and efficacy in children not established |
| Geriatric use | • Safety and efficacy same as for younger adults |
| Hepatic dysfunction | • No dosage adjustment based on liver dysfunction alone |
| Renal dysfunction | • No dosage adjustment based on renal dysfunction alone<br>• Use in end-stage disease not established |
| Drug interactions | • Formal studies not conducted<br>• Caution advised when combined with drugs affecting hemostasis |
| Warnings | • Ischemic stroke within 3 mo<br>• Intracranial AV malformation or aneurysm<br>• GI bleeding within 6 weeks<br>• Chronic severe liver disease<br>• Known bleeding diathesis<br>• Concurrent therapeutic heparin (≥15 units/kg/h)<br>• Platelet count <30,000 (even if increased posttransfusion)<br>• Antiplatelet drugs within 7 days (e.g., ASA >650 mg q.d.)<br>• Thrombolytic therapy within 3 days<br>• Oral anticoagulants or glycoprotein IIb/IIIa inhibitors<br>• PT INR >3.0<br>• Any condition with significant bleeding hazard<br>• Bleeding hazard in location difficult to manage |

Guidelines based on information current at the time of writing. Check for postmarketing updates regarding safety, indications, contraindications, and dosing recommendations.
AV, arteriovenous; GI, gastrointestinal; ASA, aspirin; PT, prothrombin time; INR, international normalized ratio.

infectious complication rates and length of intensive care unit stay in critically ill patients [153]. Hopefully, further research will identify immunonutrition formulations that are safe and efficacious and define patient subsets that clearly benefit from such intervention.

2. **CSFs,** in addition to stimulating proliferation, enhance neutrophil antimicrobial function. Currently, recombinant human G-CSF (filgrastim) and GM-CSF (sargramostim) are available commercially for clinical use in the United States. The availability of these two CSFs and the finding that they enhance neutrophil antimicrobial function kindled interest in exploring their efficacy as adjunct therapy for treating bacterial and fungal infections in nonneutropenic hosts (Table 2.1) [154]. Clinical trials of G-CSF for treating nonneutropenic patients with sepsis have yielded conflicting results [123]. As with many other potential therapeutic modalities, the heterogeneous nature of sepsis as a syndrome and nonspecific nature of terminology contribute to inconsistent data regarding the use of G-CSF for improving outcomes in patients with sepsis.

**D. IVIG** should be administered routinely when treating septic patients with underlying immunoglobulin deficiencies. IVIG has been used as in patients without documented immunoglobulin deficiency, based on the premise that this immunomodulatory therapy improves host defense. In certain countries, despite a lack of clinical efficacy data, IVIG is used regularly for treating patients with severe sepsis. To date, well-designed, large, randomized clinical trials have not been undertaken to support the use of IVIG as routine adjunct therapy in the treatment of severe sepsis. Results from a recent small nonblinded study showed that IVIG reduced mortality (**67% untreated vs. 34% treated, $p = 0.02$**) in patients with streptococcal toxic shock syndrome [155]. A recent meta-analysis involving a limited number of patients suggested that IVIG may be beneficial for treating sepsis and septic shock [156]. Pending further data to support its routine use for treating patients with severe sepsis or septic shock, IVIG is currently recommended for treating sepsis in patients with underlying immunoglobulin deficiency syndromes and streptococcal toxic shock syndrome.

**E. Antitoxin interventions.** Many components of invading microorganisms are capable of triggering the systemic inflammatory response. Antitoxin interventions include therapeutic agents or modalities directed at blocking or neutralizing or removing pathogen factors that trigger or sustain ongoing SIRS.

1. **Antiendotoxin therapy.** Antiendotoxin strategies have been studied extensively over the past two decades [157]. Several antiendotoxin monoclonal antibody preparations have been used in large clinical trials with disappointing results. Attributing earlier clinical trial "failures" to inconsistent terminology and related sepsis trial designs, the most recent large clinical trial using E5 murine monoclonal antiendotoxin was tailored to eliminate trial design problems identified in earlier studies. The study involved more than 1,000 patients with gram-negative sepsis and concluded the antiendotoxin therapy tested had no effect or an effect too small to be detected using standard approaches to sepsis trial design and sample size [158]. Lacking definitive proof of efficacy, the future for antiendotoxin therapy is questionable, despite a frustrating tendency to show beneficial effect in post-hoc analyses from large clinical trials.
2. **Bactericidal/permeability-increasing protein (BPI)** is a 55-kDa protein constituent of human neutrophil azurophilic granules with selective activity against gram-negative bacteria. BPI belongs to a family of proteins of lipid and endotoxin binding proteins. Although BPI has a high affinity for the highly conserved lipid A portion of the lipopolysaccharide shared by all gram-negative bacteria, antibacterial activity depends on the envelope structure of a particular pathogen, which determines accessibility. BPI antibacterial action mechanisms are unclear but appear related to outer membrane perturbation followed by inner membrane disruption through a number of sequential interactions [159]. Cathelicidin and defensin proteins appear to enhance the early effects of BPI on bacteria, including growth inhibition and phospholipid hydrolysis activation. Later bactericidal effects, accelerated by complement membrane attack complex and phospholipid hydrolysis, require BPI penetration to the bacterial inner membrane. Although predominantly an intracellular antibacterial agent, during inflammation neutrophils also release BPI into the extracellular environment. In the search for novel antiinfectives, a recombinant amino-terminal BPI fragment ($rBPI_{21}$) was developed as potential treatment for gram-negative sepsis. In phase II and a limited number of phase III clinical trials, $rBPI_{21}$ appears to be nontoxic and nonimmunogenic and has shown some therapeutic benefit in humans [160].

## VI. Prevention

Despite an increasing armamentarium of antimicrobial agents and remarkable technologic advances in critical care medicine, mortality rates for sepsis remain disturbingly high, de facto, due to lack of specific interventions and reliable diagnostic assays. Although molecular research is discovering intriguing details regarding cytokine gene polymorphisms associated with severe sepsis, clinical applicability for disease prevention is presently uncertain [161]. Sepsis prevention should be a major priority for all health care providers and institutions. Handwashing, barrier precautions, use of antibiotic-impregnated catheters, and other infection control measures reduce risk for nosocomial infections. Rotating empiric antibiotic therapy is associated with declines in antimicrobial resistance and holds promise for reducing infectious mortality, particularly in intensive care unit settings [162].

## REFERENCES


1. Centers for Disease Control. Increase in National Hospital Discharge Survey rates for septicemia—United States, 1979–1987. *Morb Mortal Wkly Rep MMWR* 1990;39:31–34.
2. Angus DC, Linde-Zwirble WT, Lidicker J, et al. Epidemiology of severe sepsis in the United States: analysis of incidence, outcome, and associated costs of care. *Crit Care Med* 2001;29:1303–1309.
3. Quartin AA, Roland MH, Schein MD, et al. Magnitude and duration of the effect of sepsis on survival. *JAMA* 1997;277:1058–1063.
4. Bone RC, Balk RA, Cerra FB, et al. American College of Chest Physicians/Society of Critical Care Medicine Consensus Conference: definitions for sepsis and organ failure and guidelines for the use of innovative therapies in sepsis. *Crit Care Med* 1992;20:864–874 [also published in *Chest* 1992;101:1644–1655].
5. Marshall J. Both the disposition and the means of cure: "severe SIRS," "sterile shock," and the ongoing challenge of description. *Crit Care Med* 1997;25:1765–1766.
6. Vincent JL. Dear SIRS, I'm sorry to say I don't like you. . . . *Crit Care Med* 1997;25:372–374.
7. Dellinger RP, Bone RC. To SIRS with love. *Crit Care Med* 1998;26:178–179.
8. Bossink AWJ, Groeneveld ABJ, Hack CE, et al. Prediction of mortality in febrile patients: how useful are systemic inflammatory response syndrome and sepsis criteria? *Chest* 1998;113:1533–1541.
9. Bone RC. Why new definitions of sepsis and organ failure are needed. *Am J Med* 1993;95:348–350.
10. Munford RS, Pugin J. Normal responses to injury prevent systemic inflammation and can be immunosuppressive. *Am J Resp Crit Care Med* 2001;163:316–321.
11. Mira J-P, Cariou A, Grall F, et al. Association of TNF2, a TNF-$\alpha$ promotor polymorphism, with septic shock susceptibility and mortality: a multicenter study. *JAMA* 1999;282:561–568.
12. Kumar A, Short J, Parrillo JE. Genetic factors in septic shock. *JAMA* 1999;282:570–581.
13. Waterer GW, Quasney MW, Cantor RM, et al. Septic shock and respiratory failure in community-acquired pneumonia have different TNF-polymorphism associations. *Am J Resp Crit Care Med* 2001;163:1599–1604.
14. From the bench to the bedside: the future of sepsis research. Executive summary of the American College of Chest Physicians, National Institute of Allergy and Infectious Disease, and National Heart, Lung, and Blood Institute Workshop. *Chest* 1997;111:744–753.
15. Dinarello CE. Cytokines as endogenous pyrogens. *J Infect Dis* 1999;179[Suppl 2]:S294–S304.
16. Mackowiak PA, Bartlett JG, Borden EC, et al. Concepts of fever: recent advances and lingering dogma. *Clin Infect Dis* 1997;25:119–138.
17. Johnson RM, Brown EJ. Cell-mediated immunity in host defense against infectious diseases. In: Mandell GL, Bennett JE, Dolin R, eds. *Principles and practice of infectious diseases,* 5th ed. New York: Churchill Livingstone, 2000:112–146.
18. Tramont EC, Hoover DL. Innate (general or nonspecific) host defense mechanisms. In: Mandell GL, Bennett JE, Dolin R, eds. *Principles and practice of infectious diseases,* 5th ed. New York: Churchill Livingstone, 2000:31–38.
19. Dinarello CA. Proinflammatory cytokines. *Chest* 2000;118:503–508.
20. Dajani AS, Taubert KA, Wilson W, et al. Prevention of bacterial endocarditis: recommendations by the American Heart Association, from the Committee on Rheumatic Fever, Endocarditis, and Kawasaki Disease, Council on Cardiovascular Diseases in the Young. *JAMA* 1997;277:1794–1801.
21. Torres A, Dorca J, Zalacain E, et al. Community-acquired pneumonia in chronic obstructive pulmonary disease: a Spanish multicenter study. *Am J Resp Crit Care Med* 1997;154:1456–1461.

22. Balk RA. Severe sepsis and septic shock. *Crit Care Clin* 2000;16:179–192.
23. Opal SM, Cross AS. Clinical trials for severe sepsis: past failures, and future hopes. *Infect Dis Clin North Am* 1999;13:285–297.
24. Hartung T, Döcke WD, Ganter F, et al. Effect of granulocyte colony-stimulating factor treatment on ex vivo blood cytokine response in human volunteers. *Blood* 1995;85:2482–2489.
25. Dennis EA. Phospholipase $A_2$ in eicosanoid generation. *Am J Resp Crit Care Med* 2000;161:S32–S35.
26. Funk CD. Prostaglandins and leukotrienes: advances in eicosanoid biology. *Science* 2001;294:1871–1875.
27. Hla T, Lee M-J, Ancellin N, et al. Lysopholipids—receptor revelations. *Science* 2001;294:1875–1878.
28. Nagase T, Uozumi N, Ishii S, et al. Acute lung injury by sepsis and acid aspiration: a key role for cytosolic phospholipase $A_2$. *Nature Immunol* 2000;1:42–46.
29. Das N, Asatryan L, Reddy MA, et al. Differential role of cytosolic phospholipase $A_2$ in the invasion of brain microvascular endothelial cells by *Escherichia coli* and *Listeria monocytogenes. J Infect Dis* 2001;184:732–737.
30. Bone RC. Phospholipids and their inhibitors: a critical evaluation of their role in the treatment of sepsis. *Crit Care Med* 1992;20:884–890.
31. Brower RC, Matthay MA. Treatment of ARDS. *Chest* 2001;120:1347–1367.
32. Goldsberry GT, Hurst JM. Adult respiratory distress syndrome and sepsis. *New Horizons* 1993;1:342–347.
33. Patrick DA, Moore EE, Sullivan CC, et al. Secretory phospholipase $A_2$ activity correlates with postinjury multiple organ dysfunction. *Crit Care Med* 2001;29:989–993.
34. Halushka PV, Reines HD, Barrow SE, et al. Elevated plasma 6-keto-prostaglandin $F_{1\alpha}$ in patients with septic shock. *Crit Care Med* 1985;13:451–453.
35. Quinn JV, Slotman GJ. Platelet-activating factor and arachidonic acid metabolites mediate tumor necrosis factor and eicosanoid kinetics and cardiopulmonary dysfunction during bacteremic shock. *Crit Care Med* 1999;27:2485–2494.
36. Bernard GR, Wheeler AP, Russell JA, et al. The effects of ibuprofen on the physiology and survival of patients with sepsis. *N Engl J Med* 1997;336:912–918.
37. D'Ambrosio D, Mariani M, Panina-Bordignon P, et al. Chemokines and their receptors guiding T lymphocyte recruitment in lung inflammation. *Am J Resp Crit Care Med* 2001;164:1266–1275.
38. Samuelsson B. The discovery of leukotrienes. *Am J Respir Crit Care Med* 2000; 161[Suppl]:S2–S6.
39. Rådmark O. The molecular biology and regulation of 5-lipoxygenase. *Am J Respir Crit Care Med* 2000;161[Suppl]:S11–S15.
40. Holgate ST, Sampson AP. Antileukotriene therapy: future directions. *Am J Respir Crit Care Med* 2000;161[Suppl]:S147–S153.
41. Hedqvist P, Gautam N, Lindbom L. Interactions between leukotrienes and other inflammatory mediators/modulators in the microvasculature. *Am J Respir Crit Care Med* 2000;161[Suppl]:S117–S119.
42. Anderson MR, Blumer JL. Prognostic markers in sepsis: the role of leukotrienes. *Crit Care Med* 2000;28:3762–3763.
43. Morlion BJ, Torwesten E, Kuhn KS, et al. Cysteinyl-leukotriene generation as a biomarker for survival in the critically ill. *Crit Care Med* 2000;28:3655–3658.
44. Serhan CN, Takano T, Chiang N, et al. Formation of endogenous "antiinflammatory" lipid mediators by transcellular biosynthesis: lipoxins and aspirin-triggered lipoxins inhibit neutrophil recruitment and vascular permeability. *Am J Respir Crit Care Med* 2000;161[Suppl]:S95–S101.
45. Levy BD, Clish CB, Schmidt B, et al. Lipid mediator class switching during acute inflammation: signals in resolution. *Nature Immunol* 2001;2:612–619.
46. Moncada S, Ferreira SH, Vane JR. Prostaglandins, aspirin-like drugs and the oedema of inflammation. *Nature* 1973;246:217–219.
47. Weissmann G. Prostaglandins as modulators rather than mediators of inflammation. *J Lipid Mediators* 1993;6:275–286.
48. Mathiak G, Szewczyk D, Abdullah F, et al. Platelet-activating factor (PAF) in experimental and clinical sepsis. *Shock* 1997;7:391–404.

49. Koltai M, Hosford D, Braquet PG. Platelet-activating factor in septic shock. *New Horizons* 1993;1:87–95.
50. Mackoiak PA, Plaisance KI. Benefits and risks of antipyretic therapy. *Ann NY Acad Sci* 1998;856:214–223.
51. Kluger MJ, Kozak W, Conn CA, et al. Role of fever in disease. *Ann NY Acad Sci* 1998;856:224–233.
52. Kluger MJ, Kozak W, Conn CA, et al. The adaptive value of fever. *Infect Dis Clin North Am* 1996;10:1–20.
53. Aronoff DM, Neilson EG. Antipyretics: mechanisms of action and clinical use in fever suppression. *Am J Med* 2001;111:304–315.
54. Graham RM, Stephens CJ, Silvester W, et al. Plasma degradation of platelet-activating factor in severely ill patients with clinical sepsis. *Crit Care Med* 1994;22:204–212.
55. Moncada S, Palmer RMJ, Higgs EA, et al. Nitric oxide: physiology, pathophysiology and pharmacology. *Pharmacol Rev* 1991;43:109–142.
56. Cobb JP, Danner RL. Nitric oxide in septic shock. *JAMA* 1996;275:1192–1196.
57. Symeonides S, Balk RA. Nitric oxide in the pathogenesis of sepsis. *Infect Dis Clin North Am* 1999;13:449–463.
58. Morely JJ, Kushner I. Serum C-reactive protein levels in disease. *Ann NY Acad Sci* 1982;389:406–418.
59. Tillett WS, Francins Jr T. Serological reactions in pneumonia with non-protein somatic fraction of pneumococcus. *J Exp Med* 1930;52:561–571.
60. Gabay C, Kushner I. Acute-phase proteins and other systemic responses to inflammation. *N Engl J Med* 1999;340:448–454.
61. Rangel-Frausto MS, Wenzel RP. The epidemiology and natural history of bacterial sepsis in sepsis and multi-organ failure. In: Fein AM, Abraham AM, Balk RA, eds. *Sepsis and multiorgan failure.* Baltimore: Williams & Wilkins, 1997:27–34.
62. Centers for Disease Control. Nosocomial infections surveillance, 1983. *Morb Mortal Wkly Rep MMWR* 1984;132[Suppl]:9S–22S.
63. Parillo JE, Parker NN, Natanson C, et al. Septic shock in humans—advances in the understanding of pathogenesis, cardiovascular dysfunction and therapy. *Ann Intern Med* 1990;111:227–242.
64. Scahberg DR, Culver DH, Gaynes RP. Major trends in the microbiology etiology of nosocomial infections. *Am J Med* 1991;92:72S–75S.
65. Rangel-Frausto MS. The epidemiology of bacterial sepsis. *Infect Dis Clin North Am* 1999;13:299–312.
66. Horn DL, Morrison DC, Opal SM, et al. What are the microbial components implicated in the pathogenesis of sepsis? Report on a symposium. *Clin Infect Dis* 2000;31:851–858.
67. Nau R, Helmut E. Modulation of release of proinflammatory compounds by antibacterials: potential impact on course of inflammation and outcome in sepsis and meningitis. *Clin Microbiol Rev* 2002;15:95–110.
68. Morrison DC, Silverstein R, Luchi M, et al. Structure-function relationships of bacterial endotoxins: contribution to microbial sepsis. *Infect Dis Clin North Am* 1999;13:313–340.
69. Bannon J, Visvanathan K, Zabriski JB. Structure and function of streptococcal and staphylococcal superantigens in septic shock. *Infect Dis Clin North Am* 1999;13:387–396.
70. Sriskandan S, Cohen J. Gram-positive sepsis. *Infect Dis Clin North Am* 1999;13:397–412.
71. Sparwasser AJ, Miethke G, Lipford K, et al. Bacterial DNA causes septic shock. *Nature* 1997;386:336–337.
72. Jarisch A. herapeutische Versuche bei Syphilis. *Wien Med Wochenschr* 1895;45:721–724.
73. Herxheimer K, Krause K. Ueber eine bei Syphilitischen vorkommende Quecksilberreaktion. *Dtsch Med Wochenschr* 1902;28:895–897.
74. Fekade D, Knox K, Hussein A, et al. Prevention of Jarisch-Herxheimer reactions by treatment with antibodies against tumor necrosis factor alpha. *N Engl J Med* 1996;335:311–315.

75. Raoult D, Foucault C, Brouqui P. Infections in the homeless. *Lancet Infect Dis* 2001;1:77–84.
76. Barriere SL, Lowry SF. An overview of mortality risk prediction in sepsis. *Crit Care Med* 1995;23:376–393.
77. Angus DC, Wax RS. Epidemiology of sepsis: an update. *Crit Care Med* 2001;29[Suppl]:S109–S116.
78. Rello J, Ricart M, Mirelis B, et al. Nosocomial bacteremia in a medical-surgical intensive care unit: epidemiologic characteristics and factors influencing mortality in 111 episodes. *Intensive Care Med* 1994;20:94–98.
79. Rangel-Frausto M. The epidemiology of bacterial sepsis. *Infect Dis Clin North Am* 1999;13:299–312.
80. Opal SM, Cohen J. Clinical gram-positive sepsis: does it fundamentally differ from gram-negative bacterial sepsis? *Crit Care Med* 1999;27:1608–1616.
81. Friedman G, Silva E, Vincent JL. Has the mortality of septic shock changed with time? *Crit Care Med* 1998;26:2078–2086.
82. Wheeler AP, Bernard GR. Treating patients with severe sepsis. *N Engl J Med* 1999;340:207–214.
83. Bernard GR, Wheeler AP, Russell JA, et al. Effects of ibuprofen on the physiology and survival of patients with sepsis. *N Engl J Med* 1997;336:912–918.
84. Young LS. Sepsis syndrome. In: Mandell GL, Bennett JE, Dolin R, eds. *Principles and practice of infectious diseases,* 5th ed. New York: Churchill Livingstone, 2000:806–819.
85. Levin PD, Yinnon AM, Hersch M, et al. Impact of the resin blood culture medium on the treatment of critically ill patients. *Crit Care Med* 1996;24:797–801.
86. Mermal LA, Maki DG. Detection of bacteremia in adults: consequences of culturing an inadequate volume of blood. *Ann Intern Med* 1993;119:270–272.
87. Kellogg JA, Manzella JP, McConville JH. Clinical laboratory comparison of the 10-ml isolator blood culture system with BACTEC radiometric blood culture media. *J Clin Micrbiol* 1984;20:618–623.
88. Magadia RR, Weinstein MP. Laboratory diagnosis of bacteremia and fungemia. *Infect Dis Clin North Am* 2001;15:1009–1024.
89. Kellogg JA, Manzella JP, Bankert DA. Frequency of low-level bacteremia from birth to fifteen years. *J Clin Microbiol* 2000;38:2181–2185.
90. Washington JA. Blood cultures: principles and techniques. *Mayo Clin Proc* 1975;50:91–98.
91. Weinstein MP, Reller LB, Murphy JR, et al. The clinical significance of positive blood cultures: a comprehensive analysis of 500 episodes of bacteremia and fungemia in adults. *Rev Infect Dis* 1983;5:35–53.
92. Vaisanen IT, Michelsen T, Valtonen V, et al. Comparison of arterial and venous blood samples for the diagnosis of bacteremia in critically ill patients. *Crit Care Med* 1985;13:664–667.
93. Aronson MD, Bor DH. Blood cultures. *Ann Intern Med* 1987;106:246–253.
94. Weinstein MP. Current blood culture methods and systems: clinical concepts, technology, and interpretation of results. *Clin Infect Dis* 1996;23:40–46.
95. DesJardin JA, Falagas ME, Ruthazer RR, et al. Clinical utility of blood cultures drawn from indwelling central venous catheters in hospitalized patients with cancer. *Ann Intern Med* 1999;131:641–647.
96. Li J, Plorde JL, Carlson LG. Effects of volume and periodicity on blood cultures. *J Clin Microbiol* 1994;32:2829–2831.
97. Weinstein MP, Towns ML, Quarterlty SM, et al. The clinical significance of positive blood cultures in the 1990s: a prospective comprehensive evaluation of the microbiology, epidemiology, and outcome of bacteremia and fungemia in adults. *Clin Infect Dis* 1997;24:584–602.
98. Yagupsky P, Nolte FS. Quantitative aspects of septicemia. *Clin Microbiol Rev* 1990;3:269–279.
99. Wolk D, Mitchell S, Patel R. Principles of molecular microbiology testing methods. *Infect Dis Clin North Am* 2001;15:1157–1204.
100. Louie M, Cockerill III FR. Susceptibility testing: phenotypic and genotypic tests for bacteria and mycobacteria. *Infect Dis Clin North Am* 2001;15:1205–1226.

101. Carlet J. Rapid diagnostic methods in the detection of sepsis. *Infect Dis Clin North Am* 1999;13:483–493.
102. Hausfater P, Ben Ayed S, Rosenheim M, et al. Usefulness of procalcitonin as a marker of systemic infection in emergency department patients: a prospective study. *Clin Infect Dis* 2002;34:895–901.
103. Selberg O, Hecker H, Martin M, et al. Discrimination of sepsis and systemic inflammatory response syndrome by determination of circulating plasma concentrations of procalcitonin, protein complement 3a, and interleukin-6. *Crit Care Med* 2000;28:2793–2798.
104. Brunkhorst FM, Wegscheider K, Forycki ZF, et al. Procalcitonin for early diagnosis and differentiation of SIRS, sepsis, severe sepsis, and septic shock. *Intensive Care Med* 2000;26[Suppl]:S148–S152.
105. Suprin E, Camus C, Gacouin A. Procalcitonin: a valuable indicator of infection in a medical ICU? *Intensive Care Med* 2000;26:1232–1238.
106. Enguix A, Rey C, Concha A, et al. Comparison of procalcitonin with C-reactive protein and serum amyloid for the early diagnosis of bacterial sepsis in critically ill neonates and children. *Intensive Care Med* 2001;27:211–215.
107. Brunkhorst FM, Eberhard OK, Brunkhorst R. Discrimination of infectious and noninfectious causes of early acute respiratory distress syndrome by procalcitonin. *Crit Care Med* 1999;27:2172–2176.
108. Kuse E-R, Langfeld I, Jaeger K, et al. Procalcitonin in fever of unknown origin after liver transplantation: a variable to differentiate acute rejection from infection. *Crit Care Med* 2000;28:555–559.
109. Hammer S, Meisner F, Dirschedl P, et al. Procalcitonin: a new marker for diagnosis of acute rejection and bacterial infection in patients after heart and lung transplantation. *Transpl Immunol* 1998;6:235–241.
110. Rau B, Steinbach G, Gansauge F, et al. The role of procalcitonin and interleukin-8 in the prediction of infected necrosis in acute pancreatitis. *Gut* 1997;41:832–840.
111. Reith HB, Mittelkötter U, Wagner R. Procalcitonin (PCT) in patients with abdominal sepsis. *Intensive Care Med* 2000;26[Suppl]:S165–S169.
112. Pasculle W. Update on legionella. *Clin Microbiol News* 2000;22:97–101.
113. Braley SE, Groner TR, Fernandez M-U, et al. Overview of diagnostic imaging in sepsis. *New Horizons* 1993;1:214–230.
114. Wunderink RG. Radiologic diagnosis of ventilator-associated pneumonia. *Chest* 2000;117[Suppl]:188S–190S.
115. Wood SD, Ries KR, White Jr GL, et al. Maxillary sinusitis: the focus of toxic shock syndrome in a male patient. *West J Med* 1987;147:467–469.
116. Becker W, Meller J. The role of nuclear medicine in infection and inflammation. *Lancet Infect Dis* 2001;1:326–333.
117. Dellinger RP. Current therapy for sepsis. *Infect Dis Clin North Am* 1999;13:495–509.
118. Simon D, Trenholme G. Antibiotic selection for patients with septic shock. *Crit Care Clin* 2000;16:215–231.
119. Bartlett JG, Dowell SF, Mandell LA, et al. Practice guidelines for the management of community-acquired pneumonia in adults. *Clin Infect Dis* 2000;31:347–382.
120. Niederman MS, Mandell LA. Guidelines for the management of adults with community-acquired pneumonia. *Am J Resp Crit Care Med* 2001;163:1730–1754.
121. Johanson W, Seidenfeld J, Gomez P, et al. Bacteriologic diagnosis of nosocomial pneumonia following prolonged mechanical ventilation. *Am Rev Respir Dis* 1988;137:259.
122. Task Force of the American College of Critical Care Medicine, Society of Critical Care Medicine. Practice parameters for hemodynamic support of adult patients with sepsis. *Crit Care Med* 1999;27:639–660.
123. Vincent J-L, Sun Q, Dubois M-J. Clinical trials of immunomodulatory therapies in severe sepsis and septic shock. *Clin Infect Dis* 2002;34:1084–1093.
124. Perla D, Marmorston J. Suprarenal cortical hormone and salt in the treatment of pneumonia and other serious infections. *Endocrinology* 1940;27:367–374.
125. Bone RC, Fisher CJ, Clemmer TP, et al. A controlled clinical trial of high-dose methylprednisolone in the treatment of severe sepsis and septic shock. *N Engl J Med* 1987;317:653–658.

126. The Veteran's Administration Systemic Sepsis Cooperative Study Group. Effect of high-dose glucocorticosteroid therapy on mortality in patients with clinical signs of systemic sepsis. *N Engl J Med* 1987;317:659–665.
127. Lefering R, Neugebauer EAM. Steroid controversy in sepsis and septic shock: a meta-analysis. *Crit Care Med* 1995;23:1294–1303.
128. Cronin L, Cook DJ, Carlet J, et al. Corticosteroid treatment for sepsis: a critical appraisal and meta-analysis of the literature. *Crit Care Med* 1995;23:1430–1439.
129. Auburtin M, Porcher R, Bruneel F, et al. Pneumococcal meningitis in the intensive care unit: prognostic factors of clinical outcome in a series of 80 cases. *Am J Respir Crit Care Med* 2002;165:713–717.
130. Annane D. Corticosteroids for septic shock. *Crit Care Med* 2001;29[Suppl]:S117–S120.
131. Bollaert PE, Charpentier C, Levy B, et al. Reversal of late septic shock with supraphysiologic doses of hydrocortisone. *Crit Care Med* 1998;26:645–650.
132. Briegel J, Forst H, Haller M, et al. Stress doses of hydrocortisone reverse hyperdynamic septic shock: a prospective randomized double-blind single-center study. *Crit Care Med* 1999;27:723–732.
133. Annane D. Effects of the combination of hydrocortisone (HC)-fludrocortisone (FC) on mortality in septic shock. *Crit Care Med* 2000;28:A46(abst).
134. Di Perri G, Di Perri IG, Monteiro GB, et al. Pentoxifylline as a supportive agent in the treatment of cerebral malaria in children. *J Infect Dis* 1995;171:1317–1322.
135. Akriviadis E, Botla R, Briggs W. Pentoxifylline improved short-term survival in severe acute alcoholic hepatitis. *Gastroenterology* 2000;119:1637–1648.
136. Boldt J, Brosch C, Piper SN. Influence of prophylactic use of pentoxifylline on postoperative organ function in elderly cardiac surgery patients. *Crit Care Med* 2001;29:952–958.
137. Bacher A, Mayer N, Klimscha W, et al. Effects of pentoxifylline on hemodynamics and oxygenation in septic and nonseptic patients. *Crit Care Med* 1997;25:795–800.
138. Zeni F, Pain P, Vindimian M, et al. Effects of pentoxifylline on circulating cytokine concentrations and hemodynamics in patients with septic shock: results from a a double-blind, randomized, placebo-controlled study. *Crit Care Med* 1996;25:207–214.
139. Honore PM, Jamez J, Wauthier M, et al. Prospective evaluation of short-term, high-volume isovolemic hemofiltration on the hemodynamic course and outcome in patients with intractable circulatory failure resulting from septic shock. *Crit Care Med* 2000;28:3581–3587.
140. Surgenor SD, Corwin HL. Hemofiltration in sepsis: is removal of "bad humors" enough? *Crit Care Med* 2000;28:3751–3752.
141. Looney MR, Matthay MA. The role of protein C in sepsis. *Curr Infect Dis Rep* 2001; 3:413–418.
142. Eisele B, Lamy M, Thijs B, et al. Antithrombin III in patients with severe sepsis: a randomized, placebo-controlled, double-blind, multicenter trial, plus a meta-analysis on all randomized, placebo-controlled, double-blind trials with antithrombin III in severe sepsis. *Intensive Care Med* 1998;24:663–672.
143. Abraham E. Tissue factor inhibition and clinical trial results of tissue factor pathway inhibitor in sepsis. *Crit Care Med* 2000;28[Suppl]:S31–S33.
144. Bernard GR, Vincent J-L, Laterre P-F, et al. Efficacy and safety of recombinant human activated protein C for severe sepsis. *N Eng J Med* 2001;344:699–709.
145. Matthay MA. Severe sepsis—a new treatment with both anticoagulant and anti-inflammatory properties. *N Engl J Med* 2001;344:759–762.
146. Van der Poll T. Immunotherapy of sepsis. *Lancet Infect Dis* 2001;1:165–174.
147. Abraham E, Wunderink R, Silverman H, et al. Efficacy and safety of monoclonal antibody to human tumor necrosis factor alpha in patients with sepsis syndrome: a randomized, controlled, double-blind, multicenter clinical trial. *JAMA* 1995;273:934–941.
148. Cohen J, Carlet K. INTERSEPT Study Group. INTERSEPT: an international, multicenter, placebo-controlled trial of monoclonal antibody to human tumor necrosis factor-$\alpha$ in patients with sepsis. *Crit Care Med* 1996;24:1431–1440.
149. Keane J, Gershon S, Wise R, et al. Tuberculosis associated with infliximab, a tumor necrosis factor (alpha)-neutralizing agent. *N Engl J Med* 2001;345:1098–1104.

150. Angstwurm MW, Schottdorf J, Schopohl J, et al. Selenium replacement in patients with severe systemic inflammatory response syndrome improves clinical outcome. *Crit Care Med* 1999;26:1807–1813.
151. Kirov MY, Evgenov OV, Egorina EM, et al. Infusion of methylene blue in human septic shock: a pilot, randomized, controlled study. *Crit Care Med* 2001;29:1860–1876.
152. Bower BH, Cerra FB, Bershadsky B, et al. Early enteral administration of a formula (Impact) supplemented with arginine, nucleotides, and fish oil in intensive care unit patients: results of a multicenter, prospective, randomized, clinical trial. *Crit Care Med* 1995;23:436–449.
153. Heyland DK, Novak F, Drover JW, et al. Should immunonutrition become routine in critically ill patients? A systematic review of the evidence. *JAMA* 2001;286:944–953.
154. Root RK, Dale DC. Granulocyte colony-stimulating factor and granulocyte-macrophage colony-stimulating factor: comparisons and potential for use is the treatment of infections in nonneutropenic patients. *J Infect Dis* 1999;179[Suppl 2]:S342–S352.
155. Kaul R, McGeer A, Norrby-Teglund A, et al. Intravenous immunoglobulin therapy for streptococcal toxic shock syndrome: a comparative observational study. *Clin Infect Dis* 1999;28:800–807.
156. Alejandria MM, Lansang MA, Dans LF, et al. *Cochrane Database Syst Rev* 2001;2: CD001090.
157. Vincent JL, Cohen J. Another antiendotoxin strategy to be added to the list. *Crit Care Med* 1997;25:1949–1950.
158. Angus DC, Birmingham MC, Balk RA. E5 murine monoclonal antiendotoxin antibody in gram-negative sepsis: a randomized controlled trial. *JAMA* 2000;283:1723–1730.
159. Levy O, Elsback P. Bactericidal/permeability-increasing protein in host defense and its efficacy in the treatment of bacterial sepsis. *Curr Infect Dis Rep* 2001;3:407–412.
160. Levin M, Quint P, Goldstein B, et al. Recombinant bactericidal/permeability-increasing protein (rBPI21) as adjunctive treatment for children with severe meningococcal sepsis: a randomized trial. *Lancet* 2000;356:961–967.
161. Goldfarb R. Investigations into the polydeterminant nature of sepsis. *Crit Care Med* 1999;11:2587–2588.
162. Raymond DP, Pelletier SJ, Crabtree TD, et al. Impact of rotating empiric antibiotic schedule on infectious mortality in an intensive care unit. *Crit Care Med* 2001;29:1101–1108.

# 3. NEONATAL SEPSIS AND INFECTIONS

George K. Siberry and Mark C. Steinhoff

The frequency and severity of bacterial infections are greater in the newborn period than at any time thereafter. The newborn often does not manifest the classic clinical signs of infection usually observed in children and adults. Moreover, the maturing physiology of the newborn requires that drug therapy be carefully individualized. This chapter is designed to help practitioners manage infectious diseases in these especially vulnerable patients.

I. **Background.** Infection and disease caused by bacteria and viruses are not uncommon in newborn infants (Table 3.1). Systemic bacterial infection occurs in fewer than 1% of newborns, and viral disease may occur in 6% to 8% of all neonates [1]. The rate of septicemia is 3.5 per 1,000 full-term infants [2]. Among full-term infants evaluated for suspected bacterial infection, only 2.2% have culture or clinical evidence of bacterial infection [3]. Nosocomial bacterial infection has been reported in 2% to 25% of newborns in intensive care nurseries [4]. **The mortality rate of neonates from infections varies among nurseries but has been reported as 15% to 50% for early-onset sepsis and 10% to 20% for late-onset sepsis. The mortality rate is higher still among premature infants.** Thus, even in this antibiotic era, the rates of morbidity and mortality from neonatal infections are extraordinarily high. Some of the reasons for the higher incidence and increased severity of neonatal infections are examined in the following sections.

A. **Definitions**

1. **Fetus:** from eighth week of gestation to birth.
2. **Neonate:** birth to 28 days of age.
3. **Infant:** 1 month to 1 year.
4. **Early-onset neonatal infection:** occurs within the first 7 days of life and usually is caused by organisms acquired during the intrauterine or intrapartum stages.
5. **Late-onset neonatal infection:** occurs after 7 days and frequently results from postpartum (often nosocomial) colonization.

B. **Perinatal environments.** Infections may be caused by pathogenic organisms acquired before, during, or after birth. In passing from intrauterine to independent existence, the newborn is exposed to and becomes colonized with many microrganisms.

1. **Intrauterine.** The fetus develops in a sterile ecosphere, protected from maternal microorganisms by the placenta and the amniotic membranes. Intrauterine infection can result from:
   a. **Transplacental passage of pathogens** with placentitis, as seen in **viral infection** (e.g., rubella, cytomegalovirus [CMV], herpes simplex virus [HSV], hepatitis, human immunodeficiency virus [HIV], mumps), **bacterial infections** (e.g., syphilis, tuberculosis, *Listeria,* and *Salmonella* infections), and **protozoal infections** (e.g., toxoplasmosis and malaria).
   b. **Infection that ascends** through the cervix, causing amnionitis.
2. **Intrapartum.** During normal delivery, the sterility of the amniotic space is lost when the membranes rupture. As the neonate passes through the birth canal, he or she is newly colonized with the wide variety of organisms resident in the maternal cervicovaginal canal. Common organisms include streptococci, *Escherichia coli,* and other aerobic and anaerobic enteric bacteria. The neonate also may be exposed to *Chlamydia, Neisseria gonorrhoeae,* HSV, HIV, and CMV if the mother is infected.
3. **Postpartum.** In the postpartum period, the neonate is in contact first with the hospital nursery and then with the household. If ill, the newborn will be exposed to a large number of staff as well as devices used for respiratory and metabolic support, all of which increase the likelihood of infection. Organisms that may spread in the nursery include enteroviruses, HSV, respiratory syncytial virus (RSV), and parainfluenza viruses.

II. **Ontogeny of the immune system.** In addition to movement from one environment to another, the newborn also progresses from one level of immune function to another. The

Table 3.1. Frequency of Perinatal Infections Due to Selected Microorganisms

| Microorganism | Mother (per 1,000 Pregnancies) | Fetus (Intrauterine per 1,000 Live Births) | Neonate (Intrapartum per 1,000 Live Births) |
|---|---|---|---|
| Cytomegalovirus | | | |
| During pregnancy | 16–130 | 5–15 | — |
| At delivery | 110–280 | — | 50–100 |
| Hepatitis B[a] | 1–2 acute<br>5–15 chronic | Rare | 0.1–0.3 |
| *Chlamydia* | 40–50 | — | 10–60 (conjunctivitis)<br>3–10 (pneumonia) |
| Rubella | | | |
| Epidemic | 20–40 | 4–30 | 0 |
| Interepidemic | 0.1–1.0 | — | 0.2 |
| *Toxoplasma gondii* | 1.5–6.4 | 1.3–7.0 | 0 |
| Herpes simplex | 1–10 | Rare | 0.1–0.5 |
| Hepatitis C[b] (incomplete data) | 0–43 | Unknown | Unknown |
| Human immunodeficiency virus | 1.6[c] | | |
| *Treponema pallidum* | 0.2 | 0.13[d] | 0 |
| Group B streptococcus | 50–250 | — | 0.6[e]–1.4[f] |
| *Escherichia coli* | Common | — | 0.6[f] |

Data not specifically footnoted were modified and updated from Remington JS, Klein JO. *Infectious diseases of the fetus and newborn infant.* Philadelphia: WB Saunders, 1976.
[a]Data from International Federation of Gynecology and Obstetrics. Hepatitis in pregnancy. ACOG Technical Bulletin No. 174, November 1992. *Int J Gynecol Obstet* 1993;42:189.
[b]Data from Silverman NS et al. Hepatitis C virus in pregnancy: seroprevalence and risk factors for infection. *Am J Obstet Gynecol* 1993;169:583.
[c]Data from Pizzo PA, Wilfert CM, eds. *Pediatric AIDS,* 3rd ed. Baltimore: Williams & Wilkins, 1998;3–11.
[d]Data from Congenital syphilis—United States, 2000. *MMWR* 2001;50:573–577.
[e]Data from Schrag SJ et al. Group B streptococcal disease in the era of intrapartum antibiotic prophylaxis. *N Engl J Med* 2000;342:15–20.
[f]Data from Schuchat A et al. Risk factors and opportunities for prevention of early-onset neonatal sepsis: a multicenter case-control study. *Pediatrics* 2000;105:21–26.

fetus may be viewed as a compromised host in a protected, sterile environment. Similarly, the newborn is a less compromised host whose immune function matures rapidly while in contact with the normal environment [5]. Because of the unique environment and the maturing immunocompetence of the neonate, the microorganisms that cause disease are different from those seen later in childhood or in adults.

A. **B-lymphocytes** are present by the 10th week of gestation. **Antibody production** is noted by the 20th week. Virtually all the immunoglobulin G (IgG) present at birth has been passively transferred from the maternal circulation. This transfer occurs predominantly between 32 weeks' gestation and birth; consequently, premature newborns have lower levels of IgG than do full-term infants. The half-life of this maternally derived IgG is approximately 25 days; the nadir is reached at 2 to 4 months, before the child's own production increases. Infants have a diminished antibody response to the polysaccharide antigens of the encapsulated bacteria (*Streptococcus pneumoniae, Haemophilus influenzae,* and *Neisseria meningitidis*). These are not common causes of neonatal disease, probably because of specific antibody acquired from the mother.

B. **T-lymphocytes.** There is little information about the early development of T-lymphocytes. Homograft rejection is present by the fifth month of gestation. T-cell function probably is intact at birth but may not be fully effective because the nonspecific inflammatory response is deficient in newborns.

C. **Leukocytes** are present early in gestation: granulocytes at 2 months, lymphocytes at 3 months, and monocytes at 4 to 5 months. Leukocyte bactericidal function probably is normal at birth, but there is abnormal chemotaxis and probably deficient phagocytosis.

D. **Humoral factors. Complement** is synthesized and present early in gestation but, at birth, serum **C1q, C2, C3, C4, C5, factor B,** and total hemolytic levels are **low.** The **opsonic and chemotactic activities** of the sera of premature and term neonates are decreased when compared with adult sera.

E. **Passive immunity**

1. **Transplacental transport of maternal IgG** provides some protection against the following microorganisms (if the mother has antibodies): *Streptococcus pneumoniae,* other *Streptococcus* species, *Staphylococcus* species, *Haemophilus influenzae,* and common (by natural infection or immunization) viral agents (enteroviruses, measles, rubella, chickenpox). Usually, little protection is transferred against enteric gram-negative organisms.
2. **Breast milk** is rich in **secretory IgA** directed against respiratory and enteric microorganisms. It also contains active T- and B-lymphocytes, leukocytes, macrophages, and nonspecific inhibitors of bacterial and viral replication.

## PHARMACOLOGY AND USE OF ANTIBIOTICS IN NEONATES

In addition to changes in immune function, the newborn also experiences rapid physiologic changes that are important in terms of drug dosage. **In the practice of pediatrics, all drugs are administered on the basis of surface area or weight until the child reaches adult size.**

### I. Pharmacology

A. **Route of administration.** Absorption of an oral drug may be affected by the initial decreased gastric acidity of newborns and by the decreased intestinal motility of premature infants. The vasomotor instability of neonates makes the subcutaneous and intramuscular routes unreliable. For these and other reasons, **antibiotics for severe neonatal infections should be administered intravenously.**

B. **Antibiotic distribution** in infants is unique because of the rapid changes in body composition and compartments that occur after birth.

1. **The extracellular fluid** (ECF) compartment comprises up to 50% of total body weight in neonates and decreases to 25% by 1 year and to 20% in adulthood. **Because the ECF compartment comprises such a high percentage of the neonate's total body weight, the volume of distribution of some drugs, such as the aminoglycosides, is increased, requiring larger doses relative to weight.**
2. **Serum albumin** is quantitatively and qualitatively different in neonates relative to adults, being lower in concentration and showing less affinity for the penicillins. In neonates, albumin is important as a binder of bilirubin. Drugs that displace bilirubin from albumin (sulfonamides and selected cephalosporins) must be used with care to avoid kernicterus [6,7].

C. **Antibiotic metabolism in the newborn** is different from that in adults and children and changes rapidly in the first week of life.

1. **Hepatic.** Some hepatic enzyme systems are not fully developed at birth, and drugs rendered inactive by those systems must be administered in lower doses. Because of the decreased glucuronidation of chloramphenicol, newborns require less frequent and lower doses to avoid the gray baby syndrome.
2. **Renal.** Renal blood flow, glomerular filtration, and tubular function are diminished.
   a. **The glomerular filtration rate** is only 30% of adult levels, and this increases the half-life of the aminoglycosides and chloramphenicol.
   b. **Tubular secretion** is decreased to 20% of adult levels. Thus, the half-life of the penicillin family is lengthened.

## II. Some principles of antibiotic use

**A. Dosages. Table 3.2** gives recommended dosages for selected antibiotics after consideration of body mass and physiologic maturity. **Note that drug amounts are listed per dose, not per day.**

1. **Aminoglycosides.** Because of wide individual variation in the excretion of the aminoglycosides, their prolonged use (>5 days) should be guided by serum levels to prevent development of toxic or ineffectual levels (see Chapter 27). Some experts recommend higher doses with longer intervals to attain high-normal peaks and normal troughs.
2. **Chloramphenicol** doses should be guided by **serum levels** (see section **B.3**).

**B. Adverse reactions**

1. **Penicillins.** The penicillin group of drugs is safe in neonates and infants. IgE-mediated immediate reactions are rare, even in children born to allergic mothers. Methicillin-induced renal toxicity has been reported but is rare in neonates.
2. **Aminoglycosides.** The older agents (kanamycin and gentamicin) are safe when used as recommended. Experience with amikacin and tobramycin reveals no acute toxicity in newborns when used in recommended doses and when serum levels are monitored.
3. **Chloramphenicol** is well documented as the cause of the **gray baby syndrome** in neonates. It should be used only when less toxic drugs will not suffice, and serum levels should be monitored. Careful observation for early signs of gray baby syndrome (vomiting, abdominal distention, diarrhea, poor sucking, and respiratory distress) should be undertaken with complete blood counts (CBCs) and platelet counts at least twice weekly to detect hematologic abnormalities. (See Chapter 27.)

**C. Special limitations of use of antibiotics in neonates**

1. **Sulfonamides** have only bacteriostatic effects on bacteria. They can cause kernicterus by their competition with unconjugated bilirubin for albumin binding sites. Because of this and the availability of other drugs, there is **no current indication for sulfonamides in neonates** except for treatment of toxoplasmosis and *Pneumocystis carinii* pneumonia (PCP).
2. **Tetracyclines** are bacteriostatic and have considerable toxicity. They bind to bone and teeth by chelation with calcium, causing decreased bone growth and permanent discoloration of teeth. **The use of this group of drugs should be avoided from the second trimester of gestation to the eighth year of life.**
3. **Cephalosporins.** The first-generation (e.g., cephalothin and cefazolin) and most second-generation agents (e.g., cefuroxime and cefoxitin) do not adequately penetrate the cerebrospinal fluid (CSF). The third-generation cephalosporins (cefotaxime and ceftriaxone) penetrate the CSF well and are active against many gram-negative bacilli. These agents are discussed in detail in Chapter 27. **Ceftriaxone should be avoided in the first 4 weeks of life because it affects bilirubin-albumin binding and may increase the risk of bilirubin encephalopathy in jaundiced neonates [6,8]; therefore, cefotaxime is preferred in the neonate [9,10].**
4. **Nafcillin should not be used in premature or very young infants** because its excretion is predominantly by hepatic mechanisms, which may be deficient.

## III. Antibiotic use in the pregnant or lactating woman (see Chapter 27)

**A. Placental transfer of antibiotics.** As a general rule, pregnant women should avoid **all** unnecessary drugs because of the risk of fetal toxicity. **Sulfonamides** given to mothers late in pregnancy have caused kernicterus or hemolytic anemia in infants deficient in glucose-6-phosphate dehydrogenase (G6PD). Similarly, **tetracycline** has caused dental deformities and discoloration. Of the aminoglycosides, **streptomycin** used during pregnancy has been associated with eighth nerve dysfunction in neonates. The documented fetal toxicity of these antibiotics warrants careful evaluation of their use in pregnancy [11].

**B. Antibiotics in breast milk.** There are limited data on nursing neonates regarding adverse effects associated with antibiotics administered to their mothers [11,12]. Nevertheless, nursing mothers should avoid all unnecessary drugs. In order to minimize infant exposure to necessary drugs, mothers should generally take their drugs

Table 3.2. Recommended Dosages of Selected Antibiotics for Neonates by Age and Birth Weight

| Antibiotic | Route of Administration | Dose (mg/kg[a]) at 0–7 Days of Age | | Dose (mg/kg[a]) at 8–30 Days of Age | |
|---|---|---|---|---|---|
| | | Wt <2,000 g | Wt >2,000 g | Wt <2,000 g | Wt >2,000 g |
| Acyclovir | i.v. | 20 q8–12h | 20 q8h | 20 q8h | 20 q8h |
| Amikacin[b] | i.v., i.m. | 7.5 q12h | 7.5–10 q12h | 7.5–10 q8h | 10 q8h |
| Amphotericin B | i.v. | 0.25–1.0 q24h | 0.25–1.0 q24h | 0.25–1.0 q24h | 0.25–1.0 q24h |
| Ampicillin[c] | i.v., i.m. | 25–50 q12h | 25–50 q8h | 25–50 q8h | 25–50 q6h |
| Cefotaxime[d] | i.v., i.m. | 50 q12h | 50 q8–12h | 50 q8h | 50 q6-8h |
| Ceftazidime | i.v., i.m. | 50 q12h | 50 q8–12h | 50 q8h | 50 q8h |
| Chloramphenicol[e] | i.v., orally | 25 q24h | 25 q24h | 25 q24h | 25 q12h |
| Clindamycin | i.v., i.m., orally | 5 q12h | 5 q8h | 5 q8h | 5–7.5 q6h |
| Erythromycin | orally | 10 q12h | 10 q12h | 10 q8h | 10 q8h |
| Gentamicin[f] | i.v., i.m. | 2.5 q12h | 2.5 q12h | 2.5 q8h | 2.5 q8h |
| Methicillin | i.v., i.m. | 25–50 q12h | 25–50 q8h | 25–50 q8h | 25–50 q6h |
| Nafcillin[g] | i.v. | 25 q12h | 25 q8h | 25 q8h | 25 q6h |
| Oxacillin | i.v., i.m. | 25 q12h | 25 q8h | 25 q8h | 25 q6h |
| Penicillin G[h] | i.v., i.m. | 25,000–50,000 units q12h | 25,000–50,000 units q8h | 25,000–50,000 units q8h | 25,000–50,000 units q6h |
| Penicillin benzathine | i.m. only | 50,000 units once (maximum 2.4 million) | 50,000 units once | 50,000 units once | 50,000 units once |
| Penicillin procaine | i.m. only | 50,000 units q24h (maximum 4.8 million) | 50,000 units q24h | 50,000 units q24h | 50,000 units q24h |
| Ticarcillin | i.v., i.m. | 75 q12h | 75 q8h | 75 q8h | 100 q8h |
| Tobramycin[i] | i.v., i.m. | 2.5 q12h | 2.5 q12h | 2.5 q8h | 2.5 q8h |
| Vancomycin[j] | i.v. | 10–15 q12–18h | 10–15 q8–12h | 10–15 q8h | 10–15 q8h |

i.v., intravenous; i.m., intramuscular; q8h, every 8 hours.
[a]Penicillin doses are expressed in units per kilogram.
[b]Serum antibiotic levels must be monitored. Listed doses are for initiation of therapy. Target amikacin peak drawn 30–60 minutes after dose is 20–30 mg/L, and trough drawn within 30 minutes before dose is 5–10 mg/L.
[c]Meningitis requires 300–400 mg/kg/day of ampicillin.
[d]Cefotaxime and other third-generation cephalosporins are described in detail in Chapter 27.
[e]Loading dose of 20 mg/kg i.v. or orally. Target chloramphenicol peak drawn 30 minutes after IV dose or 2 hours after PO dose is 15–25 mg/L for meningitis and 10–20 mg/L for other infections. Trough drawn within 30 minutes of i.v. or oral dose should be 5–15 mg/L for meningitis and 5–10 mg/L for other infections.
[f]Serum antibiotic levels must be monitored. Listed doses are for initiation of therapy. Target gentamicin peak drawn 30–60 minutes after dose is 6–10 mg/L and trough drawn within 30 minutes before dose is <2 mg/L. Some experts recommend higher doses with longer intervals to attain high-normal peaks and normal troughs.
[g]Excretion predominantly hepatic; use with caution in young and premature infants.
[h]Group B streptococcal sepsis requires 200,000 units/kg/day of pencillin G. Group B streptococcal meningitis requires 450,000 units/kg/day of penicillin G.
[i]Serum antibiotic levels must be monitored. Listed doses are for initiation of therapy. Target tobramycin peak drawn 30–60 minutes after dose is 6–10 mg/L and trough drawn within 30 minutes before dose is <2 mg/L.
[j]Serum antibiotic levels usually monitored. Listed doses are for initiation of therapy. Target vancomycin peak drawn 60 minutes after dose is 25–40 mg/L and trough drawn within 30 minutes before dose is <10 mg/L.

immediately after breast-feeding. Short-acting instead of long-acting drug preparations are preferred for lactating women. An important consideration is the total daily "dose" a nursing baby would receive; in many cases, this dose is not toxicologically significant.

Few drugs are absolutely contraindicated in breast-feeding (bromocriptine, cyclophosphamide, cyclosporine, doxorubicin, dextroamphetamine, ergotamine, lithium, methotrexate, phenindione, all drugs of abuse). For many drugs, however, there are case reports of adverse effects or theoretical adverse effects on the infant that warrant caution and consideration of temporary suspension of breast-feeding. Examples of such antibacterial drugs include chloramphenicol, ciprofloxacin and other quinolones, doxycycline and other tetracyclines, metronidazole, and sulfonamides (although trimethoprim-sulfamethoxazole is categorized as compatible with breast-feeding by the American Academy of Pediatrics [AAP]). The reader is referred to references 11 and 12 for a complete review of available data and concerns of drugs with breast-feeding.

## NEONATAL SEPSIS (SEPSIS NEONATORUM)

I. **Bacteriology.** The most common organisms causing neonatal sepsis and meningitis in the United States have changed over the decades. In the 1940's, the group A streptococci and, in the 1950's, the staphylococci (especially phage group I) were prominent. Since the early 1960's, *Escherichia coli* and, currently, the group B streptococci have been the major causative bacteria [1,2]. The prevalent pathogenic organisms in a single nursery change with time and may not be similar to organisms found on other wards. It is valuable to be aware of the most common pathogens in one's own nursery as well as of their antibiotic susceptibilities.

A. ***E. coli*** is one of the maternal enteric organisms that colonize the gastrointestinal (GI) tract of the newborn, and can invade the blood and meninges (see section on Neonatal Meningitis).

B. **Group B streptococci have become the most common cause of bacteremia and sepsis in many nurseries** [13].

1. **Acquisition of group B streptococci.** The organisms can be acquired **intrapartum** from the maternal cervix or vagina and colonize the skin and upper respiratory and GI tracts of the neonate. Colonization rates among pregnant women range from 5% to 40% depending on the population and culture technique. **Of infants born to colonized mothers, 40% to 75% are themselves colonized, but only 1% to 2% will develop early-onset disease.** The infants are colonized with the strains borne by their mothers. The presence of specific maternal antibody appears to protect the infant from early-onset sepsis. Determining the most efficacious and cost-effective time to screen for group B streptococcal colonization has been hampered by lack of sensitive and specific rapid diagnostic techniques, poor adherence to prenatal care, and the intermittent nature of maternal group B streptococcal colonization. **Prevention guidelines** [14] from the Centers for Disease Control, American Academy of Pediatrics, and American College of Obstetrics and Gynecology **recommend** either screening by rectovaginal culture for group B streptococci carriage at 35 to 37 weeks' gestation followed by intrapartum prophylaxis with intravenous penicillin for all carriers, or no screening but prophylaxis based on defined risk factors (Figs. 3.1 through 3.3). No economic analysis of this strategy is available, but analyses of similar prevention strategies have demonstrated cost savings [15].

2. **Syndromes caused by group B streptococci**

   a. **Early-onset disease** occurs in the first 5 to 7 days of life, often as overwhelming sepsis with apnea and shock [16,17]. This devastating presentation frequently is associated with obstetric complications and prematurity. The pulmonary manifestations may be difficult to differentiate clinically or radiologically from the respiratory distress syndrome. Meningitis occurs in 15% to 30% of cases. Mortality rates of 50% in the 1960's and 1970's have declined to 10% to 20% with early aggressive management. Recurrences occur in approximately 3% of cases.

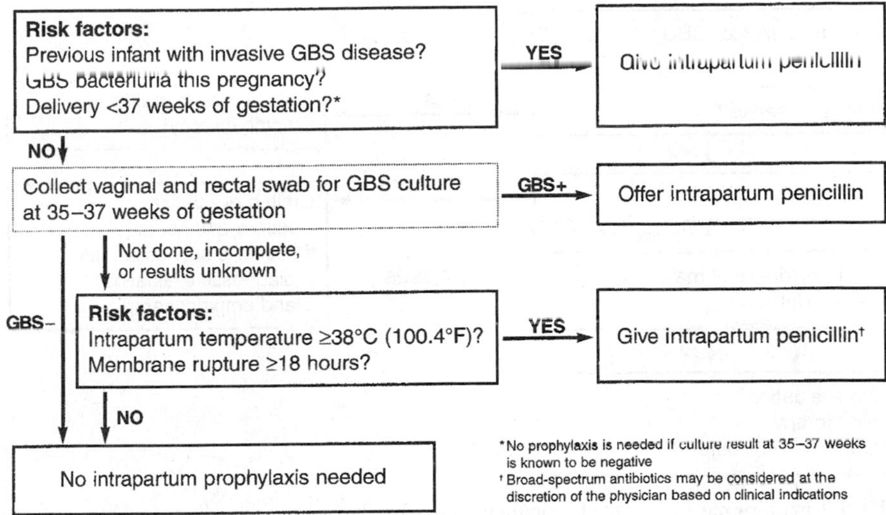


**FIG. 3.1** Prevention strategy for early-onset group B streptococcus disease using prenatal culture screening at 35 to 37 weeks of gestation.

b. **Late-onset disease** occurs after 7 days of age (to 4 months of age) and usually presents as sepsis, meningitis, or another localized infection.

C. ***Listeria monocytogenes*** is a gram-positive rod that may cause congenital disease resulting in abortion or stillbirth. It is likely that peripartum colonization leads, in some neonates, to early- or late-onset disease [18].

1. **Early-onset disease** appears in the first week of life, often in premature infants, with pneumonia, shock, and salmon-colored dermal papules. Assisted ventilation often is required, and the mortality rate may reach 50%.

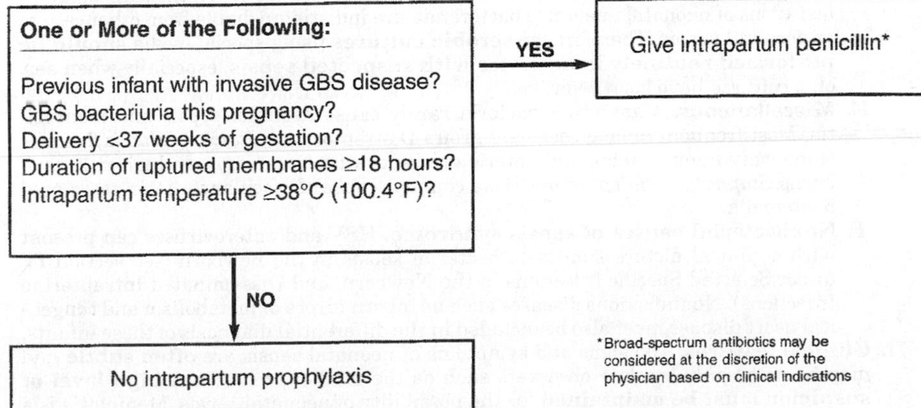


**FIG. 3.2** Prevention strategy for early-onset group B streptococcus disease using risk factors without prenatal culture screening.

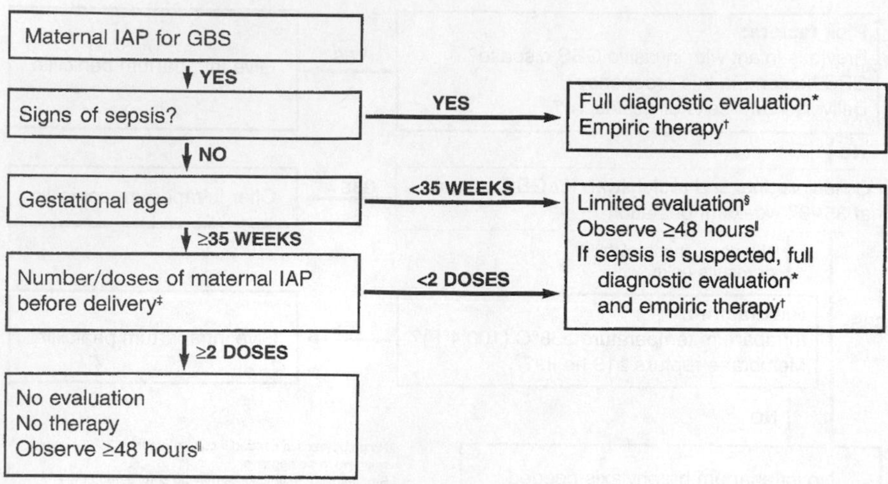


**FIG. 3.3** Empiric management of neonate born to a mother who received intrapartum antimicrobial prophylaxis (*IAP*) for prevention of early-onset group B streptococcus disease. This algorithm is suggested but is not an exclusive approach of management. *Includes CBC and differential, blood culture, and chest radiograph if respiratory symptoms. A lumbar puncture is performed at the discretion of the physician. †Duration of therapy will vary depending on results of blood culture and CSF findings (if obtained), as well as on the clinical course of the infant. If laboratory results and clinical course are unremarkable, duration may be as short as 48 to 72 hours. ‡, applies to penicillin or ampicillin chemoprophylaxis; §, CBC and differential, blood culture. ||Does not allow early discharge.

2. **Late-onset disease** often presents as meningitis in full-term infants. In some cases, the CSF is characterized by a lymphocytosis rather than polymorphonuclear leukocytes; however, this is unusual [19]. Therapy with ampicillin, alone or with gentamicin, results in a lower mortality rate than that associated with early-onset disease.

D. **Anaerobes** cause approximately 10% to 25% of all neonatal bacteremias [20], although only a portion of affected neonates will be septic. However, the clinical manifestations of neonatal anaerobic bacteremia are indistinguishable from other causes of neonatal sepsis. Therefore, **anaerobic cultures** using special media **should be performed routinely in neonates with suspected sepsis,** especially when aerobic cultures have been negative.

E. **Miscellaneous.** Many other bacteria rarely cause neonatal sepsis and meningitis. Most frequent among these are group D streptococci, *Haemophilus influenzae* (commonly nontypeable), and enteric gram-negative organisms. In high-risk newborns, *Staphylococcus epidermidis* is a common cause of vascular catheter-associated bacteremia.

F. **Nonbacterial causes of sepsis syndrome.** HSV and enteroviruses can present with a clinical picture similar to bacterial sepsis in the newborn (see section **IV** under Selected Specific Infections in the Newborn, and Disseminated Intrauterine Infections). Noninfectious diseases such as inborn errors of metabolism and congenital heart disease must also be included in the differential diagnosis of these infants.

II. **Clinical features.** The signs and symptoms of neonatal sepsis are **often subtle** and may be noted only by close observers such as the mother or nurse. **A high level of suspicion must be maintained** for the possibility of neonatal sepsis. Meningitis is a common complication.

A. **Factors associated with neonatal sepsis** are listed in Table 3.3. When any of these factors is present, at least a CBC and blood culture should be performed.

Table 3.3. Factors Associated with Neonatal Sepsis

| Source or Cause | Remarks |
|---|---|
| Early-onset sepsis | |
| Maternal perinatal infection | Fever, pyuria, and foul amniotic fluid are signs of maternal infection. |
| Prolonged rupture of the membranes | Variably defined as >12, 18, or 24 h. |
| Prolonged labor, difficult delivery | Meconium staining may reflect stress and hypoxia of infant. |
| Prematurity and low birth weight | Rate of septicemia is inversely correlated with birth weight and gestational age.[a] |
| Low Apgar score, resuscitation | Hypoxia, hypoperfusion, aspiration, and intubation are all associated with septicemia. |
| Late-onset sepsis | |
| Congenital anomalies | Meningomyelocele, sinus tracts, and the like provide routes for infection. |
| Prolonged intensive care nursery admission | Increased risk of nosocomial infection. |
| Procedures or manipulations | Fetal monitoring electrodes, umbilical vein or artery catheters, chest tubes, arterial cannulas, and such provide routes and sites for infection. |
| Gender | Male infants are more likely to become septic than are female infants. |

[a]Data from Buetow KC, Klein SW, Lane RB. Septicemia in premature infants. *Am J Dis Child* 1965; 110:20.

Most neonates with suspected sepsis are started empirically on antibiotics after appropriate laboratory studies have been performed. In some cases, the infant may simply be observed for further signs of illness before antibiotics are started.

B. **Symptoms and signs** in neonatal sepsis are shown in Table 3.4.

III. **Diagnosis. The clinician must suspect sepsis with the report of any of the signs listed in Table 3.4.** A history and physical examination will provide further information [21,22].

A. **Samples of blood, urine, and CSF** [23] must be obtained, examined, and cultured. Body surface cultures (ear canal, nasopharynx, axilla, umbilicus, groin, and gastric aspirate) are of limited value [24], except with HSV disease.

B. **Laboratory tests** may be useful in making the diagnosis.

1. **Peripheral white blood cell (WBC) count** (Table 3.5). Many infected infants, particularly premature infants, exhibit **leukopenia** rather than leukocytosis. Leukopenia should heighten concern about possible infection, although it is nonspecific. Birth asphyxia, pregnancy-induced hypertension, prematurity, low birth weight, and other conditions also may cause a low WBC count [25]. Various hematologic scoring systems have been studied, including the ratio of immature to total neutrophils, but these scoring systems are imperfect predictors of sepsis [26].
2. **Latex agglutination (LA) is not routinely recommended in the diagnosis of** group B streptococcal sepsis.
3. **Other tests,** when used individually, are unreliable indicators of neonatal sepsis. These include the erythrocyte sedimentation rate, nitroblue tetrazolium test, and levels of C-reactive protein, haptoglobin, interleukin-6, and procalcitonin. A combination of a complete leukocyte count, microerythrocyte sedimentation rate, and C-reactive protein level may be more accurate than any single test. Serial normal C-reactive protein levels over the first 1 to 3 days may be the best marker of absence of sepsis [4].

C. **Presumptive therapy.** Ultimately, the clinical condition of the baby should determine whether presumptive therapy is begun. **Because neonatal sepsis often**

Table 3.4. Symptoms and Signs of Neonatal Sepsis

| Signs and Symptoms | Approximate Percentage of Cases |
|---|---|
| Temperature | |
| Hyperthermia | 50 |
| Hypothermia | 15 |
| Pulmonary | |
| Dyspnea | 20 |
| Periodic breathing or apnea | 20 |
| Cyanosis | 25 |
| Cardiovascular (tachycardia, bradycardia, hypotension, shock) | 25 |
| Gastrointestinal | |
| Anorexia | 30 |
| Vomiting | 20 |
| Abdominal distention | 20 |
| Diarrhea | 10 |
| Hepatic | |
| Hepatomegaly | 30–50 |
| Jaundice | 30 |
| Hematologic (bleeding diathesis) | 2–10 |
| CNS | |
| Lethargy | 35 |
| Irritability or jitteriness (or both) | 15 |
| Seizure | 15 |
| Asymptomatic | 6–9 |

Data from Buetow KC, Klein SW, Lane RB. Septicemia in premature infants. *Am J Dis Child* 1965;110:29. Gluck L, Wood HF, Fousek MD. Septicemia of the newborn. *Pediatr Clin North Am* 1966;13:1131; McCracken GH Jr, Shinefield HR. Changes in the pattern of neonatal septicemia and meningitis. *Am J Dis Child* 1966;112:33; and Nyhan WL, Fousek MD. Septicemia of the newborn. *Pediatrics* 1958;22:268.

**progresses rapidly and is associated with a high mortality rate, early presumptive therapy must be instituted when this diagnosis is suspected, as soon as cultures are obtained.** Many infants are treated for minimal indications, and only a few will prove to have sepsis. In one report [27], 6.5% of 1,551 infants in two nurseries were treated with antibiotics for presumed sepsis, but only 6% of those treated had positive blood cultures. Rapid early treatment is essential, even though it is recognized that many patients may be treated unnecessarily.

Table 3.5. Range of White Blood Cell Counts ($\times 1{,}000/mm^3$) and Ratios for Normal Infants of all Weights and Gestational Ages

| Age | Total Neutrophils | Immature (Band) Neutrophils |
|---|---|---|
| Birth | 1.8–6.0 | 0–1.1 |
| 12 h | 7.8–14.5 | 0–1.4 |
| 1 day | 7.2–12.6 | 0–1.3 |
| 2 days | 3.6–8.1 | 0–0.8 |
| 5 days | 1.8–5.4 | 0–0.5 |
| 28 days | 1.8–5.4 | 0–0.5 |

Adapted from Manroe BL et al. The neonatal blood count in health and disease I. Reference values for neutrophilic cells. *J Pediatr* 1979;95:89, with permission.

Table 3.6. Suggested Initial Empiric Antibiotic Therapy of Neonatal Infections

| Clinical Syndrome | Suggested Therapy |
|---|---|
| Early-onset sepsis, meningitis | Ampicillin and either gentamicin or cefotaxime |
| Late-onset sepsis, meningitis | Ampicillin (or vancomycin) and cefotaxime |
| Early-onset pneumonia | Ampicillin and either gentamicin or cefotaxime |
| Catheter sepsis | Vancomycin and cefotaxime |
| Necrotizing enterocolitis | Ampicillin (or vancomycin), gentamicin, and clindamycin |

IV. **Therapy** (Table 3.6)

A. **Antibiotics**

1. **Early-onset disease.** Therapy must be directed against group B streptococci, other gram-positive cocci including enterococci, gram-negative enteric organisms, and *Listeria*. **Intravenous ampicillin and either an aminoglycoside** (the choice based on local susceptibility patterns) **or cefotaxime** intramuscularly or intravenously should be used initially. Culture results will guide more specific therapy [10,28,29].
2. **Late-onset disease** is caused by the same organisms listed for early-onset disease, plus hospital-acquired staphylococci and gram-negative organisms. **Ampicillin and either an aminoglycoside or cefotaxime** are most often used parenterally for initial therapy. If methicillin-resistant staphylococci are epidemiologically important in the neonatal intensive care population, **vancomycin and a third-generation cephalosporin should be used** until culture and sensitivity results are available.
3. **Duration of therapy.** Specific management must be individualized, taking into consideration maternal antibiotic therapy prepartum and intrapartum, quality of culture specimens, culture results, and the overall clinical course. In some instances, infants are treated empirically in the face of negative cultures.
   a. **If initial cultures are negative** and the infant is asymptomatic, most clinicians would stop antibiotic therapy after 3 days and observe closely.
   b. **If initial blood cultures are positive** and meningitis is not present, most authorities recommend a 10-day course of treatment, based on susceptibility data.
4. Anaerobic infection, resistant bacterial infection, viral infection (especially HSV), fungal infection and noninfectious disorders should be suspected in any infant not doing well on the recommended initial therapy.

B. **Ancillary care** is of equal importance and usually requires an intensive care nursery.

1. **Vital signs,** including blood pressure and blood gases, should be monitored.
2. **Ventilatory support** often is required because of hypoxia and hypercapnia.
3. **Fluid and electrolytes** must be monitored closely, because acidosis, hypoglycemia, and electrolyte imbalances are common in the ill neonate.
4. **Red blood cell transfusions** may be necessary to improve intravascular volume and oxygen-carrying capacity.
5. **Other blood products** such as white cells, intravenous immunoglobulin (IVIG), and fresh frozen plasma have all been used as adjuncts to antibiotic therapy [30]. IVIG has not been consistently effective or beneficial as prophylaxis in premature neonates or as adjunctive therapy for septic neonates, and is not routinely recommended [31–33]. Fresh frozen plasma should be used for infants with disseminated intravascular coagulation (DIC) and has been advocated to improve the diminished serum complement and opsonic activity of neonates. The data on the efficacy of granulocyte transfusions in neonates is mixed and incomplete, and their use varies by center.

## NEONATAL MENINGITIS

I. **Clinical features.** The presenting features of meningitis in the neonate may not be different from those listed for sepsis (see Table 3.4). In some series, convulsions,

Table 3.7. Composition of Normal Cerebrospinal Fluid in Newborns

| | Total WBC/mm$^3$ | | ANC | | Glucose (mg/dL) | | Protein (mg/dL) | |
|---|---|---|---|---|---|---|---|---|
| Age | Mean | Range | Mean | Range | Mean | Range | Mean | Range |
| Premature newborn | 9.0 | 0–29 | NR | NR | 50 | 24–63 | 115 | 65–150 |
| Full-term newborn | 8.2 | 0–22 | NR | NR | 52 | 34–119 | 90 | 20–170 |
| 0–4 wk | 11.0 | 0–50 | 0.40 | 0–7.5 | 46 | 36–61 | 84 | 35–189 |
| 4–8 wk | 7.1 | 0–50 | 0.18 | 0–2.1 | 46 | 29–62 | 59 | 19–121 |

WBC, white blood cell; ANC, absolute neutrophil count; NR, not reported.
Adapted from Bonadio WA. The cerebrospinal fluid: physiologic aspects and alterations associated with bacterial meningitis. *Pediatr Infect Dis J* 1992;11:423, with permission.

irritability, or lethargy were more prominent. Only rarely will an infant with meningitis exhibit a bulging fontanelle or nuchal rigidity.

**II. Diagnosis.** Samples of blood, CSF, and urine should be obtained, examined, and cultured. The tests listed in section **III** under Neonatal Sepsis may be useful, especially detection of antigen by counter immunoelectrophoresis (CIE) or the latex agglutination (LA) test. Table 3.7 lists normal values for CSF analysis in newborns.

**III. Bacteriology.** *E. coli* and group B streptococci cause up to 70% of neonatal meningitis, with *Listeria monocytogenes* accounting for another 5%. Eighty percent of all *E. coli* meningitides are due to organisms carrying the K1 polysaccharide capsular antigen. Approximately 30% of all newborn babies are colonized with K1 strains, and the rate of meningitis is estimated to be 1 of every 100 colonized infants. Carriage of K1 strains has been demonstrated in a high percentage of nursery personnel, so infants may be colonized postnatally as well. The severity of disease and the presence of sequelae have a positive correlation with the presence and concentration of the K1 antigen in the CSF. Other pathogens known to cause meningitis include other "typical" bacteria (*Staphylococcus aureus, S. epidermidis, Citrobacter diversus* [34]), mycobacteria (tuberculosis), syphilis, viral infections (HSV, CMV, enteroviruses), toxoplasmosis, *Candida* species, and noninfectious causes (hemorrhage, malignancy).

**IV. Therapy**

**A. Antibiotics**

1. **Initial therapy. Parenteral ampicillin and either an aminoglycoside or cefotaxime should be used. The highest doses indicated in Table 3.2 should be administered** because of the limited penetration of some of these antibiotics into the CSF. If gram-negative bacilli are seen on CSF Gram stain, some experts would use ampicillin with both an aminoglycoside and cefotaxime pending culture results [35–37].
2. **Group B streptococci (suspected or proved). Usual regimens include cefotaxime alone or a combination of penicillin or ampicillin with gentamicin for a total of 14 to 21 days.** Because of the relative resistance of group B streptococci to penicillin and reports of relapse after therapy, the recommended doses of penicillin have been raised. Aqueous penicillin should be given at 450,000 units/kg/day (see Table 3.2). If combination therapy is initiated and CSF sterilization is documented at 24 to 48 hours, gentamicin can be discontinued and therapy completed with penicillin or ampicillin alone. Some experts recommend repeat CSF examinations at 24 to 48 hours into therapy to document sterilization and again at the completion of therapy to document decrease in CSF protein (<200 mg/dL) and neutrophils (<20%–30%) [4].
3. ***Listeria monocytogenes*** should be treated with parenteral ampicillin or penicillin. The duration of therapy is as recommended for group B streptococci (see section **2**). Some experts add a parenteral aminoglycoside (e.g., gentamicin) for synergy.

4. **Enteric gram-negative bacteria** are more difficult to eradicate from the CSF than gram-positive bacteria, in part because of the low levels of aminoglycosides achieved therein. Several routes of antibiotic administration have been studied, including the intralumbar and intraventricular routes. Controlled trials have shown either no additional benefit over the intravenous route or detrimental effects [38], and appropriate parenteral antibiotics remain the standard of care.
   a. **Third-generation cephalosporins.** Cefotaxime appears useful and safe in infants [9,10,29]. It achieves good CSF levels and has broad activity against gram-negative enteric bacteria. However, this third-generation agent is not active against *Pseudomonas* species, enterococci, or *L. monocytogenes* and does not have optimum activity against most staphylococci. Ceftriaxone, although similar to cefotaxime in its spectrum of activity, affects bilirubin-albumin binding and may increase the risk of bilirubin encephalopathy in jaundiced neonates; therefore, it should be avoided if possible [6,8]. Ceftazidime has a spectrum of activity similar to that of cefotaxime, with the added benefit of antipseudomonal activity. It may be used in the setting where *Pseudomonas* is a suspected pathogen.
   b. **Aminoglycosides** remain important in the management of meningitis, particularly with penicillin-tolerant strains of group B streptococci and enteric gram-negative organisms. They are used together with another antibiotic, usually a $\beta$-lactam.
   c. **Chloramphenicol** has been used in patients with susceptible bacteria, but this is not an ideal agent. Serum levels must be carefully monitored in neonates to avoid toxicity. Furthermore, chloramphenicol is usually bacteriostatic rather than bactericidal against gram-negative bacilli.
   d. **Recommendation.** Because of the difficulties and controversies involved in treating enteric gram-negative bacilli meningitis, we **suggest an infectious disease consultation. Combination therapy with cefotaxime or ceftazidime plus gentamicin is recommended once a gram-negative organism is diagnosed by CSF gram stain or culture, pending final identification and susceptibilities.** A third-generation cephalosporin alone can be used for susceptibile *E. coli* or *Klebsiella* species. For *Pseudomonas* species and most other gram-negative bacteria, combination therapy with a $\beta$-lactam and an aminoglycoside is used for the entire course; choice of specific agents is guided by isolate susceptibilities and adequacy of CSF penetration (see Chapter 27).

      In general, repeat lumbar punctures are performed at 48 to 72 hours to document sterilization of the CSF, and therapy is continued for 14 days after sterilization or for a total of 21 days. Many experts recommend neuroimaging for cases of meningitis caused by gram-negative bacilli.

B. **Ancillary care** (see section **IV.B** under Neonatal Sepsis). It is particularly important to monitor free water intake to avoid the hyponatremia due to inappropriate secretion of antidiuretic hormone associated with meningitis. Above all, support of blood pressure and perfusion must be optimized. Corticosteroids have not been studied in the neonate and are not recommended (see Chapter 6). Other important evaluations after recovery from acute meningitis include hearing screens and careful neurodevelopmental follow-up.

## SELECTED SPECIFIC INFECTIONS IN THE NEWBORN

I. **Ophthalmia neonatorum,** or **conjunctivitis** in an infant under 4 weeks of age usually is caused by organisms acquired in the birth canal [39]. *Chlamydia trachomatis,* staphylococci, gonococci, streptococci, and viruses including HSV are all documented as etiologic agents of this disease. Prophylaxis is mandated in most of the United States. Silver nitrate drops 1% (Crede solution), tetracycline, or erythromycin ointment have efficacy against gonococcal conjunctivitis. One of these three products should be applied to the neonate's eyes within an hour of birth. The silver nitrate solution may cause an early, nonpurulent discharge that should resolve within 24 to 48 hours. Conjunctivitis due to *Neisseria gonorrhoeae* and other gram-negative organisms requires appropriate parenteral antibiotics. Ophthalmia caused by staphylococci and gonococci often is of earlier onset than conjunctivitis caused by *C. trachomatis* or adenovirus. The approach to and therapy for this problem are discussed further in Chapter 7 (section **IV** under Conjunctivitis). **The conjunctival discharge is infectious, so handwashing control measures are important to prevent spread** to attendants and other patients in the nursery.

**II. Upper respiratory tract infections. Otitis media** is common in infants with cleft palate and not uncommon in normal infants in the first month of life. This infection may present in isolated fashion or as part of a generalized septicemia. A full review of this topic is available [40]. (See also Chapter 8.)

**A. Bacteriology.** Published reports implicate gram-negative organisms such as *E.coli* and *Klebsiella* species, as well as *S. aureus, Haemophilus* species, and streptococci.

**B. Diagnosis** is based on the finding of a gray or red tympanic membrane with decreased mobility. Tympanocentesis should be attempted to confirm the diagnosis and to direct therapy, because sepsis or meningitis may be a consequence of inappropriate therapy. A full sepsis workup should be performed for all ill-appearing infants. If a tympanocentesis is not performed, close follow-up must be assured to evaluate for possible treatment failures.

**C. Therapy. Initial therapy is controversial.** We advocate tympanocentesis followed by parenteral ampicillin and either an aminoglycoside or a third-generation cephalosporin for all neonates with otitis media, until culture results are available. Others suggest that outpatient amoxicillin therapy in a well-appearing older neonate is safe and sufficient initial therapy. Treatment should continue for 7 to 10 days or longer if purulent tympanic abnormalities persist (see Table 3.2 for doses).

**III. Lower respiratory tract infections** in neonates can be classified as congenital, intrapartum, or postnatal, depending on when the pathogen was acquired. Rales, decreased breath sounds, and percussion dullness may be difficult to detect in the neonate. **The finding of respiratory distress should lead to chest radiography, which is the most useful tool in confirming or ruling out pneumonia.** A CBC and blood culture also should be performed.

**A. Congenital pneumonia** usually is part of a transplacental infection. Rubella, CMV, HSV, congenital syphilis, and *Toxoplasma gondii* can all cause this type of pneumonia.

1. **Clinical features.** Infants with transplacental congenital pneumonia are often small for gestational age and bear the other stigmata of their infection. (See the discussion under Disseminated Intrauterine Infections.)
2. **Therapy.** There is no therapy for rubella infection. Clinical trials are underway to assess the possible role of ganciclovir in congenital CMV infections. The pneumonias associated with toxoplasmosis, congenital syphilis, and herpes virus should be treated as discussed under Disseminated Intrauterine Infections.

**B. Intrapartum pneumonia** is due to the aspiration of maternal cervicovaginal organisms or of infected amniotic fluid and is manifested at birth or shortly thereafter.

1. **Clinical presentation.** Babies with bacterial pneumonia may present as asphyxiated newborns with fulminant disease. Group B streptococci may cause devastating early-onset sepsis with pneumonia and respiratory distress.
2. **Cultures.** Cultures of blood and culture and Gram stain of respiratory secretions should be obtained. The latter is best obtained by tracheal aspiration under direct vision with a laryngoscope. If a pleural effusion is present, needle aspiration should be performed for diagnostic studies.
3. **Therapy.** Intrapartum pneumonia should be treated with parenteral ampicillin and either an aminoglycoside or cefotaxime for 10 days. If group B streptococci are suspected, the higher dose of ampicillin in Table 3.2 should be doubled.

**C. Postpartum pneumonia** often is nosocomial in origin, the infant acquiring an organism from the nursery attendants or equipment.

1. **Etiology.** Of particular concern are hospital-acquired staphylococcal and gram-negative bacterial pneumonias. RSV, parainfluenza viruses, and influenza

viruses are all common causes of postnatally acquired pneumonia. Because these agents often cause respiratory tract disease that cannot, with certainty, be clinically distinguished from bacterial disease, antibiotic therapy is usually initiated in lower respiratory tract disease of acute onset in the first month of life.

2. **Clinical features.** These neonates present with the development of respiratory distress: cyanosis, tachypnea, cough, apnea, expiratory grunting, nasal flaring, and subcostal and sternal retractions.
3. **Cultures** should be performed as discussed under section **B.2.** Viral cultures also should be obtained from the skin, rectum, conjunctiva, throat, and nasopharynx. Viral antigen detection tests are available for many respiratory viruses.
4. **Therapy.** Postpartum pneumonia should be treated initially with broad-spectrum parenteral antibiotics (e.g., cefotaxime and an aminoglycoside) (Table 3.6). If the organism is either staphylococcus or a gram-negative organism, therapy with the appropriate antibiotic should continue for 3 weeks. Ribavirin is not routinely recommended for the treatment of RSV infection; monthly palivizumab or RSV-IVIG can prevent severe disease and is indicated for selected infants during respiratory season. Amantadine, rimantidine, and the neuraminidase inhibitors have not been approved for treatment of influenza in newborns.

D. **Chlamydial pneumonitis** is a clinically distinct syndrome in infants infected intrapartum. Of those neonates who are exposed, 10% to 20% develop pneumonitis (Table 3.1).

1. **Clinical features.** Symptoms usually become apparent at 4 to 12 weeks of age. Half of the infants have a history of conjunctivitis. There is a gradual worsening of cough, which may occur in staccato paroxysms that result in cyanosis. There is no whoop, and fever is rare. Inspiratory crepitations and abnormal tympanic membranes are common features found on physical examination. Radiographs show patchy alveolar infiltrates and hyperinflation. Many affected infants have eosinophilia of more than 400/mm$^3$ [41,42]. Infants may excrete *C. trachomatis* for up to 2 years [43].
2. **Diagnosis** is suggested by the history and clinical features. Swabs of conjunctivae and nasopharynx can be submitted for chlamydia culture and antigen detection tests for diagnostic confirmation.
3. **Therapy of conjunctivitis or pneumonia is with systemic antibiotics.** Regimens include 2 weeks of erythromycin 40 to 50 mg/kg/day, or sulfisoxazole 150 mg/kg/day [44]. Erythromycin therapy has been associated with pyloric stenosis; azithromycin at 20 mg/kg daily for 3 days may be an effective alternative [45].

E. ***Ureaplasma urealyticum* and *Mycoplasma hominis*** have been associated with pneumonia in the newborn. Colonization rates of up to 80% have been estimated among pregnant women, 15% to 30% of their newborns are surface-colonized at birth. The presence of these organisms in the placenta has been associated with chorioamnionitis, spontaneous abortion, prematurity, and congenital pneumonia. High antibody levels to *U. urealyticum* have been found in infants with respiratory disease and chronic lung disease [46,47].

1. **Clinical features** are not unique in pneumonia caused by these organisms.
2. **Diagnosis.** Because of high colonization rates, these pathogens should be considered when pneumonia is diagnosed. Isolation of these organisms requires special media.
3. **Therapy.** Erythromycin has been recommended for treatment of *U. urealyticum* cases [48], but no efficacy data for this agent are available.

## IV. GI infections

A. **Diarrheal disease** is more prevalent in infancy and childhood than at any later period; this may be due to the diminished immunocompetence previously mentioned. Local antimicrobial factors such as gastric pH, peristalsis, and secretory IgA are also altered and may contribute to increased susceptibility. Breast milk probably compensates for some of the deficiencies of local immunity, but only a fraction of neonates receive it. Enteric pathogens may be acquired orally, either intrapartum or postpartum.

1. **Etiology.** It is possible that a proportion of neonatal diarrheal disease is not infectious in origin, being due instead to changes in the composition and volume of the diet or to changes in bowel function. Of the infectious diarrheas, rotavirus is the most frequent; *Salmonella* and *Shigella* species and *E. coli* account for some of the remainder [49]. *Campylobacter* enteritis has occurred in neonates (see Chapter 13). *Clostridium difficile* rarely causes disease in neonates, because *C. difficile* is part of the normal neonatal flora, recovery of this organism or detection of its toxin in neonates does not indicate *C. difficile* disease. It is likely that other agents exist that are not yet identified.
2. **Evaluation.** A fresh stool smear should be examined for leukocytes by methylene blue staining to determine whether an invasive organism is responsible. Fecal leukocytes are often present in diarrhea caused by *Salmonella* and *Shigella* species or invasive *E. coli*, whereas they are usually absent in toxicogenic bacterial or viral disease. (For further discussion, see Chapter 13.) **Fresh stools should be cultured** for enteric pathogens, and blood cultures should be obtained.
3. **Therapy**
   a. **Replacement of fluid losses** is the most important aspect of treatment. Monitoring of the infant's output, weight, and vital signs must be meticulous.
   b. **Antibiotic therapy** for bacterial diarrhea is somewhat controversial. The following are suggested guidelines.
      (1) ***Salmonella* and *Shigella* species.** A neonate ill with the invasive organisms *Salmonella* and *Shigella* should be treated initially with parenteral cefotaxime (pending susceptibility data) because of the risk for systemic involvement and metastatic infection. Blood cultures and CSF cultures are recommended for infants under 3 months of age with *Salmonella* infection even in the absence of fever or toxic appearance. Antibiotic sensitivities should be determined on all bacterial isolates to guide further therapy. *Shigella* should be treated for at least 5 to 7 days. Treatment of *Salmonella* gastroenteritis may prolong the carrier state, but initially ill-appearing or febrile young infants and those infants with proven invasive *Salmonella* infection require antibiotics. Ten to fourteen days of therapy are recommended for *Salmonella* bacteremia and 4 weeks for *Salmonella* meningitis [50].
      (2) ***E. coli*.** Diarrhea in neonates and infants has been associated with certain enteropathogenic serotypes of *E. coli* (mechanism unknown), invasive *E. coli*, or strains of *E. coli* that produce an enterotoxin. Unfortunately, the tests for identification of the latter two groups of *E. coli* are not widely available. An infant with prolonged diarrhea who has an enteropathogenic serotype of *E. coli* in the stools might benefit from a course of oral neomycin (100 mg/kg/day) or colistin (15 mg/kg/day).
      (3) ***Campylobacter*.** Erythromycin therapy has been suggested (see Chapter 13).
   c. **Isolation. The affected infant should be isolated immediately to prevent nosocomial spread.** Infection control methods such as isolation, the placing of infants in cohorts, and enforced gowning and handwashing for all caregivers are paramount in the management of enteric infections in the nursery.

**B. Necrotizing enterocolitis (NEC)** [51–54] is an often severe GI disturbance of unknown primary etiology accompanied by systemic illness, and often associated with sepsis and peritonitis. Most cases (62%–94%) occur in premature infants, though it can occur in full-term infants. Age at onset is inversely proportional to gestational age. NEC occurs both sporadically and as a nursery epidemic. It has an incidence of about 10% (range 3%–22%) of all premature infants, and the mortality rate may reach 20% to 40%. Mortality is highest among infants with lower birth weights and lower gestational age, and in earlier case series. Blood cultures are positive in up to 50% of cases. The organisms found in the blood are similar to the enteric flora seen in peritoneal fluid, with *E. coli, Klebsiella,* and *Enterobacter* species predominating.

1. **Diagnosis**
   a. **Presenting systemic signs** include temperature instability, apnea, lethargy, glucose instability, DIC, and acidosis. Common GI signs include abdominal distention, feeding intolerance, increased gastric residuals, vomiting, diarrhea, and blood (occult or gross) in the stools. Physical signs in advanced disease include peritonitis and crepitance or cellulitis of the abdominal wall. Onset is generally sudden in full-term infants but can be sudden or insidious (over 1–2 days) in preterm infants.
   b. **Roentgenographic evaluation** may show ileus, bowel distention, pneumatosis intestinalis, portal vein gas, or free peritoneal gas.
   c. **Laboratory tests** are nonspecific. Thrombocytopenia and neutropenia often occur, and frank DIC may develop. The stool may exhibit reducing substances, occult blood, or gross blood. Acidosis is usually metabolic or mixed. Blood cultures may be positive up to 50% of the time.
2. **Medical therapy** should be instituted as soon as this diagnosis is suspected.
   a. **Fluids and nutrition.** Enteral feedings are immediately stopped and nasogastric suction begun. Because oral feedings must be discontinued for at least 2 weeks, intravenous alimentation by the central or peripheral route should be started as soon as the baby is stable. Infants with NEC generally require increased fluids and sodium, and a urine output of ≥1 to 2 mL/kg/h should be maintained.
   b. **Antibiotics.** Parenteral ampicillin (or vancomycin) and an aminoglycoside (or broad-spectrum cephalosporin) should be started. Some neonatologists advocate the addition of parenteral clindamycin or metronidazole, particularly if perforation is suspected, but there is no evidence that these antibiotics improve outcome [54,55] and there is some concern that routine use of clindamycin may increase the risk of strictures. Antibiotics should generally continue for *at least* 10 to 14 days, longer if surgery is required or clinical response is slow.
   c. **Transfusion** may be necessary for volume repletion, and some clinicians advocate the use of fresh frozen plasma.
   d. **Serial radiographs.** Repeat lateral and supine radiographic views of the abdomen should be obtained every 8 hours to detect advancement or perforation.
   e. **Surgical intervention** is indicated for clinical or radiographic evidence of perforation, cellulitis of the anterior abdominal wall, or clinical deterioration despite optimal medical management.

**V. Genitourinary (GU) infections.** Urinary tract infections are not uncommon in the newborn; in this period, they are more common in boys than in girls. Rates for bacteriuria range from 1% in full-term infants to 3% in premature infants. The most common causative organisms are *E. coli, Klebsiella* species, and, less commonly, enterococci [55,56].

**A. Clinical presentation.** Failure to gain weight, vomiting, fever, and jaundice are the most common symptoms. Local symptoms are rare; occasionally, a poor urinary stream in boys may draw attention to the GU tract. Bacteriuria may be the first sign of sepsis.

**B. Diagnosis.** Examination of clean-catch urines can be confused by the presence of WBCs from circumcision or vaginal discharge. Most clinicians accept that clean catch urine with 20 to 25 WBCs/mm$^3$ or more in the first week and 10 to 25 WBCs/mm$^3$ or more in the second week is abnormal. A suprapubic bladder tap or bladder catheterization provides uncontaminated urine for urinalysis, Gram staining, and culture. The presence of any bacterial growth in a bladder tap or at least 1,000 colonies/mL in a catheterized specimen may be significant and is an indication for blood cultures and the initiation of therapy.

**C. Initial treatment** should be guided by findings on Gram stain and usually consists of ampicillin and an aminoglycoside. Urine should be sterile 48 hours after initiation of therapy, and specific treatment should be continued for 10 to 14 days.

**D. Further investigation.** After control of the infection, **renal ultrasonography** and **voiding cystourethrography** are mandatory, because GU malformations are found in 5% to 10% of these patients. **Follow-up urine cultures** after completion of therapy are important because reinfection is frequent. Daily antibiotic prophylaxis (usually with amoxicillin for the first 6 to 8 weeks of life and either cotrimoxazole or nitrofurantoin thereafter) is indicated for vesicoureteral reflux and many genitourinary anomalies (see Chapter 15).

**VI. Musculoskeletal infections**

**A. Neonatal osteomyelitis** is rare but important because of its morbidity [57]. See also Chapter 5.

1. **Pathogenesis.** Pathogens gain access to the bone through bacteremia, direct inoculation (e.g., monitoring electrodes or venipuncture), or spread from adjacent infection. Because the fetal vascular connections extend from the metaphysis through the epiphyseal plate into the epiphysis and persist until 18 months of age, epiphysitis (with permanent damage of the growth plate) and secondary arthritis can result. The femur, humerus, tibia, and radius are the most commonly affected bones. Ninety percent of neonatal osteomyelitis is due to *S. aureus,* streptococci, *H. influenzae,* and pneumococci. Coliforms are rare causative agents.
2. **Clinical presentation.** Affected infants often appear well, are afebrile, and may manifest only guarding of the affected area with decreased spontaneous movement, local swelling, and tenderness. Other babies may exhibit septicemic symptoms that overshadow the local findings.
3. **Diagnosis**
   a. **X-ray findings** are very useful. Because of the rapid remodeling of bone in infants, changes may be evident within 7 days. **Bone scans** may be positive within days of onset of symptoms.
   b. **Needle aspiration** of the involved bone and secondarily infected joint space will provide material for Gram staining and culture.
4. **Therapy.** If gram-positive organisms are seen, a parenteral penicillinase-resistant penicillin should be given. If gram-negative organisms are seen, ampicillin and an aminoglycoside should be adequate. If no organisms are seen, a penicillinase-resistant penicillin and an aminoglycoside should be used. Drainage may be required if there is localization of pus. Specific parenteral therapy should continue for at least 3 weeks. If available, infectious disease and orthopedic consultations should be obtained.

**B. Septic arthritis.** A primary infectious arthritis without involvement of nearby bone may be secondary to a bacteremia or to direct inoculation (as by femoral venipuncture). *S. aureus,* gram-negative organisms (*E. coli, Pseudomonas* species, *Haemophilus* species, gonococci), and *Streptococcus* species account for most cases [58]. This presents in a manner identical to osteomyelitis in the newborn. The affected joint should be aspirated. The initial therapy and duration of therapy are similar to those suggested for osteomyelitis. Drainage and immobilization of the joint are important elements of treatment.

**VII. Skin infections.** The neonate is particularly susceptible to local skin infections because of the presence of one or two wounds (umbilical cord and circumcision), the immaturity of the stratum corneum, and the initial absence of the normal dermal bacterial flora. Only some local infections will be discussed here.

**A. Superficial pustular rashes** are usually due to streptococci or staphylococci and can be treated topically with hexachlorophene or an antibiotic ointment. Widespread or invasive lesions should be Gram-stained and cultured and treatment started with parenteral antibiotics to prevent septicemia. Cellulitis, erysipelas, folliculitis, and impetigo should all be treated with a parenteral penicillinase-resistant penicillin while awaiting cultures.

**B. Staphylococcal scalded skin syndrome** may appear in any one of its manifestations, either sporadically or as a nursery outbreak [59]. Staphylococci in phage group II that produce an exotoxin (exfoliatin) may cause (a) bullous impetigo, (b) Ritter disease in infants, (c) Lyell disease or toxic epidermal necrolysis in older children, or (d) a scarlatiniform rash (staphylococcal scarlet fever).

1. **Clinical presentation.** Initially, the rash is erythematous, and at times tender, and it often has a sandpaper texture. Skin creases may have increased erythema (Pastia lines). Within 2 days, the epidermis peels off at sites of minor trauma (Nikolsky sign), and large, flaccid bullae appear, which also may exfoliate. The areas of exfoliation dry out, and seborrhea-like flakes appear. These flakes often are found around the mouth and desquamate over 3 to 5 days, leaving normal skin underneath. During the exfoliative stage of the disease, infants are febrile, irritable, and uncomfortable, but usually not severely ill. Children with the scarlatiniform rash syndrome do not develop a strawberry tongue and do not exfoliate.
2. **Diagnosis** is made based on the clinical findings, because the toxicogenic staphylococci may not be recovered from the local lesion.
3. **Therapy.** All forms of this disease should be treated with a parenteral penicillinase-resistant penicillin. Fluid therapy may be necessary because of the increased insensible fluid loss through the damaged skin.

C. **Omphalitis** occurs when pathogenic bacteria predominate in the normally necrotic **umbilical stump.** It is manifested by oozing and purulent discharge from the stump and by local periumbilical inflammation and erythema. The most common causative organisms are staphylococci, *Streptococcus* species, and coliforms. Gram staining and culture should be performed. Because omphalitis can serve as the source of an ascending phlebitis (funisitis) leading to peritonitis or septicemia, it should be vigorously treated with local care and parenteral antibiotics, initially a penicillinase-resistant penicillin and either an aminoglycoside or cefotaxime.

D. **Circumcision wound infections** are caused by the same organisms that cause omphalitis and are treated similarly.

E. **Neonatal breast abscess** occurs in full-term infants. It is usually unilateral and occurs more often in girls. *S. aureus* is the most common pathogen, although streptococci and coliforms also have been described. Early in the course of infection, fluid should be expressed from the iodine-cleansed nipple for Gram staining and culture. In early infection, parenteral antibiotics probably will suffice for cure. Incision and drainage may be required in advanced cases. In either situation, treatment should begin with penicillinase-resistant penicillin and an aminoglycoside and should continue for 10 days with the appropriate drug (Table 3.2).

VIII. **Hepatitis B virus** (HBV) has a unique natural history in newborns, who have difficulty clearing the infection; infants have a high probability of becoming chronic carriers of the virus. Chronic carriers of HBV have an estimated 25% risk of developing cirrhosis or hepatocellular carcinoma. (See Chapter 14.) **Since 1991, universal immunization of infants with HBV vaccine has been recommended as the best approach to eliminating transmission of HBV** [60]. We will discuss the specific recommendations for prevention of perinatal transmission. (See further discussion of HBV vaccine in Chapter 23.)

A. **Infants acquire HBV from their mothers.** The probability of infection of the infant is increased if the maternal HBV infection is symptomatic or occurs late in pregnancy. Mothers who are positive for hepatitis surface or e antigen (HBsAg or HBeAg) transmit the virus to 80% of their infants. Most of these infants do not have symptomatic disease, but **90% become chronic HBV carriers, and up to 25% die of chronic liver disease in adulthood** [60].

B. **Passive protection with either HBV immunoglobulin (HBIG) or immunization with HBV vaccine** is approximately 70% effective in preventing chronic infection in the newborn. Passive and active immunization used together is 90% effective. **Current recommendations** [61] are that all infants born to HBsAg-positive mothers, regardless of the mother's HBeAg or anti-HBe status, should receive both **HBIG** (0.5 mL intramuscularly [i.m.]) and **HBV vaccine** (0.5 mL i.m. at a separate site) within 12 hours of birth, and additional vaccine doses at 1 month and 6 months of age (see Chapter 23). Immunized infants should be tested for HBsAg and anti-HBs 1 to 3 months after the final (third) vaccine dose.

C. **All pregnant women,** particularly those at increased risk, **should be routinely tested for HBsAg during an early prenatal visit in each pregnancy.** If screening has not been done during pregnancy or the results are not available, an HBsAg test should be administered at the time of admission or soon afterward. **Infants of mothers with pending tests or of mothers who did not receive prenatal care should receive HBIG and HBV vaccine** within 12 hours of birth in the dosage appropriate for infants born to HBsAg-positive mothers (5 $\mu$g Recombivax HB or 10 $\mu$g Engerix-B). In full-term infants, HBIG (but not HBV vaccine) can be safely postponed up to 7 days if maternal HBsAg results are expected by that time. The HBV vaccine dose given immediately after birth to preterm infants weighing less than 2 kg (because of positive or unknown maternal HBsAg status) should not be counted in the required three-dose schedule; three subsequent doses are still required.

D. **Infants should be managed with hepatitis precautions in the nursery.** There is no contraindication to breast-feeding.

IX. **Hepatitis C virus** (HCV) is the major cause of non-A non-B hepatitis. Mothers infected with HCV transmit the virus to their infants at an average rate of 5% to 6% (range 0%–25%). Higher maternal titers of HCV RNA have been associated with increased risk of transmission, but no threshold titer has been clearly established. Maternal infection with HCV and HIV increases the risk of transmission to 14% (5%–36%) and 17%, respectively. Although transmission is thought to occur intrapartum, vaginal and cesarean deliveries have similar transmission rates. Breast-feeding is not contraindicated because it does not appear to increase the risk of transmission [62,63]. Diagnosis of HCV infection of the infant rests on persistence of anti-HCV antibody beyond 12 months of age; however, if earlier diagnosis is needed (e.g., symptomatic infant), HCV-RNA detection in blood can be performed after 1 to 2 months of age. The natural history of perinatal HCV infection is unknown. Treatment with recombinant $\alpha$-interferon or ribavirin has not been evaluated in infancy [64]. (See Chapter 14.)

X. **Enteroviruses,** specifically **coxsackievirus,** have been implicated in neonatal disease [65]. They probably infect the neonate in the peripartum or postpartum period. Echoviruses and coxsackie B serotypes have caused nursery outbreaks during community epidemics. Most enteroviruses are capable of causing meningoencephalitis or GI disease. They can cause an undifferentiated febrile illness that leads to the consideration of sepsis in neonates. Coxsackie B serotypes have caused a serious disease consisting of encephalitis, myocarditis, and hepatitis, whereas echoviruses are associated with a hepatitis-sepsis syndrome.

**Diagnosis** is by culture or polymerase chain reaction (PCR) (of stool, urine, nasopharyngeal aspirate, CSF) or serologic evaluation, and treatment is supportive. Pleconaril is a promising orally active agent with limited safety and efficacy data for treatment of severe enteroviral illness in neonates and other age groups [66]. At this writing, the drug has not been licensed but may be obtained on a compassionate care basis from the manufacturer Viropharma (Exton, PA, 610-217-7541, *questions@viropharma.com*). A placebo-controlled trial of neonatal enterovirus sepsis is underway by the Collaborative Antiviral Study Group of the NIH. **Infants in the nursery with suspected coxsackievirus disease should be isolated** to prevent spread of this devastating infection.

XI. **Varicella** is a rare infection in the neonate but is discussed here because of the availability of therapy [67]. Infection of the fetus early in pregnancy is associated with a congenital syndrome in 2.3% of neonates, consisting of cutaneous scars, limb hypoplasia and paralysis, encephalitis, and chorioretinitis [68]. **The outcome of perinatal varicella depends on the time of exposure of the infant.** If maternal disease occurs more than 5 days before delivery, there is little or no risk of dissemination or sequelae. If maternal disease occurs within 5 days before or 2 days after delivery, approximately half the newborns will develop varicella with a risk of severe disseminated varicella and a 30% mortality rate.

**Infants in the high-risk group should receive zoster immune globulin (125 units, 1.25 mL i.m.)** as soon as possible after delivery [61]. If clinical varicella develops, **acyclovir** should be used. An infectious disease consultation is advised.

Infants born to mothers with varicella should be isolated in the nursery. Infants cannot receive the varicella vaccine.

**XII. *Candida* species** are the most common cause of fungal infection seen in newborns. True congenital candidiasis may be either local cutaneous or systemic disease, and differs from neonatal systemic candidiasis by age at onset and organ involvement. Neonatal systemic candidiasis usually involves multiple organs (rarely is skin involved) and can be divided into two forms: catheter-associated sepsis and disseminated candidiasis. Premature infants and infants with hyperalimentation catheters or with prolonged exposure to broad-spectrum antibiotics are at highest risk of disease [69,70].

**A. Diagnosis** is made by recovery of *Candida* from blood, CSF, or joint, pleural, or other normally sterile fluid. Antigen and antibody detection techniques have not been useful.

**B. Therapy.** Most authorities recommend removal of vascular catheters and administration of amphotericin B in doses of 0.5 to 1.0 mg/kg intravenously once daily over a period of 4 to 6 hours. Flucytosine (5-FC) may provide additional therapeutic benefit in selected fungal infections (100–150 mg/kg/day in three to five divided doses orally). Conclusive clinical data are available only for the use of 5-FC in *Cryptococcus neoformans* meningitis. The duration of antifungal therapy remains controversial. In disseminated infection, a total dose of 25 to 30 mg/kg of amphotericin B has been recommended. Some authorities suggest limiting the maximum maintenance dose of amphotericin B to 0.5 mg/kg/day in very-low-birth-weight (<1,500 g) infants [70,71]. Both drugs are nephrotoxic and hepatotoxic; appropriate monitoring of organ function and antifungal blood levels are recommended, as is an infectious disease consultation. (See Chapters 2 and 17.) For a review of antifungal agents in neonatal systemic candidiasis, see van den Anker et al. [72]. There is increasing experience with fluconazole in neonates, particularly for treatment of urinary candidiasis without evidence of disseminated disease.

## DISSEMINATED INTRAUTERINE INFECTIONS

The syndrome of disseminated intrauterine infection is caused by diverse organisms that generally result in distinguishable clinical conditions with overlapping features. These infections have been given the acronym TORCH (toxoplasmosis, other, rubella, cytomegalovirus, herpes), which has led to the false perception that they are clinically identical and uniformly diagnosed by serology, commonly referred to as TORCH titers. These titers usually refer to measurement of organism-specific IgG; however, an infant's IgG is maternal in origin. IgM assays for these congenital infections do not have a high enough sensitivity or specificity to make them useful single diagnostic tests. Therefore, **a single TORCH titer is not a complete laboratory evaluation.** A comprehensive evaluation for suspected perinatal infection includes consideration of epidemiologic factors, maternal history, physical examination, and laboratory and radiographic findings [73]. The laboratory investigation must be undertaken in a logical, reasoned, and timely manner. Every attempt should be made to establish a definitive diagnosis because prognosis and treatment vary by disease; however, a firm diagnosis cannot always be made immediately. Careful clinical and serologic follow-up for 6 to 15 months may be necessary before an infection can be excluded or implicated.

Intrauterine infections may present with a variety of manifestations or no clinical findings at all. **Some signs that should lead to consideration of an intrauterine infection are listed in Table 3.8.** These signs are not unique to congenital infections; therefore, other diagnostic possibilities also must be explored (e.g., cardiac disease, inherited metabolic defects, immunologic disease). **In many situations, infants with congenital infections share the following characteristics:** (a) inapparent or mild disease in the mother, (b) a wide range of severity of infection in the fetus, (c) overlapping clinical features, and (d) variability of long-term sequelae. When a congenital infection is suspected, evaluations usually include (but are not limited to) placental pathology, plotting growth parameters, cranial imaging, ophthalmologic examination, liver function tests, and CBC.

**Infectious agents that may cause congenital infections** (disseminated or localized, intrauterine or peripartum) **include but are not limited to** toxoplasmosis, syphilis, rubella, CMV, enterovirus, parvovirus B19, HIV, herpes simplex virus, varicella-zoster

Table 3.8. Common Clinical Features Associated with Intrauterine Infection in Neonates

| | |
|---|---|
| Growth retardation | Myocarditis |
| Hepatosplenomegaly | Cardiac abnormalities |
| Jaundice | Chorioretinitis |
| Hemolytic anemia | Keratoconjunctivitis |
| Petechiae, ecchymoses | Cataracts |
| Microcephaly, hydrocephalus | Glaucoma |
| Intracranial calcification | Nonimmune hydrops |
| Pneumonitis | Bone abnormalities |

virus, HBV, and HCV. A brief summary of the common causes of disseminated intrauterine infections follows. For an in-depth discussion, refer to the textbook of Remington and Klein [4].

**I. *Toxoplasma gondii*** is a protozoan that may infect the fetus by transplacental passage during maternal parasitemia. Approximately 50% of infants whose mothers seroconvert during pregnancy are infected, although only 10% of these infants have clinical manifestations. Acute maternal infection early in pregnancy is less likely to cause fetal infection but more likely to cause symptomatic disease in infected fetuses; maternal infections late in pregnancy result in infection in most fetuses, but the vast majority of cases are subclinical. The estimated frequency of clinically evident infection in the United States is 1 to 4 per 1,000 live births [4].

**A. Clinical presentation.** The affected newborn exhibits chorioretinitis, CSF pleocytosis and elevated protein, microcephaly, and cerebral calcifications. Petechiae, hepatosplenomegaly, jaundice, a maculopapular rash, and interstitial pneumonitis have been described in these infants.

**B. Diagnosis is made** using the following methods:

1. Rising toxoplasma-specific IgG titers over the first 4 to 6 months of life
2. IgM assays (double-sandwich technique, state or reference laboratory)
3. Direct demonstration of tachyzoites in placenta or infant tissue
4. Culture of toxoplasma from infant blood, cord blood, placenta, CSF, amniotic fluid
5. PCR of fetal blood, amniotic fluid, neonatal blood, and CSF under study

**C. Therapy for 1 year** should include a combination of pyrimethamine (2 mg/kg/day for 2 days with maximum of 25 mg/day, then 1 mg/kg/day for 2 to 6 months, then 1 mg/kg/day Monday, Wednesday, and Friday to finish the year of total therapy) and sulfadiazine (50 mg/kg/dose twice daily), with folinic acid (10 mg three times weekly) to prevent bone marrow toxicity. Enrollment in the National Collaborative Treatment Trial is encouraged (phone 773-834-4152). CBC and platelet counts should be monitored twice weekly. Corticosteroids (prednisone 1–2 mg/kg/day) may be added for patients with active macular chorioretinitis or a CSF protein level of greater than1 g/dL. Infectious disease consultation is recommended.

**II. Rubella.** Congenital rubella is still a problem [74]. Fetal rubella infection may result in teratogenesis or abortion if it occurs in the first 2 months of gestation. Infection after the first trimester is associated with disseminated disease.

**A. Clinical presentation.** The majority (up to 68%) of neonatal infections are subclinical. The classic presentation is of a small, full-term, "blueberry muffin" baby with thrombocytopenic purpura, cataracts, cardiac lesions, and hepatosplenomegaly. Pneumonitis, metaphyseal radiolucencies, and CNS involvement, with bulging fontanelles, are also seen. Hearing defects and mental retardation may become apparent only later in childhood.

**B. Diagnosis** is made by any one of these tests:

1. High or rising complement fixation or hemagglutination inhibition titers (IgG)
2. Elevated specific IgM
3. Viral culture from respiratory secretions or urine (notify laboratory that rubella is suspected)

C. **Therapy is symptomatic. Infected neonates may excrete the virus for months, and they should be placed in strict isolation.**

III. **Cytomegalovirus** is the most common virus of neonates [75], and may be acquired transplacentally, peripartum, or postnatally. Of pregnant women, 4% have cytomegaloviruria, and 10% to 15% have positive cervical cultures. It is likely that infants infected early *in utero* are affected more than those who acquire the agent later. Cytomegaloviruria has been demonstrated in 1% of neonates (range 0.2%–2.0%); most of these acquired the organism transplacentally. Maternal antibody does not prevent infection of the fetus, but it does ameliorate severity. Infants of mothers with primary CMV infection who presumably did not have passive antibody were more likely to have symptomatic infection and sequelae [76].

A. **Clinical presentation.** It is estimated that 95% of all babies with intrauterine CMV infection are asymptomatic. Symptomatic disseminated intrauterine disease is characterized by: (a) intrauterine growth retardation, (b) hepatosplenomegaly, (c) jaundice, (d) petechiae, and (e) pulmonary involvement. Of 106 symptomatic cases, 70% had hepatosplenomegaly, petechiae, and jaundice, and 53% had microcephaly at birth [77].

B. **Diagnosis** of CMV intrauterine disease is made using any of these tests:

1. Viral culture from urine or throat in the first 2 weeks of life
2. Persistently high complement fixation titers (IgG)
3. Persistently high IgM fluorescent antibody assay

C. **Therapy** is largely symptomatic. A trial of ganciclovir for symptomatic and asymptomatic neonatal disease is underway by the Collaborative Antiviral Study Group of the NIH. Careful hand-washing and secretion precautions are advised.

D. **Prognosis.** Mortality is 12% in those with disseminated disease [77]. Survivors may develop chorioretinitis, periventricular cerebral calcifications, and deafness. **The cytomegaloviruria may continue intermittently for years.**

IV. **Herpes simplex virus** (HSV) usually is acquired peripartum but may be transmitted transplacentally as well. Both HSV types 1 and 2 cause disease in neonates.

A. **Clinical manifestations. One should suspect this diagnosis when caring for a septic neonate** [78]. Three syndromes are recognized: skin, eyes, and mouth (SEM), CNS, and disseminated disease. However, not all exposed infants are infected. Rates of infection in newborns are 30% to 50% following exposure to primary maternal disease and 3% to 5% following recurrent maternal disease. Although there are many more women with recurrent disease than primary disease, the higher attack rate for the latter results in 50% of the neonatal cases. **Neonatal HSV disease cannot be ruled out on the basis of maternal history** [79,80].

1. **Disseminated infections.** These infants may have jaundice, hepatomegaly, pneumonitis, bleeding diathesis, and CNS manifestations. Only half develop the typical vesicular rash. Mortality is 80%, and most survivors have sequelae.
2. **Local disease** implies involvement of only one organ system: CNS, or skin, eyes, or mouth.

B. **Diagnosis** may be made by using one of the following tests:

1. Viral culture of skin, rectum, throat, nasopharynx, conjunctiva, urine, stool, and CSF (CSF PCR also available)
2. Cytologic evaluation of skin lesion (multinucleate giant cells on Tzanck smear)
3. Rising complement fixation titers
4. Elevated specific IgM titers

C. **Treatment** of all forms of HSV infection or suspected HSV infection with **acyclovir** (20 mg/kg/dose i.v. every 8 hours for 10–21 days) should be started as soon as viral cultures have been obtained [81,82]. The use of suppressive oral acyclovir therapy following intravenous therapy for disease in a neonate is controversial. Advice should be sought from a Pediatric Infectious Disease consultant. The evaluation and management of a well infant born to a mother with active herpetic lesions is also controversial (see section **D**).

D. **Prevention.** When the mother has documented active genital HSV infection, cesarean section has reduced neonatal acquisition rates from 50% to 6% in some studies. Evaluation and management of an exposed infant is controversial. Some experts recommend the use of routine surface (conjunctiva, nasopharynx, umbilicus, rectum) cultures obtained after 48 hours of life, and if positive, should lead to a full workup and consideration of therapy. Close follow-up by a physician and immediate evaluation of the infant for any signs of illness are the cornerstones of management. (See Chapter 16.)

**V. Syphilis. The number of cases of congenital syphilis has increased steadily since the 1980's, in parallel with adult primary cases,** so clinicians must again be alert for this important intrauterine infection, which has devastating sequelae if untreated. The treponema usually is acquired transplacentally, although intrapartum acquisition is possible. A mother with untreated primary or secondary syphilis is unlikely to have any normal children; half will be premature or suffer perinatal death, and the remainder will have congenital syphilis [83]. The rates of these outcomes decrease with maternal infection in late gestation to 10% perinatal death and 10% congenital syphilis.

**A. Clinical presentation.** Approximately 50% of infected newborns are initially asymptomatic. Infants with congenital infection may demonstrate a vesicular or bullous rash that includes the palms and soles; they may have chronic rhinitis (snuffles), maculopapular rash, abnormal CSF, pneumonitis, myocarditis, nephrosis, pseudoparalysis, nonimmune hydrops, condylomata lata, hepatosplenomegaly, and generalized lymphadenopathy. These manifestations may not be apparent at birth but may develop during the first few weeks of life [84,85].

**Bony lesions** appear roentgenographically at 1 to 3 months and are characteristic: symmetric metaphyseal involvement with elevation of the periosteum, and osteomyelitic lesions, most often involving the humerus and tibia. These bone changes are said to occur in 90% of infants who manifest congenital syphilis [86]. Osteochondritis and periostitis may be painful and manifested by the pseudoparalysis of a limb due to pain (pseudoparalysis of Parrot).

**B. Diagnosis may be problematic.** Therefore, appropriate treatment often is administered without a definitive diagnosis. **Because the risks of therapy with penicillin are minimal and the sequelae of untreated syphilis can be permanent, treatment is advised in doubtful cases.** Infants born to mothers with no prenatal care should be tested by VDRL or a similar serologic screening test for syphilis.

1. **Diagnosis depends on the following:**
   a. Identification of the spirochete in any of the skin lesions or in the nasal discharge by **dark-field examination,** or
   b. **Serologic evaluation** (see Chapter 16). Serum from the mother or infant is preferred over cord blood specimens for serology, because of false-positive and false-negative rates in the latter [87]. Infected infants are often asymptomatic at birth and, if maternal or infant infection occurred late in pregnancy, infected infants also may be seronegative. The RPR or VDRL test usually is used for screening, and the fluorescent treponemal antibody absorption (FTA-ABS) test is used for confirmation. Maternal antibody is transmitted to the infant, and these tests measure both IgG and IgM.
2. **All newborns suspected of having congenital syphilis on the basis of maternal history, maternal serology, or physical findings should be fully evaluated by** (a) careful examination for clinical signs of syphilis; (b) serology, including IgM if available; (c) radiologic survey of long bones; and (d) a lumbar puncture to collect CSF for cell count, protein, a dark-field examination, and a Venereal Disease Research Laboratory (VDRL) test (not a rapid plasma reagin [RPR] test). If available, the placenta should be examined for focal villitis and spirochetes.

**C. Therapy.** Recommendations account for reports of **failure of benzathine penicillin.** Initiation of therapy is based on maternal and infant serology, clinical findings, and history of maternal treatment. The mother's data are assessed first. If a serologically positive mother did not receive adequate therapy or received nonpenicillin therapy, or if adequate follow-up is not assured, her infant should be treated with penicillin at birth [85].

**Infants with proven or probable disease should receive 10 to 14 days of aqueous crystalline penicillin G.** Current Centers for Disease Control and American Academy of Pediatrics recommendations are for 10 to 14 days of intravenous therapy with crystalline penicillin G 50,000 units/kg/dose every 12 hours for the first week and every 8 hours after the seventh day [61,85]. Some authorities suggest procaine penicillin (50,000 units/kg/day i.m. in one dose) for 10 to 14 days. A few infants will manifest a Herxheimer reaction, with a fever spike 6 to 8 hours after the first penicillin dose. (See Chapter 16.)

Management of **asymptomatic infants** with normal CSF and normal long-bone radiographs is also determined by the adequacy of maternal therapy. Only if the mother received documented adequate penicillin therapy more than 1 month before delivery, and follow-up of the infant is ensured, can observation without therapy be contemplated. For all other situations (likely the majority), **10 to 14 days of intravenous aqueous crystalline penicillin is recommended.**

**D. Follow-up.** Treated infants should be seen at 3 months, and then at 6-month intervals for repeat serologic evaluation, CSF examinations (if initial CSF results are abnormal), and clinical reevaluation, until it is clear that RPR or VDRL titers are falling. Untreated or benzathine-treated infants should be seen at 1, 2, 4, 6, and 12 months. The RPR or VDRL titers should decrease by 3 months of age, and FTA-ABS titers should decrease by 6 months. If antibody titers remain stable or increase, reevaluation and therapy are mandatory.

**VI. Human parvovirus B19,** the etiologic agent of erythema infectiosum, has been associated with adverse fetal outcome following maternal infection. Case reports include spontaneous abortions, hydrops fetalis, and stillbirths, as well as normal infants. Data are not yet adequate to determine fully the risk for fetal morbidity and death following acute maternal infection with parvovirus B19. Available studies suggest that the risk of fetal death following acute maternal infection in the first 20 weeks of gestation is 3% to 9%, whereas the risk following household exposure of a woman with unknown serologic status is approximately 1% to 2% [87].

**A. Clinical presentation.** The principal adverse fetal outcome has been nonimmune hydrops with severe ascites and pericardial and pleural effusions, which result from severe anemia caused by direct infection and destruction of reticulocytes by parvovirus B19 (aplastic crisis) [73,88–90].

**B. Diagnosis** may be made by using any of the following tests:

**1.** Specific IgM determination in cord or neonatal blood

**2.** PCR for viral DNA

**3.** Persistent infant B19 IgG at 12 months of age and IgM; although these are not readily available

Until such tests and further data are available, the findings of elevated maternal α-fetoprotein levels, hydrops fetalis, and fetal aplastic crisis may be the best indicators of B19 infection.

**C. Therapy.** No specific therapy is available.

**VII. HIV** can be transmitted from mothers to infants *in utero*, intrapartum, or postpartum through breast milk. The reader is referred to the website ***www.hivatis.org*** [91] for continually updated guidelines for prevention of perinatal transmission and management of exposed and infected infants. The risk for **perinatal transmission** varies according to patient population and geographic location; in North America this is in the range of 20% to 25% for untreated patients, but only 1% to 2% when infected women receive prophylaxis. Issues of concern in the neonatal period center around early diagnosis of HIV infection, evaluation for *Pneumocystis carinii* prophylaxis, and management of associated conditions such as low birth weight, drug withdrawal, congenital syphilis, or hepatitis.

**A. Prevention [91]. All pregnant women should be offered HIV testing regardless of identifiable risk factors;** HIV testing should be sought for newborns whose mothers were not tested during the pregnancy. A placebo-controlled trial of zidovudine (ZDV; formerly azidothymidine [AZT]), in pregnant women and their newborn infants demonstrated a significantly reduced transmission rate compared with placebo (8% vs. 25%). In an African study, combined ZDV and 3TC given intrapartum and to the newborn for 1 week resulted in 10% transmission compared with 17% with placebo. A single maternal dose of nevirapine (NVP) during labor combined with a single postnatal dose reduced transmission from 21% to 12% compared with ZDV (abbreviated course) in an African study. In a developed countries study, addition of NVP to ZDV did not reduce the transmission rate below the already low rate of 2% with ZDV alone. Thus, it is recommended that the ZDV regimen (antepartum from second trimester, intrapartum, and 6 weeks in newborn) be offered to all mother-infant pairs; addition of 3TC or NVP should be considered for women presenting in labor without prior HIV treatment/diagnosis. ZDV combined with other antiretrovirals should be offered to pregnant women with high viral loads or an immunologic, virologic, or clinical indication for antiretroviral treatment. The use of resistance testing should follow standard practice, and may help guide the choice of antiretroviral drugs in these scenarios.

Higher viral loads are associated with increased risk of transmission, although transmission has been documented despite low viral loads (<1,000 HIV copies/mL). Elective cesarean section (prior to onset of labor or membrane rupture) has been shown to decrease transmission for women not receiving antiretroviral therapy or with a viral load of greater than 1,000 copies/mL. (See related discussion in Chapter 19.)

**B. Clinical presentation.** No recognizable dysmorphic syndrome has been associated with HIV infection. **Most perinatally infected infants are asymptomatic at birth.** A small number of infants may develop symptoms within the first few days or weeks of life, including PCP, active CMV disease, or acute bacterial infections. There appear to be two distinct patterns of natural history among perinatally infected children. One group develops symptoms within the first year of life, whereas the other group remains asymptomatic for 3 to 5 years or more. Ongoing studies are attempting to delineate the factors responsible for this variation in disease progression. Symptoms most commonly include oral candidiasis, failure to thrive, developmental delay, loss of developmental milestones, lymphadenopathy, recurrent or severe bacterial infections, pneumonia (PCP), lymphocytic interstitial pneumonitis, chronic or recurrent diarrhea, and hepatosplenomegaly [92].

**C. Diagnosis. The reader is referred to *hivatis.org* [90].** Because infants acquire maternal IgG transplacentally, routine HIV testing with IgG antibody-based assays (enzyme-linked immunosorbent assay, Western blot) are not diagnostically useful. It is, however, **important to establish the diagnosis by other means as early as possible for preventive, therapeutic, and prognostic reasons.** Evaluation should include HIV DNA PCR (or HIV culture) and T-cell subsets prior to discharge (<48 hours of age), at 1 to 2 months of age, and 3 to 6 months of age. A positive PCR result or abnormal T-cell subsets or clinical concern for HIV infection require prompt and thorough reevaluation for HIV infection and of immunologic status in consultation with an HIV specialist. It is currently recommended that all infected infants be offered combination antiretroviral treatment. **A referral to a local or regional pediatric HIV specialist is advised.**

**D. Therapy.** Infants should generally receive ZDV 2 mg/kg/dose orally every 6 hours (every 12 hours if preterm with change to every 8 hours at 2 to 4 weeks depending on degree of prematurity) for the first 6 weeks. At 6 weeks, all exposed infants should receive PCP prophylaxis with cotrimoxazole until HIV infection is absolutely excluded. It is currently recommended that all infected infants be offered combination antiretroviral treatment in consultation with a pediatric HIV specialist.

**E. Routine care.** Careful attention to growth and development is essential. HIV-exposed infants should not receive oral polio vaccine (not in routine use for normal infants in the United States). CBC with T-cell subsets should be followed. Any suspicious clinical or laboratory findings merit careful and close follow-up.

**VIII. Other infectious agents** should be considered when evaluating an infant with a suspected intrauterine infection. These include tuberculosis [93], *L. monocytogenes, Leptospirosis,* hepatitis B, enteroviruses, adenoviruses, varicella-zoster virus and Epstein-Barr virus. Infants with these infections have demonstrated findings included in Table 3.8. As more is learned about the pathogenesis of old and new microbial agents, identification of other agents active in intrauterine infection will undoubtedly continue.

Although much is known about neonatal infections, controlled trials of therapy are limited in number [94]. As a consequence, many recommendations are expert opinions based on limited data. Therefore, close individualized care should be afforded all ill neonates.

**IX. Infections contraindicating breast-feeding.** Breast-feeding should be discontinued for active maternal tuberculosis, maternal herpetic breast lesions, and maternal HIV infection (in the United States).

## REFERENCES


1. Gladstone IM, Ehrenkranz RA, Edberg SC, et al. A ten-year review of neonatal sepsis and comparison with the previous fifty-year experience. *Pediatr Infect Dis J* 1990;9:819.
2. Schuchat A, Zywicki SS, Dinsmoor MJ, et al. Risk factors and opportunities for prevention of early onset neonatal sepsis: a multicenter case control study. *Pediatrics* 2000;105:21–26.
3. Escobar GJ, Li DK, Armstrong MA, et al. Neonatal sepsis work ups in infants greater than 2000 grams at birth: a population based study. *Pediatrics* 2000;106:256–263.
4. Remington JD, Klein JO. *Infectious disease of the fetus and newborn infant,* 5th ed. Philadelphia: WB Saunders, 2001.
5. Wilson CB. Immunologic basis for increased susceptibility of the neonate to infection. *J Pediatr* 1986;108:1.
6. Robertson A, Fink S, Karp W. Effect of cephalosporins on bilirubin-albumin binding. *J Pediatr* 1988;112:291.
7. Fink S, Warren K, Robertson A. Effect of penicillins on bilirubin-albumin binding. *J Pediatr* 1988;113:566.
8. Martin E, et al. Ceftriaxone-bilirubin-albumin interactions in the neonate: an *in vivo* study. *Eur J Pediatr* 1993;152:530.
9. Spritzer R, Kamp HJVD, Dzoljic G, et al. Five years of cefotaxime use in a neonatal intensive care unit. *Pediatr Infect Dis* 1990;9:92.
10. Jacobs RF. Efficacy and safety of cefotaxime in the management of pediatric infections. *Infection* 1991;19(suppl 6):330.
11. Briggs GG, Freeman RK, Yaffe SJ. *A reference guide to fetal and neonatal risk: drugs in pregnancy and lactation,* 5th ed. Baltimore: Williams & Wilkins, 1998.
12. American Academy of Pediatrics. Committee on Drugs. The transfer of drugs and other chemicals into human milk. *Pediatrics* 2001;108:776.
13. Noya FJD, Baker CJ. Prevention of group B streptococcal infection. *Infect Dis Clin North Am* 1992;6:41.
14. Centers for Disease Control. Revised guidelines for prevention of early-onset group B streptococcal (GBS) infection. *Pediatrics* 1997;99:489–496.
15. Mohle-Boetani JC, et al. Comparison of prevention strategies for neonatal group B streptococcal infection. *JAMA* 1993;270:1442.
16. Yagupsky P, Menegus MA, Powell KR. The changing spectrum of group B streptococcal disease in infants: an eleven-year experience in a tertiary care hospital. *Pediatr Infect Dis J* 1991;10:801.
17. Adams WG, et al. Outbreak of early onset group B streptococcal sepsis. *Pediatr Infect Dis J* 1993;12:565.
18. Gellin BG, Broome CF. Listeriosis. *JAMA* 1989;261:1313.
19. Schwarze R, Bauermeister CD, Ortel S, et al. Perinatal listeriosis in Dresden, 1981–1986: clinical and microbiological findings in 18 cases. *Infection* 1989;17:131.
20. Noel GJ, et al. Anaerobic bacteria in a neonatal intensive care unit: an eighteen-year experience. *Pediatr Infect Dis J* 1988;7:858.
21. Gerdes JS. Clinicopathologic approach to the diagnosis of neonatal sepsis. *Clin Perinatol* 1991;18:361.
22. Polin RA, St. Geme JW III. Neonatal sepsis. *Adv Pediatr Infect Dis* 1992;7:25.
23. Wiswell TE, et al. No lumbar puncture in the evaluation for early neonatal sepsis: will meningitis be missed? *Pediatrics* 1995;95:803.
24. Evans ME, et al. Sensitivity, specificity, and predictive value of body surface cultures in a neonatal intensive care unit. *JAMA* 1988;259:248.

25. Baley JE, et al. Neonatal neutropenia: clinical manifestations, cause, and outcome. *Am J Dis Child* 1988;142:116.
26. Rodwell RL, Taylor KMCD, Tudehope DI, et al. Hematologic scoring system in early diagnosis of sepsis in neutropenic newborns. *Pediatr Infect Dis J* 1993;12:372.
27. Hammerschlag MR, et al. Patterns of use of antibiotics in two newborn nurseries. *N Engl J Med* 1977;296:1268.
28. Bradley JS. Neonatal infections. *Pediatr Infect Dis J* 1985;4:315.
29. Word BM, Klein JO. Current therapy of bacterial sepsis and meningitis in infants and children: a poll of directors of programs in pediatric infectious diseases. *Pediatr Infect Dis J* 1989;7:267.
30. Cairo MS, et al. Randomized trial of granulocyte transfusion versus intravenous immune globulin therapy for neonatal neutropenia and sepsis. *J Pediatr* 1992;120:281.
31. Baker CJ, et al. Intravenous immune globulin for the prevention of nosocomial infection in low birth-weight neonates. *N Engl J Med* 1992;327:213.
32. Fanaroff AA, et al. A controlled trial of intravenous immune globulin to reduce nosocomial infections in very-low-birth-weight infants. *N Engl J Med* 1994;330:1107.
33. Hill HR. Intravenous immunoglobulin use in the neonate: role in prophylaxis and therapy of infection. *Pediatr Infect Dis J* 1993;12:549.
34. Kline MW. *Citrobacter* meningitis and brain abscess in infancy: epidemiology, pathogenesis, and treatment. *J Pediatr* 1988;113:430.
35. McCracken GH Jr, et al. Consensus report: antimicrobial therapy for bacterial meningitis in infants and children. *Pediatr Infect Dis J* 1987;6:501.
36. Klein JO, Feign RD, McCracken GH. Report of the task force on diagnosis and management of meningitis. *Pediatrics* 1986;78:959–979.
37. Plotkin SA, et al. Meningitis in infants and children. *Pediatrics* 1988;81:904.
38. McCracken GH Jr, Mize SG, Threckeld N. Neonatal meningitis cooperative study. Intraventricular gentamicin therapy in gram-negative bacillary meningitis of infancy: report of the Second Neonatal Meningitis Cooperative Study Group. *Lancet* 1980;1:787.
39. Hammerschlag MR. Neonatal conjunctivitis. *Pediatr Ann* 1993;22:346.
40. Burton DM, Seid AB, Kearns DB, Pransky SM. Neonatal otitis media. *Arch Otolaryngol Head Neck Surg* 1993;119:672.
41. Beem MO, Saxon EM. Respiratory tract colonization and a distinctive pneumonia syndrome in infants infected with *Chlamydia trachomatis*. *N Engl J Med* 1977;296:306.
42. Rettig PJ. Perinatal infections with *Chlamydia trachomatis*. *Clin Perinatol* 1988;15:321.
43. Bell TA, et al. Chronic *Chlamydia trachomatis* infections in infants. *JAMA* 1992;267:400.
44. Centers for Disease Control. Recommendations for the prevention and management of *Chlamydia trachomatis* infections, 1993. *MMWR* 1993;42:1.
45. Hammerschlag MR, Gelling M, Roblin PM, et al. Treatment of neonatal chlamydial conjunctivitis with azithromycin. *Pediatr Infect Dis J* 1998;17:1049–1050.
46. Cassell GH, et al . *Ureaplasma urealyticum* intrauterine infection: Role in prematurity and disease in newborns. *Clin Microbiol Rev* 1993;6:69.
47. Wang EE, Matlow AG, Ohlsson A, et al. *Ureaplasma urealyticum* infections in the perinatal period. *Clin Perinatol* 1997;24:91–105.
48. Waites KB, Crouse DT, Cassell GH. Antibiotic susceptibilities and therapeutic options for *Ureaplasma urealyticum* infections in neonates. *Pediatr Infect Dis J* 1992;11:23.
49. Steinhoff MC, Smith DH. Diarrheagenic *E. coli*. In: Vaughn VC, McKay RJ, Behrman RE, eds. *Nelson textbook of pediatrics,* 11th ed. Philadelphia: WB Saunders, 1979:769.
50. St. Geme JW, et al. Consensus: management of *Salmonella* infection in the first year of life. *Pediatr Infect Dis J* 1988;7:615.
51. Kliegman RM, Walsh MC. Neonatal necrotizing enterocolitis: pathogenesis, classification, and spectrum of illness. *Curr Prob Pediatr* 1987;17:219.
52. Caplan MS, Jilling T. New concepts in necrotizing enterocolitis. *Curr Opin Pediatr* 2001;13:111–115.
53. Stoll B. Epidemiology of necrotizing enterocolitis. *Clin Perinatol* 1994;21:205–218.
54. Kanto WP, Hunter JE, Stoll BJ. Recognition and medical management of necrotizing enterocolitis. *Clin Perinatol* 1994;21:335–346.

55. Littlewood JM. Sixty-six infants with urinary tract infection in the first month of life. *Arch Dis Child* 1972;47:218.
56. Ginsburg CM, McCracken GH. Urinary tract infections in young infants. *Pediatrics* 1982;69:409.
57. Asmar BI. Osteomyelitis in the neonate. *Pediatr Infect* 1992;6:117.
58. Dan M. Septic arthritis in young infants: clinical and microbiological correlations and therapeutic implications. *Rev Infect Dis* 1984;6:147.
59. Melish ME, Glasgow LA. Staphylococcal scalded skin syndrome. The expanded clinical spectrum. *J Pediatr* 1971;78:958.
60. Centers for Disease Control. Hepatitis B virus: a comprehensive strategy for eliminating transmission in the United States through universal childhood vaccination. Recommendations of the Immunization Practices Advisory Committee (ACIP). *MMWR* 1991; 40:1.
61. American Academy of Pediatrics. Pickering LK, et al., eds. *2000 Red Book: report of the Committee on Infectious Diseases,* 25th ed. Elk Grove Village, IL: American Academy of Pediatrics, 2000. Hepatitis B, pp 289–302; Varicella-zoster infections, pp 624–638; Syphilis, pp 547–559.
62. Recommendations for prevention and control of hepatitis C virus (HCV) infection and HCV-related chronic disease. *MMWR* 1998;47:1–39.
63. Effects of mode of delivery and infant feeding on the risk of mother-to-child transmission of hepatitis C virus. European Paediatric Hepatitis C Virus Network. European Paediatric Hepatitis C Virus Network. *Br J Obstet Gynecol* 2001;108:371–377.
64. A-Kader HH, Balistreri WF. Hepatitis C virus: implications to pediatric practice. *Pediatr Infect Dis J* 1993;12:853.
65. Abzug MJ, et al. Neonatal enterovirus infection: virology, serology, and effects of intravenous immune globulin. *Clin Infect Dis* 1995;20:1201.
66. Rotbart HA, Webster AD for Pleconaril Treatment Group. Treatment of potentially life threatening enterovirus infections with pleconaril. *Clin Infect Dis* 2001;32:228–235.
67. Brunell PA. Varicella in pregnancy, the fetus, and the newborn: problems in management. *J Infect Dis* 1992;166(suppl 1):842.
68. Pastuszak AL, et al. Outcome after maternal varicella infection in the first 20 weeks of pregnancy. *N Engl J Med* 1994;330:901.
69. Butler KM, Baker CJ. *Candida:* an increasingly important pathogen in the nursery. *Pediatr Clin North Am* 1988;35:543.
70. Baley JE, Kliegman RM, Fanaroff AA. Disseminated fungal infections in very low birth weight infants: clinical manifestations and epidemiology. *Pediatrics* 1984;73:144.
71. Koren G, et al. Pharmacokinetics and adverse effects of amphotericin B in infants and children. *J Pediatr* 1988;118:559.
72. van den Anker JN, et al. Antifungal agents in neonatal systemic candidiasis. *Antimicrob Agents Chemother* 1995;39:1391.
73. Stamos JK, Rowley AH. Timely diagnosis of congenital infections. *Pediatr Clin North Am* 1994;41:1017–1033.
74. Lee SH, Ewert DP, Frederick PD, et al. Resurgence of congenital rubella syndrome in the 1990s. Report on missed opportunities and failed prevention policies among women of childbearing age. *JAMA* 1992;267:2616.
75. Brown HL, Abernathy MP. Cytomegalovirus infection. *Semin Perinatol* 1998;22:260–266.
76. Fowler KB, et al. The outcome of congenital cytomegalovirus infection in relation to maternal antibody status. *N Engl J Med* 1992;326:663.
77. Boppana SB, et al. Symptomatic congenital cytomegalovirus infection: neonatal morbidity and mortality. *Pediatr Infect Dis J* 1992;11:93.
78. Whitley RJ. Neonatal herpes simplex virus infections. *Clin Perinatol* 1988;15:903.
79. Brown ZA, et al. Neonatal herpes simplex virus infection in relation to asymptomatic maternal infection at the time of labor. *N Engl J Med* 1991;324:1247.
80. Prober CG, et al. The management of pregnancies complicated by genital infections with herpes simplex virus. *Clin Infect Dis* 1992;15:1031.
81. Whitley R, et al. A controlled trial comparing vidarabine with acyclovir in neonatal herpes simplex virus infection. *N Engl J Med* 1991;324:444.
82. Whitley RJ, Gnann JW Jr. Acyclovir: a decade later. *N Engl J Med* 1992;326:782.

83. Reyes MP, Hunt N, Ostrea EM Jr, et al. Maternal congenital syphilis in a large tertiary-care urban hospital. *Clin Infect Dis* 1993;17:1041.
84. BJ Stoll. Congenital syphilis: evaluation and management of neonates born to mothers with reactive serologic tests for syphilis. *Pediatr Infect Dis J* 1994;13:845.
85. Centers for Disease Control and Prevention. Sexually transmitted diseases treatment guidelines 2002. *MMWR* 2002;51(RR-6):1–78.
86. Hira SK, et al. Early congenital syphilis: clinicoradiologic features in 202 patients. *Sex Transm Dis* 1985;12:177.
87. Chhabra RS, et al. Comparison of maternal sera, cord blood, and neonatal sera for detecting presumptive congenital syphilis: relationship with maternal treatment. *Pediatrics* 1993;91:88.
88. American Academy of Pediatrics: Committee on Infectious Diseases. Parvovirus, erythema infectiosum, and pregnancy. *Pediatrics* 1990;85:131.
89. Centers for Disease Control and Prevention. Risks associated with human parvovirus B19 infection. *MMWR* 1989;39:81.
90. Ware R. Human parvovirus infection. *J Pediatr* 1989;114:343.
91. Guidelines for the use of antiretroviral agents in pediatric HIV-infection, 12/14/2001. Public Health Service Task Force recommendations for the use of antiretroviral drugs in pregnant HIV-1 infected women for maternal health and interventions to reduce perinatal HIV-1 transmission in the United States, February 4, 2002. *www.hivatis.org.*
92. Falloon J, et al. Human immunodeficiency virus infection in children. *J Pediatr* 1989;114:1.
93. Cantwell MY, et al. Brief report: congenital tuberculosis. *N Engl J Med* 1994;330:1051.
94. Sinclair JC, Bracken MB, eds. *Effective care of the newborn infant.* Oxford: Oxford University Press, 1992.

# 4. SKIN AND SOFT TISSUE INFECTIONS

Fred A. Lopez and Charles V. Sanders

In organizing this chapter on skin and soft tissue infections, the syndrome of fever and rash will be addressed briefly. Afterward, more limited, superficial skin problems will be addressed (e.g., impetigo, folliculitis, cutaneous abscesses), followed by more involved infections (e.g., pedal puncture wounds, bite wounds, cellulitis, necrotizing soft tissue infections). The chapter will conclude with the basic principles of surgical site infections, tetanus prophylaxis, and infectious agents of bioterrorism (i.e., anthrax, smallpox, tularemia, and plague) that can present with cutaneous manifestations.

## FEVER AND RASH

Skin and soft tissue infections are common problems confronting the physician in the office, emergency department, and inpatient hospital settings. Often, patients present with the syndrome of fever and rash. **An organized approach to this syndrome should include a meticulous history** that addresses the following points:

**I. Age of the patient.** Historically, virus-associated exanthems (i.e., measles; rubella; varicella; rubeola; roseola; hand, foot, and mouth disease; erythema infectiosum; Kawasaki syndrome) have been seen in the pediatric population. Enhanced and expanded immunization attempts have impacted significantly the epidemiology of many of these infections [1]. The most recent recommended childhood immunization schedules (***www.cdc.gov/nip/***) for the United States target hepatitis B, diphtheria, tetanus, pertussis, *Haemophilus influenzae* type b, polio, *Streptococcus pneumoniae,* measles, mumps, rubella, varicella, and hepatitis A. **Immunization histories** are important because many of these agents can cause fever and rash syndromes.

**II. Time of the year.** The season of the year may be helpful in prioritizing a differential diagnosis. Traditionally, rubella infections have been observed in the winter and spring; varicella (Color Plate 4.1) in the winter and early spring; rubeola in the winter and spring; *Coxsackievirus*-associated herpangina or hand, foot, and mouth disease (Color Plate 4.2 and 4.3) in the summer and fall; and erythema infectiosum in the winter and spring. The presence of infections can reflect when vectors for transmission are most widespread. Examples of vector-dependent diseases that are seen in the summer and fall include tick-borne diseases such as Lyme disease (Color Plate 4.4) and Rocky Mountain spotted fever. Mosquitoes are vectors for the West Nile virus infections recently seen in the northeastern United States during the summer and fall of 1999 [2]. Higher ambient temperatures seen in the summer months are responsible for sustaining growth of organisms such as *Vibrio vulnificus,* which can cause necrotizing skin infections in swimmers in Gulf Coast waters (Color Plate 4.5).

**III. Geography and travel.** An appreciation of the epidemiology of infectious diseases in different parts of the world is essential when assessing fever in the returned traveler [3]. For example, certain fungi are endemic in selected regions of the United States. *Histoplasma capsulatum* and *Blastomyces dermatitidis* (Color Plate 4.6) are found in the Mississippi and Ohio River valleys, whereas *Coccidioides immitis* is found in the southwestern United States. In contrast, a traveler to southeastern Asia would be exposed to the fungus *Penicillium marneffei.* In the United States, typhoid fever due to *Salmonella typhi* is often a consequence of travel to developing countries in Latin America, Africa, and Asia where there is decreased access to safe food and drinking water. Travelers from tropical areas of South America and Africa who present with petechiae or ecchymoses may have acquired a mosquito-borne disease such as yellow fever or dengue fever. The Centers for Disease Control and Prevention (CDC) provides a webpage that highlights infectious disease concerns for travelers (www.cdc.gov/travel/).

**IV. Medication history.** Drug-induced cutaneous reactions occur in approximately 2% to 3% of patients in the hospital [4,5]. Severe adverse cutaneous reactions to drugs occur less frequently and have been estimated to occur in approximately 1 of every 1,000 inpatients [6]. These cutaneous reactions include the Stevens-Johnson syndrome (SJS) and toxic epidermal necrolysis (TEN), disorders that are associated with more than one mucosal erosion, fever, and possible respiratory and gastrointestinal (GI) tract involvement. At least 50% of these reactions are medication related, usually developing 7 to 21 days after initiation of the offending drug. Sulfonamides, anticonvulsants, aminopenicillins, certain nonsteroidal antiinflammatory drugs, and allopurinol are more frequently reported causes of drug-induced SJS and TEN.

**V. Host immune status** [7]. Individuals with humoral- and complement-associated immunodeficiencies (e.g., splenectomy) are at increased risk for infections with encapsulated organisms such as *S. pneumoniae* (Color Plate 4.7), *Neisseria meningitidis* (Color Plate 4.8), and *Haemophilus influenzae.* Patients with cell-mediated immunodeficiency are susceptible to infections with organisms such as *Salmonella* species, *Mycobacteria* species, herpes viruses, *C. immitis, H. capsulatum, P. marneffei, Cryptococcus neoformans,* and *Strongyloides* species, to name a few. Neutropenia or neutrophil dysfunction is associated with infections due to staphylococci, enterococci, anaerobic bacteria, the Enterobacteriaceae, *Pseudomonas aeruginosa, Candida* species, and *Aspergillus* species.

**VI. Predisposition to infective endocarditis.** Risk factors for endocarditis should be sought, such as predisposing cardiac conditions [8] (see Chapter 12). Intravenous drug use is also considered a predisposition for development of infective endocarditis [9]. Skin lesions associated with endocarditis include Osler nodes (Color Plate 4.9), Janeway lesions, splinter hemorrhages, and cutaneous and subconjunctival petechiae.

**VII. Exposure history.** An exposure history is important to obtain in patients who present with fever and rash. Specific etiologies may be dictated by occupation. Healthcare workers are exposed to blood-borne diseases such as human immunodeficiency virus (HIV), hepatitis B, and hepatitis C, as well as aerosolized agents such as *N. meningitidis* and *Mycobacterium tuberculosis.* Fishermen and butchers may be exposed to *Erysipelothrix rhusiopathiae;* wilderness workers to ticks infected with rickettsial organisms; animal handlers to a broad range of microbes including *C. neoformans, Chlamydia psittaci, Bacillus anthracis, Francisella tularensis* (Color Plate 4.10), *Streptobacillus moniliformis, Yersinia pestis, Brucella* species, *Pasteurella multocida* (Color Plate 4.11), *Bartonella henselae,* and the rabies virus, to name a few.

A thorough **sexual history** is a priority. Although many of the sexually transmitted diseases manifest as localized genital diseases, some such as syphilis and gonorrhea may produce systemic symptoms and a more generalized rash. Infection-associated genital ulcer diseases include syphilis, herpes simplex, chancroid, donovanosis, and lymphogranuloma venereum. *Neisseria gonorrhoeae* and *Chlamydia trachomatis* primarily affect the urogenital tract. Reiter syndrome, manifesting as a triad of conjunctivitis, arthritis, and urethritis, can be seen after chlamydial urethritis. An underdiagnosed condition is the acute seroconversion syndrome associated with primary HIV infection. Signs or symptoms seen in more than 50% of patients presenting with acute HIV infection include fever, myalgia, rash, pharyngitis, malaise, and lymphadenopathy [10,11] (see Chapter 19).

**VIII. Specific characteristics of the rash** that should be addressed when evaluating the patient with fever and skin lesions include the following [12–15]:

**A.** History of similar rash
**B.** Description of lesions
**C.** Time of onset of the rash
**D.** Initial location of rash
**E.** Change or progression of rash
**F.** Duration of rash
**G.** Exacerbating or ameliorating interventions
**H.** Associated signs and symptoms
  **1.** Abnormal chest findings
  **2.** Headache and stiff neck
  **3.** Lymphadenopathy
  **4.** Joint pains
  **5.** Desquamation
  **6.** Mucous membrane lesions

## IMPETIGO

Impetigo is a primary pyoderma classically seen in children who are 2 to 5 years of age. Two forms of impetigo exist: nonbullous (i.e., simple superficial impetigo) and bullous.

I. **Clinical characteristics**
   A. **Nonbullous impetigo** is more common. Typically, multiple lesions initially present as a vesicle before progressing to a pustule and finally a plaque with a dried, thick, honey-colored crust (Color Plate 4.12). Traumatized and exposed areas of the face, scalp, or extremities are most frequently involved. Predisposing factors of impetigo include varicella infection, ulcers associated with trauma, reactions to insect bites or stings, burns, diabetes mellitus, hypogammaglobulinemia, HIV infection, scabies, and atopic dermatitis [16]. Patients are relatively asymptomatic, and rarely complaining of fever, pain, or itching. Local lymphadenopathy is often present. Impetigo usually resolves without any therapy.
   B. **Bullous impetigo** presents as clear to yellow-colored flaccid bullous lesions that become pustular with surrounding erythema (Color Plate 4.13). After rupturing, these lesions develop crusted centers that resemble nonbullous impetigo. Coalescence of these lesions may create lesions that are several centimeters in diameter. These lesions are typically nonpruritic and occur on the trunk, face, neck, perineum, or periumbilical areas. Local lymphadenopathy is more common in nonbullous disease. Systemic symptoms are usually absent.

II. **Epidemiology**
   A. **Nonbullous impetigo** is more common in humid, warm climates. The agents responsible for infection include *Streptococcus pyogenes* (group A streptococcus) and *Staphylococcus aureus,* often in combination [17]. Highly contagious, impetigo can spread among individuals in close living situations, for example, among infants in nursery and day-care settings or family members at home. Spread may be from infected individuals or carriers of *S. pyogenes* and *S. aureus;* carriage of these organisms also predisposes to infection.

   **Bullous impetigo** is usually caused by group II phage type 71, exfoliative toxin A–producing strains of *S. aureus.*

III. **Diagnosis and therapy**
   A. **Nonbullous impetigo**
      1. **Diagnosis** is usually based on the clinical presentation, and microbiologic workup is not recommended unless there is uncertainty about the diagnosis or failure of the infection to resolve with appropriate antibiotics. Identification in gram-stained specimens or isolation of the etiologic agent from culture of skin lesions can be used for definitive diagnosis. Histopathologic examination reveals neutrophils and lymphocytes in intracorneal and subcorneal epidermal and dermal pustules. Titers of anti-DNAse B can help document recent skin infection with group A streptococci.
      2. **Based on the microbiology of impetigo, therapy should target both streptococci and staphylococci.**
         a. Lesion-associated crusts should be debrided and cleansed with agents such as povidone-iodine or chlorhexidine.
         b. **Oral antibiotic therapy** consisting of approximately 10 days of dicloxacillin, erythromycin (equivalent dosing of clarithromycin or azithromycin), cephalexin, or clindamycin is effective and preferred for widespread disease. Some clinicians favor its use in close living situations where several members are already infected because topical agents do not eliminate streptococci from the respiratory tract [18].
         c. **Mupirocin** therapy, applied **topically** three times daily for 10 days, can be used for limited disease that does not involve the mouth or scalp and is as effective as oral regimens [19–21].
   B. **Bullous impetigo**
      1. **A clinically based diagnosis** can be made in obvious cases. Definitive diagnosis requires microbiologic studies (i.e., Gram stain and culture of bullae fluid).
      2. **Therapy. Topical mupirocin is not as effective as in nonbullous impetigo. Oral agents directed against staphylococci** are recommended. Dicloxacillin,

a first-generation cephalosporin, amoxicillin/clavulanic acid, erythromycin, clarithromycin, or clindamycin for 7 to 10 days can be used. Disseminated disease may dictate the use of an intravenous antistaphylococcal agent.

IV. **Complications. Cellulitis, osteomyelitis, septic arthritis, lymphangitis, lymphadenitis, and glomerulonephritis** are potential complications of impetigo [16]. Nephritogenic strains of group A streptococcus include M serotypes 2, 49, 55, 57, 59, 60, and 61. The latency period between the pyoderma and renal disease is approximately 3 weeks. Treatment of streptococcus-associated impetigo does not appear to change the risk for development of glomerulonephritis.

V. **Prophylaxis and control measures**

A. **Strict attention to personal hygiene** including regular bathing and clothing that protects infected areas of the body that are usually exposed can be helpful.

B. **Some experts have recommended that skin lesions such as those associated with insect bites or minor trauma with abrasions should be treated with topical antibiotic agents such as neomycin-bacitracin to prevent development of impetigo** [22].

C. **Antibiotic prophylaxis with penicillin** has been used in the management of patients with acute poststreptococcal glomerulonephritis and their family members with streptococcal colonization as well as in the control of some epidemics in other high-risk settings. However, no standard recommendations exist for prophylaxis.

D. Hospitalized patients with extensive group A streptococcal skin infections that cannot be adequately covered should be in **contact isolation** for at least 24 hours after antibiotic therapy has been initiated. Children with impetigo should refrain from close contact with others (including school) for at least 24 hours after initiation of antibiotic therapy [18].

## FOLLICULITIS

I. **Clinical characteristics**

A. **Superficial folliculitis** is best defined as a pyoderma confined to the hair follicle. Usually manifested as erythematous, pruritic papules ($\leq$5 mm in diameter) with a central pustular component, these lesions are often found on the face, scalp, back, buttocks, arms, and legs (Color Plate 4.14). Rupture of the pustule results in a crusted lesion. Predisposing factors for this superficial follicular infection include poor hygiene, warmer weather associated with high humidity, and occlusive ointments and dressings. The causative organism is usually *S. aureus.* **Hot tub folliculitis** refers to a folliculitis that develops after exposure to a high density of *P. aeruginosa* in a contaminated whirlpool, hot tub, or swimming pool. Multiple erythematous pruritic papulopustular lesions typically appear in the axillae, buttocks, legs, trunk, and waist within a couple of days of the exposure (Color Plate 4.15).

II. **Diagnosis can often be made on clinical grounds,** although organisms may be cultured from pustular lesions.

III. **Treatment**

A. **Folliculitis typically resolves without therapy.** Warm saline compresses may provide symptomatic relief, and topical agents such as erythromycin, clindamycin, or gentamicin are usually adequate for treatment.

B. **Preventative measures are most important** and include optimizing good hygiene and skin cleansing, avoiding sources of infection and in the case of "hot tub folliculitis," improved pool maintenance. Patients with recurrent staphylococcal folliculitis may benefit from monthly application of nasal mupirocin ointment (see nasal carriage of *S. aureus* below) [23].

## CUTANEOUS ABSCESSES

I. **Types**

A. **Furuncles.** Usually a result of a preceding infection of a hair follicle, a furuncle (or boil) is a tender, fluctuant, subcutaneous inflammatory nodule that extends to the dermis. Risk factors for development include defects in neutrophil function, obesity, corticosteroid use, occlusive dressings, hemodialysis-dependent renal failure, atopic dermatitis, parenteral drug use, diabetes, malnutrition, contact sports and exposure to individuals with follicular infections [16,24,25]. These lesions tend to form in areas of friction and sweating, including the back of the neck, axillae, face, groin, thighs, and buttocks. Often solitary, a furuncle can enlarge and become painful before spontaneously draining purulent material. A surrounding cellulitis may be present. Associated constitutional symptoms are not frequently observed. The causative organism is most commonly *S. aureus,* although the microbiology is dictated by the organisms that colonize involved areas. Healthy individuals with recurrent furunculosis are often nasal carriers of *S. aureus.* Abscesses consisting of aerobic and anaerobic bacteria are more prevalent in the perirectal area [26].

B. **Carbuncles.** A carbuncle refers to a series of coalescent furuncles that express pus from multiple tracts. These collections of multiple abscesses can be quite painful and are more likely to be accompanied by fever. In patients with cellulitis and fever, incision and drainage are usually required in addition to oral antibiotics.

C. **Skin abscesses other than furuncles/carbuncles** are common and typically reflect extension of superficial skin infections to the deeper dermis and subcutaneous fat. On occasion, bacteremic seeding of skin and soft tissue can result in a localized abscess. Although many patients will develop spontaneous cutaneous abscesses, predisposing risk factors include trauma, intravenous drug use, diabetes mellitus, and chronic carriage of *S. aureus.* These lesions are usually solitary, erythematous nodules associated with localized pain, swelling, and lymphadenopathy. Although bacteremia and adjacent septic arthritis and osteomyelitis can occur, these lesions often drain spontaneously and are not associated with systemic toxicity. The microbiology of these abscesses results from organisms that colonize the local mucocutaneous structures. As a result, *S. aureus* is the most common organism isolated from cutaneous abscesses, but mixed flora can be appreciated in abscesses found in perirectal, oral, and genitourinary (GU) areas [27].

II. **Evaluation of cutaneous abscesses**

A. **Clinical evaluation should include assessment for fever and other signs of systemic infection.** A complete blood count and blood cultures should be obtained if systemic signs of infection are present. Gram stains and cultures of drainage or aspirated material are also recommended.

B. **Incision and drainage**

1. **Abscesses on the lips and nose should not be drained** due to emissary venous drainage resulting in possible extension to the cavernous sinus.
2. Because incision and drainage of lesions may result in transient bacteremia with organisms associated with infective endocarditis, **prophylaxis with antibiotics should be administered to individuals with cardiac conditions that are associated with increased risk for cardiac valvular infection** [8].

III. **Treatment.** For smaller furuncles, the application of moist heat can be helpful in promoting drainage. Incision and drainage is often needed for larger cutaneous abscesses, particularly in patients with cellulitis and fever. Antibiotics are used in selected clinical circumstances.

A. **Incision and drainage** should be performed except for abscesses on the lips and nose. These lesions can be managed with warm compresses and, if indicated, antibiotics.

B. **Antibiotics** should be reserved for the following situations:

1. **Immunocompromised patients (including those with diabetes mellitus)**
2. **Fever and systemic symptoms**
3. **Surrounding cellulitis, lymphangitis, osteomyelitis, or invasion of blood stream**
4. **Infective endocarditis prophylaxis in patients with at-risk cardiac conditions**
5. **Chronic nasal carriage in patients who have recurrent furunculosis**

C. **Antibiotic regimens should be pathogen directed** based on the results of Gram stain and culture of purulent material. Recommended regimens for adults include:

1. **Gram-positive cocci**

   a. **Oral therapy.** Dicloxacillin, 250 to 500 mg every 6 hours, or cephalexin, 500 mg every 6 hours, for approximately 10 days can be used. In the penicillin- or cephalosporin-allergic patient, oral clindamycin, 300 mg every 6 hours can be used.

**b. Parenteral therapy.** Nafcillin or oxacillin, 1 to 2 g intravenously (i.v.) every 4 to 6 hours, is recommended. In the patient with a delayed penicillin allergy, cefazolin, 1 g i.v. every 8 hours, can be used. If penicillin allergy is immunoglobulin E (IgE) mediated, clindamycin, 600 to 900 mg i.v. every 8 hours, or vancomycin, 15 mg/kg i.v. every 12 hours, is recommended.

**2. Mixed cutaneous abscess (i.e., perirectal, oral, and GU areas) treatment should include coverage for *S. aureus*, streptococci, gram-negative bacilli, and anaerobic bacteria, including *Bacteroides* species.**

**a. Oral therapy.** Amoxicillin (500 mg) and clavulanate (125 mg) orally every 8 hours can be used empirically.

**b. Parenteral therapy.** Ampicillin-sulbactam 3 g i.v. every 8 hours, piperacillin-tazobactam 3.375 i.v. every 6 hours or 4.5 g i.v. every 8 hours, and ticarcillin-clavulanate 3.1 g i.v. every 4 to 6 hours can be administered.

**3. Nasal carriage of *S. aureus*.** Eradication of *S. aureus* from the nares should be pursued in individuals with recurrent furuncles. Twice daily application of 2% mupirocin for 5 days every month is often effective [23,28]. Ten days of oral rifampin 600 mg daily combined with dicloxacillin 500 mg every 6 hours also may be effective. For methicillin-resistant *S. aureus* colonization, 7 to 14 days of mupirocin is recommended. Oral clindamycin 150 mg daily for 3 months has been used successfully for prevention [29]. Patients with recurrent furuncles and impaired neutrophil function may benefit from vitamin C 1 g daily for approximately 6 weeks [30].

**IV. Prevention measures against deep follicular infections include eradication of nasal carriage of *S. aureus*,** avoidance of risk factors associated with development of furuncles/carbuncles (e.g., intravenous drug use), improved hygiene including the use of antiseptic soaps (e.g., chlorhexidine), and the use of nonirritating clothing that fits loosely.

## PUNCTURE WOUNDS OF THE FEET

**I. Clinical characteristics.** Plantar surface puncture wounds have been reported to constitute approximately 7% of lower extremity trauma cases evaluated in the emergency department [31]. Most of these injuries are due to nails and typically occur during the warmer summer months [32]. Three percent to 15% of nail puncture wounds become infected, and complications include cellulitis, localized deep soft tissue abscess, osteomyelitis, or pyoarthrosis [33]. The factors contributing to the development of infection include the presence of a foreign body, depth and location of the wound, host immune status, presence of a sneaker, type of penetrating object, and time elapsed from injury to presentation [34]. Most bone infections are due to *P. aeruginosa,* particularly when the puncture wound occurs through the inner sole of the sneaker, a site of pseudomonal colonization. Other organisms reported to cause infection include *S. aureus, S. pyogenes,* Enterobacteriaceae, and anaerobes. Polymicrobial osteomyelitis is more common in diabetic adults [35].

**II. Treatment. Initial management** of the puncture wound should include the following:

**A.** Use detergent or iodophor to clean the wound.

**B.** Trim the epidermal flap of the wound.

**C.** Consider probing the wound for depth and the presence of a foreign body.

**D.** Consider plain films of the foot when uncertain whether a foreign body remains in wound.

**E.** Tetanus assessment and administration as recommended (see section on Tetanus below).

**F. The decision to administer prophylactic antibiotics is controversial and left to the treating physician** particularly in wounded patients who are immunocompromised. Antibiotics should be administered when soft tissue infection is present.

**G. Remove foreign bodies, debride necrotic infected tissue and drain abscesses when present.** Raz and colleagues [33] have reported on the successful management of nail puncture wound infections (primarily caused by *Pseudomonas aeruginosa*) by using routine surgical incision, debridement, and drainage of abscess material. Following surgery, oral ciprofloxacin (750 mg orally twice daily) is administered for 7 days to patients with deep tissue abscess and cellulitis;

duration is 14 days for patients with early bone involvement [33]. If the microbiologic etiology is uncertain, then empiric therapy for skin and soft tissue infections is directed primarily against *S. aureus* (penicillinase-resistant semisynthetic penicillins or first-generation cephalosporins) and for bone and joint infections, *S. aureus* and *P. aeruginosa* (i.e., nafcillin and ceftazidime or levofloxacin) [36].

## ANIMAL BITES AND RABIES PREVENTION

Approximately 0.5% to 1% of all emergency room visits in the United States are due to bite wounds, an impressive statistic when one recognizes that more than 75% of individuals who receive a bite wound will not present for medical evaluation [37]. Hospitalization is required in about 1% to 5% of these visits [38].

**I. Types of bite wounds**

**A. Dog bites.** Dogs account for more than 75% of all animal bites. Children are most commonly involved, and the location of injury typically includes an extremity or the head and neck. **Almost 20% of these wounds become infected.**

1. **Bacteriology.** The microbiology of dog bite–associated infections is complex and includes streptococci, *S. aureus, Pasteurella canis* (most common isolate) and *P. multocida, Eikenella corrodens, Capnocytophaga canimorsus,* and anaerobes such as *Fusobacterium, Bacteroides, Porphyromonas,* and *Prevotella* species [39]. ***C. canimorsus,*** a gram-negative facultative anaerobic bacillus that normally colonizes the dog's oral cavity, can cause fulminant sepsis and disseminated intravascular coagulopathy in immunocompromised patients, particularly those without splenic function.
2. **Evaluation and management** [37]
   - **a.** In all types of bites, a thorough history should be obtained including the type of animal, the circumstances surrounding the bite (i.e., provoked or unprovoked), and the immune status of the individual bitten. A physical examination should include investigation for signs of infection and joint, nerve, bone, or vascular penetration. **Risk for infection is increased in puncture- or crush-associated injuries.**
   - **b.** Normal saline **irrigation of all wounds is recommended,** with the need for surgical debridement dictated by the degree of injury.
   - **c. Wound cultures** are not helpful when there are no signs of infection except in the setting of puncture wounds or tears. Cultures are recommended from all infected wounds, and radiographs can be helpful in assessing for bone involvement.
   - **d. Hand wound infections, necrotic wounds, and possible walled-off infections should precipitate a surgical consultation.** Wounds should be examined more than 1 day after a bite. Infected wounds, deep puncture wounds, and bites to the hand should not be closed primarily. With the exception of facial wounds, which may be closed primarily, no clear recommendations exist for **primary closure** of fresh wounds seen less than 6 to 8 hours after a bite. Delayed primary closure is often allowed in uninfected higher risk wounds.
   - **e.** The best use of **prophylactic antibiotics** in patients who present within 8 hours of a dog bite is unclear. Some experts recommend **prophylactic antimicrobial treatment for 3 to 5 days** after most dog bites, particularly high-risk wounds associated with deep punctures; crush injuries; hand, foot, or facial wounds; immunocompromised patients; wounds near joints or bones (particularly if prosthesis in place); and moderate and severe wounds, especially those requiring surgical debridement [37,40]. Minor wounds may not require treatment. **The duration of treatment for infected wounds is at least 10 days.** Bone or joint involvement dictates an extended course.
   - **f. The suggested empiric choice for hospitalized patients requiring parenteral therapy** is a penicillin and $\beta$-lactamase inhibitor combination such as ampicillin-sulbactam, 3 g i.v. every 6 hours. **The choice for oral outpatient therapy** is amoxicillin-clavulanate, 500 mg orally every 8 hours or 875 mg orally every 12 hours.

g. **In the penicillin-allergic patient,** options include a fluoroquinolone (such as levofloxacin or ciprofloxacin) plus clindamycin or clindamycin plus trimethoprim-sulfamethoxazole (for children).

3. **Elevation of the affected area is recommended.**
4. Tetanus prophylaxis and rabies assessment needs to be addressed.
5. **Close follow-up** of patients who are not hospitalized.

B. **Cat bites.** The incidence of infection after a cat bite is reported at 28% to 80%, considerably higher than after dog bites [39]. The increased rate of infection is due to the deep puncture wounds (potentially involving joint or bone) created by the sharp and thin teeth of cats (see also Chapter 21).

1. **Microbiology.** *P. multocida* is the most common pathogen isolated from cat bites (>50% of cases) (Color Plate 4.11); otherwise, the polymicrobial spectrum is similar to that for dog bites. However, the number of organisms isolated is usually less.
2. **Antibiotic therapy. Because of the increased incidence of infection after cat bites, prophylactic antibiotics are commonly used for 3 to 5 days.** Empiric therapy should be active against *P. multocida,* and typically includes agents used for dog bites. *Pasteurella* infections usually develop within 24 to 48 hours and are susceptible to penicillin, aminopenicillins, cefuroxime, doxycycline, and trimethoprim-sulfamethoxazole.
3. **Assessment and treatment** of infected wounds should follow the same recommendations as for dog bites.

C. **Human bite injuries** occur after a bite from another human (i.e., occlusional bites) or after a closed fist injury that usually involves the metacarpophalangeal joints. **Closed-fist injuries can be devastating** when they involve deeper soft tissues, bones, or joints, and are more susceptible to infection than animal bites. As a result, initial inpatient management is often required, and usually with the assistance of a hand surgeon.

1. **Bacteriology.** *S. aureus, E. corrodens, H. influenzae,* streptococci, and $\beta$-lactamase–producing oral anaerobes are most commonly associated with infection. Potential pathogens can include blood-borne microbes such as hepatitis B or C, herpes simplex virus, HIV and *Treponema pallidum.*
2. **Antibiotics**
   a. When patients are seen soon after their injury, **3 to 5 days of prophylactic antibiotics are often recommended. The choice for oral outpatient therapy is amoxicillin-clavulanate.**
   b. **Obvious wound infections require a more prolonged course that is dictated by the extent of injury. These patients are usually hospitalized and are administered parenteral therapy, usually a penicillin and $\beta$-lactamase inhibitor combination such as ampicillin-sulbactam, ticarcillin-clavulanic acid, or piperacillin-tazobactam.** Cefoxitin also may be used. **In the penicillin-allergic patient,** options include a fluoroquinolone (such as levofloxacin or ciprofloxacin) plus clindamycin or clindamycin plus trimethoprim-sulfamethoxazole (for children).
3. Normal saline irrigation, radiographs to assess for bone involvement, debridement when indicated, and tetanus assessment are essential.

D. **Other animal bites.** Bites from a variety of animals, including primates, pigs, horses, fish, alligators, sheep, rats, and ferrets, have been reported. Infectious disease consultation is recommended for assistance when evaluating and managing these zoonotic infections [37].

II. **Rabies prophylaxis.** In the United States, human-associated rabies infections have decreased to approximately zero to five cases per year [41]. When one examines the 36 cases of rabies in humans in the United States since 1980, more than 50% derive from bats [41]. In contrast, dogs appear to be the most common source of human-associated rabies outside the United States. This infection is incurable, mandating the need for avoidance of high-risk circumstances and rapid institution of prophylaxis when indicated. An understanding of the epidemiology of rabies and circumstances surrounding postexposure treatment is useful (Tables 4.1 and 4.2) [42].

Table 4.1. Rabies Postexposure Prophylaxis Guide: United States, 1999

| Animal Type | Evaluation and Disposition of Animal | Postexposure Prophylaxis Recommendations |
|---|---|---|
| Dogs, cats, and ferrets | Healthy and available for 10 days observation | Persons should not begin prophylaxis unless animal develops clinical signs of rabies.[a] |
| | Rabid or suspected to be rabid | Immediately vaccinate. |
| | Unknown (e.g., escaped) | Consult public health officials. |
| Skunks, raccoons, foxes, and most other carnivores; bats | Regarded as rabid unless animal proven negative by laboratory tests[b] | Consider immediate vaccination. |
| Livestock, small rodents, lagomorphs (rabbits and hares), large rodents (woodchucks and beavers), and other mammals | Consider individually | Consult public health officials. Bites of squirrels, hamsters, guinea pigs, gerbils, chipmunks, rats, mice, other small rodents, rabbits, and hares almost never require antirabies postexposure prophylaxis. |

[a] During the 10-day observation period, begin postexposure prophylaxis at the first sign of rabies in a dog, cat, or ferret that has bitten someone. If the animal exhibits clinical signs of rabies, it should be killed and immediately tested.
[b] The animal should be killed and tested as soon as possible. Holding for observation is not recommended. Discontinue vaccine if immunofluorescence test results of the animal are negative.
Reprinted from Centers for Disease Control and Prevention. Human rabies prevention—United States, 1999: recommendations of the Advisory Committee on Immunization Practices (ACIP). *MMWR* 1999;48: 1–21; with permission.

**A. Considerations prior to antirabies therapy are outlined in Table 4.1.** The cost associated with rabies prophylaxis is considerable, and prophylaxis cannot be instituted liberally after every animal bite [42].

1. **Type of animal.** Bats and wild terrestrial carnivorous animals (particularly skunks, raccoons, foxes, and coyotes) are more likely than domestic animals (i.e., dogs, cats, and ferrets), livestock, and rodents to be infected with rabies. Because the probability of rabies infections in particular animals varies geographically, consideration should be given for contacting local or state public health authorities regarding the need for postexposure prophylaxis.
2. **Characteristics of attack and animal's vaccination status.** An attack by an animal that is unprovoked and not associated with feeding or handling reflects a higher likelihood that the animal is infected with rabies. Dogs, cats, or ferrets that have been appropriately vaccinated are unlikely to be rabid.
3. **Characteristics of exposure.** Rabies virus transmission requires a rabid animal and introduction of its potentially infectious tissue material onto mucous membranes or into open wounds. Transmission of infectious material such as saliva or neural tissue is most commonly accomplished by animal bites, but contamination of nonintact skin (open wounds, scratches, abrasions) or mucous membranes represent potential nonbite exposures. Exposure to aerosols containing a high density of rabies virus in the laboratory or in caves and transplantation of rabies-infected human corneas should also be considered potentially infectious.

**B. Recommendations for wound treatment and vaccination are listed in Tables 4.1 and 4.2.** Urgent evaluation and management are needed in potential rabies exposures. Recommendations include the following [42]:

Table 4.2. Rabies Postexposure Prophylaxis Schedule: United States, 1999

| Vaccination Status | Treatment | Regimen[a] |
|---|---|---|
| Not previously vaccinated | Wound cleansing | All postexposure treatment should begin with immediate thorough cleansing of all wounds with soap and water. If available, a virucidal agent such as a povidone-iodine solution should be used to irrigate the wounds. |
| | RIG | Administer 20 IU/kg body weight. If anatomically feasible, the full dose should be infiltrated around the wound(s) and any remaining volume should be administered i.m. at an anatomic site distant from vaccine administration. Also, RIG should not be administered in the same syringe as the vaccine. Because RIG might partially suppress active production of antibody, no more than the recommended dose should be given. |
| | Vaccine | HDCV, RVA, or PCEC 1.0 mL i.m. (deltoid area),[b] one each on days 0,[c] 3, 7, 14, and 28. |
| Previously vaccinated[d] | Wound cleansing | All postexposure treatment should begin with immediate thorough cleansing of all wounds with soap and water. If available, a virucidal agent such as a povidone-iodine solution should be used to irrigate the wounds. |
| | RIG | RIG should not be administered. |
| | Vaccine | HDCV, RVA, or PCEC 1.0 mL i.m. (deltoid area),[b] one each on days 0[c] and 3. |

HDCV, human diploid cell vaccine; PCEC, purified chick embryo cell vaccine; RIG, rabies immune globulin; RVA, rabies vaccine adsorbed; i.m., intramuscularly.

[a] These regimens are applicable for all age groups, including children.

[b] The deltoid area is the only acceptable site of vaccination for adults and older children. For younger children, the outer aspect of the thigh may be used. Vaccine should never be administered in the gluteal area.

[c] Day 0 is the day the first dose of vaccine is administered.

[d] Any person with a history of preexposure vaccination with HDCV, RVA, or PCEC; prior postexposure prophylaxis with HDCV, RVA, or PCEC; or previous vaccination with any other type of rabies vaccine and a documented history of antibody response to the prior vaccination.

Reprinted from Centers for Disease Control and Prevention. Human rabies prevention—United States, 1999: recommendations of the Advisory Committee on Immunization Practices (ACIP). *MMWR* 1999; 48:1–21; with permission.

1. **Management of the wound.** Prompt and complete cleansing of the wound with water and soap and a cidal agent for viruses (e.g., povidone-iodine) is recommended. Tetanus prophylaxis and management of secondary bacterial infections should be instituted as indicated.
2. **Approach to the potentially infected animal.** A pet that is not suspected to be rabid can be isolated and observed for 10 days. If a veterinarian observes any signs of rabies during the confinement period then the pet should be killed. The intact head should be sent under refrigerated conditions to a qualified laboratory for diagnostic immunofluorescence testing. Animals that are regarded as rabid should be killed and evaluated immediately in the laboratory for the presence of the rabies virus.
3. **Postexposure prophylaxis should be initiated as soon as possible.** In the previously unvaccinated individual, vaccination includes **passive prophylaxis with rabies immunoglobulin (RIG) and active prophylaxis with rabies vaccine** (Table 4.2).

a. At the beginning of antirabies prophylaxis, **human RIG** is administered once at a dose of 20 IU/kg body weight. As much of this dose as is anatomically possible should be infiltrated around the wound and the remaining amount should be administered intramuscularly in an area remote from administration of vaccine. A different syringe for administration of RIG and vaccine is also recommended.

b. **Active immunization** should begin as soon as possible after the exposure and in conjunction with RIG. Three types of inactivated human rabies vaccine are available in the United States for postexposure prophylaxis: (a) human diploid cell rabies vaccine (HDCV); (b) rabies vaccine adsorbed (RVA); and (c) purified chick embryo cell vaccine (PCEC). These vaccines are alike in efficacy and safety, and 1-mL doses should be administered in the deltoid muscle on days 0, 3, 7, 14, and 28 in the previously unvaccinated individual. If the individual has previously received the rabies vaccine, then 1 mL of the human rabies vaccine is administered in the deltoid muscle on day 0 and day 3.

c. **Complete recommendations can be obtained from the CDC** [42]. Table 4.2 can be used as a postexposure antirabies treatment guide.

4. **Preexposure vaccination** is indicated for individuals who are frequently exposed to animals who are at risk for being infected with the rabies virus. These individuals include veterinarians, animal control handlers, investigators in rabies laboratories, spelunkers, wildlife officers, and foreign travelers to countries where contact is expected with animals in regions where dogs infected with rabies is endemic and medical care is inaccessible. Recommendations for preexposure prophylaxis include [42]:

a. HDCV, PCEC, or RVA, 1.0 mL intramuscularly (i.m.; deltoid area), administered in three separate doses on days 0, 7, and 21 or 28. Three separate doses of HDCV, 0.1 mL intradermally, can be administered over the deltoid area on days 0, 7, and 21 or 28 as an alternative to the intramuscular HDCV regimen.

b. A postvaccination rabies antibody titer should be checked every 6 months to 2 years in certain high-risk groups, in order to assess the need for preexposure booster doses of vaccine.

c. Preexposure prophylaxis eliminates the need for RIG after a rabies exposure, but 1 mL of human rabies vaccine (HDCV, RVA, or PCEC) still needs to be administered in the deltoid muscle on days 0 and 3.

## CELLULITIS AND RELATED SKIN INFECTIONS

**Cellulitis is an infectious inflammatory process involving the deepest portion of the dermis of the skin and subcutaneous fat.** This infection typically develops in the extremities and presents as a warm, erythematous, tender, swollen, and poorly demarcated skin process (Color Plate 4.16). Systemic symptoms may include fever, chills, and muscle pain. **Predisposing factors** include tinea pedis, substance abuse, diabetes mellitus, burns, trauma from puncture wound or surgery, venous insufficiency, and lymphatic interruption [43]. **Many organisms can cause cellulitis in selected circumstances.**

I. **Etiology of cellulitis**

A. ***S. pyogenes*** **and** ***S. aureus*** **are the most common causes of simple uncomplicated cellulitis.** Initial treatment should be directed against both of these bacteria and typically includes parenteral nafcillin or cefazolin when treating patients with systemic signs and symptoms or those who are immunocompromised. If the infection is mild, oral antibiotics can be used.

B. **Group B streptococci** (*S. agalactiae*) can cause skin and soft tissue infections in nonpregnant adults, especially in the elderly and in those with diabetes, a pressure ulcer, underlying malignancy, cirrhosis, or neurologic impairment, as well as in those infected with HIV [44–46]. In fact, skin and soft tissue infections are the most common manifestation of invasive disease with group B streptococci, presenting as cellulitis, ulcerations, and even necrotizing fasciitis (NF). Infections are often nosocomial, associated with the placement of an intravenous catheter, and primarily due to capsular serotypes Ia, III, and V. This organism remains sensitive to penicillin, but increasing resistance to erythromycin and clindamycin is being reported.

**For uncomplicated skin infections requiring hospitalization, penicillin G, 2 million units i.v. every 4 to 6 hours is recommended.** Vancomycin, 15 mg/kg i.v. every 12 hours can be administered to the penicillin-allergic patient. First- and third-generation cephalosporins also may be used as alternative therapy. Surgical debridement may be essential to remove devitalized skin and soft tissue.

**C. Erysipeloid** refers to a skin infection caused by a gram-positive bacillus, *Erysipelothrix rhusiopathiae,* which is found in many fish, mammals, and birds. The handling of infected material allows the organism to enter through breaks in the skin. Butchers, fisherman, and veterinarians are at increased risk for infection. The site of entry, usually the dorsum of the hand, becomes violaceous, warm, and swollen (Color Plate 4.17). Well-defined maculopapular lesions, bullous lesions, and plaques can be seen. Rarely, bacteremia and endocarditis develop in immunocompromised hosts. Skin infections are usually self-limited after 2 to 3 weeks, but the use of **penicillin G or an aminopenicillin, the drugs of choice,** can hasten recovery. A total daily dose of 12 to 20 million units of i.v. penicillin G administered every 4 to 6 hours for 4 to 6 weeks is recommended for endocarditis. Imipenem, fluoroquinolones, and third-generation cephalosporins are also active against this organism.

**D. *H. influenzae* cellulitis, primarily a bacteremic complication of children,** classically presents as a **violaceous facial cellulitis (often involving the periorbital or cheek areas).** Although much less commonly observed in adults, **H. influenzae** cellulitis is usually associated with respiratory tract infections and typically involves the upper thorax and neck [47]. The treatment of choice is a third-generation cephalosporin or ampicillin (if susceptible).

**E. Skin and soft tissue lesions are observed in up to 30% of patients with pseudomonal sepsis. Usually observed in immunocompromised hosts,** cutaneous manifestations include cellulitis, folliculitis, bullae, nodules, abscesses, and vesicles and plaques [48,49]. **Ecthyma gangrenosum** is the characteristic necrotic skin lesion reported in a significant number of patients with malignancy, neutropenia, and pseudomonal bacteremia. These lesions are usually located in the axilla or perineum. Burn wounds complicated by *Pseudomonas* infection and bacteremia often form eschars and are associated with mortality rates of greater than 75% [50]. Treatment usually includes surgical removal of necrotic tissue and combination therapy consisting of an antipseudomonal $\beta$-lactam or quinolone and an aminoglycoside (cefipime, ceftazidime, piperacillin, mezlocillin, imipenem, or ciprofloxacin plus gentamicin, tobramycin, or amikacin).

**F. Wound infections due to water exposure** can develop in patients with lacerations, puncture wounds, or marine-animal bites.

1. ***Vibrio vulnificus.*** Immunocompromised individuals, particularly those with cirrhosis, are at increased risk for infection with *V. vulnificus,* a gram-negative curved bacillus that is found in warm seawaters. Infections may occur at traumatized sites after exposure to contaminated seawater or seafood, or after ingestion of contaminated seafood. A cellulitis that progresses to an invasive NF with associated hemorrhagic bullae is characteristic (Color Plate 4.5). Optimal therapy includes aggressive surgical debridement, supportive care, and antibiotics. The choice of antibiotics includes a third-generation cephalosporin like ceftazidime (2 g i.v. every 8 hours), plus doxycycline, 100 mg orally or i.v. every 12 hours; cefotaxime, 2 g i.v. every 8 hours, also can be used. Some investigators recommend an aminoglycoside in lieu of doxycycline [51]. The organism is also susceptible to quinolones such as ciprofloxacin (400 mg i.v. every 12 h or 750 mg orally every 12 hours).
2. ***Aeromonas*** skin infections can develop in cancer patients receiving chemotherapy or in cirrhotic patients after exposure to contaminated fresh water (Color Plate 4.18). Cutaneous manifestations may be similar to *V. vulnificus*–associated infections. Surgical debridement is indicated, and antibiotic recommendations include ciprofloxacin 400 mg i.v. every 12 hours or 750 mg orally every 12 hours. Trimethoprim-sulfamethoxazole and non–first-generation cephalosporins also may be useful.
3. ***Edwardsiella tarda,*** a gram-negative bacillus in the Enterobacteriaceae family, can cause wound infections after exposure to contaminated fresh water [52].

Abscesses, hemorrhagic bullae, cellulitis, and myonecrosis have been described. Antibiotic therapy should be guided by susceptibility testing. This organism is generally susceptible to antimicrobial agents used for treatment of gram-negative bacillary infections, including ampicillin, cephalosporins, aminoglycosides, fluoroquinolones, and trimethoprim-sulfamethoxazole.

4. ***Mycobacterium marinum,*** a nontuberculous mycobacteria, is the most common cause of mycobacterial skin disease. Lesions usually develop 2 to 6 weeks after trauma-associated contact with water, including saltwater, lake water, swimming pool water, or aquarium water. Violaceous papules that develop into ulcerative plaques are frequently described, often in a sporotrichoid pattern (Color Plate 4.19). Four antimicrobial regimens are recommended by the American Thoracic Society: doxycycline, 100 mg orally twice daily; clarithromycin, 500 mg orally twice daily; trimethoprim-sulfamethoxazole (160/800 mg) orally twice daily; or ethambutol, 15 mg/kg/day orally, plus rifampin, 600 mg/day orally [53]. Treatment should continue for at least 3 months. Surgical debridement also may be necessary when the infection proves refractory to antimicrobial agents.

**II. Erysipelas.** This infection involves the upper dermis and superficial lymphatics, and **is characterized by skin lesions that are well demarcated, painful, erythematous, and elevated.** The lower extremities or face are most often involved, and the diagnosis is usually made on clinical grounds. **The microbiologic cause is almost always *S. pyogenes*,** although less commonly other $\beta$-hemolytic streptococci, *S. aureus,* and gram-negative bacilli may be involved. If systemic signs of infection are present or if the patient is immunocompromised, parenteral agents such as nafcillin oroxacillin, penicillin G, or cefazolin are indicated. Oral agents such as dicloxacillin, penicillin, or cephalexin can be given in milder cases or those in which improvement is noted. Vancomycin, clindamycin, or erythromycin can be used in the penicillin-allergic patient.

**III. Diagnosis.** The diagnosis of cellulitis and erysipelas is often made on clinical grounds based on the presence of erythema, swelling, warmth, tenderness and pain, regional lymphadenopathy, and associated tinea pedis. Systemic signs and symptoms such as fever and malaise may not always be present. Other diagnostic studies include the following:

**A. Gram staining of aspirate or biopsy** may be helpful in directing initial therapy.

**B. Results of needle aspiration or punch biopsy to obtain tissue for aerobic and anaerobic cultures** are usually negative but may be pursued. Needle aspiration cultures of the leading edge are reported to yield positive results in less than 20% of cases, but may be indicated and helpful in immunocompromised patients or when isolating the etiologic agent is necessary, antibiotic therapy is failing, or atypical etiologic agents are suspected [54]. Direct aspiration of tissue without injection of saline may increase the yield of aspirate cultures [55]. Punch biopsy cultures have been reported to have a higher yield of microbial isolation than blood cultures or needle aspirates, but add no additional microbiologic information to direct cultures from swabs of primary lesions [56].

**C. Blood cultures** are often obtained. In one recent study of more than 500 adult patients admitted to a hospital with community-acquired cellulitis, cultures were definitively positive in approximately 2% of cases and had minimal impact on the treatment prescribed [57]. The investigators concluded that blood cultures should be obtained in "unusually severe cases, such as possibly elderly patients with acute onset of illness, high grade fever and significant leukocytosis and immunocompromised patients" [57]. Similar results have been reported in the pediatric population [58].

**D. Serologic studies for the presence of group A streptococcus** may help support the diagnosis of streptococcal disease when isolation of the organism has not been achieved.

**E. Radiographic studies are usually unnecessary.** Plain films may be helpful in identifying gas, bony involvement, or the presence of foreign bodies. Computed tomography (CT) or magnetic resonance imaging (MRI) can assist in determining whether the infection is confined to skin and soft tissue or whether fascia, muscle, or bone is involved [59].

**IV. Treatment**

A. **General principles.** Clinical and initial microbiologic clues can be helpful in directing therapy while awaiting culture results.

B. **Antibiotic treatment** suggestions for adults with cellulitis.

1. **The most common bacterial causes of cellulitis are group A streptococcus and *S. aureus*.** Therapy is typically directed against both of these pathogens.
   a. **Recommended treatment regimens for hospitalized adult patients** include nafcillin or oxacillin, 2 g i.v. every 4 to 6 hours, or cefazolin, 1 to 2 g i.v. every 8 hours. Alternative parenteral agents, particularly for patients with IgE-mediated penicillin allergy, include vancomycin, 15 mg/kg i.v. every 12 hours, or clindamycin, 450 to 900 mg i.v. every 8 hours.
   b. **Mild infection** in adults can be treated orally with dicloxacillin, 500 mg every 6 hours, or cephalexin, 250 to 500 mg every 6 hours. Clindamycin, 300 to 450 mg every 6 hours, can be used in penicillin-allergic patients; oral macrolides such as erythromycin (500 mg every 6 hours) are sometimes used in this setting.
   c. **The hospitalized adult patient with uncomplicated culture-proven group A streptococcal cellulitis** can be treated with penicillin G, 1 to 2 million units i.v. every 4 to 6 hours.
   d. **Vancomycin** treatment of possible methicillin-resistant *Staphylococcus aureus* infection should be considered for **patients who reside in nursing homes or have recently been hospitalized.**
2. **Diabetes-associated, perineal, or other suspected mixed aerobic-anaerobic cellulitis** dictates the use of broad-spectrum antibiotics. In the hospitalized patient, penicillin and $\beta$-lactamase inhibitor combinations such as piperacillin-tazobactam (3.375 g i.v. every 6 hours), ampicillin-sulbactam (3 g i.v. every 6 hours), or ticarcillin-clavulanate (3.1 g i.v. every 4–6 hours) are often recommended. Imipenem (500 mg i.v. every 6 hours) or a third-generation cephalosporin such as ceftriaxone (2 g i.v. every 24 hours) in combination with metronidazole (500 mg i.v. every 6 hours) or clindamycin (600–900 mg i.v. every 8 hours) also can be considered.
3. **Antibiotic regimens for culture-proven pathogens are reviewed above in section I.**

C. **Additional issues. Surgical evaluation** is necessary when invasive skin and soft tissue infection is suspected and when cellulitis progresses despite appropriate antibiotic therapy. Approximately **10 days of antibiotic therapy is adequate** for uncomplicated infections. **Adjunctive measures** may include immobilization of involved areas and local application of moist heat.

## PYOMYOSITIS

**Pyomyositis,** a disease increasingly observed in North America, is a term used to describe a purulent infection of muscle [60,61]. Localized trauma to muscle is often observed in patients prior to the development of muscle infection.

I. **Risk factors** include HIV infection, diabetes mellitus, thiamine deficiency, scurvy, parasitic myositis, infection with leptospirosis, certain viral myositis infections, and IgM deficiency [60,61].

II. **The predominant etiologic agent** is ***S. aureus,*** although streptococci, *Neisseria gonorrhoeae, Yersinia enterocolitica, H. influenzae,* Enterobacteriaceae, *Clostridium septicum,* and *Candida albicans* also may cause pyomyositis.

III. **Clinical characteristics.** Patients typically develop muscle pain, local edema, and fever. Examination of the muscle is described as “woody” or indurated. The “purulent” stage develops later. Muscle tenderness is usually present, but fluctuance and inflammation may not be appreciated due to the depth of the infection. Leukocytosis and an elevated erythrocyte sedimentation rate are common, but the muscle enzyme levels are normal. Gram stain and culture of pus is helpful in identifying the etiologic agent. Approximately 5% to 31% of patients will have positive blood cultures [60,61].

IV. **Treatment** consists of drainage of purulent material and pathogen-directed intravenous therapy, usually targeting staphylococci.

## NECROTIZING SOFT TISSUE INFECTIONS

I. **Types.** Necrotizing infections of the soft tissues are described by a variety of terms, including Meleney synergistic gangrene, clostridial cellulitis, nonclostridial anaerobic cellulitis, gas gangrene, and NF [62]. These infections are usually characterized by rapidly spreading destruction of skin, subcutaneous fat, fascia, and muscle with associated systemic toxicity. **Most of these infections are polymicrobial and include mixed aerobic and anaerobic bacteria.**

A. **Meleney synergistic gangrene** describes a progressive and indolent necrotizing infection of the skin and epifascial soft tissues (Color Plate 4.20). This infection is typically seen in postsurgical patients, frequently in association with small bowel or large bowel ostomies. Slowly expanding ulcerations that are painful and surrounded circumferentially by necrotic skin are described. Microaerophilic streptococci, *S. aureus,* anaerobes including *Peptostreptococcus* and *Bacteroides,* and occasionally gram-negative bacilli may be isolated from this mixed infection. Surgical drainage and debridement are necessary. Antibiotics are directed against mixed aerobic and anaerobic flora. Options in adults include penicillin and $\beta$-lactamase inhibitor combinations used alone, such as piperacillin-tazobactam, 3.375 g i.v. every 6 hours; and clindamycin, 600 to 900 mg i.v. every 8 hours, or vancomycin, 15 mg/kg i.v. every 12 hours, plus ciprofloxacin, 400 mg i.v. every 12 hours.

B. **Clostridial anaerobic cellulitis,** another necrotizing infection of the epifascial soft tissue, is usually seen after trauma or surgery. The incubation period is often several days, but the infection, once established, extends quickly. Gas formation is often appreciated, although patients do not appear systemically unstable. Surgical removal of necrotic tissue is mandatory. Penicillin G, 24 million units divided doses i.v. every 24 hours, is recommended for adults. Clindamycin, 900 mg i.v. every 8 hours, or metronidazole, 500 mg i.v. every 6 hours, may be used for penicillin-allergic patients. **Nonclostridial nonaerobic cellulitis** is due to anaerobic bacteria other than clostridia, often in association with other bacteria, including staphylococci, streptococci, and aerobic gram-negative bacilli. Predisposing conditions include diabetes mellitus, and the clinical presentation is similar to clostridial cellulitis. Surgical debridement and broad-spectrum antibiotic coverage is indicated. Recommended antibiotic therapy (adult doses listed) includes imipenem, 500 mg i.v. every 6 hours; a penicillin and $\beta$-lactamase inhibitor combination such as piperacillin-tazobactam, 3.375 g i.v. every 6 hours; or ceftriaxone, 2 g i.v. every 24 hours, plus metronidazole, 500 mg i.v. every 6 hours.

C. **Clostridial gas gangrene** (i.e., clostridial myonecrosis) is caused by the inoculation of clostridial species (e.g., *Clostridium perfringens, C. histolyticum, C. novyi, C. septicum, C. fallax,* and *C. bifermentans*) into necrotic tissue. These infections are often associated with trauma or bowel-associated surgeries (Color Plate 4.21 and 4.22). A spontaneous and nontraumatic form of clostridial myonecrosis is caused by *C. septicum;* predisposing factors for bacteremia with this organism include GI abnormalities (including colon cancer, GI surgery, and diverticulitis), leukemia, lymphoma, neutropenia, and HIV infection. Clostridial myonecrosis has a sudden onset with associated systemic toxicity, hemodynamic instability, and exquisite pain. The wound is often swollen with surrounding pale-colored skin that may later change to a bronzish-discoloration. A malodorous serosanguinous discharge is often appreciated. Vesicles and bullae may develop, and gas may be detected in the affected tissue. The diagnosis should be suspected in the appropriate clinical situations. A Gram stain of tissue or associated exudate may reveal gram-positive bacilli ("box-cars") with a paucity of polymorphonuclear leukocytes. When bacteremia is present, significant hemolysis may be appreciated. Surgical removal of devitalized infected tissue is the cornerstone of therapy. Antibiotic regimens in adults include clindamycin, 900 mg i.v. every 8 hours, plus penicillin, 24 million units i.v. over 24 hours or in divided doses administered every 4 hours; or metronidazole, 500 mg i.v. every 6 hours; or chloramphenicol, 1 g i.v. every 6 hours. **The exact role of hyperbaric oxygen therapy in this setting is unclear, but its use should not preclude or delay necessary surgical debridement** [63,64].

D. **Necrotizing fasciitis** is an infectious disease emergency that refers to widespread destruction of deep subcutaneous tissue and fascia with relative sparing of muscle and skin. Patients with fulminant NF are toxic appearing and often develop multiorgan failure. Other clinical features associated with this infection include severe local pain, lack of skin findings, fever, and evidence of soft tissue gas such as crepitance [65]. Skin manifestations initially include a local cellulitis with progression to diffuse erythema and edema, dusky blue discoloration indicative of necrosis, and often associated bullae formation. By the time cutaneous, fascial, and associated nerve necrosis occurs, localized pain has been replaced by anesthesia. Two types of NF exist: type 1 and type 2 [66].

1. **Type 1 NF** is a polymicrobial infection caused by synergistic anaerobes (especially *Bacteroides* and/or *Peptostreptococcus*), gram-negative aerobic bacilli, and gram-positive aerobes such as group A streptococci and enterococci (Color Plate 4.23). Predisposing factors include surgery, diabetes mellitus, and peripheral vascular disease.
2. **Type 2 NF** is caused by streptococci, usually group A streptococcus (*S. pyogenes*) and, rarely, group B, C, and G streptococci. Predisposing factors for necrotizing infection due to these "flesh-eating bacteria" (group A streptococcus) include blunt trauma, penetrating injuries and minor cuts, varicella infection, intravenous drug use, surgical procedures, burns, exposure to an index case, trauma, and possibly nonsteroidal antinflammatory drugs [67,68]. The incidence of group A streptococcus–associated NF is increasing significantly and is often associated with a toxic shock–like syndrome.
3. **Management.** Prompt and definitive **surgical incision and debridement is essential** to optimizing the outcome. Intraoperative specimens can be used to tailor pathogen-specific therapy. In addition to supportive care, **antibiotic therapy for type 1 NF** in adults can include cefotaxime, 2 g i.v. every 8 hours or ceftriaxone, 2 g i.v. every 24 hours, plus metronidazole, 500 mg i.v. every 6 hours or clindamycin, 900 mg i.v. every 8 hours; or piperacillin-tazobactam, 3.375 g i.v. every 6 hours; or ampicillin-sulbactam, 3 g i.v. every 6 hours; or ticarcillin-clavulanate, 3.1 g i.v. every 4 to 6 hours; or imipenem, 500 mg i.v. every 6 hours. **Recommendations for treatment of type 2 NF** in adults include penicillin G, 4 million units i.v. every 6 hours or 24 million units i.v. over 24 hours plus clindamycin, 900 mg i.v. every 8 hours. Clindamycin is added because its efficacy is not affected by the inoculum or growth phase of group A streptococci, and because of its inhibition of toxin production. Some anecdotal reports also suggest that adjunctive i.v. immunoglobulin may be beneficial [69]. Hyperbaric oxygen therapy also can be considered as adjunctive therapy for NF but is not considered the standard of care [70].

E. **Fournier gangrene** is a form of type 1 NF that classically affects the male genital organs and perineum. Combinations of Enterobacteriaceae, anaerobic streptococci, *S. aureus,* enterococci, $\beta$-hemolytic streptococci, and various anaerobes can be isolated. Although this infection can occur spontaneously, predisposing factors include GU trauma, GU surgery, GU instrumentation, or extension from intraabdominal, perianal, perirectal, or urinary tract infections. Other risk factors may include diabetes, liver disease, and alcohol abuse. Characterized by severe pain and systemic toxicity, an initially localized cellulitis can spread rapidly and invasively to involve the scrotum, penis, perineum, or anterior abdominal wall. Aggressive surgical evaluation with wide debridement and drainage is essential. The testes' separate blood supply prevents necrosis of the testicles and results in a rare need for orchiectomy. Broad-spectrum antimicrobial regimens used for type 1 NF are required to address the polymicrobial nature of this mixed aerobic and anaerobic infection.

II. **Diagnosis.** Studies that may be helpful in the assessment and diagnosis of necrotizing infections of the soft tissues include the following:

A. **Vigilant and serial clinical examinations** are paramount for detecting the progression of disease, development of crepitance, and evolution of necrotic skin lesions.

B. **Soft tissue radiographs and CT scans** can reveal the presence of gas in soft tissues that is not palpable on physical examination. Enterobacteriaceae, anaerobic streptococci, *Bacteroides* species, and clostridia can generate gas within tissues. **MRI** appears to be most sensitive in distinguishing necrotizing from non-necrotizing skin and soft tissue infections [71].

C. **A high index of clinical suspicion of necrotizing skin and soft tissue infections is often needed to precipitate surgical exploration and debridement. Needle aspiration** of suspect lesions may assist with determining the etiology of infection [72]. Early performance and examination of **frozen-section full-thickness soft tissue biopsies** can expedite surgical evaluation and therapy [73]. In NF, a blunt probe typically passes without resistance along the deep fascial planes. Direct visualization of necrotic fascia during surgery is diagnostic.

D. **Gram staining and anaerobic and aerobic culturing of infected tissue or lesion-associated exudate should be performed.** In addition to microbiologic analysis, histopathologic evaluation also should be performed to assist in determining the extent of tissue destruction.

E. **Standard blood cultures also should be obtained.**

F. **Nonspecific laboratory abnormalities can include a leukocytosis with a predominance of neutrophils and its early precursor forms as well as increasing creatine phosphokinase levels.**

III. **Approach to therapy is multidimensional and includes the following:**

A. **Supportive care and hemodynamic stabilization, including adequate nutrition, electrolyte supplementation, fluid resuscitation, and maintenance of adequate organ perfusion pressures and oxygenation are required.**

B. **Early aggressive surgical debridement with possible repeat interventions** is a priority [63].

C. **Antibiotic therapy is essential.** Empiric broad-spectrum antimicrobial therapy to cover mixed aerobic and anaerobic pathogens is recommended. The regimen can be modified when further clinical and microbiologic data become available. Regimens for specific necrotizing infections are detailed earlier in this section.

## GENERAL PRINCIPLES OF WOUND INFECTION MANAGEMENT

Postsurgical and trauma-associated wound infections are well described. Approximately 2% of surgical procedures are complicated by surgical site infections (SSIs). Surgical site infections may be superficial incisional SSIs of the skin and subcutaneous tissue, deep incisional SSIs of the deep soft tissue, fascia, and muscle, or organ space SSIs. They are responsible for approximately 15% of nosocomial infections [74].

I. **Overview of surgical site/wound infections.** A detailed overview and recommendations for prevention of surgical site infections has recently been published by the Centers for Disease Control and Prevention [75]:

A. **Microbiology.** Data from the National Nosocomial Infections Surveillance System reveals that the most common organisms responsible for SSIs are (in descending order): *S. aureus,* coagulase-negative staphylococci, enterococci, *E. coli, P. aeruginosa, Enterobacter* species, *Proteus mirabilis, Klebsiella pneumoniae,* other streptococci, *Candida albicans,* nonenterococcal group D streptococci, other gram-positive aerobes, and *Bacteroides fragilis* [76]. The endogenous bacterial flora of the patient are common pathogens in surgical wound infections. The pathogens isolated are a reflection of the type of operation [75]. Gram-negative bacilli, enterococci, and anaerobes are likely pathogens after entering a GI organ. *S. aureus* and coagulase-negative staphylococci are likely pathogens after cardiac procedures, neurosurgical procedures, and procedures involving placement of grafts, prostheses, or implants. Gram-negative bacilli are likely pathogens after urologic procedures, and gram-negative bacilli, enterococci, group B streptococci, and anaerobes are likely pathogens after obstetric and gynecologic procedures. Surgical team members and instruments also may serve as exogenous sources of SSI-associated pathogens.

B. **Pathogenesis.** The risk for SSIs is directly proportional to the inoculum size and virulence of organisms contaminating the surgical site and inversely proportional to the resistance of the host patient; that is, the presence of foreign material and necrotic tissue or the use of immunosuppressive therapy increase the risk for SSIs.

C. **Patient characteristics** that may increase the risk for SSIs include smoking cigarettes, diabetes mellitus or other immunodeficient states, steroid use, malnutrition, coexistent infections at another body site, microbial colonization, more than 120% of ideal body weight, prolonged preoperative stays, preoperative nasal colonization with *S. aureus,* perioperative transfusion, and very young or very old age [75].

**D. Operation characteristics** that may dictate the risk for development of SSIs include duration of surgical scrub, antisepsis of skin, preoperative shaving and skin preparation, length of operation, perioperative antimicrobial prophylaxis, ventilation of the operating room, sterilization of surgical instruments, surgical technique, and the presence of foreign bodies including drains in the surgical site [75].

**II. Epidemiology.** Three variables are used to reliably predict the risk for development of SSIs. These risk factors include the likelihood that microbes have contaminated the wound site, the length of the surgical procedure, and the general physical status of the patient [77].

**A. Surgical wounds can be divided into the following categories** to assess the risk for microbial contamination [78]:

1. **Clean wounds (class I)** involve noncontaminated skin in which sterile technique is maintained and there is no entry into GI, respiratory or GU tracts. In general, the risk of infection is below 2%. Examples of these procedures include breast tumor excision, thyroidectomy, and herniorrhaphy. Antibiotic prophylaxis is not routinely recommended.
2. **Clean-contaminated wounds (class II)** are created under controlled circumstances when there is entry into body areas that are considered contaminated, i.e., GI, respiratory, or GU tracts. In general, the risk for infection is greater than or equal to 10% in the absence of antibiotic prophylaxis. Examples of these procedures include appendectomy and hysterectomy.
3. **Contaminated wounds (class III)** result from trauma, procedures associated with major breaks in aseptic technique, or spillage from the GI tract and entry into an area of acute inflammation that is not purulent. The risk of infection in this setting approaches 30%, and antibiotic treatment is recommended. Examples include removal of malignancies with inflammation and repair of perforated diverticulum.
4. **Dirty infected wounds (class IV)** include older trauma-associated open wounds, those with gross contamination with devitalized tissue or foreign bodies, and those associated with drainage of frankly purulent material. The risk for infection approaches 40%, and treatment with antibiotics is recommended. Examples include repair of open compound fractures and drainage of intraabdominal abscesses.

**B. The length of operation** is another important independent factor for wound infection assessment. Operations that last longer than the 75th percentile for duration of each specific surgical procedure are associated with increased risk for infection [79]. Abdominal operations also increase the risk for infection [80].

**C. The physical status of the patient** is also important in risk assessment. Patients with severe systemic disease or multiple comorbidities are at increased risk for development of infection [75].

**III. Clinical presentation and evaluation.** The diagnosis of a wound infection can be difficult. Criteria for defining superficial incisional surgical site infections have been proposed by the Centers for Disease Control and Prevention and include purulent drainage from the surgical site, isolation of organisms from aseptically obtained tissue or fluid, and the presence of wound-associated tenderness, swelling, erythema, or warmth [81]. In deep incisional SSIs, purulent drainage, dehiscence of the deep incision, fever, pain, and fluctuance indicative of an abscess are helpful criteria. Malodorous wound discharges or crepitance on physical exam also may be helpful in predicting wound infection. In patients who have systemic signs and symptoms, blood cultures should be obtained.

**IV. Treatment**

**A. Surgical drainage with debridement to remove all foreign material and necrotic, infected tissue are often required.**

**B. Initial antibiotic choices** should be guided by the likely pathogens associated with specific operations or exposures and by initial results of Gram staining from wound-associated exudate or tissue. Pathogen-directed therapy can be instituted once culture results become available. Listed below are choices and doses appropriate for adults with normal renal function.

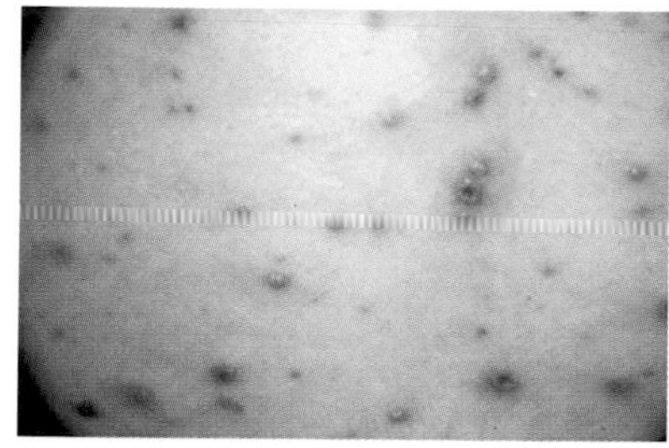

1

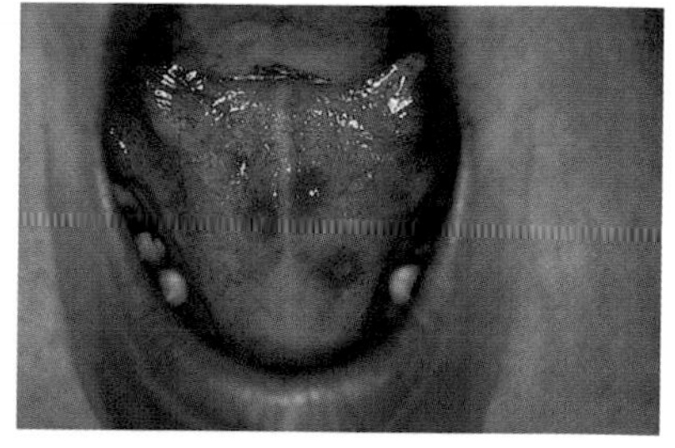

2

**COLOR PLATE 4.1 Varicella.** Close-up view of primary lesions showing vesiculopustules.

**COLOR PLATE 4.2 Hand, foot, and mouth disease.** Papuloulcerative lesions on erythematous bases of the palate.

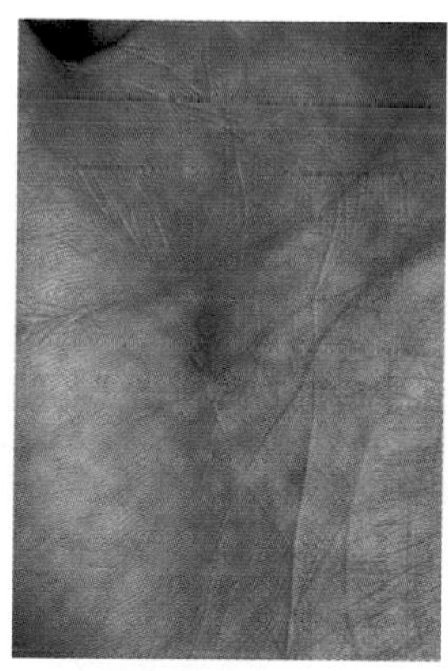

3

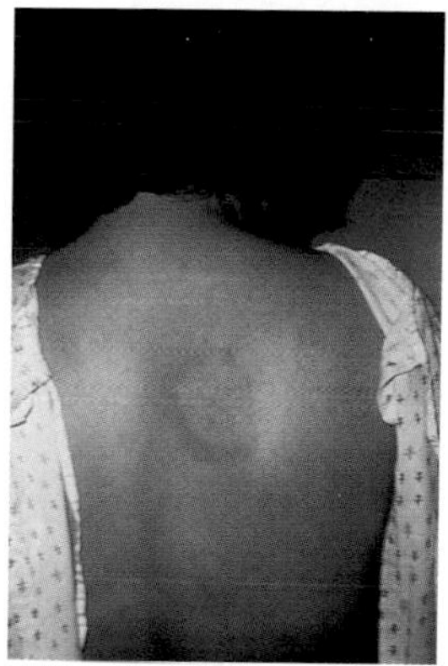

4

**COLOR PLATE 4.3 Hand, foot, and mouth disease.** Two vesicular lesions on erythematous bases on the palm.

**COLOR PLATE 4.4 Lyme disease.** Expanding red annular plaque of Lyme disease.

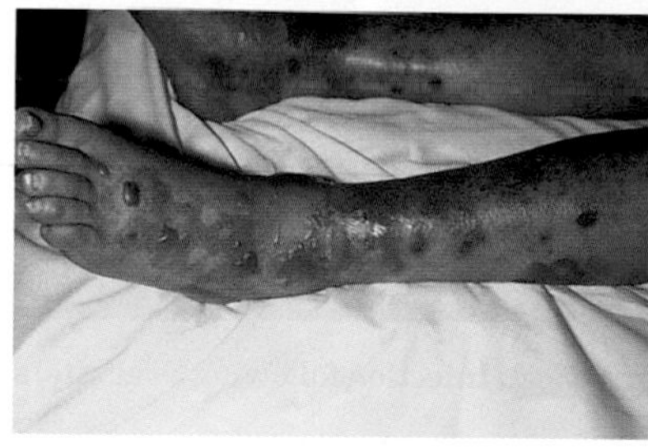

5

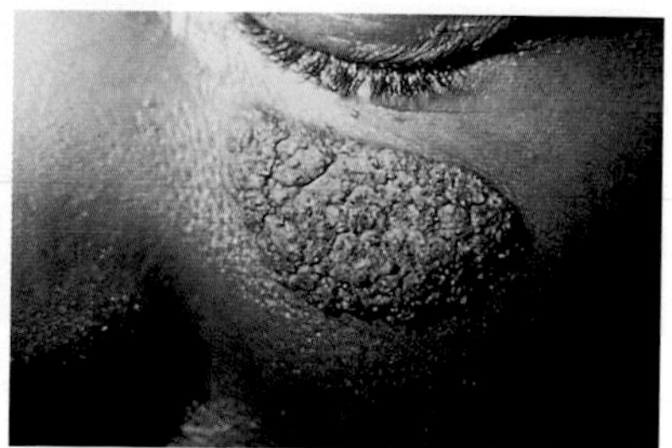

6

**COLOR PLATE 4.5 Vibrio vulnificus.** Hemorrhagic and bullous skin lesions of the feet and lower legs, also showing hemorrhagic necrosis of the dorsum of the left foot.

**COLOR PLATE 4.6 Disseminated blastomycosis.** Verrucous plaque on the upper cheek.

Figures reprinted from Sanders CV, Nesbitt LT, Jr., eds. *The skin and infection: a color atlas and text.* Baltimore: Williams & Wilkins, 1995, with permission.

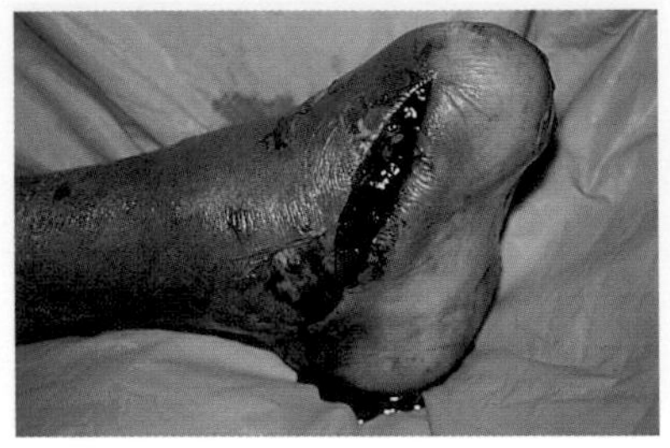
20

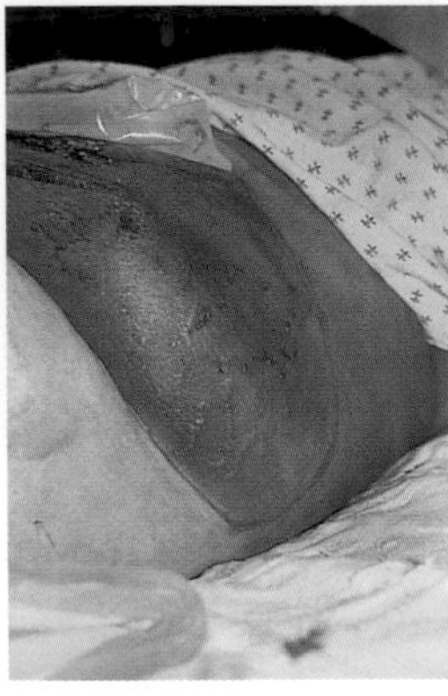
21

**COLOR PLATE 4.20 Synergistic necrotizing cellulitis.** In a patient after transmetatarsal amputation.

**COLOR PLATE 4.21 Clostridial myonecrosis.** Clostridial myonecrosis that developed after resection of a leiomyosarcoma of the rectum.

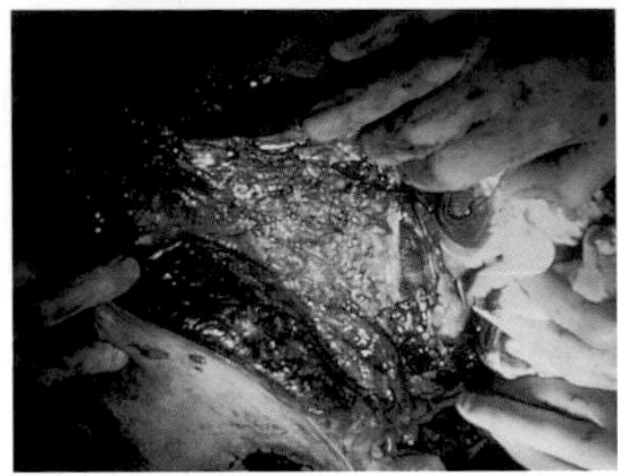
22

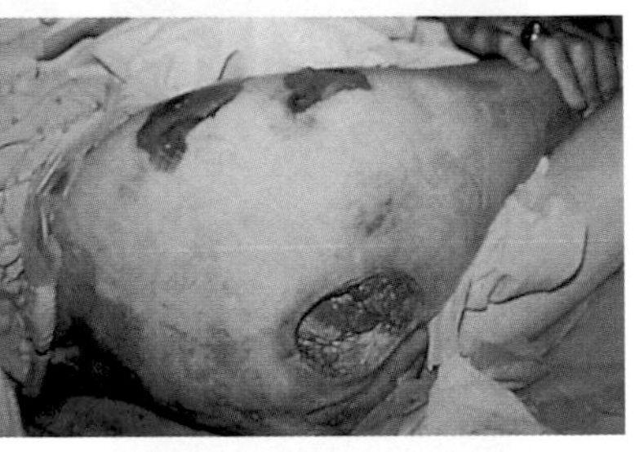
23

**COLOR PLATE 4.22 Clostridial myonecrosis.** Clostridial myonecrosis that developed after resection of a leiomyosarcoma of the rectum.

**COLOR PLATE 4.23 Necrotizing fasciitis and myonecrosis.** A mixed aerobic/anaerobic infection.

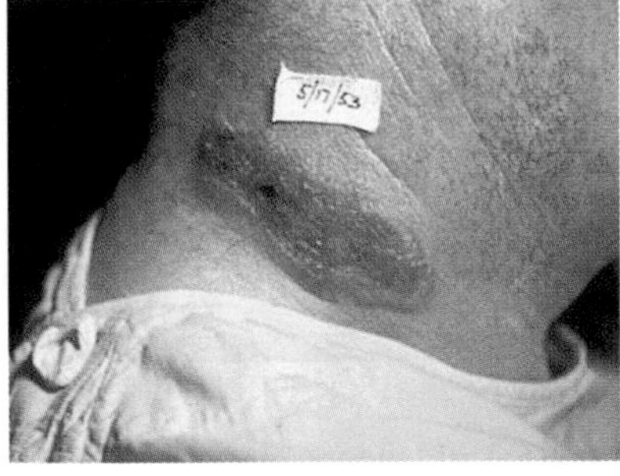

24

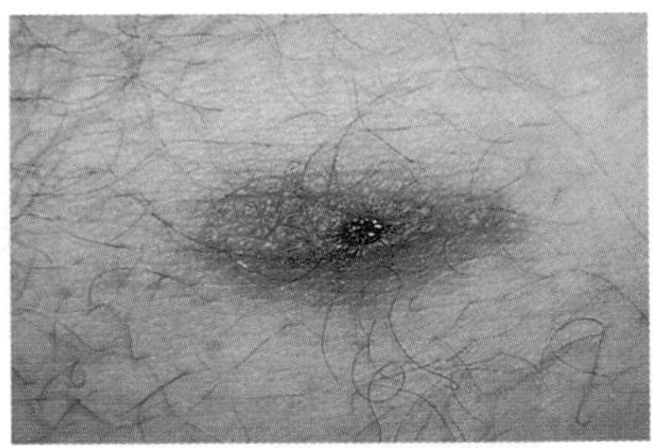
25

**COLOR PLATE 4.24 Anthrax.** Lesion on right side of neck with central eschar. (Courtesy of the Centers for Disease Control and Prevention.)

**COLOR PLATE 4.25 Tularemia.** Erythematous nodule with hemorrhagic necrotic center, close-up view.

Figures 20–23 and 25 reprinted from Sanders CV, Nesbitt LT, Jr., eds. *The skin and infection: a color atlas and text.* Baltimore: Williams & Wilkins, 1995, with permission.

1. **Traumatic wound infection, culture pending.** These infections can be due to numerous combinations of microbes, including staphylococci, streptococci, gram-negative bacilli, and anaerobes including clostridial species. Beta-lactam and $\beta$-lactamase inhibitor combinations such as piperacillin-tazobactam (3.375 g i.v. every 6 hours), ampicillin-sulbactam (3 g i.v. every 6 hours), or ticarcillin-clavulanate (3.1 g i.v. every 4 to 6 hours) are often recommended. Imipenem (500 mg i.v. every 6 hours) also can be considered. A quinolone such as ciprofloxacin (400 mg i.v. every 12 hours) also should be considered if trauma was incurred in water.
2. **Surgical site infection, culture pending**
   - **a.** If surgery involves the GU tract, GI tract, oropharynx, or esophagus, potential microbes include staphylococci, streptococci, enterococci, gram-negative bacilli, and anaerobes. In the hospitalized patient, $\beta$-lactam and $\beta$-lactamase inhibitor combinations such as piperacillin-tazobactam (3.375 g i.v. every 6 hours), ampicillin-sulbactam (3 g i.v. every 6 hours), or ticarcillin-clavulanate (3.1 g i.v. every 4 to 6 hours) are often recommended. Imipenem (500 mg i.v. every 6 hours) or a third-generation cephalosporin such as ceftriaxone (2 g i.v. every 24 hours) in combination with metronidazole (500 mg i.v. every 6 hours) also can be considered.
   - **b.** If surgery does not involve the GU tract, GI tract, oropharynx, or esophagus, potential microbes include staphylococci, streptococci, and gram-negative bacilli. In these patients, $\beta$-lactam and $\beta$-lactamase inhibitor combinations such as piperacillin-tazobactam (3.375 g i.v. every 6 hours), ampicillin-sulbactam (3 g i.v. every 6 hours), or ticarcillin-clavulanate (3.1 g i.v. every 6 hours) are often recommended. Vancomycin (15 mg/kg i.v. every 12 hours) should be considered if methicillin-resistant *Staphylococcus aureus* (MRSA) is suspected or hospital epidemiology documents its increased prevalence.

**V. Prophylaxis**

**A. Antibiotic prophylaxis to prevent SSIs** has proven effective when antibiotics are administered preoperatively. Surgical antibiotic prophylaxis is covered in Chapter 27. The use of antibiotics for management of trauma-associated wounds is less well defined and should be dictated by the clinical signs and symptoms if bacterial contamination has already occurred by the time the wound is evaluated.

**B. Tetanus prophylaxis** is discussed below.

## TETANUS

*Clostridium tetani* is a gram-positive anaerobic spore-forming bacillus that is found in the soil and intestinal contents of many farm animals and even humans. Inoculation of this organism typically occurs in wounds associated with acute injury. These injuries include puncture wounds due to nails, tattooing, body piercing, animal bites, splinters, lacerations, and abrasions. Non–acute injury conditions associated with the development of tetanus include intravenous drug use, diabetes mellitus, otitis media, and tooth infections [82]. Approximately 5% of cases are observed in chronic skin wounds or ulcers [83]. The average incubation period is usually 6 to 12 days and is inversely proportional to the distance between the inoculation site and the central nervous system. After sporulating under anaerobic conditions, this bacteria produces an exotoxin that acts at spinal synapses to interfere with neurotransmission. The resultant effect is uncontrolled muscle contractions and exaggerated reflexes. The clinical case definition for tetanus is the "acute onset of hypertonia and/or painful muscular contractions (usually of the muscles of the jaw and neck) and generalized muscle spasms without other apparent medical cause" [84]. In the United States, a total of 124 cases of tetanus were reported from 1995 through 1997, primarily affecting unvaccinated or insufficiently vaccinated individuals [82]. Individuals over 60 years of age are at increased risk for tetanus, a reflection of decreased prevalence of immunity to tetanus in this age group. Tetanus is completely preventable by effective vaccination.

**I. Prevention**

**A. Primary vaccination series and routine tetanus prophylaxis [85].** Routine recommendations for tetanus prevention include a complete primary vaccination

Table 4.3. Summary Guide to Tetanus Prophylaxis in Routine Wound Management

| History of Adsorbed Tetanus Toxoid (doses) | Clean Minor Wounds | | All Other Wounds[b] | |
|---|---|---|---|---|
| | Td[a] | TIG[a] | Td[c] | TIG |
| Unknown or <3 | Yes | No | Yes | Yes |
| >3[d] | No[e] | No | No[f] | No |

[a] Td, tetanus and diphtheria (adult type) adsorbed toxoids; TIG, human tetanus immunoglobulin (250 units i.m.). (TIG is preferred over equine antitoxin.) When tetanus toxoid and TIG are given concurrently, the adsorbed toxoid is recommended. (Separate syringes and separate sites should be used.)
[b] Such as, but not limited to, wounds contaminated with dirt, feces, soil, saliva, and so on; puncture wounds; avulsions; and wounds resulting from missiles, crushing, burns, and frostbite.
[c] For children under 7 years of age; $DT_aP$ (DT, if pertussis vaccine is contraindicated) is preferred to tetanus toxoid alone. For persons 7 years and older, Td is preferred to tetanus toxoid alone.
[d] If only three doses of fluid toxoid have been received, a fourth dose of toxoid, preferably an adsorbed toxoid, should be given.
[e] Yes, if more than 10 years since last dose.
[f] Yes, if more than 5 years since last dose. (More frequent boosters are not needed and can accentuate side effects.)
Reprinted from Centers for Disease Control. Diphtheria, tetanus, and pertussis. Recommendations for vaccine use and other preventive measures. *MMWR* 1991;40:21–22, with permission.

DTaP (diphtheria and tetanus toxoids and acellular pertussis vaccine) series administered at 2 months, 4 months, 6 months, 15 to 18 months, and 4 to 6 years of age. Subsequent routine tetanus toxoid boosters given as Td (tetanus and diphtheria toxoids) should be administered every 10 years. A complete primary vaccination series for persons greater than or equal to 7 years of age consists of three doses of Td with 4 weeks separating the first and second doses and 6 to 12 months separating the second and third doses; routine toxoid booster should then be administered every 10 years. **Protective antibodies decline over time.** Serologic surveys have shown that in the United States from 1988 to 1991, 72% of adults over 70 years of age did not have immunity to tetanus [86]. **Physicians should not administer toxoid booster to patients with a history of neurologic reaction, urticaria, or anaphylaxis with previous vaccination. Patients with Arthus-like reactions should not be given booster doses at more frequent intervals than every 10 years [85].**

B. **Tetanus prophylaxis in wound management.** Passive immunization with tetanus immunoglobulin (TIG) or active immunization with tetanus toxoid is an important consideration in wound management. U.S. Public Health Service recommendations (Table 4.3) are dictated by the patient's tetanus immunization history and the type of wound [87–90]. Wounds that are nonpenetrating, superficial, less than 6 hours old, linear in configuration, and manifest no associated tissue necrosis or contamination are classified as clean and minor.

II. **Clinical characteristics of tetanus** [88,89]. Several clinical types of tetanus have been described. **Most patients who develop tetanus are diagnosed with generalized tetanus.** Trismus (i.e., lockjaw), a reflection of rigidity of the masseters, is the most common presenting sign. Orbicularis oris rigidity produces the characteristic sardonic smile (*risus sardonicus*). Persistent contractions of the chest and back muscles with flexion of the arms and extension of the lower extremities (i.e., opisthotonos) may develop. Painful generalized muscle contractions can be precipitated by minor sensory stimuli, including noise and touch. Spasm of the larynx or glottis can impair gas exchange and swallowing; difficulty with urination and defecation is another potential complication. The overall mortality rate is approximately 30% and residual neurologic complications are not common in survivors.

**Neonatal tetanus, a form of generalized tetanus,** is seen primarily in undeveloped conditions where tetanus immunization rates for mothers are low and occurs as a result of contamination of the umbilical cord and stump. Infants develop generalized muscle spasms and irritability. **Cephalic tetanus** manifests as cranial nerve dysfunction, usually in the setting of otitis media or other head-associated injuries and infections. Although not common, **local tetanus** is characterized by muscle contractions in the area where the injury occurs.

**III. Diagnosis.** The diagnosis of tetanus is usually made on clinical grounds in patients with a recent history of injury and the new onset of characteristic neurologic findings. Common laboratory studies such as complete blood counts and chemistries are usually normal. With the exception of an elevated opening pressure, lumbar puncture and the cerebrospinal fluid profiles are normal. The microbiologic identification of *C. tetani* from wound specimens is not very sensitive or specific. Radiographic imaging of the central nervous system is unremarkable. The differential diagnosis includes dystonic reactions to neuroleptic drugs, local infection or trauma to the teeth or masseters, hysteria, hypocalcemia, and strychnine poisoning.

**IV. Treatment.** All the following treatment modalities should be instituted [88,90].

- **A. Human tetanus immunoglobulin** administered i.m. is recommended as soon as possible. In general, a single dose of 3,000 to 6,000 units is recommended for children and adults, although a dose of 500 units may be as effective as larger doses [90]. Despite the recommendations of some experts, no increased efficacy has been proven with infiltration of TIG around the area of the wound. In the event that TIG is not available, i.v. immune globulin may be used [90].
- **B.** Because natural infection does not result in immunity, a complete course of active tetanus toxoid immunization is recommended once the patient has recovered.
- **C. If possible, debridement of foreign and necrotic tissue** should be pursued.
- **D. Supportive medical care** should be provided in a quiet environment so that stimuli resulting in spasms or seizures can be minimized. Benzodiazepines and curare-like agents (vecuronium, pancuronium) are indicated for management of spasms or seizures. Mechanical ventilatory support may be required.
- **E. Antibiotic therapy. When compared with penicillin G, metronidazole appears to be more clinically effective for the treatment of tetanus** [91]. Metronidazole, 500 mg i.v. every 6 hours, for 10 to 14 days is recommended for adults. Parenteral penicillin G, 2 million units every 6 hours, is recommended as an alternative choice.

**V. Prognosis.** The overall case fatality incidence for known outcomes among 122 patients in the United States from 1995 through 1997 was 11% [82]. The case fatality incidence in patients 20 to 39 years of age was 2.3%. Patients with tetanus who were 40 to 59 years of age had a case fatality incidence of 16%, increasing to 18% in those greater than 59 years of age.

## POTENTIAL BIOLOGIC WARFARE AGENTS

Events of the new millennium have provided an impetus for physicians to be cognizant of biologic warfare agents. Several of these potential agents produce cutaneous manifestations, including *Bacillus anthracis,* variola major, *Francisella tularensis,* and *Yersinia pestis.* This list is not exhaustive, and the reader is referred to the CDC website (*www.bt.cdc.gov.*) for updated details regarding potential biologic warfare agents.

**I. Anthrax**

- **A. Clinical characteristics [92–97].** Anthrax, a gram-positive sporulating rod, can cause inhalational, GI, and cutaneous infections.
  1. **Inhalational disease** occurs after spores of *Bacillus anthracis* are inhaled. Macrophages in the lung ingest these spores and carry them to mediastinal lymph nodes where they proliferate and produce toxins that result in edema and hemorrhage. After an incubation period of 1 to 7 days, infection classically manifests as a biphasic illness with a prodrome of dry cough, muscle pains, headache, fever, and abdominal pain (i.e., flulike symptoms) followed by a short interval of improvement. Afterward, the fulminant development of severe pulmonary failure, hemodynamic instability, and, in 50% of patients, meningeal inflammation is noted.
  2. **GI disease** develops approximately 2 to 5 days after ingestion of meat that is contaminated with spores. Spores presumably enter through defects in the

mucosal lining of the gut, with ulcerations usually noted in the caecum and ileum and associated mesenteric lymph node inflammation. Patients typically present with nausea, vomiting, abdominal pain, fever, and bloody diarrhea. Ascites also has been reported.

3. **Cutaneous disease** represents the greatest proportion of anthrax infections (>95%). One to 14 days after inoculation, a pruritic, **painless** papule develops that enlarges and then vesiculates. Lesion-associated fluid discharge is often clear to serosanguinous. A brawny, nonpitting, almost gelatinous edema surrounds the vesicle. This lesion then ruptures and develops a necrotic eschar, which can be surrounded by increased edema and numerous vesicles (Color Plate 4.24). The patient presents with fever, particularly if bacteremia is present. Numerous lesions may be observed, typically occurring on the face and extremities.

**B. Epidemiology.** Endemic areas of infection include western Asia and Africa. Anyone exposed to spores can develop disease, and those at greatest risk include individuals who work in industries where there is exposure to goat hair, wool, cashmere, dying cattle, or infected meat. The spectre of bioterrorism has now placed other individuals at risk, including postal/mailroom workers, laboratorians, media personalities, and governmental figures.

**C. Diagnosis of cutaneous anthrax**

1. A complete blood count may reveal a leukocytosis with increased band forms.
2. If inhalational anthrax is suspected, a chest radiograph should be obtained (see Chapter 11).
3. Early identification can be made with Gram staining of blood, cerebrospinal fluid, or cutaneous lesion aspirates or biopsies. These organisms are large, gram positive, encapsulated, and rodlike in appearance.
4. *B. anthracis* can be isolated from routine cultures. Culture of skin lesion aspirates, blood, cerebrospinal fluid, and pleural fluid with routine media can be useful for isolation. Speciation should be pursued to differentiate from other potential pathogens associated with the *Bacillus* species (e.g., *B. cereus*).
5. Serologic antibody testing of acute and convalescent serum is helpful for epidemiologic purposes.
6. Enzyme-linked immunoassays for antigen detection and nucleic acid–based testing such as polymerase chain reaction (PCR) are rapid diagnostic tests available primarily at reference laboratories.

**D. Treatment [94,95,97]**

1. **Recommended initial treatment for inhalational anthrax in adults (including pregnant and immunocompromised patients)** includes ciprofloxacin, 400 mg i.v. every 12 hours or doxycycline, 100 mg i.v. every 12 hours plus 1 or 2 other antibiotics that are active *in vitro* against the implicated strain (i.e., ampicillin, penicillin, clindamycin, clarithromycin, imipenem, vancomycin, rifampin, chloramphenicol). Once the patient is stable, oral monotherapy with ciprofloxacin 500 mg orally twice daily or doxycycline, 100 mg orally twice daily can be used in lieu of intravenous therapy to complete a 60-day course. Steroids can be considered when meningitis or serious edema develops.
2. **Recommended treatment for cutaneous anthrax in adults (including pregnant and immunocompromised patients)** includes ciprofloxacin, 500 mg orally twice daily, or doxycycline, 100 mg orally twice daily for 60 days. If systemic symptoms, extreme edema, or facial/neck edema are present, treat as inhalational anthrax (see above).

**E. Prophylaxis [94,95,97]**

1. **Postexposure prophylaxis recommendations for adults (including pregnant and immunocompromised patients)** include ciprofloxacin, 500 mg orally every 12 hours, or doxycycline, 100 mg orally twice daily. If the isolate is susceptible, amoxicillin, 500 mg orally every 8 hours, or doxycycline, 100 mg orally twice daily, is optimal. The total duration of antibiotics should be 60 days.
2. **Vaccination.** A six-dose anthrax inactivated cell-free vaccine series is used for U.S. military personnel [98,99]. Availability is limited, and its routine use is currently not recommended. If available, vaccine can be offered to persons exposed from a bioterrorist attack along with prolonged antibiotics [95].

**II. Smallpox.** Vaccination against variola major (smallpox) was universally discontinued in 1980. Large scale use of this organism as a biologic warfare agent would likely be devastating in the United States because no American has been vaccinated in over 27 years. Unlike anthrax, person-to-person transmission occurs by droplet nuclei. The case fatality rate is greater than 30% among previously unvaccinated individuals [100,101].

**A. Clinical characteristics [100,101]. The virus is transmitted primarily via droplet nuclei** that embed in the oropharynx or respiratory tract. After an incubation phase of 7 to 17 days, infected individuals develop flulike symptoms, including fever, back pain, and headache. **A rash described initially as maculopapular then develops over 1 to 2 days on the oropharyngeal mucosa, face, and upper extremities (including palms and soles) before centrifugally involving the thorax and lower extremities. The lesions are typically most dense on the face and extremities, and all lesions appear to be at the same stage of evolution.** The rash then develops a vesiculopustular appearance that eventually crusts over after 8 to 14 days, leaving scars that are described as "pitted." Encephalitis and keratitis are possible complications.

In contrast, chickenpox has an incubation period of 2 to 3 weeks with a short prodromal period before a more superficial vesicular rash evolves in a centripetal distribution (albeit rarely involving the palms and soles). The lesions appear every few days and are classically found in different stages of evolution. Crusting of the lesions occurs within 1 week.

**B. Epidemiology.** When smallpox infections existed, occurrences were most common in winter and spring and among younger populations. With no vaccination in the United States for greater than a quarter century, even **vaccinated individuals may be susceptible to smallpox infection due to waning immunity.**

**C. Diagnosis [100].** Fluid from vesiculopustular lesions is evaluated with electron microscopy. The clinical presentation and epidemiologic background combined with the visualization of virions consistent with orthopoxvirus are useful in making a presumptive diagnosis. The diagnosis is confirmed by growth of the virus under specialized conditions and strain characterization by nucleic acid–based techniques such as PCR and restriction fragment length polymorphisms. **Laboratory investigations should be pursued in experienced laboratories with high containment capabilities.**

**D. Preexposure vaccination.** Limited supplies of smallpox vaccine and vaccinia immune globulin exist, but efforts to increase supplies of both will result in a need for reassessment of policy for use in prevention of primary infection. Currently, the CDC controls access to both of these agents. Renewed vaccine production is currently being commissioned by the CDC [100].

**E. Postexposure treatment [100].** No antiviral therapy has proven reliably effective against smallpox infection. When infection develops, care is primarily supportive. In a smallpox outbreak, **all infected individuals should be isolated to prevent human-to-human transmission.** Close contacts of these individuals should be vaccinated and observed, preferably in a domestic setting. Vaccination within 96 hours of exposure appears to prevent infection and improve outcome [102]. Because contaminated laundry from these patients can spread the smallpox virus, autoclaving of sheets and clothes is essential. Disinfection of contaminated inanimate objects with hypochlorite and ammonia is also recommended.

**III. Tularemia.** Quite virulent, only a few organisms of *Francisella tularensis* (tularemia) are required to cause infection. The etiologic agent of "rabbit fever," this small gram-negative coccobacillary organism primarily causes infections in animals. The usual mode of transmission to humans is by contact with contaminated tissues and body fluids or from the bite of an infected tick, mosquito, or deerfly. Much less commonly, the organism is transmitted from animal bites, ingestion, or inhalation.

**A. Clinical characteristics [103–105].** Contingent on numerous factors, including the route of inoculation and the inoculum size, the clinical presentations associated with tularemia are diverse. **The most common type of infection is ulceroglandular disease,** accounting for more than 75% of all tularemia infections. After an incubation period of approximately 3 to 5 days, **a painful pruritic erythematous papule or nodule** develops at the site of inoculation, which typically involves the distal upper extremities. **Localized tender lymphadenopathy** is also appreciated. **The skin lesion ulcerates with a necrotic center** (Color Plate 4.25). Disease onset is sudden, and the patient may appear toxic, with fatigue, fever, and chills. The organisms can disseminate hematogenously from lymph nodes and reside in organs of the reticuloendothelial system.

Release of this organism in an aerosolized form would be the likely transmission route in biologic warfare, and the pleuropulmonary or inhalational form of tularemia would predominate (see Chapter 11).

**B. Epidemiology [103–105].** In nonoutbreak situations, natural infection with tularemia is reported with increased frequency in summer months when ticks are most prevalent. Most cases in the United States are reported from Arkansas, Missouri, Oklahoma, Texas, Utah, and Tennessee. These infections are usually seen in men, perhaps due to increased recreational activities that include hunting or exposure to wild mammals. If used as a biologic weapon, all individuals would be susceptible to *F. tularensis* and health-care providers would need to have heightened clinical suspicion.

**C. Diagnosis [103–105].**

1. Skin and respiratory abnormalities are not specific. Clinical suspicion is important in directing further workup.
2. Gram staining of infected skin or sputum rarely reveals the organism. Direct fluorescent antibody stains are useful in rapid identification of the organism in body fluids or tissue.
3. Special media are needed for cultivation of this organism from pharyngeal, gastric, sputum, and blood specimens, and include cysteine-enriched broth and blood agar, and thioglycollate broth. Buffered charcoal-yeast and chocolate agar also can be used. Laboratorians need to be informed when the diagnosis of tularemia is suspected. Any activity resulting in aerosolization or droplet formation of culture materials mandates biosafety level 3 conditions [103].
4. Serologic tests using microagglutination, tube agglutination, or enzyme immunoassay technology can be used for diagnostic confirmation and epidemiologic studies.
5. Rapid diagnostic tests, including PCR, enzyme-linked immunosorbent assay, and antigen detection assays, exist but are usually available only in specialized reference or research laboratories [106].

**D. Treatment [103].**

1. If an individualized approach can be taken toward the infected adult with tularemia, the preferred choice for treatment is streptomycin, 1 gm i.m. twice daily; gentamicin, 5 mg/kg/day i.m. or i.v. is an acceptable alternative. Treatment length is 10 days. Alternative choices include doxycycline, 100 mg i.v. twice daily for 14 to 21 days; ciprofloxacin, 400 mg i.v. twice daily for 10 days; or chloramphenicol, 15 mg/kg i.v. four times daily for 14 to 21 days.
2. In a mass casualty situation, treatment recommendations for adults include a 14-day course of doxycycline, 100 mg orally twice daily, or ciprofloxacin, 500 mg orally twice daily. Antibiotic susceptibility testing should be pursued in order to direct further therapy. In the setting of inhalational exposure, prophylactic therapy with 14 days of oral doxycycline or ciprofloxacin is recommended.
3. Person-to-person transmission does not occur and isolation of infected individuals is not necessary.

**E. Vaccination.** A live attenuated vaccine for *F. tularensis* exists that has been used for protecting individuals who are at increased risk for infection (e.g., laboratory workers who work with the organism). It is not recommended for postexposure prophylaxis by the Working Group on Civilian Defense [103].

**IV. Plague.** *Yersinia pestis* is the etiologic agent of plague. It has been identified by the Working Group on Civilian Biodefense as a potentially serious biologic warfare agent because of its high case fatality rate, its human-to-human transmissability, and its ability to be administered as an aerosol [107]. The reservoir is typically a rodent, and the usual mode of transmission to humans is by a flea bite.

**A. Clinical characteristics [107–109].** Approximately 2 to 7 days after the bite of a plague-infected flea, approximately 90% of patients develop high fever, malaise, nausea and vomiting, chills, headache, and **tender localized matted lymphadenopathy** (usually axillary, cervical, or inguinal) with overlying erythema known as **buboes,** hence the name **bubonic plague.** Other skin lesions described in bubonic plague include a vesiculopustular lesion at the site of inoculation; petechiae, ecchymoses, and gangrene can develop as complications of bacteremia, sepsis, and disseminated intravascular coagulation.

Approximately 5% of individuals develop a **septicemia** with no development of buboes. The case fatality rate approaches 25% to 50%, and these patients also may present with ecthyma-gangrenosum–like lesions, gangrenous lesions, and petechial-purpuric lesions.

**Pneumonic plague** develops in approximately 5% of patients as a result of the hematogenous spread of bacilli in patients with bubonic or septicemic plague (secondary pneumonic plague) or as a primary process. Primary pneumonic plague occurs in patients who inhale *Y. pestis* when exposed to humans or nonhuman animals with pneumonic plague. These patients present with hemoptysis, cough, shortness of breath, chest pain, fever, malaise, and, occasionally GI disturbances. Complications in patients with a fulminant course include purpura, necrotic skin lesions, and bleeding. Case fatality rates are reported to exceed 50% [109] (see Chapter 11).

**B. Epidemiology [107,108].** Most cases of natural plague are reported from Africa, Asia, Central America, and South America. In the United States, most cases are reported in the summer and early fall from the southwestern states of New Mexico, Colorado, California, or Utah. If used as a biologic agent of terrorism, aerosolized transmission would likely be preferred, resulting in primary pneumonic plague (see Chapter 11).

**C. Diagnosis [107–109]**

1. Clinical suspicion is needed when patients present with suggestive clinical findings.
2. Chest radiography should be performed.
3. Gram staining of aspirates from buboes, sputum, or blood can be helpful in identifying bipolar safety pin–like gram-negative bacilli.
4. The organism can be isolated from standard cultures of blood, sputum, or buboe-associated aspirates. Optimal growth occurs on McConkey or blood agar at 28°C [107]. Laboratorians need to be informed when the diagnosis of plague is suspected. Any activity resulting in aerosolization or droplet formation of culture materials mandates biosafety level 3 conditions [107].
5. Rapid diagnostic confirmatory tests such as PCR, antigen detection, IgM enzyme immunoassay, and immunofluorescence staining are available at reference laboratories, including the CDC.
6. Serologic testing for antibodies is primarily useful for epidemiologic purposes.

**D. Treatment [107]**

1. If an individualized approach can be taken toward the infected adult with plague, the preferred choice for treatment is streptomycin, 15 mg/kg i.m. twice daily, or gentamicin, 5 mg/kg i.m. or i.v. once daily. Alternative choices include doxycycline, 100 mg i.v. twice daily or 200 mg/day i.v.; ciprofloxacin, 400 mg i.v. twice daily; or chloramphenicol 25 mg/kg i.v. as a loading dose followed by 15 mg/kg i.v. four times daily. Treatment length is 10 days and oral therapy can be used once the patient is stable. Gentamicin is preferred for pregnant patients.
2. In a mass casualty setting and for postexposure prophylaxis, preferred recommendations for adults include doxycycline, 100 mg orally twice daily, or ciprofloxacin, 500 mg orally twice daily. The alternative choice is chloramphenicol, 25 mg/kg orally four times daily. Treatment length for a mass casualty setting is 10 days and for postexposure prophylaxis 7 days.
3. Respiratory droplet precautions should be taken in the treatment of all patients with plague until pulmonary involvement is ruled out, or until at least 48 hours of antimicrobial therapy and clinical improvement is observed.

**E. Vaccination.** A formalin-killed vaccine existed (but is no longer available) that was not helpful in preventing primary pneumonic plague [107]. Effective immunizations against pneumonic plague are being pursued.

## ACKNOWLEDGMENT

We thank Tami Hotard, MA, Department of Medicine at Louisiana State University School of Medicine in New Orleans, for her expert editorial contributions.

## REFERENCES

1. Cherry JD. Contemporary infectious exanthems. *Clin Infect Dis* 1993;16:199–207.
2. Chiang WK. Update on emerging infections from the Centers for Disease Control and Prevention. Update: surveillance for West Nile virus in overwintering mosquitoes—New York, 2000. *Ann Emerg Med* 2000;36:61–63.
3. Magill AJ. Fever in the returned traveler. *Infect Dis Clin North Am* 1998;12:445–469.
4. Arndt KA, Jick H. Rates of cutaneous reactions to drugs: a report from the Boston Collaborative Drug Surveillance Program. *JAMA* 1976;235:918–923.
5. Bigby M, Jick S, Jick H, et al. Drug-induced cutaneous reactions: a report from the Boston Collaborative Drug Surveillance Program on 15,438 consecutive inpatients, 1975 to 1982. *JAMA* 1986;256:3358–3363.
6. Roujeau JC, Stern RS. Severe adverse cutaneous reactions to drugs. *N Engl J Med* 1994;331:1272–1285.
7. Lopez FA, Sanders CV. Dermatologic infections in the immunocompromised (nonHIV) host. *Infect Dis Clin North Am* 2001;15:1–32.
8. Dajani AS, Taubert KA, Wilson W, et al. Prevention of bacterial endocarditis: recommendations by the American Heart Association. *JAMA* 1997;277:1794–1801.
9. Durack DT, Lukes AS, Bright DK. New criteria for diagnosis of infective endocarditis: utilization of specific echocardiographic findings. *Am J Med* 1994;96:200–209.
10. Daar ES, Little S, Pitt J, et al. Diagnosis of primary HIV-1 infection. *Ann Intern Med* 2001;134:25–29.
11. Niu MT, Stein DS, Schnittman SM. Primary human immunodeficiency virus type 1 infection: review of pathogenesis and early treatment intervention in humans and animal retrovirus infections. *J Infect Dis* 1993;168:1490–1501.
12. Nesbitt LT Jr. Evaluating the patient with a skin infection—general considerations. In: Sanders CV, Nesbitt LT Jr, eds. *The skin and infection: a color atlas and text.* Baltimore: Williams & Wilkins, 1995:1–13.
13. Sanders CV. Approach to the diagnosis of the patient with fever and rash. In: Sanders CV, Nesbitt LT Jr, eds. *The skin and infection: a color atlas and text.* Baltimore: Williams & Wilkins, 1995:296–305.
14. Sumaya CV. Acute exanthematous disease. In: Pickering LK, Dupont HL, eds. *Infectious diseases of children and adults. A step-by-step approach to diagnosis and treatment.* Menlo Park, CA: Addison-Wesley, 1986:167.
15. Lopez FA, Sanders CV. Fever and rash in the immunocompetent patient. *UpToDate* 2001.
16. Sadick NS. Current aspects of bacterial infections of the skin. *Dermatol Clin* 1997;15:341–349.
17. Barnett BO, Frieden IJ. Streptococcal skin diseases in children. *Semin Dermatol* 1992;11:3–10
18. American Academy of Pediatrics. Group A streptococcal infections. In: Pickering LK, ed. *2000 Red book: report of the Committee on Infectious Diseases,* 25th ed. Elk Grove Village, IL: American Academy of Pediatrics, 2000:526–536.
19. Kaye ET. Topical antibacterial agents. *Infect Dis Clin North Am* 2000;14:321–339.
20. Britton JW, Fajardo JE, Krafte-Jacobs B. Comparison of mupirocin and erythromycin in the treatment of impetigo. *J Pediatr* 1990;117:827.
21. Sadick NS. Bacterial disease of the skin. In: Rakel RE, ed. *Conn's current therapy.* Philadelphia: WB Saunders, 1997:823–828.
22. Maddox JS, Ware JC, Dillon HC. The natural history of streptococcal skin infection: prevention with topical antibiotics. *J Am Acad Dermatol* 1985;13:207.
23. Raz P, Miron D, Colodner R, et al. A 1-year trial of nasal mupirocin in the prevention of recurrent staphylococcal nasal colonization and skin infection. *Arch Intern Med* 1996;156:1109–1112.

24. Zimakoff J, Rosdahl VT, Petersen W, et al. Recurrent staphylococcal furunculosis in families. *Scand J Infect Dis* 1988;20:403–405.
25. Rhody C. Bacterial infections of the skin. *Primary Care* 2000;27:459–473.
26. Meislin HW, Lerner SA, Graves MH, et al. Cutaneous abscesses: anaerobic and aerobic bacteriology and outpatient management. *Ann Intern Med* 1977;87:145–149.
27. Summanen PH, Talan DA, Strong C, et al. Bacteriology of skin and soft tissue infections: comparison of infections in intravenous drug users and individuals with no history of intravenous drug use. *Clin Infect Dis* 1995;20(suppl 2):279–282.
28. Scully BE, et al. Mupirocin treatment of nasal staphylococcal colonization. *Arch Intern Med* 1992;152:353–356.
29. Klempner MS, Styrt B. Prevention of recurrent staphylococcal skin infections with low-dose oral clindamycin therapy. *JAMA* 1988;260:2682–2685.
30. Levy R, Shriker O, Porath A, et al. Vitamin C for the treatment of recurrent furunculosis in patients with impaired neutrophil functions. *J Infect Dis* 1996;173:1502–1505.
31. Reinherz RP, Hong DT, Tisa LM, et al. Management of puncture wounds in the foot. *J Foot Surg* 1985;24:288–292.
32. Fitzgerald RH, Cowan JD. Puncture wounds of the foot. *Orthop Clin North Am* 1975;6:965–972.
33. Raz P, Miron D. Oral ciprofloxacin for treatment of infection following nail puncture wounds of the foot. *Clin Infect Dis* 1995;21:194–195.
34. Chisholm CD, Schlesser JF. Plantar puncture wounds: controversies and treatment recommendations. *Ann Emerg Med* 1989;18:1352–1157.
35. Lavery LA, Walker SC, Harkless LB, et al. Infected puncture wounds in diabetic and nondiabetic adults. *Diabetes Care* 1995;18:1588–1591.
36. Chudnofsky CR, Sebastian S. Special wounds. Nail bed, plantar puncture, and cartilage. *Emerg Med Clin North Am* 1992;10:801–822.
37. Goldstein EJC. Current concepts on animal bites: bacteriology and therapy. *Curr Clin Top Infect Dis* 1999;19:99–111.
38. Weiss HB, Friedman DI, Coben JH. Incidence of dog bite injuries treated in emergency departments. *JAMA* 1998;279:51–53.
39. Talan DA, Citron DM, Abrahamian FM, et al. Bacteriologic analysis of infected dog and cat bites. *N Engl J Med* 1999;340:85–92.
40. Cummings P. Antibiotics to prevent infection in patients with dog bite wounds: a meta-analysis of randomized trials. *Ann Emerg Med* 1994;23:535–540.
41. Noah DL, Drenzek CL, Smith JS, et al. Epidemiology of human rabies in the United States, 1980 to 1996. *Ann Intern Med* 1998;128:922–930.
42. Centers for Disease Control and Prevention. Human rabies prevention—United States, 1999: recommendations of the Advisory Committee on Immunization Practices (ACIP). *MMWR* 1999;48:1–21.
43. Callahan EF, Adal KA, Tomecki KJ. Cutaneous (non-HIV) infections. *Dermatol Clin* 2000;18:497–508.
44. Farley MM, et al. A population based assessment of invasive disease due to group B streptococci in nonpregnant adults. *N Engl J Med* 1995;328:1807.
45. Farley MM. Group B streptococcal disease in nonpregnant adults *Clin Infect Dis* 2001;33:556–561.
46. Jackson LA, Hilsdon R, Farley MM, et al. Risk factors for group B streptococcal disease in adults. *Ann Intern Med* 1995;123:415–420.
47. Drapkin MS, et al. Bacteremic *Haemophilus influenzae* type b cellulitis in the adult. *Am J Med* 1977;63:449–452.
48. Bodey GP. Dermatologic manifestations of infections in neutropenic patients. *Infect Dis Clin North Am* 1994;8:655–675.
49. El Baze P, Thyss A, Vinti H, et al. A study of nineteen immunocompromised patients with extensive skin lesions caused by *Pseudomonas aeruginosa* with and without bacteremia. *Acta Dermatol Venereol (Stockh)* 1991;71:411–415.
50. McManus AT, Mason AD Jr, McManus WF, et al. Twenty-five year review of *Pseudomonas aeruginosa* bacteremia in a burn center. *Eur J Clin Microbiol* 1985;4:219–223.
51. Chuang YC, Yuan CY, Liu CY, et al. *Vibrio vulnificus* infection in Taiwan: report of

28 cases and review of clinical manifestations and treatment. *Clin Infect Dis* 1992;15:271–276.

52. Slaven EM, Lopez FA, Hart SM, et al. Myonecrosis caused by *Edwardsiella tarda:* a case report and case series of extraintestinal *E. tarda* infections. *Clin Infect Dis* 2001;32:1430–1433.
53. American Thoracic Society. Diagnosis and treatment of disease caused by nontuberculous mycobacteria. *Am J Respir Crit Care Med* 1997;156(suppl):1–25.
54. Sachs MK. The optimum use of needle aspiration in the bacteriologic diagnosis of cellulitis in adults. *Arch Intern Med* 1990;150:1907–1912.
55. Traylor KK, Todd JK. Needle aspirate culture method in soft tissue injections: injection of saline vs. direct aspiration. *Pediatr Infect Dis J* 1998;17:840–841.
56. Hook EW III, Hooton TM, Horton CA, et al. Microbiologic evaluation of cutaneous cellulitis in adults. *Arch Intern Med* 1986;146:295–297.
57. Perl B, Gottehrer NP, Raveh D, et al. Cost-effectiveness of blood cultures for adult patients with cellulitis. *Clin Infect Dis* 1999;29:1483–1488.
58. Berger Sadow K, Chamberlain JM. Blood cultures in the evaluation of children with cellulitis. *Pediatrics* 1998;101:1–4.
59. Struk DW, Munk PL, Lee MJ, et al. Imaging of soft tissue infections. *Radiol Clin North Am* 2001;39:277–303.
60. Christin L, Sarosi GA. Pyomyositis in North America: case reports and review. *Clin Infect Dis* 1992;15:668–677.
61. Walling DM, Kaelin WG Jr. Pyomyositis in patients with diabetes mellitus. *Rev Infect Dis* 1991;13:797–802.
62. Bisno AL, Stevens DL. Streptococcal infections of skin and soft tissues. *N Engl J Med* 1996;334:240–245.
63. McHenry CR, Piotrowski JJ, Petrinic D, et al. Determinants of mortality for necrotizing soft-tissue infections. *Ann Surg* 1995;221:558–563.
64. Stevens DL, Bryant AE, Adams K, et al. Evaluation of therapy with hyperbaric oxygen for experimental infection with *Clostridium perfringens. Clin Infect Dis* 1993;17:231–237.
65. Green RJ, Dafoe DC, Raffin TA. Necrotizing fasciitis. *Chest* 1996;110:219–229.
66. Giuliano A, Lewis F, Hadley K, et al. Bacteriology of necrotizing fasciitis. *Am J Surg* 1977;134:52–57.
67. Stevens DL. Could nonsteroidal antiinflammatory drugs (NSAIDs) enhance the progression of bacterial infections to toxic shock syndrome? *Clin Infect Dis* 1995;21:977–980.
68. Chen JL, Fullerton KE, Flynn NM. Necrotizing fasciitis associated with injection drug use. *Clin Infect Dis* 2001;33:6–15.
69. Perez CM, Kubak PM, Cryer HG, et al. Adjunctive treatment of streptococcal shock syndrome using intravenous immunoglobulin: case report and review. *Am J Med* 1997;102:111–113.
70. Riseman JA, Zamboni WA, Curtis A, et al. Hyperbaric oxygen therapy for necrotizing fasciitis reduces mortality and the need for debridements. *Surgery* 1990;108:847–850.
71. Rahmouni A, Chosidow O, Mathieu D, et al. MR imaging in acute infectious cellulitis. *Radiology* 1994;192:493–496.
72. Uman SJ, Kunin CM. Needle aspiration in the diagnosis of soft tissue infections. *Arch Intern Med* 1975;135:959–961.
73. Stamenkovic I, Lew PD. Early recognition of potentially fatal necrotizing fasciitis: the use of frozen-section biopsy. *N Engl J Med* 1984;310:1689–1693.
74. Emori TG, Gaynes RP. An overview of nosocomial infections, including the role of the microbiology laboratory. *Clin Microbiol Rev* 1993;6:428–442.
75. Mangram AJ, Horan TC, Pearson ML, et al. Guideline for prevention of surgical site infection. *Infect Control Hosp Epidemiol* 1999;20:247–280.
76. Centers for Disease Control and Prevention. National Nosocomial Infections Surveillance (NNIS) report, data summary from October 1986-April 1996, issued May 1996. A report from the National Nosocomial Infections Surveillance (NNIS) System. *Am J Infect Control* 1996;24:380–388.

77. SHEA, APIC, CDC, SIS. Consensus paper on the surveillance of surgical wound infections. *Infect Control Hosp Epidemiol* 1992;13:599–605.
78. Simmons BP. Guideline for prevention of surgical wound infections. *Infect Control* 1982;3:185–196.
79. Culver DH, Horan TC, Gaynes RP, et al. Surgical wound infection rates by wound class, operative procedure, and patient risk index. National Nosocomial Infections Surveillance System. *Am J Med* 1991;91(suppl 3B):152–157.
80. Haley RW, Culver DH, Morgan WM, et al. Identifying patients at high risk of surgical wound infection: a simple multivariate index of patient susceptibility and wound contamination. *Am J Epidemiol* 1985;121:206–215.
81. Horan TC, Gaynes RP, Martone WJ, et al. CDC definitions of nosocomial surgical site infections: a modification of CDC surgical wound infections. *Infect Control Hosp Epidemiol* 1992;13:606–608.
82. Bardenheier B, Prevots R, Khetsuriani N, et al. Tetanus surveillance—US, 1995–1997. *MMWR* 1998;47:1–13.
83. Sanford, J. Tetanus—forgotten but not gone. *N Engl J Med* 1995;332:812.
84. Centers for Disease Control and Prevention. Case definitions for infectious conditions under public health surveillance. *MMWR* 1997;46:1–55.
85. ACIP. Update on adult immunization recommendations of the Immunization Practices Advisory Committee (ACIP). *MMWR* 1991;40;1–52.
86. Gergen PJ, McQuillan GM, Kiely M, et al. A population-based serologic survey of immunity to tetanus in the US. *N Engl J Med* 1995;332:761–766.
87. ACIP. Diphtheria, tetanus, and pertussis: recommendations for vaccine use and other preventive measures—recommendations of the Immunization Practices Advisory Committee (ACIP). *MMWR* 1991;40.
88. Weinstein L. Tetanus. *N Engl J Med* 1974;289:1293–1296.
89. Centers for Disease Control and Prevention resource page. Tetanus. In: Health Topics, 6th ed. 2000;5:57–66. Available at: *www.cdc.gov/nip/publications/pink/tetanus.pdf.* Accessed August 2, 2001.
90. American Academy of Pediatrics. Tetanus. In: Pickering LK, ed. *2000 Red book: report of the Committee on Infectious Diseases,* 25th ed. Elk Grove Village, IL: American Academy of Pediatrics, 2000:563–568.
91. Ahmadsyah I, Salim A. Treatment of tetanus: an open study to compare the efficacy of procaine penicillin and metronidazole. *BMJ* 1985;291:648–650.
92. Pile JC, Malone JD, Eitzen EM, et al. Anthrax as a potential biological warfare agent. *Arch Intern Med* 1998;158:429–434.
93. Dixon TC, Meselson M, Guillemin J, et al. Anthrax. *N Engl J Med* 1999;341:815–826.
94. Swartz MN. Recognition and management of anthrax—an update. *N Engl J Med* 2001;345:1621–1626.
95. Inglesby TV, O'Toole T, Henderson DA, Bartlett JG, et al. Anthrax as a biological weapon 2002: updated recommendations for management. *JAMA* 2002;287:2236–2252.
96. Meselson M, Guillemin J, Hugh-Jones M, et al. The Sverdlovsk anthrax outbreak of 1979. *Science* 1994;266:1202–1208.
97. Centers for Disease Control and Prevention. Update: investigation of bioterrorism-related anthrax and interim guidelines for exposure management and antimicrobial therapy, October 2001. *MMWR* 2001;50:909–919.
98. US Department of Defense. Anthrax vaccine, military use in Persian gulf region [press release]. Washington, DC: US Department of Defense, September 8, 1998.
99. Michigan Department of Public Health. Anthrax vaccine absorbed. Lansing: Michigan Dept of Public Health, 1978.
100. Henderson DA, Inglesby TV, Bartlett JG, et al. Smallpox as a biological weapon: medical and public health management. *JAMA* 1999;281:2127–2137.
101. Fenner F, Henderson DA, Arita A, et al. *Smallpox and its eradication.* Geneva, Switzerland: World Heath Organization, 1988:1460.
102. Dixon CW. *Smallpox.* London, England: J&A Churchill Ltd,1962:1460.
103. Dennis DT, Inglesby TV, Henderson DA, et al. Tularemia as a biological agent: medical and public health management. *JAMA* 2001;285:2763–2773.

104. Evans ME, Gregory DW, Schaffner W, et al. Tularemia: a 30-year experience with 88 cases. *Medicine* 1985;64:251–269.
105. Jester JD. Skin signs of infectious zoonoses. In: Sanders CV, Nesbitt LT Jr, eds. *The skin and infection: a color atlas and text.* Baltimore: Williams & Wilkins,1995:277.
106. Grunow R, Splettstoesser W, McDonald S, et al. Detection of *Francisella tularensis* in biological specimens using a capture enzyme-linked immunosorbent assay, an immunochromatographic handheld assay, and a PCR. *Clin Diag Lab Immunol* 2000;7:86–90.
107. Inglesby TV, Dennis DT, Henderson DA, et al. Plague as a biological weapon: medical and public health management. *JAMA* 2000;283:2281–2290.
108. Jester JD. Skin signs of infectious zoonoses. In: Sanders CV, Nesbitt LT Jr, eds. *The skin and infection: a color atlas and text.* Baltimore: Williams & Wilkins, 1995:278.
109. Centers for Disease Control and Prevention. Fatal human plague. *MMWR* 1997;278: 380–382.

# 5. BONE AND JOINT INFECTIONS

Rathel L. Nolan and Stanley W. Chapman

## OSTEOMYELITIS

**Osteomyelitis** is an inflammatory process in bone and bone marrow. Most often caused by pyogenic bacteria, it may also be caused by mycobacteria and fungi. Multiple classification schemes have been devised.

I. **Acute versus chronic osteomyelitis.** This clinical distinction is sometimes difficult to make. The following definitions provide a useful separation with implications in therapy and prognosis [1].
   A. **Acute** cases are those in their **first presentation.** The history may be short (days for hematogenous osteomyelitis) or long (weeks to months for contiguous osteomyelitis).
   B. **Chronic** osteomyelitis cases are those that have relapsed in a site of previously identified disease. Chronic osteomyelitis is more difficult to treat successfully and carries a poorer prognosis. Surgical intervention is usually required.

II. **Pathogenic classification.** The most useful clinical classification is based on pathogenesis, as outlined by Waldvogel et al. [1].
   A. **Hematogenous osteomyelitis** results from bacteremic seeding of bone.
   B. **Contiguous-focus osteomyelitis** is caused by spread from an adjacent area of infection, as in postoperative infections, direct inoculation from trauma, or extension from an area of soft tissue infection.
   C. **Peripheral vascular disease-associated osteomyelitis** usually occurs in patients with diabetes with or without large vessel insufficiency.

III. **Other classifications.** Other classification systems are based on special circumstances such as (a) a unique age group (neonatal osteomyelitis), (b) a unique clinical setting (e.g., intravenous drug use or sickle cell disease), (c) a microbiologic cause (gram-negative, anaerobic, etc.), or (d) an unusual anatomic location (e.g., vertebral osteomyelitis). A clinicopathologic classification proposed by Cierny et al. [2] facilitates comparison of therapeutic outcomes.

IV. **The changing spectrum of osteomyelitis.** Previously, osteomyelitis was predominantly hematogenous and caused by *Staphyloccoccus aureus.* **Presently, osteomyelitis occurs most frequently from contiguous-focus spread after an open fracture or reconstructive surgery or as a result of vascular insufficiency.** There has been an increase in nosocomial cases, as well as an increase in unusual bacterial causes, including gram-negative bacilli, anaerobes, and mixed infections. Increasing prevalence of antimicrobial-resistant bacteria markedly complicates therapy [3,4].

## HEMATOGENOUS OSTEOMYELITIS

Hematogenous osteomyelitis occurs most often in rapidly growing bone, which explains the increased frequency among children. Recent series note an increasing frequency in older patients, so that the age distribution is bimodal [5–7]. Hematogenous osteomyelitis may occur in any bone, but the long bones (i.e., femur, tibia, and humerus) are most frequently involved in children. Older patients tend to have more vertebral involvement.

I. **Pathophysiology and patient age.** The pathophysiology and clinical presentation are age related [8].
   A. **Children.** In children aged 1 to 16 years, disease is most frequent in the metaphysis of long bones (Fig. 5.1). This is believed to result from sluggish blood flow through a sinusoidal venous system, a deficiency of phagocytic cells in this region, and poor collateral circulation. The susceptibility of this region to trauma may also play a role. A history of antecedent trauma may be obtained in 30% of patients with hematogenous osteomyelitis.
      1. **Anatomic considerations.** In childhood, there are no anastomotic vascular channels between the metaphyseal and epiphyseal circulations (Fig. 5.1). The epiphyseal growth plate acts as a barrier, resulting in the spread of infection laterally and rupture of the cortex into the subperiosteal space, with subsequent subperiosteal abscess formation.

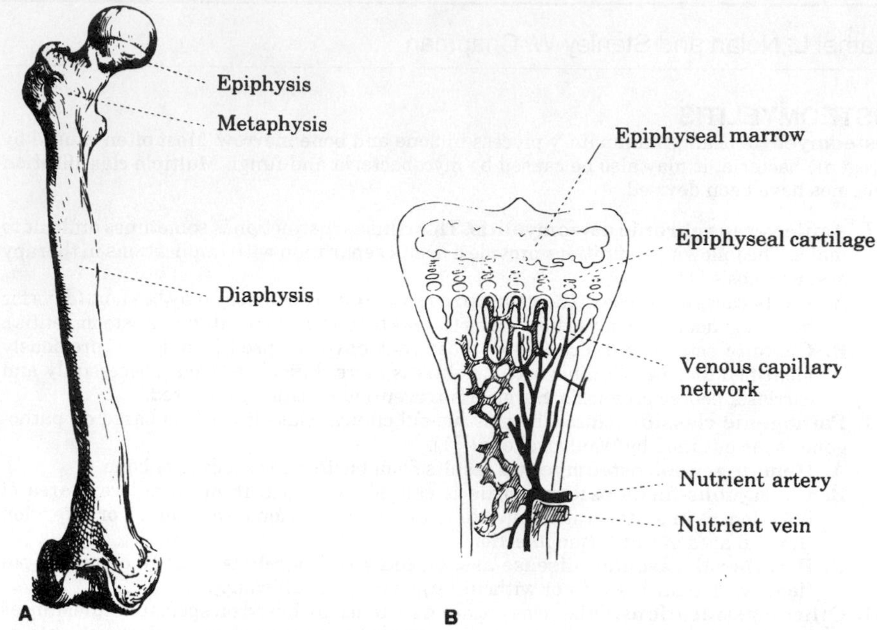


**FIG. 5.1 A:** Femur, showing diaphysis, metaphysis, and epiphysis. **B:** Vascular supply of a long bone in the area of the metaphysis and epiphysis. (From Waldvogel FA, Medoff G, Swartz MN. Osteomyelitis: a review of clinical features, therapeutic considerations, and unusual aspects. *N Engl J Med* 1970;282:198–206, with permission.)

When infection has reached the subperiosteal space, it may spread longitudinally along the shaft of the bone or rupture through the periosteum. Separation of the bone from the periosteum is accompanied by exuberant periosteal growth and new bone formation. This circumferential new bone covering is referred to as an **involucrum.**

2. **Sequestrum.** In the course of the infection, segments of bone may lose vascular supply due to such factors as increased pressure, acidic pH, and effects of leukocytic enzymes. Such an area of **devitalized bone** is referred to as a **sequestrum.** These areas must be surgically removed because they **act as foreign bodies** and will prevent effective antibiotic therapy.
3. **Associated septic arthritis.** As previously noted, the epiphyseal growth plate serves as a barrier to the spread of infection. In children, osteomyelitis complicated by septic arthritis occurs only in joints in which the metaphysis is intracapsular, such as the proximal femur and proximal humerus.

**B. Neonates and infants younger than 1 year**

1. **Septic arthritis is common.** In contrast to older children, at this age anastomotic channels exist between the metaphyseal and epiphyseal circulations. **Infection may spread rapidly to the epiphysis and joint space, resulting in septic arthritis** (Fig. 5.1).
2. Involvement of the epiphyseal growth plate may result in growth deformities.
3. The metaphyseal cortex is immature. Spreading exudate rapidly reaches the periosteum and ruptures it, infecting the surrounding periosteal tissues. This accounts for the frequent soft tissue abscesses found in this age group.

**C. Adults.** Hematogenous osteomyelitis is less common in adults. Initial localization is to the subchondral region of bone or the vertebrae.

1. **Anatomic considerations.** In adults, vascular connections between metaphyseal and epiphyseal vessels result after resorption of the growth cartilage. Spread of infection to the joint space by this route can occur. The periosteum is bound tightly to bone and has less osteoblastic activity so that subperiosteal abscess and involucrum formation are unusual.
2. **Vertebral osteomyelitis.** This is most common in adults 50 years of age and older and accounts for the bimodal age distribution of hematogenous osteomyelitis.

**D. Special considerations**

1. **Sickle cell disease.** The bone infarcts and marrow thrombosis that complicate this hemoglobinopathy predispose to bacterial localization in bone. Osteomyelitis at multiple sites is common. *Salmonella* species and *Staphylococcus aureus* are the most common pathogens [9,10].
2. **Intravenous drug users and hemodialysis patients.** Repeated intravascular injections in intravenous drug users and vascular access infections in hemodialysis patients result in an increased frequency of hematogenous osteomyelitis [11,12].

## II. Microbiologic features

**A. Staphylococci**

1. ***S. aureus*** remains the most common pathogen, but the percentage of hematogenous osteomyelitis due to *S. aureus* has declined from 80% to 90% of cases in the past to 40% to 60% in recent years [5–7].
2. ***Staphylococcus epidermidis*** causes approximately 5% or fewer cases of disease. Because inadvertent contamination of cultures by this organism is frequent, its real role as a pathogen is unknown.

**B. Streptococci**

1. **Group A** streptococcal isolates cause disease in children and occasionally in adults.
2. **Group B** streptococci are common in neonates and may be a more common pathogen in this age group than are staphylococci [13]. Group B streptococci also occur in diabetic patients.

**C. *Haemophilus influenzae*** is now an infrequent cause of osteomyelitis in the United States due to widespread usage of conjugated polysaccharide vaccine [14].

**D. Gram-negative enteric bacilli** (e.g., *Escherichia coli, Salmonella,* and *Klebsiella* species) most often occur in adults and account for 10% to 15% of cases of hematogenous osteomyelitis. **Certain patient groups are predisposed** to hematogenous osteomyelitis caused by gram-negative organisms: neonates (Enterobacteriaceae), patients with sickle cell disease *(Salmonella),* and intravenous drug users (*Pseudomonas*). Patients with underlying chronic illness, including chronic renal disease, alcoholism, diabetes, and malignancy, also have an increased risk of gram-negative infections [15].

**E. Anaerobes** are uncommon causes of hematogenous osteomyelitis [16].

**F. Polymicrobial infections** can occur [17].

**G. Mycobacteria,** particularly tuberculosis, can cause vertebral osteomyelitis. This entity is discussed in section IV under Special Forms of Osteomyelitis, below.

**H. Fungi** can cause an indolent form of osteomyelitis and may have a propensity to involve bones of the feet or hands and the vertebrae. For further discussion, see section V under Special Forms of Osteomyelitis, below. Individual fungal infections are also discussed in Chapter 17.

## III. Clinical manifestations

**A. Acute symptoms.** The classic presentation of hematogenous osteomyelitis is sudden onset of bone pain and toxicity with high fevers, rigors, and diaphoresis. Most patients present with symptoms of less than 3 weeks' duration. Children and infants may be symptomatic for less than 1 week. Extensive use of antibiotics for conditions other than osteomyelitis may modify the clinical presentation. Atypical presentations are more common and uncommon sites more frequent [5,7,18].

1. **Localized signs** include limitation of motion of the involved extremity, soft tissue swelling, erythema, warmth, and point tenderness over the involved area.

2. **Systemic manifestations** are seen in 50% or fewer patients. They may include fever, chills, night sweats, malaise, anorexia, and weight loss.
3. **Minimal vague symptoms** may be reported by as many as 40% of patients for 1 to 2 months. This indolent course is likely in the following situations:
   a. **Primary subacute pyogenic osteomyelitis (Brodie abscess).** This is characterized by the indolent formation of abscess, most frequently occurring at the metaphysis of long bones. Local pain is the most common presenting symptom [19].
   b. **Vertebral osteomyelitis** in the adult. See section II under Special Forms of Osteomyelitis, below.
   c. **Pelvic osteomyelitis.** The presenting symptoms for this condition may be unusual, including abdominal pain, gait disturbance, and sciatica [20].

B. **Neonatal osteomyelitis** is often a difficult diagnostic problem. Soft tissue swelling, localized tenderness, and decreased motion of an extremity (pseudoparalysis) are the most common findings. See Chapter 3, section VI.A under Selected Specific Infections in the Newborn, for further discussion.

C. **Sickle cell disease.** The **diagnosis** of osteomyelitis in these patients is **challenging,** because the clinical signs and symptoms mimic those associated with an acute pain crisis. For this reason, **blood cultures should always be obtained in patients presenting with an apparent acute sickle pain crisis.**

IV. **Diagnosis.** Various cultural, hematologic, serologic, and radiographic procedures are helpful in making a clinical diagnosis and substantiating the etiology of disease. In an era of increasing prevalence of unusual and antimicrobial-resistant pathogens, vigorous attempts should be made to establish the specific etiology of disease. Availability of the pathogen for susceptibility testing is essential to guide antimicrobial therapy. The diagnostic modalities described below are applicable to all forms of osteomyelitis.

A. **Blood cultures** should be drawn in all patients with suspected osteomyelitis. Approximately 50% of patients with acute hematogenous osteomyelitis have positive blood cultures. Neonatal osteomyelitis is often associated with bacteremia. Blood cultures are less likely to be positive in other forms of osteomyelitis, such as contiguous focus disease, chronic osteomyelitis, and osteomyelitis associated with peripheral vascular disease. Two to four separate sets of blood cultures should be drawn.

B. **Leukocytosis** can occur, but normal or minimally elevated leukocyte counts are common and cannot be used to exclude the diagnosis of osteomyelitis.

C. **The erythrocyte sedimentation rate** (ESR) may be normal early in the disease but will usually rise as the disease progresses. A normal ESR does not exclude the diagnosis. An elevated ESR provides an excellent parameter by which to monitor therapeutic response, becuase the ESR progressively declines with successful therapy.

D. **C-reactive protein** level is usually elevated at the time of presentation and falls with successful therapy. It is used with ESR to monitor therapeutic response [21].

E. **Radiographic evaluation** is very helpful and should be done routinely in all patients. The radiologic changes may lag days to weeks behind the clinical presentation. The usual sequence of radiologic changes is as follows:
   1. **Roentgenograms are normal** early in the disease course. Bone scans may detect abnormalities at this stage. However, if bone destruction is present, no further imaging may be necessary [22].
   2. **Soft tissue swelling and subperiosteal elevation** are the earliest abnormalities. These findings may be subtle and may not appear until 10 to 14 days after onset of symptoms. Serial radiographic examinations may be required.
   3. **Lytic changes** on roentgenography do not appear until 30% to 50% of bone is removed and usually are not detectable until 2 to 6 weeks after the onset of disease.
   4. **Sclerotic changes** appear weeks after onset of illness due to delay in mineralization after new matrix formation. Sclerotic changes associated with periosteal new bone formation (involucrum) denote a more chronic process.
   5. **Other diseases** may cause osteomyelitis-like changes on radiographs: chronic venous stasis of the lower extremities with periosteal reaction involving the tibia; osteoid osteoma; and neoplasms involving bone.

F. **Radionuclide scanning** is most helpful early in the course of acute disease, before the development of roentgenographic changes. Positive scans may be seen as early as 24 hours after the onset of symptoms.

1. Scanning with **technetium** radiophosphates is most commonly used, especially the **three-phase scans.** Radiation exposure approximates that of a standard roentgenogram and is not contraindicated in pediatric patients. Because of the possibility of referred pain or multicentric disease, whole body images should be obtained in patients with suspected osteomyelitis. More detailed radiographic examination of suspicious areas may then be obtained. Other processes, such as primary and metastatic tumor, osteonecrosis, arthritis, cellulitis, and abscess, may cause false-positive examinations.
2. Indium-labeled leukocyte scans have excellent sensitivity and specificity for diagnosis of early osteomyelitis. They are more technically challenging and result in a substantially higher radiation dose than do technetium bone scans [23].

G. **Magnetic resonance imaging (MRI)** is sensitive for the early detection of osteomyelitis. It is used to identify soft tissue infection, distinguish soft tissue from bone marrow involvement, and distinguish between abscess and cellulitis. It is the preferred modality for diagnosis of vertebral osteomyelitis. MRI is also useful in evaluation of treatment failures and in planning surgical intervention. Computed tomography (CT) provides excellent images of bone cortex and is used for biopsy localization [24].

H. **Needle aspirations** from soft tissue collections, subperiosteal abscesses, and intraosseous lesions to obtain culture material should be performed in all patients in whom an unequivocal etiologic diagnosis is not obtained by blood cultures. Needle aspiration is preferably performed before administration of antibiotics.

I. **Joint fluid analysis** should be undertaken if there is an associated joint effusion. The aspirated effusion should be analyzed for cellular content, chemistries, Gram stain, and culture.

J. **Open biopsy** should be entertained in patients in whom a specific etiology is not obtained by blood cultures or needle aspiration, especially when tuberculosis, fungi, or malignancy is suspected. Biopsy material should be submitted for histopathologic examination and appropriate cultures.

V. **Initial therapy.** Initial therapy should be aggressive. Inadequate therapy of acute osteomyelitis may result in relapse and development of chronic disease.

A. **Principles of antibiotic use.** Antibiotics are the mainstay of therapy, although few prospective comparative trials exist on which to base selection of antibiotics and determine duration of therapy. Special aspects of their use are as follows.

1. **Parenteral agents** are generally recommended as the initial treatment to ensure compliance and also to achieve optimal bone levels. Because antibiotic penetration into bone is low, these agents are usually given in high doses. Antibiotic penetration is related to bone vascularity (i.e., cancellous bone levels are higher than cortical bone). Antibiotic levels are also higher in diseased bone. The penicillins, cephalosporins, gentamicin, vancomycin, clindamycin, and ciprofloxacin achieve concentrations in bone that exceed the minimal inhibitory concentration (MIC) of most susceptible organisms causing osteomyelitis [25–27]. In relationship to serum levels achieved, clindamycin and ciprofloxacin penetrate bone especially well. As such, these latter two agents have proven useful in the treatment of all forms of osteomyelitis, whether administered intravenously or as oral therapy.
2. **Oral antibiotic therapy**

a. **Children.** It is common practice to treat acute hematogenous osteomyelitis in children with oral antibiotics after an initial course of parenteral therapy. Patients are treated with intravenous antibiotics for 5 to 10 days. After a favorable clinical response is noted, the patient is switched to high dose oral therapy, which is continued for at least 3 more weeks. **Several aspects of oral therapy deserve special emphasis.**

(1) The **causative organism** must be available for study and proven susceptible to the oral agents chosen.
(2) Appropriate surgical debridement or drainage must be performed.
(3) **Compliance must be ensured.** If there is any doubt as to the patient's

strict compliance with therapy, outpatient treatment must be abandoned [28].

(4) **Monitoring of serum bactericidal levels** is advocated by some experts to ensure adequate gastrointestinal absorption and adequate serum concentrations [29].

(5) **Patients should be without significant underlying diseases.**

(6) Prolonged follow-up is needed, because disease may recur years after an apparent cure.

**b. Adults.** It is our practice to complete a full course (i.e., 4–6 weeks) of intravenous antibiotics for the initial therapy of most adults with acute hematogenous osteomyelitis. We try to avoid oral therapy in adult patients because of the lower antibiotic concentrations that are achieved in bone. An exception to this exists, however, for the usage of oral quinolones for osteomyelitis, especially that due to gram-negative pathogens. The clinical outcomes of patients with osteomyelitis treated with ciprofloxacin and ofloxacin were reported as similar to those of patients treated with intravenous antibiotics alone [30,31]. It should be noted, however, that the patient cohorts treated were relatively small. As a result of these and other studies, oral ciprofloxacin has been recommended for "step-down" therapy for adults with osteomyelitis after 10 to 14 days of intravenous antibiotics. Before changing to oral therapy, the necessary surgical management should be performed and clinical improvement should be evident. As for osteomyelitis in children, susceptibility of the pathogen to the quinolones must be demonstrated and compliance with therapy must be assured. We usually continue oral treatment for another 4 to 6 weeks after completion of intravenous antibiotics. No *in vitro* or clinical efficacy data exist for the use of the newer quinolones (i.e., levofloxacin, gatifloxacin, and moxifloxacin) in the treatment of osteomyelitis. Some recommend the addition of rifampin to a quinolone regimen to enhance the efficacy of both agents (synergy) and to reduce the development of drug-resistant bacteria. The combination of a quinolone and rifampin has proven useful in the treatment of prosthetic joint infections as outlined later in this chapter. Other antibiotics, such as clindamycin and trimethoprim-sulfamethoxazole, have been used successfully for the oral treatment of osteomyelitis. We recommend infectious disease consultation for osteomyelitis patients being considered for oral therapy.

3. **Bactericidal agents** are preferred.
4. ***In vitro* susceptibility** studies performed against the causative organism aid in the selection of appropriate therapy. **Careful susceptibility studies are essential in this disease because of the prolonged therapy required.** Antibiotic combinations, which may have additive toxicities, are best avoided unless clearly indicated based on susceptibility data. This again emphasizes the need to obtain the etiologic pathogen for susceptibility studies.
5. **Use of serum bactericidal levels to monitor** therapeutic efficacy is advocated by some experts. In this technique the patient's serum is obtained immediately before and after antibiotic administration. Serial dilutions of the serum are then tested for bactericidal activity against the offending pathogen. It was initially anticipated that this test might predict therapeutic success or failure early in the course of treatment. The real value of the test is unknown, however, due to lack of a standardized protocol and absence of large clinical studies to support its use [29].
6. **Prolonged therapy** for acute hematogenous osteomyelitis is important. Antibiotics must be administered for a minimum of 4 to 6 weeks. Cure rates of greater than 90% are expected. Administration of oral antibiotics as follow-up therapy in patients receiving adequate courses of parenteral therapy does not improve outcome when given for acute osteomyelitis [1].
7. **Evaluation of initial therapeutic response.** Failure of the patient to show clinical improvement within 48 to 72 hours should prompt reevaluation. Diagnostic and therapeutic surgery may be necessary.

**B. Initial therapy while awaiting cultures (Table 5.1)**

1. Adults

Table 5.1. Empiric Initial Therapy of the Seriously Ill Patient with Acute Osteomyelitis

| Patient Age | Likely Pathogens | Therapy[a] |
|---|---|---|
| Neonates and infants <2 mo old | *Staphylococcus aureus,* enteric gram-negative bacilli, group B streptococci | Penicillinase-resistant semisynthetic penicillin (PRSP) (e.g., oxacillin,)[b,c] plus cefotaxime |
| Children | | |
| Without hemoglobinopathy | *S. aureus* | PRSP or first-generation cephalosporin or clindamycin or vancomycin[c] |
| With hemoglobinopathy | *S. aureus, Salmonella* species | PRSP plus cefotaxime[c] |
| Adults | *S. aureus* and enteric gram-negative bacilli in high-risk patients[d] | PRSP. In high-risk patients, add third-generation cephalosporin or aminoglycoside[c,e] |

[a]Dosages are discussed in Table 16.2 and in Chapters 3 and 28.
[b]Nafcillin should be avoided in the premature and in the very young infant, because the child's hepatic excretion may be deficient. If on Gram staining of a needle aspiration of the involved bone gram-negative organisms are seen, cefotaxime is initially suggested. See Chapter 3.
[c]In the patient with a history of delayed penicillin allergy, a first-generation cephalosporin is substituted for a PRSP. In a patient with immediate allergy to penicillin, vancomycin or clindamycin may be substituted. If MRSA is suspected, vancomycin is used.
[d]High-risk patients include intravenous drug users, hemodialysis patients, diabetics, and patients with underlying debilitating diseases.
[e]A third-generation cephalosporin (e.g., ceftriaxone) with PRSP (to ensure optimal *S. aureus* therapy) may be used in patients in whom an aminoglycoside is contraindicated or undesirable and in whom *Pseudomonas* species are not suspected. If MRSA is a concern, intravenous vancomycin can be used while awaiting susceptibility data.

a. After cultures are obtained, antistaphylococcal therapy, usually with a penicillinase-resistant semisynthetic penicillin, is recommended for cases of uncomplicated hematogenous osteomyelitis. In patients with histories of delayed penicillin reactions, a first-generation cephalosporin may be used. In patients with histories of immediate penicillin reactions, clindamycin is recommended. If methicillin-resistant *S. aureus* (MRSA) is suspected, administration of vancomycin is appropriate while awaiting susceptibility data.

b. **When gram-negative organisms are suspected** (see section II.D, above), an antistaphylococcal agent plus a third-generation cephalosporin or ciprofloxacin or an aminoglycoside may be used.

2. **Children.** In children less than 2 months of age a penicillinase-resistant penicillin plus cefotaxime is recommended for coverage of *S. aureus,* enteric gram-negative bacilli, and group B streptococci. An identical regimen is recommended in children with sickle cell disease to provide coverage for both *S. aureus* and *Salmonella* species. In children older than 2 months of age without associated hemoglobinopathy, empiric therapy is directed toward *S. aureus* with a penicillinase-resistant penicillin or first-generation cephalosporin or clindamycin or vancomycin as described in section 1.a. above.

C. **Specific antibiotics and alternatives for commonly used agents are shown in** Table 5.2.

D. **Surgery**

1. **When treated with appropriate doses of antibiotics, most cases of hematogenous osteomyelitis are cured without surgery.** Outcomes are better if therapy is begun within 3 to 5 days after the onset of symptoms. It is nonetheless important for an orthopedic surgeon to follow these patients to help assess the future need for surgery.

Table 5.2. Therapy of Osteomyelitis Directed at Specific Pathogens

| Pathogen | Antibiotic of Choice[a,b] | Alternative Antibiotics[c] |
|---|---|---|
| *Staphylococcus aureus* | | |
| Methicillin-susceptible | Penicillinase-resistant semisynthetic penicillin (e.g., nafcillin or oxacillin) (adults: 9–12 g/d; children: 200 mg/kg/d) | First-generation cephalosporin (e.g., cefazolin) (adults: 4 g/d; children: 100 mg/kg/d)[c] or clindamycin (adults: 1.8–2.4 g/d; children: 20–40 mg/kg/d) |
| Methicillin-resistant | Vancomycin (adults: 2 g/d; children 40 mg/kg/d)[d] | |
| *Streptococcus pyogenes* (group A streptococci) | Aqueous penicillin G (adults: 12–18 million units/d; children: 200,000–3000,000 units/kg/d) | First-generation cephalosporin or clindamycin[e] |
| *S. agalactiae* (group B streptococci) | Aqueous penicillin G (as for group A streptococci) | First-generation cephalosporin[e] or vancomycin[f] |
| *Salmonella* species | Ceftriaxone or cefotaxime[g] | Ciprofloxacin[h] |
| *Pseudomonas aeruginosa* | Piperacillin or similar agent plus aminoglycoside[i] | Ciprofloxacin[h] |
| *Escherichia coli* | Ceftriaxone or cefotaxime | Ciprofloxacin[h] |
| *Klebsiella pneumoniae* | Ceftriaxone or cefotaxime | Ciprofloxacin[h] |
| *Bacteroides fragilis* | Metronidazole or clindamycin | Ampicillin-sulbactam, imipenem |
| Anaerobic and microaerophilic streptococci | Aqueous penicillin G (as for Streptococci) | First-generation cephalosporin |

[a] **The daily intravenous dosage recommendations listed are for adults and children older than 4 weeks with normal renal function.** See Chapter 3 for dosage recommendations in neonates and infants younger than 4 weeks. See Chapter 27 for a further discussion of antibiotics.
[b] High-dose intravenous therapy is recommended for acute osteomyelitis.
[c] The first-generation cephalosporins are more active against *S. aureus* than are the second- and third-generation cephalosporins.
[d] Due to poor penetration of vancomycin into bone, some experts add oral rifampin in therapy of susceptible strains. (Adults, 600 mg/d; children, 20 mg/kg/d).
[e] In dosages shown for methicillin-susceptible *S. aureus.*
[f] In dosages shown for methicillin-resistant *S. aureus.*
[g] For dosages, infectious diseases consultation is suggested. See Chapter 27.
[h] Use of ciprofloxacin may prevent extended hospitalization in puncture wound osteomyelitis in adults. Flouroquinolones should not be used in children, teenagers, or pregnant females. Infectious diseases consultation is advised. See Chapter 27.
[i] An aminoglycoside and a penicillin derivative active against *P. aeurginosa* are used together for synergy.

2. **Indications for surgery** include the following:
   a. **Diagnosis.** Diagnostic aspiration should be routinely performed in osteomyelitis unless blood cultures unequivocally provide the pathogen.
   b. **Hip joint involvement** (osteomyelitis of the femoral metaphysis). Drainage must be done early in these cases because of the likelihood of rupture of the cortex and spread of infection into the hip joint.
   c. **Neurologic complications** of vertebral or cranial osteomyelitis. See section II.D.3 under Special Forms of Osteomyelitis, below.
   d. **Poor or no response to therapy.** When patients fail to respond clinically after 48 to 72 hours of therapy, a drainage procedure may be necessary. Surgical drainage most often is needed in patients with disease caused by gram-negative enteric bacilli. A subperiosteal collection of pus that does not respond to therapy also requires drainage. Cultures should be obtained on all surgical specimens.
   e. **Sequestra. These should be removed surgically.**

**E. Monitoring therapeutic response**

1. **Signs and symptoms.** Successful therapy is indicated by resolution of fever, local tenderness, and erythema.
2. **ESR.** If the ESR was elevated initially, it should decline with appropriate therapy; however, it may not return to normal on completion of successful therapy.
3. **Elevated C-reactive protein.** Elevated levels of C-reactive protein should also fall toward the normal range with successful therapy.
4. **Radiography.** Radiographic improvement may lag behind clinical improvement. Serial roentgenograms must be interpreted cautiously. We usually repeat a roentgenogram 2 to 3 weeks into the course of therapy and at the end of therapy in uncomplicated cases. A radiograph obtained 2 to 3 months after completion of antibiotic therapy provides a useful baseline if disease recurs.
5. **Serial bone scans.** These should not be used to monitor response to therapy. Bone scans may remain positive months after clinical cure because healing bones absorb radiotracers.

**VI. Prognosis.** The prognosis for cure in patients with uncomplicated acute hematogenous osteomyelitis is good. Prognosis is, however, related to a variety of factors, including the causative organism, the duration of symptoms before therapy, patient age, and the duration of antibiotic treatment.

**A. Adequate antibiotic therapy** is essential. There is a 10% to 20% recurrence rate in patients treated for acute hematogenous osteomyelitis [28]. Recurrences are more common in adult patients and also patients who have received less than optimal therapy.

**B.** Patients with hematogenous osteomyelitis due to gram-negative organisms appear to have a higher rate of recurrence [32].

**C. The best opportunity for cure is with initial therapy.** Of patients with recurrent disease, only 50% were cured after complete surgical debridement and 4 to 6 weeks of intravenous antibiotics [1]. **Acute osteomyelitis must be vigorously and adequately treated to prevent the development of chronic infection.**

## CONTIGUOUS-FOCUS OSTEOMYELITIS

Contiguous-focus osteomyelitis due to spread from an adjacent focus of infection has some special characteristics that require emphasis.

**I. Clinical setting**

**A. Postoperative infections** constitute many cases of contiguous-focus osteomyelitis.

1. **Open reduction of closed fractures** is the most common predisposing surgical procedure.
2. **Less common predisposing surgeries** include craniotomies, prosthetic hip and other reconstructive joint surgery, disk surgery, tumor resections, and sternotomy for open heart surgery. These infections can be complicated by the use of foreign materials, including metal, plastic, and bone cement, which serve as a nidus of infection that is resistant to antibiotic therapy.

**B. Contamination of bone** occurring at the time of an open fracture is also common [4].

**C. Contiguous soft tissue infections,** with spread to the bone, can involve any site.

1. Osteomyelitis also may occur by spread from an infected tooth socket or sinuses, skin ulcerations, wounds, or decubitus ulcers and from infections introduced by foreign bodies (e.g., puncture wounds).
2. Osteomyelitis frequently occurs in bone underlying pressure ulcers and is particularly difficult to diagnose. Bone biopsy may be useful [33].

**D. Puncture wounds** uncommonly cause osteomyelitis, particularly of the small bones of the feet.

**II. Microbiologic features.** These infections **often are mixed,** because the adjacent wound infections are commonly due to mixed pathogens.

**A. Staphylococci**

1. ***S. aureus*** is the most common isolate. Approximately 50% to 60% of cases involve *S. aureus,* especially when disease involves the long bones, hip, and vertebrae. However, *S. aureus* may not be the only pathogen present.
2. ***S. epidermidis*** must also be considered a pathogen, especially when associated with prosthetic joints. These infections frequently have an indolent course, manifested primarily as constant pain after implantation [34].

**B. Gram-negative bacteria** often are involved in mixed infections. *Pseudomonas* and other gram-negative bacteria are associated with the osteomyelitis secondary to puncture wounds [35]. *Pasteurella multocida* infection may occur after cat or dog bites [36].

**C. Anaerobic infections** have been underestimated because of poor culture techniques. Anaerobes may be involved in osteomyelitis of the long bones subsequent to trauma and fracture, osteomyelitis related to peripheral vascular disease, pelvic osteomyelitis due to spread from decubitus ulcers, or osteomyelitis of cranial and facial bones due to spread from a contiguous soft tissue source.

**D. Osteomyelitis after open fractures** may be due to unusual organisms. Contamination caused by soil may cause infection with *Nocardia, Clostridia,* or *Bacillus* species, whereas fresh water contamination predisposes to *Aeromonas* or *Plesiomonas* disease [4].

**III. Clinical manifestations.** Most patients follow an **indolent course** and are diagnosed within 1 to 2 months of the onset of disease. Delay in diagnosis often occurs in postoperative infections. This is related in part to the use of prophylactic or postoperative antibiotics, disease due to atypical organisms of low pathogenicity, and the presence of foreign material.

**A. Presenting symptoms** include fever, regional soft tissue swelling, erythema, and warmth. Purulent drainage from wounds and sinus tracts is common in both the acute and chronic forms.

**B. Site of involvement** may affect the presentation. Osteomyelitis of cranial bones often lacks signs or symptoms of disease, whereas infection of the long bones and pelvis often presents with fever and pain.

**IV. Diagnosis**

**A. Blood cultures** are infrequently positive. Nevertheless, two or three blood cultures should be obtained.

**B. Leukocyte counts** are commonly normal or minimally elevated.

**C.** The **ESR and C-reactive protein** levels may be elevated, but normal levels do not exclude the diagnosis.

**D. Radiographic evaluation.** In patients with osteomyelitis secondary to a contiguous focus of infection the diagnosis often is delayed, and roentgenographic changes are likely to be detectable at the time of presentation. Such findings may be difficult to interpret due to radiographic changes associated with the precipitating event (e.g., fracture, prosthetic devices, pressure-related change in bone in decubitus ulcers). Serial examinations by a radiologist usually are most helpful in these cases.

**E. Technetium radiophosphate bone scans** may be difficult or impossible to interpret in this setting because of adjacent inflammation and infection or postoperative changes [37]. Other techniques, such as MRI (if a metal prosthesis is not present), may be helpful [24].

**F. Cultures of wounds and draining sinuses are not as helpful as bone cultures.** In patients with draining sinuses or wounds, the interpretation of cultures is complicated because there may be multiple isolates or isolates of low pathogenicity or cultures may be sterile. Cultures of wounds and sinus tracts do not correlate well with those performed on underlying infected bone. A definitive bacteriologic diagnosis requires careful cultures of bone either by needle aspiration or by open biopsy. Needle biopsy for histopathologic and culture confirmation of osteomyelitis under pressure sores is preferred before instituting antibiotic therapy [33,38].

**G. Open biopsy** may be necessary in those patients who have had an unacceptable response to therapy or in whom needle aspiration is indicated but cannot be performed.

**V. Therapy.** Treatment of contiguous osteomyelitis is **less successful** than treatment of the acute hematogenous forms. Relapse may occur in 40% to 50% of cases [1,5–7,39]. **Surgery is an essential aspect of therapy in this disease.**

A. **Poor therapeutic response.** This is a result of a number of factors, including (a) the longer duration of infection before treatment; (b) the presence of foreign bodies after reconstructive orthopedic procedures; (c) the presence of devitalized bone in postfracture cases; (d) the increased frequency of mixed infections, which may not be adequately diagnosed or treated; and (e) malnutrition and chronic illness in patients with pressure ulcers.

B. **Antibiotic therapy**

1. **The basic principles** of antibiotic use (discussed under Hematogenous Osteomyelitis, above) are true also for contiguous-focus osteomyelitis. Because of the high frequency of mixed infections, **it is critical to obtain good specimens for culture** so that antibiotics can be directed against true pathogens rather than wound colonizers.
2. Selection of **specific antibiotics** depends on the results of susceptibility studies. Common dosage schedules are shown in Table 5.2.
3. The ideal **duration of therapy** for this form of osteomyelitis is unknown. Each case is affected by many variables, such as the site of involvement, the adequacy of surgical debridement, underlying chronic illness of the patient, and the presence of a foreign body and whether it can reasonably be removed.
   a. **Prosthetic device-related infections are discussed later in this chapter.**
   b. **Wound-associated infection (without prosthetic devices).** In general, we usually treat these patients with 4 to 6 weeks of parenteral antibiotics based on susceptibility studies of the causative organism. Because of the poor prognosis of this form of osteomyelitis, we frequently extend our therapy by changing to an oral agent. There is no proof, however, that longer courses of therapy improve outcome.

   As discussed in the treatment of hematogenous osteomyelitis, "step-down" to an oral antibiotic (i.e., clindamycin or ciprofloxacin, with or without rifampin) is an option in selected patients. Infectious disease consultation is recommended in these difficult cases.

C. **Surgery.** Wounds or abscesses must be adequately debrided or drained. Sequestra must be removed, because they act as foreign bodies and decrease the likelihood of cure. Surgery usually is necessary early in these cases to obtain diagnostic material. Further debridement may be necessary if clinical response is slow. Whether prosthetic devices should be surgically removed is discussed later in this chapter.

D. **Monitoring response.** See section V.D. under Hematogenous Osteomyelitis, above.

## OSTEOMYELITIS ASSOCIATED WITH PERIPHERAL VASCULAR DISEASE

Most patients with osteomyelitis associated with peripheral vascular disease are diabetic. Osteomyelitis does occur, however, in patients with severe atherosclerosis or vasculitis in the absence of diabetes. Most patients are older than 50 years, and the bones of the toes and feet are most often involved. **For a separate discussion of soft tissue infections without obvious osteomyelitis in the diabetic foot, see later in this chapter.**

I. **Pathophysiology.** Neuropathy is present in most diabetic patients with foot disease predisposing to mechanical or thermal injuries. There is **tissue ischemia** such that ulcers occurring as a result of trauma heal poorly, become chronic, and frequently extend into bone. **Antibiotics penetrate poorly into these ischemic areas, frequently necessitating surgical debridement** [40].

II. **Microbiologic features.** Most wound or sinus drainage cultures and most surgical bone specimens reveal a mixed flora of gram-positive organisms, gram-negative organisms, and anaerobes [41,42].

A. **Common mixed infections.** Staphylococci are most frequently isolated followed in frequency by streptococci and aerobic gram-negative bacilli. Polymicrobial disease is frequent.

B. **Anaerobes.** The role of anaerobes is debated. Presence of long-standing disease and tissue necrosis increases the likelihood of anaerobic disease [41,42].

III. **Clinical manifestations.** Few patients have systemic symptoms, and sepsis is rare.

A. **Local signs and symptoms predominate,** including swelling and erythema. Pain may be absent in patients with advanced neuropathy. Osteomyelitis occurs from extension from cutaneous ulcers occurring over bony prominences. Osteomyelitis is more likely the more chronic, deeper, and wider the ulcer. Crepitus of the soft tissues may be present due to either aerobic or anaerobic infection. Foul odor may be due to the presence of anaerobes or necrotic tissue [40,42].

B. **Long-standing diabetic complications** are often the predominant findings. These include neuropathy, diminished or absent arterial pulses, skin and nail changes, retinopathy, and nephropathy. The presence of such complications may adversely affect disease outcome [40,42].

IV. **Diagnosis**

A. **Blood cultures** are seldom positive. Fever occurs most often in bacteremic patients.

B. **Leukocyte counts** are usually normal.

C. **ESRs** are usually markedly elevated. A normal ESR in a diabetic patient with a toe or foot ulcer does not, however, rule out osteomyelitis.

D. On **radiographic evaluation,** diagnosis of osteomyelitis is **often difficult.** Diabetics may have bony changes on routine roentgenography as a result of peripheral vascular disease and neuropathic osteoarthropathy [40]. These changes may be difficult to differentiate from true osteomyelitis. Consultation with an experienced radiologist is indicated.

E. **Other imaging modalities**

1. **Technetium-99m bone scans** have low specificity in the presence of underlying neuropathic osteoarthropathy.
2. **Indium-111–labeled** leukocyte scanning is more specific for infection but may be difficult to interpret if there is overlying soft tissue infection.
3. **MRI** is superior to CT and probably has superior specificity and sensitivity to the above [23,24].

F. **Ulcers with bone exposed,** detected either by visualization or by use of blunt probing, should be treated as if there were underlying osteomyelitis. The ability to see bone or reach it by probing has a high specificity and positive predictive value in diagnosing osteomyelitis, but the sensitivity and negative predictive value are low. If bone cannot be detected by probing and plain radiographs do not suggest osteomyelitis, treatment can be aimed at a soft tissue infection [43].

G. **Bone biopsy** remains the definitive modality for diagnosis of osteomyelitis. Percutaneous biopsy is performed using an approach avoiding infected tissue to prevent contamination of cultures or introduction of bacteria into uninfected bone. Specimens should be submitted for histopathology and aerobic and anaerobic cultures. Cultures of the overlying wound are less satisfactory in that results frequently differ from those taken from bone [33].

H. **Doppler or angiographic studies** are necessary to detect focal vascular lesions that, if corrected, could improve macrocirculation to the involved extremity. Improvement in blood supply to the lesion promotes healing and enhances delivery of antibiotics to the diseased tissue.

V. **Therapy.** Response to antibiotics alone often is unsatisfactory. Many patients are hospitalized on multiple occasions for treatment of recurrent disease. Initial therapy is usually conservative, with prevention of major amputations the primary goal. Prolonged courses of antibiotics may improve outcomes [42], but surgical debridement is usually necessary [44].

A. **Conservative approach.** To avoid more radical surgery, the following conservative measures are undertaken, although they are time-consuming and may be unsuccessful.

1. **Limited local incision and drainage** is done to remove necrotic debris.
2. **The principles of antibiotic therapy are as** outlined in section V.A. In one report high dose parenteral antibiotics for at least 4 weeks or a combined intravenous and oral regimen for at least 10 weeks was associated with a good outcome (defined as no ablative surgical procedure) in 29 of 51 patients. A poor outcome after limited surgical drainage and antibiotics was noted in patients with abscess, necrosis, or gangrene. Others advocate more aggressive surgery [42,44].

3. **Vascular surgery** may improve the macrocirculation to the involved extremity in patients with correctable focal arterial lesions.
4. **Limited amputations** of digits or parts of digits may prevent more radical future amputations. Adjacent areas of cellulitis should be treated with antibiotics preoperatively [45].

**B. Ablative surgery.** Patients who have done poorly with the conservative approach or who have evidence of abscess or gangrene may need ablative surgical therapy. Before amputation, it is important to perform arteriography or Doppler studies to rule out a surgically correctable arterial lesion and to assess the probability of healing of the surgical wound.

## SPECIAL FORMS OF OSTEOMYELITIS

**I. Chronic osteomyelitis** is defined as a **recurrent** problem: The patient has been previously treated for osteomyelitis at the same site [1]. Chronic osteomyelitis occurs most often after contiguous-focus osteomyelitis and peripheral vascular disease-associated osteomyelitis [46].

**A. Special considerations.** Chronic osteomyelitis carries a worse prognosis than acute osteomyelitis. Treatment failure rates in chronic osteomyelitis are higher than in the acute form, and the therapy is different.

**B. Clinical manifestations.** Patients only occasionally have acute symptoms. Systemic manifestations such as fever are uncommon. Localized signs and symptoms are also less common, with the exception of sinus tract or wound drainage, which is very common.

**C. Microbiologic features. *S. aureus* is a common pathogen.** Staphylococcal infections may recur years after the initial episode. Gram-negative bacteria may also be involved. Specific therapy should be guided by cultures obtained from biopsy.

**D. Diagnosis.** Determining the extent of disease activity and identifying a causative pathogen may be difficult.

1. **Blood cultures** are not often helpful, because bacteremia is rare.
2. **White blood cell (WBC) counts** are normal in most patients.
3. The **ESR** may be elevated, but this is a nonspecific finding.
4. Radiographic evaluation is complicated by the presence of prior bony abnormalities. It may not be possible to detect new or progressive abnormalities unless older radiographs are available for comparison.
5. **Technetium radiophosphate scans** are less helpful than in cases of acute osteomyelitis. Because scans may remain positive for years in the absence of active infection, a negative scan usually excludes active disease. **Indium-labeled leukocyte scans** have shown varying sensitivity in detecting active infection [37].
6. **CT and MRI** are useful in defining sequestra, directing needle aspiration, and planning the operative approach in chronic osteomyelitis [24].
7. When deciding whether to perform **wound or sinus cultures,** it is important to remember that organisms cultured from draining sinus tracts may not represent the true bacteriology of the underlying bone infection when compared with bone biopsy cultures [46]. **Definitive bacteriologic diagnosis requires culture of bone biopsy specimens.**
8. **Needle aspiration and surgical biopsy** should be performed before any antibiotic is administered [46]. Aerobic, anaerobic, mycobacterial, and fungal cultures should be performed. Many chronic cases eventually require surgery. A diagnostic and therapeutic procedure is preferred before initiation of antibiotic therapy. Preoperative antibiotics may decrease the yield of cultures obtained at the time of surgery. Gram stains of the surgical specimens may help in the initial empiric choice of antibiotics.

**E. Therapy** is neither well established nor particularly effective. Evidence from controlled trials to guide therapeutic decisions is lacking. Goals of therapy should be thoughtfully considered and individualized. Cure of chronic osteomyelitis is hard to define because relapses are frequent and may occur months to years after the most aggressive therapy [4]. Attempts at "cure" may require extensive, sometimes limb-threatening, surgery followed by prolonged courses of sometimes toxic and expensive antibiotics. Such treatment courses are unsuitable for some patients in whom chronic symptoms are tolerable. "Suppression" of symptoms with chronic, perhaps lifelong, antibiotic therapy or treatment of exacerbations of symptoms with antibiotics may be more reasonable courses of action. Infectious disease and orthopedic consultation is recommended.

1. **Surgical intervention may be required** to remove sequestra, to debride necrotic and devitalized material, and to obtain culture material. At times, extensive debridement is done with attempts at autogenous grafting with pulverized bone to fill in all defects [47]. Protocols using combined extensive debridement, antibiotic therapy, and vascularized muscle flaps to cover the wound have shown promising results [48].
2. **Antibiotics** are used, but the best regimen is debatable. In contrast to the basic principles that guide therapy in acute osteomyelitis (see section V.A under Hematogenous Osteomyelitis, above), the **optimal approach** to antibiotic therapy in chronic cases **is unknown.**
   a. **Parenteral agents** are often used initially, but the duration of therapy is poorly defined.
   b. **Combination therapy** with an antistaphylococcal penicillin and rifampin has been successful in some patients with chronic staphylococcal osteomyelitis [4].
   c. **The long-term** (3–6 months) **use of oral agents** has reported to be successful in treating chronic osteomyelitis [49]. Although many patients had disease attributable to gram-positive cocci, the quinolone antibiotics may prove especially useful in treating chronic osteomyelitis caused by aerobic gram-negative bacilli, especially *P. aeruginosa,* which previously required parenteral antibiotics [50]. See Chapter 27 for a detailed discussion of these agents.
3. **Hyperbaric oxygen** is advocated by some clinicians in the treatment of chronic osteomyelitis. Large-scale clinical trials proving efficacy are lacking.
4. **Consultation is advised in these difficult cases.** Adequate surgical debridement is essential. A regimen of 3 to 6 weeks of parenteral antibiotics is often used initially, followed by prolonged oral or parenteral therapy.

**F. Complications of long-standing chronic osteomyelitis**

1. **Secondary amyloidosis,** although reported in some reviews, is very rare.
2. **Carcinoma,** primarily epidermoid carcinoma, occurs in the sinus tract of fewer than 1% of cases of chronic osteomyelitis. It is usually heralded by increased pain and drainage from the sinus tract. If cancer is suspected, the entire sinus tract is resected because the carcinoma may lie deep within the tract.

**II. Vertebral osteomyelitis** occurs more frequently in older patients and may result from either hematogenous seeding of the bone or as the result of a postoperative wound infection and contiguous spread. Risk factors include diabetes, immunodeficiency, and intravenous drug abuse. Although uncommon, the incidence of this disease is increasing; it accounts for about 2% to 4% of all cases of pyogenic osteomyelitis [51–53].

**A. Special considerations.** Intravertebral disk space infections (discitis) refers to an inflammatory and/or infectious process of the vertebral disk. Discitis may result from hematogenous seeding of the disk [54]. Discitis in adults has also been reported postoperatively after spine surgery [55], after discography [56], and in intravenous drug users [57]. In adults pyogenic bacteria are cultured in most cases, and early involvement of contiguous vertebral bodies is documented radiographically. As such, it is our opinion that discitis in adults clinically behaves like pyogenic vertebral osteomyelitis and should be approached as such. In contrast, discitis in children represents a unique clinical syndrome and is discussed later in this chapter [58] (see section III).

**B. Pathogenesis and clinical setting**

1. Spontaneous cases of vertebral osteomyelitis occur most often from hematogenous seeding. In addition to arterial spread of infection, retrograde spread of infection is purported to occur from a urinary tract or pelvic source via Batson plexus, a venous plexus that forms a direct connection between the vasculature of the pelvis and the spinal column. The extensive anastomoses and lack of valves in the veins of Batson plexus are believed to facilitate spread of infection to adjacent vertebrae,

particularly after urinary tract infection or genitourinary manipulation in the elderly.

2. Other cases occur by spread from the contiguous focus of infection, especially after disk surgery. Contiguous focus vertebral osteomyelitis is being increasingly reported.
3. **The incidence of vertebral osteomyelitis is highest in adults 50 years of age and older.** This increased incidence is considered to be a result of subchondral vascular changes in vertebrae from the axial stress and osteoarthritis that accompany aging.
4. When associated with intravenous drug use, vertebral osteomyelitis occurs in younger adults, with peak incidence between 20 and 50 years of age. The duration of symptoms is shorter, usually less than 3 months [57]. Pyogenic **vertebral osteomyelitis in children is uncommon** and has been reviewed elsewhere [58].
5. The lumbar vertebrae are most commonly involved, followed by thoracic and then cervical vertebrae. In drug addicts, there is a high incidence of cervical spinal involvement [51–53].
6. Nosocomial infection, usually due to intravenous cannula-related sepsis with staphylococci, has become an increasingly important problem [51].

C. **Microbiologic features.** *S. aureus* is the most common pathogen. *Salmonella* and gram-negative organisms associated with prior urinary tract infection or genitourinary manipulations also are common. *Pseudomonas* species are common in drug addicts. Tuberculosis can mimic bacterial infections (this is discussed further in section IV). MRSA has been reported, usually with nosocomial infections associated with catheter- or wound-related sepsis [59].

D. **Clinical manifestations.** There is commonly an inordinate delay between symptom onset and diagnosis.

1. **Back pain,** described as dull and continuous, is the most common symptom. In a recent series, 85% of patients presented with back pain [59]. It is present at rest and exacerbated by movement or straining but only slightly relieved by analgesics. Regional paraspinal muscle spasm, percussion tenderness of the spinal column, and point tenderness of the involved spinous processes frequently are present.
2. **Referred pain** due to nerve root irritation may mislead the examiner and direct attention from vertebral involvement. Lumbar disease, for example, can present as pain in the hip or leg.
3. **Neurologic complications** can occur. Because of the indolent nature of the illness, patients may present with late neurologic sequelae such as paraplegia and meningitis [51–53]. Limb weakness was noted in about one-half of patients in one series [59].
4. **Fever** is often absent and was reported in only 30% of patients in a recent series and has overall been noted in 20% to 50% of patients [59].

E. **Diagnosis**

1. **Blood cultures** should be obtained but often are negative. Blood cultures have been reported positive in 24% to 50% of patients and when positive for a pathogen are assumed to be the etiologic agent [59].
2. The **WBC** count is elevated in most patients [59].
3. The **ESR** is usually elevated (80–90 mm/h) and is considered a useful test supporting the diagnosis of vertebral osteomyelitis. A normal ESR makes the diagnosis of vertebral osteomyelitis open to question. C-reactive protein levels are also usually elevated [52].
4. **Radiographic evaluation** (i.e., spinal films) is essential. Intervertebral disk involvement favors the diagnosis of pyogenic infection or tuberculosis. Findings are often nonspecific [59].
5. **Bone scans** are helpful but have the limitations previously discussed.
6. **MRIs** are highly sensitive and specific in the diagnosis of spinal infection and **provide more accurate anatomic information than bone scans. They have largely supplanted CTs** in the evaluation of vertebral osteomyelitis [52].
7. **Needle biopsy or open biopsy** is essential to substantiate the diagnosis and provide culture material [52,59] if blood cultures are negative. Unfortunately,

bone biopsy cultures may be negative in up to 25% of cases. When this occurs, histologic examination of the biopsy may confirm inflammatory changes compatible with osteomyelitis. A second needle biopsy is suggested if the first sample is culture negative. If the second needle biopsy is culture negative, an open surgical biopsy should be considered [52].

**F. Therapy**

**1. Antibiotics**

**a.** The principles of **antibiotic therapy** are as outlined in section V under Hematogenous Osteomyelitis, above.

**b.** When infection is due to MRSA, combination therapy with rifampin and intravenous vancomycin is indicated. This recommendation is based on studies of animal models that have shown the combination of vancomycin plus rifampin is superior to vancomycin alone for bone sterilization [59].

**c. Duration.** Antibiotics usually are given for at least 4 weeks and often for 6 weeks [52]. Often, prolonged intravenous antibiotics are given at home (see Chapter 27). If the patient is very compliant and reliable and susceptibility data allow for an oral agent (e.g., oral quinolones for susceptible gram-negative bacteria), a combination of initial intravenous antibiotics followed by oral antibiotics is used.

The contribution of oral antibiotics after the initial 4 to 6 weeks of therapy is controversial. Some reviewers recommend them for 3 months after 1 month of intravenous therapy; other investigators believe that if parenteral therapy is given for 6 weeks, subsequent oral therapy is not required [59].

**d.** Because of the importance of eradicating this infection with the initial regimen and lack of clear-cut guidelines, infectious disease consultation is advised to help select intravenous and oral antibiotic regimens for these difficult problems.

**e.** The ESR and C-reactive protein are good tools to monitor the success of therapy; with proper antibiotic therapy, they should be expected to fall toward the normal range [52].

**2.** The role of **surgery** is debated. Definite indications include (a) neurologic complications such as cord compression, (b) drainage of paravertebral abscess, (c) failure to make a bacteriologic diagnosis after repeated needle biopsies, (d) poor clinical response, and (e) the presence of gross bone destruction, leading to significant deformity or instability [52].

**3. Adjunctive therapy** includes bed rest and a half-shell cast or body brace if the spine is unstable.

**G. Prognosis.** When early diagnosis is combined with adequate antibiotic therapy, prognosis is generally good. Reviews cite a mortality of less than 5% to 7%, with residual neurologic deficits occurring in 7% to 12%. Between 80% and 90% of patients recovered uneventfully with appropriate antibiotic therapy alone or with antibiotics combined with surgery [52,53]. If, while on antibiotic therapy for vertebral osteomyelitis, the patient develops symptoms of a compressive neuropathy, MRI can be performed to determine whether there is a collection of pus that may require neurosurgical drainage.

Relapses can occur. In one series, 15% of patients (three patients) had relapses, and in two of the three patients the infecting organism was MRSA [59].

**III. Intervertebral disk space infection (discitis)** is most frequently reported in children less than 5 years of age. It occurs almost exclusively in the lumbar region and presents with a painful gait and refusal to walk. The pathophysiology and pathogenesis of discitis in children remains poorly understood and is controversial [58].

**A. Pathogenesis.** Substantial controversy exists in the pediatric literature concerning the role of inflammation versus infection in the pathogenesis of discitis [59–61]. Some studies report positive blood or disk biopsy cultures (usually *S. aureus*) in more than half of the patients sampled. Other studies, however, have found few positive cultures and have reported resolution of illness without antimicrobial therapy. A number of cases have been reported temporally associated with a viral illness in which no bacterial etiology can be documented. Finally, antecedent trauma has been described in up to one-third of cases, but its role in causation of discitis is uncertain. Discitis in children is probably due to a variety of causes, including trauma, viral disease, and bacteria. **However, we believe that the prevailing clinical evidence supports a low grade bacterial infection** as the cause of most cases of discitis and that the failure to obtain positive cultures may be due to sterilization of the area by host defenses between the onset of symptoms and biopsy.

**B. Presentation.** Fever and other systemic signs of infection are absent in more than 50% of the patients. When present fever can vary from low grade to high spiking temperatures. In most children the **onset** of discitis is **gradual and subtle.** The presenting symptom is most commonly **back pain,** occasionally with associated difficulties in ambulation. In the very young irritability or refusal to ambulate may be as specific a presentation as can be expected. Children may complain of pain referred to the hip or leg or may show signs suggesting meningeal irritation or an abdominal pathology severe enough to prompt laparotomy.

**C. Diagnosis.** There are two useful investigations in suggesting the likelihood of intervertebral disk space infection: the ESR and roentgenographic examination. Needle aspiration can establish the diagnosis.

**1. ESR and complete blood count**

**a. Elevation of the ESR occurs in 90% to 100% of cases** in both children and adults and is commonly the earliest, and sometimes the only, laboratory abnormality seen. **Any postdiscectomy patient with increasing back pain and an ESR greater than 50 at 2 or more weeks after surgery should be considered to have discitis until proven otherwise.** The ESR may be used as an indicator of therapeutic response but occasionally remains elevated for months.

**b.** The total leukocyte and differential blood cell counts are normal in 50% or more of patients. Marked elevations suggest extension of infection to structures contiguous to the disk space.

**2. Roentgenography.** The **hallmark** of intervertebral disk space infection is the roentgenographic finding of **disk space narrowing.** This change may not be present until 2 to 3 weeks after onset of infection [60]. If roentgenograms are negative, either the examination should be repeated after an additional 2 to 3 weeks or a radionuclide scan should be performed. Displacement of vertebrae may occur, and oblique views as well as routine views of the spine should be obtained. Erosion of the vertebral endplates usually follows the narrowing, occurring by 3 to 5 weeks after onset.

**3. Scans**

**a.** $^{99m}$**Tc** bone scans are useful in establishing an early and accurate diagnosis; such scans are positive in many cases within 7 days of onset and in nearly all cases after 2 weeks of back pain. But $^{67}$**Ga bone scanning has also proven beneficial** [62].

**b.** There are conflicting reports as to the usefulness of **CT** in making an early diagnosis of discitis [63,64]. Disk space narrowing and adjacent bone involvement may be detected before changes on plain roentgenograms. CT offers greater accuracy than radionuclide scanning in depicting adjacent soft-tissue pathologic processes.

**c.** Discitis also gives rise to characteristic changes on **MRI,** with an accuracy of diagnosis similar to radionuclide scans. MRI also provides anatomic information about the adjacent thecal sac and spinal cord not shown by radionuclide scans. A recent prospective blinded study using gadolinium-enhanced MRI found that changes in signal intensity in the intervertebral disk space and adjacent marrow are uncommon after routine discectomy. In seven biopsy and culture-proven discitis patients, gadolinium enhancement of the adjacent vertebral bone marrow, disk space, and posterior annulus fibrosus was identified. None of 15 asymptomatic postdiscectomy patients exhibited these changes [64]. **MRI may also be superior to CT** in providing finer resolution of the interface between the disk and adjacent bone.

**4. Blood cultures** should be routinely obtained. They are more likely to be positive if the patient is seen early in the course. If they are positive, especially in a child with *S. aureus* infection, a diagnostic needle aspiration may be avoided.

5. **Needle aspiration** of the disk space is the preferred way to obtain material for culture (aerobic, anaerobic, and mycobacterial), **particularly in postoperative discitis.** In some studies, this procedure has provided an etiologic agent for as many as 85% of cases in which it was performed. Aspirations should be performed before antibiotic therapy is started. However, it has now become common practice to treat children with uncomplicated discitis without first performing a culture [61]. A skin test for tuberculosis is recommended.

D. **Microbiologic features.** In those cases in which a bacterial etiology is established, more than 90% are due to *S. aureus.* Streptococci are implicated occasionally.

E. **Differential diagnosis includes acute pyogenic osteomyelitis, trauma, tuberculous vertebral osteomyelitis, paraspinal abscess, and spinal cord tumor.**

F. **Therapy**

1. Although discitis in children is presumed to be of bacterial etiology in most cases, outcome has generally been reported to be the same whether or not the patient receives antibiotics [58,60,65]. **Because no controlled prospective studies have been done, recommendations for treatment remain controversial.**
   a. Many authorities now recommend **a trial of immobilization of the spine,** generally with a body cast, as the key to providing relief of pain [58,61]. The duration of immobilization is guided primarily by improvement of the pain and secondarily, by favorable changes in the ESR and roentgenograms, but is generally in the range of 4 weeks.
   b. A reasonable recommendation is that **a child who fails to respond to immobilization should receive intravenous antibiotic therapy,** usually with a first-generation cephalosporin or semisynthetic penicillinase-resistant penicillin for 5 to 7 days, followed by 7 to 14 days of a similar oral antistaphylococcal antibiotic [61]. Generally, 3 to 4 weeks of antibiotic therapy have been successful.

G. **Prognosis.** The clinical data indicate that discitis in children is generally short-lived and carries a good prognosis [65].

IV. **Infection associated with prosthetic devices** occurs in 1% to 5% of cases [66]. These infections are particularly difficult to manage, but prosthesis removal is not necessary in all cases. Some infections respond to antibiotic management alone.

A. **Special considerations.** Prosthetic devices act as foreign bodies. The question routinely arises as to whether the prosthesis must be removed or whether prolonged antibiotic therapy alone will be adequate.

B. **The approach to these infections** is discussed later in this chapter under Prosthetic Joint Infections.

C. **Intramedullary fixation nails.** These nails represent a unique situation, because their premature removal, even when they are infected, will often result in an unstable fracture, nonunion, and persistent infection. The device must usually be left in place and the infection treated with parenteral antibiotics and careful local surgery for debridement and drainage. The nail is removed when union is achieved [67].

V. **Tuberculous osteomyelitis** should be suspected in any case of vertebral osteomyelitis or osteomyelitis at any site that has not responded to antibiotic therapy. In the United States one-fifth of tuberculosis cases occur at extrapulmonary sites. One-third of human immunodeficiency virus (HIV)-infected individuals with tuberculosis have extrapulmonary disease with or without pulmonary involvement [68].

A. **Pathogenesis.** Bone involvement results primarily from hematogenous spread, most commonly from the lung. Extension from a caseating lymph node or lymphatic drainage also may occur. There is a predilection for the coexistence of renal and skeletal tuberculosis. In almost all cases, the organism is *Mycobacterium tuberculosis,* although rare cases of atypical mycobacteria have been reported [69].

B. **Clinical manifestations.** Tuberculous osteomyelitis is seen primarily in adults. Skeletal tuberculosis, like pulmonary tuberculosis, is less common in children.

1. **Signs and symptoms.** These cases usually have a long indolent course.
   a. **Asymptomatic** bone lesions may be discovered on roentgenograms taken for other reasons. As with pyogenic organisms, patients with tuberculosis of the

spine may have a paucity of symptoms and may not present until development of paravertebral abscess or neurologic complications including paraplegia and meningitis (see section II).

b. **Fever** may or may not be present. Tuberculous osteomyelitis should always be considered, however, in the patient with fever of unknown origin and an asymptomatic bone lesion.

c. **Pain** is the most common complaint and may be accompanied by local swelling and tenderness.

d. **Chronic draining sinuses** may be present.

2. **Bones involved.** Although any bone may be involved, 50% of cases involve the spine (50% thoracic, 25% cervical, 25% lumbar); 12% pelvis; 10% hip and femur; 10% knee and tibia; 7% ribs; 2% ankle, shoulder, elbow, or wrist; and 3% at multiple sites [68].

C. **Diagnosis.** In addition to the usual methods of diagnosing bacterial osteomyelitis, the following diagnostic tests are important in patients with suspected tuberculous bone disease.

1. **Chest roentgenography** is necessary to look for evidence of pulmonary tuberculosis. Because only approximately 50% of patients with skeletal tuberculosis have roentgenographic evidence of pulmonary tuberculosis, a negative chest radiograph cannot disprove the diagnosis [70]. Sputum cultures (or gastric cultures if sputum is not available) are necessary if active pulmonary infection is suspected.

2. A **tuberculin skin test** is part of the workup of any destructive bone or joint lesion, especially when it is monoarthritic or involves the spine. A negative skin test must never be used to rule out disease (see Chapter 11).

3. **Needle or open biopsy** is important. In chronic infections in which tuberculosis is suspected and in all cases of vertebral osteomyelitis of unknown etiology, **tissue for histopathologic analysis and culture is crucial.** Special stains and cultures for bacteria, mycobacteria, and fungi should be performed.

D. **Treatment**

1. See Chapter 11. Therapy is similar to that given for pulmonary disease, that is, a four-drug regimen of isoniazid, rifampin, pyrazinamide, and ethambutol for 2 months followed by two drugs, rifampin and isoniazid, for an additional 4 months. Infectious diseases consultation is advised [71].

2. **Surgery**

a. **Nonvertebral disease.** Except in far advanced disease, surgery is seldom necessary. Surgery is indicated to prevent deformity, to improve joint function, and to control disease that has not responded to chemotherapy. Surgery usually is delayed until after 2 to 3 months of chemotherapy [68].

b. **Vertebral disease.** In the past, spinal tuberculosis (Pott disease) commonly required surgical fusion. More recent studies show successful treatment in uncomplicated cases by chemotherapy alone. Spinal fusion usually occurs spontaneously with the healing process. Indications for surgery include marked neurologic deficit, drainage of large abscesses, worsening neurologic deficit despite adequate chemotherapy, and progression of kyphosis or instability despite adequate chemotherapy [71,72].

E. **Prognosis.** With appropriate chemotherapy, the prognosis with skeletal tuberculosis is good.

1. **Nonvertebral disease.** Coexistent joint involvement is frequent. Residual sequelae are often the result of deformity and functional impairment of the involved joint. Most patients, however, do recover normal function after chemotherapy alone [68].

2. **Vertebral disease.** Central nervous system involvement, including meningitis or paraplegia, is the most serious complication of tuberculous infection of the spine. Spinal deformities, kyphosis, and scoliosis also occur as a result of destruction of vertebrae. In children, these deformities may be progressive [71,72].

VI. **Fungal osteomyelitis.** Osteomyelitis can result from invasive infections due to a number of fungal pathogens, including *Candida* species, *Aspergillus* species, *Sporothrix schenckii, Coccidioides immitis, Blastomyces dermatitidis, Histoplasma capsulatum,*

*Cryptococcus neoformans,* and a variety of less commonly encountered pathogens. Fungal osteomyelitis should be considered in any indolent osteomyelitis that has not responded to routine measures or in any patient with evidence of disseminated fungal disease. Therapy is generally complex and prolonged. Adequate discussion of the subject is beyond the scope of this chapter. We refer the reader to a recent review of the subject [73] (see also Chapter 17).

## DIABETIC FOOT INFECTIONS

Foot infections are a common cause of morbidity and mortality in patients with diabetes. Twenty-five percent of all diabetics develop severe foot or leg problems. Foot infections account for fully 20% of diabetic hospitalizations. At least 50% of all nontraumatic lower extremity amputations occurring in the United States are performed on diabetics [74].

**I. Pathophysiology**

**A. Peripheral neuropathy.** Peripheral neuropathy is likely the most important risk factor for development of foot lesions in diabetic patients. Neuropathy is present in over 80% of diabetics with foot lesions [75].

**1.** Loss of protective pain sensation due to peripheral neuropathy leads to loss of awareness of traumatic injury and subsequent breaks in the skin and skin ulceration [74]. The initial lesion occurs at weight-bearing points, frequently under the first or fifth metatarsal heads or on the heel. These painless ulcers may go unnoticed and unattended for days to weeks. Bacteria may then invade the base of these neglected ulcers and either spread along fascial planes or penetrate fascia and soft tissue to reach the periosteum.

**2.** Motor nerve involvement leads to weakness in muscles of the foot, causing a cavus deformity and clawing of the toes. This leads to maldistribution of weight while walking, predisposing to traumatic injury, skin ulceration, and infection.

**3.** Autonomic neuropathy causes interference with sweating, resulting in dry cracked skin that may allow invasion of microorganisms [75].

**B. Ischemia.** Arteriosclerosis occurs at a rate 20 times higher in type 2 diabetics than in nondiabetic control subjects matched for sex and age. Peripheral vascular disease is common in patients with diabetes, producing ischemia that contributes to the development of as many as one-third of foot ulcers [75]. Lack of adequate blood supply impedes delivery of antibiotics to infected tissue and impairs tissue healing.

**C. Other factors.** Other factors leading to ulceration and infection include pressure due to faulty fitting shoes [76], superficial fungal infections, improper trimming of toenails, overgrown nails, or thermal injury due to lack of awareness of heat [75].

**II. Microbiologic features.** The organisms isolated are related in part to the severity of underlying disease, which has been divided into mild non–limb-threatening infections and more severe limb-threatening infections [44,77] (see discussion in section III). Patients in both groups frequently receive multiple courses of different antibiotics. Recent receipt of antibiotics increases the likelihood of recovery of atypical or drug-resistant organisms, particularly MRSA [78] but also enterococcus and *Pseudomonas aeruginosa* [79]. Recent hospitalization also predisposes to presence of these pathogens [80]. Severity and chronicity of disease, culture technique, and laboratory capabilities also affect culture results.

**A. Mild non–limb-threatening infections** are caused primarily by *S. aureus* (more than 50% of patients) and aerobic streptococci. Facultative gram-negative bacilli and anaerobic organisms are less frequent. **In half** of these patients, the infections are **monomicrobial** [44].

**B. Severe limb-threatening infections usually are polymicrobial.** Deep tissue cultures that avoid surface contamination usually yield a mixed culture of aerobes and anaerobes.

**1. Aerobes**

**a.** ***S. aureus*** **and coagulase-negative staphylococci** are the most common aerobic isolates [80,81]. Staphylococci are found in approximately two-thirds of patients in whom only a single organism is isolated [41].

**b.** Approximately 20% of isolates are **streptococci** (including group B) **and enterococci** [41,81]. The pathogenic role of coagulase-negative staphylococci, enterococci, and corynebacteria often is difficult to discern, particularly when these organisms are cultured along with more typical pathogens. These organisms can be viewed as skin contaminants and not pathogens (unless they are isolated in pure culture or the patient is not responding to therapy that is not aimed at these organisms) [44]. Prior administration of antibiotics or prior hospitalization complicates interpretation of cultures yielding these organisms, as noted above.

c. **Enterobacteriaceae** account for 24% to 27% of organisms isolated. Common isolates include *Proteus, Klebsiella,* and *Enterobacter* species *Morganella morganii,* and *E. coli* [41,81]. *Pseudomonas* and *Acinetobacter* species are common contaminants in specimens from ulcers or open draining lesions but are infrequently isolated from deep tissue cultures [41].

2. **Anaerobes** are isolated from 40% to 80% of patients with severe or advanced disease. They usually are present in cultures yielding multiple organisms [41,81,82].
   a. The presence of anaerobes is associated with a higher frequency of fever and foul-smelling lesions [81].
   b. Common anaerobic isolates include anaerobic streptococci (14% to 17%), *Bacteroides* species (9%–14%), and *Clostridium* species (2%–7%). *Bacteroides* species are more frequently found in necrotizing infections and osteomyelitis than in abscesses [41]. Although rare, infection due to *Clostridium* species may be rapidly progressive. Lack of an inflammatory response on Gram stain in the presence of gram-positive organisms should raise suspicion that *Clostridium* is present.

III. **Clinical manifestations.** Meaningful comparison of the many different studies on diabetic foot infections is hindered by the lack of a uniform grading system accounting for neuropathy, ischemia, and wound depth, all thought to be major predictors of poor outcome. Both the Wagner and the University of Texas wound classification systems hold promise in this regard [83].

A. **Non–limb-threatening versus limb-threatening infections.** Reviewers have suggested a practical clinical classification of infections [44] that appears to be a useful approach.

1. **Non–limb-threatening infections.** Patients have superficial infection and minimal cellulitis (<2 cm of extension from portal of entry) and lack systemic toxicity. If an ulcer is present, it does not penetrate fully through the skin. These patients do not have bone or joint involvement or significant underlying ischemia.
2. **Limb-threatening infections.** Patients have more extensive cellulitis (>2 cm of extension from the portal of entry) and lymphangitis. Full-thickness ulcers often are present. Infection of contiguous bones or joints occurs frequently.

   Significant ischemia with or without gangrene may be present. Fever is seen in only some patients and is more common in those with extensive soft tissue involvement, deep plantar abscesses, bacteremia, or hematogenously seeded remote sites of infection.

B. **Local signs and symptoms** predominate and include those related to infection, vasculopathy, and neuropathy.

1. **Infection.** The anatomic location of the infection affects prognosis. Proximal infections (along metatarsals, at the heel, or above the ankle) are associated with lower limb salvage and higher mortality [84].
   a. Most cases of lower extremity infection in diabetics begin as chronic perforating ulcers.
   b. Infection is heralded by warmth, redness, swelling, and purulent exudate. **Tenderness is often minimal or absent due to neuropathy** [42,85].
   c. Gas in the soft tissues may be visualized by roentgenography or detected as crepitus on physical examination. Gas usually is from mixed infection with gram-negative bacilli and anaerobes rather than *Clostridium* species infection. A foul odor may be present due to necrosis or anaerobic infection [81]. Gangrene due to infection or ischemia may be seen.
   d. It is important to determine the extent of deep tissue destruction and possible bone and joint involvement by unroofing all encrusted areas and inspecting

the wound carefully [86]. **Surgical consultation should be obtained routinely. Osteomyelitis underlying diabetic ulcers is common.** Incidence of clinically silent osteomyelitis is as high as 68% when sought with bone biopsy and cultures [87].

2. **Vascular disease.** Patients may complain of intermittent claudication or resting pain relieved by dependency. Pulses may be decreased or absent. Bruits, shiny cold skin, decreased hair and nail growth, atrophy of subcutaneous fat, and a rapid decrease of Doppler pressures may also be present. Other findings include delayed capillary filling time, ischemic rubor, and collapsed veins [75].
3. **Neuropathy.** This is most prominent in the lower extremities. Commonly, the forefoot may have significant neuropathy, whereas the hindfoot and lower leg have relatively normal sensation. A simple method of identifying patients who have lost protective sensation is to press a nylon monofilament against the skin of the foot; the inability of the patient to feel the force of the monofilament correlates with an increased risk of neuropathic foot injury [88].

C. **Systemic signs and symptoms** often occur late and indicate severe infection.

1. Uncontrolled hyperglycemia may indicate uncontrolled infection [86].
2. Fever occurs with undrained pus, when a virulent organism is involved, or when bacteremia is present. Otherwise, fever is relatively uncommon. Even in patients with limb-threatening sepsis, only 36% had fever exceeding 100°F (37.8°C) during the first day of admission [82], except in bacteremia and in cases in which anaerobes were recovered from deep cultures [44,81] (see section **A.2**).

## IV. Diagnosis

A. **Leukocytosis** may be minimal or absent even with severe infection. Even with limb-threatening sepsis, leukocytosis (WBC count > 10,000/mm$^3$) was noted in only 53% of patients at admission [82].

B. The **ESR** is usually elevated.

C. **Blood cultures** are positive in approximately 10% to 15% of patients but should be obtained in all patients. The highest rates of positive cultures are seen in febrile patients [39].

D. The **best method for** obtaining **wound or tissue cultures** from diabetic foot infections **is still debated** [89]. These wounds are chronic and are often colonized superficially with organisms that are not causative (e.g., staphylococci or enterococci).

**Several methods are used. Aerobic and anaerobic cultures should be performed** before antibiotics are started.

1. **With debridement.** When debridement is performed, cultures of deep tissue or necrotic tissue, including bone, can be obtained. Routine aspirate or biopsy of unexposed bone is not advised.
2. **Direct ulcer culture.** The open ulcer can be cleaned carefully (usually with Betadine, which is allowed to dry and then removed with alcohol sponges) and any overlying eschar debrided; a swab can then be inserted through the opening of the ulcer deeply into the wound to obtain a deep culture. The swab can then be plunged into anaerobic transport media and brought quickly to the laboratory for processing.
3. Bullae or fluctuant collections should be aspirated and cultured [44].

E. **Gram stains** usually reveal mixed flora and may not be especially helpful; however, the lack of an inflammatory response and the presence of gram-positive rods may indicate a clostridial infection, which may be rapidly progressive [84].

F. **Radiographs**

1. Radiolucent areas within the soft tissues may occur due to dissection of air into open ulcers or as a result of debridement. **Presence of air** in the soft tissue also occurs as a result of gas-forming bacterial infection [90]. Gas formation is usually due to other anaerobes, coliforms, streptococci, and, rarely, *Clostridia* species. Because air in the soft tissues can occur secondary to a number of benign causes, its presence alone should not be used as justification for amputation. The differentiation of osteomyelitis from diabetic osteopathy may be difficult [90]. Sequential radiographs may help. Radiographs may be normal in early osteomyelitis [40,42].

(See section IV.D under Osteomyelitis Associated with Peripheral Vascular Disease, above.)

**G. Indium-labeled leukocyte scans are the most sensitive method to detect occult osteomyelitis.** In one study, these scans proved more sensitive than either roentgenograms or bone scans [87] (see Section IV.E under Osteomyelitis Associated with Peripheral Vascular Disease, above).

**H. MRI** is also highly accurate in the diagnosis of occult osteomyelitis and is used to detect soft tissue abscess [24].

**I. Probing the base of the ulcer** to detect bone is a useful technique to identify osteomyelitis, as discussed in section IV.G under Osteomyelitis Associated with Peripheral Vascular Disease, above. Because necrotic debris frequently masks the ulcer floor, this technique may be the only way to accurately assess ulcer depth and to identify involvement with contiguous bone [43].

**V. Therapy.** Early surgical and infectious disease consultation is recommended.

**A. Medical therapy**

1. **Antibiotics** are the mainstay of treatment and are recommended in the presence of an ulcer with surrounding cellulitis, a foul-smelling lesion, fever, or deep tissue infection.

   a. **Empiric antibiotic therapy is necessary until culture results are available.** Few well-controlled comparative trials exist on which to base recommendations for therapy [91]. Recommendations for empiric therapy are increasingly problematic in an era of increasing incidence of antimicrobial resistance. Risk of infection with drug-resistant pathogens is increased with recent prior use of antibiotics and recent hospitalization, as previously noted. Antibiotics are given in full dose due to the potential for poor penetration into diseased tissue. Nephrotoxic antibiotics should be avoided. Possible antibiotic options are summarized in Table 5.3.

      (1) **For non–limb-threatening infection,** therapy is directed at staphylococci and streptococci. Outpatient regimens using 2 weeks of oral cephalexin or clindamycin are generally effective. In some patients who have cellulitis surrounding the superficial ulcer, hospitalization for a short course of intravenous antibiotics is warranted. Although the optimal therapy is unknown, empiric monotherapy with cefazolin, cefoxitin, cefotetan, ceftizoxime, clindamycin, ticarcillin-clavulanic acid, ampicillin-sulbactam, or piperacillin-tazobactam are appropriate [41,42,74,81]. Therapy is modified based on results of deep tissue cultures. Patients may be stepped down to oral therapy when clinical improvement is evident.

      (2) **For more severe limb-threatening infections,** broad-spectrum antibiotics are used to treat anticipated polymicrobial infection. Options include piperacillin-tazobactam, combination of ceftriaxone and clindamycin (or metronidazole), combination of ciprofloxacin and clindamycin (or metronidazole), imipenem-cilastatin, or ampicillin-sulbactam [80]. Therapy, again, must be modified based on results of deep tissue culture.

      (3) **For life-threatening infections,** imipenem-cilastatin or combination regimens are recommended. Some experts include coverage against enterococci in this setting. Short courses of aminoglycosides in combination with other broad-spectrum agents may be used in the setting of gram-negative sepsis. Short-term use minimizes risk of aminoglycoside nephrotoxicity [82]. Vancomycin is included if MRSA is a concern because of recent hospitalization or recent antibiotic exposure. Less toxic agents are substituted once culture results become available.

   b. **The results of deep tissue cultures are used to direct continued antibiotic choices.**

      (1) If the patient is doing well clinically and is improving on an empiric antibiotic regimen not active against a particular isolate from a deep ulcer culture, the clinical response suggests the organism may be just a colonizer and therefore needs no directed antibiotic therapy.

      (2) By contrast, if bacteria are isolated that are resistant to the current antibiotic regimen but the patient is not doing well clinically, it is reasonable

Table 5.3. Selected Empiric Antimicrobial Regimens for Foot Infections in Patients with Diabetes Mellitus

| Regimen |
|---|
| Non–limb-threatening infection |
| Oral regimen |
| Cephalexin[a] |
| Clindamycin |
| Dicloxacillin |
| Amoxicillin-clavulanate |
| Parenteral regimen |
| Cefazolin |
| Oxacillin or nafcillin |
| Clindamycin |
| Cefoxitin |
| Cefotetan |
| Ceftizoxime |
| Ticarcillin-clavulanic acid |
| Ampicillin-sulbactam |
| Piperacillin-tazobactam |
| Limb-threatening infection |
| Oral regimen |
| Fluoroquinolone and clindamycin (or metronidazole) |
| Parenteral regimen |
| Ampicillin-sulbactam |
| Ticarcillin-clavulanate |
| Piperacillin-tazobactam |
| Cefoxitin or cefotetan |
| Fluoroquinolone and clindamycin (or metronidazole) |
| Imipenem-cilastatin |
| Ceftriaxone and clindamycin (or metronidazole) |
| Life-threatening infection |
| Parenteral regimen |
| Imipenem-cilastatin |
| Vancomycin, metronidazole, and aztreonam |
| Ampicillin-sulbactam and an aminoglycoside |
| Piperacillin-tazobactam and an aminoglycoside |

Note: Regimens require adjustment if the patient has a history of allergies. Consider use of aminoglycosides in the setting of gram-negative sepsis. Consider addition of vancomycin if MRSA suspected due to recent hospitalization or prior recent treatment with antibiotics. Doses are commensurate with the severity of infection, with appropriate modification for impaired renal function.

[a]Authors' note: We favor full doses of cephalexin, i.e., 750–1,000 mg qid, in the adult. In severe renal failure, doses must be adjusted as described in Chapter 27.

Modified from Caputo GM, et al. Assessment and management of foot disease in patients with diabetes. *N Engl J Med* 1994;331:854, with permission.

to expand antibiotic coverage to include these pathogens. At times, unnecessarily broad antibiotic coverage is unavoidable [41].

**c.** The optimal **duration of antibiotic therapy** for soft tissue diabetic infections **is unknown** [44].

**(1)** For osteomyelitis, prolonged courses are needed as discussed earlier in this chapter. In patients with pedal osteomyelitis, if all infected bone has not been removed, prolonged antibiotics (e.g., 6–12 weeks) may be reasonable.

**(2)** For infections limited to soft tissue, intravenous therapy has often been given for 10 to 14 days. In patients who do well, oral therapy can be used to complete a 2-week course.

**(3)** Courses longer than 2 weeks are usually not required in non–limb-threatening infections. After resolution of cellulitis, ulcer care depends primarily on local care.

(4) Foot infections with a secondary bacteremia, commonly *S. aureus* or *Bacteroides* species, require protracted therapy (see Chapter 2).

(5) Decisions regarding amputation versus continued medical management remain controversial. Conservative management with culture-directed antibiotics and local care is successful in most patients without gangrenous tissue [92].

2. **Glycemic control** should be strict. Insulin is used for immediate glycemic control even in non–insulin-dependent patients [86]. An excellent monitor of the adequacy of debridement is blood sugar control, which improves as the infection is controlled [93].
3. **Weight-bearing of neuropathic ulcers** must be eliminated to allow healing. Various strategies exist from crutches, bed rest, and wheel chairs to casts, braces, and shoe cutouts [94].
4. **After adequate debridement and antibiotic management,** use of topical recombinant human platelet-derived growth factor (becaplermin) may speed time to complete healing of foot ulcers [95].

**B. In severe infection, early surgical consultation should be obtained.** Simple debridement of soft tissues, wide incision and drainage of pedal compartments, or open amputations may be appropriate. Removal of necrotic tissue and drainage of pus should not be delayed while awaiting medical stabilization [94].

1. **Nonablative procedures. Surgical considerations include the following:**
   - **a.** Deep infections do not respond to small stab wounds and drains.
   - **b.** The procedure should ensure later reconstruction, conserving as much healthy tissue as possible.
   - **c.** The initial procedure is rarely definitive. Follow-up procedures are usually required.
2. **Amputations.** If the infection is acutely life-threatening or if the architecture of the foot has been destroyed, amputation may be necessary [42]. Amputation may be preferable in patients who have undergone long courses of unsuccessful treatment. Amputation and rehabilitation may improve quality of life in this situation [96].
3. **Revascularization.** Adequacy of arterial circulation should be assessed in all patients with foot infection [44]. Arterial insufficieny is a factor in 60% of nonhealing ulcers and 46% of major amputations [97]. Appropriate noninvasive studies include Doppler segmental arterial pressures, wave form analysis, ankle-brachial indices, toe pressures, and transcutaneous oxygen tension [94]. Evidence of vascular insufficiency should prompt vascular surgery consultation. Aggressive surgical correction of arterial insufficiency may speed healing and allow management of infection without amputation [44].

**VI. Prevention.** Diabetic foot infections are best prevented by preventing ulcers. Comprehensive diabetic foot care programs reduce the incidence of ulcers and subsequent infections [98]. Effective programs involve multiple disciplines and should include the following.

**A.** Tight glycemic control is necessary to slow onset of neuropathy.

**B.** Examination of the foot is performed during any patient contact. At a minimum the examiner should look for skin breaks, increased temperature, and callus formation.

**C.** Calluses should be promptly removed and bony deformities corrected.

**D.** Patients should be taught to avoid extreme bath water temperature, avoid foot soaks, and dry the foot thoroughly after bathing. Nails should be trimmed correctly. Tinea pedis should be treated promptly. Formal educational programs are desirable, with frequent reinforcement during clinic follow-up.

**E.** Patients should be instructed in selection of appropriate footwear that reduces abnormal pressures on the foot. New shoes should be broken in slowly and ill-fitting shoes avoided. Athletic running shoes are beneficial. Custom-made footwear or sole inserts are preferable.

## SEPTIC (INFECTIOUS) ARTHRITIS

Septic (infectious) arthritis usually begins acutely in a single joint. Symptoms of inflammation may include pain, erythema, tenderness, swelling, and limitation of motion of the joint.

Occasionally, multiple joints are involved. **A noninfectious inflammatory joint process such as crystal-induced arthritis (gout or pseudogout) may mimic a septic joint.** Early diagnosis with rapid institution of therapy is necessary to minimize joint damage [99–104].

Most cases occur due to hematogenous seeding of bacteria from a distant site. Synovial tissue is susceptible to seeding by bacteria due to lack of a basement membrane and vascularity. After infection, the body's inflammatory response damages the ground substance of the articular surface. Lack of appropriate therapy causes erosion of cartilage and joint space narrowing. Patients with chronic arthritis, particularly those receiving intraarticular injections, are predisposed to joint infections. In patients without chronic arthritis there is frequently a history of antecedent trauma to the joint [101].

**I. Clinical presentation.** Risk factors for joint infection include rheumatoid arthritis, sickle cell disease, immunosuppression, prior sexually transmitted disease, narcotic use, or presence of a prosthetic joint. Prior or current remote site of infection should be sought during a careful history and physical.

**A. History**

1. **Multiple joint involvement** occurs in around 10% of patients [101].
2. **Prior joint damage** predisposes to infection. In a patient with rheumatoid arthritis, an inflamed joint that is out of phase with other joints (i.e., especially tender or warm) may be infected.
3. The usual **signs of inflammation** (tenderness, erythema, and swelling) are minimal in some patients.
4. **Systemic symptoms.** Fever occurs in 90% to 95% of patients but may be low grade, especially in immunosuppressed or rheumatoid arthritis patients. Chills are infrequent.
5. **Duration of symptoms** varies. In bacterial infections, symptoms occur usually over a few days unless patients have preexisting joint disease. Mycobacterial or fungal infections may be insidious, with symptoms present for months [103].
6. Most **commonly involved joints** are the knee, elbow, wrist, shoulder, hip, or ankle. In children, 79% occur in the hip, knee, or ankle [105]. Presenting complaint with hip infection may be only pain on motion.
7. **Prosthetic joint infections** are discussed in detail in a separate section in this chapter.
8. **Gonococcal disease is the most common cause of septic arthritis in the 15- to 40-year-old group.** The disseminated gonococcal syndrome occurs predominantly during the second or third trimester of pregnancy or during menstruation.
9. **Viral syndromes,** including rubella, rubella vaccination, hepatitis B, hepatitis C, varicella-zoster, and human parvovirus, can be associated with arthritis [104,106,107].
10. **Joint tuberculosis** classically presents as a subacute monoarthritis of a weight-bearing joint. Fungal infections have a variable presentation but are frequently of gradual onset [103,108,109].
11. **Postinfectious, or reactive, arthritis** is associated with gastrointestinal tract infection with *Shigella, Salmonella, Campylobacter,* and *Yersinia* species in patients with the HLA-B27 histocompatibility antigen [110].
12. **Lyme disease** (see Chapter 21).

**B. Physical examination**

1. **Joint inflammation** should be carefully sought.
2. **Range of motion** is markedly decreased due to pain.
3. **Tenosynovitis** (inflammation of the tendon sheath) occurs in rheumatoid arthritis, gout, and trauma but is also a common manifestation of gonococcal disease. Pain due to tenosynovitis occurs with active motion or when the involved joint is flexed to stretch the tendon.
4. **Concurrent infections** at other sites occur in 50% to 75% of cases.
5. **Skin rashes** commonly occur in disseminated gonococcal infections. Lesions may be macular, vesicular, or pustular, often with a necrotic center and are seen most frequently on the distal extremities. Rash occurs during the early bacteremic

Table 5.4. Examination of Joint Fluid

| Measure | Normal | Group 1 (Noninflammatory) | Group 2 (Inflammatory) | Group 3 (Septic) |
|---|---|---|---|---|
| Volume (mL) (knee) | >3.5 | Often >3.5 | Often >3.5 | Often >3.5 |
| Clarity | Transparent | Transparent | Translucent-opaque | Opaque |
| Color | Clear | Yellow | Yellow-opalescent | Yellow-green |
| Viscosity | High | High | Low | Variable |
| WBC/mm$^3$ | >200 | 200–2,000 | 2,000–100,000 | >100,000[a] |
| Polymorphonuclear leukocytes | >25% | >25% | ≥50% | ≥75%[a] |
| Culture | Negative | Negative | Negative | Often positive |
| Mucin clot | Firm | Firm | Firm | Friable |
| Glucose (mg/dL) | Nearly equal to blood | Nearly equal to blood | >25, lower than blood | >25, much lower than blood |

[a]Lower with infections caused by partially treated or low-virulence organisms.
From Rodnan GP, McEwen C, Wallace SL, eds. Primer on the rheumatic diseases. *JAMA* 1973;224 [Suppl.]:661, with permission.

phase with migratory arthralgias and variable degrees of joint inflammation. Cultures of blood are frequently positive with negative cultures of joints. Within 1 or 2 days, classic joint inflammation is present, but cultures and Gram stains are positive in only some cases. Similar skin lesions are infrequently seen in streptococcal and meningococcal arthritis [104].

6. **Prosthetic joints** may not appear inflamed. Passive range of motion may be preserved, whereas active range of motion is limited by pain.
7. **Joint tuberculosis** is associated with swelling, limitation of movement, muscle spasm, and regional lymphadenopathy. Erythema is often absent [104,108,109].

II. **Laboratory aids.** Examination of the joint fluid is the most important test.

A. **Direct joint aspiration** should be performed in every case of suspected infection. As a therapeutic maneuver, as much fluid should be removed as possible without risking damage to the synovial lining. Orthopedic or rheumatologic consultation is recommended in difficult cases or in suspected prosthetic joint infection. The characteristics of synovial fluid in pyogenic and other forms of arthritis are shown in Table 5.4. **Joint fluid analysis should include the following:**

1. **The total differential cell count and the leukocyte count are the most sensitive and specific synovial fluid tests for pyarthrosis.** Total WBC count generally exceeds 40,000/mm$^3$ with polymorphonuclear neutrophils in excess of 75% [110]. Rarely, crystal-induced and rheumatoid flares can cause a similar picture.
2. **Synovial fluid glucose and protein levels** are neither sensitive nor specific indicators of bacterial arthritis. Glucose levels may be 50% of blood glucose levels but may be normal, particularly in gonococcal arthritis [102,110].
3. **Gram stains** are positive in 35% to 65% of bacterially infected joints [99–102]. Gram stains are of particular importance in patients who have received antibiotic therapy before evaluation because cultures may have been rendered negative.
4. **Cultures and stains** should be performed on all inflammatory joints. Aerobic and anaerobic culture should be done on all fluid specimens. In suspected gonococcal disease, **fluid should be plated directly on to chocolate agar media.** Mycobacterial and fungal cultures and smears should be obtained in chronic or ill-defined inflammatory joint problems. In tuberculous arthritis, smears are positive in 20% to 25% of cases and cultures in 80%.
5. **Crystal examination** under polarized light is important to detect gout or pseudogout. Acute crystal-induced arthritis may mimic bacterial processes, or both processes can occur simultaneously.

6. **Detection of a pathogen by polymerase chain reaction** is helpful in Lyme arthritis due to *Borrelia burgdorferi* [111].

B. **Blood cultures** may be positive in 10% of cases. A minimum of two sets drawn 20 minutes apart should be obtained in all patients.

C. **Cultures of other sites** may reveal an associated infection. If gonococcal disease is suspected, cultures of cervix, urethra, pharynx, and rectum should be obtained.

D. **Radiography**

1. **Early** in the course of disease, radiographs show only soft tissue changes (e.g., swelling, fascial plane obliteration, or increased volume of the joint) that suggest an effusion [112].
2. **Late** changes in contiguous bony structures occur no sooner than 10 to 14 days after infection. Follow-up radiographs are helpful in detection of intercurrent osteomyelitis [112].
3. **Ultrasound** may be useful to demonstrate a joint effusion and guide needle aspiration of the joint.
4. **Radioisotope scans** usually three or four phase $^{99m}$Tc bone scans are the most rapid method of determination of site and distribution of joint infections.
5. **CT** is used mainly to guide needle aspiration. MRI is highly sensitive for detection of early septic arthritis and is much more specific than conventional radiographs or CT [113].

E. **Miscellaneous. Peripheral blood leukocytosis** occurs in 60% to 70% of cases but may be absent in immunosuppressed patient or prosthetic joint infections. ESRs are usually elevated [102]. **Tuberculin skin testing** should be performed in all cases of chronic monoarticular arthritis.

F. **Synovial tissue biopsy** for culture and histologic examination should be considered in chronic arthritis in which routine joint fluid examination has not yielded a diagnosis [114].

III. **Microbiologic features of septic joints**

A. **Bacterial infection.** Almost any organism can cause septic arthritis; however, certain bacteria are implicated in most cases. Age and predisposing factors predict likely pathogens [99,103]. In the 15- to 40-year-old group, gonococcus remains the most common etiology, although its incidence may be declining. Gonococcal arthritis occurs primarily in women (>75% of cases) and in homosexual men, both of whom are more likely to have asymptomatic or unrecognized infection at other sites [115]. Arthritis due to other agents is seen primarily in men.

1. **Neonates.** In infants younger than 3 months, adjacent bone is involved in as many as two-thirds of cases [116].
2. **Children** [117–121]. In pediatric patients, *S. aureus, H. influenzae,* and streptococci are the most important pathogens. However, *H. influenzae* is uncommon after 5 years of age. **Since the introduction and use of the *H. influenzae* b conjugate vaccine, there has been a continuous and marked decline in the percent of cases due to this pathogen in young children** [123]. Before the introduction of this vaccine, staphylococci caused as many as 40% of the cases of these infections [117–121], but in a recent series, in part due to the decline of *H. influenzae* b disease, staphylococci and streptococci accounted for 70% of culture-confirmed cases [122]. Development of sequelae is significantly associated with (a) infection in infants younger than 6 months, (b) delay of 4 or more days in instituting medical or surgical treatment, (c) infection due to *S. aureus,* and (d), most strikingly, involvement of the hip or shoulder with concomitant presence of osteomyelitis [117–121].
3. **Adults with nongonococcal arthritis**
   a. ***S. aureus* is implicated in most cases.** In some reported series more than 90% of patients with underlying rheumatoid arthritis and septic arthritis had *S. aureus* infection [100]. **Local prevalence rates of MRSA should be considered in choosing therapy** [123].
   b. ***Streptococcus* species** are important etiologies in all age groups. Reports emphasize the importance of routine serologic typing of streptococcal isolates from joint fluid. The incidence of infections with groups G and B streptococci appears to be increased in patients with several chronic underlying conditions,

such as cirrhosis and diabetes [101,124]. Arthritis caused by these streptococci may be marked by a slow response to therapy, with persistent synovitis and joint destruction [125,126]. Enterococcal infections are unusual but have recently been reviewed [127].

c. **Gram-negative bacilli** are uncommon but warrant **special consideration in certain patients,** such as those with malignancies; medical immunosuppression; narcotic use; underlying chronic debilitating diseases, especially in the elderly; or prior noninfectious joint disease [99,100,101,103]. Gram-negative bacillary septic arthritis is occasionally seen in young and generally healthy hosts [128]. In heroin addicts with septic arthritis, *Serratia* and *Pseudomonas* species are relatively common. Brucella arthritis may be seen in immigrants to the United States who usually present with involvement of the sacroiliac, knee, or hip joint. The diagnosis is made either by blood cultures or serology [101].

d. **Anaerobic bacteria** are uncommon but have received increasing recognition as etiologic agents in septic arthritis. The predominant species are *Propionibacterium acnes,* anaerobic gram-positive cocci, and *Bacteroides* species [129]. Coinfection with facultative or aerobic organisms occurred in only 11% of cases. **Predisposing factors** include trauma, contiguous infection, prosthetic joint, prior surgical or needle entry into the joint, and diabetes. Such factors were present in 75% of cases.

e. **Prosthetic joint infections** are associated with a wide spectrum of implicated bacteria. Although staphylococci (both *S. aureus* and *S. epidermidis*) may be involved in more than half the cases, streptococci, gram-negative enteric bacilli, and anaerobic bacteria often are isolated in this setting (see also Prosthetic Joint Infections, below).

f. **Polyarticular septic arthritis** occurs in approximately 10% of adult patients with nongonococcal septic arthritis. **Many of these patients do poorly.** In a recent review [130] of 25 patients with nongonococcal polyarticular septic arthritis, all patients were older than 50 years, 52% had concurrent rheumatic diseases (generally rheumatoid arthritis), blood cultures were positive in 86%, and the mortality was 32%. **At presentation, many patients were mistakenly believed to be manifesting flares in their underlying rheumatoid arthritis or systemic lupus erythematosus and 20% were afebrile.** *S. aureus* accounted for 80% of cases, and streptococci, including *S. pneumoniae,* and gram-negative organisms accounted for approximately 20%.

g. **Bite wounds** with contiguous joint involvement may be associated with mixed flora (see detailed discussion in Chapter 4).

B. **Reactive arthritis** is a term used to describe a sterile but inflammatory process of the synovium preceded or triggered by an infection occurring anywhere outside the joint. Infectious agents that have been implicated include *Salmonella, Shigella, Yersinia, Campylobacter,* group A $\beta$-hemolytic streptococci, *Staphylococcus,* and, most especially, *Chlamydia* [131–133]. The latter has been strongly associated with the subsequent development of Reiter syndrome. Some reports suggest that long-term antimicrobial therapy of chlamydia may favorably impact the course of the associated Reiter syndrome [134].

C. **Nonbacterial disease**

1. **Viral infections generally are distinguished by the sudden onset of severe joint pain with or without effusion. Various types of exanthems occur in almost all.** The most common viral causes of arthritis are **human parvovirus B19 (fifth disease),** natural **rubella** infection, rubella vaccination, **hepatitis B** virus, and HIV [103,106,107,135]. In outbreaks of **fifth disease,** women present with symmetric arthritis in late winter and in the spring. The onset of joint symptoms in adults occurs with the rash or shortly after the eruption; small joints of the hands are most frequently involved with a self-limited course [136]. **With hepatitis B,** patients may have a history of urticaria for 1 to 6 weeks along with the onset of joint symptoms, resolving commonly with the onset of jaundice. The arthritis is symmetric. Hands are affected most often, followed by knees and ankles. Joint effusions are scanty [101].

HIV **has been associated with a variety of arthritis syndromes, including** an acute symmetric polyarthritis affecting the small joints of the hands and wrists, a disabling subacute oligoarticular arthritis affecting mainly knees and ankles, and a "painful articular syndrome," lasting fewer than 24 to 48 hours, involving the knees, elbows, or shoulders characterized by severe intermittent arthralgia without synovitis, often requiring narcotic analgesics. Psoriatic arthritis, Reiter syndrome, and a variety of other syndromes are also associated with HIV. Arthritis can be a manifestation of infection with mumps (especially in men), influenza, arboviruses, Epstein-Barr virus (infectious mononucleosis), and varicella. Reviews of viral arthritis have been published [106,135,137].

2. **Mycobacterial and fungal arthritis is characterized by slow evolution** of physical and radiographic findings [101]. Fungal arthritis is seen mainly in immunocompromised patients. Evidence of disseminated disease is common [109]. Among the fungi, sporotrichotic, candidal, and coccidioidal arthritis are the most common, but arthritis can also occur with blastomycosis, cryptococcosis, and histoplasmosis. Bayer and Guze [138] reviewed fungal arthritis in detail. See further discussion in Chapter 17. *Coccidioides immitis* monoarticular infection typically occurs in non-white immunosuppressed men from endemic areas. Joint infections in patients with blastomycosis primarily spread from a contiguous focus of osteomyelitis. Candidal infections of peripheral joints generally are of acute onset due to hematogenous spread [101].

   *M. tuberculosis* and atypical mycobacteria are uncommon but important causes of chronic indolent infectious arthritis [108,109]. These have been reviewed by Meier and Hoffman [139].

   **Cultures of synovial tissue produce a higher yield** than cultures of joint fluid **in cases of mycobacterial and fungal infection** [101].
3. **Lyme disease** [140–143], caused by the tickborne spirochete *B. burgdorferi*, characteristically occurs in summer. It frequently is characterized by a unique skin lesion, erythema chronicum migrans, and often is accompanied by systemic flu-like symptoms. From several days to as long as 2 years later, approximately 60% of untreated patients develop brief recurring episodes of either an asymmetric oligoarthritis affecting primarily large joints or a migratory polyarthritis [140,142]. Diagnostic issues, problems with serologic testing [140,143], and therapy [140,144] are **discussed in detail in Chapter 21.**

**IV. Differential diagnosis**

**A.** Conditions that may be associated with joint effusion are listed in Table 5.5. Infectious arthritis (group 3) would more commonly have to be distinguished from the inflammatory joint diseases listed in group 2 than from diseases in the other categories. It must be remembered that **bacterial arthritis may complicate, and in part be obscured by, the inflammatory conditions listed in group 2. The laboratory approach outlined** in section II should help sort out such possibilities, including crystal-induced synovitis.

**B.** Arthritis in the presence of bacterial endocarditis is due to bacterial seeding of one or more joints or to immune complex disease. The development of arthritis in an unusual site suggests the possibility of endocarditis.

**C. Acute transient synovitis of the hip,** sometimes called **"toxic synovitis** of the hip" or "acute transient epiphysitis," is the most common cause of a painful hip in children under 10 years of age [145]. Boys are most frequently affected, especially between 3 and 6 years, but the disorder can occur in infancy and early adolescence. The etiology is unknown. The onset of hip pain with motion and weight-bearing may be acute or gradual. There may be a slight fever, usually not higher than 100°F to 101°F [145]. There are no changes of the bone on conventional radiographs; scintigraphy with $^{99m}$Tc studies are normal or show slight diffuse increase in uptake. The peripheral WBC count and ESR are normal. **Aspiration of the hip joint will yield clear fluid that is sterile on culture.** Antibiotics are not indicated if synovial fluid cultures are negative. Corticosteroids are not effective, but antiinflammatory drugs may be useful. This entity is reviewed in more detail elsewhere [145].

**D. Postinfectious (reactive) arthritis,** usually with multiple joints involved, can be seen as an immunologic response during infection with certain agents (e.g.,

Table 5.5. Differential Diagnosis by Joint Fluid Groups

| Group 1 (Noninflammatory) | Group 2 (Inflammatory) | Group 3 (Septic) | Hemorrhagic |
|---|---|---|---|
| Degenerative joint disease | Rheumatoid arthritis | Bacterial infections | Hemophilia or other hemorrhagic diathesis |
| Trauma[a] | Acute crystal-induced synovitis (gout and pseudogout) | | Trauma with or without fracture |
| Osteochondritis dissecans | Reiter syndrome | | Neuropathic arthropathy |
| Osteochondromatosis | Ankylosing spondylitis | | Pigmented villonodular synovitis |
| Neuropathic arthropathy[a] | Psoriatic arthritis | | Synovioma |
| Subsiding or early inflammation | Arthritis accompanying ulcerative colitis and regional enteritis | | Hemangioma and other benign neoplasm |
| Hypertrophic osteoarthropathy[b] | Rheumatic fever[b] | | |
| Pigmented villonodular synovitis[a] | Systemic lupus erythematosus | | |
| | Progressive systemic sclerosis (scleroderma)[b] | | |

[a]May be hemorrhagic.
[b]Group 1 or 2.
From Rodnan GP, McEwen C, Wallace SL, eds. Primer on the rheumatic diseases. *JAMA* 1973;224 [Suppl.]:661, with permission.

hepatitis B); see section III.C.1. Postinfectious arthritis also can develop after meningococcal infections, sexually transmitted diseases, or enteric infections due to *Shigella, Salmonella, Campylobacter,* and *Yersinia* species. The presence of the specific histocompatibility antigen HLA-B27 increases the likelihood of postinfectious arthritis and appears to predispose to more severe disease [101] (see related discussion in section III.B). Joint fluid cultures are sterile.

V. **Therapy for bacterial joint infections requires both** removal of purulent material (i.e., **adequate drainage**) from the joint and administration of appropriate **antibiotics.** Weight-bearing should be avoided, but immobilization of the joint is unnecessary [103]. In most cases, medical management will be successful if symptomatic improvement occurs within 48 hours.

A. **Drainage of purulent material.** By needle aspiration, as much purulent material as possible should be removed without damage to the synovial membrane. Frequent aspiration (daily or more often), as fluid reaccumulates, is an essential adjunct to antibiotic therapy.

1. **Purposes of joint aspiration**
   - **a.** To provide drainage of the enclosed space, which functionally is acting like an abscess.
   - **b.** To provide symptomatic relief.
   - **c.** To relieve joint pressure and remove inflammatory debris including enzymes that cause destruction of articular cartilage.
   - **d.** To ensure that therapy is effective by doing follow-up smears, cultures, and leukocyte counts.
2. **Frequency and duration.** The infected joint fluid must be removed by needle aspiration or open drainage whenever fluid reaccumulates or in certain special

settings noted later. Repeated aspirations within the first 48 hours of antibiotic therapy usually provides adequate drainage.

**B. Repeated aspirations versus open drainage.** This remains a controversial subject, with little experimental evidence to support either viewpoint. Several studies [117,118,121,146] support the concept that early drainage is more important than the method of drainage for all joints except the hip, where an initial surgical approach is required (i.e., open drainage). As such, there is no clear-cut benefit to open surgical drainage versus drainage by repeated aspirations [121,146,147]. Whereas repeated needle aspirations (i.e., daily, or more often if fluid accumulates rapidly) of the infected joint are appropriate for most cases of septic arthritis, surgical drainage is to be considered early in the course in certain situations, as follows:

1. **Lack of response to appropriate antibiotic therapy and repeat needle aspirations.** The precise time one should wait is controversial. Some authorities favor open drainage if adequate response has not occurred within 48 to 72 hours of antibiotic therapy and serial aspirations [101]; others allow up to 1 week.
2. **Inability to drain the joint adequately by needle aspiration** due to large amounts of debris, fibrin, or loculations [146].
3. **Infection of a prosthetic joint** (see under Prosthetic Joint Infections, below).
4. **Relative inaccessibility of the joint** or advanced disease and necrosis, as might be the case in an infected hip [103]. The need for surgical (open) drainage of an infected hip often is stated but not established by controlled studies. In the absence of such a study, **most clinicians believe that hip joint infections,** except perhaps gonococcal infections, **require surgical drainage.** Suppurative arthritis of the shoulder also requires either radiographically guided aspiration or surgical drainage [101].
5. **Gram-negative bacillary arthritis.** These patients have a poorer prognosis. Most patients with gram-positive joint infections attain complete recovery of the joint. However, only some patients with gram-negative arthritis achieve such a result. Some authors advocate early explorative arthrotomy in these patients to ensure adequate drainage, to assess and drain perisynovial abscesses, and to debride any contiguous osteomyelitis [128].

**C. Antibiotic therapy**

1. **Instillation of antibiotics directly into the joint is unnecessary and unwise.** Most antibiotics diffuse readily into the synovial fluid [148,149], and intraarticular injections of antibiotics may induce a chemical synovitis.
2. **Parenterally administered antibiotics** usually are indicated in the treatment of septic arthritis.
   a. **Penetration of antibiotics into synovial fluid.** According to studies, the following antibiotics are reported to reach levels in synovial fluid that would be adequate in therapy: penicillin G, ampicillin, nafcillin, carbenicillin, cephalothin, cefazolin, cefuroxime, clindamycin, chloramphenicol, tetracycline, sulfonamides, vancomycin, gentamicin, amikacin, ceftriaxone, ceftazidime, aztreonam, imipenem, and probably cefotaxime. It is likely that penetration into synovial fluid is greater earlier in the course of septic arthritis, when the degree of inflammation is greater. This suggests caution regarding too rapid a change in antibiotic therapy to lower doses of parenteral therapy or to oral therapy in nongonococcal infections. Oral ciprofloxacin is a potential agent for susceptible pathogens.
   b. **Specific recommendations for treatment of nongonococcal arthritis.** Initial antibiotic therapy is based on results of the synovial fluid Gram stain, as **shown in Table 5.6.** When the culture and sensitivity results are available, the initial regimens are modified to include the least toxic effective antibiotic.
   c. **Gonococcal arthritis.** Treatment of gonococcal infections in the United States is complicated by the spread of infections due to antibiotic-resistant *N. gonorrhoeae* and the high frequency of intercurrent chlamydial infections in persons with gonorrhea; guidelines for therapy have recently been revised [150]. If an organism is isolated from joint fluid cultures, antimicrobial

Table 5.6. Antibiotic Therapy of Bacterial Arthritis Based on Initial Gram Stain

| Gram Stain | Drug of Choice | Dosage | Alternatives[a] |
|---|---|---|---|
| Gram-positive cocci | Nafcillin (or oxacillin) or vancomycin (if oxacillin-resistant *S. aureus* is deemed a significant risk) | 9 g/d i.v. in divided doses q4h in adults; 100–200 mg/kg/d i.v. in divided doses q4h in children (for vancomycin, 1 g q12h in adults, with modifications based on creatinine clearance; see Chapter 28) | First-generation cephalosporin (e.g., cefazolin or cephalothin), clindamycin |
| Gram-negative cocci | | | |
| Adult | Ceftriaxone[b,c] | 1 g i.v. once daily in adults | Cefotaxime[b,c] ceftizoxime[b,c] or spectinomycin[b] |
| Young child (>6 yr) | Ceftriaxone[b,c,d] | 50 mg/kg/d (max. 2 g) i.v. once daily | Cefotaxime 50 mg/kg/d i.v. in individual doses q8h |
| Gram-negative bacilli | Gentamicin[e] plus ticarcillin[f] | 4.5–5.0 mg/kg/d i.m. or i.v. in divided doses 8qh if renal function is normal<br>15–18 g/d i.v. in divided doses q4h in adults; 200–300 mg/kg/d i.v. in divided doses q4h in children | Gentamicine and third-generation cephalosporin |
| No organisms seen | | | |
| Young adult, healthy | Ceftriaxone | As above | Cefoxitin |
| Patient with risk factors (see text) | Nafcillin and gentamicin | As above | Third-generation cephalosporin[g] |
| Young child (>6 yr) | Ceftriaxone[g] | As above | Cefuroxime or ampicillin[h] and nafcillin |
| Neonate,[i] infant (>3 mo) | Cefotaxime[g,j] or cefotaxime and gentamicin[k] | See Chapters 3 and 28. | Oxacillin, cefotaxime,[g] and an aminoglycoside[k] |

[a]Specific doses of alternative agents are discussed in Chapter 27. In the penicillin-allergic patient with a delayed reaction, cephalosporins often are used as alternative agents. In patients with an immediate, severe reaction to a penicillin cephalosporins should not be used without skin testing (see Chapter 24).

[b]See discussion in text (section **V.C.2.c**) under Infectious Arthritis.

[c]When susceptibility data are not available for gonococcal infections, a third-generation cephalosporin now is preferred [51].

[d]May be coccobacillary forms of *Haemophilus influenzae,* which are susceptible to third-generation cephalosporins (e.g., ceftriaxone, cefotaxime), as are gonococci.

[e]Local aminoglycoside susceptibility patterns must be considered. If gentamicin resistance is common, tobramycin or amikacin is preferred.

[f]Or mezlocillin or piperacillin (see Chapter 27).

[g]In the past, the third-generation cephalosporins were believed to have significantly less antistaphylococcal activity than the semisynthetic penicillinase-resistant penicillins and first-generation cephalosporins, so some clinicians added an antibiotic (e.g., oxacillin) to ensure **optimal** antistaphylococcal activity while awaiting culture data. However, more recent data suggest that some third-generation cephalosporins (e.g., ceftriaxone and cefotaxime) may have adequate antistaphylococcal activity. See Chapter 27 discussion of cephalosporins. Some experts still favor an antistaphylococcal agent (e.g., oxacillin) added to a third-generation cephalosporin for enhanced *S. aureus* activity.

[h]If ampicillin-resistant *H. influenzae* is common, a third-generation cephalosporin (e.g., ceftriaxone) or cefuroxime is preferred while awaiting culture and susceptibility data (see footnote d).

[i]See Chapter 3 for dosages and other options.

[j]If community-acquired infection. See text.

[k]If hospital-acquired infection. See text.

Modified from Goldenberg DL, Cohen AS. Acute infectious arthritis: a review of patients with nongonococcal joint infections (with emphasis on therapy and prognosis). *Am J Med* 1976;60:369, with permission.

susceptibility testing should be performed. Patients should be initially hospitalized for therapy and examined for evidence of endocarditis or meningitis, both of which are rare. The treatment of gonococcal arthritis is similar to that for disseminated gonococcal infection [150].

3. **Duration of parenteral therapy**
   a. **Gonococcal arthritis** (see Chapter 16).
   b. **Nongonococcal arthritis**
      (1) **Adults.** Therapy is continued until the arthritis appears to be resolved. The usual duration of therapy is 2 weeks for infections due to *H. influenzae,* streptococci, or gram-negative cocci [101], if there is no underlying joint disease and if the patient does well with initial therapy. Longer courses of therapy (e.g., 3 weeks) are indicated in patients with gram-negative infections, slowly responding infections (despite adequate drainage), or infections with virulent organisms such as *S. aureus* [101]. Whether additional oral therapy is indicated after full courses of parenteral therapy is controversial, although patients with prosthetic joint infections often receive prolonged courses, as noted under Prosthetic Joint Infections (see below).
      When an effective oral regimen is available (e.g., trimethoprim-sulfamethoxazole or oral quinolone very active against the pathogen), oral therapy often is used to complete a full course of therapy (see section (3)).
      (2) **Initial parenteral therapy followed by oral treatment of children.** Short courses of parenteral therapy (i.e., 5–7 days) followed by 10 to 21 days of oral antibiotics in children appears generally successful if the initial clinical response is favorable and adequate serum bactericidal activity is demonstrated (i.e., >1:8) [151]. However, some guidelines and precautions should be heeded.
         (a) The serum bactericidal titer (peak) on the day after the initiation of oral therapy should be at least 1:8 when the pathogen is a gram-negative bacillus, *S. aureus,* or *H. influenzae,* and at least 1:32 when the organism is a streptococcus. Therefore, the pathogen causing the septic arthritis must be isolated so the laboratory can provide information on bactericidal levels necessary to eliminate it.
         (b) If the bactericidal level is suboptimal, the dosage of antibiotic must be increased. Usually, the oral dose is two to three times that used for minor infections. These higher doses were well tolerated in children [151].
         (c) Ideally, the entire course of oral agents should be given in the hospital, especially if there is any doubt about patient compliance. If the therapy is given at home, three precautions must be taken:
            (i) There must be an **adequate bactericidal titer** of the antibiotic in the serum before discharge.
            (ii) **Compliance** with the oral regimen at home **must be ensured** after careful discussion with the patient and family.
            (iii) The patient should be **followed up weekly** to check on his or her clinical condition and to monitor the serum bactericidal level.
         (d) The **duration of therapy** will depend on the organism and the patient's clinical response. For *H. influenzae,* streptococci, or gram-negative cocci, a minimum of 2 weeks of therapy is suggested. For *S. aureus* or gram-negative bacilli, a minimum of 3 weeks is suggested. If the clinical response is slow or the ESR remains elevated, more prolonged therapy and reevaluation are necessary. Cases must be individualized, especially when *S. aureus* is involved (see Chapter 27). In gram-negative infections, if susceptible to trimethoprim-sulfamethoxazole or ciprofloxacin, an oral agent may be used.
      (3) **In adults, there is far less experience with parenteral short-course therapy followed by oral therapy.** One group [152] suggests the bactericidal level should be a trough measurement and should be at least a 1:8 against the isolated pathogen. (See Chapter 25 for additional discussion of bactericidal levels.)

D. **Prosthetic joint infections** (see Prosthetic Joint Infections, below)

E. **Repeated aspirations to monitor therapy.** Repeated joint aspirations, within the first 5 to 7 days of therapy [101], serve to monitor effectiveness of the antimicrobial therapy and to remove debris that may be destructive to the joint. Within a few days of adequate therapy, the joint fluid should become sterile; for example, serial cultures of joint fluid that become negative within 5 days of the initiation of therapy have been considered to be indicative of a good clinical response [101]. Within 1 week, the leukocyte count should be substantially lowered if a good outcome is to be expected with the therapeutic regimen in use. In addition, fluid reaccumulation should be markedly decreasing. **In the absence of such indications of response,** despite appropriate antibiotic therapy as determined by cultures and sensitivity testing, **open surgical drainage is to be considered,** as discussed in section B.

F. **Therapy for nonbacterial joint infections.** Infectious disease consultation is advised for treatment of mycobacterial and fungal infections. See Chapters 11 and 17 for therapeutic options for fungal and mycobacterial infections, respectively.

VI. **Prognosis.** The prognosis in infectious (septic) arthritis varies greatly. In older children and adults without other comorbidities and for whom a large single joint is infected, the overall prognosis for survival and full return of joint function is excellent. In contrast, infants and neonates in whom the hip joint is involved may have permanent sequelae, including leg length discrepancy [153]. Similarly, in the elderly, permanent sequelae and accompanying osteomyelitis are more common, and death rates approaching 20% have been reported [154]. In a recent review, characteristics of patients with bacterial arthritis associated with a poor outcome included age of at least 60 years, preexisting (rheumatoid) arthritis, infection of the hip or shoulder, duration of symptoms of more than 1 week before treatment, involvement of more than four joints, and persistently positive cultures after a 7-day course of appropriate antibiotics [101].

## PROSTHETIC JOIN INFECTIONS

Under optimal conditions, the overall rate of total joint replacement infections has decreased in recent years to 1% to 2% [155], although precise rates of infection may be difficult to obtain and depend on the joint replaced and the extent of time after the operation [156]. **Risk factors that appear to be associated with the development of infection in prosthetic joints include** advanced age, malnutrition, rheumatoid arthritis, diabetes mellitus, use of corticosteroids, and preexisting infection at another site. Additional risks include prior surgery in the affected joint, location and design of the implanted prosthesis (with knee arthroplasties having a higher incidence of infection than hips), and occurrence of a local hematoma or superficial wound infection in the postoperative period [155,157]. In a recent review, prior joint surgery, perioperative wound complications, and underlying rheumatoid arthritis were the most well-established risk factors [156]. Prosthetic joint infections have been recently reviewed elsewhere [156,158].

I. **Initiation of infection.** Bacterial contamination of the joint may be initiated either during or after implantation. Despite aseptic surgical techniques, intraoperative contamination can occur via air contamination, generally caused by dispersion of desquamated skin scales from individuals in the operating room; it may also occur from the patient's own skin or contact with the surgeon's hand through a punctured glove [159]. Significantly fewer infections have been found in operating rooms using ultraclean as opposed to conventional air circulation systems [160]. In contrast, deep infection initiated after surgery is caused by hematogenous spread of bacteria from distant sites. Most of these are believed to originate from cutaneous lesions, the respiratory tract, urinary tract, and oral cavity [102,105].

Most series have demonstrated that 80% to 90% of prosthetic joint infections, evident in the first 2 years after operation, originate in the operating room, with later hematogenously acquired infections accounting for the remainder [159].

II. **Biopathogenesis.** Within hours of implantation, the surface of the prosthesis is covered by a layer of glycoproteins, some of which act as receptors that facilitate the adherence of both tissue cells and bacteria. After adherence has taken place, many bacteria produce a slime, the glycocalyx, which renders adherence irreversible, permits optimal concentration of nutrients, and provides protection against both phagocytosis

Table 5.7. Microbiology of 1,033 Prosthetic Joint Infections[a] Seen at Mayo Clinic from 1969 to 1991

| Microorganism(s) | No. (%) of Prosthetic Joint Infections |
|---|---|
| Coagulase-negative staphylococci | 254 (25) |
| *S. aureus* | 240 (23) |
| Polymicrobial | 147 (14) |
| Gram-negative bacilli | 114 (11) |
| Streptococci[b] | 79 (8) |
| Unknown[c] | 83 (8) |
| Anaerobes | 62 (6) |
| Enterococci | 29 (3) |
| Other microorganisms | 25 (2) |
| Total | 1,033 (100) |

[a] All cases met case definition of definite infection. See text for discussion section **IV.D.**
[b] Includes $\beta$-hemolytic streptococci and viridans group streptococci.
[c] Includes cases in which there was no growth on routine bacterial cultures, routine bacterial cultures were not obtained, or microbiological information was not available.
From Steckelberg JM, Osman DR. Prosthetic joint infections. In: Bisno AL, Waldvogel FA, eds. *Infections associated with indwelling medical devices,* 2nd ed. Washington, DC: American Society for Microbiology, 1994:266, with permission.

by leukocytes and antibiotics. After the initial invasion of bacteria into tissue, host defenses react within 2 to 5 hours to localize the infection and prevent spread to adjacent tissues. During this decisive period, antibiotics are successful in reducing the total number of bacteria and tilting the balance in favor of host defenses, but after this time their effect is very limited [159].

**III. Microbiologic features.** More than 50% of prosthesis-related infections are caused by gram-positive organisms. Most of these appear to be due to staphylococci, with coagulase-negative staphylococcal species outnumbering *S. aureus* in some series. Streptococci, including the anaerobic *Peptococcus* species, cause most of the rest of such infections. Enteric gram-negative bacteria account for 10% to 28% of infections in various series [159]. Many of these agents are skin commensals or transient skin contaminants (Table 5.7).

**IV. Diagnosis**

**A. Clinical presentation. A high degree of clinical suspicion** is required because the presentation is generally indolent and the degree of pain and systemic symptoms often are considerably less pronounced than in septic arthritis of a native joint. In addition, pain due to mechanical loosening (not due to infection) and that due to sepsis can present with a similar clinical picture. In joint sepsis, **pain is a prominent feature,** usually is constant, is exacerbated by weight-bearing, and increases over time. It occurs in 90% of patients, although such hallmarks of infection as fever, localized edema and erythema, and sinus tract drainage each occur in only 30% to 40% of patients. An acute or fulminant presentation is more common with virulent organisms such as *S. aureus* or pyogenic $\beta$-hemolytic streptococci, whereas a chronic indolent course is more typical of infection with less virulent organisms, for example, coagulase-negative staphylococci [156].

**B. Radiographic studies**

1. **Serial radiograph findings.** Loosening or dislocation of the prosthesis in association with cortical bone resorption or periosteal reaction is suggestive of infection but may also be seen with mechanical loosening alone [161].
2. **Bone scans.** Recent studies of traditional three-phase $^{99m}$Tc bone imaging concluded that this test was "limited in its ability to discern between infection and aseptic loosening as the incidence of false negative results is unacceptably high" [162].
3. A summary of seven studies using **$^{111}$In-labeled autologous leukocytes** reported somewhat better results, with an average sensitivity of 79% and a

specificity of 81% [163]. $^{111}$In-labeled nonspecific IgG scintigraphy may be slightly better still (i.e., overall sensitivity of 97% and specificity of 85%), but both false-positive and false-negative results occur.

4. **Conclusion. Although useful, none of these tests is entirely satisfactory in defining whether joint sepsis is present in all cases.** Therefore, technetium bone scanning alone cannot usefully distinguish septic and aseptic loose prostheses [158]. However, a positive scan may be highly suggestive of infection, which can then be confirmed by aspiration and/or biopsy. Gallium scanning has a high reported specificity, indicating that a positive result correlates well with confirmation of infection at aspiration or biopsy but has a low sensitivity [158].

C. **Laboratory studies**

1. **Aspiration of joint fluid and subsequent histologic and microbiologic examination of tissue samples obtained at surgery remain the tests of choice for a definitive diagnosis of prosthetic joint infection.** In one recent study, the sensitivity of fine-needle aspiration for detecting the infecting microorganism was 87% and its specificity was 95%, compared with biopsy cultures obtained at the time of surgery [164].
   a. **Cultures should be obtained without recent antibiotic therapy.** Because of the critical importance of making a microbiologic diagnosis, in most nonacute cases, antimicrobial therapy should be withheld until all aspirate and/or intraoperative specimens have been obtained. If antimicrobial therapy has already been started, it should be stopped when possible for 10 to 14 days before any diagnostic procedure to avoid false-negative culture results [156].
   b. **Good aerobic and anaerobic cultures** should be routinely processed. As much fluid for culture as possible should be obtained at the time of a diagnostic joint aspiration [156]. For chronic indolent infections, fungal and mycobacterial cultures are advised.
   c. When prosthesis debridement or removal is performed, the surgeon should obtain multiple tissue samples for culture and histopathology. Intraoperative cultures should include **tissue** from the bone–cement interface, if possible, and samples of any purulence [156]. In chronic infections, mycobacterial and fungal cultures are also advised.
   d. **Histopathologic examination** for inflammation, granulomas, and tissue stains for organisms can be very useful.
   e. Careful susceptibility studies should be performed on any isolated bacterial pathogens.
   f. The predictive value of a single positive surveillance culture at the time of a revision arthroplasty for a failed prosthesis is unknown; such a result requires careful correlation with the clinical context [156].
   g. Cultures of drainage from sinus tracts do not reliably identify the etiologic microorganisms [156,158].
2. **Blood cultures** should routinely be obtained (e.g., two or three samples drawn 30–60 minutes apart).
3. Nonspecific tests such as the ESR and C-reactive protein may be of limited value in raising the clinician's level of suspicion and diagnosing the initial infection or in monitoring the response to therapy.

D. In the recent Mayo Clinic summary, **a definite prosthetic joint infection** was defined by at least one of the following criteria: (a) two or more cultures from sterile joint aspirates or intraoperative cultures were positive for the same organism, (b) purulence was observed at the time of surgical inspection, (c) acute inflammation consistent with infection was present on histopathologic examination of intracapsular tissue, or (d) a sinus tract that communicates with the joint spaces was present [156].

V. **Therapy.** The **optimal approach** to treatment of the infected arthroplasty **remains unclear.** There are few randomized prospective studies reported, and virtually none compares different treatment arms within a single well-controlled study.

A detailed discussion of the infectious disease considerations of the different surgical approaches appears elsewhere [156,158]. To consistently achieve microbiology cure, it is necessary to remove the prosthesis and all associated cement and completely debride devitalized tissue and bone. Issues about reimplantation that remain controversial include the optimal time to reimplantation, the role of antibiotic impregnated cement, the need for antibiotic-impregnated polymethylmethacrylate spacers (e.g., in two-stage reimplantation for total knee prosthetic infections), and the optimal type and duration of administration of intravenous and oral antimicrobials [156]. **Therefore, we suggest close cooperation of the orthopedic surgeon and the infectious disease consultant in managing these patients.**

**A.** Nonetheless **two-stage replacement,** involving removal of the hip or knee prosthesis and a 6- to 8-week course of intravenous antibiotic therapy followed by reimplantation has been widely recommended [156,161,165]. Antibiotic-impregnated cement spacers commonly are used as adjunctive therapy in arthroplasty for replacement of the infected knee, in preparation for reimplantation. Success rates for microbiologic cure with this technique vary but average approximately 80% to 90%.

**B.** A growing number of reports have suggested that **implant salvage,** using either antibiotic therapy alone or antibiotics plus surgical debridement, may be feasible in selected patients. This approach has evolved out of multiple concerns, not the least of which are the potential surgical and medical complications attending joint removal and reimplantation in the generally elderly patients, many of whom have other underlying medical illnesses and the risk factors outlined earlier.

1. In addition, new antimicrobial regimens may cure infections that previously were believed to be untreatable without removal of the device [166]. Data from both animal models [166,167] and human clinical trials now are available to support consideration of this approach. Treatment regimens combining rifampin with either quinolone or $\beta$-lactam antibiotics can be particularly effective with reported success rates of more than 80% in some studies [166,167], although such success also has been reported in some series not using such combinations [155,168,171]. Treatment durations have generally been prolonged (e.g., $\geq$6–12 months).
2. **As encouraging as these recent studies may be, enthusiasm must be tempered by numerous other studies demonstrating poorer outcomes (success rates only in the 20%–40% range)** [155,169,170,172–174]. The treatment of these infections is clearly evolving.
3. **In our opinion, patients who might be considered for an attempt at implant salvage must meet at least the following criteria:**
   - **a.** A loosened prosthesis is not present.
   - **b.** The microorganism is susceptible to antibiotics, including oral antibiotics that the patient can tolerate.
   - **c.** The patient is not septic, requiring immediate removal of the infected prosthesis. It should be recognized that cure rates using this approach appear to be higher with acute (generally defined as symptoms of less than 2–4 weeks' duration) as opposed to chronic infections.
   - **d.** Finally, the patient must understand that failure may necessitate, but does not preclude, standard therapy, including prosthesis removal and subsequent reimplantation, arthrodesis, resection arthroplasty, or other treatment options. In contradistinction to others [160,169], we do not believe that infection with *S. aureus* represents a contraindication to this approach. Experience with gram-negative organisms is more limited.

**C. Debridement with retention of the prosthesis** procedures usually have been unsuccessful for chronic well-established infections [156]. For early acute infections (i.e., within less than 3 months of the primary surgery) in the presence of a draining infected hematoma without cellulitis, thorough open surgical debridement, irrigation, and antibiotics may salvage up to 70% of prosthetic hip or knee replacements [158]. Recently, delivery of high concentrations of antibiotic via implantable pumps has been used with promising success in acute prosthetic infections [158]. Further evaluation and experience with this technique is needed.

**D. Suppressive antimicrobial therapy** without concomitant surgical intervention **is not considered standard therapy** for prosthetic joint infection because satisfactory functional outcomes are so low [158]. In some situations, antibiotic suppression (long term) is combined with initial surgical debridement with the goal of suppression of symptoms and maintenance of a functioning joint. This may be rational, and often the only option, in some carefully selected patients when (a) removal of the prosthesis is not feasible, (b) the organism is of low virulence and highly susceptible to oral antimicrobial agents, (c) the patient is not systemically ill, (d) the patient is compliant, and (e) the prosthesis is not loose [156].

VI. **Postoperative superficial wound infection, a major risk for subsequent prosthesis infection.** Aggressive early local care and intravenous antibiotic therapy of these infections have been highly successful in preventing the involvement and removal of the prosthesis [173]. In view of the rapid evolution of treatment options in infections of prosthetic joints, infectious disease consultation is advised.

VII. **Prophylaxis** Antibiotic prophylaxis reduces the frequency of deep wound infection after total joint replacement, and short courses of cefazolin commonly are recommended [175] (see Chapter 27). The use of operating rooms with ultraclean air has a similar effect [160]. Antibiotic-impregnated cement may be equally as effective, but these data are more preliminary. **See related discussion in Chapter 27.**

## INFECTIOUS BURSITIS

I. **Clinical presentation.** Septic bursitis most commonly involves the prepatellar or olecranon bursa.

A. **History.** The common background of patients is a history of either acute or chronic repetitive trauma to the knee or elbow. A history of concurrent superficial skin infection near to the involved area is frequently elicited. Infection is thought to occur due to local spread from the skin.

1. **Pain** and **swelling,** usually acute over a few hours, occurs in the vast majority.
2. **Fever** occurs in one-half of cases.
3. **History of recent intrabursal steroid injection** is frequent in misdiagnosed cases [176].

B. **Physical examination**

1. **There is usually bursal swelling** with maximal tenderness over the center of the bursa. There is a varying degree of local inflammatory reaction.
2. **Peribursal cellulitis** is frequent.
3. **Range of motion** of the joint is preserved, unlike septic arthritis.

II. **Diagnostic aids. Definitive diagnosis is via aspiration of bursal fluid that should be performed in all cases. Frequently, sympathetic joint effusions occur with septic bursitis. These effusions must also be sampled to ensure no concurrent joint infection exists.**

A. **Bursal fluid aspiration.** Grossly, fluid may vary from appearance from thin serous to frank pus.

1. **Leukocyte counts** are frequently less than 20,000 cell/mm$^3$ and may range from 1,500 to more than 400,000 cells/mm$^3$ with predominance of polymorphonuclear leukocytes.
2. **Glucose levels** and protein levels are not helpful.
3. **Gram stains** are positive around 50% of the time. It is of particular importance to guide therapy in patients who have received prior antibiotics in whom fluid cultures may have been rendered negative.
4. **Urate crystal examination** should be performed because gout may mimic or occur with septic bursitis.
5. **Aerobic and anaerobic cultures** should be obtained on all specimens [176].

B. **Blood cell count.** The peripheral WBC count and ESR range from normal to markedly elevated and a leukocytosis greater than 10,000 cells/mm$^3$ is seen in approximately 60% of cases.

C. **Radiography** is infrequently helpful.

D. **Blood cultures** are rarely positive when a single bursa is involved.

III. **Bacteriology of septic bursitis.** ***S. aureus*** **is involved in as many as 90% of cases.** Streptococcal species, particularly *Streptococcus pyogenes,* is the next most frequent. Coagulase-negative staphylococci account for 1% or 2%. Gram-negative bacteria, mycobacteria, and fungi are infrequently reported.

IV. **Differential diagnosis** includes septic arthritis, gout, trauma, or hemorrhagic olecranon bursitis in patients with uremia.

V. **Therapy** includes appropriate antibiotics and drainage, usually via repeated needle aspirations.

A. **Antibiotics.** Most empiric therapy should be directed against *S. aureus.* Further therapy is guided by results of culture and Gram stain. Oral therapy may be used in immunocompetent patients without significant systemic symptoms (e.g., fever) or overlying cellulitis.

1. **For therapy of methicillin-susceptible *S. aureus***

a. **Parenteral therapy.** A semisynthetic penicillinase-resistant penicillin such as nafcillin or oxacillin, 1.0 to 1.5 g every 4 to 6 hours, can be given to adults. In children, 100 to 150 mg/kg/day in divided doses is given every 4 to 6 hours.

In the patient with a delayed penicillin reaction, a first-generation cephalosporin (e.g., cefazolin, 1 g every 8 hours in adults) is recommended. In patients with immediate type hypersensitivity to penicillin, clindamycin is recommended.

b. **Oral therapy.** Antistaphylococcal agents such as dicloxacillin or cloxacillin, 500 mg four times a day in adults, can be given. In the adult patients with delayed type penicillin hypersensitivity, an oral cephalosporin such as cephalexin or cephradine, 500 mg to 1 g four times day, can be used. Oral clindamycin may be used in patients with immediate type hypersensitivity to penicillin.

2. **If MRSA** is suspected due to recent hospitalization or in patients receiving chronic hemodialysis, **vancomycin** is used.

3. **Duration of therapy.** In immunocompetent patients with uncomplicated disease, therapy may be continued for 1 week after sterilization of bursal fluid as determined by culture performed at the time of repeated aspiration. Immunocompromised patients require more prolonged therapy, generally in excess of 10 days of parenteral therapy before sterilization of the bursa.

B. **Adequate drainage is essential** and should be performed via needle aspiration every 1 to 3 days. Indications for surgical intervention include failure of needle aspiration to provide adequate drainage, bursa inaccessible to needle drainage, pointing abscess, foreign body or necrotic tissue removal, or recurrent or refractory disease.

VI. **Response to therapy** is determined by clinical improvement and demonstration of conversion of bursal cultures from positive to negative [176].

## REFERENCES


1. Waldvogel FA, Medoff G, Swartz MN. Osteomyelitis: a review of clinical features, therapeutic considerations, and unusual aspects. *N Engl J Med* 1970;282:198.
2. Cierny G, Mader JT, Pennick JJ. A clinical staging system for adult osteomyelitis. *Contemp Orthop* 1985;10:17.
3. Lew DP, Waldvogel FA. Osteomyelitis. *N Engl J Med* 1997;336:999.
4. Haas DW, McAndrew MP. Bacterial osteomyelitis in adults: evolving considerations in diagnosis and treatment. *Am J Med* 1996;101:550.
5. Waldvogel FA, Vasey H. Osteomyelitis: the past decade. *N Engl J Med* 1980;303:360.
6. Weinstein AJ. Osteomyelitis: microbiologic, clinical and therapeutic considerations. *Prim Care* 1981;8:557.
7. Gentry LO. Overview of osteomyelitis. *Orthop Rev* 1987;16:255.
8. Kahn DS, Pritzker KPH. The pathophysiology of bone infection. *Clin Orthop* 1973; 96:12.
9. Wald ER. Risk factors for osteomyelitis. *Am J Med* 1985;78[Suppl. 6B]:206.
10. Piehl FC, Davis RJ, Prugh SI. Osteomyelitis in sickle cell disease. *J Pediatr Orthop* 1993;13:225.
11. Chandrasekar PH, Narula AP. Bone and joint infections in intravenous drug abusers. *Rev Infect Dis* 1986;8:904.
12. Leonard A, et al. Osteomyelitis in hemodialysis patients. *Ann Intern Med* 1973;78: 651.
13. Edwards MS, et al. An etiologic shift in infantile osteomyelitis: the emergence of the group B streptococcus. *J Pediatr* 1978;93:578.
14. Howard AW, Viskontas D, Sabbagh C. Reduction in osteomyelitis and septic arthritis related to haemophilus influenzae type B vaccination. *J Pediatr Orthop* 1999;19:705.

15. Meyers BR, et al. Clinical patterns of osteomyelitis due to gram-negative bacteria. *Arch Intern Med* 1973;131:228.
16. Brook I, Frazier EH. Anaerobic osteomyelitis and arthritis in a military hospital: a 10-year experience. *Am J Med* 1993;94:21.
17. Pichichero ME, Friesen HA. Polymicrobial osteomyelitis: report of three cases and a review of the literature. *Rev Infect Dis* 1982;4:86.
18. Craigen MAC, Watters J, Hackett JS. The changing epidemiology of osteomyelitis in children. *J Bone Joint Surg* 1992;74:541.
19. Miller WB Jr, Murphy WA, Gilula LA. Brodie abscess: reappraisal. *Radiology* 1979; 132:15.
20. Edwards MS, et al. Pelvic osteomyelitis in children. *Pediatrics* 1978;61:62.
21. Roine I, et al. Serial serum C-reactive protein to monitor recovery from acute hematogenous osteomyelitis in children. *Pediatr Infect Dis J* 1995;14:40.
22. Jaramillo D, et al. Osteomyelitis and septic arthritis in children: appropriate use of imaging to guide treatment. *AJR Am J Roentgenol* 1995;165:399.
23. Sammack B, et al. Osteomyelitis: a review of currently used imaging techniques. *Eur Radiol* 1999;9:894.
24. Tehranzadeh J, et al. Imaging of osteomyelitis in the mature skeleton. *Radiol Clin North Am* 2001;39:223.
25. Pancoast SJ, Neu HC. Antibiotic levels in human bone and synovial fluid used in the evaluation of antimicrobial therapy of joint and skeletal infections. *Orthop Rev* 1980;9:49.
26. Wacha H, Wagner D, Schafer V, et al. Concentration of ciprofloxacin in bone tissue after single parenteral administration to patients older than 70 years. *Infection* 1990; 18:173.
27. Meissner A, Borner K, Koeppe P. Concentrations of ofloxacin in human bone and cartilage. *Antimicrob Chemother* 1990;26:69.
28. Karwowska A, Daries D, Jadavji T. Epidemiology and outcome of osteomyelitis in the era of sequential intravenous-oral therapy. *Pediatr Infect Dis J* 1998;17: 1021.
29. Weinstein MP, et al. Multicenter collaborative evaluation of a standardized serum bactericidal test as a predictor of therapeutic efficacy in acute and chronic osteomyelitis. *Am J Med* 1987;83:218.
30. Gentry LO, Rodriguez GG. Oral ciprofloxacin compared with parenteral antibiotics in the treatment of osteomyelitis. *Antimicrob Agents Chemother* 1990;34:40.
31. Gentry LO, Rodriguez-Gomez G. Ofloxacin versus parenteral therapy for chronic osteomyelitis. *Antimicrob Agents Chemother* 1991;35:538.
32. Meyers BR, et al. Clinical patterns of osteomyelitis due to gram-negative bacteria. *Arch Intern Med* 1973;131:228.
33. Khatri G, Wagner DK, Sohnle P. Effect of bone biopsy in guiding antimicrobial therapy of osteomyelitis complicating open wounds. *Am J Med Sci* 2001;321:367.
34. Gillespie WJ. Prevention and management of infection after total joint replacement. *Clin Infect Dis* 1997;25:1310.
35. Brook JW. Management of pedal puncture wounds. *J Foot Ankle Surg* 1994;33:463.
36. Bell DB, Marks MI, Eickhoff TC. *Pasteurella multocida* arthritis and osteomyelitis. *JAMA* 1969;210:343.
37. Turpin S, Lambert R. Role of scintigraphy in musculoskeletal and spinal infections. *Radiol Clin North Am* 2001;39:169.
38. Mader JT, Mohan D, Calhoun J. A practical guide to the diagnosis and management of bone and joint infections. *Drugs* 1997;54:253.
39. Darouiche RO, Landon GC, Klima M, et al. Osteomyelitis associated with pressure sores. *Arch Intern Med* 1994;154:753.
40. Lipsky BA. Osteomyelitis of the foot in diabetic patients. *Clin Infect Dis* 1997;25: 1318.
41. Wheat LJ, et al. Diabetic foot infections: bacteriologic analysis. *Arch Intern Med* 1986;146:1935.
42. Bamberger DM, Daus GP, Gerding DN. Osteomyelitis in the feet of diabetic patients. Long-term results, prognostic factors, and the role of antimicrobial and surgical therapy. *Am J Med* 1987;83:653.

43. Grayson ML, Gibbons GW, Levin E, et al. Probing to bone in infected pedal ulcers. *JAMA* 1995;27:721.
44. Caputo GM, et al. Assessment and management of foot disease in patients with diabetes. *N Engl J Med* 1994;331:834.
45. Ger R. Prevention of major amputation in the diabetic patient. *Arch Surg* 1985; 120:1317.
46. Gentry LO. Approach to the patient with chronic osteomyelitis. *Curr Clin Top Infect Dis* 1987;8:62.
47. Overton LM, Tully WP. Surgical treatment of chronic osteomyelitis in long bones. *Am J Surg* 1973;26:736.
48. Hansel DP. Vascularized tissue transfer: an adjunct to the treatment of osteomyelitis. *Orthop Rev* 1989;18:595.
49. Mader JT, Shirtliff ME, Berquist SC, et al. Antimicrobial treatment of chronic osteomyelitis. *Clin Orthop Relat Res* 1999;360:47.
50. Gentry LO, Rodriguez-Gomez G. Ofloxacin versus parenteral therapy for chronic osteomyelitis. *Antimicrob Agents Chemother* 1991;35:538.
51. Belzunegui J, et al. Hematogenous vertebral osteomyelitis in the elderly. *Clin Rheumatol* 2000;19:344.
52. Huang T, Bendo JA. Vertebral osteomyelitis. *Butt Hosp Joint Dis* 2000;59:211.
53. Carragee EJ. Pyogenic vertebral osteomyelitis. *J Bone Joint Surg [Am]* 1997;79A:874.
54. Honan M, et al. Spontaneous infectious discitis in adults. *Am J Med* 1996;100:85.
55. Dall BE, et al. Postoperative discitis. Diagnosis and management. *Clin Orthop* 1987; 224:138.
56. Fraser RD, Osti OL, Vernon-Roberts B. Discitis after discography. *J Bone Joint Surg [Br]* 1987;69:26.
57. Sapico FL, Montgomerie JZ. Vertebral osteomyelitis in intravenous drug abusers: report of three cases and review of the literature. *Rev Infect Dis* 1980;2:196.
58. Fernandez M, Carrol CL, Baker CJ. Discitis and vertebral osteomyelitis in children: an 18-year review. *Pediatrics* 2000;105:1299.
59. Torda AJ, Gottlieb T, Bradbury R. Pyogenic vertebral osteomyelitis: analysis of 20 cases and review. *Clin Infect Dis* 1995;20:320.
60. Boston HC Jr, Bianco AJ Jr, Rhodes KH. Disc space infections in children. *Orthop Clin North Am* 1975;6:953.
61. Cushing AH. Diskitis in children. *Clin Infect Dis* 1993;17:1.
62. Nolla-Sole JM, et al. Role of technetium-99m diphosphonate and gallium-67 citrate bone scanning in the early diagnosis of infectious spondylodiscitis. A comparative study. *Ann Rheum Dis* 1992;51:665.
63. Price AC, et al. Intervertebral disk-space infection: CT changes. *Radiology* 1983; 149:725.
64. Boden SD, et al. Postoperative diskitis: distinguishing early MR imaging findings from normal postoperative disk space changes. *Radiology* 1992;184:765.
65. Jansen BR, Hart W, Schreuder O. Discitis in childhood:12–35 year follow up of 35 patients. *Acta Orthop Scand* 1993;64:33.
66. Gillespie WJ. Prevention and management of infection after total joint replacement. *Clin Infect Dis* 1997;25:1310.
67. Patzakis MJ, Wilkins J, Wiss DA. Infection following intramedullary nailing of long bones. Diagnosis and management. *Clin Orthop* 1986;212:182.
68. Watts HG. Lifeso RM. Current concepts review: tuberculosis of bone and joints. *J Bone Joint Surg [Am]* 1996;78A:288.
69. Wolinsky E. Nontuberculous mycobacteria and associated diseases. *Am Rev Respir Dis* 1979;119:107.
70. Davidson PT, Horowitz I. Skeletal tuberculosis: a review with patient presentations and discussion. *Am J Med* 1970;48:77.
71. Pertuiset E, et al. Spinal tuberculosis in adults: a study of 103 cases in a developed country, 1980–1994. *Medicine (Baltimore)* 1999;78:309.
72. Thirteenth report of the Medical Research Council Working Party on Tuberculosis of the Spine. A 15 year assessment of controlled trails of the management of tuberculosis of the spine in Korea and Hong Kong. *J Bone Joint Surg [Br]* 1998;80B:456.

73. Johnson MD, Perfect JR. Fungal infections of the bones and joints. *Curr Infect Dis Rep* 2001;3:450.
74. Cunha BA. Antibiotic selection for diabetic foot infections: a review. *J Foot Ankle Surg* 2000;39:253.
75. Laing P. The development and complications of diabetic foot ulcers. *Am J Surg* 1998;176[Suppl A]:115.
76. Corson JD, et al. The diabetic foot. *Curr Probl Surg* 1986;23:721.
77. Grayson ML. Diabetic foot infections. *Infect Dis Clin North Am* 1995;9:143.
78. Tentoloaris N, et al. Methicillin-resistant *Staphylococcus aureus:* an increasing problem in a diabetic foot clinic. *Diabet Med* 1999;16:767.
79. Goldstein EJC, Citron DM, Nesbit CA. Diabetic foot infections. Bacteriology and activity of 10 oral antimicrobial agents against bacteria isolated from consecutive cases. *Diabetes Care* 1996;19:638.
80. Grayson ML, et al. Use of ampicillin/sulbactam versus imipenem/cilastatin in the treatment of limb-threatening foot infections in diabetic patients. *Clin Infect Dis* 1994;18:683.
81. Sapico FL, et al. The infected foot of the diabetic patient: quantitative microbiology and analysis of clinical features. *Rev Infect Dis* 1984;6[Suppl 1]:S171.
82. Grayson ML. Diabetic foot infections. *Infect Dis Clin North Am* 1995;9:143.
83. Oyibo SO, et al. A comparison of two diabetic foot ulcer classification systems. *Diabetes Care* 2001;24:84.
84. Kaufman J, Breeding L, Rosenberg N. Anatomic location of acute diabetic foot infection: its influence on the outcome of treatment. *Am Surg* 1987;53:109.
85. Taylor LM, Porter JM. The clinical course of diabetics who require emergent foot surgery because of infection or ischemia. *J Vasc Surg* 1987;6:454.
86. Gibbons GW. The diabetic foot: amputations and drainage of infection. *J Vasc Surg* 1987;5:791.
87. Newman LG, et al. Unsuspected osteomyelitis in diabetic foot ulcers. *JAMA* 1991; 266:1246.
88. Mayfield JA, Sugarman JR. The use of the Semmes-Weinstein monofilament and other threshold tests for preventing foot ulcerations and amputation in persons with diabetes. *J Fam Prac* 2000;49:517.
89. Pellizzer M, et al. Deep tissue biopsy vs. superficial swab culture monitoring in the microbiological assessment of limb-threatening diabetic foot infection. *Diabetes Med* 2001;18:822.
90. Zlatkin MB, et al. The diabetic foot. *Clin North Am* 1987;25:1095.
91. Mason J, et al. A systematic review of foot ulcers in patients with type II diabetes mellitus II: treatment. *Diabetes Med* 1999;16:889.
92. Pittet D, et al. Outcome of diabetic foot infections treated conservatively. *Arch Intern Med* 1999;159:851.
93. Gibbons GW, Habershaw GM. Diabetic foot infections: anatomy and surgery. *Infect Dis Clin North Am* 1995;9:131.
94. Frykbert RG, et al. Diabetic foot disorders: a clinical practice guideline. *J Foot Ankle Surg* 2000;39:S1.
95. Weiman JT, Smeill JM, Yachin S. Efficacy and safety of a topical gel formulation of recombinant human platelet-derived growth factor-bb (becaplermin) in patients with chronic neuropathic diabetic ulcers. *Diabetes Care* 1998;21:822.
96. American Diabetes Association consensus development conference on diabetic foot wound care. *Diabetes Care* 1999;22:1354.
97. Pomposelli FB, et al. Efficacy of the dorsal pedal bypass for limb salvage in diabetic patients: short term observations. *J Vasc Surg* 1990;11:745.
98. Mayfield JA, Reiber GE, Sanders LJ, et al. Technical review: preventive foot care in people with diabetes. *Diabetes Care* 1998;21:2161.
99. Garcia-Kutzbach A, Masi AT. Acute infectious agent arthritis (IAA): a detailed comparison of proved gonococcal and other blood-borne bacterial arthritis. *J Rheumatol* 1974;1:93.
100. Goldenberg DL, Reed JL. Bacterial arthritis. *N Engl J Med* 1988;312:764.
101. Smith JW, Piercy EA. Infectious arthritis. *Clin Infect Dis* 1995;20:225.

102. Kraft SM, Panush RS, Longley S. Unrecognized staphylococcal pyarthrosis with rheumatoid arthritis. *Semin Arthritis Rheum* 1985;14:196.
103. Ward JR, Atcheson SG. Infectious arthritis. *Med Clin North Am* 977;61:313
104. Epstein JH, Zimmermann B, Ho G. Polyarticular septic arthritis. *J Rheumatol* 1986; 13:1105.
105. Fink CW, Nelson JD. Septic arthritis and osteomyelitis in children. *Clin Rheum Dis* 1986;12:423.
106. Saag KG, Naides SJ. Practical management for suspected viral arthritis. *Contemp Intern Med* 1993;5:35.
107. Naides SJ. Parvovirus B19 infection. *Rheum Dis Clin North Am* 1993;19:457.
108. Enarson DA, et al. Bone and joint tuberculosis: a continuing problem. *Can Med Assoc J* 1979;120:139.
109. Mahowald ML, Messner RP. Arthritis due to mycobacteria, fungi, and parasites. In: Koopman WJ, ed. *Arthritis and allied conditions: a textbook of rheumatology,* 13th ed. Philadelphia: Lea & Febiger, 1993:2305–2320.
110. Shmerling RH, et al. Synovial fluid tests: what should be ordered? *JAMA* 1990; 264:1009.
111. Nocton JJ, et al. Detection of *Borrelia burgdorferi* DNA by polymerase chain reaction in synovial fluid from patients with Lyme arthritis. *N Engl J Med* 1994;330:229.
112. Hendrix RW, Fisher MR. Imaging of septic arthritis. *Clin Rheum Dis* 1986;12:459.
113. Greenspan A, Tehranzadeh J. Imaging of infectious arthritis. *Radiol Clin North Am* 2001;39:267.
114. Goldenberg DL, Cohen AS. Synovial membrane histopathology in the differential diagnosis of rheumatoid arthritis, gout, pseudogout, systemic lupus erythematosus, infectious arthritis, and degenerative joint disease. *Medicine (Baltimore)* 1978;57:239.
115. Angulo JM, Epinoza LR. Gonococcal arthritis. *Comp Ther* 1999;25:155.
116. Dan M. Septic arthritis in young infants: clinical and microbiologic correlations and therapeutic implications. *Rev Infect Dis* 1984;6:147.
117. Welkon CJ, et al. Pyogenic arthritis in infants and children: a review of 95 cases. *Pediatr Infect Dis* 1986;5:669.
118. Wilson NIL, DiPaola M. Acute septic arthritis in infancy and childhood. *J Bone Joint Surg [Br]* 1986;68:584.
119. Nade S. Acute septic arthritis in infancy and childhood. *J Bone Joint Surg [Br]* 1983; 65:234.
120. Green NE, Edwards K. Bone and joint infections in children. *Orthop Clin North Am* 1987;18:555.
121. Herndon WA, et al. Management of septic arthritis in children. *J Pediatr Orthop* 1986; 6:576.
122. Jackson MA, et al. The changing face of childhood pyogenic arthritis: implications for therapy. Presented at the 33rd Annual Meeting of the Infectious Disease Society of America, San Francisco, Calif., Sept. 1995 (abstract 433).
123. Baker DG, Schumacher HR Jr. Acute monoarthritis. *N Engl J Med* 1993;329:1013.
124. Jackson LA, et al. Risk factors for group B streptococcal disease in adults. *Ann Intern Med* 1995;123:415.
125. Lam K, Bayer AS. Serious infections due to group G streptococci. Report of 15 cases with in vitro-in vivo correlations. *Am J Med* 1983;75:561.
126. Small CB, et al. Group B streptococcal arthritis in adults. *Am J Med* 1984;76:367.
127. Raymond NJ, Henry J, Workowski KA. Enterococcal arthritis: case report and review. *Clin Infect Dis* 1995;21:516.
128. Bayer AS, et al. Gram-negative bacillary septic arthritis: clinical, radiographic, therapeutic, and prognostic features. *Semin Arthritis Rheum* 1977;7:123.
129. Brook I, Frazier EH. Anaerobic osteomyelitis and arthritis in a military hospital: a 10-year experience. *Am J Med* 1993;94:21.
130. Dubost J-J, et al. Polyarticular septic arthritis. *Medicine (Baltimore)* 1993;72: 296.
131. Deighton C. B-haemolytic streptococci and reactive arthritis in adults. *Ann Rheum Dis* 1993;52:475.
132. Kingsley GH. Reactive arthritis: a paradigm for inflammatory arthritis. *Clin Exp Rheumatol* 1993;11[Suppl 8]:529.

133. Rahman MU, Schumacher HR, Hudson AP. Recurrent arthritis in Reiter's syndrome: a function of inapparent chlamydial infection of the synovium? *Semin Arthritis Rheum* 1992;21:259.
134. Silveira LH, et al. Chlamydia-induced reactive arthritis. *Rheum Dis Clin North Am* 1993;19:351.
135. Calabrese LH. Human immunodeficiency virus (HIV) infection and arthritis. *Rheum Dis Clin North Am* 1993;19:477.
136. Gran JT, et al. The variable clinical picture of arthritis induced by human parvovirus B19: report of seven adult cases and review of the literature. *Scand J Rheumatol* 1995;24:174.
137. Rynes RI. Painful rheumatic syndromes associated with human immunodeficiency virus infection. *Rheum Dis Clin North Am* 1991;17:79.
138. Bayer AS, Guze LB. Fungal arthritis. *Semin Arthritis Rheum* 1978–1979;8:142, 200 and 1979–1980;9:66, 145, 218.
139. Meier JL, Hoffman GS. Mycobacterial and fungal infections. In: Kelley WN, et al., eds. *Textbook of rheumatology,* 4th ed. Philadelphia: Saunders, 1993:1467–1483.
140. Kalish R. Lyme disease. *Rheum Dis Clin North Am* 1993;19:399.
141. Rahn DW. Lyme disease—where's the bug? [editorial]. *N Engl J Med* 1994;330:282.
142. Shrestha M, Grodzicki RL, Steere AC. Diagnosing early Lyme disease. *Am J Med* 1985;78:235.
143. Lyme disease—Connecticut. *MMWR Morb Mortal Wkly Rep* 1988;37:1.
144. Dattwyler RJ, et al. Treatment of late Lyme borreliosis—randomized comparison of ceftriaxone and penicillin. *Lancet* 1988;1:1191.
145. Tachdjian MO. Acute transient synovitis of the hip. In: *Pediatric orthopedics,* 2nd ed. Philadelphia: Saunders, 1990:1461–1465.
146. Broy SB, Schmid FR. A comparison of medical drainage (needle aspiration) and surgical drainage (arthrotomy or arthroscopy) in the initial treatment of infected joints. *Clin Rheum Dis* 1986;12:501.
147. Cooper C. Bacterial arthritis in the elderly. *Gerontology* 1986;32:222.
148. Nelson JD. Antibiotic concentrations in septic joint effusions. *N Engl J Med* 1971;284: 349.
149. Parker RH, Schmid FR. Antibacterial activity of synovial fluid during therapy of septic arthritis. *Arthritis Rheum* 1971;14:96.
150. Centers for Disease Control and Prevention. 2002 Sexually transmitted diseases treatment guidelines. Published May 10, 2002 and available on website www.cdc.gov/std treatment.
151. Syrogiannopoulos GA, Nelson JD. Duration of antimicrobial therapy for acute suppurative osteoarticular infections. *Lancet* 1988;1:37.
152. Black J, et al. Oral antimicrobial therapy for adults with osteomyelitis or septic arthritis. *J Infect Dis* 1987;155:968.
153. Mikhail IS, Alarcon GS. Nongonococcal bacterial arthritis. *Rheum Dis Clin North Am* 1993;19:311.
154. Vincent GM, Amirault JD. Septic arthritis in the elderly. *Clin Orthop* 1990;251:241.
155. Wilde AH. Management of infected knee and hip prostheses. *Curr Opin Rheum* 1993;5:317.
156. Steckelberg JM, Osman DR. Prosthetic joint infection. In: Bisno AL, Waldvogel FA, eds. *Infections associated with indwelling medical devices,* 2nd ed. Washington, DC: American Society of Microbiology, 1994:259–290.
157. Wymenga AB, et al. Perioperative factors associated with septic arthritis after arthroplasty: prospective multicenter study of 362 knee and 2,651 hip operations. *Acta Orthop Scand* 1992;63:665.
158. Norden C, Gillespie WJ, Nade S. Infections in total joint replacement. In: *Infections in bones and joints.* Boston: Blackwell, 1994:291–319.
159. Wymenga AB, et al. Prosthesis-related infection: etiology, prophylaxis and diagnosis (a review). *Acta Orthop Belg* 1990;56:463.
160. Lidwell OM, et al. Effect of ultraclean air in operating rooms on deep sepsis in the joint after total hip or knee replacement: a randomised study. *Br Med J* 1982;285:10.
161. Paya CV, Wilson WR, Fitzgerald RH Jr. Management of infection in total knee replacement. *Curr Clin Top Infect Dis* 1988;9:222–240.

162. Levitsky KA, et al. Evaluation of the painful prosthetic joint. *J Arthroplasty* 1991; 6:237.
163. Cuckler JM, et al. Diagnosis and management of the infected total joint arthroplasty. *Orthop Clin North Am* 1991;22:523.
164. Ross AC. Infections complicating joint replacement and other orthopedic conditions. *Curr Opin Rheum* 1993;5:461.
165. Fitzgerald RH Jr. Infections of hip prostheses and artificial joints. *Infect Dis Clin North Am* 1989;3:329.
166. Widmer AF, et al. Antimicrobial treatment of orthopedic implant-related infections with rifampin combinations. *Clin Infect Dis* 1992;14:1251.
167. Drancourt M, et al. Oral rifampin plus ofloxacin for treatment of *Staphylococcus*-infected orthopedic implants. *Antimicrob Agents Chemother* 1993;37:1214.
168. Davenport K, Traina S, Perry C. Treatment of acutely infected arthroplasty with local antibiotics. *J Arthroplasty* 1991;6:179.
169. Hartman MB, et al. Periprosthetic knee sepsis: the role of irrigation and debridement. *Clin Orthop* 1991;273:113.
170. Rand JA. Alternatives to reimplantation for salvage of the total knee arthroplasty complicated by infection. *J Bone Joint Surg [Am]* 1993;75-A:282.
171. Goulet JA, et al. Prolonged suppression of infection in total hip arthroplasty. *J Arthroplasty* 1988;3:109.
172. Schoifet SD, Morrey BF. Treatment of infection after total knee arthroplasty by debridement with retention of the components. *J Bone Joint Surg [Am]* 1990;72-A:1383.
173. Rasul AT Jr, Tsukayama D, Gustilo RB. Effect of time of onset and depth of infection on the outcome of total knee arthroplasty infections. *Clin Orthop* 1991;273:98.
174. Burger RR, Basch T, Hopson CN. Implant salvage in infected total knee arthroplasty. *Clin Orthop* 1991;273:105.
175. Norden CW. Antibiotic prophylaxis in orthopedic surgery. *Rev Infect Dis* 1991;13[Suppl 10]:5842.
176. Zimmermann B, Mikolich DJ, Ho G. Septic bursitis. *Semin Arthritis Rheum* 1995;24; 391.

# 6. CENTRAL NERVOUS SYSTEM INFECTIONS

Allan R. Tunkel and W. Michael Scheld

## MENINGITIS

**Meningitis** is inflammation of the meninges identified by an abnormal number of white blood cells in the cerebrospinal fluid (CSF). The meningitis syndrome may be caused by a wide variety of infectious and noninfectious diseases (Table 6.1). Here we review the common infectious causes of meningitis.

**I. Epidemiology and etiology**

A. **Viruses** are the major cause of the **acute aseptic meningitis syndrome,** a term used to define any meningitis, particularly one with a lymphocytic pleocytosis, for which a cause is not apparent after initial evaluation and routine stains and cultures of CSF [1]. The common viral agents that cause the acute aseptic meningitis syndrome are as follows.

1. **Enteroviruses** are currently the leading recognizable cause of the aseptic meningitis syndrome, accounting for 80% to 85% of all cases in which a pathogen is identified [1,2]. Enteroviruses are worldwide in distribution and spread by the fecal–oral, and perhaps respiratory, routes; periods of warm weather and sparse clothing may facilitate spread. Enteroviruses may also be recovered from houseflies, wastewater, and sewage [1]. The predominant enteroviruses isolated from patients with meningitis during the years 1970 to 1983 in the United States were (in decreasing order) echovirus 11; echovirus 9; coxsackievirus 115; echoviruses 30, 4, and 6; coxsackieviruses B2, B4, B3, and A9; echoviruses 3, 7, 5, and 21; and coxsackievirus B1 [2]. In addition, the newly numbered enteroviruses 70 and 71 have been reported to commonly cause central nervous system (CNS) disease [3–5].

   Infants and young children are most susceptible because there is absence of previous exposure and immunity, although enteroviruses are also the most common causes of aseptic meningitis among adults [6]. In one large cohort study from Finland, children younger than 1 year of age had an annual incidence of viral meningitis of 219 cases per 100,000 population versus an incidence of 19 cases per 100,000 population in children between the ages of 1 and 4 years [7]. Immunodeficiency and possibly physical exercise also predispose to enteroviral meningitis [1].

2. **Arboviruses.** The most common vector-transmitted cause of aseptic meningitis is St. Louis encephalitis virus, a flavivirus [1]. Aseptic meningitis accounts for approximately 15% of all symptomatic cases of St. Louis encephalitis and may be as high as 35% to 60% in children. These infections are more common in warmer months when contact with the insect vector is more likely. Other arboviruses reported to cause aseptic meningitis include the California encephalitis group of viruses (e.g., La Crosse, Jamestown Canyon, and Snowshoe hare viruses, which are bunyaviruses) and the agent of Colorado tick fever, an orbivirus, which is seen in mountain and western regions of the United States and Canada.

3. **Mumps virus** infection commonly occurs in the winter and spring months. CNS disease caused by mumps virus can occur in patients without evidence of parotitis; 40% to 50% of patients with meningitis have no evidence of salivary gland enlargement at presentation. **In an unimmunized population, mumps is one of the most common causes of aseptic meningitis and encephalitis,** with symptomatic meningitis occurring in 10% to 30% of patients [8]. Males are affected two to five times more often than females, and the peak incidence is in children aged 5 to 9 years. Although the incidence of mumps has decreased markedly with widespread use of the attenuated live virus vaccine [1,8], vaccine-associated mumps meningitis also has been reported [9].

4. **Lymphocytic choriomeningitis virus** was one of the earliest viruses associated with human aseptic meningitis, although it now is reported rarely [1]. It is transmitted to humans by contact with rodents (e.g., hamsters, rats, mice) or their excreta through ingestion of contaminated food or exposure of open wounds

Table 6.1. Differential Diagnosis of the Meningitis Syndrome

**Infectious etiologies**

Bacteria
- *Haemophilus influenzae*
- *Neisseria meningitidis*
- *Streptococcus pneumoniae*
- *Listeria monocytogenes*[a]
- *Streptococcus agalactiae*
- Aerobic gram-negative bacilli
- Staphylococci
- Enterococci
- Other streptococci
- Anaerobes
- *Pasteurella multocida*
- *Leuconostoc* species
- *Stomatococcus mucilaginosus*
- *Brucella* species[a]
- *Chlamydia psittaci*
- *Chlamydia trachomatis*
- *Mycoplasma pneumoniae*[a]
- *Mycoplasma hominis*[a]
- *Ureaplasma urealyticum*
- *Nocardia* species[a]
- *Actinomyces* species[a]
- *Mycobacterium tuberculosis*[a]
- Nontuberculous mycobacteria
- *Tropheryma whippelii*
- *Bartonella* species

Viruses
- Nonpolio enteroviruses[a,b]
- Mumps virus[a]
- Arboviruses[a,c]
- Herpesviruses[a,d]
- Lymphocytic choriomeningitis virus[a]
- Human immunodeficiency virus[a]
- Adenovirus[a]
- Influenza A and B viruses[a]
- Parainfluenza viruses
- Measles virus (rubella)[a]
- Rubella virus (German measles)[a]
- Poliovirus[a]
- Rotavirus
- Encephalomyocarditis virus
- Vaccinia virus (cowpox)[a]
- Rabies virus
- Parvovirus B19
- Sandfly fever virus serotype Toscana
- West Nile virus[a]
- Hedraviruses (e.g., Nipah virus)[a]

Fungi
- *Cryptococcus neoformans*[a]
- *Candida* species[e]
- *Coccidioides immitis*[e]
- *Histoplasma capsulatum*[a,e]
- *Aspergillus* species[e]
- *Blastomyces dermatitidis*[e]
- *Sporothrix schenckii*[e]
- *Paracoccidioides brasiliensis*[e]
- *Pseudallescheria boydii*[e]
- *Cladosporium* species[e]
- *Zygomycetes* species
- *Pneumocystis carinii*

Spirochetes
- *Treponema pallidum* (syphilis)[a]
- *Borrelia burgdorferi* (Lyme disease)[a]
- *Leptospira* species[a]
- *Borrelia recurrentis* (relapsing fever)[a]
- *Spirillum minor* (rat-bite fever)

Rickettsiae
- *Richettsia rickettsii* (Rocky Mountain spotted fever)[a]
- *Rickettsia conorii*
- *Coxiella burnetii* (Q fever)
- *Rickettsia prowazekii* (epidemic or louse-borne typhus)[a]
- *Rickettsia typhi* (endemic or murine typhus)[a]
- *Rickettsia tsutsugamushi* (scrub typhus)[a]
- *Ehrlichia* species[a]

Protozoa and helminths
- *Naegleria fowleri*[a]
- *Acanthamoeba* species[a,e]
- *Angiostrongylus cantonensis*
- *Baylisascaris procyonis*
- *Toxoplasma gondii*[a,e]
- *Taenia solium* (cysticercosis)[e]
- *Trichinella spiralis*[e]
- *Trypanosoma* species[a,e]
- *Paragonimus* species[e]
- *Echinococcus granulosus*[e]
- *Strongyloides stercoralis* (hyperinfection syndrome)[e]
- *Schistosoma* species
- *Entamoeba histolytica*[e]
- *Gnathostoma spinigerum*[e]
- *Multiceps multiceps*[e]

Algae
- *Prototheca wickerhamii*

Other infectious syndromes
- Parameningeal foci of infection[f]
- Infective endocarditis[a]
- Bacterial toxins[g]
- Viral postinfectious syndromes
- Postvaccination[h]

**Noninfectious etiologies and diseases of unknown etiology**

Systemic illnesses
- Systemic lupus erythematosus
- Sarcoidosis
- Behçet disease[a]
- Sjögren syndrome
- Mixed connective tissue disease

Table 6.1. *Continued.*

| | |
|---|---|
| Rheumatoid arthritis | Intrathecal injections[m] |
| Polymyositis | Chymopapain injection |
| Wegener granulomatosis | Miscellaneous |
| Lymphomatoid granulomatosis | Seizures |
| Polyarteritis nodosa | Migraine or migraine-like syndromes |
| Granulomatous angiitis | Mollaret's meningitis |
| Other cerebral vasculitides | Serum sickness |
| Familial Mediterranean fever | Heavy metal poisoning |
| Kawasaki syndrome | Malignancies |
| Vogt-Koyanagi-Harada syndrome | Lymphomatous meningitis |
| Medications | Carcinomatous meningitis |
| Antimicrobial agents[i] | Leukemia |
| Nonsteroidal antiinflammatory agents[j] | Intracranial tumors and cysts |
| Muromonab-CD3 (OKT3) | Craniopharyngioma |
| Azathioprine | Dermoid or epidermoid cyst |
| Cytosine arabinoside (high-dose) | Pituitary adenoma |
| Carbamazepine[k] | Astrocytoma |
| Immunoglobulin[l] | Glioblastoma multiforme |
| Phenazopyridine | Medulloblastoma |
| Ranitidine | Pinealoma |
| Procedure related | Ependymoma |
| Postneurosurgery | Teratoma |
| Spinal anesthesia | |

[a] May also present as encephalitis.
[b] Primarily echoviruses and coxsackieviruses.
[c] In the United States the major etiologic agents are the mosquito-borne California, St. Louis, Eastern equine, Western equine, and Venezuelan equine encephalitis viruses and the tick-borne Colorado tick fever.
[d] Primarily herpes simplex virus type 2 but also herpes simplex virus type 1, varicella-zoster virus, cytomegalovirus, Epstein-Barr virus, and human herpesvirus-6.
[e] More commonly presents as chronic meningitis or focal central nervous system lesions.
[f] Brain abscess, sinusitis, otitis, mastoiditis, subdural abscess, epidural abscess, venous sinus thrombophlebitis, pituitary abscess, cranial osteomyelitis.
[g] Scarlet fever, streptococcal pharyngitis, toxic shock syndrome, pertussis, diphtheria.
[h] Mumps, measles, polio, pertussis, rabies, vaccinia.
[i] Trimethoprim, sulfamethoxazole, trimethoprim-sulfamethoxazole, ciprofloxacin, penicillin, isoniazid.
[j] Ibuprofen, sulindac, naproxen, tolmetin.
[k] In patients with connective tissue diseases.
[l] Aseptic meningitis can occur after high-dose intravenous immunoglobulin.
[m] Air, dyes, isotopes, antimicrobial agents, antineoplastic agents, steroids, dyes.

to dirt. The greatest risk is in pet owners, persons living in impoverished and nonhygienic situations, and laboratory workers [10]. Human-to-human transmission does not occur.

**5.** **Herpesviruses** include herpes simplex viruses (HSVs) types 1 and 2, varicella-zoster virus, cytomegalovirus (CMV), Epstein-Barr virus, human herpesvirus 6, and human herpesvirus 7. Neurologic complications associated with the **HSVs are the most significant** [11]. HSVs account for 0.5% to 3.0% of all cases of aseptic meningitis. HSV aseptic meningitis is **most commonly associated with primary genital infection with HSV type 2 [12] and is less likely with recurrences of genital herpes [13].** Primary genital infection with HSV type 1 and nonprimary genital infection with HSV of either type rarely result in meningitis [12]. Cases of Mollaret recurrent meningitis have been associated with HSV types 1 and 2 [14,15].

Acute aseptic meningitis has also been associated with herpes zoster in patients with or without typical skin lesions [16,17]. Single cases of Mollaret recurrent meningitis have been associated with Epstein-Barr virus [18]. Meningitis from human herpesvirus 6 has been associated with roseola infantum [19], encephalitis [20], recurrent seizures in children [21], and after bone marrow transplantation [22]. CMV and Epstein-Barr virus may cause aseptic meningitis with a mononucleosis syndrome, particularly in immunocompromised hosts.

6. **Human immunodeficiency virus (HIV)** can infect the meninges early and persist in the CNS [23,24]. Meningitis associated with HIV may occur as part of the primary infection or in an already infected patient; HIV has been isolated from the CSF in some cases [25]. However, CNS infection often is clinically silent. Retrospective studies have noted that 5% to 10% of HIV-infected patients develop an acute meningoencephalitis during or after the mononucleosis-like syndrome that heralds initial infection [23,26].

**B. Bacteria.** Bacterial meningitis is an important problem worldwide [27]. The overall annual attack rate for bacterial meningitis in the United States from 1978 through 1981 was approximately 3.0 cases/100,000 population [28], although this varied based on age, race, and gender. This compares with an attack rate of 45.8 cases per 100,000 population in approximately 4,100 cases in Salvador, Brazil from 1973 through 1982 [29]. Bacterial meningitis is also a significant problem in hospitalized patients. Forty percent of 493 episodes in adults aged 16 years or older at the Massachusetts General Hospital from 1962 through 1988 were nosocomial, and these episodes had a high mortality [30].

1. ***Haemophilus influenzae.*** In the early 1980's *H. influenzae* caused 45% to 48% of bacterial meningitis in the United States, with an overall mortality of 3% to 6% [28,31]. Most cases occurred in infants and children younger than 6 years, and more than 90% were caused by capsular type b strains. **The widespread use of conjugate vaccines has profoundly reduced the incidence of invasive *H. influenzae* type b childhood infections** (see section **VII.B.1.b)** [32], and it now causes 7% of bacterial meningitis in the United States. During 1995 in 22 counties of four states, the overall incidence of bacterial meningitis also was dramatically decreased to 0.2 cases per 100,000 population [33]. *H. influenzae* meningitis in older children and adults should suggest the presence of certain underlying conditions, including sinusitis, otitis media, epiglottitis, pneumonia, diabetes mellitus, alcoholism, splenectomy or asplenia, head trauma with CSF leak, and immunodeficiency (e.g., hypogammaglobulinemia) [34,35].
2. ***Neisseria meningitidis*** causes 25% of cases of bacterial meningitis in the United States, most commonly in children and young adults, with an overall mortality of 3% to 13% [28,31,35]. Serotype B strains usually occur in sporadic outbreaks, serogroups A and C may occur in epidemics, and type Y strains may be associated with pneumonia. The incidence of serogroup C disease has been increasing, with several recent outbreaks reported in the United States, Canada, and Europe [36–38]; most cases have been caused by one strain of the electrophoretic type 37, termed ET-15. **Patients with deficiencies in the terminal complement components** (C5-C8, and perhaps C9), the so-called membrane attack complex, **have a markedly increased incidence of neisserial infections,** although their meningococcal case fatality rate of 3% is lower than the rate of 19% for the general population [39].
3. ***Streptococcus pneumoniae.*** Pneumococcal meningitis is most frequently observed in adults, accounting for 47% of total cases in the United States and carrying a mortality of 19% to 26% [28,31,35]. Patients often have contiguous or distant foci of infection such as pneumonia, otitis media, mastoiditis, sinusitis, and endocarditis. Risk factors for serious infection include splenectomy or functional asplenia, multiple myeloma, hypogammaglobulinemia, alcoholism, malnutrition, chronic liver or renal disease, malignancy, Wiskott-Aldrich syndrome, thalassemia major, and diabetes mellitus [40,41]. The pneumococcus is the most common etiologic agent of meningitis in patients who have a basilar skull fracture with CSF leak [42].
4. ***Listeria monocytogenes*** causes 8% of cases of bacterial meningitis in the United States [35] but has a high mortality of 15% to 29% [28,31,35]. Serotypes 1/2b and

4b have been implicated in up to 80% of meningitis cases. Listerial infection is **most common in neonates** (up to 10% of cases); pregnant women may harbor the organism asymptomatically in their genital tract and rectum and transmit the infection to their infants. **Other predisposing conditions include** older age (≥50 years), alcoholism, malignancy, immunosuppression (e.g., renal transplant recipients), corticosteroid therapy, diabetes mellitus, liver disease, chronic renal disease, collagen vascular diseases, and conditions associated with iron overload [43,44]. *Listeria* meningitis is found only infrequently in patients with HIV infection [45,46], despite its increased incidence in patients with deficient cell-mediated immunity. Meningitis can also occur in previously healthy adults.

5. ***Streptococcus agalactiae.*** In the United States, this organism accounts for 12% of bacterial meningitis, with a mortality ranging from 7% to 23% [28,31,35]. The group B streptococcus is a **common** cause of meningitis **in neonates** [47], with 52% of cases reported during the first month of life [35]. The risk of transmission from mother to infant is increased when the inoculum of organisms and number of sites of maternal colonization is high; group B streptococcus has been isolated from vaginal or rectal cultures of 15% to 40% of asymptomatic pregnant women. Horizontal transmission has also been documented from the hands of nursery personnel to the infant. Most cases of neonatal meningitis are caused by subtype III organisms and occur after the first week of life. Group B streptococcal meningitis in adults appears to be increasing in frequency, often is associated with severe underlying diseases, and has a high mortality rate of 27% to 34% [48–50]. Risk factors for adults include age older than 60 years, diabetes mellitus, parturient women, cardiac disease, collagen vascular diseases, malignancy, alcoholism, hepatic failure, renal failure, and corticosteroid therapy; no underlying illnesses were found in 43% of patients in one study [49].
6. **Aerobic gram-negative bacilli** (e.g., *Klebsiella* species, *Escherichia coli, Serratia marcescens, Pseudomonas aeruginosa, Salmonella* species) have become increasingly important etiologic agents for bacterial meningitis [30,51]; mortality rates range from about 30% to 80%. Meningitis has occurred **after head trauma or neurosurgical procedures** and may also be found **in neonates, the elderly, immunosuppressed patients, and patients with gram-negative septicemia.** Some cases have been associated with disseminated strongyloidiasis in the hyperinfection syndrome, in which meningitis caused by enteric bacteria occurs secondary to seeding of the meninges during persistent or recurrent bacteremias associated with the migration of infective larvae [52]. Alternatively, larvae that invade the meninges may carry enteric organisms on their surfaces or within their own gastrointestinal tracts.
7. **Staphylococci.** *Staphylococcus aureus* accounts for 1% to 9% of cases of bacterial meningitis and is usually found in early postneurosurgical or posttrauma patients and in those with CSF shunts [53,54]. Rarely, *S. aureus* meningitis occurs as a complication of a temporary epidural catheter [55]. Other underlying conditions include diabetes mellitus, alcoholism, chronic renal failure requiring hemodialysis, injection drug use, and malignancies. Thirty-five percent of cases occur in the setting of head trauma or neurosurgery, and an additional 20% have infective endocarditis or paraspinal infection. Community-acquired sources also include sinusitis, osteomyelitis, and pneumonia. Mortality from *S. aureus* meningitis has ranged from 14% to 77%. *Staphylococcus epidermidis* is the most common cause of meningitis in patients with CSF shunts [54], accounting for 47% to 64% of cases.
8. **Other bacteria.** ***Nocardia*** **meningitis** usually occurs in the setting of predisposing conditions such as immunosuppressive drug therapy, malignancy, head trauma, CNS procedures, chronic granulomatous disease, and sarcoidosis [56]. **Enterococci** are unusual pathogens [57], generally seen in pediatric patients with CNS pathology and in adults with underlying illness (especially immunosuppressive therapy). **Anaerobic meningitis** is unusual, often polymicrobial, and generally associated with a contiguous focus (e.g., otitis, sinusitis, pharyngitis, brain abscess, head and neck malignancy, recent head and neck surgery

or wound infection, posttrauma, postneurosurgery) [58,59]. **Diphtheroids** may cause CNS shunt infections [54]. Streptococcal meningitis has complicated diagnostic myelography [60].

**C. Tuberculosis.** Virtually all mycobacterial infections of the CNS are caused by *Mycobacterium tuberculosis.* Tuberculous meningitis accounts for approximately 15% of extrapulmonary cases or approximately 0.7% of all clinical tuberculosis in the United States [61]. A disproportionately increased rate of CNS tuberculosis occurs in the U.S. homeless population and in nonwhite Americans. Most childhood cases occur during the first 5 years of life, although it is uncommon among those younger than 6 months. Other factors such as advanced age, immunosuppressive drug therapy, lymphoma, gastrectomy, pregnancy, diabetes mellitus, and alcoholism may lead to reactivation tuberculosis [62]. It is estimated that **HIV infection** accounts for almost 6,000 to 9,000 new cases of tuberculosis annually in the United States [63]. Extrapulmonary disease occurs in over 70% of patients with acquired immunodeficiency syndrome (AIDS) but in only 24% to 45% with less advanced HIV infection [64].

**D. Spirochetes**

1. ***Treponema pallidum*** disseminates to the CNS during early infection and can be isolated from the CSF of patients with primary syphilis. CSF laboratory abnormalities are detected in 5% to 9% of patients with seronegative primary syphilis [65]. However, the actual rate of CNS invasion during the early stages is likely to be considerably higher. Clinical neurosyphilis can be divided into four distinct syndromes: syphilitic meningitis, meningovascular syphilis, parenchymatous neurosyphilis, and gummatous neurosyphilis. The incidence of syphilitic meningitis is greatest in the first 2 years after initial infection and is estimated to occur in only 0.3% to 2.4% of patients. In contrast, meningovascular syphilis occurs months to years after syphilis acquisition (peak incidence is at approximately 7 years) and is found in 10% to 12% with CNS involvement [65]. Parenchymatous neurosyphilis has two variants, general paresis and tabes dorsalis, which are relatively rare and do not become apparent until 10 to 20 years after acquisition of infection. Gummata are late manifestations of tertiary syphilis and may occur anywhere, although gummatous neurosyphilis is rare.

   **The overall incidence of neurosyphilis has increased in association with HIV infection** [66,67]. In one report, 44% of patients with neurosyphilis had AIDS and 1.5% of AIDS patients were found to have neurosyphilis at some point during their disease [68]. In a review of neurosyphilis cases in San Francisco from 1985 to 1992, 75% were either infected with HIV or in a high-risk group for HIV [69] (see Chapters 16 and 18).
2. ***Borrelia burgdorferi*** is the etiologic agent of Lyme disease. The nervous system is involved clinically in at least 10% to 15% of patients with Lyme disease [70,71], either while erythema migrans is still present or 1 to 6 months later. Using polymerase chain reaction (PCR), spirochetal DNA was detected in CSF samples from 8 of 12 patients with acute (<2 weeks) disseminated Lyme borreliosis [72], indicating that *B. burgdorferi* usually invades the CNS early in infection (see Chapter 21).

**E. Fungi**

1. ***Cryptococcus neoformans*** is associated with bird droppings but can also be found in fruits, vegetables, milk, and soil. *C. neoformans* is the most common fungal cause of meningitis, usually occurring in persons who are immunosuppressed. Risk factors include reticuloendothelial malignancies (e.g., lymphoma), sarcoidosis, collagen vascular diseases (e.g., systemic lupus erythematosus), diabetes mellitus, chronic hepatic failure, chronic renal failure, organ transplantation, and corticosteroids [73]. *C. neoformans* meningitis also occurs in apparently healthy individuals. **Patients with AIDS currently constitute the highest risk group [74];** 5% to 10% of AIDS patients eventually develop cryptococcal meningitis [75–77].
2. ***Candida*** are normal commensals of humans. Tissue invasion usually occurs in persons with altered host defenses, including those with malignancies, neutropenia, chronic granulomatous disease, diabetes mellitus, thermal injuries, or

a central venous catheter and in those receiving corticosteroid therapy, broad-spectrum antimicrobial agents, or hyperalimentation [78,79]. *Candida* meningitis is uncommon, occurring in fewer than 15% of patients with CNS candidiasis [80–82]. *C. albicans* is the species most commonly isolated in CNS disease.

3. ***Coccidioides immitis*** is endemic in the semiarid regions and deserts of the southwestern United States (California, Arizona, New Mexico, Texas), where approximately one-third of the population is infected [83]. Less than 1% of patients will subsequently develop disseminated disease, usually within the first 6 months after infection. Of those with disseminated disease, one-third to one-half have meningeal involvement [84,85]. Disseminated disease has been associated with extremes of age, male gender, nonwhite race, pregnancy, and immunosuppression (e.g., corticosteroid therapy, organ transplantation, and HIV infection) [83].

**F. Protozoa and helminths**

1. **Amebae.** *Naegleria fowleri* is the main cause of primary amebic meningoencephalitis in humans [86,87]. Strains have been recovered from lakes, puddles, pools, ponds, rivers, sewage, sludge, tap water, air-conditioner drains, and soil. Sporadic cases of primary amebic meningoencephalitis occur when persons, usually children and young adults, swim or play in water containing the amebae or when swimming pools or water supplies have become contaminated, often through failure of chlorination. Several cases (often caused by *Acanthamoeba* species or leptomyxid amebae) have been reported in patients [88–90] with advanced HIV.
2. ***Angiostrongylus cantonensis.*** Infection of humans by the larvae of the nematode *A. cantonensis* can lead to an eosinophilic meningitis [52,91]. *A. cantonensis* is widespread, and human infections are fairly common in many parts of the world (e.g., Thailand, India, Malaysia, Vietnam, Indonesia, Papua New Guinea, and the Pacific Islands, including Hawaii). The definitive hosts are rats, and they may spread the parasites from port to port on ships. Larvae invade the brain either directly from the bloodstream or after migrating through other organs. Once there, they mature into adult worms that migrate through the brain. *Baylisascaris procyonis* is a newly recognized cause of eosinophilic meningoencephalitis (see Chapter 21).

**II. Clinical presentation**

**A. Viral meningitis**

1. **Enteroviruses.** The clinical manifestations of enteroviral meningitis depend on host age and immune status [1].
   - **a. In neonates** fever is ubiquitous and usually accompanied by vomiting, anorexia, rash, or upper respiratory symptoms and signs. Neurologic involvement may be associated with nuchal rigidity and a bulging anterior fontanelle, although infants younger than 1 year are less likely to demonstrate meningeal signs. Mental status may be altered, but focal neurologic signs are uncommon. Meningoencephalitis in neonates may be severe, with morbidity and mortality as high as 74% and 10%, respectively [92].
   - **b. In contrast,** the clinical findings of enteroviral meningitis **beyond the neonatal period** are rarely those of severe disease and poor outcome [1,93]. The onset usually is sudden, with fever present in 76% to 100% of patients. More than half have nuchal rigidity. Headache (often severe and frontal) is nearly always present in adults; photophobia also is common. Nonspecific symptoms and signs include vomiting, anorexia, rash, diarrhea, cough, upper respiratory findings (especially pharyngitis), and myalgias. Other clues to enteroviral disease, in addition to time of year and known epidemic disease, include the presence of exanthems, myopericarditis, conjunctivitis, and specifically recognizable enteroviral syndromes such as pleurodynia, herpangina, and hand-foot-and-mouth disease [6]. The duration of enteroviral meningitis is usually less than 1 week, and many patients are improved after the lumbar puncture [94], probably as a result of reduced intracranial pressure. In contrast, a recent outbreak of enterovirus 71 infection in Taiwan involved patients 3 months to 8.2 years of age, the chief neurologic complaint was rhombencephalitis in 90%, and the case fatality rate was 14% [4].

c. In children and adults with absent or deficient humoral immunity (e.g., agammaglobulinemia), which impairs clearance of enteroviruses, chronic enteroviral meningitis or meningoencephalitis may develop and last several years, often with a fatal outcome [95].

2. **Mumps virus.** The most frequent clinical presentation of mumps CNS infection is the nonspecific triad of fever, vomiting, and headache [8]. The fever usually is high and lasts 3 to 4 days. Salivary gland enlargement is present in only 50% or so of patients. Other findings include neck stiffness, lethargy or somnolence, and abdominal pain. Most patients have signs of meningitis without evidence of cortical dysfunction and, in uncomplicated cases, recover within 7 to 10 days. Mumps virus rarely causes encephalitis, seizures, polyradiculitis, polyneuritis, cranial nerve palsies, myelitis, Guillain-Barré syndrome, and fatality.
3. **Lymphocytic choriomeningitis virus** infection begins with nonspecific symptoms. After a brief improvement, approximately 15% of patients develop severe headache, photophobia, lightheadedness, lumbar myalgias, and pharyngitis. Late manifestations such as orchitis, arthritis, myopericarditis, and alopecia are also seen.
4. **Herpesviruses.** Meningitis caused by HSV type 2 usually is characterized by stiff neck, headache, and fever [12]. Neurologic complications were found in 37% of 27 patients with HSV type 2 meningitis and consisted of urinary retention, dysesthesias, paresthesias, neuralgia, motor weakness, paraparesis, concentration difficulties of nearly 3 months' duration, and impaired hearing [13]. All neurologic findings, however, subsided within 6 months. Recurrent meningitis was documented in five patients. Pharyngitis, lymphadenopathy, and splenomegaly should suggest Epstein-Barr virus infection. A diffuse vesiculopustular rash may be seen in patients with meningitis caused by varicella-zoster virus.
5. **Human immunodeficiency virus.** Acute HIV infection may cause a typical aseptic meningitis syndrome [23,25,26]. In addition, some patients may present with an atypical syndrome that is chronic, tends to recur, and often is associated with cranial neuropathies (usually V, VII, and VIII) or long tract findings. The most common features are headache, fever, and meningeal signs. Illness is self-limited or recurrent rather than progressive. HIV may occasionally cause a dramatic self-limited encephalitis or encephalopathy during the acute phase of infection.

**B. Bacterial meningitis**

1. **Clinical presentation.** Most patients have fever, headache, meningismus, and signs of cerebral dysfunction (i.e., confusion, delirium, or a declining level of consciousness ranging from lethargy to coma) [27,40,96]. In one review of community-acquired bacterial meningitis in adults, the classic triad of fever, nuchal rigidity, and change in mental status was found in only two-thirds of patients [30]. Another review found the absence of fever, neck stiffness, and altered mental status effectively eliminated the likelihood of acute meningitis in adults (sensitivity of 99% to 100% for the presence of one finding in the diagnosis of acute meningitis) [97].
2. **Meningismus** may be subtle, marked, or accompanied by Kernig or Brudzinski signs. These signs are elicited in only 50% or so of adult patients with bacterial meningitis, and their absence does not rule out the diagnosis.
   a. **Kernig sign** is elicited with the patient in the supine position. The thigh is flexed on the abdomen with the knee also flexed, and the leg then is passively extended. The patient resists leg extension if there is meningeal inflammation.
   b. **Brudzinski sign** is best known as the nape-of-the-neck sign in which passive neck flexion results in flexion of the hips and knees.
3. **Cranial nerve palsies** (especially III, IV, VI, and VII) and **focal cerebral signs** are seen in 10% to 20% of cases. **Seizures** occur in approximately 30% of patients. Signs of increased intracranial pressure may develop, including coma, hypertension, bradycardia, and palsy of cranial nerve III. Papilledema is seen in fewer than 5% of cases early in infection, and its presence should suggest an alternative diagnosis.

4. **A specific etiologic diagnosis may be suggested by certain symptoms or signs.**
   a. **Characteristic skin rash.** Nearly 50% of patients with meningococcemia, with or without meningitis, present with a prominent rash located principally on the extremities [27,96]. The rash is typically **erythematous and macular early** in the course of illness but quickly **evolves into a petechial phase** and then further coalesces into a purpuric form (see Color Plate 4.8). The rash often matures rapidly, with new petechial lesions appearing during the physical examination. A similar rash may also be seen in patients who have undergone splenectomy with rapidly overwhelming sepsis caused by *S. pneumoniae* (Color Plate 4.7) or *H. influenzae* type b.
   b. **Rhinorrhea or otorrhea due to a CSF leak** may result from a basilar skull fracture that produces a dural fistula between the subarachnoid space and nasal cavity, the paranasal sinuses, or middle ear. In these patients, meningitis may be recurrent and is most commonly caused by *S. pneumoniae.*
   c. Patients with *L. monocytogenes* meningitis have an increased tendency to experience seizures and focal deficits early in the course of infection. Some have ataxia, cranial nerve palsies, or nystagmus due to rhombencephalitis [43,44], although there may be no evidence of parenchymal brain involvement.
5. **Some patients may not manifest the classic symptoms and signs of bacterial meningitis. For example, elderly patients,** especially those with underlying conditions (e.g., diabetes mellitus or cardiopulmonary disease), may present insidiously with lethargy or obtundation, no fever, and variable signs of meningeal inflammation [97]. **In patients with head trauma,** the symptoms and signs of meningitis may be present as a result of the underlying injury [42]. In all these patients, an altered or changed mental status should not be ascribed to other causes until bacterial meningitis has been excluded by CSF examination.

C. **Tuberculous meningitis**
   1. **Children** with tuberculous meningitis commonly **present with** nausea, vomiting, and behavioral changes [61]. Headache is observed in fewer than 25% of cases. Seizures are infrequent (10% to 20% of cases) before hospitalization, although more than 50% may develop seizures during hospitalization. Some children develop an encephalitic course, characterized by stupor, coma, and convulsions without signs of meningitis.
   2. **Adults.** In contrast, the clinical presentation in adults is usually **more indolent,** with an insidious prodrome characterized by malaise, lassitude, low grade fever, intermittent headache, and changing personality [98]. A meningitic phase develops within 2 to 3 weeks characterized by protracted headache, meningismus, vomiting, and confusion. **A history of prior tuberculosis is obtained in fewer than 20% of cases** [99]. Adult patients may also present with a rapidly progressive acute meningitis syndrome indistinguishable from bacterial meningitis [62].
   3. **On physical examination,** fever is an inconstant finding, observed in 50% to 98% of cases [61,100]. Meningismus and signs of meningeal irritation are absent in 25% to 40% of children and adults with tuberculous meningitis, although 88% of patients admitted to an intensive care unit had meningeal findings in a review [101]. Up to 30% of patients have focal neurologic signs on presentation, usually unilateral or, less commonly, bilateral cranial nerve palsies; most often affected is cranial nerve VI, followed by cranial nerves III, IV, and VIII. Hemiparesis may result from ischemic infarction, usually in the middle cerebral artery territory. Chorea, hemiballismus, athetosis, myoclonus, and cerebellar ataxia are seen less frequently. Choroidal tubercles may be observed on funduscopic examination (~10% of cases).
   4. **Coexisting HIV infection.** The clinical manifestations are not modified significantly by HIV infection [102,103]. Fever, headache, and altered mentation are the most frequent presenting symptoms; meningeal signs are absent in up to 50% of patients.

**D. Spirochetal meningitis**

1. ***Treponema pallidum.*** Syphilitic **meningitis** usually presents with headache, nausea, and vomiting. In one series these were present in 91% of patients [65]. Meningismus was seen in 59% and fever in fewer than half of patients. Seizures occurred in 17% of patients, whereas cranial nerve palsies were found in 45% of cases (most commonly cranial nerves VII and VIII, followed by II, III, V, and VI). Focal abnormalities such as hemiplegia, aphasia, or mental status changes were less common.

   **Meningovascular syphilis** is distinguished temporally and on the basis of focal neurologic findings as a result of focal syphilitic arteritis, which almost always occurs in association with meningeal inflammation [65]. Most patients experience weeks to months of an episodic prodrome that includes headache or vertigo, personality changes (e.g., apathy or inattention), behavioral changes (e.g., irritability or memory impairment), insomnia, or occasional seizures. Focal deficits may also occur and, if untreated, may progress to a stroke syndrome with irreversible neurologic deficits.

   **Coinfection with HIV may modify the clinical course of syphilis** [66–68]. Patients with HIV infection are more likely to progress to neurosyphilis and to show accelerated disease courses. However, in one study of HIV-infected and noninfected patients with syphilis at sexually transmitted disease clinics in Baltimore [104], no significant differences were observed in clinical stage or in disease progression.

2. ***Borrelia burgdorferi.*** Meningitis is the most important neurologic abnormality of acute disseminated Lyme disease. Headache is the single most common symptom (30% to 90% of patients), whereas neck stiffness is seen in only 10% to 20% [70]. Photophobia, nausea, and vomiting are intermediate in frequency. Approximately two-thirds of patients have systemic symptoms, including malaise, fatigue, myalgias, fever, arthralgias, and involuntary weight loss. If untreated, symptoms last from 1 to 9 months. Patients typically experience recurrent attacks of meningeal symptoms lasting several weeks, alternating with similar periods of milder symptoms.

   Approximately half of all patients with Lyme meningitis have mild cerebral symptoms, usually consisting of somnolence, emotional lability, depression, impaired memory and concentration, and behavioral symptoms [70]. These symptoms may fluctuate in severity in untreated patients before they resolve. Transverse myelitis, spastic paraparesis or quadriparesis, disturbances of micturition, and Babinski sign are reported rarely during this stage. Approximately 50% of patients have cranial neuropathies. Facial nerve palsy is the most common (80% to 90%), is rapid in onset (often 1 to 2 days), and often is accompanied by slight ipsilateral facial numbness or tingling or ipsilateral ear or jaw pain. It is bilateral in 30% to 70% of cases, although the two sides are affected asynchronously in most cases. Other cranial nerves affected less commonly are cranial nerves II and III, the sensory portion of nerves V and VI, and the acoustic portion of nerve VIII. Recovery usually occurs within 2 months.

**E. Fungal meningitis**

1. ***Cryptococcus neoformans.*** Cryptococcal meningitis **presents differently in non-AIDS and in AIDS patients** [73,75–77].
   - **a. In non-AIDS patients** the **presentation** is typically **subacute** over days to weeks. The most frequent complaint is headache; fever, meningismus, and personality changes also occur. Approximately 50% have confusion, irritability, and other personality changes reflecting meningoencephalitis. Ocular abnormalities (e.g., papilledema and cranial nerve palsies) occur in nearly 40% of cases; direct invasion of the optic nerve also may occur.
   - **b.** In contrast, the **presentation in AIDS** patients may be very subtle. The only clinical findings may be headache, fever, and lethargy. Meningeal signs occur in some patients. Photophobia and cranial nerve palsies often are absent. On the African continent, AIDS patients with cryptococcal meningitis have higher rates of neurologic compromise [105,106], possibly because of the advanced stage of illness at the time of presentation.

2. ***Candida*** meningitis may be abrupt or insidious in onset [80–82]. The most common symptoms are fever, headache, and meningismus. Depressed mental status, confusion, cranial nerve neuropathies, and focal neurologic signs may also be seen.
3. ***Coccidioides immitis*** meningitis may present acutely, although it most often follows a subacute or chronic course [84,85]. Complaints include headache, low grade fever, weight loss, and mental status changes. Approximately 50% of patients develop disorientation, lethargy, confusion, or memory loss. Signs of meningeal irritation usually are absent, although they have been reported in as many as one-third of cases. Nausea, vomiting, focal neurologic deficits, and seizures may also occur.

**F. Protozoal and helminthic meningitis**

1. **Amebae.** Primary amebic meningoencephalitis presents in two forms [86,87].
   a. **Acute form.** After an incubation period of 3 to 8 days, there is the sudden onset of high fever, photophobia, headache, and progression to stupor or coma. This is usually indistinguishable from acute bacterial meningitis, although focal signs and seizures are more common in amebic meningoencephalitis. Early symptoms of abnormal smell or taste may be reported because of olfactory involvement. Confusion, irritability, and restlessness progress to delirium, stupor, and coma. Death in untreated patients generally occurs within 2 to 3 days from the onset.
   b. **Subacute or chronic form.** Patients present more insidiously with low grade fever, headache, and focal signs (e.g., hemiparesis, aphasia, cranial nerve palsies, visual field disturbances, diplopia, ataxia, seizures); the olfactory bulbs usually are spared. Deterioration occurs over a period of 2 to 4 weeks until death. However, longer durations of illness have also been reported (range, 5 to 18 months).
2. ***Angiostrongylus cantonensis.*** Symptoms of meningitis begin 6 to 30 days after ingestion of raw mollusks or other sources of the parasite [52,91]. Findings include severe headache (90%), stiff neck (56%), paresthesias (54%), and vomiting (56%). Moderate fever is present in approximately half of the cases.

**III. Diagnosis.** The diagnosis of meningitis ultimately is based on the findings in the CSF.

**A. Viral meningitis**

1. **Enteroviruses.** CSF pleocytosis is almost always present in enteroviral meningitis [1]. The cell count is usually 100 to 1,000/mm$^3$, although counts in the several thousands have also been reported; higher CSF white blood cell counts have been associated with a greater likelihood of isolating the causative enterovirus. **Neutrophils may dominate the CSF profile early in infection, although this quickly gives way to a lymphocytic predominance over the first 6 to 48 hours.** However, in a recent retrospective chart review of 158 cases of meningitis (138 aseptic and 20 bacterial), 51% of 53 patients with aseptic meningitis and duration of illness of more than 24 hours had a neutrophil predominance in CSF [107], suggesting that a CSF neutrophil predominance is not useful as a sole criterion in distinguishing between aseptic and bacterial meningitis. An elevated CSF protein and decreased CSF glucose, if present, are usually mild, although extremes of both have been reported. A specific virologic diagnosis depends on virus isolation from the CSF in tissue culture, although the sensitivity for enteroviral serotypes is only 65% to 75%. Isolation of a non-polio enterovirus from the throat or rectum of a patient with aseptic meningitis is suggestive, but the mean shedding periods from those sites after infection are 1 week and several weeks, respectively, so shedding from a past infection cannot be ruled out. In addition, viral shedding can occur in 7.5% of healthy control subjects during enterovirus epidemics [1]. Rapid diagnosis by immunoassay techniques has been hampered by the lack of a common antigen among the various serotypes and the low concentrations of virus in body fluids. Recent advances in PCR technology promise to greatly facilitate diagnosis and are 94% to 100% specific for the diagnosis of enteroviral meningitis [6,108–110].

2. **Mumps virus.** In mumps meningitis, there is almost always a **CSF pleocytosis** (usually < 500/mm$^3$) **that is primarily mononuclear cells** (>80% lymphocytes in 80% to 90% of patients) [8]. The CSF protein is normal in more than half of patients. The CSF glucose may be decreased in up to 25% of cases. A fourfold rise in mumps antibody titer by complement fixation or hemagglutination inhibition testing of paired acute and convalescent sera is diagnostic. Mumps virus can be grown from CSF in tissue culture for at least a week after the onset of disease, but sensitivity of this technique is highly variable (30% to 50% if collected from CSF early during the course of mumps CNS infection). Use of molecular diagnostic techniques, such as PCR, may have applicability in the diagnosis of mumps meningitis in the future.
3. **Lymphocytic choriomeningitis virus.** The CSF typically shows a lymphocytic pleocytosis (usually <750/mm$^3$, although counts up to several thousand may be seen). Hypoglycorrhachia is seen in up to 25% of cases. No rapid detection method is available. The virus may be cultured from blood and CSF early in infection and later from urine. The diagnosis usually is made by a fourfold rise from acute to convalescent sera.
4. **Herpesviruses.** With HSV type 2 meningitis, there is a lymphocytic pleocytosis (<500/mm$^3$) and a normal glucose. The virus has been cultured from the CSF and buffy coat of some patients. Using PCR, HSV type 2 was strongly associated with typical cases of Mollaret meningitis in patients without symptoms or signs of genital infection [15]. PCR also has confirmed the presence of varicella zoster DNA in the CSF of patients with herpes zoster meningitis [111].
5. **Human immunodeficiency virus.** The CSF in HIV-infected patients typically shows a mild lymphocytic pleocytosis (20 to 300/mm$^3$), mildly elevated protein, and normal or slightly decreased glucose [26]. HIV has been isolated from the CSF in some patients with neurologic disease, although it can be isolated from HIV-infected patients without neurologic symptoms or signs as well [112,113]. A few mononuclear cells and elevated protein in CSF are common in HIV-positive patients throughout the course of infection. There is a correlation between CSF concentrations of HIV RNA (the "CSF viral load") and severity of AIDS dementia complex [114,115], although there is considerable overlap in CSF values of HIV RNA in relation to clinical neurologic severity. Thus, CSF viral load cannot be used alone for diagnosis or to predict severity of AIDS dementia complex [24].

**B. Bacterial meningitis**

1. **Cerebrospinal fluid. The diagnosis of bacterial meningitis rests on CSF examination by lumbar puncture** [27,96,116]. The opening pressure is elevated in virtually all cases, with values exceeding 600 mm $H_2O$ suggesting the presence of cerebral edema, intracranial suppurative foci, or communicating hydrocephalus.
   a. **The white blood cell count usually is elevated in untreated bacterial meningitis**—commonly 1,000 to 5,000/mm$^3$ (range of <100 to >10,000/mm$^3$) **with a neutrophilic predominance**—although approximately 10% of patients with acute bacterial meningitis present with a lymphocytic predominance in CSF. This is more common in neonatal gram-negative bacillary meningitis and *L. monocytogenes* meningitis (approximately 30%). Patients with very low CSF white blood cell counts (0 to 20/mm$^3$), despite high CSF bacterial concentrations, have a poor prognosis. **In up to 4% of cases, CSF pleocytosis will be absent [117]. This is most common in premature neonates** (up to 15% of cases) **and in infants younger than 4 weeks** (17% of cases). Normal CSF white blood cell counts also have been seen with meningococcal meningitis [118], accounting for almost 10% of cases in one study [119]. **Therefore, a Gram stain and culture should be performed on all CSF specimens even if the white blood cell count is normal.** A decreased CSF glucose concentration (<40 mg/dL) is found in approximately 60% and a CSF-serum glucose ratio less than 0.31 in nearly 70% of patients [120]. The CSF protein is elevated in virtually all patients.

b. **Gram staining of CSF** permits a rapid accurate identification of the causative microorganism in 60% to 90% of patients; the specificity is nearly 100% [121]. The likelihood of detecting the organism by Gram stain correlates with the specific pathogen and the concentration of bacteria in CSF: Concentrations of no more than $10^3$ colony-forming units/mL yield positive Gram stains approximately 25% of the time, whereas CSF concentrations of at least $10^5$ colony-forming units/mL yield positive microscopy in up to 97% of cases. The yield of Gram stain also depends on the bacterial pathogen [122]. Bacteria are observed in 90% of cases of meningitis caused by *S. pneumoniae,* 86% of cases caused by *H. influenzae,* 75% of cases caused by *N. meningitidis,* and 50% of cases caused by gram-negative bacilli; the CSF Gram stain is positive in only one-third of patients with *L. monocytogenes* meningitis [44]. The probability of identifying organisms decreases with prior antimicrobial therapy (40% to 60% and <50% positivity on Gram stain and culture, respectively). In infants and children with bacterial meningitis, CSF cultures became sterile in 90% to 100% within 24 to 36 hours of "appropriate" antimicrobial therapy [117].

c. **Rapid diagnostic tests** [122]. **Counterimmunoelectrophoresis** (CIE) on CSF detects specific antigens of meningococci (serogroups A, C, Y, or W135), *H. influenzae* type b, pneumococci (83 serotypes), type III group B streptococci, and *Escherichia coli* K1. The sensitivity of CIE ranges from 50% to 95%, although the test is highly specific. CIE is rarely used today because it requires high-quality antisera, stringent quality control, special equipment, and an experienced technician for optimal sensitivity. Staphylococcal coagglutination and latex agglutination tests are more rapid (<15 minutes) and 10-fold more sensitive than CIE. **Latex agglutination techniques** detect the antigens of *H. influenzae* type b, *S. pneumoniae, N. meningitides, E. coli* K1, and the group B streptococci in CSF. However, many of the kits do not include tests for group B meningococcus, and other kits probably are poor detectors of this antigen because of its limited immunogenicity. **One of these tests should be performed on all CSF specimens from patients with presumed bacterial meningitis, if the CSF formula is consistent with the diagnosis and the CSF Gram stain is negative.** However, a negative test does not rule out infection by a specific pathogen. The routine use of CSF bacterial antigen tests has been questioned [123], because positive results have not modified therapy and false-positive and false-negative results may occur.

**PCR** can amplify DNA from the common meningeal pathogens. In one small study of meningococcal meningitis [124], the sensitivity and specificity of CSF PCR were both 91%. A semi-nested PCR strategy for simultaneous detection of *N. meningitidis, H. influenzae,* and streptococci in 304 clinical CSF samples [125] had a diagnostic sensitivity and specificity of 94% and 96%, respectively, although some false-positive results occurred. Refinements in PCR may improve its usefulness in the diagnosis of bacterial meningitis, particularly when the CSF Gram stain, bacterial antigen tests, and cultures are negative.

Serum C-reactive protein has a high sensitivity (96%), high specificity (93%), and high negative predictive value (99%) in distinguishing Gram stain negative bacterial meningitis from viral meningitis on admission [126]. Elevated serum concentrations of procalcitonin also are useful in distinguishing between bacterial and viral meningitis; a serum procalcitonin concentration of more than 0.2 ng/mL has a sensitivity and specificity of 100% for bacterial meningitis [127].

2. **Radiography.** Cranial computed tomography (CT) and magnetic resonance imaging (MRI) do not aid in the acute diagnosis but should be considered in patients who have persistent or prolonged fever, clinical evidence of increased intracranial pressure, focal neurologic findings or seizures, enlarging head circumference (in neonates), persistent neurologic dysfunction, or persistently abnormal CSF parameters or cultures [47,114]. Radiographic studies may be

particularly useful in patients with meningitis as a result of a basilar skull fracture with CSF leak [42,54], and CT may detect air-fluid levels, opacification of the air sinuses, or intracranial air; CT with reconstruction can also be used to document or localize fracture sites. Radioisotope cisternography, with cottonoid pledgets placed at the outlet of the nasal sinuses, can be used to document a CSF leak, although high-resolution CT with water-soluble contrast enhancement of the CSF (metrizamide cisternography) is the best currently available test for defining the site of leakage.

**C. Tuberculous meningitis.** Routine blood tests are not helpful in the diagnosis. A **syndrome of inappropriate antidiuretic hormone secretion,** resulting in hyponatremia, hypochloremia, and elevated urine osmolality and sodium, was documented in 17 of 24 children with tuberculous meningitis [128]. **Chest radiographic abnormalities** (usually reflecting primary tuberculosis) are common in children with CNS tuberculosis, whereas in adults the changes usually include apical scarring, calcified Ghon complexes, and nodular upper lobe disease [61]. Miliary radiographic disease has been documented in 25% to 50% of adults with tuberculous meningitis. Children with CNS tuberculosis usually have reactive tuberculin skin tests (positivity rates of 85% to 90%), although 35% to 60% of adults thought to have tuberculous meningitis do not react to first- or second-strength purified protein derivative (PPD) [99,100]. The rates of tuberculin reactivity are low in HIV-infected patients with active disease, ranging from 33% to 71% [64].

**1. CSF examination.** The CSF appearance in tuberculous meningitis is typically clear or opalescent. When the CSF is permitted to remain at room temperature or in a refrigerator for a short time, however, a cobweb-like clot, the classic **"pellicle" of tuberculosis,** may form secondary to the high fibrinogen content and presence of inflammatory cells [61]. **A moderate CSF pleocytosis** of more than 5 cells/mm$^3$ is present in 90% to 100% of patients, although the counts seldom exceed 500/mm$^3$ [100]. The initial differential count contains both lymphocytes and neutrophils, with conversion to a lymphocytic predominance over several weeks. Conversely, in patients receiving antituberculous chemotherapy, an initial lymphocytic predominance may become neutrophilic on subsequent CSF examinations [62], the so-called therapeutic paradox. The **CSF glucose concentration usually is modestly depressed** (median value, 40 mg/dL); hypoglycorrhachia has correlated with more advanced disease. Most patients have elevated CSF protein concentrations (median values of 150–200 mg/dL); values higher than 1,000 to 2,000 mg/dL have been reported usually in association with spinal block. In contrast, normal CSF protein concentrations were found in 43% of 37 HIV-infected patients with tuberculous meningitis [102].

Because of the low number of organisms in CSF, **identification by specific stains is difficult.** In many series, fewer than 25% of specimens are smear positive [61,99,101]. Staining any pellicle, layering the centrifuged sediment of large CSF volumes onto a single slide with repeated applications until the entire pellet can be stained at once, and obtaining repeated specimens may increase yield. One study demonstrated an 86% rate of acid-fast smear positivity when up to four separate CSF specimens were examined for each patient [100], although this rate has not been duplicated consistently. False-negative CSF cultures are common; even with four CSF specimens, almost 20% of patients have negative CSF cultures.

**Based on the inadequate yield of CSF stains and cultures, several newer diagnostic modalities are being developed for the rapid diagnosis of tuberculous meningitis [61].** Some use biochemical assays to measure some feature of the organism or the host response (e.g., bromide partition test, adenosine deaminase assay), whereas others are immunologic tests that detect mycobacterial antigen or antibody in CSF (e.g., tuberculostearic acid antigen, enzyme-linked immunosorbent assay, latex agglutination). Despite the promise of these immunodiagnostic tests for rapid diagnosis of tuberculous meningitis, there are problems with cross-reacting antibodies against nonpathogenic mycobacteria and with the presence of bacterial or fungal antigenic moieties. **PCR** to detect fragments of mycobacterial DNA in CSF is an equally promising tool

[129]. The usefulness of these tests in the diagnosis of tuberculous meningitis requires large-scale confirmatory studies.

2. **Radiography. No radiologic changes are pathognomonic** for tuberculous meningitis [61]. On CT of the head, hydrocephalus frequently is present at diagnosis or develops during the course of infection. Contrast enhancement of the basal cisterns, with widening and blurring of the basilar arterial structures, also may be seen. Periventricular lucencies represent tuberculous exudate and tubercle formation adjacent to the choroid and ependyma. MRI may be superior to CT in identifying basilar meningeal inflammation and small tuberculoma formation. MR angiography has been used to detect the characteristic vascular narrowing and the rare complication of aneurysm formation [130].

**D. Spirochetal meningitis**

1. ***Treponema pallidum.*** For diagnosis of CNS syphilis, no single routine laboratory test is definitive. Common nonspecific CSF abnormalities in syphilitic meningitis include a mononuclear pleocytosis (>10 cells/mm$^3$ in most patients), elevated CSF protein concentrations (78% of patients), and mild decrease in CSF glucose concentrations (<50 mg/dL in 55% of patients) [65]. Oligoclonal bands and intrathecally produced antitreponemal antibodies frequently are present.

   **Serologic testing** has been used to aid in the diagnosis of neurosyphilis, although testing of CSF specimens in patients with syphilis is problematic [67]. For example, CSF is subject to blood contamination in approximately 10% of lumbar punctures, which may lead to a false-positive CSF serologic test result; the likelihood of a false-positive test depends on the relative amount of contamination, the antibody titer in blood, and the sensitivity of the test. For patients with a serum venereal disease research laboratory test (VDRL) of less than 1:256, sufficient blood contamination to be visible to the naked eye is required to cause false-positive CSF VDRL results. **The specificity of the CSF VDRL for neurosyphilis is high, but the sensitivity is low (reactive tests in only 50% to 85% of patients).** Therefore, a reactive CSF VDRL test in the absence of blood contamination is sufficient to diagnose neurosyphilis, and a nonreactive result does not exclude the diagnosis. A nonreactive CSF fluorescent treponemal antibody absorption test effectively rules out neurosyphilis, although the specificity of the test is much less than the CSF VDRL because of the possibility of leakage of small amounts of antibody from the serum into CSF. Furthermore, the significance of a reactive CSF fluorescent treponemal antibody absorption as a diagnostic tool for neurosyphilis is undefined. **PCR** can detect *T. pallidum* DNA in CSF from patients with acute symptomatic neurosyphilis [131], although further large-scale studies are needed to determine the sensitivity and specificity of this technique. Based on the difficulties in the diagnosis of neurosyphilis, elevation of CSF concentrations of white blood cells or protein in the appropriate clinical and serologic setting should lead to initiation of therapy (see Chapter 16).

2. ***Borrelia burgdorferi.*** Typical CSF changes in Lyme meningitis are a pleocytosis (usually <500 cells/mm$^3$), with more than 90% lymphocytes in 75% of cases [70]; plasma cells may also be present. There is usually an elevated CSF protein (up to 620 mg/dL) and a normal glucose, although the glucose can be low with illness of longer duration.

   The best available laboratory test for diagnosis is demonstration of specific serum antibody to *B. burgdorferi,* which in a patient with a compatible neurologic abnormality is strong evidence for the diagnosis [70,71]. Specific IgM, IgG, or IgA antibody against *B. burgdorferi* also appears in CSF and indicates intrathecal antibody synthesis [71]. However, antibody tests are poorly standardized, and there is marked interlaboratory variability [132]. When the pretest probability of Lyme disease is 0.20 to 0.80, sequential testing with enzyme-linked immunosorbent assay and Western blot is recommended (see Chapter 21) [133,134]. PCR has occasionally identified *B. burgdorferi* DNA in CSF from patients with Lyme neuroborreliosis [71,72]. Culture of CSF is insensitive [71].

**E. Fungal meningitis**

1. ***Cryptococcus neoformans.*** Most non-AIDS patients with cryptococcal meningitis have a CSF pleocytosis (range, 20–500 cells/mm$^3$), with the proportion of

neutrophils usually lower than 50% [73]. **AIDS patients may have very low or even normal CSF leukocyte counts during active infection; as many as 65% have fewer than 5 white blood cells/mm$^3$** [75–77]. CSF protein concentrations usually are elevated, with concentrations in excess of 1,000 mg/dL, suggesting subarachnoid block. CSF glucose concentrations may be normal in two-thirds of AIDS patients. CSF India ink examination is a rapid effective test (if the laboratory has significant experience) that is positive in 50% to 75% of patients with cryptococcal meningitis. This yield increases up to 88% in AIDS patients. Cryptococcal meningitis with completely normal CSF parameters has been described in AIDS patients [135]; normal indices were found in 17% of HIV-infected patients in one study from South Africa [105]. The yield of CSF culture is excellent in both non-AIDS and AIDS patients.

**Diagnosis is aided by the latex agglutination test** for detection of cryptococcal polysaccharide antigen [75–77]. The test is both sensitive and specific when samples are first heated to eliminate rheumatoid factor. The cryptococcal polysaccharide antigen may be positive in early infection even when the CSF culture is negative. In smaller laboratories, it may be a more reliable test than the India ink examination. A presumptive diagnosis is made with a CSF titer of 1:8 or higher. **Serum cryptococcal polysaccharide antigen may also be detected, particularly in severely immunosuppressed patients** (i.e., those with AIDS) [77], although the value of the serum polysaccharide antigen for screening patients suspected of having meningeal disease has not been established. Antigen titers generally are higher in serum than in CSF of patients with cryptococcal meningitis. Furthermore, extremely high CSF polysaccharide antigen titers have been reported in AIDS patients; early reports suggested that titers of 1:10,000 or higher predicted a poor outcome [76], although some patients have responded well to antifungal therapy despite high initial titers.

2. ***Candida.*** Patients with *Candida* meningitis usually have a CSF pleocytosis, with a mean of 600 cells/mm$^3$; lymphocytes or neutrophils may predominate [80,81]. Direct microscopy of CSF detects yeast cells in approximately 50% of cases. Organisms are readily grown from CSF in most cases. A single positive culture from a patient with risk factors or symptoms is considered significant when CSF indices are compatible with meningitis and the fungus is isolated in pure culture [79].
3. ***Coccidioides immitis.*** CSF pleocytosis is seen in coccidioidal meningitis and may occasionally reveal a prominent eosinophilia [85,136]. Only 25% to 50% of patients have positive CSF cultures. Serum complement-fixing antibody titers in excess of 1:32 to 1:64 suggest dissemination [84,85]. CSF complement-fixing antibodies are present in at least 70% of cases of early meningitis and from virtually all patients as disease progresses. In fact, the antibody titers parallel the course of meningeal disease, although in patients who relapse CSF pleocytosis, elevated protein, or decreased glucose usually develop before detectable CSF antibody recurs. Complement-fixing antibodies may fail to develop in serum or CSF in patients with immunodeficiencies.

**F. Protozoal and helminthic meningitis**

**1. Amebae**

- **a. Acute form.** The CSF formula in patients with the acute form of primary amebic meningoencephalitis reveals a neutrophilic pleocytosis, low glucose, elevated protein, and red blood cells [86,87]. The Gram stain is always negative. However, examination of fresh warm CSF specimens can reveal the motile trophozoites.
- **b. Subacute or chronic form.** In patients with the subacute or chronic form of the illness, the CSF inflammatory response is less florid with a predominant mononuclear leukocytosis [86]. The CSF protein concentration is elevated, and the glucose is often normal or slightly reduced. Because amebae are not found in CSF, the diagnosis usually requires examination of a biopsy or necropsy specimen revealing the characteristic cysts. The value of serologic tests is variable. Serum immunofluorescence, amebic immobilization titers, and complement-fixing antibodies support the diagnosis, although

demonstration of rising titers is necessary as some normal persons have circulating antibodies.

2. ***Angiostrongylus cantonensis.*** The combination of history of ingesting suspected food, moderate to high peripheral eosinophilia, and CSF eosinophilia suggests angiostrongyloidiasis [86]. The CSF leukocytosis is moderate, with 16% to 72% eosinophils and increased protein concentration; CSF larvae are found occasionally.

**IV. Approach to the patient with meningitis.** Initial management of presumed bacterial meningitis includes lumbar puncture to determine whether the CSF formula is consistent with that diagnosis [27,96,137]. If purulent meningitis is present, empiric antimicrobial therapy should be instituted based on results of Gram staining or rapid bacterial antigen tests. However, if no etiologic agent can be identified by these means or if there is a delay in performance of the lumbar puncture, empiric antimicrobial therapy should be instituted based on the patient's age and underlying disease status. Antimicrobial therapy should be ordered on initial clinical impression; in critically ill patients, the first dose may precede lumbar puncture. There are no prospective clinical data on the optimal timing of antimicrobial therapy in bacterial meningitis. In a recent retrospective study of 269 patients with community-acquired bacterial meningitis [138], delayed initiation of antimicrobial therapy was associated with adverse clinical outcome when the patient's condition advanced from a low- or intermediate-risk stage to a high-risk stage of prognostic severity, supporting the assumption that treatment of bacterial meningitis before it advances to a high level of clinical severity improves outcome. **In patients with a focal neurologic examination or papilledema and suspected bacterial meningitis, a CT of the head should be performed before lumbar puncture** to rule out the presence of an intracranial mass lesion because of the risk of herniation [120]. The true incidence of this problem is unclear but has been suggested to be much lower than 1.2% in patients with papilledema and approximately 12% in patients without papilledema but with elevated intracranial pressure. However, the time involved in waiting for a CT significantly delays initiation of antimicrobial therapy, with the potential for increased morbidity and mortality. Therefore, **emergent empiric antimicrobial therapy should be initiated before the CT. Blood cultures should be obtained before empiric antibiotic therapy.** Although CSF cultures may be sterile after initiation of antimicrobial therapy, pretreatment blood cultures and the CSF formula, Gram stain, or bacterial antigen tests will likely provide evidence for or against bacterial meningitis. Our choices of **empiric antimicrobial therapy** are shown in **Table 6.2.** Once the pathogen is isolated and susceptibility testing is known, antimicrobial therapy can be modified for optimal treatment (Table 6.3). Recommended dosages for CNS infections in adults are shown in Table 6.4; dosages for infants and children are shown in Table 6.5.

**V. Antimicrobial therapy**

**A. Viral meningitis.** Currently, **there is no specific antiviral chemotherapy for the enteroviruses; treatment is supportive** [2]. However, pleconaril has recently been shown to have beneficial effects on the clinical, virologic, laboratory, and radiologic parameters in patients with severe enterovirus infections [139]. Recovery of patients with HSV type 2 meningitis usually is complete without neurologic sequelae; it is not clear whether antiviral treatment alters the course of mild HSV type 2 meningitis. However, treatment with acyclovir generally is indicated for primary genital herpes infection [11]. Specific antiretroviral therapy should be considered for acute HIV infection.

**B. Bacterial meningitis**

**1. *Haemophilus influenzae***

**a.** Therapy for *H. influenzae* type b meningitis has been altered by the emergence of $\beta$-lactamase–producing strains. Resistance to chloramphenicol has also been described, more commonly from areas such as Spain (>50% of isolates) than from the United States (<1% of isolates) [27,96]. A prospective study found chloramphenicol to be bacteriologically and clinically inferior to ampicillin, ceftriaxone, or cefotaxime in the treatment of childhood bacterial meningitis caused predominantly by *H. influenzae* type b, even with chloramphenicol-sensitive isolates. The third-generation cephalosporins

Table 6.2. Empiric Therapy for Purulent Meningitis[a]

| Predisposing Factor | Common Bacterial Pathogens | Antimicrobial Therapy |
|---|---|---|
| Age | | |
| 0–4 wk | *Streptococcus agalactiae, Escherichia coli, Listeria monocytogenes, Klebsiella pneumoniae* | Ampicillin plus cefotaxime; *or* ampicillin plus an aminoglycoside (see Chap. 3) |
| 1–23 mo | *Streptococcus pneumoniae, Haemophilus influenzae, S. agalactiae Neisseria meningitidis, E. coli* | Third-generation cephalosporin[b]; or ampicillin plus chloramphenicol[c] |
| 2–50 yr | *S. pneumoniae, N. meningitidis* | Third-generation cephalosporin[b] ± ampicillin[c] |
| >50 yr | *S. pneumoniae, N. meningitidis, L. monocytogenes,* aerobic gram-negative bacilli | Ampicillin plus a third-generation cephalosporin[b] |
| Immunocompromised host | *S. pneumoniae, N. meningitidis, L. monocytogenes,* aerobic gram-negative bacilli (including *Pseudomonas aeruginosa*), *S. aureus* | Vancomycin + ampicillin + either ceftazidime or cefepime |
| Basilar skull fracture | *S. pneumoniae, H. influenzae,* group A β-hemolytic streptococci | Third-generation cephalosporin[b] |
| Head trauma; postneurosurgery | *Staphylococcus aureus, Staphylococcus epidermidis,* aerobic gram-negative bacilli (including *P. aeruginosa*) | Vancomycin + either ceftazidime or cefepime |
| Cerebrospinal fluid shunt | *S. epidermidis, S. aureus,* aerobic gram-negative bacilli (including *P. aeruginosa*), diphtheroids | Vancomycin + either ceftazidime or cefepime |

[a] Vancomycin should be added to empiric therapeutic regimens when highly penicillin-resistant or cephalosporin-resistant strains of *S. pneumoniae* are suspected; see text for details.
[b] Cefotaxime or ceftriaxone.
[c] See text for details.

(cefotaxime or ceftriaxone) are as effective as the combination of ampicillin plus chloramphenicol for bacterial meningitis. Thus, the **third-generation cephalosporins (cefotaxime or ceftriaxone) are recommended as empiric therapy for children with bacterial meningitis** [137].

**b.** Several comparative trials have documented a slower rate of CSF sterilization and a higher incidence of hearing impairment in patients receiving cefuroxime for bacterial meningitis [140,141]. Furthermore, there have been cases of *H. influenzae* meningitis in patients receiving cefuroxime for nonmeningeal *H. influenzae* disease. Therefore, **cefuroxime is not recommended** as first-line treatment of bacterial meningitis. In addition, there have been case reports of delayed CSF sterilization in *H. influenzae* meningitis treated with ceftizoxime or ceftazidime. However, *in vitro* resistance of *H. influenzae* to the third-generation cephalosporins and fluoroquinolones has not yet been described.

**c.** In a prospective randomized comparison of cefepime with cefotaxime for treatment of bacterial meningitis in infants and children, cefepime was found to be safe and therapeutically equivalent to cefotaxime [142] and is a suitable alternative.

Table 6.3. Specific Antimicrobial Therapy for Meningitis

| Microorganism | Standard Therapy | Alternative Therapies |
|---|---|---|
| Bacteria | | |
| *Haemophilus influenzae* | | |
| $\beta$-Lactamase negative | Ampicillin | Third-generation cephalosporin[a], cefepime; chloramphenicol; aztreonam |
| $\beta$-Lactamase positive | Third-generation cephalosporin[a] | Chloramphenicol; cefepime; aztreonam; fluoroquinolone |
| *Neisseria meningitidis* | Penicillin G or ampicillin[b] | Third-generation cephalosporin[a]; chloramphenicol; fluoroquinolone; meropenem |
| *Streptococcus penumoniae* | | |
| Penicillin MIC <0.1 $\mu$g/mL | Penicillin G or ampicillin | Third-generation cephalosporin[a]; chloramphenicol |
| Penicillin MIC 0.1–1.0 $\mu$g/mL | Third-generation cephalosporin[a] | Meropenem; cefepime |
| Penicillin MIC $\geq$2.0$\mu$g/mL | Vancomycin + a third-generation cephalosporin[a,c] | Meropenem; fluoroquinolone[d] |
| *Enterobacteriaceae* | Third-generation cephalosporin[a] | Aztreonam; meropenem; fluoroquinolone; trimethoprim-sulfamethoxazole |
| *Pseudomonas aeruginosa* | Ceftazidime[e] or cefepime[e] | Aztreonam[e]; meropenem[e]; fluoroquinolone[e] |
| *Listeria monocytogenes* | Ampicillin or penicillin G[e] | Trimethoprim-sulfamethoxazole; meropenem |
| *Streptococcus agalactiae* | Ampicillin or penicillin G[e] | Third-generation cephalosporin[a]; vancomycin |
| *Staphylococcus aureus* | | |
| Methicillin sensitive | Nafcillin or oxacillin | Vancomycin |
| Methicillin resistant | Vancomycin | |
| *Staphylococcus epidermidis* | Vancomycin[c] | |
| Mycobacteria | | |
| *Mycobacterium tuberculosis* | Isoniazid + rifampin + pyrazinamide | Ethambutol[f]; ethionamide[f]; streptomycin |
| Spirochetes | | |
| *Treponema pallidum* | Penicillin G | Doxycycline[g]; ceftriaxone[g] |
| *Borrelia burgdorferi* | Third-generation cephalosporin[a] | Penicillin; doxycycline |
| Fungi | | |
| *Cryptococcus neoformans* | Amphotericin B[h] | Fluconazole; itraconazole[g] |
| *Candida* species | Amphotericin B[h] | Fluconazole[g] |
| *Coccidiodes immitis* | Fluconazole | Amphotericin B[i] |
| Protozoa and helminths | | |
| *Naegleria fowleri* | Amphotericin B[i] + rifampin + doxycycline | |

[a] Cefotaxime or ceftriaxone.
[b] Some would use a third-generation cephalosporin for meningococcal strains that demonstrate intermediate sensitivity to penicillin; see text for details.
[c] Addition of rifampin should be considered.
[d] Currently under investigation in patients with pneumococcal meningitis; value has not been established.
[e] Addition of an aminoglycoside should be considered.
[f] Add to standard therapy in cases of suspected drug resistance; see text for details.
[g] Value of these antimicrobial agents has not been established.
[h] Addition of 5-flucytosine should be considered.
[i] Intravenous and intraventricular administration.
MIC, minimum inhibitory concentration.

Table 6.4. Maximum Recommended Dosages of Antimicrobial Agents for Central Nervous System Infections in Adults with Normal Renal and Hepatic Function[a]

| Antimicrobial Agent | Total Daily Dose | Dosing Interval (hr) |
|---|---|---|
| Amikacin[b] | 15 mg/kg | 8 |
| Amphotericin B[c] | 0.6–1.0 mg/kg | 24 |
| Amphotericin B lipid complex | 5 mg/kg | 24 |
| Ampicillin | 12 g | 4 |
| Aztreonam | 6–8 g | 6–8 |
| Cefepime | 6 g | 8 |
| Cefotaxime | 8–12 g | 4–6 |
| Ceftazidime | 6 g | 8 |
| Ceftriaxone | 4 g | 12–24 |
| Chloramphenicol[d] | 4–6 g | 6 |
| Ciprofloxacin | 800–1,200 mg | 8–12 |
| Doxycycline | 200–400 mg | 12 |
| Ethambutol[e,f] | 15–25 mg/kg | 24 |
| Ethionamide[e] | 1 g | 12 |
| Fluconazole | 400–800 mg | 24 |
| Flucytosine[e,g] | 100 mg/kg | 6 |
| Gentamicin[b] | 3–5 mg/kg | 8 |
| Imipenem | 2 g[n] | 6 |
| Isoniazid[e,h] | 300 mg | 24 |
| Itraconazole | 800 mg | 12 |
| Liposomal amphotericin B | 3–5 mg/kg | 24 |
| Meropenem | 6 g | 8 |
| Metronidazole | 30 mg/kg | 6 |
| Miconazole | 1.5–3.0 g | 8 |
| Nafcillin | 9–12 g | 4 |
| Oxacillin | 9–12 g | 4 |
| Penicillin G | 24 million units | 4 |
| Pyrazinamide[e,i] | 15–30 mg/kg | 24 |
| Rifampin | 600 mg | 24 |
| Streptomycin[j,k] | 15 mg/kg | 24 |
| Sulfadiazine[e] | 4–6 g | 6 |
| Tobramycin[b] | 3–5 mg/kg | 8 |
| Trimethoprim-sulfamethoxazole[l] | 10–20 mg/kg | 6–12 |
| Vancomycin[b,m] | 2–3 g | 8–12 |

[a] Unless otherwise indicated, therapy is administered intravenously.
[b] Need to monitor serum concentrations to ensure adequate peaks. See Chapter 27.
[c] Can increase dosage to 1.5 mg/kg/day in severely ill patients.
[d] Higher dose recommended for pneumococcal meningitis.
[e] Oral administration.
[f] Maximum daily dosage of 2.5 g.
[g] Maintain serum concentrations of 50–100 $\mu$g/mL.
[h] Initiate therapy at a dosage of 10 mg/kg/day (up to 600 mg/day).
[i] Maximum daily dosage of 2 g.
[j] Intramuscular administration.
[k] Maximum daily dosage of 1 g.
[l] Dosage based on trimethoprim component.
[m] May need to monitor cerebrospinal fluid concentrations in severely ill patients.
[n] In a patient with normal renal function, some clinicians may consider a higher dose. See Chapter 27.

Table 6.5. Recommended Dosages of Antimicrobial Agents for Central Nervous System Infections in Infants and Children with Normal Renal and Hepatic Function[a,b]

| Antimicrobial Agent | Total Daily Dose in Infants and Children (Dosing Interval in hr) |
|---|---|
| Amikacin[c] | 20–30 mg/kg (8) |
| Amphotericin B | 0.25–1.0 mg/kg (24) |
| Ampicillin | 200–300 mg/kg (6) |
| Cefepime | 50 mg/kg (8) |
| Cefotaxime | 200 mg/kg (6–8) |
| Ceftazidime | 125–150 mg/kg (8) |
| Ceftriaxone | 80–100 mg/kg (12–24) |
| Chloramphenicol | 75–100 mg/kg (6) |
| Ethambutol[d,e] | 15–25 mg/kg (24) |
| Ethionamide[d,f] | 10–20 mg/kg (12) |
| Flucytosine[d,g] | 100 mg/kg (6) |
| Gentamicin[c] | 7.5 mg/kg (8) |
| Isoniazid[d,h,i] | 10–20 mg/kg (12–24) |
| Metronidazole | 30 mg/kg (12) |
| Nafcillin | 200 mg/kg (6) |
| Penicillin G | 0.25 mU/kg (4–6) |
| Pyrazinamide[d,j] | 15–30 mg/kg (12–24) |
| Rifampin[d,k] | 10–20 mg/kg (12–24) |
| Streptomycin[l] | 20–40 mg/kg (12) |
| Tobramycin[c] | 7.5 mg/kg (8) |
| Trimethoprim-sulfamethoxazole[m] | 10–20 mg/kg (6–12) |
| Vancomycin[c] | 50–60 mg/kg (6) |

[a] Unless otherwise indicated, therapy is administered intravenously.
[b] **See Table 3.2 for neonate dosages.**
[c] Need to monitor peak and trough serum concentrations.
[d] Oral administration.
[e] Maximum daily dosage of 2.5 g.
[f] Maximum daily dosage of 1 g.
[g] Maintain serum concentrations of 50–100 μg/mL.
[h] Some clinicians initiate therapy at 30 mg/kg for the first several weeks.
[i] Maximum daily dosage of 300 mg.
[j] Maximum daily dosage of 2 g.
[k] Maximum daily dosage of 600 mg.
[l] Intramuscular administration.
[m] Dosage based on trimethoprim component.

2. ***Neisseria meningitidis.*** The antimicrobial agents of choice for *N. meningitidis* meningitis are **penicillin G or ampicillin,** although these recommendations may change in future years [27]. Meningococcal strains have been reported from several areas (particularly Spain) that are relatively resistant to penicillin G, with a minimum inhibitory concentration (MIC) range of 0.1 to 1.0 μg/mL, due to altered penicillin-binding proteins 2 and 3 [143]. In one U.S. population-based surveillance study for invasive meningococcal disease, 3 of 100 isolates had penicillin MICs of 0.12 μg/mL [144]. In another active population-based surveillance study in seven geographically dispersed areas of the United States during 1997, 3 of 90 isolates were intermediately resistant to penicillin (MIC 0.12 μg/mL) [145]; 49 of the remaining 87 isolates had penicillin MICs of 0.06 μg/mL. The clinical significance of these isolates is unclear because patients with meningitis caused by these organisms recovered with standard penicillin therapy. However, isolated reports of penicillin treatment failure have been described [146,147]. Based on these data, some authorities would treat meningococcal meningitis with a third-generation cephalosporin (either cefotaxime or ceftriaxone)

pending results of *in vitro* susceptibility testing. Chloramphenicol is the standard treatment for meningococcal meningitis in developing countries because of its low cost and ease of administration. However, high-level chloramphenicol resistance (MIC $\geq$ 64 $\mu$g/mL) has recently been described [148], indicating the importance of continued surveillance for resistant strains. Trovafloxacin was found to be equivalent to ceftriaxone in children with meningococcal meningitis in one report [149], although concerns of liver toxicity preclude its use in the therapy of bacterial meningitis.

3. **Streptococcus pneumoniae**
   a. **The therapy for meningitis caused by pneumococci has been modified based on current pneumococcal susceptibility patterns.** Numerous reports from throughout the world have documented strains relatively resistant to penicillin, with an MIC range of 0.1 to 1.0 $\mu$g/mL, as well as strains highly resistant to penicillin (MIC $\geq$ 2.0 $\mu$g/mL) [27,137,150–152]. The overwhelming majority of resistant strains are serotypes 6, 14, 19, and 23. The mechanism of this resistance is alterations in the structure and molecular size of penicillin-binding proteins. Most multiresistant strains in the United States have disseminated from a multiresistant serotype 23F clone of *S. pneumoniae* isolated in Spain as early as 1978.

      Based on these antimicrobial susceptibility trends and because sufficient CSF concentrations of penicillin are difficult to achieve with standard high parenteral dosages (initial CSF penicillin concentrations of approximately 1 $\mu$g/mL), **penicillin is no longer recommended as empiric antimicrobial therapy when *S. pneumoniae* is considered a likely infecting pathogen. Indeed, early reports documented clinical failure in most patients with penicillin-nonsusceptible *S. pneumoniae* who were treated with penicillin [153]. For patients in whom relatively resistant strains are found, a third-generation cephalosporin (ceftriaxone or cefotaxime) should be used [27]; vancomycin plus a third-generation cephalosporin (either cefotaxime or ceftriaxone) should be used when highly resistant strains are suspected or isolated** (see Chapter 27).
   b. Although a third-generation cephalosporin is the antimicrobial agent of choice for pneumococcal meningitis caused by isolates with intermediate penicillin resistance, pneumococcal strains resistant to the third-generation cephalosporins (MIC $\geq$ 2 $\mu$g/mL) have also been reported [27,154–156]. For the third-generation cephalosporins, pneumococcal meningitis strains with MICs no more than 0.5 $\mu$g/mL are defined as susceptible, 1.0 $\mu$g/mL as intermediate, and at least 2.0 $\mu$g/mL as resistant. However, some patients have been treated successfully with only high-dose cefotaxime or ceftriaxone when the MIC to the third-generation cephalosporin is no more than 1.0 $\mu$g/mL. Clinical failures with chloramphenicol have been reported in patients with penicillin-resistant isolates [157], likely due to poor bactericidal activity against these strains. In one study, 20 of 25 children had an unsatisfactory outcome (i.e., death, serious neurologic deficit, poor clinical response). Chloramphenicol alone is not recommended for empiric therapy. **These data indicate the need to perform susceptibility testing of all pneumococcal isolates,** at which time optimal antimicrobial therapy can be chosen.
   c. **Vancomycin may not be optimal therapy for patients with pneumococcal meningitis [158].** Of 11 consecutive patients with pneumococcal meningitis caused by relatively resistant strains who were treated with intravenous vancomycin, all improved and 10 were eventually cured, but 4 failed vancomycin therapy [159]. Reasons for failure may have included variability in serum vancomycin concentrations or impaired CSF vancomycin penetration as a result of adjunctive dexamethasone administration. In addition, there are recent descriptions of *S. pneumoniae* strains that are tolerant to vancomycin [160,161]; tolerance may be a precursor phenotype to the development of resistance. **These data indicate the need for careful**

**monitoring of, and perhaps even measurement of CSF vancomycin concentrations in, adult patients receiving vancomycin therapy for pneumococcal meningitis.** Infectious disease consultation is advised. The addition of intrathecal or intraventricular vancomycin should be considered for treatment of unresponsive cases. Some investigators have recommended the addition of rifampin (if the organism is susceptible) to vancomycin for treatment of meningitis caused by highly resistant pneumococcal strains [153], although there are no firm data to support this. Meropenem, a new carbapenem with less proconvulsive activity than imipenem, yields microbiologic and clinical outcomes similar to either cefotaxime or ceftriaxone [162,163]. The newer fluoroquinolones (levofloxacin, moxifloxacin, gatifloxacin) are active *in vitro* against resistant pneumococci and in animal models of penicillin-resistant pneumococcal meningitis [27,164] but have not been studied in humans with this disease (see Chapter 27).

4. ***Listeria monocytogenes.*** **The third-generation cephalosporins are inactive in meningitis caused by *L. monocytogenes.*** Therapy for patients with *Listeria* meningitis should consist of ampicillin or penicillin G [43,44]; the addition of an aminoglycoside should be considered in proven infection because of *in vitro* synergy and enhanced killing in a variety of animal models. In the penicillin-allergic patient, trimethoprim-sulfamethoxazole, which is bactericidal against *Listeria in vitro,* should be used. Chloramphenicol has been associated with an unacceptably high failure rate in patients with *Listeria* meningitis. Vancomycin is also unsatisfactory for *Listeria* meningitis, despite favorable *in vitro* susceptibility results. However, intraventricular administration of vancomycin was successful in a case of recurrent *L. monocytogenes* meningitis [165]. Meropenem is active *in vitro* and in experimental animals and was successfully used in a pediatric renal transplant patient with *Listeria* meningitis [166]; meropenem may be a useful alternative in the future (see also Chapter 3).
5. ***Streptococcus agalactiae.*** Standard therapy for meningitis caused by the group B streptococcus is the combination of ampicillin plus an aminoglycoside [47]. This combination is recommended due to *in vitro* synergy and recent reports detailing the presence of penicillin-tolerant strains [49,50]. Alternative agents are the third-generation cephalosporins. Vancomycin is reserved for penicillin-allergic patients in whom cephalosporins are contraindicated (see also Chapter 3).
6. **Aerobic gram-negative bacilli**
   a. The treatment of bacterial meningitis caused by enteric gram-negative bacilli has been revolutionized by the availability of the **third-generation cephalosporins** [27,137], with cure rates of 78% to 94%. Ceftazidime has enhanced activity against *P. aeruginosa,* and ceftazidime-containing regimens have successfully cured adult and pediatric patients with *P. aeruginosa* meningitis [167,168]. Concomitant intrathecal or intraventricular aminoglycoside therapy should be considered in patients who are not responding to conventional parenteral therapy. Although this rarely is needed at present, it was associated with a higher mortality than systemic therapy alone in infants with gram-negative meningitis and ventriculitis.
   b. **Other antimicrobial agents.** Aztreonam attains excellent CSF concentrations and has been efficacious in the treatment of gram-negative meningitis [169]. Imipenem was effective in one case of *Acinetobacter* meningitis and eradicated bacteria from CSF in a study of 21 children (most cases caused by *H. influenzae* type b and *N. meningitidis*) [170]. However, a high rate of seizure activity (33%) limits its usefulness for bacterial meningitis. High-dose meropenem (2 g every 8 hours) given for 18 weeks was successful in a lymphoma patient with *P. aeruginosa* meningitis in whom therapy with ceftazidime plus gentamicin had failed [171] and in another patient with posttraumatic *P. aeruginosa* meningitis [172]. Intravenous meropenem was also successfully used in combination with intraventricular polymyxin B in a patient with ventriculoperitoneal shunt-associated ventriculitis caused by a ceftazidime-resistant *K. pneumoniae* [173]. The development of meropenem

resistance during treatment of *Acinetobacter* meningitis [174] indicates the need to consider emergence of resistance in patients who fail to respond despite initially appropriate antimicrobial therapy.

The fluoroquinolones (e.g., ciprofloxacin, pefloxacin) have been used successfully in some patients with gram-negative meningitis [27]. Their primary usefulness is for treatment of multidrug-resistant gram-negative organisms (e.g., *P. aeruginosa*) or when the response to conventional $\beta$-lactam therapy is slow (e.g., meningitis caused by *Salmonella* species). These agents should never be used as first-line empiric therapy in meningitis of unknown etiology because of their variable *in vitro* activity against pneumococci and *L. monocytogenes.*

7. **Staphylococci.** *S. aureus* meningitis should be treated with nafcillin or oxacillin [53], with vancomycin reserved for patients allergic to penicillin or when methicillin-resistant organisms are suspected or isolated. The addition of rifampin should be considered in patients not responding to therapy. Meningitis caused by coagulase-negative staphylococci, the most commonly encountered organism in CSF shunt infections, should be treated with vancomycin; rifampin should be added if the patient fails to improve [54]. Removal of the shunt often is necessary. Intraventricular teicoplanin, an investigational glycopeptide antimicrobial agent, was successful in seven patients with staphylococcal neurosurgical shunt infection [54,175].
8. **Duration of therapy.** Traditionally, the duration of antimicrobial therapy in patients with bacterial nonmeningococcal meningitis has been 10 to 14 days [176]. However, 7 days of therapy are safe and effective for *H. influenzae* type b meningitis, although treatment must be individualized and some patients may require longer courses. Meningococcal meningitis can be treated for 7 days with intravenous penicillin, though some authors have suggested that 4 days of therapy are adequate. In adults with meningitis caused by enteric gram-negative bacilli, treatment should be continued for 3 weeks to minimize relapses. Ten to 14 days are recommended for treatment of meningitis caused by *S. pneumoniae,* 14 to 21 days for *S. agalactiae,* and at least 21 days for *L. monocytogenes,* although these regimens are based more on tradition and anecdotes than on rigidly standardized clinical trials.

   Completion of intravenous therapy for bacterial meningitis may be accomplished in the outpatient setting if several criteria are met: inpatient therapy for 6 days; afebrile 24 to 48 hours before discharge; no significant neurologic dysfunction, seizure activity, or focal findings; clinically stable or improving; taking all fluids by mouth; received first dose of the outpatient antimicrobial agent under medical supervision and without reaction; access to home health nursing; reliable intravenous line and infusion device, if needed; daily examination by a physician and reliable follow-up; patient and/or family compliance with the program; and a safe environment with access to a telephone, utilities, food, and a refrigerator [177,178].

C. **Tuberculous meningitis.** Until the advent of effective chemotherapy, CNS tuberculosis was a uniformly fatal disease. Even now, the optimal drug regimen, dosage, route of administration, and duration of therapy remain undefined (for recommendations, see Tables 6.3 through 6.5). Therapy for tuberculous meningitis should be initiated on the basis of a strong clinical suspicion and should not be delayed until proof of infection is obtained. The principles of therapy for tuberculous meningitis are similar to those for treatment of tuberculosis elsewhere [61,62]. Isoniazid, rifampin, and pyrazinamide have very good CSF penetration; in the presence of meningeal inflammation, the peak CSF concentrations of isoniazid, rifampin, and pyrazinamide are approximately 90%, 20%, and 100%, respectively, of peak serum concentrations (see Chapter 11).

1. **Isoniazid-rifampin–susceptible strains.** In non-immunocompromised patients, a 6-month treatment regimen is recommended, consisting of isoniazid, rifampin, and pyrazinamide for the first 2 months and isoniazid and rifampin for an additional 4 months. Several studies have demonstrated the efficacy of this short-course regimen in patients with tuberculous meningitis [179,180].

However, some authors recommend 9 months of treatment, and we favor this approach [62]. Furthermore, HIV-infected patients usually require longer courses of therapy [64]. Several studies have reported similar outcomes in patients with or without HIV infection who have tuberculous meningitis. However, therapy for tuberculous meningitis may need to be individualized, with longer durations of therapy used in patients with a higher severity of illness.

2. **Multidrug-resistant strains and empiric therapy.** Drug-resistant tuberculosis has been increasing in frequency worldwide [61]. Risk groups include immigrants from countries in Asia, Africa, and the Americas; known contacts of drug-resistant cases; homeless and impoverished individuals; and residents of certain geographic areas in the United States, particularly adjacent to the Mexican border. In addition, secondary resistance may develop during chemotherapy if adherence is poor. In cases of suspected drug resistance or when the rate of isoniazid resistance is not known to be less than 4%, **ethambutol or streptomycin should be added to the three-drug regimen outlined in section 1 until susceptibility results have been obtained** (see Chapter 11).

   Therapy of tuberculous meningitis caused by resistant organisms should also be guided by drug penetration into CSF [61]. Ethambutol penetrates poorly into CSF except when the meninges are inflamed. There is good evidence, however, that ethionamide crosses both healthy and inflamed meninges, with peak CSF concentrations comparable with those achieved in serum. The fluoroquinolones (e.g., ciprofloxacin and ofloxacin) also penetrate well into CSF and have good *in vitro* activity against *M. tuberculosis.* Amoxicillin-clavulanate or imipenem has been used in individual cases of meningitis caused by multidrug-resistant *M. tuberculosis.* Meningitis suspected to be caused by multidrug-resistant *M. tuberculosis* should be treated with at least five drugs until susceptibility studies are performed. Infectious disease consultation is advised. Preliminary data suggest that HIV-infected patients with meningitis caused by rifampin- or multidrug-resistant *M. tuberculosis* are more likely to die in the 60 days after collection of CSF than HIV-infected patients with fully susceptible or other resistant isolates [181].

**D. Spirochetal meningitis**

1. ***Treponema pallidium.*** With neurosyphilis, the goals are to arrest disease progression and to reverse clinical symptoms and signs [65]. Except for cranial nerve abnormalities, syphilitic meningitis usually resolves without therapy. The general prognosis for meningovascular syphilis after therapy is very good, except for patients with larger neurologic deficits before therapy; in this situation, therapy may halt progression and prevent further ischemic events caused by neurosyphilis.

   **The preferred treatment of CNS syphilis is intravenous penicillin G, 18 to 24 million units/day divided every 4 hours for 10 to 14 days** [65,67,181a]. Alternatively, procaine penicillin, 2.4 million units intramuscularly daily, plus probenecid (500 mg orally four times a day) for 10 to 14 days can be used. Some experts recommend follow-up therapy with three weekly injections of benzathine penicillin G, although there are no data to support this practice. No large studies have been performed to evaluate alternative antimicrobial agents for neurosyphilis. On the basis of case reports, clinical experience, and extrapolations from animal studies, other agents with potential utility in the penicillin-allergic patient include the tetracyclines, chloramphenicol, and ceftriaxone. Erythromycin is not recommended based on treatment failures. HIV-infected patients with neurosyphilis need careful monitoring for response to therapy [67,182]. Follow-up lumbar puncture should be performed every 6 months in all patients until CSF changes have normalized. Standard therapy for neurosyphilis has failed in HIV-infected patients, probably because immunologic responses play an important role in controlling infection even with adequate antimicrobial therapy **(see Chapters 16 and 18).**

2. ***Borrelia burgdorferi.*** Intravenous ceftriaxone (2 g once daily) for 14 to 28 days is preferred for the neurologic manifestations of Lyme disease, including meningitis; cefotaxime (2 g every 8 hours) or penicillin G (20 to 24 million units/day)

are acceptable alternatives [70,71]. Acute meningeal and systemic symptoms resolve within days or weeks, whereas chronic disease takes months to improve [71]. CNS abnormalities are arrested by treatment, but some residual deficits may occur. There is no evidence to support treatment durations of longer than 4 weeks. However, no regimen has proven to be universally effective (see Chapter 21).

**E. Fungal meningitis**

**1. *Cryptococcus neoformans***

**a. Non-AIDS patients. Combination therapy with amphotericin B plus 5-flucytosine (5-FC) for 4 to 6 weeks is preferred.** Untreated, cryptococcal meningitis was nearly always fatal. Amphotericin B improved the prognosis dramatically, although morbidity, mortality, and relapse rates remained high, especially in immunocompromised patients (cure rates $\leq$ 52% after the first course of therapy). A large prospective trial in the pre-AIDS era compared combination therapy with amphotericin B (0.3 mg/kg/day) plus 5-FC (150 mg/kg/day) for 6 weeks to amphotericin B (0.4 mg/kg/day) alone for 10 weeks [183]. Combination therapy produced fewer failures, fewer relapses, more rapid CSF sterilization, and less nephrotoxicity than amphotericin B alone; cure or improvement occurred in 67% of patients given the combination versus 41% given only amphotericin B. Mortality between the two groups was not different. However, this study was criticized because of the low dose of amphotericin B used in the single-agent arm. A later trial compared a 4-week with a 6-week regimen of amphotericin B plus 5-FC therapy [184]. **The 4-week regimen could be used in** the subset of patients who, at presentation, had no neurologic complications, no underlying diseases or immunosuppressive therapy, a pretreatment CSF white blood cell count more than $20/mm^3$, and a serum cryptococcal antigen titer less than 1:32 and who, at 4 weeks, had a negative CSF India ink test and a CSF cryptococcal antigen titer less than 1:8. 5-FC toxicity was common (38%), indicating that 5-FC concentrations may need to be monitored (keep levels of 50 to 100 $\mu$g/mL) [185].

**The optimal use of fluconazole is unclear.** In a recently published report of 157 non–HIV-infected patients with CNS cryptococcosis [186], patients were more likely to receive an induction regimen with amphotericin B (~90%) and subsequent fluconazole (65%), suggesting a role for fluconazole in consolidation therapy for this population. **However, pending further data non-AIDS patients should receive 4 to 6 weeks of amphotericin B plus 5-FC** (see Chapter 17).

**b. AIDS patients.** A double-blind multicenter trial randomly assigned patients with a first episode of AIDS-associated cryptococcal meningitis to amphotericin B (0.7 mg/kg/day) without or with 5-FC (100 mg/kg/day) for 2 weeks, followed by 8 weeks of treatment with either itraconazole (400 mg/day) or fluconazole (400 mg/day) [187]. At 2 weeks, there were no significant differences in clinical outcome or CSF sterilization. At 10 weeks, 72% of the fluconazole recipients versus 60% of the itraconazole recipients had negative CSF cultures, although the clinical response rate was similar in both groups. In a multivariate analysis, the addition of 5-FC during the initial 2 weeks and treatment with fluconazole for the next 8 weeks were independently associated with CSF sterilization. **The preceding data support the initial use of amphotericin B, with or without 5-FC, for a period of approximately 2 weeks; this period may need to be prolonged in patients who are severely ill. This initial treatment period then is followed by fluconazole (400 mg/day) to complete a 10-week course.** Dosages of fluconazole up to 800 mg/day have benefited some AIDS patients with cryptococcal meningitis who failed primary therapy or who relapsed [188]. Lipid formulations of amphotericin B have been studied in AIDS patients with cryptococcal meningitis [189,190]. When liposomal amphotericin (4 mg/kg/day) was compared with amphotericin B (0.7 mg/kg/day), the median time to CSF sterilization was shorter with amphotericin B and, at 14 days, significantly more patients had sterile CSF [190], although the time to clinical response and the failure rate did not differ between groups. **Further studies are needed before liposomal amphotericin B can be recommended.**

**AIDS patients with cryptococcal meningitis have a high rate of relapse once antifungal therapy is discontinued** [75,76]; the prostate gland may represent a sequestered reservoir for relapse. **Fluconazole (200 mg/day) is** superior to amphotericin B (1 mg/kg/wk) and itraconazole (200 mg/day) in preventing relapses [191,192], **and is the agent of choice for secondary prevention (see Chapter 18).**

2. ***Candida.*** The treatment of choice for *Candida* meningitis is amphotericin B with or without 5-FC [80,81]. Although there are no studies comparing the efficacy of single and combination therapy, some investigators recommend combination therapy based on more rapid CSF sterilization and possible reduction of long-term neurologic sequelae in newborns. Cure rates with amphotericin B alone have ranged from 67% to 89% in adults and 71% to 100% in neonates. However, up to 56% of surviving neonates had psychomotor retardation and 50% had hydrocephalus [80,81]. Increased mortality in adult patients is associated with a delay of more than 2 weeks from the onset of symptoms to diagnosis, a CSF glucose concentration less than 35 mg/dL, intracranial hypertension, and focal neurologic deficits. Fluconazole may be an acceptable alternative agent for the therapy of *Candida* meningitis [193,194].
3. ***Coccidioides immitis.*** Based on the results of a collaborative study [195], **fluconazole is recommended as first-line therapy** for coccidioidal meningitis. Fluconazole (400 mg once daily) was given to 50 consecutive patients with coccidioidal meningitis (including 9 with HIV) for up to 4 years (median of 37 months). Of the 47 assessable patients, 37 (79%) responded to treatment, with most improvement occurring within 4 to 8 months. However, 24% had a persistent CSF pleocytosis, indicating a need for careful follow-up. In nonresponders, increasing the dose of fluconazole (commonly done by physicians in endemic areas) or instituting intrathecal amphotericin B might be required. Fluconazole therapy may need to be continued indefinitely.

   Amphotericin B was previously used, usually both intravenously and intrathecally [84,85]. Intrathecal administration may be via the lumbar, cisternal, or ventricular routes (i.e., through an Ommaya reservoir); the usual dosage is 0.5 mg three times weekly for 3 months, although 1.0 to 1.5 mg combined with hydrocortisone can be used. Mortality of 50% has been reported, although one study found a survival rate of 91% over after 75 months if larger doses of intrathecal amphotericin B (1.0 to 1.5 mg) were used [196]. Amphotericin is discontinued once the CSF has been normal for at least 1 year on an intrathecal regimen of once every 6 weeks. However, intrathecal amphotericin B is poorly tolerated, often leading to arachnoiditis.

**F. Protozoal and helminthic meningitis**

1. **Amebae.** Many antimicrobial agents have *in vitro* activity against free-living amebae [87]. These include amphotericin B, the tetracyclines, the imidazoles, qinghaosu, and rifampin. Only four patients reported in the literature have survived after therapy for primary amebic meningoencephalitis [86,87,197]. All received amphotericin B along with various other antimicrobial agents. The best-documented survivor received amphotericin B and miconazole intravenously and intrathecally, as well as rifampin, sulfisoxazole, and dexamethasone. However, no effective regimen has been established. Therapy with parenteral and intracisternal amphotericin B combined with rifampin and tetracycline for 2 to 3 weeks has been suggested.
2. ***Angiostrongylus cantonensis.*** Symptomatic treatment is indicated for eosinophilic meningitis caused by *A. cantonensis* [86]. Most patients recover within 1 to 2 weeks. Thiabendazole has been used in the early stages of larvae migration, but the drug fails as soon as the worm reaches the CNS.

**VI. Adjunctive therapy**

**A. Viral meningitis.** Adjunctive measures have been used in seriously ill patients with enteroviral meningitis [1]. Administration of gamma globulin by multiple routes (including directly into the CNS) has led to stabilization or improvement of agammaglobulinemic patients with chronic enteroviral meningitis or meningoencephalitis. Neonates with overwhelming enteroviral sepsis and meningitis have received intravenous gamma globulin, maternal plasma, and exchange transfusions, with occasional successes [198].

**B. Bacterial meningitis**

**1. Antiinflammatory agents.** Despite effective bactericidal antimicrobial agents, morbidity and mortality from bacterial meningitis remain unacceptably high.

**a. Animal models.** Studies in animal models have demonstrated that development of a subarachnoid space inflammatory response is a major factor contributing to morbidity and mortality [27,96,136,199]. Therefore, investigators have examined whether attenuation of this response would improve outcome. In an experimental rabbit model of *H. influenzae* type b meningitis, treatment with ceftriaxone plus dexamethasone consistently reduced brain water content, CSF pressure, and CSF lactate to a greater degree than ceftriaxone alone, although the differences were not statistically significant. However, it was suggested that adjunctive dexamethasone might be more beneficial if administered early or even before the occurrence of antibiotic-induced bacterial lysis and release of microbial products. Using the same animal model, ceftriaxone administration led to a significant increase in CSF endotoxin concentrations followed by a rise in CSF tumor necrosis factor concentrations. Simultaneous administration of dexamethasone and ceftriaxone did not affect release of endotoxin into CSF but markedly attenuated CSF concentrations of tumor necrosis factor. Adjunctive dexamethasone therapy also resulted in a significant decrease in CSF leukocytosis and a trend toward earlier improvement in CSF concentrations of glucose, lactate, and protein. These parameters improved without any decrease in bacterial killing.

**b. Clinical trials.** Based on observations in animal models, several clinical trials were undertaken in the late 1980's and early 1990's to determine the effects of adjunctive corticosteroids on outcome in patients with bacterial meningitis [27].

**(1) A recently published meta-analysis of clinical trials from 1988 to 1996 [200] supported the routine use of adjunctive dexamethasone (0.15 mg/kg every 6 hours for 2 to 4 days) in infants and children with *H. influenzae* type b meningitis and, if commenced with or before antimicrobial therapy, suggested a benefit for pneumococcal meningitis of childhood.** Evidence was strongest for hearing outcomes. In contrast, a retrospective nonrandomized study of children with pneumococcal meningitis found that adjunctive dexamethasone was not beneficial [201], although the dexamethasone was administered before or within 1 hour of the first antibiotic dose and children in the dexamethasone group had a higher severity of illness. **When dexamethasone is used, the timing of administration is crucial. Administration of dexamethasone before or concomitant with antimicrobial therapy is recommended** for optimal attenuation of subarachnoid space inflammation; patients should be carefully monitored for the possibility of gastrointestinal hemorrhage.

However, vaccination against *H. influenzae* type b in infancy has decreased the incidence of serious infections due to *H. influenzae* type b by more than 90%. Therefore, most future cases of bacterial meningitis in the United States will be caused by bacteria for which there are only limited data regarding the benefit of adjunctive steroid therapy [202].

**(2) In adults or in patients with meningitis caused by other bacterial organisms, the routine use of adjunctive dexamethasone is not recommended pending results of ongoing studies.** However, some authors recommend its use in all cases of meningitis with a likely bacterial etiology (i.e., demonstrable bacteria on CSF Gram stain, which may predict the patients at greatest risk of bacteriolysis-induced exacerbation of inflammation) [199], although there are no supportive clinical data. In adults with severely impaired mental status (stupor or coma) documented cerebral edema (e.g., by CT), or markedly elevated intracranial pressure (i.e., high opening pressure on lumbar puncture, palsy of cranial nerve VI), dexamethasone may be beneficial. Use of **dexamethasone is of particular concern in patients treated with vancomycin** for pneumococcal meningitis, because this may significantly reduce CSF vancomycin penetration (see section (4) following).

(3) **In neonates,** clinical trials on the role of corticosteroids in meningitis have not been performed. Therefore, their use is not suggested (see Chapter 3).

(4) **Penetration of antibiotics into the CSF** is becoming a greater concern in treating meningitis caused by penicillin-resistant *S. pneumoniae* (see section **V.B.3** and Chapter 27). In particular, vancomycin penetrates the CSF quite poorly. Furthermore, in a rabbit model, penetration of vancomycin into the CSF was reduced with concomitant dexamethasone therapy, with delayed CSF sterilization. Therefore, in areas where high-level penicillin-resistant *S. pneumoniae* are prevalent and empiric vancomycin is used, steroid therapy may prove harmful [202]. **For any patient receiving adjunctive dexamethasone who is not improving as expected or who has a pneumococcal isolate for which the cefotaxime or ceftriaxone MIC is at least 2.0 μg/mL, a repeat lumbar puncture 36 to 48 hours after initiation of therapy is recommended** to document the sterility of CSF [152].

2. **Reduction of intracranial pressure.** Several methods are available to reduce intracranial pressure [203], including elevation of the head of the bed to 30 degrees to maximize venous drainage with minimal compromise of cerebral perfusion, the use of hyperosmolar agents (e.g., mannitol) to move water from brain tissue into the intravascular compartment, and the use of corticosteroids. In addition, hyperventilation to maintain the $Pa_{CO_2}$ between 27 and 30 mmHg, which causes cerebral vasoconstriction and reduction in cerebral blood volume, has also been used, although some experts have questioned its routine use to reduce intracranial pressure in patients with bacterial meningitis [204]. Infants and children with bacterial meningitis who have initially normal CTs of the head can be treated with hyperventilation to reduce elevated intracranial pressure safely because it is unlikely that cerebral blood flow would be reduced to ischemic thresholds. However, in children with cerebral edema on head CT, cerebral blood flow is more likely to be normal or reduced. Therefore, hyperventilation might decrease intracranial pressure at the expense of cerebral blood flow, possibly reducing the latter to ischemic thresholds. These patients would likely benefit more from early use of diuretics, osmotically dehydrating agents (provided that intravascular volume is protected), and corticosteroids, although controlled trials have yet to be performed. Glycerol, an osmotic dehydrating agent that can be given orally, has been evaluated in 122 infants and children with bacterial meningitis [205]; 7% of the glycerol-treated patients and 19% of those not given glycerol had audiologic or neurologic sequelae ($p = 0.052$). However, further trials are needed before glycerol can be recommended.

   Patients in whom elevated intracranial pressures continue despite these measures may be treated with high-dose barbiturates to decrease cerebral metabolic demands and cerebral blood flow [203]. Vasoconstriction in normal tissue also occurs during barbiturate therapy, thereby shunting blood to ischemic tissue and protecting the brain from ischemia. This is of unproven benefit, however, for meningitis and elevated intracranial pressure and must be considered experimental.

3. **Basilar skull fracture.** Patients who have suffered a basilar skull fracture with CSF leak may have persistent dural defects associated with recurrent episodes of bacterial meningitis. Although many will cease spontaneously, surgery is indicated for leaks that persist for several weeks or in patients who present with

delayed or recurrent infection [42]. Surgery is not indicated in the acute phase (<7 days) of leakage because there is no difference in outcome when patients with acutely repaired leaks are compared with those whose leaks stop spontaneously within 7 days.

4. **Cerebrospinal shunt infections.** All components of an infected CSF shunt should be removed at the beginning of antimicrobial therapy [54] and an external ventriculostomy placed to clear the ventriculitis and monitor CSF parameters. Many organisms can adhere to the prostheses and survive antimicrobial therapy with the shunt left *in situ.* Furthermore, the propensity for the entire shunt to be contaminated when one portion is infected argues against partial revisions. With externalization, treatment success is usually greater than 90% [54].

C. **Tuberculous meningitis.** Despite chemotherapy inflammation often continues at the base of the brain, with subsequent organization of necrotic tissue and exudate, fibroblastic proliferation, and formation of dense fibrocollagenous tissue compressing adjacent structures and impeding circulation of CSF. **Corticosteroids** are the most commonly advocated adjunctive agents for tuberculous meningitis [61,62,98]; patients frequently defervesce, with clearing of sensorium and improvement in well-being even after only a few doses. Their primary value may be their ability to treat or avert the development of spinal block, possibly by lowering the CSF protein content; an improvement in overall mortality has been ascribed to their effect on this poor prognostic sign. However, an increase in significant neurologic sequelae has been observed in survivors who received corticosteroids. In contrast, a study from Egypt found reduced neurologic complications and case fatality rates in patients who received dexamethasone with antituberculous chemotherapy [206]. Another prospective, controlled, randomized study from the republic of South Africa found that corticosteroids improved survival and intellectual outcome in children with tuberculous meningitis [207]. Despite the controversy, **most authorities advocate the use of corticosteroids in selected cases** with extreme neurologic compromise, elevated intracranial pressure, impending herniation, or impending or established spinal block [61,62]. Some authors also recommend corticosteroids in patients with CT evidence of either hydrocephalus or basilar meningitis. Prednisone (approximately 1 mg/kg/day, tapered over 1 month) often is given, although other doses of dexamethasone or hydrocortisone have been used.

D. **Fungal meningitis.** Patients with cryptococcal meningitis may have several complications despite antifungal therapy. Increased intracranial pressure and hydrocephalus has been noted in AIDS patients with cryptococcal meningitis, possibly due to increased CSF outflow resistance. Ventriculoperitoneal shunting, frequent high-volume lumbar punctures, acetazolamide, and corticosteroids have been used for these complications. However, the precise roles of these adjunctive measures (particularly corticosteroids) in the treatment of cryptococcal meningitis remain to be established. Shunting procedures can ameliorate the sequelae of elevated intracranial pressure in AIDS patients with cryptococcal meningitis [208–210].

## VII. Prevention

A. **Viral meningitis.** The cornerstone of **prevention of mumps is active immunization** with the live attenuated mumps vaccine [8]. Widespread use of the mumps vaccine has greatly reduced the incidence of mumps and mumps meningoencephalitis. Mumps meningitis has been reported in children 11 days to 2 months after vaccine administration, although it is not clear whether these cases represented vaccine failure or meningitis due to the vaccine strain of mumps virus.

B. **Bacterial meningitis**

1. ***Haemophilus influenzae***

a. **Chemoprophylaxis.** Several studies have documented the transmission to household contacts. Most secondary cases (75%) of *H. influenzae* type b meningitis occur within 6 days of onset of the index case, although untreated household contacts remain at increased risk for at least 1 month. The risk is markedly age dependent and highest for children younger than 2 years. Daycare outside the home may be another risk factor for transmission [27].

The **rationale for the use of chemoprophylaxis** to prevent secondary disease is eradication of nasopharyngeal colonization of *H. influenzae* type b, thereby preventing transmission to young susceptible contacts [27]. The chemoprophylactic agent of choice is rifampin (20 mg/kg/day, with a maximum dose of 600 mg, for 4 days) for all individuals, including adults, in households with at least one unimmunized or incompletely immunized child younger than 48 months or with an immunocompromised child of any age. Chemoprophylaxis is not recommended for daycare contacts 2 years or older unless two or more cases occur in the daycare center within a 60-day period. For children younger than 2 years, the determination of whether to administer prophylaxis needs to be individualized and should be considered more strongly in daycare centers that resemble households where children have prolonged contact. Rifampin is not recommended for pregnant women, because the risk of rifampin to the fetus has not been established. The index patient should also receive rifampin because some antibiotics (e.g., ampicillin) given for therapy do not eliminate nasopharyngeal colonization. Unimmunized or partially immunized children also should receive a dose of vaccine and be scheduled for completion of the required series.

b. **Immunoprophylaxis.** The Immunization Practices Advisory Committee [27] recommends that all children should be vaccinated with one of the licensed *H. influenzae* type b conjugate vaccines (see Chapter 23).

2. ***Neisseria meningitidis***

a. **Chemoprophylaxis is recommended for close contacts of the index case, defined as** household contacts, daycare contacts, nursery school contacts, contacts who sleep or eat in the same dwelling, close contacts in a closed community such as a military barracks or boarding school, and anyone directly exposed to the patient's oral secretions (e.g., kissing, mouth-to-mouth resuscitation, endotracheal intubation, or endotracheal tube management) [27,211]. Chemoprophylaxis should be administered to the index case before hospital discharge unless ceftriaxone or cefotaxime were used for therapy.

b. **Chemoprophylaxis regimens**

(1) **Rifampin.** The Centers for Disease Control and Prevention currently recommends **rifampin** at 12-hour intervals for 2 days in the following dosages [27,211]: adults, 600 mg; children beyond the neonatal period, 10 mg/kg; and infants younger than 1 month, 5 mg/kg. However, there are several problems with rifampin chemoprophylaxis, including efficacy of only 80% or so, adverse events, need for multiple doses over 2 days, and emergence of resistant organisms (up to 10%–27% of isolates).

(2) **Alternatives. Ceftriaxone** (250 mg intramuscularly in adults and 125 mg in children) was shown to eliminate the meningococcal serogroup A carrier state in 97% of patients in one study for up to 2 weeks [212], although parenteral administration is required. A single dose of **oral ciprofloxacin** (500 or 750 mg in adults) is also very effective in eliminating the nasopharyngeal carriage of *N. meningitidis;* ciprofloxacin may well supplant rifampin for chemoprophylaxis in adults. Ciprofloxacin is not recommended for persons younger than 18 years because of concerns regarding cartilage damage. **In pregnant patients, ceftriaxone is the safest agent for chemoprophylaxis.**

c. **Immunoprophylaxis.** The quadrivalent meningococcal vaccine (serogroups A, C, Y, and W135) is currently recommended for certain high-risk patients, including those who are close contacts of the primary case as an adjunct to chemoprophylaxis [27,211], although this is controversial and of unproven efficacy. The vaccine is not recommended for routine use in the United States because of the overall low risk of infection, inability to protect against serogroup B disease, and inability to provide lasting immunity to young children. However, because of an increase in invasive meningococcal disease in adolescents and young adults of high school and college age in the United States, the Advisory Committee on Immunization Practices recommends that college freshman dormitory residents and their parents are given information about meningococcal vaccination and that other undergraduate students wishing to reduce their risk can also choose to be vaccinated [213] (see Chapter 23).

Conjugate vaccines against serogroups A and C meningococci have been developed. The United Kingdom became the first country to implement routine immunization with a monovalent serogroup C conjugate vaccine (three doses for children aged 2 to 4 months, two doses for children older than 4 months but younger than 1 year, and one dose for all others). In the first 9 months of use in a catch-up immunization program [214], vaccine efficacy was 92% in toddlers and 97% in teenagers.

3. ***Streptococcus pneumoniae***
   a. **Chemoprophylaxis.** The risk of secondary pneumococcal disease in contacts of infected patients has not been defined, although outbreaks have been described in closed populations such as gold miners, military recruits, and jail inmates [27]. Further studies are needed before chemoprophylaxis is recommended for contacts of patients with pneumococcal meningitis. Prophylaxis with oral penicillin in patients with sickle cell disease is not usually needed with the availability of the conjugate vaccine.
   b. **Immunoprophylaxis.** The efficacy of the 23-valent pneumococcal vaccine in preventing pneumococcal meningitis has never been documented, although its use in high-risk patients would seem prudent. Vaccination for persons traveling to an area with a significant incidence of resistant pneumococci may also be warranted. The pneumococcal conjugate vaccine is 97.4% effective in preventing invasive pneumococcal disease in children caused by vaccine serotypes and is recommended for all infants less than 2 years of age [215,216]. See further discussion of the pneumococcal vaccine in Chapter 11.
4. **Basilar skull fracture.** Despite conflicting studies, a recent meta-analysis [217] suggested that **use of prophylactic antibiotics is not recommended** for patients with basilar skull fracture and CSF leak because they do not change the incidence of meningitis and may result in selection of resistant organisms (see Chapter 27).

## ENCEPHALITIS

The syndrome of acute encephalitis shares many features with acute meningitis, although the likelihood of mental status changes early in disease before the onset of obtundation or coma is more common in encephalitis. Clinically, seizures are more likely to occur with encephalitis, and associated systemic illness is more prominent [218–221]. Numerous infectious and noninfectious agents have been reported to cause acute encephalitis (see Table 6.1 for agents of meningitis that may also cause encephalitis). Here **we concentrate on encephalitis caused by the herpesviruses, especially HSV, because these represent the most common and only currently treatable forms of viral encephalitis.** For a general review of viral encephalitis, see Whitley [221]; for a discussion of CMV infections of the CNS (which can include an encephalitis) in patients with AIDS, see McCutchan [221a].

I. **Epidemiology and etiology**
   A. **Herpes simplex virus.** HSV infections of the CNS are among the most common (10%–20% of encephalitis viral infections in the United States) and most severe of all human viral infections of the brain and are associated with significant morbidity and mortality (>70% with ineffective or no therapy) [218]. HSV encephalitis occurs throughout the year (i.e., is nonseasonal) and in patients of all age groups, with whites accounting for 95% of patients with biopsy-proven disease. Most cases (94%–96%) are caused by HSV type 1.
   B. **Varicella-zoster virus.** The actual incidence of CNS involvement during varicella is unknown, although it has ranged from 0.1% to 0.75% [219]. Herpes zoster is a consequence of reactivation of latent varicella-zoster virus; a direct correlation exists between cutaneous dissemination and visceral involvement, including meningoencephalitis. In general, the CNS complications of herpes zoster are associated with a higher morbidity and mortality than those of acute varicella, possibly due to the patient's advanced age and underlying disease status. A variety of varicella-zoster

virus–induced neurologic disorders have been described in AIDS patients, including multifocal leukoencephalitis, ventriculitis, myelitis, myeloradiculitis, and focal brainstem lesions [222].

**II. Clinical presentation**

**A. Herpes simplex virus.** Most patients with biopsy-proven HSV encephalitis present with an encephalopathic process characterized by **altered mentation and decreasing levels of consciousness with focal neurologic findings,** including dysphasia, weakness, and paresthesias [218]. **Fever and personality changes** are uniformly present. Approximately two-thirds of patients with biopsy-proven disease develop either focal or generalized **seizures.** HSV encephalitis may progress slowly or with alarming rapidity; commonly, there is progressive loss of consciousness leading to coma. Although clinical evidence of a temporal lobe lesion often is believed to be a result of HSV encephalitis, a variety of other diseases has been shown to mimic this condition, including various infections (abscess/subdural empyema), tuberculosis, cryptococcosis, toxoplasmosis, CMV, tumor, and subdural hematoma [177]. Immunocompromised patients with HSV encephalitis may develop more diffuse nonnecrotizing encephalitis involving the cerebral hemispheres and brainstem [223].

**B. Varicella-zoster virus.** The most common neurologic abnormality associated with varicella-zoster virus is cerebellar ataxia; although meningoencephalitis and cerebritis are less common, they frequently are more severe [222]. Headache, fever, and vomiting often are accompanied by altered sensorium, with seizures occurring in 29% to 52% of patients. Focal neurologic abnormalities, including cranial nerve dysfunction, aphasia, and hemiplegia, have also been described. Encephalitis, the most common CNS abnormality associated with herpes zoster, is most common in patients of advanced age, after immunosuppression, and in those with disseminated cutaneous zoster. Some patients with ophthalmic zoster present with contralateral hemiplegia; this finding is seen in up to one-third of CNS abnormalities in herpes zoster. The zoster ophthalmicus usually precedes the hemiplegia by several weeks, although it has been reported to occur as late as 6 months after the rash.

**III. Diagnosis**

**A. Herpes simplex virus**

1. **Routine studies of CSF** in patients with HSV encephalitis are **not diagnostic** [218,221]. The CSF white blood cell count is elevated (mean of 100 cells/mm$^3$) in 97% of patients with biopsy-proven disease, with a lymphocytic predominance. The presence of **red blood cells in CSF suggests** the diagnosis but is not definitive. The CSF protein is elevated also (averaging approximately 100 mg/dL). Approximately 5% to 10% of patients with HSV encephalitis have normal CSF studies on first evaluation. Virus is isolated from CSF only 4% or so of the time.
2. **PCR to detect HSV DNA is highly sensitive and specific for** the diagnosis of HSV encephalitis [224,225]. In one study, the sensitivity and specificity of PCR were 91% and 92%, respectively, in patients with biopsy-proven disease [225]; specificity would have been higher except that some tissue specimens were fixed in formalin, which killed the infectious virus. **The PCR test for HSV in CSF is now the optimal way to diagnose HSV encephalitis** [218].
3. **Noninvasive studies may be useful** [218,221].
   a. **Electroencephalography** is a sensitive test (approximately 84%) that reveals characteristic spike-and-slow wave activity and periodic lateralizing epileptiform discharges located predominantly over the temporal and frontotemporal regions.
   b. **CTs** show low density areas with mass effect localized to the temporal lobe in 50% to 75% of patients at some time during the course of their illness.
   c. **MRI (with enhancement)** demonstrates lesions earlier and is superior to CT in localizing these lesions to the orbital–frontal and temporal lobes; MRI is considered by experts to be the most important and specific imaging technique for HSV encephalitis [226–228]. HSV encephalitis typically affects the temporal lobes, predominantly their inferior aspects. Involvement is usually asymmetric, and the deep white matter may demonstrate the earliest abnormalities. Some believe a normal MRI would be unusual even in early HSV encephalitis [226].

d. **Radionuclide brain scans** may reveal increased uptake in both temporal lobes; brain scan is more sensitive than CT early in the disease course.

e. However, despite the availability of these diagnostic modalities, **none** is uniformly **satisfactory for the diagnosis of HSV encephalitis.**

4. In the past, the most specific means of diagnosing HSV encephalitis was a **brain biopsy** [218]. The presence of Cowdry type A intranuclear inclusions supports the diagnosis of viral infections, although these are found only in approximately 50% of cases. Brain tissue should also be subjected to immunofluorescence, which is a rapid, sensitive, and reliable method for detecting herpes antigen; virus can also be isolated from brain tissue. With the availability of PCR studies on CSF, brain biopsy now is seldom indicated (see section 2).

**B. Varicella-zoster virus.** The CSF often is abnormal in varicella-associated encephalitis with a lymphocytic pleocytosis and elevated protein [222]. The electroencephalogram usually reveals diffuse abnormalities (e.g., diffuse slowing), although focal abnormalities may occur even without seizure activity. With herpes zoster-associated encephalitis, the CSF also usually reveals a lymphocytic pleocytosis and elevated protein; however, up to 40% to 50% of patients with uncomplicated herpes zoster (i.e., without CNS involvement) may have a mild CSF pleocytosis or elevated protein. The virus has been cultured from brain tissue and CSF, detected by PCR, and viral inclusions are well-described in autopsy series. In patients with zoster ophthalmicus with contralateral hemiplegia, a unilateral arteritis or thrombosis of involved vessels may be seen on cerebral angiography and cerebral infarction may be seen on CT or MRI.

**IV. Approach to the patient with viral encephalitis.** Despite the number of viral organisms that may cause encephalitis, herpes simplex remains the only viral CNS infection for which therapy (i.e., acyclovir) is beneficial. Based on the ease of administration and good safety profile of acyclovir, an empiric course should be administered for patients with presumed viral encephalitis [221]. The availability of PCR will eliminate the need for biopsy in most instances, although in unusual cases it may be indicated. MRI is important when encephalitis is suspected [226,228]. Infectious disease consultation is advised.

**V. Antimicrobial therapy**

**A. Herpes simplex virus.** In biopsy-proven HSV encephalitis, **acyclovir** reduced mortality (19%) compared with vidarabine (55%), the previously accepted therapy [229]. Furthermore, 38% of patients in the acyclovir group returned to a normal level of functioning compared with only 15% to 20% of patients in the vidarabine group. In a recent study of 42 patients with HSV encephalitis, 30% died or had a severe neurologic deficit [230]; of the remaining 70%, most had persistent neurologic signs and/or symptoms. Acyclovir should be administered intravenously at a dosage of 10 mg/kg every 8 hours in patients with normal renal function. Although many patients have been treated for 14 days, many experts now prefer a 14- to 21-day course [231].

**B. Varicella-zoster virus.** Intravenous acyclovir is also the drug of choice for patients with varicella-zoster virus–associated CNS infection who are at high risk for progressive disease [232]. Although no clinical trial has established the value of antiviral therapy of herpes zoster-associated encephalitis, we believe acyclovir should be used in this setting.

**C. Other viruses.** Although ganciclovir or foscarnet commonly is given to HIV-infected patients with CNS symptoms, proof of efficacy against cytomegaloviral CNS disease is lacking. No therapy is of proven benefit for Epstein-Barr virus disease. The treatment of arboviral infections (e.g., eastern or western equine encephalitis, St. Louis encephalitis) is supportive.

## BRAIN ABSCESS

**I. Epidemiology and etiology**

**A. Bacteria.** The likely bacterial species responsible for brain abscess formation depends on the pathogenic mechanism involved [233–235]. The most common are streptococci (aerobic, anaerobic, and microaerophilic), isolated in 60% to 70% of abscesses. These bacteria, particularly the *S. milleri* (also called *S. intermedius*) group, are normal inhabitants of the oral cavity, appendix, and female genital tract and have a proclivity for abscess formation. *S. aureus* is isolated from brain abscess in 10% to 15% of patients, usually those with endocarditis or cranial trauma. The isolation of anaerobes has increased with use of proper techniques; *Bacteroides* species are isolated in 20% to 40% of cases, often in mixed culture. The enteric gram-negative bacilli (e.g., *E. coli, Klebsiella* species, *Pseudomonas* species) are isolated in 23% to 33% of cases; these usually are seen with otitic foci of infection or in the immunocompromised patient. Other bacterial species are isolated much less frequently (<1% of cases) and include *H. influenzae, S. pneumoniae,* and *L. monocytogenes.* In addition, *Nocardia* species are more often isolated in patients with defects in cell-mediated immunity, as in patients receiving corticosteroid therapy, in organ transplant recipients, and in patients with neoplastic disorders; some *Nocardia* cases have also been described in patients with AIDS.

**B. Fungi.** Many of the etiologic agents of fungal meningitis (see section I.E under Meningitis) may also cause brain abscesses [185]. For example, although *Candida* species may produce meningitis, focal CNS disease is more common. Indeed, *Candida* is the most common fungal species to cause brain abscess (often multiple, not macroscopic). However, several other fungal species need to be considered, especially in the immunocompromised host. For further discussion see Chapter 17.

1. ***Aspergillus* species.** Intracranial seeding of *Aspergillus* species occurs during dissemination of the organism from the lungs or by direct extension from a site anatomically adjacent to the brain [236]. The brain is involved in 40% to 70% of cases with disseminated disease. Most patients with *Aspergillus* brain abscesses are neutropenic and have an underlying hematologic malignancy. Other risk groups include patients with Cushing syndrome, diabetes mellitus, hepatic disease, and chronic granulomatous disease. Injection drug users, postcraniotomy patients, organ transplant recipients, HIV-infected patients, and patients receiving chronic corticosteroid therapy are also at risk.
2. **Mucormycosis.** Mucormycosis is one of the most fulminant fungal infections known [236]. Predisposing conditions include diabetes mellitus (70% of cases), usually in association with acidosis; acidemia from other profound systemic illness; hematologic neoplasia; renal transplantation; injection drug use; and use of deferoxamine. Fewer than 5% of cases involve otherwise normal healthy patients. CNS disease may result from direct extension (i.e., the rhinocerebral form) or by hematogenous dissemination from other sites of infection. Most infections are caused by the genus *Rhizopus,* and the genera *Absidia* and *Mucor* also have been isolated.
3. ***Pseudallescheria boydii.*** CNS disease may occur in both normal and immunocompromised hosts. This organism is being increasingly referred to as *Scedosporium apiospermum,* the asexual form of *P. boydii.* The organism may enter the CNS by direct trauma, by hematogenous dissemination from a primary site of infection, via an intravenous catheter, or by direct extension from infected sinuses [236,237]. Because of the presence of *P. boydii* in contaminated water and manure, there is an association between near-drowning and subsequent illness [238,239].

**II. Clinical presentation**

**A. Bacterial brain abscess** may have either an indolent or fulminant course [233–235].

1. **The clinical manifestations occur secondary to the presence of a space-occupying mass lesion** rather than systemic signs of infection. Findings include **headache (70%),** which may be moderate to severe and hemicranial or generalized; **nausea and vomiting (50%),** presumably due to increased intracranial pressure; **seizures (25%–35%),** which usually are generalized; and **nuchal rigidity and papilledema (25%).** Most patients also have **mental status changes,** ranging from lethargy to coma. **Focal neurologic deficits** are seen in approximately 50% of cases and will vary depending on the location of brain involved.
2. **Fever is observed in only 45% to 50% of cases.** Only approximately half of patients present with the triad of headache, fever, and focal neurologic deficit.
3. The clinical **presentation of brain abscess also depends on the intracranial location** [233]. For example, frontal lobe abscess often presents with headache, drowsiness, inattention, and deterioration of mental status; hemiparesis with

unilateral motor signs and a motor speech disorder also are common. Patients with cerebellar abscesses present with ataxia, nystagmus, vomiting, and dysmetria. Temporal lobe abscesses may cause headache, aphasia, or a visual field defect (e.g., upper homonymous quadrantanopia). Abscesses of the brainstem usually present with facial weakness, fever, headache, hemiparesis, dysphagia, and vomiting [190].

**B. Fungal brain abscess.** The clinical presentation of fungal brain abscess is similar to that caused by bacteria and depends on the intracranial location of the abscess and the fulminant nature of the organisms [236]. However, patients with certain fungal pathogens may present with specific symptoms and signs.

1. ***Aspergillus* species.** Patients most commonly present with signs of a stroke referable to the area of involved brain. Headache, encephalopathy, and seizures have also been described. Fever is not a constant finding, and meningeal irritation is rare.
2. **Mucormycosis.** Symptoms from rhinocerebral mucormycosis are referable to the eyes or sinuses and include headache (often unilateral), facial pain, diplopia, lacrimation, and nasal stuffiness or discharge; fever and lethargy have also been described [236]. Signs include development of a nasal ulcer, facial swelling, nasal discharge, proptosis, and external ophthalmoplegia. Orbital involvement is seen in two-thirds of patients. Cranial nerve abnormalities are also common. Because of the proclivity of the organism for blood vessel invasion, thrombosis is a striking feature of disease. Focal neurologic findings (e.g., hemiparesis, seizures, monocular blindness) suggest far-advanced disease. Invasion and occlusion of the cavernous sinus and carotid artery can occur as the disease progresses.
3. ***Pseudallescheria boydii.*** CNS infection with *P. boydii* usually becomes manifest 15 to 30 days after an episode of near-drowning but has varied [237–239]. Clinical presentation depends on localization in the CNS and includes seizures, altered consciousness, headache, meningeal irritation, focal neurologic deficits, abnormal behavior, and aphasia.

## III. Diagnosis

**A. Bacterial brain abscess. The diagnosis of brain abscess was revolutionized by the availability of CT,** which is excellent for examining the brain parenchyma and the paranasal sinuses, mastoids, and middle ear [233,234]. Typically, CT reveals a hypodense lesion with a peripheral uniform ring of contrast enhancement. There may also be a surrounding hypodense area of brain edema. **MRI is now the first imaging procedure of choice** for patients suspected of having this disorder [240]. MRI offers significant advantages over CT, including the early detection of cerebritis, detection of cerebral edema with greater contrast between edema and brain, more conspicuous spread of inflammation into the ventricles and subarachnoid space, and earlier detection of satellite lesions. Administration of the paramagnetic agent gadolinium diethylenetriamine penta-acetic acid permits clear differentiation of the central abscess, surrounding enhancing rim, and cerebral edema.

**B. Fungal brain abscess.** Noninvasive studies (e.g., CSF examination, CT, MRI) for the diagnosis of fungal brain abscess usually are nonspecific, although some exceptions do exist [236]. For example, the finding of a cerebral infarct in a patient with risk factors for invasive aspergillosis suggests that diagnosis; such an infarction typically develops into either single or multiple abscesses. In rhinocerebral mucormycosis, CT and MRI typically show sinus opacification, erosion of bone, and obliteration of deep fascial planes; cavernous sinus involvement may also be seen on MRI. In injection drug abusers with cerebral mucormycosis, the most frequent site of CNS disease is the basal ganglia.

**Definitive diagnosis of fungal brain abscess requires biopsy** with appropriate fungal stains [236]. The mucicarmine stain will specifically identify *C. neoformans. Aspergillus* species appear as septate hyphae with acute-angle dichotomous branching, whereas typical nonseptate hyphae with right-angle branching are seen in mucormycosis. *P. boydii* appears as septate hyphae in clinical specimens, although the hyphae are narrower and do not show the dichotomous branching seen in aspergillosis. Fluorescent antibody staining is also a sensitive method for identifying *P. boydii.*

Table 6.6. Empiric Antimicrobial Therapy for Bacterial Brain Abscess

| Predisposing Condition | Usual Bacterial Isolates | Antimicrobial Regimen |
|---|---|---|
| Otitis media or mastoiditis | Streptococci (anaerobic or aerobic), *Bacteroides* spp., Enterobacteriaceae | Metronidazole + a third-generation cephalosporin[a] |
| Sinusitis (frontoethmoidal or sphenoidal) | Streptococci, *Bacteroides* spp., Enterobacteriaceae, *Staphylococcus aureus, Haemophilus* spp. | Vancomycin + metronidazole + a third-generation cephalosporin[a] |
| Dental sepsis | Mixed *Fusobacterium* and *Bacteroides* spp., streptococci | Penicillin + metronidazole |
| Penetrating trauma or postneurosurgery | *S. aureus,* streptococci, Enterobacteriaceae, *Clostridium* | Vancomycin + a third-generation cephalosporin[a] |
| Congenital heart disease | Streptococci, *Haemophilus* spp. | Penicillin + a third-generation cephalosporin[a] |
| Lung abscess, empyema, bronchiectasis | *Fusobacterium, Actinomyces, Bacteroides* spp., streptococci, *Nocardia asteroides* | Penicillin + metronidazole + a sulfonamide[b] |
| Bacterial endocarditis | *S. aureus,* streptococci | Vancomycin + gentamicin *or* nafcillin + ampicillin + gentamicin |

[a] Cefotaxime or ceftriaxone; ceftazidime or cefepime is used if *Pseudomonas aeruginosa* is suspected.
[b] Trimethoprim-sulfamethoxazole; include if *N. asteroides* is suspected.

**IV. Approach to the patient with brain abscess**

**A. Microbiologic diagnosis.** When a brain abscess is suggested by radiologic studies, a microbiologic diagnosis ideally should be made to guide antimicrobial therapy. CT has made it possible to perform stereotactically guided abscess aspiration. Specimens should be sent for Gram stain, aerobic and anaerobic cultures, Ziehl-Neelsen stain for *Mycobacteria,* modified acid-fast stain for *Nocardia,* and silver stains for fungi. Cultures for *Mycobacteria, Nocardia,* and fungi should also be performed.

**B. Empiric antibiotic therapy.** In patients with bacterial brain abscess, once a diagnosis is made either presumptively by radiologic studies or by CT-guided aspiration of the lesion, antimicrobial therapy should be initiated [233–235]. If an aspiration cannot be performed or if Gram staining is unrevealing, **empiric therapy should be initiated based on the presumed pathogenic mechanism of abscess formation** (Table 6.6).

1. **Streptococci.** Because of the high rate of isolation of streptococci, especially the *S. milleri* group, from brain abscesses of different etiologies, high-dose intravenous **penicillin G** or another drug active against these organisms (e.g., a third-generation cephalosporin, either cefotaxime or ceftriaxone) should be included.
2. **Anaerobes.** Although penicillin G is active also against most anaerobes, *Bacteroides fragilis* is an exception that may be isolated in a high percentage of cases. **Metronidazole** is the agent of choice against *B. fragilis* in this setting. Metronidazole attains high concentrations in brain abscess pus, and its entry into brain abscesses is not altered by concomitant administration of corticosteroids.
3. **Enterobacteriaceae. A third-generation cephalosporin** or trimethoprim-sulfamethoxazole should be used when members of the Enterobacteriaceae family are suspected. Ceftazidime or cefepime is the agent of choice for *P. aeruginosa* brain abscess.
4. ***S. aureus.*** Nafcillin should be used when *S. aureus* is considered likely (e.g., staphylococcal endocarditis, cranial trauma); vancomycin is reserved for patients allergic to penicillin or when methicillin-resistant organisms are suspected or isolated.

Table 6.7. Antimicrobial Therapy for Brain Abscess

| Organism | Standard Therapy | Alternative Therapies |
|---|---|---|
| *Actinomyces* species | Penicillin G | Clindamycin |
| *Aspergillus* species | Amphotericin B[a] | Itraconazole[b], voriconazole[c] |
| *Bacteroides fragilis* | Metronidazole | Chloramphenicol, clindamycin, ampicillin-sulbactam |
| *Candida* species | Amphotericin B[a] | Fluconazole[b] |
| *Cryptococcus neoformans* | Amphotericin B[a] | Fluconazole |
| Enterobacteriaceae | Third-generation cephalosporin[d] | Aztreonam, trimethoprim-sulfamethoxazole, fluoroquinolone, meropenem |
| *Fusobacterium* species | Penicillin G | Metronidazole |
| *Haemophilus* species | Third-generation cephalosporin[d] | Aztreonam, trimethoprim-sulfamethoxazole |
| *Listeria monocytogenes* | Ampicillin or penicillin G[e] | Trimethoprim-sulfamethoxazole |
| *Nocardia asteroides* | Trimethoprim-sulfamethoxazole or sulfadiazine | Minocycline, imipenem, a third-generation cephalosporin[d], fluoroquinolone[b] |
| *Pseudallescheria boydii* | Voriconazole | Fluconazole[b], itraconazole[b], miconazole |
| *Pseudomonas aeruginosa* | Ceftazidime[e] or cefepime[e] | Aztreonam[b], fluoroquinolone[b], meropenem[b] |
| *Staphylococcus aureus* | | |
| Methicillin-sensitive | Nafcillin or oxacillin | Vancomycin |
| Methicillin-resistant | Vancomycin | |
| *Streptococcus milleri*, other streptococci | Penicillin G | Third-generation cephalosporin[d], vancomycin |

[a] Addition of flucytosine should be considered.
[b] Efficacy not yet proven in brain abscess due to this organism.
[c] May become the agent of choice.
[d] Cefotaxime or ceftriaxone.
[e] Addition of an aminoglycoside should be considered.

5. ***Nocardia.*** When a *Nocardia* species is suspected or proven, trimethoprim-sulfamethoxazole should be used [233]. Alternative agents include minocycline, amikacin, imipenem, the third-generation cephalosporins, and the fluoroquinolones. Combination therapies have been used in *Nocardia* brain abscess, and combination regimens containing a third-generation cephalosporin or imipenem along with a sulfonamide should be considered for immunocompromised patients or those in whom therapy fails [234] (see Chapter 17).

C. **Modification of antibiotics after culture data.** If positive cultures are obtained, antimicrobial therapy can be modified for optimal treatment (Table 6.7). Dosages of antimicrobial agents for CNS infections are shown in Tables 6.4 and 6.5.

D. **Surgical therapy**

1. **Most bacterial brain abscesses require surgical excision for optimal therapy** (see section 2 below for exceptions) [233,234]. Abscess aspiration by stereotactic CT guidance affords the surgeon rapid, accurate, and safe access to virtually any intracranial location and allows for swift relief of increased intracranial pressure. However, **aspiration has the major disadvantage of incomplete drainage of multiloculated lesions.** Complete abscess excision can be used when aspiration is unsuccessful and when abscesses exhibit gas on radiologic evaluation. Emergent surgery is indicated in patients developing worsening neurologic deficits. Excision is contraindicated in the early stages before a capsule is formed. All brain abscesses more than 2.5 cm in diameter should be aspirated or excised for optimal management [241].

2. **Certain patients may require only medical therapy** [242,243]. Among these are patients with medical conditions that increase risk of surgery, multiple abscesses, abscesses in a deep or dominant location, concomitant meningitis or ependymitis, early abscess reduction with clinical improvement after antimicrobial therapy, and an abscess measuring less than 3 cm.

E. **Duration of antibiotic therapy.** High-dose intravenous antimicrobial therapy should be continued for 6 to 8 weeks; this often is followed by oral antimicrobial therapy if appropriate agents are available. A shorter course of therapy (i.e., 3 to 4 weeks) may be appropriate for patients who have undergone complete surgical excision of the abscess.

Nocardial brain abscess should be treated for 3 to 12 months [233]. Surgical excision should also be performed for optimal therapy.

F. **Fungal brain abscess.** A combined medical and surgical approach usually is required for optimal treatment of fungal brain abscesses.

1. ***Aspergillus* species.** Successful management for *Aspergillus* brain abscess includes excisional surgery or drainage in combination with antifungal therapy. Medical therapy is amphotericin B 0.8 to 1.25 mg/kg/day, with doses up to 1.5 mg/kg/day depending on the clinical response [244], although few instances of survival have been reported. Total doses of 3 g or more of amphotericin B are required. The addition of 5-FC may increase success rates, although no controlled trials have demonstrated the efficacy of this approach. Itraconazole has *in vitro* activity against *Aspergillus,* and high-dose therapy (800 mg daily for 5 months followed by 400 mg daily for 4.5 months) resulted in resolution of cerebral abscesses caused by *A. fumigatus* in an elderly asthmatic patient who was treated with corticosteroids [245]. Voriconazole has had mixed (though favorable when compared with historical data) results in open label trials [246].
2. **Mucormycosis.** Therapy of mucormycosis includes amphotericin B, correction of underlying metabolic derangements, and aggressive surgical debridement [235]. Surgery is essential because of the propensity of this organism to invade blood vessels and impede delivery of antifungal agents to the sites of infection. A possible adjunct to therapy is hyperbaric oxygen, although no prospective controlled studies have been performed to assess its efficacy. Anecdotal experience with use of granulocyte colony-stimulating factor has shown benefit; granulocyte colony-stimulating factor needs to be explored as potential adjunctive therapy in this disease.
3. ***Pseudallescheria boydii.*** *P. boydii* exhibits *in vitro* resistance to amphotericin B. Miconazole has been the antifungal agent of choice [236,237], although intravenous or intrathecal administration is required and relapses are common. One case of *P. boydii* brain abscess was successfully treated with voriconazole and aggressive surgical intervention [247]. We consider voriconazole to be the agent of choice (Table 6.7). Surgical drainage is the cornerstone of effective therapy.

## REFERENCES


1. Rotbart HA. Viral meningitis and the aseptic meningitis syndrome. In: Scheld WM, Whitley RJ, Durack DT, eds. *Infections of the central nervous system,* 2nd ed. Philadelphia: Lippincott-Raven Publishers, 1997:23–46.
2. Strikas RA, Anderson LJ, Parker RA. Temporal and geographic patterns of isolates of nonpolio enterovirus in the United States, 1970–1983. *J Infect Dis* 1986;153:346–351.
3. Ho M, Chen ER, Parker RA. An epidemic of enterovirus 71 infection in Taiwan. *N Engl J Med* 1999;341:929–935.
4. Huang CC, Liu CC, Chang UC, et al. Neurologic complications in children with enterovirus 71 infection. *N Engl J Med* 1999;341:936–942.
5. Dolin R. Enterovirus 71: emerging infections and emerging questions. *N Engl J Med* 1999;341:984–985.
6. Rotbart HA, Brennan PJ, Fife KH, et al. Enterovirus meningitis in adults. *Clin Infect Dis* 1998;27:896–898.
7. Rantakallio P, Leskinen M, von Wendt L. Incidence and prognosis of central nervous

system infections in a birth cohort of 12,000 children. *Scand J Infect Dis* 1986;18:287–294.
8. Gnann JW Jr. Meningitis and encephalitis caused by mumps virus. In: Scheld WM, Whitley RJ, Durack DT, eds. *Infections of the central nervous system,* 2nd ed. Philadelphia: Lippincott-Raven Publishers, 1997:169–180.
9. Miller E, Goldacre M, Pugh S, et al. Risk of aseptic meningitis after measles, mumps, and rubella vaccine in UK children. *Lancet* 1983;341:979–982.
10. Dykewicz CA, Dato VM, Fisher-Hoch, SP, et al. Lymphocytic choriomeningitis outbreak associated with nude mice in a research institute. *JAMA* 1992;267:1349–1353.
11. Corey L, Spear PG. Infections with herpes simplex viruses (second of two parts). *N Engl J Med* 1986;314:749–757.
12. Corey L, Adams HG, Brown ZA, et al. Genital herpes simplex virus infection: clinical manifestations, course, and complications. *Ann Intern Med* 1983;98:958–972.
13. Bergström T, Vahlne A, Alestig K, et al. Primary and recurrent herpes simplex virus type 2-induced meningitis. *J Infect Dis* 1990;162:322–330.
14. Yamamoto LJ, Tedder DG, Ashley R, et al. Herpes simplex virus type 1 DNA in cerebrospinal fluid of a patient with Mollaret's meningitis. *N Engl J Med* 1991;325:1082–1085.
15. Tedder DG, Ashley R, Tyler K, et al. Herpes simplex virus infection as a cause of benign recurrent lymphocytic meningitis. *Ann Intern Med* 1994;121:334–338.
16. Mayo DR, Booss J. Varicella zoster-associated neurologic disease without skin disease. *Arch Neurol* 1989;46:313–315.
17. Barnes DW, Whitley RJ. CNS diseases associated with varicella zoster virus and herpes simplex virus infection. Pathogenesis and current therapy. *Neurol Clin* 1986;4:265–283.
18. Graman PS. Mollaret's meningitis associated with acute Epstein-Barr virus mononucleosis. *Arch Neurol* 1987;44:1204–1205.
19. Huang LM, Lee CY, Lee PI, et al. Meningitis caused by human herpesvirus-6. *Arch Dis Child* 1991;66:1443–1444.
20. McCullers JA, Lakeman FD, Whitley RJ. Human herpesvirus 6 is associated with focal encephalitis. *Clin Infect Dis* 1995;21:571–576.
21. Kondo KH, Nagafuji A, Hata C, et al. Association of human herpesvirus 6 infection of the central nervous system with recurrence of febrile convulsions. *J Infect Dis* 1993;167:1197–1200.
22. Wang FZ, Linde A, Hagglund H, et al. Human herpesvirus 6 DNA in cerebrospinal fluid specimens from allogeneic bone marrow transplant patients: does it have clinical significance? *Clin Infect Dis* 1999;28:562–568.
23. Berger JR, Simpson DM. Neurological complications of AIDS. In: Scheld WM, Whitley RJ, Durack DT, eds. *Infections of the central nervous system,* 2nd ed. Philadelphia: Lippincott-Raven Publishers, 1997:255–271.
24. Price RW. Neurologic complications of HIV infection. *Lancet* 1996;348:445–452.
25. McArthur JC. Neurologic manifestations of AIDS. *Medicine (Baltimore)* 1987;66:407–437.
26. Hollander H, Stringari S. Human immunodeficiency virus-associated meningitis. Clinical course and correlations. *Am J Med* 1987;83:813–816.
27. Tunkel AR, Scheld WM. Acute meningitis. In: Mandell GL, Bennett JE, Dolin R, eds. *Principles and practice of infectious diseases,* 5th ed. Philadelphia: Churchill Livingstone, 2000:959–997.
28. Schlech WF III, Ward JI, Band JD, et al. Bacterial meningitis in the United States, 1978 through 1981. The national bacterial meningitis surveillance study. *JAMA* 1985;253:1749–1754.
29. Bryan JP, de Silva HR, Tavares A, et al. Etiology and mortality of bacterial meningitis in northeastern Brazil. *Rev Infect Dis* 1990;12:128–135.
30. Durand ML, Calderwood SB, Weber DJ, et al. Acute bacterial meningitis in adults. A review of 493 episodes. *N Engl J Med* 1993;328:21–28.
31. Wenger JD, Hightower AW, Facklam RR, et al. Bacterial meningitis in the United States, 1986: report of a multistate surveillance study. *J Infect Dis* 1990;162:1316–1323.

32. Centers for Disease Control and Prevention. Progress toward elimination of *Haemophilus influenzae* type b disease among infants and children—United States, 1987–1997. *Mortal Morb Wkly Rep MMWR* 1998;47:993–998.
33. Schuchat A, Robinson K, Wenger JD, et al. Bacterial meningitis in the United States in 1995. *N Engl J Med* 1997;337:970–976.
34. Spagnuolo PJ, Ellner JJ, Lerner PI, et al. *Haemophilus influenzae* meningitis: the spectrum of disease in adults. *Medicine (Baltimore)* 1982;61:74–85.
35. Farley MM, Stephens DS, Brachman PS, et al. Invasive *Haemophilus influenzae* disease in adults. A prospective, population-based surveillance. *Ann Intern Med* 1992;116:806–812.
36. Jackson LA, Schuchat A, Reeves MW, et al. Serogroup C meningococcal outbreaks in the United States: an emerging threat. *JAMA* 1995;273:383–389.
37. Whalen CM, Hockin JC, Ryan A, et al. The changing epidemiology of invasive meningococcal disease in Canada, 1985 through 1992. *JAMA* 1995;273:390–394.
38. Berron S, La Fuente LD, Martin E, et al. Increasing incidence of meningococcal disease in Spain associated with a new variant of serogroup C. *Eur J Clin Microbiol Infect Dis* 1998;17:85–89.
39. Ross SC, Densen P. Complement deficiency states and infection: epidemiology, pathogenesis and consequences of neisserial and other infections in an immune deficiency. *Medicine (Baltimore)* 1984;64:243–273.
40. Geiseler PJ, Nelson KE, Levin S, et al. Community-acquired purulent meningitis: a review of 1,316 cases during the antibiotic era, 1954–1976. *Rev Infect Dis* 1980;2:725–745.
41. Musher DM. Infections caused by *Streptococcus pneumoniae:* clinical spectrum, pathogenesis, immunity, and treatment. *Clin Infect Dis* 1992;14:801–809.
42. Tunkel AR, Scheld WM. Acute infectious complications of head trauma. In: Braakman R, ed. *Handbook of clinical neurology, head injury.* Amsterdam: Elsevier Science, 1990:317–326.
43. Lorber B. Listeriosis. *Clin Infect Dis* 1997;24:1–11.
44. Mylonakis E, Hohmann E., Calderwood SB. Central nervous system infection with *Listeria monocytogenes:* 33 years' experience at a general hospital and review of 776 episodes from the literature. *Medicine (Baltimore)* 1998;77:313–336.
45. Decker CF, Simon GL, DiGioia RA, et al. *Listeria monocytogenes* infections in patients with AIDS: report of five cases and review. *Rev Infect Dis* 1991;13:413–417.
46. Berenguer J, Solera J, Diaz MD, et al. Listeriosis in patients infected with human immunodeficiency virus. *Rev Infect Dis* 1991;13:115–119.
47. Saez-Llorens X, McCracken GH Jr. Bacterial meningitis in neonates and children. *Infect Dis Clin North Am* 1990;4:623–644.
48. Farley MM, Harvey RC, Stull T, et al. A population-based assessment of invasive disease due to group B streptococci in nonpregnant adults. *N Engl J Med* 1993;328:1807–1811.
49. Dunne DW, et al. Quagliarello V. Group B streptococcal meningitis in adults. *Medicine (Baltimore)* 1993;72:1–10.
50. Domingo P, Barquet N, Alvarez M, et al. Group B streptococcal meningitis in adults: report of twelve cases and review. *Clin Infect Dis* 1997;25:1180–1187.
51. Unhanand M, Mustafa MM, McCracken GH Jr, et al. Gram-negative enteric bacillary meningitis: a twenty-one-year experience. *J Pediatr* 1993;122:15–21.
52. Cameron ML, Durack DT. Helminthic infections of the central nervous system. In: Scheld WM, Whitley RJ, Durack DT, eds. *Infections of the central nervous system,* 2nd ed. Philadelphia: Lippincott-Raven Publishers, 1997:845–878.
53. Schlesinger LS, Ross SC, Schaberg DR. *Staphylococcus aureus* meningitis: a broad-based epidemiologic study. *Medicine (Baltimore)* 1987;66:148–156.
54. Kaufman BA. Infections of cerebrospinal fluid shunts. In: Scheld WM, Whitley RJ, Durack DT, eds. *Infections of the central nervous system,* 2nd ed. Philadelphia: Lippincott-Raven Publishers, 1997:555–577.
55. Pegues DA, Carr DB, Hopkins CC. Infectious complications associated with temporary epidural catheters. *Clin Infect Dis* 1994;19:970–972.
56. Bross JE, Gordon G. Nocardial meningitis: case reports and review. *Rev Infect Dis* 1991;13:160–165.

57. Stevenson KB, Murray EW, Sarubbi FA. Enterococcal meningitis: report of four cases and review. *Clin Infect Dis* 1994;18:233–239.
58. Heerema MS, Ein ME, Musher DM, et al. Anaerobic bacterial meningitis. *Am J Med* 1979;67:219–227.
59. Law DA, Aronoff SC. Anaerobic meningitis in children: case report and review of the literature. *Pediatr Infect Dis J* 1992;11:968–971.
60. Gelfand MS, Abolnik IA. Streptococcal meningitis complicating diagnostic myelography: three cases and review. *Clin Infect Dis* 1995;20:582–587.
61. Zugar A, Lowy FD. Tuberculosis of the central nervous system. In: Scheld WM, Whitley RJ, Durack DT, eds. *Infections of the central nervous system,* 2nd ed. Philadelphia: Lippincott-Raven Publishers, 1997:417–443.
62. Leonard JM, Des Prez RM. Tuberculous meningitis. *Infect Dis Clin North Am* 1990; 4:769–787.
63. Markowitz N, Hansen NI, Hopewell PC, et al. Incidence of tuberculosis in the United States among HIV-infected persons. *Ann Intern Med* 1997;126:123–132.
64. Barnes PF, Block AB, Davidson PT, et al. Tuberculosis in patients with human immunodeficiency virus infection. *N Engl J Med* 1991;324:1644–1650.
65. Hook EW III. Central nervous system syphilis. In: Scheld WM, Whitley RJ, Durack DT, eds. *Infections of the central nervous system,* 2nd ed. Philadelphia: Lippincott-Raven Publishers, 1997:669–684.
66. Musher DM, Hamill RJ, Baughn RE. Effect of human immunodeficiency virus (HIV) infection on the course of syphilis and on the response to treatment. *Ann Intern Med* 1990;113:872–881.
67. Hook EW III, Marra CM. Acquired syphilis in adults. *N Engl J Med* 1992;326:1060–1069.
68. Katz DA, Berger JR. Neurosyphilis in acquired immunodeficiency syndrome. *Arch Neurol* 1989;46:895–898.
69. Flood JM, Weinstock HS, Guroy ME, et al. Neurosyphilis during the AIDS epidemic, San Francisco, 1985–1992. *J Infect Dis* 1998;177:931–940.
70. Reik L Jr. Lyme disease. In: Scheld WM, Whitley RJ, Durack DT, eds. *Infections of the central nervous system,* 2nd ed. Philadelphia: Lippincott-Raven Publishers, 1997:685–718.
71. Steere AC. Lyme disease. *N Engl J Med* 2001;345:115–125.
72. Luft BJ, Steinman CR, Neimark HC, et al. Invasion of the central nervous system by *Borrelia burgdorferi* in acute disseminated infection. *JAMA* 1992;267:1364–1367.
73. Sabetta JR, Andriole VT. Cryptococcal infection of the central nervous system. *Med Clin North Am* 1985;69:333–345.
74. Mitchell TG, Perfect JR. Cryptococcosis in the era of AIDS 100 years after the discovery of *Cryptococcus neoformans. Clin Microbiol Rev* 1998;8:515–548.
75. Kovacs JA, Kovacs AA, Polis M, et al. Cryptococcosis in the acquired immunodeficiency syndrome. *Ann Intern Med* 1985;103:533–538.
76. Zugar A, Louie E, Holzman RS, et al. Cryptococcal disease in patients with the acquired immunodeficiency syndrome. Diagnostic features and outcome of treatment. *Ann Intern Med* 1986;104:234–240.
77. Chuck SL, Sande MA. Infections with *Cryptococcus neoformans* in the acquired immunodeficiency syndrome. *N Engl J Med* 1989;321:794–799.
78. Crislip MA, Edwards JE Jr. Candidiasis. *Infect Dis Clin North Am* 1989;3:103–133.
79. Geers TA, Gordon SM. Clinical significance of *Candida* species isolated from cerebrospinal fluid following neurosurgery. *Clin Infect Dis* 1999;28:1139–1147.
80. Bayer AS, Edwards JE Jr, Seidel JS, et al. *Candida* meningitis. Report of seven cases and review of the English literature. *Medicine (Baltimore)* 1976;55: 477–486.
81. Lipton SA, Hickey WF, Morris JH, et al. Candidal infection in the central nervous system. *Am J Med* 1984;76:101–108.
82. Walsh TJ, Hier DB, Caplan LP. Fungal infections of the central nervous system: comparative analysis of risk factors and clinical signs in 57 patients. *Neurology* 1985;35:1654–1657.

83. Galgiani JN. Coccidioidomycosis: a regional disease of national importance. Rethinking approaches to control. *Ann Intern Med* 1999;130:293–300.
84. Bouza E, Dreyer JS, Hewitt WL, et al. Coccidioidal meningitis. An analysis of thirty-one cases and review of the literature. *Medicine (Baltimore)* 1981;60:139–172.
85. Ampel NM, Wieden MA, Galgiani JN. Coccidioidomycosis: clinical update. *Rev Infect Dis* 1989;11:897–911.
86. Niu MT, Duma RJ. Meningitis due to protozoa and helminths. *Infect Dis Clin North Am* 1990;4:809–841.
87. Durack DT. Amebic infections. In: Scheld WM, Whitley RJ, Durack DT, eds. *Infections of the central nervous system,* 2nd ed. Philadelphia: Lippincott-Raven Publishers, 1997:831–844.
88. Gardner HAR, Martinez AJ, Visvesvara GS, et al. Granulomatous amebic encephalitis in an AIDS patient. *Neurology* 1991;41:1993–1995.
89. Di Gregorio C, Rivasi R, Mongiardo N, et al. *Acanthamoeba* meningoencephalitis in a patient with acquired immunodeficiency syndrome. *Arch Pathol Lab Med* 1992;116:1363–1365.
90. Gordon SM, Steinberg J, DuPuis MH, et al. Culture isolation of *Acanthamoeba* species and leptomyxid amebas from patients with amebic meningoencephalitis, including two patients with AIDS. *Clin Infect Dis* 1992;15:1024–1030.
91. Koo J, Pien F, Kliks MM. *Angiostrongylus (Parastrongylus)* eosinophilic meningitis. *Rev Infect Dis* 1988;10:1155–1162.
92. Kaplan MH, Klein SW, McPhee J, et al. Group B coxsackievirus infections in infants younger than three months of age: a serious childhood illness. *Rev Infect Dis* 1983;5:1019–1032.
93. Wilfert CM, Lehrman SN. Enteroviruses and meningitis. *Pediatr Infect Dis* 1983;2:333–341.
94. Jaffe M, Srugo I, Tirosh E, et al. The ameliorating effect of lumbar puncture in viral meningitis. *Am J Dis Child* 1989;143:682–685.
95. McKinney RE Jr, Katz SL, Wilfert CM. Chronic enteroviral meningoencephalitis in agammaglobulinemic patients. *Rev Infect Dis* 1987;9:334–356.
96. Roos KL, Tunkel AR, Scheld WM. Acute bacterial meningitis in children and adults. In: Scheld WM, Whitley RJ, Durack DT, eds. *Infections of the central nervous system,* 2nd ed. Philadelphia: Lippincott-Raven Publishers, 1997:335–401.
97. Gorse GJ, Thrupp LD, Nudleman KL, et al. Bacterial meningitis in the elderly. *Arch Intern Med* 1989;149:1603–1606.
98. Kent SJ, Crowe SM, Yung A, et al. Tuberculous meningitis: a 30-year review. *Clin Infect Dis* 1993;17:987–994.
99. Ogawa SK, Smith MA, Brennessel DJ, et al. Tuberculous meningitis in an urban medical center. *Medicine (Baltimore)* 1987;66:317–326.
100. Kennedy DH, Fallon RJ. Tuberculous meningitis. *JAMA* 1979;241:264–268.
101. Verdon R, Chevret S, Laissy JP, et al. Tuberculous meningitis in adults: review of 48 cases. *Clin Infect Dis* 1996;22:982–988.
102. Berenguer J, Moreno S, Laguna F, et al. Tuberculous meningitis in patients infected with the human immunodeficiency virus. *N Engl J Med* 1992;326:668–672.
103. Dube MP, Holtom PD, Larsen RA. Tuberculous meningitis in patients with and without human immunodeficiency virus infection. *Am J Med* 1992;93:520–524.
104. Hutchinson CM, Rompalo AM, Reichart CA, et al. Characteristics of patients with syphilis attending Baltimore STD clinics: multiple, high-risk subgroups and interactions with human immunodeficiency virus infection. *Arch Intern Med* 1991;151:511–516.
105. Moosa MYS, Coovadia YM. Cryptococcal meningitis in Durban, South Africa: a comparison of clinical features, laboratory findings, and outcome for human immunodeficiency virus (HIV)-positive and HIV-negative patients. *Clin Infect Dis* 1997;24:131–134.
106. Heyderman RS, Gangaidzo IT, Hakim JG, et al. Cryptococcal meningitis in human immunodeficiency virus-infected patients in Harare, Zimbabwe. *Clin Infect Dis* 1998; 26:284–289.
107. Negrini B, Kelleher KJ, Wilfert CM. Cerebrospinal fluid findings in aseptic versus bacterial meningitis. *Pediatrics* 2000;105:316–319.

108. Ahmed A, Brito F, Goto C, et al. Clinical utility of polymerase chain reaction for diagnosis of enteroviral meningitis in infancy. *J Pediatr* 1997;131:393–397.
109. Gorgievski-Hrisoho M, Schumacher JD, Vilimonovic N, et al. Detection of PCR of enteroviruses in cerebrospinal fluid during a summer outbreak of aseptic meningitis in Switzerland. *J Clin Microbiol* 1998;36:2408–2412.
110. Van Vliet KE, Glimaker M, Lebon P, et al. Multicenter evaluation of the Amplicor enterovirus PCR test with cerebrospinal fluid from patients with aseptic meningitis. *J Clin Microbiol* 1998;36:2652–2657.
111. Echevarria JM, Cases I, Tenoirio A, et al. Detection of varicella-zoster virus-specific DNA sequences in cerebrospinal fluid from patients with acute aseptic meningitis and no cutaneous lesions. *J Med Virol* 1994;43:331–335.
112. Hollander H, Levy JA. Neurologic abnormalities and recovery of human immunodeficiency virus from cerebrospinal fluid. *Ann Intern Med* 1987;106:692–695.
113. Chalmers AC, Aprill BS, Shephard H. Cerebrospinal fluid and human immunodeficiency virus. Findings in healthy, asymptomatic, seropositive men. *Arch Intern Med* 1990;150:1538–1540.
114. Ellis RJ, Hsia K, Spector SA, et al. Cerebrospinal fluid human immunodeficiency virus type 1 RNA levels are elevated in neurocognitively impaired individuals with acquired immunodeficiency syndrome. *Ann Neurol* 1997;42:679–688.
115. McArthur JC, McClernon DR, Cronin MF, et al. Relationship between human immunodeficiency virus-associated dementia and viral load in cerebrospinal fluid and brain. *Ann Neurol* 1997;42:689–698.
116. Feigin RD, McCracken GH Jr, Klein JO. Diagnosis and management of meningitis. *Pediatr Infect Dis J* 1992;11:785–814.
117. Bonadio WA. The cerebrospinal fluid: physiologic aspects and alterations associated with bacterial meningitis. *Pediatr Infect Dis J* 1992;11:423–432.
118. Sivakmaran M. Meningococcal meningitis revisited: normocellular CSF. *Clin Pediatr* 1997;36:351–355.
119. Coll MT, Uriz MS, Pineda V, et al. Meningococcal meningitis with "normal" cerebrospinal fluid. *J Infect* 1994;29:289–294.
120. Marton KI, Gean AD. The spinal tap: a new look at an old test. *Ann Intern Med* 1986;104:840–848.
121. La Scolea LJ Jr, Dryja D. Quantitation of bacteria in cerebrospinal fluid and blood of children with meningitis and its diagnostic significance. *J Clin Microbiol* 1984;19:187–190.
122. Gray LD, Fedorko DP. Laboratory diagnosis of bacterial meningitis. *Clin Microbiol Rev* 1992;5:130–145.
123. Finlay FO, Witheerow H, Rudd PT. Latex agglutination testing in bacterial meningitis. *Arch Dis Child* 1995;73:160–161.
124. Ni H, Knight AI, Cartwright K, et al. Polymerase chain reaction for diagnosis of meningococcal meningitis. *Lancet* 1992;340:1432–1434.
125. Radstrom P, Backman A, Qian N, et al. Detection of bacterial DNA in cerebrospinal fluid by an assay for simultaneous detection of *Neisseria meningitidis, Haemophilus influenzae* and streptococci using a seminested PCR strategy. *J Clin Microbiol* 1994;32:2738–2744.
126. Sormunen P, Kallio MJT, Kilpi T, et al. C-reactive protein is useful in distinguishing Gram stain-negative bacterial meningitis from viral meningitis in children. *J Pediatr* 1999;134:725–729.
127. Viallon A, Zeni F, Lambert C, et al. High sensitivity and specificity of serum procalcitonin levels in adults with bacterial meningitis. *Clin Infect Dis* 1999;28:1313–1316.
128. Cotton MF, Donald PR, Schoeman JR, et al. Plasma arginine vasopressin and the syndrome of inappropriate antidiuretic hormone secretion in tuberculous meningitis. *Pediatr Infect Dis J* 1991;10:837–842.
129. Bonington A, Strang JIG, Klapper PE, et al. Use of Roche AMPLICOR *Mycobacterium tuberculosis* PCR in early diagnosis of tuberculous meningitis. *J Clin Microbiol* 1998;36:1251–1254.
130. Gupta RK, Gupta S, Singh D, et al. MR imaging and angiography in tuberculous meningitis. *Neuroradiology* 1994;36:87–92.

131. Noordhoek GT, Wolters EC, de Jonge MEJ, et al. Detection by polymerase chain reaction of *Treponema pallidum* DNA in cerebrospinal fluid from neurosyphilis patients before and after antibiotic treatment. *J Clin Microbiol* 1991;29:1976–1984.
132. Corpuz M, Hilton E, Lardis MP, et al. Problems in the use of serologic tests for the diagnosis of Lyme disease. *Arch Intern Med* 1991;151:1837–1840.
133. American College of Physicians. Guidelines for laboratory evaluation in the diagnosis of Lyme disease. *Ann Intern Med* 1997;127:1106–1108.
134. Tugwell P, Dennis DT, Weinstein A, et al. Laboratory evaluation in the diagnosis of Lyme disease. *Ann Intern Med* 1997;127:1109–1123.
135. Shaunak S, Schell WA, Perfect JR. Cryptococcal meningitis with normal cerebrospinal fluid. *J Infect Dis* 1989;160:912.
136. Schermoly MJ, Hinthorn DR. Eosinophilia in coccidioidomycosis. *Arch Intern Med* 1988;148:895–896.
137. Tunkel AR, Wispelwey B, Scheld WM. Bacterial meningitis: recent advances in pathophysiology and treatment. *Ann Intern Med* 1990;112:610–623.
138. Aronin SI, Peduzzi P, Quagliarello VJ. Community-acquired bacterial meningitis: risk stratification for adverse clinical outcome and effect of antibiotic timing. *Ann Intern Med* 1998;129:862–869.
139. Rotbart HA, Webster AD, The Pleconaril Treatment Registry Group. Treatment of potentially life-threatening enterovirus infections with pleconaril. *Clin Infect Dis* 2001;32:228–235.
140. Lebel MH, Hoyt MJ, McCracken GH Jr. Comparative efficacy of ceftriaxone and cefuroxime for treatment of bacterial meningitis. *J Pediatr* 1989;114:1049–1054.
141. Schaad UB, Suter S, Gianella-Borradori A, et al. A comparison of ceftriaxone and cefuroxime for the treatment of bacterial meningitis in children. *N Engl J Med* 1990;322:141–147.
142. Saez-Llorens X, Castano E, Garcia R, et al. Prospective randomized comparison of cefepime and cefotaxime for treatment of bacterial meningitis in infants and children. *Antimicrob Agents Chemother* 1995;39:937–940.
143. Saez-Nieto JA, Lujan R, Berron S, et al. Epidemiology and molecular basis of penicillin- resistant *Neisseria meningitidis* in Spain: a 5-year history (1985–1989). *Clin Infect Dis* 1992;14:394–402.
144. Jackson LA, Tenover FC, Baker C, et al. Prevalence of *Neisseria meningitidis* relatively resistant to penicillin in the United States, 1991. *J Infect Dis* 1994;169:438–441.
145. Rosenstein NE, Stocker SA, Popovic T, et al. Antimicrobial resistance of *Neisseria meningitidis* in the United States, 1997. *Clin Infect Dis* 2000;30:212–213.
146. Casado-Flores J, Osona B, Comingo P, et al. Meningococcal meningitis during penicillin therapy for meningococcemia. *Clin Infect Dis* 1995;25:1479.
147. Goldani LZ. Inducement of *Neisseria meningitidis* resistant to ampicillin and penicillin in a patient with meningococcemia treated with high doses of ampicillin. *Clin Infect Dis* 1998;26:772.
148. Galimand M, Gerbaud G, Guibourdenche M, et al. High-level chloramphenicol resistance in *Neisseria meningitidis*. *N Engl J Med* 1998;339:868–874.
149. Hopkins S, Williams D, Dunne M, et al. A randomized, controlled trial of oral or IV trovafloxacin vs. ceftriaxone in the treatment of epidemic meningococcal meningitis. In: *Program and Abstracts of the 36th Interscience Conference on Antimicrobial Agents and Chemotherapy.* Washington, DC: American Society for Microbiology, 1996.
150. Hofmann J, Cetron MS, Farley MM, et al. The prevalence of drug-resistant *Streptococcus pneumoniae* in Atlanta. *N Engl J Med* 1995;333:481–486.
151. Campbell GD, Silberman R. Drug-resistant *Streptococcus pneumoniae*. *Clin Infect Dis* 1998;26:1188–1195.
152. Rocha P, Baleeiro C, Tunkel AR. Impact of antimicrobial resistance on the treatment of invasive pneumococcal infections. *Curr Infect Dis Rep* 2000;2:399–408.
153. Kaplan SL, Mason EO. Management of infections due to antibiotic-resistant *Streptococcus pneumoniae*. *Clin Microbiol Rev* 1998;11:628–644.
154. Ruiz-Irastorze GR, Garea C, Alonso JJ, et al. Failure of cefotaxime treatment in a patient with penicillin-resistant pneumococcal meningitis and confirmation of

nosocomial spread by random amplified polymorphic DNA analysis. *Clin Infect Dis* 1995;21:234–235.

155. Florez C, Silva G, Martin E. Cefotaxime failure in pneumococcal meningitis caused by a susceptible isolate. *Pediatr Infect Dis J* 1996;15:723–724.
156. Pacheco TR, Cooper CK, Hardy DJ, et al. Failure of cefotaxime in an adult with *Streptococcus pneumoniae* meningitis. *Am J Med* 1997;102:303–305.
157. Friedland IR, Klugman KP. Failure of chloramphenicol therapy in penicillin-resistant pneumococcal meningitis. *Lancet* 1992;339:405–408.
158. Ahmad A. A critical evaluation of vancomycin for treatment of bacterial meningitis. *Pediatr Infect Dis J* 1997;16:895–903.
159. Viladrich PF, Gudiol F, Linares J, et al. Evaluation of vancomycin for therapy of adult pneumococcal meningitis. *Antimicrob Agents Chemother* 1991;35:2467–2472.
160. Novak R, Henriques B, Charpentier E, et al. Emergence of vancomycin tolerance in *Streptococcus pneumoniae. Nature* 1999;399:590–593.
161. McCullers JA, English BK, Novak R. Isolation and characterization of vancomycin-tolerant *Streptococcus pneumoniae* from the cerebrospinal fluid of a patient who developed recrudescent meningitis. *J Infect Dis* 2000;181:369–373.
162. Bradley JS, Scheld WM. The challenge of penicillin-resistant *Streptococcus pneumoniae* meningitis: current antibiotic therapy in the 1990s. *Clin Infect Dis* 1997;24:S213–S221.
163. Odio CM, Puig JR, Feris JM, et al. Prospective, randomized, investigator-blinded study of the efficacy and safety of meropenem vs. cefotaxime therapy in bacterial meningitis in children. *Pediatr Infect Dis J* 1999;18:581–590.
164. Chowdhury MH, Tunkel AR. Antibacterial agents in infections of the central nervous system. *Infect Dis Clin North Am* 2000;14:391–408.
165. Richards SJ, Lambert CM, Scott AC. Recurrent *Listeria monocytogenes* meningitis treated with intraventricular vancomycin. *J Antimicrob Chemother* 1992;29:351–353.
166. Weston VC, Punt J, Vloebeghs M, et al. *Listeria monocytogenes* meningitis in a penicillin-allergic paediatric renal transplant patient. *J Infect* 1998;37:77–78.
167. Fong IW, Tomkins KB. Review of *Pseudomonas aeruginosa* meningitis with special emphasis on treatment with ceftazidime. *Rev Infect Dis* 1985;7:604–612.
168. Rodriguez WJ, Khan WN, Cocchetto DM, et al. Treatment of *Pseudomonas* meningitis with ceftazidime with or without concurrent therapy. *Pediatr Infect Dis J* 1990;9:83–87.
169. Kilpatrick M, Girgis N, Farid Z, et al. Aztreonam for treating meningitis caused by gram-negative rods. *Scand J Infect Dis* 1991;23:125–126.
170. Wong VK, Wright HT Jr, Ross LA, et al. Imipenem/cilastatin treatment of bacterial meningitis in children. *Pediatr Infect Dis J* 1991;10:122–125.
171. Donnelly JP, Horrevorts AM, Sauerwein RW, et al. High-dose meropenem in meningitis due to *Pseudomonas aeruginosa. Lancet* 1992;339:1117.
172. Chmelik V, Gutvirth J. Meropenem treatment of post-traumatic meningitis due to *Pseudomonas aeruginosa. J Antimicrob Chemother* 1993;32:922–923.
173. Segal-Maurer S, Mariano N, Qavi A, et al. Successful treatment of ceftazidime-resistant *Klebsiella pneumoniae* ventriculitis with intravenous meropenem and intraventricular polymyxin B: case report and review. *Clin Infect Dis* 1999;28:1134–1138.
174. Nunez ML, Martinez-Toldos C, Bru M, et al. Appearance of resistance to meropenem during treatment of a patient with meningitis by *Acinetobacter. Scand J Infect Dis* 1998;30:421–423.
175. Cruciani M, Navarra A, Di Perri G, et al. Evaluation of intraventricular teicoplanin for the treatment of neurosurgical shunt infections. *Clin Infect Dis* 1992;15:285–289.
176. Radetsky M. Duration of treatment in bacterial meningitis: a historical inquiry. *Pediatr Infect Dis J* 1990;9:2–9.
177. Waler JA, Rathore M.H. Outpatient management of pediatric bacterial meningitis. *Pediatr Infect Dis J* 1995;14:89–92.
178. Tice AD, Strait K, Ramey R, et al. Outpatient parenteral antimicrobial therapy for central nervous system infections. *Clin Infect Dis* 1999;29:1394–1399.

179. Alarcon F, Escalante L, Perez Y, et al. Tuberculous meningitis. Short course of chemotherapy. *Arch Neurol* 1990;47:1313–1317.
180. Jacobs RF, Sunakorn P, Chotpitayasunonah T, et al. Intensive short course chemotherapy for tuberculous meningitis. *Pediatr Infect Dis J* 1992;11:194–198.
181. Tunkel AR. Chronic meningitis. *Curr Infect Dis Rep* 1999;1:160–165.
181a. Centers for Disease Control and Prevention. Sexually transmitted diseases treatment guidelines 2002. *MMWR* 2002;51(RR-6):18–25.
182. Hook EW III. Management of syphilis in human immunodeficiency virus-infected patients. *Am J Med* 1992;93:477–479.
183. Bennett JE, Dismukes WE, Duma RJ, et al. A comparison of amphotericin B alone and combined with flucytosine in the treatment of cryptococcal meningitis. *N Engl J Med* 1979;301:126–131.
184. Dismukes WE, Cloud G, Gallis HA, et al. Treatment of cryptococcal meningitis with combination amphotericin B and flucytosine for four as compared with six weeks. *N Engl J Med* 1987;317:334–341.
185. Stamm AM, Diasio RB, Dismukes WE, et al. Toxicity of amphotericin B plus flucytosine in 194 patients with cryptococcal meningitis. *Am J Med* 1987;83:236–242.
186. Pappas PG, Perfect JR, Cloud GA, et al. Cryptococcosis in HIV-negative patients in the era of effective azole therapy. *Clin Infect Dis* 2001;33:690–699.
187. Van der Horst CM, Saag MS, Cloud GA, et al. Treatment of cryptococcal meningitis associated with the acquired immunodeficiency syndrome. *N Engl J Med* 1997;337:15–21.
188. Berry AJ, Rinaldi MG, Graybill JR. Use of high-dose fluconazole as salvage therapy for cryptococcal meningitis in patients with AIDS. *Antimicrob Agents Chemother* 1992;36:690–692.
189. Sharkey PK, Graybill JR, Johnson ES, et al. Amphotericin B lipid complex compared with amphotericin B in the treatment of cryptococcal meningitis in patients with AIDS. *Clin Infect Dis* 1996;22:315–321.
190. Leendera ACAP, Reiss P, Portegies P, et al. Liposomal amphotericin B (AmBisome) compared to amphotericin B both followed by oral fluconazole in the treatment of AIDS-associated cryptococcal meningitis. *AIDS* 1997;11:1463–1471.
191. Powderly WG, Saag MS, Cloud GA, et al. A controlled trial of fluconazole or amphotericin B to prevent relapse of cryptococcal meningitis in patients with the acquired immunodeficiency syndrome. *N Engl J Med* 1992;326:793–798.
192. Saag MS, Cloud GA, Graybill JR, et al. A comparison of itraconazole versus fluconazole as maintenance therapy for AIDS-associated cryptococcal meningitis. *Clin Infect Dis* 1999;28:291–296.
193. Casado JL, Quereda C, Oliva J, et al. Candidal meningitis in HIV-infected patients: analysis of 14 cases. *Clin Infect Dis* 1997;25:673–676.
194. Rodriguez-Arrondo F, Aguirrebengoa K, De Arce A, et al. Candidal meningitis in HIV-infected patients: treatment with fluconazole. *Scand J Infect Dis* 1998;30:417–418.
195. Galgiani JN, Catanzaro A, Cloud G, et al. Fluconazole therapy for coccidioidal meningitis. *Ann Intern Med* 1993;119:28–35.
196. Labadie EL, Hamilton RH. Survival improvement in coccidioidal meningitis by high-dose intrathecal amphotericin B. *Arch Intern Med* 1986;146:2013–2018.
197. Brown RL. Successful treatment of primary amebic meningoencephalitis. *Arch Intern Med* 1991;151:1201–1202.
198. Abzug MJ, Keyserling HL, Lee ML, et al. Neonatal enterovirus infection: virology, serology, and effects of intravenous immune globulin. *Clin Infect Dis* 1995;20:1201–1206.
199. Quagliarello V, Scheld WM. Bacterial meningitis: pathogenesis, pathophysiology, and progress. *N Engl J Med* 1992;327:864–872.
200. McIntyre PB, Berkey CS, King SM, et al. Dexamethasone as adjunctive therapy in bacterial meningitis: a meta-analysis of randomized clinical trials since 1988. *JAMA* 1997;278:925–931.
201. Arditi M, Mason EO Jr, Bradley JS, et al. Three-year multicenter surveillance of pneumococcal meningitis in children: clinical characteristics, and outcome related to penicillin susceptibility and dexamethasone use. *Pediatrics* 1998;102:1087–1097.

202. Prober CG. The role of steroids in the management of children with bacterial meningitis. *Pediatrics* 1995;95:29–31.
203. Lyons MK, Meyer FB. Cerebrospinal fluid physiology and the management of increased intracranial pressure. *Mayo Clin Proc* 1990;65:684–707.
204. Ashwal S. Neurologic evaluation of the patient with acute bacterial meningitis. *Neurol Clin* 1995;13:549–577.
205. Kilpi T, Peltola H, Jauhiainen T, et al. Oral glycerol and intravenous dexamethasone in preventing neurologic and audiologic sequelae of childhood bacterial meningitis. *Pediatr Infect Dis J* 1995;14:270–278.
206. Girgis NI, Farid Z, Kilpatrick ME, et al. Dexamethasone adjunctive treatment for tuberculous meningitis. *Pediatr Infect Dis J* 1991;10:179–183.
207. Schoeman JF, Van Zyl LE, Laubscher JA, et al. Effect of corticosteroids on intracranial pressure, computed tomographic findings, and clinical outcome in young children with tuberculous meningitis. *Pediatrics* 1997;99:226–231.
208. Bach MC, Tally PW, Godofsky EW. Use of cerebrospinal fluid shunts in patients having acquired immunodeficiency syndrome with cryptococcal meningitis and uncontrollable intracranial hypertension. *Neurosurgery* 1997;41:1280–1283.
209. Fessler RD, Sobel J, Guyot L, et al. Management of elevated intracranial pressure in patients with cryptococcal meningitis. *J Acquir Immune Defic Syndr* 1998;17:137–142.
210. Park NK, Hospenthal DR, Bennett JE. Treatment of hydrocephalus secondary to cryptococcal meningitis by use of shunting. *Clin Infect Dis* 1999;28:629–633.
211. Centers for Disease Control and Prevention. Control and prevention of meningococcal disease and control and prevention of serogroup C meningococcal disease: evaluation and management of suspected outbreaks. *Morb Mortal Wkly Rep MMWR* 1997;46:1–11.
212. Schwartz B, Al-Tobaiqi A, Al-Ruwais A, et al. Comparative efficacy of ceftriaxone and rifampicin in eradicating pharyngeal carriage of group A *Neisseria meningitidis*. *Lancet* 1988;1:1239–1242.
213. Harrison LH. Preventing meningococcal infection in college students. *Clin Infect Dis* 2000;30:648–651.
214. Ramsey ME, Andrews N, Kaczmarski EB, et al. Efficacy of meningococcal serogroup C conjugate vaccine in teenagers and toddlers in England. *Lancet* 2001;357:195–196.
215. Black S, Shinefield H, Fireman B, et al. Efficacy, safety and immunogenicity of heptavalent pneumococcal vaccine in children. *Pediatr Infect Dis J* 2000;19:187–195.
216. American Academy of Pediatrics, Committee on Infectious Diseases. Policy statement: recommendations for the prevention of pneumococcal infections, including use of pneumococcal conjugate vaccine (Prevnar), pneumococcal polysaccharide vaccine, and antibiotic prophylaxis. *Pediatrics* 2000;106:362–366.
217. Villalobos T, Arango C, Kubilis P, et al. Antibiotic prophylaxis after basilar skull fracture. *Clin Infect Dis* 1998;27:364–369.
218. Whitley RJ. Herpes simplex virus. In: Scheld WM, Whitley RJ, Durack DT, eds. *Infections of the central nervous system,* 2nd ed. Philadelphia: Lippincott-Raven Publishers, 1997:73–89.
219. Barnes DW, Whitley RJ. CNS diseases associated with varicella zoster virus and herpes simplex virus infection: pathogenesis and current therapy. *Neurol Clin* 1986;4:265–283.
220. Whitley RJ, Cobbs CG, Alford CA Jr, et al. Diseases that mimic herpes simplex encephalitis: diagnosis, presentation, and outcome. *JAMA* 1989;262:234–239.
221. Whitley RJ. Viral encephalitis. *N Engl J Med* 1990;323:242–250.
221a. McCutchan JA. Cytomegalovirus infections of the nervous system in patients with AIDS. *Clin Infect Dis* 1995;20:747–754.
222. Gnann JW Jr, Whitley RJ. Neurologic manifestations of varicella and herpes zoster. In: Scheld WM, Whitley RJ, Durack DT, eds. *Infections of the central nervous system,* 2nd ed. Philadelphia: Lippincott-Raven Publishers, 1997:91–105.
223. Johnson M, Valyi-Nagy T. Expanding the clinicopathologic spectrum of herpes simplex encephalitis. *Hum Pathol* 1998;29:207–210.

224. Rowley A, Lakeman R, Whitley RJ, et al. Diagnosis of herpes simplex encephalitis by DNA amplification of cerebrospinal fluid cells. *Lancet* 1990;335:440–441.
225. Lakeman FD, Whitley RJ, and the National Institute of Allergy and Infectious Diseases Collaborative Antiviral Study Group. Diagnosis of *Herpes simplex* encephalitis: application of polymerase chain reaction to cerebrospinal fluid from brain-biopsied patients and correlation with disease. *J Infect Dis* 1995;171:857–863.
226. Bleck TP. Imaging for Central nervous system infections. In: Mandell GL, Bennett JE, Dolin R, eds. *Principles and practice of infectious diseases: update.* 1995;4:1–13.
227. Schlesinger Y, Buller RS, Brunstrom JE, et al. Expanded spectrum of herpes simplex encephalitis in childhood. *J Pediatr* 1995;126:234–241.
228. Johnson RT. Acute encephalitis. *Clin Infect Dis* 1996;23:219–226.
229. Whitley RJ, Alford CS, Hirsch MS, et al. Vidarabine versus acyclovir therapy of herpes simplex encephalitis. *N Engl J Med* 1986;314:144–149.
230. McGrath N, Anderson NE, Croxson MC, et al. Herpes simplex encephalitis treated with acyclovir: diagnosis and long-term outcome. *J Neurol Neurosurg Psychiatry* 1998;63:321–326.
231. Medical Letter. Drugs for non-HIV viral infections. *Med Lett Drugs Ther* 1994;36:27.
232. Shepp D, Dandliker PS, Meyers JD. Treatment of varicella-zoster virus in severely immunocompromised patients: a randomized comparison of acyclovir and vidarabine. *N Engl J Med* 1986;314:208–212.
233. Tunkel AR, Wispelwey B, Scheld WM. Brain abscess. In: Mandell GL, Bennett JE, Dolin R, eds. *Principles and practice of infectious diseases,* 5th ed. Philadelphia: Churchill Livingstone, 2000:1016–1028.
234. Mathisen GE, Johnson JP. Brain abscess. *Clin Infect Dis* 1997;25:763–781.
235. Heilpern KL, Lorber B. Focal intracranial infections. *Infect Dis Clin North Am* 1996;10:879–898.
236. Sepkowitz K, Armstrong D. Space-occupying fungal lesions. In: Scheld WM, Whitley RJ, Durack DT, eds. *Infections of the central nervous system,* 2nd ed. Philadelphia: Lippincott-Raven, 1997:741–762.
237. Berenguer J, Diaz-Mediavilla J, Urra D, et al. Central nervous system infection caused by *Pseudallescheria boydii. Rev Infect Dis* 1989;11:890–896.
238. Dworzack DL, Clark RB, Borkowski WJ, et al. *Pseudallescheria boydii* brain abscess: association with neardrowning and efficacy of high-dose, prolonged miconazole therapy in patients with multiple abscesses. *Medicine (Baltimore)* 1989;68:218–224.
239. Wilichowski E, Christen H-J, Schiffmann H, et al. Fatal *Pseudallescheria boydii* panencephalitis in a child after near-drowning. *Pediatr Infect Dis J* 1996;15:365–370.
240. Zimmerman RA, Girard NJ. Imaging of intracranial infections. In: Scheld WM, Whitley RJ, Durack DT, eds. *Infections of the central nervous system,* 2nd ed. Philadelphia: Lippincott-Raven Publishers, 1997:923–944.
241. Mamelak AN, Mampalam TJ, Obana WG, et al. Improved management of multiple brain abscesses: a combined medical and surgical approach. *Neurosurgery* 1995;36:76–86.
242. Carpenter JL. Brain stem abscesses: cure with medical therapy, case report, and review. *Clin Infect Dis* 1994;18:219–226.
243. Boom WH, Tuazon CU. Successful treatment of multiple brain abscesses with antibiotics alone. *Rev Infect Dis* 1985;7:189–199.
244. Denning DW, Stevens DA. Antifungal and surgical treatment of invasive aspergillosis: review of 2,121 published cases. *Rev Infect Dis* 1990;12:1147–1201.
245. Sanchez C, Mauri E, Dalmau D, et al. Treatment of cerebral aspergillosis with itraconazole: do high doses improve the prognosis? *Clin Infect Dis* 1995;21:1485–1487.
246. Denning DW, Ribaud P, Milpied N, et al. Efficacy and safety of voriconazole in the treatment of acute invasive aspergillosis. *Clin Infect Dis* 2002;34:563–571.
247. Nesky MA, McDougal EC, Peacock JE Jr. *Pseudallescheria boydii* brain abscess successfully treated with voriconazole and surgical drainage: case report and literature review of central nervous system pseudallescheriasis. *Clin Infect Dis* 2000;31:673–677.

# 7. EYE INFECTIONS

Marlene L. Durand

Eye infections include infections of the globe of the eye (e.g., keratitis, endophthalmitis) and infections of the surrounding tissues (e.g., lid infections, orbital cellulitis). The primary care physician is often the first physician to see a patient with an eye infection, but for conditions other than simple conjunctivitis, an ophthalmologist should be consulted. Many eye infections produce loss of vision if not correctly diagnosed and treated.

## EYELID INFECTIONS

**I. Anatomy.** Each eyelid contains glands of Zeis (sebaceous) and Moll (sweat) adjacent to eyelash follicles (Fig. 7.1) and meibomian glands (sebaceous) within the tarsal plate (Fig. 7.2). The tarsal plate is the fibrous "skeleton" of each eyelid.

**II. Hordeolum**

**A. Clinical characteristics.** A hordeolum is an acute infection of either a meibomian gland (internal hordeolum) or a gland of Zeis (external hordeolum, also called a stye). An internal hordeolum is a painful erythematous papule that points to the inner surface of the lid, whereas a stye forms at the lid margin. The most common pathogen is *Staphylococcus aureus.*

**B. Treatment**

1. Apply warm compresses every 4 to 6 hours.
2. Apply topical antibiotic ointment (e.g., bacitracin) daily at bedtime.
3. If no response, incision and drainage should be considered.

**III. Chalazion**

**A. Clinical characteristics.** A chalazion is a firm painless papule on the inner surface of the eyelid. It arises within a meibomian gland as a result of a sterile inflammatory response to a previous hordeolum or to inspissated sebum. Most resolve within 1 month, but some require an intralesional injection of steroids. A sebaceous cell carcinoma of the eyelid may be mistaken for a recurrent chalazion.

**B. Treatment.** Intralesional steroids (triamcinolone acetonide) or surgical excision may be required.

**IV. Marginal blepharitis.**

**A. Clinical characteristics.** Marginal blepharitis is a diffuse inflammation of the eyelid margins. It is usually due to hypersecretion of sebum by the meibomian glands; superinfection with *S. aureus* may play a role. It may be mild, with only hyperemia and scaling at the lid margins (seborrheic blepharitis), or more severe, with destruction of the lash follicles and tiny lid margin ulcerations (ulcerative blepharitis). It is typically chronic and remitting and may be associated with seborrheic dermatitis or rosacea. Chronic blepharitis is one of the most common conditions seen by ophthalmologists [1].

**B. Treatment.** Gently scrub eyelids with warm water and baby shampoo twice daily. With acute inflammation, apply bacitracin ointment twice daily for 1 to 2 weeks. If there is associated rosacea, give oral tetracycline, 250 mg once daily for several months.

## INFECTIONS OF THE LACRIMAL SYSTEM

**I. Anatomy.** Tears are produced primarily by the **lacrimal gland** (Fig. 7.3). They drain through **canaliculi** into the **lacrimal sac** and then drain into the nose beneath the inferior turbinate.

**II. Dacryoadenitis**

**A. Clinical characteristics.** Dacryoadenitis, or infection of the lacrimal gland, is rare. Acute dacryoadenitis presents as a tender, warm, red swelling of the lateral portion of the upper eyelid. Etiologies include *S. aureus, Streptococcus pneumoniae, Haemophilus influenzae, Moraxella catarrhalis,* and Epstein-Barr virus, mumps, and adenovirus. Epstein-Barr virus can cause unilateral or bilateral dacryoadenitis [2]. Chronic dacryoadenitis is very rare and presents as a painless swelling of the gland. It is most often caused by viruses (e.g., mumps, Epstein-Barr virus, cytomegalovirus, coxsackievirus) but may be due to tuberculosis or syphilis. More common causes of

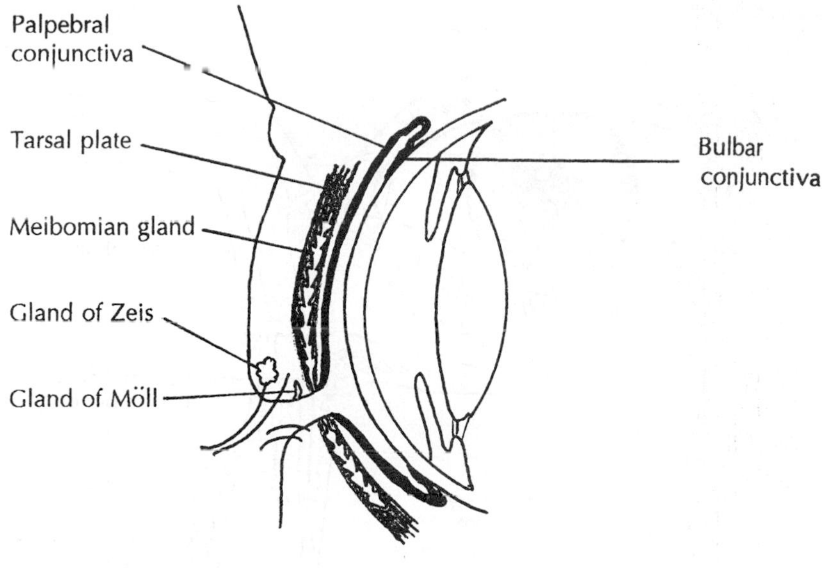


**FIG. 7.1** Sagittal section of the eyelids and anterior eyeball.

chronic enlargement of the lacrimal gland are autoimmune disorders (e.g., Sjögren syndrome or sarcoidosis) and tumors.

**B. Treatment.** For probable bacterial infections, an intravenous (i.v.) antibiotic (e.g., cefuroxime) active against the bacteria listed above is used for the first few days, followed by an oral antibiotic (e.g., cefuroxime or amoxicillin-clavulanate) to complete 10 to 14 days of therapy.

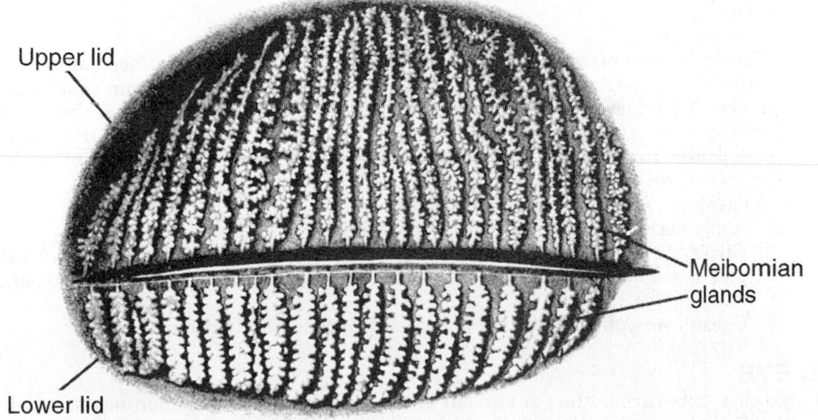


**FIG. 7.2** The meibomian, or tarsal, glands of the eyelids. (From Last RJ. *Eugene Wolff's anatomy of the eye and orbit.* Edinburgh: Churchill Livingstone, 1976, with permission.)

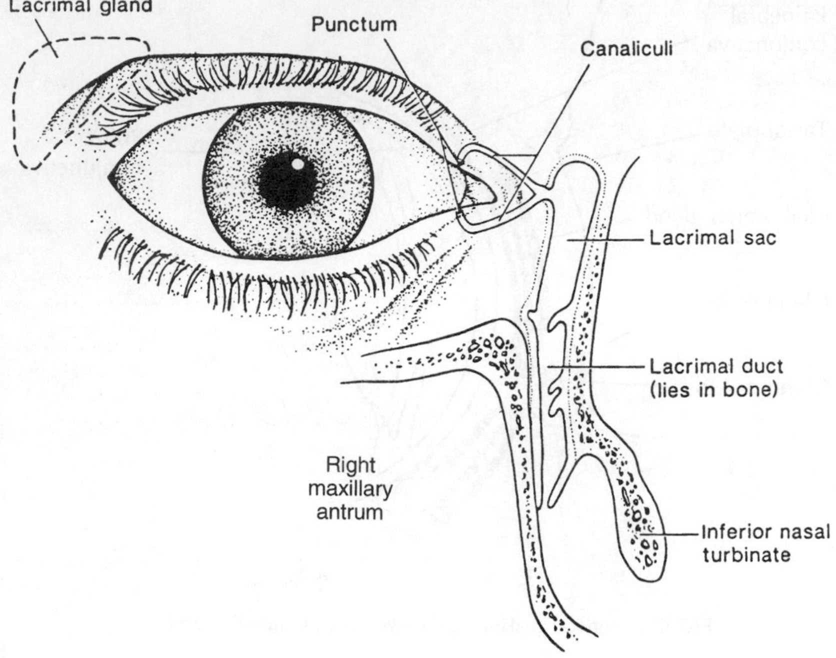


**FIG. 7.3** The lacrimal system. (Modified from Barza M, Baum J. Ocular infections. *Med Clin North Am* 1983;67:131–152, with permission.)

**III. Canaliculitis**

**A. Clinical characteristics.** Canaliculitis is an inflammation of the canaliculi. The puncta are swollen, red, and pruritic ("pouting punctum"), and the involved eye has **epiphora** (excessive tearing). The most common pathogen is *Actinomyces israelii*. Yellow "sulfur granules" composed of aggregates of these organisms may be expressed from the puncta.

**B. Treatment.** Irrigation through the involved punctum (performed by an ophthalmologist).

**IV. Dacryocystitis**

**A. Clinical characteristics.** The most common infection of the lacrimal system is acute dacryocystitis (lacrimal sac infection). It usually results from obstruction of the lacrimal duct. The patient typically has epiphora for several months and then develops a painful, red, swollen, fluctuant area in the nasal corner of the eye. Common causes are *S. aureus, Streptococcus pyogenes, S. pneumoniae* (in infants), and *H. influenzae* (in children).

**B. Treatment**

1. Apply warm compresses every 2 to 4 hours.
2. Give systemic antibiotics for *S. aureus* and streptococci and, in children, for those plus *S. pneumoniae* and *H. influenzae* (e.g., Augmentin or i.v. Unasyn, depending on severity).
3. Consult an ophthalmologist for possible incision and drainage.

## RED EYE

**Red eye** is a sign rather than a clinical entity. It is the most common ocular condition presenting to primary care physicians. Although it may be due to nonspecific conjunctivitis, a red eye may be the first sign of a serious eye condition. Conjunctivitis is **not** characterized by a decrease in vision or deep eye pain. If these symptoms are present, the patient should

Table 7.1. Differential Diagnosis of the Common Causes of an Acute Red Eye

| | Conjunctivitis | Iritis[a] | Glaucoma[b] | Corneal Trauma/Infection |
|---|---|---|---|---|
| Incidence | Extremely common | Common | Uncommon | Common |
| Discharge | Moderate to copious | None | None | Watery or purulent |
| Vision | No effect | Slightly blurred | Markedly blurred | Usually blurred |
| Pain | None | Moderate | Severe | Moderate to severe |
| Conjunctival injection | Diffuse; more toward fornices | Mainly circumcorneal | Diffuse | Diffuse |
| Cornea | Clear | Usually clear | Steamy | Change in clarity related to cause |
| Pupil size | Normal | Small | Moderately dilated and fixed | Normal |
| Pupillary light response | Normal | Poor | None | Normal |
| Intraocular pressure | Normal | Normal | Elevated | Normal |
| Smear | Causative organisms | No organisms | No organisms | Organisms found only in corneal ulcers due to infection |

[a] Acute anterior uveitis.
[b] Angle-closure glaucoma.
From Vaughan D, Asbury T, Riordan-Eva P, eds. *General ophthalmology*, 13th ed. Norwalk, CT: Appleton & Lange, 1992, with permission.

see an ophthalmologist immediately. Table 7.1 lists the differential diagnoses of an inflamed eye. Note the redness of conjunctivitis, due to dilation of the superficial conjunctival vessels, is most intense peripherally. Redness that is most intense centrally around the corneal edge (paralimbal injection or "ciliary flush") is due to dilation of a deeper episcleral vascular plexus and indicates serious eye disease.

## CONJUNCTIVITIS

Infectious conjunctivitis is the most common eye infection seen by the primary care physician. Distinguishing viral from bacterial conjunctivitis is difficult. Equally important is distinguishing these from other causes of red eye, as noted earlier. Most cases of acute conjunctivitis occur in young children, in whom *H. influenzae, S. pneumoniae,* and adenoviruses account for most cases [3]. Chlamydiae are intracellular bacteria, but for purposes of clarity chlamydial and bacterial infections are considered separately below.

I. **Anatomy.** The conjunctiva (Fig. 7.1) is a thin translucent mucous membrane that lines the eyelids (palpebral conjunctiva) and covers the anterior sclera, or "whites of the eyes" (bulbar conjunctiva). It does not cover the cornea but merges with the corneal epithelium at the **limbus** (corneal–scleral border). Goblet cells scattered in the conjunctiva add mucus to the tear film that lubricates the eye.

II. **General clinical characteristics.** Symptoms of conjunctivitis are similar regardless of etiology. Initially, there is mild to moderate unilateral discomfort—itching, burning, and discharge—that within a few days spreads to the other eye (except in hyperacute conjunctivitis, when symptoms progress rapidly).

 A. **Significant pain is not present.** A painful red eye suggests a different diagnosis.
 B. **True visual impairment is not present.** A thick conjunctival discharge may cloud vision, but this clears with blinking.

**C. Distinction between viral and bacterial conjunctivitis.** Viral conjunctivitis typically has a minimal conjunctival discharge that is clear, has follicles that are visible in the palpebral conjunctiva, and often has preauricular adenopathy. In bacterial conjunctivitis, discharge is thick and causes lids to stick together in the morning, the palpebral conjunctiva has papillae but not follicles, and preauricular adenopathy is absent.

1. **Follicles** are foci of lymphoid hyperplasia within the palpebral conjunctiva that give it a pebbly appearance. They are typical of viral or chlamydial infections. Children younger than 3 years lack conjunctival lymphoid tissue. Follicles do not form.
2. **Papillae** may be similar to follicles in appearance, but papillae have a central tuft of blood vessels seen with magnification and follicles are encircled by a blood vessel. Fine papillae, characteristic of bacterial or chlamydial infection, give the palpebral conjunctiva a smooth, red, velvety appearance. Giant papillae suggest a type of allergic conjunctivitis (vernal keratoconjunctivitis) or a reaction to contact lenses.

**III. Viral conjunctivitis**

**A. Clinical characteristics.** Viral is more common than bacterial conjunctivitis in developed countries. Preauricular lymphadenopathy, conjunctival follicles, and a thin watery discharge are characteristic of viral conjunctivitis.

1. **Adenovirus** is the most common cause of viral conjunctivitis. There are three manifestations. **Nonspecific follicular conjunctivitis** is the typical mild adenoviral conjunctivitis that resolves in 7 to 10 days. **Pharyngoconjunctival fever** is most often caused by serotypes 3, 4, and 7. It is transmitted through respiratory droplets, fomites, or through poorly chlorinated swimming pools. After an incubation period of 5 to 12 days, patients develop fever, pharyngitis, and conjunctivitis first in one eye followed in 1 to 3 days by disease in the other. **Epidemic keratoconjunctivitis (EKC)** is most often caused by serotypes 8 and 19. It is highly contagious. Outbreaks have originated in eye clinics [4]. Virus may by transmitted by unwashed hands [5] and can persist on doorknobs for up to 2 months. Incubation period is about 8 days. EKC usually affects young adults during fall and winter months, and in contrast with pharyngoconjunctival fever, conjunctivitis is unilateral in two-thirds of patients. There are no associated systemic symptoms. EKC is often painful due to corneal involvement (keratitis) in (80%) that occurs after 6 to 10 days [6]. Although conjunctivitis and pain resolve in 2 to 3 weeks, the keratitis may cause photophobia and decreased vision for months.
2. **Herpes simplex virus** (HSV) is a rare cause of follicular conjunctivitis alone, because it usually involves the cornea as well. It may be mistaken for EKC in the acute stage [7]. However, in HSV herpetic vesicles may often be found on the eyelids and lid margins (see section III under Infectious Keratitis and Chapter 4).
3. **Acute hemorrhagic conjunctivitis** is caused primarily by highly contagious enterovirus type 70 and a variant of coxsackievirus type A24. Recent outbreaks have occurred primarily in humid climates (e.g., India, Singapore). A large outbreak occurred in fall 1998 in the U.S. Virgin Islands [8]. The incubation period is short (8 to 48 hours), and disease lasts 5 to 7 days. It is characterized by subconjunctival hemorrhages, marked eyelid edema, tearing, and foreign body sensation.
4. **Molluscum contagiosum** is caused by an unidentified pox virus and is more common in patients infected with human immunodeficiency virus. The umbilicated lesions are common on the eyelids and may cause a chronic follicular conjunctivitis.
5. **Miscellaneous.** Conjunctivitis may be a component of other viral infections, such as influenza, varicella, rubella, rubeola, infectious mononucleosis, cytomegalovirus, and herpes zoster ophthalmicus. The conjunctival inflammation in these conditions, however, is usually a minor manifestation of a more generalized infection.

**B. Diagnosis** is based on clinical features (Table 7.2), although distinguishing viral from bacterial conjunctivitis may be difficult. Viral cultures are rarely indicated in

Table 7.2. Features That Distinguish the Common Causes of Conjunctivitis

| Feature | Bacterial Conjunctivitis | Viral Conjunctivitis | Chlamydial Conjunctivitis |
|---|---|---|---|
| Conjunctival injection | Moderately severe | Minimal | Absent or minimal |
| Exudate | Moderate to profuse (polymorphonuclear) | Minimal (usually mononuclear) | Minimal in adults, copious in newborns |
| Sticking of lids on awakening | Yes | No | Absent in adults, present in newborns |
| Papillae (palpebral conjunctiva) | Present | Usually absent | May be present |
| Follicles (palpebral conjunctiva) | Usually absent | Present | Present in adults, absent in newborns |
| Preauricular lymphadenopathy | Absent | Present | Present in adults, absent in newborns |
| Response to antibiotic therapy | Yes | No | Yes |
| Duration of untreated disease | Up to several weeks | Several weeks | Persistent |

From Baum J, Barza M. Infections of the eye. In: Gorbach SL, Bartlett JG, Blacklow NR, eds. *Infectious diseases*. Philadelphia: Saunders, 1992, with permission.

nonspecific viral conjunctivitis but may be helpful in suspected HSV conjunctivitis. In EKC, viral cultures are positive in 80% of patients during the first week of symptoms.

C. **Treatment.** Except for HSV conjunctivitis, viral conjunctivitis without corneal involvement warrants no specific therapy. These conditions usually are self-limited, lasting 7 to 10 days unless bacterial superinfection occurs. Patients should be advised to return immediately if symptoms worsen or if any eye pain develops. They should also be educated about the importance of good hand-washing in preventing spread of the disease to others. Patients with EKC should be advised that the infection is highly transmissible, and they should stay out of work for 2 weeks. They should also be reminded to wash their hands frequently and use a separate washcloth and towel.

**HSV conjunctivitis** may last 2 to 3 weeks. Patients with this diagnosis should be followed by an ophthalmologist. Antiviral therapy, both topical (e.g., trifluridine drops every 2 hours) and systemic (e.g., acyclovir 200 mg five times a day), is indicated.

IV. **Bacterial conjunctivitis**

A. **Hyperacute (purulent)**

1. **Clinical characteristics.** Hyperacute bacterial conjunctivitis is the most severe form of conjunctivitis and usually caused by *Neisseria gonorrhoeae* and rarely by *N. meningitidis*. The patient presents with a purulent exudate that is so copious it reaccumulates as soon as it is wiped away. There is usually marked eyelid edema, chemosis (conjunctival edema), and tender preauricular nodes. A large series of **gonococcal conjunctivitis** found bilateral eye involvement in over one-third and keratitis (corneal infection) in two-thirds [9]. Keratitis may lead to corneal perforation. **Meningococcal conjunctivitis** may mimic gonococcal conjunctivitis but is followed by systemic meningococcal disease in nearly 20% of patients [10].
2. **Diagnosis.** In a patient with hyperacute conjunctivitis, a Gram stain of conjunctival exudate that shows gram-negative diplococci, many intracellular, should prompt immediate therapy for *Neisseria* as soon as cultures are taken. Cultures of exudate should be plated directly onto chocolate and Thayer-Martin plates and these placed in a 5% carbon dioxide atmosphere as soon as possible. If delay in transport is anticipated, use a "Jembec" Thayer-Martin plate and a $CO_2$-generating tablet.

3. **Treatment.** For treatment of neonates, see section VI. For gonococcal conjunctivitis in adults, the Centers for Disease Control and Prevention [11] recommends a single 1-g dose of ceftriaxone (intramuscular or i.v.). For highly penicillin-allergic patients, single-dose therapy with 500 mg oral ciprofloxacin will treat genital or pharyngeal infection and would presumably be adequate therapy for conjunctival disease in adults, although efficacy data are not available. Saline eye drops may be given to clear the exudate. We would also culture and treat for possible coexisting chlamydiae with either doxycycline (100 mg twice a day for 7 days) or azithromycin (1 g orally once) in adults. Patients with meningococcal conjunctivitis should be evaluated and treated for systemic meningococcal disease (see Chapter).

**B. Acute**

1. **Clinical characteristics** include a thick mucopurulent exudate that causes the eyelashes to stick together when the patient awakens. Symptoms usually begin in one eye but become bilateral 1 to 2 days later. In children, the most common etiologies are *H. influenzae* and *S. pneumoniae*. The average age of one large series was 2 years, and conjunctivitis with acute otitis media was seen in 40% of patients [12]. *H. influenzae* was the most common pathogen (60%) in conjunctivitis-otitis cases. Outbreaks of bacterial conjunctivitis may occur, and *S. pneumoniae* that cannot be typed is a common cause. Sporadic cases may be related genetically to outbreak strains [13]. In adults, *S. aureus, S. pneumoniae, and H. influenzae* are etiologic. In one study of adults in a chronic care facility, bacteria were isolated in 38% of acute episodes, and *S. aureus* was the most common pathogen [14]. Gram-negative bacillary infections are rare except in patients with abnormal corneas or patients in intensive care units; *Pseudomonas* is particularly destructive. Unusual causes include *Borrelia burgdorferi* and *Bartonella hensleae*.
2. **Diagnosis.** Conjunctival cultures and Gram stains may be helpful in suspected bacterial conjunctivitis and should always be obtained in patients with severe or hyperacute conjunctivitis and in patients who fail to respond to initial therapy. They should also be obtained in patients who have a filtering bleb from prior glaucoma surgery, because these patients are at increased risk for endophthalmitis (see section VI under Endophthalmitis).
3. **Treatment.** Except for *Pseudomonas,* treatment is topical only (Table 7.3). Ointments can be given less frequently (every 4 to 6 hours) than eye drops (every 2 to 4 hours) and therefore are useful at bedtime but may transiently blur vision after each application during the day. Therapy may be stopped 48 to 72 hours after clearing of signs and symptoms (usually 7–10 days). Patients should be advised to avoid contamination of the ointment tube or dropper tip and to return if they are no better in 2 to 3 days.
   a. **Empiric.** Begin broad-spectrum topical therapy while awaiting culture results. Erythromycin or bacitracin ointments are inexpensive and may be used for mild infection in adults (these cover only gram-positive organisms). Polytrim (trimethoprim and polymixin B) ophthalmic solution is a useful broad-spectrum agent; Polysporin ointment (bacitracin and polymixin B) and sulfonamides (e.g., 10% sulfacetamide or 4% sulfisoxazole) also provide broad-spectrum coverage. Topical gentamicin or tobramycin eye drops have a narrower spectrum and are more irritating to the corneal surface. Quinolone eye drops (e.g., ofloxacin) are well tolerated and provide broad-spectrum coverage but are very expensive. Their use for trivial conjunctival infections is discouraged because of concern for emerging bacterial resistance.
   b. **Gram-positive** infections. Bacitracin (500 units/g) or erythromycin (0.5%) ointments, or any of the broad-spectrum agents listed, may be used for mild infections. Pneumococcal infections may be resistant to erythromycin and may require ofloxacin or levofloxacin eye drops. In severe pneumococcal conjunctivitis due to a highly resistant strain, vancomycin eye drops are indicated, but these must be compounded by the pharmacy because they are not commercially available.

Table 7.3. Some Commercially Available Antibiotic Eye Drops and Ophthalmic Ointments

| Antibiotic | Trade Name[a] | Concentration |
|---|---|---|
| Bacitracin[b] | AK-TRACIN | 500 units/g |
| Ciprofloxacin[c] | Ciloxan | 0.3% |
| Ofloxacin | Ocuflox | 0.3% |
| Levofloxacin | Quixin | 0.5% |
| Erythromycin[b] | (generic) | 0.5% |
| Gentamicin[b,c] | Genoptic, Gentacidin | 0.3% |
| Sulfacetamide sodium[b] | AK-SULF, Cetamide | 10% |
| Sulfacetamide sodium[c] | Ocu-Sul-10,-15; 30 | 10%, 15%, 30% |
| Sulfisoxazole diolamine[c] | Gantrisin | 4% |
| Tetracycline[b,c] | Achromycin | 1% |
| Tobramycin[b,c] | Tobrex | 0.3% |
| Combinations | | |
| Bacitracin and polymyxin B[b] | Polysporin | — |
| Neomycin, polymyxin B, and bacitracin[b] *or* gramicidin[c] | Neosporin | — |
| Trimethoprim and polymyxin B[c] | Polytrim | — |

[a] The trade name list is not all-inclusive. In addition, most of these antibiotics are available also as generic preparations.
[b] Ointment available.
[c] Solution (eyedrops) available.

c. **Gram-negative** infections. Use ciprofloxacin or an aminoglycoside. Because of high local concentrations achieved by topical application, aminoglycosides also provide some coverage of *S. aureus* (but not streptococci).

C. **Chronic**

1. **Clinical characteristics.** Chronic conjunctivitis may be divided into follicular and nonfollicular. Nonfollicular is usually caused by *S. aureus* or occasionally *Moraxella lacunata*. It is often associated with chronic blepharitis. Anaerobes are a rare cause of chronic conjunctivitis. Chronic follicular conjunctivitis is usually caused by *Chlamydia trachomatis* (see below). Chronic conjunctivitis may also have a noninfectious etiology, such as allergic conjunctivitis.
2. **Diagnosis.** Gram staining and cultures (including anaerobic) will identify the underlying pathogen.
3. **Treatment** should be guided by culture results (see section B.3). Eyelid hygiene is important if there is blepharitis. Evaluation of the lacrimal system (for organism reservoir) may be indicated if symptoms recur.

V. **Chlamydial conjunctivitis.** ***C. trachomatis*** is responsible for two distinct ocular syndromes: trachoma, a blinding disease, and inclusion conjunctivitis, a relatively benign infection. Trachoma is caused by serotypes A–C, inclusion conjunctivitis by types D–K. Inclusion conjunctivitis occurs in sexually active adults and neonates; the neonatal disease is discussed in section VI.

A. **Trachoma**

1. **Clinical characteristics.** Trachoma blinds 4.9 million people and is the second most common cause (after cataracts) of blindness in the world [15]. It is endemic in areas of Africa (e.g., Egypt, The Gambia, Tanzania), the Middle East (e.g., Saudi Arabia), and northern India. Initial infection may heal spontaneously, but blindness occurs only after many years of infection and reinfection that causes corneal vascularization and scarring. Person-to-person contact and flies are the major modes of transmission. Young children are the main reservoir for infection, and women are much more likely to have severe trachoma than men, probably because of their contact with children.

   Trachoma has four stages: conjunctivitis, corneal vascularization, scarring, and scar retraction. Chronic recurrent follicular conjunctivitis, involving the upper eyelid and extending to the cornea, is typical of trachoma and is rare in other ocular conditions.

2. **Diagnosis.** Giemsa stain, but not Gram stain, shows typical basophilic cytoplasmic inclusion bodies in conjunctival epithelial cells. However, the direct fluorescent monoclonal antibody stain [6] (e.g., MicroTrak), enzyme immunoassay (e.g., Chlamydiazyme), or DNA probe (e.g., ligase chain reaction) are more sensitive (87%–100%). Reference laboratories can isolate organisms but not routine media.
3. **Treatment.** The World Health Organization Global Alliance for the Elimination of Trachoma by the Year 2020 has adopted the "SAFE" strategy: surgery, antibiotic treatment, promotion of facial cleanliness, and environmental changes [16]. Village-wide treatment with azithromycin, one dose weekly for 3 weeks, resulted in a 64% to 93% decrease in village-wide prevalence rates at 1 year follow-up in three villages, a reduction superior to that achieved by 6-week daily therapy with 1% topical tetracycline [17].

**B. Adult inclusion conjunctivitis**

1. **Clinical characteristics.** Occurring in sexually active adolescents and adults, adult inclusion conjunctivitis is typically a low-grade, chronic, bilateral follicular conjunctivitis with a minimal mucopurulent discharge. It begins 2 to 19 days after exposure to infected genital or urinary tract secretions and occurs in approximately 1 in 300 patients with genital chlamydial infections. Indirect transmission in poorly chlorinated swimming pools may occur. Conjunctival follicles are present as in trachoma, but there is greater involvement of the **lower palpebral conjunctiva,** and preauricular adenopathy is more common. Moreover, the macropannus and scarring of trachoma are not present.
2. **Diagnosis.** See section V.A.2.
3. **Treatment.** Use oral erythromycin (500 mg four times a day) or a doxycycline (100 mg twice a day) for 2 weeks in adults. Azithromycin has been used as single-dose therapy for genital infections, but efficacy data for treating conjunctivitis are unavailable. Untreated inclusion conjunctivitis may lead to chronic follicular conjunctivitis lasting 3 to 12 months and to subepithelial corneal infiltrates.

**VI. Ophthalmia neonatorum.** Ophthalmia neonatorum (ON) refers to any conjunctival inflammation in the newborn. Most cases occur in the first 2 weeks of life. Chlamydiae are the most common infectious cause of ON, but gonococci are the most serious. Silver nitrate eye drops, tetracycline ointment, or erythromycin ointment all are equally effective in preventing gonococcal ON and equally poor at preventing chlamydial ON. In a study from Kenya, a 2.5% ophthalmic solution of povidone-iodine as prophylaxis against ON was more effective, less toxic, and less expensive than silver nitrate or erythromycin [18].

**A. General guidelines.** Because gonococcal infections are rapidly **destructive, consider conjunctivitis in the newborn as an ophthalmic emergency and obtain prompt ophthalmologic consultation.** Do not rely on the timing of the infection or the clinical appearance alone to make a specific diagnosis: There is too much overlap with other conditions. Obtain Gram stain, immunofluorescent stain for chlamydiae, routine cultures, and culture on chocolate and Thayer-Martin media for *N. gonorrhoeae.* If the stains are not diagnostic, begin topical erythromycin empirically while awaiting culture results.

**B. Chlamydial conjunctivitis** (neonatal inclusion conjunctivitis)

1. **Clinical characteristics.** Onset is classically 5 to 14 days after birth. There may be unilateral or bilateral involvement, with conjunctival hyperemia, eyelid edema, and profuse exudate. Newborns lack lymphoid tissue and fail to develop an acute follicular conjunctivitis, which is typical of the adult infection. *C. trachomatis* types D–K are responsible (as is true for adult inclusion conjunctivitis).
2. **Diagnosis.** See section V.A.2. Polymerase chain reaction may be as sensitive and specific as culture, though much faster, in detecting *C. trachomatis* in conjunctival and nasopharyngeal specimens from infants with conjunctivitis [19].
3. **Treatment.** Oral erythromycin (50 mg/kg/day in divided doses) for 10 to 14 days is the preferred agent. It eradicates nasopharyngeal carriage 80% of the time, and a second course may be necessary [11]. Topical erythromycin therapy may be

omitted if it is not tolerated. Parents should be treated for presumed chlamydial genital infection.

C. **Gonococcal conjunctivitis**
   1. **Clinical characteristics.** Onset is on days 2 to 5. Initially, the exudate may be serosanguineous, frequently bilateral, with marked purulence and chemosis. Complications are rare with adequate therapy but include corneal ulceration and endophthalmitis.
   2. **Diagnosis.** If the Gram stain shows gram-negative diplococci (many intracellular), the infant should be hospitalized, immediately evaluated for systemic disease (arthritis, meningitis, sepsis), and started on therapy as soon as cultures are obtained.
   3. **Treatment.** Although a single-dose of ceftriaxone (25 to 50 mg/kg intramuscularly or intravenously; maximum 125 mg) is effective for gonococcal ON, we recommend daily therapy at this dose for at least 72 hours to ensure that cerebrospinal fluid and blood cultures are negative. Cefotaxime (50 to 100 mg/kg/day divided every 12 hours) may be used instead of ceftriaxone in neonates with hyperbilirubinemia. Prompt ophthalmologic consultation should be obtained in all cases. Parents should be evaluated and treated for genital disease.

D. **Other infections.** ***S. aureus*** infection has a variable onset (usually days 4 to 7) and results in an acute purulent conjunctivitis that is diagnosed by culture and Gram stain (in the absence of other detectable ocular pathogens). Topical erythromycin generally is effective for minor infections. For more serious infections, a systemic semisynthetic penicillin (e.g., oxacillin) for 7 days is suggested. (See Chapter 3, Table 3.2 for dosages of systemic antibiotics in neonates.) **HSV type 2** may cause a bilateral conjunctivitis in 15% to 20% of infected infants and may precede or follow dissemination. Onset occurs on days 2 to 14 postpartum. Treatment is with systemic acyclovir and topical antiviral therapy.

E. **Chemical conjunctivitis** is the most common noninfectious cause of ON, occurring in 90% of infants treated with prophylactic silver nitrate drops. The appearance of inflammation (eyelid edema, conjunctival hyperemia, watery discharge) within 24 hours of prophylaxis is diagnostic. Smears and cultures are negative. It resolves (without treatment) in 24 to 48 hours.

## INFECTIOUS KERATITIS (INFECTION OF THE CORNEA)

**Infectious keratitis,** or infection of the cornea, can lead to loss of vision either because of the resulting corneal scarring or because of progression to perforation and endophthalmitis. These infections **should be managed by an ophthalmologist.** Recognition of corneal disease is the primary function of the generalist.

I. **Anatomy.** The cornea is the 1-mm-thick clear "window" of the eye that has a major role in focusing light: It accounts for almost three-fourths of the total refractive power of the eye. It has no blood vessels but has many sensory nerve fibers (cranial nerve V). It is composed of three layers: the epithelium, stroma or interstitium, and endothelium. The corneal epithelium is five cell layers thick and serves as a barrier to infection. Breaks in the epithelium may lead to bacterial invasion of the corneal stroma.

II. **General principles.** Keratitis may involve only the epithelium (epithelial keratitis), the stroma (interstitial keratitis), or both (ulcerative keratitis). The **major signs and symptoms** of acute keratitis are a **unilateral red eye** with **pain, photophobia, tearing, decreased vision, and a corneal defect.** A **hypopyon** (visible layer of pus in the anterior chamber) may be present and, in keratitis but not endophthalmitis, represents a sterile inflammatory response rather than intraocular infection. The cornea often appears cloudy due to corneal edema. In eyes with large corneal ulcers, the ulcer appears as a white defect in the corneal surface and may be seen with a flashlight. Some corneal ulcers, however, can only be seen with a slit lamp.

III. **Viral keratitis**
   A. **Herpes simplex.** HSV is the most common cause of keratitis in the United States, with 500,000 cases diagnosed annually. Herpetic keratitis is third or fourth most common diagnosis in patients requiring corneal transplants [6]. Most (95%) cases of HSV keratitis are due to HSV type 1, with the exception of neonatal herpetic

keratitis. HSV 1 is usually acquired in childhood and remains latent in the trigeminal ganglion, which innervates the eye.

1. **Clinical characteristics**
   a. **Primary HSV** keratitis is rare, and the term refers to the first infection with HSV in a nonimmune patient. Patients present with multiple herpetic vesicles on the eyelids and periorbital area of one eye, and keratitis develops in approximately two-thirds of these patients.
   b. **Recurrent HSV** accounts for nearly all cases of HSV keratitis, including **initial episodes.** Patients complain of eye irritation (foreign-body sensation), photophobia, and decreased vision. Initial episodes usually involve only the corneal epithelium. On slit-lamp examination of the fluorescein-stained cornea, the typical branchlike dendritic forms can be seen in the epithelium. There is less discomfort than expected because diminished corneal sensation is part of this condition. **Recurrent episodes** occur in one-third of patients within 2 years of the initial attack. Recurrences may involve only the epithelium, but repeated attacks increase the risk of stromal involvement, which may result in permanent corneal scarring. In one large study, previous episodes of stromal keratitis increased the risk of subsequent stromal keratitis 10-fold [20]. Long-term acyclovir prophylaxis decreases this risk [21].
2. **Diagnosis.** The typical morphologic appearance of a dendritic ulcer (seen best with fluorescein dye) will usually allow a diagnosis, but its absence does not exclude HSV infection (especially in children). Viral cultures or direct fluorescent antibody tests on corneal scraping may confirm the diagnosis.
3. **Treatment.** The patient should be followed by an ophthalmologist. Patients with epithelial keratitis should be treated with oral antiviral agents active against HSV (e.g., acyclovir, valacyclovir, or famciclovir). Topical antiviral agents, such as 1% solution of trifluridine (Viroptic eye drops every 2 hours), idoxuridine (Herplex eye drops every 1 hour), and vidarabine (Vira-A 3% ointment five times daily) may also be used; trifluridine is the most effective. Topical 3% acyclovir ophthalmic ointment, not yet available in the United States, appears to be as effective as trifluridine. Topical steroids are contraindicated in epithelial keratitis but, when used with topical trifluridine, may be helpful in treating HSV stromal hepatitis [22]. Oral acyclovir does not seem to be effective in treating stromal keratitis [23]. Patients with frequent recurrences of HSV keratitis, or with stromal keratitis, should be given chronic prophylaxis with acyclovir 400 mg orally twice a day, because this decreases the risk of stromal recurrences [21].

B. **Herpes zoster ophthalmicus** is defined as herpes zoster involvement of the first (ophthalmic) division of the trigeminal nerve. It is due to reactivation of latent varicella and is most often seen in the elderly. Involvement of the eye occurs in approximately 75% of cases, corneal involvement in 55% [24].

1. **Clinical characteristics.** In 25% of cases, the disease begins with severe unilateral neuralgia. This is followed by typical skin lesions along the distribution of the first division of the trigeminal nerve. A rash on the tip of the nose (Hutchinson sign) signifies involvement of the nasociliary branch of this division. This is said to increase the risk of corneal involvement, although this has not been substantiated by some studies [24]. Involvement of the cornea is often stromal (deep), unlike HSV, which primarily involves the corneal epithelium. Pseudodendrites may occur and may be confused with HSV dendrites. The keratitis often is accompanied by an anterior uveitis (inflammatory cells in the anterior chamber; see under Uveitis, section III). Loss of corneal sensation is common and may persist for months. Herpes zoster and varicella-zoster virus infections are discussed further in Chapter 4.
2. **Treatment.** Oral acyclovir for 10 days decreases the incidence of keratitis and uveitis in patients with herpes zoster ophthalmicus while also decreasing the duration of skin lesions [25]. Acyclovir should be dosed at 800 mg orally five times daily, assuming normal renal function. Valacyclovir 1 g three times a day or famciclovir 500 mg orally three times a day may be used in place of acyclovir.

The role of topical antiviral agents in herpes zoster ophthalmicus is unclear. Topical steroids should not be used except by an ophthalmologist.

**IV. Bacterial keratitis**

**A. Etiology.** More than 30,000 cases of ulcerative keratitis occur in the United States annually [26]. Major risk factor for keratitis in a recent Swiss study were contact lens wear (36%), blepharitis (21%), trauma (20%), and xerophthalmia (15%) [27]. Overnight wear of soft contact lenses increases the risk of keratitis 10- to 15-fold [28,29].

Over 40% of keratitis cases are culture-negative but presumed bacterial. Most culture-positive cases are due to gram-positive organisms (75%–80%) and gram-negative bacilli in 20% to 25% [30]. However, a high proportion of gram-positive isolates in these series are coagulase-negative staphylococci, diphtheroids, and *Propionibacterium acnes,* organisms that may be an ocular surface colonizers rather than pathogens in keratitis. Assuming these are pathogens, the most common organisms are coagulase-negative staphylococci (39%), *S. aureus* (16%), *P. acnes* (9%), *Pseudomonas* (6%), *Serratia* (6%), viridans streptococci (6%), and *S. pneumoniae* (3%) [30]. *Pseudomonas aeruginosa* is the most common pathogen in contact lens-related cases.

**B. Clinical characteristics.** Bacterial keratitis usually presents as a corneal ulcer that is readily apparent as a gray–white well-circumscribed defect in the corneal surface. Patients present acutely with a painful red eye; usually the redness is most intense at the limbus rather than peripherally as in conjunctivitis.

**C. Diagnosis.** When bacterial keratitis is suspected, an ophthalmologist should see the patient immediately and scrape the cornea (under slit-lamp visualization) for Gram stain and culture (aerobic, fungal, and anaerobic, if possible). Because of the paucity of material, the scrapings should be placed directly on slides and culture media in the office and sent to the microbiology laboratory (rather than swabs). Many culture-negative cases will respond to broad-spectrum antibacterial therapy. However, failure of response to therapy in culture-negative cases warrants repeat corneal scrapings or biopsy for culture of organisms including aerobes, anaerobes, fungi, mycobacteria, and *Acanthamoeba* [31].

**D. Treatment.** The patient should be started on empiric broad-spectrum fortified antibiotic eye drops given for the first 24 to 48 hours every half-hour or hour around the clock. Severe cases should be admitted because they may require this regimen for several days. If two different antibiotic drops are used, the second should be given 5 minutes after the first to prevent washout. Frequency can be decreased (especially at night) as the eye improves.

Nearly all antibiotic eye drops used for treating keratitis must be made up by the hospital pharmacy, because they are more concentrated than commercially available preparations (Table 7.4). The exceptions are the quinolone eye drops. These are recent additions (ciprofloxacin eye drops approved 1990, ofloxacin 1996, levofloxacin 2000). It is controversial whether initial empiric therapy should include traditional combination therapy with cefazolin plus fortified tobramycin or a quinolone such as ofloxacin alone. Several studies have shown success rates of 85% to 90% with either regimen [30,32]. The topical quinolones have demonstrated safety and efficacy in adults [32]; safety in children younger than 12 years has not been established. However, we prefer initial empiric combination therapy (e.g., vancomycin plus tobramycin) for severe cases requiring hospitalization, particularly if the patient is using a quinolone eye drop at the time of admission. Ciprofloxacin-resistant bacterial keratitis cases have been reported, and resistance may be increasing [33]. Once cultures are positive, therapy can be tailored to the organism (Table 7.5).

Systemic antibiotics are rarely indicated, except for deep corneal ulcers with impending perforation or extension into the sclera. Choice of antibiotic should be made based on culture result.

**V. Fungal keratitis**

**A. Etiology.** Fungal keratitis (keratomycosis) is rare in the United States and Europe but common in tropical countries such as India. In the United States keratomycosis comprises less than 2% of infectious keratitis cases, and most cases of mold keratitis

Table 7.4. Concentration of Fortified Topical Antibiotic Solutions (Eye Drops) Used to Treat Bacterial Corneal Ulcers (Keratitis)

| Antibiotic[a] | Concentration |
|---|---|
| Amikacin | 20 mg/mL |
| Cefazolin | 33, 50, or 133 mg/mL |
| Chloramphenicol[b] | 5 mg/mL (0.5%)[c] |
| Ciprofloxacin[b] | 3 mg/mL (0.3%) |
| Gentamicin | 14 mg/mL |
| Levofloxacin | 5 mg/mL (0.5%) |
| Ofloxacin | 3 mg/mL (0.3%) |
| Ticarcillin | 6 mg/mL |
| Tobramycin | 14 mg/mL |
| Vancomycin | 14 or 25 mg/mL |

[a] Start with a loading dose of 1 drop/min for 5 min, then 1 drop q30 min.
[b] Available commercially at this concentration. All others must be made up by the hospital pharmacist.
[c] Concentrations may be expressed either as milligrams per milliliter or as a percentage: 10 mg/mL = 1%.

occur in the South. Many different fungi cause keratitis; *Aspergillus, Fusarium,* and *Candida* have been most commonly reported, with *Candida* predominating in northern climates and *Fusarium* in the southern United States. Mold keratitis is more likely after corneal trauma with vegetable matter trauma (including from use of nylon-line lawn trimmers) [34], whereas *Candida* species are more likely pathogens in abnormal corneas (e.g., keratoconjunctivitis sicca), where they are often colonizers, especially in eyes receiving topical steroids.

**B. Clinical characteristics.** Fungal ulcers are indolent and usually have a different slit-lamp appearance than bacterial ulcers. Typically, there is a gray plaque-like infiltrate and ulcer with an irregular border, often with several smaller satellites and a sterile hypopyon.

**C. Diagnosis.** It may be difficult to isolate the causative organism. A fungal stain (e.g., calcofluor) should be performed, and corneal scraping should be plated on Sabouraud media for fungal cultures. If initial cultures are negative, repeat scrapings must be done and a corneal biopsy may be necessary.

**D. Treatment.** Mold keratitis is much more difficult to cure than yeast or bacterial keratitis. Topical antifungal therapy should be coordinated with the ophthalmologist (Table 7.6). For *Aspergillus,* give topical amphotericin, possibly with the

Table 7.5. Suggested Therapeutic Regimen for Bacterial Corneal Ulcers

| Etiology | Topical Drops (q30 min) | Systemic (i.v.) |
|---|---|---|
| Empiric therapy | Cefazolin or vancomycin plus ciprofloxacin or tobramycin | If spread into sclera |
| *S. aureus* | Vancomycin or cefazolin (if oxacillin-sensitive strain) | |
| *S. pyogenes* | Cefazolin or vancomycin | |
| *S. viridans* | Cefazolin or vancomycin | |
| *S. pneumoniae* | Vancomycin (or cefazolin if penicillin-sensitive strain) | |
| *N. gonorrhoeae* | Ciprofloxacin | Ceftriaxone |
| *Pseudomonas* | Ciprofloxacin *plus* tobramycin | Ceftazidime or Ticarcillin plus |
| *Moraxella* | Ciprofloxacin plus gentamicin | |
| *Nocardia* | Sulfacetamide | |

Table 7.6. Topical Treatment of Fungal Corneal Ulcers

| Organism | Drug | Topical Concentration |
|---|---|---|
| *Candida* | Amphotericin | 1.5 or 3 mg/mL (0.15% or 0.3%) |
| | Flucytosine | 10 mg/mL |
| | Fluconazole | 2 mg/mL |
| *Aspergillus* | Amphotericin | 1.5 or 3 mg/mL |
| | Flucytosine | 10 mg/mL |
| *Fusarium* | Natamycin | 5% |

addition of 5-flucytosine. For *Fusarium,* natamycin has been more successful than amphotericin. In England, topical econazole has proved useful, but this azole is not available in the United States. Systemic therapy with amphotericin is *not* indicated (benefit uncertain and significant toxicity). Oral itraconazole penetrates the cornea and eye poorly but may prevent scleral extension in peripherally located ulcers due to molds. For *Candida* keratitis, topical amphotericin is recommended, possibly with the addition of 5-flucytosine. Oral fluconazole achieves excellent corneal penetration, and both oral and topical therapy may be useful in treating *Candida albicans* keratitis. If lesions progress on topical and systemic therapy, corneal transplantation (keratoplasty) may be considered early by the corneal specialist.

**VI. Parasitic keratitis**

**A. Etiology.** *Acanthamoeba* is an amoeba that lives in tap water and is the most common cause of parasitic keratitis in industrialized countries. Over 90% of patients with *Acanthamoeba* keratitis wear contact lenses [35]. Patients who wear soft contact lenses or omit contact lens disinfection are especially at risk. The keratitis is usually chronic. Typically, the patient has been treated for several weeks with antibiotics before the diagnosis is considered. Hallmarks include a ring corneal infiltrate, a lack of corneal neovascularization despite chronicity, and severe pain, out of proportion to clinical findings. A ring infiltrate is a late sign, but nearly pathognomonic. Earlier signs include a dendritiform keratitis similar to HSV or a linear infiltrate starting near the center of the cornea and radiating to the limbus (radial keratoneuritis).

**B. Diagnosis. Cultures require special techniques.** Corneal scrapings should be placed in special transport media (Page saline) and on glass slides. In the microbiology laboratory, slides should be stained with calcofluor white to show the cysts and trophozoites. Page saline solution should be plated on nonnutrient agar that is overlain with an *Escherichia coli* "lawn." The amoebae will grow on this media after 48 to 72 hours and may be readily viewed under a light microscope. If these techniques fail, a corneal biopsy should be obtained for pathology and repeat culture.

**C. Treatment.** *Acanthamoeba* keratitis is difficult to cure, and advanced infections may fail medical therapy. Corneal transplant should be avoided in active infection, if possible, as recurrence in the corneal graft is common [36]. The therapy of choice is polyhexamethalene biguanide 0.02% (Baquacil), a cationic disinfectant used as a swimming pool cleaner. Initially, this should be given hourly around the clock. Ideally, a second topical solution, Brolene (propamidine isethionate 0.1%), should be added hourly for double therapy [37]. Brolene 0.15% ointment is useful at night after the patient has improved, when hourly treatment is no longer necessary. Unfortunately, Brolene is almost impossible to obtain in the United States, where it is investigational, but it is readily available in Great Britain. Neosporin drops (neomycin-polymixin-gramicidin) may be used as a second agent in place of Brolene but are much less effective.

**VII. Interstitial keratitis** refers to infection of the corneal stroma (interstitium). There is no surface ulceration, and the corneal appears diffusely cloudy. Only limited agents cause this type of keratitis. The most common are recurrent herpes simplex and syphilis. In the early 1900's, interstitial keratitis was a classic manifestation of congenital syphilis; patients often had no other stigmata of the disease. Interstitial keratitis may occur in either secondary or tertiary syphilis. Therefore, both a nonspecific (rapid plasma reagin [RPR]) and a specific (fluorescent treponemal antibody absorption [FTA-ABS] or trepenema pallidum passive agglutination [TPPA]) test should be obtained, because late syphilis frequently has a negative RPR (all cases will have positive TPPA tests). All patients with ocular syphilis should be tested for human immunodeficiency virus. Interstitial keratitis also occurs in tuberculosis, leprosy, and Lyme disease.

## ENDOPHTHALMITIS

Endophthalmitis means intraocular infection, but in general usage it refers to bacterial or fungal infection of the vitreous or aqueous. In nearly all cases, the vitreous is involved. Because the vitreous is in contact with the retina, retinal destruction may follow. Bacterial endophthalmitis usually presents over 12 to 24 hours, whereas fungal endophthalmitis is typically more indolent. Any type of endophthalmitis can cause loss of vision and should be treated as a medical emergency.

**I. Anatomy.** The vitreous body is a clear gel that fills the posterior segment of the eye (Fig. 7.4). It has a volume of approximately 4 mL. It is not regenerated but may be removed by vitrectomy and replaced with fluid. The aqueous occupies a smaller volume (0.25 mL) and is continuously regenerated, with a turnover time of 100 minutes. Probably because of this rapid turnover, the aqueous is more resistant to infection than the vitreous. The aqueous and vitreous are separated by the posterior capsule of the lens. Breaks in this can lead to "wicking" of the vitreous into the anterior segment of the eye, increasing the risk of endophthalmitis.

**II. Etiology.** Endophthalmitis is divided into six categories. The most common pathogens for each category are noted in Table 7.7 [38]. Organisms gain entry either through surgery, trauma, a filtering bleb, or the bloodstream, most commonly after cataract surgery.

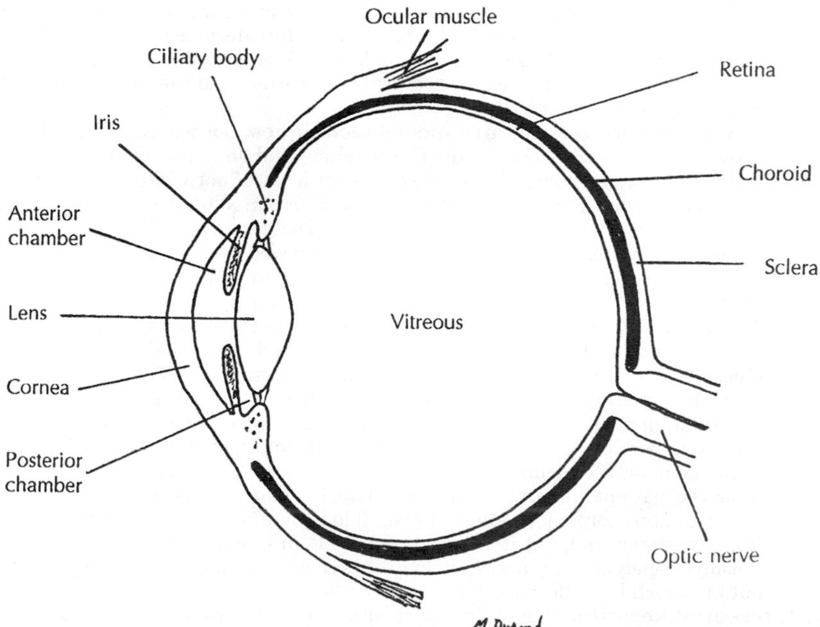


**FIG. 7.4** The globe of the eye.

Table 7.7. Endophthalmitis: The Most Common Pathogens and Recommended Initial Empiric Intravitreal Antibiotics

| Category | Pathogens | Empiric Intravitreal Antibiotics |
|---|---|---|
| Postcataract | Coagulase-negative *Staphylococcus S. aureus*, streptococci | Vancomycin 1 mg plus ceftazidime 2 mg or amikacin 0.4 mg (400 μg) |
| Chronic pseudophakic | P. acnes | Vancomycin 1 mg |
| Bleb related | *H. influenzae*, *S. pneumoniae*, viridans streptococci | Vancomycin 1 mg plus ceftazidime 2 mg |
| Posttraumatic | *Bacillus cereus*, coagulase-negative staphylococci | Vancomycin 1 mg plus ceftazidime 2 mg |
| Endogenous | *S. aureus*, streptococci, gram-negative bacilli | Vancomycin 1 mg plus ceftazidime 2 mg or amikacin 0.4 mg (400 μg) |
| Fungal | *Candida, Aspergillus, Fusarium* | Amphotericin 10 μg |

**III. Diagnosis**

**A. Sampling techniques: vitrectomy versus needle aspirate.** The aqueous can be aspirated by an ophthalmologist (usually a retina specialist) in the office or emergency room by inserting a needle into the aqueous and aspirating 0.1 mL of fluid for culture. The vitreous may also be sampled in the office by needle aspirate, using a 22- to 27-gauge needle, yielding 0.2 mL of vitreous gel for Gram stain and culture. Alternatively, the vitreous gel may be "debrided" through a vitrectomy procedure in the operating room. In this procedure, a 20-gauge vitrector, attached to a ventrui-aspiration vitrectomy machine, cuts and aspirates the vitreous into a collecting cannister, whereas a separate cannula provides continuous infusion of balanced salt solution to maintain eye pressure. A vitrectomy can provide an initial undiluted vitreous sample if a syringe is attached by three-way stopcock to the vitrector tubing, but most of the vitreous is contained in dilute washings in the collecting cannister.

**B. Culture techniques.** Vitreous and aqueous samples are cultured on blood agar, chocolate agar, meat broth, and Sabouraud media. Samples sent in a syringe (usually 0.1–0.2 mL) should be plated directly, whereas the dilute washings (30–50 mL) obtained at vitrectomy surgery should be vacuum filtered through a 0.45-μg filter and the filter paper divided and placed on culture plates. An unusual feature of Gram stains of the vitreous or aqueous is that they may contain **pigment granules** (a "dust" believed to come from the iris in inflammation or trauma). These may **resemble gram-positive cocci on Gram staining,** although they appear more refractile than bacteria and are more often football-shaped than spherical. Gram stains of the vitreous are positive in 50% of cases. Vitreous cultures are more often positive than aqueous cultures, and cultures of vitrectomy washings are more often positive than vitreous needle aspirate cultures (76% vs. 43%) [39].

**IV. Acute postcataract endophthalmitis.** There are over 2 million cataract operations performed in the United States annually, and endophthalmitis occurs in 0.1% to 0.2% of cases. Nearly all cases are due to bacteria that normally colonize the conjunctiva and are introduced into the aqueous during surgery.

**A. Clinical characteristics.** Symptoms develop over 12 to 48 hours, within 1 week of surgery in 75% and within 1 month in nearly all cases. Most patients present with blurred vision (94%), red eye (82%), and eye pain or discomfort (74%) [40]. Patients are otherwise well, afebrile, and have a normal or only slightly elevated white blood count. The eye is injected and has decreased vision. In most eyes (85%), a hypopyon is visible. The view of the retina is poor, obscured by a cloud of intravitreal cells.

**B. Bacteriology.** With rare exception, all cases are bacterial. About 30% have negative cultures. Of the culture-positive cases, 94% are due to gram-positive bacteria: coagulase-negative staphylococci (70%), *S. aureus* (10%), streptococci (9%), and other gram-positives (5%). Gram-negative bacilli cause only 6% of cases [40].

**C. Treatment.** Endophthalmitis is a medical emergency that requires initial empiric therapy as soon as cultures are obtained. Note that the synthetic intraocular lens placed at the time of cataract surgery does not need to be removed. There are three components of therapy, and some remain controversial. Most ophthalmologists have changed their practice of treating endophthalmitis since 1995 as a result of the Endophthalmitis Vitrectomy Study (EVS) [40], a multicenter, randomized, prospective trial involving 420 patients. However, major flaws in this study's design have prompted some to question the results [41].

1. **Intravitreal antibiotics.** The need for intravitreal injection of antibiotics is unquestioned. Vancomycin 1 mg plus either ceftazidime 2 mg or amikacin 0.4 mg are given empirically, each antibiotic diluted by 0.1 mL and injected separately into the vitreous after a vitreous sample is obtained (or at the end of the vitrectomy case). Ceftazidime is less toxic to the retina than amikacin, so is favored by many.

   A single intravitreal injection of antibiotic may not kill all bacteria, however. In the EVS, all patients received intravitreal vancomycin plus amikacin, but some patients who were recultured several days later had persistently positive cultures. Cultures were much less likely to be persistently positive (13% vs. 71%) if the patient's initial procedure was a vitrectomy rather than an aspirate biopsy [42].

2. **Vitrectomy vs. needle aspirate.** Vitrectomy (see section III) debrides the vitreous, analogous to draining an abscess. Until the EVS was published, ophthalmologists performed emergency vitrectomies on nearly all suspected cases for therapeutic reasons. Now, however, most ophthalmologists perform vitrectomies only for patients who present with the worst vision, "light perception," and perform needle aspirates on all others. The EVS randomized patients to receive either a VIT (vitrectomy) or a TAP (aspirate-biopsy) and concluded that in light perception patients, VIT was clearly beneficial. Only 20% of light perception patients in the VIT group were left with severe visual loss, versus 47% in the TAP group. In patients presenting with better vision, there was no apparent difference between VIT and TAP groups. However, this result of the EVS has been questioned because the TAP group was not homogeneous. Only one-third of the TAP group received a needle aspirate, whereas two-thirds had a vitreous "biopsy," performed using a vitrector in the operating room. Critics point out that this biopsy was really a mini-vitrectomy, so that the VIT group and most TAP patients were treated in a similar manner [41]. Of note, within the TAP group, patients who received the mechanized "biopsy" had a much better visual outcome than did patients who received needle aspirate alone [43]. We suspect that if the EVS had randomized vitrectomy versus needle aspirate, vitrectomy may have proven to be beneficial for many patients with endophthalmitis.

3. **Systemic antibiotics.** A blood–eye barrier exists that is similar to the blood–brain barrier. There are numerous studies in animal models of antibiotic penetration after intravenous therapy but few in humans. As in meningitis, inflammation greatly increases antibiotic penetration. Systemic antibiotics that penetrate the inflamed eye well include vancomycin [44], ceftazidime (better than other cephalosporins), and the quinolones (ciprofloxacin and ofloxacin have been studied). Aminoglycosides do not achieve therapeutic vitreous levels. Therefore, before the EVS, i.v. vancomycin plus i.v. ceftazidime had been standard empiric antibiotic coverage for endophthalmitis. The EVS randomized patients to receive either i.v. amikacin plus ceftazidime or no i.v. antibiotics and found there was no difference between the two groups. As a consequence, ophthalmologists rarely give systemic antibiotics for endophthalmitis, and most

publications report that they are not necessary. However, we believe systemic amikacin plus ceftazidime were poor choices for postcataract endophthalmitis (80% of culture-positive EVS cases were caused by staphylococci) and that the benefit of systemic antibiotics is therefore still unknown. One approach would be to treat all patients (after vitrectomy and intravitreal antibiotics) with i.v. vancomycin plus ceftazidime for 48 hours until vitreous culture results are known [45]. If cultures are negative or grow only coagulase-negative staphylococci and the eye is improving, systemic antibiotics could be stopped. If streptococci, *S. aureus,* or gram negative bacilli grow, a 7-day course of systemic antibiotics might be appropriate.

4. **Other therapies.** Topical antibiotic drops are relatively harmless, although their value in endophthalmitis is unknown. Subconjunctival antibiotic injections are also of unknown benefit but carry risk so are not recommended.

## V. Chronic pseudophakic endophthalmitis

**A. Clinical characteristics.** The term "pseudophakic" refers to the synthetic intraocular lens placed during cataract surgery. This type of endophthalmitis is very rare. Unlike acute postcataract endophthalmitis, patients present with weeks to months of mild eye discomfort and mild decrease in vision. Examination reveals mild intraocular inflammation and a white plaque in the residual lens capsular sac.

**B. Etiology.** *Propionibacterium acnes* cause nearly all cases but often fail to grow even with anaerobic cultures.

**C. Treatment.** Vitrectomy and intravitreal injection of vancomycin 1 mg are standard therapy. Systemic antibiotics are not necessary. Removal of the intraocular lens and remnant lens capsule are often required for cure.

## VI. Bleb-related endophthalmitis

**A. Clinical characteristics.** A filtering bleb is created during glaucoma surgery to allow excess aqueous humor to leak out of the eye and to be resorbed by the overlying conjunctiva. This bleb is a defect in the sclera in which only the conjunctiva serves as a barrier between the aqueous and outside world. Occasionally blebs are created as a complication of other types of eye surgery. A bleb is visible on gross examination as a small swelling on the surface of the eyeball, usually beneath the upper lid. Endophthalmitis results when virulent bacteria gain entry into the eye via this thin-walled bleb. "Blebitis" may be the first sign of danger. Endophthalmitis usually develops acutely, often months to years after bleb surgery. Patients present with typical signs of acute endophthalmitis (eye pain, decreased vision). Because of the virulence of the usual pathogens, visual outcome is poor [46].

**B. Etiology.** About 50% of cases are caused by *H. influenzae* or streptococci (viridans streptococci, *S. pneumoniae*); *Moraxella catarrhalis* is a less common pathogen.

**C. Treatment.** Vitrectomy, intravitreal, and i.v. vancomycin plus ceftazidime is used. Simplify once culture results are known.

**D. Prevention.** Because some cases are due to *S. pneumoniae,* we recommend that all patients with blebs are vaccinated with the pneumococcal vaccine.

## VII. Posttraumatic endophthalmitis

**A. Clinical characteristics.** Endophthalmitis develops acutely in 4% to 13% of patients who suffer penetrating eye trauma ("ruptured globe") [47]. To prevent endophthalmitis, prophylactic systemic antibiotics (e.g., i.v. vancomycin and ceftazidime) are usually given for several days after the laceration has been repaired. Risk of endophthalmitis is much higher in lacerations caused by metal objects than by glass or after blunt trauma. Risk is also increased if primary closure is delayed more than 24 hours and if the lens has been disrupted [48]. With patients who develop endophthalmitis, symptoms and signs are the same as for postcataract endophthalmitis (see section IV.A). Onset is usually in the first 3 days for virulent organisms (*Bacillus,* gram-negative bacilli) but may be weeks to months for fungi. *Bacillus cereus* typically produces a ring-shaped corneal infiltrate and a fulminant endophthalmitis, with rapid loss of vision in the affected eye.

**B. Bacteriology.** *Bacillus* species are uniquely important in posttraumatic endophthalmitis, accounting for 15% to 30% of cases. Coagulase-negative staphylococci cause as many or more cases, but infection is much milder. Gram-negative bacilli (e.g., *Klebsiella, Pseudomonas*) or fungi usually cause fewer than 20% of cases. Streptococci were the major pathogens in children in one series [49].

**C. Treatment.** See section IV. **Because of the virulence of the usual pathogens,** we believe all patients should receive vitrectomy, intravitreal vancomycin plus amikacin, and i.v. vancomycin plus either ceftazidime or ciprofloxacin for the first 48 to 72 hours. Vancomycin is effective for *B. cereus*. Once cultures are finalized, antibiotics may be simplified and continued for 7 to 10 days if a virulent organism grows. A repeat intravitreal injection of vancomycin or ceftazidime (depending on culture result) at 48 hours may be necessary for persistent inflammation.

**VIII. Endogenous endophthalmitis**

**A. Clinical characteristics.** Patients with endogenous **bacterial** endophthalmitis complain of eye discomfort and decreased vision; 17% [50] have bilateral eye involvement. Although endophthalmitis may be the initial manifestation of bacteremia, there are often signs and symptoms related to the source of the bacteremia as well (e.g., endocarditis, urinary tract infection, gastrointestinal abscess, cellulitis, meningitis). However, systemic symptoms (fever, chills, weight loss, malaise) were present in only about half of the patients in one recent series [50]. Endocarditis was the most common source of infection (approximately 40% of cases) in this series. Endogenous **fungal** endophthalmitis, usually caused by *Candida,* is discussed below (see section IX).

**B. Diagnosis.** Multiple **blood cultures** should be drawn. Unlike postcataract or posttraumatic endophthalmitis, blood cultures are frequently positive (in 72% of cases [50]).

**C. Bacteriology.** The single most common bacterial pathogen in a recent series [50] was *S. aureus,* causing one-fourth of cases, whereas streptococci (including pneumococci) and gram-negative bacilli each caused about one-third of cases.

**D. Treatment.** Patients should receive vitrectomy and intravitreal antibiotics, in addition to the systemic antibiotics that are indicated for their underlying infection.

**IX. Fungal endophthalmitis**

**A. Clinical characteristics.** Endophthalmitis due to *Candida* usually occurs in the setting of candidemia and is usually due to *C. albicans*. The term "ocular candidiasis" includes both endophthalmitis, in which the vitreous is infected and cloudy, and the more common chorioretinitis, in which tiny white "fluff balls" can be seen in the retina but the vitreous is clear. The distinction is important, because treatment differs. Symptoms are similar, and in both the onset is usually subacute, and patients have decreased vision but rarely eye pain. The eye may be seeded during unrecognized candidemia in hospitalized patients, but the patient may be asymptomatic initially. In one prospective study, 9% of 118 patients with candidemia had chorioretinitis on a screening exam (patients were asymptomatic); no patients had endophthalmitis [51]. Symptoms may not become apparent until weeks later in untreated ocular candidiasis.

Endophthalmitis due to molds (e.g., *Aspergillus, Fusarium*) is very rare and occurs after penetrating trauma, eye surgery, or extension of fungal keratitis. Onset is often weeks after the event. Patients complain of eye pain and decreased vision. The vitreous is cloudy and appears to contain "cotton balls."

**B. Diagnosis.** Vitreous cultures should be sent for fungal stain (e.g., calcofluor) and culture.

**C. Therapy.** For patients with *Candida* chorioretinitis, treatment of the candidemia with systemic antifungals nearly always cures the intraocular infection as well. In *Candida* endophthalmitis, however, a vitrectomy plus intravitreal injection of amphotericin (10 $\mu$g) is indicated in addition to systemic therapy. Systemic amphotericin is indicated for candidemia until the species of yeast is known and then can be changed to oral fluconazole if the isolate is a sensitive species (e.g., *C. albicans*). Treatment with fluconazole should be high dose (400 to 600 mg/day orally) for 6 weeks, with monitoring of liver function tests. In patients with mold endophthalmitis, a vitrectomy should be performed, any intraocular lens removed, and intravitreal amphotericin (10 $\mu$g) injected. Weekly injections of amphotericin may be required. Successful therapy is rare, but systemic amphotericin therapy is

Table 7.8. Uveitis: Classification and the Most Common Infectious Etiologies

| Category | Infection |
|---|---|
| Anterior uveitis | Herpes simplex |
| Iritis | Herpes zoster |
| Iridocyclitis | Syphilis |
| | Tuberculosis |
| Intermediate uveitis | Lyme disease |
| Cyclitis | |
| Vitritis | |
| Pars planitis | |
| Posterior uveitis | Toxoplasmosis |
| Choroiditis | Tuberculosis |
| Chorioretinitis | Candida |
| Retinitis | Herpes simplex, zoster (ARN) |
| | Cytomegalovirus |
| Panuveitis | Syphilis |
| | Tuberculosis |
| | Leptospirosis |

Note that most causes of uveitis are not infectious but are autoimmune or idiopathic. The list of infectious agents refers to each category rather than subcategory.

not indicated because of lack of efficacy. Systemic azoles have not proved useful. Fluconazole has good penetration into the eye but very poor activity against filamentous fungi, whereas itraconazole has good *in vitro* activity against molds but does not cross the blood–eye barrier.

## UVEITIS

**I. Anatomy.** The eye has three concentric coats (Fig. 7.4): (a) a fibrous protective outermost coat composed of sclera (posterior five-sixths) and cornea (anterior one-sixth); (b) the highly vascular **uvea,** composed of iris, ciliary body, and choroid; and (c) the retina. The retina is in direct contact with the choroid, and inflammation of the choroid often involves the retina as well (chorioretinitis).

**II. Classification.** Uveitis classification is confusing because there are different classification schemes [52] and because retinitis is usually included in posterior uveitis, even though the retina is not part of the uvea. Table 7.8 gives one classification. Anterior uveitis includes inflammation of the iris (iritis) or iris and ciliary body (iridocyclitis) and accounts for 50% to 90% of uveitis cases. Intermediate uveitis includes cyclitis (inflammation of the ciliary body), vitreitis (inflammation of the vitreous), and pars planitis (pars plana is the pigmented posterior zone of the ciliary body). It accounts for about 5% of uveitis cases. Posterior uveitis includes inflammation of the choroid (choroiditis) or retina (retinitis) or both (chorioretinitis) and accounts for 15% of uveitis cases. Panuveitis occurs in less than 10% of uveitis patients [52].

**III. Anterior uveitis (iritis, iridocyclitis)**

**A. Clinical characteristics.** Patients usually present with a **painful red eye and decreased vision.** There may be pupillary constriction, photophobia, and tearing. On slit-lamp examination, there are cells and "flare" (protein) in the anterior chamber. The inner surface of the cornea may be speckled with keratic precipitates that are either fine ("granular") or globular ("granulomatous" or "mutton fat" keratic precipitates). The term "granulomatous" is descriptive and does not refer to finding granulomas on pathology. Granulomatous keratic precipitates are less common than granular keratic precipitates and more often associated with sarcoidosis, syphilis, or tuberculosis. Note that topical steroids may change granulomatous keratic precipitates to granular keratic precipitates.

**B. Etiology.** Almost 90% of cases are idiopathic or have a rheumatologic etiology (e.g., sarcoidosis, ankylosing spondylitis, Reiter syndrome). The most common infectious cause is herpes (simplex and zoster), which accounts for 10% of anterior uveitis cases. Rarely, anterior uveitis is associated with syphilis, tuberculosis, or Lyme disease.

1. **HSV** type I causes recurrent anterior uveitis in up to 40% of patients with a history of herpetic keratitis. The virus may cause recurrent iritis or iridocyclitis without active corneal disease. Disease is thought due mainly to the immune reaction to the virus, and treatment with topical steroids and topical trifluridine is effective. The benefit of adding oral acyclovir for iridocyclitis was not clear in a prospective trial [53], although chronic suppressive therapy with acyclovir 400 mg orally twice a day reduced frequency of recurrence. **Herpes zoster virus** may cause an anterior chamber inflammation from iridocyclitis as part of **herpes zoster ophthalmicus,** and treatment is the same as for keratitis (see Infectious Keratitis, section III).
2. **Syphilis** in the acquired form may cause an anterior uveitis, is usually bilateral, and most often associated with secondary syphilis. In two-thirds of cases, the patient has granulomatous rather than granular keratic precipitates. Syphilis may also cause a posterior uveitis (see below) or panuveitis. **This diagnosis should be considered in any patient with uveitis and a positive RPR.** Syphilitic uveitis may also occur in latent and tertiary syphilis, so an FTA-ABS or TPPA should be requested, because many of these cases will have negative RPRs. A TPPA is preferred, as FTA-ABS may rarely be falsely positive in rheumatologic diseases [54]. In patients with ocular syphilis, a lumbar puncture is indicated to rule out coexistent neurosyphilis. Treatment for ocular syphilis is the same as for neurosyphilis (10 days of intravenous penicillin at 24 million units/day) (see also Chapter 16).
3. **Tuberculosis** may cause an anterior uveitis, but a more common manifestation is multifocal choroiditis (see below).

**IV. Intermediate uveitis.** Most cases are idiopathic (70%) or due to sarcoidosis (20%) or multiple sclerosis (8%). Lyme accounts for 0.6% of cases.

**A. Lyme disease.** Lyme disease is rarely associated with uveitis. Some reported cases may be suspect because diagnosis is often based on serology. Uveitis usually occurs in the later stages of the disease. Lyme can cause anterior uveitis, neuroretinitis, retinal vasculitis, choroiditis, and panuveitis, but intermediate uveitis—especially vitreitis—may be the most common manifestation [55]. The vitreitis is often severe and accompanied by a granulomatous anterior chamber reaction and inflammation of the optic disk (papillitis).

**V. Posterior uveitis (including retinitis)**

**A. Clinical characteristics.** Unlike patients with anterior uveitis, patients with posterior uveitis usually have no pain and present with subacute decrease in vision. Toxoplasmosis is the most common cause, accounting for 25% of posterior uveitis cases, whereas cytomegalovirus was common in patients with acquired immunodeficiency syndrome (AIDS) before highly active antiretroviral treatment (HAART).

**B. Viral etiologies**

1. **Cytomegalovirus** produces a retinitis in immunocompromised patients. Though now uncommon, it affected over 30% of patients with AIDS before the advent of HAART (see Chapter 18,19).
2. **Other herpesvirus infections. HSV and varicella-zoster virus** can cause a retinitis but more typically cause a keratouveitis (see section III.B). They are the most common causes of **acute retinal necrosis** . First described 30 years ago, acute retinal necrosis often starts as an iritis and then causes a fairly rapid (days to weeks) destruction of the retina [56]. The retinal destruction characteristically starts in the periphery. In one-third of patients, the other eye will become involved. Treatment with high-dose i.v. acyclovir (10 mg/kg every 8 hours for 2 to 3 weeks) is followed by oral therapy (e.g., valacyclovir for 4 to 6 weeks) to prevent disease in the other eye.

**C. Bacterial etiologies**

1. **Syphilis** was the leading cause of chorioretinitis in the early 1900's but is now uncommon. The most common ocular finding in congenital syphilis is a bilateral

chorioretinitis, whereas a patchy neuroretinitis with retinal hemorrhage is most common in acquired syphilis (seen mainly in latent or tertiary stages). Treatment is as described for syphilitic anterior uveitis (see section III.B.2).

2. **Tuberculosis** was once a common cause of posterior uveitis but is now rare. The most common ocular manifestation is a multifocal choroiditis, with multiple (five to several hundred) discrete lesions in the deep choroid. Vitreitis and an anterior granulomatous uveitis may also be seen. The diagnosis of ocular disease is not difficult in patients with evidence of tuberculosis elsewhere (e.g., in the lungs, lymph nodes, or renal system), because diagnosis may be confirmed by biopsy and/or culture from these other sites. However, ocular disease often occurs in patients with no other manifestations of tuberculosis. In these patients, diagnosis is a dilemma. There is no good diagnostic test for ocular tuberculosis. Cultures of the aqueous or vitreous are negative, and polymerase chain reaction of the vitreous has an unknown sensitivity and specificity. In four of the six cases in the literature with positive polymerase chain reaction for tuberculosis, there were no other manifestations of the disease and diagnosis was presumptive [57]. Biopsy of the choroid can be done but is not indicated because the procedure carries a high risk for loss of the eye. At present, diagnosis in patients with no other evidence of tuberculosis must be based on clinical judgment. Not all patients with a positive purified protein derivative (PPD) and uveitis have ocular tuberculosis, but some do. The diagnosis should be considered in patients with a positive PPD who have classic manifestations of ocular tuberculosis (e.g., multifocal choroiditis). Treatment for ocular tuberculosis should be for 12 months (see Chapter 11).

**D. Fungal etiologies**

1. ***Candida*** In a recent prospective study (see under Endophthalmitis), chorioretinitis developed in 9% of patients with candidemia. Treatment of the candidemia (see Chapter 17) will also treat the chorioretinitis.
2. ***Cryptococcus*** may cause a chorioretinitis. This is almost always seen in patients who also have cryptococcal meningitis (see Chapter 17).
3. **Presumed ocular histoplasmosis syndrome** is a syndrome of bilateral chorioretinal scars ("histo spots"), peripapillary atrophy, and maculopathy seen predominantly in patients who live in the Ohio and Mississippi River valleys of the United States. Although presumed to be due to *Histoplasma capsulatum*, there is no proof of this. No antifungal therapy is indicated.

**E. Parasitic etiologies**

1. ***Toxoplasma gondii*** is the leading cause of posterior uveitis. It produces a retinochoroiditis, usually as a result of reactivation of latent infection. The classic finding of ocular toxoplasmosis is of a yellow-white lesion adjacent to a brown-black retinal scar. The view of the retina is often hazy due to accompanying vitreal inflammation, so the funduscopic exam may have a "headlight in the fog" appearance. In contrast, vitreal inflammation is almost never seen in cytomegalovirus retinitis. In immunosuppressed patients, especially patients with AIDS, the retinal lesions are multifocal and often bilateral, and there may be associated central nervous system lesions. The diagnosis of ocular toxoplasmosis is clinical (i.e., by the appearance of the ocular lesions). There are no good laboratory tests. Serology is usually positive, but this is nonspecific because of the high prevalence of seropositivity in the general population. Serology may also be falsely negative.

   Peripheral lesions that do not threaten vision may not require treatment. Treatment for vision-threatening lesions in adults includes sulfa drugs (e.g., sulfadiazine 1 g orally every 6 hours), pyrimethamine (25 mg/day orally) with folinic acid "rescue" (5 mg/day orally), and clindamycin (300 mg orally four times a day). Prednisone is often added in cases with severe vitreous inflammation and lesions threatening the macula. Sulfadiazine probably is superior to trimethoprim-sulfamethoxazole, although the latter (one Bactrim DS tablet orally twice a day) has been used successfully in immunocompetent patients. Note that patients should have frequent complete blood counts while on pyrimethamine. Recently, atovaquone has been successfully used to treat ocular toxoplasmosis [58].

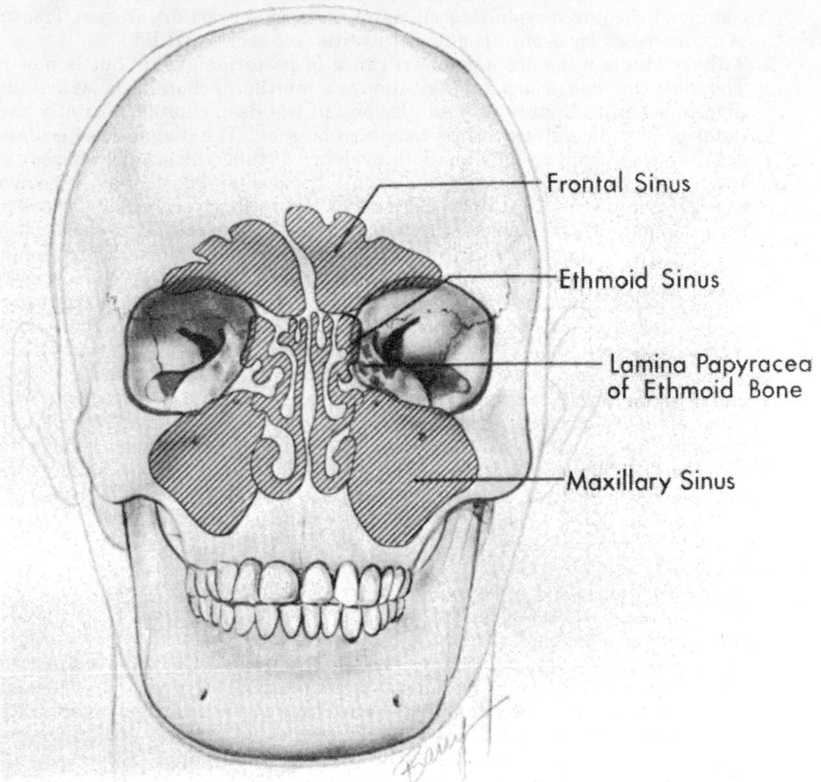


**FIG. 7.5** The paranasal sinuses. (Modified from Lessner A, Stern GA. Preseptal and orbital cellulitis. *Infect Dis Clin North Am* 1992;6:933–952, with permission.)

Because all available therapies treat only the tachyzoites but not the tissue cysts, treatment suppresses but does not cure the infection, and recurrence of ocular toxoplasmosis occurs in two-thirds of patients.

**VI. Other infectious causes of uveitis.** Very rare causes of uveitis include leptospirosis, brucellosis, *Pneumocystis carinii,* Whipple disease, and *Toxocara canis*.

## ORBITAL AND PERIORBITAL INFECTIONS

**I. Anatomy.** The orbit is surrounded by the paranasal sinuses (Fig. 7.5) and the bones of the orbit and the sinuses are shared (e.g., the medial wall of the orbit is the very thin lateral wall of the ethmoid sinus). The globe of the eye fills most of the anterior portion of the orbit, whereas loose fatty tissue and muscle fill most of the posterior part. The **orbital septum** is a fascial layer extending from the orbital rim periosteum to the tarsal plates in the eyelids, and it is a major barrier preventing superficial (**preseptal**) infection from extending posteriorly into the orbit. The orbital veins drain into the cavernous sinus. They have no valves so they freely communicate with the veins of the face and paranasal sinuses.

**II. Etiology.** Most orbital infections (50%–80%) are secondary to sinusitis, usually involving the ethmoid or frontal sinuses. Other orbital infections may follow trauma, surgery, dacryocystitis, or eyelid infections. Figure 7.6, adapted from the classic study by

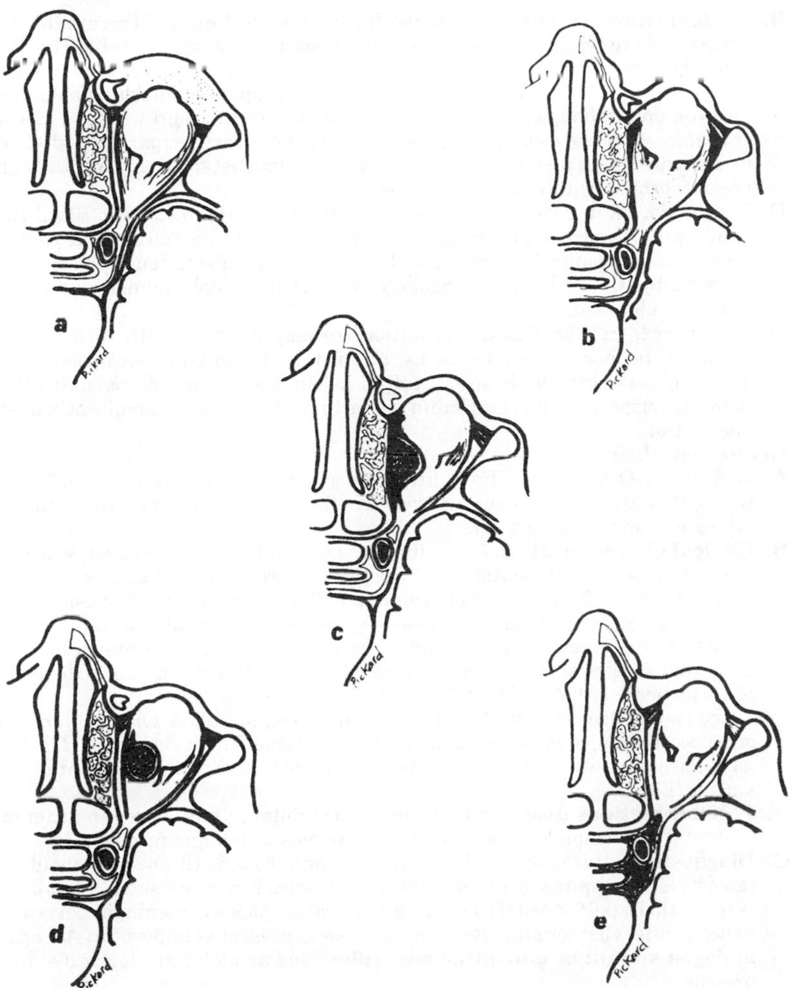


**FIG. 7.6** The five main categories of orbital infection: (a) Preseptal cellulitis, (b) orbital cellulitis, (c) subperiosteal abscess, (d) orbital abscess, (e) cavernous sinus thrombosis. (Modified from Chandler JR, Langenbrunner DJ, Stevens FR. The pathogenesis of orbital complications in acute sinusitis. *Laryngoscope* 1970;80:1414, with permission.)

Chandler, Langenbrunner, and Stevens [59], illustrates the five main categories of orbital infection. With the exception of cavernous sinus thrombosis, ocular findings are nearly always unilateral.

**III. Preseptal ("periorbital") cellulitis**

**A. Definition.** Preseptal cellulitis is an infection that **involves the entire eyelid and surrounding tissues anterior to the orbital septum** but does not extend to the deeper contents of the orbit. Infection is secondary to sinusitis or upper respiratory infection in more than 50% of patients and to eye trauma in 25% [59]. Most patients are children younger than 10. *S. aureus,* streptococci, and *H. influenzae* are the most common pathogens. A mixed infection including oral anaerobes may occur after an animal or human bite to the lid area.

**B. Clinical characteristics. Pain, swelling, and erythema of the eyelid** and low grade fever are typical, although one-third of patients remain afebrile. The distensibility of the periorbital tissues results in severe eyelid edema. It is important to note that there are no signs of orbital involvement: no proptosis (anterior displacement of the eye), ophthalmoplegia (limitation of eye movement), pain with eye movement, or change in visual acuity. Proptosis may not be grossly apparent and should be measured with an instrument (Hertel exophthalmometer). If any orbital signs are present, orbital cellulitis must be considered.

**C. Diagnosis.** As in most cases of cellulitis, there is little to culture. Blood cultures should be obtained, and any draining wound should be cultured. If there is no obvious source, sinus disease should be excluded by sinus radiographs or computed tomography (CT) or by otolaryngology evaluation. An ophthalmology consultation should be obtained.

**D. Treatment.** In mild cases, oral antibiotics may be given with close (e.g., daily) follow-up. In more severe cases, i.v. antibiotics should be given initially and the patient observed in the hospital. Initial i.v. antibiotics include nafcillin (if a skin source is suspected) and ampicillin-sulbactam (if there is concomitant sinusitis or bite wound).

**IV. Orbital cellulitis**

**A. Definition.** Orbital cellulitis is diffuse infection of the orbital contents. Most infections follow sinusitis, but they may occur after trauma, preseptal cellulitis (and its etiologies), or, rarely, surgery.

**B. Clinical characteristics.** In addition to the eyelid swelling, redness, warmth, and tenderness seen in preseptal cellulitis, there is proptosis and pain with eye movement. There is often orbital pain, conjunctival hyperemia, and chemosis (conjunctival edema). Most patients are febrile and have elevated white blood cell counts. As the infection progresses, there is limitation of ocular motility. Orbital abscess or subperiosteal abscess should be considered if there is inferior and lateral displacement of the globe (i.e., the eye looks downward and outward).

The major pathogens are *S. aureus,* group A streptococci, *S. pneumoniae,* viridans streptococci (e.g., *S. intermedius*), and *H. influenzae.* The incidence of *H. influenzae* as a cause of orbital cellulitis has decreased markedly since the advent of the HiB vaccine [60].

1. **Noninfectious diseases** that can mimic orbital cellulitis are rapidly enlarging orbital neoplasms such as rhabdomyosarcoma or malignant melanoma.

**C. Diagnosis.** Cultures of blood, conjunctiva, and wounds (if present) should be obtained. Needle aspiration of the orbital soft tissues is not indicated. A lumbar puncture should be performed if there is any clinical suspicion of meningitis. A cranial CT to determine whether sinusitis or an abscess is present is important. **An ophthalmologist should be consulted regardless** and an otolaryngologist if sinusitis is present.

**D. Treatment.** Intravenous antibiotics should be started as soon as cultures are obtained. Antibiotics that penetrate the blood–brain barrier should be chosen even in the absence of signs of meningitis. Delay in treatment or inadequate antibiotics may result in loss of vision or even death.

1. **Posttraumatic.** A semisynthetic penicillin (e.g., nafcillin).
2. **Postsurgical.** Broad-spectrum coverage (e.g., nafcillin and cefotaxime).
3. After **bite wounds or anaerobic infection.** Ampicillin-sulbactam is suggested. See related discussion in Chapter 4 under Animal Bites.
4. **Sinusitis-related** (or nontraumatic). Nafcillin plus a third-generation cephalosporin (e.g., cefotaxime or ceftriaxone).

**E. Mucormycosis** is a rapidly progressive necrotizing fungal infection of the paranasal sinuses that may present initially as a bacterial orbital cellulitis. There are subtle differences in presentation, however. In bacterial orbital cellulitis, the lids are red, hot, and tender; pain is usually limited to the orbit; and there are no paresthesias (except possibly decreased sensation in very swollen lids). In mucormycosis, the lids are often very edematous, may be faintly pink, but are often not red or hot. Patients with mucormycosis often have pain or paresthesias in the cheek, temple, or forehead where there is no sign of cellulitis, and these symptoms may occur 1 to 2 days before any evidence of ocular or facial abnormality. Mucormycosis is very rare, and most cases occur in insulin-dependent diabetics (70% of cases) or immunocompromised hosts. Patients receiving desferrioxamine chelation therapy are also at risk. The fungus invades blood vessels, causing ischemic necrosis of tissues. It spreads rapidly (in days) from sinus focus to involve the orbit, followed by the cavernous sinus and brain. The **diagnosis** is suspected in the appropriate host by the appearance of an area of necrosis (e.g., black eschar) in the nasal mucosa on endoscopic examination. However, very rarely and in early disease, the mucosa may look normal, but deep surgical biopsy of the middle turbinate will show the invading hyphae [61]. Diagnosis must be confirmed by biopsy of tissue (usually intranasal or sinus), showing the characteristic nonseptate hyphae invading tissue. Therapy is with aggressive surgical debridement and intravenous amphotericin (or liposomal amphotericin).

**V. Subperiosteal abscess**

**A. Definition.** A subperiosteal abscess is a collection of pus between the periosteal lining and the bony wall of the orbit. If pus ruptures into the orbit itself, it is an orbital abscess (see section VI). A subperiosteal abscess usually results from the extension of an infection within a sinus.

**B. Clinical characteristics.** As in orbital cellulitis there is redness and swelling of the eyelids, proptosis, orbital pain, and usually a fever and an elevated white blood cell count. In addition, there is ophthalmoplegia and **displacement of the globe.** Because the ethmoid or frontal sinuses are most commonly involved, displacement tends to be downward and laterally ("down and out"). *S. aureus,* streptococci, and *H. influenzae* are the most common pathogens.

**C. Diagnosis.** Blood cultures should be obtained. Emergency consultations with an ophthalmologist and an ear, nose, and throat surgeon should be obtained as well as an emergency CT (the relative merits of CT vs. magnetic resonance imaging in this setting have not been defined). Sinus cultures obtained endoscopically may be helpful if surgery is delayed. At the time of surgery, aerobic and anaerobic cultures should be obtained and the material should be Gram stained.

**D. Treatment.** As in orbital cellulitis, delay in treatment may result in loss of vision. In most patients, immediate surgical drainage of the subperiosteal abscess and involved sinus should be performed. Intravenous antibiotics should include a semisynthetic penicillin and a third-generation cephalosporin (e.g., nafcillin and ceftriaxone) and should be started as soon as initial blood and sinus cultures have been taken.

**VI. Orbital abscess**

**A. Definition.** An orbital abscess is a collection of pus within the orbit. It results either from a consolidation of infection in orbital cellulitis or from rupture of a subperiosteal abscess. Progression of infection in the patient with orbital cellulitis despite adequate intravenous antibiotics or a decrease in either visual acuity or extraocular movement suggests development of an intraorbital abscess.

**B. Clinical characteristics.** The eyelids are red, warm, and swollen, and there is often marked chemosis. As in subperiosteal abscess, the **globe often is displaced downward and laterally. Eye mobility is severely limited,** and there is usually a marked decrease in vision. Fever and leukocytosis are common. *S. aureus* and streptococci are the most common pathogens. The distinction between orbital and subperiosteal abscess may be difficult to make clinically.

**C. Diagnosis.** Blood cultures should be drawn. **An emergency CT and emergency consultations with an ophthalmologist and an ear, nose, and throat surgeon** should be obtained. At surgery, the abscess material should be sent for Gram stain and aerobic and anaerobic cultures. In immunocompromised patients, smears and cultures for acid-fast bacilli and fungus should also be done.

**D. Treatment.** In this condition, as in subperiosteal abscess, emergency surgical drainage of the abscess is the most important component of therapy. Empiric i.v. antibiotics should be given as soon as possible, however, while awaiting this surgery. Delay in treatment may result in loss of vision. After blood cultures have been taken, empiric i.v. therapy with a semisynthetic penicillin and a third-generation cephalosporin (e.g., nafcillin and ceftriaxone) should be started. Antibiotics should be adjusted when culture results are available.

**VII. Cavernous sinus thrombosis.** Cavernous sinus thrombosis is a very rare but life-threatening complication of orbital infection that can occur when a septic phlebitis of the veins draining the orbit leads to thrombosis of the cavernous sinus. Because the cavernous sinus drains both orbits, thrombosis leads to bilateral eye findings (proptosis, periorbital edema, ophthalmoplegia). Because of the proximity of the cavernous sinus to the meninges, meningeal signs and frank meningitis can also occur. The patient appears very ill and may have papilledema in addition to "frozen" globes. The major pathogens are *S. aureus* and streptococci. Meningeal doses of broad-spectrum antibiotics (e.g., nafcillin, metronidazole, ceftriaxone) should be used. The use of anticoagulants is controversial.

## REFERENCES


1. McCulley JP, Shine WE. Changing concepts in the diagnosis and management of blepharitis. *Cornea* 2000;19:650–658.
2. Rhem MN, Wilhelmus KR, Jones DB. Epstein-Barr virus dacryoadenitis. *Am J Ophthalmol* 2000;129:372–375.
3. Wald ER. Conjunctivitis in infants and children. *Pediatr Infect Dis J* 1997;16 [2 Suppl]:S17–S20.
4. Montessori V, Scharf S, Holland S, et al. Epidemic keratoconjunctivitis outbreak at a tertiary referral eye care clinic. *Am J Infect Control* 1998;26:399–405.
5. Azar MJ, Dhaliwal DK, Bower KS, et al. Possible consequences of shaking hands with your patients with epidemic keratoconjunctivitis. *Am J Ophthalmol* 1996;121:711–712.
6. Pavan-Langston D. Viral diseases of the cornea and external eye. In: Albert DM, Jakobiec FA, eds. *Principles and practice of ophthalmology,* 2nd ed. Philadelphia: Saunders, 2000:847.
7. Uchio E, Takeuchi S, Itoh N, et al. Clinical and epidemiological features of acute follicular conjunctivitis with special reference to that caused by herpes simplex virus type 1. *Br J Ophthalmol* 2000;84:968–972.
8. Center for Disease Control. Acute hemorrhagic conjunctivitis—St. Croix, U.S. Virgin Islands, September–October 1998. *MMWR Morb Mortal Wkly Rep* 1998;47:899–901.
9. Wan WL, et al. The clinical characteristic of the course of adult gonococcal conjunctivitis. *Am J Ophthalmol* 1986;102:572.
10. Barquet N, Gasser I, Domingo P, et al. Primary meningococcal conjunctivitis: report of 21 patients and review. *Rev Infect Dis* 1990;12:838–847.
11. Centers for Disease Control and Prevention. 1998 Guidelines for the treatment of sexually transmitted diseases. *MMWR Morb Mortal Wkly Rep* 1998;47(RR-1):60.
12. Block SL, Hedrick J, Tyler R, et al. Increasing bacterial resistance in pediatric acute conjunctivitis (1997–1998). *Antimicrob Agents Chemother* 2000;44:1650–1654.
13. Barker JH, Musher DM, Silberman R, et al. Genetic relatedness among nontypeable pneumococci implicated in sporadic cases of conjunctivitis. *J Clin Microbiol* 1999;37:4039–4041.
14. Boustcha E, Nicolle LE. Conjunctivitis in a long-term care facility. *Infect Control Hosp Epidemiol* 1995;16:210–216.
15. Whitcher JP, Srinivasan M, Upadhyay MP. Corneal blindness: a global perspective. *Bull World Health Organ* 2001;79:214–221.
16. Pruss A, Mariotti SP. Preventing trachoma through environmental sanitation: a review of the evidence base. *Bull World Health Organ* 2000;78:258–266.
17. Schachter J, West SK, Mabey D, et al. Azithromycin in control of trachoma. *Lancet* 1999;354:630–635.
18. Isenberg SJ, Apt L, Wood M. A controlled trial of povidone-iodine as prophylaxis against ophthalmia neonatorum. *N Engl J Med* 1995;332:562–566.
19. Hammerschlag MR, Roblin PM, Gelling M, et al. Use of polymerase chain reaction for the detection of *Chlamydia trachomatis* in ocular and nasopharyngeal specimens from infants with conjunctivitis. *Pediatr Infect Dis J* 1997;16:293–297.
20. Herpetic Eye Disease Study Group. Predictors of recurrent herpes simplex virus keratitis. *Cornea* 2001;20:123–128.
21. Herpetic Eye Disease Study Group. Acyclovir for the prevention of recurrent herpes simplex virus eye disease. *N Engl J Med* 1998;339:300–306.

22. Wilhelmus KR, et al. Herpetic eye disease study. A controlled trial of topical corticosteroids for herpes simplex stromal keratitis. *Ophthalmology* 1994;101:1883.
23. Barron BA, Gee L, Hauck WW, et al. Herpetic Eye Disease Study. A controlled trial of oral acyclovir for herpes simplex stromal keratitis. *Ophthalmology* 1994;101:1871–1872.
24. Womack LW, Liesegang TJ. Complications of herpes zoster ophthalmicus. *Arch Ophthalmol* 1983;101:42.
25. Cobo LM. Oral acyclovir in the treatment of acute herpes zoster ophthalmicus. *Ophthalmology* 1986;93:763.
26. Pepose JS, Wilhelmus KR. Divergent approaches to the management of corneal ulcers. *Am J Ophthalmol* 1992;114:630–632.
27. Schaefer F, Bruttin O, Zografos L, et al. Bacterial keratitis: a prospective clinical and microbiological study. *Br J Ophthalmol* 2001;85:842–847.
28. Schein OD, et al. The relative risk of ulcerative keratitis among users of daily-wear and extended-wear soft contact lenses: a case-control study. *N Engl J Med* 1989;321:773.
29. Schein OD, et al. The impact of overnight wear on the risk of contact lens-associated ulcerative keratitis. *Arch Ophthalmol* 1994;112:186.
30. O'Brien TP, Maguire MG, Fink NE, et al. and the Bacterial Keratitis Study Research Group. Efficacy of ofloxacin vs cefazolin and tobramycin in the therapy for bacterial keratitis. *Arch Ophthalmol* 1995;113:1257–1265.
31. Ficker L, et al. Microbial keratitis—the false negative. *Eye* 1991;5:549.
32. Panda A, Ahuja R, Srinivas Sastry S. Comparison of topical 0.3% ofloxacin with fortified tobramycin plus cefazolin in the treatment of bacterial keratitis. *Eye* 1999;13: 744–747.
33. Goldstein MH, Kowalski RP, Gordon YJ. Emerging fluoroquinolone resistance in bacterial keratitis: a five-year review. *Ophthalmology* 1999;106:1313–1318.
34. Clinch TE, et al. Fungal keratitis from nylon lawn trimmers. *Am J Ophthalmol* 1992;114:437.
35. Radford CF, Lehmann OJ, Dart JKG, et al. for the National *Acanthamoeba* Keratitis Study Group. *Acanthamoeba* keratitis: multicentre survey in England 1992–6. *Br J Ophthalmol* 1998;82:1387–1392.
36. Ficker LA, Kirkness C, Wright P. Prognosis for keratoplasty in *Acanthamoeba* keratitis. *Ophthalmology* 1993;100:105.
37. Lindquist TD. Treatment of *Acanthamoeba* keratitis. *Cornea* 1998;17:11–16.
38. Durand ML, Heler JS. Endophthalmitis. *Curr Clin Topics Infect Dis* 2000;20:271–297.
39. Donahue SP, Kowalski RP, Jewart BH, et al. Vitreous cultures in suspected endophthalmitis. Biopsy or vitrectomy? *Ophthalmology* 1993;100:452–455.
40. Endophthalmitis Vitrectomy Study Group. Results of the Endophthalmitis Vitrectomy Study: a randomized trial of immediate vitrectomy and of intravenous antibiotics for the treatment of postoperative bacterial endophthalmitis. *Arch Ophthalmol* 1995;113:1479.
41. Flynn HW, Meredith TA. The Endophthalmitis Vitrectomy Study [Letter]. *Arch Ophthalmol* 1996;114:1027–1028.
42. Doft BH, Kelsey SF, Wisniewski SR. the EVS Study Group. Additional procedures after the initial vitrectomy or tap-biopsy in the Endophthalmitis Vitrectomy Study. *Ophthalmology* 1998;105:707–716.
43. Han DP, Wisniewski SR, Kelsey SF, et al. Microbiologic yields and complication rates of vitreous needle aspiration versus mechanized vitreous biopsy in the Endophthalmitis Vitrectomy Study. *Retina* 1999;19:98–102.
44. Meredith TA, et al. Vancomycin levels in the vitreous cavity after intravitreous administration. *Am J Ophthalmol* 1995;119:774.
45. Durand ML. Management of endophthalmitis in the post-Endophthalmitis Vitrectomy Study era [Letter]. *Arch Ophthalmol* 2002;120:233–234.
46. Ciulla TA, Beck AD, Topping TM, et al. Blebitis, early endophthalmitis, and late endophthalmitis after glaucoma-filtering surgery. *Ophthalmology* 1997;104:986–995.
47. Duch-Samper AM, et al. Endophthalmitis following open-globe injuries. *Curr Opin Ophthalmol* 1998;9:59–65.
48. Thompson WS, Rubsamen PE, Flynn HW Jr, et al. Endophthalmitis after penetrating ocular trauma: risk factors and visual acuity outcomes. *Ophthalmology* 1995;102:1696–1671.

49. Alfaro DV, Roth DB, Laughlin RM, et al. Paediatric post-traumatic endophthalmitis. *Br J Ophthalmol* 1995;79:888–891.
50. Okada AA, et al. Endogenous bacterial endophthalmitis: report of a ten year retrospective study. *Ophthalmology* 1994;101:832.
51. Donahue SP, Greven CM, Zuravleff JJ, et al. Intraocular candidiasis in patients with candidemia: clinical implications derived from a prospective multicenter study. *Ophthalmology* 1994;101:1302–1309.
52. Shafik S, Foster CS. Definition, classification, etiology, and epidemiology. In: Foster CS, Vitale AT, eds. *Diagnosis and treatment of uveitis.* Philadelphia: W.B. Saunders, 2002:17.
53. The Herpetic Eye Disease Study Group. A controlled trial of oral acyclovir for iridocyclitis caused by herpes simplex virus. *Arch Ophthalmol* 1996;114:1065–1072.
54. Murphy FT, George R, Kubota K, et al. The use of Western blotting as the confirmatory test for syphilis in patients with rheumatic disease. *J Rheumatol* 1999;26:2448–2453.
55. Baer JC. Borreliosis. In: Foster CS, Vitale AT, eds. *Diagnosis and treatment of uveitis.* Philadelphia: WB Saunders, 2002:245.
56. Walters G, James TE. Viral causes of the acute retinal necrosis syndrome. *Curr Opin Ophthalmol* 2001;12:191–195.
57. Samson CM, Foster CS. Tuberculosis. In: Foster CS, Vitale AT, eds. *Diagnosis and treatment of uveitis.* Philadelphia: WB Saunders, 2002:264.
58. Pearson PA, Piracha AR, Sen HA, et al. Atovaquone for the treatment of toxoplasma retinochoroiditis in immunocompetent patients. *Ophthalmology* 1999;106:148–153.
59. Chandler JR, Langenbrunner DJ, Stevens FR. The pathogenesis of orbital complications in acute sinusitis. *Laryngoscope* 1970;80:1414.
60. Donahue SP, Schwartz G. Preseptal and orbital cellulitis in childhood. A changing microbiologic spectrum. *Ophthalmology* 1998;105:1902–1905.
61. Case Records of the Massachusetts General Hospital: case 9-2002. *N Engl J Med* 2002;346:924–929.

# 8. UPPER RESPIRATORY TRACT INFECTIONS

Robert F. Betts

With the exception of $\beta$ streptococcus group A, viruses cause most cases of upper respiratory tract infection (URI). The term URI is somewhat of a misnomer. The respiratory viruses infect all of the respiratory epithelial-lined respiratory system, producing rhinitis, pharyngitis, otitis, laryngitis, and bronchitis. Clinical manifestations vary by age and somewhat by specific virus subtype. However, any one of the many respiratory viruses can produce any one of the several syndromes listed. Most of these syndromes are self-limited. What makes them so important in the United States is that they consume so much medical attention and so much of our medical resources. Approximately 20 million office prescriptions per year in the United States are written for URIs [1,2]. The most common reason has been otitis media, but bronchitis and sinusitis are not far behind [1]. These infections accounted for more than 75% of prescriptions written annually in physicians' offices [1]. Therefore, a practical approach to these common problems is essential.

I. The **"common cold"**: definition and pathophysiology
   A. **Definition.** Although we strive to define this syndrome, there is certainly not common agreement as to its definition, certainly not by the lay public. Some include only a stuffy nose and a sore throat in the definition and call facial pain sinusitis and cough bronchitis, believing they are somehow different. Others include all the above. Virus in pure culture has been isolated from sinus puncture [3,4], from the middle ear [5], and in animals from the trachea.
   B. **Pathophysiology.** Over the last several years a great deal of information has accumulated indicating that respiratory symptoms are caused by elaboration of inflammatory mediators in response to viral infection [6,7]. The viruses themselves, with the exception of influenza and perhaps adenovirus, are not cytotoxic. Observations indicate that rhinovirus can be detected in the nasal secretions without any symptoms whatsoever. When cytokines are produced, the syndrome takes shape [6,7].
   C. **Anatomic changes.** Computed tomographic studies on subjects with rhinovirus caused by URI reveal **abnormalities of the sinuses in more than 85% of cases.** These abnormalities resolve without antibiotics [8,9]. **Mucopurulent rhinitis** (thick, opaque, or discolored nasal discharge) **frequently develops 1 to 3 days after the onset of the common cold.** Desquamated epithelial and polymorphonuclear cells in the nasal secretions provide this color change in the absence of virulent bacteria [9].

II. **Specific syndromes**
   A. Nasopharyngitis **is characterized by rhinorrhea, sneezing, sore throat, cough, and, in children, low-grade fever.**
      1. **Frequency.** Children may have three to eight and adults one to three colds per year [9].
      2. **Etiology.** Rhinoviruses and coronaviruses account for most infections in children; rhinoviruses are especially important in adults.
      3. **Course.** The **usual duration is 6 to 7 days** with peak symptoms on the second and third days. It often begins with a mild sore throat, and within 24 hours clear and copious nasal discharge develops, by which time the sore throat has decreased. Accompanying the discharge is frequent sneezing with obstruction of one or the other of the nasal passages. Mucopurulent discharge mentioned above then evolves. Cough occurs by the second or third day due to release of inflammatory mediators [7]. Systemic symptoms, but rarely fever, are present on days 2 to 4.
      4. **Management: symptomatic therapy in rhinovirus colds (and probably other etiologies).**
         a. **Naproxen,** and other nonsteroidal antiinflammatory drugs (NSAIDs), begun at the very first symptoms in young adults significantly reduces symptoms of headache, malaise, myalgia, and cough [10]. Virus shedding is not altered. This suggests an important role for prostaglandin or cyclooxygenases in cough and in systemic symptoms [7,10].

b. **First-generation antihistamines.** Based on earlier studies, the role of antihistamines in the therapy of common colds was controversial [11]. However, if first-generation antihistamines are initiated at the onset of the very first symptoms, they are very beneficial in adults. First-generation antihistamines appear more beneficial than second generation [12]. **Clemastine fumarate** reduces sneezing and rhinorrhea [13]. Likewise, **brompheniramine maleate** (e.g., the antihistamine in Dimetapp) was similarly efficacious, and it also reduced cough [14]. Mild drowsiness, dry mouth, and dry throat are potential side effects in some patients. The combination of naproxen and a first-generation antihistamine are highly effective. It is hoped that a similar approach in children would reduce otitis manifestations, but that awaits further study.

c. **Intranasal ipratropium bromide (Atrovent) used for 4 days** provides specific relief of rhinorrhea and sneezing with common colds in adults [15,16].

d. **Pseudoephedrine plus acetaminophen** when given to subjects who had cold symptoms for less than 48 hours led to improvement of "sinus" pain, pressure, and congestion when compared with control subjects in a preliminary report. The combination was well tolerated, except that 4% of the pseudoephedrine-acetaminophen subjects complained of nervousness [17].

e. **Other.** Acetaminophen in children and acetaminophen or aspirin in adults have been used, but these have not proven as effective as other NSAIDs. Cold-water vaporization has been used.

f. **Antimicrobial agents should not be given for the common cold.** Controlled trials of antibiotics have shown that treatment fails to change the course and the outcome of the illness. Furthermore, they do not prevent bacterial complications [9]. One well-conceived study (none in the study had received the above outlined symptomatic therapy) indicated that a third of antibiotic recipients and a third of placebo recipients were better in a week. However, a higher percentage of the 10% from whom respiratory pathogens were isolated pretreatment and had received placebo had progression of symptoms at 1 week [18]. The results from this study support the approach of waiting 7 days before using antibiotics. By so doing, only the 5% to 10% with progression would receive therapy.

g. **Antiviral agents** At the moment, there is no clear evidence that treatment of common cold with an antiviral agent is useful. This may be because symptoms are more due to host response than to viral replication. Prophylaxis during either the season of heightened activity (September and May) or in the family setting may prove more useful [19].

5. **Complications.** Otitis media or **bacterial sinusitis** may follow a cold that sometimes merits antibiotics. See below for specific discussions of these entities.

6. **Transmission** is from person to person, requires close contact, and probably involves transfer of the virus from the hands of an infected person to an intermediate surface or directly to the hands of a susceptible person [20]. **Therefore, good handwashing can help prevent the spread of these viral infections.** Illness in one family member should prepare others to initiate symptomatic therapy outlined above at the earliest symptoms.

**B. Acute pharyngitis and tonsillitis**

1. **Definitition.** The onset of pain in the throat manifested especially on swallowing, sometimes associated with tonsil exudates.

2. **Etiology.** Most pharyngitis is due to virus (usually >70%) and is not exudative. Pharyngitis produced by Epstein-Barr virus (EBV) is often the only respiratory manifestation of this disease (see Chapter 9). The earliest manifestation of both *Mycoplasma pneumoniae* and *Chlamydia pneumoniae* infection is pharyngitis without rhinitis. Group A *Streptococcus pyogenes* (GAS) are the major cause of bacterial pharyngitis. Arcanobacterium are an uncommon cause of bacterial pharyngitis, and *Corynebacterium diphtheriae* is rare in the highly vaccinated.

3. **Clinical presentation [21]. See Table 8.1.**

a. **Pharyngitis caused by viruses** is suggested by a rapid progression to include rhinorrhea, obstruction of the nasal passage(s), cough, conjunctivitis, hoarseness (which have up to 80% negative predictive value), and absence

Table 8.1. Differentiating Features of Pharyngitis Caused by Group A Streptococci and Viruses

| | "Classic" Streptococcal Pharyngitis | Viral Pharyngitis |
|---|---|---|
| Season | Late winter or early spring | All seasons |
| Age | Peak: 5–11 yr | All ages |
| Symptoms | Sudden onset<br>Sore throat, may be severe<br>Headache<br>Abdominal pain, nausea, vomiting | Onset varies<br>Sore throat, often mild<br>Fever varies<br>Myalgia, arthralgia<br>Abdominal pain may occur with influenza A or Epstein-Barr virus |
| Signs | Pharyngeal erythema and exudate<br>Tender enlarged anterior cervical nodes<br>Palatal petechiae<br>Tonsillar hypertrophy<br>Scarlet fever rash<br>Absence of cough, rhinitis, hoarseness, conjunctivitis, and diarrhea | Characteristic enanthems<br>Characteristic exanthems<br>**Often with cough, rhinitis, hoarseness, conjunctivitis, or diarrhea** |

Modified from Tanz RR, Shulman ST. Pharyngitis. In: Long-SS, Pickering LK, Prober CG, eds. *Principles and practice of pediatric infectious diseases.* New York: Churchill/Livingstone, 1997:202, with permission.

of fever. Viral infection is especially common in children less than age 3 [22]. Adenovirus can cause a syndrome that largely presents as pharyngitis with associated conjunctivitis. Exudate is commonly detected. EBV has exudates and tonsil enlargement as a major component of its presentation (see Chapter 9).

**b.** The **"classic" clinical features of GAS** are onset in winter or spring; school-aged child; abrupt onset of fever, sore throat, headache, and abdominal pain; pharyngeal tonsil inflammation, often (but only 50% of the time) with yellowish exudates; swollen uvula; and tender anterior cervical lymph nodes.

**c. Differential diagnosis.** Several experts have tried to differentiate the clinical presentation of GAS versus viral infections (Table 8.1).

**4. Laboratory testing should be performed when clinical and epidemiologic features suggest GAS infection but not if viral infection is considered likely** (see section II.B.3). The exception would be for acute EBV infection.

**a. Throat culture for GAS infection.** The sensitivity of a single throat culture is approximately 95%. Plates that are negative at 24 hours should be reexamined at 48 hours [21]. Specimens should be obtained from the surface of both tonsils (or tonsil fossae) and the posterior pharyngeal wall. Other areas of the oropharynx and mouth are unacceptable [21].

About 50% of subjects with EBV mononucleosis harbor GAS in their pharynx. In the winter, 30% to 35% of asymptomatic grade-school children are colonized with group A streptococci. If these carriers acquire viral pharyngitis, a throat culture will show GAS. This type of patient is assumed to have GAS infection and is often treated. This is one reason those patients with a sore throat and characteristics of viral illness only should not be cultured.

**b. Rapid streptococcal antigen test.** This test has excellent specificity (>95%), so a **positive test for clinical purposes establishes the diagnosis.** However, the sensitivity of the antigen test is only positive in 80% to 90% or even lower of those with a positive culture, so a **negative antigen test should be confirmed with conventional blood agar plate culture [21,22].** An area of debate is whether those who are antigen negative and culture positive may simply be colonized. Rapid identification and treatment of GAS pharyngitis can reduce the risk of spread of GAS infection, allowing these patients to return to school, day care, or work sooner and can reduce morbidity associated with this illness [21,22] (see section 4.d).

c. **Antibody studies** (antistreptolysin O [ASO], streptozyme) are **not advised** except to confirm prior GAS infections in suspected acute rheumatic fever or acute glomerulonephritis. It is also helpful in prospective epidemiologic studies conducted to separate patients with acute infections from those who are carriers [21]. Monospot serology for EBV is very helpful to confirm that infection (see Chapter 9).

d. **When to treat.** To provide any symptomatic relief from the treatment, it must be initiated immediately. However, prior studies have shown that therapy can be safely postponed up to 9 days after onset of symptoms and still prevent acute rheumatic fever [21,22]. In those with signs and symptoms highly suggestive of GAS infection, empiric therapy can be started, and if the cultures are negative, therapy can be discontinued. If the ill individual has a history of rheumatic fever, treatment is indicated immediately. However, if not, GAS infection is usually a self-limited disease: Fever and constitutional symptoms disappear spontaneously within 3 to 4 days of onset even without therapy [21], which has resulted in difficulty reaching statistical significance for penicillin therapy in small placebo-controlled studies. Therefore the clinician has considerable flexibility in initiating therapy.

e. **Regimens.** Unless contraindicated, **penicillin remains the treatment of choice** for GAS pharyngitis [21,23], and twice daily regimens, if taken, are effective and may help improve compliance. Resistance to penicillin has not been described. Amoxicillin is an acceptable alternative to penicillin and is often used because it is more palatable and the cost is comparable. However, because of its broader antimicrobial spectrum, use of amoxicillin results in greater selective pressure for resistant bacteria [22]. Family members are not usually treated unless they exhibit symptoms and have positive cultures or strep screens or they have rheumatic heart disease [24]. Cultures after treatment do not need to be obtained if symptoms clear with treatment. **Common regimens are shown in Table 8.2. In the penicillin-allergic patient, erythromycin is the major alternative,** or clindamycin can be used. The more expensive second- and third-generation cephalosporins are 10 to 20 times more expensive than penicillin, excessively broad spectrum, and, although sometimes encouraged by the pharmaceutical industry, seldom indicated [25]. Tetracycline and sulfonamides are not used both because of resistance and because even with susceptible strains sulfonamides do not prevent rheumatic fever.

f. **Recurrent streptococcal pharyngitis** [21,23,26]. Some individuals will improve with penicillin but do not clear the organism and symptoms recur. One explanation has been that $\beta$-lactamase–positive organisms present in the oropharynx inactivate penicillin. If the organism is susceptible to clindamycin, use of that drug leads to successful eradication. Outbreaks of GAS and "ping-pong" spread within a family are discussed elsewhere [21].

C. **Acute otitis media** (AOM) **can be classified as AOM or otitis media with effusion. The natural history of** appropriately treated **AOM includes persistent middle ear effusions for several weeks in most children.**

1. **Definition. AOM is fluid** in the middle ear **in association with signs or symptoms of** otalgia or otorrhea usually with fever [27]. **A middle ear effusion is virtually always present,** except in rare circumstances when the practitioner may observe signs of acute inflammation in the hours before fluid accumulates in the middle ear [27]. **Pneumatic otoscopy is used** to assess position, color, translucency, and mobility of the tympanic membrane [27].

2. **Physical findings in AOM**

a. **Local signs** such as otorrhea with evidence of middle ear origin, bulging tympanic membrane with cloudy or yellow fluid behind it or if tympanic membrane is distinctly red, or local ear pain should be sought.

Table 8.2. Treatment Regimens for Acute Streptococcal Pharyngitis in Children

| | Regimen | Cost of Course[a] |
|---|---|---|
| **Oral agents** | | |
| Penicillin V | 125 mg (if <27 kg) to 250 mg[b] (if >27 kg) b.i.d. for 10 days | $3 |
| Erythromycin | | |
| Ethylsuccinate | 40 mg/kg/day (to max. of 1,000 mg/day) in two to four divided doses for 10 days | $20 |
| Estolate | 20–40 mg/kg/day (to max. of 1,000 mg/day) in two to four divided doses for 10 days | $11–22[c] |
| Cephalexin or Cephradine (first-generation cephalosporin) | 25–50 mg/kg/day in two or three divided doses for 10 days | $10–80[d] |
| Clarithromycin | 15 mg/kg/day (to max. of 500 mg/day) divided b.i.d. for 10 days | $30–55[c] |
| Azithromycin | 12 mg/kg once daily (with max. 500 mg on first day, 250 mg subsequent days) for 5 days | $28 |
| Clindamycin[e] | 20 mg/kg day (max. 1.8 g/day) divided t.i.d. for 10 days | $17.50 |
| **Parenteral agent** | | |
| Benzathine penicillin G[f] | 600,000 units if <27 kg and 1.2 million units if >27 kg IM once only | $6 |

[a] Actual wholesale costs (rounded off). 1999 Redbook.
[b] 500 mg bid for adolescents.
[c] Depending on weight.
[d] Wide range depending on weight and whether generic or trade.
[e] Clindamycin has been used in patients with multiple antibiotic allergies and to eradicate the group *Astreptococcus* "carrier state."
[f] The single i.m. dose eliminates the problem of compliance, but the shot is painful.
Courtesy of Joseph S. Bertino, Jr. Pharm.D., Bassett Healthcare, Cooperstown, NY.

b. **Fever** is presumably indicative of AOM **when there are associated local signs;** in the absence of these local signs, fever often may be unrelated to middle ear effusion.
c. **Nonspecific signs and symptoms** that do not help make the diagnosis of AOM include rhinorrhea, cough, irritability, anorexia, headache, vomiting, or diarrhea.

3. Physical examination (PE) in otitis media with effusion. **Fluid in the middle ear in the absence of signs or symptoms of acute infection.**
4. **Diagnosis**
   a. **Myringotomy** is carried out by incision of the tympanic membrane. That or tympanocentesis leads to recovery of the organisms [28].
   b. **Physical findings.** Both redness and bulging should be present. Merely immobility is not sufficient to make the diagnosis because this can be present in secretory otitis media.
5. **Etiology [27,28].** Bacteria are isolated from 50% to 60% of cases and include *S. pneumoniae* (25%–50%), *Haemophilus influenzae* **(most cannot be typed)** (15%–30%), and *Moraxella catarrhalis* **(most are β-lactamase positive)** (3%–20%). Viruses have also been isolated in pure culture, including respiratory syncitial virus (RSV), rhinovirus, parainfluenza, and influenza [5]. *Mycoplasma pneumoniae* is a consideration and has been associated with bullous myringitis.
6. **Treatment** One of the most hotly debated topics is if, or when, to treat AOM. Controlled trials show nearly identical outcome in treated or untreated subjects.

There is spontaneous clearance of bacteria in at least 40% and perhaps as high as 80% of cases [27,28]. *Haemophilus* is more likely to clear spontaneously than is *S. pneumoniae* [29]. Additionally, virus in pure culture is isolated from the middle ear, and these cases would not benefit from antibiotics [5]. Another factor is the increasing incidence of pneumococcus with minimal inhibitory concentrations (MIC) to penicillin of at least 1 μg/mL (see Chapter 11). Not only are these organisms resistant to penicillin, they are also resistant to macrolides (erythromycin/azithromycin), trimethoprim-sulfamethoxazole (TMP-SMZ), oral cephalosporins, and tetracycline. Whereas the resistance to amoxicillin (amoxicillin/clavulanate) is relative and can be overcome with higher doses [30], the resistance to the macrolides is absolute.

Careful evaluation in prospective studies has raised the question of whether antibiotics should be used at all [31,32]. Recognizing the high rate of spontaneous resolution, investigators from Holland believed that lack of pain control rather than persistent fever was the reason for apparent failure in most studies. The rational for using antibiotics, to prevent mastoiditis or meningitis, is not supported by data [33]. Thus, newer thinking is to use acetaminophen for 72 hours and consider antibiotics if symptoms persist or consider continued observation [31–35]. Exceptions to that rule would be for those children with severe symptoms or perforation of the ear drum, which provides physicians some leeway [35]. Against this background, a consensus group gathered by the Centers for Disease Control and Prevention has made recommendations for treatment [36].

a. **Amoxicillin** is the antibiotic of choice. Most experts believe that the pneumococcus not only is the most common pathogen in AOM, but also is the most likely to cause severe or persistent symptoms or suppurative and systemic complications if treated inappropriately [29]. Consequently, treatment regimens must be active against *S. pneumoniae.* The dose recommended has been increased from 40 to 80 or even 90 mg/kg because of the number of relatively resistant pneumococcus with high MICs has been increasing (Table 8.3). This was done without benefit of good studies, but in a trial comparing azithromycin to amoxicillin, Dagan et al. [37,38] showed that amoxicillin at that dose eradicated carriage of pneumococcus more frequently than did azithromycin, regardless of the MIC. In addition, also without benefit of good studies, a dose for adults of 1.0 g every 8 hours has been suggested. Uncomplicated AOM may be treated with a short course (5–7 days) in selected patients [28,39].
b. **Amoxicillin clavulanate** Because β-lactamase + *Haemophilus* and *Moraxella* are etiologic possibilities, this drug is often chosen. It is more effective than azithromycin in eradicating *Haemophilus* species. [30,37]. If used

Table 8.3. Antibiotics for Acute Otitis Media in Children (e.g., Child Weighing 18.5 kg)

| Drug | Daily Dosage[a] | Cost (10–Days Therapy)[b] |
|---|---|---|
| Amoxicillin | 60–90 mg/kg in three doses | $14[c] |
| Amoxicillin-clavulanate | 90/12.5 mg/kg** in two doses | $128[c] |
| Cefprozil | 30 mg/kg in two doses | $64 |
| Erythromycin-sulfisoxazole | 50/150 mg/kg in four doses | $25 |
| Trimethoprim-sulfamethoxazole | 8/40 mg/kg in two doses | $19 |
| Clarithromycin[d] | 15 mg/kg in two doses | $30 |
| Ceftriaxone | Single i.m. dose, 50 mg/kg (not to exceed 1 g) | $40 |

Courtesy of Joseph S. Bertino, Jr. Pharm.D., Bassett Healthcare, Cooperstown, NY.
[a]Daily dose usually divided up into two or three doses each day.
[b]Actual wholesale costs (rounded off), 1997 Redbook.
[c]Actual costs will vary, depending on weight of child.
[d]Azithromycin is used in acute otitis media.

at 90 mg/kg or 1.5 g every 12 hours, the incidence of diarrhea is less than with a dose of 1.0 g every 8 hours. Amoxicillin remains first line because the above two organisms are far more likely to clear spontaneously and are less virulent.

c. **Cephalosporins** Parenteral ceftriaxone has a high cure rate. Many pediatricians administer a single dose intramuscularly in the office (50 mg/kg maximum dose) [40]. By contrast, many of the oral cephalosporins have insufficient activity against the pneumococcus to be effective [41]. For example, in the ferret model, amoxicillin is superior to cefuroxime [42]. Furthermore, oral cephalosporins are relatively expensive.

d. **Other. The macrolides** have been used for the last several years. However, the absolute resistance mentioned above [43] has led to two problems. First, although macrolides eradicate susceptible pneumococcus quite well, they have no effect on resistant organisms and failure results. Second and more importantly, in day-care settings, macrolide susceptible organisms (that are also susceptible to penicillin) are eradicated and replaced by macrolide absolute resistant organisms (that are also relatively resistant to penicillin) [38]. This does not happen with amoxicillin use. **TMP-SMZ** resistance has become so frequent that its failure rate is predicted to be unacceptable [44]. **Quinolone** antibiotics (moxifloxacin, gatifloxacin) have excellent activity against all the middle ear organisms but are not approved for children because of the theoretical interference with cartilage development.

7. **Persistent middle ear effusion** 2 to 8 weeks after therapy does not require retreatment [27]. Middle ear effusion persists for weeks to months (i.e., 70% of children have fluid in the middle ear at 2 weeks, 50% at 1 month, 20% at 2 months, and 10% at 3 months, despite appropriate therapy) [27]. If that child presents with another fever, their effusion will still be present. To justify antibiotics, focal signs should be present.

8. **For chronic otitis media with effusion** (lasting >3 months) accompanied by significant bilateral hearing loss, bilateral myringotomy with insertion of tympanotomy tubes is effective [27,45].

9. **Antibiotic prophylaxis.** Because of the potential consequences of the emergence of penicillin-resistant pneumococcus, experts advise prophylaxis only in special settings.

   a. **Indications.** Children with three or more well-documented and separate episodes in the preceding 6 months or four or more episodes in the preceding 12 months is the only indication for which beneficial effects of prophylaxis is persistent and persuasive [27]. **Duration** of prophylaxis should be no longer than 6 months, because longer courses are less effective and may be more likely to promote colonization with resistant bacteria [27]. **Agents** that have been used include **sulfisoxazole** (75 mg/kg/day in one or two divided doses). This **is the preferred agent** and may be less likely than amoxicillin to produce colonization with $\beta$-lactamase–producing bacteria or resistant pneumococcus. Amoxicillin (e.g., 20 mg/kg once daily) has been used. Oral cephalosporins have not been shown to be effective.

10. **Other interventions** that may reduce the incidence of AOM without the risks of antibiotic exposure should be undertaken [27]: eliminating smoking at home, eliminating pacifiers, and using influenza and conjugated pneumococcus vaccines [46].

D. **Acute bronchitis accompanies acute viral URI.** Even though most of these cases are viral in origin, antibiotics are commonly and unnecessarily prescribed for 66% of adults and 75% of children with uncomplicated acute bronchitis [2,47].

1. **Definitions/clinical diagnosis.** Bronchitis is inflammation of the bronchial mucosa, resulting in a productive cough. The **definition in normal children** is not well established. Most clinicians believe that a child with **cough, with or without fever or sputum production, excluding pneumonia, bronchiolitis, and asthma [48], has bronchitis.** Similarly, **in adults without underlying chronic lung disease,** acute productive cough, no or low-grade temperature, and no evidence of pneumonia on physical examination or chest x-ray makes the

diagnosis of bronchitis. However, the lack of consensus regarding nomenclature and clinical definition of cough illnesses leads to difficulty in comparing patient populations and results in reported studies.

2. **Etiology. Viruses cause most cases. In adults,** rhinoviruses, influenza, parainfluenza, and adenoviruses are common. **In children** parainfluenza, RSV, and influenza virus are especially important. The role for *Bordetella pertussis* (whooping cough) as a cause of protracted cough in adults is undergoing study. **In children** most prolonged-cough illnesses are allergic, postinfectious, or viral and do not require antibiotics. Because reactive airway disease is common, even in the absence of wheezing, many of these patients respond well to bronchodilator therapy [48]. Sputum or nasopharynx colonizers (e.g., *S. pneumoniae, H. influenzae, S. aureus*) can be isolated in the laboratory even when the underlying process is viral in origin.

   Viruses can cause a protracted cough, but a protracted cough is less likely to be viral in origin. In the absence of purulent sputum, *M. pneumoniae* and *Chlamydia pneumoniae* should also be considered in older children, teenagers, and adults, especially adults exposed to school-aged children or teenagers with prolonged respiratory illnesses (i.e., >10 days).
3. **Clinical findings.** Fever is common in viral bronchitis, especially when caused by influenza and RSV, and in and of itself does not predict the need for antibiotics [48]. However, if fever persists in adults it may be a clue to bacterial superinfection. Examination of the chest may reveal sibilant rhonchi but no areas of consolidation. Chest roentgenograms reveal no densities.
4. **Diagnosis.** Historical clues pointing to a virus are the simultaneous presence of similar illness in close contacts. If the individual who seems to be the index case for the presenting patient was ill 2 weeks earlier, that points to *M. pneumoniae* and *C. pneumoniae.* Viral identification, especially by rapid diagnostic methods, supports an etiology and may delay un-needed antibiotic therapy. Gram stain of expectorated sputum may demonstrate organisms consistent with *S. pneumoniae.* If fever has persisted, isolation of a pathogenic bacteria supports the use of antibiotics and susceptibility studies directs therapy, but merely isolating an alleged respiratory pathogen does not mandate use of antibiotics. Children with chronic cough (>4 weeks) should be evaluated for reactive airway disease, tuberculosis, pertussis, cystic fibrosis, aspiration of a foreign body, or sinusitis.
5. **Therapy for normal subjects.** Principles are published for children [48], and these principles also apply to adults. Because bronchitis is part of the acute viral URI, the principles of early use of antihistamines and NSAIDs discussed under URI apply here and have the same clinical benefit.
   a. **Nonspecific cough** in normal children or adults rarely warrants antibiotics [48]. Studies of acute bronchitis in adults and cough illness/bronchitis in children have shown no benefit of antibiotics. Furthermore, prophylactic use of antibiotics in these patients does not prevent or decrease the severity of bacterial complications after viral URI. Neither the character nor the culture results of sputum or nasopharyngeal secretions is helpful in determining the need for antibiotics. Virus- and bacteria-induced airway inflammatory changes can cause "purulent" sputum with leukocytes. **For protracted cough (>10 days) antibiotics may be indicated.** However, 20% of adults with culture-confirmed rhinovirus colds continue to have cough for more than 14 days after onset of symptoms if they do not receive antihistamines and NSAIDs at the time of first symptoms [48]. If the clinical history supports mycoplasma or chlamydia, an empiric course of a macrolide or doxycycline (in children >8 years of age) is suggested. In children, pertussis and *M. pneumoniae* (see section D.2) benefit from antibiotics.
6. **Patients with underlying lung disease** receive empiric antibiotics more commonly. **Children** with cystic fibrosis and other severe lung disease (e.g., bronchopulmonary dysplasia, lung hypoplasia, chronic aspiration) are more likely to benefit from antibiotics, and therapy must be individualized [48]. **Adults** with structural lung disease (e.g., bronchiectasis or obstructive lung disease/emphysema) also may benefit from antibiotics.

**E. Acute exacerbations of chronic bronchitis.** Chronic bronchitis typically is defined as the production of sputum on most days for at least 3 months per year for more than 2 years.

1. **Clinical presentation.** An acute exacerbation of chronic bronchitis is a clinical syndrome associated with an increase in cough and an increase of sputum (both amount and purulence or a change in color). There is increased breathlessness without evidence of clinical or chest roentgenographic pneumonia. Most do not have systemic symptoms.
2. **Causes of acute exacerbations** include environmental factors, such as exposure to cigarette smoke, pollutants, fumes, pollens, and the like; these are important cofactors. Respiratory viruses appear to play a more important role in these acute illnesses than does *M. pneumoniae.* Many of these patients are chronically colonized with *S. pneumoniae* and *H. influenzae.* Presumably, these colonizing bacteria become minimally invasive, and therefore patients are more symptomatic, in the setting of sluggish white blood cell function caused by the virus infection. **Viral and bacterial etiologies cannot be distinguished clinically.**
3. **Diagnosis.** Physical examination reveals wheezing and rhonchi but no evidence of consolidation. The role of sputum cultures in this setting is unclear. Often empiric antibiotics are used without a sputum culture. If in selected patients cultures are desirable (e.g., the patient with multiple antibiotic allergies), a sputum culture should be obtained **before** starting antibiotics, because cultures obtained after antibiotics are difficult to interpret.
4. **Therapy.** The precise role of antibiotics in acute flare-ups is unclear [49,50]. Because minimally invasive bacterial infections are not well tolerated in patients with chronic lung disease, antibiotics are often initiated. **Many of these patients seem to respond clinically,** and some studies have shown that in the most severely symptomatic patients, antibiotics help [49,50]. Therapy is directed primarily against *S. pneumoniae* and *H. influenzae.* Various regimens have been recommended for adults (Table 8.4). Duration of therapy varies, but typically **5 days of therapy** is sufficient to reestablish host bacteria "equilibrium." **For recurrent bouts, antibiotic regimens can be rotated** with the hope of minimizing the selection of resistant pathogens.

**F. Acute sinusitis.** As previously discussed, in adults, and presumably in children, well-documented common colds are associated with changes of the sinuses, as revealed by computed tomography (CT) [8]. (See the earlier discussion under URI.) These changes reverse spontaneously in 80% of cases. Quite often, facial pain blamed on sinusitis is instead an atypical migraine syndrome and responds to Imitrex or other similar medications.

1. **Pathogenesis.** For viral respiratory infection (e.g., rhinovirus), the exact mechanisms that lead to disease in the sinus cavity are not known, but it is speculated

Table 8.4. Antibiotic Options in Adults with Acute Exacerbations of Chronic Bronchitis

| Drug | Daily Dosage (for 5 days) | Comments |
|---|---|---|
| Amoxicillin | 250 mg p.o. t.i.d. | Commonly used |
| Trimethoprim-sulfamethoxazole | 1 DS tab b.i.d. | Good sputum levels, commonly used |
| Erythromycin[a] | 250 mg q.i.d. | Not as active against *H. influenzae* |
| Cefuroxime axetil | 250 mg b.i.d. | Expensive |
| Tetracycline hydrochloride | 250 mg p.o. q.i.d. | On empty stomach |
| Doxycycline | 100 mg b.i.d. | Compliance is better |

[a]For patients who cannot tolerate the more cost-effective erythromycin preparations, azithromycin (500 mg on day 1 and then 250 mg once daily on days 2–5) or clarithromycin (250–500 mg b.i.d.) can be used.

that it is similar to that which causes rhinitis. Presumably, a virus stimulates inflammatory pathways and the parasympathetic nervous system, resulting in engorgement of the capacitance vessels in the venous erectile tissue of the nasal turbinate. Simultaneously, intercellular leakage of plasma into the nose and (presumably) sinuses, discharge of seromucous glands and goblet cells, and stimulation of pain nerve and sneeze and cough reflexes occurs [51]. Abnormalities are commonly seen on CT. Mucus and transudation of plasma into the sinus cavity presumably add to the viscosity of the material accumulating within the sinuses. Sinus disease may result from malfunction of the normal mucociliary clearance process, in part due to the very viscous secretions and partial/total obstruction (because of inflammation) of the usual drainage pathways of the sinuses. Furthermore, the opening of the osteomeatal complex is very narrow, and the walls of the passage are bone and thus not compliant. Natural drainage is very slow.

2. **Diagnosis.** Physical examination, if the disease is in the maxillary sinus, will illicit facial tenderness accompanied by pain on striking the upper molars. Postnasal drip may be conspicuous, and transillumination of the sinuses may be inhibited by fluid. However, the latter is unreliable. Coronal CT of sinuses may reveal fluid and/or thickened membranes, but this finding is present in both bacterial and viral sinusitis.
3. **Symptoms.** Excess nasal secretions, posterior nasal drip, facial pain, and pain in the vertex of the head are the classic complaints. If antihistamines and NSAIDs are initiated early, these complaints are reduced in frequency and severity.
4. **Complications.** Acute bacterial sinusitis has been reported to follow viral URI (sinusitis) in 0.5% to 5% of instances. Most cases of acute sinusitis resolve without antibiotic treatment [8,51,52]. The specific factors that determine whether bacterial invasion of the sinus will occur after a viral URI are unknown. Sneezing, coughing, and nose blowing may create pressure differentials that cause deposition of bacteria-containing nasal secretions into the sinus. Once bacteria are deposited into the cavity of an obstructed sinus, bacterial growth conditions are favorable; granulocyte phagocytosis may be impaired by the reduced oxygen tension in the obstructed sinus. This complication usually manifests about 7 days after onset. This process may take weeks to resolve [51].
   a. **Other risk factors for acute bacterial sinusitis.** Swimming and nasal obstruction due to polyps, foreign bodies, and tumor precede this process in a few cases. **An allergic cause** can usually be established by a history of paroxysmal sneezing, itching eyes, allergen exposure, and similar prior episodes. Patients can often self-diagnose the problem [51]. Dental infection can be the source. Other less common risk factors include acquired immunodeficiency syndrome, abnormalities of white blood cell function, cleft palate, cystic fibrosis, and immune deficiencies such as agammaglobulinemia [51].
   b. **Symptoms and signs.** Fever occurs in only 40% to 50%. Facial pain and tenderness (along with tenderness of an upper molar) are often found. Although some clinicians interpret **mucopurulent rhinitis** (thick, opaque, or discolored nasal discharge), especially in children, as indicating the presence of bacterial sinusitis, this sign is simply part of the natural course of a nonspecific uncomplicated URI. The nasal discharge in a cold changes from clear to purulent during the first few days of illness. In addition, the color and characteristics of the discharge do not predict whether bacteria will be isolated [52]. Cough is common in children and adults. Hyposomia (decreased smell sensation) is common. When the sinusitis follows a dental infection, a foul odor of the breath and molar pain are additional characteristics [51].
   c. **Separating viral versus bacterial** versus mixed is not possible, by clinical parameters alone. **CTs are not recommended** because of their lack of specificity. Patients with a common cold have sinus abnormalities most of the time [8]. In his excellent review, **Gwaltney [51] emphasized that clinical parameters define classic bacterial sinusitis: "Classic"** acute bacterial sinusitis will have **fever, facial pain, marked tenderness** (over the involved sinus), **erythema, or swelling.** Also in this group are patients with molar pain or other evidence of an odontogenic cause of the infection. In

children, fever more than 39°C, periorbital swelling, and facial pain or dental pain is suggestive [52].

d. **Rarely, sinusitis can be complicated by meningitis, brain abscess, or orbital infections.**

e. **Etiologic organisms.** Nasopharyngeal cultures do not reflect the bacteriology of the sinuses [52]. The **gold standard** is identification of organisms by puncture of the sinuses. However, this is generally used only in complex cases, and only about 60% of sinus aspirates in suspected cases of acute sinusitis yield bacteria. [52]. Puncture studies have shown that *S. pneumoniae* and *H. influenzae* account for 50% of cases in adults and children. *M. catarrhalis* is more common in children (about 20% of isolates) than in adults. A recent reviewer emphasizes that in children, acute sinusitis is usually caused by the same bacterial pathogens that cause AOM [52]. *S. aureus* and streptococcus group A cause less than 5% of cases. Anaerobic infections are infrequent in children. In adults, most anaerobic sinusitis arises from infection of the roots of premolar teeth, thus representing a pure bacterial infection [51]. Viruses alone may account for 10% to 15% [51,52]. The etiology of the cases that are negative on the bacterial culture has not been fully studied, but presumably viruses are important in most. The role of *C. pneumoniae* and *M. pneumoniae* has not been well established [51]. Fungi occasionally cause sinusitis and usually present with pressure changes, such as proptosis, and bony erosion [51].

f. **Roentgenographic studies** are indicated when (a) episodes of sinusitis are recurrent, (b) complications are suspected, (c) the diagnosis is unclear, (d) the patient is responding poorly, or (e) sinus surgery is contemplated [52]. Most clinicians have moved to coronal CTs or magnetic resonance imaging but only after acute URI has resolved. Abnormalities include air-fluid levels, opacification, or mucosal thickening of more than 4 mm [52]. **Loss of bony markings medially *should not* be interpreted as osteomyelitis.** These changes are simply pressure necrosis on a very thin wall. **A classic air-fluid level usually means an acute bacterial sinusitis** [51]. Opacification and mucosal thickening are often nonspecific and may be chronic or due to prolonged URIs. Until about ages 5 to 6, the frontal and sphenoid sinuses do not appear and may not be fully developed until adolescence. Misinterpretation of absent sinuses as opacified can lead to the overdiagnosis of sinusitis. In particular, films should be read with great caution in children less than 1 year of age [52].

5. **Therapy.** As with otitis media, acute sinusitis will often resolve even without antimicrobial therapy [52]. **Therefore only "classic" cases, or those with protracted symptoms (>8–10 days), or complex cases should be treated. Protracted sinonasal symptoms (>8–10 days) suggest that bacterial infection has complicated a viral URI.** The latter should have resolved or at least improved by 10 days. In children, prolonged nonspecific URI signs and symptoms without improvement for more than 10 to 14 days merit therapy, whereas children with symptoms improving by 7 to 10 days of onset probably have an uncomplicated viral URI.

   a. **Antibiotics. (See Table 8.5)** Randomized placebo-controlled trials of antibiotics for acute community-acquired bacterial sinusitis with the use of pretreatment and posttreatment sinus aspirate cultures have not been conducted. In several nonrandomized studies, appropriate doses of antibiotics are highly effective in eradicating or substantially reducing bacterial titers in the sinus cavity. When 10-day regimens are used, a bacteriologic cure rate of more than 90% has been achieved [51].

      (1) **Amoxicillin for initial management of acute uncomplicated is successful in sinusitis as it is in otitis in most** children [34–36,52], and probably most adults, despite $\beta$-lactamase production by most isolates of *M. catarrhalis* and some *H. influenzae* [52]. For adolescents and adults, 500 mg orally three times a day and for children 60 to 80 mg/kg/day can be used.

      (2) **For those unresponsive to amoxicillin in 48 to 72 hours or for whom amoxicillin is contraindicated or who are experiencing recurrent**

Table 8.5. Alternative Antibiotics for Sinusitis

| Antibiotics | Oral Dose in Adults | Oral Dose in Children | Comment |
|---|---|---|---|
| Amoxicillin-clavulanate | 875 mg b.i.d. | [a] | Some view as an optimal agent of choice for penicillin-resistant *S. pneumoniae* in children (or adults) |
| TMP-SMZ | 1 DS b.i.d. | [a] | Misses some *S. pneumoniae* |
| Cefuroxime axetil | 250 mg b.i.d. | [a] | Expensive[b] |
| Cefprozil | 250 mg b.i.d. | [a] | Expensive[b] |
| Azithromycin | 5-day course (Z pack) | [a] | Macrolide with fewest gastrointestinal side effects[b] |
| Clarithromycin | 250 mg b.i.d. | [a] | [b] |
| Advanced fluoroquinolone (e.g., levofloxacin) | 500 mg q.d. | Avoid | Effective against penicillin-resistant *S. pneumoniae,* useful in adults allergic to penicillin/cephalosporins. Expensive |

[a] For dosages in sinusitis, use same regimens as in acute otitis media. See Table 8.3.
[b] May miss some penicillin-resistant *S. pneumoniae.* See Chapter 11.

**infections,** a $\beta$-lactamase stable agent (e.g., amoxicillin-clavulanate) or a $\beta$-lactamase stable cephalosporin active against pneumococci (e.g., cefuroxime axetil) is suggested [30,37,51].

(3) **See Table 8.5. Antibiotics are usually given for 10 days** [51] or for 7 days beyond the point of substantial improvement. Recently, in a report from the Netherlands, adults with acute maxillary sinusitis and abnormal conventional radiographs (mucosal swelling of more than 5 mm, complete shadowing, or a fluid level) were randomized to receive either amoxicillin 750 mg three times a day for 7 days or placebo. Amoxicillin (used because most of the organisms that they had identified in a preliminary study were susceptible) did not improve clinical outcomes [53]. This preliminary study is difficult to interpret because the critically important duration of sinus-like symptoms was not specified, the number of patients with diagnostic radiographic abnormalities (air-fluid level) was not specified, and it is well known that some improve without antibiotics. However, at least it implies that therapy in acute disease is not indicated.

(4) **In severely ill patients** with intracranial or orbital extension, intravenous therapy with ceftriaxone and vancomycin (to cover high-level penicillin-resistant *S. pneumoniae*) should be started. Infectious disease consultation is advised.

b. **Ancillary therapy** is directed at drainage of the nasal passages and sinuses and relief of sneezing, coughing, and systemic symptoms [51].

(1) **Decongestants.** Although serial CTs show that decongestants have little or no effect in promptly draining the sinuses, they are commonly used. **Oral decongestants are preferred over topical** nasal decongestants, which are often associated with rebound vasodilatation and obstruction and pharyngeal irritation. Oral decongestants are safe for patients with stable hypertension who are receiving appropriate antihypertensive treatment [17,51].

(2) **Topical steroids are useful** if there is evidence of an **allergic component** to the patient's illness. The use of topical (or oral) steroids as decongestants has not been rigorously evaluated. In volunteers with rhinovirus-induced rhinosinusitis, topical steroids had little, if any, beneficial effect on nasal symptoms [51].

(3) **Mucoevacuant drugs** (e.g., guaifenesin) are used on theoretical grounds, but their usefulness has not been **established** [51].

(4) **NSAIDs** are useful in treating systemic symptoms such as fever and malaise and may be helpful in reducing cough [51]. Acetaminophen is also used as an analgesic.

(5) **Cough suppressants** with dextromethorphan or codeine may be needed to control cough.

(6) **Antihistamines.** Although there may be a reluctance to use first-generation antihistamines because of their anticholinergic activity and the possibility of their drying secretions and impairing drainage, testing under randomized, controlled, blinded conditions has shown a reduction of about 50% in sneezing and a reduction of about 30% in rhinorrhea and nasal mucus weights in volunteers with experimental rhinovirus colds. There was no evidence of other symptoms or prolongation of the overall illness, indicating that drying of secretions and impairment of drainage were not problems [51]. Therefore **the use of antihistamines (in adults) for symptomatic improvement in the early phase seems reasonable.** Whether antihistamines, by reducing sneezing and nasal secretions, are truly beneficial has not been proven. See related discussion under the common cold.

c. **Prevention [51]**

(1) Prevention of **viral URI may be minimized** by avoiding contact with people with colds. Carrying out handwashing when contact occurs between infected and noninfected persons is useful. Covering the mouth with disposable nasal tissues when coughing or sneezing is desirable.

(2) **Influenza vaccine** reduces attack rate in all age groups and reduces severity in the elderly, but it is effective only against influenza and not other viruses that cause respiratory illness.

(3) **Prophylactic antibiotics** to prevent recurrent acute bacterial sinusitis are **not recommended** and will add to the selection of resistant pathogens.

**G. Chronic sinusitis (defined as symptoms persisting for 6 months).** Patients with chronic sinusitis need to be referred to an otolaryngologist for nasal endoscopy and/or CT study and consideration for drainage procedures.

1. **Etiology.** The organisms isolated from chronic sinusitis patients differ substantially from those isolated in acute sinusitis. In a small percent, *Haemophilus* species are isolated but coagulase-negative staphylococcus, *Pseudomonas aeruginosa,* anaerobic bacteria, and fungi are more common [54]. Thus, although antibiotics discussed in the section on acute sinusitis are used at times with protracted courses of 3 to 4 weeks, the rationale for that cannot be justified based on the organisms identified. However, many times when there is an acute infection, no attempt at isolation of the etiologic organism is carried out and antibiotics are administered with apparent response. No randomized studies have been conducted to ascertain the value of such treatment, which leaves the matter largely unresolved.

2. **Management.** Mechanical measures are the most important part of care of these patients. Irrigation with normal saline three times a day is one of the most important steps. If this simple step is unsuccessful, endoscopic enlargement of the openings will often prove useful. Unfortunately, loss of ciliary function is part of the disease process so that even this step may not prove entirely successful. However, overall, such procedures have proven to be quite cost-effective.

**H. External otitis**

1. External otitis is usually a superficial infection of the external auditory canal that is typically initiated by moisture and is often referred to as "swimmer's ear." It is most commonly caused by *Pseudomonas* species. Avoiding swimming and/or keeping the ears dry and using topical treatment usually suffice. Often the condition responds to careful cleaning of the canal by gentle suction or irrigation. In other instances, antibiotic drops (polymyxin, neomycin, and hydrocortisone [e.g., Cortisporin otic]) or dilute acetic acid or boric acid solutions (to lower the pH) suffice. This topic has been reviewed in detail elsewhere [55].

2. **Malignant external otitis** is an important infection caused by *P. aeruginosa* and is associated with a high mortality (20%), if untreated. This disease process begins as an external otitis that may progress to involve the cartilaginous tissue and may penetrate to the base of the brain. Cranial nerve (especially facial), sigmoid sinus thrombosis, and meningitis have resulted in death [56]. This disease occurs almost exclusively in elderly diabetics but has been described in nondiabetic patients who have underlying malignancy or are immunocompromised, including patients with acquired immunodeficiency syndrome. Ear, nose, and throat and infectious disease consultation are advised.

   a. **Diagnosis is often difficult.** One must have a high index of suspicion. Patients complain of progressively increasing pain and tenderness of the tissues around the ear and mastoid region. They seldom have fever or systemic symptoms or a peripheral leukocytosis. Cranial nerve abnormalities may develop. Often there is persistent drainage from the external canal that yields *P. aeruginosa* on culture. The presence of granulation tissue at the junction of the osseous and cartilaginous portions of the external ear is a highly suggestive finding [56]. CTs can help detect early bone involvement and extent of the disease process. However, technetium phosphate radionucleotide bone scans can identify early bony involvement when there is no destruction on CTs; gallium-67 citrate scans are also a sensitive indicator of infection [56].

   b. **Treatment.** Topical therapy is ineffective. Most patients require hospitalization and, at least initially, for well-established infection combination parenteral antibiotics to achieve synergy against *P. aeruginosa.* Ticarcillin or piperacillin is often combined with tobramycin (or another aminoglycoside to which the pathogen is susceptible). In the penicillin-allergic patient, ceftazidime can be combined with an aminoglycoside. Ciprofloxacin may be useful [56,57] in selected cases (i.e., early disease or for completion of therapy if the organism is susceptible). Serial gallium scans have been used to monitor response to therapy [56].

**I. Epiglottitis/supraglottitis.** Epiglottitis is an acute and severe inflammation of the epiglottis; some use the term supraglottitis for this condition, indicating inflammation not only of the epiglottis but also of the surrounding tissue [58]. Before the early 1990's, epiglottitis was primarily an illness of children and due usually to invasive *H. influenzae* b. Since the early 1990's and widespread use of *H. influenzae* b vaccinations in children in the United States, studies have shown a significant change in the epidemiology; epiglottitis now occurs almost exclusively in adults [58]. Although invasive *H. influenzae b* remains an important etiologic pathogen in adults, *S. pneumoniae* cause a significant number of cases; group A streptococci have also been isolated [59].

1. **Clinical presentation [57,60]. In children,** the onset of epiglottitis with *H. influenzae b* is classically abrupt, with sore throat, fever, and toxicity. The symptoms usually progress rapidly in such a manner that dysphagia, drooling, and respiratory distress with stridor become apparent. This diagnosis is still a concern in children who have not been adequately vaccinated against *H. influenzae*. **In adults,** recent series note that symptoms and signs may be more subacute: sore throat, painful or difficulty with swallowing, and muffled voice occur in most, and fever or chills, drooling, stridor, sitting erect, dyspnea, cough, and ear pain can also occur [58,60].
2. **Clinical diagnosis. This disease is a** potential medical emergency **and** requires a high index of suspicion **on the basis of the history and clinical findings. The diagnosis can be** confirmed by visualization of the epiglottis and supraglottic area. This should only be performed by well-trained personnel; emergency equipment must be available **for maintaining the airway.**
3. **Laboratory and radiologic features.** Lateral neck roentgenograms may be useful early in less toxic patients who are not in respiratory difficulty. The epiglottis appears as an enlarged rounded shadow resembling a thumb. **Leukocyte count is usually elevated to more than 15,000/mm$^3$, often with a pronounced left shift. Blood cultures should be obtained.**
4. **Management.** Swift and careful management is essential in this disease and directly correlates with the outcome. In the acutely ill patient, valuable time may be unnecessarily wasted obtaining roentgenograms. Ensuring an adequate airway must take priority. **In young children, nasotracheal intubation and thus emergency consultation (e.g., otolaryngology, anesthesia) is often necessary. In adults, need for intubation is less pressing.** Factors predictive of the need for airway intervention were stridor and sitting erect in one study [60].
5. **Antibiotics.** Parenteral cephalosporin (second- or third- generation agents; i.e., cefuroxime, ceftriaxone), which is effective against ampicillin-resistant *H. influenzae* or ampicillin-sulbactam or parenteral chloramphenicol in the patient in whom penicillins and cephalosporins are contraindicated, should be initiated immediately. If not contraindicated, we favor ceftriaxone or ampicillin-sulbactam, which are also very active against group A streptococcus, mostly *S. pneumoniae* and *S. aureus.* In a critically ill adult and/or in an area with a high incidence of high-level penicillin-resistant *S. pneumoniae,* we would add intravenous vancomycin (along with ceftriaxone) until at least blood culture data are available because more than 20% of adult cases may be due to *S. pneumoniae.* Corticosteroids may be used briefly to help reduce the postintubation edema that develops, but their efficacy has not been proven in this setting [60].

## REFERENCES

1. McCaig LF, Hughes JM. Trends in antimicrobial drug prescribing among office-based physicians in the United States. *JAMA* 1995;273:214.

2. Gonzales R, Steiner JF, Sande MA. Antibiotics prescribing for adults with colds, upper respiratory tract infections, and bronchitis by ambulatory care physicians. *JAMA* 1997;278:901.
3. Evans FO, et al. Sinusitis of the maxillary antrum. *N Engl J Med* 1975;293:735.
4. Gwaltney JM Jr, Syndor A Jr, Sande MA. Etiology and treatment of acute sinusitis *Ann Otol Rhinol Laryngol* 1981;90[Suppl](3 Pt 3):68–71.
5. Heikkinen T, Thint M, Chonmaitree T. Prevalence of various respiratory viruses in middle ear during acute otitis media. *N Engl J Med* 1999;340:260.
6. Yoon HG, Zhu Z, Gwaltney JM Jr, et al. Rhinovirus regulation of IL-1 receptor antagonist in vivo and in vitro: a potential mechanism of symptom resolution. *J Immunol* 1999;162:7461–7469.
7. Seymour ML, Gilby N, Bardin PG, et al. Rhinovirus infection increase 5-lipoxygenase and cyclooxygenase-2 in bronchial biopsy specimens from nonatopic subjects. *J Infect Dis* 2002;185:540–544.
8. Gwaltney JM Jr, et al. Computed tomographic study of the common cold. *N Engl J Med* 1994;330:25.
9. Rosenstein N, et al. The common cold—principles of judicious use of antimicrobial agents. *Pediatrics* 1998;101[Suppl]:181.
10. Sperber SJ, et al. Effects of naproxen on experimental rhinovirus colds: a randomized, double-blind controlled trial. *Ann Intern Med* 1992;117:37.
11. Smith MB, Feldman W. Over-the-counter cold medications: a critical review of clinical trials between 1950 and 1991. *JAMA* 1993;269:2258.
12. Muether PS, Gwaltney JM Jr. Variant effect of first-and second-generation antihistamines as clues to their mechanism of action on the sneeze reflex in the common cold. *Clin Infect Dis* 2001;33:1483–1488.
13. Turner RB, Sperber RJ, Sorrentino JV, et al. Effectiveness of clemastine fumarate for treatment of rhinorrhea and sneezing associated with the common cold. *Clin Infect Dis* 1997;25:824.
14. Gwaltney JM, Druce HM. Efficacy of brompheniramine maleate for treatment of rhinovirus colds. *Clin Infect Dis* 1997;25:1188.
15. Hayden FG, et al. Effectiveness and safety of intranasal ipratropium bromide in common colds: a randomized, double-blind, placebo-controlled trial. *Ann Intern Med* 1996;125:89.
16. Diamond L, et al. A dose-response study of the efficacy and safety of ipratropium bromide nasal spray in the treatment of the common cold. *J Allergy Clin Immunol* 1995;95:1139.
17. Sperber SJ, Turner RB, Sorrentino JV, et al. Effectiveness of pseudoephedrine plus acetaminophen for treatment of symptoms attributed to the paranasal sinuses associated with the common cold. *Arch Fam Med* 2000;9:979–985.
18. Kaiser L, Lew D, Hirschel B, et al. Effect of antibiotic treatment in the subset of common cold patients who have bacteria in their naso-pharyngeal secretions. *Lancet* 1996;347:1507–1510.
19. Rotbart HA. Treatment of picornavirus infections. *Antiviral Res* 2002;53:83–98.
20. Gwaltney JM Jr, Hendley JO. Transmission of experimental rhinovirus infection by contaminated surfaces. *Am J Epidemiol* 1982;116:828–833.
21. Bisno AL, et al. Diagnosis and management of group A streptococcal pharyngitis: a practice guideline. *Clin Infect Dis* 1997;25:574.
22. Schwartz B, et al. Pharyngitis: principles of judicious use of antimicrobial agents. *Pediatrics* 1998;101[Suppl]:171.
23. American Academy of Pediatrics. *1997 Red book,* 25th ed. Elk Grove, IL: 2000:526–536.
24. Dajani AS, et al. Treatment of acute streptococcal pharyngitis and prevention of rheumatic fever: a statement of health professionals by the Committee on Rheumatic Fever, Endocarditis, and Kawasaki Disease of the Council on Cardiovascular Disease in the Young, the American Heart Association. *Pediatrics* 1995;96:758.
25. Markowitz M, Gerber MA, Kaplan EL. Treatment of streptococcal pharyngotonsillitis: reports of penicillin's demise are premature. *J Pediatr* 1993;123:679.
26. Gerber MA. Treatment of failures and carriers: perceptions or problems. *Pediatr Infect Dis J* 1994;13:576.
27. Dowell SF, et al. Otitis media: principles of judicious use of antimicrobial agents. *Pediatrics* 1998;101[Suppl]:165.

28. Pichichero ME. Changing the treatment paradigm for acute otitis media. *JAMA* 1998;279:1748.
29. Poole MD. Implications of drug-resistant *Streptococcus pneumoniae* for otitis media. *Pediatr Infect Dis J* 1998;17:953.
30. Dagan R, Hoberman A, Johnson C, et al. Bacteriologic and clinical efficacy of high dose amoxicillin/clavulanate in children with acute otitis media. *Pediatr Infect Dis J* 2001;20:829.
31. Hirschmann JV. Methods for decreasing antibiotic use in otitis media. *Lancet* 1998;352:672.
32. Congeni BL. Therapy of acute otitis media in an era of antibiotic resistance. *Pediatr Infect Dis J* 1999;18:371.
33. Van Buchem FL, Peeters MF, Van't Hof MA. Acute otitis media: a new treatment strategy. *BMJ* 1985;290:1033.
34. Froom J, et al. Antimicrobials for acute otitis media? A review from the International Primary Care Network. *BMJ* 1997;315:98.
35. Gorbach SL. Reducing antibiotic resistance by less use of antibiotics for otitis media. *Infect Dis Clin Pract* 1999;8:ii.
36. American Academy of Pediatrics. *1997 Red book,* 25th ed. Elk Grove Village, IL: 2000:647–648.
37. Dagan R, Johnson CE, McLinn S, et al. Bacteriological and clinical efficacy of amoxicillin/clavulanate vs. azithromycin in acute otitis media. *Pediatr Infect Dis J* 2000;19:95.
38. Dagan R, Leibovitz F, Cheletz G, et al. Antibiotic treatment in acute otitis media promotes superinfection with resistant Streptococcus pneumoniae carried before initiation of treatment. *J Infect Dis* 2001;183:880–886.
39. Kozyrskyj AL, et al. Treatment of acute otitis media with a shortened course of antibiotics: a meta-analysis. *JAMA* 1998;279:1736.
40. Varsano I, Volovitz B, Horev Z, et al. Intramuscular ceftriaxone compared with oral amoxicillin-clavulanate for treatment of acute otitis media in children. *Eur J Pediatr* 1997;156:858–863.
41. Dagan R, Abramson O, Leibobitz E, et al. Bacteriologic response to oral cephalosporins: are established susceptibility break points appropriate in the case of acute otitis media? *J Infect Dis* 1997;176:1253–1259.
42. Cenjor C, Ponte C, Parra A, et al. In vivo efficacy of amoxicillin and cefuroxime against penicillin-resistant *Streptococcus pneumoniae* in a gerbil model of acute otitis media *Antimicrob Agents Chemother* 1998;42:1361–1364.
43. Dagan R, Leibovitz E, Fliss DM, et al. Bacteriologic efficacies of oral azithromycin and oral cefaclor in treatment of acute otitis media in infants and children. *Antimicrob Agents Chemother* 2000;44:43–50.
44. Leiberman A, Leibovitz E, Piglansky L, et al. Bacteriologic and clinical efficacy of trimethoprim-sulfasoxazole for treatment of acute otitis media. *Pediatr Infect Dis* 2001;20:26.
45. Stool SE, et al. Managing otitis media with effusion in young children: clinical practice guideline no. 12. U.S. Department of Health and Human Services. Public Health Service. Agency for Health Care Policy and Research Publications no. 94-0622, 1994.
46. Klugman KP. Efficacy of pneumococcal conjugate vaccines and their effect on carriage and antimicrobial resistance. *Lancet Infec Dis* 2001;1:85–91.
47. Nyquist AC. Antibiotic prescribing for children with colds, upper respiratory tract infections, and bronchitis. *JAMA* 1998;279:875.
48. O'Brien KL, et al. Cough illness/bronchitis: principles of judicious use of antimicrobial agents. *Pediatrics* 1998;101[Suppl]:178.
49. Anthonisen NR. Antibiotic therapy in exacerbations of chronic obstructive pulmonary disease. *Ann Intern Med* 1987;106:196.
50. Ball P, Make B. Acute exacerbations of chronic bronchitis: an international comparison. *Chest* 1998;113[Suppl]:199S.
51. Gwaltney JM Jr. Acute community-acquired sinusitis. *Clin Infect Dis* 1996;23: 1209.
52. O'Brien KL, et al. Acute sinusitis: principles of judicious use of antimicrobial agents. *Pediatrics* 1998;101[Suppl]:174.

53. Van Buchem FL, et al. Primary-care-based randomized placebo-controlled trial of antibiotic treatment in acute maxillary sinusitis. *Lancet* 1997;349:683.
54. Schlosser RJ, London SD, Gwaltney JM Jr, et al. Microbiology of chronic frontal sinusitis. *Laryngoscope* 2001;111:1330–1332.
55. Bojrab DI, Bruderly T, Abdulrazzak Y. Otitis externa. *Otolaryngol Clin North Am* 1996;29:761.
56. Slattery WH, Brackmann DE. Skull base osteomyelitis: malignant external otitis. *Otolaryngol Clin North Am* 1996;29:795.
57. Gehanno P. Ciprofloxacin in the treatment of malignant external otitis. *Chemotherapy* 1994;40[Suppl 1]:35.
58. Mayo-Smith MF, et al. Acute epiglottitis: an 18-year experience in Rhode Island. *Chest* 1995;108:1640.
59. Trollfors B, et al. Aetiology of acute epiglottitis in adults. *Scand J Infect Dis* 1998;30:49.
60. Frantz TD, et al. Acute epiglottitis in adults: analysis of 129 cases. *JAMA* 1994;272:1358.

# 9. INFECTIOUS MONONUCLEOSIS AND PRIMARY EPSTEIN-BARR VIRUS INFECTION

John W. Cixboy

Infectious mononucleosis (IM) is an acute illness common in adolescents characterized by the classic triad of fever, pharyngitis, and lymphadenopathy; serologically by the transient appearance of heterophile antibodies (sheep or horse erythrocyte agglutinins); and hematologically by an absolute lymphocytosis reflecting the unusually strong T-cell response elicited by virally infected B-lymphocytes. The Epstein-Barr virus (EBV), or human herpesvirus 4, is the primary etiologic agent. Acute infection is accompanied by immunoglobulin M (IgM) antibodies specific to EBV. The exaggerated nature of the T-cell response suggests that the **syndrome is largely immunopathogenic** in nature. Atypical cases highlight the protean manifestations of EBV infection that can confound clinical diagnosis. Furthermore, other infectious agents, specifically cytomegalovirus (CMV), acute human immunodeficiency virus 1 (HIV-1), and *Toxoplasma gondii,* can cause an IM-like syndrome that must be distinguished. A clear understanding of **age-related patterns of the disease,** combined with knowledge of **serologic profiles characteristic of acute EBV infection,** facilitates a diagnosis of IM and institution of appropriate therapeutic measures [1,2].

**I. Etiology.** EBV is a DNA virus of the gammaherpesvirus subfamily. Its discovery in Burkitt lymphoma, together with a demonstrated biologic capability to confer unlimited growth potential on infected B cells in culture, led to its designation as the first **human tumor virus** [3]. EBV manipulates the different phases of B-cell development to establish lifelong infection of its host while promoting successful transmission to new individuals. Aside from IM, the virus has a causal role in Burkitt lymphoma, Hodgkin disease, nasopharyngeal carcinoma, posttransplantation lymphoproliferative disease, gastric carcinoma, and oral hairy leukoplakia of acquired immunodeficiency syndrome (AIDS). EBV's ability to infect both lymphocytes and epithelial cells provides a pathobiologic basis for these diverse disease associations.

- **A.** The EBV link to IM was discovered serendipitously when a technician in the Henle laboratory, who devised immunofluorescent assays to EBV-specific antibodies, seroconverted after an episode of IM [4]. The finding was confirmed by large seroepidemiologic studies in college students [5–8]. Heterophile-positive IM occurred in patients without preexisting EBV antibody, and was followed by acquisition of EBV-specific antibodies.
- **B.** IM, from an evolutionary standpoint, is a **disease of delayed primary infection** distinctive to upper socioeconomic groups. Most children in developing countries become infected with EBV during the first 3 years of life, and 100% are infected at the end of their first decade. Early primary infections, which are almost always asymptomatic, probably reflect parent-to-child oral transmission of EBV. By contrast, up to half of the children in Western countries are EBV seronegative at the end of their first decade of life, and some 5% of adults are seronegative.

**II. Clinical features of IM**

- **A. Age at primary infection.** Patient age can have a major impact on clinical manifestations of primary EBV infection [9–16]. Most young children acquire the virus asymptomatically, with fewer than 10% developing a syndrome resembling IM. When primary EBV infection is delayed until adolescence, clinical manifestations occur in up to 50% of cases. Primary infection of the elderly is uncommon, if only because 90% to 97% of all population groups studied have seroconverted by adulthood. However, cases in adults can be severe, with atypical clinical manifestations that may mislead the clinician and provide a diagnostic challenge.
- **B. Viral acquisition and incubation period.** EBV is an ubiquitous agent that, paradoxically, is not highly contagious or efficiently spread. For instance, susceptible college roommates of students with IM undergo seroconversion at no greater frequency than the general student population [7,17]. Transmission requires intimate personal contact. Viral inoculation generally occurs via saliva passed between a susceptible individual and an asymptomatic oropharyngeal shedder of EBV (hence, the "kissing

disease"). **In healthy EBV-seropositive adults** followed prospectively over 15 months, **90% shed EBV in their saliva** at least once, with 25% shedding virus on every occasion [18]. Immunocompromised patients have still higher rates of shedding. Symptomatic infection at adolescence may relate to a larger inoculum of transmitted virus and the ensuing T-cell reaction. In young children the route of transmission may be more indirect, with smaller virus inoculums and inapparent symptomatology. Although EBV can be detected in the male and female genital tract, the implications of this distribution for person-to-person spread has not been demonstrated [19–22]. IM also has occurred subsequent to blood transfusion as well as bone marrow and organ transplantation.

No seasonal pattern has been documented. The incubation period for primary EBV infection is estimated to be 30 to 50 days. Little is known about early events of infection since timing of an exposure to an asymptomatic shedder is difficult to document. Onset of IM is usually preceded by several days of nonspecific prodromal symptoms that include chills, sweats, fever, and malaise.

**C. Signs and symptoms.** The **classical clinical triad** in IM is prolonged **fever** (10–14 days; 38°–40°C), **sore throat, and lymphadenopathy.** Additional common symptoms include malaise, headache, myalgias, sweats, and anorexia. Clinical findings that help support a bedside diagnosis include the following:

1. **Tonsillar enlargement, exudative tonsillitis, and pharyngeal inflammation.** Tonsillar enlargement is common, with tonsils occasionally meeting at midline. The pharynx is erythematous with an exudate present in a third of cases. The pharyngitis is indistinguishable from that caused by group A streptococcus or other viruses. Palatal petechiae occur in up to half.
2. **Lymphadenopathy.** Posterior and anterior cervical lymphadenopathy occurs in 80% to 90%, with submandibular, axillary, and inguinal nodes frequently enlarged.
3. **Hepatomegaly** is present in approximately 25%, with abnormal liver function tests in 80% of patients. Clinical jaundice may occur in up to 5% of cases.
4. **Splenomegaly** is present in more than half the cases over the course of illness. **Vigorous abdominal palpation during examination** should be avoided. Abdominal pain due to splenic enlargement is relatively uncommon and should alert one to the possibility of splenic rupture.
5. **Rash.** A rash, occurring in 5% to 10% of patients, is variable in presentation (maculopapular, petechial, scarlitinaform, urticarial, or erythema multiforme-like). **Ampicillin administration** produces a pruritic, maculopapular rash in 90% to 100% of patients, and may appear after cessation of the drug.

**D. Hematologic abnormalities**

1. **Lymphocytes.** The central hematologic manifestation of IM is an absolute and relative lymphocytosis, with monocytes and lymphocytes accounting for 60% to 70% of the total white cell count, some 10% to 20% of which are **atypical lymphocytes.** Atypical lymphocytes represent activated T cells (EBV typically infects B cells), are larger than the mature lymphocyte normally found in the circulation, and have a vacuolated cytoplasm, lobulated and eccentrically placed nuclei, with a cell membrane that is often indented by neighboring erythrocytes. Atypical lymphocytes are a hematologic hallmark of IM, but they are not pathognomonic; they are also found in CMV infection, viral hepatitis, toxoplasmosis, rubella, mumps, roseola, and drug reactions.
2. **Total white blood cell (WBC) count.** WBC counts generally range between 12,000 and 20,000/mm$^3$, but WBCs up to 50,000/mm$^3$ may occasionally be seen. A mild, self-limited neutropenia (2,000–3,000 granulocytes/mm$^3$) is present in a majority of cases, although profound granulocytopenia also has been reported.
3. **Thrombocytopenia** (<140,000/mm$^3$) may occur in half of the cases due to increased destruction by an enlarged spleen or antiplatelet antibodies.

**E. Heterophile antibodies and elevated serum inmmunoglobulins.** The early phase of acute IM is associated with mildly elevated levels of total serum IgG, IgM, and IgA, consistent with a **virus-driven polyclonal activation of the B-cell system.** Paralleling this general increase is the transient appearance of a

Table 9.1. Divergent Features of Epstein-Barr Virus–Induced Infectious Mononucleosis Related to Age at Onset

| | Age in Years | | | |
|---|---|---|---|---|
| Feature | <4[a] (%) | 14–35[b] (%) | >40[c] (%) | >60[b] (%) |
| Fever | 92 | 95 | 95 | 85 |
| Pharyngitis | 68 | 76 | 43 | 26 |
| Lymphadenopathy | 94 | 98 | 47 | 33 |
| Hepatomegaly | 64 | 23 | 42 | 33 |
| Jaundice | NR | 8 | 27 | 26 |
| Splenomegaly | 82 | 65 | 33 | 15 |
| Rash | 34 | NR | 12 | NR |
| Upper respiratory symptoms | 51 | NR | NR | NR |
| Eyelid edema | 14 | NR | NR | NR |

[a]Data from Sumaya CV, Ench Y. Epstein-Barr virus infectious mononucleosis in children. I. Clinical and general laboratory findings. *Pediatrics* 1985;75:1011–1019.
[b]Data from Schmader KE, van der Horst CM, Klotman ME. Epstein-Barr virus and the elderly host. *Rev Infect Dis* 1989;11:64–73.
[c]Data from Axelrod P, Finestone AJ. Infectious mononucleosis in older adults. *Am Fam Physician* 1990;42:1599–1606.
NR, not reported.

mix of heterophile and autoantibodies, usually of the IgM class. **Heterophile antibodies** occur as a **by-product of primary EBV infection** in about 90% of cases but **do not react with EBV antigens.** Originally described by Paul and Bunnell as sheep erythrocyte agglutinins, they form the basis for the commonly used rapid spot assays diagnostic for IM. Agglutinating antibodies to horse, goat, and camel erythrocytes as well as beef erythrocyte hemolysins are also demonstrable in serum of patients with IM. Other nonspecific antibody responses observed in patients include rheumatoid factors, antinuclear factors, antiplatelet and antineutrophil antibodies, cryoglobulins, and cold reactive antibodies to i antigen on RBCs.

F. **Atypical presentations.** Primary infection with EBV has been defined largely by the syndrome of IM. The spectrum of illness is quite broad, however, and individual cases may have all, some, or none of the classic triad mentioned above (Table 9.1) [23]. Attempts to exclude cases with unusual features or those that fail to meet all the classic criteria for IM may result in delayed diagnosis or misdiagnosis, particularly in **infants and the elderly** [9–16].

Although generally asymptomatic in younger children, primary EBV infection can produce symptomatology that when present is atypical for acute IM. Among 17 infants reported by Fleisher with serologic evidence of primary EBV infection, none developed signs or symptoms that were suggestive of acute IM [11]. Initial diagnoses varied from respiratory tract infection (43%) to otitis media (29%), pharyngitis (21%), and gastroenteritis (7%). Sumaya and Ench noted that in children under 4 years of age signs of upper respiratory tract infection were found in 51% versus 15% of older children [9]. Cutaneous rashes occur more frequently in younger children as does eyelid or periorbital swelling. A palpable spleen and liver were more frequent in children under 4 years of age.

Of the well-known triad of fever, pharyngitis, and lymphadenopathy, elderly patients are much less likely to have lymphadenopathy and pharyngitis than are younger patients [13–16]. Fever is present in almost all older patients, and abdominal pain, hepatomegaly, and liver function abnormalities occur in substantial numbers, frequently leading to an initial clinical impression of hepatitis. Older adults have fewer atypical lymphocytes and less significant lymphocytosis. Splenomegaly is less evident. The illness tends to be more prolonged in older adults.

**III. Diagnosis.** The clinical manifestations of fever, sore throat, lymphadenopathy together with atypical lymphocytosis and a positive heterophile test establish the diagnosis of EBV-induced IM.

**A. Differential diagnosis.** A variety of infectious agents can produce some of the clinical signs and symptoms of EBV-induced IM. Because they do not invoke a heterophile antibody response, these entities have been dubbed heterophile-negative mononucleosis and constitute some 10% to 15% of all cases. With careful attention to clinical and serologic features of the illness, IM-like entities can generally be differentiated from primary EBV infection.

1. **CMV infection.** CMV is responsible for about 8% of IM cases, or approximately half of the heterophile-negative cases. By comparison to those with EBV-induced disease, patients with the CMV mononucleosis-like syndrome tend to be older (25–35 years, although the syndrome also occurs in children [24]), pharyngitis and cervical lymphadenopathy is less frequent, and atypical lymphocytosis may be less intense. Acute CMV infection can be diagnosed by testing for the presence of IgM antibody to CMV.
2. **Acute retroviral syndrome.** Differentiating acute retroviral syndrome from IM is crucial and has obvious public health implications. Because acute HIV-1 infection may be particularly contagious, initiation of counseling may prevent further transmission. Early treatment also may reduce the incidence of HIV-1 complications. Acute retroviral syndrome presents with a broad array of signs and symptoms, with less than 20% of cases having classic features of IM [25]. A more acute onset and absence of exudative tonsillitis or tonsillar hypertrophy may help differentiate the syndrome from IM. A maculopapular rash (40%–80% of patients) and mucocutaneous ulceration are more characteristic of the acute retroviral syndrome. On the likelihood that health-care providers would perform testing for heterophile antibodies on patients that actually had acute retroviral syndrome, 563 heterophile antibody negative patient samples were retrospectively tested for HIV-1 RNA and p24 antigen. Approximately 1% were determined to have primary HIV-1 infection [26]. A rare false-positive heterophile test has been reported during the acute retroviral syndrome, probably as a consequence of EBV reactivation [27,28]. Clinicians considering a diagnosis of IM should also evaluate the patient's HIV risk behaviors and at least consider the diagnosis of primary HIV infection.
3. **Toxoplasmosis.** In the mononucleosis-like syndrome caused by acute toxoplasmosis, pharyngitis is not a prominent feature, the degree of lymphocytosis is mild, and liver functions are normal even in the presence of hepatomegaly. A history of ingestion of raw or undercooked meat or exposure to oocysts from cat feces may provide clues implicating this etiologic agent. The IgM immunofluorescent antibody test for *Toxoplasma gondii* is useful in diagnosing this disease.
4. **Streptococcal pharyngitis** may mimic IM in early stages. Throat cultures for $\beta$-hemolytic streptococci are positive in up to 30% of patients with IM. Therefore, isolation of this organism does not exclude a diagnosis of IM. Splenomegaly is absent in streptococcal sore throat, and normal hepatic enzymes serve as a differentiating factor.
5. **Hepatitis A.** Atypical lymphocytosis is of a lesser magnitude (<10% atypicals). Transaminase enzymes are disproportionately higher than levels of alkaline phosphatase, whereas the reverse is true of EBV and CMV hepatitis. Generally in EBV-induced disease, liver function test results are elevated two to three times the upper limit of normal (>10 times normal suggests another diagnosis).
6. **Rubella virus.** Rubella may be manifested by fever, sore throat, lymphadenopathy, and a mild atypical lymphocytosis, but the characteristic exanthem and shorter clinical course are generally not confused with IM.
7. **Other miscellaneous causes** include human herpes virus 6, adenovirus, diphtheria, *Mycoplasma* species, *Bartonella henselae* (cat scratch disease), leptospirosis, and brucellosis. Various hematologic neoplasms can present with features mimicking IM.

**B. Serologic diagnosis.** Laboratory diagnosis of acute EBV infection depends primarily on serologic testing. EBV-induced IM results in the production of antibodies against both unrelated antigens as well as EBV-specific antigens.

1. **Heterophile antibodies** are detected as sheep and horse red cell agglutinins and beef cell hemolysins. The classic heterophile antibody titer is read as the greatest serum dilution at which sheep erythrocytes agglutinate, after preabsorption of test serum against guinea pig kidney to eliminate cross-reaction with Forssman and serum sickness antibodies. Commercially available spot tests (Monospot, Mono-Test, Mono-Latex, Monosticon) and solid-phase immunoassays (Immunocard Mono, Monolert) have largely replaced the classic Paul-Bunnell sheep cell agglutination assay because of ease of use.
   - **a.** Heterophile antibody responses are generally present in 80% to 90% of cases by the third week of illness. **Repeat testing at weekly intervals** may be necessary in some patients, since up to 15% may not have detectable levels of heterophile antibody at presentation, then become positive on retesting in the second or third week of illness. Titers remain elevated for 3 to 6 months, but occasionally for as long as 1 year.
   - **b.** False-negative rates with the rapid test kits are 10% to 15 % [29]. **False-negative results are common in children under 4 years of age,** with fewer than 20% testing positive by the rapid slide test [9]. Hence, age of the patient is a critical consideration in the evaluation of heterophile-negative IM.
   - **c.** False-positive results, although rare, have been reported in patients with lymphoma, hepatitis, and other viral infections.
2. **EBV-specific antibody studies** should be reserved for the approximately 10% of cases of IM that are heterophile-negative, for diagnosis in children under 4 years of age, or for diagnosis in patients with atypical presentations. The antibodies are measured either by immunofluorescence or enzyme-linked immunosorbent assay. Antibody profiles allow the differentiation of recent from remote infection.
   - **a.** Presence of **IgM antibodies to viral capsid antigen (VCA)** is virtually diagnostic of acute EBV infection and is the most useful titer for general clinical purposes. VCA IgM usually disappears within 1 to 2 months. VCA IgG is also apparent at clinical presentation and is maintained for life. Detection of VCA IgG on a single sampling indicates only that infection with EBV has occurred sometime in the past.
   - **b.** Antibodies to **Epstein-Barr nuclear antigen 1 (EBNA1)** appear later in the course of IM (2–4 weeks) and persist for life. **VCA IgM/VCA IgG in the absence of EBNA1 antibodies,** followed by the appearance of EBNA1 antibodies in convalescent serum (at 4–6 weeks), is diagnostic of acute EBV infection. Failure to develop EBNA1 antibodies, or loss of a preexisting titer, has been associated with chronic active EBV infection.
   - **c.** Antibody to EBV early antigen (EA) may be detected in the majority of patients with IM, then falls to a low or undetectable level.
   - **d.** **Healthy carriers** of virus are consistently VCA IgG and anti-EBNA1 positive. A significant number of virus carriers also maintain antibodies to EA. **Titers can differ markedly** among healthy individuals, and differences tend to be stable over time.

**C. Virus isolation and molecular diagnostic techniques.** Culture of Epstein-Barr virus from oropharyngeal secretions or peripheral blood is possible, but impractical in the clinical laboratory. The lymphocyte transformation assay requires 4 to 6 weeks, and viral isolation does not necessarily indicate acute infection, given the life-long carrier state established in all infected individuals. Quantitative PCR for estimating viral load in peripheral blood has been shown to be useful in the diagnosis and management of aberrant EBV infections, with high viral burdens demonstrated in peripheral blood of patients with chronic active EBV and posttransplantation lymphoproliferative disease [30,31]. The technique is unlikely to be helpful for the routine diagnosis of IM.

**IV. Complications.** Diagnostic confusion can result from the varied complications accompanying primary EBV infection, manifestations that in some cases are the sole presentation of illness. Most complications resolve fully, although rare fatalities do occur.

**A. Hematologic.**

1. **Autoimmune hemolytic anemia** occurs in up to 3% of cases, generally mediated by cold-agglutinin antibodies of anti-i specificity. The anemia resolves without treatment over a 1- to 2-month period in most individuals. Hemophagocytic syndrome also has been described.
2. Mild **thrombocytopenia** is common, but platelet counts of less than 1,000/mm$^3$ with associated intracerebral bleeding can occur.
3. **Granulocytopenia** is usually mild and self-limiting, but deaths associated with bacterial sepsis have been reported.

**B. Neurologic manifestations** (<1% of cases) can be the first (and sometimes the only) manifestation of IM, with the heterophile antibody often being negative. **Nerve palsies and encephalitis** are the most common neurologic complications. Encephalitis seen with IM is acute in onset, rapidly progressive, and severe, but is usually associated with complete recovery. An "Alice-in-Wonderland" syndrome, characterized by metamorphopsia (distortion of size, shape, and spatial relations of objects), has been described. Aseptic meningitis, Guillain-Barré syndrome, Bell palsy, and transverse myelitis also have been reported.

**C. Splenic rupture** (0.2% of cases) must be considered whenever abdominal pain occurs. History of preceding trauma can be elicited in only half the cases, suggesting spontaneous rupture.

**D. Upper airway obstruction** is estimated to occur in up to 1% of cases.

**E. Other complications** rarely observed include myositis, myocarditis, pneumonitis, pancreatitis, acute renal failure, and death. Death is most commonly associated with neurologic complications, splenic rupture, or airway obstruction. A familial syndrome passed in an X-linked–recessive pattern (X-linked lymphoproliferative disease or Duncan syndrome) may result in overwhelming infection at primary infection with death (typically from a fulminant hepatic failure) in up to 40% of affected males.

**V. Management. No therapy is indicated for the vast majority of cases** of EBV-induced IM. Treatment is primarily supportive, but corticosteroid or antiviral therapy may be considered in special settings.

**A. Specific antiviral therapy is not indicated** for most cases of IM. Acyclovir (ACV), a nucleoside analogue that blocks EBV replication through inhibition of viral DNA polymerase, has little if any effect on the disease course, but is capable of preventing viral shedding from the oropharynx [32,33]. Symptoms are therefore unlikely to be the result of viral replication per se, and IM most likely represents an immunopathologic disease. (Contrast this to the effect of drug in oral hairy leukoplakia of AIDS, where ACV effectively resolves lingual lesions associated with exuberant EBV replication [34]). Use in immunocompromised patients at risk for EBV-induced lymphoproliferative disease with the idea of limiting additional B-cell recruitment by infectious virus may be ineffective. Elimination of EBV replication as an endogenous source of infectious virus does not translate into a reduced load of latently infected B cells in the circulation [35]. However, other considerations favoring therapy of primary EBV infections in specific immunocompromised hosts may exist [36]. Ganciclovir and cidofovir have demonstrated *in vitro* activity against EBV, but there are no clinical indications for their use in IM.

**B. Salicylates or other analgesics** are appropriate for control of fever, headache, and sore throat.

**C. Corticosteroids** have been useful in management of specific complications, although their value has not been confirmed in controlled studies. Prednisone at a dosage of 40 to 60 mg/day for 7 to 10 days, to be rapidly tapered once a clinical response is achieved, can be considered for the following complications:

1. **Impending airway obstruction** due to severe tonsillitis and pharyngeal edema
2. **Severe thrombocytopenia**
3. **Acute hemolytic anemia**
4. **Myocarditis**
5. **Neurologic complications**

**D. Precautionary measures** to protect against splenic rupture in the first few weeks after diagnosis might include care in splenic palpation and attention to constipation. Contact sports should be avoided until the spleen has resumed normal size.

E. **Control measures**

1. **Physical isolation of patients** is not indicated in hospital or home settings, given that intimate contact is required for virus transmission. Standard precautions are sufficient.
2. Individuals with acute EBV infection **should not be** selected as **tissue or blood donors** when possible, due to the enhanced cell-associated viral load accompanying primary infection.

VI. **Prognosis** Most cases of IM resolve spontaneously over a 3- to 6-week period, with periods of well-being interrupted by recrudescence of symptoms. Associated malaise is more gradual in its resolution, lasting up to 3 to 4 months in some individuals. As with all human herpesviruses, primary infection is followed by establishment of a life-long carrier state characterized by asymptomatic oropharyngeal shedding and the possibility for reactivation disease.

A. Self-assessed **failure to recover** completely from IM has been reported by 38% of patients at 2 months and 12% at 6 months, with persistent symptoms characterized mainly as fatigue and impaired functional status but without objective markers of disease [37].

B. **Chronic active EBV infection** [38–40] is a rare outcome of primary EBV infection that is characterized by **severe illness** lasting greater than 6 months and is associated with fever, **major organ involvement** (interstitial pneumonitis, bone marrow hypoplasia, hepatosplenomegaly, persistent hepatitis and hepatic failure, lymphadenitis, uveitis), a **highly unusual serologic profile to EBV** (IgG to VCA >1:5120, EA >1:640, and a low to undetectable EBNA1 titer), persistently high EBV loads in peripheral lymphocytes, and occasional development of natural killer cell or T-cell lymphoproliferative disease.

C. The **chronic fatigue syndrome** is not specifically related to EBV infection [41,42].

D. **Reinfection,** or serial acquisition of EBV strains, does occur [43,44]. Whether there are clinical manifestations or serologic responses characteristic of repeat infections remains to be resolved [45].

E. A history of IM has been linked epidemiologically to a threefold increased **risk for Hodgkin disease in younger adults** [46]. Although about half of all Hodgkin disease tumors contain EBV-positive Reed-Sternberg cells, a history of IM has not been predictive of which tumors will contain the virus [47].

## REFERENCES


1. Schooley RT. Epstein-Barr virus (infectious mononucleosis). In: Mandell GL, Bennett JE, Dolin R, eds. *Principles and practice of infectious diseases,* 5th ed. New York: Churchill Livingstone, 2000:1599–1612.
2. Rickinson AB, Kieff E. Epstein-Barr virus. In: Fields BN, Knipe DM, Howley PM, et al., eds. *Field's virology,* 4th ed. Philadelphia: Lippincott-Raven, 2001:2575–2627.
3. Pagano JS. Epstein-Barr virus: the first human tumor virus and its role in cancer. *Proc Assoc Am Physicians* 1999;111:573–580.
4. Henle G, Henle W, Diehl V. Relation of Burkitt's tumor associated herpestype virus to infectious mononucleosis. *Proc Natl Acad Sci USA* 1968;59:94–101.
5. Niederman JC, McCollum RW, Henle G, et al. Infectious mononucleosis: clinical manifestations in relation to EB virus antibodies. *JAMA* 1968;203:205–209.
6. Evans AS, Niederman JC, McCollum RW. Seroepidemiologic studies of infectious mononucleosis with EB virus. *N Engl J Med* 1968;279:1121–1127.
7. Sawyer RN, Evans AS, Niederman JC, et al. Prospective studies of a group of Yale University freshman. I. Occurrence of infectious mononucleosis. *J Infect Dis* 1971;123:263–270.
8. University Health Physicians and PHLS Laboratories. A joint investigation of infectious mononucleosis and it relationship to EB virus antibody. *BMJ* 1971;4:643.
9. Sumaya CV, Ench Y. Epstein-Barr virus infectious mononucleosis in children. I. Clinical and general laboratory findings. *Pediatrics* 1985;75:1003–1010.
10. Sumaya CV, Ench Y. Epstein-Barr virus infectious mononucleosis in children. II. Heterophil antibody and viral specific responses. *Pediatrics* 1985;75:1011–1019.
11. Fleisher G, Henle W, Henle G, et al. Primary infection with Epstein-Barr virus in infants in the United States: clinical and serologic observations. *J Infect Dis* 1979;139:553–558.

12. Hickey SM, Strasburger VC. What every pediatrician should know about infectious mononucleosis in adolescents. *Pediatr Clin North Am* 1997;44:1541–1556.
13. Auwaerter PG. Infectious mononucleosis in middle age. *JAMA* 1999;281:454–459.
14. Axelrod P, Finestone AJ. Infectious mononucleosis in older adults. *Am Fam Physician* 1990;42:1599–1606.
15. Hurwitz CA, Henle W, Henle G, et al. Infectious mononucleosis in patients aged 40 to 72 years: report of 27 cases, including 3 without heterophil-antibody responses. *Medicine* 1983;62:256–262.
16. Schmader KE, van der Horst CM, Klotman ME. Epstein-Barr virus and the elderly host. *Rev Infect Dis* 1989;11:64–73.
17. Hallee TJ, Evans AS, Niederman JC, et al. Infectious mononucleosis at the United States Military Academy. A prospective study of a single class over 4 years. *Yale J Biol Med* 1974;47:182–195.
18. Yao QY, Rickinson AB, Epstein MA. A re-examination of the Epstein-Barr virus carrier state in healthy seropositive individuals. *Int J Cancer* 1985;35:35–42.
19. Sixbey JW, Lemon SM, Pagano JS. A second site for Epstein-Barr virus shedding: the uterine cervix. *Lancet* 1986;2:1122–1122.
20. Sisson BA, Glick L. Genital ulceration as a presenting manifestation of infectious mononucleosis. *J Pediatr Adolesc Gynecol* 1998;11:185–187.
21. Portnoy J, Ahronheim GA, Ghibu F, et al. Recovery of Epstein-Barr virus from genital ulcers. *N Engl J Med* 1984;311:966–968.
22. Naher H, Gissmann L, Freese UK, et al. Subclinical Epstein-Barr infection of both the male and female genital tract: indication for sexual transmission. *J Invest Dermatol* 1992;98:791–793.
23. Taga K, Taga H, Tosato G. Diagnosis of atypical cases of infectious mononucleosis. *Clin Infect Dis* 2001;33:83–88.
24. Lajo A, Borque C, del Castillo F, et al. Mononucleosis caused by Epstein-Barr virus and cytomegalovirus in children: a comparative study of 124 cases. *Pediatr Infect Dis J* 1994;13:56–60.
25. Vanhems P, Allard R, Cooper DA, et al. Acute human immunodeficiency virus type 1 disease as a mononucleosis-like illness: Is the diagnosis too restrictive? *Clin Infect Dis* 1997;24:965–970.
26. Rosenberg ES, Caliendo Am, Walker BD. Acute HIV infection among patients tested for mononucleosis [Letter]. *N Engl J Med* 1999;340:969.
27. Vidrih JA, Walensky RP, Sax PE, et al. Positive Epstein-Barr virus heterophile antibody tests in patients with primary human immunodeficiency virus infection. *Am J Med* 2001;111:192–194.
28. Walensky RP, Rosenberg ES, Ferraro MJ, et al. Investigation of primary human immunodeficiency virus infection in patients who test positive for heterophile antibody. *Clin Infect Dis* 2001;33:570–572.
29. Linderholm M, Boman J, Juto P, et al. Comparative evaluation of nine kits for rapid diagnosis of infectious mononucleosis and Epstein-Barr virus-specific serology. *J Clin Microbiol* 1994;32:259–261.
30. Stevens SJ, Pronk I, Middeldorp JM. Toward standardization of Epstein-Barr virus DNA load monitoring: unfractionated whole blood as preferred clinical specimen. *J Clin Microbiol* 2001;39:1211–1216.
31. Ohga S, Nomura A, Takada H, et al. Epstein-Barr virus (EBV) load and cytokine gene expression in activated T cells of chronic active EBV infection. *J Infect Dis* 2001;183: 1–7.
32. Andersson J, Britton S, Ernberg I, et al. Effect of acyclovir on infectious mononucleosis: a double-blinded, placebo-controlled study. *J Infect Dis* 1986;153:283–290.
33. Torre D, Tambini R. Acyclovir for treatment of infectious mononucleosis: a meta-analysis. *Scand J Infect Dis* 1999;31:543–547.
34. Walling DM, Flaitz CM, Nichols CM, et al. Persistent productive Epstein-Barr virus replication in normal epithelial cells in vivo. *J Infect Dis* 2001;184:1499–1507.
35. Yao QY, Ogan P, Rowe M, et al. Epstein-Barr virus-infected B cells persist in the circulation of acyclovir-treated virus carriers. *Int J Cancer* 1989;43:67–71.
36. Mañez R, Breinig MC, Linden P, et al. Posttransplant lymphoproliferative disease in

primary Epstein-Barr virus infection after liver transplantation: the role of cytomegalovirus disease, *J Infect Dis* 1997;176:1462–1467.
37. Buchwald DS, Rea TD, Katon WJ, et al. Acute infectious mononucleosis: characteristics of patients who report failure to recover. *Am J Med* 2000;109:531–537.
38. Rickinson AB. Chronic symptomatic Epstein-Barr virus infections. *Immunol Today* 1986;7:13–14.
39. Straus SE. The chronic mononucleosis syndrome. *J Infect Dis* 1988;157:405–412.
40. Ishihara S, Okada S, Wakiguchi H, et al. Chronic active Epstein-Barr virus infection in children in Japan. *Acta Paediatr* 1995;84:1271–1275.
41. Mawle AC, Nisenbaum R, Dobbins JG, et al. Seroepidemiology of chronic fatigue syndrome: a case control study. *Clin Infect Dis* 1995;21:1386–1389.
42. McKenzie R, Straus SE. Chronic fatigue syndrome. *Adv Intern Med* 1995;40:119–153.
43. Sixbey JW, Shirley P, Chesney PJ, et al. Detection of a second widespread strain of Epstein-Barr virus. *Lancet* 1989;2:761–765.
44. Yao QY, Croom-Carter DSG, Tierney RJ, et al. Epidemiology of infection with Epstein-Barr virus types 1 and 2: lessons from the study of a T cell immunocompromised hemophiliac cohort. *J Virol* 1998;72:4352–4363.
45. Pichler R, Berg J, Hengstschlager A, et al. Recurrent infectious mononucleosis caused by Epstein-Barr virus with persistent splenomegaly. *Milit Med* 2001;166:733–734.
46. Glaser SL, Jarrett RF. The epidemiology of Hodgkin's disease. In: Diehl V, ed. *Hodgkin's disease.* London: Bailliere Tindall, 1996:401–416.
47. Sleckman BG, Mauch PM, Ambinder RF, et al. Epstein-Barr virus in Hodgkin's disease: correlation of risk factors and disease characteristics with molecular evidence of viral infection. *Cancer Epidemiol Biomarkers Prevent* 1998;7:1117–1121.

# 10. INFLUENZA AND INFECTIONS OF THE TRACHEA, BRONCHI, AND BRONCHIOLES

John J. Treanor and Caroline Breese Hall

## INFLUENZA

Influenza is a relatively specific syndrome resulting from infection with any influenza A or B virus. Infection with other respiratory viruses occasionally may result in influenza-like illness, but other viruses do not cause epidemics that affect all age groups. Infection with influenza A or B virus may result in any of the other viral syndromes discussed in this chapter. Influenza C virus infection results in only a small proportion of common cold illnesses and is not discussed in this chapter.

I. **Etiology.** Influenza viruses are medium-sized enveloped viruses with a segmented RNA genome and are classified into types A, B, and C. The envelope of influenza A and B viruses contains two glycoproteins: the hemagglutinin (H) and the neuraminidase (N). Multiple subtypes of H and N exist for influenza A viruses, and standard nomenclature for these viruses includes the type, location, and year of isolation, strain designation, and H and N subtype for influenza A viruses.

II. **Epidemiology.** Influenza occurs in yearly epidemics, with occasional worldwide epidemics referred to as pandemics. In a community, an epidemic due to a single subtype generally lasts 5 to 6 weeks, but more prolonged epidemics may occur. Attack rates may be as high as 10% to 20% and are usually highest in young children, whereas hospitalization rates are highest in the elderly. Yearly epidemic activity is manifested by increases in school absenteeism, visits to health- care facilities, admissions to hospitals for pneumonia, and deaths [1].

   Influenza viruses have a high degree of antigenic variability, which allows for recurrent epidemics despite widespread prior exposure to influenza viruses in the population. Two forms of this antigenic variation are recognized: antigenic drift and antigenic shift.

   A. **Antigenic drift, which occurs in both A and B viruses,** is a relatively **minor antigenic change** within the H or N due to the accumulation of point mutations. The antigenically variant virus is able to infect individuals and spread within the population despite the presence of antibody to previous strains of virus, and epidemics of variable extent result.

   B. **Antigenic shift** refers to **major antigenic change** within the H or N, resulting in a new subtype. These viruses enter a population that is immunologically naïve. Worldwide pandemics result (Table 10.1). Antigenic shift occurs only with influenza A viruses.

III. **Clinical manifestations.** Characteristically, the onset of influenza is abrupt after an **incubation period** of 1 to 2 days. Many patients can recall the exact hour of onset.

   A. **Symptoms. Systemic symptoms** predominate and include feverishness, chilliness or occasionally frank shaking chills, headaches, myalgias, malaise, and anorexia [2]. Malaise and fatigue may be quite prolonged. Myalgias may involve the extremities or the long muscles of the back, and may be accompanied by arthralgias. **Respiratory symptoms,** particularly dry cough or nasal discharge, also are usually present at the onset, but they are overshadowed by the systemic symptoms. Nasal obstruction, hoarseness, and dry or sore throat may be present as well, and these symptoms tend to become more prominent as the disease progresses. **Ocular symptoms,** although less commonly present, are helpful diagnostically and include photophobia, tearing, burning, and pain on moving the eyes. **In the young infant,** influenza mimics sepsis (fever and no localizing findings). Even in older children, influenza may be manifest occasionally as an undifferentiated febrile illness without respiratory or localizing symptoms. **In the elderly,** fever may be low grade or absent, and myalgias and feverishness minimal. The presentation is dominated by severe fatigue, malaise, and listlessness.

   B. **Signs.** Early in the course of illness, the patient appears toxic, the face is flushed, and the skin is hot and moist. Eyes are watery and reddened.

Table 10.1. Major Antigenic Shifts and Pandemic Influenza

| Year | Interval (years) | Designation | Changes in Indicated Surface Proteins | Results |
|---|---|---|---|---|
| 1889 | — | H3N2 | — | Moderate pandemic |
| 1918 | 29 | H1N1 | H, N | Most severe pandemic |
| 1957 | 39 | H2N2 | H, N | Severe pandemic |
| 1968 | 11 | H3N2 | H | Moderate pandemic |
| 1977 | 9 | H1N1 | H, N | Mild |

H, hemagglutinin; N, neuraminidase.

1. **Fever** is the most important finding. It usually rises rapidly to a peak of 100° to 106°F (38°–41°C) within 12 hours of onset of systemic symptoms. It usually is continuous but may be intermittent, especially if antipyretics are administered. On the second and third days of illness, the fever is usually 0.5° to 1.0°F (0.5°C) lower, and as the fever subsides, so do the systemic symptoms. Fever may last from 1 to 5 or more days.
2. **Nasal and other respiratory findings.** Clear **nasal discharge** is common. Nasal obstruction occurs less frequently. The mucous membranes are hyperemic, but exudate is not observed. Small, tender cervical lymph nodes may be present. Transient, scattered rhonchi or localized areas of rales are found in fewer than 20% of cases.

   As systemic signs and symptoms diminish, respiratory complaints and findings become more apparent. **Cough** is the most frequent and troublesome symptom and may be accompanied by substernal discomfort or burning. Nasal obstruction and discharge and pharyngeal pain and injection also are common. Such symptoms and signs usually persist 3 to 4 days after fever subsides. Cough, lassitude, and malaise may last 1 to 2 weeks after disappearance of other manifestations.

**IV. Laboratory findings** are nonspecific. Leukocytosis of up to 15,000 cells/mm$^3$ may be observed early in the illness, usually without a shift to the left. Mild leukopenia may be observed later. Pulmonary findings seen on radiography are described in section **VII.A.**

**V. Diagnosis**

**A. Viral cultures. Specific diagnosis is best made by viral culture techniques.** Separate swab specimens of throat and nose are ideal and should be placed immediately into viral transport media for good results. In cases of tracheobronchitis or pneumonia, sputum constitutes the best specimen in adults, whereas in children a nasal wash is best. Specimens tested in cell cultures or embryonated chicken eggs may yield positive results as early as 3 days. For isolated or complicated cases, viral diagnosis is essential.

**B. Direct antigen detection tests** have become available in which the presence of influenza-specific antigens in respiratory secretions is detected immunologically. These tests include the Directigen Flu A + B (Becton-Dickinson), Quickvue Flu (Quidel Corporation), and Flu OIA (Biostar). In addition, the Zstat Flu test (Zymtek) identifies influenza through detection of viral neuraminidase activity. Each of these tests has a turnaround time of 30 minutes or less, with reported sensitivities of 60% to 90% compared with cell culture [3]. Generally, performance is better with nasopharyngeal swabs, washes, or sputum than with throat gargles or swabs [4,5].

**C. Epidemiologic data are sufficient to make the diagnosis in most uncomplicated cases in adults.** If influenza is prevalent in the community, most adults and older children with acute febrile respiratory illness, especially with nonproductive cough, have influenza [6]. However, in children, multiple respiratory viruses such as respiratory syncytial virus (RSV) and parainfluenza,virus which may be present concurrently, confound the clinical diagnosis. Elderly patients may not manifest the systemic symptoms seen in younger adults. A specific viral diagnosis should always be sought in hospitalized patients with complications of influenza.

## VI. Treatment

**A. Symptomatic.** Symptomatic therapy such as that described for common colds, pharyngitis, and tracheobronchitis may be advised for fever, headache, myalgias, and cough. **Salicylates and salicylate-containing medications are not advised for children with influenza. The use of salicylates in children has been associated with Reye syndrome.** Acetaminophen and ibuprofen are commonly used as antipyretic agents.

**B. Antiviral agents**

1. **Neuraminidase inhibitors: oseltamivir and zanamivir.** These agents work through inhibition of the viral neuraminidase, an enzyme with critical roles in penetration of respiratory tract mucus and in the release of virus from infected cells. The neuraminidase inhibitors are active against both influenza A and influenza B viruses at millimolar concentrations or less [7]. Activity against influenza viruses include avian viruses with all nine known neuraminidase subtypes.

   Both zanamivir and oseltamivir have been shown to be effective in the treatment of uncomplicated influenza of healthy adults, resulting in an approximately 30% more rapid resolution of illness and a more rapid return to normal activities [8,9]. Both drugs also have resulted in significantly reduced rates of influenza complications, such as pneumonia and bronchitis, and early treatment with oseltamivir also may result in less frequent subsequent hospitalizations. Treatment should be begun within 48 hours of symptom onset, and continued for 5 days, at dosages shown in Table 10.2.

   Oseltamivir therapy in children results in more rapid resolution of fever and clinical symptoms, and reduced rates of otitis media [10]. Oseltamivir is approved for children as young as 1 year. Studies of neuraminidase inhibitors in elderly individuals and those with high-risk conditions have also generally shown a trend toward more rapid reduction of symptoms and possibly reduced complications.

   Both oseltamivir and zanamivir are well tolerated when used for therapy. Approximately 10% of treated individuals experience mild nausea with the first dose of oseltamivir, particularly when administered on an empty stomach. Because food does not interfere with absorption, when possible, oseltamivir should be administered with food. In controlled trials of zanamivir, side effects have not been different from placebo. However, there have been multiple reports of significant bronchospasm when zanamivir has been administered to patients with acute influenza.

   Resistance to neuraminidase inhibitors arises in approximately 3% of treatment courses with oseltamivir and less often with zanamivir. Resistance arises either through mutations within the neuraminidase site, which decreases binding, or through mutations in the hemagglutinin, which decrease the affinity of the virus for its receptor [11–13]. Both types of resistance appear to decrease the replication efficiency of the virus, and the resistant viruses have attenuated virulence in animals.

2. **M2 inhibitors: amantadine and rimantadine.** These chemically related agents act by inhibiting the influenza A virus M2 protein, an ion channel that is critical for viral uncoating. **Both drugs are active only against influenza A viruses** [14]. Treatment should be begun within 48 hours of symptom onset, and continued for 2 to 5 days, at dosages shown in Table 10.2.

   Controlled trials of uncomplicated influenza in healthy adults showed that both drugs resulted in more rapid reductions in symptoms, more rapid return to normal activities, and reduced levels and duration of viral shedding when compared with placebo, aspirin, or acetaminophen [15,16]. The efficacy of the two drugs is similar. Treatment of children with either drug also has been shown to reduce the duration and severity of fever and other symptoms, but only amantadine is approved for this indication in the United States. Neither drug has

Table 10.2. Properties of Antiviral Agents for Influenza

| | M2 Inhibitors | | Neuraminidase Inhibitors | |
|---|---|---|---|---|
| Agents | Amantadine | Rimantadine | Zanamivir | Oseltamivir |
| Spectrum of activity | A only | A only | A and B | A and B |
| Metabolism/excretion | | | None | Hepatic deesterification<br>Renal tubular excretion |
| Drug interactions | Antihistamines, anticholinergics increase CNS side effects | None | None | None (probenecid reduces renal clearance) |
| Usual adult dose | | | | |
| Therapy | 100 mg orally b.i.d. | 100 mg orally b.i.d. | 10 mg (2 inhalations) b.i.d. | 75 mg orally b.i.d. |
| Prophylaxis | 100 mg orally b.i.d. | 100 mg orally b.i.d. | NA | 75 mg/day orally |
| Dosing in children | | | | |
| Therapy | ≤40 kg: 5 mg/kg/day | ≤40 kg: 5 mg/kg/day | NA (≥7 years of age: adult dose) | <40 kg: 2 mg/kg orally b.i.d. |
| Prophylaxis | ≤40 kg: 5 mg/kg/day | ≤40 kg: 5 mg/kg/day | NA | NA (≥13 years of age: adult dose) |
| Dosage modifications | | | | |
| Renal dysfunction | Reduce if CrCl ≤50 mL/min | 100 mg/day if CrCl ≤10 mL/min | No change | Half dose for CrCl <10–30 mL/min |
| Hepatic dysfunction | No change | 100 mg/day orally if severe | Not studied | Not studied |
| Elderly | 100 mg/day orally | 100 mg/day orally | No change | No change |
| Main side effects | CNS (major)<br>GI (minor) | CNS (minor)<br>GI (minor) | Bronchospasm (not recommended in asthma) | GI (observed in 10–14% of prescribed courses) |

CNS, central nervous system; b.i.d., twice daily; NA, not applicable; GI, gastrointestinal; CrCl, creatine clearance.

Adapted from Centers for Disease Control and Prevention. Prevention and control of influenza: recommendations of the Advisory Committee on Immunization Practices (ACIP). *MMWR* 2001;50(RR-4):1–32; with permission.

been evaluated in high-risk subjects or for treatment of complicated influenza (e.g., hospitalized patients or those with pneumonia).

Both amantadine and rimantadine are generally well tolerated when used for treatment, although minor central nervous system (CNS) disturbances such as difficulty concentrating and sleeping may be seen with amantadine. Amantadine may lower the seizure threshold and should be avoided in individuals with a history of seizures or seizure potential. Dosage reductions are recommended in the elderly (Table 10.2).

Viruses may become resistant to M2 inhibitors through single point mutations in the M2 protein [17], and such resistant viruses arise frequently (~30% of treatment courses or more) in treated individuals [18]. Resistant viruses are fully virulent in animal models and can be transmitted to and cause typical influenza in contacts.

C. **Antibiotics should not be used in uncomplicated influenza because they are of no benefit and potentially harmful by causing resistant secondary bacterial infections to occur.** Antibiotic therapy should be reserved for confirmed bacterial infections.

VII. **Complications.** The majority of influenza cases are not associated with any significant complications. However, a spectrum of complications has been well described.

A. Two kinds of **pulmonary complications** are well recognized: primary influenza viral pneumonia and secondary bacterial pneumonia. Comparative features of the secondary pulmonary complications of influenza are shown in Table 10.3.

1. **Primary influenza viral pneumonia** occurs predominantly in persons with cardiovascular disease (especially rheumatic heart disease with mitral stenosis) or in pregnant women. Cases rarely occur in young healthy adults, however.

a. **Clinical manifestations.** Following onset of symptoms, there is rapid progression of fever, cough, dyspnea, hypoxemia, and cyanosis [20]. Physical examination and chest radiography reveal bilateral findings, consistent with pulmonary edema, but no consolidation is seen. There are no pathognomonic findings.

b. **Course and prognosis.** These patients often show **a progressive downhill course unresponsive to antibiotics.** Serial arterial blood gases show progressive hypoxemia. Despite supportive care with artificial ventilation (including extracorporeal oxygenation), the mortality rate is high. At autopsy, findings include tracheitis, bronchitis, diffuse hemorrhagic pneumonia, hyaline membrane lining alveolar ducts and alveoli, and a paucity of inflammatory cells within the alveoli.

c. **A relatively mild form of viral interstitial pneumonia may occur in young children** that is clinically similar to the lower respiratory tract disease produced by other common respiratory viruses in infants, such as respiratory syncytial and parainfluenza viruses. These infants may present with a fever, mild cough, and upper respiratory tract symptoms, and may be admitted with the diagnosis of possible sepsis. Chest radiography typically shows interstitial infiltrates in one or more lobes. This type of lower respiratory tract involvement is part of the acute influenza syndrome rather than a secondary complication.

2. **Secondary bacterial pneumonia is more common** than primary viral pneumonia.

a. **Clinical manifestations.** This is encountered more frequently in the elderly or those with preexisting pulmonary disease. It starts with a typical influenza illness, often followed by a period of improvement lasting 1 to 4 days, and then a relapse. New fever is associated with symptoms and signs of bacterial pneumonia such as cough, sputum production, and often consolidation on physical examination and chest radiography. However, the period of improvement may not occur, and the course is variable. Gram stains and cultures of sputum may reveal predominance of a pathogen, most often *Streptococcus pneumoniae* or *Haemophilus influenzae.* Mixed bacterial pneumonias and *Staphylococcus aureus* secondary pneumonia also occur more frequently after influenza [21].

Table 10.3. Comparative Features of Pulmonary Complications of Influenza

| Clinical Parameter | Primary Viral Pneumonia | Secondary Bacterial Pneumonia | Mixed Viral-Bacterial Pneumonia | Localized Viral Pneumonia |
|---|---|---|---|---|
| Setting | Cardiovascular disease; pregnancy; young adult (Hsw1N1) | Elderly age; pulmonary disease | Same as for primary viral or secondary bacterial pneumonia | ?Normal host |
| Clinical history | Relentless progression from classic 3-day influenza | Improvement, then worsening after 3-day classic influenza | Picture of A or B | Continuation of cough after classic 3-day syndrome |
| Physical examination | Bilateral findings, no consolidation | Consolidation | Consolidation | Area of rales |
| Sputum Bacteriologic evaluation | Negative | Pneumococci Staphylococci, *H. influenzae* | Pneumococci Staphylococci, *H. influenzae* | Negative |
| Chest roentgenogram | Bilateral findings | Consolidation | Consolidation | Segmental infiltrate |
| WBC count | Leukocytosis with shift to left | Leukocytosis with shift to left | Leukocytosis with shift to left | Usually normal |
| Isolation of influenza virus | Yes | No | Yes | Yes |
| Response to antibiotics | No | Yes | Yes | No |
| Mortality | High | Low | Low | Very low |

b. **Course and prognosis.** These patients **respond to specific antibiotic therapy** and supportive measures.
c. **Therapy.** Therapy should be guided by the results of sputum Gram stain and culture. Because the spectrum of bacterial etiologies is similar to that seen with community- acquired pneumonia (CAP), guidelines for CAP are reasonable [22]. This includes an oral macrolide such as azithromycin or clarithromycin or an oral fluoroquinolone with antipneumococcal activity in outpatients, and intravenous (i.v.) ceftriaxone (1 g every 24 hours), in hospitalized adults with normal renal function. In children, therapy should be directed against *S. pneumoniae* and group A streptococcus.

3. **Other pulmonary complications.** During an outbreak of influenza, **many cases are observed that do not fit clearly into either of the preceding categories.** Many of these patients have mixed viral and bacterial infection of the lung (Table 10.3), and most of these mixed infections respond to antibiotics. In addition, milder forms of influenza viral pneumonia involving only one lobe or segment have been described, which do not invariably lead to death and are often confused with pneumonia due to *Mycoplasma pneumoniae.*
4. **Otitis media** occurs in up to 30% of children 3 to 4 days after onset of influenza.

B. **Reye syndrome** is a rare hepatic and CNS complication occurring primarily in children who ingest salicylates **after influenza B** viral infection, but also after varicella and influenza A infection. It presents as encephalopathy and fatty degeneration of the liver. Since intensive educational campaigns began, the syndrome has almost disappeared.

C. **Myositis and myoglobinuria** with tender leg muscles and elevated serum creatine phosphokinase levels have been reported (mostly in children) after influenza A and influenza B infection, most commonly the latter. Symptoms may be sufficiently severe to prevent walking, but neurologic changes are not evident.

D. **Guillain-Barré syndrome (GBS)** has been reported to occur after influenza A infection, numerous other infections, and rarely after influenza immunization.

E. Both **myocarditis** and **pericarditis** have been associated rarely with influenza A and B viral infection. However, neither myocarditis nor pericarditis is observed commonly on autopsy of those dying of primary influenza viral pneumonia.

F. **Neurologic complications** besides Reye syndrome also may occur with influenza, such as encephalopathy and ataxia. Febrile convulsions are a relatively frequent complication of influenza in preschool children. A rapidly progressive encephalopathy with bilateral thalamic necrosis has been reported in children in Japan [23,24].

## VIII. Prevention

A. **Inactivated influenza vaccines** are 70% to 90% effective in the prevention of influenza illness when there is a good antigenic match between vaccine and epidemic viruses [25–27]. Vaccination of young adults is also associated with decreased absenteeism from work or school and is significantly cost saving in working adults [28]. Inactivated vaccine also is effective in prevention of influenza in children, with prevention of asthma exacerbations [29] and reductions in the rate of acute otitis media [30], and has substantial economic benefit in this age group [31,32]. Relatively few prospective trials of protective efficacy have been conducted in high- risk populations. In one recent randomized placebo-controlled trial in an elderly population, inactivated vaccine was approximately 58% effective in preventing laboratory-documented influenza [33]. In addition, numerous retrospective case-control studies have documented the effectiveness of inactivated influenza vaccines in these individuals. Vaccine is protective against influenza and pneumonia-related hospitalization in the elderly, and is accompanied by a decrease in all-cause mortality [34].

1. **Formulation.** Inactivated influenza vaccines consist of inactivated whole virus, disrupted virus (split-product), or purified H and N (subunit) vaccines. The immunogenicity of each is similar. Because of the frequent antigenic changes, the virus strains to be included in the vaccine must be updated regularly. The trivalent formulation of influenza vaccine contains one H3N2, one H1N1, and one B virus.

Table 10.4. Target Groups for Influenza Vaccination

| |
|---|
| Groups at increased risk for influenza-related complications |
| Persons ≥65 years of age |
| Residents of nursing homes and other chronic-care facilities that house persons of any age who have chronic medical conditions |
| Adults and children who have chronic disorders of the pulmonary or cardiovascular systems, including asthma |
| Adults and children who have required regular medical follow-up or hospitalization during the preceding year because of chronic metabolic diseases (including diabetes mellitus), renal dysfunction, hemoglobinopathies, or immunosuppression (including immunosuppression caused by medications or by human immunodeficiency [HIV] virus) |
| Children and teenagers (6 months to 18 years of age) who are receiving long-term aspirin therapy and therefore might be at risk for developing Reye syndrome after influenza infection |
| Women who will be in the second or third trimester of pregnancy during the influenza season. |
| Persons 50–64 years of age and those who can transmit influenza to those at high risk |
| Physicians, nurses, and other personnel in both hospital and outpatient-care settings, including emergency response workers |
| Employees of nursing homes and chronic-care facilities who have contact with patients or residents |
| Employees of assisted living and other residences for persons in groups at high risk |
| Persons who provide home care to persons in groups at high risk |
| Household members (including children) of persons in groups at high risk |

Adapted from Centers for Disease Control and Prevention. Prevention and control of influenza: recommendations of the Advisory Committee on Immunization Practices (ACIP). *MMWR* 2001;50(RR-4):1–32; with permission.

2. **Indications.** Target groups for influenza vaccination [19] include (a) those who are at increased risk for influenza-related complications, (b) persons who can transmit influenza to those at high risk, and (c) individuals between the ages of 50 and 64. This last group contains a significant proportion of the individuals under the age of 65 who have high-risk conditions. An age-based strategy represents the most effective way to reach these patients, and vaccination beginning at age 50 is consistent with recommendations for annual physician visits (Table 10.4). In addition, vaccine may be used in any individual who wishes to avoid an unpleasant influenza illness.
3. **Administration. A single dose of vaccine is sufficient for most individuals, but two doses of vaccine are required in those who have not been primed by previous infection** or vaccination with similar antigen type, such as children under 9 years of age, or in the event of antigenic shift. Whole-virus vaccine should not be used in children under 12 years of age because of increased systemic reactions. Because the duration of protective immunity afforded by influenza vaccine appears to be limited and vaccine formulations change frequently, annual vaccination, usually in the late fall (e.g., late October or November) is recommended. Vaccine may be administered at the same visit as pneumococcal vaccine, which, although not given yearly, is also recommended for many of the same groups of individuals.
4. **Side effects** of influenza vaccine **are minimal,** consisting of mild soreness at the injection site in a minority of recipients. Systemic symptoms following vaccination are rare and occurred at approximately the same rate in vaccine and placebo recipients in controlled trials. In some years, GBS has been associated with influenza vaccine. The risk of GBS following vaccination is estimated at approximately one excess case of GBS for every million doses of vaccine [35].

B. **A live attenuated influenza vaccine** (FluMist) is also being considered for licensure in the United States for use in children and healthy adults. This vaccine has excellent efficacy in children under 6 years of age, in which a two-dose vaccine schedule provided 96% protection against influenza A and 90% protection against influenza B [36]. The vaccine also protected against a significant antigenic variant [37], suggesting that the live attenuated vaccine induces a broadly cross-reactive antibody response in children. Efficacy studies of FluMist have not been conducted in adults. However, a trial of a related monovalent vaccine in adults showed approximately equal efficacy to inactivated vaccine in the prevention of laboratory-confirmed influenza illness [38]. In addition, FluMist reduced the rates of severe febrile illness in adults during the influenza season [39]. Although the vaccine is well tolerated in high-risk and elderly subjects, there are insufficient data suggesting efficacy to recommend use in these populations.

C. **Chemoprophylaxis** with the drugs described in section VI.B above is also effective for prevention of influenza. All four agents appear to have similar levels of efficacy, with the proviso that amantadine and rimantadine are only effective against influenza A viruses, and that zanamivir, while shown to be effective for prevention of influenza in controlled studies, is not licensed for this indication in the United States. Studies of chemoprophylaxis have generally dealt with two situations: seasonal prophylaxis, in which an antiviral agent is administered throughout the influenza season, and postexposure prophylaxis, in which drug is given for a relatively shorter period of time following a known exposure to an influenza-infected person. Antiviral prophylaxis cannot substitute for vaccination, but can be considered for several situations listed below:

1. **Seasonal prophylaxis.** Administration of amantadine, rimantadine, zanamivir, or oseltamivir for 4 to 6 weeks during influenza epidemics results in reductions of 70% to 90% in the rates of laboratory confirmed influenza [40–42]. In a comparative trial, the efficacies of amantadine and rimantadine were identical, but rimantadine was associated with a lower frequency of CNS side effects than was amantadine [40]. Zanamivir and oseltamivir have not been compared directly. Although seasonal prophylaxis has been the basis for many clinical trials, the circumstances in which this would be used clinically are rare. However, seasonal prophylaxis can be considered in high-risk patients in whom vaccination is not possible or is contraindicated, for immunodeficient individuals who do not respond to vaccination, or for unvaccinated individuals who care for high-risk patients.
2. **Postvaccination prophylaxis.** Development of a protective immune response following influenza vaccine can take as long as 2 weeks, so short-term prophylaxis should be used in high-risk patients who are not vaccinated until after influenza epidemic activity has begun. None of the four available agents are known to interfere with the immune response to inactivated vaccine.
3. **Family prophylaxis.** Many studies have demonstrated that short-term prophylaxis of family members with amantadine [43], rimantadine [44,45], zanamivir [46], or oseltamivir [47] following identification of an index case can reduce the rate of secondary family cases during the period in which prophylaxis is administered. An important observation of these studies has been that resistant influenza A viruses have emerged rapidly and have been transmitted to contacts when amantadine or rimantadine were used both for treatment of index cases and prophylaxis of contacts [48]. In contrast, resistant viruses have not been isolated in studies where the index case has received treatment and contacts have received prophylaxis with either zanamivir or oseltamivir.
4. **Outbreak prophylaxis in chronic care institutions.** Where a volatile mix of high- risk populations and crowding exists, explosive and devastating outbreaks of influenza can occur. Thus, once an outbreak of influenza is recognized, potentially exposed individuals should receive prophylaxis with an appropriate antiviral agent for a minimum of 2 weeks, or for 1 week after the last recognized case [49]. Amantadine-resistant viruses emerge rapidly in this setting, and where possible, amantadine- (or rimantadine-) treated patients should be isolated from those receiving prophylaxis. The neuraminidase inhibitors may

offer some advantages in this setting because of the less frequent resistance [50], but they are significantly more expensive.

5. **Dosing and administration.** Dosing and administration of available chemotherapeutic agents are described in Table 10.8.

## LARYNGITIS AND CROUP (ACUTE LARYNGOTRACHEOBRONCHITIS)

I. **Acute viral laryngitis** is an afebrile, self-limited illness characterized by **hoarseness** or sometimes loss of voice. Visualization of the larynx reveals erythema and some edema, with little involvement of the pharynx and nose. As an isolated syndrome, acute viral laryngitis occurs much less frequently than does acute viral rhinitis or pharyngitis. However, some degree of laryngitis occurs in 10% to 20% of patients with common colds, and a somewhat higher incidence exists in patients with acute viral pharyngitis. The viruses most frequently isolated are parainfluenza virus types 1, 2, and 3. Although presumably all the remaining respiratory viruses occasionally may be involved, none of these has been isolated regularly. **Bacteria are not a cause** of this syndrome. There is **no specific treatment,** but resting the voice and inhalation of steam or cold-water vapor often are helpful.

II. **Acute viral laryngotracheobronchitis (croup)** [51]. Acute laryngotracheobronchitis, or viral croup, is a clinically distinctive syndrome characterized by respiratory distress, inspiratory stridor, and subglottic swelling that occurs predominantly in children 6 months to 5 years of age.

A. **Etiology.** As discussed in Chapter 8, parainfluenza virus type 1 is the most frequent cause of croup [52]. Parainfluenza viruses types 2 and 3 and influenza A also are major agents. Influenza A is particularly important, for although it is a less frequent cause of croup than parainfluenza type 1, it tends to cause more severe disease. Less common causes of croup are RSV, influenza B virus, rhinoviruses, adenoviruses, enteroviruses, rubeola virus, and *M. pneumoniae.* Overall, viruses may be recovered from croup cases more frequently (40%–75%) than from other types of respiratory illnesses.

B. **Epidemiology** of croup mirrors that of its major viral agents, occurring when parainfluenza type 1 is prevalent, which often is in the fall of every other year. Fewer upsurges of croup are seen with parainfluenza type 2 activity, which, although less predictable than type 1, also occurs in the fall [53]. The number of croup cases may increase with influenza A outbreaks (which usually occur between December and April). In contrast, parainfluenza type 3 viruses often cause outbreaks of infection in spring [54].

C. **Clinical manifestations** [51]. An upper respiratory tract infection usually precedes the onset of croup, which is heralded by a **distinctive cough** with a deep, brassy tone, called a seal's bark. Laryngitis and fever are common, particularly with influenza A and parainfluenza viral infections.

1. **Stridor.** The development of **inspiratory** stridor is usually abrupt, often occurring at night, and is associated with respiratory distress. Obstruction of air flow occurs during both inspiration and expiration but is greater on inspiration because the negative inspiratory pressure tends to further narrow the subglottic area.
2. **Respiratory findings.** Retractions of the accessory muscles of the chest wall are common, and the **respiratory rate is increased** but usually to no more than 50 to 60 breaths per minute. Inspiration is prolonged and, on auscultation, rales, wheezes, and rhonchi may be heard. With increasing obstruction, the breath sounds may diminish and cyanosis may appear. The course of croup is variable and fluctuating.
3. **Hypoxemia** occurs in the hospitalized patients with croup. It arises from involvement of the lung parenchyma. Subglottic inflammation, which is most evident clinically, does not contribute to the hypoxemia until fatigue and hypercapnia ensue.

D. **Diagnosis.** The diagnosis is made on the basis of the characteristic clinical features and can be confirmed by a posteroanterior radiograph of the neck, which in viral croup shows the narrowing of the tracheal air shadow in the subglottic region. Viral cultures can be performed on respiratory secretions. It is important to distinguish this syndrome from other causes of airway obstruction, such as epiglottitis.

E. **Treatment.** Many and varied therapies have become legendary, their success being based on grandmothers' trials and the characteristic fluctuating course of croup.

1. **Oxygen is the mainstay** of treatment for the severely affected.
2. **The value of mist therapy has not been proved.** Water from the standard home- use vaporizer cannot reach the lower respiratory tract because of the large particle size.
3. **Nebulized racemic epinephrine** gives symptomatic relief by diminishing airway obstruction. However, the clinical improvement is transitory (<2 hours) and generally is not associated with an improvement in the arterial oxygen saturation. Side effects such as tachycardia may occur. Recommended doses are 0.25 mL of a 2.25% solution for children less than 6 months of age, and 0.5 mL for older children.
4. **Corticosteroids.** Steroids have been shown to confer significant benefits in the management of mild, moderate, and severe croup, including more rapid improvement in symptoms, reduced length of hospital stay, and reduced rates of intubation. Parenteral dexamethasone in doses over 0.3 mg/kg, nebulized corticosteroids, and oral dexamethasone (0.15–0.6 mg/kg) have all been shown to be equally effective [55]. Administration of single-dose steroid therapy in this setting has not been associated with significant side effects, and should probably be used on any patient with significant enough illness to require an emergency room or clinic visit [56].
5. Croup is largely a viral illness, so **antibiotics are not beneficial** and should only be used when concomitant bacterial infection is present.
6. **Ventilatory support** may be necessary for the rare hospitalized patients with significant obstruction not responsive to corticosteroids.

## BACTERIAL TRACHEITIS

I. **Bacterial tracheitis** is a relatively rare syndrome that mimics epiglottitis or severe viral croup [57]. Although this syndrome has been recognized only recently, and has been described mostly in children, it may occur at any age. It is important to differentiate bacterial tracheitis from viral croup because of its potential for rapid progression that necessitates intubation and because of the need for prompt antibiotic therapy.

II. **Etiology.** Bacterial tracheitis usually is caused by *S. aureus* and *H. influenzae* type b, but group A streptococci and *S. pneumoniae* also have been associated with this syndrome.

III. **Clinical manifestations.** Bacterial tracheitis affects those who have had previous tracheal injury or compromise, such as by intubation or sometimes by a preceding viral infection. The onset is acute, with stridor, dyspnea, and sometimes high fever. Abundant purulent sputum or secretions are usually evident and may cause rapid airway obstruction as in epiglottitis.

IV. **Diagnosis is made by direct laryngoscopy,** which shows localized inflammation and membranous exudate in the subglottic area, and sometimes by a lateral soft tissue radiograph of the neck, demonstrating the subglottic narrowing with a shaggy, exudative membrane. The epiglottis is usually normal, however. Blood cultures are generally negative.

V. **Treatment.** Therapy should be initiated as soon as possible with antibiotics for the most likely organisms, such as ceftriaxone. Cultures of the exudative membrane should subsequently allow the antibiotic regimen to be narrowed to cover the isolated pathogen.

## BRONCHIOLITIS

**Bronchiolitis** is confined to children (mainly ages 1–24 months). It is **due primarily to infection with RSV** [58], **but occurs** with other viruses.

I. **Symptoms.** After several days of typical upper respiratory tract illness, the infant develops a deepening cough and the onset of dyspnea and wheezing.

II. **Signs.** The infant's respiratory rate increases, and retraction of the intercostal muscles is seen due to respiratory obstruction. On auscultation, rales, rhonchi, and expiratory wheezing are present and may fluctuate in intensity. Cyanosis may be present; even without overt cyanosis, however, hypoxemia is commonly present [59].

III. **Chest radiography** shows hyperaeration with or without infiltrates. The infiltrates result either from the atelectasis, which is part of the pathology of bronchiolitis, or from a concomitant viral pneumonia, which is frequently also present.

**IV. Diagnosis. Rapid diagnostic tests of** respiratory secretions to detect RSV as well as other respiratory viruses such as parainfluenza and influenza viruses are widely available (see Chapter 25). Lacking those, a clinical diagnosis can be made, particularly during an outbreak of RSV infections, by the characteristic findings of acute respiratory signs with wheezing and hyperaeration in a child in the first 2 years of life. The major entities in the differential diagnosis are asthma, gastroesophageal reflux, and aspiration of a foreign body.

**V. Therapy.**

**A. Antiviral therapy** is available for some of the viruses responsible for bronchiolitis, but the use of such therapy for the most common etiology, RSV, remains controversial. Ribavirin therapy has resulted in diminished clinical severity and improved oxygenation in all of the randomized, placebo-controlled studies in which these outcomes were assessed. However, the numbers of subjects in such studies have been small, and studies have not confirmed significant long-term benefits in treated children. The high cost, difficult aerosol administration, and concern about potential toxicity among exposed health-care workers, combined with the conflicting results of clinical trials, have contributed to the controversy over its use. The American Academy of Pediatrics currently recommends that ribavirin be considered, primarily in selected high-risk infants, with the decision individualized according to the particular clinical circumstances [60].

**B. Bronchodilators** may produce modest short-term clinical improvements, but their use is controversial because benefit is not consistently observed in all infants and treatment may be associated with side effects such as tachycardia. Because a subgroup of infants with bronchiolitis appear to benefit from nebulized bronchodilators, a monitored trial may be warranted in infants with moderate to severe disease.

**C. Corticosteroids** are generally ineffective and are not indicated in previously healthy infants with bronchiolitis [61,62].

**D. Antibiotics are not warranted, and bacterial suprainfections are rare.** The mainstay of supportive therapy is the monitoring and maintenance of adequate oxygenation.

**VI. Prevention.** Prophylaxis against RSV lower respiratory tract disease, including bronchiolitis, may be provided by i.v. administration of RSV-IGIV (intravenous immune globulin), which contains high titers of RSV neutralizing antibody from selected donors, or intramuscular administration of palivizumab, a humanized mouse monoclonal antibody to RSV. Controlled studies of these agents have demonstrated significant reductions in hospital admissions in infants receiving monthly prophylaxis for 5 months during RSV season [63,64]. The American Academy of Pediatrics recommends that palivizumab or RSV-IGIV prophylaxis should be considered for infants under 2 years of age with chronic lung disease who required medical therapy within 6 months prior to the onset of the RSV season. Palivizumab is preferred because of its easy intramuscular administration and safety. Infants born at 32 weeks' gestation or earlier who do not have chronic lung disease also may be considered for such prophylaxis depending on other risk factors [65]. In general, decisions for use within both groups of infants must be individualized.

## VIRAL PNEUMONIA

Pneumonia is covered in Chapter 11. However, because **viral pneumonia** is due to the same viruses responsible for other respiratory tract syndromes, see Chapter 8 for further discussion.

**I. Infants and children.** In infants and children under 5 years of age (especially under age 2), **viruses are the most common cause of pneumonia.** RSV, the parainfluenza viruses, and influenza A virus are the most important pathogens.

**II. Otherwise healthy adults** seldom have true viral pneumonia [66].

**A. Young adults.** The majority of cases are associated with influenza viruses (see section **VIII**). Adenoviruses also have been described as causes of significant outbreaks of atypical pneumonia in military recruits, and less often, in civilians. Adenovirus illness is typically mild, but more severe disseminated infections and deaths have been reported [67]. Chest radiographs taken in adults with varicella reveal infiltrates in 10% to 20%, most frequently with a nodular infiltrate with peribronchial distribution involving both lungs. RSV occasionally causes pneumonia in otherwise healthy adults [68]. Clinical features of the hantavirus pulmonary syndrome include onset of severe pulmonary dysfunction after a 2- to 3-day prodrome of nonspecific influenza-like symptoms, fever, myalgias, cough, gastrointestinal symptoms, and headache [69]. Laboratory abnormalities include leukocytosis, increased hematocrit due to hemoconcentration, and thrombocytopenia with coagulopathy.

**B. Older adults** are much more likely to have bacterial pneumonia, although influenza virus can cause pneumonia, and RSV has recently been associated with pneumonia and exacerbations of chronic lung disease in the elderly [70]. It has been estimated that 2% to 4% of pneumonia deaths among the elderly in the United States may be due to RSV [71]. Parainfluenza viruses also have been reported as occasional causes of pneumonia in adults and in the elderly [72].

**C. Patients infected with the human immunodeficiency virus.** Cytomegalovirus (CMV) often is isolated from the respiratory secretions (or lung biopsies) of these patients. How often CMV is a primary pathogen (if ever) in this setting is unclear (see Chapter 18).

**D. Other immunosuppressed patients** may develop severe, life-threatening pulmonary infections with RNA and DNA viruses, including both viruses that are typical causes of lower respiratory tract disease in normal hosts, and other, more opportunistic viral pathogens. CMV is etiologic, particularly in lung and marrow transplant recipients. The highest risk is 1 to 3 months posttransplantation, with the peak incidence at 8 weeks. The presence of neutropenia, abnormalities of liver function test results, and mucosal ulcerations may be clinical clues to the diagnosis. Herpes simplex pneumonia has been reported largely in immunocompromised or debilitated individuals. The majority of cases present as a focal pneumonia as a result of contiguous spread from the upper respiratory tract; diffuse interstitial disease resulting from hematogenous spread occurs in up to 40% of cases [73]. Varicella-zoster virus is an important problem in individuals with hematologic malignancies and others with iatrogenic immunosuppression, with the greatest risk seen in organ transplantation. Adenoviruses are significant causes of morbidity and mortality in immunocompromised patients, particularly after transplantation. In contrast to infection in normal hosts, infection in immunocompromised subjects tends to be disseminated, with isolation of virus from multiple body sites including lung, liver, gastrointestinal tract, and urine [74].

RNA viruses have also received increasing recognition as potential causes of significant morbidity and mortality in this population [75]. RSV is well recognized as a cause of pneumonia in recipients of bone marrow [76] and solid organ transplantation [77]. Many cases are nosocomial. The illness typically begins with upper respiratory tract infection symptoms that progress over several days to severe, life-threatening lower respiratory tract involvement. Mortality rates of 50% or higher are typical if pneumonia supervenes, particularly if disease occurs in the preengraftment period [78]. Parainfluenza viruses also have been reported as a less frequent lower respiratory tract pathogen in both solid organ and bone marrow transplantation [75]. Influenza virus also may cause severe disease in transplant recipients [79] and leukemics. Rhinovirus infections in this population are also common, but tend to be associated less frequently with lower respiratory tract disease [80]. Measles giant cell pneumonia is a severe, usually fatal form of pneumonia in immunosuppressed individuals [81], who may present without rash or other typical manifestations of measles, and a high index of suspicion must be maintained.

## REFERENCES


1. Glezen WP, Couch RB. Interpandemic influenza in the Houston area, 1974–1976. *N Engl J Med* 1978;298:587–593.
2. Nicholson KG. Human influenza. In: Nicholson KG, Webster RG, Hay AJ, eds. *Textbook of influenza.* Oxford: Blackwell, 1998:219–266.
3. Newton DW, Treanor JJ, Menegus MA. Clinical and laboratory diagnosis of influenza virus infections. *Am J Managed Care* 2000;6(suppl):265–275.
4. Ryan-Pourier KA, Katz JM, Webster RG, et al. Application of directagen FLU-A for the detection of influenza A virus in human and non-human specimens. *J Clin Microbiol* 1992;30:1072–1075.

5. Covalciuc KA, Webb KH, Carlson CA. Comparison of four clinical specimen types for detection of influenza A and B viruses by optical immunoassay (FLU OIA test) and cell culture methods. *J Clin Microbiol* 1999;37:3971–3974.
6. Monto AS, Gravenstein S, Elliott M, et al. Clinical signs and symptoms predicting influenza infection. *Arch Intern Med* 2000;160:3243–3247.
7. Gubareva LV, Kaiser L, Hayden FG. Influenza virus neuraminidase inhibitors. *Lancet* 2000;355:827–835.
8. Hayden FG, Osterhaus ADME, Treanor JJ, et al. Efficacy and safety of the neuraminidase inhibitor zanamivir in the treatment of influenzavirus infections. *N Engl J Med* 1997;337:874–880.
9. Treanor JJ, Hayden FG, Vrooman PS, et al. Efficacy and safety of the oral neuraminidase inhibitor oseltamivir in treating acute influenza: a randomized, controlled trial. *JAMA* 2000;283:1016–1024.
10. Whitley RJ, Hayden FG, Reisinger KS, et al. Oral oseltamivir treatment of influenza in children. *Pediatr Infect Dis J* 2001;20:127–133.
11. Gubareva LV, Matrosovich MN, Brenner MK, et al. Evidence for zanamivir resistance in an immunocompromised child infected with influenza B virus. *J Infect Dis* 1998;178:1257–1262.
12. Gubareva LV, Bethell R, Hart GJ, et al. Characterization of mutants of influenza A selected with the neuraminidase inhibitor 4-guanidino-Neu5Ac2en. *J Virol* 1996;70:1818–1827.
13. Blick TJ, Sahasrabudhe A, McDonald M, et al. The interaction of neuraminidase and hemagglutinin mutations in influenza virus in resistance to 4-guanidino-neu5ac2en. *Virology* 1998;246:95–103.
14. Douglas RG Jr. Prophylaxis and treatment of influenza. *N Engl J Med* 1990;322:443–450.
15. Younkin SW, Betts RF, Roth FK, et al. Reduction in fever and symptoms in young adults with influenza A/Brazil/78 H1N1 infection after treatment with aspirin or amantadine. *Antimicrob Agents Chemother* 1983;23:577–582.
16. Van Voris LP, Betts RF, Hayden FG, et al. Successful treatment of naturally occurring influenza A/USSR/77 H1N1. *JAMA* 1981;245:1128–1131.
17. Hay AJ, Wolstenholme AJ, Skehel JJ, et al. The molecular basis of the specific anti-influenza action of amantadine. *EMBO J* 1985;4:3021–3024.
18. Hall CB, Dolin R, Gala CL, et al. Children with influenza A infection: treatment with rimantadine. *Pediatrics* 1987;80:275–282.
19. Centers for Disease Control and Prevention. Prevention and control of influenza: recommendations of the Advisory Committee on Immunization Practices (ACIP). *MMWR* 2001;50(RR-4):1–32.
20. Louria DB, Blumenfeld HL, Ellis JT, et al. Studies on influenza in the pandemic of 1957–1958. II. Pulmonary complications of influenza. *J Clin Invest* 1959;38:213–265.
21. Schwarzmann SW, Adler JL, Sullivan RFJ, et al. Bacterial pneumonia during the Hong Kong influenza epidemic of 1968–1969. *Arch Intern Med* 1971;127:1037–1041.
22. Bartlett JG, Dowell SF, Mandell LA, et al. Practice guidelines for the management of community-acquired pneumonia in adults. *Clin Infect Dis* 2000;31:347–382.
23. Sugaya N. Influenza-associated encephalopathy in Japan: pathogenesis and treatment. *Pediatr Int* 2000;42:215–218.
24. Shinjoh M, Bamba M, Jozaki K, et al. Influenza A–associated encephalopathy with bilateral thalamic necrosis in Japan. *Clin Infect Dis* 2000;31:611–613.
25. Meiklejohn G, Eickhoff TC, Graves P, et al. Antigenic drift and efficacy of influenza virus vaccines, 1976–1977. *J Infect Dis* 1978;138:618–624.
26. Meiklejohn G. Viral respiratory disease at Lowry Air Force Base in Denver, 1952–1982. *J Infect Dis* 1983;148:775–783.
27. Ruben FL. Prevention and control of influenza: role of vaccine. *Am J Med* 1987;82:31–33.
28. Nichol KL, Lind A, Margolis KL, et al. The effectiveness of vaccination against influenza in healthy, working adults. *N Engl J Med* 1995;333:889–893.
29. Kramarz P, Destefano F, Gargiullo PM, et al. Does influenza vaccination prevent asthma exacerbations in children? *J Pediatr* 2001;138:306–310.

30. Clements DA, Langdon L, Bland C, et al. Influenza A vaccine decreases the incidence of otitis media in 6- to 30-month old children in day care. *Arch Pediatr Adolesc Med* 1995;149:1113–1117.
31. Cohen GM, Nettleman MD. Economic impact of influenza vaccination in preschool children. *Pediatrics* 2000;106:973–976.
32. White T, Lavoie S, Nettleman MD. Potential cost savings attributable to influenza vaccination of school-aged children. *Pediatrics* 1999;103:e73.
33. Govaert TM, Thijs CT, Masurel N, et al. The efficacy of influenza vaccination in elderly individuals. A randomized double-blind placebo-controlled trial. *JAMA* 1994;272:1956–1961.
34. Fedson DS, Wajda A, Nicol JP, et al. Clinical effectiveness of influenza vaccination in Manitoba. *JAMA* 1993;270:1956–1961.
35. Lasky T, Tarracciano GJ, Magder L, et al. The Guillain-Barrè syndrome and the 1992–1993 and 1993–1994 influenza vaccines. *N Engl J Med* 1998;339:1797–1802.
36. Belshe RB, Mendelman PM, Treanor J, et al. The efficacy of live attenuated cold- adapted trivalent, intranasal influenzavirus vaccine in children. *N Engl J Med* 1998;358:1405–1412.
37. Belshe RB, Gruber WC, Mendelman PM, et al. Efficacy of annual vaccination with live attenuated, cold-adapted, trivalent, intranasal influenza virus vaccine against a variant (A/Sydney) not contained in the vaccine. *J Pediatr* 2000;136:168–175.
38. Edwards KM, Dupont WD, Westrich MK, et al. A randomized controlled trial of cold-adapted and inactivated vaccines for the prevention of influenza A disease. *J Infect Dis* 1994;169:68–76.
39. Nichol KL, Mendelman PM, Mallon KP, et al. Effectiveness of live, attenuated intranasal influenza virus vaccine in healthy, working adults: a randomized controlled trial. *JAMA* 1999;282:137–144.
40. Dolin R, Reichman RC, Madore HP, et al. A controlled trial of amantadine and rimantadine in the prophylaxis of influenza A in humans. *N Engl J Med* 1982;307:580–584.
41. Monto AS, Robinson DP, Herlocher ML, et al. Zanamivir in the prevention of influenza among healthy adults: a randomized controlled trial. *JAMA* 1999;282:31–35.
42. Hayden FG, Atmar RL, Schilling M, et al. Use of the selective oral neuraminidase inhibitor oseltamivir to prevent influenza. *N Engl J Med* 1999;341:1336–1346.
43. Galbraith AW, Oxford JS, Schild GC. Protective effect of 1-adamantanamine hydrochloride on influenza A2 in the family environment. *Lancet* 1969;2:1026–1028.
44. Clover RD, Crawford SA, Abell TD, et al. Effectiveness of rimantadine prophylaxis of children within families. *Am J Dis Child* 1986;140:706–709.
45. Crawford SA, Clover RD, Abell TD, et al. Rimantadine prophylaxis in children: a follow-up study. *Pediatr Infect Dis J* 1988;7:379–383.
46. Hayden FG, Gubareva LV, Monto AS, et al. Inhaled zanamivir for the prevention of influenza in families. *N Engl J Med* 2000;343:1282–1289.
47. Welliver R, Monto AS, Carewicz O, et al. Effectiveness of oseltamivir in preventing influenza in household contacts: a randomized controlled trial. *JAMA* 2001;285:748–754.
48. Hayden FG, Belshe RB, Clover RD, et al. Emergence and apparent transmission of rimantadine-resistant influenza A virus in families. *N Engl J Med* 1989;321:1696–1702.
49. Drinka PJ, Gravenstein S, Schilling M, et al. Duration of antiviral prophylaxis during nursing home outbreaks of influenza A: a comparison of two protocols. *Arch Intern Med* 1998;158:2155–2159.
50. Gravenstein S, Drinka P, Osterweil D, et al. A multicenter prospective double-blind randomized controlled trial comparing the relative safety and efficacy of zanamivir to rimantadine for nursing home influenza outbreak control. Options for the Control of Influenza IV. Crete, 2000.
51. Hall CB, McBride JT. Acute laryngotracheobronchitis. In: Mandell GL, Bennet JE, Dolin R, eds. *Principles and practice of infectious diseases.* Philadelphia: Churchill Livingstone, 2000:663–669.
52. Denny FW, Murphy TF, Clyde WAJ, et al. Croup: an 11-year study in a pediatric practice. *Pediatrics* 1983;71:871–876.

53. Knott AM, Long CE, Hall CB. Parainfluenza viral infections in pediatric outpatients: seasonal patterns and clinical characteristics. *Pediatr Infect Dis J* 1994;13:269–273.
54. Glezen WP, Frank AL, Taber LH, et al. Parainfluenza virus type 3: seasonality and risk of infection and risk of infection in young children. *J Infect Dis* 1984;150:851–857.
55. Johnson DW, Jacobson S, Edney PC, et al. A comparison of nebulized budesonide, intramuscular dexamethasone, and placebo for moderately severe croup. *N Engl J Med* 1998;339:498–503.
56. Jaffe DM. The treatment of croup with glucocorticoids. *N Engl J Med* 1998;339:553–554.
57. Donnelly BW, McMillan JA, Weiner LB. Bacterial tracheitis: report of eight new cases and review. *Rev Infect Dis* 1990;12:729–735.
58. Wright AL, Taussig LM, Ray CG, et al. The Tucson Children's Respiratory study. II. Lower respiratory tract illness in the first year of life. *Am J Epidemiol* 1989;129:1232–1236.
59. Wohl MEB, Chernick V. Bronchiolitis. *Am Rev Respir Dis* 1978;118:759–781.
60. American Academy of Pediatrics. Reassessment of the indications for ribavirin therapy in respiratory syncytial virus infections. *Pediatrics* 1996;97:137–140.
61. Goebel J, Estrada B, Quinonez J, et al. Prednisolone plus albuterol versus albuterol alone in mild to moderate bronchiolitis. *Clin Pediatr* 2000;39:213–220.
62. Cade A, Brownlee KG, Conway SP, et al. Randomized placebo controlled trial of nebulised corticosteroids in acute respiratory syncytial viral bronchiolitis. *Arch Dis Child* 2000;82:126–130.
63. Connor E, PREVENT Study Group. Reduction of respiratory syncytial virus hospitalization among premature infants and infants with bronchopulmonary dysplasia using respiratory syncytial virus immune globulin prophylaxis. *Pediatrics* 1997;99:93–99.
64. IMpact RSV Study Group. Palivizumab, a humanized respiratory syncytial virus monoclonal antibody, reduces hospitalization from respiratory syncytial virus infection in high-risk infants. *Pediatrics* 1998;102:531–537.
65. American Academy of Pediatrics. Prevention of respiratory syncytial virus infections: indications for the use of palivizumab and update on the use of RSV-IGIV. *Pediatrics* 1998;102:1211–1216.
66. Greenberg SB. Viral pneumonia. *Infect Dis Clin North Am* 1991;5:603–621.
67. Klinger JR, Sanchez MP, Curtin LA, et al. Multiple cases of life-threatening adenovirus pneumonia in a mental health care center. *Am J Respir Crit Care Med* 1998;157:645–649.
68. Dowell SF, Anderson LJ, Gary HE, Jr., et al. Respiratory syncytial virus is an important cause of community-acquired lower respiratory infection among hospitalized adults. *J Infect Dis* 1996;174:456–462.
69. Duchin JS, Koster FT, Peters CJ, et al. Hantavirus pulmonary syndrome: a clinical description of 17 patients with a newly recognized disease. *N Engl J Med* 1994;330:949–955.
70. Falsey AR. Respiratory syncytial virus infection in older persons. *Vaccine* 1998;16:1775–1778.
71. Han LL, Alexander JP, Anderson LJ. Respiratory syncytial virus pneumonia among the elderly: an assessment of disease burden. *J Infect Dis* 1999;179:25–30.
72. Marx A, Gary HE Jr, Marston BJ, et al. Parainfluenza virus infection among adults hospitalized for lower respiratory tract infection. *Clin Infect Dis* 1999;29:134–140.
73. Ramsey PG, Fife KH, Hackman RC, et al. Herpes simplex virus pneumonia: clinical, virologic, and pathologic features in 20 patients. *Ann Intern Med* 1982;97:813–820.
74. La Rosa AM, Champlin RE, Mirza NB, et al. Adenovirus infections in adult recipients of blood and marrow transplants. *Clin Infect Dis* 2001;32:871–875.
75. Sable CA, Hayden FG. Orthomyxoviral and paramyxoviral infections in transplant recipients. *Infect Transplant* 1995;9:987–1003.
76. Hertz MI, Englund JA, Snover D, et al. Respiratory syncytial virus–induced acute lung injury in adult patients with bone marrow transplants: a clinical approach and review of the literature. *Medicine* 1989;68:269–281.

77. Englund JA, Sullivan CJ, Jordan MC. Respiratory syncytial virus infection in immunocompromised adults. *Ann Intern Med* 1988;109:203–208.
78. Ghosh S, Champlin RE, Englund J, et al. Respiratory syncytial virus upper respiratory tract illnesses in adult blood and marrow transplant recipients: combination therapy with aerosolized ribavirin and intravenous immunoglobulin. *Bone Marrow Transplant* 2000;25:751–755.
79. Whimbey E, Eling LS, Couch RB, et al. Influenza A virus infection among hospitalized adult bone marrow transplant recipients. *Bone Marrow Transplant* 1994;13:437–440.
80. Bowden RA. Respiratory virus infections after marrow transplant: the Fred Hutchinson Cancer Research Center experience. *Am J Med* 1997;102:27–30.
81. Kaplan LJ, Daum RS, Smaron M, et al. Severe measles in immunocompromised patients. *JAMA*. 1992;267:1237–1241.

# 11. LOWER RESPIRATORY TRACT INFECTIONS (INCLUDING TUBERCULOSIS)

Robert L. Penn and Robert F. Betts

Virtually any type of infectious agent can cause pneumonia. It develops when the host is confronted by a virulent organism for which he or she has no specific defense, or when the usual lung defense mechanisms are impaired regardless of the virulence of the organism.

Pneumonia can be induced by aspiration of minute quantities of virulent organisms, or by aspiration of larger quantities of virulent or nonvirulent organisms. In addition, aspiration of noninfectious gastric contents or inhalation of toxic fumes can produce an inflammatory pneumonitis that is sometimes followed by secondary bacterial infection. Another mechanism is inhalation of microorganisms in small-particle aerosols, as occurs in tuberculosis.

Occasionally microorganisms can embolize to the lung through the bloodstream, and frequently without evidence of airway disease. This most often occurs from right-sided endocarditis or from sites drained by the inferior or superior vena cava, for example the jugular vein.

## GENERAL CONCEPTS OF ORGANISM–HOST INTERACTION

**I. The organism**

- **A. Availability.** Colonization by an organism or acute exposure to an organism in the environment is an essential precondition for the development of pneumonia.
- **B. Virulence.** The virulence of most bacterial respiratory pathogens is related to their ability to **adhere to receptor sites** on respiratory epithelial cells and pneumocytes, and to **resist natural host defenses in the lung.**
  - **1.** The virulence of the pneumococcus is related to its ability to adhere to receptor sites on respiratory epithelial cells and pneumocytes. **Receptor sites** on the pneumocyte for the pneumococcus increase twofold when there is associated inflammation (e.g., influenza).
  - **2. Importance of the capsule.** The ability of the pneumococcus to **resist phagocytosis via its capsule** enables it to survive and replicate in the alveolus. All species of *Streptococcus pneumoniae* that cause disease are encapsulated, and frequency and severity of disease are related to the quantity of capsule. Encapsulated *Haemophilus influenzae* type b can cause pneumonia that is associated with bacteremia, whereas nonencapsulated *H. influenzae* usually causes only exacerbations of bronchitis and occasionally bronchopneumonia. Its capsule and its ability to adhere to respiratory epithelium probably explain why *Klebsiella pneumoniae* causes pneumonia. *Klebsiella* species also elaborate cytotoxic enzymes.
- **C. Other factors.** Unencapsulated organisms can cause pneumonia if the quantity aspirated is sufficiently high. For example, decaying teeth harbor high titers of anaerobic bacteria. Impairment of host defenses also favors the establishment of infection. Loss of ciliary activity is an important risk factor, as may occur from viral infection of the lower respiratory tract, drugs such as alcohol, airway obstruction from a tumor or a foreign body, or exposure to an irritant such as cigarette smoke.

**II. Host defense mechanisms** [1]

- **A. Upper airway defenses**
  - **1. Mechanical defenses** such as air filtration, the epiglottic reflex, upper airflow turbulence, cough, and mucociliary clearance protect the lower airway. Neurologic or esophageal diseases enhance access to the bronchial tree. Inhaled toxins, abnormal bronchial secretions (e.g., cystic fibrosis), viral infections, endobronchial tumors, or foreign bodies (e.g., an endotracheal tube) impair these mechanical defenses.
  - **2. Secretory immunoglobulin A (IgA)** impairs microbial adherence and neutralizes viruses.
- **B. Lower respiratory defenses**
  - **1. IgG and secretory IgA antibodies** both diffuse into mucosal secretions, while IgG predominates in the alveolar milieu. Vaccines or previous infections stimulate

antibody production. Mucosal applied vaccines more effectively stimulate IgA. Absence of antibodies is a risk factor, as occurs in multiple myeloma and agammaglobulinemia. Deficiencies of $IgG_2$ or $IgG_4$ predispose to recurrent sinus and bronchial infections, especially if combined with IgA deficiency.

2. **Complement** activation generates opsonins, chemotactic molecules, and lytic activity. The functional absence of complement in sickle cell disease and certain inherited deficiency states leads to increased incidence of sinopulmonary infections.
3. **Phagocytic defenses consist of alveolar macrophages and neutrophils.** Alveolar macrophages are the initial phagocytic defense and play a central role in recruiting neutrophils and other aspects of lung inflammation [1]. Either a quantitative or a qualitative defect in phagocytes may contribute to pyogenic infection. Impaired migration of phagocytes is a risk factor. For example, high alcohol concentrations impair neutrophil migration. Organisms such as *Legionella* and *Mycobacterium* species can survive within nonimmune alveolar macrophages. Optimal defense against facultative intracellular pathogens requires activation of macrophages via specific T-lymphocyte immunity.
4. **Other antibacterial substances** in the lower airways include lysozyme, fibronectin, free fatty acids, iron-binding proteins, defensins, cathelicidins, and collectins, including surfactant proteins [1].

## CLINICAL APPROACH TO COMMUNITY-ACQUIRED PNEUMONIA (CAP)

I. **Important history and epidemiologic data** include the following points, as well as the season of the year [2–6]. Influenza, pneumococcal, and haemophilus etiologies are more prevalent in the winter.

A. **Family history.** Respiratory syncytial virus, influenza, *Mycoplasma pneumoniae,* and *Chlamydophila (Chlamydia) pneumoniae* are just a few examples of pneumonia that may spread within families, although *Mycoplasma* and *Chlamydophila* spread more slowly than the viruses.

B. **Travel history.** A history of travel to or residence in certain areas of the country is essential for acquisition of coccidioidomycosis, histoplasmosis, or blastomycosis (see Chapter 17). Travel to Southeast Asia or the South Pacific at any time should raise the possibility of infection with *Pseudomonas pseudomallei,* for illness can develop years after exposure.

C. **Unusual contacts.** Occupational exposures, outdoors activities, or contact with animals and birds or their excreta suggest such entities as hantavirus pulmonary syndrome, histoplasmosis, Legionnaires disease, plague, psittacosis, Q fever, and tularemia.

D. **Recent hospitalization, institutionalization, or antibiotic therapy.** Gram-negative pneumonias and infections caused by antibiotic-resistant organisms, including resistant pneumococci, are much more frequent in these patients.

E. **Infection with the human immunodeficiency virus (HIV) or the presence of HIV risk factors** suggests the possibility of both gram-negative and gram-positive bacterial pneumonias [7], as well as a variety of opportunistic pathogens such as *Pneumocystis carinii* and *Rhodococcus equi* (see Chapter 18).

F. **Age** is an important factor.

1. In the **neonatal period,** *Streptococcus agalactiae* is an important cause of pneumonia acquired through contact in the birth canal (see Chapter 3).
2. **The infant**
   a. **Respiratory syncytial virus** (RSV), parainfluenza, and influenza are common in infancy and may occur in epidemics.
   b. **Encapsulated bacteria.** Both *S. pneumoniae* and *H. influenzae* type b may cause pneumonia in children 5 to 18 months of age. This is related both to loss of maternal antibody and to the failure of children in this age group to form antibody to polysaccharide antigens. The incidence of invasive *H. influenzae* type b infections has declined among infants since the introduction of the *H. influenzae* type b conjugate vaccines in 1988. Hopefully, the pneumococcal conjugate vaccine will have the same effect on *S. pneumoniae* infections.

3. In **children** (3 months old to teenagers) with CAP, the most frequently identified causes are *S. pneumoniae, M. pneumoniae,* RSV, *Chlamydophila pneumoniae,* nontypable *H. influenzae,* and *Moraxella catarrhalis* [8]. RSV is more common in children under 5 years of age, and *M. pneumoniae* and *C. pneumoniae* are more common in older children. Recent studies have found the frequent occurrence of mixed infections [8].
4. In **young adults** (18–45 years) *Mycoplasma* species and *Chlamydophila pneumoniae* are the most common causes year round, but influenza predominates during epidemics.
5. **Older ambulatory adults** are just as likely as younger adults to have pneumococcal pneumonia and influenza [9]. However, one review noted an increased proportion of haemophilus, staphylococcal, and gram-negative pneumonias in the elderly [10].
6. **Institutionalized older adults** are often colonized with gram-negative rods. Thus, when pneumonia develops, gram-negative pneumonia is more likely, although pneumococcal disease still is prevalent. Staphylococci (including methicillin-resistant strains), haemophilus, moraxella, anaerobes, viruses, and *Mycobacterium tuberculosis* also regularly cause pneumonia in this group [9].

**G. Predisposing conditions**

1. **In alcoholics,** *S. pneumoniae* is the most prevalent organism, but anaerobes, *H. influenzae, K. pneumoniae,* and *M. tuberculosis* also are regularly encountered.
2. **Aspiration pneumonia** occurs in patients with alcoholism, drug abuse, recent general anesthesia, trauma, other causes for mental obtundation, stroke, swallowing problems, esophageal dysmotility (e.g., scleroderma, stricture, or achalasia), tracheoesophageal fistula, gastroparesis, feeding tubes, tracheotomy, seizure disorders, and other serious underlying diseases. Anaerobes are common pathogens in this setting, often as part of a mixed infection, unless the patient is edentulous. Nosocomial aspiration pneumonias also may involve aerobic gram-negative bacilli and *Staphylococcus aureus.* (See section **II** under Specific Therapy and Special Considerations.)
3. **Chronic obstructive pulmonary disease** (COPD) is associated with *H. influenzae, S. pneumoniae, M. catarrhalis,* and *Legionella* pneumonias.
4. **Cystic fibrosis** predisposes to staphylococcal, mucoid strains of *Pseudomonas aeruginosa, Stenotrophomonas maltophilia,* and *Burkholderia cepacia* infection. The latter gram-negative organisms usually appear after repeated courses of antibiotics.
5. **Postinfluenza bacterial pneumonias** are commonly caused by staphylococci, *H. influenzae,* or *S. pneumoniae.*
6. **Sickle cell disease** is an important risk factor for pneumococcal pneumonia.
7. **Immunosuppression** predisposes to a wide variety of potential organisms.

**H. Hospital-acquired pneumonias** [11,12]. Oropharyngeal colonization by gram-negative organisms, especially *Klebsiella* species, increases in the infirm elderly, and with severe acute illness, prolonged hospitalization, diabetes, renal failure, intubation, or prior antibiotic exposure. **Gram-negative organisms must be considered when pneumonia develops in these settings.** Other important nosocomial pathogens include *S. aureus,* anaerobes from aspiration, *Legionella* species, fungi, and some viruses.

**II. Symptoms and signs.** For CAP, the individual often has had a recent, mild upper respiratory tract infection and then develops chills, fever, cough associated with pleuritic chest pain, dyspnea, and purulent sputum. However, the complete spectrum of these symptoms may be lacking, depending on the host and the organism.

**A. Host considerations**

1. **Neonates** with *Chlamydia* pneumonia usually are mildly ill and do not have fever (see Chapter 3).
2. **Young infants** with viral pneumonia almost always present with respiratory distress and fever but, at times, infants may appear septic.
3. **Elderly** patients often develop a change in eating habits or mental function with a minimum of respiratory symptoms [9]. Other important clues include

unexplained diminished activity, a fall, new incontinence, or the decompensation of an underlying medical problem. Fever may be minimal or absent. Tachypnea or tachycardia may be the first evidence of pulmonary involvement. Abnormalities on the chest radiograph may be difficult to interpret because of underlying heart and lung disease.

4. **Patients with chronic bronchitis** may exhibit a change in the quantity and type (color and general appearance) of sputum as the first sign of pneumonia.
5. **Neutropenic patients** may not produce sputum and may have few chest radiograph abnormalities.

**B. Special considerations by organism**

1. Anaerobic infections, tuberculosis, and pulmonary mycoses usually have a more gradual onset of symptoms than pyogenic bacterial pneumonias.
2. Some pneumonias characteristically have scant and nonpurulent sputum production, although this has proven to be nonspecific [2,6].
   a. ***M. pneumoniae*** **and** ***C. pneumoniae*** usually have a gradual onset characterized by fever, protracted cough, and minimal sputum.
   b. **Legionnaires disease** characteristically causes only a modest amount of sputum production and nonspecific systemic symptoms [13]. Other manifestations include relative bradycardia, renal abnormalities, delirium, diarrhea, and hyponatremia.
   c. **Q fever, psittacosis, and viral pneumonias** are nonbacterial pneumonias discussed in section **V** under Specific Therapy and Special Considerations. A history of occupational or other exposure to animals and birds or a local epidemic of influenza may help increase one's index of suspicion for these diagnoses.

**III. Physical examination.** In addition to examination of the chest, special emphasis should be placed on a search for signs of nonpneumonic infection such as endocarditis, meningitis, and salpingitis. Evidence of an associated pleural effusion should be sought. Other relevant findings include deep venous thrombosis leading to pulmonary embolism, lymphadenopathy, or clubbing, suggesting neoplasia.

**IV. Radiologic evaluation** [14]. Chest radiography is always indicated [2]. Although the x-ray film yields useful clues, **it seldom identifies a specific etiologic diagnosis.**

**The compromised host, the very young, and the very old pose special diagnostic problems.** In some, the physical findings may be minimal, but the radiograph may clearly reveal the pneumonia. In others, particularly neutropenic patients, the initial radiograph may fail to show any infiltrates despite clinical findings of pneumonia.

**A. Location of infiltrates**

1. Infiltrates in the **apical segment of the lower lobe or in the posterior segment of the upper lobe suggest aspiration while recumbent,** whereas infiltrates in the **basal segment of the lower lobe suggest aspiration while more upright** [15]. However, aspiration in different postures may lead to pneumonia in other dependent locations.
2. **Upper lobe** involvement can occur in any pneumonia, but it is particularly common **in tuberculosis,** *Klebsiella* infection, and melioidosis. Lower lobe infiltrates in an immunocompetent host make tuberculosis less likely, but do not exclude this possibility. Involvement of the anterior segment of an upper lobe by itself usually is considered nontuberculous and possibly related to other infection or tumor.

**B. Cavitation.** Cavities must be distinguished from pneumatoceles or infiltration around a bulla. Comparison with the uninvolved lung can be helpful in the latter instance.

1. Cavities **without air-fluid levels** are **suggestive of tuberculosis,** but also may occur in fungal infections.
2. Cavities **with air-fluid levels** suggest abscess formation from staphylococci, anaerobes, gram-negative bacilli, coccidioidomycosis, nocardiosis, or melioidosis. **Occasionally, loculated pleural effusion in association with a bronchopleural fistula can mimic an abscess.**

**C. Volume loss.** If there is evidence of associated volume loss, correctable bronchial obstruction must be excluded.

**D. Pleural fluid.** Sampling pleural fluid may lead to a specific diagnosis and chest tube drainage. In addition, the presence of an effusion is suggestive of certain pathogens. (See the discussion on pleural effusions later in this chapter under Pleural Effusion versus Empyema.)

1. Pleural effusion without pneumonia suggests tuberculosis, tumor, or a subdiaphragmatic process.
2. *M. pneumoniae* and *C. pneumoniae* infections may have small effusions that are not readily detected.
3. Pneumococcal pneumonia frequently is associated with effusion. The fluid may be sterile or may represent a frank empyema. Thoracentesis is indicated to exclude an associated empyema if the effusion volume is sufficient.
4. Anaerobic organisms, *Streptococcus pyogenes,* and *Escherichia coli,* as well as staphylococcal pneumonia in children, commonly produce pleural fluid.
5. *M. tuberculosis* that has produced cavities, *K. pneumoniae,* and *P. pseudomallei* may be associated with pleural fluid.
6. Influenza viral infections rarely are associated with effusion.
7. Legionnaires disease may cause a pleural effusion, although large effusions are uncommon [13,16].

**E. Mediastinal adenopathy** is seen with lung cancer, and in acute pneumonias caused by tuberculosis, fungal infections, tularemia, and *M. pneumoniae* in children.

**F. Miscellaneous findings.** Pericardial effusion, widening of the mediastinum, evidence of a bronchopleural fistula, and free air under the diaphragm require further evaluation. Chemotherapy, radiation, drug reactions, pulmonary embolism, heart failure, vasculitis, and cancer can mimic the radiographic appearance of pneumonia [3,17].

**G. Follow-up chest radiography. Rapid changes in infiltrates** (e.g., over 5–36 hours) **seldom occur in pneumonia, and suggest pulmonary edema or atelectasis.** Although repeat radiologic evaluation may assist in management, this is often overused.

1. **If the patient is clinically improving,** follow-up radiography should be postponed. **Infiltrates due to pneumonia often take a month to clear completely,** and this varies with host factors and the microbial etiology [17]. Clearing may take **even longer in the elderly** (1–12 weeks). Therefore, it is wise to postpone a follow-up radiographic examination in the patient whose clinical response is appropriate. If at least partial clearing does not occur after 6 weeks, or pneumonias recur in the same location, then fiberoptic bronchoscopy should be considered [17].

   Fibrosis or scarring may be present despite clearing of the infiltrate, particularly after aerobic gram-negative or anaerobic infections. More extensive scarring often is associated with tuberculosis and histoplasmosis.
2. **If the patient is not improving** or develops a new fever, increasing pulmonary symptoms, or sputum production, **follow-up radiography is important** [17]. **Radiographs** may identify bronchial obstruction, a new pulmonary infection, an associated effusion that may be infected, an abscess, or noninfectious complications.

**V. Identification of the pathogen.** Recent guidelines for CAP support empiric management without diagnostic studies for those otherwise healthy adults with mild illness who are being treated as outpatients [2,4,6]. **However, identifying the pathogen provides a diagnosis and is of primary importance in further management [2]. Every effort should be made to obtain diagnostic specimens** (not be left to the untrained) **before initiating antibiotic therapy** [2]. Sputum for smear and culture, blood cultures, culture of any pleural fluid, and cerebrospinal fluid (CSF) if meningitis is a possible complication should be obtained.

**A. Normal mouth flora.** Common, normal colonizers of the oropharynx are listed in Table 11.1. These are often observed on Gram staining and routinely recovered on sputum cultures. **Isolation of these organisms from expectorated sputum**

Table 11.1. Common Colonizers of the Oropharynx

| Organism | Incidence Range (%) |
|---|---|
| *Staphylococcus aureus* | 35–40 |
| *Streptococcus pyogenes* (group A) | 0–9 |
| *Streptococcus pneumoniae* | 0–50 |
| *Neisseria meningitidis* | 0–15 |
| *Haemophilus influenzae* | 5–20 |
| Gram-negative aerobic bacilli | 2[a] |

[a]Approximate percentage isolated by using routine culture techniques. With special broth cultures, more than 10% of normals may have gram-negative colonizers. Of elderly nursing home patients, 6%–40% may be found to be colonized with gram-negative organisms (as revealed by routine culture techniques).

Adapted from Sommers HM. The indigenous microbiota of the human host. In: Youmans GP et al., eds. *The biologic and clinical basis of infectious diseases* 2nd ed. Philadelphia: WB Saunders, 1980; with permission.

**does not prove they are pathogens in the lower respiratory tract.** (See the discussion of colonization vs. infection in section **VIII.**)

B. **Methods of sputum collection** [2,4,6]
   1. **Coughed specimens. Sputum from a deep cough,** not saliva, must be studied to minimize contamination by oropharyngeal colonizers. In at least 20% to 30% of cases, adequate sputum is not available; this is particularly true in the elderly and the acutely ill [18].
   2. **Nasotracheal aspirations** are always contaminated with some oral colonizers. However, the procedure may stimulate deep expectorations that produce an adequate specimen.
   3. **Bronchoscopy.** Passing the bronchoscope through the upper airway picks up colonizers unless special techniques are used (see further discussion in section **VI**).
   4. **Other.** Transtracheal aspiration (TTA), direct lung aspiration, and open lung biopsy bypass normal oropharyngeal colonizers. Thus, these specimens are suitable for anaerobic cultures. **Organisms seen in or cultured from these specimens usually represent lower respiratory tract pathogens.** (See further discussion in section **VI.**)

C. **Gram staining of sputum**[19]. The technique and interpretation of Gram stains is discussed in Chapter 25. This helpful procedure always should be attempted, although this view is not held by all clinicians [2,4,6]. The sputum Gram stain assists in several ways.
   1. Gram staining helps **assess the adequacy of the sputum specimen. If more than 10 squamous epithelial cells are seen per low-power field, the sample is contaminated with oral secretions.** A repeat sputum should be obtained, or an invasive method of specimen collection should be considered.
   2. A predominance of gram-positive cocci or gram-negative bacilli is helpful.
   3. Gram staining of pleural fluid, TTA, protected brush specimens, or percutaneous lung aspirates are even more valuable, because normal colonizers are absent.

D. **Acid-fast smears and cultures** should be obtained when upper lobe disease is present or when tuberculosis is otherwise suspected. The methods are described in Chapter 25.

E. **Sputum: special studies.**
   1. During epidemics, virus identification should be attempted.
   2. In a normal young adult, attempts at isolation of viruses and *M. pneumoniae* are reasonable. Viruses other than influenza are rare in normal adults.
   3. The compromised host usually should undergo mycobacterial, fungal, and viral studies.

4. *Legionella* studies should be performed on appropriate specimens when this is a possible diagnosis [3]. (See section **VI** under Specific Therapy and Special Considerations.)
5. Fungal smears and cultures should be sent when patients from endemic regions present with compatible illness.

F. **If sputum is not available** and the patient is not ill enough for an invasive procedure, the clinician must use empiric antibiotics (see section **B** above and section **IX**) [2,4,6].

VI. **Invasive procedures** [20]. Fiberoptic bronchoscopy with a protected specimen brush (PSB) or bronchoalveolar lavage (BAL) is most widely used. **Their diagnostic value is significantly reduced by prior antibiotic therapy.** Percutaneous thin-needle lung aspiration is best reserved for accessible enigmatic lesions [21]. Open lung biopsy usually is considered only after other methods have proven nondiagnostic or in immunocompromised hosts.

A. **Indications. Most patients with CAP are successfully managed without an invasive procedure** [2,4,6]. The value of these tests for nosocomial and ventilator-associated pneumonias is unclear [12,22]. **Consider an invasive procedure if the severity of the illness or its rate of progression is significant enough to warrant the risks, and when:**
1. Adequate specimens are unobtainable using noninvasive techniques.
2. The resulting specimens will be properly and quickly processed.
3. There are no absolute contraindications present.

B. **Transtracheal aspiration** is used only infrequently at present and **should be performed only by experienced personnel.**

C. **Fiberoptic bronchoscopy methods.** Fiberoptic bronchoscopy has become widely available. **Oral contamination is unavoidable using fiberoptic bronchoscopy alone** without additional appropriate culture techniques.
1. **The PSB** consists of a double-sheathed tube sealed at the distal end [20]. After the bronchoscope is positioned, the whole PSB is pushed through the inner channel several centimeters beyond the bronchoscope. The inner sheath then is pushed beyond the plug, and a sterile brush is advanced through the open inner sheath, collecting 0.001 mL of secretions.
   a. **Quantitative cultures are necessary** because contamination is inevitable. Organisms, including anaerobes, growing at $\geq 10^3$/mL are considered significant.
   b. **This procedure is useful in diagnosing acute nosocomial pneumonia in the mechanically ventilated patient** [23–25].
   c. The **risks** are low and include pneumothorax, transient fever or infiltrates, and decreased oxygenation.
2. **Bronchoalveolar lavage** [20]. BAL is performed by wedging the fiberoptic bronchoscope in a distal airway and injecting and aspirating 50 mL (mini-BAL) to 150 mL (standard BAL) of sterile normal saline through the bronchoscope. BAL samples a larger area of lung than the PSB and thus offers a theoretic advantage.
   a. **Quantitative cultures of BAL fluid are necessary** to distinguish infecting from contaminating bacteria. Organisms, including anaerobes, growing at $\geq 10^4$/mL are considered significant.
   b. **Gram stain of BAL fluid sediment to detect intracellular organisms may provide a rapid indication of potential pathogens** [26]. Cytology and other stains also should be performed on samples from immunocompromised patients.
   c. **BAL is useful in evaluating immunocompromised patients with pulmonary infiltrates, and in the diagnosis of ventilator-associated pneumonia** [24,26,27].
   d. **Risks** include fever, infiltrates, and decreased oxygenation.

D. **Nonbronchoscopic methods** of bronchial aspiration, BAL, and PSB sampling in ventilated patients offer promise [28]. These blinded (nonvisualized) procedures are performed through an endotracheal tube without radiographic guidance, and require quantitative cultures. Their diagnostic yield and risks are similar to those for bronchoscopic methods [28].

**VII. Other laboratory testing** depends in part on the site of care and the likely potential etiologies, and often is needed to determine the need for hospitalization (see section **IX.A**).

**A. Patients who are otherwise healthy and suitable for outpatient care** may be managed with no additional testing [2,4,6].

**B. Patients requiring emergency room evaluation or hospitalization** should routinely have additional tests [2,4,6].

1. **White blood cell (WBC) and differential count.** Leukocytosis or left shift is nonspecific. Leukopenia has been linked to a poor prognosis.
2. **Abnormal renal or liver function tests** have been associated with bacterial and nonbacterial types of infection, and have implications for medication use.
3. **Oxygen saturation. Pulse oximetry** should be performed on all patients requiring emergency room evaluation or hospitalization. **Arterial blood gas levels** should be determined on patients with severe illness or underlying obstructive lung disease [4,6].
4. **HIV testing** may be indicated.

**C. Serologic studies** may be useful for epidemiologic purposes, to retrospectively determine an etiology, or to evaluate chronic pneumonia.

1. **Mycoplasmal pneumonia. Cold agglutinins are not specific for *Mycoplasma*,** as discussed in section **V.D.2** under Specific Therapy and Special Considerations. **Antibodies to *M. pneumoniae*** reach a diagnostic titer only after a delay.
2. ***Chlamydophila pneumoniae*** **and *Legionella*.** Diagnostic antibody titers develop only weeks after the patient is symptomatic. (See Specific Therapy and Special Considerations.)
3. **Influenza.** Changes in antibody titers between acute and convalescent specimens can make a retrospective diagnosis. (See Chapters 10 and 25.)
4. **Fungal serologic studies.** These may help to support a diagnosis of a pulmonary mycosis, especially in patients with a chronic pneumonia (see Chapter 17).
5. **Q fever and psittacosis** are often diagnosed serologically.

**D. Antigen detection.** A positive antigen test establishes a specific etiology, but a negative test does not exclude a possible etiology. (See Chapter 25 for discussion of these techniques.)

1. **Latex agglutination test results to detect bacterial antigens in urine and serum are infrequently positive in patients with pneumonia.** Detection of antigen in pleural fluid may be helpful in patients pretreated with antibiotics. A commercial immunochromatographic test for pneumococcal antigen in urine may be helpful as an adjunct to smears and cultures for rapid diagnosis, but there is limited experience with this assay at present [2,29]. The Quellung reaction also is useful for the rapid diagnosis of *S. pneumoniae,* but the required expertise and reagents are not generally available [2].
2. ***Legionella*** **urine antigen test** is useful for the rapid diagnosis of *Legionella pneumophila* serogroup I infection.
3. **Influenza, RSV,** and other respiratory viruses may be rapidly diagnosed with commercially available antigen assays [2].
4. **Serum cryptococcal antigen** is helpful in compromised hosts, including HIV infection (see Chapter 18).

**E. Nucleic acid detection.** Polymerase chain reaction (PCR) and probe techniques offer promise for rapidly identifying *Mycoplasma, Chlamydophila (Chlamydia), Legionella,* tuberculosis, hantavirus, and some agents of biologic warfare. However, their utility for routine use in clinical laboratories for the rapid diagnosis of pneumonia is untested [30].

**F. Tuberculosis skin test.** The tuberculosis skin test **is not particularly helpful in a patient with CAP.** A positive test result does not mean that the pneumonia is tuberculous, and a negative test result does not rule out tuberculosis. (See section **III** under Tuberculosis: Basic Concepts for additional discussion of skin testing.)

**VIII. Colonization versus infection.** ***Colonization* refers to the presence of organisms that are not causing disease.** The clinician must determine which organisms growing from a sputum or tracheal aspirate culture are colonizers so as to avoid unnecessary antibiotic therapy.

**A. Clinical settings in which respiratory colonization must be distinguished from infection**

1. **Elderly patients** have an increased incidence of colonization by *S. aureus* and gram-negative organisms, making it difficult to ascertain the true cause of a pneumonia [9].
2. **Debilitated hospitalized patients.**
   a. **Fever not due to pneumonia is frequent** in patients who are hospitalized for another reason (e.g., surgery or myocardial infarction) or who require intensive care [12].
   b. **The chest radiograph often is abnormal but not because of a pneumonia.** Atelectasis, congestive heart failure (CHF), and pulmonary infarction may mimic pneumonia.
3. **After antibiotics have been given.** Sputum cultures from febrile patients being treated with antibiotics frequently grow gram-negative organisms or staphylococci. In this circumstance **culture data alone should not dictate therapy in the absence of supportive clinical findings.**

**B. Key points to help differentiate colonization from superinfection**

1. **Findings that support sputum colonization are** a clinical course that is stable or improving, and an absence of marked sputum production [31]. If the recovering individual develops fever or leukocytosis and yet has stable respiratory signs with no increase in sputum, there will usually be another explanation such as phlebitis, line infection, candidemia, urinary tract infection, wound infection, *Clostridium difficile,* drug fever, or myocardial infarction.
2. **Findings that support respiratory superinfection** are fever, leukocytosis, and worsened respiratory status [31].
   a. **Respiratory changes are the key findings.**
      (1) **Ventilatory status.** Even minor additional pulmonary infection can precipitate respiratory deterioration [31], and when absent, superinfection is unlikely. However, respiratory deterioration also may result from other causes such as distant infection, CHF, or embolism.
      (2) **Production of nonpurulent sputum.** If sputum is nonpurulent **without many polymorphonuclear leukocytes,** bacterial superinfection is unlikely unless the patient is leukopenic [31].
   b. **A chest radiograph** that reveals a new infiltrate in the presence of worsened respiratory status and fever supports the diagnosis of pulmonary superinfection. However, **in practice the radiograph is not always helpful.** New infiltrates may not be noticeable because of diffuse lung injury, may lag behind the onset of superinfection, or may have a noninfectious cause.
3. **Specific microbiologic diagnosis.** When superinfection is suspected, blood cultures and sputum smears and cultures should be obtained. If not contraindicated, **an invasive procedure may help** differentiate between colonization and infection (see section **VI**).

**IX. General concepts of therapy.** Treatment of pneumonia usually is started prior to defining a specific etiology, and the clinician must consider several key factors when planning the initial management. The reader is referred to the latest versions of several published guidelines for adults with CAP for further information [2,4,6,32]. These guidelines exclude immunoincompetent patients, including those with HIV.

**A. When to hospitalize.** The Pneumonia Patient Outcomes Research Team (PORT) study defined a prediction rule for mortality in CAP [33]. This and other studies identified **certain factors associated with a poor outcome from CAP** (Table 11.2). **When present, particularly if multiple factors are present**

Table 11.2. Risk Factors for a Poor Outcome from Pneumonia

| |
|---|
| Age ≥65 years |
| Serious underlying conditions |
| Chronic lung, heart, liver, or renal disease |
| Malignancy |
| Diabetes mellitus |
| Malnutrition |
| Cerebrovascular disease, or recurrent aspiration |
| Alcoholism |
| Cystic fibrosis, or bronchiectasis |
| Immunodeficiency (including splenectomy) |
| Hospitalization for pneumonia within 1 year |
| Physical findings |
| Tachypnea ≥30 breaths/min |
| Hypotension |
| Fever ≥40°C (104°F) |
| Hypothermia <35°C (95°F) |
| Distant sites of infection |
| Altered level of consciousness |
| Laboratory findings |
| Leukocytosis >30,000 cells/$mm^3$ |
| Leukopenia <4,000 cells/$mm^3$ |
| Neutropenia <1,000 cells/$mm^3$ |
| Hypoxemia (room air $Pa_{O_2}$ <60 mm Hg) |
| Hypercapnia (room air $Pa_{CO_2}$ >50 mm Hg) |
| Anemia |
| Renal insufficiency |
| Complications |
| Mechanical ventilation required |
| Adult respiratory distress syndrome |
| Sepsis syndrome |
| Radiographic findings |
| Two or more lobes involved |
| Significant pleural effusion |
| Cavitation |
| Rapid spread |

These factors have been associated with either death or a complicated course, particularly if multiple ones are present simultaneously [6].

**together, hospitalization should be strongly considered** [6]. However, **prediction rules should not override the judgment of the clinician about the need for hospitalization** [2,4,6]. Other considerations include emesis, risks for complications (increased by splenectomy, neuromuscular disorders, and immunosuppression), ability to follow instructions, home support, substance abuse, likelihood of follow-up, and patient preference. Furthermore, we strongly consider hospitalization for the clinical diagnosis of influenza-related pneumonia because of the risk for rapid deterioration.

**B. Antibiotic principles. Antibiotics should be started as soon as possible** [2,6]. Initial therapy is based on the clinical presentation, site of care, certain patient risk factors, and any organisms seen on Gram stains of sputum and pleural fluid.

**1. Narrow-spectrum versus broad-spectrum initial coverage.** Antibiotics with narrow coverage are indicated for patients who are only mildly ill and at least risk. Broader empiric coverage may be necessary for severely ill patients, those at greatest risk for complications (see Table 9.2), or those with nondiagnostic smears and infection of uncertain etiology. **Antibiotics should be modified based on cultures, susceptibility data,** other diagnostic studies, and the initial response.

- **a. If the initial evaluation suggests pneumococcal pneumonia** the possibility of drug-resistant *S. pneumoniae* (DRSP) must be kept in mind. Unless there is a high level of penicillin resistance, mild DRSP pneumonia usually responds to appropriate $\beta$-lactam therapy [32]. However, a macrolide or antipneumococcal fluoroquinolone should be added for moderate or severe infections. Gatifloxacin, moxifloxacin, and levofloxacin are the fluoroquinolones considered to have enhanced pneumococcal activity [32]. However, **treatment failures associated with levofloxacin resistance have been reported** [34].
  - **(1) Outpatients** may be given an oral $\beta$-lactam with reliable antipneumococcal activity such as amoxicillin, amoxicillin-clavulanate, cefuroxime, or cefpodoxime.
  - **(2) Inpatients not critically ill** may be given parenteral ceftriaxone or cefotaxime. Cefuroxime and ampicillin-sulbactam also may be used but are less active than the third-generation cephalosporins against DRSP [32].
  - **(3) Critically ill inpatients** should be given parenteral ceftriaxone or cefotaxime because of their superior activity against DRSP, plus a macrolide or an antipneumococcal fluoroquinolone. This is because **combination therapy may be superior to a $\beta$-lactam alone for severe pneumococcal pneumonia** [35]. Vancomycin should not be used routinely except in patients with suspected meningitis [32].
- **b. If gram-negative pneumonia is suggested,** then broad-spectrum coverage for resistant organisms such as *Pseudomonas aeruginosa* should be given (e.g., piperacillin-tazobactam or cefepime).
- **c.** If the clinical presentation is highly suggestive of mycoplasmal pneumonia, a macrolide (e.g., erythromycin) or tetracycline is sufficient.

**2. Site-of-care and patient risk factors**

- **a. Outpatients.** A macrolide, doxycycline, or an antipneumococcal fluoroquinolone are appropriate because they cover the most commonly identified pathogens: pneumococci, *M. pneumoniae,* and *C. pneumoniae.* Clarithromycin or azithromycin are recommended over erythromycin if *H. influenzae* is suspected [2]. For patients under 50 years of age without comorbidities, a macrolide or doxycycline is preferred. For patients over 50 or those with comorbidities, an antipneumococcal fluoroquinolone is suggested. Because of concerns about the development of resistance, the fluoroquinolones are best reserved for this latter group. A combination of a reliable oral antipneumococcal $\beta$-lactam (amoxicillin, amoxicillin- clavulanate, cefuroxime, or cefpodoxime) plus a macrolide or doxycycline is an alternative [6].
- **b. Inpatients receiving care on a routine ward.** A third-generation cephalosporin (cefotaxime or ceftriaxone) or a $\beta$-lactam/$\beta$-lactamase inhibitor (ampicillin-sulbactam or piperacillin-tazobactam) plus either an antipneumococcal fluoroquinolone or a macrolide are recommended for this group [2,6]. An antipneumococcal fluoroquinolone alone is an alternative. Patients without risk factors for DRSP or enteric gram-negative bacilli may be given intravenous (i.v.) followed by oral azithromycin as monotherapy [36,37]. However, macrolide resistance is increasing among pneumococci, making this regimen less attractive [32].
- **c. Inpatients requiring intensive care.** Intravenous therapy with an extended- spectrum cephalosporin (cefotaxime or ceftriaxone) or $\beta$-lactam/$\beta$-lactamase inhibitor (ampicillin-sulbactam or piperacillin-tazobactam) plus a macrolide or an antipneumococcal fluoroquinolone is usually sufficient [2,6]. Patients with risk factors for pseudomonas infection (structural lung diseases including bronchiectasis and cystic fibrosis, >10 mg/day of prednisone, broad-spectrum antibiotics for at least 1 week during the prior month, and malnutrition) should be given a fluoroquinolone plus either piperacillin,

piperacillin-tazobactam, a carbapenem, or cefepime. When piperacillin-tazobactam is chosen, the dose must be increased to assure adequate antipseudomonal activity. (Aspiration is discussed in section **II** and *Legionella* in section **VI** under Specific Therapy and Special Considerations.)

**3. Reevaluating initial regimens**

**a. Response to therapy** varies with the infecting organisms. In addition, host factors such as increasing age, underlying illnesses, extent of lung involvement, bacteremia and immunosuppression lengthen this process [2,6]. Many patients remain ill or even continue to worsen within the first 48 to 72 hours despite appropriate therapy, but once improvement begins, it should progress without complications [6]. **The expected responses** in an otherwise healthy adult with CAP are listed below.

(1) **Subjective feelings of improvement** usually occur within 1 to 3 days [2].

(2) **Fever** usually responds within 2 to 4 days in nonbacteremic pneumococcal pneumonia. Patients with *Mycoplasma* may become afebrile within 1 to 2 days, whereas patients with *Legionella* may take 5 days or longer to become afebrile [2].

(3) **Abnormal chest examination findings** may persist for longer than a week in up to 40% of patients [6].

(4) **Leukocytosis** usually has begun to resolve within the first 3 to 4 days.

(5) **Bacteremia** should no longer be present after 24 to 48 hours of appropriate antibiotics [2].

(6) **Radiographic improvement takes longer to occur than does clinical improvement,** and radiographs may initially progress even though clinical improvement has begun [2,6]. The role for follow-up radiographs is discussed in section **IV.G** under Clinical Approach to Community-Acquired Pneumonia.

**b. Known etiology.** Isolates from blood, pleural fluid, or lower respiratory tract secretions are presumed etiologic agents. **Once a specific cause of pneumonia has been identified, therapy should be adjusted to the most effective narrow-spectrum regimen with the least toxicity and cost** [2,4,6]. This is true even for patients who initially responded to an empiric broad-spectrum regimen [38].

**c. Unknown etiology.** Initial diagnostic studies are negative in up to 50% of cases [6].

(1) **If patients have responded to empiric therapy, it may be continued.** Pneumococci and several other treatable causes (*Mycoplasma, Chlamydophila,* and *Legionella*) are difficult to prove with standard sputum studies.

(2) **If gram-negative bacteria were not isolated from well-collected sputum, the diagnosis of endobronchial gram-negative pneumonia essentially has been excluded.** In these patients it is safe to stop specific gram-negative therapy after only a few days [38]. The exceptions are neutropenic patients and those with embolic pneumonia. In embolic pneumonia the blood cultures are often positive even when the sputum is negative.

**d. Patients not responding to initial therapy** should be further evaluated for the following circumstances [2,4,6]:

(1) **The diagnosis of pneumonia was incorrect** and another illness is present, such as heart failure, atelectasis, adult respiratory distress syndrome (ARDS), or infarction.

(2) **The diagnosis of pneumonia was correct, but the chosen antibiotics failed.** This could be from **inadequate dosing** caused by patient nonadherence, poor absorption, vomiting, or drug interactions. In addition, there may be a **resistant pathogen,** such as DRSP, methicillin-resistant *S. aureus* (MRSA), many gram-negative bacilli, *Nocardia, Mycobacterium* species, and viral or fungal pathogens that do not respond to antibiotics.

(3) **Thoracic complications** may delay the clinical response. These include lung necrosis or abscess formation, empyema, and airway obstruction from tumor, secretions, or a foreign body. Suppurative pericarditis is an uncommon complication.

(4) **Metastatic infections** from the lung include meningitis, septic arthritis, peritonitis, endocarditis, and solid organ abscess.

(5) **A new nosocomial infection** may cause deterioration. Examples are urinary infection, i.v. catheter–related sepsis, and *C. difficile* colitis.

4. **Switching from i.v. to oral therapy,** usually by day 3, is endorsed by the published guidelines [2,4,6]. Eligible patients must be improved, stable, taking oral agents, and have normal gastrointestinal function. The American Thoracic Society (ATS) recommends that four specific criteria be met: improved cough and dyspnea, decreasing WBC count, a functioning gastrointestinal tract, and no fever; however, patients do not have to be afebrile if they meet the other criteria [6].

   **Antibiotics chosen for oral therapy should achieve levels adequate for the suspected or proven pathogens,** and when possible are based on susceptibility test results. **If the etiology is unidentified, providing similar oral coverage is easiest when a single agent or a narrow-spectrum i.v. regimen was chosen at the outset.** Otherwise, an antipneumococcal fluoroquinolone or a combination of oral agents usually is required. **Patients may be discharged the same day that oral therapy is instituted** [6]. Follow-up is used to reinforce adherence, identify side effects or intolerance, and to assure continued clinical improvement.

5. **Duration of therapy. There is a paucity of data to guide the optimal duration of therapy for patients without an identified etiology,** and the published guidelines do not specifically address this issue [2,4,6]. Suggestions range from 7 to 14 days for CAP based on the clinical response [4], 3 afebrile days [2] to 7 to 10 days [6] for pneumococcal pneumonia, and 10 to 14 days [6] to a minimum of 14 days [2] for other bacterial pneumonias, *M. pneumoniae, C. pneumoniae,* or Legionnaires disease in immunocompetent hosts [2].

## SPECIFIC THERAPY AND SPECIAL CONSIDERATIONS

I. **Pneumococcal pneumonia** is the most common bacterial pneumonia in adults. Transient bacteremia occurs in 20% to 30% of patients.

A. **Risk groups** [39]. Cigarette smoking is a major risk factor for invasive disease in immunocompetent adults [40]. Immunosuppression from any cause is important, including acquired immunodeficiency syndrome (AIDS) [41], asplenia, and sickle cell disease. The elderly (particularly institutionalized), children under 2 years of age (particularly in day care), and patients with alcoholism, uncontrolled diabetes, and chronic lung, heart, or kidney diseases are at increased risk. Influenza may predispose to pneumococcal pneumonia (see Chapter 10).

B. **Clinical manifestations.** Pneumococcal pneumonia is the prototype of acute lobar pneumonia. Although there may be a preceding upper respiratory infection, **"classic" pneumococcal pneumonia** is usually so abrupt in onset that patients recall the exact time their pneumonia began. They initially experience chills, rigor, fever, dyspnea, dry cough, and pleuritic chest pain. There usually is a single rigor unless intermittent antipyretics are taken. Cough becomes productive of purulent sputum within the first 6 to 24 hours; a pinkish or rusty coloration indicates alveolar bleeding and is common. Examination reveals an acutely ill patient in obvious respiratory distress, with splinting of the involved chest and signs of consolidation with or without a friction rub. Radiographs show alveolar filling with air bronchograms in the affected lobes, unless there is significant underlying emphysema. Subsegmental infiltrates are less common.

   **This classic presentation is not the most common.** A subacute presentation may occur more frequently [42], and in many cases it is difficult to clinically distinguish pneumococcal pneumonia from "atypical" pneumonia. Increased sputum production, pleural involvement, and leukocytosis favor a pneumococcal etiology [43].

1. **Complications** include shock, respiratory failure, empyema, meningitis, septic arthritis, purulent pericarditis, and endocarditis.
2. **The differential diagnosis** includes other bacteria, including *S. aureus, S. pyogenes, H. influenzae, K. pneumoniae,* and other gram-negative bacilli. Gram stains of sputum and pleural fluid help to rapidly identify the most likely organism.

**C. Prognosis.** Pneumococcal pneumonia continues to be associated with a significant rate of mortality [44]. In their study of bacteremic pneumonia, Austrian and Gold [45] found that overall mortality exceeded 15%. Those with preexisting cardiac disease, carcinoma, cirrhosis, and hematologic malignancies had a mortality rate of approximately 30%, compared with 7% among those without these comorbidities. Risk also was increased in patients over 50 years of age and those with multilobe involvement. Feikin et al. [44] found that $\beta$-lactam resistance did not increase mortality unless the organism had a penicillin minimum inhibitory concentration (MIC) of 4.0 $\mu$g/mL or higher.

**D. Antibiotic therapy. Antibiotic selection is critical because penicillin-resistant pneumococci, due to altered penicillin-binding proteins, are prevalent and there is evidence that combination therapy is superior to a $\beta$-lactam alone** [35,46]. A survey of United States strains in 1999 to 2000 found intermediate penicillin resistance (a penicillin MIC of 0.12–1.0 $\mu$g/mL) in 12.7% and high-level resistance (MIC = 2.0 $\mu$g/mL) in 21.5% [47]. High-level resistance is associated with resistance to cephalosporins, chloramphenicol, trimethoprim- sulfamethoxazole (TMP-SMX), erythromycin, and clindamycin [46,47]. **Infections with penicillin-resistant pneumococci are associated with** the extremes of age, residence in or exposure to an institutional setting, including nursing homes and day care, close exposure to an infected person, recent antimicrobial therapy, comorbidities including immunosuppression, and alcoholism [6,48]. (See **Chapter 27.**)

1. **Empiric treatment** recommendations are summarized in section **IX.B.1.a.** under Clinical Approach to Community-Acquired Pneumonia, and should not routinely include vancomycin [32].
2. **Subsequent therapy should be based on susceptibility tests.**
   a. **For penicillin-susceptible strains,** 2.4 million units per day of i.v. penicillin G is suggested; cefazolin (500 mg every 12 hours) or ceftriaxone once daily are alternatives for patients with a delayed penicillin reaction.
   b. **For strains with a penicillin MIC of less than 4 $\mu$g/mL,** a penicillin or cephalosporin can be successful if the dose is raised to provide higher levels of drug [32].
   c. **Infections caused by *S. pneumoniae* with an MIC of 4 $\mu$g/mL** or higher can be treated with vancomycin, gatifloxacin, or moxifloxacin. There is limited outcome data using a fluoroquinolone for highly resistant infections.
3. **Patients with significant penicillin allergy** should be treated with vancomycin, gatifloxacin, or moxifloxacin. Alternatives with limited clinical experience include linezolid and quinupristin/dalfopristin [2].
4. **Meningeal infections** caused by pneumococci with any degree of penicillin resistance should be treated with vancomycin.
5. **Resistance to fluoroquinolones has been found** at a low rate in the United States, but the isolates also often are resistant to penicillin and other drugs [47,49,50]. Fluoroquinolone resistance seems to be increasing in Canada and may increase in the United States with increasing prescriptions for fluoroquinolones [49]. Resistance is based on mutations in DNA gyrase or topoisomerase subunits, or reduced drug penetration [49,50]. Ofloxacin, levofloxacin, and ciprofloxacin are least active *in vitro* against *S. pneumoniae,* whereas gatifloxacin and moxifloxacin are more active [47]. Because levofloxacin resistance has been associated with treatment failures and death [34], gatifloxacin or moxifloxacin is preferred.
6. For therapy of meningitis, see Chapter 6.

**E. Vaccines**

1. **Rationale for pneumococcal vaccination**
   a. **Prevention of disease** is important because of its frequent occurrence, associated mortality, and **increasing** antibiotic resistance [51,52].
   b. *S. pneumoniae* contains an **antiphagocytic capsule** of highly polymerized polysaccharides, and there are at least 90 distinct antigenic serotypes. Specific humoral immunity that leads to opsonophagocytosis is an important host defense against the pneumococcus. This is the basis for the current vaccines, which **stimulate the production of type-specific antibodies** against the capsule.
2. **Vaccine composition.** Two types of vaccine are currently available.
   a. The two **purified polysaccharide vaccines** contain the same 23 polysaccharide antigens (25 $\mu$g each). These 23 serotypes have been shown to cause approximately 87% of bacteremic pneumococcal pneumonia in adults, virtually 100% of childhood bacteremia and meningitis, and 85% of acute otitis media [53]. The polysaccharide antigens are not immunogenic in children age 2 years and younger, and some serotypes are not reliably immunogenic until age 5 years [54]. In addition, the polysaccharide vaccine has not reduced nasopharyngeal carriage of the pneumococcus [52].
   b. The 7-valent **protein conjugate vaccine** was licensed in February 2000. It includes serotypes that, together with cross-reacting serotypes, accounted for 86% of bacteremia, 83% of meningitis, and 65% of acute otitis media in children age 5 years and younger [54]. The protein conjugate vaccine can be administered to infants as young as 6 weeks of age [54]. It reduces mucosal carriage of pneumococcal serotypes contained in the vaccine [51,52,54].
   c. **Both types of vaccine include important serotypes associated with antibiotic resistance,** although resistance is increasing among strains not contained in the protein conjugate vaccine [51,52].
3. **Antibody response**
   a. **Purified polysaccharide vaccines.** Because responsiveness to purified polysaccharide antigens is T-cell independent and under genetic control, it is not associated with long-term memory cells, children age 2 years and younger do not respond, and some healthy adults do not respond even after repeat immunization [39]. **Antibody responses comparable with most healthy young adults,** and with presumed partial protection for disease, have been demonstrated **in patients with asplenia caused by splenectomy or sickle cell disease** [39].

      **Lower antibody responses occur in** the elderly, and patients with nephrotic syndrome or chronic renal failure, COPD, and insulin-dependent diabetes [39]. In general, **patients who are immunocompromised from any cause have a poor or absent response;** this includes patients with leukemia, lymphoma, multiple myeloma, and transplantation [39]. If patients with **Hodgkin disease** are **vaccinated at least 2 weeks before** splenectomy, radiation therapy, or chemotherapy, they manifest a better antibody response, although it declines during subsequent chemotherapy [39]. **Response in HIV-infected patients relates to the degree of immunosuppression**; those with AIDS or $CD4^+$ counts of less than 500 cells/$\mu$L have reduced antibody responses [39] that are improved by at least 1 month of zidovudine. **Thus, persons with HIV should be vaccinated as soon as possible in the natural course of their infection.** Vaccination together with antiretroviral therapy may improve responsiveness to the purified polysaccharide vaccine [52].
   b. **Protein conjugate vaccine.** This vaccine is more immunogenic in inducing type- specific antibody responses in healthy young children, and results in an anamnestic response to subsequent purified polysaccharide vaccine [52,54]. Similar good responses occur in children with sickle cell disease and HIV infection, and in Alaska Native and American Indian children [54].

4. **Effectiveness**
   a. **Purified polysaccharide vaccines.** Their **overall effectiveness in preventing invasive pneumococcal disease in immunocompetent persons ranges from 56% to 81%** [39]. Protection varies markedly within certain populations, and **a protective effect in immunocompromised patients was difficult to measure** [55]. Efficacy is highest in immunocompetent adults under 55 years of age (93% protective), and declines with age at vaccination and time since vaccination [55]. **Vaccine efficacy averages 75% in immunocompetent patients 65 years and older, and is cost effective** [39]. **Efficacy has ranged from 65% to 84% among patients with moderate risk** from underlying medical conditions such as diabetes, CHF, COPD, and asplenia [39,52].
   b. **Protein conjugate vaccine.** This vaccine was **97.4% effective in preventing invasive disease from vaccine serotypes** in a prelicensing trial [54]. A large Finnish trial in children found that vaccine reduced all pneumococcal otitis media episodes by 34%, serotype- specific pneumococcal episodes by 57%, and cross-reactive serotype pneumococcal episodes by 51% [56]. However, episodes from other serotypes of pneumococci increased by 33% [56].
5. **Side effects**
   a. **Purified polysaccharide vaccines.** Their **safety has been well established** [39]. **Mild local reactions** of pain, erythema, or discomfort occur in approximately 50% of recipients and last less than 48 hours. **Systemic reactions are rare** and include transient chills, fever to 40°C (104°F), and weakness. When current guidelines are followed, reactions to repeat vaccination are similar in type and frequency to initial vaccination [39,54]. There is no increase in reactions when purified polysaccharide vaccine is given after protein conjugate vaccine [54].
   b. **Protein conjugate vaccine [54].** In prelicensing evaluations, 10% to 13% of **infants** given a full four-injection vaccine series had erythema, 10% to 12% had induration, and 15% to 23% had local tenderness. Only erythema increased in size with subsequent doses. Fever of greater than 100.4°F occurred in 15% to 24%, and fever of greater than 102.2°F ranged from 0.9% after the first dose to 2.5% after the second dose. The rate of seizures within the first 72 hours was 1 per 7,000 doses, well below the rate previously seen with whole-cell pertussis vaccine. **Older children** generally had higher rates of local reactions, fussiness was their most common systemic effect, and fever of greater than 100.4°F after one dose occurred in 7% to 37%. Experience with the safety of giving protein conjugate vaccine after purified polysaccharide vaccine is limited.
6. **Precautions and contraindications**
   a. **Purified polysaccharide vaccines.** Their **safety has not been adequately studied during the first trimester of pregnancy,** but no adverse outcomes have been reported [39]. Therefore, vaccine should be given to high-risk women prior to pregnancy. They are contraindicated in patients with a prior hypersensitivity reaction to the vaccine or one of its components.
   b. **Protein conjugate vaccine.** It is best to delay vaccine until resolution of moderate or severe illness, although it may be given with minor illness [54]. Vaccine is contraindicated in patients with a prior hypersensitivity reaction to the vaccine or one of its components. Simultaneous administration of the protein conjugate vaccine with a purified polysaccharide vaccine is not recommended [54]. The current formulation (Prevnar, Wyeth Lederle Vaccines) should be used with caution in patients with latex sensitivity because its packaging contains natural rubber. There is no published information about the use of this vaccine in pregnancy.
7. **Indications for use.** Recipients should be informed that the vaccine does not entirely eliminate the risk of pneumococcal pneumonia.
   a. **Purified polysaccharide vaccines** are approved for use in adults and children at least 2 years of age at risk for invasive pneumococcal disease and who

are capable of responding [39,52]. Note that the protein conjugate vaccine should be used initially in children up to age 5 years (see section **I.E.7.b**).

(1) **Persons 65 years of age or older.** Everyone in this group should be vaccinated, including those with an unknown vaccination status and those who received vaccine before reaching 65 years of age but who have not been revaccinated in the prior 5 years.

(2) **Splenectomized patients,** including autosplenectomy from sickle cell anemia. Vaccine should be given at least 2 weeks prior to an elective splenectomy.

(3) **Patients with alcoholism, COPD, CHF, cyanotic congenital heart disease, cirrhosis, diabetes, nephrotic syndrome, or renal failure.**

(4) **HIV-infected adults and adolescents.**

(5) **Immunocompromised patients,** including those with leukemia, lymphoma, Hodgkin disease, multiple myeloma, generalized malignancy, solid organ or bone marrow transplants, immunosuppressive chemotherapy, and long-term steroid use. Both the physician and the patient must recognize that response to the vaccine may be limited. **Patients** with Hodgkin disease and others **about to undergo immunosuppression should be vaccinated at least 2 weeks before immunosuppressive therapy** (see section **I.E.3.a**).

(6) **In special settings or populations with a known increased risk, such as** residents of nursing homes or long-term care facilities, Alaska Natives and American Indians, and those with CSF leak.

(7) **Children 24 to 59 months of age previously given the protein conjugate vaccine and who are in one of the above high-risk groups** [54]. The purified polysaccharide vaccine should be given at least 2 months after the last dose of the protein conjugate vaccine.

**b. Protein conjugate vaccine is indicated for infants and children between 2 and 59 months of age** [54]. Note that the protein conjugate vaccine should not replace purified polysaccharide vaccine for adults and children age 5 years and older.

(1) **All children up to 23 months of age.**

(2) **High-risk children 24 to 59 months of age.** This includes those with sickle cell hemoglobinopathies, anatomic or functional asplenia, HIV infection, congenital immunodeficiencies, renal failure, nephrotic syndrome, chronic cardiac diseases, chronic lung diseases, CSF leaks, diabetes, and immunocompromising conditions such as leukemia, lymphoma, Hodgkin disease, chemotherapy, radiation therapy, long-term steroid use, and solid organ transplants.

(3) **Other children 24 to 59 months of age who should be considered for vaccination** include all those 24 to 35 months of age, Alaska Native or American Indians, African Americans, and those who attend day-care centers.

(4) **High-risk children 24 to 59 months of age previously given a purified polysaccharide vaccine.** The protein conjugate vaccine should be started at least 2 months after the purified polysaccharide vaccine.

**8. Dosage [39,54]**

**a. Purified polysaccharide vaccines.** The usual dose is a single 0.5-mL intramuscular (i.m.) or subcutaneous injection given at any time during the year. **The pneumococcal vaccine may be given simultaneously with influenza vaccination** at separate sites.

**b. Protein conjugate vaccine.** Each dose is 0.5 mL administered i.m., given in schedule with other recommended vaccines. **Children who begin vaccination up to 6 months of age** are given a primary series of three doses at least 1 to 2 months apart, followed by an additional dose at 12 to 15 months of age and at least 2 months after the primary series. **Children who begin vaccination at 7 to 11 months of age** are given a primary series of two doses at least 1 to 2 months apart, followed by an additional dose at 12 to 15 months of age and at least 2 months after the primary series. **Children who begin vaccination at 12 to 23 months of age** are given only a primary series of two doses at least 2 months apart. **High-risk children who begin vaccination at 24 to 59 months of age** are given only a primary series of two doses at least 2 months apart. **Healthy children who begin vaccination at 24 to 59 months of age** are given only a single dose.

9. **Revaccination** currently is recommended only with the purified polysaccharide vaccines [39,54]. Candidates are highest risk patients and those with a poor antibody response (asplenia, HIV infection, leukemia, lymphoma, Hodgkin disease, multiple myeloma, malignancy, nephrotic syndrome, renal failure, organ or bone marrow transplants, and immunosuppression from chemotherapy or corticosteroids). All those 65 years of age and older who received the vaccine at least 5 years previously and were under 65 years old when initially vaccinated also should be revaccinated. The interval between doses should be at least 5 years, except in high-risk children age 10 years and under, who should be revaccinated 3 years after a prior dose of purified polysaccharide vaccine. Revaccination is contraindicated if there was a severe reaction to the initial dose.

II. **Aspiration pneumonia** [15] refers to pneumonia caused by macroaspiration. Patients with obtundation or a defective cough-epiglottic reflex are at highest risk.

A. **Aspiration pneumonitis** develops after sterile gastric acid aspiration, resulting in a chemical injury to the lung.

1. **No antibiotic therapy is usually required.** Institution of pulmonary drainage and careful observation are indicated. Early therapy does not prevent infection but instead selects for resistant organisms.
2. **For patients at risk for gastric colonization with pathogenic bacteria (those with small-bowel obstruction, antacid or antisecretory use, gastroparesis, and gastric tube feedings),** antibiotic therapy may be considered after specimens for Gram stain and culture are obtained. An invasive diagnostic procedure may help.

B. **Community-acquired aspiration pneumonias account for 5% to 15% of CAP.** The typical patient risk factors are discussed in section I.G.2 under Clinical Approach to Community-Acquired Pneumonia. Oral anaerobes, penicillin-sensitive pneumococci [57], and many other aerobic organisms are involved. **Clindamycin is a traditional agent for anaerobic aspiration pneumonia.** If used, at least 10 to 15 million units/day of i.v. aqueous penicillin G should be given because of increasing penicillin resistance among non-fragilis *Bacteroides* species, fusobacteria, other oral anaerobes, and the pneumococci [32,58–62]. However, the optimal dosage of penicillin for aspiration pneumonia is unknown. Although Marik [15] recommends levofloxacin or ceftriaxone, this is controversial [63]. Gatifloxacin and moxifloxacin, but not levofloxacin, have anaerobic activity and should be adequate for these infections, but there is little clinical experience with their use for this purpose. Seriously ill patients should be given a broad-spectrum regimen that includes coverage for anaerobes.

C. **Hospital-acquired aspiration pneumonia.** Hospitalized patients are at risk for gram-negative pneumonia. **Gastric and pharyngeal colonization by gram-negative bacilli and *S. aureus* may be important in the pathogenesis** [11,64]. Continuous gastric feedings or prophylaxis for stress ulcers with antacids or histamine ($H_2$) blockers are risk factors by overcoming the normal gastric acid barrier permitting bacterial growth in the stomach. Stress-ulcer prophylaxis with sucralfate, as compared with agents that raise gastric pH, has lowered the incidence of nosocomial pneumonia in some but not all studies [65,66]. Initial empiric therapy for patients hospitalized longer than 4 days or with severe illness should include an antipseudomonal $\beta$-lactam (e.g., piperacillin-tazobactam, cefepime, or imipenem) plus either an aminoglycoside or a fluoroquinolone to cover enteric gram-negative bacilli and pseudomonas [11,67]. Anaerobic coverage should be included for any patient with severe gum or dental disease, foul sputum, necrotizing pneumonia, or lung abscess [15]. If an antipseudomonal drug without useful anaerobic activity (ceftazidime, cefepime, and aztreonam) is chosen, then clindamycin or metronidazole should be added. See section **IX** for further discussion of nosocomial pneumonias.

**III.** ***H. influenzae*** causes bronchitis in patients with chronic lung disease (see Chapter 8). Primary pneumonia usually occurs in the elderly, patients with chronic lung diseases, and in HIV infection. Rapidly fatal pneumonia in younger adults with normal immune systems and ventilator-associated pneumonia also have been described [68,69]. In children under 5 years of age, the incidence of invasive disease has dramatically decreased since the introduction of the conjugated *H. influenzae* type b vaccines. However, in developing countries *H. influenzae* type b is still an important problem [70].

**A. Diagnosis.** A positive blood culture for *H. influenzae* confirms the diagnosis. In addition to type b, other encapsulated non–type b and nontypable strains occur and may be complicated by bacteremia [71]. Thus, latex agglutination for type b antigen in serum and urine is insensitive.

**B. Therapy.** Beta-lactamase production accounts for the frequent occurrence of ampicillin resistance.

1. **Unknown ampicillin susceptibility or known ampicillin resistance.** If a well-obtained sputum shows pleomorphic gram-negative rods on Gram stain, ceftriaxone or cefotaxime should be used because they are active against $\beta$-lactamase–positive strains. Therapy can be modified when cultures become available.
2. **Known ampicillin-susceptible strains.** If the isolate is $\beta$-lactamase negative, penicillin or ampicillin is satisfactory. Most authorities recommend ampicillin, 1 to 2 g i.v. every 4 hours in adults, because of clinical experience. Therapy usually is continued for 10 to 14 days, and may be completed with oral amoxicillin. Cefuroxime, ceftriaxone, and cefotaxime also are very active. Fluoroquinolones, clarithromycin, azithromycin, and TMP-SMX are alternatives for the penicillin-allergic patient. (See further discussion in Chapter 27.)

**C. Prognosis.** In bacteremia, mortality may approach 36% in older adults [71]. The mother usually survives infection during pregnancy, but fetal loss is common [71].

**IV. Gram-negative pneumonias.** Most are hospital acquired, although community-acquired gram-negative pneumonias occur.

**A. Setting and etiology.** Important etiologies include the Enterobacteriaceae (*Klebsiella, Enterobacter,* and *Serratia*), *P. aeruginosa,* and other *Pseudomonas* species, and less common pathogens such as *Acinetobacter* species. Although uncommon overall, *K. pneumoniae* is the most commonly identified community-acquired gram-negative pneumonia [72].

1. **Community-acquired** gram-negative pneumonias occur in the elderly from nursing homes, and patients with underlying lung disease, alcoholism, or chronic debilitating disease.
2. **Hospital-acquired** gram-negative pneumonia usually occurs with mechanical ventilation or aspiration, and in compromised hosts.

**B. Diagnosis.** Diagnosis can be difficult, and the clinician must distinguish colonization from true infection. (See section **VIII** under Clinical Approach to Community-Acquired Pneumonia.)

**C. Therapy.** Most authorities use two agents known to be synergistic *in vitro,* although definitive studies are lacking (see **Chapter 27**). We believe this is essential for patients with necrotizing infections or abscess formation. Partially because of poor antibiotic activity in sputum, **treatment is given for at least 2 weeks.** (See also section **IX.E.2.**) Empiric antibiotics should cover *Pseudomonas aeruginosa,* and may be narrowed when an organism is recovered.

1. ***Klebsiella.*** Ceftriaxone, cefotaxime, and cefepime are active against *K. pneumoniae in vitro,* and monotherapy can be used [12]. Other potentially useful agents include imipenem, meropenem, piperacillin-tazobactam, the fluoroquinolones, and aztreonam. Nosocomial *Klebsiella* species can be multiply resistant; imipenem is often active against these isolates. (See discussion in **Chapter 27.**)
2. ***Pseudomonas.*** **Combination i.v. therapy commonly is used** to prevent the development of resistance, and to achieve synergy if possible. Recommendations

for suspected *Pseudomonas* pneumonia are given in section **IX.B.2.c** under Clinical Approach to Community-Acquired Pneumonia [2,4,6]. Hatchette et. al. [73] made similar recommendations based on their review of community-acquired *Pseudomonas* pneumonia. Monotherapy with an antipseudomonal $\beta$-lactam or quinolone is not optimal initial therapy (see related discussions in Chapter 27). When the infection is under good control, oral ciprofloxacin may be used for susceptible organisms to complete therapy. When aminoglycosides are used, serum levels should be monitored carefully as much to ensure adequate levels as to avoid toxicity.

3. **Compromised hosts with pneumonia** are discussed separately in section **VIII.**

V. **"Atypical pneumonia"** [74]

A. **Historical view. Atypical pneumonia** originally referred to those pneumonias that had clinical features distinct from classic lobar pneumonia.

1. **A subacute illness,** with onset over several days.
2. **Early nonspecific systemic manifestations** of fever, headache, and myalgias.
3. **Cough is often the most prominent early respiratory symptom and initially nonproductive.** Dyspnea and pleuritic chest pain are rare.
4. **Initially scant and mucoid sputum,** which may be purulent as illness progresses.
5. **Chest physical findings** that often underestimate the extent of radiographic changes.
6. **Leukocytosis** usually less than or equal to 15,000/mm$^3$.

B. **Distinguishing between atypical and typical etiologies on the basis of clinical and radiographic features alone is not reliable** [2,6,74]. Thus, the clinician must be familiar with many possible etiologies to appropriately manage CAP [74].

C. **There are numerous potential etiologies** for atypical pneumonia. *M. pneumoniae* and *C. pneumoniae* are discussed in detail since they cause the syndrome most frequently, and a few of the others are briefly reviewed [74]. *Legionella* species are discussed in section VI.

D. ***Mycoplasma pneumoniae*** is the most common cause of "atypical pneumonia" [75]. The illness spreads in families with an incubation period of 2 to 3 weeks. **Those at greatest risk for infection are 5 to 20 years of age, although it occurs in all age groups** [76]. Outbreaks may occur in the community or in institutional settings [77,78]. **Only partial immunity follows infection,** and repeated infections in the same patient have been documented. In addition, patients with hypogammaglobulinemia have an increased susceptibility [79].

1. **Clinical manifestations** [80]

a. **Pharyngitis** is much more prominent than rhinitis and may be the earliest symptom. **Protracted cough with minimal sputum production is the most common symptom,** although occasional individuals will produce significant quantities of sputum. Bullous myringitis is a traditional clue in the diagnosis, but it is infrequent and may be present in other pneumonias. Pleurisy and easily demonstrable pleural effusions are unlikely to be due to mycoplasmal pneumonia. **Occasionally, *M. pneumoniae* produces severe illness,** especially in patients with sickle cell disease.

b. **Extrapulmonary manifestations** may occur either with or without the respiratory component [80,81]. These include vomiting or diarrhea, morbilliform skin rashes, erythema multiforme, arthritides, and several central nervous system (CNS) syndromes such as aseptic meningitis.

c. **A history of a similar illness 2 weeks earlier in a family member** may be elicited. In contrast, with viral illness contacts are usually ill at the same time.

d. **Radiographic findings** include segmental and subsegmental infiltrates that may be bilateral [14]. Features suggesting mycoplasmal pneumonia include the absence of consolidation, limited progression, relatively rapid resolution, and in some reports hilar adenopathy [82]. Computed tomography

(CT) scans may show ground-glass infiltration and nodules not readily seen on plain films [83].

2. **Diagnosis.** The organism grows slowly and is difficult to isolate, so most laboratories do not offer cultures for *Mycoplasma.* The diagnosis most often is made serologically.
   a. **Cold agglutinins** develop in approximately half of patients, but **are not specific.** They have been seen in influenza, mononucleosis, other infections, and lymphoproliferative diseases. A titer of 1:128 or more is suggestive of *Mycoplasma* infection. Hemolytic anemia is an uncommon complication.
   b. Commercially available **enzyme immunoassay** has replaced complement fixation (CF) as the preferred serologic test [77,84]. Major disadvantages to serodiagnosis are that information is unavailable during the acute illness, IgM antibodies may persist for prolonged periods, and reinfection may result in a poor IgM response. A fourfold or greater antibody increase occurring between acute and convalescent sera collected 4 weeks apart is diagnostic.
   c. **Rapid diagnostic tests** undergoing evaluation include antigen capture assays, nucleic acid hybridization, and PCR. Particularly intriguing is the use of multiplex PCR for the simultaneous testing of multiple respiratory pathogens on the same specimen [85]. Studies to clarify their usefulness are needed because they can detect the carrier state that exists in the absence of active disease.
3. **Differential diagnosis.** It may not be possible to differentiate between other infections, such as *C. pneumoniae,* Legionnaires disease, and even atypical presentations of bacterial pneumonia. Clinical features suggesting *Mycoplasma* infection include spread in family members or close contacts, the extrapulmonary findings cited previously, and absence of pleuritic symptoms [86].
4. **Therapy.** Either **erythromycin or tetracycline for 14 to 21 days** will shorten the duration of illness and reduce the frequency of relapse. However, the organism may be shed for up to 4 months even with therapy. Erythromycin and tetracycline are equally effective; the adult doses are either 250 mg four times daily or 500 mg three times daily. Erythromycin 30 to 50 mg/kg/day in divided doses is given to children weighing under 25 kg, and no more than 1 g daily to those weighing over 25 kg. Clarithromycin and azithromycin have fewer side effects, but are much more expensive. Tetracycline should not be used during pregnancy, in nursing mothers, or in children under 8 years of age. Doxycycline can be used in place of tetracycline; the adult dose is 100 mg twice daily, and for children age 8 years and older 1 to 2 mg/kg twice daily. Levofloxacin and other newer fluoroquinolones are active *in vitro,* but they are more expensive and should not be used in children. Prophylactic antibiotics have been suggested during outbreaks in closed populations; five days of azithromycin helped control an outbreak in a long-term care facility [78]. (See Chapter 27.)

E. ***Chlamydophila (Chlamydia) pneumoniae. C. pneumoniae*** **is the second most common cause of atypical pneumonia.** It occurs year round, is worldwide in its distribution, and may cause outbreaks [87,88]. Antibodies to *C. pneumoniae* are rare in preschool-aged children but increase rapidly in prevalence through adolescence and young adulthood. Seropositivity is high, up to 75%, among the elderly [88]. Aerosol transmission from human to human predominates, but environmental contamination and fomite spread also is possible [88]. The average person may have several infections over their lifetime [87], although these may represent reactivation of latent *C. pneumoniae* during another infection.

1. **Clinical manifestations. Most infections are asymptomatic or produce only mild illness.** *C. pneumoniae* accounts for **approximately 10% of CAP,** and nosocomial pneumonia is also possible. Combined infections have been frequent [87], but these may represent reactivation of *C. pneumoniae* during an unrelated pneumonia. Pneumonia, bronchitis, pharyngitis, otitis, and sinusitis are the most common syndromes. Many patients have a "biphasic" illness with early fever, and may be afebrile when they eventually seek medical care. Initial symptoms may include gradual onset of sore throat, pharyngitis, and hoarseness [87]. Pneumonia with nonproductive cough is delayed by 1 to 4 weeks in

primary infection, and approximately 1 week longer in reinfection [87]. Bronchitis with or without pneumonia may be subacute in onset, and may have a prolonged recovery phase. Pharyngitis and sinusitis, with or without otitis, also may occur by themselves or as part of pneumonia [87,88].

An elevated erythrocyte sedimentation rate (ESR) and a normal WBC count are the rule. The most common radiographic picture is unilateral subsegmental or segmental infiltrates indistinguishable from mycoplasmal infection or other etiologies for CAP that resolve rapidly [87]. Convalescence may be prolonged, but most patients recover. Severe pneumonia is more likely with increasing age and mixed infections; death is rare and occurs most frequently in the elderly and in those with underlying illness or mixed infection [88].

*C. pneumoniae* has been implicated in several other clinical syndromes. These include bronchospastic disease, endocarditis, myocarditis, and atherosclerosis [88].

2. **Diagnosis.** Cultures are not available in most centers. **Serologic diagnosis** uses the microimmunofluorescence test for *C. pneumoniae* IgM and IgG antibodies [88]. In primary infection IgM antibodies appear after a 2- to 4-week delay, so that acute and convalescent specimens should be separated by no less than 4 weeks. In reinfection cases IgM may not appear but IgG titers increase within 1 to 3 weeks. The older chlamydial CF test is nonspecific. Rapid diagnosis by specific antigen or DNA detection is not widely available [87,88].
3. **Differential diagnosis.** Prospective studies have not identified any feature distinctive of *C. pneumoniae* infection. Hoarseness and sore throat may be a consistent finding with illness, but many other prevalent respiratory agents also cause these symptoms.
4. **Therapy.** Clinical experience suggests that **macrolides, tetracyclines, and newer fluoroquinolones** are effective [2]. We favor doxycycline in adults, 100 mg twice daily, for 10 to 14 days. Clarithromycin, azithromycin, and the newer fluoroquinolones are active *in vitro.* Treatment failures and relapses occur. Relapses are treated with either the same or a different antibiotic. Excretion of the organism for up to 1 year after therapy has been described [88].

F. ***Chlamydia psittaci*** causes psittacosis. Psittacosis (or ornithosis) is a **systemic infection acquired from occupational or home contact with infected birds,** including parrots, parakeets, turkeys, and others. The onset may be abrupt, and the illness is potentially fatal. Diagnosis depends on acute and convalescent serologic studies. Tetracyclines are the agents of choice [89], and are given for 1 to 2 weeks after clinical improvement to minimize relapses.

G. ***Coxiella burnetii.*** This obligate intracellular parasite causes **Q fever** [90].

1. **Epidemiology.** Although *C. burnetii* is found on five continents and in at least 51 countries, the rates of Q fever vary widely from region to region [90]. Q fever is endemic to Nova Scotia, accounting for 5% of ambulatory patients with an identified cause of CAP [75]. Infections occur most commonly after exposure (often occupational) to infected aerosols from products of conception or from milk, wool, or fresh cheese from infected animals. Several outbreaks have occurred that were unrelated to traditional animal reservoirs for *C. burnetii,* involving exposure to stillborn kittens or parturient cats, sheep used in research, wild rabbits, manure, and living along a road used for a sheep drive [91,92].
2. **Clinical findings. Acute Q fever** may include pneumonia, hepatitis, or both. Illness begins abruptly with rigors, fever, headache, and myalgias. Nonproductive cough is present in at least half of the patients with pneumonia. There may be relative bradycardia for the degree of fever. Chest examination often is unremarkable despite obvious radiographic infiltrates. Hepatomegaly indicates liver involvement; splenomegaly is much less frequent. Radiographic infiltrates usually are subsegmental or segmental, may have a pleural base, and are indistinguishable from other types of CAP. However, **rounded opacities** should suggest the possibility of Q fever pneumonia. Other laboratory findings are equally nonspecific. **Chronic Q fever** may rarely involve the lungs, presenting as pseudotumor or fibrosis [90]. **Serologic methods are the mainstay of diagnosis** [93].

3. **Treatment is suggested for all symptomatic acute *C. burnetii* infections** because of the potential for later chronic Q fever. **In adults,** 2 weeks of oral **doxycycline,** 100 mg twice daily, is the regimen of choice. Chloramphenicol is an alternative, but the newer fluoroquinolones are also effective [90]. Erythromycin treatment failures for pneumonia have occurred, but the addition of rifampin has been effective [94].

H. **Viral pneumonia. In infants and children,** RSV, parainfluenza viruses, adenoviruses, influenza, and varicella-zoster virus are most common. **In adults, viral pneumonia is uncommon but influenza is the most important cause.** Adenovirus may cause outbreaks in military recruits and sporadic community cases. Respiratory infections in adults that cause hospitalization include RSV and influenza, particularly in the elderly and in contacts of children with RSV infection (e.g., adult family members and hospital personnel). In addition, nursing home outbreaks of RSV illness have been documented. For further discussion, see Chapter 10.

I. ***Pneumocystis carinii* pneumonia** should be considered in patients with HIV infection.

VI. **Legionnaires' and related diseases.** A great deal has been learned about *Legionella* since the July 1976 outbreak of Legionnaires disease at the American Legion convention in Philadelphia [13].

A. **Microbiology.** There are at least 42 species and 64 serogroups of Legionellaceae, and at least 20 of them are proven human pathogens [95–97]. However, *L. pneumophila* serogroup 1 is responsible for 70% to 80% of *Legionella* pneumonias in the United States, and *L. micdadei* is the next most common cause [74,96]. Thus, the clinical aspects of these two species will be stressed.

1. ***Legionella pneumophila*** is an aerobic, gram-negative, fastidious organism that grows best in 2.5% to 5.0% carbon dioxide on special media (e.g., charcoal yeast extract agar supplemented with $\alpha$-ketoglutarate) containing cysteine [97]. Visible growth may take up to 10 days. Although this is a gram-negative bacillus, it does not stain well with ordinary Gram stain. **Special silver stains** (e.g., Dieterle) **are used to demonstrate the organism in tissue.**
   a. The organism produces a $\beta$-lactamase and is resistant to penicillins and cephalosporins. It contains an endotoxin (not highly active biologically), and produces many enzymes and potential toxins whose role in virulence is uncertain [97].
   b. **At least 15 serologic types** have been identified [96].
2. ***Legionella micdadei*** is recognized as causing "Pittsburgh pneumonia" and infections previously believed to be due to *Rickettsia*-like organisms (i.e., the Tatlock and HEBA organisms) [95]. These organisms also grow on charcoal yeast extract agar. ***L. micdadei* is weakly acid-fast,** which may lead to a mistaken diagnosis of tuberculosis. It does not regularly produce $\beta$-lactamases.
3. ***Legionella longbeachae*** infection has been associated with gardening and the use of potting soil [98].
4. **Other *Legionella* species** causing disease in humans continue to be retrieved from new infections or recovered from samples of previously unidentified pneumonias [95].

B. **Incidence.** The exact incidence of infections due to *L. pneumophila* and related species is unknown; estimates show wide variation with locale and time. Overall, **2% to 9% of CAP** is due to these bacteria [13]. **The rates of hospital-acquired pneumonias** caused by *Legionella* also **vary,** depending on the medical center and the patient population.

1. ***L. pneumophila*** causes 2% to 15% of pneumonias requiring hospitalization, and an even higher proportion of severe pneumonias requiring admission to the intensive care unit (ICU) [13].
2. ***L. micdadei* causes nosocomial infections in the compromised host,** although community-acquired infections and outbreaks may occur [95,99,100]. Predisposing factors include transplantation, hematologic malignancy, high doses of corticosteroids, previous surgery, and underlying chronic lung disease or other serious illness.

**C. Epidemiology.** *Legionella* are aquatic organisms transmitted by water and air through airborne droplets or microaspiration [13,101]. Human-to-human transmission does not occur. Environmental reservoirs frequently contain algae that provide nutrients and amebae and protozoa that support intracellular multiplication; growth in water is further favored by elevated temperatures, iron, and limited bacterial competition.

Soil excavation, air-conditioning systems, water evaporative condensers, and potable water have been point sources for outbreaks, especially in summer months. Sporadic cases occur year round. Following environmental exposure, the pneumonia attack rate is low and in the range of 0.1% to 5% [102], but the attack rate for Pontiac fever is higher [99].

**D. Host factors.** Legionellosis is seen in any age group. **Elderly or compromised patients may develop fatal infection.** Patients at greatest risk [13,95,97] are as follows:

1. **Immunocompromised patients,** including organ transplant recipients and persons receiving chemotherapeutic agents, radiation therapy, or corticosteroids **are at risk for nosocomial *Legionella* infection.** Legionellosis is uncommon in HIV- infected individuals.
2. **Dialysis patients.**
3. **Late-middle-aged to elderly men.**
4. **Hosts with chronic underlying disease** (e.g., organic heart disease, lung disease, renal disease, and diabetes).
5. **Alcoholics and smokers, particularly in the presence of COPD.**
6. **Patients undergoing major surgery.**
7. **Neonates with ventilator-associated pneumonia.**

**E. Clinical manifestations** [13,95,97]. There is a **broad spectrum** of disease due to *L. pneumophila* and *L. micdadei.*

1. **Asymptomatic infection** is well described, including in the outbreak setting [102].
2. **Pontiac fever** is a non-pneumonic disease named after an outbreak in Pontiac, Michigan, in 1968. After a 1- to 2-day incubation period, there is an abrupt onset of fever, chills, headache, myalgias, and malaise. Acute symptoms usually last less than a week, the illness being self-limited even without specific therapy.
3. **Pneumonia** is the most common symptomatic problem. **Clinical and laboratory manifestations of *Legionella* pneumonia are not distinctive,** although a scoring system has been used at one institution to identify patients with legionellosis [3]. Mixed infections have been reported.
   a. **Pulmonary manifestations.** The spectrum of disease is **highly variable.** Mild to moderate illness (e.g., bronchitis or an atypical pneumonia syndrome) or moderate to severe pneumonia with adult respiratory distress syndrome may occur. Illness usually begins with nonspecific symptoms of malaise, myalgias, headache, and fever, after an incubation period of 2 to 10 days. An initially dry and nonproductive cough is present in approximately 90% of patients, and often progresses to produce purulent sputum. Temperatures of 39° to 40°C (102°–104°F) are common, as are shaking chills. Pulmonary symptoms steadily progress over several days. Chest pain and hemoptysis may falsely suggest pulmonary embolism. Early physical findings are often nonspecific and may include a pulse-temperature deficit [3] that may have been overemphasized [13]. Signs of consolidation develop, but pleural friction rubs are uncommon. **Radiologic findings are nonspecific.** Infiltrates that are initially unilateral and patchy frequently progress to bilateral consolidation. Nodular lesions, diffuse alveolar patterns, cavitation, and abscess formation may be seen. Small pleural effusions may develop, but large effusions are uncommon.
   b. **Other manifestations** of pneumonic infections may include abdominal pain, nausea, vomiting, and diarrhea. Neurologic findings include headache, confusion, disorientation, delirium, and, although rare, focal neurologic findings. Results of lumbar puncture studies are normal. **Hyponatremia is**

**found more commonly** in *Legionella* pneumonia than with other etiologies of pneumonia.

c. **Miscellaneous findings.** Hepatomegaly and liver function test abnormalities, disseminated intravascular coagulation, hypophosphatemia, and hematuria occur no more frequently than in other types of pneumonia.

4. **Extrapulmonary infections** have included bacteremia, lymphadenitis, **prosthetic valve endocarditis,** sinusitis, osteomyelitis, hemodialysis shunt infections, peritonitis, pancreatitis, pericarditis, myocarditis, cellulitis, wound infection, and abscesses in organs and soft tissues. These can result from hematogenous seeding or from direct inoculation with contaminated water.

F. **Diagnosis [96,103]. Legionellosis should be sought in any at-risk hospitalized patient with limited sputum, sputum Gram stain showing leukocytes but few organisms, or a poor response to $\beta$-lactam antibiotics [13].**

1. **Routine Gram stains of sputum** frequently show moderate to large numbers of polymorphonuclear leukocytes (and monocytes), often with no bacteria.
2. **Cultures for *Legionella*** have a diagnostic specificity of 100%, and should be performed whenever possible. They require special media, so the laboratory should be alerted to their possibility, and **growth takes several days.** In centers with experience sputum culture has a sensitivity of 80% [13]; however, in routine clinical practice it may be 10% or less [96]. Bronchial washings, bronchoalveolar lavage, and lung tissue have sensitivities similar to sputum or higher [97]. The yield from pleural fluid culture is less. *Legionella* organisms also have been isolated from blood but the yield is low.
3. **Direct fluorescent antibody** (DFA) testing of respiratory secretions, pleural fluid, or lung tissue is technically difficult. Results may not be reliable in inexperienced laboratories or when the screened serogroups do not reflect the locally prevalent *Legionella* [96]. Thus, the sensitivity of this test ranges from 33% to 68% [96]. Organisms may remain detectable by DFA for several days after starting antibiotics. Although specific, false-positive results have occurred in the presence of other bacteria, and from *Legionella* contamination of test reagents [96].
4. **Antigen detection in urine of serogroup 1 only** is commercially available in kits. These tests have high specificity and a sensitivity of approximately 70% [13]. They may be positive well into the patient's illness and even after therapy has been started. Antigenuria may be prolonged so that a positive test may result from an unrelated prior infection. Also, false-negative results may be obtained from infection with other *Legionella* species. The tests can be used with other specimens, including pleural fluids [97].
5. **PCR is promising** but not widely available [96]. PCR is capable of detecting any *Legionella* species, is very sensitive, and is rapid enough to affect empiric therapy.
6. **Serologic studies** (immunofluorescence assay, enzyme-linked immunosorbent assay [ELISA], counterimmunoelectrophoresis, or agglutination tests) are 40% to 60% sensitive and have good specificity [13]. Sensitivity is highest for *L. pneumophila* (75%–80%), and is 50% or less for non-pneumophila species [96]. Because serum antibody may be delayed, samples should be obtained every 2 to 3 weeks for 4 to 12 weeks. False-positive results have been reported from cross-reaction with other organisms [96]. Thus, **serology is useful for epidemiologic purposes but does not influence initial patient management.**

   With paired sera, a fourfold increase in either IgM or IgG titer to 1:128 or more is considered diagnostic of disease. **A single titer** of 1:256 or more has a low positive predictive value and **should not be used for diagnosis in an individual patient.**

G. **Therapy.** *In vitro* antibiotic susceptibility tests for *Legionella* do not reliably predict clinical efficacy [16,95,97]. Thus, most therapeutic information has come from clinical experience, animal studies, or *in vitro* models of intracellular infection. In these models, erythromycin, tetracycline, rifampin, TMP-SMX, and the fluoroquinolones are effective; erythromycin is bacteriostatic. The penicillins, cephalosporins, and aminoglycosides are ineffective. **In fact, a pneumonia that progresses during treatment with the latter should suggest the possibility of *Legionella* infection.** Treatment failures and relapses have been reported with erythromycin but also may occur with other agents.

1. **Isolation.** Special precautions are not required.
2. **Mildly ill** and previously healthy individuals may receive outpatient treatment with any of the alternatives listed below.
3. **In hospitalized adults, i.v. therapy should be given initially** but may be finished orally. **Most authorities no longer consider erythromycin the drug of choice** [2]. Recommended agents include the following:
   a. **Azithromycin** 1,000 mg on the first day and 500 mg daily for the next 4 days can be given [13]. The duration is extended to 10 to 14 days with life-threatening infection or in immunocompromised hosts.
   b. **A fluoroquinolone** (ciprofloxacin, levofloxacin, or gatifloxacin) may be given for 10 to 14 days, and extended to 21 days for life-threatening infection or in immunocompromised hosts. A quinolone is preferred in transplant patients to avoid potential drug interactions with cyclosporine or tacrolimus [95,104].
   c. **Doxycycline** is given in a dose of 100 mg i.v. every 12 hours after a single 200-mg loading dose. The duration of therapy is the same as for the fluoroquinolones.
   d. **Rifampin** is active *in vitro* and in animals, but **is never used alone.** It may be added (300–600 mg every 12 hours) when azithromycin or a fluoroquinolone are not used for immunocompromised hosts or severe infections; there is no benefit to adding rifampin to azithromycin or a fluoroquinolone [104]. The potential for drug interactions should be evaluated before using rifampin.
   e. **Other agents** with reports of success include TMP-SMX (adult dose of 160 mg TMP and 800 mg SMX every 8–12 hours), imipenem, and clindamycin [13].

H. **Prognosis** is related to the underlying disease and the early institution of appropriate therapy. In nonimmunosuppressed patients, the mortality rate is low. In immunosuppressed patients, mortality may be as high as 50% if specific therapy is delayed [97].

I. **Prevention.** There is no vaccine for legionellosis. Routine cultures of the hospital water supply have been recommended, particularly in institutions caring for transplant and other immunosuppressed patients [97,100].

VII. **Hantavirus pulmonary syndrome (HPS)** [105]. Found worldwide, hantaviruses are enveloped negative-sense RNA viruses in the family Bunyavirudae. Hantavirus illnesses are most common in Asia and Europe and include syndromes of hemorrhagic fever with renal failure (e.g., Korean hemorrhagic fever) and nephropathia epidemica. In May 1993, an outbreak of unexplained ARDS in otherwise healthy adults was reported in the Four Corners area of Arizona, Colorado, New Mexico, and Utah. Intense investigation revealed a new hantavirus, the Sin Nombre virus. HPS has since been caused by at least four other new hantaviruses (New York, Monongahela, Bayou, and Black Creek Canal viruses) in different areas of the United States [106].

A. **Epidemiology**

1. **Rodents are the primary reservoir** for HPS viruses, including the deer mouse, white-footed mouse, rice rat, and cotton rat. The **predominant modes of transmission** to humans are ingestion or inhalation of aerosolized rodent excreta, and direct contact with rodents, rodent excreta, or rodent saliva. The majority of exposures have occurred in and around the home [106].
2. **Human-to-human spread has not occurred in the United States,** but has been implicated in an outbreak in Argentina [107].
3. **As of April 2001 there were a total of 283 cases from 31 states,** and since then the first case was reported from Vermont [106]. Most cases have occurred in the Southwest, and 60% have occurred in men. Ages ranged from 10 to 75 years with a mean of 37 years. **Case fatality since the 1993 outbreak has been 38%.** Updated information is available at *www.cdc.gov/ncidod/diseases/hanta/hantvrus.htm.*

**B. Clinical manifestations.** Classic HPS is described, although mild and asymptomatic infections occur.

1. **A brief prodrome usually lasts 3 to 6 days.** Common symptoms include fever, chills, myalgias, headache, dizziness, abdominal discomfort, nausea, and vomiting. Cough is not prominent initially. **Pharyngitis and coryza are not common features** of this syndrome.
2. **Pulmonary involvement is marked by the onset of cough, dyspnea, and tachypnea.** There may be rapid progression to respiratory failure. Fever, hypoxia, hypotension, and volume depletion become prominent. **Noncardiogenic pulmonary edema and depressed myocardial function** occur. Radiographs show bilateral interstitial edema, and pleural effusions are common.
3. **Laboratory abnormalities** have included leukocytosis with early myeloid forms and atypical lymphocytes, **hemoconcentration, thrombocytopenia,** proteinuria, microscopic hematuria, hypoalbuminemia, elevated blood urea nitrogen and creatinine, elevated lactate dehydrogenase (LDH) and transaminases, coagulopathy, and lactic acidosis [105,106].
4. **Improvement** is marked by diuresis, resolution of hemoconcentration, and increased oxygenation. Recovery may proceed rapidly, or may take weeks [105,106].

**C. Diagnosis must rest on clinical suspicion** early in the hantavirus pulmonary syndrome. HPS should be considered for patients with a febrile illness and unexplained respiratory failure. Information about diagnostic tests is available from local and state public health agencies, and the Centers for Disease Control and Prevention (CDC).

1. Culture is difficult and not readily available.
2. **Serology.** Specific IgM and IgG are detected in acute and convalescent samples using an ELISA. Either acute-phase IgM or a fourfold increase in IgG titer is diagnostic.
3. **Immunohistochemical staining** of tissue detects hantavirus antigens in tissue.
4. **PCR** can identify virus in tissue, serum, or blood and may be positive very early.

**D. Therapy**

1. Rapid institution of **supportive therapy in an ICU** has been critical to survival. Extracorporeal membrane oxygenation has been helpful in two of three reported cases.
2. There is **no evidence that ribavirin is effective** but a trial is underway.

**E. Prevention** involves minimizing exposure to rodents and their excreta. No vaccine is available.

**VIII. Pneumonia in the compromised host** [108–112]. Pneumonia is common in the compromised host, rapid deterioration may occur, and mortality of 40% to 50% is frequently reported. Patients at risk include those on immunosuppressive chemotherapy or moderate- to high-dose corticosteroids; those with transplants; patients with congenital or acquired immune deficits; HIV-infected patients; and those with malignancy, especially myeloproliferative or lymphoproliferative disorders (see Chapters 18 and 20).

**A. The clinical dilemma**

1. **Urgent problem.** Rapid evaluation before the patient deteriorates is necessary.
2. **Multiple infectious and noninfectious causes** may have the same clinical presentation. An invasive procedure often is necessary for diagnosis.
3. **Routine laboratory data often are nonspecific.** Many of the infectious agents causing the pneumonia cannot be diagnosed from routine sputum samples. Radiography cannot provide specific diagnoses.
4. **Multiteam approach.** Management requires the cooperative efforts of subspecialists in oncology, infectious disease, pulmonary disease, thoracic surgery, and pathology. If facilities are not available for such a multiteam approach, consideration should be given to transferring such patients to another institution.

**B. Host factors**

1. **Humoral deficiencies** include congenital or acquired hypogammaglobulinemias and hypocomplementemias. Humoral deficiencies commonly accompany

multiple myeloma, chronic lymphocytic leukemia, bone marrow transplantation, and cancer chemotherapies. These patients are at highest risk for infections caused by *S. pneumoniae* and *H. influenzae,* among other pyogenic bacteria.

2. **Neutropenia. The neutropenic host may not produce sputum, exhibit the expected findings on physical examination, or initially demonstrate radiographic abnormalities.** Frequent bacterial pathogens include streptococci, staphylococci, Enterobacteriaceae, and *P. aeruginosa.* Zygomycetes and *Aspergillus* species are common after prolonged antibiotic therapy.
3. **Impaired cell-mediated immunity** may be part of a congenital immunodeficiency or may be acquired as a result of lymphomas, cytotoxic drugs, corticosteroids, radiation therapy, HIV infection, and malnutrition. Defective cellular immunity predisposes to *Nocardia* species, *Legionella* species, mycobacteria, *Cryptococcus neoformans, Histoplasma capsulatum,* cytomegalovirus (CMV), varicella-zoster virus, *Pneumocystis carinii,* and *Strongyloides stercoralis.* **Corticosteroids** are an important predisposing factor for many pathogens but particularly for *Nocardia, Legionella, M. tuberculosis,* most fungi, *P. carinii,* and *S. stercoralis.*
4. **Combinations** of the conditions cited in sections **VIII.B.1–3,** in addition to impairments to nonimmune pulmonary defenses, are commonly present.

C. **Differential diagnosis** is extensive. The major considerations include the following:

1. **Infection.** With the exception of some viruses, most infections can be treated specifically if a particular organism or agent can be demonstrated.
   a. **Bacteria.** Aerobic gram-negative bacteria (*Klebsiella* species, *E. coli, Pseudomonas* species) are common pathogens. *S. aureus* may be increasing in relative frequency as initial therapies have focused on gram-negative bacilli [108]. *L. pneumophila* and *L. micdadei* (see section **VI**) also must be considered.
   b. **Tuberculosis** may reactivate during immunosuppression.
   c. ***Pneumocystis carinii* pneumonia** occurs in AIDS, lymphocytic leukemia, Hodgkin disease, systemic lupus erythematosus, bone marrow or organ transplants, and newborns with agammaglobulinemia.
   d. **Fungi**
      (1) ***Aspergillus* species and Zygomycetes (including *Mucor* species)**
         (a) **Most patients are granulocytopenic and often are febrile despite broad-spectrum antibiotic therapy.** Other clues to the diagnosis include pleuritic chest pain, bloody sputum, nasal and sinus abnormalities, and rapidly progressive nodular or cavitary infiltrates.
         (b) Fungal elements invade vascular channels and cause thrombosis and pulmonary infarction. Dissemination to other organ systems, particularly the CNS, occurs. Aspergillus invasive tracheobronchitis is seen in lung transplant patients, and occasionally in heart, renal, or liver transplants [112].
         (c) Repeated isolation of aspergilli from sputum is sufficient to initiate antifungal therapy, although false-negative results are common. Because there may be commensal organisms in the airways, particularly if there is underlying chronic lung disease, **demonstration of invasion of tissue by transbronchial biopsy or open lung biopsy is necessary to establish a definitive diagnosis.** However, this is often difficult in these very ill and frequently thrombocytopenic patients. In the bone marrow transplant patient, a positive sputum culture is 95% predictive for invasive disease [109].
         (d) **Early therapy,** including amphotericin B and surgical debridement, is essential to increasing survival.
      (2) Other fungi, such as *C. neoformans, H. capsulatum,* and *Coccidioides immitis* can cause pulmonary infection but are less common (see Chapter 17).

e. **Viruses**

(1) **CMV** is commonly reactivated in the compromised host, and almost always in transplant recipients [113]. However, reactivation is far more commonly asymptomatic than symptomatic. Thus, one needs to distinguish CMV infection from CMV disease. CMV is transmitted by fresh blood transfusion, WBC transfusion, or allografts. If an individual has no previous immunity, a primary infection develops. CMV pneumonia is most common in recipients of allogeneic bone marrow transplants, heart transplants, and liver transplants (see Chapter 20).

(2) **RSV, varicella-zoster virus, influenza, parainfluenza, and adenoviruses** are other important causes of viral pneumonias in compromised patients. Herpes simplex virus pneumonia is rare.

f. ***Nocardia*** causes pulmonary infection in patients with cardiac or renal transplantation and steroid use, among others (see Chapter 17).

g. **Other infectious agents.** *Toxoplasma gondii* and certain roundworms, especially *S. stercoralis,* may cause pneumonia in the compromised host.

2. **Tumor infiltration** can mimic pneumonia [114], particularly from lymphomas, leukemias, and alveolar cell carcinoma. **Leukostasis** with subsequent vascular occlusion in the lung can occur with high WBC counts.

3. **Drug-induced infiltrates** must be considered. Drugs that can induce lung disease include bleomycin, busulfan, methotrexate, mitomycin (with or without vinca alkaloids), the nitrosoureas (e.g., carmustine), cyclophosphamide, and the taxanes. Pulmonary edema may result from the use of i.v. cytosine arabinoside, or from cardiac toxicity secondary to anthracyclines.

4. **CHF** may, at times, be difficult to distinguish from diffuse interstitial pneumonia.

5. **Alveolar hemorrhage** may cause an infiltrate and predispose the patient to develop a superimposed bacterial pneumonia. Most patients are thrombocytopenic, with or without other coagulopathies.

6. **Idiopathic interstitial fibrosis** of any type may be present, including bronchiolitis obliterans with organizing pneumonia. Blood and bone marrow transplant patients also may have the **idiopathic pneumonia syndrome** with bilateral interstitial infiltrates and no cardiac or infectious cause [114].

7. **Radiation pneumonitis** may mimic an infectious process.

8. **Pulmonary infarction** is difficult to distinguish from acute infection.

9. **Collagen vascular diseases.** Pulmonary involvement mimicking pneumonia is most common in systemic lupus erythematosus, Goodpasture syndrome, and Wegener granulomatosis. It may be difficult to differentiate disease progression from infection, particularly if patients are receiving immunosuppressive therapy.

10. **Lung transplant patients** have noninfectious pulmonary infiltrates for several other reasons. Reperfusion injury in the donor lung may occur in the first few days after transplantation. Acute rejection usually presents within the first 3 months, and may recur during the first 1 to 2 years. Bronchiolitis obliterans usually presents later after transplantation and is marked by airway obstruction and not by lung infiltrates.

D. **Initial clinical approach.** The possibility of an infectious process should be assessed quickly because early effective therapy may be life saving [109,110].

1. **Diagnostic studies** have recently been reviewed [111].

a. **Spontaneous or induced sputum stains** for ***Pneumocystis*** **and smears and cultures** for bacteria, mycobacteria, fungi, and *Legionella* should be performed.

b. **An invasive procedure** to obtain lower respiratory tract secretions may be required (see section **VI** under Clinical Approach to Community-Acquired Pneumonia).

(1) **Bronchoscopy with BAL, PSB, or transbronchial biopsy** provides a specific diagnosis in many patients (25%–98%) [111], but is contraindicated in patients requiring mechanical ventilation or with severe

hypoxemia, and in those with bleeding diatheses. Major complications occur in fewer than 5% when biopsy is not performed, but increase significantly with biopsy; significant complications from biopsy include hemorrhage and pneumothorax [111].

(2) **Open lung biopsy** has a diagnostic yield of 37% to 85% [111]. Open lung biopsy may be preferred for focal infiltrates not accessible by transthoracic biopsy or in whom the latter is contraindicated, in patients suspected of having certain noninfectious diagnoses (e.g., interstitial pneumonitis or drug reactions), in those with a rapidly advancing illness, and when other biopsies (e.g., transbronchial) are nondiagnostic. Open lung biopsy permits control of ventilation and bleeding, and provides a larger tissue sample that can be processed for rapid interpretation (e.g., frozen sections). In some patient populations, however, the results have infrequently influenced therapy or improved the eventual outcome, so **appropriate patient selection is critical** [111].

(3) An alternative to open lung biopsy is **video-assisted thoracoscopic surgery (VATS).** VATS has a similar yield to open lung biopsy and may be particularly useful to assess pleural involvement. It can be performed after platelet transfusion if the patient is thrombocytopenic [111].

c. **Blood cultures** should be obtained for every patient and, for some patients (e.g., those with AIDS), special media for mycobacteria and fungi may be included.

d. **Pleural fluid** should be examined when present if it can safely be obtained.

e. **Mucocutaneous lesions** should be scraped or examined via biopsy for microorganisms.

f. **Other specimens** (e.g., bone marrow, joint fluid, CSF, and urine) may be helpful.

g. **Serologic studies** may be obtained for *Legionella, Mycoplasma,* fungi, and viruses, but are rarely helpful in choosing initial therapy.

h. **Serial evaluations** of respiratory status should be monitored, including chest roentgenograms and arterial blood gases or oximetry. Progressive hypoxia may be the only early clue to the presence of *Pneumocystis* infection or other interstitial pneumonias.

2. **Host factors and the setting** in which the infection arose can help to narrow the possible etiologies. The specific underlying disease may predispose to specific pathogens, as discussed in section **VIII.B.**

3. **The tempo of the illness and the type of radiographic abnormality** may be of some help in narrowing the diagnostic possibilities [110]. An acutely progressive illness favors gram-positive and gram-negative bacteria, pulmonary edema, embolism, hemorrhage, and leukoagglutinin reactions. A subacute to chronic illness should suggest CMV, *Pneumocystis, Mycoplasma, Nocardia, and Mycobacterium* species, and fungi, among other infections; radiation pneumonitis and drug toxicity would be among the noninfectious possibilities. Radiographic patterns (e.g., consolidative, nodular, or diffuse infiltrates) may help support certain infectious and noninfectious etiologies, but many pathogens are associated with more than one pattern. Thus, the roentgenographic appearance is best used in conjunction with an assessment of the tempo of the illness. A "wedge defect" or nodular defect in a febrile leukopenic patient, despite broad-spectrum antibiotics, raises the possibility of an invasive fungus, especially *Aspergillus* species.

E. **Initial therapy. It is imperative that a specific diagnosis is reached as quickly as possible. Empiric antiinfectives** should be started while awaiting the results of cultures. If the results of sputum stains and other rapid diagnostic studies are negative, therapy is based on host factors, setting, tempo of illness progression, and radiographic pattern.

1. **Neutropenic patients with pneumonia require combination therapy directed against gram-negative bacilli.** A $\beta$-lactam or newer fluoroquinolone plus an aminoglycoside is appropriate. Coverage for *Legionella* can be assured by adding a macrolide to regimens not including a fluoroquinolone. Vancomycin

may be added where MRSA is frequent. In patients already on antibiotics, adding amphotericin should be considered. When a cause is identified, specific therapy is substituted.

2. **In the very ill patient with diffuse infiltrates,** we empirically add TMP-SMX for *P. carinii* to an antibiotic combination directed against common bacteria and *Legionella.* If the infiltrate is focal and the patient is very ill, *Legionella* coverage is essential. Amphotericin B also may be given if *Aspergillus* or other fungal infections are likely. **An invasive diagnostic procedure should be planned within the first 24 to 48 hours.**

F. **Reassessment of the management plan.**

1. **If the initial studies are nondiagnostic and there is no response to empiric therapy** within 48 to 72 hours, then an invasive diagnostic procedure should be performed if not already done. An early multidisciplinary approach will help prevent unnecessary delays in this evaluation. Whether to perform an open lung biopsy or VATS initially, rather than begin with a transthoracic or transbronchial biopsy and then proceed to an open lung biopsy if negative, requires case-by-case assessment.
2. **If patients have clearly and quickly responded to the initial regimen and an alternative noninfectious diagnosis (e.g., pulmonary edema) is not established,** then continuing empiric therapy without an invasive procedure is acceptable. This also may be appropriate for patients with far-advanced underlying disease expected to be rapidly fatal even in the absence of infection, for patients in whom invasive procedures are contraindicated, or in patients who refuse the procedures.

G. **Prevention.** Prevention of pneumonia in the compromised host generally has involved strategies to prevent colonization, prophylactic antibiotics to prevent clinical infection, immunoprophylaxis, and modulation of the immune system. Avoidance of situations that lead to aspiration also is of value.

1. **Hand-washing** is the most important measure to prevent colonization in hospitalized immunocompromised hosts. Total protected environments with HEPA (high-efficiency particulate air) filtration of room air are useful for bone marrow transplant patients and others with prolonged neutropenia.
2. **TMP-SMX prophylaxis** has been shown to be of value in **preventing *P. carinii pneumonia*** in HIV-infected patients and in children with lymphatic leukemia. It has been more difficult to establish that antibacterial prophylaxis is reliably effective in preventing other pulmonary infections.
3. **Antifungal prophylaxis** with oral fluconazole has reduced invasive yeast infections, but resistant yeasts and *Aspergillus* infections may emerge.
4. **Antiviral agents** are effective as prophylaxis in certain specific populations such as kidney and bone marrow transplant recipients.
5. **Immunization** is important and should be given before immunosuppressive chemotherapy. Pneumococcal vaccine is indicated for elderly, asplenic, and other compromised hosts. Influenza vaccines, by reducing the frequency of influenza, should help prevent the secondary complication of pneumonia. Immunoglobulin may be given to patients with immunoglobulin deficiency or impairment, particularly from chronic lymphocytic leukemia, myeloma, or bone marrow transplantation in the postengraftment period.
6. **Growth factors,** such as granulocyte colony-stimulating factor (G-CSF) or granulocyte-macrophage colony-stimulating factor (GM-CSF), speed recovery from cytopenias and can reduce the frequency of infections by shortening the period of neutropenia.

IX. **Nosocomial pneumonia, pneumonia that develops after at least 72 hours of hospitalization,** has the highest mortality rate of all hospital-acquired infections [11,12,64,65,115,115a].

A. **Etiologies**

1. **Bacteria** are the most frequent cause, and many infections are polymicrobial. Aerobic gram-negative bacilli are found in at least 55% to 85% of cases gram-positive cocci in 20% to 30% of cases, and 40% to 60% are mixed infections [11]. *H. influenzae* and *S. pneumoniae* have been recognized as causes of early

nosocomial pneumonia. Anaerobic bacteria are important in nursing home-associated pneumonia [116] and aspiration, but not in ventilator-associated pneumonias [117]. The incidence of *Legionella* infection varies, depending on the hospital and patient population. (See section **VI.**)

2. **Fungi** are important in immunocompromised hosts. *Aspergillus* species and other filamentous fungi are the most common isolates in this population.
3. **Viral** etiologies for nosocomial pneumonia often are unrecognized because special studies for their detection are performed only infrequently. RSV, influenza A and B, parainfluenza, and adenovirus are most important.

**B. Pathogenesis.** Nosocomial bacteria gain access to the lungs most often through endotracheal tubes and aspiration. Inhalation of contaminated aerosols, hematogenous spread, and direct inoculation also occur but are less frequent.

1. **Colonization of the pharynx by gram-negative bacilli** is more common in aged, debilitated, or institutionalized patients, and this accounts for the high incidence of these organisms in nosocomial pneumonias (see also section **II.C**).
   **Clinical conditions that increase the pharyngeal carriage of gram-negative bacilli include** endotracheal intubation, coma, acidosis, alcoholism, uremia, diabetes mellitus, prior antimicrobial therapy, and nasogastric tubes [65]. An increase in the adherence of gram-negative bacilli to oropharyngeal and tracheal cells may accompany many of these conditions; this can arise in part from antibiotic-induced reduction in normal flora, reduced salivary flow, increased salivary protease content, and changes in cellular surface carbohydrates.
2. **Gastric colonization** also may be an important reservoir for gram-negative bacilli and *S. aureus* (see section **II.C**). This is **associated with conditions that raise intragastric pH over 4.0,** including aging, achlorhydria, enteral feedings, antacids, and $H_2$-blockers.
3. **Bacteria in aerosols from** contaminated nebulizers, certain types of humidifiers, and anesthesia equipment may be directly inhaled into the lower airways.

**C. Risk factors** for bacterial nosocomial pneumonia have been identified [11,64,65, 115a]. **Endotracheal tubes** impair coughing and provide access to the lung. They also become coated with a biofilm of organisms that may be a reservoir for potential pathogens.

1. **Host-related factors** include age over 65 to 70 years, obesity, smoking, and underlying illnesses such as COPD, alcoholism, malnutrition, and prior immunosuppression.
2. **Type of illness** also influences the risk for nosocomial pneumonia. **Thoracic and abdominal surgical procedures** are important predisposing events [118]. Other risk factors include a depressed level of consciousness, neurosurgical trauma, admission to an ICU, shock, and need for **mechanical ventilation.**
3. **Other management practices and devices,** in addition to endotracheal intubation, increase risk. These include stress-ulcer prophylaxis that increases intragastric pH, insertion of a nasogastric tube, large-volume tube feedings, reflux of ventilator tube condensate into the trachea, changing ventilator tubing on a daily basis, improper care of respiratory devices, **breaks in common infection-control practices** that carry organisms from one patient to another, **and inappropriate use of antibiotics.**

**D. Diagnosis.** The steps differ depending on whether there is underlying lung disease and whether the patient is intubated. **A diligent search for noninfectious causes of fever and pulmonary infiltrates,** particularly in ventilated patients, must be made.

1. Clinical criteria often are used in **nonintubated patients.** These include the presence of fever, leukocytosis, cough, purulent sputum, and a new or progressive radiographic infiltrate. Caution must be used when applying these clinical criteria to patients with underlying lung diseases, because the criteria are nonspecific [12].

2. The **diagnosis of ventilator-associated pneumonia (VAP) may be very difficult,** particularly in patients with accompanying ARDS [67]. VAP should be suspected and a chest radiograph obtained if at least two of the following are present: fever or hypothermia, leukocytosis or leukopenia, purulent sputum, and decreased oxygenation [22]. If the chest radiograph is abnormal, the patient should be treated for VAP [22]. We feel that if oxygenation is unchanged, another cause should be vigorously sought. Because clinical and radiographic criteria are nonspecific [119,120], expert practitioners apply additional diagnostic methods when available [115a,121].
   a. **Quantitative cultures of tracheal aspirates.** Direct tracheal aspirate cultures cannot be used to make this distinction in the diagnosis of ventilator-associated nosocomial pneumonia. Using threshold concentrations of $10^5$ or $10^6$ organisms per milliliter or greater, quantitative tracheal aspirate cultures have varied and low sensitivity and specificity [122]. Because of the problems with false-positive and false-negative results and an incomplete understanding of the effects of antibiotic therapy on interpreting results, quantitative (and nonquantitative) cultures of tracheal aspirates are of limited value [122].
   b. The detection of microscopic **elastin fibers in sputum** may be associated with any cause of lung necrosis. Thus, this study is not recommended [122].
   c. **Quantitative cultures of PSB or BAL specimens offer the most promise** [23,25,26,28,121]. Gram stain to detect intracellular organisms on BAL specimens is specific but not as sensitive. Techniques are available to obtain these specimens with or without bronchoscopy. The effects of prior antibiotics are incompletely understood, but overall they have not been shown to alter the diagnostic yield. However, in an individual patient they may result in a false-negative culture by suppressing growth of true pathogens. For these reasons, quantitative cultures of PSB or BAL specimens should be obtained before making any changes in antibiotic therapy. It has not been demonstrated that the use of these procedures has an impact on patient outcome, although they may help promote the prudent use of antibiotics [115a].
   d. **Open lung biopsy** is almost never necessary.

E. **Therapy.** Effective therapy involves ensuring airway patency and adequate oxygenation, using pressors and other supportive measures, draining secretions, and administering antibiotics. **Administration of empiric antibiotics should not be delayed,** and must take into consideration local resistance patterns [115a,121]. **The best outcome occurs when initial antibiotics are active against the infecting organisms** [11,67]. Gram stains of reliable specimens are useful to help direct initial therapy. Whenever possible, **specific antibiotics should be substituted as specific pathogens become known. The ATS has published recommendations** for empiric therapy [115], **but these must be individualized to the specific institution, setting, patient characteristics, and local resistance patterns** [121,123]. Most regimens should have activity against *S. pneumoniae, H. influenzae,* and the gram-negative bacilli noted in section **IX.A.** (See also section **IV.C.**)
   1. **Early illness (<5 days) in patients without risk factors for resistant organisms** may be treated with ticarcillin-clavulanate, piperacillin-tazobactam, carbapenems, or an antipneumococcal fluoroquinolone. Ciprofloxacin monotherapy should not be used because it is less active against pneumococci and anaerobes. See Chapter 27 for a discussion of inducible $\beta$-lactamase resistance from cephalosporin overuse.
   2. **Patients with risk factors for resistant organisms and those with severe illness or necrotizing infection** should be treated **with a combination regimen.** Preliminary results suggest an improved outcome for an aminoglycoside plus piperacillin-tazobactam when compared with the aminoglycoside plus either ceftazidime or imipenem, particularly for *Pseudomonas aeruginosa* infections [11,67]. If *S. maltophilia* is a concern, then TMP-SMX is used.

3. Nafcillin or vancomycin should be included when *S. aureus* is suspected. Vancomycin is preferred if MRSA is possible.
4. A macrolide or fluoroquinolone should be added whenever *Legionella* organisms are possible. See section **VI.G** for treatments of legionellosis.

**F. Prevention.** Strategies to prevent nosocomial pneumonias are based on an understanding of their pathogenesis and risk factors (see sections **IX.B** and **XI.C**). **Guidelines for the prevention of nosocomial pneumonia have been published** [64,65].

1. **The use of systemic antibiotics for pneumonia prophylaxis is not recommended.**
2. **Hand washing and other routine infection-control practices are essential.**
3. If possible, **elevate the head of the bed** to 30 to 45 degrees to prevent aspiration. Discontinue tube feedings, nasogastric tubes, and endotracheal tubes as soon as possible. **Continuous aspiration of subglottic secretions** in intubated patients should be considered. **Chlorhexidine oral care** is also effective [64].
4. **Effective pain control and chest physiotherapy** (e.g., coughing, deep breathing, incentive spirometry) **should be priorities in postoperative patients.**
5. **Stress-ulcer prophylaxis that does not elevate gastric pH** (e.g., sucralfate) is preferred.
6. **Immunizations** should be **updated** and smoking curtailed, particularly prior to elective surgery.
7. **Sterile equipment and water** should be used for procedures that contact mucous membranes. The internal parts of mechanical ventilators do not need to be sterilized.
8. **Ventilator tubing condensate should not be allowed to drain into the patient's airway,** and tubing should be changed no more frequently than every 48 hours.
9. Small-volume nebulizers should be filled with sterile fluids and not used for more than one patient unless sterile or high-level disinfected.
10. **Selective decontamination** remains a promising strategy [124], but is not recommended for routine use because of lack of standardization and concern about promoting resistant organisms [125].

**X. Pneumonia in children** (1-month-olds to teenagers). Certain aspects of childhood pneumonia warrant emphasis [5,8,126,127]. For example, a very young child may have only fever and tachypnea, and rarely produces sputum. Neonates are discussed in Chapter 3.

**A. Age is of great importance in the likely etiologies** and their mode of presentation.

1. **Infants 1 to 3 months of age** are most likely to have pneumonia of viral origin (RSV, parainfluenza virus). Occasionally, the etiology will be bacterial, including group B streptococci, *H. influenzae, S. pneumoniae, S. aureus, S. pyogenes,* and *Bordetella pertussis.* Afebrile pneumonia in infants 1 to 3 months of age usually is caused by *Chlamydia trachomatis.* This illness is indolent and marked by poor feeding, failure to thrive, a chronic cough, conjunctivitis, tachypnea, and diffuse rales.
2. **Between the ages of 3 months and 5 years,** *S. pneumoniae* and viruses predominate. RSV, parainfluenza virus, influenza types A and B, and adenovirus are most important. Mixed infections are common in younger children hospitalized with pneumonia. Encapsulated organisms (*S. pneumoniae, H. influenzae,* and *Neisseria meningitidis*) are more frequent in children over 3 months of age as maternal antibodies wane. Other bacteria and *Mycoplasma* are occasional pathogens in this age group. *H. influenzae* type b is important in unimmunized children.
3. The causes of pneumonia **in children over 5 years of age** are more like those in young adults. Pneumococcal, mycoplasmal, and *Chlamydophila* predominate. As in adults, anaerobes occur in patients prone to aspiration. Group

A streptococci, *M. catarrhalis,* and *Legionella* species are less common in childhood pneumonias.

**B. Radiographic clues**

1. **Pneumonia with effusion** most likely has **a bacterial etiology** unless the tuberculin skin test is positive or there is a contact history for tuberculosis.
2. **Lobar consolidation** implies a **bacterial process.** *S. pneumoniae* is the most likely pathogen, although *S. pyogenes* and *K. pneumoniae* may produce a similar picture.
3. **Abscesses** are caused by staphylococci or, if putrid, anaerobic infection. **Pneumatoceles** may be seen with staphylococcal and other bacterial childhood pneumonias, and gram-negative infection in newborns.
4. **Bronchopneumonias** (diffuse, patchy infiltrates) are usually **nonbacterial** in origin.

**C. Management often is empiric** because clinical, laboratory, and radiographic features often cannot be used to distinguish between the possible causes.

1. **Diagnosis**
   a. **Sputum culture is not useful in infants and young children.**
   b. Nasopharyngeal secretions are used for **antigen detection** and **viral cultures.** Tests to detect bacterial antigens in the urine are not useful because they lack both sensitivity and specificity. **PCR** is promising but not widely available.
   c. **Serologic studies** can provide a retrospective diagnosis.
   d. **Cultures of blood and pleural fluid** are specific, but infrequently positive.
   e. **Bronchoscopy** is reserved for those with serious illness, underlying diseases such as immunosuppression, and suspected obstruction or foreign body aspiration.
2. **Hospitalization.** The decision to hospitalize often is difficult. It should be considered for the very young, and those with immunosuppression, serious underlying disease, toxicity or hypoxemia, multilobar bacterial infection, significant pleural effusion, inadequate oral intake, failed outpatient care, or a family that is unable to cope.
3. **Antibiotic selection** is based on the chest radiograph, age of the child, host characteristics, and the Gram stain results of any pleural fluid or other available material. Amoxicillin, amoxicillin-clavulanate, a macrolide, or cefuroxime are appropriate for outpatients. Hospitalized patients should be given i.v. cefotaxime or cefuroxime; high-dose ampicillin and ampicillin-sulbactam are alternatives. Vancomycin is used if high-level penicillin-resistant pneumococci (see section **I.C**), MRSA, or meningitis are suspected [32]. A macrolide is added if atypical pathogens are suspected. Tetracyclines should not be used in children under 8 years of age, and the fluoroquinolones should not be given to patients under 18 years of age [128]. **If viral infection is suspected, antibiotics should be withheld.**
4. Children with recurrent severe bacterial infections or infection with an unusual organism may need to be evaluated for the presence of an immunologic defect.

**XI.** ***S. aureus*** causes only 1% to 10% of CAP, but up to 16% of hospital-acquired pneumonias [129]. It deserves emphasis because of its high mortality.

**A. Settings**

1. Most cases of staphylococcal **CAP** occur as a complication of influenza (see Chapter 10), in the elderly, or in those with significant underlying pulmonary or other illness; some patients may be nursing home residents.
2. **Nosocomial** ***S. aureus*** **pneumonia** occurs in hospitalized, debilitated patients. **Risk factors favoring MRSA** are prolonged hospitalization, serious underlying cardiopulmonary disease, and prior antibiotic use [129].

**B. Radiographic manifestations** of staphylococcal pneumonia are varied. **Children with a rapidly progressive pneumonia, pneumatoceles or abscesses, and early pleural involvement** are likely to have staphylococcal infections. In adults, infiltrates are often bilateral and multilobar. Pleural effusions are common, as are empyemas. **Embolic pneumonias** often have a circular appearance and may progress to central cavitation.

**C. Therapy** is given i.v. for 2 to 3 weeks. Vancomycin is used initially, but proven methicillin-sensitive *S. aureus* infection should be treated with oxacillin or nafcillin, 9 to 12 g/day in the adult and 200 mg/kg/day in children divided every 4 to 6 hours. Cefazolin may be used if it is not contraindicated for penicillin-allergic patients (see Chapter 27). Vancomycin is used for serious penicillin allergy or MRSA, which generally responds less well [129]. Linezolid and quinupristin/dalfopristin are alternatives to vancomycin.

**D. Isolation.** Droplet precautions are indicated during the first 24 to 48 hours of therapy.

## PNEUMONIA AND BIOTERRORISM

**The United States suffered its first use of anthrax for bioterrorism in the wake of the terrible events of September 11, 2001 [130]. Although this event used the mail to target journalists and politicians, future episodes may not be confined to the same risk groups.** This section briefly reviews the features of those bacterial respiratory infections most likely to be used as part of a bioterrorist event [2]. Updated information is available on the CDC website (*www.bt.cdc.gov*), and local authorities.

**I. Anthrax** is caused by the spore-forming aerobic gram-positive rod *Bacillus anthracis.* Aerosol delivery provides the most danger, with the majority of cases presenting as **inhalational anthrax.** Cutaneous (see Chapter 4) and gastrointestinal anthrax also occur.

**A. Pathogenesis [131,132]. Inhalation of *B. anthracis* endospores** does not usually cause a true pneumonia [2]. The minimal infectious dose is unknown but must be relatively low, particularly when compared with the median lethal dose ($LD_{50}$) of 2,500 to 55,000 inhaled spores [132]. Spores are 1 to 5 $\mu$m in diameter, and if processed correctly may be dispersed for long distances by wind or other air currents. After gaining access to the alveoli they are transported to mediastinal and other regional nodes by alveolar macrophages. Germination and bacterial multiplication ensue, and hematogenous dissemination may lead to sepsis and meningeal involvement. The organism possesses an antiphagocytic capsule, protective antigen, lethal factor, and edema factor. Lethal toxin, formed by lethal factor binding to protective antigen, stimulates the release of inflammatory mediators and inhibits intracellular signaling by inactivating mitogen-activated protein kinase. Edema toxin, formed by edema factor binding to protective antigen, impairs cellular water homeostasis and can inhibit neutrophil function. Hemorrhage, edema, and necrosis ensue.

**B. The incubation period** is variable, but **may be prolonged.** Most cases that followed the accidental airborne release of anthrax spores in the 1979 outbreak in Sverdlovsk occurred 9 to 10 days after exposure [133]. However, fatal cases also occurred up to 6 weeks later. This and primate data led to recommendations of 60 days of prophylactic or therapeutic antibiotics [130].

**C. Clinical manifestations** [131,134–136]. Inhalational anthrax is a biphasic illness.

1. **Early signs and symptoms suggest an influenza-like illness (ILI).** Combinations of fever, chills, fatigue or malaise, nonproductive cough, nausea or vomiting, weakness, and chest discomfort predominate. Laboratory studies are equally nonspecific. Clinical features, in addition to the epidemiologic setting, help distinguish ILI from anthrax [137]. **Sore throat and rhinorrhea are common in ILI,** whereas chest discomfort, pleuritic chest pain, and nausea or vomiting are more frequent in anthrax. Chest radiographs are usually normal in ILI, but abnormal in anthrax (see section **I.D**).
2. **The next phase is heralded by progressive respiratory signs and symptoms,** which may occur after a short period of improvement. Patients have **dyspnea, worsened cough, and diaphoresis.** Sepsis syndrome and evidence of meningitis may be present. Laboratory studies may reveal **leukocytosis with left shift, elevated transaminases, and hypoxemia.** In this phase **death may occur within hours or days.**

**D. Radiographic studies provide important diagnostic clues** and may be abnormal early.

1. **Chest radiographs were abnormal on admission** in each of the initial 10 bioterrorism-related cases in the United States, although abnormalities may be overlooked [135]. Characteristic findings include **mediastinal widening, paratracheal or hilar enlargement, and pleural effusions.** Infiltrates may be present, particularly in the sickest patients [134,135]. Effusions or infiltrates may occur initially without mediastinal widening.
2. **Chest CT is more sensitive than chest radiography in detecting the extent of mediastinal involvement.** Based on the initial experience, **early CT scanning is encouraged** when inhalational anthrax is considered possible [130,136].

**E. Diagnosis** [138]. Inhalational anthrax can be diagnosed quickly only with a high degree of suspicion.

1. **Blood cultures** should be obtained on all patients before the initiation of antibiotics.
2. **Gram stain of buffy coat smears** may provide a rapid clue to the diagnosis, but the sensitivity of this procedure is unknown [134].
3. **Pleural fluid** should be obtained when effusions are present, and Gram stained and cultured. Fluid is characteristically hemorrhagic with elevated protein and relatively few leukocytes. A positive Gram stain rapidly suggests the diagnosis. PCR is performed and a cell block for immunohistochemistry analysis is taken if results of other studies are negative.
4. **CSF** should be obtained when there is a question of meningeal involvement. Fluid is frequently bloody with positive Gram stains [131].
5. **Bronchoscopy** may provide a diagnosis if there are radiographic infiltrates [135].
6. **Special studies for nonculture diagnosis,** including immunohistochemistry and PCR, are available through local public health authorities and the CDC. Serologic testing for IgG antibodies to the protective antigen is also available at the CDC and may be helpful in difficult cases.
7. **Rapid diagnostic tests for influenza** should be considered.
8. **Nasal swab cultures are of no value** for diagnosis or exclusion of this disease [139].

**F. Therapy for inhalational anthrax.** Early effective therapy is essential in improving outcome. The choice of antibiotics depends on the extent of illness and the susceptibility profile of the infecting strain. All the strains involved in the fall of 2001 had the same sensitivity pattern. This is in part the basis for the following recommendations [132,140].

1. A cephalosporinase and an inducible penicillinase are included in the *B. anthracis* genome, so that **cephalosporins and penicillins should not be used alone** [130].
2. **Initial therapy. Combination i.v. antibiotics are recommended for initial treatment** of all patients with inhalational anthrax. The same treatment regimens listed below also are indicated for immunocompromised and pregnant hosts [132,140]. With mass casualties, oral therapy may be the only option [132].
   - a. **Adults** [140]
     - (1) **Either ciprofloxacin 400 mg every 12 hours or doxycycline 100 mg every 12 hours** should be used with one or two additional drugs (see below). Ciprofloxacin is preferred if meningitis is present because of better penetration.
     - (2) **Other active agents** that may be used in combination with ciprofloxacin or doxycycline include rifampin, vancomycin, penicillin, ampicillin, chloramphenicol, imipenem, clindamycin, and clarithromycin. It has been suggested but not proven that clindamycin has an antitoxigenic effect [136].
     - (3) **A successful initial regimen** is ciprofloxacin, rifampin, and clindamycin [136].
   - b. **Children** [132,141]. Because of the gravity of the infection and potential for penicillin failure, i.v. ciprofloxacin or doxycycline are also recommended for children.

(1) **Either ciprofloxacin 10 to 15 mg/kg every 12 hours (maximum of 1 g/day) or doxycycline** should be used with one or two additional drugs [see section **I.F.2.a.(2)**]. Ciprofloxacin is preferred if meningitis is present, as noted above. The **dose of doxycycline** is 100 mg every 12 hours for children over 8 years of age and weighing over 45 kg, and 2.2 mg/kg every 12 hours for children weighing less than 45 kg or those under 8 years of age (maximum dose of 100 mg).

(2) Experience with other fluoroquinolones in children is limited.

3. **Continued therapy and duration.** All patients should receive antibiotics **for a total of 60 days** because of the potential for late germination of persistent spores.
   a. **Adults may be switched to oral therapy** when there has been continued clinical improvement [140]. Ciprofloxacin 500 mg twice daily or doxycycline 100 mg twice daily to finish the 60 days is acceptable alone [135] or with rifampin [141].
   b. **Children also may be switched to oral therapy** when there has been clinical improvement [141]. **Either ciprofloxacin** 10 to 15 mg/kg every 12 hours (maximum of 1 g/day) **or doxycycline** (oral doses equivalent to i.v. doses above) **should be continued for the first 14 to 21 days,** with or without another agent. **Amoxicillin may be used for sensitive isolates to finish the remainder of the 60 days** because of the potential for side effects with prolonged use of ciprofloxacin or doxycycline in children [141].
4. **Adjunctive measures** include drainage of pleural effusions, and mechanical ventilation or other support in an intensive care unit. Steroids have been used for patients with extensive edema, respiratory compromise, and meningitis [140].
5. Since **person-to-person transmission does not occur,** patients with inhalation anthrax may be cared for in routine hospital rooms using standard precautions.

G. **Prognosis.** The outcome from inhalational anthrax has been dismal, with a mortality rate in prior reports of 86% to 97% [130]. However, only 4 of the initial 10 United States patients in 2001 died [135]. Possible reasons for the improved survival rate include heightened awareness, use of newer diagnostic studies, early antibiotic combination therapy, and modern supportive care [135]. Patients who postpone seeking therapy, who are seriously ill at presentation, or who have effective treatment delayed have a worse prognosis [134].

H. **Antibiotic prophylaxis is indicated following airborne exposure** because of the serious nature of this illness. **The standard duration of prophylaxis is 60 days for individuals with a proven exposure risk** because of the potential for a prolonged incubation period. Because the inoculum is low, **penicillins are expected to be effective for prophylaxis** even though they are not recommended for treatment [141]. At least 32,000 individuals began prophylaxis after September 2001, and 5,000 were candidates for the full 60-day course [142]. **Appropriate law enforcement and public health authorities should be notified** [139].

1. **Adults** may be given either **ciprofloxacin 500 mg orally twice daily or doxycycline 100 mg orally twice daily** [143]. However, some prefer doxycycline because of concern about fluoroquinolone resistance with long-term and widespread ciprofloxacin use.
2. **Pregnant women should be given ciprofloxacin** in the doses above, and doxycycline should be avoided [144]. **If the isolate is penicillin sensitive, then amoxicillin** 500 mg orally three times daily is an alternative.
3. **Infants and children should be given oral amoxicillin** 80 mg/kg/day in three divided doses (maximum of 500 mg per dose) for penicillin-sensitive isolates [141].
4. **Breast-feeding women should be given amoxicillin** 500 mg orally three times daily if the isolate is penicillin susceptible [141]. If amoxicillin is contraindicated, then ciprofloxacin or doxycycline may be used and the breast milk discarded [141].
5. Initial surveillance efforts found **adherence and side effects with prophylaxis** to be similar to prior reported experience [142].

6. **Three options can be offered at the end of the 60-day course,** particularly for those individuals with high-level exposure and who were adherent with antibiotics [145]:
   a. **Monitoring for illness after finishing 60 days of antibiotic prophylaxis.**
   b. **Continued antibiotic until day 100,** with monitoring for illness and adverse drug reactions, because of the theoretic risk for illness up to 100 days after exposure.
   c. **Anthrax vaccine** (three doses given over 4 weeks) **plus an additional 40 days of antibiotic prophylaxis.** Vaccine is available only as an "investigational new drug" through designated clinics. Informed consent and follow-up investigations are required.
7. **Future events may result in modification of these recommendations;** up-to-date information should be obtained from local, state, and federal public health officials.

II. **Plague is caused by the gram-negative coccobacillus *Yersinia pestis*.** Pneumonic plague is a potentially lethal disease that can be transmitted from person to person. This makes it useful for bioterrorism, which was recognized long before the biology of plague was understood [146]. Other forms of the disease are septicemic and bubonic plague.

A. **Pathogenesis of pneumonic plague.** Plague persists as a worldwide enzootic infection of rats and other rodents [146]. *Y. pestis* is transmitted to its human host as **bubonic plague** through the bite of a flea. The majority of cases develop fever with acutely inflamed regional lymph nodes (buboes) 2 to 8 days after the original flea bite. A few patients develop primary septicemic plague with or without buboes. **Direct inhalation of the organism, from bioterrorism** or via droplets from a patient with plague pneumonia, **leads to primary pneumonic plague. Secondary pneumonic plague** occurs when the lung is involved by **hematogenous spread** from either bubonic or septicemic plague.

B. **Clinical manifestations** [147]. Primary pneumonic plague usually has an incubation period of 2 to 4 days, ranging from 1 to 6 days [147]. **Illness begins abruptly,** and may have a fulminant course. Patients may have fever, chills, rigors, dyspnea, cough, malaise, and myalgias. Nausea, vomiting, diarrhea, or abdominal pain may be prominent in some patients. **Sputum is often bloody.** Physical examination would be expected to reveal a bubo only in secondary pneumonic plague. **Chest radiographs are nonspecific, showing patchy infiltrates or consolidation** that may be bilateral. Progression to death may be rapid, with sepsis, disseminated intravascular coagulation, and multisystem organ failure; this is not specific for plague but may be seen in any severe pneumonia.

C. **Diagnosis of primary plague pneumonia** depends on a high index of suspicion.
   1. **Clinical clues** to the possibility of plague pneumonia as the result of bioterrorism include the clustered occurrence of severe pneumonias, the presence of hemoptysis and sepsis, and the rare finding of a cervical bubo [147].
   2. **Microbiological studies are very helpful. Gram stains** (or Wright, Giemsa, and Wayson stains) of sputum, blood, or bubo aspirate may reveal the characteristic bipolar staining of this small gram-negative bacillus or coccobacillus. The organism grows on standard media and in routine blood cultures.
   3. **Immunofluorescent stains** are diagnostic when available through public health laboratories. Immunoassay to detect the F1 antigen also may be helpful but is not readily available. PCR can be diagnostic as well but is not standardized.

D. **Management [147]. Presumptive therapy should be started as quickly as possible for exposed patients who have a compatible illness.** Failure to respond may be an indication of antibiotic resistance, rare in natural infection.
   1. **With contained casualties, streptomycin** (30 mg/kg/day in 2 i.m. doses) **or gentamicin** (5 mg/kg/day i.v. or i.m., or 2 mg/kg load followed by 1.7 mg/kg every 8 hours i.v. or i.m.) **are preferred for** adults and children with normal renal function. Acceptable alternatives include i.v. doxycycline, ciprofloxacin, or chloramphenicol. Gentamicin is preferred in pregnancy. Immunocompromised patients are given one of these same treatment regimens. The duration of therapy

is 10 days, and may be finished orally (see section **II.D.2**) after the patient has clearly improved.

2. **With mass casualties, only oral therapy may be available.** Ten days of **doxycycline or ciprofloxacin** should be used to treat adults and children, with chloramphenicol an alternative except in children under 2 years of age. The doxycycline dosage is 100 mg twice daily for adults and children weighing at least 45 kg, and 2.2 mg/kg twice daily for children weighing less than 45 kg [147]. Ciprofloxacin dosage is 500 mg twice daily in adults, and 20 mg/kg twice daily in children. Doxycycline should be avoided if possible in children under 8 years of age. Doxycycline is preferred for the treatment of pregnant women in the setting of mass casualties.
3. **Prophylactic oral antibiotics should be given to all asymptomatic exposed individuals.** Doxycycline is preferred for this purpose, with the same restrictions and alternatives as listed for treatment of mass casualties. Patients should take prophylaxis for 7 days, and immediately report any fever or cough. The same prophylaxis is recommended for immunocompromised patients [147].
4. **All patients with plague should be placed in droplet isolation until after the first 48 hours of effective therapy and there is clinical improvement, or until pulmonary involvement is excluded.**
5. Supportive care in a critical care setting is often required.
6. **Public health authorities should be notified immediately** so that contacts may be traced and any needed vector control measures instituted.

**III. Tularemia** is caused by the pleomorphic gram-negative coccobacillus *Francisella tularensis.* The United States and former Soviet Union weaponized this agent, although the United States destroyed its biologic weapons arsenal by 1973 [148]. Clinical forms include ulceroglandular, glandular, oculoglandular, typhoidal, pneumonic, and oropharyngeal [149].

**A. Pathogenesis.** Tularemia is a widespread zoonosis of small mammals, including rabbits. The organism may be transmitted to a human host by the bite of a tick or fly, and by direct contact with or ingestion of infected animals, excreta, water, soil, and vegetation. Tularemia pneumonia may result from direct inhalation of the organism (primary pneumonia), or from hematogenous spread to the lungs as a consequence of one of the other clinical forms. **Bioterrorist use would result in aerosol exposure, and most subsequent cases are expected to be primary pneumonic tularemia** [148]. However, such an exposure also could result in other forms of tularemia by the organism penetrating the skin (ulceroglandular, glandular, or typhoidal), conjunctivae (oculoglandular), or oral mucosa (oropharyngeal). Natural outbreaks of primary tularemia pneumonia are more likely to occur in a rural setting [148,150].

**B. Clinical manifestations from a bioterrorism aerosol exposure** [148]. The incubation period for primary tularemia pneumonia is expected to be 3 to 5 days, and ranges from 1 to 14 days [148]. There would be a cluster of patients with the **abrupt onset** of a nonspecific febrile illness. **Progression to frank clinical pulmonary involvement may be rapid or subacute,** with the onset of dyspnea, cough without prominent sputum, and pleuritic chest pain. **Chest radiographs often show subsegmental or lobar infiltrates** that may involve more than one lobe, **pleural effusions, and hilar adenopathy.** Rounded densities, miliary changes, or cavitation are less common [149]. Pleural fluid studies are often similar to those found in tuberculous effusions [149]. Respiratory failure, sepsis, multisystem organ failure, and death may occur.

**C. Diagnosis.** Results from routine laboratory studies are nonspecific, and rapid diagnostic tests for tularemia are not readily available [149].

1. **Clinically,** the occurrence of a cluster of patients with unexplained atypical pneumonia, pleural involvement, and hilar adenopathy should raise suspicion.
2. **Routine microbiologic specimens** including blood cultures should be submitted, and the laboratory alerted to the possibility of *F. tularensis* infection because it is fastidious and potentially dangerous to them. **Gram-stained smears of respiratory secretions** may help differentiate this illness from inhalational

anthrax and plague pneumonia [148]. Definitive diagnosis is established by culture identification of the organism in clinical specimens.

3. Fluorescent antibody stains, antigen detection, and PCR techniques are available in only a few specialized laboratories but can provide a specific and rapid diagnosis [148].
4. **Serologic assays are not useful acutely,** because increasing titers require 10 or more days. With a longer duration of illness, a diagnostic fourfold or greater increase in titer may occur between acute and convalescent specimens. A single tube agglutination titer of at least 1:160 or a microagglutination titer of at least 1:128 supports the diagnosis in the presence of a compatible clinical illness.

D. **Management of tularemia resulting from a bioterrorism event** [148]. Treatment regimens may need to be adjusted if susceptibility studies reveal antibiotic resistance.

1. **With contained casualties, therapy is similar to that listed for plague.** The total duration of treatment is 10 days with the aminoglycosides or ciprofloxacin, and is 14 days with doxycycline or chloramphenicol to reduce relapses. Treatment may be finished orally.
2. **With mass casualties, oral therapy with doxycycline or ciprofloxacin is similar to that listed for plague,** except the duration is 14 days. Ciprofloxacin is preferred for the treatment of pregnant women in the setting of mass casualties [148]. Streptomycin or gentamicin is preferred for immunocompromised patients if possible.
3. **Asymptomatic exposed individuals seen in the incubation period for tularemia should receive prophylaxis** with 14 days of either doxycycline or ciprofloxacin, with the same restrictions as listed for treatment of mass casualties. However, delayed discovery of a covert tularemia bioterrorism event may be more likely. In this circumstance prophylaxis is withheld and antibiotic treatment begun if a potentially exposed person develops an unexplained fever or flu-like illness within 2 weeks of the last presumed exposure [148].
4. **Person-to-person transmission does not occur,** so standard precautions are used.
5. **Hospital infection control and local public health authorities should be notified immediately** of any case of suspected or confirmed tularemia.

## PARAPNEUMONIC EFFUSION AND EMPYEMA

**Parapneumonic pleural effusion** is pleural fluid found in association with pneumonia, lung abscess, or bronchiectasis [151]. An **empyema** is grossly infected or purulent fluid (pus) in the pleural space. **All complicated parapneumonic effusions and empyemas require drainage.**

I. **Parapneumonic effusions**

A. **Parapneumonic effusions progress through three pathologic stages** [151]. The initial stage is the exudative stage, when fluid is free-flowing and with relatively low numbers of neutrophils. Early exudative parapneumonic effusions are often sterile, and appropriate therapy in this stage will avoid the necessity for tube drainage. The fibropurulent stage occurs next with an increase in fluid, the influx of neutrophils, and an increasing chance for bacterial invasion. Glucose and pH decrease, and LDH increases. Fibrin is deposited on pleural surfaces with a tendency for fluid loculation, making effective bedside drainage very difficult. The final stage is organization. Pleural fluid is thick, and fibroblast growth into loculations results in a visceral pleural peel entrapping lung and requiring surgical decortication.

B. **Thoracentesis should be performed when there is at least 10 mm of pleural fluid on a lateral decubitus film,** and fluid sent for the following studies [151].

1. **Differential cell counts.** High counts of **polymorphonuclear leukocytes suggest bacterial infection,** and an alternative etiology should be sought if this is not found [151]. A high percentage of small lymphocytes may be seen in tuberculosis and malignancies. Mesothelial cells are uncommon in tuberculous effusions. Uncommonly, 5% to 20% eosinophils are seen, but this is a nonspecific finding

associated with pneumothorax, hemothorax, Hodgkin disease, Churg-Strauss syndrome, benign asbestos effusion, drug reactions, and paragonimiasis.

2. **Chemistries. Glucose** may be reduced with pneumonia, malignancy, tuberculosis, hemothorax, paragonimiasis, and Churg-Strauss syndrome; it may be very low in effusions from rheumatoid arthritis. Tuberculous effusions may, on occasion, have normal glucose levels. **LDH** levels help classify parapneumonic effusions [151].
3. **pH.** The pH of the pleural fluid may help distinguish complicated from benign effusions (see section **D**). Pleural fluid samples should be placed in wet ice, transported to the laboratory, and processed immediately. **A pleural fluid pH of less than 7.2 occurs in** effusions associated with bacterial infections, tuberculosis, esophageal rupture, malignancy, rheumatoid arthritis, hemothorax, urinothorax, paragonimiasis, Churg-Strauss syndrome, and systemic acidosis. The cause of pleural fluid acidosis in the absence of systemic acidosis is primarily leukocyte metabolism, but bacterial metabolism also may contribute. In empyemas caused by some *Proteus* species, the pH may be normal or high because of the urea-splitting activity of the bacteria.
4. **Cultures. Gram stains with aerobic and anaerobic** cultures should be performed routinely. If tuberculosis and fungal infections are considered, one should obtain and centrifuge large volumes of fluid and then culture the sediment.

**C. Thoracic CT** scanning will help determine whether fluid is loculated or whether pleural fibrosis has occurred, localize fluid for drainage, and assess the underlying lung.

**D. Classification and management** [151,152]. Parapneumonic effusions are classified using radiographic and pleural fluid results. All effusions at least 10 mm thick on the lateral decubitus film require thoracentesis.

1. **Class 1 effusions are termed nonsignificant.** These are free-flowing effusions that are less than 10 mm thick on the lateral decubitus film. No thoracentesis is indicated.
2. **Class 2 effusions are termed typical parapneumonic.** Fluid is free flowing and not purulent, with negative smears and cultures, a glucose level of greater than 40 mg/dL, pH greater than 7.2, and LDH less than 1,000 IU/L. **Therapeutic thoracentesis** should be done, and repeated if fluid rapidly recurs or the patient remains ill with a significant effusion.
3. **Class 3 effusions are termed borderline complicated.** These have **either** a fluid pH between 7.0 and 7.2, an LDH of greater than 1,000 IU/L, or loculations even though the glucose level is greater than 40 mg/dL and smears and cultures are negative. **Serial therapeutic thoracentesis should be performed if the fluid is not loculated.** Tube drainage is indicated if the pH and glucose levels decrease and the LDH level increases, but not if these values normalize. **If a previously loculated fluid persists or the patient remains ill after an initial therapeutic thoracentesis, then chest tube drainage is required.** A **thrombolytic can be instilled into the tube** to try to improve tube drainage.
4. **Class 4 effusions are termed simple-complicated.** These effusions are not loculated and do not appear purulent. However, the glucose level is less than 40 mg/dL, pH is less than 7.0, and results of Gram stain or culture are positive. **Either repeated thoracentesis or chest tube drainage is indicated.** If glucose, pH and LDH are improving on repeat thoracentesis, then serial thoracentesis can suffice. If glucose and pH remain low, tube drainage is needed.
5. **Class 5 effusions are termed complex-complicated.** They are loculated, but otherwise meet the description of simple-complicated effusions. They should be **managed with chest tube insertion and intrapleural thrombolytics.** If drainage is not complete after one to two thrombolytic doses, surgical intervention is needed.
6. **Class 6 effusions are termed simple empyemas.** These are either free flowing or confined to a single loculus. **Large-bore chest tube drainage** is indicated. Surgical decortication will be needed if an empyema cavity persists despite tube drainage.

7. **Class 7 effusions are termed complex empyemas.** Initial management of these multiloculated empyemas includes multiple large-bore chest tubes with intrapleural thrombolytics. Nonetheless, **thoracoscopy or thoracotomy is often required.**

**II. Pleural empyema** [153,154]. An empyema is **pus in the pleural space.** Some patients may be very toxic with an empyema, while others may have only low-grade fever. When frank pus is found, pleural fluid gram stain and cultures are important but glucose, pH, and LDH are not needed.

A. **The underlying causes** for empyemas include the following:
   1. **Pulmonary infections** (pneumonia, aspiration pneumonia, and lung abscess)
   2. **Postthoracotomy**
   3. **Direct spread of infection** (e.g., from an abdominal or orofacial source)
   4. **Esophageal rupture,** suggested by a fluid pH less than 6.0 or an increased amylase [155]
   5. **Idiopathic,** believed to be the result of a pneumonia that has since resolved
   6. **Hematogenous spread** (uncommon in adults but more frequent in children)

B. **Bacteriology.** Bacteria vary with age and predisposing conditions. Mixed infections are frequent, and organisms producing $\beta$-lactamases are often isolated.
   1. **Anaerobes** play a significant role in empyemas complicating aspiration pneumonia, lung abscess, oropharyngeal infection, and intestinal infection. These include *Bacteroides* species, *Prevotella* species, *Fusobacterium nucleatum,* and *Peptostreptococcus* species, often in combination. Mixed aerobic and anaerobic infections are common.
   2. **Aerobic bacteria.** Although once common, *S. pyogenes* is now seen less frequently. In contrast, pneumococci continue to be an important cause of empyema. *S. aureus* and aerobic gram-negative bacilli are common pathogens in postthoracotomy patients and in patients with nosocomial pneumonias. The importance of *H. influenzae* type b empyemas in children has been diminished by the protein-conjugate vaccine.

C. **Management.** The principles of empyema management are to control infection, minimize morbidity and hospitalization, and maximize resultant lung function.
   1. **Adequate drainage.** Because pus in the pleural cavity represents infection in a closed space, **drainage is always necessary.** Only rarely is adequate drainage achieved by daily thoracentesis. Usually fluid is too thick or loculated, and image-guided chest tube drainage is necessary. If there is poor response in the first 24 hours and the patient is stable, then instillation over 2 to 3 days of intrapleural thrombolytics may be tried. Repeat imaging studies should be followed to assure complete drainage and a reduction in the cavity size. When this fails, early surgical intervention is indicated.

      **Video-assisted thoracoscopy** may help break down loculations, provide for thorough irrigation, allow visual placement of drainage tubes, and may obviate the need for open thoracotomy. Even with careful patient selection, 10% to 20% of VATS procedures need to be converted to thoracotomy [154].
   2. **Antibiotics** are initiated on the basis of the Gram stain findings and the clinical setting, and altered on the basis of culture results [153,155]. Empiric regimens for empyemas associated with pneumonia should provide aerobic and anaerobic coverage, while postthoracotomy empyemas require coverage for *S. aureus, P. aeruginosa,* and other aerobic gram-negative bacilli. In general, if adequate drainage can be achieved quickly, the authors will use i.v. antibiotics for approximately 14 days. However, the actual duration of therapy will depend on the underlying source, causative organisms, clinical response, and duration of significant pleural drainage or effusion. Because antibiotics achieve adequate levels, there is no need for intrapleural antibiotics [153]. However, bioavailability of aminoglycosides and some $\beta$-lactams in empyema fluid is poor [153,155]. Thus, it is best that aminoglycosides not be used alone to treat gram-negative empyemas.
   3. **Bronchopleural fistula** may occur in association with empyemas or complicated parapneumonic effusions. **Rapid adequate percutaneous drainage is essential to prevent escape of purulent material into the bronchial tree** and for cure. **The initial clue is an air-fluid level in the pleural cavity.** Other

causes of an air-fluid level in infection include a ruptured esophagus and rupture of an underlying lung abscess. Gas formation from microbial growth is an uncommon cause, so that another explanation should be sought. CT scans are helpful in separating pleural from intraparenchymal air-fluid levels. Confirmation is achieved by placing the chest tube to water seal (i.e., bubbling is seen). Thoracic **surgical consultation is advised.**

## LUNG ABSCESS

Lung abscess is a suppurative cavitary lesion in the lung parenchyma surrounded by inflammation and necrosis. Most lung abscesses are at least 2 cm in diameter when recognized, and may not contain an air-fluid level. Necrotizing pneumonia, an earlier manifestation of the same pathophysiologic process, consists of multiple small cavities within areas of acute consolidation. Pulmonary gangrene, the extreme manifestation of this process, is distinguished by extensive lung necrosis [156]. Mycobacteria and fungi (e.g., histoplasmosis and coccidioidomycosis) also can cause cavitating lung disease. Tuberculosis is discussed later in this chapter, and fungal infections are discussed in Chapter 17.

I. **Types of lung abscesses.** Primary lung abscess is due to a primary necrotizing lung infection. Secondary lung abscess is the result of an extrapulmonary infection that has spread to involve the lung, such as embolic abscesses from right-sided endocarditis. Lung abscesses can be further separated into the following categories:
   A. **Anaerobic.** These are **due to aspiration of oropharyngeal organisms.** Most involve two to three anaerobes, and may include a nonanaerobic species. *Bacteroides* species, *Prevotella intermedia, P. melaninogenica,* other *Prevotella* species, *F. nucleatum, Veillonella,* and peptostreptococci are common. Frequent nonanaerobes are *Streptococcus intermedius,* and other microaerophilic and aerobic streptococci.
   B. A **specific** abscess follows a necrotizing pneumonia **due to a single organism,** such as *K. pneumoniae, P. aeruginosa,* other gram-negative bacilli, *Legionella* species, *S. aureus, Nocardia* species, or *Actinomyces.* Melioidosis and paragonimiasis are more important causes of lung abscess in parts of the world other than the United States.
   C. **Septic emboli** may result in abscess formation. Important sources include intravascular, pelvic, orofacial, gastrointestinal, and urinary infections. Organisms include *Fusobacterium necrophorum* from septic jugular vein phlebitis (Lemierre syndrome), *Bacteroides fragilis* from pelvic or intraabdominal infections, and *E. coli* from urinary, biliary, or gastrointestinal tract infections.
   D. **Infected lung bullae** pose a special clinical problem [157]. Infection is a secondary phenomenon and does not cause lung necrosis. Illness is milder than with lung abscess; duration of symptoms is shorter, putrid sputum is rare, and normal leukocyte counts are common. The radiographic hallmark is an air-fluid level in a preexisting emphysematous bulla with minimal surrounding infiltrate. Response to penicillin suggests that oral anaerobic and aerobic bacteria are the causative organisms. Improvement with oral antibiotics and chest physiotherapy is prompt, and bronchoscopy and other invasive procedures are not indicated [157].

II. **Clinical presentation and microbiology**
   A. **Anaerobic lung abscesses** often occur with poor dental hygiene and **risks for aspiration** (see section **I.G.2** under Clinical Approach to Community-Acquired Pneumonia).
      1. **Poor dental hygiene** allows for a high-titered inoculum **with aspiration** [158]. After aspiration, chest film evidence of an abscess takes 7 to 16 days to appear. **Anaerobic abscess is uncommon in the edentulous patient** unless there is a predisposing pulmonary disorder.
      2. **Predisposing pulmonary disorders** include bronchogenic carcinoma or other bronchial obstructions, bronchiectasis, and pulmonary infarction [158]. COPD does not predispose to anaerobic lung infections.
      3. **Symptoms** of cough, production of sputum (which often has a foul odor), weight loss, and malaise may be present for several days to weeks or months. Symptoms are **insidious and prolonged** compared with those of the typical bacterial pneumonia.

4. The patient with a lung abscess on roentgenography that does not fit the preceding description may have one of the secondary forms discussed next.

B. **Aerobic lung abscesses** most often result from necrotizing pneumonia. Patients with *S. aureus* or gram-negative pneumonias (which may be nosocomial) are usually acutely ill. Occasionally, the presentation is indolent and similar to an anaerobic abscess.

C. **Embolic pneumonias** are suggested by the clinical setting and blood culture results.

D. **Other causes.** Unusual bacteria, tuberculosis, other mycobacteria, fungi, and noninfectious causes are considered when patients do not fit the preceding categories.

III. **Diagnosis.** Useful diagnostic studies are those that verify the clinical impression and help identify infections due to resistant or unusual organisms.

A. **Radiographic appearance.** Aspiration-induced **anaerobic abscesses** involve the right lung more often than the left, and usually are found in dependent segments. These are the posterior segments of the upper lobes and the superior segments of the lower lobes when supine, and the basal segments of the lower lobes when upright. **Embolic abscesses** are suggested by multiple round cavities in the lower lobes (higher blood flow). **Airway obstruction** is suggested by atelectasis, a mass, or a foreign body. Hilar adenopathy, parapneumonic effusions, empyemas, and bronchopleural fistulas occur with any type. Prior films may demonstrate evolution of acute infiltrates to abscess formation.

**Concealed lung abscesses** are not evident on routine chest radiographs because of extensive infiltrates or effusions, inadequate drainage, or failure to obtain an upright view. They comprise up to 18% of lung abscesses, and are found by CT scan, surgery, or autopsy [159,160]. Delay in recognizing the true nature of the lung pathology may prove fatal [159].

B. **Elastin fibers in sputum** indicate a necrotizing infection [122], but this has not found wide clinical utility. One cannot predict which pneumonia will lead to a lung abscess.

C. **Sputum collection and evaluation**

1. **Expectorated sputum**

a. Sputum and breath often have a **foul odor in anaerobic** lung abscess.

b. **Gram-stained smears of expectorated sputum are useful.** Findings with anaerobic abscess include neutrophils, and a mixture of gram-positive and gram-negative organisms with no predominant type. In contrast, aerobic abscesses show a predominant morphology (e.g., *S. aureus* or aerobic gram-negative bacilli).

c. **Cultures of expectorated sputum are of little value** because they are inadequate for anaerobes and often contaminated with potentially pathogenic aerobes [158].

d. **Specimens for mycobacteria, fungi, and *Legionella*** studies may be necessary in selected patients with an unclear etiology or an atypical clinical course.

2. **Invasive procedures.** Transtracheal aspirates, bronchoscopy with PSB or BAL for quantitative cultures, and percutaneous lung or abscess puncture provide specimens suitable for both anaerobic and aerobic cultures. Appropriate specimen handling is critical [158].

**Invasive procedures usually are unnecessary** with anaerobic abscess because the clinical diagnosis is reliable and the microbiology is predictable [161]. They may be helpful if an adequate expectorated specimen is unobtainable, if a delay in specific therapy is potentially life threatening, or if an unusual or resistant organism is suspected. Pulmonary consultation is advised.

D. **Blood cultures** should be obtained in febrile patients or when embolic pneumonia is possible (e.g., addicts, endocarditis, and intraabdominal or pharyngeal space infections).

E. **Acid-fast smears** help exclude *Mycobacterium,* although air-fluid levels are infrequent in tuberculosis. Some patients at risk for aspiration are also at risk for tuberculosis (e.g., alcoholics). The diagnosis of fungal pneumonia is discussed in Chapter 17.

F. **Thoracentesis** should be performed if sufficient quantities of pleural fluid are detected.

G. **Fiberoptic bronchoscopy** should not be routine [162], but is indicated for suspected cavitating carcinoma or bronchial obstruction, and significant hemoptysis. Absence of fever or systemic symptoms, no predisposing factors for lung abscess, no leukocytosis, and minimal or no surrounding infiltrate suggest underlying lung cancer [162].

IV. **Management. Successful treatment is initially indicated by** a rapid decrease in any foul odor to the sputum, an improved appetite, and the return of a subjective sense of well-being. Fever from anaerobic abscess should abate within the first week [58], but this may take up to 2 weeks. Large amounts of purulent sputum may continue for several weeks, but Gram stains should reveal a marked decrease in organisms. Chest radiographs first show a reduction in the surrounding infiltrate and a decrease in cavity fluid, but initially the cavity may enlarge as necrotic lung is expectorated.

A. **Abscess drainage** is essential.

1. **Drainage usually occurs through the tracheobronchial tree.** If the patient is raising sputum and is improving clinically and radiologically, drainage is adequate. Cautious chest physiotherapy and postural drainage should be reserved for patients having difficulty with secretions to minimize the risk for endobronchial spread of infection and respiratory failure.
2. **Percutaneous catheter drainage** [163]. This is particularly suitable when urgent drainage is needed because of life-threatening sepsis or a large fluid-filled abscess ($\geq$4–6 cm) with a significant risk for aspiration of cavity contents, cough is ineffective, medical therapy fails, or the risk of surgical intervention is too great. Image guidance permits placement to avoid uninvolved pleura and lung, the detection of loculations, and an assessment of the drainage.
3. **Surgery** is required in only a few circumstances. Common indications include significant hemoptysis, suspected or proved lung cancer, abscess rupture with pyopneumothorax, and failure of medical therapy or catheter drainage.
4. **Obstruction to drainage** is suspected with unexplained deterioration, abrupt decrease in sputum production or tube output, or increasing amounts of cavity fluid.

B. **Antibiotics** are the mainstay of therapy (adult doses shown below).

1. **Anaerobic abscess.** Many oral anaerobes are **increasingly resistant to penicillin** due to penicillinase production.
   a. **Penicillin G alone has proven inferior** in prospective, randomized trials [58].
   b. **Clindamycin** resistance occurs in some *Peptostreptococcus, Sutterella, Fusobacteria,* non-perfringens *Clostridia,* and *Bacteroides* species [158].
   c. **Metronidazole should not be used alone** because of a high clinical failure rate [58,158]. Metronidazole is relatively inactive for some *Sutterella,* anaerobic cocci, microaerophilic streptococci, *Actinomyces,* and *Proprionobacterium* strains [158]. Long-term metronidazole may be complicated by its disulfuram-like interaction with alcohol, and peripheral neuropathy (see **Chapter 27**).
   d. **Alternative agents active against anaerobes** but with less published clinical experience include ampicillin-sulbactam, amoxicillin-clavulanate, ticarcillin-clavulanate, piperacillin-tazobactam, cefoxitin, imipenem, meropenem, gatifloxacin, moxifloxacin, and chloramphenicol. Disadvantages include their very broad coverage, expense, and potential for uncommon but serious toxicities (e.g., seizures with imipenem, and aplasia with chloramphenicol).
   e. **Drugs that have limited anaerobic activity** include the antistaphylococcal penicillins, ceftazidime, erythromycin and other macrolides, fluoroquinolones other than gatifloxacin and moxifloxacin, TMP-SMX, the tetracyclines, aztreonam, and the aminoglycosides [58,158].
   f. **Suggested regimens** include higher doses of i.v. penicillin G (10–20 million units/day) to cover relatively resistant organisms [158]) plus either oral or i.v. metronidazole (500 mg every 6 hours) or i.v. clindamycin (600 mg every 8 hours). In one study 21% of anaerobes were resistant to penicillin, 12%

resistant to metronidazole, and 5% resistant to clindamycin; however, almost all the anaerobes were susceptible to the combination of penicillin and metronidazole [161]. When the patient has been afebrile for at least 3 to 5 days, one can switch to oral therapy with penicillin V (750 mg four times daily), and either metronidazole or clindamycin (300–450 mg four times daily).

2. **Aerobic lung abscesses. Combination i.v. therapy is used initially for aerobic gram-negative necrotizing lung infections,** and based on local resistance patterns. Infectious disease consultation is advised. Coverage for MRSA and resistant gram-negative bacilli such as *P. aeruginosa* are often necessary. Antibiotic therapy should be narrowed when susceptibility studies are available. Therapy for embolic abscesses depends on the organism and the underlying focus (i.e., endocarditis).
3. **Duration of therapy. Oral therapy may be substituted** when there is clear and sustained improvement. In general, aerobic abscesses require longer i.v. therapy than anaerobic abscesses. **Antibiotics are continued** until there is a return to the usual state of health, sputum is minimal and not purulent, there is no infiltrate surrounding the cavity, the cavity has healed or is a stable thin-walled scar, and the ESR or C-reactive protein is normalized. **The optimal duration of total antibiotic therapy must be individualized,** and several months may be required to meet these goals.

**C. Complications and outcome**

1. **Empyema** can complicate lung abscess, with or without a **bronchopleural fistula.**
2. **Hemorrhage into the cavity** is suggested by hemoptysis and rapidly fluctuating air-fluid levels. An obstructing blood clot may be present, although hemorrhage alone may mimic obstruction.
3. **Aspiration of abscess contents** can cause rapid deterioration or sudden death.
4. Brain abscess, clubbing, and amyloidosis are rare in the antibiotic era.
5. **Prognosis** depends on the underlying conditions and etiologic agents. In anaerobic lung abscess, mortality has been as low as 4% in the antibiotic era; the average time to maximum cavity closure is estimated at 65 days [58]. Mortality in aerobic lung abscess is higher, particularly in immunocompromised hosts. Risk factors for a worse outcome include multiple abscesses, an abscess larger than 6 cm, prolonged symptoms, obstruction, old age, and debilitating chronic disease.

## TUBERCULOSIS: BASIC CONCEPTS

Tuberculosis remains a worldwide health problem and presents with sufficient variability to cause diagnostic confusion [164,165]. The focus of this chapter is on *Mycobacterium tuberculosis* in the United States and four important presentations: primary pneumonia, postprimary disease, pleurisy, and disseminated disease. Other extrapulmonary manifestations, therapeutic agents and their toxicity, and chemoprophylaxis also are discussed.

### I. Epidemiology

**A. In the United States,** *M. tuberculosis* infects an estimated 15 million persons. Tuberculosis reemerged between 1985 and 1992, and approximately 67,000 more cases occurred than would have been anticipated had the earlier rate of decline continued [166]. **Each year since 1992 the number of tuberculosis cases have declined,** to 16,377 cases in the year 2000 for a rate of 5.8 cases per 100,000 population [164,166]. **At the same time the numbers of foreign-born persons with tuberculosis, and their proportion of the total cases, have continued to increase.** Disease risk is highest within the first years after immigration [167]. Thus, control of tuberculosis in foreign-born individuals will be of major importance in meeting the goals for eliminating tuberculosis in this country [167,168].

**B. Outside the United States,** tuberculosis remains a tremendous problem. It is estimated that one-third of the world's population, almost 2 billion persons, is infected with *M. tuberculosis.* From this reservoir come 8 million new tuberculosis patients and approximately 3 million deaths each year [164]. Thus, 95% of tuberculosis disease occurs in developing countries, where there are few medical or public health resources and where concomitant HIV infection is common [164].

## II. Pathogenesis of tuberculosis

### A. Overview

1. **Reservoir.** Although some animals are susceptible to *M. tuberculosis* infection, **humans** are the only important natural reservoir for this organism.
2. **Transmission.** Spread of *M. tuberculosis* is almost exclusively **by small-particle aerosols termed droplet nuclei,** and rarely by contaminated dust or fomites. Airborne particles bearing organisms are generated by coughing, sneezing, and even speaking or singing [164]. Inhaled droplet nuclei, each containing two to three bacilli, are of sufficiently small size (1–5 $\mu$m) to be deposited into the alveolar space [164]. Although a single organism is sufficient to infect animals, most human infections follow exposures to many more droplet nuclei and bacilli. Transmission depends on the numbers of bacilli expelled, their concentration in the air over time, the duration of an exposure to contaminated air, and host immunity [164].
3. **Primary infection** results from exposure to airborne organisms produced by someone with active pulmonary tuberculosis. Organisms reach the alveoli (most often in the middle or lower lung zones), multiply intracellularly in alveolar macrophages, and **silently spread through lymphatics to hilar or other regional lymph nodes, and then through the bloodstream** to many sites [169]. *M. tuberculosis* bacilli continue to grow at some of these sites for 2 to 12 weeks until, in an immunocompetent host, **cell-mediated immunity develops** [164]. At this time granulomas are formed and growth of organisms is inhibited, but they are not killed. Consequently, organisms that have been dormant can become reactivated [170]. **In approximately 5% of normal hosts the original infection cannot be contained, and clinical disease develops rapidly or within the first 2 years** [164]. In the remaining 95% the original infection is controlled and remains subclinical.
4. **Postprimary reactivation infection.** Clinical disease develops in 5% of immunocompetent persons at a time remote from the initial infection as a result of endogenous reactivation of a previously established quiescent focus [164]. The **preferential sites for reactivation are those of persistently high oxygen tension.** These include the **superior lung segments (except anterior), kidneys, bones, and CNS.**
5. **Postprimary exogenous reinfection** occurs because protection following a previous infection is incomplete and may wane over time, even in immunocompetent patients [171]. The frequency of exogenous reinfection varies with the risk for infection [172]. With low risk, postprimary tuberculosis almost always is reactivation disease [172]. However, reinfections contribute to tuberculosis in HIV-infected persons, and may account for a significant proportion of adult disease in areas of the world with high rates of tuberculosis [173,174].

### B. The role of cellular immunity.

**Impairment of cellular immunity predisposes to development of clinical disease** due to progressive primary infection, exogenous reinfection, or from reactivation infection. The **major host defense against *M. tuberculosis* is the macrophage-lymphocyte system,** which is influenced by host genetic factors [169,175,176]. *M. tuberculosis* infection elicits a **Th1-type immune response** involving interferon-$\gamma$ and tumor necrosis factor $\alpha$ (TNF-$\alpha$) that activates macrophages to become more bactericidal through the generation of reactive nitrogen intermediates, and leads to granuloma formation [169,170]. The importance of TNF-$\alpha$ has been emphasized by the recognition that use of infliximab, an anti–TNF-$\alpha$ monoclonal antibody, is associated with the development of active tuberculosis, including extrapulmonary and disseminated disease [177]. **Analogous immunologic events also are responsible for many of the clinical findings in tuberculosis** [169]. Fever, anorexia, and weight loss may be mediated by cytokines induced by the infection. Tissue destruction and caseous necrosis are caused by altered cellular reactivity to the organism, or tissue delayed-type hypersensitivity. Understanding the critical differences in the pathways leading to protective immunity and tissue destruction will be essential for vaccine development.

C. **Organism factors** play a role in the development of disease, but these are poorly understood. Strains vary in their ability to be transmitted and cause infection, elicit cytokines, and grow in animals and macrophages [178–180]. However, genetic analysis of at least one hypertransmissible *M. tuberculosis* strain has not yielded clues to strain virulence [178].

III. **Purified protein derivative (PPD) skin test** [164,181]. Cellular immunity is inferred from a positive reaction to an intradermal antigen (delayed-type hypersensitivity). Antigen stimulates memory cells, which elaborate factors that attract uncommitted mononuclear cells to the area. These begin to accumulate at 24 hours and are fully manifest after 48 and 72 hours, accounting for the time the test is read.

A. **The recommended method for skin testing is intradermal inoculation into the forearm of tuberculin PPD.** This is available in only the 5-TU strength. In the United States and Canada, this strength is measured in tuberculin units (TU) and is based on achieving a biologic equivalence to the standard PPD preparation, PPD-S.

1. **Intermediate-strength PPD** contains 5 TU in the 0.1 mL injected. **All recommendations for interpreting skin testing are based on using this strength.**
2. Multiple puncture devices should not be used for diagnostic purposes [164].

B. **The maximum diameter of induration at 48 to 72 hours is measured transversely to the long axis of the forearm using palpation and inspection in oblique and direct light.** A ballpoint pen method may be used to reduce interobserver variation [164].

C. **Interpreting the reaction. False-negative responses occur on initial testing in up to 25% of patients with active pulmonary tuberculosis** [164]. False-positive reactions may result from infection with nontuberculous mycobacteria or from recent bacille baliéde Calmette-Guerin (BCG) vaccination. Thus, **three separate cut points for positivity have been defined** to optimize sensitivity and specificity for the test in different patient populations.

1. **Five millimeters or more of induration is considered positive in persons with the highest likelihood of developing active disease.** These include patients with close contact with active tuberculosis, radiographic findings consistent with old tuberculosis, HIV infection, organ transplants, and immunosuppression equivalent to taking more than 15 mg of prednisone daily for at least 4 weeks.
2. **Ten millimeters or more of induration is considered positive in those who do not meet the preceding criteria but who are at high risk for tuberculosis.** These include recent (<5 years) immigrants from countries where tuberculosis is prevalent; HIV-negative injection drug users; residents and employees of high-risk congregate settings such as prisons, nursing homes, health-care facilities, residential facilities for persons with HIV/AIDS, drug treatment centers, and homeless shelters; mycobacteriology laboratory personnel; persons with high-risk medical conditions, including silicosis, diabetes, chronic renal failure, leukemias and lymphomas, carcinoma of the head or neck and lung, more than 10% loss of ideal body weight, gastrectomy, and jejunoileal bypass; children under 4 years of age; infants, children, and adolescents exposed to high-risk adults; those with a recent (within 2 years) conversion of their skin test result; and any other locally identified high-prevalence population.
3. **Fifteen millimeters or more of induration is considered positive in anyone.**

D. **Booster effect.** A prior skin test in a previously sensitized individual may provide an immunologic boost that leads to an increase in induration from a negative to a positive interpretation (see section **III.C**), and thus mimic a skin-test conversion from recent infection. The booster effect may be seen within 1 week of an initial test, and the effect may persist for 1 year or longer. It may be found in individuals who have latent tuberculosis and waned PPD responsiveness, those who have previously received the BCG vaccine, or those previously exposed to nontuberculous mycobacteria [164]. It rarely occurs in children and becomes more important with increasing age. **The clinician needs to be particularly aware of the booster effect in** annual screening programs involving serial skin tests, and serial skin tests performed for diagnostic or other purposes.

A two-step skin test to detect the booster effect is recommended for use in programs where repeated skin testing is anticipated [164]. If the initial PPD skin test result is negative, it is repeated in 1 to 3 weeks. The second skin test serves as the baseline response.

E. **Causes of negative skin test reactions** [164]. Subcutaneous or other inadequate injections, and use of impotent tuberculin preparations, should be excluded.
   1. **The most common cause is the absence of infection with *M. tuberculosis*.**
   2. **False-negative skin test results may occur with** recent or overwhelming tuberculosis; tuberculous pleurisy; acute nontuberculous infections (especially acute viral infection); live virus vaccinations; lymphoma or leukemia; sarcoidosis; other immunosuppressive diseases or drugs; renal disease; poor nutrition; newborn or advanced age; surgery; and burns.
   3. **Anergy testing is no longer recommended** to identify tuberculosis infection or to help interpret a negative PPD test result [164,181].

F. **Skin-test conversion**
   1. Conversion from a negative to positive reaction is an **increase of 10 mm or greater induration on a subsequent test** [164,181]. For persons who undergo repeated testing (e.g., health-care workers), **recent conversion** is defined as an increase of 10 mm or greater induration **within a 2-year period** and indicates recent tuberculous infection [164,181].
   2. **False skin test conversion** may occur from the booster effect (see section **III.D**), concurrent infection with *Brucella* or other intracellular organisms resulting in nonspecific enhancement of tuberculin skin test reactivity, or correction of the cause for a prior false-negative skin test result giving the erroneous impression of skin test conversion even when there has simply been a return to baseline skin test reactivity.

G. **Skin testing is targeted for populations at high risk for tuberculosis** and thus candidates for preventive therapy [164,181]. These include groups at risk for recent *M. tuberculosis* infection, and those at increased risk for progression to active disease no matter the duration of infection (see sections **III.C.1** and **III.C.2**). It also is appropriate for patients with findings compatible with tuberculosis but no definitive diagnosis. **Skin testing is discouraged for low-risk persons.**

IV. **Diagnosis.** The cornerstone of diagnosis is the presence of acid-fast bacilli (AFB) on smears from sputum and other clinical specimens, and the isolation of *M. tuberculosis* on culture.

A. **Smears and cultures** [164]. **Early morning sputum is best, and three specimens are sufficient.** All specimens usually test positive in untreated patients.
   1. **Sputum induction using nebulized saline** is helpful for those unable to expectorate.
   2. **Fiberoptic bronchoscopy** with bronchial washings, BAL, or biopsy may be needed when spontaneous or induced sputums fail to provide diagnostic specimens. **Expectorated sputums also should be collected in the immediate postbronchoscopy period, the next morning, and on subsequent days when available** because they may be the only positive samples.
   3. **AFB smears** are discussed in Chapter 25. At least three AFB must be seen to consider a smear positive, using either a fluorochrome or a carbol-fuchsin method. **Screening with the fluorochrome stain is preferred** because it is easier and faster to read.

      Sputum must contain 5,000 to 10,000 bacilli/mL before smears are reliably positive [164]. The estimated organism burden is $10^2$ to $10^4$ in fibronodular lesions, and $10^7$ to $10^9$ in cavitary lesions. Thus, **cavitary disease is usually smear positive and contagious.**
   4. **Gastric aspirates and urines for smear and culture.** Aspiration of early morning gastric contents before the patient has eaten or arisen from bed may be used for children and adults from whom sputum cannot be obtained. The

first voided morning urine is the preferred specimen, and should be repeated on three separate days [164]. Because smears cannot distinguish saprophytic from pathogenic mycobacteria, smears of gastric aspirates and urines usually are not used. A review of a 10-year experience that excluded HIV-infected patients found only one possible false-positive urine smear and no false-positive smears of gastric aspirates, suggesting that positive acid-fast smears of gastric aspirates or urines are helpful [182]. However, smears from urine frequently test negative and may not be cost effective [164].

5. **Cultures may be positive when smears test negative** because cultures require only 10 to 100 viable organisms to become positive [164]. Thus, patients with negative smear results but positive cultures are four to five times less infectious than patients with positive smear results [183]. Nonetheless, smear-negative patients may still transmit tuberculosis [183].
6. **Time delay of cultures**
   a. **Solid media.** Approximately **3 to 8 weeks are required** for visible growth on traditional solid media, and another 3 to 4 weeks for susceptibility test results.
   b. **Automated liquid culture systems reduce the average detection time to 1 to 3 weeks** [164]. These systems also provide results for susceptibility testing to commonly used drugs in much shorter times than when using solid media [164].
7. **Rapid identification of any acid-fast growth** is generally accomplished using DNA probes to hybridize with mycobacterial ribosomal RNA. Probes are commercially available that identify the *M. tuberculosis* complex, the *M. avium* complex, *M. kansasii,* and *M. gordonae.* High-performance liquid chromatography also may be used but is not as widely available. Investigational techniques include spoligotyping, polymerase chain restriction analysis, and DNA sequence analysis [164].

B. **Newer rapid diagnostic methods** include nucleic acid amplification techniques, immunologic techniques, and tests to detect mycobacterial cellular components [164,184].

1. **Nucleic acid amplification (NAA) tests** are available to detect *M. tuberculosis* directly in clinical specimens [164,184,185]. The amplified mycobacterium tuberculosis direct test (MTD, Gen-Probe) and the Amplicor mycobacterium tuberculosis test (Roche Diagnostic Systems) use different techniques but have similar utility. Both detect nearly all sputum smear-positive and half of the smear-negative cases of culture-proven pulmonary tuberculosis [164,184]; only the MTD test has been approved by the U.S. Food and Drug Administration (FDA) for use with smear-negative sputum specimens [185]. Although a negative NAA test never excludes the possibility of tuberculosis, patients whose sputum is repeatedly AFB smear positive and NAA negative may be presumed to have nontuberculous mycobacterial infection if inhibitors are not found [185].

   **NAA tests should not replace routine AFB smears and cultures** or clinical judgment [185]. The best way to use these expensive and technically demanding tests has not been defined, but the CDC and others have made preliminary proposals [184,185]. NAA may yield positive results even after successful chemotherapy because they can amplify nucleic acids from dead organisms [164]. Thus, they should be used only for diagnosis and not to follow therapy.
2. **Immunologic techniques for diagnosis** are being pursued in order to improve on the detection of both latent and active tuberculosis. These techniques include developing improved antigen mixtures for skin testing, identifying *in vitro* lymphocyte responses to *M. tuberculosis,* and developing improved methods of serodiagnosis [184,186]. It is hoped that current investigations will lead to improved immunodiagnosis for tuberculosis, and that this will help in future vaccine trials [186].

V. **Clinical forms of tuberculosis.** Four important forms of tuberculosis are discussed below: primary tuberculous pneumonia, postprimary (reactivation) disease, pleurisy, and disseminated (miliary) disease. Some of these can appear in combination. Therapy is discussed in section **VII.**

A. **Primary tuberculous pneumonia.** After initial inhalation (see section **II.A.3**), a symptomatic **primary pneumonia,** often with ipsilateral hilar adenopathy, occasionally develops, particularly at the extremes of age. Atelectasis may result from lymph node enlargement, particularly in young children. If the primary pneumonia progresses despite delayed hypersensitivity, it may be associated with cavitation or dissemination infection (progressive primary disease) [164,169].

1. **Clinical manifestations.** Patients may have only a cough or may be very ill with high fever and inanition, depending on their age [169]. Sputum volume may be large and often contains abundant polymorphonuclear leukocytes.
2. **Diagnosis.** Skin test results frequently are negative. **Sputum AFB smear results often are highly positive.** Radiographic features may include lobar consolidation, cavitary disease with middle or lower zone infiltration, hilar adenopathy, and atelectasis.
3. **Communicability is potentially high** because of the large numbers of organisms in the sputum. Thus, **proper respiratory isolation is essential.**

B. **Postprimary (reactivation) tuberculosis is marked by upper lobe disease that often includes cavitation.** This usually occurs many months or years after the primary infection. Upper lobe disease also may quickly follow a primary infection if host immunity is insufficient, either with or without lower lobe involvement [169]. Infiltration is most common in the apical and posterior segments of the upper lobes and the apical segments of the lower lobes, and usually evolves to include air-filled cavities. Noncavitary nodules or infiltrates are more common in the elderly and the immunosuppressed. At this stage, the process almost always steadily progresses unless treated. Bronchogenic spread may involve lower and middle lobes, and may be bilateral.

1. **Clinical manifestations.** Most individuals are moderately ill with anorexia, fatigue, productive cough, night sweats, fever, weight loss, and weakness. Sputum may be blood streaked. In some, the illness can be very severe, whereas in others with extensive parenchymal involvement, symptoms are minimal or nonexistent. Physical findings are nonspecific, and abnormalities in the chest may be minimal despite extensive disease. Large cavities may produce amphoric breath sounds.
2. **Diagnosis.** The chest roentgenogram may not readily show early infiltrates or distinguish active from inactive disease, and cannot yield a specific diagnosis; chest CT can provide further supportive information in difficult cases. A first-morning sputum sample should be sent for acid-fast smear and cultures (see Chapter 25); if the initial smear is negative, then a total of three (but no more than five) specimens should be examined. Sputum should be induced using nebulized hypertonic saline when spontaneous specimens are not produced. If this is unsuccessful, then fiberoptic bronchoscopy should be considered (see section **IV.A**). If bronchoscopy is not an option, then gastric aspirates should be sent. Three first-morning urine specimens also should be obtained when genitourinary involvement is suspected or when sputum smears are negative.
3. **Communicability is high** before therapy because of the large numbers of organisms in cavitary disease. **These patients should be placed in respiratory isolation.**

C. **Tuberculous pleurisy** may be a manifestation of either primary infection or postprimary disease. It also occurs as part of disseminated disease either alone or with simultaneous effusions in the pericardial and peritoneal spaces (tuberculous polyserositis). In the past, tuberculous pleurisy was more common in younger individuals as a consequence of recent infection. However, at present it is more common in older individuals [169]. Tuberculous pleural effusions are due to the breakdown of a subpleural focus releasing its contents into the pleural space, followed by acute inflammation from a cell-mediated hypersensitivity reaction [187]. In contrast, tuberculous empyema results when a bronchopleural fistula spills the contents of a cavity or other parenchymal focus into the pleural space [164].

1. **Clinical manifestations.** Onset of pleural involvement may be insidious or abrupt, and occasionally patients are very ill. **Symptoms may be minimal or include some combination of cough, fever, pleuritic chest pain, and dyspnea** [187]. Evidence for pleural effusion may be present on chest examination, although a pleural friction rub is usually not present. On chest radiography the effusion usually is unilateral and small, and infiltrates are not seen in approximately 30% of patients [164].

   Tuberculous pleural effusions are self-limited, resolving spontaneously within several months. Without treatment the risk of subsequent clinical tuberculosis is high, developing in up to two-thirds of patients within the next 5 years [187]. Thus, **antituberculous chemotherapy is always indicated** to prevent active disease at other sites even though it may not shorten illness from pleurisy. A short course of corticosteroids has been proposed to speed recovery and fluid resorption, and prevent pleural fibrosis [169]. However, a recent systematic literature review failed to find sufficient evidence of a benefit from steroids [188], and complete thoracoscopic drainage leads to rapid improvement independent of corticosteroid use [189]. For these reasons **we do not recommend the routine use of corticosteroids for tuberculous pleurisy.**
2. **Diagnosis.** Unless pulmonary tuberculosis is also present, diagnosis of tuberculous pleurisy requires thoracentesis and usually a pleural biopsy. Diagnosis may be delayed if the patient has other potential causes for an effusion [190].
   a. **Pleural fluid** is an exudate with a predominance of lymphocytes; neutrophils may be prominent, however, particularly early in the illness [169,187]. Mesothelial cells should not constitute more than 5% of the total cell count. Glucose levels are most often normal but may be low. **Acid-fast smears of the pleural fluid are almost always negative.** The yield from pleural fluid cultures is usually less than 25%, but is highest when large-volume specimens are submitted and centrifuged [164,187].
   b. **Pleural biopsy.** A single biopsy procedure (collecting three or four tissue samples) **sent for histology, and acid-fast stains and cultures** will provide positive findings in approximately 67% of cases. This increases to approximately 90% after a second biopsy [190]. A combination of pleural fluid studies plus pleural biopsies for histology, acid-fast stains, and cultures should establish the diagnosis in 90% to 95% of patients. Biopsy directed by **pleuroscopy increases the yield** from a single procedure [164].
   c. **Skin tests.** The **intermediate PPD** is usually positive but **may be negative in up to 30% of patients** [187]. However, most patients with an initial negative test result eventually develop a positive reaction during therapy.
   d. **Other pleural fluid diagnostic tests** that have been proposed include PCR, measurement of adenosine deaminase levels, and interferon-$\gamma$ levels [191]. These tests are not generally available and their value is uncertain, particularly in the United States where tuberculosis accounts for only a small proportion of exudative pleural effusions [164,187].
3. **Communicability** depends on the presence of concomitant pulmonary tuberculosis.

D. **Disseminated (miliary) tuberculosis** implies widespread disease due to failure to contain the organism. This can occur either as part of a primary infection or as a manifestation of postprimary tuberculosis. In the former, *M. tuberculosis* hematogenously spreads from the primary lung focus and continues to grow in multiple organs. In the latter, previously contained foci break down and allow hematogenous dissemination (see section **II**). On pathologic examination these sites are granulomatous nodules 1 to 2 mm in size that grossly resemble millet seeds, and thus the term *miliary tuberculosis* was applied to mean disseminated disease [164]. **Factors predisposing to dissemination include** extremes of age, minority race, malnutrition, measles, pertussis, AIDS, alcoholism, diabetes, pregnancy, malignancies, and immunosuppressive diseases or therapies [169].

1. **Clinical aspects.** There are no pathognomonic clinical features of disseminated disease, and the **onset of illness may be abrupt or very insidious.** Although cough and other respiratory symptoms may be present, **constitutional**

**symptoms usually predominate.** Patients may simply exhibit fever, night sweats, anorexia, weight loss, and weakness [164]. Prominent headache suggests meningitis, pleuritic chest pain suggests pleurisy, and abdominal pain suggests peritonitis. Physical findings are variable, but common abnormalities (in decreasing order) are fever, wasting, hepatomegaly, chest findings, lymphadenopathy, and splenomegaly [164]. The presence of skin lesions, and scrotal or genital masses should be sought. Choroidal tubercles may be seen on retinal examination and are very supportive of the diagnosis (see Chapter 7). Occasional patients will be profoundly ill and may have respiratory failure or other signs of sepsis.

**2. Diagnosis**

**a. Chest radiography**

**(1) The miliary radiographic pattern is diffuse, 2- to 4-mm nodular lesions,** but this may not be visible initially. Thus, repeat chest films should be obtained if the initial film is unremarkable.

**(2) Nondiagnostic chest films. Overall 15% of patients with disseminated tuberculosis do not have the classic miliary pattern,** but in some series this has been as high as 50% [164]. **Unfortunately, the diagnosis is often delayed because it is not considered unless the miliary radiographic pattern is present.** This frequently has been observed in older patients with reactivation of a nonpulmonary focus (late generalized tuberculosis) presenting with fevers and no clear etiology [169].

**b. Acid-fast smears and cultures.** Because the organism is often growing in inaccessible sites, invasive procedures are frequently required. See Chapter 25.

**(1) Sputum AFB smear results are positive in** approximately 33% and, at best, sputum cultures are positive in only 50% to 76% of patients with disseminated disease. Bronchoscopy with transbronchial biopsy should be considered in patients with abnormal chest radiographs but negative sputums.

**(2) Gastric cultures** are positive in 33% to 75% of patients.

**(3) Urine cultures** are positive in 25% to 59%, even with a normal urinalysis.

**(4) Results of bone marrow biopsy** for cultures may be positive in up to 33% of patients. Histopathologic examination may reveal granulomas in more than 80%.

**(5) Liver biopsy cultures are helpful, as is histologic appearance.** Supportive diagnostic material usually is found, provided there is some abnormality suggesting hepatic involvement prior to biopsy.

**(6) Lymph node biopsy** should be considered whenever accessible adenopathy is present. This procedure is associated with little morbidity and frequently reveals caseating granulomas or positive acid-fast smears.

**(7) CSF examination** should be performed in patients with headaches or neurologic symptoms suggestive of tuberculous meningitis (see Chapter 6).

**c. Histologic study** of organs sampled for biopsy may be very helpful. Typical granulomas with central necrosis may be seen, and acid-fast organisms may be visible.

**d. Skin test results are often negative.**

**e. Blood tests.** The WBC count is usually normal [169], but can range from leukopenia to a leukemoid reaction so striking as to suggest leukemia. Monocytosis, lymphopenia, thrombocytopenia, and anemia also may be present. Alkaline phosphatase and transaminases may be elevated, but jaundice is uncommon. Hyponatremia occurs with meningeal involvement or adrenal insufficiency.

**3. Relationship to fever of unknown origin** (FUO). Disseminated tuberculosis should be considered in the evaluation of FUO (see Chapter 1).

4. **Communicability** depends on the presence of significant pulmonary involvement.

VI. **Extrapulmonary tuberculosis.** When extrapulmonary tuberculosis occurs **in the absence of disease in the lung, the extrapulmonary infection is responsible for the major clinical manifestations.** It also may occur with simultaneous pulmonary tuberculosis or as part of disseminated infection (see section **V.D**). Extrapulmonary tuberculosis did not decline in frequency when pulmonary disease was declining. It is found most often in children, ethnic and racial minorities, women, foreign-born individuals, and patients with HIV infection.

A. **Clinical presentation**

1. **Symptoms or signs usually are localized,** with minimal or absent constitutional symptoms. Often the diagnosis is reached during evaluation of a specific problem such as pyuria, ascites, pericardial effusion, or lymphadenopathy.
2. **Systemic illness.** A small percentage of patients have constitutional symptoms associated with extrapulmonary disease. These patients usually have more widespread disease, or also have pulmonary involvement.
3. **Chest radiographic evidence of pulmonary disease is not always seen** when active infection is present in an extrapulmonary focus. Fewer than 50% of patients with lymph node, renal, CNS, or bone tuberculosis have chest film changes.

B. **Forms of extrapulmonary disease.** Pleural and disseminated tuberculosis are discussed in section **V.**

1. **Meningitis.** See Chapter 6.
2. **Pericarditis.** See Chapter 12 under Pericarditis and Myocarditis.
3. **Renal disease.** See Chapter 15 under Genitourinary Tuberculosis.
4. **Bone disease.** See Chapter 5 under Special Forms of Osteomyelitis.
5. **Lymph node disease.** Lymphatic tuberculosis is found in all age groups, although it is most common in children under 15 years of age, women, and foreign-born individuals.

a. **Clinical manifestations** vary with the extent of nodal involvement and underlying host characteristics [192].

(1) **Isolated lymph nodes** are usually nontender and firm, although there may be overlying erythema. The most common sites of involvement are the cervical (scrofula) and supraclavicular areas, but mediastinal, mesenteric, or retroperitoneal nodal tuberculosis is also possible [164,169]. Cervical lymph node disease, including breakdown and drainage, can occur with either minimal or no constitutional symptoms. Hilar adenopathy can develop without obvious lung disease, and patients are usually symptomatic [193].

(2) **Generalized lymph node involvement** usually is part of disseminated disease. Constitutional symptoms, fever, and weight loss are common. The initial clinical impression may be of a lymphoreticular neoplastic process.

(3) **Lymph node involvement due to drainage of an infected organ** is a more common cause of lymph node infection than is primary lymph node disease. Children with hilar or other mediastinal adenopathy may develop atelectasis.

(4) **Lymph node involvement with atypical mycobacteria** is more common than with *M. tuberculosis.* Submandibular or cervical adenopathy is often due to *M. scrofulaceum* in young children, and to *M. avium* complex in older children. This is distinct from lymph node involvement with disseminated *M. avium* complex infection in AIDS (see Chapter 18).

b. **Diagnosis. Fine-needle aspiration biopsy** is now advocated over total excisional biopsy as the initial procedure because it frequently supports a presumptive diagnosis with limited risk for complications when combined with modern chemotherapy. However, the microbiologic yield is low [164,169].

(1) **Histologic features.** Biopsy and culture of the lymph nodes often reveal the diagnosis. Although fine-needle aspiration may reveal epithelioid cells and granuloma, AFB stains are usually negative. PCR may

improve the ability to demonstrate *M. tuberculosis* in fine-needle aspiration specimens [194].

(2) **Tuberculin skin test.** Lymph node disease is more common in younger than in older patients, and the skin test result is often positive.

6. **Serous surface involvement** (pleural effusion, pericardial effusions, and peritonitis) usually results from breakdown of a contiguous focus with discharge of its contents into the serous cavity of a previously sensitized individual. A significant inflammatory reaction ensues despite the presence of relatively few intact organisms.

a. **Clinical manifestations.** Serous involvement can mimic serositis of unexplained etiology. The peritoneum, the pericardial sac, and, as already mentioned, the pleura may be involved either singly or in any combination.

(1) **Pleural effusions** are discussed in section **V.B.**

(2) **Pericardial effusions** are discussed in Chapter 12.

(3) **Peritonitis.** Patients with tuberculous peritonitis usually present with insidious onset of fever, abdominal pain or swelling, anorexia, weight loss, and an exudative ascites. The ascitic fluid protein content usually exceeds 2.5 g/100 mL, the serum ascites albumin gradient (SAAG) is less than 1.1 g/100 mL, and the ascites contains fewer than 3,000 white cells with a lymphocyte predominance. Many patients with tuberculous peritonitis have preexisting ascites from liver cirrhosis so that symptoms are attributed to that process and the diagnosis delayed [164,169]. In cirrhotic patients with tuberculous peritonitis the ascitic fluid may retain many of the characteristics of ascites due only to portal hypertension (e.g., total protein <2.5 g/100 mL and SAAG >1.1 g/100 mL); however, an elevated ascitic fluid LDH level may be a useful clue [195]. It also should be considered in chronic peritoneal dialysis patients with refractory peritonitis [196]. In women, tuberculous peritonitis may mimic ovarian carcinomatosis, including elevation of CA-125 [197].

b. **Spontaneous resolution.** Serous effusions that develop in tuberculosis may resolve spontaneously and, at least temporarily, leave no evidence of overt disease. However, very frequently (usually within a few months but occasionally as long as a few years) additional focal disease develops.

c. **Diagnosis**

(1) **Pleural effusions.** See section **V.C.**

(2) **Pericardial effusions.** See Chapter 12 under Pericarditis and Myocarditis.

(3) **Peritonitis.** Organisms are seldom seen on smears of peritoneal fluid. Large volumes of fluid can be centrifuged and cultured, but even this method results in a suboptimal yield. The diagnosis depends on demonstration of caseous granulomas in peritoneal tissue. Laparoscopy to obtain peritoneal biopsy specimens is the procedure of choice [164]. Associated pulmonary parenchymal abnormalities are seen in fewer than 50% of patients, although coexisting pleural effusions are not uncommon. Results of liver function tests usually are normal, and liver biopsies generally are not helpful. The PPD skin test result may or may not be positive. Therefore, **tuberculous peritonitis should be considered in any unexplained exudative ascites** regardless of the skin test result. Adenosine deaminase activity in ascitic fluid and PCR may be useful adjuncts to the diagnosis of tuberculous peritonitis.

7. **Skin.** Most often the skin is involved by direct spread from an underlying tuberculous focus such as epididymitis or adenitis. Hematogenous involvement of the skin is rare and usually occurs in patients with AIDS [169].

VII. **Tuberculosis and HIV Infection.** HIV-infected patients are at increased risk for reactivation infection, progressive primary infection, and reinfection [173]. **Thus, counseling and HIV antibody testing should be considered for almost all patients diagnosed with *M. tuberculosis* infection.** This is particularly true for patients with extrapulmonary disease or unusual manifestations of pulmonary tuberculosis. Furthermore, documentation of a positive PPD test result in an asymptomatic patient should serve as a stimulus to assess the risks for HIV, and to offer HIV education, counseling, and antibody testing. **See Chapter 18 for a further discussion of mycobacterial infections in HIV-infected patients.**

**VIII. Tuberculosis in the elderly** [198,199]. The growing elderly segment of our population contains a significant reservoir of latent tuberculosis acquired when the disease was more prevalent. Reactivation of these infections accounts for approximately 90% of tuberculosis disease in the elderly, although reinfections and new infections are also possible [199].

- **A.** Several **risk factors** for active tuberculosis may be present in the elderly. These include immunosenescence and concomitant predisposing diseases or conditions. Another risk is confinement in a nursing home, where reactivation tuberculosis occurs in 2% to 3% of skintest–positive individuals.
- **B. Atypical clinical manifestations and delayed diagnosis are common in the elderly. Awareness of the possibility of tuberculosis is essential to prompt diagnosis.** Symptoms often are poorly articulated, and coexistent illness may provide alternative explanations for anorexia, cough, and weight loss. Radiographic findings are frequently atypical and misinterpreted, including midlung or basal infiltrates. Miliary disease and many of the forms of extrapulmonary tuberculosis are more frequent in the elderly than in younger patients, and the mortality rate is higher in the elderly.

**IX. Tuberculosis in pregnancy** poses special problems. It is current opinion that pregnancy does not increase the risk for active tuberculosis, alter the manifestations of infection, change the outcome from clinical infection, or change the response to chemotherapy [200]. Active tuberculosis may have an adverse impact on maternal morbidity and pregnancy outcome if there is delayed diagnosis, advanced pulmonary disease, extrapulmonary disease in sites other than lymph nodes, and no or inadequate therapy [200]. However, **with early diagnosis and effective treatment the outcome for both mother and child is equal to that for nonpregnant patients.** Thus, tuberculosis during pregnancy is not an indication for therapeutic abortion. Congenital tuberculosis is rare; most neonates with tuberculosis acquire their infection in the postpartum period from an adult.

**Skin testing is the mainstay of screening** during pregnancy because of the need to avoid radiographic studies. **Skin testing is recommended in pregnancy only for women with risk factors for latent infection or for progression to active disease** [181]. Pregnancy does not significantly alter the skin test response, and tuberculin is safe during gestation [181]. A chest radiograph with appropriate shielding is indicated if the skin test result is positive. See also section **X.**

**X. Management of tuberculosis.** Practice guidelines have been published by the Infectious Diseases Society of America [201] for implementing recommended antituberculous therapy [166,181,202]. Current treatment is based on the observations that certain combinations of agents given for shorter periods of time are as effective as older regimens, and intermittent dosing is an effective alternative to daily therapy. **Directly observed therapy is important to achieve adherence** and reduce the risk for developing drug resistance.

- **A. Principles of tuberculosis therapy**
  1. **Comprehensive management must include public health efforts.** These involve monitoring for adherence, toxicity, efficacy, and relapse; tracing contacts and evaluating the home; and community surveillance for outbreaks and drug resistance.
  2. **Importance of combination therapy. Mutations causing resistance to antituberculous agents are** infrequent, unlinked phenomena. The rate of spontaneous resistance is approximately 1 in $10^6$ organisms for INH (INH), 1 in $10^8$ organisms for rifampin, only 1 in $10^{14}$ organisms to both INH and rifampin simultaneously, 1 in $10^4$ organisms for ethambutol, and 1 in $10^6$ organisms for streptomycin. Thus, resistance is avoided by using combination regimens.
  3. **Microbiologic diagnosis should be attempted on all patients, and *M. tuberculosis* isolates should routinely undergo susceptibility studies** [164,201].
  4. **Drug resistance.** Inadequate therapy is the most common explanation.

a. **Factors favoring the development of resistance** include the use of a single agent for active infection, erratic adherence to proper therapy, suboptimal drug dosing, malabsorption of drugs, or the failure to include enough active agents for partially resistant organisms. **Patients previously treated with regimens not containing both INH and rifampin are presumed to harbor strains of *M. tuberculosis* resistant to the previously used drugs until proven otherwise** [202].

b. **Detecting resistance** may be done using agar media (results take many weeks) or using the liquid BACTEC method for faster results. With the agar proportion method, resistance is defined as the growth on drug-containing media of 1% or more of the number of organisms growing on control media [164]. Laboratories may report results at both a "critical concentration" of drug (the concentration that reliably inhibits wild-type bacilli but not resistant mutants in the same inoculum) and a higher concentration. Although resistance is determined at the critical concentration, results at the higher concentration may be useful to assess the degree of resistance [164]. Rapid methods to identify genetic resistance determinants have been developed, and an assay detecting the *rpoB* gene mutations for rifampin resistance is commercially available in Europe [184]. However, resistance genotyping is not ready for clinical application in the United States at present [164].

5. **Multidrug-resistant (MDR) tuberculosis in the United States has declined** since 1993, both in patients previously untreated and in those with prior tuberculosis [203]. However, MDR tuberculosis is prevalent and increasing in other parts of the world [204].

   a. **Definitions. MDR refers to organisms resistant to both INH and rifampin.** In **primary resistance,** the patient from whom the isolate is obtained has never received the involved drugs. In **secondary resistance,** the patient has been treated with the drugs to which the isolate is resistant.

   b. **Epidemiology.** Contributing to MDR strains are poor adherence to therapy, homelessness, crowding in jails and other institutions, the HIV epidemic, diminished public health resources, and immigration from areas with high rates of drug resistance. Past outbreaks of MDR tuberculosis have occurred in hospitals, prisons, congregate settings (e.g., homeless shelters), and other facilities. Nosocomial MDR tuberculosis in major urban areas has centered around HIV-infected patients (see Chapter 18). Failure to identify and isolate patients promptly, as well as premature discontinuation of isolation, has contributed to outbreaks.

   c. **At least three active new agents should be used** when MDR tuberculosis is suspected or proven [202].

6. **Directly observed therapy (DOT) is optimal** for all patients [166]. In DOT a health-care worker or other reliable person watches the patient take his or her medications.

B. **Treatment regimens.** The choice of agents depends on the local incidence of drug resistance. A four-drug regimen is used initially for the first 8 weeks of therapy when INH resistance is 4% or greater [202]. The continuation phase of therapy should include INH and rifampin for susceptible organisms. Recommended treatment regimens are effective for pulmonary and extrapulmonary forms of tuberculosis.

1. **Regimens for initial empiric therapy**

   a. **Four drugs are preferred** for almost all patients [169]. INH, rifampin, pyrazinamide, and either ethambutol or streptomycin are given for the first 8 weeks.

   b. **Three drugs** may be used when local INH resistance rates are lower than 4% [202]. INH, rifampin, and pyrazinamide are given for the first 8 weeks.

   c. **When resistance to multiple agents is prevalent,** five or six drugs should be used based on the known patterns of susceptibility in the community.

2. **Options to continue therapy for susceptible organisms** (i.e., organisms susceptible to INH, rifampin, and standard drugs)

a. INH and rifampin may be used for the remaining 4 months of a minimum 6-month regimen. See section **IX.C.2** for the use of intermittent therapy.
b. Intermittent therapy with the initial four-drug regimen may be used to complete a minimum of 6 months of treatment (see section **IX.C.2**).

3. **Continuation therapy when susceptibilities are unavailable** is based on the clinical and radiographic response to treatment and the probability for resistance. Consultation with a tuberculosis expert is advised.
4. **Treatment for resistant organisms must be individualized.** Patients with isolated INH resistance may be treated with rifampin, pyrazinamide, and ethambutol for a minimum of 6 months [166]. Patients with isolated rifampin resistance may be treated with INH, pyrazinamide, and streptomycin for a minimum of 9 months, or INH and ethambutol for a minimum of 18 months [166]. Isolated resistance to pyrazinamide is rare in *M. tuberculosis,* and should suggest infection with *M. bovis* because this organism is inherently resistant to this agent. However, *M. tuberculosis* strains resistant only to pyrazinamide have been reported recently in North America [205]. **Resistance to both INH and rifampin poses particular difficulties** because simultaneous resistance to other drugs is common. Most cases of MDR tuberculosis can be cured with intensive and prolonged chemotherapy combined with surgery when needed [166,206]. **Consultation with an expert in the therapy of MDR tuberculosis is advised.**
5. **Addition of drugs to an existing regimen.** When there is concern about resistance or an inadequate response, at least two, and preferably three, new drugs should be added together. The addition of only one drug to a regimen to which resistance has occurred may result in resistance to the new drug as well.

C. **Frequency of drug administration**

1. **Daily therapy** was the standard for many years. Oral agents usually are given once daily in the fasting state in the morning.
2. **Intermittent therapy may be given 2 or 3 times weekly.** Because fewer doses of medications are used, **all patients receiving intermittent regimens must be carefully supervised using DOT to ensure adherence.** The toxicities of intermittent and daily regimens appear similar. Because fewer doses and less monitoring for efficacy are needed, the cost of intermittent regimens usually is less than that of daily therapy. There are three options for intermittent therapy [166,202].
   a. After daily therapy for the first 8 weeks with three or four drugs (see section **X.B.1**), INH and rifampin may be given two or three times weekly for a minimum of 16 weeks. This is used only when isolates are known to be susceptible to both of these drugs.
   b. After daily therapy for the first 2 weeks, the four-drug regimen may be given twice weekly for the next 6 weeks. Twice-weekly INH and rifampin may be continued for a minimum of 16 more weeks, when isolates are known to be susceptible to both of these drugs.
   c. The four-drug regimen may be given three times per week for a minimum of 6 months when isolates are known to be susceptible to INH and rifampin.

D. **Duration and type of therapy**

1. **Standard short-course regimens.** These have replaced longer courses as the **treatments of choice for tuberculosis for organisms susceptible to INH and rifampin.** The success of the 9-month regimen depends on the use of INH and rifampin together, and the 6-month regimen depends on the inclusion of pyrazinamide for the initial 2 months. The optimal use of short-course therapy requires familiarity with those situations for which it is not suitable (see section **X.D.2**).
   a. **Six-month therapy.** The ATS and CDC have adopted minimum 6-month regimens as standard therapy for pulmonary tuberculosis [202]. This duration also is suggested for most cases of extrapulmonary tuberculosis. Treatment is given for a minimum of 6 months and for at least 3 months after sputum cultures become negative.

b. **Nine-month therapy.** Experience with the 9-month regimen has shown it to be effective for pulmonary and most extrapulmonary tuberculosis. It is used for susceptible organisms when INH and rifampin must be given alone or without the initial use of pyrazinamide.

2. **Exceptions. Standard regimens should not be used in the following circumstances:**

   a. **Suspected or proved INH resistance.** This may include patients from countries with a high incidence of primary INH resistance, those failing standard therapy, those who relapse after taking INH without rifampin, and close contacts of a patient with INH-resistant tuberculosis [202].

   b. **When rifampin is not used.** An older regimen should be chosen for these patients when isolates are susceptible (see section **X.D.4**).

   c. **When INH is not used.** Rifampin plus ethambutol for a minimum of 12 months is recommended for susceptible organisms [202].

   d. **When neither INH nor rifampin is used.** Three or four drugs to which the organism is susceptible are required for a minimum of 18 months.

   e. **In the presence of significant hepatic disease.** In such a case, ethambutol plus either INH or rifampin may be chosen. However, studies to date indicate minimal additive hepatic toxicity when patients with lesser degrees of liver disease are treated with INH plus rifampin [202].

   f. **With renal insufficiency.** Pyrazinamide is not recommended in patients with severe renal insufficiency, and blood levels of INH or ethambutol may be required [202]. Drugs to be avoided in patients with any impairment of renal function include streptomycin, kanamycin, capreomycin, and cycloserine.

   g. **When symptoms persist or sputum smears or cultures remain positive after 2 months of therapy,** this indicates treatment failure. Patients should be assessed for adherence and drug resistance. Expert consultation is advised [202].

   h. **When severe illness, miliary tuberculosis, or tuberculous osteomyelitis and arthritis are present** at any age, treatment is extended to a minimum of 12 months [202]. Infants and children with meningeal tuberculosis should be treated for at least 12 months [202]. Infectious disease consultation is advised.

   i. **In immunosuppressed patients.** These patients may receive any of the preceding options for initial and follow-up therapy, including intermittent regimens [169]. However, the **duration of therapy must be determined by the individual response to treatment.** See Chapter 18 for therapy of HIV-infected patients.

3. **MDR tuberculosis** is treated for longer periods, depending on the extent of resistance and the clinical response [206].

4. **Older (traditional) regimens.** Before the advent of the short-course regimens just outlined, combinations used for susceptible organisms had to be given for longer periods of time. Previously, therapy consisted of INH and ethambutol given for at least 18 months; streptomycin was added for the first 1 to 2 months. INH and streptomycin given for the full 18 months of treatment is an acceptable alternative but is potentially more toxic and requires many injections. Either of these regimens may be administered daily or twice weekly.

5. **Pregnancy.** The 9-month regimen should be chosen in a pregnant patient, and ethambutol is added initially to INH and rifampin. Pyrazinamide is not advised for use in the United States during pregnancy because its teratogenic potential is undefined, although it is recommended elsewhere [200,202]. Pyridoxine should be given with any INH-containing regimen. Streptomycin has documented harmful effects on the fetus and should not be used (see **Chapter 27**). Kanamycin, capreomycin, cycloserine, and ethionamide also should be avoided because of their potential risk to the fetus [202]. Breast-feeding is permissible during treatment. Steps should be taken to prevent and detect transmission of maternal tuberculosis to the neonate. See also section **IX**.

E. **Infection control aspects.** Nosocomial tuberculosis is a recognized risk to patients and employees in health-care facilities. Transmission is most likely to occur from patients who have unrecognized pulmonary or laryngeal tuberculosis, are not on effective antituberculous therapy, and have not been placed in proper (respiratory) isolation. Patients who have MDR tuberculosis can remain infectious for prolonged periods, increasing the risk for nosocomial or occupational transmission [207].

1. **Guidelines for preventing the transmission of *M. tuberculosis*in health-care facilities** have been presented in detail elsewhere [207].
2. **Isolation should be continued until the patient is noninfectious** [201].
   - **a.** The length of time required for a patient to become noninfectious after starting antituberculous therapy varies considerably. Isolation should be discontinued only when the patient is on effective therapy, is improving clinically, and has had three consecutive negative sputum smears collected on three separate days [207].
   - **b.** Patients who are improving may go home with positive smear results if public health authorities have completed their household evaluation, no continued contact is at increased risk for tuberculosis (e.g., immunosuppressed persons or infants), the patient agrees not to have any outside contacts with potentially susceptible persons, and arrangements for DOT and follow-up have been completed [201].
   - **c.** Isolation can be discontinued if the diagnosis of tuberculosis is ruled out.

**F. Specific agents** [166,202,208,209]. Although there is significant experience with older agents, new drugs are needed to further improve efficacy, reduce toxicity, and shorten therapy [210].

1. **INH** remains the single most important antituberculous agent. It is bactericidal and penetrates tissue well, including the CNS. It is metabolized primarily by the liver. Doses are reduced only in advanced renal failure, and ideally guided by serum levels.
   - **a. Dosage.** The **usual daily dosage in adults** is 5 mg/kg up to 300 mg orally given once each day. An intramuscular form is available. In life-threatening disease (e.g., meningitis or miliary disease), dosages of 10 mg/kg/day (up to 600 mg/day) often are recommended. The **usual daily dosage in children** is 10 mg/kg once each day (300 mg maximum), although higher doses in meningitis may be used [208]. **Dosages for intermittent regimens are** 15 mg/kg two or three times weekly for adults, and 20 to 30 mg/kg twice weekly for children, up to a maximum of 900 mg [202,208].
   - **b. Side effects**
     - **(1) Hepatitis is the major side effect** of INH. Ten percent or more of patients on INH have transaminase elevations, but only 1% overall have significant hepatitis (deaths have been reported). Risk factors for the development of hepatitis include alcoholic liver disease, increasing over age 30 years, being a woman of a minority race, malnutrition, pregnancy and the post-partum period, and acetaminophen use [209]. There is a fourfold increased risk of hepatitis when INH and rifampin are used together [169].

       **Any patient on INH should be warned about the symptoms of hepatitis.** Mild hepatic dysfunction (e.g., alcoholism) does not preclude the use of INH (and rifampin). If possible, we avoid INH (and rifampin) when baseline transaminases are six to eight times the normal level until these levels improve. Most experts advocate monthly testing of high-risk patients and those with abnormal test results prior to the start of therapy. Liver function tests should be performed if suggestive symptoms occur, and the drug discontinued if hepatitis is present. Monitoring of serial aspartate aminotransferase (AST) and alanine aminotransferase (ALT) levels may help prevent serious sequelae of INH-induced hepatitis prior to symptoms. Elevations of the transaminases more than three to five times normal should lead to consideration of stopping INH [202].
     - **(2) Neurologic toxicity** can occur but is uncommon at the usual INH dose of 5 mg/kg [202]. Peripheral neuropathies usually can be prevented by

the concomitant administration of pyridoxine 10 to 25 mg/day. After an INH-induced neuropathy has occurred, pyridoxine 50 to 100 mg/day can be used as treatment. Routine prophylactic use of **pyridoxine with INH should be reserved for** patients predisposed to neurologic toxicity because of higher INH doses, pregnancy, diabetes, uremia, alcoholism, malnutrition, or prior seizures [181]. Children and adolescents on milk- and meat-deficient diets also should be given pyridoxine [208]. Seizures, optic neuritis, encephalopathies, and the hand-shoulder syndrome rarely occur.

(3) **Hypersensitivity reactions** with fever, rash, and rheumatoid syndromes occur. Positive antinuclear antibodies and lupus erythematosus cell preparations may be seen.

(4) **Concomitant phenytoin use.** Doses of phenytoin may have to be reduced when INH is used because INH delays renal clearance of phenytoin sodium. Levels of phenytoin should be measured and doses adjusted [202].

2. **Rifampin** is bactericidal for *M. tuberculosis,* and it penetrates tissues well, including the CNS. The spectrum of activity, pharmacokinetics, and adverse reactions are discussed in detail in **Chapter 27.**

a. **Dosages**

(1) The **usual daily adult dosage** is 10 mg/kg up to 600 mg once daily (two 300-mg capsules), 1 hour before or 2 hours after meals. In children, the dosage is 10 to 20 mg/kg once daily, not to exceed 600 mg. Dosages are the same for the intermittent regimens [202,208]. In renal failure, the dose is not reduced.

(2) **Fixed-dose combinations.** A combination of rifampin 120 mg, INH 50 mg, and pyrazinamide 300 mg (Rifater) has FDA approval for the initial 2 months of daily therapy. The dosage is four tablets each day for patients weighing 44 kg or less, five tablets for those weighing 45 to 54 kg, and six tablets for those weighing 55 kg or more. The combination of rifampin 300 mg and INH 150 mg (Rifamate) has been licensed in the United States since 1975.

b. **Adverse reactions.** Patients should be warned in advance that their **urine, tears, sweat, and saliva may have a red-orange, harmless discoloration;** soft contact lenses may become permanently discolored [202]. Other side effects include hepatotoxicity, which is the major concern; adverse drug interactions with a variety of agents; immunologic reactions, including hypersensitivity reactions and a flulike illness with sporadic use; and renal failure, thrombocytopenia, or hemolysis, which occur rarely. These are discussed in detail in **Chapter 27.** Rifampin may reduce the effectiveness of oral contraceptives.

The **potential for hepatotoxicity** deserves comment. Rifampin can cause mild liver function abnormalities and, at times, severe hepatitis. Severe hepatotoxicity may develop rapidly after the start of INH in combination with rifampin [169]. Risk for rifampin-induced hepatitis is increased in patients with preexisting alcoholic liver disease [209]. If hepatitis develops in a patient on INH and rifampin, both agents must be stopped. A primarily cholestatic pattern is most likely caused by rifampin, whereas either drug may cause transaminase elevations. See also section **XI.B.3.**

c. **Other rifamycins.** Two other agents related to rifampin are available in the United States. Rifapentine, approved in 1998, is a long-acting analogue of rifampin that can be given once or twice weekly. Rifabutin has less effect on the hepatic cytochrome P-450 system, and is used in place of rifampin for treatment of HIV-infected patients taking protease inhibitors (see Chapter 18).

3. **Ethambutol** is an oral agent that penetrates tissue well. Although CSF levels are 10% to 50% of plasma levels in the presence of meningeal inflammation, they are low relative to the critical concentration of ethambutol. Ethambutol is bacteriostatic.

a. **Dosages.** Tablets are available in 100- and 400-mg strengths. In prolonged therapy, 15 mg/kg to a maximum of 2.5 g, given once daily, usually is recommended. Some authorities use 25 mg/kg/day for no longer than the first 2 months of therapy and then reduce the dosage to 15 mg/kg/day. The twice-weekly dose for children and adults is 50 mg/kg, and for three times per week in adults is 25 to 30 mg/kg, up to a maximum of 2.5 g [202,208]. Doses must be reduced in renal failure.

b. **Side effects.** Ethambutol can cause retrobulbar optic neuritis. The first manifestation may be loss of color vision. Thus, ethambutol should be avoided when possible in children too young to assess color discrimination [208]. This appears to be dose related and rarely occurs when the 15-mg/kg/day regimen is used. Hypersensitivity reactions, hyperuricemia, and gastrointestinal intolerance can occur.

4. **Pyrazinamide** has been used in both initial therapy and retreatment regimens. It is bactericidal and works well in an acid environment and intracellularly [202]. It is well absorbed orally and penetrates the CNS when the meninges are inflamed.

   a. **Dosages.** The usual dosage in children is 20 to 40 mg/kg given once daily, up to a maximum of 2 g [208]. One recommended daily dosing schedule for adults is 1.5 g for those weighing 50 kg or less, 2 g for those weighing 51 to 74 kg, and 2.5 g for those weighing 75 kg or more [166]. Suggested twice weekly doses for adults are 2.5 g for those weighing 50 kg or less, 3 g for those weighing 51 to 74 kg, and 3.5 g for those weighing 75 kg or more; suggested three times weekly doses for adults are 2 g for those weighing 50 kg or less, 2.5 g for those weighing 51 to 74 kg, and 3 g for those weighing 75 kg or more [166]. The twice-weekly dose in children is 50 mg/kg up to a maximum of 2 g/dose [208].

   b. **Toxicity.** Nausea and vomiting are the most common adverse effects. Pyrazinamide does not significantly increase the risk for hepatotoxicity when used for the first 2 months in short-course regimens, and hepatotoxicity is less common with the currently recommended doses [202,209]. Hyperuricemia is common and may be used as an indication of compliance; acute gout is uncommon, although arthralgias may occur in adolescents and adults [202,208].

5. **Streptomycin.** This injectable agent is bactericidal at an alkaline pH and, like other aminoglycosides, poorly penetrates into the CNS.

   a. **Dosages.** The dosage for adults is 15 mg/kg i.m. once daily, up to 1 g; 10 mg/kg up to a maximum of 500 to 750 mg is used for patients over 60 years of age. The daily and twice-weekly dose for children is 20 to 40 mg/kg i.m. up to a maximum of 1 g [208]. The intermittent dose for adults is 25 to 30 mg/kg up to a maximum of 1.5 g for twice-weekly and thrice-weekly regimens [202]. The total amount administered should be less than 120 g [202]. Doses must be reduced in renal failure.

   b. **Side effects.** Ototoxicity is the most serious side effect, and vestibular damage is more common than auditory loss. Renal toxicity is much less common than with other aminoglycosides. Hypersensitivity reactions can occur. (See **Chapter 27.**)

6. **Second-line drugs.** Paraaminosalicylic acid (PAS), cycloserine, ethionamide, capreomycin, kanamycin, amikacin, ciprofloxacin, ofloxacin, levofloxacin, rifabutin, and rifapentine are all useful drugs under appropriate circumstances [166,202,208]. Some are particularly useful for resistant forms of tuberculosis, and in treating atypical mycobacterial infections. Because side effects are common, the reader is advised to seek consultation before using these agents.

G. **Therapy for specific problems**

1. **Smear-negative, culture-negative pulmonary tuberculosis** presents with clinical and radiographic tuberculosis and a positive PPD skin test but negative smear results and cultures. Although their mycobacterial burden is low, these patients, if untreated, have a high rate of disease progression over the ensuing 5 years. Patients with negative smear results should begin standard therapy

while awaiting culture results. If cultures are negative and there is no concern about drug resistance, then it is appropriate to continue INH and rifampin for a total of 4 months of therapy [202].

2. **Extrapulmonary disease.** Extrapulmonary tuberculosis due to susceptible organisms can be treated in the same way as pulmonary tuberculosis if INH and rifampin can be used [166,202]. Extrapulmonary sites usually contain smaller numbers of bacilli than do pulmonary sites, and INH and rifampin penetrate these sites well. Exceptions that require longer therapy have been discussed in section **X.D.2.h,** and infectious disease consultation is advised. HIV infection should be considered in any patient presenting with extrapulmonary tuberculosis (see Chapter 18).
3. **Drug-resistant cases.** Drug resistance should be suspected in patients who relapse after receiving a regimen not containing both INH and rifampin [202]. At least two, and preferably three, new agents should be used pending the results of susceptibility tests. Relapses that follow INH with rifampin in short-course therapy for susceptible organisms often are caused by susceptible organisms and are retreated using the same regimen [202]. Complicating the decision regarding treatment options is evidence that reinfection may occur, particularly in immunosuppressed patients. Treatment of patients who are close contacts of persons with proven drug-resistant tuberculosis, of those who contracted the disease in countries with a high incidence of drug resistance, and of those who fail therapy is best guided by the results of susceptibility tests. See related discussions in sections **X.A** and **X.B.**
4. **HIV-infected patients.** Therapy for tuberculosis should be started whenever acid-fast bacilli are found in patients with HIV infections, because it is impossible to distinguish between *M. tuberculosis* and *M. avium* complex without cultures. The use of rifampin will increase the methadone dose needed to prevent withdrawal symptoms in patients on methadone maintenance. See Chapter 18.
5. **Tuberculosis in pregnancy.** The risks from tuberculosis during pregnancy to the mother and fetus far outweigh the risks from chemotherapy. See section **X.D.5** and section **IX.**
6. **Tuberculosis in children.** Following the principles in adult therapy, short course therapy has been recommended for use in children [202,208].
7. **Therapy in renal failure.** Antituberculous medications cleared by the kidney include streptomycin, kanamycin, capreomycin, ethambutol, and cycloserine. If one needs to use these drugs in renal failure, dosage should be adjusted and levels monitored.

**H. Miscellaneous issues related to therapy**

1. **Adjunctive corticosteroids** have been used in various forms of tuberculosis but are controversial. They are beneficial for outcome in tuberculous meningitis and pericarditis [211]. They are useful in patients with associated adrenal insufficiency, and also may provide a short-term benefit in severely toxic patients (e.g., with disseminated tuberculosis) [211]. Preliminary evidence from endemic areas suggests a benefit in patients with tuberculous peritonitis, but their routine use for this problem is not recommended until any benefit is proven to outweigh risks [212,213].
2. **Hospitalization is often necessary** for diagnostic evaluation and initiation of therapy, particularly for patients with severe disease or suspected drug resistance. Hospitalization also is necessary in severe drug reactions, life-threatening infections, coexisting illnesses requiring hospital care, and the rare circumstance in which there is a special threat to the community. Uncomplicated pulmonary disease occasionally can be managed entirely as an outpatient. See section **X.E** for duration of isolation.
3. **Follow-up cultures.** Guidelines for follow-up are available from state or county health departments. Usually sputum smears and cultures are performed monthly until three specimens test negative, and then cultures monitored at 2- to 3-month intervals during therapy. Patients successfully completing a standard regimen of INH and rifampin for susceptible organisms do not need routine follow-up [202].

4. **Follow-up radiography.** A repeat chest radiograph after 2 to 3 months of therapy helps assess response to treatment. More frequent films may be needed to adequately follow patients whose initial sputum smears were negative. In addition, a film taken at completion of therapy provides a useful baseline for future comparison. Routine annual radiography is not recommended for patients who remain well.
5. **Public health follow-up.** The local public health department should screen contacts of index cases, arrange for DOT, and follow up on discharged patients.

**XI. Treatment of latent tuberculosis.** Patients with a positive intermediate PPD test result but without active disease are considered to have latent tuberculosis, meaning that persistent dormant and viable bacilli are present with the potential for later reactivation. **Both skin testing and treatment for latent tuberculosis are indicated only in patients with a high risk for developing active tuberculosis [181]. This includes those with recent infection and those at increased risk for progression to active disease regardless of the duration of latent infection** (see section **III.C**). Recommendations recently have been updated [181,214,215].

**A. Hepatotoxicity**

1. **INH.** Before one initiates INH, the potential risks of INH-related hepatitis must be considered [see section **X.F.1.b.(1)**]. Hepatotoxicity increases with age and alcohol consumption. Patients with active liver disease, end-stage liver disease, or documented INH-related hepatotoxicity should not receive INH. We withhold INH if transaminases are three times normal or higher in patients with symptoms, and five times normal or higher in patients without symptoms [181].
2. **Rifampin plus pyrazinamide for 2 months.** Severe and fatal liver injury has been reported in HIV-negative patients receiving this regimen [181,214,215]. A few patients were given this regimen after recovering from INH-induced hepatitis. Fatal cases had onset of hepatitis in the second month of treatment.

**B. Current treatment options** may be given using DOT [181,215].

1. **INH for 9 months. This regimen is preferred for most adults and children,** including those with HIV. The daily dose is 5 mg/kg in adults and 10 to 20 mg/kg in children, up to a maximum of 300 mg. The twice-weekly dose is 15 mg/kg in adults and 20 to 40 mg/kg in children, up to a maximum of 900 mg. Pyridoxine (10 to 25 mg/day) may be given simultaneously to selected patients (see section **X.F.1.b.(2)**).
2. **INH for 6 months.** This regimen, dosed as above, provides a shorter option that may be used in selected patients at the discretion of public health authorities and providers. **It is not recommended for children, those with radiographic changes of prior tuberculosis, and HIV-infected patients.**
3. **Rifampin plus pyrazinamide daily for 2 months.** Trials in HIV-infected persons showed that 2 months of this combination is effective and safe. However, the potential for hepatotoxicity precludes its widespread use at present [215]. **Caution is urged,** particularly in those taking other potentially hepatotoxic drugs and those with alcoholism. It should not be used in children, patients with underlying liver disease, or for patients with previous INH-induced hepatitis. It may be considered for patients judged unlikely to complete a longer regimen, if monitoring can be assured. The pyrazinamide dose is 15 to 20 mg/kg and not more than 20 mg/kg, to a maximum of 2 g daily [215]. The rifampin dose is 10 mg/kg to a maximum of 600 mg daily. **Close monitoring is required, and no more than 2 weeks of medication should be dispensed at any one visit.** Treatment should be stopped permanently for transaminase elevation over five times normal without symptoms, any transaminase elevation with hepatitis symptoms, or any bilirubin elevation [215]. Women taking oral contraceptives with rifampin should use an additional form of contraception.
4. **Rifampin daily for 4 months.** This regimen may be used as an alternative for patients intolerant to INH, and for contacts of patients with INH-resistant and rifampin-susceptible isolates. The dose is 10 mg/kg to a maximum of 600 mg daily in adults, and is 10 to 20 mg/kg to a maximum of 600 mg daily in children. Rifabutin in adjusted doses may be substituted for rifampin in HIV-infected patients taking certain antiretroviral agents [181]. However, rifapentine use is

not recommended at this time [181]. Women taking oral contraceptives with rifampin should use an additional form of contraception.

C. **Monitoring.** Patients receiving INH or rifampin should be seen at least monthly [181], and every 2 weeks if receiving rifampin plus pyrazinamide [215].

1. **Patients should be cautioned about the symptoms of hepatitis** (anorexia, nausea, vomiting, malaise, abdominal pain, jaundice, etc.), **and advised to interrupt therapy and seek medical evaluation if these symptoms develop** [181,215]. This is especially important in patients who drink alcoholic beverages daily.
2. **Baseline liver function tests** should be performed in patients whose initial evaluation suggests an underlying liver disorder, those with a known liver disease, those with HIV infection, pregnant women and those within 3 months of delivery, regular users of alcohol, and anyone judged at risk for chronic liver disease [181].
3. **Serial monitoring** of liver tests should be performed in all patients whose baseline levels were elevated, and for patients at risk for hepatotoxicity (see section **XI.C.2**). Transaminases and bilirubin should be checked every other week in patients receiving rifampin plus pyrazinamide [215].
4. **Liver function tests should be checked in patients with hepatitis-like symptoms.**
5. Uric acid may be checked in patients with arthritis while receiving pyrazinamide.

D. **Special considerations**

1. **HIV infection.** The 9-month INH regimen is preferred. HIV-infected persons with negative skin tests do not benefit from treatment for latent tuberculosis unless they are contacts of an active case of tuberculosis [181]. See Chapter 18.
2. **Pregnancy.** Because the risk for active tuberculosis is not increased by pregnancy, many patients can safely wait until after delivery and the early postpartum period. This will prevent the increased risk for INH hepatitis during this time [181]. Women with recent infection and those with HIV, however, should receive treatment for latent tuberculosis during pregnancy [181]. An INH regimen is preferred; rifampin is considered an acceptable alternative despite limited experience [181]. Breast-feeding can continue during treatment. Pyridoxine is indicated for all pregnant and nursing women taking INH, and for nursing infants whose mothers are taking INH [208].
3. **Children who are contacts of contagious tuberculosis** should be evaluated for active disease. If the initial PPD is negative and active disease is excluded, then INH is given for 3 months. At this time the child should be reevaluated for active disease and the PPD repeated. If the repeat PPD remains negative, INH may be stopped [208]. If the repeat PPD is positive and active disease is excluded, then INH is continued to finish a total of 9 months of therapy [208].
4. **Immunosuppressed patients who are contacts of active tuberculosis cases** should receive full treatment for latent tuberculosis (after active disease is excluded) even if repeat skin test results remain negative [181].
5. **Contacts of patients with INH-resistant tuberculosis** that is susceptible to rifampin should receive the 4-month regimen of rifampin (or rifabutin) [181].
6. **Contacts of patients with MDR tuberculosis** will not benefit from treatment with INH or rifampin. Their treatment should be individualized on the basis of susceptibility results. High-risk patients may be given pyrazinamide and ethambutol, or pyrazinamide and a fluoroquinolone for 6 to 12 months; the longer duration should be used for immunosuppressed patients [181]. Pyrazinamide and ethambutol are preferred in children because of the need to avoid long-term treatment with fluoroquinolones in this age group [181]. Consultation with an expert in resistant tuberculosis is advised.

E. **BCG vaccine.** BCG vaccination **has very limited usefulness in the United States** [216].

1. **It is considered for** infants and children with negative skin tests who are repeatedly exposed to infectious cases of tuberculosis and cannot receive preventive therapy or cannot be separated from the index patient, or are repeatedly

exposed to a patient with infectious MDR tuberculosis and they cannot be separated from the index patient [208,216]. BCG vaccine should be considered for health-care workers in settings where exposure and transmission of MDR tuberculosis is likely and this cannot be controlled by other measures [216]. BCG is contraindicated in immunosuppressed hosts (including those with HIV infection) and pregnant women [216].

2. **A history of previous BCG vaccination** does not alter the interpretation of the PPD skin test result or the decision process to give treatment for latent tuberculosis [181].
3. New vaccines being developed include attenuated, subunit, and DNA vaccines. They are needed to help eliminate tuberculosis as a worldwide problem [217].

**XII. Nontuberculous mycobacteria (NTM).** Although NTM are less virulent than *M. tuberculosis,* their importance has been highlighted by the frequent occurrence of *M. avium* complex infections in patients with AIDS (see Chapter 18). It often is difficult for the clinician to determine whether the isolation of these mycobacteria is clinically significant. The ATS has published guidelines to help with their management [218]. A few general points warrant emphasis.

A. **Incidence.** Infections caused by NTM are not reportable in the United States. In association with the AIDS epidemic, NTM isolates became more common than isolates of *M. tuberculosis* [218]. In the pre-AIDS era, approximately 2% to 10% of all mycobacterial infections in the United States were due to NTM.

B. **Classification.** At least 50 species of NTM are considered potential pathogens.
   1. **Bacteriologic methods** for classification traditionally have used growth rates and pigment production (e.g., Runyon group). The time needed for a mycobacterium to grow may provide the first clue to the presence of NTM infection.
   2. NTM also can be **grouped clinically according to their likelihood of causing different types of infection** [219]. For example, *M. avium* complex and *M. kansasii* are common causes of chronic pulmonary infections, whereas *M. fortuitum, M. chelonae, M. abscessus,* and *M. marinum* are common causes for skin infections.
   3. **Molecular methods** will become more important in the future.

C. **Epidemiology and pathogenesis**
   1. **Sources.** Environmental sources are the likely reservoir for NTM infections. These include water for *M. avium* complex, *M. marinum, M. kansasii,* and many rapid growers [218]. Most NTM also have been isolated from soil.
   2. **Transmission. Person-to-person spread does not occur.** Humans presumably acquire disease by inhalation or aspiration, which leads to pulmonary disease; local inoculation, which causes skin or subcutaneous infections; and ingestion, leading to mucosal entry with cervical adenitis or disseminated disease in AIDS.
   3. **There is usually some underlying host defense impairment,** either local or systemic, in patients with NTM infection. Many, but not all, chronic pulmonary infections from *M. avium* complex and *M. kansasii* occur in patients with underlying structural lung disease, and those from rapid growers are associated with esophageal disorders predisposing to aspiration [220]. Cystic fibrosis patients with structural lung changes are also at risk for pulmonary NTM infection. With the exception of the strong association of AIDS with disseminated *M. avium* complex infections, however, specific immunodeficiencies have been postulated but not proven [220].

D. **Diagnosis can be difficult** because these organisms are both saprophytes and true pathogens. Furthermore, underlying disease can account for the presenting symptoms.
   1. **Skin tests.** Antigens similar to the PPD previously prepared for some species showed considerable cross-reactivity and are not readily available. Most experts believe that they **were not useful in diagnosing the individual patient.** However, preliminary results using the *M. avium* sensitin antigen for skin testing are promising [220].
   2. **Acid-fast smears.** One cannot reliably distinguish *M. tuberculosis* from an NTM or identify a specific NTM by smear characteristics.

3. ***Mycobacterium* studies.** Cultures should be performed as discussed in Chapter 25. Commercial probes are available for identifying *M. avium* complex, *M. kansasii,* and *M. gordonae* growing in cultures.
4. **Clinical criteria for the diagnosis of infection** caused by NTM have been published [218]. These are most relevant for pulmonary infections caused by *M. avium* complex, *M. kansasii,* and *M. abscessus* and may not fit the diagnosis of infections caused by other species. The diagnosis of pulmonary NTM infection requires fulfillment of clinical, radiographic, and microbiologic criteria.
   a. **A compatible clinical illness and the exclusion of other diseases.**
   b. **Compatible persistent or progressive changes on chest radiograph or high-resolution chest CT.**
   c. **Supportive microbiological results** consisting of at least three sputums or bronchial washes within 1 year with positive cultures and negative AFB smear results, or two sputums or bronchial washes within 1 year with positive cultures and 1 with a positive AFB smear result; or, a single bronchial wash with at least 2+ growth or at least 2+ AFB smear-positive results; or, a lung biopsy showing any degree of growth, or showing granulomas or AFB on smear with at least one culture-positive sputum or bronchial wash, or a normally sterile site outside the lung showing any growth on biopsy [218]. These criteria are the same for immunosuppressed patients except that 1+ or greater growth is accepted.

E. **Clinical syndromes.** These are briefly summarized tc emphasize the variety of possible clinical presentations [218,219].
1. **Mycobacterial lymphadenitis in children** is usually caused by *M. avium* complex, and less often by *M. scrofulaceum,* which together account for 90% of cases; the remainder are caused by *M. tuberculosis.* However, in adults *M. tuberculosis* causes at least 90% of cases and NTM the remainder.
2. **Pulmonary NTM infections** may not be distinguishable from tuberculosis. Patients usually complain of cough, sputum production, and fatigue but also may have fever, weight loss, and hemoptysis. *M. kansasii* and *M. avium* complex are most frequently involved. Many patients with chronic cavitary changes have underlying COPD, bronchiectasis, or other structural lung disorders. Older patients, often women, without underlying lung disease are more likely to have midzone nodular infiltrates.
3. **Cutaneous infections,** for example from *M. marinum,* can present with slowly enlarging papules or verrucae, which may go on to ulcerate.
4. **Bone and joint infections** may occur as a result of trauma, surgery, or other sources of direct inoculation.
5. **Disseminated disease** similar to miliary tuberculosis may occur and is more likely to be seen in immunocompromised patients, particularly those with AIDS in whom *M. avium* complex can be isolated from blood or bone marrow cultures (see Chapter 18).
6. **Nosocomial NTM infections** often involve rapid growers and are device-related, such as peritoneal and central i.v. catheters and indwelling CNS shunts.

F. **Therapy** is individualized based on the species involved, susceptibility results, and host characteristics. Localized disease (e.g., a single lymph node or skin nodule) usually is treated by complete surgical excision alone. Documented pulmonary infections require multidrug regimens. **Review of recent guidelines and expert consultation is advised.** Treatment of *M. avium* complex in AIDS patients is discussed in Chapter 18.

## REFERENCES

1. Zhang P, Summer WR, Bagby GJ, et al. Innate immunity and pulmonary host defense. *Immunol Rev* 2000;173:39–51.
2. Bartlett JG, Dowell SF, Mandell LA, et al. Practice guidelines for the management of community-acquired pneumonia in adults. Infectious Diseases Society of America. *Clin Infect Dis* 2000;31:347–382.
3. Cunha BA. Community-acquired pneumonia. Diagnostic and therapeutic approach. *Med Clin North Am* 2001;85:43–77.

4. Mandell LA, Marrie TJ, Grossman RF, et al. Canadian guidelines for the initial management of community-acquired pneumonia: an evidence-based update by the Canadian Infectious Diseases Society and the Canadian Thoracic Society. The Canadian Community-Acquired Pneumonia Working Group. *Clin Infect Dis* 2000;31:383–421.
5. McCracken GH Jr. Etiology and treatment of pneumonia. *Pediatr Infect Dis J* 2000;19:373–377.
6. Niederman MS, Mandell LA, Anzueto A, et al. Guidelines for the management of adults with community-acquired pneumonia. Diagnosis, assessment of severity, antimicrobial therapy, and prevention. *Am J Respir Crit Care Med* 2001;163:1730–1754.
7. Afessa B, Green B. Bacterial pneumonia in hospitalized patients with HIV infection: the Pulmonary Complications, ICU Support, and Prognostic Factors of Hospitalized Patients with HIV (PIP) Study. *Chest* 2000;117:1017–1022.
8. McIntosh K. Community-acquired pneumonia in children. *N Engl J Med* 2002;346:429–437.
9. Marrie TJ. Community-acquired pneumonia in the elderly. *Clin Infect Dis* 2000;31:1066–1078.
10. Woodhead M. Pneumonia in the elderly. *J Antimicrob Chemother* 1994;34(suppl A):85–92.
11. Lynch JP 3rd. Hospital-acquired pneumonia: risk factors, microbiology, and treatment. *Chest* 2001;119(suppl):373–384.
12. Cunha BA. Nosocomial pneumonia. Diagnostic and therapeutic considerations. *Med Clin North Am* 2001;85:79–114.
13. Stout JE, Yu VL. Legionellosis. *N Engl J Med* 1997;337:682–687.
14. Katz DS, Leung AN. Radiology of pneumonia. *Clin Chest Med* 1999;20:549–562.
15. Marik PE. Aspiration pneumonitis and aspiration pneumonia. *N Engl J Med* 2001;344:665–671.
16. Edelstein PH. Legionnaires' disease. *Clin Infect Dis* 1993;16:741–747.
17. Kuru T, Lynch JP 3rd. Nonresolving or slowly resolving pneumonia. *Clin Chest Med* 1999;20:623–651.
18. Fein AM. Pneumonia in the elderly: overview of diagnostic and therapeutic approaches. *Clin Infect Dis* 1999;28:726–729.
19. Roson B, Carratala J, Verdaguer R, et al. Prospective study of the usefulness of sputum Gram stain in the initial approach to community-acquired pneumonia requiring hospitalization. *Clin Infect Dis* 2000;31:869–874.
20. Torres A, el-Ebiary M. Invasive diagnostic techniques for pneumonia: protected specimen brush, bronchoalveolar lavage, and lung biopsy methods. *Infect Dis Clin North Am* 1998;12:701–722.
21. Vuori-Holopainen E, Salo E, Saxen H, et al. Etiological diagnosis of childhood pneumonia by use of transthoracic needle aspiration and modern microbiological methods. *Clin Infect Dis* 2002;34:583–590.
22. Grossman RF, Fein A. Evidence-based assessment of diagnostic tests for ventilator-associated pneumonia. Executive summary. *Chest* 2000;117(suppl):177–181.
23. Baughman RP. Protected-specimen brush technique in the diagnosis of ventilator-associated pneumonia. *Chest* 2000;117(suppl):203–206.
24. Fagon JY, Chastre J, Wolff M, et al. Invasive and noninvasive strategies for management of suspected ventilator-associated pneumonia. A randomized trial. *Ann Intern Med* 2000;132:621–630.
25. Mayhall CG. Ventilator-associated pneumonia or not? Contemporary diagnosis. *Emerg Infect Dis* 2001;7:200–204.
26. Torres A, El-Ebiary M. Bronchoscopic BAL in the diagnosis of ventilator-associated pneumonia. *Chest* 2000;117(suppl):198–202.
27. Baselski V, Mason K. Pneumonia in the immunocompromised host: the role of bronchoscopy and newer diagnostic techniques. *Semin Respir Infect* 2000;15:144–161.
28. Campbell GD, Jr. Blinded invasive diagnostic procedures in ventilator-associated pneumonia. *Chest* 2000;117:207–211.
29. Murdoch DR, Laing RT, Mills GD, et al. Evaluation of a rapid immunochromatographic test for detection of *Streptococcus pneumoniae* antigen in urine samples from adults with community-acquired pneumonia. *J Clin Microbiol* 2001;39:3495–3498.

30. Ieven M, Goossens H. Relevance of nucleic acid amplification techniques for diagnosis of respiratory tract infections in the clinical laboratory. *Clin Microbiol Rev* 1997;10:242–256.
31. Tillotson JR, Finland M. Bacterial colonization and clinical superinfection of the respiratory tract complicating antibiotic treatment of pneumonia. *J Infect Dis* 1969;119:597–624.
32. Heffelfinger JD, Dowell SF, Jorgensen JH, et al. Management of community-acquired pneumonia in the era of pneumococcal resistance: a report from the Drug-Resistant *Streptococcus pneumoniae* Therapeutic Working Group. *Arch Intern Med* 2000;160:1399–1408.
33. Fine MJ, Auble TE, Yealy DM, et al. A prediction rule to identify low-risk patients with community-acquired pneumonia. *N Engl J Med* 1997;336:243–250.
34. Davidson R, Cavalcanti R, Brunton JL, et al. Resistance to levofloxacin and failure of treatment of pneumococcal pneumonia. *N Engl J Med* 2002;346:747–750.
35. Waterer GW, Somes GW, Wunderink RG. Monotherapy may be suboptimal for severe bacteremic pneumococcal pneumonia. *Arch Intern Med* 2001;161:1837–1842.
36. Plouffe J, Schwartz DB, Kolokathis A, et al. Clinical efficacy of intravenous followed by oral azithromycin monotherapy in hospitalized patients with community-acquired pneumonia. The Azithromycin Intravenous Clinical Trials Group. *Antimicrob Agents Chemother* 2000;44:1796–1802.
37. Vergis EN, Indorf A, File TM Jr, et al. Azithromycin vs. cefuroxime plus erythromycin for empirical treatment of community-acquired pneumonia in hospitalized patients: a prospective, randomized, multicenter trial. *Arch Intern Med* 2000;160:1294–1300.
38. McGehee JL, Podnos SD, Pierce AK, et al. Treatment of pneumonia in patients at risk of infection with gram-negative bacilli. *Am J Med* 1988;84:597–602.
39. Prevention of pneumococcal disease: recommendations of the Advisory Committee on Immunization Practices (ACIP). *MMWR* 1997;46:1–24.
40. Nuorti JP, Butler JC, Farley MM, et al. Cigarette smoking and invasive pneumococcal disease. Active Bacterial Core Surveillance Team. *N Engl J Med* 2000;342:681–689.
41. Nuorti JP, Butler JC, Gelling L, et al. Epidemiologic relation between HIV and invasive pneumococcal disease in San Francisco County, California. *Ann Intern Med* 2000;132:182–190.
42. Musher DM. Infections caused by *Streptococcus pneumoniae:* clinical spectrum, pathogenesis, immunity, and treatment. *Clin Infect Dis* 1992;14:801–807.
43. Bochud PY, Moser F, Erard P, et al. Community-acquired pneumonia. A prospective outpatient study. *Medicine (Baltimore)* 2001;80:75–87.
44. Feikin DR, Schuchat A, Kolczak M, et al. Mortality from invasive pneumococcal pneumonia in the era of antibiotic resistance, 1995–1997. *Am J Public Health* 2000;90:223–229.
45. Austrian R, Gold J. Pneumococcal bacteremia with special reference to bacteremic pneumococcal pneumonia. *Ann Intern Med* 1964;60:759–776.
46. Whitney CG, Farley MM, Hadler J, et al. Increasing prevalence of multidrug-resistant Streptococcus pneumoniae in the United States. *N Engl J Med* 2000;343:1917–1924.
47. Doern GV, Heilmann KP, Huynh HK, et al. Antimicrobial resistance among clinical isolates of *Streptococcus pneumoniae* in the United States during 1999–2000, including a comparison of resistance rates since 1994–1995. *Antimicrob Agents Chemother* 2001;45:1721–1729.
48. Kellner JD, Gibb AP, Zhang J, et al. Household transmission of *Streptococcus pneumoniae,* Alberta, Canada. *Emerg Infect Dis* 1999;5:154–158.
49. Resistance of *Streptococcus pneumoniae* to fluoroquinolones—United States, 1995–1999. *MMWR* 2001;50:800–804.
50. Urban C, Rahman N, Zhao X, et al. Fluoroquinolone-resistant *Streptococcus pneumoniae* associated with levofloxacin therapy. *J Infect Dis* 2001;184:794–798.
51. Giebink GS. The prevention of pneumococcal disease in children. *N Engl J Med* 2001;345:1177–1183.
52. Poland GA. The prevention of pneumococcal disease by vaccines: promises and challenges. *Infect Dis Clin North Am* 2001;15:97–122.
53. American Academy of Pediatrics. Pneumococcal infections. In: Pickering LK, ed. *2000*

*Red Book: Report of the Committee on Infectious Diseases* 25th ed. Elk Grove Village, IL: American Academy of Pediatrics, 2000:452–460.

54. Preventing pneumococcal disease among infants and young children. Recommendations of the Advisory Committee on Immunization Practices (ACIP). *MMWR* 2000;49:1–35.
55. Shapiro ED, Berg AT, Austrian R, et al. The protective efficacy of polyvalent pneumococcal polysaccharide vaccine. *N Engl J Med* 1991;325:1453–1460.
56. Eskola J, Kilpi T, Palmu A, et al. Efficacy of a pneumococcal conjugate vaccine against acute otitis media. *N Engl J Med* 2001;344:403–409.
57. Mier L, Dreyfuss D, Darchy B, et al. Is penicillin G an adequate initial treatment for aspiration pneumonia? A prospective evaluation using a protected specimen brush and quantitative cultures. *Intens Care Med* 1993;19:279–284.
58. Bartlett JG. Anaerobic bacterial infections of the lung and pleural space. *Clin Infect Dis* 1993;16(suppl 4):248–255.
59. Finegold SM, Wexler HM. Present studies of therapy for anaerobic infections. *Clin Infect Dis* 1996;23(suppl 1):9–14.
60. Marina M, Strong CA, Civen R, et al. Bacteriology of anaerobic pleuropulmonary infections: preliminary report. *Clin Infect Dis* 1993;16(suppl 4):256–262.
61. Rasmussen BA, Bush K, Tally FP. Antimicrobial resistance in anaerobes. *Clin Infect Dis* 1997;24(suppl 1):110–120.
62. Snydman DR, McDermott L, Cuchural GJ Jr, et al. Analysis of trends in antimicrobial resistance patterns among clinical isolates of *Bacteroides fragilis* group species from 1990 to 1994. *Clin Infect Dis* 1996;23(suppl 1):54–65.
63. Dreyfuss D, Mier L. Aspiration pneumonia. *N Engl J Med* 2001;344:1868–1869; discussion 1869–1870.
64. Kollef MH. The prevention of ventilator-associated pneumonia. *N Engl J Med* 1999;340:627–634.
65. Centers for Disease Control and Prevention. Guidelines for prevention of nosocomial pneumonia. *MMWR* 1997;46:1–79.
66. Cook D, Guyatt G, Marshall J, et al. A comparison of sucralfate and ranitidine for the prevention of upper gastrointestinal bleeding in patients requiring mechanical ventilation. Canadian Critical Care Trials Group. *N Engl J Med* 1998;338:791–797.
67. Morehead RS, Pinto SJ. Ventilator-associated pneumonia. *Arch Intern Med* 2000;160:1926–1936.
68. Eveloff SE, Braman SS. Acute respiratory failure and death caused by fulminant *Haemophilus influenzae* pneumonia. *Am J Med* 1990;88:683–685.
69. Rello J, Ricart M, Ausina V, et al. Pneumonia due to *Haemophilus influenzae* among mechanically ventilated patients. Incidence, outcome, and risk factors. *Chest* 1992;102:1562–1565.
70. Shann F. *Haemophilus influenzae* pneumonia: type b or non-type b? *Lancet* 1999;354:1488–1490.
71. Farley MM, Stephens DS, Brachman PS Jr, et al. Invasive *Haemophilus influenzae* disease in adults. A prospective, population-based surveillance. CDC Meningitis Surveillance Group. *Ann Intern Med* 1992;116:806–812.
72. Carpenter JL. *Klebsiella* pulmonary infections: occurrence at one medical center and review. *Rev Infect Dis* 1990;12:672–682.
73. Hatchette TF, Gupta R, Marrie TJ. *Pseudomonas aeruginosa* community-acquired pneumonia in previously healthy adults: case report and review of the literature. *Clin Infect Dis* 2000;31:1349–1356.
74. File TM Jr, Tan JS, Plouffe JF. The role of atypical pathogens: *Mycoplasma pneumoniae, Chlamydia pneumoniae,* and *Legionella pneumophila* in respiratory infection. *Infect Dis Clin North Am* 1998;12:569–592.
75. Marrie TJ, Peeling RW, Fine MJ, et al. Ambulatory patients with community-acquired pneumonia: the frequency of atypical agents and clinical course. *Am J Med* 1996;101:508–515.
76. Marrie TJ. Bacteremic community-acquired pneumonia due to viridans group streptococci. *Clin Invest Med* 1993;16:38–44.
77. Outbreak of community-acquired pneumonia caused by *Mycoplasma pneumoniae*—Colorado, 2000. *MMWR* 2001;50:227–230.

78. Klausner JD, Passaro D, Rosenberg J, et al. Enhanced control of an outbreak of *Mycoplasma pneumoniae* pneumonia with azithromycin prophylaxis. *J Infect Dis* 1998;177:161–166.
79. Roifman CM, Rao CP, Lederman HM, et al. Increased susceptibility to *Mycoplasma* infection in patients with hypogammaglobulinemia. *Am J Med* 1986;80:590–594.
80. Clyde WA, Jr. Clinical overview of typical *Mycoplasma pneumoniae* infections. *Clin Infect Dis* 1993;17(suppl 1):32–36.
81. Taylor-Robinson D. Infections due to species of *Mycoplasma* and *Ureaplasma*: an update. *Clin Infect Dis* 1996;23:671–682; quiz 683–674.
82. Macfarlane JT, Miller AC, Roderick Smith WH, et al. Comparative radiographic features of community acquired Legionnaires' disease, pneumococcal pneumonia, mycoplasma pneumonia, and psittacosis. *Thorax* 1984;39:28–33.
83. Reittner P, Muller NL, Heyneman L, et al. Mycoplasma pneumoniae pneumonia: radiographic and high-resolution CT features in 28 patients. *AJR* 2000;174:37–41.
84. Thacker WL, Talkington DF. Analysis of complement fixation and commercial enzyme immunoassays for detection of antibodies to *Mycoplasma pneumoniae* in human serum. *Clin Diagn Lab Immunol* 2000;7:778–780.
85. Grondahl B, Puppe W, Hoppe A, et al. Rapid identification of nine microorganisms causing acute respiratory tract infections by single-tube multiplex reverse-transcription PCR: feasibility study. *J Clin Microbiol* 1999;37:1–7.
86. Plouffe JF. Importance of atypical pathogens of community-acquired pneumonia. *Clin Infect Dis* 2000;31(suppl 2):35–39.
87. Kauppinen M, Saikku P. Pneumonia due to *Chlamydia pneumoniae*: prevalence, clinical features, diagnosis, and treatment. *Clin Infect Dis* 1995;21(suppl 3):244–252.
88. Kuo CC, Jackson LA, Campbell LA, et al. *Chlamydia pneumoniae* (TWAR). *Clin Microbiol Rev* 1995;8:451–461.
89. Medical Letter. The Choice of Antibacterial Drugs. *Med Lett Drugs Ther* 2001;43: 69–78.
90. Maurin M, Raoult D. Q fever. *Clin Microbiol Rev* 1999;12:518–553.
91. Marrie TJ. *Coxiella burnetii* (Q fever) pneumonia. *Clin Infect Dis* 1995;21(suppl 3): 253–264.
92. Raoult D, Marrie T. Q fever. *Clin Infect Dis* 1995;20:489–495; quiz 496.
93. Fournier PE, Marrie TJ, Raoult D. Diagnosis of Q fever. *J Clin Microbiol* 1998;36:1823–1834.
94. Marrie TJ. *Coxiella burnetii* (Q Fever). In: Mandell GL, Bennett JE, Dolin R, eds. *Principles and practice of infectious diseases,* 5th ed. Philadelphia: Churchill Livingstone, 2000:2043–2050.
95. Muder RR. Other *Legionella* species. In: Mandell GL, Bennett JE, Dolin R, eds. *Principles and practice of infectious diseases,* 5th ed. Philadelphia: Churchill Livingstone, 2000:2435–2441.
96. Waterer GW, Baselski VS, Wunderink RG. Legionella and community-acquired pneumonia: a review of current diagnostic tests from a clinician's viewpoint. *Am J Med* 2001;110:41–48.
97. Yu VL. *Legionella pneumophila* (Legionnaires' disease). In: Mandell GL, Bennett JE, Dolin R, eds. *Principles and practice of infectious diseases,* 5th ed. Philadelphia: Churchill Livingstone, 2000:2424–2435.
98. Legionnaires' disease associated with potting soil—California, Oregon, and Washington, May–June 2000. *MMWR* 2000;49:777–778.
99. Fields BS, Haupt T, Davis JP, et al. Pontiac fever due to *Legionella micdadei* from a whirlpool spa: possible role of bacterial endotoxin. *J Infect Dis* 2001;184:1289–1292.
100. Muder RR, Stout JE, Yu VL. Nosocomial *Legionella micdadei* infection in transplant patients: fortune favors the prepared mind. *Am J Med* 2000;108:346–348.
101. Fiore AE, Nuorti JP, Levine OS, et al. Epidemic Legionnaires' disease two decades later: old sources, new diagnostic methods. *Clin Infect Dis* 1998;26:426–433.
102. Boshuizen HC, Neppelenbroek SE, van Vliet H, et al. Subclinical *Legionella* infection in workers near the source of a large outbreak of legionnaires disease. *J Infect Dis* 2001;184:515–518.

103. Marrie TJ. Diagnosis of legionellaceae as a cause of community-acquired pneumonia—"... continue to treat first and not bother to ask questions later"—not a good idea. *Am J Med* 2001;110:73–75.
104. Edelstein PH. Antimicrobial chemotherapy for Legionnaires disease: time for a change. *Ann Intern Med* 1998;129:328–330.
105. Fabbri M, Maslow MJ. Hantavirus pulmonary syndrome in the United States. *Curr Infect Dis Rep* 2001;3:258–265.
106. Hantavirus pulmonary syndrome—Vermont, 2000. *MMWR* 2001;50:603–605.
107. Padula PJ, Edelstein A, Miguel SD, et al. Hantavirus pulmonary syndrome outbreak in Argentina: molecular evidence for person-to-person transmission of Andes virus. *Virology* 1998;241:323–330.
108. Baughman RP. The lung in the immunocompromised patient. Infectious complications part 1. *Respiration* 1999;66:95–109.
109. Collin BA, Ramphal R. Pneumonia in the compromised host including cancer patients and transplant patients. *Infect Dis Clin North Am* 1998;12:781–805.
110. Cunha BA. Pneumonias in the compromised host. *Infect Dis Clin North Am* 2001;15:591–612.
111. Santamauro JT, Mangino DA, Stover DE. The lung in the immunocompromised host: diagnostic methods. *Respiration* 1999;66:481–490.
112. Tamm M. The lung in the immunocompromised patient. Infectious complications part 2. *Respiration* 1999;66:199–207.
113. Betts RF, Freeman RB, Douglas RG Jr, et al. Transmission of cytomegalovirus infection with renal allograft. *Kidney Int* 1975;8:385–392.
114. Crawford SW. Noninfectious lung disease in the immunocompromised host. *Respiration* 1999;66:385–395.
115. Hospital-acquired pneumonia in adults: diagnosis, assessment of severity, initial antimicrobial therapy, and preventive strategies. A consensus statement, American Thoracic Society, November 1995. *Am J Respir Crit Care Med* 1996;153:1711–1725.
115a. Chastre J, Fagon JY. Ventilator-associated pneumonia. *Am J Respir Crit Care Med* 2002;165:867–903.
116. Lentino JR. Nosocomial pneumonia: more than just ventilator-associated. *Curr Infect Dis Rep* 2001;3:266–273.
117. Marik PE, Careau P. The role of anaerobes in patients with ventilator-associated pneumonia and aspiration pneumonia: a prospective study. *Chest* 1999;115:178–183.
118. Arozullah AM, Khuri SF, Henderson WG, et al. Development and validation of a multifactorial risk index for predicting postoperative pneumonia after major noncardiac surgery. *Ann Intern Med* 2001;135:847–857.
119. Wunderink RG. Clinical criteria in the diagnosis of ventilator-associated pneumonia. *Chest* 2000;117(suppl):191–194.
120. Wunderink RG. Radiologic diagnosis of ventilator-associated pneumonia. *Chest* 2000;117:188–190.
121. Rello J, Paiva JA, Baraibar J, et al. International Conference for the Development of Consensus on the Diagnosis and Treatment of Ventilator-Associated Pneumonia. *Chest* 2001;120:955–970.
122. Cook D, Mandell L. Endotracheal aspiration in the diagnosis of ventilator-associated pneumonia. *Chest* 2000;117(suppl):195–197.
123. Fiel S. Guidelines and critical pathways for severe hospital-acquired pneumonia. *Chest* 2001;119(suppl):412–418.
124. Bergmans DC, Bonten MJ, Gaillard CA, et al. Prevention of ventilator-associated pneumonia by oral decontamination: a prospective, randomized, double-blind, placebo-controlled study. *Am J Respir Crit Care Med* 2001;164:382–388.
125. Pittet D, Eggimann P, Rubinovitch B. Prevention of ventilator-associated pneumonia by oral decontamination: just another SDD study? *Am J Respir Crit Care Med* 2001;164:338–339.
126. McCracken GH Jr. Diagnosis and management of pneumonia in children. *Pediatr Infect Dis J* 2000;19:924–928.
127. Nelson JD. Community-acquired pneumonia in children: guidelines for treatment. *Pediatr Infect Dis J* 2000;19:251–253.

128. American Academy of Pediatrics. Antimicrobial agents and related therapy. In: Pickering LK, ed. *2000 Red Book: Report of the Committee on Infectious Diseases,* 25th ed. Elk Grove Village, IL: American Academy of Pediatrics, 2000:645–646.
129. Gonzalez C, Rubio M, Romero-Vivas J, et al. Bacteremic pneumonia due to *Staphylococcus aureus:* A comparison of disease caused by methicillin-resistant and methicillin-susceptible organisms. *Clin Infect Dis* 1999;29:1171–1177.
130. Lane HC, Fauci AS. Bioterrorism on the home front: a new challenge for American medicine. *JAMA* 2001;286:2595–2597.
131. Dixon TC, Meselson M, Guillemin J, et al. Anthrax. *N Engl J Med* 1999;341:815–826.
132. Inglesby TV, Henderson DA, O'Toole T, et al. Anthrax as a biological weapon 2002: updated recommendations for management. *JAMA* 2002;287:2236–2252.
133. Meselson M, Guillemin J, Hugh-Jones M, et al. The Sverdlovsk anthrax outbreak of 1979. *Science* 1994;266:1202–1208.
134. Borio L, Frank D, Mani V, et al. Death due to bioterrorism-related inhalational anthrax: report of 2 patients. *JAMA* 2001;286:2554–2559.
135. Jernigan JA, Stephens DS, Ashford DA, et al. Bioterrorism-related inhalational anthrax: the first 10 cases reported in the United States. *Emerg Infect Dis* 2001;7:933–944.
136. Mayer TA, Bersoff-Matcha S, Murphy C, et al. Clinical presentation of inhalational anthrax following bioterrorism exposure: report of 2 surviving patients. *JAMA* 2001;286:2549–2553.
137. Considerations for distinguishing influenza-like illness from inhalational anthrax. *MMWR* 2001;50:984–986.
138. Update: Investigation of bioterrorism-related anthrax and interim guidelines for clinical evaluation of persons with possible anthrax. *MMWR* 2001;50:941–948.
139. Interim guidelines for investigation of and response to *Bacillus anthracis* exposures. *MMWR* 2001;50:987–990.
140. Update: Investigation of bioterrorism-related anthrax and interim guidelines for exposure management and antimicrobial therapy, October 2001. *MMWR* 2001;50:909–919.
141. Update: Interim recommendations for antimicrobial prophylaxis for children and breastfeeding mothers and treatment of children with anthrax. *MMWR* 2001;50:1014–1016.
142. Update: Investigation of bioterrorism-related anthrax and adverse events from antimicrobial prophylaxis. *MMWR* 2001;50:973–976.
143. Update: Investigation of anthrax associated with intentional exposure and interim public health guidelines, October 2001. *MMWR* 2001;50:889–893.
144. Updated recommendations for antimicrobial prophylaxis among asymptomatic pregnant women after exposure to *Bacillus anthracis. MMWR* 2001;50:960.
145. Additional options for preventive treatment for persons exposed to inhalational anthrax. *MMWR* 2001;50:1142, 1151.
146. Christopher GW, Cieslak TJ, Pavlin JA, et al. Biological warfare. A historical perspective. *JAMA* 1997;278:412–417.
147. Inglesby TV, Dennis DT, Henderson DA, et al. Plague as a biological weapon: medical and public health management. Working Group on Civilian Biodefense. *JAMA* 2000;283:2281–2290.
148. Dennis DT, Inglesby TV, Henderson DA, et al. Tularemia as a biological weapon: medical and public health management. *JAMA* 2001;285:2763–2773.
149. Cross JT Jr, Penn RL. *Francisella tularensis* (tularemia). In: Mandell GL, Bennett JE, Dolin R, eds. *Principles and practice of infectious diseases,* 5th ed. Philadelphia: Churchill Livingstone, 2000:2393–2402.
150. Feldman KA, Enscore RE, Lathrop SL, et al. An outbreak of primary pneumonic tularemia on Martha's Vineyard. *N Engl J Med* 2001;345:1601–1606.
151. Light RW, Rodriguez RM. Management of parapneumonic effusions. *Clin Chest Med* 1998;19:373–382.
152. Colice GL, Curtis A, Deslauriers J, et al. Medical and surgical treatment of parapneumonic effusions: an evidence-based guideline. *Chest* 2000;118:1158–1171.
153. Bryant RE, Salmon CJ. Pleural effusion and empyema. In: Mandell GL, Bennett

JE, Dolin R, eds. *Principles and practice of infectious diseases,* 5th ed. Philadelphia: Churchill Livingstone, 2000:743–750.
154. Heffner JE. Infection of the pleural space. *Clin Chest Med* 1999;20:607–622.
155. Bryant RE, Salmon CJ. Pleural empyema. *Clin Infect Dis* 1996;22:747–762; quiz 763–744.
156. Penner C, Maycher B, Long R. Pulmonary gangrene. A complication of bacterial pneumonia. *Chest* 1994;105:567–573.
157. Peters JI, Kubitschek KR, Gotlieb MS, et al. Lung bullae with air-fluid levels. *Am J Med* 1987;82:759–763.
158. Finegold SM. Lung abscess. In: Mandell GL, Bennett JE, Dolin R, eds. *Principles and practice of infectious diseases,* 5th ed. Philadelphia: Churchill Livingstone, 2000:751–755.
159. Boon ES, Grupa N, Langenberg CJ, et al. Concealed lung abscess in critically ill, mechanically ventilated patients. *Neth J Med* 1996;48:100–104.
160. Groskin SA, Panicek DM, Ewing DK, et al. Bacterial lung abscess: a review of the radiographic and clinical features of 50 cases. *J Thorac Imaging* 1991;6:62–67.
161. Hammond JM, Potgieter PD, Hanslo D, et al. The etiology and antimicrobial susceptibility patterns of microorganisms in acute community-acquired lung abscess. *Chest* 1995;108:937–941.
162. Sosenko A, Glassroth J. Fiberoptic bronchoscopy in the evaluation of lung abscesses. *Chest* 1985;87:489–494.
163. Erasmus JJ, McAdams HP, Rossi S, et al. Percutaneous management of intrapulmonary air and fluid collections. *Radiol Clin North Am* 2000;38:385–393.
164. Diagnostic Standards and Classification of Tuberculosis in Adults and Children. This official statement of the American Thoracic Society and the Centers for Disease Control and Prevention was adopted by the ATS Board of Directors, July 1999. This statement was endorsed by the Council of the Infectious Disease Society of America, September 1999. *Am J Respir Crit Care Med* 2000;161:1376–1395.
165. Rao VK, Iademarco EP, Fraser VJ, et al. Delays in the suspicion and treatment of tuberculosis among hospitalized patients. *Ann Intern Med* 1999;130:404–411.
166. Small PM, Fujiwara PI. Management of tuberculosis in the United States. *N Engl J Med* 2001;345:189–200.
167. Centers for Disease Control and Prevention. Recommendations for prevention and control of tuberculosis among foreign-born persons. Report of the Working Group on Tuberculosis among Foreign-Born Persons. *MMWR* 1998;47:1–29.
168. Progress toward the elimination of tuberculosis—United States, 1998. *MMWR* 1999;48:732–736.
169. Haas DW. *Mycobacterium tuberculosis.* In: Mandell GL, Bennett JE, Dolin R, eds. *Principles and practice of infectious diseases,* 5th ed. Philadelphia: Churchill Livingstone, 2000:2576–2607.
170. Flynn JL, Chan J. Tuberculosis: latency and reactivation. *Infect Immun* 2001;69:4195–4201.
171. Shafer RW, Singh SP, Larkin C, et al. Exogenous reinfection with multidrug-resistant *Mycobacterium tuberculosis* in an immunocompetent patient. *Tuber Lung Dis* 1995;76:575–577.
172. Fine PE, Small PM. Exogenous reinfection in tuberculosis. *N Engl J Med* 1999; 341:1226–1227.
173. Small PM, Shafer RW, Hopewell PC, et al. Exogenous reinfection with multidrug-resistant *Mycobacterium tuberculosis* in patients with advanced HIV infection. *N Engl J Med* 1993;328:1137–1144.
174. van Rie A, Warren R, Richardson M, et al. Exogenous reinfection as a cause of recurrent tuberculosis after curative treatment. *N Engl J Med* 1999;341:1174–1179.
175. Ellner JJ, Hirsch CS, Whalen CC. Correlates of protective immunity to *Mycobacterium tuberculosis* in humans. *Clin Infect Dis* 2000;30(suppl 3):279–282.
176. Flynn JL, Chan J. Immunology of tuberculosis. *Annu Rev Immunol* 2001;19:93–129.
177. Keane J, Gershon S, Wise RP, et al. Tuberculosis associated with infliximab, a tumor necrosis factor alpha-neutralizing agent. *N Engl J Med* 2001;345:1098–1104.
178. Bishai W. Tuberculosis transmission—rogue pathogen or rogue patient? *Am J Respir Crit Care Med* 2001;164:1104–1105.

179. Valway SE, Sanchez MP, Shinnick TF, et al. An outbreak involving extensive transmission of a virulent strain of *Mycobacterium tuberculosis. N Engl J Med* 1998;338:633–639.
180. Zhang M, Gong J, Yang Z, et al. Enhanced capacity of a widespread strain of *Mycobacterium tuberculosis* to grow in human macrophages. *J Infect Dis* 1999;179:1213–1217.
181. Targeted tuberculin testing and treatment of latent tuberculosis infection. This official statement of the American Thoracic Society (ATS) was adopted by the ATS Board of Directors, July 1999. This is a Joint Statement of the ATS and the Centers for Disease Control and Prevention (CDC). This statement was endorsed by the Council of the Infectious Diseases Society of America (IDSA), September 1999, and the sections of this statement as it relates to infants and children were endorsed by the American Academy of Pediatrics (AAP), August 1999. *Am J Respir Crit Care Med* 2000;161(suppl):221–247.
182. Klotz SA, Penn RL. Acid-fast staining of urine and gastric contents is an excellent indicator of mycobacterial disease. *Am Rev Respir Dis* 1987;136:1197–1198.
183. Behr MA, Warren SA, Salamon H, et al. Transmission of *Mycobacterium tuberculosis* from patients smear-negative for acid-fast bacilli. *Lancet* 1999;353:444–449.
184. Schluger NW. Changing approaches to the diagnosis of tuberculosis. *Am J Respir Crit Care Med* 2001;164:2020–2024.
185. Update: Nucleic acid amplification tests for tuberculosis. *MMWR* 2000;49:593–594.
186. Gennaro ML. Immunologic diagnosis of tuberculosis. *Clin Infect Dis* 2000;30(suppl 3): 243–246.
187. Morehead RS. Tuberculosis of the pleura. *South Med J* 1998;91:630–636.
188. Matchaba PT, Volmink J. Steroids for treating tuberculous pleurisy. *Cochrane Database Syst Rev* 2000;2:CD001876.
189. Wyser C, Walzl G, Smedema JP, et al. Corticosteroids in the treatment of tuberculous pleurisy. A double- blind, placebo-controlled, randomized study. *Chest* 1996;110:333–338.
190. Epstein DM, Kline LR, Albelda SM, et al. Tuberculous pleural effusions. *Chest* 1987;91:106–109.
191. Villegas MV, Labrada LA, Saravia NG. Evaluation of polymerase chain reaction, adenosine deaminase, and interferon-gamma in pleural fluid for the differential diagnosis of pleural tuberculosis. *Chest* 2000;118:1355–1364.
192. Shriner KA, Mathisen GE, Goetz MB. Comparison of mycobacterial lymphadenitis among persons infected with human immunodeficiency virus and seronegative controls. *Clin Infect Dis* 1992;15:601–605.
193. Ayed AK, Behbehani NA. Diagnosis and treatment of isolated tuberculous mediastinal lymphadenopathy in adults. *Eur J Surg* 2001;167:334–338.
194. Singh KK, Muralidhar M, Kumar A, et al. Comparison of in house polymerase chain reaction with conventional techniques for the detection of *Mycobacterium tuberculosis* DNA in granulomatous lymphadenopathy. *J Clin Pathol* 2000;53:355–361.
195. Shakil AO, Korula J, Kanel GC, et al. Diagnostic features of tuberculous peritonitis in the absence and presence of chronic liver disease: a case control study. *Am J Med* 1996;100:179–185.
196. Talwani R, Horvath JA. Tuberculous peritonitis in patients undergoing continuous ambulatory peritoneal dialysis: case report and review. *Clin Infect Dis* 2000;31:70–75.
197. Stout JE, Woods CW, Alvarez AA, et al. *Mycobacterium bovis* peritonitis mimicking ovarian cancer in a young woman. *Clin Infect Dis* 2001;33:14–16.
198. Packham S. Tuberculosis in the elderly. *Gerontology* 2001;47:175–179.
199. Rajagopalan S. Tuberculosis and aging: a global health problem. *Clin Infect Dis* 2001;33:1034–1039.
200. Ormerod P. Tuberculosis in pregnancy and the puerperium. *Thorax* 2001;56:494–499.
201. Horsburgh CR Jr, Feldman S, Ridzon R. Practice guidelines for the treatment of tuberculosis. *Clin Infect Dis* 2000;31:633–639.
202. Bass JB Jr, Farer LS, Hopewell PC, et al. Treatment of tuberculosis and tuberculosis infection in adults and children. American Thoracic Society and the Centers for Disease Control and Prevention. *Am J Respir Crit Care Med* 1994;149:1359–1374.

203. Centers for Disease Control and Prevention. Reported tuberculosis in the United States, 2000. *www.cdc.gov/nchstp/tb/surv/surv2000/*, 2001. Accessed December 1, 2001.
204. Espinal MA, Laszlo A, Simonsen L, et al. Global trends in resistance to antituberculosis drugs. World Health Organization-International Union against Tuberculosis and Lung Disease Working Group on Anti-Tuberculosis Drug Resistance Surveillance. *N Engl J Med* 2001;344:1294–1303.
205. Hannan MM, Desmond EP, Morlock GP, et al. Pyrazinamide-monoresistant *Mycobacterium tuberculosis* in the United States. *J Clin Microbiol* 2001;39:647–650.
206. Tahaoglu K, Torun T, Sevim T, et al. The treatment of multidrug-resistant tuberculosis in Turkey. *N Engl J Med* 2001;345:170–174.
207. Centers for Disease Control and Prevention. Guidelines for preventing the transmission of *Mycobacterium tuberculosis* in health-care facilities, 1994. *MMWR* 1994;43:1–132.
208. American Academy of Pediatrics. Tuberculosis. In: Pickering LK, ed. *2000 Red Book: Report of the Committee on Infectious Diseases,* 25th ed. Elk Grove Village, IL: American Academy of Pediatrics, 2000:593–613.
209. Wallace RJ Jr. Antimycobacterial agents. In: Mandell GL, Bennett JE, Dolin R, eds. *Principles and practice of infectious diseases,* 5th ed. Philadelphia: Churchill Livingstone, 2000:436–448.
210. O'Brien RJ, Nunn PP. The need for new drugs against tuberculosis. Obstacles, opportunities, and next steps. *Am J Respir Crit Care Med* 2001;163:1055–1058.
211. Dooley DP, Carpenter JL, Rademacher S. Adjunctive corticosteroid therapy for tuberculosis: a critical reappraisal of the literature. *Clin Infect Dis* 1997;25:872–887.
212. Alrajhi AA, Halim MA, al-Hokail A, et al. Corticosteroid treatment of peritoneal tuberculosis. *Clin Infect Dis* 1998;27:52–56.
213. Haas DW. Is adjunctive corticosteroid therapy indicated during tuberculous peritonitis? *Clin Infect Dis* 1998;27:57–58.
214. Fatal and severe hepatitis associated with rifampin and pyrazinamide for the treatment of latent tuberculosis infection—New York and Georgia, 2000. *MMWR* 2001;50: 289–291.
215. Update: Fatal and severe liver injuries associated with rifampin and pyrazinamide for latent tuberculosis infection, and revisions in American Thoracic Society/CDC recommendations—United States, 2001. *MMWR* 2001;50:733–735.
216. The role of BCG vaccine in the prevention and control of tuberculosis in the United States. A joint statement by the Advisory Council for the Elimination of Tuberculosis and the Advisory Committee on Immunization Practices. *MMWR* 1996;45:1–18.
217. Development of new vaccines for tuberculosis. Recommendations of the Advisory Council for the Elimination of Tuberculosis (ACET). *MMWR* 1998;47:1–6.
218. Diagnosis and treatment of disease caused by nontuberculous mycobacteria. This official statement of the American Thoracic Society was approved by the Board of Directors, March 1997. *Am J Respir Crit Care Med* 1997;156(suppl):1–25.
219. Brown BA, Wallace RJ Jr. Infections due to nontuberculous *Mycobacterium.* In: Mandell GL, Bennett JE, Dolin R, eds. *Principles and practice of infectious diseases,* 5th ed. Philadelphia: Churchill Livingstone, 2000:2630–2636.
220. Holland SM. Nontuberculous mycobacteria. *Am J Med Sci* 2001;321:49–55.

# 12. CARDIAC INFECTIONS

Deborah E. Sentochnik and Adolf W. Karchmer

## INFECTIVE ENDOCARDITIS

*Infective endocarditis* (IE) is a microbial infection of an endothelial surface of the heart. Valves are the most commonly involved structures, but infection may occur at the site of a septal defect, on chordae tendonae, or on mural endocardium. The term *infective endocarditis* includes infections of vascular endothelium such as may occur with patent ductus arteriosus, arteriovenous fistulas, and coarctation of the aorta. The syndrome can be caused by a broad array of bacterial species, fungi, mycobacteria, chlamydia, rickettsia, and mycoplasma. Bacterial endocarditis (BE) is the most commonly recognized form of the disease and is often characterized as acute (ABE) or subacute (SBE) on the basis of clinical presentation. Streptococci, staphylococci, enterococci, and fastidious gram-negative coccobacilli are responsible for the majority of cases of IE.

Endocarditis in intravenous drug users (IVDU) or in association with prosthetic heart valves presents special clinical and microbiologic features and is discussed in separate sections in this chapter. Antibiotic prophylaxis to prevent bacterial endocarditis is discussed in Chapter 27, section B.

I. **Pathogenesis** [1,2]. The characteristic lesion of IE is the **vegetation,** a variably sized amorphous mass of platelets and fibrin in which a dense population of bacteria and only a few inflammatory cells are enmeshed.
   A. **Endothelial damage.** The hydrodynamics leading to endothelial damage include the impact of a high-velocity jet, flow from a high to low pressure chamber, and high-velocity flow across a narrow orifice. A platelet and thrombin complex forms at the site in response to the damage. It is at the same location as this sterile thrombus formation that principles of hydrodynamics also allow the maximum deposition of bacteria during bacteremia, that is, just beyond the low-pressure side of the orifice, or at the site of jet stream impact on the endothelium. IE is uncommon in association with low-pressure flow abnormalities such as an isolated atrial septal defect or pure mitral stenosis.
   B. **Bacteremia.** Bacteremia allows the conversion of the sterile thrombus to a vegetation. Bacteremia rates are highest for events that traumatize the oral mucosa, especially the gingiva, and progressively decrease with procedures involving the genitourinary tract and the gastrointestinal tract [3]. A further increased risk of bacteremia occurs in the presence of a diseased mucosal surface, especially an infected one.
   C. **Bacterial factors.** Bacterial adherence to the thrombus is crucial in order for infection to occur. Multiple factors that enhance adherence, including the ability to produce dextran, cause aggregation of platelets, and bind to fibronectin, appear to be important for most of the gram-positive organisms that commonly cause IE. Resistance to host defense mechanisms is also pivotal. The ability of many gram-negative bacilli to cause IE is limited by complement-mediated bactericidal activity of serum [2].
   D. **Intact endothelium.** *Staphylococcus aureus* is the most common gram-positive organism of ABE able to infect intact vascular endothelium. The reasons for this are incompletely understood.

II. **Clinical presentation**
   A. **Patient population**
      1. **Underlying heart disease.** Fifty-five percent to 75% of patients with IE of native valves have predisposing conditions, including rheumatic heart disease, congenital heart disease, mitral valve prolapse, degenerative heart disease, asymmetric septal hypertrophy, or intravenous (i.v.) drug abuse [4–6]. As the population at risk has been decreasing in recent decades, rheumatic heart disease has become a less important predisposing condition, accounting for fewer than 20% of cases [7]. Mitral valve prolapse accounts for 7% to 30% of IE in native valves not related to drug abuse or nosocomial infection. The frequency of this underlying etiology for IE likely reflects the high frequency of the lesion in the

general population (2%–4% of healthy persons and 20% among young women). Increased risk of IE in patients with mitral valve prolapse occurs in those with both prolapse and a mitral regurgitation murmur [8]. Congenital heart disease is identified in approximately 10% of patients with IE. One-fourth to one-half of all cases of IE occur in patients with no identifiable underlying heart lesion. It is possible that clinically undetectable degenerative change is present.

2. **Nosocomial risk.** A substantial number of cases of nosocomial endocarditis associated with bacteremia from i.v. catheters, postoperative wound infections, genitourinary manipulation, hyperalimentation lines, and hemodialysis shunts have been described in patients hospitalized or treated for a variety of other illnesses [9].
3. **Age.** The median age range of patients with IE has increased to 47 to 69 years in recent decades compared with 30 to 40 years in the preantibiotic and early antibiotic eras [2]. This likely reflects a larger number of older persons at risk and a smaller number of young people with rheumatic heart disease.

**B. Signs and symptoms** [10]. The presenting signs and symptoms of BE **are variable and often nonspecific.** The possibility of this diagnosis should be considered whenever a patient presents with **fever** of more than several days' duration with no other apparent cause and in association with a significant heart murmur. The **type of clinical presentation** can have practical implications with regard to probable bacterial etiology and the degree of urgency in instituting therapy; it is therefore useful to attempt to classify suspected BE as acute or subacute.

1. **SBE.** Patients with typical SBE have an insidious and poorly defined onset of a variety of symptoms that may include weakness, fatigue, anorexia, night sweats, weight loss, arthralgias, myalgias, fever, and neurologic symptoms. Symptoms may be present for weeks or months at the time of presentation. The onset may be related to antecedent events such as dental work, although in most cases no definite antecedent event is apparent.
2. **ABE.** In contrast, patients with ABE usually have a more circumscribed and acute onset of chills, fever, back pain, arthralgia, and myalgia, and often look acutely ill. The patient may be seen within several days to a week from the onset of illness. Infections that antedate the onset of endocarditis may be identified, although, as in SBE, they often are not apparent. Some patients fall between these extremes and cannot be classified easily.
3. **Peripheral signs** of BE, many of which are immunologically mediated, can include splenomegaly, petechiae, clubbing, and retinal and subungual (splinter) hemorrhage. Janeway lesions are small hemorrhagic or erythematous, nontender macules on the palms and soles due to septic emboli. They occur more often in ABE. Osler nodes are small, subcutaneous, tender nodules found on the pulp of digits and are due to septic emboli or, possibly, vasculitis. Roth spots are pale-centered, oval, retinal hemorrhages, usually near the optic disk. More common in the preantibiotic era, these signs, which increase in incidence with increasing duration of untreated illness, are now seen in fewer than 20% of cases of BE.
4. **Fever.** Because fever is almost always present in the patient who is not on antipyretics or antiinflammatory agents, a normal temperature pattern under reliable observation makes the diagnosis doubtful. Occasional exceptions to this rule occur in elderly patients or those with debilitating illness.
5. **Cardiac signs**
   a. **Murmurs.** A heart murmur is apparent in 85% or more of cases, and the absence of both fever and murmur makes the probability of BE slight, although it does not rule out the possibility entirely.
      (1) **Valvular lesions.** The distribution of valvular lesions, as expected, varies with the type of underlying heart disease reported. If IVDUs are excluded, the vast majority of patients have either aortic or mitral valve involvement (in approximately equal proportions), or both. Tricuspid involvement is rare except in IVDUs, in whom it is common. Occasional cases of right-sided endocarditis have been described secondary to infected central venous catheters or pulmonary artery catheterization [11].

(2) **Changing murmurs.** New murmurs or striking changes in the intensity of murmurs are the **exception** rather than the rule in patients with BE. Some change in intensity due to tachycardia, anemia, or fever is fairly common. If new murmurs or significant changes in murmur intensity occur, they are likely to represent either aortic or mitral insufficiency and are frequently associated with congestive heart failure (CHF).

(3) **BE without a murmur** tends to be seen (a) early in the course of acute endocarditis that involves previously normal valves, (b) with infection that involves mural endocardium rather than valves, (c) with congenital bicuspid aortic valves, (d) in isolated tricuspid valve involvement, and (e) in some elderly patients.

**b. Other cardiac signs**

(1) **CHF** results primarily from progressive valvular insufficiency, although associated myocarditis also may contribute.

(2) **Heart block and arrhythmias** might occur if there is involvement of the conducting system.

(3) **Pericarditis** rarely complicates BE but can result from extension of a mural or valvular ring abscess.

6. **Embolic phenomena.** In either ABE or SBE, signs and symptoms of embolic phenomena may occur. These manifest as episodes of vascular occlusion that cause pain in the abdomen (mesenteric or splenic arterial involvement), chest (coronary or pulmonary emboli), or extremities. Hematuria may result from emboli to the kidneys, blindness from retinal artery involvement, and acute neurologic symptoms (including stroke) from cerebrovascular involvement. These signs and symptoms in combination with fever or a murmur should always suggest the strong possibility of underlying BE.

7. **Central nervous system. Approximately one-third of patients with BE exhibit neurologic disturbances as a major presenting symptom or as a later complication of BE** [12,13]. Stroke is a common presenting neurologic problem, and toxic encephalopathy manifesting as a variety of severe mental disturbances without focal neurologic defects also is common. Meningitis, headache, visual impairment, mononeuritis, convulsions, brain abscess, mycotic aneurysm, and intracerebral bleeds also are seen. **The possibility of BE should be considered in patients of any age when fever or a murmur accompany these neurologic signs or symptoms.**

8. **Rheumatologic manifestations.** Twenty-five percent to 40% of patients with BE have myalgias, especially low back pain, or arthralgias as a presenting or predominant symptom [14]. Arthritis is less common and is typically a nonspecific inflammatory response. Septic arthritis can be seen in ABE, especially with *S. aureus* infection.

9. **The elderly.** Within this large group of patients, the diagnosis of BE is particularly prone to be missed or inordinately delayed. CNS or cardiac signs and symptoms frequently are ascribed to progression of underlying arteriosclerotic disease, and the possibility of BE thus is overlooked. The onset of symptoms often is insidious, fever may not be prominent, and a murmur may be absent [15,16]. The systolic murmurs that are common in elderly individuals may be erroneously regarded as insignificant.

## III. Diagnosis.
With the exception of microbiologic studies, laboratory findings are variable, nonspecific, and of little definitive value in the diagnosis of endocarditis.

### A. Nonspecific findings

1. **Erythrocyte sedimentation rate and C-reactive protein are elevated** in almost all patients with SBE [17].
2. A mild to moderate normocytic-normochromic **anemia** is common. The severity tends to be related to the duration of the illness, and patients with ABE often are not anemic.
3. **Peripheral leukocyte counts** usually are normal or moderately elevated, although prominent leukocytosis may be seen in acute infection.
4. **Thrombocytopenia** may be seen in patients with ABE and in those with splenomegaly accompanying more chronic infections.

5. On **urinalysis,** microscopic hematuria and proteinuria are common, whereas red blood cell casts may appear if glomerulonephritis complicates the course.

B. **Blood cultures and bacteremia.** Blood cultures must be obtained whenever the diagnosis of BE is suspected; they will be positive in 85% to 95% of cases. (See Chapter 25 for the technique of obtaining blood cultures.) In endocarditis, as in other intravascular infections, bacteremia (when present) is persistent in the great majority of cases. The finding of intermittent bacteremia in a suspected case of endocarditis should suggest some other focus as a source.

1. **In suspected ABE.** When acute endocarditis is suspected and prompt therapy is believed to be indicated, three blood cultures, taken from separate venipuncture sites at 15- to 30-minute intervals over 1 to 2 hours, are adequate for identifying more than 90% of bacteremic patients with ABE; at the same time, they provide enough samples to minimize confusion over possible contamination.
2. **In suspected SBE.** When the presentation of endocarditis is subacute and the need for therapy is not so urgent, three blood cultures over a 24-hour period are sufficient. If these cultures remain negative after 24 to 48 hours, another two or three sets should be obtained [18,19]. Culture of arterial blood or bone marrow offers no advantage over culture of venous blood.
3. **In suspected fungal endocarditis.** Blood cultures for fungi should be obtained using a specific method such as lysis-centrifugation.
4. **Laboratory involvement.** The laboratory should be advised that endocarditis is a possible diagnosis and told if any unusual bacteria are suspected that might require special processing. In addition, once a causative organism is identified, the laboratory should be requested to save the isolate until therapy has been completed. **Special culture** techniques that may help in diagnosis are discussed in Chapter 25.
5. **Serologic tests** may be useful in diagnosis of IE due to *Bartonella* species, *C. burnetii, Chlamydia* species, *Legionella* species, or *Brucella* species.

C. **Resected emboli.** Resection of large emboli may be of diagnostic as well as therapeutic value in patients with suspected endocarditis and with negative blood cultures. Resected emboli should be cultured and examined histologically for bacteria and fungi. Polymerase chain reaction may be especially useful in this circumstance [20].

D. **Spinal fluid.** Purulent meningitis is rare in BE but can be seen in ABE due to a virulent organism such as *S. aureus* or *Streptococcus pneumoniae.* Spinal fluid in BE due to other organisms with signs of meningeal irritation typically has an aseptic profile, albeit with a slight predominance of polymorphonuclear cells, and cerebrospinal fluid (CSF) cultures are typically negative. With neurologic involvement, the CSF may show a mild pleocytosis (predominantly leukocytic), elevated protein level, and normal glucose level.

E. **Echocardiography.** Among patients with clinical and microbiologic evidence of endocarditis, two-dimensional echocardiography (2D echo) used across the chest wall (transthoracic echo, or TTE) identifies vegetations in approximately 65% of patients. In contrast, 2D echo with biplane imaging from the esophagus (transesophageal echo, or TEE) visualizes vegetations in 85% to 90% of these patients [21]. The ability to identify vegetations varies with vegetation size and location as well as body habitus and underlying diseases. TEE is particularly useful in patients with suboptimal TTE (e.g., those with pulmonary disease, obesity, chest wall deformities, and ventilator dependency). Furthermore, TEE is the approach of choice for evaluating the tricuspid and pulmonic valves and a prosthesis in the mitral position. In his editorial, Jameison concludes that TEE is better than TTE in finding evidence of vegetations, quantifying valvular dysfunction, and diagnosing the spread of infection; this advantage is especially noted in patients with prosthetic valve endocarditis [22]. Nevertheless, 2D echo, regardless of the approach, cannot distinguish between marantic and infective endocarditis (healed vs. actively infected vegetations) or thrombus and vegetation. Furthermore, in some patients 2D echo may not distinguish between vegetations and noninfective valve abnormalities (i.e., valve thickening or calcification). Given its less than 100% sensitivity for detecting vegetations as well as these other limitations, 2D echo **cannot be used**

**to exclude BE, especially when the diagnosis is likely based on clinical information** [21]. It also is generally an inadequate approach to screening for BE among patients in whom the clinical index of suspicion is not high. Whereas 2D echo–demonstrated vegetations are not required to establish the diagnosis of BE in a patient with positive blood cultures and a clinical syndrome indicative of endocarditis, the echocardiogram may provide clinically useful information among patients with a BE syndrome and negative blood cultures. The major utility of TEE over TTE in the diagnosis of native valve endocarditis arises when the TTE is a technically inadequate study or indicates an intermediate likelihood of endocarditis [22a,22b]. In patients with suspected endocarditis involving prosthetic valves, TEE is a superior diagnostic test. In patients with a moderate probability of endocarditis but with chest configuration or lung disease limiting the utility of TTE or those with relatively low probability of endocarditis (6%–10% likelihood), for example *S. aureus* catheter-related bacteremia, initial evaluation by TEE is cost effective [23]. Furthermore, 2D echo, particularly using the transesophageal approach, supplemented by pulsed, continuous, and color flow Doppler, may provide information regarding intracardiac complications of BE and cardiac hemodynamic status that is important in assessing prognosis and the role of surgical intervention in therapy [21,24] (see section **VIII.H**). See related discussions in section **IV.D** and section **V.B,** under Endocarditis Associated with Prosthetic Valves.

F. **Diagnostic criteria.** The von Reyn criteria established in 1981 to assist in diagnosis of infective endocarditis have largely been replaced by the now well-accepted Duke criteria [25], which have recently been modified by Li et al. [26]. These are summarized in Tables 12.1 and 12.2.

1. **In 1981 von Reyn and colleagues** published a set of criteria to help diagnose "definite," "probable," "possible," and "rejected" cases of infective endocarditis. Limitations include the criteria's retrospective nature and lack of prospective validation, the lack of inclusion of echocardiographic findings, the nonrecognition of i.v. drug use as an important predisposing condition for infective endocarditis, and the requirement for histopathologic confirmation of infective endocarditis [27].

Table 12.1. Definition of Infective Endocarditis According to the Modified Duke Criteria, with Modifications Shown in Italics

Definite infective endocarditis
- Pathologic criteria
  - Microorganisms: demonstrated by culture or histologic examination of a vegetation, a vegetation that has embolized, or an intracardiac abscess specimen; *or*
  - Pathologic lesions: vegetation or intracardiac abscess confirmed by histologic examination showing active endocarditis
- Clinical criteria
  - 2 major criteria, *or*
  - 1 major and 3 minor criteria, *or*
  - 5 minor criteria

Possible infective endocarditis
- *1 major criterion and 1 minor criterion; or*
- *3 minor criteria*

Rejected
- Firm alternate diagnosis for manifestations of endocarditis; *or*
- Resolution of infective endocarditis syndrome with antibiotic therapy for ≤4 days; *or*
- No pathologic evidence of infective endocarditis at surgery or autopsy, with antibiotic therapy for ≤4 days; *or*
- Does not meet criteria for possible infective endocarditis, as above

Adapted from Li JS, et al. Proposed modifications to the Duke criteria for the diagnosis of infective endocarditis. *Clin Infect Dis* 2000;30:633–638; with permission.

Table 12.2. Definition of Terms Used in the Modified Duke Criteria for the Diagnosis of Infective Endocarditis (IE), with Modifications Shown in Italics

- Major criteria
  - Blood culture positive for IE
    - Typical microorganisms consistent with IE from 2 separate blood cultures:
      - Viridans streptococci, *Streptococcus bovis,* HACEK group[a] *Staphylococcus aureus; or*
      - Community-acquired enterococci, in the absence of a primary focus; *or*
    - Microorganisms consistent with IE from persistently positive blood cultures, defined as follows:
      - At least 2 positive cultures of blood samples drawn >12 h apart; *or*
      - All of 3 or a majority of ≥4 separate cultures of blood (with first and last sample drawn at least 1 h apart)
    - *Single positive blood culture for* Coxiella burnetii *or anti-phase I IgG antibody titer >1:800*
  - Evidence of endocardial involvement
  - Echocardiogram positive for IE *(TEE recommended in patients with prosthetic valves, rated at least "possible IE" by clinical criteria, or complicated IE [paravalvular abscess]; TEE as first test in other patients),* defined as follows:
    - Oscillating intracardiac mass on valve or supporting structures, in the path of regurgitant jets, or on implanted material in the absence of an alternative anatomic explanation; *or*
    - Abscess; *or*
    - New partial dehiscence of prosthetic valves
  - New valvular regurgitation (worsening or changing or preexisting murmur not sufficient)
- Minor criteria
  - Predisposition, predisposing heart condition or injection drug user
  - Fever, temperature >38°C
  - Vascular phenomena: major arterial emboli, septic pulmonary infarcts, mycotic aneurysm, intracranial hemorrhage, conjunctival hemorrhages, and Janeway lesions
  - Immunologic phenomena: glomerulonephritis, Osler nodes, Roth spots, and rheumatoid factor
  - Microbiologic evidence: positive blood culture but does not meet a major criterion as noted above[b] or serologic evidence of active infection with organism consistent with IE
  - *Echocardiographic minor criteria eliminated*

[a]HACEK, *Haemophilus* species *Actinobacillus actinomycetemcomitans, Cardiobacterium hominis, Eikenella* species, and *Kingella kingae.*
[b]Excluding single positive cultures for coagulase-negative staphylococci and organisms that do not cause endocarditis.
Adapted from Li JS, et al. Proposed modifications to the Duke criteria for the diagnosis of infective endocarditis. *Clin Infect Dis* 2000;30:633–638; with permission.

2. **Modified Duke criteria for infective endocarditis** are summarized in Tables 12.1 and 12.2. When used carefully over the entire clinical evaluation period (i.e., not limited to initial findings only), the criteria appear to be sensitive and specific.
   - **a.** Erroneous rejection of the diagnosis of endocarditis is unlikely.
   - **b.** When using these criteria to guide therapy in an individual patient, patients who are categorized as having possible infective endocarditis should be treated as having infective endocarditis. This may lead to treatment of some individuals who do not have the infection. The potential for overdiagnosis and excess treatment has been reduced by modifications that now require at least one major criterion or three minor criteria to designate possible endocarditis [26].
   - **c.** The findings of echocardiography are important major criteria in the Duke diagnostic schema. TEE compared with TTE improved the sensitivity of the Duke criteria to establish definite endocarditis by 25%. The enhanced diagnostic effect of TEE was greatest when prosthetic valve endocarditis

was suspected and when the clinical likelihood of endocarditis was intermediate. In 4% the TEE finding resulted in alterations in therapy (rejected diagnoses became definite) [28]. See related discussion of echocardiography in section **III.E** and related discussions under Endocarditis Associated with Prosthetic Valves.

**IV. Microbiologic features**

**A. Organisms**

1. **Streptococci** account for approximately 55% of all cases of native valvular BE in the nonaddict population [2].
   - **a.** Approximately 35% of all cases are due to viridans streptococci, the single most common organism.
   - **b.** Approximately 10% are caused by enterococci.
   - **c.** Approximately 10% are caused by other nonhemolytic, microaerophilic, anaerobic, or nonenterococcal group D streptococci. Group A $\beta$-hemolytic streptococci are a rare cause.
2. **Staphylococci** (approximately 35% of cases) [2]. Most staphylococci causing BE are coagulase-positive. Coagulase-negative staphylococci are common in prosthetic valve endocarditis but infrequently cause disease on native valves.
3. **Miscellaneous organisms** (10% of cases). This includes HACEK organisms (*Haemophilus, Actinomyces, Cardiobacterium, Eikenella, Kingella*), pseudomonas [29], gram-negative enteric bacilli [30], pneumococci [31], and gonococci. Reports can be found of endocarditis caused by almost any bacterium [2,32]. *Bartonella* species [33] and *C. burnetii* [34,35] have emerged as causative organisms. *Tropheryma whippelli,* the cause of Whipple disease, can rarely cause IE [36,37].

**B. Culture-negative endocarditis** [38,39]. A small proportion of patients with BE have persistently negative blood cultures. In some series, this comprised 15% or more of all patients; however, the true proportion is probably less than 5%. The diagnosis usually is suspected in patients with fever of undetermined cause who have underlying heart disease or a newly discovered murmur.

**The usual cause is prior antibiotic therapy,** the effect of which can last for days and, if therapy was prolonged, even for weeks, rendering blood cultures negative. Fungi and organisms that are difficult to culture might also be responsible. A search for pathogens such as *C. burnetii, Chlamydia* species, *Bartonella* species and *Legionella* species may be worthwhile. Diagnosis may require serologic or other nonculture techniques.

**C. Fungi** [40]. Fungal IE can be seen in prosthetic valve endocarditis (PVE), where the most common cause is *Candida albicans,* and in the IVDU population, where nonalbicans *Candida* infections are most often seen.

**D. Microbiologic and clinical correlations.** Although overlap exists, there is a correlation between clinical presentation and the infecting organism. Bacteria with low inherent virulence such as viridans streptococci usually infect previously damaged heart valves. Damage due to infection tends to progress slowly, and patients are likely to have a subacute or chronic course.

More virulent organisms, such as *S. aureus,* may infect previously normal valves, and tend to produce acute systemic toxicity as well as rapid valve destruction. ***S. aureus* is the most commonly isolated organism in patients presenting with ABE.**

**V. Treatment: basic principles**

**A. General considerations.** Prolonged administration of relatively high doses of bactericidal antibiotics is indicated. Dense populations of metabolically dormant organisms exist on vegetations. The avascularity of the center of the lesion also contributes to the difficulty in achieving its permanent sterilization.

**B. Laboratory aids**

1. **Serum bactericidal titer (SBT).** The SBT is the highest dilution of the patient's serum during antibiotic therapy that kills 99.9% of the standard inoculum of the patient's infecting organism *in vitro.* Peak titers of 1:64 or 1:32 and trough titers of 1:32 obtained with a standardized SBT method correlate with bacteriologic cure. SBT is a poor predictor of bacteriologic failure. When using regimens

considered optimal on the basis of clinical experience, monitoring therapy using the SBT is not recommended [41]. It may be useful when treating patients with IE caused by organisms for which optimal therapy is not established or when using unconventional antimicrobial regimens.

2. **Antibiotic levels.** Vancomycin and aminoglycoside levels should be monitored.

C. **Initiating treatment.** When a patient has suspected BE, a decision must be made as to the urgency of initiating therapy on a presumptive basis before blood culture results are available. In the severely ill patient in whom ABE is suspected, it is reasonable to take three blood cultures over a 1-hour period and to institute therapy promptly because of the rapid progression of this disease. **In the patient who has a subacute or chronic illness and a nonspecific clinical picture, it often is best to await blood culture results before starting antibiotics.**

D. **Outpatient therapy** [42,43]. Patients who have responded to initial therapy and are afebrile, who are not experiencing threatening complications, who will be compliant with therapy, and who have a suitable home situation can be considered for outpatient therapy. Close laboratory and clinical monitoring should continue. Antibiotic choices should not be compromised.

VI. **Antibiotic therapy for specific types of endocarditis. The following recommendations assume normal renal function;** drug doses may have to be adjusted for renal insufficiency, as is described in Chapter 27. The doses given here are for adult patients. Treatment in penicillin-allergic patients is discussed in section **VII.** Consensus recommendations for therapy from the American Heart Association writing group are published elsewhere [41].

A. **Viridans streptococci**

1. **Penicillin-susceptible viridans streptococci and *Streptococcus bovis* (minimum inhibitory concentration [MIC] ≤ 0.1 μg/mL).**

a. **Penicillin alone.** A four-week course of aqueous penicillin G 12 to 18 million units per day i.v. by continuous infusion or divided into doses given every 4 hours achieves bacteriologic cure in up to 99% of patients.

b. **Short course (2-week) combination therapy with penicillin (see a) and gentamicin 1mg/kg every 8 hours** has been associated with bacteriologic cure rates as high as 98% [43]. This regimen is appropriate for uncomplicated cases of endocarditis due to highly penicillin susceptible viridans streptococci occurring in patients at low risk for aminoglycoside toxicity. **This course is not recommended for patients with complications** such as shock, intracardiac abscess, or extracardiac foci of infection.

c. **Ceftriaxone once daily.** Ceftriaxone 2 g once daily plus either gentamicin (3 mg/kg) [44] or netilmicin (4 mg/kg) [45] given as a single daily dose for 14 days has been shown to be effective. However, experience with single daily dosing of aminoglycosides in the treatment of IE is limited, and these regimens are not currently recommended.

2. **Viridans streptococci relatively resistant to penicillin (MIC >0.1 to <0.5) is treated with penicillin plus an aminoglycoside.** This combination synergistically kills viridans streptococci *in vitro.* Although streptomycin has been used in classic studies, gentamicin is the standard in clinical practice. An appropriate course consists of aqueous penicillin G 18 million units daily by continuous infusion or divided into six equal doses and gentamicin 1 mg/kg intramuscularly (i.m.) or i.v. every 8 hours for 2 weeks, followed by penicillin alone for an additional 2 weeks.

3. **Abiotrophia species (previously called nutritionally variant streptococci), *Streptococcus adjacens,* and *Streptococcus defectivus.*** These organisms are generally more resistant to penicillin than are other viridans streptococci [46]. They should be treated with enterococcal IE regimens. Bacteriologic cure may be difficult, and relapse rates high.

4. **Viridans streptococci with penicillin MIC of ≥0.5** [47]. Enterococcal IE regimens should be followed.

B. ***Streptococcus bovis*** is treated the same as viridans streptococci.

C. ***Streptococcus pyogenes, Streptococcus pneumoniae,* and groups B, C, and G streptococci.** IE caused by these organisms has been either refractory to antibiotic therapy or associated with extensive valvular damage. Penicillin G 3 million units i.v. every 4 hours for 4 weeks is recommended for treatment of endocarditis due to group A streptococci and pneumococci. Until a pneumococcus has been demonstrated to be sensitive to penicillin (MIC $< 0.1$ μg/mL) treatment with ceftriaxone plus vancomycin may be preferable [48]. Endocarditis due to group G, C, or B streptococci is more difficult to treat than that due to penicillin-susceptible viridans streptococci. Therefore, the addition of gentamicin to the first 2 weeks of a 4-week high-dose penicillin regimen is often recommended [49]. Surgery is commonly required.

**D. Enterococci.** Ninety percent of enterococcal endocarditis [50] is due to *Enterococcus faecalis,* with the remainder due almost entirely to *Enterococcus faecium.* Enterococci are less susceptible to killing by penicillin alone than are other streptococci and are resistant to clinically applicable levels of gentamicin. **Effective bactericidal therapy requires the use of a cell wall–active agent such as penicillin, ampicillin, or vancomycin with an aminoglycoside to achieve synergy.** Gentamicin 1 mg/kg i.v. or i.m. every 8 hours should be combined with one of these agents. Synergistic combination therapy results in cure rates of approximately 85% [41].

1. MICs to penicillin vary from 1 to 2 μg/mL, with most in the range of 1.0 to 4.0 μg/mL. Eighteen to 30 million units of i.v. penicillin G daily is appropriate when renal function is normal (see Chapter 27). Ampicillin 12 g per 24 hours i.v. given by continuous infusion or every 4 hours in six equally divided doses may be substituted. **Peak gentamicin levels need only be in the range of 3 μg/mL for synergy to occur.** Although there is ample *in vitro* evidence for the role of gentamicin, most clinical evidence comes from using streptomycin in combination with penicillin. However, the ototoxicity of streptomycin, the need for intramuscular administration, and the substantial percentage of *in vitro* resistance has led to the standard use of gentamicin instead. The recommended duration of therapy is at least 4 weeks with both agents and 6 weeks if the symptoms were present for more than 3 months before appropriate antibiotic therapy was begun or in complicated disease [41].
2. The incidence of **high-level gentamicin-resistant strains of enterococci** (MIC $\geq$500 μg/mL) [51] **warrants routine laboratory screening of clinically significant isolates.** This characteristic is seen in 25% of *E. faecalis* and 50% of *E. faecium* infections. Of isolates with this gentamicin resistance, 30% to 40% are sensitive to streptomycin, whose resistance is mediated by a distinct genetic element. There are few well-documented cases of endocarditis due to aminoglycoside-resistant enterococci. Infectious disease consultation is advised. Optimal duration of antibiotic therapy is unknown. Successful therapy may include valve replacement. If high-level resistance to both gentamicin and streptomycin are found, therapy can be attempted with an 8- to 12-week course of a cell wall–active agent alone if susceptibility is demonstrated. See section **D.4** below for other therapeutic considerations.
3. **High-level penicillinase production,** especially among *E. faecium,* has been documented [52]. Screening for the production of this β-lactamase should be undertaken if therapy is to include ampicillin or penicillin. Vancomycin activity is not influenced by the enzyme. Unfortunately, many penicillinase-producing strains are also highly resistant to aminoglycosides, thus precluding the use of a known synergistic combination.
4. **Enterococci resistant to vancomycin** and variably resistant to other glycopeptides are reported [53], as are isolates resistant to all available antibiotics. (See related discussion in Chapter 27.) There is some experience in the use of newer agents such as quinupristin/dalfopristin (susceptible *E. faecium* only) [54] and linezolid [55,56].

**E. Staphylococci** [41]

1. **Penicillinase-resistant semisynthetic penicillins.** Oxacillin or nafcillin 2 g i.v. every 4 hours is indicated. If the organism is ultimately found to be susceptible to penicillin (MIC $\leq$ 0.1 μg/mL), aqueous penicillin G 18 to 24 million units per 24 hours should be used instead.

2. **Combination therapy.** There is *in vitro* and experimental *in vivo* evidence that low-dose gentamicin in combination with a semisynthetic penicillin effects more rapid killing of staphylococci and sterilization of valves than does penicillin alone. This suggests that addition of gentamicin 1 mg/kg every 8 hours for the first few days of treatment may be of value. Because clinical trials have failed to show an improved outcome with combined therapy [57], gentamicin generally should be omitted in patients with relative contraindications to its use, as is described for gentamicin use in cases of viridans streptococci (see section **A.1.b**).

   From a practical standpoint, it may be reasonable to use combination therapy (if not contraindicated) for the first 3 to 5 days, in an attempt to clear the bacteremia rapidly and minimize damage to the heart valve [41]. The more long-term addition of gentamicin (1 mg/kg i.v. or i.m every 8 hours) or rifampin (300 mg orally every 8 hours), or both, in patients who are not responding to a $\beta$-lactam alone has been suggested [57]. Determination of serum bactericidal levels may be useful in this circumstance.
3. **Methicillin-resistant *S. aureus*** (MRSA) BE is treated with vancomycin. The usual initial dose is 1.0 g every 12 hours (see Chapter 27). Infectious diseases consultation is suggested.
4. **Coagulase-negative staphylococci** account for 1% to 3% of native valve endocarditis [58]. Therapeutic options are similar to those for *S. aureus,* and there may be a role for combination therapy. Sensitivity testing should guide treatment decisions.
5. **Duration of therapy.** Treatment should be continued for 4 to 6 weeks. The 6-week course often is suggested for patients with an initial delayed clinical response or complicated course.
6. **Indications for surgery** are discussed in section **VIII.G.1.**

F. **Other forms of BE.** Infectious disease consultation is recommended.
1. **HACEK** organisms usually are treated with ampicillin or ceftriaxone plus gentamicin for 4 weeks. Ceftriaxone alone can be used [41].
2. **Enteric gram-negative** BE is difficult to treat. The most potent agent, as determined by *in vitro* sensitivity testing, should be used and serum bactericidal levels followed. It is wise to combine most agents, especially the $\beta$-lactams, with gentamicin. Duration of therapy is 4 to 6 weeks [30].
3. ***Pseudomonas aeruginosa*** endocarditis is seen almost exclusively in IVDUs. Tobramycin 5 to 8 mg/kg/day combined with an antipseudomonal penicillin (e.g., mezlocillin or piperacillin), ceftazidime, or ciprofloxacin for 6 weeks is usual therapy [29]. (See section **VIII.G.2.**)
4. **Miscellaneous.** The reader is referred to recent articles dealing with endocarditis due to *C. burnetii* [34,35] and therapy for *Bartonella* species infections [33]. Published experience in the form of case reports or small series dealing with a specific causative agent should be reviewed when dealing with endocarditis due to unusual organisms.

G. **Initial treatment of suspected ABE prior to culture results.** Therapy should be directed to *S. aureus* because it is the most common organism in patients who have ABE. Vancomycin plus gentamicin is appropriate and also provides coverage for possible enterococcal infection. Oxacillin or nafcillin 2 g every 4 hours may be substituted for vancomycin in the patient at increased risk for nephrotoxicity. Antibiotic therapy aimed at both staphylococci and enterococci will cover, with few exceptions, any other bacteria that are likely to be present.

H. **Blood culture–negative endocarditis** [39]. Recommended therapy includes ampicillin plus an aminoglycoside as outlined in section **D.1** on treatment of enterococcal endocarditis. Given that in the absence of confounding antibiotic therapy enterococci and staphylococci are unlikely to be causes of culture-negative IE, ceftriaxone may be used instead of ampicillin. (See section **VIII.G.3.**)

I. **Fungi.** Fungal endocarditis **almost always requires a combined chemotherapeutic and surgical approach** [59]. Amphotericin B is administered at 0.5 mg/kg/day. Most *Candida* and *Torulopsis* species are sensitive to flucytosine, and 150 mg/kg/day orally may be added to the amphotericin; flucytosine, however, should not be used alone. The best results have been reported with early surgical intervention and prolonged postoperative antifungal therapy (see Chapter 17). Prolonged or indefinite fluconazole has been suggested for patients treated either medically or surgically [40,60]. There are reports of a subset of patients with candida IE cured by prolonged fluconazole administration. Infectious disease consultation is advised.

**VII. Treatment of patients with a history of penicillin allergy.** If the results of properly performed skin tests for penicillin allergy are negative, the chance of a serious immediate or accelerated reaction to penicillin administration is negligible. Most patients with a history of penicillin allergy have negative skin test results and can receive penicillin. Cephalosporins are often a useful alternative in penicillin-allergic patients, but a possibility of cross-reactivity does exist. This subject is covered in detail in Chapter 24. The doses outlined here are for adults who have normal renal function.

**A. Sensitive viridans streptococci.** For some patients it may be preferable to perform skin tests for penicillin allergy and to give penicillin G if the results are negative. If the patient has a history of a delayed penicillin allergy, cephalosporins can usually be administered (see Chapter 24). In these patients, ceftriaxone 2 g i.v. once daily can be used [41]. If the patient has a history of an immediate, severe reaction to penicillins, or if skin tests to a cephalosporin also are positive, or if one is waiting for skin tests to be performed, vancomycin 0.5 g every 6 hours or 1 g every 12 hours can be given. (See Chapter 27 for dosing regimens for vancomycin.) Therapy should continue for 4 weeks.

**B. Penicillin G–susceptible *S. aureus*.** Proceed in the same manner as for viridans streptococci. However, if a cephalosporin can be administered, a first-generation cephalosporin (e.g., cefazolin) should be used.

**C. Penicillin G–resistant *S. aureus*.** Most patients can be treated with semisynthetic penicillin after appropriate skin tests. If alternative drugs are necessary, either a first-generation cephalosporin, for example, cefazolin 2 g every 8 hours (in the patient with delayed allergy) [41] or vancomycin 0.5 g every 6 hours or 1 g every 12 hours (see Chapter 27), can be used. Therapy should continue for 6 weeks if possible. Some clinical failures are observed when vancomycin has been used as an alternate therapy in *S. aureus* endocarditis [61]. Therefore, in the penicillin-allergic patient, infectious disease consultation is advised to help determine the optimal antibiotic regimen.

**D. Enterococci and other highly penicillin-resistant streptococci.** Every effort should be made, including appropriate skin testing and consideration of desensitization procedures if necessary (see Chapter 24), to give penicillin or ampicillin to patients with endocarditis due to these pathogens. If neither of these drugs can be given, vancomycin 0.5 g every 6 hours or 1 g every 12 hours (see Chapter 27 for dosing regimens) for 6 weeks, is the best alternative. Although the MIC of vancomycin for enterococci averages approximately 3 $\mu$g/mL or less, it usually is not bactericidal *in vitro* against enterococci, and the addition of gentamicin or streptomycin is advisable. The toxic effects of vancomycin plus an aminoglycoside may be additive, and it is important to observe the patient closely for any evidence of renal or eighth nerve toxicity. Should these occur, the aminoglycoside should be stopped. Serum levels should be monitored (see Chapter 27).

**E. Streptococci with penicillin MIC between 0.2 and 0.5 $\mu$g/mL.** Patients with immediate hypersensitivity reactions to penicillin should be treated with vancomycin alone for 4 weeks. For those with nonimmediate hypersensitivity, either vancomycin or ceftriaxone for 4 weeks combined with gentamicin for the first 2 weeks are appropriate regimens.

**F. Other infections.** The general principles outlined in sections A through D are applicable. The choice of alternative drugs should be guided by results of *in vitro* testing. Bactericidal antibiotics or antibiotic combinations should be used, and serum bactericidal levels should be monitored, if possible, when *in vitro* MBCs imply that it may be difficult to achieve adequate blood levels. For unusual or resistant bacteria, infectious disease consultation is advised.

**VIII. Role of surgery in endocarditis** [22]. Clinical judgment is an integral part of decisions regarding surgery.

A. **Progressive or significant heart failure that does not resolve with medical therapy.** Severe CHF in this setting carries a very high mortality rate with medical therapy alone. Heart failure that resolves with medical therapy is not considered an absolute criterion for prompt surgical intervention, although in conjunction with other problems it may contribute to a decision for surgical intervention.

B. **Fungal endocarditis** is a strong indication for surgery.

C. **Persistent bacteremia** (7–10 days) despite appropriate antibiotic therapy is considered a strong indication for surgery. Metastatic extracardiac foci of infection such as osteomyelitis, septic pulmonary emboli, and intraabdominal abscesses should be excluded. A TEE is indicated to look for a perivalvular or myocardial abscess [62].

D. **Emboli.** A single major embolic episode raises the question of surgery, and some have suggested that two major embolic episodes are a strong indication. However, the risk of further embolization in these patients is unknown, and precise recommendations are difficult. The size of the residual vegetation by echocardiography and the presence or absence of other clinical and ehcocardiographic findings that would benefit from surgery should weigh heavily in this decision.

E. **Relapse of infection.** Surgery may be indicated if relapse occurs after a single course of antibiotic therapy, particularly if infection involves a prosthetic valve and maximal therapy has been given. It is almost certainly indicated if relapse occurs after a second extended therapeutic course.

F. **Evidence of extension of infection. The development of persistent heart block or bundle branch block strongly suggests extension of infection** (see section **IX.C.2**); the onset of pericarditis suggests rupture of an annular abscess into the pericardial space. These, as well as detection of valvular ring or myocardial abscesses, left-to-right shunts with septal infection, and ruptured chordae tendineae or papillary muscle, all suggest the need for surgery, although they may not individually be absolute indications. See related discussion of myocardial abscess in section **V.B.1** under Endocarditis Associated with Prosthetic Valves.

G. **Microbiologic considerations**

1. ***Staphylococcus aureus*** endocarditis often is complicated by heart failure and periannular abscess [62,63]. It is also an independent predictor of in-hospital mortality [64]. **Early surgery should be considered in the presence of CHF or a perivalvular abscess or if bacteremia fails to clear within 7 to 10 days.**
2. ***Pseudomonas aeruginosa*** has been difficult to cure with medical therapy alone and has been regarded as an indication for early valve replacement [65]. However, with the advent of more potent antipseudomonal antibiotics, particularly the fluoroquinolones, this tenet is no longer absolute. (See section **VI.F.3.**)
3. **Culture-negative endocarditis.** Persistent unexplained fever while on empiric antibiotics likely represents ineffective antimicrobial therapy or unappreciated perivalvular infection.

H. **Echocardiographic findings as indications for cardiac surgery.** The echocardiogram can provide information regarding hemodynamic status and intracardiac complications of endocarditis, which is very useful in assessing the potential role of surgery in the therapy of BE [21,24]. See related discussion under section **III.E.**

1. Echocardiographic quantitation of regurgitant flow across valves damaged by BE, combined with echocardiographic assessment of left ventricular function and clinical findings, allows accurate identification of patients who will benefit from surgical correction of valve dysfunction.
2. Similarly, judgment regarding the timing of surgical intervention is facilitated by echocardiographic findings. Simultaneous reading of the electrocardiogram (EKG) and an M-mode image of the mitral valve can identify premature closure (before the onset of systole) of the valve, which is a sign of left ventricular overload with cardiac decompensation and indicates a need for prompt surgical intervention.
3. The Doppler studies can reveal aberrant flow through fistulous connections, thereby identifying patients with invasive extravalvular disease. Similarly, the

TEE has been shown to be highly sensitive and specific, in comparison with TTE, for identifying paravalvular and septal myocardial abscesses (see section **III.E**) [62]. Also, by identifying pericarditis and pericardial effusion in patients with aortic valve BE, a finding often associated with aortic ring abscess, the echocardiogram may call attention to this intracardiac complication. These findings suggest the need for surgical intervention.

4. The demonstration of vegetations, especially large ones in patients with BE, often raises anxiety about serious emboli and the advisability of valve replacement. In many studies, patients with vegetations detectable by echocardiography have had higher rates of CHF and systemic embolization than patients without detectable vegetations, and in some series these rates are particularly increased when vegetations are greater than 10 mm in diameter.

   Vegetation mobility and valve location also may be important factors in the rate of embolization [66,67]. However, studies relating imaged vegetations to embolic complications have not routinely distinguished whether complications preceded or followed echocardiography. In some studies echocardiography does not demonstrate vegetation characteristics that are associated with subsequent embolization [68]. Furthermore, the rate of embolic events in endocarditis decreases rapidly (over 2–3 weeks) with effective antimicrobial therapy. Additionally, decision analyses that weigh the risks of surgical intervention against the hazards of continued medical therapy are not available for these situations.

   **As a result, there is no general agreement as to the predictive value of demonstrable vegetations,** whatever the size or location, in terms of the need for prompt surgical intervention. Decisions for surgery are based primarily on assessment of valve dysfunction, hemodynamics, antibiotic efficacy, and intracardiac complications, although the presence, size, mobility, and location of vegetations may be important additional considerations when, despite the primary assessment, the role of surgery remains uncertain [69].

**I. Timing of surgery**

1. **Hemodynamic considerations.** If there is valvular regurgitation and significant impairment of cardiac function, surgical intervention before the development of severe intractible hemodynamic dysfunction is recommended regardless of the duration of preceding antimicrobial therapy [65,70]. In those patients with valvular dysfunction but in whom infection is controlled and cardiac function maintained, surgery can be put off until a course of antibiotics is completed. If a patient will require a valve replacement in the near future and has a large vegetation that will put him or her at risk for systemic embolization, early surgery is indicated. (See section **H.4.**)
2. **Neurologic considerations.** The presence of recent neurologic injury may require modification of a planned surgery schedule. When control of infection and maintenance of cardiac function permit, it has been suggested that cardiac surgery should be delayed for 2 to 3 weeks after a significant embolic infarct and for at least a month after intracerebral hemorrhage [71]. Not all authorities agree [72], however, and the reader is referred elsewhere for a more complete discussion [2].

**J. Postoperative antibiotics.** Duration of antibiotic therapy following valve replacement is not clearcut. It has been suggested that the full course of antibiotics be given postoperatively if cultures of the blood or the valve are positive at the time of operation or if results of Gram staining of resected tissue are positive. Otherwise, the usual course should be completed, but a minimum of 2 weeks of postoperative antibiotic therapy should be given.

**K. Survival after surgery** for culture-positive active endocarditis has recently been reviewed [73–75]. Mortality rates of 20% to 30% or more have commonly been reported in the acute perioperative phase. However, the long-term outcome of hospital survivors is excellent. Subsequent reoperations for periprosthetic leak are common, but recurrent infection is uncommon.

**L.** See related discussions about the indications for surgery in section **V.B** under Endocarditis Associated with Prosthetic Valves.

**IX. Course and complications of BE** [76]

**A. General.** When appropriate antibiotic therapy is begun, symptomatic improvement, decline in fever, and reversion of blood cultures to negative are usually prompt. With sensitive organisms, this is likely to occur in 24 to 48 hours, but with more resistant ones, such as *S. aureus,* it may take several days to a week before definite improvement is noted, and it may be 2 weeks or more before the patient is afebrile. Many patients who have become afebrile will continue to be so through a course of therapy, without further difficulty.

**Anemia** usually persists during the course of therapy, and it may take weeks or months for the hematocrit to return to normal. **Splenomegaly** also tends to resolve very slowly. Some patients will continue to have petechiae or Osler nodes during or after a course of successful therapy. The occurrence of these does not necessarily reflect antibiotic failure. Significant **arterial emboli also may occur up to months after completion of therapy,** in the absence of any bacteriologically active disease.

**B. Fever.** One of the most common problems seen during the course of therapy is persistence or recurrence of fever after an afebrile period [77,78]. If the infecting organism is known to be sensitive and appropriate doses of antibiotics are being administered, simple bacteriologic failure is rarely the cause.

1. **Causes of recurrent or persistent fever**
   a. **Failure to control infection.** If the infecting organism has a relatively high degree of antibiotic resistance, fever and positive blood cultures may persist despite optimal antimicrobial therapy. Failure to control infection in this circumstance indicates that valve replacement is necessary.

      In one study, extensive cardiac infection with discrete abscesses extending from the valvular ring or with widespread tissue destruction without localized abscesses was the most common cause of persistent or recurrent fever; valve replacement was required [78]. More than half the cases were caused by viridans streptococci, and most were not accompanied by pericarditis or conduction defects.

   b. **Intravenous-related phlebitis** (sterile or septic) can occur, particularly with indwelling catheters.
   c. **Metastatic abscess formation** is more likely to occur in staphylococcal infection than in infection by other organisms. Splenic abscess occurs in 3% to 5% of patients with IE [76]. Drainage, which can often be accomplished percutaneously, is generally necessary for successful therapy [79]. It is desirable to treat abscesses as completely as possible before valve replacement [27].
   d. **Recurrent emboli** from the endocardium or from deep venous thrombosis can occur.
   e. **Superimposed infections** involving the urinary tract, respiratory tract, or other sites are not uncommon.
   f. **Drug fever is a common cause of recurrent fever in this setting** (see Chapters 1 and 24).
2. **Approach to the patient with recurrent or persistent fever**
   a. A careful **reevaluation of symptoms and physical findings,** aided by appropriate laboratory and other diagnostic procedures directed toward the possibilities listed in section 1, is indicated.
   b. **Drug fever** is reviewed in Chapter 1.

**C. Cardiac effects**

1. **CHF** occurring during or after treatment of endocarditis is the most common serious cardiac complication of the disease and the major cause of mortality. CHF usually results from destruction of valves during the course of active disease or from subsequent shrinkage or scarring of valves or their supporting structures, although myocarditis also may contribute. Patients who develop aortic insufficiency are especially prone to rapid and severe cardiac decompensation. The role of surgery in these circumstances has been discussed previously.
2. **Conduction abnormalities** may occur. The appearance of new or changing conduction block suggests extension of infection to the myocardium and is associated with aortic valve involvement in most cases. It has been recommended

that valve replacement be considered in patients who develop conduction abnormalities that persist for more than a week during medical therapy and that are not secondary to drugs or ischemic heart disease [80].

3. **Coronary embolization** with myocardial infarction can occur and may contribute to CHF.
4. **Valvular obstruction** due to large vegetations occasionally is seen and generally involves the mitral valve.

D. **Mycotic aneurysms** can be seen in 5% to 10% of cases of BE in autopsy series [81]. These can occur at any site in the arterial vasculature, usually at points of bifurcation. There is a 1% to 3% incidence of intracranial mycotic aneurysms [82]. There may be prodromal symptoms, such as headache before rupture, that warrant investigation such as arteriography. Mycotic aneurysms may resolve during antibiotic therapy. They should be monitored angiographically. Urgent repair should be considered for those that enlarge during or after antibiotic therapy. Repair of a ruptured aneurysm is indicated if anatomically feasible [2].

E. **Renal complications** [83,84]—specifically, focal or diffuse glomerulonephritis—may be seen in the course of endocarditis. Both types of glomerulonephritis are probably immunologically mediated by renal deposition of circulating immune complexes, often with decreased levels of serum complement.

1. **Focal glomerulonephritis** is the more common form and results in proteinuria and hematuria but rarely in renal insufficiency.
2. **Diffuse glomerulonephritis** can cause significant renal failure. The picture sometimes is complicated by concomitant administration of nephrotoxic antibiotics or by the possibility of interstitial nephritis from penicillins. The occurrence of diffuse glomerulonephritis is related to duration of disease and is less common today than in the preantibiotic era. Renal insufficiency secondary to diffuse glomerulonephritis is likely to improve with appropriate therapy, although it may not respond well after extensive damage has occurred.

F. **Complications of antibiotic therapy**

1. **Drug fever** is discussed in Chapter 1.
2. **Allergic drug reactions.** In addition to fever, prolonged administration of high-dose penicillins or cephalosporins results in a significant rate of allergic drug reactions (see Chapter 24).
3. **Aminoglycoside toxicity** is discussed in Chapter 27.
4. **Acute interstitial nephritis,** often accompanied by renal insufficiency, may be seen with the use of almost any penicillin or cephalosporin, although the incidence is much higher with methicillin (see Chapter 27).
5. **Neutropenia** is relatively common secondary to $\beta$-lactams, especially after 15 days of therapy [85].

X. **Evaluating sustained bacteremia.** Diagnostic criteria should be applied to assess the likelihood of IE (see section **III.F**). Among patients with *S. aureus* bacteremia, the risk of IE is highest in community-acquired infection, in the absence of a peripheral focus, in IVDUs, in diabetics with chronic skin infections, and in patients with preexisting valve abnormalities [2,86,87]. The risk of nosocomial IE due to *S. aureus* bacteremia secondary to an i.v. catheter is significant [88]. Patients with *S. aureus* bacteremia who have known cardiac valve disease, develop a new significant murmur, or have persistent fever or bacteremia for 3 or more days after removal of a presumed primary focus of infection (e.g., intravascular catheter or abscess) and initiation of therapy merit echocardiographic evaluation because they are at high risk for IE [2].

A review found IE in 12 of 34 cases of enterococcal bacteremia that were community acquired, but in only 1 of 118 that were of nosocomial origin [89].

See section **IV. B** under Endocarditis Associated with Prosthetic Valves for discussion involving prosthetic valves.

## ENDOCARDITIS ASSOCIATED WITH PROSTHETIC VALVES

The incidence of PVE is highest during the initial 6 to 12 months after valve replacement but continues at a low rate thereafter. By 4 to 5 years postoperatively, as many as 3% to 6% of patients may have had PVE. In most series, the rate of infection in mechanical and bioprosthetic valves is similar. Rates of infection are similar for prostheses at the mitral or aortic position [90].

**I. Time of onset of PVE**

**A. PVE occurring within 12 months** (especially that within 2 months) of valve replacement presumably is likely to have been acquired at the time of operation or in the early postoperative period. Potential sources of contamination accounting for these cases are the heart-lung machine itself, coronary suction lines, other sources of intraoperative contamination, postoperative i.v. and urinary catheters, postoperative pneumonias, and sternal wound infections. In individual cases, however, a definite source of infection often is not identified.

**B. PVE presenting more than 12 months postoperatively.** Late infections presumably are caused by bacteremia unrelated to the initial surgical procedure and often occurring in a community setting.

**II. Pathologic features.** With mechanical valves, infection involves the valve annulus at the site of attachment, resulting in ring abscesses, with frequent extension to adjacent structures [90]. With **aortic valve** involvement, prosthetic detachment often leads to severe regurgitation, and extension of infection to conducting tissue may cause serious conduction defects. With **mitral prosthesis** involvement, severe regurgitation or conduction defects are less common, but obstruction by vegetative material may be encountered. With **bioprosthetic valves,** ring abscesses occur when infection arises in the year after valve replacement. Infection beginning later is more typically (but not always) confined to the valve leaflets. Infection may destroy the leaflets of bioprosthetic valves or may cause delayed-onset leaflet stiffness with later development of stenosis [90].

**III. Microbiologic features.** *S. epidermidis* and *S. aureus* together account for almost half the total cases of PVE. The microbiologic profile of PVE within 12 months of surgery differs from that of later onset.

**A. In early PVE,** *S. epidermidis* is the most common organism, with occasional infections by *S. aureus,* diphtheroids, gram-negative rods, and fungi.

**B. In later-onset PVE,** viridans streptococci, enterococci, *S. aureus,* and fastidious gram-negative coccobacilli often are encountered. Coagulase-negative staphylococci may cause 20% of these later infections. **Importantly, coagulase-negative staphylococci that cause PVE within 12 months of surgery often are methicillin resistant (>75%),** whereas those causing later-onset PVE are less commonly methicillin resistant (<30%) [90,91].

**C. Culture-negative PVE** occurs occasionally. Most often, it is the result of recent antimicrobial therapy. However, PVE due to *Legionella* species, mycelial fungi, *C. burnetii, Mycoplasma* species, mycobacteria, and occasional fastidious bacteria may cause PVE with negative routine blood cultures [90].

**IV. Diagnosis**

**A. Clinical features.** The clinical picture may be nonspecific or atypical, and precise diagnosis may be difficult, particularly during the initial weeks after surgery.

1. **Fever.** An unexplained and persistent fever in patients with prosthetic valves always raises the possibility of endocarditis. Therefore, serial blood cultures should routinely be drawn in febrile patients with prosthetic valves.
2. **Cardiac findings** of either a new regurgitant murmur (indicating a paravalvular leak) or unexplained refractory heart failure are important clues to the diagnosis of PVE.
3. **The presence of embolic phenomena** or immunologically mediated vasculitic lesions helps support the diagnosis, but their absence does not exclude the diagnosis.

**B.** As the time after surgery increases (>6 months), the clinical features usually are similar to those of BE in patients without prosthetic valves. However, the diagnosis of endocarditis in the early postoperative period often presents considerable difficulties, with multiple other nosocomial events confounding the evaluation of postoperative bacteremia. Patients with no cardiac or peripheral evidence of endocarditis are particularly problematic in this respect.

1. If sustained bacteremia is caused by relatively avirulent organisms that are not otherwise expected to be invasive (e.g., *S. epidermidis,* micrococci, or diphtheroids)

or if there is no apparent extracardiac source for bacteremia, the patient should be treated for endocarditis.

2. Transient bacteremia, with gram-negative rods especially, may or may not indicate endocarditis in this setting. It has been suggested that the postoperative patient with gram-negative rod bacteremia associated with an obvious extracardiac focus of infection and no clinical evidence of endocarditis need not be placed on prolonged therapy for presumed valvular infection. If bacteremia recurs after a course of therapy sufficient to eradicate the extracardiac focus, endocarditis must be seriously considered.

   Some prefer to treat all valve recipients with bacteremia for presumed endocarditis. In one study, only 16% of valve recipients with nosocomial bacteremia (not due to PVE itself) went on to develop subsequent PVE [92]. Staphylococcal bacteremia and the presence of a prosthetic mitral valve was associated with an increased risk for PVE [92]. Infectious disease consultation is advisable.

3. Sustained *S. aureus* bacteremia should be treated as endocarditis.

4. Nosocomial candidemia in patients with prosthetic valves is not always associated with nor results in PVE. In one study of 44 patients, approximately 15% had obvious PVE when candidemia was identified and another 10%, often with early postoperative candidemia, subsequently developed PVE. The interval from candidemia to overt PVE may be long (26–690 days) [93].

**C. Blood cultures**

1. In the absence of antibiotic therapy, most patients with prosthetic valve BE (85%–95%) have positive blood cultures [90].

2. With some causes of PVE, however, blood cultures may be negative (see section **III.C**). Infections with *Candida* species can occasionally result in intermittent fungemia or negative cultures. With *Aspergillus* or other mycelial fungi causing PVE, blood cultures are usually negative. Fungal PVE may result in emboli to large vessels, and the diagnosis often depends on the demonstration of fungi in resected large emboli (see Chapter 17).

3. It is important that the etiology of PVE not be obscured by premature antibiotic treatment [90].

   a. Indolent endocarditis, in the absence of hemodynamic instability that mandates surgical intervention, does not require immediate antimicrobial therapy. Antibiotics should be withheld briefly pending the isolation of an organism from blood culture [90].

   b. If oral antibiotics that might render initial blood cultures sterile have been given, this delay (3–5 days) is particularly important because it allows blood cultures to be repeated without the interference of additional therapy [90].

   c. Presentations of PVE that are acute or complicated by hemodynamic instability due to prosthetic valve dysfunction require that blood cultures be obtained and antibiotics administered promptly.

**D. Other aids to diagnosis. EKG** demonstration of conduction defects, such as increasing P-R interval, complete heart block, or left bundle branch block, suggest infection invading the conduction system. **Echocardiography** may be useful in detecting large vegetations, prosthesis detachment, perivalvular abscess, or pericarditis. TEE, which is exceptionally useful in evaluating prostheses in the mitral position, is indicated when investigating patients with possible PVE. TEE provides excellent views of the posterior portion of the aortic prosthesis; the anterior aortic root area is better visualized from a transthoracic approach. In patients at high risk of PVE, repeat studies may detect abnormalities not noted on the initial echocardiogram. TEE is strikingly more sensitive in the detection of myocardial abscess in patients with PVE than is TTE [90]. Nondiagnostic TTE evaluations are insufficient to exclude the diagnosis of PVE [21,24,67].

**V. Therapy for PVE**

**A. Antibiotic therapy** follows the same general principles previously outlined for native valve endocarditis [90]. Bactericidal antibiotics are used and administered parenterally. Because antibiotics are often given for 6 weeks, recovery of the causative organism and careful determination of susceptibility data are essential [90] (see section **IV.C**).

1. ***S. epidermidis.*** Most *S. epidermidis* isolates from patients with PVE are resistant to semisynthetic penicillins such as methicillin (see section **III**), although this may not be apparent by routine disk diffusion tests or automated MIC tests using a low bacterial inoculum. Careful evaluation of these isolates using proper methods is necessary [90]. Strains that are resistant to methicillin are also resistant to cephalosporins and other $\beta$-lactam antibiotics when studied carefully.

   The best results have been obtained with a combination antimicrobial regimen that includes rifampin and gentamicin if the organism is sensitive to these agents. The usual recommended dosages, assuming normal renal function, are vancomycin (see Chapter 27 for dosage regimens); rifampin 300 mg orally every 8 hours; and gentamicin 1.0 to 1.3 mg/kg every 8 hours. To prevent emergence of rifampin resistance, it has been suggested that vancomycin be adjusted to give peak levels of 25 to 35 $\mu$g/mL and trough levels of 10 to 15 $\mu$g/mL and that gentamicin dosage be adjusted to give a 5-$\mu$g/mL peak and 1-$\mu$g/mL trough [41,90]. Additive nephrotoxicity may result from simultaneous vancomycin and gentamicin administration; therefore, renal function should be monitored carefully (see Chapter 27). Ideally, the vancomycin and rifampin are given for 6 weeks and the gentamicin (if the strain is susceptible) for the first 2 weeks. If a strain is resistant to gentamicin and other aminoglycosides, a fluoroquinolone with enhanced gram-positive activity (if the strain is susceptible to it) may be used in lieu of the aminoglycoside [90]. **Most patients require valve replacement in addition to antibiotic therapy.**

   For treatment of PVE caused by methicillin-susceptible *S. epidermidis,* a $\beta$-lactam antibiotic should be substituted for vancomycin in the combination regimen [41,58,90].

   The treatment of PVE caused by *S. aureus* uses the same regimens recommended for treatment of *S. epidermidis* PVE. The decision to use vancomycin or a semisynthetic penicillinase-resistant penicillin is based on whether the isolate is methicillin resistant or whether the patient has a therapy-limiting penicillin allergy.

2. **Other organisms** are treated with high doses of i.v. antibiotics guided by sensitivities, as discussed earlier in section **VI** under Infective Endocarditis. Antibiotics usually are administered for at least 6 weeks; a longer course may be required for patients who do not respond promptly. **In the setting of PVE, every effort should be made to attain maximum bactericidal blood levels.** For example, it probably is best to add an aminoglycoside to penicillin for sensitive viridans streptococci infection, even though this may not be necessary for native valve infection.

3. **Initial therapy while awaiting culture results.** The decision to start antibiotic therapy before a microbiologic diagnosis has been established should be based on the clinical findings. Of particular importance is the possible need for urgent surgical intervention. In selecting antibiotics for empiric therapy, the clinical and epidemiologic circumstances must be weighed. The time that has elapsed since valve replacement may provide insight into potential causes of PVE (see section **III**) and should be carefully considered. In general, therapy should include vancomycin, gentamicin, and to provide coverage for HACEK organisms, a third-generation cephalosporin.

   Antibiotics are adjusted when culture results become available. If blood cultures remain negative, the causes of culture-negative PVE should be sought. For patients with culture-negative PVE who remain febrile during empiric therapy, surgery should be considered. Infectious disease consultation is advised.

**B. Surgery**

1. **Indications for surgery** in PVE are similar to those previously discussed for native valve endocarditis [22,65] (see section **VIII** under Infective Endocarditis), and they **have been summarized in Table 12.3.** Some of these indications are not absolute but rather serve to prompt careful consideration of surgical therapy.

   Because invasive infection unlikely to respond to antibiotics alone is often a feature of PVE beginning within 12 months after valve implantation, these patients often benefit from surgical intervention. Evidence of invasive disease

Table 12.3. Indications for Cardiac Surgery in Patients with Prosthetic Valve Endocarditis (PVE)

| |
|---|
| Moderate to severe heart failure due to prosthesis dysfunction (incompetence or obstruction) |
| Invasive and destructive paravulvular infection |
| Partial valve dehiscence |
| New or progressive conduction system disturbances |
| Fever persisting 10 or more days during appropriate antibiotic therapy |
| Purulent pericarditis |
| Sinus of Valsalva aneurysm or intracardiac fistula |
| Uncontrolled bacteremic infection during therapy |
| Infection caused by selected organisms |
| Fungi |
| *Staphylococcus aureus*[a] |
| Coagulase-negative staphylococci[a] |
| *Pseudomonas aeruginosa* |
| Relapse after appropriate antimicrobial therapy |
| Persistent fever during therapy for culture-negative PVE in absence of other causes of fever |
| Recurrent arterial emboli[b] |
| Renal failure with severe aortic regurgitation[c] |

[a]Although not a uniformly accepted indication for surgical treatment of PVE, several investigators favor surgical therapy for PVE caused by *S. aureus* or coagulase-negative staphylococci [90,95]. This may especially apply to patients who do not respond rapidly to antibiotic therapy.
[b]Rather than an indication for surgery, the potential for additional systemic emboli is often viewed as a factor that, in combination with other considerations, might help to justify surgery. Reviews suggest that recurrent emboli are rare in patients who are receiving appropriate antibiotics [90].
[c]The presence of deteriorating renal function in patients with endocarditis associated with severe aortic regurgitation is indicative of low cardiac output and should, in itself, stimulate urgent operation [22].
Modified from Karchmer AW. Infections of prosthetic heart valves. In: Bisno AL, Waldvogel FA, eds. *Infections associated with indwelling medical devices.* 3rd ed. Washington, DC: American Society for Microbiology, 2000: 145–72; Jamieson SW. Surgical therapy for infective endocarditis. *Mayo Clin Proc* 1995;70:598; with permission.

even in the absence of CHF warrants surgery [90,94]. PVE caused by *S. aureus* is unusually lethal, with low cure rates attributed to antibiotic therapy alone; affected patients should be considered for early surgical intervention [90]. Failure to achieve an afebrile status with appropriate antibiotic therapy, assuming drug fever and metastatic infection have been ruled out, is evidence of invasive disease and should prompt consideration of surgery.

Similarly, relapse after appropriate medical therapy usually is due to invasive disease; patients who experience such a relapse should be treated surgically. Failure of a patient with culture-negative PVE to become afebrile in 10 days indicates either inappropriate empiric therapy or invasive disease. Such patients should undergo surgery to clarify the etiology of PVE and debride invasive infection. Surgical intervention is appropriate and probably beneficial in as many as 40% to 50% of patients with PVE [90].

2. **Results of PVE surgery** have been reviewed elsewhere, and operative mortality rates range from 20% to 30% [73]. However in a recent series, those who survived the surgical period had a good 5- to 10-year survival rate with about 70% at 5 years and 60% at 10 years [73]. There appears to be no striking difference in survival whether a valve replacement is with tissue or mechanical prostheses [22,73].

   In a recent report, operative mortality was related to the presence of an abscess at the time of operation. Formation of an abscess cavity was commonly associated with staphylococcal infections, PVE, and the aortic site [22,73].

**VI. Prevention of PVE.** See Chapter 27.

## ENDOCARDITIS IN INTRAVENOUS DRUG USERS

**I. Clinical characteristics and diagnosis.** Symptoms of endocarditis in IVDUs are usually of 1 to 2 weeks' duration at the time of presentation, and fever is almost always observed. Endocarditis often is difficult to predict on clinical grounds in the febrile IVDU, and it differs from that in nonaddicts in several respects [96,97].

- **A.** Preexisting valvular abnormalities are usually absent.
- **B.** Tricuspid valve involvement approximates 50% to 75% of episodes. Repeated injections of particulate foreign material may damage the tricuspid endothelium, predisposing it to infection during a bacteremic episode. With isolated tricuspid involvement, a murmur is often undetectable. Neurologic and peripheral manifestations of endocarditis are relatively infrequent. Symptoms of cough, hemoptysis, dyspnea, and pleuritic chest pain associated with pneumonia or septic pulmonary emboli are common.
- **C.** Aortic or mitral valves are involved in roughly 25% to 33% of patients. Pulmonic valve involvement is rare. Left-sided endocarditis produces a clinical pattern similar to that seen in nonaddicts.
- **D.** There is a high rate of recurrence, presumably due to continued parenteral drug use [98].

**II. Microbiologic features.** *S. aureus,* the single most common organism responsible for endocarditis in IVDUs, accounts for approximately 60% of the total isolates and 80% of those in right-sided disease. Streptococci and enterococci comprise approximately 20% and cause left-sided endocarditis in the great majority of cases. *P. aeruginosa* and other aerobic gram-negative bacilli account for 10% to 15% and can display marked regional variation. Fungi, mainly *Candida* species, cause predominantly left-sided endocarditis and account for approximately 5%. Polymicrobial blood cultures are reported in nearly 5% and negative blood cultures in fewer than 10%.

**III. Treatment.** Antimicrobial therapy for endocarditis in drug addicts follows the same principles outlined earlier for the nonaddict population, except that presumptive therapy should include gram-negative coverage; indications for a surgical approach to left-sided disease also are similar. A short course (2 weeks) of a penicillinase-resistant penicillin and an aminoglycoside has been effective in uncomplicated right-sided IE caused by methicillin-sensitive *S. aureus* in drug users [99]. Dosing is as for standard staphylococcal IE therapy. Vancomycin should not be substituted in this setting [99]. Cloxacillin alone for 2 weeks also has been effective [100]. Patients with *S. aureus* tricuspid valve involvement usually do well, but occasional cases that are refractory to antimicrobial therapy require valvulectomy with or without valve replacement.

**IV. Prognosis.** The mortality rate among addicts with staphylococcal endocarditis is considerably lower than that of the general population. This probably reflects the younger population involved, a lower incidence of underlying heart or other serious diseases, and the frequency of isolated tricuspid valve involvement. However, the mortality for repeated bouts of endocarditis and of gram-negative or fungal endocarditis remains high.

The course of BE in IVDUs who are HIV positive is similar to that in HIV-negative patients [101]. However, mortality is increased for those with a CD4 count below 200/mm [102].

## PERICARDITIS AND MYOCARDITIS

**I. Pericarditis** [103]

**A. Clinical characteristics.** Pericarditis, sometimes accompanied by clinically significant myocarditis, may present as the sole or major manifestation of an infectious illness, or it may occur as a minor or incidental finding. The patient is usually febrile, and the diagnosis is suggested by symptoms of substernal pain or discomfort, which sometimes is relieved by sitting up and leaning forward; the presence of a pericardial rub is confirmatory. Occasionally, pericarditis may present with signs and symptoms of cardiac tamponade. Roentgenographic findings of an enlarged cardiac silhouette may be seen. Typical EKG changes are generalized ST segment elevations without reciprocal ST depression except in leads $V_1$ and aVR. Low-voltage QSR complexes may be seen with sizable pericardial effusions. Echocardiography is a sensitive and reliable noninvasive procedure for demonstrating the presence of significant amounts of pericardial fluid.

**B.** The **cause** often is difficult to establish. Numerous noninfectious as well as infectious causes must be considered.

**1. Noninfectious causes.** Among these are uremia, neoplasm, trauma, myocardial infarction, postmyocardial infarction (Dressler syndrome), connective tissue diseases (e.g., lupus erythematosus, rheumatoid arthritis), and rheumatic fever. History, physical examination, and appropriate laboratory studies should be directed toward ruling these out.

**2. Infectious causes** [104,105]. Although their true incidence is not known, **viral agents probably are the most common** cause of infectious pericarditis in the United States. Among proved or highly suspect viral agents, the most important are enteroviruses, especially coxsackievirus B, coxsackievirus A, and echovirus. Numerous other viral agents have been implicated. The most common diagnosis, especially in young patients without other apparent cause, is idiopathic or nonspecific pericarditis. This is often equated with viral pericarditis, although in most cases a definite viral cause cannot be proved. Much less common are cases of pyogenic or tuberculous pericarditis; nonetheless, it is important to rule these out in suggestive clinical settings. Other infectious agents known or suspected to cause pericarditis are fungi, rickettsiae, chlamydiae, mycoplasmas, protozoa, and *Legionella pneumophila.*

**C. Differential diagnosis.** Although the patient's history, physical findings, and ancillary diagnostic tests may help, specific diagnosis of presumed infectious pericarditis usually will depend on examination of pericardial fluid or on pericardial biopsy. However, these procedures often are not diagnostic and, in most patients, are not indicated. In a case of pericarditis in which the cause is still unknown after the usual diagnostic studies, one often needs to decide whether pericardiocentesis or pericardial biopsy should be performed. This decision must be individualized. Should any evidence of impending tamponade appear, a procedure is necessary for therapeutic purposes, and diagnostic information can be obtained at the same time.

In the case of the typical idiopathic pericarditis that appears to follow a relatively benign course, it usually is best to observe the patient and treat symptomatically. Should fever persist for more than a few weeks, or should the clinical course appear to be one of continued toxemia or deterioration, open drainage of the pericardium, with pericardial biopsy, may be indicated.

**D. Specific infections**

**1. Viral, idiopathic, or nonspecific pericarditis**

**a. Presentation.** In the case of viral, idiopathic, or nonspecific pericarditis, the illness tends to present acutely. In some cases, a history is obtained suggesting a viral respiratory or gastrointestinal infection that began 2 to 3 weeks previously. Signs and symptoms may be those of pericarditis alone, or there may be accompanying pleural effusions or pulmonary infiltrates.

**b. Course and complications.** The illness usually follows a benign course, resolving in 2 to 6 weeks, but symptoms may recur in 15% to 30% or more of patients [106]. The latent period between the preceding viral infection and the first symptoms of pericarditis, as well as the continued relapsing course observed in some patients, suggests a postinfectious, immunologically mediated process. Associated myocarditis, reflected by EKG changes, is frequent and occasionally is severe enough to cause cardiomegaly and CHF. Chronic cardiomyopathies have been observed in some patients. Hemorrhagic pericardial effusions, cardiac tamponade, and chronic constrictive pericarditis also have been described.

**c. Diagnosis.** The diagnosis often is presumptive and depends on observation of the clinical course after specific etiologies have been ruled out as carefully as possible.

**(1) Cultures and serologic studies.** Viral cultures of the pharynx, fecal specimens, and pericardial fluid may be performed, but in most cases the results are negative. Examination of acute and convalescent sera for a fourfold or greater increase in antiviral antibody may be helpful if a specific virus has been isolated. Screening for antibody to all possible viruses is not practical.

(2) **Pericardial drainage and biopsy** may be indicated in some patients for diagnostic purposes. Cardiac tamponade, or impending tamponade, occurs occasionally and requires drainage through an open surgical procedure or pericardiocentesis. Open drainage, which is preferred by many, offers an opportunity for examination of pericardial tissue. This is useful primarily in ruling out nonviral causes such as tuberculosis or tumor. The fluid and tissue can be cultured for virus and the tissue examined by histologic and immunofluorescent techniques. Histology is nonspecific, however, and viruses are isolated infrequently.

(3) **Treatment.** Other than pericardial drainage when indicated, management for idiopathic and viral pericarditis consists of bed rest, pain control, and monitoring for evidence of hemodynamic compromise. Animal model data suggests nonsteroidal antiinflammatory agents, and prednisone may exacerbate the myocarditis that can accompany viral pericarditis [104]. These agents should thus be avoided if there is any clinical suspicion or chemical evidence of myocarditis. Idiopathic and viral pericarditis typically run a benign and self-limited course. Relapses may occur. Colchicine may be useful in these settings [107]. Steroids and other immunosuppressive regimens are sometimes used [108].

2. **HIV-related pericarditis** [109,110] is common enough that risk factors should be assessed in the presentation of pericarditis. When large symptomatic pericardial effusions in patients with HIV were aggressively investigated, two-thirds were found to have an identifiable cause [111]. Approximately one-third of HIV-positive patients with tamponade will have mycobacterial disease (*M. tuberculosis* or *M. avium-intracellulare*) [111].

3. **Purulent pericarditis** [112,113].

   a. **Presentation.** Purulent pericarditis almost always occurs in the setting of other serious disease or a surgical procedure and results from postoperative infections after thoracic surgery (commonly open heart surgery); contiguous spread of infection from pleural, mediastinal, or pulmonary foci; contiguous spread from intracardiac infections (endocarditis, myocardial abscess); or hematogenous spread of infection from distant foci. Although the patient is obviously ill, specific signs of pericarditis such as chest pain, pericardial rub, or EKG changes often are absent. The disease is likely to follow a rapidly progressive course and carries a high mortality rate.

   b. **Microbiologic features.** In the preantibiotic era, *Streptococcus pneumoniae,* usually associated with pneumonia, caused more than 50% of cases of purulent pericarditis; staphylococci and streptococci were the next most common causative agents. More recently, staphylococci and gram-negative bacilli account for the majority of cases, usually occurring after major surgery or in patients with uremic pericarditis, cancer, myocardial infarction, diabetes, and immunosuppressed states. Meningococci, streptococci, gonococci, *H. influenzae,* and a variety of other bacteria as well as fungi [114] also are reported.

   c. **Diagnosis and treatment. Prompt drainage of pericardial fluid is essential for diagnostic and therapeutic purposes.** This may be attempted with pericardiocentesis, but surgical intervention with drainage through a pericardial window usually is preferable due to the thick nature of the infected fluid and should not be delayed. Antibiotic therapy is guided by results of Gram stains and cultures of pericardial fluid or tissue. High doses of parenteral antibiotics, equivalent to endocarditis regimens, are used. The role of early pericardiectomy is controversial.

4. **Tuberculous pericarditis** [115]

   a. **Presentation.** Tuberculous pericarditis may occur as the only clinically evident manifestation of tuberculosis, or it may be accompanied by pulmonary or other (extrapulmonary) disease. Tuberculous pericarditis has its origins in extension from adjacent pulmonary, bone, or lymph node disease; retrograde lymphatic spread from tracheobronchial nodes; or hematogenous dissemination. The presentation may be acute, subacute, or chronic. The acute disease may be productive and granulomatous, with little effusion, or it may present with abrupt accumulation of fluid and may cause tamponade. The presentation usually is insidious, however, with slow accumulation of pericardial fluid. Chronic constrictive pericarditis may result.

b. **Diagnosis.** If pericarditis occurs in association with proven active pulmonary or extrapulmonary tuberculosis, the presumptive diagnosis usually is made and the patient is treated accordingly. Otherwise, specific diagnosis depends on examination of pericardial fluid or on pericardial biopsy. Acid-fast organisms usually are not seen in pericardial fluid, and diagnosis is made mainly on the basis of cultures of fluid and pericardial tissue and histologic examination of biopsy material. Granulomatous pericarditis should be regarded as tuberculous if no other cause can be found, even if acid-fast bacilli are not demonstrable histologically.

c. **Treatment is with specific antituberculous agents.** Optimal regimens have not been clearly established. Data reviewed in Chapter 11 suggest that extrapulmonary tuberculosis due to susceptible organisms can be treated in the same way as pulmonary tuberculosis if isoniazid and rifampin are not contraindicated. (If alternate drugs must be used, infectious disease consultation is advised.) For additional discussion and specific dosage regimens, see Chapter 11 under Tuberculosis.

**The indications for corticosteroid therapy and pericardiectomy are controversial.** Steroids may hasten symptom resolution and decrease fluid reaccumulation [116].

II. **Myocarditis** [117]

A. **Viral.** Most infectious myocarditis in the United States is of viral origin. Coxsackie B virus is the most common specific organism. It is suspected that many cases of myocarditis that are classified as idiopathic are also due to an undiagnosed viral etiology. Numerous other viruses have been reported to cause myocarditis.

1. **Pathophysiology.** In recent years, it has been concluded that the myocardial injury stems not from the virus itself, but from immunologic responses initiated by the virus. The responses leading to the immune-mediated injury are incompletely defined. Some individuals may be especially prone because of inherent immunoregulatory defects.

2. **Clinical presentation.** Sixty percent of individuals complain of an antecedent flulike illness. The spectrum of presenting symptoms ranges from malaise and mild chest pain to cardiogenic shock. Typical complaints include palpitations and chest pain that may be pericardial, ischemic, or atypical sounding by description. Heart block and syncope may be seen.

3. **Diagnosis.** No blood tests are diagnostic, and viral testing has the same limitations as in pericarditis. Nonspecific ST and T-wave changes on **EKG** are common. Supraventricular and ventricular arrhythmias are frequently seen. **Echocardiography** can show a broad array of abnormalities, including wall thickening and segmental wall motion abnormalities. **Indium 111–labeled antimyosin antibody** imaging can detect myocardial necrosis. **Contrast-enhanced magnetic resonance imaging** may be helpful.

The gold standard for diagnosis has long been the endomyocardial biopsy, but many experts now feel it is not routinely warranted [118].

4. **Treatment.** Neither immunosuppression nor immunomodulation have been of consistent benefit. At present, therapy consists of control of symptoms and potential cardiac complications.

5. **Prognosis.** One-third of patients may have persistent abnormalities ranging from mild EKG changes to CHF. Although the association between acute myocarditis and dilated cardiomyopathy has almost been taken for granted for many years, the causal relationship has not been proven. It is unknown if any of those individuals with dilated cardiomyopathy represent end-stage viral myocardial infection.

B. **Lyme disease.** The carditis associated with Lyme disease typically presents as conduction abnormalities. Related dilated cardiomyopathy has not been demonstrated outside of Europe [119]. See Chapter 21.

C. **Chagas disease.** American trypanosomiasis is the world's leading cause of CHF. In the United States, it needs to be considered in immigrant populations from South America. [120].

**D. HIV-related myocarditis** [121]. Dilated cardiomyopathy is a well-recognized feature of HIV. It may be due to HIV infection of myocardial cells, coinfection with other viruses such as CMV, or an immune-related response. Cardiotoxicity from illegal substances or HIV-related therapy also may play a role [122,123].

## INFECTIONS OF PERMANENT CARDIAC PACEMAKERS AND IMPLANTABLE CARDIOVERTER DEFIBRILLATORS

**I. Permanent cardiac pacemaker infections** [124,125]. Pacemaker systems consist of a generator, which sits in a surgically created pocket below the subcutaneous or subfascial tissue in the chest or abdominal wall, and electrode leads, which may be epicardial or, more commonly, transvenous (in which case the electrodes are attached to the endocardium). The generator pocket and the intravascular and intracardiac portions of the leads eventually become encased in dense layers of endothelialized fibrous tissue.

**A. Location**

1. **Generator units or the lead wires in their subcutaneous position.** These infections are commonly seen soon after pacemaker placement or generator exchange. Later infections may be seen as a result of necrosis of the skin overlying the generator or trauma to the generator. There may be signs of swelling, erythema, and pain over the generator. Drainage is more commonly seen in infections soon after implantation. Systemic signs and bacteremia may be present.
2. **Epicardial electrodes** may become infected from spread from the generator pocket or direct contamination at placement. In addition to clinical findings noted above, pericarditis and mediastinitis may occur.
3. **Intravascular portion of the transvenous electrode (pacemaker endocarditis)** [126,127]. This usually arises because of intravascular tracking of infection of the subcutaneous portion of the pacing device. An incidence of 0.5% has been noted. Bacteremic seeding from a remote site of infection can lead to this process. Unless infection occurs after recent pacemaker implantation or manipulation with obvious acute pocket infection and systemic toxicity, the diagnosis can be elusive. TEE is especially useful in demonstrating vegetations on the electrodes, tricuspid valve, or ventricular endocardium. Symptoms can range from fever and chills to overt septic shock.

**B. Predisposing factors** [128].

1. **Skin necrosis** overlying the generator can predispose to infection. This is less common with subfascial than subcutaneous placement of the generator. Skin erosion can occur for multiple reasons, including body build, shift in generator placement, or poor nutrition.
2. **Self-induced trauma,** such as from heavy lifting, repetitive movements involving the chest wall, or a direct blow to the generator pocket area, can occur.
3. **Bacteremia** from a source other than an infected pacemaker can cause infection of the system in rare circumstances. **The pacemaker is at greatest risk for infection associated with bacteremia during the first few weeks after insertion.** The offending organisms would typically be staphylococci or streptococci from a remote site of infection. Therefore, it is important to treat promptly any infections, especially those of the skin or teeth, in patients with a pacemaker. Antibiotic prophylaxis to prevent pacemaker infection is not recommended.
4. **Dermatologic conditions** may predispose the patient to pacemaker infection if the skin overlying the generator is not intact as a consequence [129].
5. **Replacement or repositioning of the generator or electrodes** appeared to be a predisposing factor for infection in older studies. However, more recent studies have not borne this out, perhaps because current generators are smaller and lighter.

**C. Microbiologic features**

1. *S. aureus* and *S. epidermidis* are responsible for about 75% of generator pocket infections. Other common skin flora as well as Enterobacteriaceae and *Candida* species can be seen. Infections in the initial 2-week postoperative period are most commonly due to *S. aureus* and are frequently associated with bacteremia [129].

2. Pacemaker endocarditis is also most frequently caused by staphylococcal species, but a wide variety of organisms can be seen. Of note, in the early postoperative period, an *S. aureus* bacteremia from a remote site is likely to cause pacemaker endocarditis. However, bacteremia with any organism months and years after placement can be treated as the uncomplicated bacteremia itself would be because pacemaker endocarditis would be unlikely [130].

**D. Diagnosis** [131] is based on the clinical picture as well as culture results from blood or a generator pocket abscess. Criteria include the following:

1. Local inflammation or abscess of the pocket, *or*
2. Secondary infection of the skin after erosion of the generator, *or*
3. Fever and positive blood culture results in a patient with a pacemaker and no other identifiable source of infection. TEE is a useful diagnostic tool [132].

**E. Therapy** [124,125]

1. **Explantation and reimplantation.**
   - **a.** When infection is limited to the generator pocket or subcutaneous electrode without bacteremia, a one-step direct exchange of the pacing system can be performed while the patient is on antibiotics. In some cases, a two-step procedure is performed wherein the infected device is removed and the new pacer inserted at a different time while the patient is maintained with a temporary transvenous device.
   - **b.** Pacemaker endocarditis or bacteremia accompanying pacemaker infection is best treated by removing the generator and the electrodes. This may be accomplished by traction or, in more difficult cases, by the Cooks electrode extraction system. However, surgical removal requiring cardiotomy may be necessary. A temporary pacing system should be used. Antibiotics aimed at the causative organism and dosed for endocarditis should be given for a minimum of 2 weeks before a new permanent electrode is placed. There should be evidence of clinical response. If a patient's health status does not permit manipulations necessary to remove the entire system, prolonged courses of initial i.v. therapy followed by chronic suppressive oral antibiotics can be tried.
2. **Antibiotics.** Empiric choice of therapy should include an antistaphylococcal drug. If the patient is extremely ill, it is prudent to include gram-negative coverage while awaiting culture results.

**II. Implantable cardioverter defibrillator (ICD) infections** [124,125]. The technology of ICD systems continues to evolve. The technique of surgical placement of the pulse generator, extrapericardial or epicardial defibrillation patches, and a transvenous rate-sensing electrode has been largely supplanted by the use of a transvenously planted rate-sensing lead and a superior vena caval coil electrode as well as subcutaneous or epicardial electrodes all connected to a pulse generator that is placed subcutaneously or submuscularly. Infection rates have decreased from 2% to 11% [132] with the older technology to 0.8% to 1.5% with the newer systems [133,134].

**A. Timing.** The majority of ICD infections typically present within 6 months, and specifically within the initial 3 months, after placement.

**B. Symptoms.** Pain and erythema around the generator occur. Fluid collection or drainage may be present. These same findings may occur at the infraclavicular wound or subcutaneous patch wound. Epicardial patch infection may be accompanied by systemic toxicity and evidence of pericarditis.

**C. Bacteriology.** Patients are frequently bacteremic, especially if infection is due to *S. aureus* [135]. Cultures of the generator pocket may be positive even if the site looks normal. *S. aureus* and coagulase-negative staphylococci are the most frequently infecting organisms [133,135,136]. Multiple other bacteria, and on rare occasion atypical mycobacteria or yeast, can be the causative organisms. Polymicrobial infection occurs [135,136].

**D. Therapy.** Guidelines regarding therapy do not exist and management is complex. Removal of the entire ICD system appears necessary to eliminate infection, especially in the presence of systemic toxicity, bacteremia, or infection due to *S. aureus*. Infections involving only the generator site have been managed much as in the parallel situation in pacemaker infections. In cases where a patient's health status precludes removing the entire system and no virulent organisms are responsible for the infection, i.v. antibiotics followed by continuous oral suppressive antibiotic regimens has been advocated [137–139]. Duration of parenteral therapy beyond that typically needed for soft tissue infection, regardless of whether the entire system is removed or not, should be determined by the potential for endocardial involvement and the implications of bacteremia (e.g., sustained *S. aureus* bacteremia). Decisions about replacing the ICD system after complete removal need to consider the risks and benefits of reimplantation versus antiarrhythmic drug therapy. Timing of replacement is in reality generally determined by the perceived threat of persistence of inducible arrhythmias.

## REFERENCES


1. Sullam PM, Drake TA, Sande MA. Pathogenesis of endocarditis. *Am J Med* 1985;78:110.
2. Karchmer AW. Infective endocarditis. In: Braunwald E, Zipes DP, Libby P, eds. *Heart disease,* 6th ed. New York: WB Saunders, 2001:1723–1748.
3. Dankert J, et al. Involvement of bactericidal factors from thrombin-stimulated platelets in clearance of adherent viridans streptococci in experimental infective endocarditis. *Infect Immun* 1995;63:633.
4. Watanakunakorn C, Burkert T. Infective endocarditis at a large community teaching hospital, 1980–1990. *Medicine* 1993;72:90.
5. Hogevik H, et al. Epidemiologic aspects of infective endocarditis in an urban population. *Medicine* 1995;74:324–338.
6. Sandre RM, Shafran SD. Infective endocarditis. *Clin Infect Dis* 1996;22:276–286.
7. Michel PL, Acar J. Native cardiac disease predisposing to infective endocarditis. *Eur Heart J* 1995;16(suppl B):2.
8. Danchin N., et al. Mitral valve prolapse as a risk factor for infective endocarditis. *Lancet* 1989;8641:743.
9. Fernandez-Guerrero ML, et al. Hospital-acquired infectious endocarditis not associated with cardiac surgery: an emerging problem. *Clin Infect Dis* 1995;20:16.
10. Mylonakis MD, Calderwood SB. Infective endocarditis in adults. *N Engl J Med* 2001;18:1318–1330.
11. Robbins MJ, et al. Right-sided valvular endocarditis. *Am Heart J* 1986;111:128.
12. Roder BL, et al. Neurologic manifestations of *Staphylococcus aureus* endocarditis. *Am J Med* 1997;102:376–386.
13. Heiro M, et al. Neurologic manifestations of infective endocarditis. *Arch Intern Med* 2000;160:2781–2787.
14. Gonzales-Juanatey C, et al. Rheumatic manifestations of infective endocarditis in non-addicts. *Medicine* 2001;80:9–19.
15. Werner AS, et al. Infective endocarditis in the elderly in the era of transesophageal echocardiography. *Am J Med* 1996;100:90–97.
16. Giagliardi JP, et al. Native valve endocarditis in elderly and younger adult patients. *Clin Infect Dis* 1998;26:1165–1168.
17. Olaison L, Hogevik H, Alestig K. Fever, C-reactive protein, and other acute-phase reactants during treatment of infective endocarditis. *Arch Intern Med* 1997;157:885–892.
18. Washington JA. The role of the microbiology laboratory in the diagnosis and antimicrobial treatment of infective endocarditis. *Mayo Clin Proc* 1982;57:22.
19. Auckenhalter RW. Laboratory diagnosis of infective endocarditis. *Eur Heart J* 1984;5(suppl C):49.
20. Goldenberger D, et al. Molecular diagnosis of bacterial endocarditis by broad-range PCR amplification and direct sequencing. *J Clin Microbiol* 1995;20:501–506.
21. Mugge A. Echocardiographic detection of cardiac valve vegetations and prognostic implications. *Infect Dis Clin North Am* 1993;7:877.
22. Jameison SW. Surgical therapy for infective endocarditis. *Mayo Clin Proc* 1995;70:598.

22a. Lindner JR, et al. Diagnostic value of echocardiography in suspected endocarditis. *Circulation* 1996;93:730–736.

22b. Irani WN, Grayburn PA, Afridi I. A negative transthoracic echocardiogram obviates the need for transesophageal echocardiography in patients with suspected native valve active infective endocarditis. *Am J Cardiol* 1996;78:101–103.

23. Heidenreich PA, et al. Echocardiography in patients with suspected endocarditis: a cost-effective analysis. *Am J Med* 1999;107:198–208.
24. Jaffe WM, et al. Infective endocarditis, 1983–1988: echocardiographic findings and factors influencing morbidity and mortality. *J Am Coll Cardiol* 1990;15:1227.
25. Durak DT, et al. New criteria for diagnosis of infective endocarditis: utilization of specific echocardiographic findings. *Am J Med* 1994;96:200.
26. Li JS, et al. Proposed modifications to the Duke criteria for the diagnosis of infective endocarditis. *Clin Infect Dis* 2000;30:633–638.
27. Bayer AS, et al. Diagnosis and management of infective endocarditis and its complications. *Circulation* 1998;98:2836–2848.
28. Roe MT, et al. Clinical information determines the impact of transesophageal echocardiography on the diagnosis of infective endocarditis by the Duke criteria. *Am Heart J* 2000;139:945–951.
29. Komshian SV, et al. Characteristics of left-sided endocarditis due to *Pseudomonas aeruginosa* in the Detriot Medical Center. *Rev Infect Dis* 1990;12:693–702.
30. Hessen MT, Abrutyn E. Gram-negative bacterial endocarditis. In: Kaye D, ed. *Infective endocarditis,* 2nd ed. New York:Raven, 1992:251.
31. Aronin SI, et al. Review of pneumococcal endocarditis in adults in the penicillin era. *Clin Infect Dis* 1998;26:165–171.
32. Berbari EF, Cockerill FR III, Steckerberg JM. Infective endocarditis due to unusual or fastidious organisms. *Mayo Clin Proc* 1997;72:532–542.
33. Raoult D, et al. Diagnosis of 22 new cases of *Bartonella* endocarditis. *Ann Intern Med* 1996;125:646–652.
34. Raoult D, et al. Q fever 1985–1988: clinical and epidemiologic features of 1383 infections. *Medicine* 2000;79:109–123.
35. Fenollar F, et al. Risk factors and prevention of Q fever endocarditis. *Clin Infect Dis* 2001;33:312–316.
36. Jacques DH, et al. Whipple endocarditis without overt gastrointestinal disease. *Ann Intern Med* 1999;131:112–116.
37. Fenollar F, Lepidi H, Raoult D. Whipple's endocarditis: review of the literature and comparisons with Q fever, *Bartonella* infection, and blood culture-positive endocarditis. *Clin Infect Dis* 2001;33:1309–1316.
38. Hoen B, et al. Infective endocarditis in patients with negative blood cultures. *Clin Infect Dis* 1995;20:501–506.
39. Kupferwasser LI, Bayer AS. Update on culture-negative endocarditis. *Curr Clin Top Infect Dis* 2000;20:113–133.
40. Ellis ME, et al. Fungal endocarditis. *Clin Infect Dis* 2001;32:50–62.
41. Wilson WR, et al. Antibiotic treatment of adults with infective endocarditis due to streptococci, enterococci, staphylococci, and HACEK microorganisms. *JAMA* 1995;274:1706–1713.
42. Andrews M, von Reyn CF. Patient selection criteria and management guidelines for outpatient parental antibiotic therapy for native valve infective endocarditis. *Clin Infect Dis* 2001;33:203–209.
43. Roberts SA, Land SDR, Ellis-Peyler RB. Short-course treatment of penicillin-susceptible viridans streptococcal infective endocarditis with penicillin and gentamicin. *Infect Dis Clin Pract* 1993;2:191.
44. Sexton DJ. Ceftriaxone once daily for four weeks compared with ceftriaxone plus gentamicin once daily for two weeks for treatment of endocarditis due to penicillin-susceptible streptococci. *Clin Infect Dis* 1998;27:1470–1474.
45. Franciolo P, Ruch W, Stamboulian D. The International Infective Endocarditis Study treatment of streptococcal endocarditis with a single daily dose of ceftriaxone and netilmicin for 14 days. *Clin Infect Dis* 1995;21:1406–1410.
46. Bouvet A. Human endocarditis due to nutritionally variant streptococci. *Eur Heart J* 1995;16(suppl B):24.
47. Doern GV, et al. Emergence of high rates of antimicrobial resistance among viridans group streptococci in the United States. *Antimicrob Agents Chemother* 1996;40:891–894.
48. Whitby S, et al. Infective endocarditis caused by *Streptococcus pneumoniae* with high level resistance to penicillin and cephalosporin. *Clin Infect Dis* 1996;23:1176–1177.

49. Baddour LM. Infective endocarditis caused by beta-hemolytic streptococci. *Clin Infect Dis* 1998;26:66–71.
50. Morgan DW. Enterococcal endocarditis. *Clin Infect Dis* 1992;15:63.
51. Eliopoulos GM. Aminoglycoside resistant enterococcal endocarditis. *Infect Dis Clin North Am* 1993;7:117.
52. Bush LM. High-level penicillin resistance among isolates of enterococci. *Ann Intern Med* 1989;150:515.
53. Gold HS. Vancomycin-resistant enterococci. *Clin Infect Dis* 2001;33:210–219.
54. Akins RL, Rybak MJ. Bactericidal activities of two daptomycin regimens against clinical strains of glycopeptide intermediate-resistant *Staphylococcus aureus,* vancomycin-resistant *Enterococcus faecium,* and methicillin-resistant *Staphylococcus aureus* isolates in an *in vitro* pharmacodynamic model with simulated endocardial vegetations. *Antimicrob Agents Chemother* 2001;45:454–459.
55. Patel R, et al. Linezolid therapy of vancomycin-resistant *Enterococcus faecium* experimental endocarditis. *Antimicrob Agents Chemother* 2001;45:621–623.
56. Babcock HM, et al. Successful treatment of vancomycin-resistant *Enterococcus* endocarditis with oral linezolid. *Clin Infect Dis* 2001;30:1375–1375.
57. Karchmer AW. Staphylococcal endocarditis: laboratory and clinical basis for antibiotic therapy. *Am J Med* 1985;78(suppl 6B):116.
58. Whitener A. Endocarditis due to coagulase-negative staphylococci. *Infect Dis Clin North Am* 1993;7:81.
59. Mayer DV, Edwards JE Jr. Fungal endocarditis. In: Kaye D, ed. *Infective endocarditis.* New York: Raven, 1992:299.
60. Rex JH, et al. Practice guidelines for the treatment of candidiasis. *Clin Infect Dis* 2000;30:662–678.
61. Karchmer AW. *Staphylococcus aureus* and vancomycin. *Ann Intern Med* 1991;115:739.
62. Daniel WA, et al. Improvement in the diagnosis of abscesses associated with endocarditis by transesophageal echocardiography. *N Engl J Med* 1991;324:795.
63. Roder BL, et al. Clinical features of staphylococcal aureus endocarditis. *Arch Intern Med* 1999;159:532–539.
64. Fowler VG, et al. Infective endocarditis due to *Staphylococcus aureus. Clin Infect Dis* 1999;28:106–114.
65. Alsip SG, et al. Indications for cardiac surgery in patients with active infective endocarditis. *Am J Med* 1985;78:138.
66. Sanfilippo AJ, et al. Echocardiographic assessment of patients with infectious endocarditis: prediction of risk for complications. *J Am Coll Cardiol* 1991;18:1191.
67. Mugge A, et al. Echocardiography in infective endocarditis: reassessment of prognostic implications of vegetation size determined by the transthoracic and the transesophageal approach. *J Am Coll Cardiol* 1989;14:631.
68. DeCastro S, et al. Role of transthoracic and transesophageal echocardiography in predicting embolic events in patients with active infective endocarditis involving native cardiac valves. *Am J Cardiol* 1997;80:1030–1034.
69. Parker JD, Sutton MG, Karchmer AW. Echocardiography in the management of patients with suspected or proven endocarditis. *Curr Clin Top Infect Dis* 1989;11:248.
70. Reinhartz O, et al. Timing of surgery in patients with acute infective endocarditis. *J Cardiovasc Surg* 1996;37:397–400.
71. Gillinov AM, et al. Valve replacement in patients with endocarditis and acute neurologic defect. *Ann Thorac Surg* 1996;65:1125–1130.
72. Parrino PE. Does a focal neurologic deficit contraindicate operation in a patient with endocarditis? *Ann Thorac Surg* 1999;67:59–64.
73. Mullany CJ, et al. Early and late survival after surgical treatment of culture-positive active endocarditis. *Mayo Clin Proc* 1995;70:517–525.
74. Alexiou C, et al. Surgery for active culture-positive endocarditis: determination of early and late outcome. *Ann Thorac Surg* 2000;69:144–154.
75. Mansur AJ, et al. Relapses, recurrences, valve replacements, and mortality during the long-term follow-up after infective endocarditis. *Am Heart J* 2001;141:78–86.
76. Mansur AJ, et al. The complications of infective endocarditis: a reappraisal in the 1980's. *Arch Intern Med* 1992;152:2428.

77. Blumberg EA, et al. Persistent fever in association with infective endocarditis. *Clin Infect Dis* 1992;15:983.
78. Douglas A, Moore-Gillon J, Eykyn S. Fever during treatment of infective endocarditis. *Lancet* 1986;8494:1341.
79. Allan JD Jr. Splenic abscess. *Curr Clin Top Infect Dis* 1994;14:23.
80. Dinubile MJ. Cardiac conduction abnormalities complicating native valve active infective endocarditis. *Am J Cardiol* 1986;58:1213.
81. Weinstein L, Schlesinger JJ. Pathoanatomic, pathophysiologic and clinical correlation in endocarditis. *N Engl J Med* 1974;291:832.
82. Wilson WR, et al. Management of complications of infective endocarditis. *Mayo Clin Proc* 1982;57:152.
83. Feinstein EI, et al. Renal complications of bacterial endocarditis. *Am J Nephrol* 1985;5:457.
84. Conlon PJ, et al. Predictors of prognosis and risk of acute renal failure in bacterial endocarditis. *Clin Nephrol* 1997;49:96–101.
85. Olaison L, Belin L, Hogevik H, et al. Incidence of beta-lactam–induced delayed hypersensitivity and neutropenia during treatment of infective endocarditis. *Arch Intern Med* 1999;159:607–615.
86. Martera LA, Bayer AS. *Staphylococcus aureus* bacteremia and endocarditis. *Infect Dis Clin North Am* 1992;7:53.
87. Mylotte JM, McDermott C, Spooner JA. Prospective study of 114 consecutive episodes of *Staphylococcus aureus* bacteremia. *Rev Infect Dis* 1987;9:891.
88. Mermel LA, et al. Guidelines for the management of intravascular catheter–related infections. *Clin Infect Dis* 2001;32:1249–1272.
89. Gullberg RM, Homan SR, Phair JP. Enterococcal bacteremia. *Rev Infect Dis* 1989;11:74.
90. Karchmer AW. Infections of prosthetic heart valves. In: Bisno AL, Waldvogel FA, eds. *Infections associated with indwelling medical devices,* 3rd ed. Washington, DC: American Society for Microbiology, 2000:145–172.
91. Calderwood SB, et al. Risk factors for the development of prosthetic valve endocarditis. *Circulation* 1985;72:31.
92. Fang A, et al. Prosthetic valve endocarditis resulting from nosocomial bacteremia. *Ann Intern Med* 1993;119:560.
93. Nasser RM, et al. Incidence and risk of developing fungal prosthetic valve endocarditis after nosocomial candidemia. *Am J Med* 1997;103:25–32.
94. Calderwood SB, et al. Prosthetic valve endocarditis: analysis of factors affecting outcome of therapy. *J Thorac Cardiovasc Surg* 1986;92:776.
95. John MDV, et al. *Staphylococcus aureus* prosthetic valve endocarditis: optimal management and risk factors for death. *Clin Infect Dis* 1998;26:1302–1309.
96. Mathew J, et al. Clinical features, site of involvement, bacteriologic findings, and outcome of infective endocarditis in intravenous drug users. *Arch Intern Med* 1995;155:1641–1648.
97. Pulvirenti JJ, et al. Infective endocarditis in injection drug users. *Clin Infect Dis* 1996;22:40–45.
98. Baddour LM. Twelve year review of recurrent native valve infective endocarditis. *Rev Infect Dis* 1988;10:1063.
99. Fortun J, et al. Short-course therapy for right-side endocarditis due to *Staphylococcus aureus* in drug abusers. *Clin Infect Dis* 2001;33:120–125.
100. Ribera E, et al. Effectiveness of cloxacillin with and without gentamicin in short-term therapy for right-sided *Staphylococcus aureus* endocarditis. *Ann Intern Med* 1996;125:969–974.
101. Pulvirenti JJ, et al. Infective endocarditis in injection drug users: importance of human immunodeficiency virus serostatus and degree of immunosuppression. *Clin Infect Dis* 1993;158:2043–2050.
102. Ribera E, et al. Influence of human immunodeficiency virus I infection and degree of immunosuppression in the clinical characteristics and outcome of infective endocarditis in intravenous drug users. *Arch Intern Med* 1998;138:2043–2050.
103. Hoit BD. Pericardial heart disease. *Curr Prob Cardiol* 1997;22:353–400.
104. Savoia MC, Oxman MN. Myocarditis, pericarditis. In: Mandell GL, Bennett JE, Dolin R,

eds. *Principles and practice of infectious disease,* 5th ed. New York: Churchill Livingstone, 2000:925–941.
105. Zayas R, et al. Incidence of specific etiology and role of methods for specific etiologic diagnosis of primary acute pericarditis. *Am J Cardiol* 1995;75:378.
106. Fowler NO. Recurrent pericarditis. *Cardiol Clin* 1990;8:621.
107. Adler Y, et al. Colchicine treatment for recurrent pericarditis. *Circulation* 1998;97:2183–2185.
108. Marcolongo R, et al. Immunosuppressive therapy prevents recurrent pericarditis. *J Am Coll Cardiol* 1995;26:1276–1279.
109. Silva-Cardoso J, et al. Pericardial involvement in human immunodeficiency virus infections. *Chest* 1999;115:418–422.
110. Chen Y, et al. Human immunodeficiency virus–associated pericardial effusion. *Am Heart J* 1999;137;516–521.
111. Estok L, Wallach F. Cardiac tamponade in a patient with AIDS. A review of pericardial disease in patients with HIV infection. *Mt Sinai J Med* 1998;65:33–39.
112. Park S, Bayer AS. Purulent pericarditis. *Curr Clin Top Infect Dis* 1989;12:57.
113. Sagrista-Sauleda, et al. Purulent pericarditis: review of a 20-year experience in a general hospital. *J Am Coll Cardiol* 1993;22:1661–1665.
114. Schrank JH, Dooley DP. Purulent pericarditis caused by *Candida* species. *Clin Infect Dis* 1995;21:182–187.
115. Trauter BW, Darouiche RO. Tuberculous pericarditis. *Clin Infect Dis* 2001;33:954–961.
116. Dooley DP, Carpenter JL, Rademacher S. Adjunctive corticosteroid therapy for tuberculosis. *Clin Infect Dis* 1997;25:872–887.
117. Feldman AM, McNamara D. Myocarditis. *N Engl J Med* 2000;343:1389–1398.
118. Wu LA, Lapeyre AC III, Cooper LT. Current role of endomyocardial biopsy in the management of dilated cardiomyopathy and myocarditis. *Mayo Clin Proc* 2001;76:1030–1038.
119. Steere AC. Lyme disease. *N Engl J Med* 2001;345:115–125.
120. Hager JM, Rahimtoola SH. Chagas' heart disease. *Curr Prob Cardiol* 1995;20:825.
121. Flotats A, Domingo P, Carrio I. Dilated cardiomyopathy in HIV-infected patients. *N Engl J Med* 1999;340:732.
122. Michaels AD, Lederman RJ, MacGregor JS. Cardiovascular involvement in AIDS. *Curr Prob Cardiol* 1997;23:113–148.
123. Yunis NA, Stone VE. Cardiac manifestations of HIV/AIDS. *J AIDS* 1998;18:145–154.
124. Eggiman P, Waldvogel F. Pacemaker and defibrillator infections. In: Bisno AL, Waldvogel FA, eds. *Infections associated with indwelling medical devices,* 3rd ed. Washington, DC: American Society for Microbiology, 2000:247–264.
125. Karchmer AW. Infections of prosthetic valves and intravascular devices. In: Mandell AI, Bennett JE, Dolin R, eds. *Principles and practice of infectious diseases,* 5th ed. New York: Churchill Livingstone, 2000:903–917.
126. Klug D, et al. Systemic infection related to endocarditis in pacemaker leads. *Circulation* 1997;95:2098–2107.
127. Cacoub P, et al. Pacemaker infective endocarditis. *Am J Cardiol* 1998;82:480–484.
128. Wade JS, Cobbs CG. Infections in cardiac pacemakers. *Curr Clin Top Infect Dis* 1988;9:44.
129. Lewis AB, et al. Update on infections involving permanent pacemakers. *Thorac Cardiovasc Surg* 1985;89:758.
130. Camus C. Sustained bacteremia in 26 patients with a permanent endocardial pacemaker. *Clin Infect Dis* 1993;17:46–55.
131. Heimberger TS, Duma RJ. Infections of prosthetic heart valves and cardiac pacemakers. *Infect Dis Clin North Am* 1989;3:221.
132. Vilacosta I, et al. Infected transvenous permanent pacemakers: role of transesophageal echocardiography. *Am Heart J* 1993;125:904.
133. Arber N, et al. Pacemaker endocarditis. *Medicine* 1994;73:299–305.
134. Trappe HJ, Pfitzner P, Klein H. Infections after cardioverter-defibrillator implantation. *Br Heart J* 1995;73:20–24.

135. Spinler SA, et al. Clinical presentation an analysis of risk factors for infectious complications of implantable cardioverter-defibrillator implantations at a university medical center. *Clin Infect Dis* 1998;26:111–116.
136. Smith PN, Vidaillet HJ, Hayes JJ. Infections with non-thoracotomy implantable cardioverter-defibrillators: can these be prevented? *Pacing Clin Electrophysiol* 1998; 21:42–55.
137. O'Nunian S, et al. The treatment of patients with infected implantable cardioverter-defibrillator systems. *J Thorac Cardiovasc Surg* 1997;113:121–129.
138. Lai KK, Fontecchio SA. Infections associated with implantable cardioverter-defibrillators placed transvenously and via thoracotomies: epidemiology, infection control and management. *Clin Infect Dis* 1998;27:265–269.
139. Chua JD, et al. Diagnosis and management of infections involving implantable electrophysiologic cardiac devices. *Ann Intern Med* 2000;133:604–608.

# 13. GASTROINTESTINAL AND INTRAABDOMINAL INFECTIONS

Paul S. Graman and Robert F. Betts

## GASTROENTERITIS AND FOOD POISONING

Acute onset of diarrhea is a common complaint. Whether a patient needs special evaluation, antibiotic therapy, or hospitalization must be routinely evaluated. Several reviews of this topic are available [1–10].

**Adapted from a chapter by Richard E. Reese and Jerome F. Hruska.**

**I. Background**

**A. Prevalence and impact**

1. In **developing countries,** diarrheal illness is the most common infectious disease, primarily affecting children under 5 years of age. Up to 1 billion cases occur annually in this age group, with an associated 4 to 6 million deaths worldwide [5]. Children experience approximately six bouts of diarrhea per year, and an estimated 10% of these episodes result in dehydration that requires therapy [4,10].
2. In the **United States,** it is estimated that there are up to 99 million cases of diarrhea or vomiting per year with an associated 10,000 deaths. Each child has two to three episodes of acute diarrhea annually [2,4]; the incidence among adults in developed countries averages one episode per year [6]. Among the total U.S. population, approximately 50% of persons with diarrhea or gastroenteritis restrict their activities for more than a full day, 8.2 million seek medical attention, and 250,000 require hospitalization. Despite the far greater number of episodes of diarrheal illness among children compared with adults, most deaths from diarrheal illness in the United States occur in the elderly. The death rate due to gastroenteritis is 2 to 3 per 100,000 population among children and young adults and approximately 15 per 100,000 for persons over age 74 [4].

**B. Definitions**

1. **Acute diarrhea** is defined as illness of less than 2 weeks' duration. Diarrhea lasting 2 to 4 weeks is considered **persistent.** Infectious agents commonly cause acute and persistent episodes. The term **chronic diarrhea** is often restricted to illness lasting at least 1 month [6].
2. **Mild diarrhea is** three or fewer stools per day without abdominal or systemic symptoms, resulting in little or no alteration in daily activities [10].
3. **Moderate or severe diarrhea** is four or more loose stools per day, usually associated with abdominal symptoms (cramps, nausea, vomiting, tenesmus, or systemic symptoms of fever, malaise, dehydration), and causing significant restriction of normal activity [6].
4. **Dysentery** is a **generic term** that refers to a variety of disorders marked by cramping abdominal pain, tenesmus, and frequent stools, often of small volume. Stools contain blood and mucus, indicative of invasion or injury of the mucosa by a pathogen or its toxin (e.g., amebic, bacillary, *Shigella* dysentery) [10].
5. **Gastroenteritis** refers to enteric infection characterized by vomiting as a predominant symptom with or without diarrhea.
6. **Tenesmus** refers to straining, especially painful or ineffectual straining with a bowel movement or straining on defecation owing to spasms of an inflamed rectal sphincter as occurs in shigellosis [11].

**C. Pathogenesis in infectious diarrhea.** See reports published elsewhere [1–6,10] for a detailed discussion of this topic. However, a **few basic points deserve emphasis** for understanding clinical presentations and evaluations of patients with acute bacterial diarrhea. **Many pathogens use more than one mechanism** to overcome host defenses and cause illness.

1. **Adherence.** Bacteria colonize the bowel by resisting the clearing action of peristalsis. Some pathogens circumvent this by attaching or adhering to the mucosal surface. Attachment may increase the toxicity of enterotoxins by decreasing the distance they have to travel to reach target intestinal cells [2].

a. **Bacterial surface protein structures** (pili or fimbria) bind to specific ligands or receptors on intestinal epithelial cells. This is an **important mechanism for enterotoxigenic** *Escherichia coli* (ETEC) [2].

b. **Adherence factor.** A distinctly different mechanism of enteroadherence is seen with **enteropathogenic *E. coli*** (EPEC). Bacteria intimately adhere to intestinal epithelial cells based on a plasmid-conferred EPEC adherence factor, with effacement and destruction of microvilli and disruption of the cytoskeleton of underlying cells. No extensive intracellular invasion occurs, and the exact mechanism of diarrhea with EPEC remains unknown [2,3].

2. **Invasion.** Certain enteroinvasive organisms can adhere to and invade mucosal epithelial cells. Invasion and multiplication elicits an **intense inflammatory response followed by cell death.** The mucosal inflammatory reaction is not clearly understood but probably involves the release of inflammatory mediators, including kinins, interleukins, leukotrienes, and other vasoactive agents. Clinically, one sees fever, abdominal cramps, malaise, and dysentery.

   *Shigella* (which also forms a toxin called Shiga toxin) is the classic example. Enteroinvasive *E. coli* and *Salmonella* may use similar mechanisms [2].

3. **Enterotoxin production.** *Vibrio cholerae* binds to the intestinal mucosa and produces **cholera toxin,** which stimulates an increased amount of intracellular adenosine 3′ 5′-monophosphate (cyclic adenosine monophosphate) through the adenylate cyclase system. In response, an active secretion of electrolytes and fluid into the intestinal lumen occurs. It is the classic prototype enterotoxin and stimulates production of voluminous quantities of watery stools, leading to potentially life-threatening dehydration. The **intestinal mucosa appears morphologically intact** and is believed to be capable of absorbing electrolytes in a normal behavior because of the empiric observation that oral solutions supplemented with glucose can be used to treat these patients. The overall effect leads to marked increase in the luminal small-bowel fluid that is delivered to the colon, and this fluid overwhelms colonic absorption capacity, thereby causing watery diarrhea [2]. **ETEC** has a similar mechanism.

4. **Cytotoxins.** Some organisms secrete a toxin that causes cytotoxicity in tissue culture.

   a. ***Shigella dysenteriae.* Shiga toxin is the classic prototype cytotoxin.**

   b. **Enterohemorrhagic *E. coli*** (EHEC) of **serotype 0157:H7** produce Shiga-like toxins that cause hemorrhagic colitis with bloody diarrhea. The toxin cleaves adenosine from host cell ribosomal RNA and inhibits protein synthesis [1]. Absorption of toxin into the systemic circulation also may mediate the associated hemolytic-uremic syndrome (HUS) [12].

   c. **Enteropathogenic *E. coli*** and ***Vibrio parahemolyticus*** also secrete Shiga toxin.

D. **Intestinal factors** that may help prevent acquisition of diarrheal disease include gastric acidity and the normal bacterial flora.

1. **Gastric acid** destroys enteric bacteria and is an important factor in decreasing susceptibility to infection. Patients with gastric resections and achlorhydria have increased susceptibility to infection. In addition, bicarbonate taken orally has been documented to increase the attack rate of experimental *Shigella, E. coli,* and cholera.

2. **Normal bacterial flora** of the bowel is believed to compete for space and nutrients with pathogenic organisms. In addition, short-chain fatty acids produced by many intestinal flora may be inhibitory of pathogens. It has been demonstrated that pretreatment with streptomycin lowers the required infective dose of experimental *Salmonella typhi* infections [1], presumably by changing bowel flora. See also the discussion of antibiotic-related diarrhea in Chapter 27, section A.

## II. Clinical approach to the patient with diarrhea

A. **History.** A careful history may provide clues to the type of infection involved [9].

1. **High-risk groups or settings.** There are several settings in which patients are at greater risk than the general population for developing diarrhea [2,4].

a. **Recent travel,** especially **international** travel and **camping** (e.g., using water from mountain streams), or travel to **coastal** areas, is a risk factor. For a discussion of travelers' diarrhea, see Chapter 22.
b. **Day-care children or family members** are at risk because there is close contact between children who are not toilet trained. The mode of transmission appears to be either from child to child or through fomites such as toys. Currently in the United States, it is estimated that more than 10 million children attend day-care centers [2]. Viruses commonly are identified in outbreaks, as are organisms that colonize at a low inoculum (e.g., *Shigella, Giardia,* and *Cryptosporidium* [4].
c. **Chronic care facilities.** Patients appear to be at increased risk, often due in part to their debilitated state, fecal incontinence, or suppressed immune response [2].
d. **Homosexuals and patients with acquired immunodeficiency syndrome (AIDS)** are at especially high risk for infectious diarrheas. See Chapter 18 for a detailed discussion of diarrhea in AIDS patients.
e. **Other family members or very close contacts of an index case** of acute infectious gastroenteritis are at risk for similar illness.

2. **Medication exposure**
   a. Antibiotic use currently or in the preceding 4 to 6 weeks can be associated with *Clostridium difficile* diarrhea.
   b. Excessive use of **laxatives, antacids,** or **alcohol.** Chemotherapy causes diarrhea.
3. **Common-source outbreak.** The clinician should inquire about picnics, banquets, fast-food restaurants, and associates with similar illnesses.
4. **Pets.** Turtles, iguanas, and dogs have been implicated in cases of infectious diarrhea.
5. **Seafood** or **shellfish** may have been improperly handled or prepared.
6. **Certain symptoms may be helpful.** Even the number of episodes and type of diarrhea may provide clues to the pathogens involved (Table 13.1) [9].
   a. **When vomiting is the predominant symptom,** viral gastroenteritis or a food-borne illness is suggested. Food poisoning due to preformed toxin (e.g., *Staphylococcus aureus, Bacillus cereus*) causes vomiting within 4 hours of ingesting the food [4]; see section **IV.**
   b. **Mucus in the stool,** if in small amounts, raises the question of irritable bowel syndrome, but large amounts can be seen with invasive bacterial diarrheas.

Table 13.1. Clinical Features of Acute Diarrhea

| Clinical Observation | Anatomic Consideration | Pathogens to Consider |
|---|---|---|
| Passage of few, voluminous stools | Diarrhea of small bowel origin | *Vibrio cholerae,* enterotoxigenic *Escherichia coli, Shigella* strains early in the infection, *Giardia* |
| Passage of many small-volume stools | Diarrhea of large bowel origin | *Shigella, Salmonella, Campylobacter, Entamoeba histolytica* |
| Tenesmus, fecal urgency, dysentery | Colitis | *Shigella, Salmonella, Campylobacter, E. histolytica* |
| Vomiting as the predominant symptom | Gastroenteritis | Viral agents (rotavirus, calicivirus, e.g., Norwalk virus) or intoxication (*Staphylococcus aureus, Bacillus cereus*) |
| Fever as a predominant finding | Mucosal invasion | *Shigella, Salmonella, Campylobacter,* viral agents (rotavirus, calicivirus) |

Adapted from Bandres JC, Dupont HL. Approach to the patient with diarrhea. In: Gorbach SL, Bartlett JG, Blacklow NR, eds. *Infectious diseases.* Philadelphia: WB Saunders, 1992:572–575; with permission.

c. **Blood in the stool** indicates the possibility of inflammatory mucosal disease of the colon. EHEC (*E. coli* O157:H7) is the most common cause of bloody diarrhea in the United States [5]. Blood often is evident on gross examination of the stool. Usually there is no fever with 0157:H7. Occult blood testing is more sensitive but less specific. Noninfectious causes, such as ischemic bowel disease, diverticulitis, ulcerative colitis, and radiation injury, are in the differential diagnoses.

Organisms that produce enterotoxins and are invasive such as *Campylobacter* species, *Aeromonas* species, *Shigella* species, and *V. parahemolyticus,* may initially cause watery diarrhea followed by bloody diarrhea.

d. **Watery diarrhea** is more likely seen in those infections in which organisms adhere, infect, or colonize but do not destroy the epithelium (parasites, EPEC, enteric viruses) [4], and when the small bowel is affected.

e. **Fever** suggests a mucosal invasive pathogen.

f. **Systemic illness with HUS,** characterized by acute hemolytic anemia, renal failure with uremia, and disseminated intravascular coagulation, occurs with shigellosis and EHEC [5].

7. **A prior history of inflammatory bowel disease** should be assessed in case the acute symptoms represent an exacerbation of this prior, more chronic problem.

B. Physical examination does not usually help determine the cause of the diarrhea.

1. **Fever** suggests an invasive bacterial organism.
2. **Signs of dehydration** in severe cases, especially in children, include dry mucous membranes, lethargy, postural hypotension, tachycardia, sunken fontanelles, skin with decreased turgor, and dry eyes [5]. Severe dehydration requires hospitalization.
3. **Stool occult blood.** In the patient with multiple episodes of diarrhea and mucosal irritation, occult blood might be present without representing a true invasive process.

C. **Laboratory aids** in diagnosis [8,13]

1. **Gram staining** of the stool usually is not helpful because most pathogens cannot be differentiated from the normal gram-negative bowel flora. *Campylobacter* may be suggested by Gram stain findings in stool specimens (see section **V.D.2**). Rarely is *S. aureus* a cause of colitus, but if it is, Gram stain is helpful. Stool culture also should be performed if the latter is suspected.
2. **Fecal leukocytes** give a clue as to the cause. Mucus can be examined. The presence of only a few leukocytes usually is an indeterminate result.

   a. **Fecal leukocytes occur in (a) bacterial infections that invade the intestinal wall,** such as invasive *E. coli* and *Shigella* and *Salmonella* species; (b) **ulcerative colitis and Crohn disease;** and (c) **C. difficile diarrhea,** in which fecal leukocytes appear in nearly 50% of cases.

   b. **Fecal leukocytes are not seen** in (a) **viral gastroenteritis,** (b) **parasitic diarrhea,** (c) **enterotoxigenic bacterial diarrheas** (*V. cholerae, Bacillus cereus,* ETEC, etc.), or (d) ***Salmonella* carrier states.**

   c. **Fecal lactoferrin** is a sensitive marker for fecal leukocytes. A simple, rapid latex agglutination test for lactoferrin is available [5].

3. **Stool cultures.** Special media are needed to culture many of the bacterial agents that cause diarrhea. **If one suspects a particular pathogen, discussion with the microbiology laboratory supervisor leads to appropriate studies.** Special enriching techniques or media are required to isolate other agents such as *V. cholerae and V. parahemolyticus* (e.g., after exposure to coastal areas or seafood), *Yersinia enterocolitica, Campylobacter jejuni, and EHEC.* In addition, one should carefully mark the suspected agents on the laboratory specimen sheet [8].
4. **Rotavirus detection** is particularly useful for children under 3 years of age.
5. **Ova and parasite (O&P) examination** are discussed in section **D** and in section **II.A** under Gastrointestinal Parasites. In patients with chronic diarrhea, international travelers, homosexual men, and contacts of day-care centers with protracted symptoms, these specimens are especially useful to examine.

6. ***Clostridium difficile* toxin** assay is useful for patients who are on or who have been on antibiotics in the preceding 4 to 6 weeks.
7. **Proctosigmoidoscopy** examinations seldom are indicated except as follows:
   a. In homosexual men and in some cases of AIDS-related illness (see Chapter 10).
   b. In chronic or recurrent diarrhea for possible inflammatory bowel disease.
   c. In possible *C. difficile* diarrhea to provide an immediate answer.
   d. In a potential case of *Entamoeba histolytica,* because ulcerations of the intestinal wall may be characteristic in this setting. Rectal mucosal biopsy also may help [5].
8. **Radiographic studies** usually are not indicated.
   a. If toxic megacolon is a potential concern as a complication—for example, with *C. difficile* diarrhea—radiographic plain films are useful.
   b. In chronic diarrhea, pancreatic calcifications suggest chronic pancreatitis.
   c. Results of barium contrast studies of stool samples are nondiagnostic for the presence of O&P [5].
9. **Miscellaneous studies**
   a. **Peripheral white blood cell (WBC) counts** are nonspecific. Although it may be elevated in acute infectious diarrhea (e.g., *Salmonella* or *Shigella*) or *C. difficile* colitis, the WBC count also may be elevated in patients with dehydration due to nonbacterial processes.
   b. **Blood cultures.** In the febrile patient with gastroenteritis, blood cultures may be positive when other sources, including stool cultures, are negative.
   c. **Bone marrow cultures.** Biopsy specimens often are positive in typhoid fever. This may be useful in the workup of an unclear chronic fever.
   d. **Rose spots** (the transient skin rash of typhoid fever) can be sampled for biopsy and cultured.
   e. **Serologic studies.** In acute gastroenteritis, serologic studies **offer little help** except in the following special circumstances:
      (1) **Amebiasis. Indirect hemagglutination** and other antiamebic antibody tests are a useful adjunct in the diagnosis of extraintestinal amebiasis (99%+ by day 7) or active intestinal infection (80%–90% positive) but **not for the asymptomatic** patient who is passing cysts (see section **IV.E** under Gastrointestinal Parasites).
      (2) ***Salmonella* O antigen** applies only to *S. typhi.* [14]. Of infected patients, 50% convert to seropositivity after 1 week and only by the fourth week do 90% to 95% of patients show an elevated titer. Often acute *Salmonella* gastroenteritis remits before there is any seroconversion making the test not useful in most cases. They may be helpful when persistent infection has allowed time for a host antibody response. The carrier state produces very little response.

      Caution should be exercised in the interpretation of a single value. Previous seroconversion, typhoid immunization, and cross-reaction with Enterobacteriaceae O antigens can cause an isolated antibody elevation.

D. **Diagnostic workup.** Because pathogens are recovered from fewer than 10% of unselected stool samples, the cost per positive stool culture exceeds $1,000, an extremely cost-ineffective workup. See reports published elsewhere [1,2,4,5] for a rational approach. After laboratory workup, 20% to 40% of all acute infectious diarrheas remain undiagnosed [4].
   1. If the history suggests a food-borne toxin–related illness, with nausea and vomiting a few hours after eating, see Table 13.2 for a summary of important pathogens and presentation. Food-borne toxins are discussed in section **IV.**
   2. Afebrile stable patients with nonbloody diarrhea of short duration can be observed and treated conservatively with oral hydration and no extensive laboratory workup.
   3. Determine risk factors (e.g., travel, camping, day care, antibiotic use, seafood exposure, sexual contact, etc.) that may suggest a specific etiology.

Table 13.2. Clinical Features of Agent-Specific Food-Borne Disease with Symptom Onset of Less Than 12 Hours

| Organism or Agent | Incubation Period | Duration of Illness (range) | Diarrhea | Fever | Vomiting | Enterotoxin | Invasion | Foods Most Commonly Implicated | Comments |
|---|---|---|---|---|---|---|---|---|---|
| *Staphylococcus aureus* | 1–8 h | 24 h (8–18 h) | + (infrequent) | – | +++ | ++ | – | Salads, cream-filled pastries, meats (pork, beef, poultry) | High attack rates (80%–100%)<br>Outbreaks most frequent during summer |
| *Bacillus cereus* | | | | | | | | | |
| Emetic illness | 1–6 h | 9 h (2–10 h) | + | – | +++ | ++ | – | Fried rice | Abdominal cramps often experienced<br>Vomiting occurs more often than diarrhea |
| Diarrheal illness | 6–14 h | 20 h (16–48 h) | +++ | – | + | + | – | Meats, vanilla sauce, cream-baked goods, salads, chicken soup | Diarrhea occurs more often than vomiting<br>Organism may be found in stool of healthy person |
| *Clostridium perfringens* | 8–24 h | 24 h (8–72 h) | +++ | – | ± | ++ | – | Improperly stored beef, fish, or poultry dishes (after preparation); pasta salads, dairy products; Mexican foods | "Pig-bel" or necrotizing enterocolitis is a rare variant<br>Stool has no white blood cells or blood<br>Commercial kit available for detection of toxin in stool |
| Non O:1 *Vibrio cholerae* | 6–72 h | 2 days (2–12 days) | ++ | ± | ± | + (a minority produce cholera toxin) | ± | Seafood, grated eggs, potatoes | 25% can have bloody diarrhea<br>Illness similar to cholera but with much less dehydration |
| Puffer fish | <2 h | Variable | + | – | + | + Tetrodotoxin (i.e., a neurotoxin) | – | Fugu (especially prepared Japanese puffer fish), other puffer fish, vividly colored frogs of South America, blue-ringed octopus | Symptoms include paresthesias, ataxia, hypotension, seizures, cardiac arrhythmias, respiratory and skeletal muscle paralysis<br>Mortality 30%–60%<br>Treatment: gastric lavage and cardiorespiratory support<br>Prognosis greatly improves if patient survives first 6 h |

| | | | | | | | | | | |
|---|---|---|---|---|---|---|---|---|---|---|
| Paralytic shellfish | 1–3 h | 3 days (0.5–7 days) | – | – | + | + | Saxitoxin (i.e., a neurotoxin) | – | Most bivalved mollusks (shellfish), especially from endemic waters experiencing red tide blooms | Symptoms and treatment similar to puffer fish poisoning<br>Mortality rate 5%–18%<br>Etiology is concentration of toxic dinoflagellates in mollusks during red tide season (spring and fall) |
| Ciguatera | 1–6 h | Variable (can persist for months) | + | – | + | + | Ciguatoxin (i.e., a neurotoxin) | – | Barracuda, grouper, snapper, jacks, reef sharks | Most common form of fish intoxication in United States<br>Commonly seen in Florida, Hawaii, and the Caribbean<br>Symptoms similar to puffer fish poisoning<br>ELISA available for detection of toxin<br>Treatment suggested with amitriptyline |
| Scombroid fish | <2 h | Variable (2–10 h) | ± | – | + | – | (preformed histamine causes symptoms; not an allergic reaction) | – | "Blood fish" (tuna, albacore, mackerel, skip jacks) under spoiling conditions | Symptoms: flushing, generalized or localized erythema, vertigo, generalized burning sensation<br>Histamine levels can be assayed in implicated fish<br>Treatment with antihistamines very effective<br>Fish with unpleasant odor or clouded eyes should be avoided |

ELISA, enzyme-linked immunosorbent assay.
Modified from Miranda AG, DuPont HL. Small intestine: infections with common bacterial and viral pathogens. In: Yamada T, ed. *Textbook of gastroenterology*. New York: JB Lippincott, 1991:1452–1453.

4. **Further medical evaluation is indicated in patients with more severe diarrheal illness,** as evidenced by one or more of the following [6]:
   a. Fever (≥38.5°C)
   b. Profuse watery diarrhea with dehydration
   c. Bloody diarrhea or dysentery
   d. Passage of at least six unformed stools over 24 hours
   e. Prolonged diarrhea (lasting >48 hours)
   f. Severe abdominal pain
   g. Age at least 70 years
   h. Immunocompromised state (AIDS, transplantation, cancer chemotherapy)
5. **Laboratory evaluation may proceed in a stepwise fashion:**
   a. **Step 1: If the patient has mucus or blood in the stool or if fecal leukocytes (or lactoferrin) is present,** a stool culture that looks for *Shigella, Salmonella,* and *Campylobacter* is indicated. This screening approach can dramatically increase the yield of positive stool cultures and decrease the cost of workup [1,4]. Bloody diarrheal stools also should be cultured for *E. coli* O157:H7.

      **The clinician should alert the microbiology laboratory** (see section **II.C**). With a history of antibiotic use, either currently or in the preceding 4 to 6 weeks, obtain a stool for *C. difficile* toxin before obtaining the stool culture. This is particularly important in the patient with onset of diarrhea more than 72 hours after admission to the hospital.
   b. **Step 2: If stools do not contain blood, mucus, or fecal leukocytes (or lactoferrin), examination for O&P is suggested if history is supportive.**
      (1) It is usual to obtain three stools for O&P examination.
      (2) If *Giardia* species are likely, the *Giardia* antigen test should be performed (see section **IV.A.2**).
      (3) In children under 3 years of age in whom the fecal leukocyte test result is negative, an early examination for **rotavirus** is suggested (see section **VI.A**).
   c. **Step 3: If no parasites are found, then the differential diagnosis is narrowed to include viruses and certain difficult-to-culture bacteria** (e.g., *Yersinia, V. cholerae,* ETEC, EPEC, *Aeromonas hydrophila, Plesiomonas shigelloides*).
      (1) Special media for *V. cholerae* should be used only for travelers to endemic areas.
      (2) Discuss the microbiology workup with your laboratory supervisor.

## III. Therapy. In most cases of infectious diarrhea, therapy consists of supportive care.

### A. Fluid replacement

1. **Oral fluids** will suffice in most patients [15]. The World Health Organization has developed an oral solution that is inexpensive, easy to administer, and effective in all types of diarrhea and all age groups. The formula is based on the principle that glucose absorption in the small bowel facilitates sodium and fluid resorption from the intestinal lumen into the intravascular compartment [1,16].
   a. See Table 13.3. Premeasured packets of dry salts with a long shelf life, available in developing countries, are mixed with water to reconstitute the solution.
   b. Commercially available premixed oral electrolyte solutions (Pedialyte, others) are available in the United States for use in infants and children with mild to moderate diarrhea. A comparable solution can be made with 3 tablespoons corn syrup, 3/4 teaspoon salt, and 1/2 teaspoon sodium bicarbonate in 1 cup orange juice diluted with water to make 1 liter (1.05 quart) [5]. When there is associated nausea and vomiting, the patient can often be given small volumes of oral fluids on an hourly basis [16–17].
   c. Otherwise healthy persons with acute diarrhea and minimal or no dehydration will do well with sport drinks, dilute fruit juices, and other flavored soft drinks supplemented with saltine crackers, soups, and broth [6].

Table 13.3. Composition of World Health Organization Oral Rehydration Solution for Diarrheal Illness

| Ingredient | Amount |
|---|---|
| Sodium chloride | 3.5 g/L |
| Potassium chloride | 1.5 g/L |
| Glucose | 20.0 g/L |
| Trisodium citrate[a] | 2.9 g/L |

[a]An earlier formulation used sodium bicarbonate 2.5 g/L, had a shorter shelf life, but was physiologically equivalent and may still be produced in some countries.
Data from Centers for Disease Control. *Health information for international travel 2001–2002.* (the "Yellow Book"). Atlanta, GA: U.S. Department of Health and Human Services. Also available online at *www.cdc.gov/travel/yb/index.htm.*

**d.** Oral replacement therapy is contraindicated only in patients with uncontrolled vomiting, with ileus, or where hospitalization and intravenous (i.v.) fluid are indicated.

**2. Intravenous fluids** (normal saline with potassium chloride supplementation or Ringer solution) are used in patients who are severely dehydrated.

**B. Antimotility agents** [18–20]

**1.** Natural opiates such as paregoric or tincture of opium, diphenoxylate, or loperamide **provide symptomatic relief of acute diarrhea and cramps.** The latter are safer, come in convenient dosage forms, and are generally preferred. **They should be used only in adults with noninflammatory diarrhea and not with high fever or bloody stools** because these agents may potentiate the effects of bacterial disease by delaying clearance of the pathogen or its toxin. However, when used in conjunction with ciprofloxacin for bacillary dysentery in adults, loperamide has proved to be safe and effective. Treatment with diphenolyate prolongs fever in shigellosis. HUS occurs more often in *E. coli* O157:H7 following antimotility drugs, and the neurologic manifestations may be more severe.

**2. Loperamide** (Imodium) **as short-course therapy for adult travelers' diarrhea** (see Chapter 22) has a good safety record, expected efficacy in reducing stool number by approximately 80%, and availability over the counter. **Diphenolylate with atropine** (Lomotil) has central opiate effects that may endanger children who accidentally ingest the drug, and atropine side effects that may be unpleasant [6,17].

**3.** These agents are not recommended for infants and young children.

**C. Antibiotics generally are not indicated.** The need depends on (a) the clinical course superimposed on underlying medical problems and age and (b) the pathogen involved.

**1.** In the patient who is **toxic** and **profoundly dehydrated** without evidence of a self-limited process, empiric antibiotics are indicated while awaiting cultures. Antibiotics are essential for patients whose history suggests a bacteremia. Fever, bloody stool, and fecal leukocytes suggest a bacterial cause that warrants treatment. Very young and very old patients should receive empiric therapy if they are toxic or significantly dehydrated. Ceftriaxone or fluoroquinolones are options.

**2.** For further discussion of therapy of individual pathogens, see section **V.**

**D. Miscellaneous agents**

**1. Antisecretory agents.** The gastrointestinal (GI) peptide **somatostatin** and its synthetic analogues **(octreotide** and **vapreotide)** are powerful inhibitors of intestinal secretion. These agents have been used in controlling chronic

AIDS-related diarrhea of unknown etiology or diarrhea caused by microsporidia or cryptosporidiosis [6] (see Chapter 18).

2. **Absorbent agents.** Cholestyramine is a nonabsorbable exchange resin that has been used to absorb toxin, in *C. difficile* and chronic diarrhea.

E. **Bismuth subsalicylate** (Pepto-Bismol) has been used primarily in the prevention and therapy of travelers' diarrhea (see Chapter 22) or in conjunction with oral rehydration for diarrhea in young children [21], or for vomiting in patients with viral gastroenteritis [6].

F. **Antiemetics** used orally, parenterally, or rectally. Some examples are as follows:

1. **Prochlorperazine** (Compazine). For adults, 25 mg rectal suppository twice daily, or 5- or 10-mg tablets three or four times daily; or 5 to 10 mg intramuscularly (i.m.) every 4 hours not to exceed 40 mg/day when given i.m.
2. **Trimethobenzamide** (Tigan). For adults, 200 mg rectal suppository three or four times daily; oral capsules, 250 mg three or four times daily; or 200 mg i.m. three or four times daily.

IV. Agents causing rapid onset of illness (**<12 hours after ingestion**) (see Table 13.2)

A. **Staphylococcal food poisoning** is due to **a preformed enterotoxin** that is heat stable and **not destroyed by ordinary rewarming. Foods implicated are** cream-filled pastries, custards, milk products, and meats that have been improperly refrigerated.

1. **Symptoms.** Severe nausea, vomiting, abdominal pain, diarrhea, and prostration occur 1 to 6 hours after ingestion, last less than 1 day, and remit spontaneously.
2. **Diagnosis** is confirmed by isolation of *S. aureus* in the contaminated food.
3. **Therapy is supportive.** No antibiotic is indicated for this self-limited disease.

B. ***Bacillus cereus*** contamination resembles staphylococcal food poisoning and is caused by preformed enterotoxin in foods such as cereal (especially rice), dried foods, and dairy products. Illness is self-limited (abates in <24 hours) and not severe.

1. **B cereus contamination can lead to two syndromes**[22]. **The emetic syndrome** is caused by a high temperature–stable toxin. Fried rice subsequently held at room temperature is the leading cause. **The diarrheal syndrome** is mediated by a heat-and acid-labile enterotoxin.
2. **Diagnosis** of *B. cereus* contamination can be confirmed by the isolation of at least $10^5$ *B. cereus* organisms per gram from implicated food [22,23]. Special cultures are necessary.

C. ***Clostridium perfringens* food poisoning** results from ingestion of foods harboring the organisms. The ingested *C. perfringens* multiply in the small intestine and produce the diarrhea-forming enterotoxin. **Treatment is supportive.** Anaerobic **cultures and Gram staining of the incriminated food will establish the diagnosis.**

D. **Fish and shellfish poisoning** is caused by toxins present in the tissues of fish. The topic has been reviewed elsewhere [24]. **See Table 13.2 for a summary.**

In ciguatoxic fish (barracuda, red snapper, and grouper), the toxin is acquired in the food chain of the fish; large fish weighing more than 2.8 kg are more likely to be toxic [25]. Scombroid fish poisoning (tuna, mackerel, bonito, skipjack) is due to production of a histamine-like toxin by marine bacteria that grow when these fish are improperly refrigerated or preserved [26]. Shellfish poisoning (mussels, clams, oysters, and scallops) occurs because toxic dinoflagellates usually associated with red tide are ingested by the mollusks and concentrated in their tissues. **All these toxic substances have no effect on the fish or shellfish and are heat stable to cooking temperatures.**

1. **Symptoms** including abdominal cramps, nausea, vomiting, and diarrhea occur within minutes to several hours after ingestion. Neurologic symptoms in ciguatera and shellfish poisoning include numbness, paresthesia, and nerve palsies. Case fatalities, which in some series are as high as 10%, have been due to respiratory paralysis.
2. **Diagnosis is suggested by the epidemiologic features.**
3. **Therapy is primarily symptomatic.** Inducing emesis, performing gastric lavage, and administering a cathartic agent should remove unabsorbed toxin.

**V. Diseases causing delayed onset** of GI symptoms (Table 13.4) [7]

**A. *Salmonella* infections** [14,27]. *Salmonella* organisms are motile, flagellated, aerobic or facultative anaerobic, gram-negative bacilli that do not ferment lactose or sucrose.

**1. Nomenclature and serotyping.** Serotyping is relevant both clinically and epidemiologically. Certain serotypes are associated with specific clinical syndromes, and serotyping of isolates serves as an important tool in defining and controlling epidemics [8,14]. *Salmonella* serotype typhimurium is conveniently written as *Salmonella typhimurium.* Alternatively, all nontyphoidal *Salmonella* organisms are classified as *Salmonella enterica* and further identified by serotype (e.g., *Salmonella enterica* serotype typhimurium). *Salmonella* organisms possess both somatic O antigens and flagella H antigens serotypes. More than 2,300 *Salmonella* serotypes are found in nature. Many are named for the city in which they were defined.

**2. Epidemiology. Cases of salmonellosis must be reported to the state health department.** In the United States, 800,000 to 4 million cases of salmonellosis occur each year, and approximately 500 are fatal [28]. An increasing number of cases are attributable to an increase in outbreaks associated with the mass production of food products and to an increase in reporting.

**a. More than 98% of isolates are nontyphoidal,** with important animal sources of human food (e.g., meat, poultry, eggs, dairy products) frequently contaminated with these organisms. Infection results from consumption of foods that are undercooked or cross-contaminated with these products [29].

***S. enteritidis* and *S. typhimurium*** are the most common serotypes in the United States. Chickens may transmit *S. enteritidis* through infected oviducts that contaminate the egg before the shell is formed [30]. About 0.01% to more than 0.1% of eggs contain *S. enteritidis,* although the percentage may be higher in the northeastern United States [31]. When these eggs are used raw (such as in dressing for Caesar salad) or are undercooked (such as in "soft" scrambled eggs) the *Salmonella* organisms proliferate in the food. Eggs have been associated with 82% of *S. enteritidis* outbreaks in the United States [32].

**b.** Other common serotypes include *S. heidelberg, S. newport,* and *S. agona.*

**c.** The incidence of cases peaks during the summer and fall picnic season. Contamination of food-processing equipment and manufactured food products can result in large outbreaks of disease. About 224,000 persons developed *S. enteritidis* gastroenteritis in 1994 after eating a nationally distributed ice cream [33]. Less commonly, person-to-person spread via the fecal-oral route can occur.

**d. Exotic pets,** especially reptiles (snakes, turtles, iguanas), are a growing source of human salmonellosis, accounting for an estimated 3% to 5% of all cases [34]. Up to 90% of reptiles may be carriers of *Salmonella* organisms.

**e. Antibiotic-resistant *Salmonella* organisms.** Subtherapeutic concentrations of antibiotics put in the animal feed as nonspecific growth factors promote the emergence of antibiotic-resistant bacteria, including *Salmonella* species. During slaughtering this antibiotic-resistant gut flora contaminates the animal meat. A recent survey of ground meats in supermarkets found *Salmonella* organisms in 20% of samples, with 84% of the isolates resistant to at least one antibiotic and 53% resistant to three or more agents [35,36]. Multidrug-resistant strains of *S. typhimurium* (DT104) in the United States increased from 0.6% of isolates in 1980 to 34% in 1996 [28].

**f. *S. typhi*** is the most frequent isolate in developing countries but is uncommon in the United States. Animals do not serve as a reservoir of *S. typhi.* Food is infectious only if contaminated by humans during processing. In developing countries, transmission occurs primarily by direct fecal-oral spread between individuals or by fecal contamination of drinking water or food. In the United States, transmission is primarily by contamination of foodstuffs with human feces. In the United States, more than half of the cases occur in travelers.

**3. Clinical syndromes** of *Salmonella* disease include gastroenteritis, enteric fever, metastatic infection, and the carrier state.

Table 13.4. Clinical Features of Agent-Specific Food-Borne Disease with Symptom Onset of Greater Than 12 Hours

| Organism or Agent | Incubation Period | Duration of Illness (range) | Diarrhea | Fever | Vomiting | Enterotoxin | Invasion | Foods Most Commonly Implicated | Comments |
|---|---|---|---|---|---|---|---|---|---|
| *Salmonella* | 8–48 h | 3 days (1–14 days) | +++ | ++ | + | + | + (little mucosal damage) | Eggs, poultry, beef, dairy products | Infection with some serotypes can lead to severe complications in certain patients (those with malignancy, atherosclerosis, and AIDS)<br>Treatment not recommended except in severe or disseminated disease because it prolongs carriage of organism<br>Stool contains white blood cells and may contain blood |
| *Shigella* | 24–72 h (up to 7 days) | 3 days (1–14 days) | +++ | +++ | ± | + | ++ | Salads (egg, tuna, poultry), milk | Low infective dose ($10–10^2$ organisms). Person-to-person transmission common<br>Stools often contain blood, mucus, and pus<br>Systemic symptoms (headache, malaise, lethargy) common |
| *Yersinia* | 24–72 h (up to 6 days) | 7 days (2–30 days) | +++ | ++ | ± | + | + | Milk (raw or chocolate), tofu | Abdominal pain is a prominent feature of illness and may be confused with appendicitis<br>Presence of pharyngitis common in children<br>Rheumatologic postinfectious complications have been reported |
| *Campylobacter* | 2–11 days | 3 days (2–30 days) | +++ | ++ | ± | + | + | Raw, milk, poultry, beef, clams, pet animals | Stool contains red and white blood cells<br>Mostly resistant to trimethoprim-sulfamethoxazole |

| | | | | | | | | |
|---|---|---|---|---|---|---|---|---|
| | | | | | | | | Complications include meningitis and Guillain-Barré syndrome |
| *Escherichia coli* (enterotoxigenic) | 24–72 h | 3 days (1–14 days) | +++ | + | – | + | – | Salads, peeled fruits, meat dishes, pastries | At least two toxins elaborated: heat-labile (similar to choleratoxin) and heat-stable<br>Most common bacterial agent of traveler's diarrhea |
| *Vibrio parahemolyticus* | 4–96 h | 3 days (2–10 days) | ++ | ± | + | + | – (not documented in humans) | Oysters, crabs shellfish, sea water, contaminated food | Antimicrobials do not shorten illness<br>Fecal white blood cells and blood uncommon |
| *Clostridium botulinum* | 12–36 h (may be as long as 8 days) | Weeks to months | ± | – | ± | ++ (neurotoxin) | – | Raw honey (infants), improperly canned products | Neurologic symptoms are results of parasympathetic and neuromuscular blockade<br>Fatality rate 15%<br>Treatment is early administration of antitoxin<br>Infants under 1 yr of age should not be fed raw honey |
| Rotavirus | 48–72 h | 5 days (3–14 days) | +++ | + (low grade) | ++ | – | – (superficial damage to mucosa) | Fresh water, seafood | Primarily an illness of infants and children<br>Endemic in nature<br>Respiratory symptoms common<br>Can cause severe dehydration in children |
| Calicivirus (Norwalk and Norwalk-like viruses) | 24–48 h | 1 day (1–3 days) | ++ | + (low grade) | ++ | – | – (superficial damage to mucosa) | Shellfish, drinking water | Affects primarily older children and adults<br>Endemic in nature |

AIDS, acquired immunodeficiency syndrome.
Modified from Miranda AG, DuPont HL Small intestine: infections with common bacterial and viral pathogens. In: Yamada T, ed. *Textbook of gastroenterology.* New York: JB Lippincott, 1991: 1453–1455.

**a. Gastroenteritis.** *S. enteritidis, S. newport,* and *S. anatum* usually cause gastroenteritis. *Salmonella* organisms cause 10% to 15% of food poisoning cases in the United States [14]. There is an intestinal invasion with the production of fecal leukocytes and low-grade fever. In addition, an enterotoxin causes intestinal fluid secretion.

**(1) Symptoms** develop 8 to 48 hours after ingestion of contaminated food; they include colicky abdominal pain, nausea and vomiting, and then loose, watery diarrhea. There may be fever to 38° to 39°C. Symptoms usually subside spontaneously in 2 to 5 days without sequelae. Certain underlying conditions (AIDS, achlorhydria, prior gastric surgery, and inflammatory bowel disease) predispose the patient to more severe disease [14].

**(2) Diagnosis** is made by isolating the organism from the stool or the ingested food. Stool leukocytes often are seen.

**(3) Treatment of uncomplicated gastroenteritis** due to nontyphoidal *Salmonella* species is primarily supportive. The disease is usually self-limited. Antibiotics have no proven value and use **may result in a higher rate of chronic carriage and relapse** [37,38]. **Bacteremia occurs in fewer than 5% of patients with *Salmonella* gastroenteritis. Use of antibiotics should be limited to preemptive therapy among patients at high risk for invasive disease:** (a) newborn infants, probably up to 3 months of age; (b) the elderly, because of the high risk for atherosclerosis or aneurysms; (c) those with AIDS, organ transplants, lymphoproliferative disease, or other immunosuppression; (d) patients with prosthetic joints, prosthetic vascular grafts, aneurysms, or prosthetic heart valves; and (e) those with underlying sickle cell disease [14,27]. A brief course of treatment (72 hours or until resolution of fever), usually with an oral fluoroquinolone, is appropriate.

**b. Enteric (typhoid) fever** usually is caused by *S. typhi* but, infrequently, other *Salmonella* organisms, such as *S. paratyphi* or *S. choleraesuis,* are etiologic.

**(1) Symptoms.** Enteric fever is characterized by **sustained fever,** often of 2 to 4 weeks duration, hepatosplenomegaly, headaches, abdominal tenderness, and rose spots, which are slightly raised, discrete, irregular, blanching pink macules 2 to 4 mm wide and often seen on the anterior thorax. Leukopenia may be seen, as may sustained bacteremia without endothelial or endocardial seeding, but sometimes with metastatic seeding and immune complex deposition that leads to multiorgan dysfunction. Intestinal hemorrhage or perforation may result from the hyperplasia of the Peyer patches in the terminal ileum [14,27]. Surprisingly, **diarrhea occurs in as few as 50% of cases,** and then only as an early symptom. **Constipation may be a frequent complaint later in the illness.**

**(2) Diagnosis.** Culture of stool specimens, blood, bone marrow, or rose spots for *S. typhi* or other *Salmonella* species is useful. A serologic increase of febrile agglutinins against the somatic or O antigen for group D *Salmonella* is supportive. Serologic studies may be useful in epidemiologic evaluation.

**(3) Therapy.** The current agent of choice for *S. typhi* and *Salmonella* species is a fluoroquinolone or third-generation cephalosporin (e.g., ceftriaxone or cefotaxime) [39]. Alternative agents include trimethoprim-sulfamethoxazole (TMP-SMX), amoxicillin, and ampicillin after susceptibility studies return. Drug resistance is a recognized problem in countries such as Mexico. Azithromycin is effective in treating children with typhoid fever [40,41].

Treatment for uncomplicated enteric fever is 10 to 14 days, with extension to 4 weeks for metastatic foci. Oral ciprofloxacin 500 mg twice daily may obviate the need for prolonged i.v. therapy (see Chapter 27G).

**(4) Prevention.** Oral or parenteral typhoid vaccine are available (see Chapter 22).

**c. Metastatic infection.** *Salmonella* organisms metastasize to distant sites, particularly to intravascular lesions, the skeletal system, and the meninges [14,27].

(1) **High-grade bacteremia** (>50% of three or more blood cultures) strongly suggests focal **intravascular infection.** *Salmonella* organisms have a predilection for arterial atherosclerotic plaques and aneurysms. Infectious disease consultation is advised.

(2) **Osteomyelitis or suppurative arthritis** can occur at any skeletal site. Patients with sickle cell anemia or skeletal prostheses are predisposed.

(3) **Meningitis** occurs principally in young children, especially newborn infants. **Hence, in young children with salmonella gastroenteritis, early therapy is indicated** [14].

(4) **Antibiotic** therapy is the same as for enteric fever except that therapy is prolonged for endocarditis, osteomyelitis, or abscesses. Failures have occurred with oral fluoroquinolone therapy for these conditions, particularly when drainage is not optimal.

d. **Chronic carriers.** The chronic carrier state **(i.e., positive stool or urine cultures for more than 12 months)** develops in approximately 1% to 4% of adults with typhoid fever. In other *Salmonella* infections, the development of the carrier state occurs much less frequently (0.2%–0.6%). The carrier state may follow symptomatic disease or may be the only manifestation of infection; it may be the consequence of the ingestion of a small inoculum [27].

(1) The persistence of the organism, in many cases, is due to **biliary tract carriage.** If biliary calculi are present, cholecystectomy and a 10- to 14-day course of antibiotics most often is required to cure the carrier state. This invasive approach eradicates infection in 90% of cases and may be appropriate for food handlers, medical personnel, and individuals with poor personal hygiene, and for other public health reasons. Antibiotics alone are unlikely to eradicate infection in patients with biliary calculi [14].

If gallbladder function is normal, cure of the carrier state may be attempted with a 4- to 6-week course of amoxicillin (6 g/day for 28 days) [42] or ciprofloxacin (500–750 mg orally twice daily for 28 days) [43]. Other fluoroquinolones such as norfloxacin (400 mg orally twice daily for 28 days), ofloxacin (200 mg twice daily), or TMP-SMX (160 mg TMP and 800 mg SMX twice daily in adults) have been used successfully [14]. However, even with use of the fluoroquinolones, eradication of the carrier state may be impossible (see Chapter 27G).

(2) **Chronic urinary tract** carriage can occur. Predisposing factors include obstructive uropathy from renal stones, strictures, hydronephrosis, tumors, and schistosomiasis.

e. **Special considerations**

(1) *Salmonella* causes severe infection with repeated recurrences in patients with AIDS (see Chapter 18).

(2) Other patients with an increased susceptibility to *Salmonella* infections include patients with leukemia, lymphoma, renal transplants, underlying inflammatory bowel disease, and underlying schistosomiasis.

B. **Shigellosis (bacillary dysentery).** *Shigella* are nonmotile, gram-negative bacilli that do not ferment lactose. There are four serogroups: group A (*S. dysenteriae*), group B (*S. flexneri*), group C (*S. boydii*), and group D (*S. sonnei*). Most disease in the United States is produced by *S. sonnei* or *S. flexneri*.

1. **Pathogenesis and epidemiology.** Shigellosis is highly communicable; ingestion of as few as 200 viable bacteria will produce illness. This organism is spread in a family setting or in confined settings, such as a day-care center. Food-borne or waterborne transmission, although less common, is associated with large outbreaks [44] *Shigella* strains invade mucosal epithelial cells (see section **I.C.2**). The HUS that occasionally follows *S. dysenteriae* is due to *Shigella* toxin.

2. **Symptoms.** Many patients will have the classic biphasic illness in which initially a small-bowel type of diarrhea occurs, characterized by passage of a small number of voluminous watery stools. Approximately 24 to 48 hours after ingestion of the microbe, abdominal pain, high fever, and diarrhea occur, marking large bowel involvement. In a large percentage of cases, gross blood in the stool develops. Stools containing blood and mucus are passed accompanied by tenesmus [44].

3. **Diagnosis** usually is **made by stool cultures. Bacteremia is rare.** A sigmoidoscopic examination may be suggestive of this diagnosis when diffuse inflammation and shallow ulcers are seen. Leukocytes often are seen in stool smears.
4. **Therapy.** Although mild disease often has responded to supportive care, **antibiotics are indicated** because they shorten the duration of illness and decrease the relapse rate. *In vitro* susceptibility tests should be performed because of the increasing problem of resistance to ampicillin and TMP-SMX. Currently, the agents of choice are the fluoroquinolones [39] (see Chapter 27G). Recommended duration of therapy ranges from one dose to 5 days of therapy [45]. Ciprofloxacin (500 mg twice daily for 3–5 days) can be used in adults. A single dose is effective in mild illness. Alternative regimens include TMP-SMX (160 mg TMP and 800 mg SMX twice daily in adults), ampicillin, azithromycin [46], and ceftriaxone [41,44].

**C. *Yersinia enterocolitica*** is a gram-negative coccobacillus formerly classified as a *Pasteurella* species. Although first recognized in 1933 in New York State, disease caused by this organism is more frequently reported in Scandinavia, northern Europe, Japan, and Canada than in the United States. Because the culture requires special techniques, the incidence of disease in the United States probably is underestimated [47–49].

1. **Symptoms.** Fever, abdominal pain, and diarrhea commonly appear together, but the latter **is present only 50% of the time.** Erythema nodosum, reactive arthritis, exudative pharyngitis, septicemia, and terminal ileitis or mesenteric lymphadenitis also occur. **The latter two mimic appendicitis.** However, at operation the appendix appears normal. A clustering of cases of mesenteric lymphadenitis should lead to the suspicion of *Y. enterocolitica* infection. The diarrheal illness is indistinguishable from that of other enteric pathogens. Symptoms commonly last 2 weeks on average.
2. **Diagnosis. Special cold enrichment of cultures** is necessary to increase the isolation of *Yersinia*. Even then, isolation may take several days or may be missed. **The laboratory must be alerted.** Appendiceal tissue also can be cultured.
3. **Treatment.** In most cases, resolution occurs spontaneously. The value of antimicrobial agents in *Y. enterocolitica* diarrhea or mesenteric adenitis has not been established. Therapy for mesenteric adenitis is symptomatic [47].
   a. **Intestinal infection usually is self-limited,** and there have been few clinical studies of efficacy. Treatment of diarrhea should focus on appropriate management of fluid replacement.
   b. **Treatment of extraintestinal disease or complications** should be based on *in vitro* susceptibility data. Most isolates have been shown to be sensitive to TMP-SMX, third-generation cephalosporins, aminoglycosides, fluoroquinolones, and tetracyclines [47]. In a retrospective review of 43 cases of bacteremic patients, fluoroquinolones alone or third-generation cephalosporins plus aminoglycosides or fluoroquinolones constituted the most effective treatment [50].
4. **Epidemiology.** Infection occurs by ingestion of contaminated food or water. Natural reservoirs include pigs, sheep, cattle, horses, dogs, and cats. The ability of *Yersinia* to grow at low temperatures potentiates its ability to contaminate refrigerated meats and other food products. Isolates have been cultured from meat, mussels, poultry, oysters, cheese, and ice cream. Food-borne outbreaks of *Yersinia* in the United States have been associated with contaminated chocolate milk and pasteurized milk. Person-to-person transmission also may occur [47–49].

**D. *Campylobacter*.** *Campylobacter* is the most common bacterial cause of acute gastroenteritis in the United States, identified two to seven times more frequently than *Salmonella, Shigella,* or *E. coli* O157:H7. An estimated 2.4 million cases occur annually in the United States, affecting nearly 1% of the population [51]. *C. jejuni* is the most frequently isolated species (>99%). Most cases of *Campylobacter* diarrhea are sporadic, but outbreaks can occur. **Special techniques are required for isolation.** This may account for the failure in the past to discover the organism by routine culture [8].

1. **Symptoms. Diarrhea,** cramping abdominal pain, fever, and constitutional symptoms predominate. **Grossly bloody stools or occult blood** may be seen

in the majority of patients. Most patients are symptomatic only for a few days, although enteric symptoms may last up to several weeks. The incubation period is usually 48 to 72 hours after ingestion of the organism. Less than 1% of patients have bacteremia. The clinical presentation mimics other forms of acute bacterial diarrhea, and the diagnosis can be established only by culture. Guillain-Barré syndrome is a rare postinfectious complication of *C. jejuni* infection, estimated to occur fewer than 0.1% of cases [51,52].

2. **Diagnosis.** A special selective medium is required to identify *Campylobacter jejuni* from stool cultures (which may take 72 to 96 hours), but routine blood cultures support growth of the organism. Methylene blue **fecal smears** commonly **show leukocytes.**

   Fresh stools can be screened for *Campylobacter* by direct microscopy. Leukocytes and red blood cells (RBCs) in the presence of bacteria with characteristic darting motility lead to a presumptive diagnosis. On Gram staining of stool, the presence of many small curved rods and reduced amounts of normal flora suggests *Campylobacter.*

3. **Treatment.** Gastroenteritis is usually self-limited, and antibiotic treatment is not required for the majority of cases.
   a. Treatment should be considered in patients with high fevers, bloody stools, prolonged illness (>1 week), pregnancy, human immunodeficiency virus (HIV) infection, and other immunocompromised states. In patients with protracted symptoms, treatment with antibiotic appears to shorten the illness and prevent relapses [51].
   b. **Treatments of choice are oral erythromycin** (500 mg twice daily for 5 days in adults), azithromycin (500 mg on day 1; 250 mg on days 2–5), or clarithromycin. Alternatives include fluoroquinolones, clindamycin, aminoglycosides, or imipenem [39,41,51].
   c. Rapidly increasing resistance to fluoroquinolones has been observed worldwide; 10% of isolates in the United States were resistant in 1998. Fluoroquinolones should not be used unless susceptibility is confirmed [53].
   d. Bacteremic patients deserve full therapeutic courses.

4. **Epidemiology.** *C. jejuni* is a known enteric pathogen in cattle, dogs, and fowl. Animals, symptomatic and nonsymptomatic, are the source of most human infections. In developed countries, 50% to 70% of infections are attributed to undercooked chicken. Cross-contamination during food preparation easily occurs. Sporadic infections from red meats, contaminated water, and contact with pets also occur. Large outbreaks, although unusual, have been associated with consumption of unpasteurized milk. Person-to-person transmission is unusual [51,52].

E. ***E. coli* O157:H7.** *E. coli* has emerged as an **important cause of both bloody diarrhea and HUS,** the most common cause of acute renal failure in children [54–59]. In the United States alone, *E. coli* O157:H7 is estimated to cause more than 20,000 infections and as many as 250 deaths each year [57]. The organism has been referred to as an enterohemorrhagic strain (EHEC) because of its frequent production of bloody diarrhea in infected patients [55]. The *E. coli* serotype O157:H7 is designated by its somatic (O) and flagella (H) antigens.

1. **Pathogenesis.** These *E. coli* produce large amounts of toxins (Shiga-like) that are specified by bacteriophages that have infected the bacterial cells. A multistate epidemic in the western United States in 1993 was traced to **contaminated hamburger** patties that were undercooked by a fast-food restaurant chain. Subsequent U.S. Food and Drug Administration (FDA) recommendations call for increasing internal temperature for cooked hamburgers to 155°F such that the interior is no longer pink [54]. In addition to undercooked ground beef, foods such as roast beef, unpasteurized milk, lettuce, and apple cider have been implicated, as well as poorly chlorinated municipal water [56], person-to-person transmission in child day-care centers [60], and swimming in a fecally contaminated lake [57,61].

   *E. coli* O157:H7 live in the intestines of about 1% of healthy cattle and can contaminate meat during slaughter. Grinding of beef is likely to transfer contamination from the surface to the interior of the meat [54,57].

2. **Clinical syndrome.** The incubation period usually is 3 to 5 days. **Although asymptomatic carriage occurs, watery diarrhea,** often **bloody,** is the prominent symptom in 90% of cases. Vomiting can occur. **Fever is infrequent.** The absence of fever may lead clinicians to suspect a noninfectious cause for the diarrhea [57]. Abdominal cramps or pain can be severe in some patients, and most illness resolves in 5 to 7 days. ***E. coli* O157:H7** also **causes a spectrum of other illnesses, including** HUS in 6% to 14% of patients under 10 years of age. It causes some cases of thrombotic thrombocytopenia purpura in adults, which has features similar to those of HUS in children. These clinical syndromes have been reviewed elsewhere [12,55,57,59]. HUS develops on average 1 week after the onset of diarrhea. Because patients clear the organism from the GI tract rapidly, up to two thirds of patients with HUS will not have *E. coli* O157:H7 in stools [55]. Children and the elderly are at highest risk for **complications,** with 5% to 10% of patients developing HUS. This is characterized by hemolytic anemia, thrombocytopenia, and renal failure, with a fatality rate of 3% to 5% [58].
3. **Diagnosis** is made by culture on special sorbitol-MacConkey agar, which is commercially available. Colonies of *E. coli* O157:H7, which does not ferment the sorbitol, can readily be identified and confirmed by serotyping with specific antisera [55]. **Most laboratories do not culture for this organism unless requested to do so.** Because of the increasing importance of this pathogen, microbiology laboratories now are encouraged to routinely culture for this organism in bloody and nonbloody diarrheal specimens [55,57]. Tests for rapid detection of *E. coli* O157:H7 antigens and Shiga-like toxin in stool are being developed. Antibodies to O157 lipopolysaccharide are positive in the first several months after the onset of HUS, although serologic testing is currently performed only in research laboratories [55].
4. **Therapy is supportive. Antibiotic-treated patients may be more likely to develop HUS** [57]. Even though most strains of *E. coli* O157:H7 are sensitive to antibiotics used to treat infective gastroenteritis, no clinical benefit has been demonstrated.
   a. **Most experts suggest antibiotics not be used** [12,55,57,62]. In a recent prospective study of *E. coli* O157:H7 in 71 children under 10 years of age, HUS developed in 56% of children treated with antibiotics and in 8% of untreated children [12,59].
   b. **Antimotility agents or narcotics are contraindicated** because they may delay clearance of the pathogen and toxin. Use of antimotility agents has been associated with increased risk for the development of HUS and increased severity of neurologic manifestations of the syndrome [57].
   c. **Intravenous hydration** with isotonic saline is advised to correct hypovolemia that in turn may reduce toxemic injury to the kidneys. Oral fluid increases crampy abdominal pain, whereas i.v. fluid administration reduces symptoms [55].
5. **Prevention**
   a. Thorough cooking kills *E. coli* O157:H7. Optimally, **ground beef should be cooked thoroughly** until the interior is no longer pink and the juices are clear [45,58].
   b. **Patients infected** with *E. coli* O157:H7 should be considered **highly contagious** and should not return to day care or school unless illness has resolved. Some authorities have recommended that infected children be excluded until two consecutive stool cultures are negative for *E. coli* O157:H7. However, shedding of the organism may be intermittent. Supervised handwashing is the most important preventive measure [55,57,60]. The dose of *E. coli* O157:H7 that leads to symptomatic infection, like *Shigella,* is low.
   c. **All cases of confirmed *E. coli* O157:H7 infection should be reported immediately to appropriate public health authorities.** Early detection can lead to measures that will help prevent additional cases from occurring.

F. ***Vibrio parahemolyticus*** is a gram-negative, halophilic, marine organism that was first isolated in 1950 as a cause of self-limited gastroenteritis [3,63]. It is common in

Japan, where it may account for up to 70% of recognized causes of gastroenteritis. It occurs rarely in the United States, in such coastal areas as eastern Maryland, the gulf coast of Louisiana and Florida, and on cruise ships sailing between Florida and the Caribbean [64].

1. **Symptoms.** Diarrhea, cramps, weakness, nausea, chills, headache, fever, and vomiting occur 3 to 76 hours **after ingestion of contaminated raw or improperly cooked shellfish.** The mean duration of illness is approximately 3 days [63].
2. **Diagnosis.** Isolation is achieved on special media. Stool specimens may be tinged with blood and contain fecal leukocytes indicative of invasive disease. Sigmoidoscopy demonstrates superficial ulceration in some cases.
3. **Treatment.** Resolution occurs spontaneously in most cases and therapy is not indicated. No studies on the efficacy of antibiotics in gastroenteritis have been reported, but most are sensitive to tetracycline and TMP-SMX.

G. ***Clostridium difficile*** (antibiotic-related) diarrhea. **This diagnosis should be considered in any patient with a new onset of diarrhea while taking antibiotics or within 4 to 6 weeks after completing a course of antibiotics.** Fever, abdominal tenderness, leukocytosis, and fecal leukocytes are common findings.

H. **Travelers' diarrhea** is discussed in Chapter 22.

I. **Miscellaneous**

1. Other *Vibrio* species can cause diarrhea and may be linked epidemiologically to the consumption of raw or undercooked shellfish [64].
2. **Cholera,** infection due to *V. cholerae,* is rare in the United States. Domestically acquired cholera has been reported from an endemic Gulf Coast focus involving shellfish or imported foods; international travelers also can acquire cholera [64–66].
3. *Aeromonas hydrophila* may be pathogenic at times and is found in fresh water in the United States, coastal waters, shellfish, and even farm animals [3,63,67, 68].
4. *Plesiomonas shigelloides* also may cause diarrhea from contaminated shellfish (e.g., raw oysters). Rare waterborne outbreaks occur in the United States [3,63, 69–71].

J. **Parasitic disease** may mimic bacterial gastroenteritis, *Giardia* species, and *Entamoeba histolytica.* See related discussions under Gastrointestinal Parasites.

VI. **Viral gastroenteritis occurs commonly,** producing an estimated **30% to 40% of the cases of infectious diarrhea in the United States.** A study of diseases affecting families in Cleveland over a 10-year period found that infectious nonbacterial gastroenteritis was second in frequency to the common cold and accounted for 16% of illnesses [71,72].

A. **Etiology.** Four major categories of human gastroenteritis viruses have been defined since the discovery of the Norwalk virus in 1972. Well-established medically important pathogens include **rotavirus, enteric adenovirus, calicivirus (including Norwalk or Norwalk-like viruses), and astrovirus** (Table 13.5). The specific cause of many bouts of gastroenteritis cannot be determined [3,8,72–74].

1. **Rotavirus** is the agent **responsible for 30% to 60% of all cases of severe watery diarrhea in children.** It is a double-stranded RNA virus that can undergo gene reassortment, leading to new serotypes. There are at least seven distinct antigenic groups (A to G), four of which cause most disease. Group A rotavirus is most common and is the **single most important cause of dehydrating diarrhea necessitating hospitalization in children under 2 years of age** in both developed and less developed countries. Virtually all children are infected in the first 3 to 5 years of life. In the United States approximately 1 million cases of rotavirus infection occur annually, resulting in over 50,000 hospitalizations of children and 20 to 40 deaths per year [3,75]. Mild disease is seen in older children, and at times adults may acquire disease, especially after close contact with infected infants. Infants under 3 months of age seem less likely to be infected, presumably because of immunity by passive transplacental transfer of maternal antibody. Breast-feeding has not been proven to prevent infection but may be associated with milder disease and should be encouraged [76].

Table 13.5. Medical Importance, Clinical and Epidemiologic Characteristics, and Diagnosis of Human Gastroenteritis Viruses

| Virus | Medical Importance Demonstrated | Epidemiologic Characteristics | Clinical Characteristics | Laboratory Diagnostic Tests[a] |
|---|---|---|---|---|
| Rotavirus | | | | |
| Group A | Yes | Major cause of endemic severe diarrhea in infants and young children worldwide (in winter in temperate zone) | Dehydrating diarrhea for 5–7 days; vomiting and fever common | Immunoassay, electron micros copy, PAGE |
| Group B | Partially | Large outbreaks in adults and children in China | Severe watery diarrhea for 3–5 days | Electron microscopy, PAGE |
| Group C | Partially | Sporadic cases in young children worldwide | Similar to characteristics of group A rotavirus | Electron microscopy, PAGE |
| Enteric adenovirus | Yes | Endemic diarrhea of infants and young children | Prolonged diarrhea lasting 5–12 days; vomiting and fever | Immunoassay, electron microscopy with PAGE |
| Calicivirus (Norwalk virus; Norwalk-like viruses) | Yes | Epidemics of vomiting and diarrhea in children and adults; occurs in families, communities, and nursing homes; often associated with shellfish, other food, or water | Acute vomiting, diarrhea, fever, myalgia, and headache lasting 1–2 days | Immunoassay, immune electron microscopy |
| Astrovirus | Partially | Pediatric diarrhea; reported in nursing homes | Watery diarrhea, often lasting 2–3 days, occasionally longer | Immunoassay, electron microscopy |

PAGE, polyacrylamide-gel electrophoresis and silver staining of viral nucleic acid in stool.
[a]Laboratory diagnostic tests, other than those for rotavirus group A, usually are available only in specialized research or diagnostic referral laboratories. Immunoassays are usually enzyme-linked immunosorbent assay or radioimmunoassays.
Adapted from Blacklow NR, Greenberg HB. Viral gastroenteritis. *N Engl J Med* 1991;325:252; with permission.

a. **Transmission is** probably by the **fecal-oral route.** Rotavirus is shed in large numbers in the feces, and fecal infiltrates are infectious to volunteers [72]. Rotavirus can be found on toys and hard surfaces in day-care centers, suggesting fomites as a mechanism of spread. Respiratory transmission also may play a role. Waterborne transmission may occur in less developed countries [76].

b. **Infection is more common** in cooler, **winter** months in the United States, with spread typically from the Southwest to the Northeast each year.

c. **Clinical syndrome.** Rotavirus infection frequently is asymptomatic. In symptomatic infection, the incubation period is 1 to 3 days, with illness lasting 5 to 7 days in normal hosts, but the course may be more protracted in the immunocompromised host. **It is not possible to differentiate rotavirus-associated gastroenteritis from illness caused by other enteric pathogens on the basis of clinical criteria. Vomiting is common,** as is dehydration.

d. **Diagnosis.** Because large amounts of the rotavirus are in the stool, a wide variety of assays able to detect **rotavirus antigen in the stool** are sensitive and specific. Enzyme immunoassays (EIAs) and latex agglutinations assays are commercially available.

e. **Treatment** is symptomatic, preferably with oral rehydration fluids.

f. **Vaccine** to prevent rotavirus infection and disease is not currently available. A rhesus rotavirus tetravalent vaccine was incorporated into the routine childhood immunization schedule in 1999, but was withdrawn from the market the same year because of an association of this vaccine and intussusception [75,76].

2. **Enteric adenovirus** is second to the rotavirus in causing pediatric gastroenteritis, especially in children under 1 year of age. Estimates suggest that this virus accounts for 4% to 10% of pediatric diarrhea in children under 2 years of age [72].

a. **Transmission** is from person to person.

b. No seasonal peak occurs.

c. Serotypes 40 and 41 cause diarrheal disease, usually without respiratory symptoms.

d. **Clinical syndrome.** The incubation period is 8 to 10 days. Asymptomatic infection may be observed, but watery diarrhea may last 5 to 12 days, with 1 to 2 days of vomiting. Low-grade fever and dehydration occur. Nosocomial and day-care center outbreaks are common, during which high rates of asymptomatic infections occur; spread to adults is uncommon.

e. A presumptive **diagnosis** can be made if large numbers of adenoviral particles are seen on electron microscopic examination of diarrheal stool; the virus cannot be cultured with conventional cell culture. Immunoassays and dot blot hybridization assays for adenoviruses 40 and 41 are available [74].

f. **Treatment** is symptomatic.

3. **Calicivirus** (including **Norwalk virus** and serologically related **Norwalk-like** viruses) **cause approximately 40% of the outbreaks of gastroenteritis** that occur in every situation where people gather in social, health-related, or recreational circumstances. Outbreaks also result from the ingestion of contaminated drinking or swimming water, poorly cooked clams and oysters from contaminated waters, and contaminated foods such as salads and cake frosting. These viruses cause explosive epidemics of diarrhea that can sweep through a community with a high attack rate, affecting all age groups [3,72,74,77,78].

a. **Transmission** is by the fecal-oral route.

b. **Clinical syndrome.** The incubation period is 12 to 48 hours. Nausea and vomiting are common but watery diarrhea is the main symptom. Mild degrees of small intestinal malabsorption can persist for 2 weeks after the acute episode [72]. Disease caused by calicivirus in infants and young children is clinically indistinguishable from mild rotavirus illness, typically with vomiting and diarrhea lasting 1 to 2 days. Approximately 3% of the cases of diarrhea among infants and young children at U.S. day-care centers are caused by calicivirus.

c. **Diagnosis.** Because the calicivirus cannot be cultivated in the laboratory, the diagnosis can be established only by identifying viral antigen in the stool, and these tests are available only in research laboratories. Virus can be seen in fecal effluent by immune electron microscopy using serum from a convalescent subject. A monoclonal antibody–based enzyme-linked immunoabsorbent assay (ELISA) and a polymerase chain reaction (PCR) assay have been developed that can detect Norwalk virus in stool specimens, but these are not yet commercially available [74,78].

d. **Nomenclature.** Caliciviruses are often named after the locations of outbreaks of diarrheal illness attributed to these viruses (e.g., Norwalk, Hawaii, Snow Mountain).

4. **Astrovirus** is a single-stranded RNA virus that is **a major cause of diarrheal illness in children** from infancy to 7 years of age. Antibody develops to many of the seven viral serotypes by about 4 years of age, indicating that this virus probably causes frequent infections in childhood. Although similar to rotavirus illness, it is less severe. The incubation period is 1 to 4 days. Nausea, vomiting, and occasionally fever may occur, but watery diarrhea lasting 2 to 3 days is the prominent symptom. Outbreaks have been described in residential homes for the elderly. Serum antibodies whose levels may decline with age may protect young adults. The virus can be recognized in stool specimens by means of electron microscopy, specific immunoassays, RNA probe hybridization, and PCR [3,72,74].

B. **Diagnosis**

1. **In adults,** the diagnosis of viral gastroenteritis is, for all practical purposes, **a diagnosis of exclusion** because techniques are not routinely available to isolate the virus from stool [8].
   a. **History.** There is no obvious history suggesting a bacterial or parasitic process (e.g., no recent international travel, no high fever or rigors, no recent seafood ingestion). The patient may well have been exposed to a friend or family member with similar GI symptoms.
   b. **Stool examination.** The diagnosis of a viral process is supported, although not proven, by the absence of fecal leukocytes. The results of stool culture or O&P examination will be negative, and the decision of whether to order these tests must be individualized.
2. **In children,** similar principles hold, but stools can be examined for rotavirus and, at times, enteric adenovirus.

C. **Therapy is supportive** with fluid replacement.

## *HELICOBACTER PYLORI* AND PEPTIC ULCER DISEASE

*Helicobacter pylori* (formerly called *Campylobacter pylori*) has emerged as a major causative factor in the pathogenesis of peptic ulcer disease. Most peptic ulcers not caused by nonsteroidal antiinflammatory drugs (NSAIDs) are now thought to be associated with *H. pylori* infection. The organism's clinical role has been reviewed extensively [79–83].

I. **The organism** *H. pylori* is a curved, motile, microaerophilic gram-negative bacillus with flagella at one end that is found in the mucous layer overlying the epithelium of the gastric mucosa, and within the epithelial cells.

A. ***H. pylori* infection is found worldwide.** Prevalence of infection increases with age and is highest in disadvantaged socioeconomic groups. In developing countries, the prevalence of *H. pylori* colonization of gastric mucosa is nearly universal by the age of 20. Developed countries typically have a lower prevalence of *H. pylori,* particularly among younger persons. In North America more than 50% of asymptomatic persons over 60 years of age show evidence of active or past *H. pylori* infection [79]. Patients with active or inactive peptic ulcer disease, especially duodenal but also gastric, have *H. pylori* infection more often than age-matched controls, with an odds ratio of approximately 3:1 to 4:1 [84]. The only known important reservoir of *H. pylori* is humans. Although *H. pylori* has been cultured from domestic cats, there is no evidence that it is transmitted to humans from cats or other pets. Transmission is thought to occur person to person by fecal-oral or oral-oral exposures, although the route of transmission has not been confirmed. A higher prevalence of *H. pylori* antibodies has been found among institutionalized adults relative to age-matched controls, suggesting person-to-person transmission in the institutional setting [85].

**B.** Virtually all persons with *H. pylori* infection in the antral mucosa have focal epithelial cell damage and inflammation in the lamina propria.

1. *H. pylori* produces urease, which seems important in colonization and is cytotoxic to human epithelial cells.
2. Other cytotoxins produced by certain strains of *H. pylori* may function as virulence factors that damage epithelial cells and exacerbate the inflammatory process in susceptible hosts [81,86].

**C.** The importance of ***H. pylori*** **in the pathogenesis of peptic ulcer disease** is evident in the high incidence of infection among patients with peptic ulcer disease and the lower relapse rates of ulcers after eradication of *H. pylori*.

1. *H. pylori* infection is present in greater than 90% of patients with duodenal ulcers and 70% to 90% of those with gastric ulcers, excluding patients taking NSAIDs [81].
2. **The strongest evidence for the pathogenic role of *H. pylori* in peptic ulcer disease is the marked decrease in recurrence rates of ulcers following the eradication of *H. pylori*** [82,83]. Among patients with duodenal ulcer and *H. pylori* infection, ulcer recurred in only 12% of those treated with triple antibiotics plus ranitidine, compared with recurrence in 95% of those treated with ranitidine alone [87].
3. Overall, *H. pylori* appears to be a strong risk factor for development of ulcer disease, but its presence is not sufficient to cause ulcers. **Only 15% to 20% of people infected with *H. pylori* develop an ulcer during their lifetime.** Why *H. pylori* infection leads to peptic ulcer disease in a minority of infected persons is not known [81].
4. The mechanism whereby infection with *H. pylori* results in peptic ulcer disease is not well understood. Physiologic factors in the host, such as increased acid secretion in response to infection, may enhance mucosal injury. Other host factors, such as concomitant smoking, the use of NSAIDs, and stress, may play synergistic roles [81,86].

**II. Diagnosis of *H. pylori* infection** [81]

**A. Invasive techniques require endoscopy.**

1. **Culture is not indicated** for diagnosis. Culturing for *H. pylori* involves obtaining the sample by endoscopy, and culture techniques are difficult. Culture is less sensitive than routine histologic analysis of tissue. Cultures are used in research studies to determine the susceptibility of *H. pylori* to antimicrobial agents.
2. **Endoscopy with biopsy**
   a. **The organism may have a patchy distribution in the stomach,** especially in the body and fundus. Taking multiple biopsy samples improves the diagnostic yield.
   b. ***Campylobacter*-like organism (Clo) test on endoscopic biopsy samples.** Mucosal tissue is directly inoculated into medium containing urea and phenol red, which turns pink if the pH rises above 6.0. This change occurs when urea in the gel is metabolized to ammonia by the urease produced by *H. pylori*. The test is commercially available and inexpensive, and can provide a diagnosis within 1 hour of inoculation of the biopsy specimen. Sensitivity and specificity are as high as 90% and 100%, respectively. **The low cost and excellent reliability of this test make it the endoscopic method of choice for diagnosis** [81,83].
   c. **Histologic examination.** Experienced pathologists can diagnose *H. pylori* on hematoxylin and eosin staining, but false-negative results occur. Giemsa and Warthin-Starry stains permit easier visualization [83]. Histology is much more expensive than urease (Clo) testing; it is reasonable to obtain biopsy samples and perform the histologic examination only if results of the Clo test are negative [81,83].

**B. Noninvasive tests**

1. **The urea breath test is a sensitive, specific, noninvasive test to detect** *H. pylori* infection. A carbon 13– or 14–labeled urea solution is ingested. If

*H. pylori* is present in the stomach, urease produced by the organism will hydrolyze the urea to form ammonia and radiolabeled carbon dioxide. The latter is absorbed rapidly into the bloodstream and can be detected in the expired breath [81,88].

a. The urea breath test is sensitive and specific in the initial diagnosis of *H. pylori* infection and the assessment of response to antimicrobial therapy.

b. Because antimicrobial drugs and proton pump inhibitors temporarily cause false-negative results, an interval of at least 4 weeks after completion of anti–*H. pylori* therapy should be allowed before breath tests are used for confirmation of cure.

2. **Serologic tests** are available, based on ELISA and other methods, which have very high sensitivity and specificity for detecting immunoglobulin G (IgG) antibody to *H. pylori.*

a. **An elevated antibody titer to *H. pylori* indicates current infection in the untreated patient,** because spontaneous clearance of infection is rare.

b. **Serology is not useful for early follow-up testing after therapy.** Although the antibody titer decreases after eradication of *H. pylori,* the rate of decline is uncertain. Titers must be followed for at least 6 months to determine a decline [81].

3. Because of their excellent accuracy and low cost, **serology and urea breath test are the methods of choice to document infection with *H. pylori* in patients who do not otherwise require endoscopy.**

C. **The optimal strategy for evaluation and management of patients with dyspepsia, only 15% to 30% of whom have peptic ulcer disease, remains controversial** [80,83,89].

1. **Noninvasive tests for *H. pylori* are commonly used in conjunction with endoscopy.** Some experts advocate that patients with dyspepsia undergo noninvasive testing for *H. pylori* followed by anti–*H. pylori* antibiotic therapy in *H. pylori*–positive subjects. Endoscopy is reserved for nonresponders. The safety and cost effectiveness of this approach are under investigation [80,83,90].

2. Endoscopy is still required to establish a diagnosis of ulcer disease. Endoscopy is indicated in patients with dyspepsia associated with "alarm" markers for gastric or esophageal neoplasia (e.g., anemia, GI bleeding, anorexia, early satiety, vomiting, dysphagia, weight loss, or onset after age 50) [83,89].

## III. Treatment of *H. pylori* associated with peptic ulcer disease

A. **Consensus has evolved that *H. pylori* is:**

1. **A cause of acute and chronic active gastritis.**

2. **A cofactor in the pathogenesis and recurrence of peptic ulcer diseases** (see section **I.A**).

3. **A Possible cofactor in gastric carcinoma.** However, there is no evidence that treatment of *H. pylori* infection prevents development of gastric carcinoma [91].

4. **Not conclusively established as a factor in nonulcer dyspepsia.** Eradication of *H. pylori* does not consistently result in resolution of symptoms [92,93].

B. **Treatment to eradicate *H. pylori* is advocated for selected patients** [79–83].

1. **All patients with gastric or duodenal ulcers who are infected with *H. pylori*** should receive antimicrobials, whether on initial presentation or on recurrence.

2. *H. pylori*–infected patients with peptic ulcer disease who are receiving maintenance therapy with antisecretory agents or who have a history of complicated or refractory disease should be treated.

C. **Do not treat asymptomatic carriers and nonulcer dyspepsia.**

1. Prophylactic antibiotics are **not** recommended to prevent future ulcers or gastric neoplasia in asymptomatic infected patients without ulcers.

2. Treatment is not routinely advised for patients with nonulcer dyspepsia. Patients may be tested for *H. pylori* on a case-by-case basis, and treatment offered to those with a positive result [80,92,93].

3. Mucosa-associated lymphoid tumors (MALTomas) of the stomach appear to regress in patients treated for *H. pylori* with antibiotics (see section **IV.B.**)

D. **Treatment regimens.** The optimal regimen has not been defined.
   1. Attempts to eradicate *H. pylori* with single agents have not been effective and may lead to antimicrobial resistance [80,82].
   2. **Multidrug regimens** are suggested. Antimicrobials used to treat *H. pylori* include bismuth subsalicylate (Pepto-Bismol), amoxicillin, metronidazole, clarithromycin, and tetracycline in various combinations of two or three agents, usually in addition to a histamine ($H_2$)-blocker (e.g., ranitidine) or a proton pump inhibitor (e.g., omeprazole). Regimens given for 7 to 14 days have been successful in eradicating *H. pylori* in 60% to 95% of cases. The longer duration of treatment is usually more efficacious. Obstacles to effective treatment include the presence of antibiotic-resistant *H. pylori,* poor patient compliance with complex regimens, and occurrence of side effects [79–83,94,95].
      a. **Antimicrobial resistance** of *H. pylori* to metronidazole and clarithromycin is reported frequently; resistance to tetracycline and to amoxicillin is rare.
      b. The **topical action** of effective antibiotics is important.
      c. The **efficacy of many antibiotics is enhanced at increased gastric pH levels,** which may help to explain the higher rates of eradication of *H. pylori* when antimicrobial agents are combined with $H_2$-blockers or proton pump inhibitors.
      d. **Reinfection** after eradication is uncommon and appears to occur at rates as low as 1% annually in developed counties [81].
      e. **Side effects** are common with a triple-drug regimen and occur in up to 30% of recipients [82]. **Nausea and vomiting** may be seen in 20%. Alcohol should be avoided. Oropharyngeal or vaginal fungal infections can occur and may require topical therapy. **Diarrhea** may be reduced if tetracycline is used instead of amoxicillin. **Rash** is seen in 5% or fewer patients. *C. difficile* diarrhea has been reported in less than 1% of treated patients. Clarithromycin can cause a disturbance in taste that some patients find intolerable.
   3. **Examples of common treatment regimens** are provided below. Options for treatment continue to evolve. See earlier reports [79–81,83,94,95] for a more detailed discussion.
      a. Clarithromycin 500 mg twice daily plus metronidazole 500 mg twice daily (or amoxicillin 1 g twice daily) plus omeprazole 20 mg twice daily (or lansoprazole 30 mg twice daily) for 7 to 14 days.
      b. Clarithromycin 500 mg twice daily plus metronidazole 500 mg twice daily (or amoxicillin 1 g twice daily or tetracycline 500 mg twice daily) plus ranitidine bismuth citrate (Tritec) 400 mg twice daily for 7 to 14 days.
      c. Bismuth subsalicylate (Pepto-Bismol) two tablets (525 mg) four times daily plus metronidazole 250 mg four times daily plus tetracycline 500 mg four times daily for 14 days.
      d. Regimen c plus omeprazole 20 mg twice daily for 7 days.

IV. **Relationship of *H. pylori* to other GI diseases**

A. **Gastric carcinoma.** Several prospective and retrospective studies of gastric cancer have identified *H. pylori* colonization as a risk factor for this disease. This finding is not surprising, because chronic gastritis and atrophic gastritis, which are known to be associated with *H. pylori,* are also recognized risk factors for gastric carcinoma. However, the presence of *H. pylori* colonization is neither necessary nor sufficient for oncogenesis, and other factors also must be involved in the pathogenesis of gastric carcinoma [79,91].

B. **Mucosa-associated lymphoid tumors** are non-Hodgkin lymphomas of the stomach that arise from B-lymphocytes. *H. pylori* colonization is strongly associated with gastric MALTomas. Recent studies suggest that eradication of *H. pylori* results in tumor regression in most patients [79].

## GASTROINTESTINAL PARASITES

A detailed discussion of the epidemiology, clinical features, and treatment of intestinal parasitic diseases is beyond the scope of this book. However, basic concepts of diagnosis and therapy of the most common pathogens are presented here. Table 13.6 lists the vectors, most common clinical symptoms, sites of involvement in the host, and laboratory tests

Table 13.6. Helminth and Protozoan Infections of Human Gastrointestinal Tract

| | Common Name of Parasite or Disease | Site in Host | Source of Infection, Intermediate Host, or Vector | Most Common Clinical Symptoms | Laboratory Diagnosis | Remarks |
|---|---|---|---|---|---|---|
| Nemathelminths (roundworms) | | | | | | |
| *Ancylostomaa duodenale*[a] *Necator americanus*[a] | Old world hookworm; ancylostomiasis New world or tropical hookworm; uncinariasis | Small intestine (attached) | Infective filariform larvae in soil | Anemia growth retardation, GI symptoms | Eggs in stool | Prophylaxis by excreta disposal. Iron therapy important in blood regeneration. |
| *Ascaris lumbricoides*[b] | Large roundworm | Small intestine | Eggs from soil or vegetables | Vague abdominal distress | Eggs in stool | Worms migrate into bile, pancreatic duct, and peritoneum. Intestinal obstruction. |
| *Enterobius vermicularis*[b] | Pinworm, seatworm; *Oxyuris* | Large intestine, appendix | Eggs in environment; autoinfection | Anal pruritus | Eggs in perianal region, cellophane tape swab | Entire family frequently infected. Personal hygiene important. |
| *Strongyloides stercoralis*[a] | Cochin, Viet Nam diarrhea | Wall of small intestine | Larvae in soil | Abdominal discomfort, diarrhea | Larvae in stool | Autoinfection occurs. |
| *Trichinella spiralis*[b] | Trichinosis | Intestinal wall; cyst in striated muscle | Infected pork, cyst (rarely bear) | Orbital edema, muscle pain, eosinophilia | Skin test, serology, muscle biopsy | Thorough cooking of pork and pork products to kill cysts. |
| *Trichuris trichiura*[b] | Whipworm, threadworm | Cecum of large intestine, ileum | Eggs from soil or vegetables | Abdominal discomfort, anemia, bloody stools | Eggs in stool | Frequently with hookworm and *Ascaris;* adults seldom symptomatic. |
| *Toxocara canis, T. cati*[b] | Visceral larva migrans | Liver, lung, brain, eye | Eggs from soil | Pneumonitis, eosinophilia | Serology | Eosinophilia, anemia, hyperglobulinemia. |
| Platyhelminths (Tapeworms) | | | | | | |
| *Diphyllobothrium latum*[b] | Fish or broad tapeworm | Small intestine | Plerocercoid in freshwater fish | Anemia very rare | Eggs in stool | Prophylaxis by excreta disposal. Cook fish well. |
| *Hymenolepsis nana*[b] | Dwarf tapeworm | Adults and cysts in small intestine | Eggs from feces in soil; autoinfection | Abdominal discomfort | Eggs in stool | Numerous worms, infection of children. |
| *Taenia saginata*[b] | Beef tapeworm | Small intestine | Cysts in beef | Usually no symptoms | Eggs and segments in stool | Usually only one worm. |

| | | | | | | |
|---|---|---|---|---|---|---|
| *Taenia solium*[b] | Pork tapeworm | Small intestine | Cysts in pork | Usually no symptoms | Eggs and segments in stool | Uncommon in USA. Frequent in Mexico South America, Central America. |
| *T. solium* (cysts)[b] | Cysticercosis; verminous epilepsy | Muscle, brain, eye | Eggs from feces | Intracranial pressure, epilepsy | Biopsy, radiograph of calcified cysts; CT scan; serology | Autoinfection possible. Uncommon in USA. |
| *Echinococcus granulosus*[b] | Hydatid cyst | Liver, lungs, brain, bones | Eggs from dog feces | Symptoms due to pressure in affected organs | Serology, CT scan; skin test | Uncommon in USA. |
| Platyhelminths (flukes) | | | | | | |
| *Schistosoma haematobium*[a] | Schistosomiasis (bilharzia) | Veins of urinary bladder | Cercaria in fresh water, from snail | Urinary disturbances, hematuria | Eggs in urine, cystoscopy | Africa, Middle East. |
| *Schistosoma japonicum*[a] | Schistosomiasis | Veins of small intestine | Cercaria in fresh water, from snail | Dysentery, hepatic cirrhosis | Eggs in stool, liver biopsy | China, Japan, Philippines. |
| *Schistosoma mansoni*[a] | Schistosomiasis | Veins of large intestine | Cercaria in fresh water, from snail | Chronic dysentery, hepatic cirrhosis | Eggs in stool, rectal or liver biopsy | Africa, South America, common in Puerto Rico. |
| Protozoa | | | | | | |
| *Entamoeba histolytica*[b] | Intestinal amebiasis | Lumen and wall of large intestine | Cysts in food and water, from feces | Mild to severe GI distress, dysentery | Cysts or trophozoites in stool; serology | Consider possibility of hepatic infection |
| *E. histolytica*[b] | Amebic hepatitis, amebic liver abscess | Liver | Cysts in food and water, from feces | Enlarged, tender liver; fever; leukocytosis | CT scan or ultrasonography; serology; cysts or trophozoites in stool | Treat intestinal amebic infection |
| *Giardia lamblia*[b] | Flagellate diarrhea | Upper small intestine | Cysts in food and water, from feces | Mild GI distress and diarrhea, weight loss | Enzyme immunoassay of stool; cysts and trophozoites in stool | More common in children than adults |

GI, gastrointestinal; CT, computed tomography.
[a]Portal of entry is the skin.
[b]Portal of entry is the mouth.
Adapted from Brown HW, Neva FA. *Basic clinical parasitology,* 5th ed. New York: Appleton-Century-Crofts, 1983:8–17; with permission.

commonly used to make the diagnosis of intestinal parasitic infestation. For details, the reader is referred to texts and recent reviews devoted to this topic [96–98].

I. Pathogenesis of symptoms usually is related to one of the following:
   A. **Physical presence** of organisms in the GI tract with loss of nutrients or blood (as in hookworm, *Ascaris, Strongyloides,* fluke, and protozoa infestations)
   B. **Inflammatory reaction** by the host to some parasite-related protein (as in schistosomiasis and trichinosis)
   C. **Migration of parasite** (as in creeping eruption and visceral larva migrans)

II. **Diagnosis**
   A. **Stool examination is the most common means of identifying the pathogen.**
      1. **The clinician should contact the diagnostic parasitology or microbiology laboratory** for assistance.
      2. **Fresh stool specimens** are required to preserve the trophozoites of some parasites such as *E. histolytica*. The diagnostic laboratory often will reject a specimen unless it is fresh or placed in appropriate fixatives.
      3. **Many drugs and materials interfere** with the stool examination for parasites. **Iron,** Bismuth, castor oil or mineral oil, and particulate substances such as **Metamucil,** can interfere for up to 1 week after ingestion. **Barium,** gallbladder dye, **antibiotics,** iodine preparations, bismuth, antiamebic drugs, and some antimalarial drugs may make the stool difficult to examine correctly for as long as 3 weeks after ingestion.
      4. **Stool specimens should be collected before any medications or purgatives for radiologic procedures are given.**
      5. **Macroscopic examination** of the stool may reveal nematodes or proglottids. Adult worms may be washed in warm sodium chloride and examined fresh or fixed. Proglottids may be visualized clearly by mounting in 5% acetic acid [96].
      6. Saline and iodine **wet mounts** for microscopic examination are useful for trophozoites, cysts, ova, and certain helminth larvae.
      7. **Three stool samples for O&P** microscopic examination are suggested in selected patients, because a single examination may yield false-negative results. The specimen should be collected in a clean dry surface such as a bedpan or collection cup and should not be taken from the toilet or be contaminated with urine. O&P microscopic examination is time consuming and requires a skilled clinical parasitologist. O&P examination is recommended only in selected patients:
         a. **EIAs for detection of *Giardia lamblia* and *Cryptosporidium* antigen in stool have largely replaced O&P examination. O&P examination should be reserved for patients in whom there is a high clinical suspicion of parasitic infection caused by organisms other than *Giardia* or *Cryptosporidium.*** These would include immigrants or returning travelers from tropical regions that have a high prevalence of endemic parasitic disease, or immunocompromised patients or others with persistent diarrhea in whom exclusion of other causes has been accomplished by laboratory testing [8,99].
         b. **O&P examination is usually not appropriate in patients who develop diarrhea after 3 days of hospitalization.** In this setting, *C. difficile* colitis or antibiotic-associated diarrhea are far more common than parasites [8,99].
      8. **Artifacts or other objects can be mistaken for parasites.** This is especially true in old specimens. It is best to confirm one's observation by consulting with an expert.
      9. **Diagrams of common helminth eggs** are shown in Figure 13.1 and in Neva's text [96].
   B. **Geographic exposure** is useful when considering a parasitic diagnosis. For example, hookworms survive poorly in cold, northern environments, and *Echinococcus* cysts are found primarily in sheepherders of Basque origin in the western United States. The Centers for Disease Control and Prevention conducted a survey of stool specimens examined by public health laboratories in 1987. A total of 216,275 specimens were examined; parasites were found in 20.0%. Percentages were highest for protozoans: *Giardia lamblia* (7.2%), *Entamoeba coli* and *E. nana* (4.2% each),

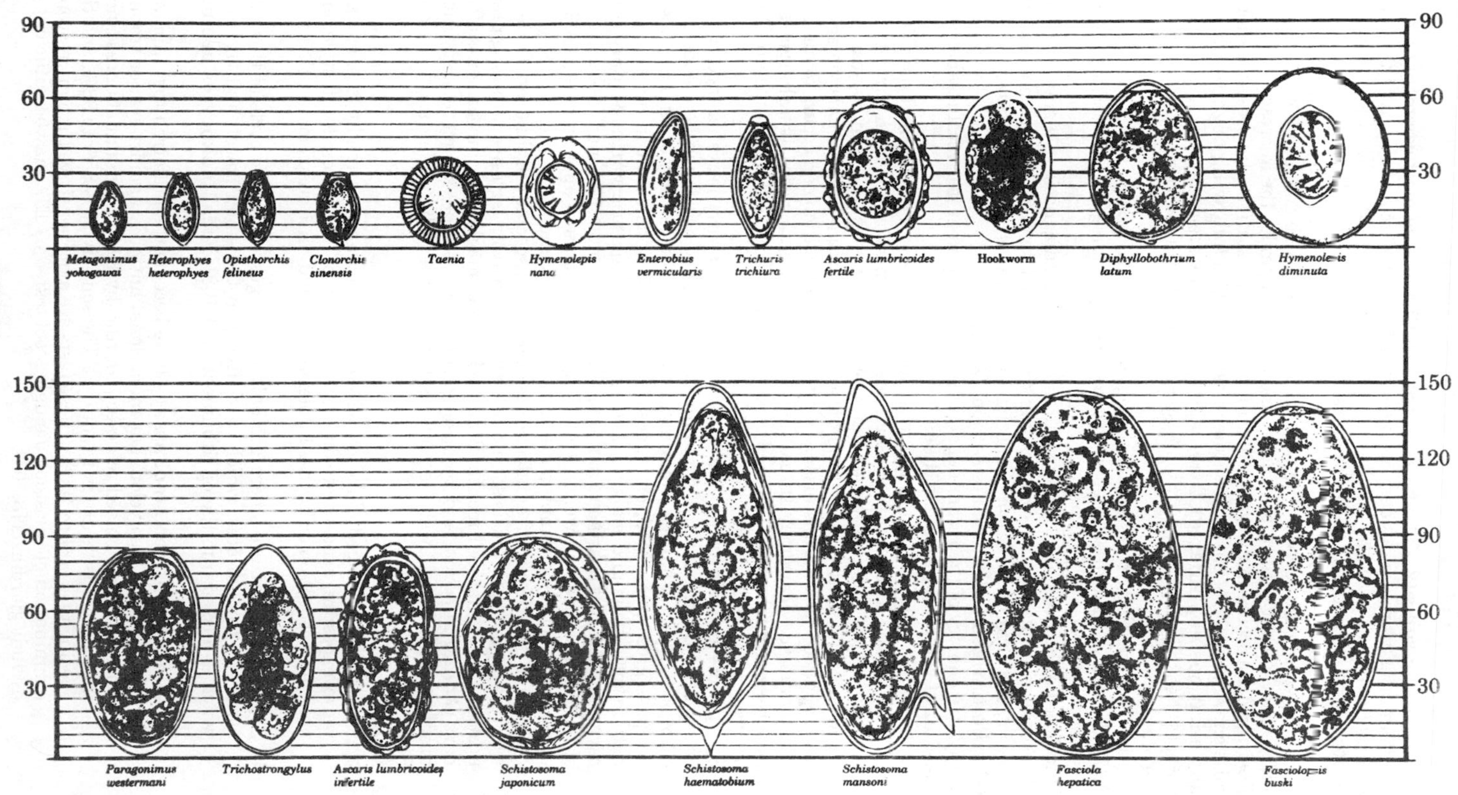


**FIG. 13.1** Relative size of helminth eggs. (Reprinted from Brooke MM, Melvin DM. *Morphology of diagnostic stages of intestinal parasites of man.* Publication No. (HSM) 72-8116. Atlanta: U.S. Department of Health, Education, and Welfare, 1972.)

*Blastocystis hominis* (2.6%), and *E. histolytica* (0.9%). The most commonly identified helminths were nematodes: hookworm (1.5%), *Trichuris trichiura* (1.2%), and *Ascaris lumbricoides* (0.8%) [100].

C. **Scotch tape** technique for **pinworms** is the test of choice for *E. vermicularis* infestations. The sticky side of clear tape is pressed against several areas of the perineum of a child with pruritus. Next the tape is placed sticky side down onto a clean glass slide, smoothed out with cotton gauze, and examined under the microscope.

D. **Eosinophilia** occurs in many, but not all, parasitic infestations. Its presence should raise one's suspicion of parasitic tissue infestation. **The following organisms usually elicit eosinophilia:** (a) *Trichinella* species, (2) visceral larva migrans, (3) filaria, (4) hookworms, (5) *Schistosoma* species, and (6) whipworms.

E. **Serologic tests**
   1. Amebiasis serologic tests are discussed in section **IV.E.4.**
   2. *Trichinella spiralis* infection can be confirmed by sending a blood specimen to the state or reference laboratory.

F. **Duodenal aspirates** have been useful in making the diagnosis in a small number of cases of giardiasis and strongyloidiasis when stool specimens were not positive for cysts, trophozoites, or larvae, and the diagnosis was strongly suspected.

G. ***Giardia* antigen** is discussed in section **IV.A.2.**

III. **Therapy.** A summary of the recommended drugs for treatment is given in Table 13.7.

IV. **Discussion of selected parasitic diseases**

A. **Giardiasis.** *Giardia lamblia* is the most frequently isolated intestinal parasite in the United States. The most common mode of transmission has been through contaminated surface water. However, person-to-person transmission in day-care centers and custodial institutions, transmission between male homosexuals via sexual contact, and food-borne transmission via fecal contamination can occur. Young children attending day care may spread infection to a parent or caregiver. Large-scale waterborne outbreaks have occurred in Leningrad, Colorado, New Hampshire, New York, Oregon, Utah, and Washington [97,101–103].

1. **Symptoms and life cycle.** Chlorination does not destroy the cystic stage, A week or two after the ingestion of contaminated water, explosive diarrhea, abdominal cramps, flatulence, nausea, vomiting, and low-grade fever may occur. Patients do not pass gross pus, blood, or mucus. Chronic infections result in milder, intermittent symptoms and malaise. The **spectrum** of disease **varies widely** from asymptomatic cyst passing to patients with acute symptoms to patients with persistent steatorrhea and weight loss. Weight loss occurs in approximately 50% of patients with chronic symptoms and averages 10 pounds [101].

   **Lactase deficiency** after infection is **common,** especially in children. Patients who recover from giardiasis should be counseled to avoid lactose-containing products for approximately 1 month. Because hypogammaglobulinemic patients often have *Giardia* infection, and because achlorhydria patients are more susceptible to infection, it is believed that IgG and stomach acid both play a role in host defense.

2. **Diagnosis**
   a. **History** of prolonged diarrhea without blood or mucus, weight loss, surface water exposure, exposure to day-care children, or a homosexual lifestyle, and mild malabsorption or lactose intolerance should raise suspicion for this diagnosis.
   b. **Stool examination.** There are only two stages in the life cycle of this parasite: the trophozoites, which exist freely in the small bowel, and the cyst, which is passed into the environment [101,103]. **Fecal leukocytes are not present.**
      (1) ***Giardia* antigen stool assays** have become the preferred test in many laboratories. A polyclonal or monoclonal antibody against cyst or trophozoite antigens is used to detect *Giardia* by EIAs or immunofluorescence; intact organisms are not required. The sensitivity is 85% to 98%, and the specificity is 90% to 100%. These tests are more sensitive than microscopic examination of the stool; a single stool tested by EIA may be sufficient to exclude giardiasis [8,101].

Table 13.7. Treatment of Common Parasitic Infections

| Organism | Drug Choice | Adult Dose | Pediatric Dose |
|---|---|---|---|
| *Giardia lamblia* | Metronidazole[a,b] | 250 mg t.i.d. for 5 days | 15 mg/kg/day in 3 doses for 5 days |
| | Furazolidone | 100 mg q.i.d for 7–10 days | 6 mg/kg/day in 4 doses for 7–10 days |
| | Paromomycin[b,c] | 25–35 mg/kg/day in 3 doses for 7 days | |
| *Trichuris trichiura* | Mebendazole *or* | 100 mg b.i.d for 3 days or 500 mg once | Same |
| | Albendazole[b] | 400 mg once[d] | Same |
| *Ascaris lumbricoides* | Mebendazole *or* | 100 mg b.i.d for 3 days or 500 mg once | Same |
| | Pyrantel pamoate[b] *or* | 11 mg/kg once (max 1 g) | Same |
| | Albendazole[b] | 400 mg once | Same |
| *Enterobius vermicularis* | Pyrantel Pamoate *or* | 11 mg/kg once (max 1 g); repeat after 2 wk | Same |
| | Mebendazole *or* | 100 mg once; repeat after 2 wk | Same |
| | Albendazole[b] | 400 mg once; repeat after 2 wk | Same |
| *Entamoeba histolytica* | | | |
| Asymptomatic | Iodoquinol[e] *or* | 650 mg t.i.d. for 20 days | 30–40 mg/kg/day in 3 doses for 20 days (max 2 g/day) |
| | Paromomycin | 25–35 mg/kg/day in 3 doses for 7 days | Same |
| Intestinal disease[f] | Metronidazole[a] | 500–750 mg t.i.d. for 10 days | 35–50 mg/kg/day in 3 doses for 10 days |
| Hepatic abscess[f] | Metronidazole[a] | 750 mg t.i.d. for 10 days | 35–50 mg/kg/day in 3 doses for 10 days |
| *Dientamoeba fragilis* | Iodoquinol[g] *or* | 650 mg t.i.d. for 20 days | 40 mg/kg/day in 3 doses for 20 days (max 2 g/day) |
| | Tetracycline[b,h] *or* | 500 mg q.i.d for 10 days | 40 mg/kg/day in 4 doses for 10 days (max 2 g/day) |
| | Paromomycin[b] | 25–30 mg/kg/day in 3 doses for 7 days | 25–30 mg/kg/day in 3 doses for 7 days |
| *Blastocystis hominis*[h] | Iodoquinol[e] *or* | 650 mg t.i.d. for 20 days | — |
| | Metronidazole[a] | 750 mg t.i.d. for 10 days | — |

t.i.d., three times daily; q.i.d., four times daily; b.i.d., twice daily.
[a]Avoid in pregnant women, especially first trimester.
[b]Approved drug but considered investigational in this condition by the U.S. Food and Drug Administration.
[c]Not absorbed. May be useful for treatment in pregnancy.
[d]In heavy infection, it may be necessary to extend therapy to 3 days.
[e]Dosage and duration of administration should not be exceeded because of the possibility of causing optic neuritis. Maximum dose 2 g/day.
[f]Treatment should be followed by a course of iodoquinol or paromomycin (intraluminal drugs) in the dosage used to treat asymptomatic amebiasis.
[g]Contraindicated in patients under 8 years of age and in pregnant women.
[h]Whether this organism is a true pathogen is controversial.
Adapted from The Medical Letter. Drugs for parasitic infections. *Med Lett Drugs Ther* 1998;40:1–12; with permission. (See this source for details of drug use, regimens for less common parasites, and summary of adverse effects of antiparasitic drugs.)

(2) **O&P examinations** are appropriate for evaluating an international traveler. Three serial liquid stools, if examined properly, will demonstrate the organism in 90% of cases. Three stools over several days are preferred because cysts may be shed intermittently. Fresh and preserved specimens are examined. Because the organisms reside in the small bowel, in a minority of patients symptoms may precede stool positivity by 1 to 2 weeks [101].

c. **Duodenal sampling.** Occasionally patients with persisting symptoms suggestive of *Giardia* infestation have negative antigen tests and negative O&P examination results. In these patients, a string test or Entero-Test (HDC Corporation, San Jose, CA), duodenal aspirate, or duodenal biopsy may be considered [101].

d. **Serum anti-*Giardia* antibody tests** usually are not available and are used more in epidemiologic studies.

3. **Therapy. All symptomatic patients deserve treatment.** Although some cases resolve spontaneously over 3 to 4 days, most persist until intervention with treatment.

a. **Metronidazole, although not FDA approved** for this indication, is the drug of choice for treatment of giardiasis. Efficacy is 80% to 95% (see Table 13.7).

b. **Furazolidone,** available in liquid suspension, is an alternative for children. It is well tolerated. Because it is only 80% effective, follow-up is important. It causes mild hemolysis if there is glucose-6-phosphate dehydrogenase deficiency [101].

c. **Tinidazole** (Fasigyn) is effective in a single dose of 2 g (not available in the United States).

d. **Albendazole** has been shown to have efficacy similar to metronidazole and fewer side effects, but clinical experience with this agent is limited [103].

e. **Therapy in pregnancy** remains an unclear issue. The suggested approach is as follows [101]:

(1) Avoid treatment altogether in the first trimester if possible.

(2) Women with mild disease may delay therapy until after delivery. Nutrition and hydration must be maintained.

(3) For women with persisting symptoms of weight loss, nausea, or dehydration necessitating therapy, use of paromomycin, an oral aminoglycoside that is excreted in the feces nearly 100% unchanged, is advised, although its efficacy may be in the 60% to 70% range [101] (see Chapter 27I). The use of metronidazole in pregnancy remains debated (see Chapter 27Q), but it is a potential option in the third trimester (see Table 13.7).

f. **Persisting symptoms** may be due to lactose intolerance, and this warrants therapy as well as careful repeat stool examination.

4. **Therapy of asymptomatic infection** (asymptomatic cyst passer) is **controversial.** Therapy may be indicated in the setting of an outbreak (e.g., in a child-care center or custodial institution) if reinfection is unlikely. Asymptomatic food handlers and day-care workers should be treated [97].

5. **Empiric therapy** sometimes is used in situations where the clinical suspicion is high but stool examinations are negative.

6. **Prevention** requires proper handling and treatment of community water supplies, appropriate disposal of human and animal waste, and good personal hygiene [102].

a. **Wilderness hikers or international travelers** must pay attention to preparing drinking water. Water needs to be boiled for at least 1 minute. An alternative is to use a filter system, but the pore size should be 1 $\mu$m or less. Halogenation of water with chlorine or iodine tablets is a less reliable treatment because it is highly dependent on the temperature, pH, and cloudiness of the water [102,103].

b. Handwashing is important before handling food and after every diaper change.

B. ***Trichuris trichiura* (whipworm) infestation**

1. **Life cycle.** Infection occurs in humans by ingestion of embryonated eggs on contaminated hands, food, soil, or fomites. After a 10- to 30-day period in

the small intestine, the larvae migrate primarily to the cecum and appendix, where they embed their anterior end into the mucosa, with the posterior end free to "whip" in the lumen. These mature adults lay eggs, which pass to the soil and repeat the cycle. The distribution of whipworm is similar to that of *A. lumbricoides.*

2. **Symptoms** are correlated with the worm burden in the large bowel. Light infections may be asymptomatic. Infections produce their damage by mechanical and lytic damage to the mucosa, with petechial hemorrhages and disruption of integrity of the GI tract by bacteria. Heavy worm burdens produce diarrhea, abdominal pain, anemia, weight loss, weakness, and even rectal prolapse.
3. **Diagnosis** is made **by examination of fecal specimens** by direct smear, formalin-ether centrifugal sedimentation, or flotation techniques. Sigmoidoscopy can demonstrate adult worms attached to the colonic mucosa in severe infection.
4. **Treatment** (see Table 13.7). Stool examination should be performed 3 weeks after treatment to confirm eradication. A second treatment course should be undertaken if necessary.

**C. *Ascaris lumbricoides* infestation**

1. **Life cycle.** Infection results from ingestion of second-stage larvae that usually are contaminants of hands or soil. The larvae hatch in the small intestine, penetrate the intestinal wall, and are carried to the lungs through the portal vein or indirectly through the lymphatics. In the lung, they live and molt in the alveoli for 10 to 14 days. Subsequently, they migrate up the bronchi to the pharynx, are swallowed, and mature sexually in the small intestine 6 to 10 weeks later. The adult phase persists for approximately 9 months. Eggs are laid daily during this period. To become infectious to humans these eggs must be deposited in an external environment with adequate shade and moisture and a temperature conducive to hatching. **In the United States, the endemic areas include** southeastern parts of the Appalachian mountain range and areas of the southern and Gulf Coast states.
2. **Symptoms are related** primarily to the **mechanical presence of the parasites.** During the transient pulmonary stage, **Loffler syndrome** (pulmonary infiltrates with eosinophilia, dyspnea, cough, and fever) may occur. The adult worm's presence in the intestine usually is asymptomatic, except in cases where the worm **migrates into** various organs, causing obstruction of the common bile duct, pancreatic duct, appendix, or even the bowel itself if the mass of worms is large. At times, a patient, especially a child, may report having coughed up a worm or passed one through the rectum.
3. **Diagnosis.** Identification of *Ascaris* **eggs in the stool** is the primary means of diagnosis. Direct smears usually are sufficient, although concentration techniques may have to be used occasionally. In the patient with partial bowel obstruction due to a mass of *Ascaris* organisms, an upper GI barium study may demonstrate small bowel worms.
4. **Treatment** is summarized in Table 13.7.

**D. *Enterobius vermicularis* (pinworm) infestation**

1. **Symptoms.** Intense **pruritus ani** and, occasionally, **pruritus vulvae** are caused by the presence of adult worms and embryonic eggs. The 15-day life cycle is initiated by the ingestion of eggs on contaminated hands or in food or drink. Because the eggs are infectious when laid, autoinoculation can occur from anal scratching then oral transmission. The larvae emerge in the upper intestine, temporarily attach themselves, copulate in the lower small intestine, and then migrate to the anus to deposit their sticky eggs on the perianal skin. Irritability, restlessness, anorexia, and insomnia (in children) with enterobiasis have been attributed to a heavy worm infestation.
2. **Diagnosis.** Eggs are not found in stool. The **Scotch tape test is used** (section **II.C**) for diagnosis. Occasional worms may be seen on the perineum and identified.
3. **Treatment** is summarized in Table 13.7. Often, pinworm is epidemic among the entire family, and it is judicious to **consider treating all members simultaneously.**

E. ***Entamoeba histolytica*** **infestation** [97,104].

1. **Life cycle.** Amebiasis is **acquired by the ingestion of cysts in contaminated water or in food that has been soiled** by a cyst carrier or contaminated by houseflies or cockroaches that have fed on human feces. The cysts undergo excystation in the small bowel. The trophozoites reach the large bowel and divide by binary fission. Some trophozoites may invade the colon and produce the characteristic flask-shaped ulcers. Others may invade the portal vein, lodge in the liver, and form a hepatic abscess. The trophozoites metamorphose into cysts as they are passed in the stools. If the diarrhea is loose and intestinal transit short, trophozoites may be seen in the stool.
2. **Pathophysiology.** Virulent strains of *E. histolytica* have significant cytopathic properties *in vitro,* consistent with their ability to cause invasive colitis *in vivo.* The majority of individuals infected with *E. histolytica* are asymptomatic. The difference between commensal and invasive *E. histolytica* infection is attributable to the existence of distinct pathogenic and nonpathogenic strains. Nonpathogenic strains (*E. histolytica* variant *dyspar*) have never been found to cause amebic colitis or liver abscess. Nearly 10% of persons infected with *E. histolytica* harbor pathogenic strains. Although almost all these patients will mount a serum antibody response to pathogenic *E. histolytica* infection, only 1 of 10 patients with pathogenic strains have symptomatic disease [104].
3. **Clinical symptoms** vary widely [104].
   a. *E. histolytica* has a number of diverse clinical presentations (Table 13.8).
   b. **The most common finding is asymptomatic intestinal infection without evidence of tissue invasion,** as defined by the absence of serum antibodies, blood in the stool, and mucosal ulcerations on colonoscopy.
   c. **Amebic colitis** has a subacute onset of bloody, mucoid diarrhea (onset over 7 days, duration 3–4 weeks), with abdominal pain, tenesmus, **fecal leukocytes,** fever, and positive serology for antiamebic antibodies (in 90% by day 7 of illness). **Fecal occult blood** test results are positive.
   d. **Liver abscess** classically presents with fever, right upper quadrant abdominal pain, and liver tenderness. Returning international travelers usually present within 5 months of their exposure. Diarrhea is seen in only 30% to 40% of those with liver abscess, and finding amebae in the stool is even less common [104].

Table 13.8. Clinical Syndromes Due to Infection by *Entamoeba Histolytica*

| |
|---|
| Intestinal |
|   Asymptomatic cyst passers (colonization) |
|   Symptomatic cyst passers |
|   Acute rectocolitis |
|   Fulminant colitis |
|     Toxic megacolon |
|     Perforation with peritonitis |
|   Chronic nondysenteric colitis |
|   Ameboma |
| Extraintestinal |
|   Liver abscess |
|   Lung abscess, empyema |
|   Pericarditis |
|   Brain abscess |
|   Venereal disease |
|   Cutaneous disease |

Reprinted from Aucott JN, Ravdin JI. Amebiasis and "nonpathogenic" intestinal protozoa. *Infect Dis Clin North Am* 1993;7:467–485; with permission.

4. **Diagnosis of amebic colitis**
   a. **A freshly passed liquid stool is examined** to identify the motile **trophozoites** of *E. histolytica*. Refrigeration at 4°C or storage in a fixative may allow some preservation (check with the parasitology laboratory). Three separate specimens should be examined (see section **II.A.3**). **Formed stools in saline** and iodine preparations are examined for amebic cysts. The formalin-ether concentration technique may help increase the yield.
   b. **Serum antiamebic antibodies** develop only with pathogenic strains, and the absence of antibodies after 7 days of infection is strong evidence against invasive amebiasis.
   c. **Colonoscopy** with scraping or biopsy of mucosal ulcers provides definitive diagnosis. Special stains (e.g., periodic acid-Schiff [PAS]) demonstrate the organism. A tissue diagnosis is especially indicated if corticosteroid therapy is being considered for the patient who has inflammatory bowel disease.
5. **Diagnosis of amebic abscess** [104]
   a. **Ultrasonography** of the liver and biliary tract is suggested. Computed tomography (CT) can be used in patients with nondiagnostic findings.
   b. **Serum antiamebic antibodies** are **present** in 99% of patients with amebic abscess within 7 to 10 days of onset of illness.
   c. If the clinical setting and evaluation are nondiagnostic, **fine-needle aspiration** under ultrasonographic or CT guidance can be performed. **Aspiration** of a liver abscess yields an "anchovy paste" fluid containing neither polymorphonuclear leukocytes nor amebae. The amebae occasionally are seen in the wall of the abscess.
6. **Therapy.** Treatment is summarized in Table 13.7 [104].
   a. **Asymptomatic *E. histolytica* infection.** It is unclear whether this condition routinely requires therapy. Treatment is recommended in asymptomatic persons from nonendemic areas, especially if the patient has underlying HIV infection or a positive test result for serum antiamebic antibodies that suggests infection with a pathogenic strain [104].
   b. If metronidazole is the preferred agent (see Table 13.7) but is contraindicated or not tolerated, alternative regimens are available [104].
   c. **Amebic abscess** usually responds to metronidazole therapy without the need to drain the abscess. It should be noted that metronidazole has excellent antibacterial activity against anaerobes, and several reports have warned that a metronidazole therapeutic trial cannot be used to differentiate an amebic abscess from an anaerobic liver abscess. (See the discussion in section **V.C** under Intraabdominal Infection.)
7. **Prevention.** Avoiding fecal-oral contamination is the only effective means of preventing *E. histolytica* infection. Boiling is the only certain means of eradicating *E. histolytica* cysts in water [104].

F. ***Cryptosporidium parvum*** is a protozoan that has emerged as a major cause of chronic diarrhea in patients with AIDS and a common cause of waterborne outbreaks of diarrhea in immunocompetent persons. Transmission occurs by ingestion of oocysts that are excreted in the feces of infected humans or animals. Ingestion of as few as 30 oocysts is known to cause infection. Because infection is ubiquitous in mammals, and the oocysts are chlorine resistant, small, and difficult to filter, contamination of water sources for drinking or recreation may readily occur, resulting in large outbreaks of illness [97,105,106].

1. **In patients with AIDS,** *Cryptosporidium, Microsporidia, Isospora belli,* cytomegalovirus (CMV), and *Mycobacterium avium* complex infections are causes of chronic, often intractable, diarrhea. These are discussed in Chapter 18.
2. **Outbreaks of cryptosporidiosis are most often waterborne.** In recent outbreaks of gastroenteritis associated with drinking water in the United States, *Cryptosporidium* caused 20% of the epidemics in which an infectious agent was identified. *Cryptosporidium* was also implicated in 50% of gastroenteritis outbreaks associated with recreational swimming pools, wade pools, lakes, or fountains [107,108]. A huge waterborne outbreak of cryptosporidiosis in Milwaukee

in 1993 resulted from contamination of municipal water supplies, affecting an estimated 403,000 persons (attack rate of 52%). Watery diarrhea was the predominant symptom (93%), but abdominal pain, low-grade fever, and vomiting were not uncommon, and 75% of infected immunocompetent patients experienced weight loss averaging 10 pounds. The mean duration of illness was 12 days [105,109]. Food-borne outbreaks have been attributed to contaminated apple cider, chicken salad, and uncooked vegetables. Person-to-person transmission is evidenced in numerous outbreaks of cryptosporidiosis in day-care centers and institutions, and secondary cases within households [105] (see related discussion in Chapter 18).

a. **Diagnosis.** Many laboratories use an immunofluorescent assay or EIA to detect *Cryptosporidium* in stool. Microscopic examination is also performed.

b. **Treatment.** Illness in immunocompetent patients is self-limited, and treatment is symptomatic.

G. ***Dientamoeba fragilis*** is an intestinal protozoan parasite that infects the cecum and ascending colon. Only the trophozoite forms are found in stool samples, and the organism does not invade tissue. Symptoms have been reported more frequently in children than in adults, although the pathogenic role of *D. fragilis* has been controversial. Surveys indicate prevalence of infection ranging from 0.5% in the United States (highest on the West Coast) to 4% in Canada. Asymptomatic carriers exist. *D. fragilis* is transmitted by the fecal-oral route. It has been hypothesized that *D. fragilis* is transmitted by the pinworm, *Enterobius vermicularis,* because *D. fragilis* has been observed in *E. vermicularis* eggs [97].

1. **Clinical manifestations**

a. **Acute dysentery** with mild to moderate diarrhea, abdominal pain, anorexia, nausea, vomiting, occasional fever, and malaise can occur.

b. **Chronic,** vague, nonspecific, **abdominal pain** that is dull, crampy, colicky, and usually in the lower abdomen can occur. It may occur after meals and last for hours. Symptoms may persist for months to years.

2. **Diagnosis**

a. **Stool specimens.** The diagnosis relies on observation of the binucleate trophozoites in a stained sample of fresh or preserved stool. At least three stool samples should be examined before any barium studies are performed. An immunofluorescence assay is being developed.

b. **Routine laboratory and radiographic studies are nonspecific.** No serologic test is available for diagnosis. Peripheral eosinophilia has been observed in 50% of cases. Concomitant *E. vermicularis* infection should be ruled out [97].

3. **Therapy** is summarized in Table 13.7. Stool specimens should be examined 3 to 4 weeks after therapy to determine whether the parasite has been eliminated.

H. ***Blastocystis hominis*** may be found in up to 25% of stool specimens examined. Only occasional patients have mild diarrhea. It is unknown whether *B. hominis* is a true pathogen or a commensal organism, or both. Controlled studies of an association between *B. hominis* and diarrhea are lacking [97,110–112].

Rarely, *B. hominis* has been implicated as a pathogen in AIDS patients, or patients on corticosteroids. Symptoms are nonspecific, including diarrhea, flatulence, abdominal pain, and anorexia. A trial of therapy in this setting may be reasonable if no other pathogen has been demonstrated (see Table 13.7).

## INTRAABDOMINAL INFECTION

I. **Clinical findings.** In patients who present with abdominal pain, fever, abdominal tenderness, and leukocytosis, the question of an intraabdominal infection is raised.

A. The **history and physical examination** provide important clues. The reader is referred to basic surgical texts for detailed information on this topic [113]. A few points:

1. **Percussion tenderness** on examination is a useful indicator of focal infection. Right upper quadrant percussion tenderness suggests biliary source. Right lower quadrant tenderness suggests appendicitis or, in women, a focal pelvic infection. Left lower quadrant tenderness suggests diverticulitis; and so on.

Diffuse abdominal percussion tenderness, often with rebound tenderness, reflects a diffuse peritoneal irritation. Corticosteroids and analgesia may mask these findings.

2. **A rectal and, in women, a pelvic examination** should routinely be performed, especially in patients with mid- to lower abdominal pain.
3. **Fever** may be modified by analgesics, NSAIDs, corticosteroids, and old age.
4. **Leukocytosis** and a left shift are commonly, but not always, present.

**B. Serial clinical evaluations and surgical evaluation are indicated.**

**C. Empiric antibiotic therapy** is started before a specific diagnosis has been established, to help contain the infection and prevent the clinical septic syndrome described in Chapter 2.

Knowledge of the normal flora of the colon helps determine empiric regimens for peritonitis (see section **II**). Knowledge of the flora in the obstructed biliary tract helps to determine antibiotic regimens for cholangitis (see section **I.D.3.a.** under Biliary Tract Infections).

**D. Cultures**

1. **Blood cultures.** Three sets drawn at 10- to 30-minute intervals often help.
2. **Peritoneal fluid cultures.** Adequate quantities of infected fluid or tissue should have aerobic and anaerobic cultures. Immediately after the abdominal cavity has been opened, a syringe is used to take up as much pus and fluid free of air as can be obtained. If air bubbles are present, they should be removed from the syringe by injection into a sponge saturated with alcohol. **Pus is the best transport medium to maintain viability of bacteria. Dry or wet swabs should be used only if pus or fluid is not available** from the peritoneal cavity. The syringe containing pus can be taken immediately to the laboratory for processing, or 3 to 4 mL can be injected into the proper anaerobic culture tube (e.g., Port-a-Cult) and sent to the laboratory.

**E. Diagnostic studies** are reviewed later. See section **III.D.4** and section **IV.C.2** under Peritonitis for the role of abdominal CT scanning.

**II. Antibiotic therapy for intraabdominal infections** has recently been reviewed [114–116].

**A. Microbiology.** The source of infecting microorganisms in most patients with intraabdominal infection is the microflora of the GI tract.

1. **Normal GI flora.** More than 400 different species of bacteria are found in a single fecal specimen. Under healthy conditions, the stomach and small bowel harbor a sparse microflora generally not exceeding $10^5$ bacteria per milliliter of contents. The number of bacteria increases in the middle and lower ileum, and there is an even greater augmentation across the ileocecal valve. **The colon harbors approximately $10^{11}$ organisms per milliliter, a number that approaches the theoretic limit that can fit into a given mass** [114].
2. Damage to the intestinal wall, either spontaneous perforation, sharp injury, or surgery with a later anastomotic leak, leads to contamination of the abdominal cavity.
   a. **Cultures** typically **reveal a mixture of organisms**—on average, two aerobes and three anaerobes. Common bacterial isolates are shown in Table 13.9. Animal model studies show that *E. coli* is responsible for the initial peritonitis and septicemia phase that causes high mortality initially if not treated appropriately. **Abscess is** caused primarily by the anaerobes, particularly *Bacteroides* species. They have both a virulence factor (a polysaccharide capsule) and resistance to peroxide that could explain the emergence of these organisms as important pathogens in abscess formation [117].
   b. The site of perforation of the GI tract is significant because an injury to the large bowel carries a high risk of abscess but so does injury to other parts of the intestinal tract [114].

**B. Antibiotic therapy** [114–122]. This should be directed at both aerobic and anaerobic bacteria. Otherwise, clinical failure is common. Monotherapy [114,117,119,120] is effective.

1. **Piperacillin-tazobactam.** This treatment is effective because it is active against the majority of infecting organisms [120]. **Ticarcillin-clavulanate**

Table 13.9. Bacteriology of Intraabdominal Infections

| | Frequency of Isolation (%) |
|---|---|
| Aerobes | |
| *Escherichia coli* | 65 |
| *Proteus* species | 25 |
| *Klebsiella* species | 20 |
| *Pseudomonas* species | 15 |
| Enterococci | 15 |
| *Streptococcus* species (other than group A or D) | 10 |
| Anaerobes | |
| *Bacteroides fragilis* | 80 |
| *Bacteroides* species (other) | 30 |
| *Clostridium* species | 65 |
| *Peptostreptococcus* species[a] | 25 |
| *Peptococcus* species[a] | 15 |
| *Fusobacterium* species | 20 |

[a]Sometimes grouped as anaerobic gram-positive cocci.
Reprinted from Gorbach SL. Treatment of intra-abdominal infections. *J Antimicrob Chemother* 1993; 31 (suppl A): 67; with permission.

(Timentin) has been used in this setting also. See the discussion of this agent in Chapter 27E.

2. **Cefoxitin** alone has been most widely studied. It was compared with either an aminoglycoside-containing regimen or a single broad-spectrum antibiotic regimen in 13 studies, which showed that cefoxitin alone is as effective as the comparative regimen [114,117]. Fewer studies have been conducted with **cefotetan,** which presumably is a reasonable alternative to cefoxitin. See Chapter 27 for a discussion of these two agents.
3. **Cefotaxime** has been shown to be superior to cefoxitin in one large series [119].
4. **Imipenem** in eight studies has been shown to be as good or even better than regimens containing an aminoglycoside [177,122]. However, it is not superior to piperacillin/tazobactam [120] nor to ciprofloxacin plus metronidazole [121]. The newer agent, ertapenem, is more appropriate for community acquired infection because its spectrum includes all of the enterobacteriaceae but not *Pseudomonas aeruginus* and other nosocomial organisms [123]. This saves imipenem for the hospital-acquired infections.
5. **Ampicillin-sulbactam** should not be used in this setting. A significant percentage of community-acquired *E. coli* are resistant to this agent; in the very ill patient, it may be more appropriate to use combination therapy (e.g., metronidazole and cefazolin). Ampicillin-sulbactam is reviewed in Chapter 27.
6. **Aminoglycosides.** Although historically ampicillin, clindamycin, or metronidazole, and an aminoglycoside were commonly used [124], **the current trend is away from this** [119–122]. See Chapter 27I for details about aminoglycosides.
   a. **Limitations.** Ampicillin's only use is for enterococci that may be unimportant. Gentamicin is relatively inactive under conditions of reduced pH. Associated nephrotoxicity is an unacceptable risk, and the potential for inadequate serum levels because of the underdosing that is used to "protect" the kidney [114,117,124] yields inferior antibiotic activity. In addition, for community-acquired organisms, cephalosporins and broad-spectrum penicillin agents with $\beta$-lactamase inhibitors offer better options.
   b. Gorbach in a review [117] concluded, **"There is now sufficient evidence to support the position that aminoglycosides are not needed and**

**should not be used for the initial treatment of uncomplicated intra-abdominal infection."** Other reviewers have reached similar conclusions [124], and we concur with these recommendations.

c. **Aminoglycosides are indicated in the therapy for intraabdominal infection when resistant gram-negative bacilli are suspected** [117]. In that situation, adequate serum levels must be achieved. These exceptions represent the minority of cases. They include (a) previous use of antibiotics, especially broad-spectrum antibiotics, in the past 30 days; (b) isolation of gram-negative bacilli resistant to $\beta$-lactam antibiotics and susceptible to aminoglycosides; (c) reoperation or recurrence of infection; and (d) prolonged hospitalization or nursing home stay preoperatively. The latter is especially important if these institutions have a background incidence of resistant gram-negative bacilli.

7. **Clindamycin and metronidazole** both have excellent anaerobic activity and have been **used** extensively **in combination** regimens for intraabdominal infection. In several comparative studies, both clindamycin and metronidazole performed equally well [117]. These agents are reviewed in detail in Chapter 27. Metronidazole may be a more cost-effective agent and possibly is associated with less *C. difficile* toxin diarrhea. Metronidazole is also more consistently active *in vitro* against *B. fragilis* than clindamycin (see Chapter 27Q). Metronidazole should be avoided in the first trimester of pregnancy and probably throughout pregnancy. In the past, these agents commonly have been combined with aminoglycosides. More recently, they have been combined with a first-generation cephalosporin (cefazolin) or a third-generation cephalosporin (e.g., ceftriaxone, ceftazidime, or cefotaxime) or aztreonam, but the aztreonam and metronidazole combination lacks activity against gram-positive organisms [115,125]. See Table 13.10.

8. **Coverage for enterococci.** There is debate about whether empiric regimens should cover enterococci. If enterococci are isolated from an intraabdominal source in a mixed culture, is specific therapy needed?

   a. Gorbach and others [114,116,118] have recently reviewed this question. Although enterococci are relatively common isolates (see Table 13.9), a review of multiple studies using combination therapy **without** specific activity against enterococci did not reveal clinical failure due to persistent enterococcal infection. Feliciano observed a low rate of complications caused by enterococcus when he used cephalosporins with no activity against enterococcus [119]. However, Barie argued to the contrary [126].

   Based on his review of accumulated studies, Gorbach [114,117] concluded, **"There appears to be no justification for the inclusion of specific**

Table 13.10. Empiric Antibiotics in Intraabdominal Infection, Including Peritonitis

| Severity and Setting | Antibiotic Regimen (Assumes Normal Renal Function) |
|---|---|
| Community-acquired | |
| Mild-moderate | Cefazolin (1 g q8h) + metronidazole (500 mg q6h)[a] |
| | Cefoxitin (2 g q6h–q8h) |
| Severe | Piperacillin-tazobactam (3.75 g q6h) |
| | Ceftriaxone (2 g q24h) + metronidazole (500 mg q6h) |
| | Clindamycin (600 mg q8h) + gentamicin |
| | Imipenem (500 mg q6h or 1 g q8h) |
| Hospital-acquired | Piperacillin (3 g q4h or 4 g q6h) + metronidazole + an aminoglycoside |
| | Imipenem ± an aminoglycoside |

q8h, every 8 hours; q6h, every 6 hours; q4h, every 4 hours.
[a]Cost-effective regimen.

**anti-enterococcal therapy in the initial treatment of mixed infections.** Furthermore, **even the isolation of enterococcus in mixed cultures initially does not necessitate specific enterococcal antibiotic therapy."**

The triple antibiotic regimen of ampicillin, clindamycin, and gentamicin discussed above was used because of activity against enterococci as well as other bowel flora, but enterococcal therapy is not necessary. Inclusion of enterococci, in fact, leads to reduced activity against the more important gram-negative organisms for reasons discussed in section 6.a–c above. Gorbach stated that clinicians have "almost mythical adherence to the belief that this organism has some special pathogenic powers in intra-abdominal infections," [117] and, therefore, it is hard not to want to "cover" for this pathogen.

**b. When should one cover enterococci** [114,116,117]? The following clinical situations serve as a guide:

**(1)** Patients with **persistent positive cultures** of these organisms in the absence of clinical improvement on nonenterococcal treatment regimens.

**(2)** Patients with multiple enterococcal positive blood cultures.

**(3)** Other reviewers suggest life-threatening intraabdominal sepsis with *Enterococcus* species isolated in pure culture or a predominance of gram-positive cocci in chains on the Gram stain of peritoneal fluid [115].

**c.** The role that vancomycin-resistant enterococci (VRE) may play in nosocomially acquired intraabdominal sepsis is not well defined but is of potential concern in the patient at risk for VRE (see related discussions in Chapter 27P).

**9. When should one cover for *Candida* species?** *Candida* is considered normal flora of the GI tract and consequently is commonly isolated. Its precise role in infection has been debated and recently reviewed [115,118].

**a.** When *Candida* is the sole isolate, or *Candida* is isolated from cultures of both peritoneal (or abscess) fluid and blood, or *Candida* invasion is identified on histologic examination of tissue, antifungal therapy is essential [115]. Other clinicians suggest that if *Candida* is isolated in high concentrations or increasing concentrations with sequential cultures, treatment is indicated, especially when host defenses are impaired [115,118]. Isolation of *Candida* from the peritoneum in acute pancreatitis also probably warrants specific therapy because these patients are more likely to have invasive disease than simple contamination [115].

**b.** When *Candida* is one of the multiple organisms contaminating the peritoneum after surgical repair of a perforated viscus, antifungal therapy is not required.

**c.** Therapeutic options include amphotericin B or fluconazole (see Chapter 17). Infectious disease consultation is advised.

**10. Significance of *Pseudomonas aeruginosa* isolated from appendiceal specimens or specimens collected after penetrating trauma.** Rates of isolation vary from 5% to 20%. Clinical significance of the data is unclear, as is the need for antipseudomonal antibiotic therapy. Further data are needed [117].

**11. Summary.** For empiric antibiotics for intraabdominal infection, many options are possible based on the principles and data presented here. **See the summary in Table 13.10.**

**a.** Monotherapy with cefoxitin or combination therapy with cefazolin plus metronidazole is rationale for mild to moderate community-acquired infection.

**b.** For severe community-acquired infection, a broader combination such as piperacillin-tazobactam and metronidazole seems rational.

**c.** For hospital-acquired infection or complex recurrent infections, aminoglycosides often are used in combination (see section **II.B.6.C**).

**III. Peritonitis** is a localized or general inflammation of the peritoneum. Microorganisms (e.g., bacteria, fungi) and irritating chemicals (bile salts, gastric contents, or talc) are the causes.

**A. Classification.** A classification system commonly used is shown in Table 13.11.

**B.** The **pathogenesis** of peritonitis is complex [127]. Some of the common ways it can occur are listed here.

1. **Primary peritonitis** refers to inflammation of the peritoneum from a suspected extraperitoneal source, often via hematogenous spread.
   a. **Spontaneous peritonitis** usually occurs in patients with underlying ascites and is seen most frequently in patients with cirrhosis, nephrotic syndrome, and systemic lupus erythematous (see section **F.1**).
   b. Peritonitis in patients with continuous ambulatory peritoneal dialysis (CAPD) is discussed in section **F.2.**
   c. Tuberculous peritonitis. See Chapter 11, section VI, under Tuberculosis: Basic Concepts.
2. **Rupture of a viscus** can occur by innumerable means, including the following:
   a. **Traumatic injury** to the abdomen, including both sharp and blunt trauma
   b. **Ulcerated lesions** of the colon or upper tract, typhoid fever, necrotizing enterocolitis, or perforation of colonic diverticula
   c. **Ischemia,** vascular insufficiency, incarcerated hernias, volvulus, or neoplasia
   d. Ingestion of foreign bodies (e.g., toothpicks, bones, pins)
3. **Pelvic inflammatory disease,** including salpingitis and endometritis, can produce localized lower abdominal peritonitis indistinguishable from appendicitis.

Table 13.11. Classification of Intraabdominal Infections

I. Primary peritonitis
  A. Spontaneous peritonitis in children
  B. Spontaneous peritonitis in adults
  C. Peritonitis in patients with CAPD
  D. Tuberculous, fungus and other granulomatous peritonitis
  E. Other forms
II. Secondary peritonitis[a]
  A. Acute perforation peritonitis (acute suppurative peritonitis)
    1. Gastrointestinal tract perforation
    2. Bowel wall necrosis (intestinal ischemia)
    3. Pelvic peritonitis
    4. Other forms
  B. Postoperative peritonitis—surgical anastomotic breakdown
  C. Posttraumatic peritonitis–blunt versus penetrating
III. Tertiary peritonitis—no clear pathogenic organism
IV. Other forms of peritonitis
  A. Aseptic or sterile peritonitis
  B. Granulomatous peritonitis
  C. Metabolic such as drug or hyperlipemic-related peritonitis
  D. Periodic peritonitis or porphyric peritonitis
V. Intraabdominal abscess
  A. Associated with primary peritonitis
  B. Associated with secondary peritonitis

CAPD, continuous ambulatory peritoneal dialysis.
[a] Secondary peritonitis is often defined as the presence of purulent exudate in the abdominal cavity from an enteric source.
Adapted from Wittman DH, Walker AP, Condon RE. Peritonitis and intra-abdominal infection. In: Schwartz SI et al., eds.) *Principles of surgery,* 6th ed. New York: McGraw-Hill, 1994:1449; with permission.

4. **Surgical postoperative** leaks and anastomotic breakdowns can occur.
5. **Tertiary peritonitis** [113] occurs after successful elimination of bacteria by antibiotics. Normally activated host defense systems continue to act through failure of autoregulation, resulting in an autoaggressive devastation of organ system functions. The clinical picture mimics occult sepsis. There is no effective therapy.
6. **Noninfectious forms** of peritonitis are reviewed elsewhere [113].
7. **Rupture of an abscess** can occur, such as of the pancreas or rarely a distended gallbladder.

**C. Flora.** Bacterial peritonitis typically is caused by multiple organisms of the large bowel (see section **II** and Table 13.9).

**D. Diagnosis**

1. **The patient's history,** remote and recent, is useful in delineating the present problem.
   a. **A remote medical history** of diverticulitis, past surgery, and so forth should be noted.
   b. **Travel** and family history with exposure to typhoid fever or tuberculosis should be noted.
   c. **Accidents with blunt trauma,** such as a steering wheel–related injury should be noted.
   d. **Recent surgical procedures** should be noted.
   e. **History of appendectomy** will help eliminate the appendix as the cause.
2. **Symptoms** can be grouped into two classes: **reflex** and **toxic. Corticosteroid use by a patient may mask typical signs and symptoms.**
   a. **Reflex symptoms** include localized or generalized pain, nausea and vomiting (especially with an obstruction), and muscular rigidity. Rigidity commonly is seen in the early stages of an acute peritonitis.
   b. **Toxic symptoms** from bacterial toxins, exudates, and intraperitoneal fluid include the following: distention, intestinal paresis, fever, and general toxemia.
3. **For physical examination,** see section **I.**
4. **Laboratory tests** that should be evaluated are as follows:
   a. **Leukocyte count** usually is elevated but is nonspecific.
   b. **Liver function tests should be performed and the serum amylase level determined.**
   c. **Radiographic examination of the abdomen** may reveal air under the diaphragm (in the case of a ruptured viscus), paralytic ileus, intestinal obstruction, volvulus, or intussusception (barium enema). Findings suggestive of paralytic ileus are common [113]. A chest radiograph should be obtained to rule out any chest process that may be causing peritoneal signs and to demonstrate air.
   d. **Scans.** Although it may only delay needed operative management [113], CT is indicated when there is suspicion of an intraabdominal abscess.
   e. **Aspiration of peritoneal fluid** is a routine part of the workup of peritonitis in the setting of ascites or if trauma with hemorrhage into the peritoneal cavity is a concern. Fluid should be examined for leukocytes (with a differential count), bacterial and fungal organisms, amylase, gastric acid, and RBCs, as indicated by the particular case. Aerobic and anaerobic cultures of the fluid **should be obtained.**
   f. **Laparoscopy** is used by some surgeons to avoid unnecessary open surgery. In some patients with superficial stab wounds, blunt trauma, or suspected pelvic inflammatory disease or appendicitis, it also may help localize an ectopic pregnancy or a ruptured spleen.
5. The **differential diagnosis** of peritonitis is complex and reflects the many diagnoses raised in Table 13.11.

**E. Treatment principles**

1. **Supportive care** is necessary in the patient with peritonitis. Use of nasogastric suction and i.v. fluid are routine.
2. **Cause of the peritonitis.** Surgical consultation is imperative.

a. Surgical repair of a ruptured viscus is essential.
b. Contaminating secretions, pus, or fecal material should be drained, and then the peritoneal cavity should be lavaged copiously.

3. **Systemic antibiotics (see section II)** to cover coliforms and anaerobes should be started preoperatively. Nonbacteremic patients receive 7 to 10 days of antibiotics, first intravenously and then orally. Shorter regimens may be effective in uncomplicated cases. In penetrating trauma–related peritonitis, 2 days of treatment may sometimes be adequate [117]. Another approach is to continue antibiotic therapy until fever is absent for 48 to 72 hours, all systemic signs of sepsis have resolved, and appetite and sense of well-being have returned [113]. Bacteremic patients receive a total of 14 days of i.v. and oral therapy to prevent complications at metastatic sites.

**F. Special considerations**

1. **Spontaneous bacterial peritonitis** (SBP). Spontaneous peritonitis is now more common in adults than in children and shows no predilection for one gender or the other. **Formerly, children (girls < 10 years of age) with nephrosis were the most commonly affected due to pneumococci or hemolytic streptococci. Now adults with cirrhosis or systemic lupus erythematosus are afflicted more commonly** [128].
   a. **Adults.** Spontaneous peritonitis usually is seen in patients with ascites, primarily with underlying cirrhosis [129]. Single organisms are the rule, with *E. coli* and *Klebsiella* species the major pathogens, accounting for 70% of infections. Gram-positive cocci may be seen in 10% to 20% and anaerobes in less than 5% [128,129]. (See section **II.**)
   b. **Pathogenesis** [130]. The balance between host defenses and transmigration of enteric organisms, primarily gram-negative bacilli, determines whether SBP develops. There is a decreased ability to kill bacteria in low-protein, low complement ascites in these patients.
   c. **Clinical features of SBP: a high index of suspicion is necessary.**
      (1) Fever and abdominal pain are seen in 60% to 80% of patients.
      (2) Onset or worsening of hepatic encephalopathy (60% of patients).
      (3) Abdominal tenderness or rebound tenderness occurs in **only** 50%.
   d. **Diagnosis.** A peritoneal tap is the most useful diagnostic test [128].
      (1) **Peritoneal fluid cell count.** An absolute neutrophil count of greater than 250 cells/mm$^3$ is a likely indication of peritoneal infection. However, patients with other inflammatory disease of the abdomen, such as tuberculous peritonitis, pancreatitis, secondary bacterial peritonitis due to perforation, and even cancer also will show elevated granulocyte counts.
         (a) **SBP classically has been defined** by an ascitic neutrophil count of at least 250 cells/mm$^3$, a positive ascitic fluid culture, and no obvious intraabdominal source of infection.
         (b) **Culture-negative neutrocytic ascites** (CNNA) **is a variant** of SBP. An ascitic fluid neutrophil count of at least 500 cells/mm$^3$, negative ascitic cultures with no prior antibiotics in the preceding month, absence of an intraabdominal source of infection, and no alternative explanation of the elevated neutrophils in the ascitic fluid defines CNNA. About one-third of patients with suspected SBP have CNNA. Response to antibiotics and mortality rates showed no statistically significant differences between SBP and CNNA. **Therefore, CNNA patients should be treated aggressively with i.v. antibiotics as would be done for SBP patients** [128].
      (2) **Ascitic fluid pH** is low in spontaneous peritonitis, whereas in sterile ascitic fluid the pH is the same as for serum [113].
      (3) **Gram stains of ascitic fluid** reveal organisms in only one-third of fluids that are subsequently culture positive [113,128]. If either gram-positive cocci or gram-negative rods are seen as single pathogen types, the diagnosis of spontaneous peritonitis is supported. If mixed gram-positive and gram-negative bacteria are seen, an intestinal perforation is more likely.

(4) **Cultures of peritoneal fluid;** both aerobic and anaerobic cultures are essential. To maximize results, 10 mL of ascitic fluid should be routinely inoculated at the bedside in blood culture media.

(5) **Blood cultures** are positive in about one-third of patients with spontaneous peritonitis. **Urine cultures** are routinely suggested (see section **b**).

(6) **Protein content is not very useful** in diagnosing SBP because it is usually less than 2.5 g/dL. However, protein content may be a useful parameter in the differential diagnosis of pancreatic ascites and tuberculous peritonitis because these conditions generally are associated with ascitic protein levels of 3.0 g/dL or greater.

e. **Therapy** [128]. Once the diagnosis of SBP is made or highly suspected, i.v. antibiotics are indicated. See Chapter 27 for details.

(1) **Cefotaxime** in adult patients with normal creatinine clearance (2 g every 8 hours) is suggested [128]. **Ceftriaxone** is also a useful agent (e.g., 1–2 g every 24 hours).

(2) **Cefoxitin or piperacillin/tazobactam** are other options. Ciprofloxacin has been effective [131].

(3) Monotherapy with aztreonam is **not recommended** because it does not cover gram-positive organisms, nor is ampicillin/sulbactam because 30% of *E. coli* are resistant. **Aminoglycosides** produce excess nephrotoxicity in liver disease.

(4) **A repeat paracentesis at** 48 hours to document decreased cell counts and negative cultures is often suggested [128,132].

(5) **Duration of antibiotic therapy.** Standard therapy has been 10 to 14 days, but a 5- to 7-day course of i.v. antibiotics appears to be effective. Some clinicians advocate determination of ascitic fluid polymorphonuclear count at 48 hours of treatment to determine duration of therapy [132].

f. **Prognosis.** A mortality rate of 30% to 40% has been observed in SBP. The probability of recurrence at 1 year is 70%, and recurrent episodes are associated with high mortality rates [128]. Many patients with SBP may be candidates for liver transplantation [129].

g. **Prevention of recurrent episodes of SBP** [128,129,133–135]. Norfloxacin (400 mg orally daily) and ciprofloxacin 750 mg weekly have reduced the 1-year recurrence rate. TMP-SMX also has been used in this setting [133]. There is no proven value for prophylaxis to prevent the initial case of SBP, although short-term prophylaxis has been useful in cirrhotic patients with an acute GI bleed [134].

2. **For peritonitis in CAPD,** see reviews published elsewhere [113,136–138]. Several points deserve emphasis.

a. **Incidence.** An overall average is 1.3 episodes per patient per year.

b. **Clinical presentation.** Abdominal pain, abdominal tenderness (often with rebound), and a cloudy appearance of the drainage dialysate fluid are common. Dialysate turbidity is often the earliest sign and sometimes the only sign. Fever is present in a few patients.

c. **Bacteriology.** *Staphylococcus* organisms (coagulase-negative) and *S. aureus* (often methicillin resistant) predominate. *Streptococcus* species are isolated 10% to 15% of the time. Gram-negative bacteria or yeast occur in patients with recurrent episodes. A single organism usually is isolated. Gram stains of the effluent generally are negative, with 9% to 40% reported positive in several series. If multiple species or anaerobes are isolated, bowel perforation should be suspected.

d. **Diagnosis.** Peritonitis can be assumed when the dialysate contains more than 100 leukocytes/mm$^3$. This dialysate should be cultured and almost always is positive. Blood cultures usually are negative.

e. **Therapy.** Intraperitoneal instillation of antibiotics helps facilitate outpatient therapy (Fig. 13.2) [138]. Some clinicians prefer the i.v. route. While awaiting cultures, a single i.v. dose of cefepime and vancomycin could be

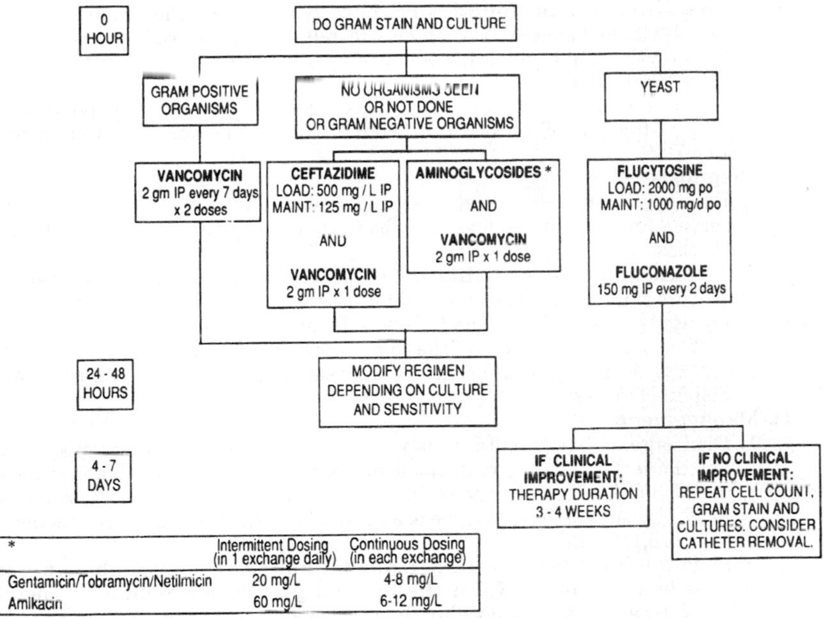


| * | Intermittent Dosing (in 1 exchange daily) | Continuous Dosing (in each exchange) |
|---|---|---|
| Gentamicin/Tobramycin/Netilmicin | 20 mg/L | 4-8 mg/L |
| Amikacin | 60 mg/L | 6-12 mg/L |

**FIG. 13.2** Treatment of peritonitis, 1993 update. *IP,* intraperitoneal administration; *MAINT,* maintenance dose. (Reprinted from the Ad Hoc Advisory Committee on Peritonitis Management. Peritoneal dialysis–related peritonitis treatment recommendations. *Perit Dial Int* 1993;13:14; with permission.)

used. See Chapter 27A for antibiotics in renal failure. The catheter should be removed for severe skin catheter site infection, if peritonitis persists despite adequate therapy, or for fungal or *Pseudomonas aeruginosa* peritonitis [113,136–138].

**f. Sclerosing encapsulating peritonitis** occurs in 1% to 5% of patients with recurrent prior bouts of bacterial peritonitis, although the exact cause is unknown. Treatment is directed at such complications as bowel obstruction [113].

**IV. General concepts of intraabdominal abscesses** [139]. Onset may be insidious. The mortality rate associated with undrained hepatic, pancreatic, and retroperitoneal abscesses is 45% to 100%. The clinician should always search for intraabdominal abscess in febrile patients without any obvious cause of fever, especially in those who have a potential predisposing cause such as inflammatory bowel disease, diverticulitis, or a history of abdominal surgery or abdominal trauma.

**A. Etiology and pathophysiology.** The GI lesions or events that typically predispose to secondary peritonitis and intraabdominal abscess include Crohn disease, **perforation of a viscus, extension of preexisting infection** (e.g., secondary to pancreatitis), **surgical procedure or trauma** (e.g., anastomotic leak stab wound,) or **intraabdominal ischemia.** Many abscesses are postoperative complications of biliary tract or GI surgery [139]. The use of laproscopic procedures has led to a higher incidence of abscess after appendectomy [140] or due to spilled stones after laparoscopic cholecystectomy [141].

**1.** Abscess formation creates an environment that readily supports the proliferation of anaerobic bacteria and produces conditions that impair the microbial activity of infiltrating neutrophils and of humoral factors, such as complement. Antibiotic transport to the suppurative focus is inhibited, and drugs within the abscess often are inactivated by a reduced local pH (e.g., aminoglycosides) [139].

2. **Abscesses can be found anywhere** within the abdomen, including the retroperitoneal space. Location may correlate with the original contamination, but may develop at distant sites such as subphrenic from a perforated appendicitis (Fig. 13.3).

B. **Microbiology.** Intraabdominal abscess reflects both quantitative and qualitative aspects of the microflora of the intestinal tract. This was discussed earlier in section **II.A.**

C. **Diagnosis**

1. Fever, chills, anorexia, weight loss, and, in some patients, abdominal pain are observed. An unexplained fever may be the only sign of an occult intra-abdominal abscess.
2. **An abdominal CT examination** is the most efficient means of diagnosing an abscess [113]. Because of the technical aspects and time delays, indium scans are used less frequently than CT scans. In an unusual setting (e.g., in the patient with an abnormal CT scan of the spleen in which multiple abscesses vs. multiple infarcts is the major differential diagnosis), a gallium or indium scan may be helpful [115,142].

D. **Management.**

1. **Drainage,** either percutaneously or operatively, is the primary mode of therapy. Patients with an undrained abscess do not do as well and may even die. The risk of complications due to delayed rupture of the abscess increases markedly. Abscesses cannot be eradicated by antibiotics alone (see section **A.1**) [113,115,118,143].
   a. **Percutaneous aspiration, using CT and ultrasonographic guidance, is usually successful if the following criteria are met:** (a) There is a well-established, unilocular fluid collection; (b) a safe percutaneous route of access is available (e.g., abscess adjacent to the body wall); and (c) joint evaluation by a surgeon and a radiologist is performed so that there is immediate operative backup available in case of failure or complications [113]. The catheter is placed for drainage via gravity on low suction until the drainage volume is minimal (<10 mL/24 hours). Percutaneous **is preferred** to operative drainage of most intraabdominal abscesses [144]. Repeat scanning should show complete collapse of the abscess cavity [115].
   b. **Pelvic abscesses** are drained through the rectum or vagina [113] (see Chapter 16).
   c. **Open surgical drainage** is indicated when (a) percutaneous drainage cannot be accomplished safely; (b) percutaneous drainage fails; (c) infected pancreatic necrosis or carcinomatous abscess is present; (d) the abscess is associated with a bowel fistula; (e) multiple isolated, interloop abscesses are present [113]; or (f) there is a coagulopathy.
   d. **Cultures** should be taken carefully at the time of drainage, with special attention to culturing anaerobically as well as aerobically.
2. **Empiric antibiotics** [113–122,124,125]. When an intraabdominal abscess is drained, empiric therapy should cover most of the common abdominal flora, until the culture results return. **Several regimens have been summarized previously** (see section **II.B** and Table 13.10). Most experts use antibiotics active against anaerobes as well as gram-negative aerobes. **The optimal duration of therapy for a drained abscess is not well defined.** Antibiotic administration should continue until all systemic signs of sepsis have resolved and the patient's appetite and sense of well-being have returned. It is not necessary to continue antibiotic therapy simply because drains remain in place. Oral therapy can be used to complete a course of therapy. Although some surgical reviews suggest that in uncomplicated cases, antibiotics can be stopped 48 to 72 hours after drainage has been established [113], a combination of i.v. and oral antibiotics for 7 to 10 days after drainage to ensure that contiguous soft-tissue cellulitis has been adequately treated is usually chosen. In bacteremic patients, a 14-day course is used to prevent complications at sites of metastatic spread.
3. **Nutritional support.** Often these patients are nutritionally depleted and may need parenteral or enteral nutrition. The enteral route is preferred, if possible.

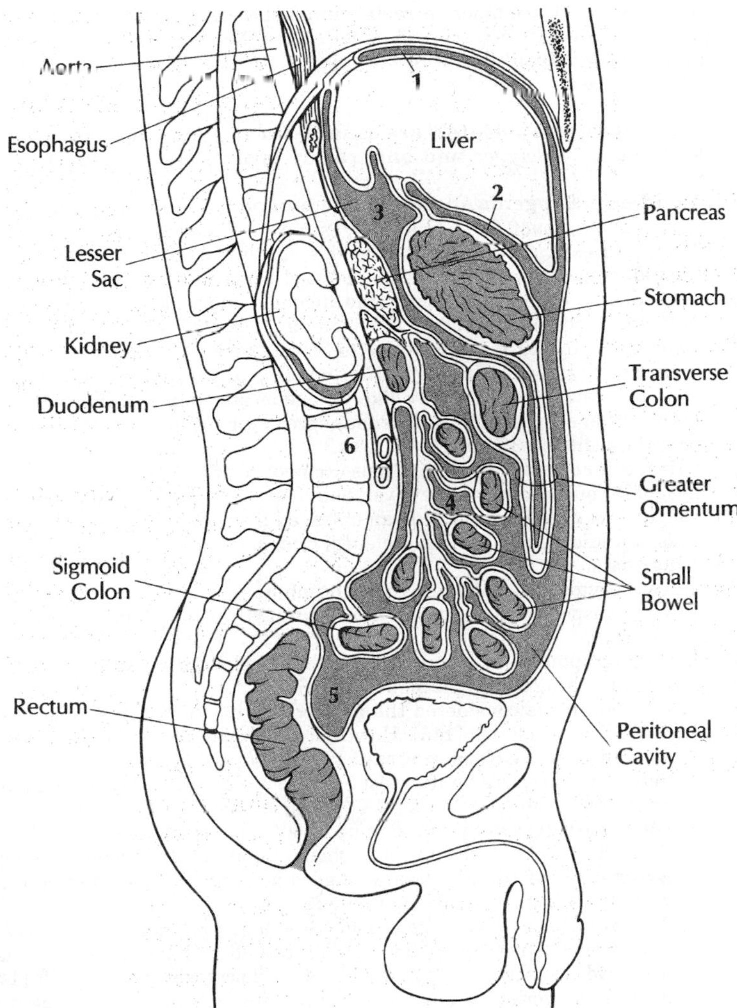


**FIG. 13.3** Areas of abscess formation within and adjacent to the peritoneal cavity are noted. They include the subphrenic space (*1*) and the subhepatic space (*2*); the lesser sac (*3*); interstices between loops of the small and large intestine (*4*); and the pelvic space (*5*). In the retroperitoneal space, abscesses may be perinephric (*6*); they also may be adjacent to or involve the pancreas, duodenum, or rectum. Because of intraabdominal circulation of infected material, abscesses may develop far from the original site of contamination. (Reprinted from Murray HW. Secondary peritonitis and intra-abdominal abscess. *Hosp Pract* 1990;25:109; with permission. Illustration by Laura Duprey.)

E. **Special issues.** Uncommon intraabdominal abscesses are discussed in section **V.**

F. **Pancreatic abscess** is discussed under section **X.**

**V. Special types of intraabdominal abscess**

A. **Diverticulitis-related abscess.**

B. **Pancreatic abscess.**

C. **Hepatic abscesses [145–147] are usually due to pyogenic bacteria** (discussed below) or to *E. histolytica* **and only rarely** to other organisms such as chlamydia.

1. **Incidence. Pyogenic abscess is uncommon.** Its incidence in hospital admissions ranges from 0.013% to 0.035% in reported series.
2. **Pathogenesis.** Liver abscess develops as a metastatic infection from an intraabdominal source to the liver, as a blood-borne infection, or from biliary tract ascending infection. Historically, the appendix and colon were the major sources of pyogenic abscesses, seeding the liver via the portal vein [145]. Recent reviews implicate the biliary tract in 20% to 35% of cases; appendicitis, diverticulitis, and so forth in approximately 25%; and idiopathic causes in 30% to 35%. Multiple liver abscesses are more likely to generate from the biliary duct system [148]. Other sources of hematogenous spread include urinary tract, pneumonia, or endocarditis in 3% to 25% of cases.
3. **Clinical presentation.** Symptoms are nonspecific or secondary to the original pyogenic source and include fever, chills, anorexia, nausea and vomiting, and weight loss. Signs may include an enlarged liver, right upper quadrant tenderness, jaundice, and right-sided pleural effusion.
4. **Diagnosis**
   a. Leukocytosis, elevated alkaline phosphatase, and other liver function tests are nonspecific. **Results of liver function studies may be absolutely normal.**
   b. Radiographic chest examination may show elevation or paralysis of the right hemidiaphragm or right pleural effusion.
   c. **CT usually is** considered the **procedure of choice,** with a sensitivity of 100% in some series [145]. However, a CT scan may be falsely interpreted as malignancy. **Ultrasonography** has a sensitivity of 82% to 96% [145]. It may be the preferred initial test because it often identifies associated biliary tract abnormality.
   d. **Blood cultures** are positive in up to 60% of patients but may not reflect all the bacterial pathogens involved when compared with liver abscess aspirates.
   e. **Aspiration of the abscess** with good aerobic and anaerobic cultures provides both diagnostic and therapeutic roles.
   f. **Amebic abscesses** are seen more frequently in men born abroad and in international travelers. These patients tend to have more focal right upper quadrant abdominal pain and less leukocytosis and left shift [146,149]. A serologic workup is diagnostically helpful (e.g., amebic hemagglutination test). (See section **IV.E** under Gastrointestinal Parasites.)
5. **Microbiology.** Either CT-guided or ultrasonographically guided aspiration will provide material for aerobic and anaerobic culture. Bacteria include aerobes and anaerobes in mixed or pure cultures [145,147]. *E. coli, Klebsiella,* and *Enterobacter* are the most common aerobic gram-negative rods. *Proteus* species, and *P. aeruginosa* are less common. *Klebsiella* is particularly common in Taiwan and Singapore [150]. Streptococci include enterococci, viridans streptococci, and microaerophilic species. *Streptococcus milleri* is an important pathogen [151]. *S. aureus* also can be isolated, usually in bacteremic patients. Anaerobic organisms, especially *Fusobacterium* and *Bacteroides* species are found in as many as 45% [145,152].
6. **Treatment.** Drainage of the abscess is critical. Antibiotics are adjunctive [153,154].
   a. **Drainage of abscess.** The **optimal approach by which to drain the abscess is debated.** In recent years, ultrasonographically guided or CT-guided percutaneous catheter drainage has been favored. Surgical drainage

may be needed in selected patients and in patients who fail attempts at percutaneous drainage [145,148,153,154].

The mortality rate associated with multiple small abscesses is higher than with a solitary large abscess. Attempts should be made to drain all abscesses, including the small satellite abscesses through the larger ones, if feasible.

b. **Antibiotics** [113–125]. Empiric therapy uses regimens aimed at mixed aerobic- anaerobic GI-biliary flora. See options in Table 13.10 and section II.B.1–11.

For protracted therapy, antibiotic regimens should be individually fashioned according to the results of the cultures and sensitivities. Many clinicians recommend prolonged therapy (1–2 months) for a drained solitary abscess and no less than 4 months' therapy for multiple liver abscesses, to prevent relapses [145]. Many of these patients may be candidates for home i.v. antibiotic regimens if a good oral agent is not available.

7. **Prognosis.** Mortality rates for hepatic abscesses have been reported to be in the 10% to 20% range, depending on underlying conditions.

D. **Splenic abscesses** are **rare** [155–159]. The incidence in autopsy series ranged from 0.2% to 0.7%, being higher in immunocompromised patients and those with AIDS [156].

1. **Pathogenesis.** The causes can be divided into (a) metastatic infections associated with bacteremia, (b) contiguous infection, (c) embolic noninfectious events causing ischemia and subsequent super infection (e.g. sickle cell anemia), (d) trauma with subsequent infection of a hematoma, and (e) immunodeficiency.
2. **Clinical presentation** often is **subtle,** regardless of the cause. **Fever** (93% of cases), **vague abdominal pain** (58%), and pain, often pleuritic in nature in the left hypochondria (40%), occur. Splenomegaly is seen in slightly more than half of patients. **Unexplained thrombocytosis in a septic intensive care unit patient with persistent left pleural effusion is suggestive** of splenic abscess.
3. **Diagnosis**
   a. **Leukocytosis** usually is seen but is nonspecific.
   b. The **chest radiograph** is surprisingly sensitive, showing abnormalities in 82%. Findings include left pleural effusion, elevation of the left hemidiaphragm, left lower lobe infiltrate, and mass effect in the left upper quadrant.
   c. **Blood cultures.** Approximately 50% of blood cultures are positive.
   d. **CT scanning** has a sensitivity of 96%, which proved significantly superior to ultrasonography (76% sensitivity) and gallium scanning (71%).
   e. The entity of hepatosplenic candidiasis is reviewed in Chapters 17 and 20.
4. **Microbiology** [156,158]. Approximately 30% of cases are due to gram-positive aerobes (staphylococci, streptococci); up to 25% to fungi (usually *Candida*), varying according to the number of immunocompromised patients in the series; 20% to 30% to gram-negative bacteria, including *Salmonella;* 20% to anaerobes; and up to 10% of specimens may be sterile.
5. **Treatment**
   a. **Splenectomy is the treatment of choice** [156–158]. Radiologically guided percutaneous drainage has been used, but treatment failure occurred in 30% in one series [156], though it was more successful in other small series [160].
   b. **Antibiotic therapy** is directed against the isolated organisms. Duration of therapy should be sufficient to treat the original source of the bacteremia. The treatment of fungal abscesses (e.g., **hepatosplenic candidiasis**) involves long-term systemic antifungal therapy (see Chapters 17 and 20). *Mycobacterium avium-intracellulare* treatment in AIDS patients is discussed in Chapter 18.
6. **Potential complications.** The most frequent complication of splenic abscess is rupture into the peritoneal cavity that causes an acute peritonitis [156,158].

E. **Retroperitoneal abscesses** are uncommon [161,162]. Because of their insidious presentation and delays in diagnosis, the mortality rate in modern series ranges from 25% to 45%.

1. **Etiology and pathogenesis.** The kidneys, ureters, pancreas, abdominal aorta, and inferior vena cava are in the retroperitoneum. The ascending colon courses through the retroperitoneum, and the duodenum and descending colon are contiguous with it. The bladder, uterus, and rectum are located in the pelvic extraperitoneal space. The most common causes of isolated retroperitoneal space abscess are renal infections and postoperative infections. Other causes include osteomyelitis of the spine with rupture into the retroperitoneal space, seeding of posttraumatic pelvic hematoma, acute cholecystitis, perforated appendicitis, diverticulitis, perforated colon carcinoma, ischiorectal abscess with penetration to the pelvic retroperitoneum, and a cryptogenic origin [162]. Tuberculosis is now uncommon.
2. **Nonspecific presentation** with nonlocalized abdominal pain and variable GI symptoms occurs in the majority of cases. Chills occur in approximately 20%; fever is documented in nearly 80%. Abdominal tenderness is noted in the majority of cases.
3. **Diagnosis** [162]
   a. **Routine laboratory tests are not specific.** Even with a renal origin, results of urinalysis are often normal.
   b. **Blood cultures** are positive in approximately 25% of cases, *E. coli* and *Bacteroides* species being the most common isolates.
   c. **CT scanning** is the **most useful test.** The role of magnetic resonance imaging (MRI) awaits further clinical experience.
4. **Microbiology** reflects the primary process.
5. **Treatment** involves drainage and i.v. antibiotics [162,163].
   a. The retroperitoneal approach (flank incision) and the pelvic approach (presacral) are more effective surgical approaches than the transperitoneal approach.
   b. **Percutaneous drainage may be the preferred** approach for drainage.
   c. **Antibiotic coverage** is based on blood and drainage cultures, as well as on clinical setting. Aerobic and anaerobic cultures should be performed on any percutaneous or surgical specimens. Infectious disease consultation is advised.

F. **Psoas abscesses** are uncommon [164–166]. These were formerly synonymous with tuberculous disease of the spine or sacroiliac joint. Now most cases are a complication of intestinal disorders. **The psoas muscle is subject to any infectious process of** the ureters, renal pelvis, spine, appendix, and ascending colon.

1. **Etiology** [164,165]. In the United States, **adults** with psoas abscess have an underlying intestinal disease, **especially Crohn disease,** but also diverticulitis, osteomyelitis, or intraabdominal abscess. In fewer than 10%, there is a primary staphylococcal psoas abscess. **In children,** staphylococcal psoas abscess is more likely (up to 75% of cases). Children are more likely to have a history of preceding trauma or cutaneous staphylococcal abscess, which may seed the psoas.
2. **Pathogenesis.** Organisms may enter the retrofascial space **directly by extension** from adjacent infection (e.g., in Crohn disease). In primary psoas abscess, hematogenous spread of staphylococci is most likely, with trauma playing a role in some cases [165].
3. **Clinical presentation** [164–166]
   a. **In adults,** symptoms often are nonspecific, but pain in the iliac fossa, groin, or hip, and tenderness of the iliac fossa are clues. Fever and leukocytosis may not be present. A positive psoas sign (pain on extension and elevation of the leg) is common, especially if there is underlying Crohn disease. The patient may complain of a limp. Frequently, the patient will lie with the hip flexed at all times. Weight loss is common. Psoas abscess rarely occurs in the elderly, and secondary abscesses usually are seen in 10- to 40-year-old patients.
   b. **In children,** often there is hip or abdominal pain, more on the right than the left side. Many have fever and a limp or decreased use of the affected leg, and some have malaise, anorexia, or history of trauma. Usually there is

no discomfort on flexion or rotation of the hip. Children present similarly to adults.

4. **Diagnosis. CT and ultrasonography** are the most accurate tests for diagnosis, although neither reliably differentiates abscess in the muscle from hematoma or neoplasm. Clinical correlation and ultrasonographically guided or CT-guided **aspiration** of the mass with culture (aerobic and anaerobic) is useful diagnostically and therapeutically [88–90]. The role of MRI awaits definition by further clinical experience.
5. **Treatment** [164–166]
   a. **Open or percutaneous drainage** is necessary. An open surgical procedure is required if the underlying pathogenesis is gastrointestinal (e.g., Crohn disease). A primary psoas abscess responds well to percutaneous drainage.
   b. **Antibiotics.** For known or highly suspected primary abscesses, antibiotics aimed at *S. aureus* are used (see Chapter 27D and P). If it is unknown whether the abscess is primary or secondary or if a secondary abscess is present, broad-spectrum antibiotics for the underlying condition can be used until specific culture results are available. For example, if an underlying GI source is suspected or known, Table 13.10 suggests antibiotic options.
6. **Prognosis.** With appropriate therapy, the prognosis is generally good, especially with a primary psoas abscess. Secondary psoas abscesses have been associated with mortality rates as high as 18%, primarily because of delayed or inadequate therapy.

**VI. Appendicitis and perforation.** Appendicitis is best treated by surgical removal of the appendix before perforation occurs. Diagnosis is made primarily on clinical grounds. It is of interest that the incidence of acute appendicitis in the United States has decreased significantly in the past two to four decades. The reasons for this are unclear [167].

A. **Pathogenesis.** Obstruction predisposes the appendiceal wall to bacterial invasion by intraluminal bacteria. The common obstructions include fecaliths, enlarged lymphatic follicles, tumors, inspissated barium, and other foreign bodies such as worms. With distention, the mucosal lining is susceptible to impairment of its blood supply, and bacterial invasion of deeper tissues occurs. As this sequence worsens, tissue infarction can occur, with the potential for perforation at the antimesenteric border [167].

B. **Microbiologic features.** Cultures reveal polymicrobial involvement, with 5 to 10 different species typically isolated. *Bacteroides fragilis* and *E. coli* are almost universally isolated. *Pseudomonas* species may be seen in up to 40% of cultures [167] (see section **II.B.10**).

C. **Clinical presentation is reviewed elsewhere** [167]. **Acute appendicitis in the elderly is a much more serious disease than in younger adults:** 60% to 90% of elderly patients are found to have a ruptured appendix at operation. Fewer than 10% of patients undergoing surgery for acute appendicitis are over 60 years of age, but more than 50% of all deaths from appendicitis are in this age group. This is due to the delay in definitive treatment, greater frequency of progressive uncontrolled infection, and the high incidence of concomitant disease. The clinical presentation may be subtle, and fever or leukocytosis may be blunted in the elderly. Diagnostic accuracy for acute appendicitis is considerably lower in children than in adults. **Appendicitis in pregnancy** does not occur frequently, but diagnosis may be difficult because of displacement of the appendix [167]. **Appendicitis in AIDS patients** may not be associated with leukocytosis.

D. **Ultrasonography** has reduced the unnecessary appendectomy rate to 7% and the delay in operation beyond 6 hours to 2%. An inflamed appendix is visualized in 86% of cases. Enlarged mesenteric nodes and mural thickening of the ileum suggest bacterial enteritis due to *Y. enterocolitica* and *C. jejuni*. Laparoscopy is used to distinguish gynecologic disease and ileitis from appendicitis [167]. Laproscopic appendectomy is associated with a higher rate of abscess formation than open appendectomy [140].

E. **Complications.** The major complication is appendiceal rupture. This occurs in 20% to 30% of city hospital patients versus approximately 15% in private hospitals. The incidence of rupture is higher in two population groups: geriatric and pediatric. Patients with appendiceal rupture tend to be quite ill, toxic, and dehydrated, with persisting local peritonitis. Usually there is obvious percussion and rebound tenderness of the right lower quadrant [167].

**F. Therapy**

1. **Surgical intervention is routinely indicated** for acute appendicitis and its complications. Schwartz cautions that to attempt to treat appendicitis with antibiotics alone is misguided because it ignores the obstructive cause of appendicitis. The timing of surgical intervention is discussed by Schwartz [167].
2. **Antibiotics**
   a. **For acute appendicitis without rupture,** short courses of antibiotics to prevent wound infection (e.g., either a single dose of cefoxitin [2 g in adults] or up to three doses) are adequate in uncomplicated cases [113–125,167, 168].
   b. **For appendiceal rupture with local peritonitis,** see section **II** for antibiotic options. The optimal duration of therapy is unclear [117], but it seems prudent that the patient be treated until he or she is afebrile for 47 to 72 hours and is clinically improving. Oral antibiotics can be used to complete the course.

**VII. Intraabdominal infections in the immunocompromised host** (e.g., acute abdomen) have been reviewed elsewhere [115,169]. Certain issues deserve special emphasis.

**A. Processes that can occur in any host** (e.g., appendicitis) may occur. Peptic ulcer disease after renal transplantation is common if excess corticosteroids are used or $H_2$-blockers are not used. Acalculous cholecystitis (see section **IX.E** under Biliary Tract Infections) and acute cholecystitis with perforation appear with increased frequency in immunocompromised hosts [169]. Diverticulitis or CMV infection with colon perforation may be seen more frequently after renal transplantation. Appendicitis infrequently occurs in the immunocompromised host, except perhaps in children [169].

**B. Special conditions in immunocompromised hosts**

1. **Neutropenic enterocolitis** is a rare but well-recognized GI complication during therapy for acute and chronic leukemia, lymphoma, and solid tumors. It is the most **common cause of acute abdomen in patients with acute leukemia** [169]. The diagnosis is based on a high index of suspicion in patients with profound neutropenia, abdominal pain, and fever. Plain abdominal radiographs may show thickened air-filled loops of bowel, an obstructive pattern, or pneumatosis intestinalis (see section **8**). In most patients the condition does not progress to necrosis, perforation of the bowel, or peritonitis. Medical management consists of bowel rest, i.v. fluids, and broad-spectrum antibiotics. Indications for operation include persistent or worsening abdominal tenderness or a worsening clinical course.
2. **Acute graft-versus-host disease** [169] **may present as an acute abdomen** in bone marrow recipients. The syndrome of acute graft-versus-host disease usually starts 3 to 4 weeks (range 2–10 weeks) after marrow transplantation and consists of dermatitis (a red maculopapular rash on the trunk, palms, soles, and ears), crampy abdominal pain that may be aggravated by food, and profuse watery diarrhea. Abdominal features usually follow skin manifestations, but they can precede them. Patients may have abdominal distention and peritoneal signs on examination, probably due to transmural edema of the small intestine. Free perforation is rare. The treatment is increased doses of immunosuppressive agents.
3. **Venoocclusive disease.** See Chapter 20.
4. **Hepatitis** with right upper quadrant abdominal pain can occur. Hepatitis C virus, CMV, and Epstein-Barr virus may be seen in these patients.
5. **Cytomegalovirus GI disease** can occur [170].
6. **Hepatosplenic candidiasis** is discussed in Chapters 17 and 20 and is associated with persisting fever, despite broad-spectrum antibiotics and resolution of leukopenia.

7. **Liver transplantation** recipients may experience surgical technical complications (see Chapter 20).
8. **Pneumatosis intestinalis** is an uncommon problem consisting of multiple gas-filled cysts in the wall of the small or large intestine. Radiologically, translucencies are found parallel to and just outside the gas-filled bowel lumen. Pneumoperitoneum can result if the cysts burst into the intestinal cavity. The patient is asymptomatic because no peritonitis results from the sterile gas. This condition is associated with a variety of conditions, including GI infections, lymphoma, leukemia, ischemic bowel disease, and intestinal obstruction. Surgical consultation is advised.
9. **Polymicrobial sepsis** in the immunocompromised host suggests possible intraabdominal pathology (e.g., abscess), and CT is recommended.
10. **Cholangitis** is caused by *Cryptosporidium,* by microsporidia such as *Enterocytozoon bieneusi* or *Encephalitozoon intestinalis,* or by CMV [170–173].

## VIII. Diverticulitis and related complications [173,174]

Diverticulosis is common. It afflicts approximately 30% of the population over 45 years of age and 60% of those over 70. It is estimated that approximately 10% to 20% of these people with diverticulosis will develop either hemorrhage or diverticulitis.

### A. Pathogenesis [173,174]

1. **Diverticula form as outpouchings** of mucosa through weak portions of the colonic wall where branches of the marginal artery penetrate the colonic tunica muscularis.
2. **The pathogenesis** of diverticular disease **is unknown.** Aging, elevation of colonic intraluminal pressure, decreased dietary fiber, and increased dietary beef fat appear to be related. Decreased luminal fiber requires more colonic segmentation to propel the material aborally. Diverticula are seen in the right colon of Asians and the sigmoid and left colon of Occidentals.
3. **Forms of the disease**
   a. **Simple diverticulosis** is generally asymptomatic. Although there may be shortening and narrowing of the bowel, there is no muscle thickening, and the diverticula frequently are reducible.
   b. **Spastic colon diverticulosis** and **painful diverticular disease** are names given to symptomatic diverticulosis. Pathologic findings show a thickened sigmoid wall but no inflammation.
   c. **Diverticulitis** results from a large or small perforation in the fundus that produces pericolic inflammation. Some perforated diverticula proceed to spontaneous healing, with fibrosis and granuloma formation next to a diverticulum.

### B. Clinical presentation and evaluation [173,174]. See Table 13.12.

1. **Clinical presentation.** Diverticulitis presents like left-sided appendicitis. Inflamed diverticula of the transverse colon may simulate ulcer pain, whereas diverticulitis of the cecum and redundant sigmoid may mimic appendicitis.
   a. The severity and persistence of pain, fever, leukocytosis, and elevated erythrocyte sedimentation rate (ESR), help to distinguish diverticulitis from benign conditions. It may be difficult to distinguish mild diverticulitis from irritable bowel syndrome with coincidental diverticula. However, the WBC count and ESR may be within normal limits.
   b. True diverticulitis in patients under 40 years of age occurs and may be severe.
   c. Abdominal findings may be minimal in the elderly and in those on corticosteroids.
   d. Diverticulosis can present with GI hemorrhage, but **bleeding usually is not seen in diverticulitis** [173].
   e. **Signs** of diverticulitis include left lower quadrant tenderness, tenderness on rectal examination in the left cul-de-sac, and occasionally a tender mass if an abscess or phlegmon has formed.
2. **Diagnosis.** In the face of known diverticulosis, fever, left lower quadrant abdominal pain and tenderness, leukocytosis, and an elevated sedimentation rate, a clinical diagnosis can often be made (see section **I.A**).

Table 13.12. A Practical Approach to the Evaluation and Diagnosis of Acute Diverticulitis

| |
|---|
| Clinical |
| Usually >60 years of age |
| Left lower quadrant localized tenderness and unremitting abdominal pain |
| Fever, leukocytosis |
| Differential diagnosis |
| Elderly |
| Ischemia, Penetrating ulcer |
| Carcinoma |
| Volvulus |
| Obstruction |
| Nephrolithiasis or urosepsis |
| Middle-aged and younger |
| Appendicitis |
| Salpingitis |
| Inflammatory bowel |
| Penetrating ulcer |
| Urosepsis |
| Qualifiers |
| Extremes of age (more virulent), oriental ancestry (right-sided symptoms), |
| Corticosteroids, immunosuppressives, and chronic renal failure (abdominal examination insensitive) |
| Evaluations |
| Plain radiographs: Good first step; may show ileus, obstruction, mass effect, perforation. |
| Contrast enema: In mild to moderate disease when the diagnosis uncertain. Use water-soluble contrast. Otherwise delay examination for 6–8 wk. |
| Endoscopy: Relative contraindication. Perform only if necessary to exclude ischemic bowel, carcinoma, or perforation. |
| CT scan: Very helpful in staging, evaluating for other diseases. Should be considered in all cases of diverticulitis with a palpable mass or clinical toxicity, failure of medical therapy, and corticosteroid use. The test of choice to evaluate acute diverticulitis in most centers. |
| Ultrasonography: Can be a safe and helpful noninvasive test to evaluate acute diverticulitis. Examinations suboptimal due to intestinal gas in 15%, very examiner dependent. |

Reprinted from Freeman SR McNally PR. Diverticulitis. *Med Clin North Am* 1993;77:1149–1167; with permission.

a. **Plain films of the abdomen** are useful to exclude extracolonic air in an abscess or evidence of colonic obstruction.

b. **CT scanning** has become the **test of choice, especially if the clinical diagnosis is not clear or a complication is suspected** [173] or if there is poor response to medical care [98]. **Any patient with a palpable abdominal mass should have a CT scan.** CT diagnostic criteria include localized colonic wall thickening (>5 mm) and inflammation of pericolic fat (poorly marginated, stranding, increased attenuation) or localized wall thickening and presence of periodic abscess [173]. CT scanning has the additional advantage of delineating extraluminal complications of diverticulitis and suggesting other diseases: tuboovarian abscess, colonic ischemia, mesenteric thrombosis, and pancreatitis, which at times may present like diverticulitis.

c. **Contrast enema.** The **safety and utility** of a contrast enema to evaluate acute diverticulitis is **controversial.** Water-soluble contrast, but not barium, may be safe and useful in patients with mild to moderate diverticulitis [173]. No preparation of the bowel should precede a water-soluble contrast enema. Communication with the radiologist to limit the study to the segment of colon in question with careful attention to the amount of pressure being applied is essential [174].

d. **Endoscopy.** Most authorities consider uncomplicated diverticulitis a contraindication because of the risk of diverticular perforation with insufflations of the bowel during the procedure [173].

e. **Ultrasonography.** False-negative results were noted in 15% of the 54 patients examined. The effectiveness of this examination is very examiner dependent [173].

f. **Blood cultures** should be obtained in hospitalized patients to detect bacteremia.

3. **Complications** [173]

a. **Fistulas.** With repeated attacks of diverticulitis, a fistulous tract can form among the bowel, bladder, integument, pelvic floor, and vagina.

b. **Obstruction** occurs usually after repeated episodes of subclinical diverticulitis. The colon becomes fixed, fibrotic, and stenosed. It is important to rule out other causes of colonic stricture such as carcinoma, Crohn disease, and ischemia.

c. **Perforation** of a diverticulum may cause peritonitis, although free peritoneal air on plain films is uncommon because the perforations are walled off.

d. **Abscess.** Failure of response to medical therapy within 24 to 48 hours or the palpation of an abdominal mass should prompt CT scanning.

e. **Frank rectal bleeding is not seen with diverticulitis.** If it is observed, other causes should be investigated.

C. **Microbiologic evaluation** of diverticulitis and related abscesses is reflective of colon flora (see section **II.A** under Intraabdominal Infection).

D. **Therapy** depends on severity and duration of illness, as well as on comorbid disease [96,98].

1. **Asymptomatic diverticulosis.** A high-fiber diet and bulk laxatives such as Metamucil are recommended. This type of diet reduces intraluminal pressure and usually produces a satisfactory subjective response. Foods with high-fiber content include fruits, vegetables, lettuce, and unrefined wheat. Unprocessed, or miller's, bran can be added to water, cereal, or milk. Harsh laxatives and high enemas should be avoided.

2. **Mild acute diverticulitis can often be handled on an outpatient basis.** Typically, these involve patients with recurrent mild symptoms [173].

a. **Clear liquid diets** are suggested until symptoms improve.

b. **Oral antibiotics** are based on GI flora. TMP-SMX and metronidazole or ciprofloxacin and metronidazole (or clindamycin) are an alternative combination. A 1-week course often is effective (see Table 13.9).

3. **Moderately to severely ill patients should be hospitalized.**

a. **GI rest.** Nothing should be taken by mouth for 48 to 72 hours or until symptoms improve, then liquid and semisolid foods may be taken as tolerated. Nasogastric suctioning is used if the patient is vomiting or has abdominal distention or obstruction.

b. **Intravenous fluids.**

c. **Antibiotics** aimed at mixed aerobic-anaerobic abdominal flora should be given (see options in Table 13.10). In moderately severe diverticulitis, cefoxitin appears to be as effective as gentamicin plus clindamycin [175]. The optimal duration is unclear, but some clinicians suggest 1 week [174].

d. **Pain control.** Meperidine may be used for severe pain. Morphine should be avoided because it increase intracolonic pressure.

e. **Clinical course.** Most patients improve in 48 to 72 hours, with a decrease in abdominal pain, leukocytosis, and fever. Failure to improve or worsening is an indication for possible surgical intervention. If not done initially, CT is indicated to determine if an abscess that could be drained is present.

f. **Surgery** for the initial attack is required in 20% to 30% of cases. **Indications** are reviewed elsewhere [173,174] but **include** failure to improve or deterioration with medical therapy; complications such as sepsis, fistula, or obstruction; and recurrent disease. Early surgery is recommended for those under 40 years of age, for the immunocompromised, and for those with presumed right-sided diverticulitis [173].

**IX. Biliary tract infections**

**A. Introduction.** The anatomy of the gallbladder and the extrahepatic biliary system and the microbiology of the obstructed biliary system are important to the understanding of biliary tract infections.

**B. Anatomic considerations** are reviewed in detail elsewhere [176], but a few important features are highlighted here (Fig. 13.4).

1. **The gallbladder** is richly innervated and lies on the undersurface of the liver adjacent to the duodenum, pylorus, hepatic flexure of the right colon, and kidney. Diseases of these adjacent organs may clinically mimic diseases of the gallbladder-biliary system.
2. **The cystic duct** connects the gallbladder to the common bile duct. Its configuration and length are variable, and anomalies in this structure are common.
3. **Bile ducts.** The extrahepatic biliary tree begins with the Y-shaped **right and left hepatic ducts,** which join at the hilum of the liver, forming the **common hepatic duct.**

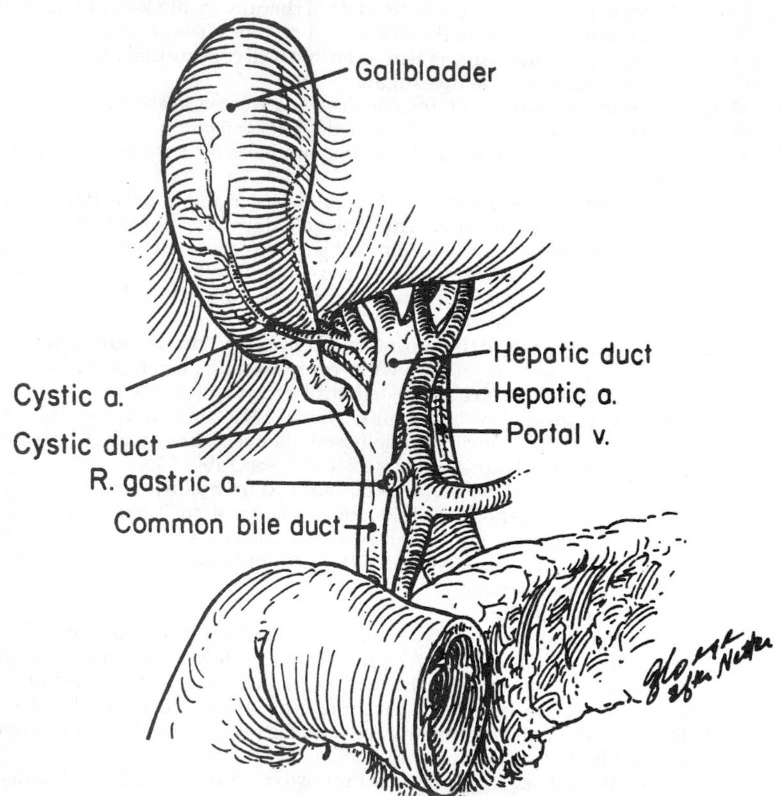


**FIG. 13.4** Normal anatomy. The diagram depicts the relationships in the porta hepatis. The triangle of Calot is bordered by the edge of the liver, the cystic duct, and the hepatic duct. (Reprinted from Roslyn JJ, Zinner MJ. Gallbladder and extrahepatic biliary system. In: Schwartz SI, et al., eds. *Principles of surgery,* 6th ed. New York: McGraw-Hill, 1994:1368; with permission.)

**The common bile duct** is approximately 8 cm long and begins at the juncture of the cystic duct and the common hepatic duct and courses through the pancreas. It can be the site of involvement for benign and malignant disease. **It empties into the duodenum** at the papilla of Vater. Typically there is a common channel, created by the joining of the pancreatic and the distal common bile duct, which empties through a single orifice into the duodenum. This is important in the pathogenesis of gallstone pancreatitis.

4. **Related terminology**
   a. **Cholelithiasis:** the presence of gallstones in the gallbladder.
   b. **Choledocholithiasis:** the presence of stones in the common bile duct.

C. **Diagnostic tests** [176–179]

1. **Plain roentgenograms** of the abdomen are of limited value. Only 15% to 20% of gallstones comprise enough calcium to show up on routine films.
2. **Ultrasonography** has a diagnostic accuracy of 95%. The patient should be fasted for at least 6 hours prior to examination. Obesity interferes with adequate visualization. **Ultrasonography** is useful in identifying intrahepatic and extrahepatic ductal dilatation as well as masses that may cause biliary obstruction. **Sonographic signs** include gallstones (impacted in the neck or cystic duct), a thickened gallbladder wall, and intraluminal sludge. A positive Murphy sign, maximum tenderness over the ultrasonographically localized gallbladder, plus gallstones have a positive predictive value of more than 90%. The sensitivity of ultrasonography for acute cholecystitis is not as great as for stones. The presence of stones does not diagnose acute cholecystitis. Dimethyl iminodiacetic acid (HIDA) scans can be more helpful (see section **5**).
3. **CT scanning** is only sensitive in identifying gallstones if thin cuts are used. However, it demonstrates biliary dilatation and masses in and around the biliary tract and pancreas. It is more useful than ultrasonography for evaluating the jaundiced patient.
4. **MRI's** role in the evaluation of hepatobiliary disease is still being analyzed.
5. **Biliary scintigraphy.** The HIDA scan uses technetium 99 labeling to **assess cystic duct patency. It is sensitive in diagnosing acute cholecystitis.**
   a. **The patient must fast for at least 4 hours because two-thirds of** nonfasted normal individuals have a contracted gallbladder and decreased gallbladder flow of tracer.
   b. **Patterns.** In a **normal** pattern, the gallbladder, common bile duct, and duodenum are all visualized within 60 minutes. In a **nonvisualization** pattern, the gallbladder is not seen, even on delayed views or after morphine sulfate administration. This **strongly implies acute cholecystitis** because it indicates cystic duct obstruction. The gallbladder may not be visualized in 60% to 90% of alcoholics, or among those on parenteral nutrition or the severely ill. Active hepatitis or pancreatitis also may yield a false-positive scan [178]. In **delayed visualization,** the gallbladder is seen after 1 to 4 hours despite intestinal visualization at 1 hour. This **suggests chronic cholecystitis,** although such a test is fairly insensitive in this setting and is abnormal only 45% of the time. This pattern also can be seen in acute cholecystitis. In the **persistent hepatocyte phase,** nonvisualization of the gallbladder and common bile duct and absent or delayed bowel activity is seen most commonly with common duct obstruction [178].
   c. **An HIDA scan** is a functional test, whereas ultrasonography is an anatomic test [176].
6. **Cholangiography** [178]. Endoscopic retrograde cholangiopancreatography (ERCP) and percutaneous transhepatic cholangiography have replaced i.v. cholangiograms.
   a. **ERCP** uses a side-viewing endoscope, permitting the biliary tract and pancreatic duct to be cannulated and visualized. ERCP has been especially useful in obstructive jaundice, in both benign and malignant disease.
   b. **Percutaneous transhepatic cholangiography** is useful in patients with more complex problems, including duct strictures or tumors.

**D. Acute cholecystitis**

**1. Pathogenesis**

**a. Calculi** lead to inflammation in 85% to 95% of cases. Pathogenesis includes stone obstruction of the cystic duct. Pressure on the mucosa by a calculus presumably causes impairment of venous return, ischemic necrosis, ulceration, gangrene, or perforation.

**b. Bacteria** have been cultured from 50% to 70% of acute cholecystitis cases. The origin of inflammation in the 30% or so without bacteria is felt to be chemical or physical.

**2. Clinical presentation.** Acute onset of right upper quadrant pain, nausea, vomiting, and fever are the most frequently presenting symptoms. Right upper quadrant tenderness, fever, and leukocytosis are common. Elevated liver function tests are less common.

**3. Microbiology** [179–181]. Healthy biliary tracts usually are sterile. In acute cholecystitis, infection appears to be a secondary phenomenon. Most bile cultures usually reveal a mixture of organisms [179]. Frequency is higher in the elderly, with jaundice in acute cholecystitis (vs. chronic), and when the common duct is obstructed.

**a. Microbiology.** GI bacteria predominate (see Table 13.9). Polymicrobial infections are the rule [180,181]. Isolation of *Klebsiella* or *Enterobacter* species plus enterococci point to the gallbladder. Anaerobes are more frequent after common duct or complex prior biliary procedures (especially biliary-intestinal anastomosis) and in the elderly.

**b. The source of bacteria** is assumed to be ascending spread from the duodenum.

**4. Antibiotic therapy.**

**a. Empiric antibiotic regimens** are aimed primarily at gram-negative bacteria. Cefazolin, ceftriaxone, and piperacillin/tazobactam are all equally effective. The need for antienterococci therapy is unclear. Anaerobes, when isolated, are in a low inoculum compared with the high inoculum associated with colon perforation. Therefore, in mild to moderately ill patients, antibiotics with optimal bowel anaerobic activity are not required. In the elderly or critically ill patient and the patient with prior common bile duct or complex biliary procedures, a therapeutic regimen that includes anaerobic activity is reasonable (Table 13.13).

**b.** Antibiotic regimens can be tailored on the basis of susceptibility data.

**5. Management** [179–181]

**a. Initial therapy** consists of fluids, nothing by mouth, parenteral analgesics, and antibiotics. If the patient is vomiting or there is gastric distention or

Table 13.13. Empiric Antibiotic Therapy in Biliary Tract Infections (When Renal Function Is Normal)

| Setting | Antibiotic Regimen |
|---|---|
| Mild-moderate | Cefazolin (1–2 g q8h)<br>Cefoxitin (2 g q6h–q8h)<br>Piperacillin-tazobactam (3.75 g q6h)<br>Ceftriaxone 2g q24h |
| Severe[a] | Ceftriaxone + metronidazole[b]<br>Piperacillin-tazobactam + gentamicin<br>Imipenem (500 mg q6h or 1 g q8h) |
| Complex nosocomial | Piperacillin, an aminoglycoside, + metronidazole or clindamycin; imipenem + an aminoglycoside |

q8h, every 8 hours; q6h, every 6 hours; q24h, every 24 hours.
[a]Fever >102.5 bilirubin >3.
[b]Needed for anaerobic organisms.

ileus, placement of a nasogastric tube is indicated. Most patients respond to this treatment in 24 to 48 hours.

b. **Cholecystectomy** remains the treatment of choice for acute cholecystitis. Timing and the potential role of laproscopic cholecystectomy are reviewed elsewhere [176,181].

E. **Acalculous cholecystitis.** Acute inflammation of the gallbladder can occur without stones (5%–15% of cholecystitis cases) [181–183]. It has been recognized with increased frequency in recent years. **Risks include debilitated hospitalized patients** who have had major surgical procedures, major trauma, burns, sepsis, multiple transfusions, hyperalimentation, inadequate nutrition or multiorgan failure, or associated disease such as diabetes or malignancy.

1. **Etiology and pathogenesis.** The cause *may* involve bile stasis, cholecystoparesis, or gallbladder ischemia [182]. Histologically, there is intense injury to the blood vessels of the gallbladder tunica muscularis and serosa, possibly due to activation of Hageman factor, which occurs after transfusions, in endotoxemia, and after trauma [182,183].
2. **Symptoms and findings** are similar to those of calculous cholecystitis.
3. **Diagnosis.** HIDA scanning, ultrasonography, and CT scanning are used. Because each test has certain limitations, multiple complementary techniques may be necessary [183].

   **Preoperative diagnosis is difficult,** and therapeutic intervention often is delayed with subsequently high morbidity and mortality [181].
4. **Therapy.** Urgent temporizing percutaneous transhepatic cholecystostomy or, preferably, cholecystectomy is advised [176]. Broad-spectrum antibiotics are used.
5. **Prognosis.** High mortality results from underlying disease, multiorgan failure, and sepsis.

F. **Ascending cholangitis** is due to infection of the biliary duct system. It is a **potentially lethal disorder requiring prompt treatment** [181,184].

1. **Etiology. Obstruction is an important feature** [181,185].
   a. **Choledocholithiasis.** Stones that have migrated from the gallbladder and infection associated with stones are the most common causes of acute cholangitis.
   b. **Obstruction also** can be due to pancreatic cancer, cholangiocarcinoma, cancer of the papilla of Vater, portahepatic metastases, biliary stricture, pancreatitis, and ***A. lumbricoides.***
2. **Pathogenesis. Bacteria** enter the bile duct from the intestine or the bloodstream and infect the bile under pressure. Bile in a normal-pressure bile duct is difficult to infect.
3. **Clinical presentation.** Abdominal pain, fever, and jaundice are common symptoms. Charcot's triad of fever, right upper quadrant pain, and jaundice occurs in only 50% to 60% of patients. Septic shock is common, especially if therapy is delayed [186].
4. **Diagnosis**
   a. Leukocytosis and elevated liver function tests (obstructive pattern) are common.
   b. Blood cultures should be drawn.
   c. **Radiologic diagnosis. See IC 1–6 above.**
5. **Therapy**
   a. **Supportive care** includes i.v. fluids.
   b. **Broad-spectrum antibiotics** may be administered, with optimal regimens for very ill patients (see Chapter 2).
   c. **Surgical consultation** for **biliary decompression.** Approximately 85% to 90% of patients respond to antibiotics and supportive care alone. Those who fail or who deteriorate on medical therapy or even those who respond may require urgent bile duct decompression. Options for decompression include the following [177,181]:

1. **Percutaneous transhepatic biliary drainage** (PTBD) is not definitive and is associated with significant complications, including bleeding, bile leak,

fistulous communications between the biliary tree and vascular tree, and sepsis.

2. **Endoscopic sphincterotomy** in conjunction with decompression or biliary drainage with a nasobiliary catheter or endoprosthesis may be used when endoscopic extraction of a stone has failed.
3. **Surgical decompression** with bile duct exploration, with or without cholecystectomy, T-tube drainage, or biliary-enteric anastomosis, also may be used.
4. **Summary.** PTBD or endoscopic sphincterotomy is believed to be the treatment of choice in the seriously ill and high-risk patient. Elective surgery can be performed once the patient has stabilized; endoscopy treatment may be definitive for patients with previous cholecystectomy and retained common bile duct stones [181].

**G. Miscellaneous infections**

1. **Gallstone pancreatitis.** See the discussion under section X.
2. **Emphysematous cholecystitis** affects primarily diabetic men [176,187]. Gas within the wall or lumen of the gallbladder is characteristic. Pathogenesis is felt to be due to obstruction of the cystic duct with subsequent development of acute ischemia and proliferation of gas-forming bacteria. Patients are acutely ill and septic appearing. Plain abdominal radiographs show gas bubbles in the right upper quadrant or outlining the biliary tract. CT scans may be the most accurate study. Early surgery is indicated to control sepsis and avoid gallbladder perforation.
3. **Perforation of the gallbladder** [176] occurs in 3% to 10% of cases of acute cholecystitis. Local ischemia, advanced age, and immunosuppression may be contributing factors.
   a. **Free perforation** (rare), an acute abdomen, and septic presentation can occur.
   b. **With pericholecystic abscess** formation, subacute presentation is common.
   c. **Secondary fistula.** Communication between the gallbladder fundus and duodenum can occur, especially in chronic cholecystitis. This may be asymptomatic unless a gallstone enters the GI tract via the fistula and causes obstruction (**gallstone ileus**), usually in the terminal ileum. The combination of small bowel obstruction and air in the biliary tract is characteristic. Treatment consists of enterotomy proximal to the obstruction, removal of the impacted stone, and cholecystectomy [176].
4. **Acute cholecystitis as a postoperative complication.** Many different antecedent operations are associated and need not be bowel procedures. Bile stasis and inspissation of the bile in the gallbladder leads to gallstones followed by obstruction. Disease occurs with the resumption of oral feedings, suggesting that contractions of the gallbladder in response to food may be a contributing factor. See section **IX.E.**
5. **Post-ERCP cholangitis** sometimes occurs [188]. Presumably the procedure may introduce bacteria along with contrast media. The risk for sepsis is higher for patients with malignant causes of biliary obstruction. Antibiotics should include therapy for *P. aeruginosa* and other nosocomial pathogens while awaiting culture data.
6. **Ceftriaxone** can cause gallbladder crystals and symptoms mimicking cholecystitis. Symptoms resolve after ceftriaxone therapy is discontinued. See Chapter 27F.

**X. Acute necrotizing pancreatitis, pancreatic abscess, and infected pancreatic pseudocyst. Acute pancreatitis** is usually a sterile inflammatory process caused by autodigestion of the pancreas. This section emphasizes infectious complications of acute pancreatitis [189–192].

**A. Etiology** [189–192]. In up to 10% of cases, the cause may not be recognized.

1. **Alcohol.** Seven to ten years of drinking usually occurs before pancreatitis develops.
2. **Gallstones** or biliary sludge are etiologic more frequently in private hospitals, whereas alcohol is more common in Veterans' Administration hospitals.

3. **Miscellaneous causes**
   a. **Hypertriglyceridemia.** Pancreatitis is associated with triglyceride levels usually in excess of 1,000 mg/dL. Appropriate therapy can prevent recurrences.
   b. **Abdominal trauma** (e.g., automobile accident) can result in pancreatitis.
   c. **Postoperative pancreatitis** occurs after upper abdominal, renal, or cardiovascular surgery. Perioperative medications, not pancreatic trauma, are strongly implicated.
   d. **Hypercalcemia** has been associated with pancreatitis.
   e. **Pregnancy.** In the third trimester and in the first 6 weeks postpartum, pancreatitis can occur and probably is related to alcohol abuse or gallstone disease.
   f. **Anatomic causes.** Tumors of the ampulla or pancreas, pancreatic or ampullary strictures, and periampullary diverticula can precipitate pancreatitis. Pancreatitis is the initial clinical presentation of 3% of patients with pancreatic cancer and 1.3% of patients with acute pancreatitis are found to have pancreatic carcinoma. Therefore, for patients over 45 years of age with idiopathic pancreatitis, duct visualization is mandatory.
   g. **Infections.** Viruses (including mumps, rubella, coxsackie B virus, Epstein-Barr virus, CMV, and acute hepatitis A, B, and C), parasites (e.g., *Ascaris*), and *Mycoplasma pneumoniae* have been associated with pancreatitis. Acute pancreatitis for patients with AIDS is most often secondary to drug use [189] (see section **9**).
   h. **Complications of ERCP.**
   i. **Drugs.** NSAIDs, erythromycin, thiazides, didanosine (ddI), pentamidine, estrogens, sulfonamides, and L-asparaginase are among the agents implicated [189].
   j. **Systemic vasculitis** can be the cause of pancreatitis.

B. **Prognosis of acute pancreatitis.** Criteria have been developed (e.g., Ranson criteria, APACHE [Acute Physiology and Chronic Health Evaluation II] criteria) to help predict the survival of a given patient based on the severity of acute pancreatitis. They are reviewed elsewhere [189,190,192]. Patients with three or more Ranson signs either have severe pancreatitis or are at risk for severe disease. Related points deserve special emphasis.
   1. **Approximately 80% of patients have mild disease;** most of these patients recover uneventfully. Pancreatic and peripancreatic necrosis are minimal [189].
   2. **Approximately 20% have severe pancreatitis** with pancreatic or peripancreatic **necrosis or pancreatic fluid collections** [192]. **Necrosis of either the duct system or the pancreatic parenchyma is the initiating event in most of the complications of acute pancreatitis and occurs in the absence of bacteria.** Necrosis occurs early in the clinical course, typically on the first day of symptoms.
      a. About 10% of patients have fluid collections due to extravasation from the ductal system.
      b. Another 10% of the total group has extensive necrosis (>10%–15% of the gland). Of these, nearly 50% (5% of the total group) will become infected. In the absence of necrosis, infection is rare, but the more extensive the necrosis, the higher is the risk for infection. Between 40% and 70% of patients with more than 30% necrosis will become infected. Infection increases until the third week and peaks in the fourth week. A high mortality rate (**80% of all deaths result from these difficult-to-treat infections**) occurs with early infection, with extensive necrosis, and in the very ill.

C. **Assessing infection**
   1. Sterile pancreatitis or peripancreatic necrosis causes leukocytosis and fever. Clinically it is uncertain when or if there is superimposed infection. Also, 50% of patients with infection may not show clinical signs of an active infection [193].
   2. **CT scan with contrast** predicts who is at risk for infection. Poorly enhanced pancreatic tissue correlates well with the presence of pancreatic necrosis [193]. If gas bubbles are seen in the pancreatic region on the scan, infection is

Table 13.14. Frequency of Bacteria in Pancreatic Infection

| | |
|---|---|
| *Escherichia coli* | 25% |
| *Pseudomonas* species | 15% |
| *Staphylococcus aureus* | 17% |
| *Klebsiella* species | 9% |
| *Proteus* species | 9% |
| *Streptococcus faecalis* | 3% |
| *Enterobacter* species | 3% |
| Anaerobes | 16% |
| *Candida* species | 3% |
| Monomicrobial | 76% |
| Polymicrobial | 24% |

Reprinted from Schmid SW, et al. The role of infection in acute pancreatitis. *Gut* 1999; 45:311–316; with permission.

presumed to be present. CT scan–guided aspirations of necrotic tissue for Gram stains and aerobic and anaerobic cultures will clarify whether infection actually exists. Commonly isolated organisms are shown in Table 13.14 [194]. Organisms resemble intestinal flora.

3. The mechanism by which colonic bacteria reach the injured pancreatic tissues is unclear. Infection of the injured pancreatic tissues appears to be a secondary phenomenon, thus raising the possibility that prophylactic antibiotics can prevent or limit infection [195].

**D. Prophylactic antibiotics to prevent infectious complications.** Recent studies suggest a benefit but the topic is complex [195–200].

1. **Mild pancreatitis.** Because most cases of pancreatitis are mild and there is no necrosis, antibiotics are not necessary in the majority of cases of pancreatitis.
2. **Moderate to severe pancreatitis includes those cases associated with necrosis.**
   a. **Timing of antibiotic initiation.** The approach that has been argued is to initiate antibiotics early, before infection develops [195]. Although this approach is logical, there are two factors that need to be weighed. First, the frequency of infection increases over the first 3 weeks and peaks at week 4 (see section X.B above). Second, almost a third of infecting organisms are not the typical bowel flora and those (including *Pseudomonas* species, *S. aureus,* and *Candida* species) are more difficult to treat. Perhaps they became a factor because typical gut flora was suppressed by early prophylaxis, allowing them to overgrow and invade. This issue is not resolved and needs further evaluation.
   b. **Antibiotic penetration into pancreatic tissue** [194].
      (1) **Piperacillin, cefotaxime, and ceftizoxime** penetrate pancreatic tissue and are active against the gram-negative bacteria that occur but less so against anaerobes.
      (2) **Imipenem** penetrates pancreatic tissue well and is active against common bacterial isolates.
      (3) The **fluoroquinolones** (e.g., ciprofloxacin) penetrate well and are active against the colonic gram-negative bacteria but not the anaerobic isolates.
      (4) **Aminoglycosides** do not penetrate pancreatic tissue well in usual dosage regimens and therefore are **not preferred agents.**
      (5) **Metronidazole** shows good penetration into pancreatic tissue. Because it is active against anaerobes, it is often combined with an antibiotic effective against the gram-negative bacteria.
   c. **Efficacy trials. Imipenem** recently was studied in a randomized multicenter clinical trial of antibiotic prophylaxis in 74 patients with a Ranson mean score of 3.7 [196] due to severe necrotizing pancreatitis. Disease originated in the biliary tract in 37, from alcoholism in 24, and from miscellaneous causes

in 13. Forty-one patients received medical therapy plus 500 mg of imipenem every 8 hours for 14 days, beginning at the time of CT demonstration of pancreatic necrosis. The other 33 patients received medical therapy alone. Pancreatic infection was proven by percutaneous aspiration or intraoperative cultures. The incidence of pancreatitis related sepsis was much lower in treated patients (12.2 vs. 30.3%, $p < 0.01$) [196]. Neither the incidence of multiorgan failure that developed in 25 patients nor mortality nor the need for surgical intervention was affected by antibiotic therapy. That there is no effect on change of management has led some to conclude that prophylaxis is not beneficial [197]. Several other analyses found benefit [198–200].

d. **Commentary.** Because patients with severe necrotizing pancreatitis with infectious complications are prone to have protracted courses and often require repeated surgical intervention, they may acquire infections due to resistant bacteria [197]. Hence, one might want to save a broad-spectrum antibiotic such as imipenem for later use rather than early use in these high-risk patients. Studies comparing imipenem to other agents would be worthwhile. **A compromise approach** may be to use prophylactic antibiotics (e.g., a third-generation cephalosporin and metronidazole) in severe cases of necrotizing pancreatitis for 7 to 10 days and save imipenem for future infectious complications when resistant bacteria may be a problem.

**E. Related issues**

1. **Surgical intervention.** The optimal approaches are still being evaluated [189,192,193], but when infection occurs, surgery is usually indicated. Typically, a surgical team directs the management of these patients. Aggressive surgical debridement (often requiring serial procedures) with open drainage in selected patients with extensive pancreatic and peripancreatic necrosis is advised. Enhanced CT scanning is very useful [192]. Percutaneous drainage of an area of infected necrosis, as a primary therapy, is believed by some to be an exercise in futility [192]. Further discussion of surgical indications is published elsewhere [193].
2. **Large fluid collections** can occur early in acute pancreatitis, within days or weeks of the onset of symptoms [192]. These fluid collections, unlike a pseudocyst, lack a wall of granulation or fibrous tissue. More than 50% of these collections disappear spontaneously. Therefore, aspirating before 4 to 6 weeks is unnecessary. Percutaneous CT-guided aspiration is a useful technique if infection is a concern.
3. **Fluid resuscitation** is important. Monitoring with a Swan-Ganz catheter often is essential in the care of the severely ill patient [192]. Acute renal failure is a common consequence of poor fluid resuscitation in pancreatitis. The hyperdynamic cardiovascular state is similar to that seen in patients with the septic syndrome (see Chapter 2). Patients with severe pancreatitis have diminished peripheral vascular resistance and decreased intravascular volume. Blood flow to the pancreas is reduced. It is believed that trypsin released into the surrounding tissues and the circulation triggers the complement cascade and kinin release. Furosemide should not be used because this leads to organ hypoperfusion followed by multiple organ failure [192].
4. **Biliary pancreatitis.** Patients with severe biliary pancreatitis and persistent signs and symptoms of obstruction or with cholangitis should undergo endoscopic or surgical relief of the biliary obstruction within the first 48 hours. Many clinicians prefer the endoscopic approach if skilled personnel are available [193]. Some clinicians feel that ERCP is indicated in all cases of biliary pancreatitis.
5. **Associated complications.** Fistulas from the bowel or pancreas, or bleeding from the retroperitoneal structures, are common. Multiorgan system failure, often as a consequence of underlying sepsis, is a common complication and is frequently associated with a fatal outcome. The overall mortality rate varies from 0% to 25%.

**F. Pancreatic abscess.** It may be difficult to distinguish between infected necrosis and early abscess formation. A true pancreatic abscess is a collection of pus

Table 13.15. Bacteriology of Pancreatic Abscesses

| Organism | No. of Patients/Total | Percentage | Range (%) |
|---|---|---|---|
| *Escherichia coli* | 164/494 | 33 | 11–49 |
| *Enterobacter* | 60/284 | 21 | 7–43 |
| *Klebsiella* | 26/189 | 14 | 7–42 |
| *Proteus* | 50/430 | 12 | 5–21 |
| *Serratia* | 8/162 | 5 | 2–11 |
| *Pseudomonas* | 16/386 | 4 | 3–29 |
| *Enterococcus* | 57/260 | 22 | 6–18 |
| *Streptococcus* | 58/323 | 18 | 4–36 |
| *Staphylococcus* | 69/499 | 14 | 0–38 |
| *Bacteroides* | 31/285 | 11 | 5–29 |
| *Candida* (yeast) | 15/158 | 9 | 2–9 |
| Polymicrobial | 140/380 | 37 | 21–57 |
| Monomicrobial | 207/380 | 54 | 29–78 |

Summary of 16 series from specimens obtained intraoperatively or by percutaneous needle aspiration. Anaerobic cultures may not have been optimal.
Reprinted from Witt MD, Edwards JE Jr. Pancreatic abscess and infected pancreatic pseudocyst: diagnosis and treatment. *Curr Clin Top Infect Dis* 1992;12:111; with permission.

and necrotic pancreatic tissue surrounded by an ill-defined wall (capsule), which occurs either within the pancreatic parenchyma or expands into the lesser sac and retroperitoneum. Although not common, pancreatic abscess is associated with a high mortality rate, between 2% and 5% [191,201–206].

1. **Etiology.** The cause of pancreatitis that led to the abscess was alcohol in 32%, biliary tract in 25%, postoperative causes in 19%, and miscellaneous causes in 25% [203].
2. **Pathogenesis.** As with infected pancreatitis, risk increases with the degree of necrosis.
3. **Clinical presentation is nonspecific.** Following the episode of pancreatitis, there may be improvement and then deterioration. The presentation may be indolent, and some patients may not be febrile or have leukocytosis [204]. However, pancreatic abscess should be suspected in any patient with an acute or resolving pancreatitis whose course is complicated by persistent fever, abdominal pain, and leukocytosis, especially about 3 to 4 weeks after the onset of the initial attack [202].
4. **Diagnosis**
   a. **CT scanning** is the best method to demonstrate the abscess [203,205]. CT may reveal a fluid collection that is indistinguishable from a pseudocyst. The presence of air within fluid collections or within the pancreas itself is strongly suggestive of a pancreatic abscess harboring gas-forming organisms. However, retroperitoneal air within peripancreatic fluid also may be seen in uninfected patients who develop a fistulous tract between the pancreas and an adjacent viscus. It is also seen in the postoperative patient, or in patients with a perforated duodenal ulcer [203].
   b. **CT-guided thin-needle aspiration** and culture of the fluid will clarify the diagnosis. Aerobic and anaerobic cultures should be performed routinely.
   c. The **role of MRI** is undergoing clinical evaluation. Only limited data are available with this technique [203].
   d. **Blood cultures** may occasionally be positive.
5. **Microbiology** in pancreatic abscesses are only partially studied (Table 13.15). Many infections are polymicrobial, and the infrequency of anaerobic isolations may reflect poor culture technique [203].
6. **Therapy**
   a. **Surgical drainage is essential** for a true pancreatic abscess [203–206].

In Altemeier's series in 1963 [206], 86% of those whose abscesses were drained surgically and treated with antibiotics survived. By contrast, if the diagnosis was missed and no surgical drainage was performed, 100% died. More recent data confirm a near 100% death rate without surgical drainage.

(1) **Percutaneous catheter drainage** at times is regarded as a temporary maneuver until patients can tolerate definitive surgery. However, if the abscess fluid is thin in consistency and there is little particulate matter in it, percutaneous drainage may be adequate treatment.

(2) **Open surgical drainage** is indicated if the fluid is thick, if rapid improvement does not occur after percutaneous drainage, or if there is CT evidence of considerable surrounding tissue necrosis in addition to the abscess [202].

b. **Nutritional support** with enteral or total parenteral nutrition is favored.

c. **Antibiotics** are useful to prevent bacteremia and aid in healing, and when used in conjunction with surgical drainage. The antibiotics should be selected on the basis of sensitivity testing against any organism isolated from blood or the abscess cavity at the time of surgery or on the basis of prior aspiration culture data. In the absence of culture data, therapy should be instituted as outlined in section **II.B.**

7. **Prognosis.** Despite aggressive surgical therapy coupled with antibiotics and nutritional support, the mortality rate in patients with pancreatic abscess is still 20% or more [201–203].

G. **Pancreatic pseudocysts** [203]. Despite considerable information generated by CT scanning and ultrasonography over the past 20 years, the natural history of pancreatic pseudocysts remains poorly understood, their classification system remains vague, and their nomenclature is controversial. Classically, the term *pancreatic pseudocyst* has been used to refer to all intrapancreatic and peripancreatic fluid collections, usually within a nonepithelialized capsule, arising in the setting of acute or chronic pancreatitis.

Fluid collection should be followed for change in size or the development of signs of infection. Such changes will determine appropriate therapy.

1. **Epidemiologic features.** Pseudocysts almost always arise in the setting of acute or chronic pancreatitis. In a summary of 11 series, the underlying condition was alcohol in 65%, biliary disease alone in 10%, both alcohol and biliary disease in 9%, postoperative trauma in 9%, and miscellaneous conditions in 14%.

2. **Pathogenesis.** The origin is not well understood. Presumably, pseudocysts develop as a result of the disruption of the ductal system, with subsequent leakage of activated pancreatic enzymes leading to necrosis of the gland and surrounding tissue. This is accompanied by the production of large volumes of exudate that dissect along retroperitoneal planes. Multiple pseudocysts occur in 10% of cases.

3. **Clinical presentation** [203]

a. Abdominal pain (60%–100%), nausea or vomiting (20%–70%), weight loss (30%–60%), palpable abdominal mass (20%–50%), jaundice (10%–20%), and abdominal tenderness (10%–60%) are seen. Probably 50% of cysts are nonpalpable, and up to 50% of palpable masses in patients with pancreatitis simply represent inflammation and edema rather than a pseudocyst.

b. **Routine laboratory tests** (WBC count, amylase levels, etc.) are nondiagnostic.

4. **Diagnosis. CT scanning** is the most accurate imaging technique, although the CT scan does not differentiate between a sterile and an infected fluid collection.

5. **Natural history of pancreatic cysts.** When serial ultrasonography or CT scanning is performed, **8% to 43% of the pseudocysts undergo spontaneous resolution,** usually within 6 weeks after onset. Therefore, it is suggested that drainage procedures be postponed until either the pseudocyst persists for more than 6 weeks or a complication arises. Some clinicians suggest prolonged observation unless the patient is symptomatic.

6. **Complications of pancreatic pseudocysts** [203]
   a. **Obstructive jaundice.** Pseudocysts at the head of the pancreas may obstruct the duodenum or compress the common bile duct.
   b. **Chemical pancreatitis** can occur if the pseudocyst ruptures acutely. This is associated with a high mortality rate.
   c. **Pancreatic ascites** can occur with a slow leak into the peritoneal cavity.
   d. **Hemorrhage** can occur, either within the cyst itself or as a result of the cyst eroding into a major artery or perforating into the GI tract.
   e. **Chronic pancreatic cysts** may be drained internally (e.g., cystogastrostomy, Roux-en-Y cystojejunostomy, anastomosis, or cystoduodenostomy).
   f. **Secondary cyst infection** can occur (see section **C**).

H. **Infected pancreatic pseudocyst** [203]
1. **Incidence.** The exact incidence is unclear; 0 to 25% of pseudocysts become infected. Further data gleaned from good aspiration culture studies are needed. Overall, this is believed to be an uncommon complication [203].
2. **Pathogenesis.** Secondary infection presumably results from (a) hematogenous seeding, (b) direct transmural passage of bacteria from adjacent bowel, and (c) possibly bacterial seeding after ERCP.
3. **Diagnosis.** Although persisting fevers, abdominal pain, and an abdominal mass in a patient with a known pseudocyst is suggestive, not all patients with infected pancreatic pseudocysts have these features. Laboratory tests are nondiagnostic.
   a. **CT scanning** will demonstrate whether a pseudocyst exists.
   b. **CT-guided or ultrasonographically guided percutaneous needle aspiration with aerobic and anaerobic cultures** will clarify whether the fluid is infected.
4. **Bacteriologic** data are limited [203]. Polymicrobial infection due to GI gram-negative and gram-positive organisms are typical.
5. **Therapy** [203]. When planning appropriate therapy for an infected pancreatic fluid collection, it is critically important to differentiate an infected pseudocyst from a pancreatic abscess. Whereas an infected pseudocyst can be treated successfully by drainage alone, this intervention would be completely inadequate for an abscess, for which open drainage and extensive debridement often are necessary.
   a. **External drainage** is preferred if the cyst is infected. A large-bore catheter is placed into the infected cyst cavity, and the catheter then is brought out the abdominal wall. Percutaneous drainage has been used as an alternative.
   b. **Internal drainage** may be a consideration in selected patients [207].

I. **Pancreatic disease in AIDS** (see Chapter 18).
1. **Drug-induced pancreatitis** can occur (see section **I.A.3.i**).
2. **Neoplasms** of the pancreas, including Kaposi sarcoma and lymphoma, have been seen in up to 8% of patients in autopsy series.
3. **Infectious agents** have been demonstrated in autopsy series, and microorganisms involved include CMV, *Cryptosporidium,* cryptococci, *T. gondii, Candida* species, and *M. tuberculosis.* These are typically seen in the setting of disseminated infections.

## REFERENCES

1. Guerrant RL, Bobak DA. Bacterial and protozoal gastroenteritis. *N Engl J Med* 1991;325:327–337.
2. Cheney CP, Wong RKH. Acute infectious diarrhea. *Med Clin North Am* 1993;77:1169–1196.
3. Greenberg HB, Matsui SM, Loutit JS. Small intestine: infections with common bacterial and viral pathogens. In: Yamada T, ed. *Textbook of gastroenterology,* 3rd ed. New York: JB Lippincott, 1999:1611–1640.
4. Powell DW. Approach to the patient with diarrhea. In: Yamada T, ed. *Textbook of gastroenterology,* 3rd ed. New York: JB Lippincott, 1999:858–901.
5. Guerrant RL, Steiner TS. Principles and syndromes of enteric infection. In: Mandell GL,

Bennett JE, Dolin R, eds. *Principles and practice of infectious diseases,* 5th ed. New York: Churchill Livingstone, 2000:1076–1090.

6. DuPont HL. Guidelines on acute infectious diarrhea in adults. The Practice Parameters Committee of the American College of Gastroenterology. *Am J Gastroenterol* 1997;92:1962–1975.
7. Surawicz CM, ed. Infectious diarrhea. *Gastroenterol Clin North Am* 2001;30:599–861.
8. Procop GW. Gastrointestinal infections. *Infect Dis Clin North Am* 2001;15:1073–1108.
9. Centers for Disease Control and Prevention. Diagnosis and management of foodborne illnesses: a primer for physicians. *MMWR* 2001;50:1–66.
10. DuPont HL. Diarrhea and gastroenteritis. In: Root RK, ed. *Clinical infectious diseases.* New York: Oxford University Press, 1999:581–588.
11. DuPont HL. Shigella. *Infect Dis Clin North Am* 1988;2:599–605.
12. Wong CS, Jelacic S, Habeeb RL, et al. The risk of the hemolytic-uremic syndrome after antibiotic treatment of *Escherichia coli* O157:H7 infections. *N Engl J Med* 2000;342:1930–1936.
13. Turgeon DK, Fritsche TR. Laboratory approaches to infectious diarrhea. *Gastroenterol Clin North Am* 2001;30:693–707.
14. Goldberg MB, Rubin RH. The spectrum of *Salmonella* infection. *Infect Dis Clin North Am* 1988;2:571–598.
15. Avery ME, Snyder JD. Oral therapy for acute diarrhea: the underused simple solution. *N Engl J Med* 1990;323:891–893.
16. Centers for Disease Control. The management of acute diarrhea in children: oral rehydration, maintenance, and nutritional therapy. *MMWR* 1992;41:1–20.
17. DuPont HL, Ericsson CD. Prevention and treatment of travelers' diarrhea. *N Engl J Med* 1993;328:1821–1827.
18. DuPont HL, Hornick RB. Adverse effect of Lomotil therapy in shigellosis. *JAMA* 1973;226:1525–1528.
19. Boyce TG, Swerdlow DL, Griffin PM. *Escherichia coli* O157:H7 and the hemolytic-uremic syndrome. *N Engl J Med* 1995;333:364–368.
20. Murphy GS, Bodhidatta L, Echeverria P, et al. Ciprofloxacin and loperamide in the treatment of bacillary dysentery. *Ann Intern Med* 1993;118:582–586.
21. Figueroa-Quintanilla D, Salazar-Lindo E, Sack B, et al. A controlled trial of bismuth subsalicylate in infants with acute watery diarrheal disease. *N Engl J Med* 1993;328:1653–1658.
22. Centers for Disease Control and Prevention. *Bacillus cereus* food poisoning associated with fried rice at two child day care centers—Virginia, 1993. *MMWR* 1994;43:177–178.
23. Luby S, Jones J, Dowda H, et al. A large outbreak of gastroenteritis caused by diarrheal toxin-producing *Bacillus cereus. J Infect Dis* 1993;167:1452–1455.
24. Underman AE, Leedom JM. Fish and shellfish poisoning. *Curr Clin Top Infect Dis* 1993;13:203–225.
25. Centers for Disease Control and Prevention. Ciguatera fish poisoning—Texas, 1997. *MMWR* 1998;47:692.
26. Centers for Disease Control and Prevention. Scombroid fish poisoning—Pennsylvania, 1998. *MMWR* 2000;49:398–400.
27. Miller SL, Pegues DA. *Salmonella* species, including *Salmonella typhi.* In: Mandell GL, Bennett JE, Dolin R, eds. *Principles and practice of infectious diseases,* 5th ed. New York: Churchill Livingstone, 2000:2344–2359.
28. Glynn MK, Bopp C, Dewitt W, et al. Emergence of multidrug-resistant *Salmonella enterica* serotype typhimurium DT104 infections in the United States. *N Engl J Med* 1998;338:1333–1338.
29. Hohmann EL. Nontyphoidal salmonellosis. *Clin Infect Dis* 2001;32:263–269.
30. Mishu B, Griffin PM, Tauxe RV, et al. *Salmonella enteritidis* gastroenteritis transmitted by intact chicken eggs. *Ann Intern Med* 1991;115:190–194.
31. Mishu B, Koehler J, Lee LA, et al. Outbreaks of *Salmonella enteritidis* infections in the United States, 1985–1991. *J Infect Dis* 1994;169:547–552.
32. Centers for Disease Control and Prevention. Outbreaks of *Salmonella* serotype Enteritidis infection associated with eating raw or undercooked shell eggs—United States, 1996–1998. *MMWR* 2000;49:73–79.

33. Hennessy TW, Hedberg CW, Slutsker L, et al. A national outbreak of *Salmonella enteritidis* infections from ice cream. *N Engl J Med* 1996;334:1281–1286.
34. Woodward DL, Khakhria R, Johnson WM. Human salmonellosis associated with exotic pets. *J Clin Microbiol* 1997;35:2786–2790.
35. White DG, Zhao S, Sudler R, et al. The isolation of antibiotic-resistant salmonella from retail ground meats. *N Engl J Med* 2001;345:1147–1154.
36. Gorbach SL. Antimicrobial use in animal feed—time to stop. *N Engl J Med* 2001; 345:1202–1203.
37. Aserkoff B, Bennett JV. Effect of antibiotic therapy in acute salmonellosis on fecal excretion of salmonellae. *N Engl J Med* 1969;281:636–640.
38. Neill MA, Opal SM, Heelan J, et al. Failure of ciprofloxacin to eradicate convalescent fecal excretion after acute salmonellosis: experience during an outbreak in health care workers. *Ann Intern Med* 1991;114:195–199.
39. Medical Letter. The choice of antimicrobial drugs. *Med Lett Drug Ther* 2001;43:69–78.
40. Frenck RW Jr, Nakhla I, Sultan Y, et al. Azithromycin versus ceftriaxone for the treatment of uncomplicated typhoid fever in children. *Clin Infect Dis* 2000;31:1134–1138.
41. Nataro JP. Treatment of bacterial enteritis. *Pediatr Infect Dis J* 1998;17:420–421.
42. Nolan CM, White PC Jr. Treatment of typhoid carriers with amoxicillin: correlates of successful therapy. *JAMA* 1978;239:2352–2354.
43. Ferreccio C, Morris JG Jr, Valdivieso C, et al. Efficacy of ciprofloxacin in the treatment of chronic typhoid carriers. *J Infect Dis* 1988;157:1235–1239.
44. DuPont HL. *Shigella* species (bacillary dysentery) In: Mandell GL, Bennett JE, Dolin R, eds. *Principles and practice of infectious diseases,* 5th ed. New York: Churchill Livingstone, 2000:2363–2369.
45. Bennish ML, Salam MA, Khan WA, et al. Treatment of shigellosis. III. Comparison of one or two doses ciprofloxacin with standard 5-day therapy: a randomized, blinded trial. *Ann Intern Med* 1992;117:727–734.
46. Khan WA, Seas C, Dhar U, et al. Treatment of shigellosis. V. Comparison of azithromycin and ciprofloxacin. A double-blind, randomized, controlled trial. *Ann Intern Med* 1997;126:697–703.
47. Black RE, Slome S. *Yersinia enterocolitica. Infect Dis Clin North Am* 1988;2:625–641.
48. Cover TL, Aber RC. *Yersinia enterocolitica. N Engl J Med* 1989;321:16–24.
49. Lee LA, Taylor J, et al. *Yersinia enterocolitica* O:3: an emerging cause of pediatric gastroenteritis in the United States. *J Infect Dis* 1991;163:660–663.
50. Gayraud M, Scavizzi MR, Mollaret HH, et al. Antibiotic treatment of *Yersinia enterocolitica* septicemia: a retrospective review of 43 cases. *Clin Infect Dis* 1993;17:405–410.
51. Allos BM, Blaser MJ. *Campylobacter jejuni* and the expanding spectrum of related infections. *Clin Infect Dis* 1995;20:1092–1101.
52. Allos BM. *Campylobacter jejuni* infections: update on emerging issues and trends. *Clin Infect Dis* 2001;32:1201–1206.
53. Smith KE, Besser JM, Hedberg CW, et al. Quinolone-resistant *Campylobacter jejuni* infections in Minnesota, 1992–1998. *N Engl J Med* 1999;340:1525–1532.
54. Centers for Disease Control Prevention. Update: multi-state outbreak of *Escherichia coli* O157:H7 infections from hamburgers—Western United States, 1992–1993. *MMWR* 1993;42:258–263.
55. Tarr PI. *Escherichia coli* 0157:117: clinical, diagnostic and epidemiologic aspects of human infection. *Clin Infect Dis* 1995;20:1–10.
56. Swerdlow DL, Woodruff BA, Brady RC, et al. A waterborne outbreak in Missouri of *Escherichia coli* O157:H7 associated with bloody diarrhea and death. *Ann Intern Med* 1992;117:812–819.
57. Boyce TG, Swerdlow DL, Griffin PM. *Escherichia coli* O157:H7 and the hemolytic uremic syndrome. *N Engl J Med* 1995;333:364–368.
58. Centers for Disease Control and Prevention. *Escherichia coli* O157:H7 outbreak linked to home-cooked hamburger—California, July 1993. *MMWR* 1994;43:213–216.
59. Tarr PI, Neill MA. *Escherichia coli* O157:H7. *Gastroenterol Clin North Am* 2001;30:735–751.
60. Belongia EA, Osterholm MT, Soler JT, et al. Transmission of *Escherichia coli* 0157:H7 infection in Minnesota child day-care facilities. *JAMA* 1993;269:883–888.

61. Slutsker L, Ries AA, Maloney K, et al. A nationwide case-control study of *Escherichia coli* O157:H7 infection in the United States. *J Infect Dis* 1998;177:962–966.
62. Zimmerhackl LB. *E. coli,* antibiotics, and the hemolytic-uremic syndrome. *N Engl J Med* 2000;342:1990–1991.
63. Holmberg SD. *Vibrios* and *Aeromonas. Infect Dis Clin North Am* 1988;2:655–676.
64. Hlady WG, Klontz KC. The epidemiology of *Vibrio* infections in Florida, 1981–1993. *J Infect Dis* 1996;173:1176–1183.
65. Hellinger WC, Alvarez S. Cholera in the United States. *Dig Dis* 1995;13:190–198.
66. Raufman JP. Cholera. *Am J Med* 1998;104:386–394.
67. Mathewson JJ, Dupont HL. Aeromonas species: role as human pathogens. *Curr Clin Top Infect Dis* 1992;12:26–36.
68. Jones BL, Wilcox MH. *Aeromonas* infections and their treatment. *J Antimicrob Chemother* 1995;35:453–461.
69. Centers for Disease Control and Prevention. *Plesiomonas shigelloides* and *Salmonella* serotype Hartford infections associated with a contaminated water supply—Livingston County, New York, 1996. *MMWR* 1998;47:394–396.
70. Soweid AM, Clarkston WK. *Plesiomonas shigelloides:* an unusual cause of diarrhea. *Am J Gastroenterol* 1995;90:2235–2236.
71. Centers for Disease Control and Prevention. Viral agents of gastroenteritis: public health importance and outbreak management. *MMWR* 1990;39:1–24.
72. Blacklow NR, Greenberg HB. Viral gastroenteritis. *N Engl J Med* 1991;325:252–263.
73. Goodgame RW. Viral causes of diarrhea. *Gastroenterol Clin North Am* 2001;30:779–795.
74. Hamer DH, Gorbach SL. Viral diarrhea. In: Feldman, ed. *Sleisenger & Fordtran's gastrointestinal and liver disease,* 6th ed. Philadelphia: WB Saunders, 1998:1614–1616.
75. Dennehy PH, Bresee JS. Rotavirus vaccine and intussusception. Where do we go from here? *Infect Dis Clin North Am* 2001;15:189–207.
76. American Academy of Pediatrics. Rotavirus infections. In: *2000 Red Book: Report of the Committee on Infectious Diseases,* 25th ed. Elk Grove Village, IL: American Academy of Pediatrics, 2000:493–495.
77. Glass RI, Noel J, Ando T, et al. The epidemiology of enteric caliciviruses from humans: a reassessment using new diagnostics. *J Infect Dis* 2000;181(suppl):254–261.
78. Centers for Disease Control and Prevention. Norwalk-like viruses: public health consequences and outbreak management. *MMWR* 2001;50:1–17.
79. Blaser MJ. *Helicobacter pylori* and related organisms. In: Mandell GL, Bennett JE, Dolin R, eds. *Principles and practice of infectious diseases,* 5th ed. New York: Churchill Livingstone, 2000:2285–2293.
80. Howden CW, Hunt RH. Guidelines for the management of *Helicobacter pylori* infection. Ad Hoc Committee on Practice Parameters of the American College of Gastroenterology. *Am J Gastroenterol* 1998;93:2330–2338.
81. Walsh JH, Peterson WL. The treatment of *Helicobacter pylori* infection in the management of peptic ulcer disease. *N Engl J Med* 1995;333:984–991.
82. National Institutes of Health Consensus Development Panel on *Helicobacter pylori* in Peptic Ulcer Disease. *Helicobacter pylori* in peptic ulcer disease. *JAMA* 1994;272:65–69.
83. Soll AH, for the Practice Parameters Committee of the American College of Gastroenterology. Medical treatment of peptic ulcer disease: practice guidelines. *JAMA* 1996;275:622–629.
84. Nomura A, Stemmermann GN, Chyou PH, et al. *Helicobacter pylori* infection and the risk for duodenal and gastric ulceration. *Ann Intern Med* 1994;120:977–981.
85. Everhart JE. Recent developments in the epidemiology of *Helicobacter pylori. Gastroenterol Clin North Am* 2000;29:559–578.
86. Cohen H. Peptic ulcer and *Helicobacter pylori. Gastroenterology Clin North Am* 2000;29:775–789.
87. Graham DY, Lew GM, Klein PD, et al. Effect of treatment of *Helicobacter pylori* infection on the long-term recurrence of gastric or duodenal ulcer. A randomized, controlled study. *Ann Intern Med* 1992;116:705–708.
88. Graham DY, Klein PD. Accurate diagnosis of *Helicobacter pylori*. 13C-urea breath test. *Gastroenterol Clin North Am* 2000;29:885–893.

89. Bytzer P, Talley NJ. Dyspepsia. *Ann Intern Med* 2001;134:815–822.
90. McColl KE, Murray LS, Gillen D, et al. Randomized trial of endoscopy with testing for *Helicobacter pylori* compared with non-invasive *H pylori* testing alone in the management of dyspepsia. *Br Med J* 2002;324:999–1002.
91. Uemura N, Okamoto S, Yamamoto S, et al. *Helicobacter pylori* infection and the development of gastric cancer. *N Engl J Med* 2001;345:784–789.
92. Talley NJ, Vakil N, Ballard ED 2nd, et al. Absence of benefit of eradicating *Helicobacter pylori* in patients with nonulcer dyspepsia. *N Engl J Med* 1999;341:1106–1111.
93. Laine L, Schoenfeld P, Fennerty MB. Therapy for *Helicobacter pylori* in patients with nonulcer dyspepsia. A meta-analysis of randomized, controlled trials. *Ann Intern Med* 2001;134:361–369.
94. Graham DY. Therapy of *Helicobacter pylori:* current status and issues. *Gastroenterology* 2000;118(suppl):2–8.
95. Medical Letter. Drugs for treatment of peptic ulcers. *Med Lett Drugs Ther* 1997;39:1–4.
96. Neva FA. *Basic clinical parasitology,* 6th ed. New York:Appleton & Lange, 1994.
97. Katz DE, Taylor DN. Parasitic infections of the gastrointestinal tract. *Gastroenterol Clin North Am* 2001;30:797–815.
98. Maguire JH, Keystone JS, eds. Parasitic diseases. *Infect Dis Clin North Am* 1993;7:467–738.
99. Morris AJ, Murray PR, Reller LB. Contemporary testing for enteric pathogens: the potential for cost, time, and health care savings. *J Clin Microbiol* 1996;34:1776–1778.
100. Kappus KD, Lundgren RG Jr, Juranek DD, et al. Intestinal parasitism in the United States: update on a continuing problem. *Am J Trop Med Hyg* 1994;50:705–713.
101. Hill DR. *Giardia lamblia.* In: Mandell GL, Bennett JE, Dolin R, eds. *Principles and practice of infectious diseases,* 5th ed. New York: Churchill Livingstone, 2000:2888–2894.
102. Center for Disease Control and Prevention. Giardiasis surveillance United States, 1992–1997. CDC Surveillance Summaries. *MMWR* 2000;49:1–13.
103. Ortega YR, Adam RD. *Giardia:* overview and update. *Clin Infect Dis* 1997;25:545–550.
104. Aucott JN, Ravdin JI. Amebiasis and "nonpathogenic" intestinal protozoa. *Infect Dis Clin North Am* 1993;7:467–485.
105. Guerrant RL. Cryptosporidiosis: an emerging, highly infectious threat. *Emerg Infect Dis* 1997;3:51–57.
106. Juranek DD. Cryptosporidiosis: sources of infection and guidelines for prevention. *Clin Infect Dis* 1995;21(suppl 1):57–61.
107. Centers for Disease Control and Prevention. Protracted outbreaks of cryptosporidiosis associated with swimming pool use—Ohio and Nebraska, 2000. *MMWR* 2001;50:406–410.
108. Centers for Disease Control and Prevention. Surveillance for waterborne-disease outbreaks—United States, 1997–1998. *MMWR* 2000;49:1–35.
109. MacKenzie WR, Hoxie NJ, Proctor ME, et al. A massive outbreak in Milwaukee of *Cryptosporidium* infection transmitted through the public water supply. *N Engl J Med* 1994;331:161–167.
110. Senay H, MacPherson D. *Blastocystis hominis:* epidemiology and natural history. *J Infect Dis* 1990;162:987–990.
111. Udkow MP, Markell EK. *Blastocystis hominis:* prevalence in asymptomatic versus symptomatic hosts. *J Infect Dis* 1993;168:242–244.
112. Stenzel DJ, Boreham PF. *Blastocystis hominis* revisited. *Microbiol Rev* 1996;9:563–584.
113. Wittmann DH, Walker AP, Condon RE. Peritonitis and intra-abdominal infection. In: Schwartz SI, et al., eds. *Principles of surgery,* 6th ed. New York: McGraw-Hill, 1994:1449.
114. Gorbach SL. Treatment of intra-abdominal infections. *J Antimicrob Chemother* 1993;31(suppl A):67.
115. McClean KI, et al. Intra-abdominal infection: a review. *Clin Infect Dis* 1994;19:100.
116. Elsakr R, Johnson DA, Younges Z, et al. Antimicrobial treatment of intra-abdominal infections. *Dig Dis* 1998;16:47–60.
117. Gorbach SL. Intra-abdominal infections. *Clin Infect Dis* 1993;17:961.

118. Bartlett J. Intra-abdominal sepsis. *Med Clin North Am* 1995;79:599.
119. Feliciano DV, Gentry LO, Bitondo CG, et. al. Single agent prophylaxis for penetrating abdominal trauma. Results and comments on emergence of enterococcus. *Am J Surg* 1986;152:674–681.
120. Brismar B, Malmborg AS, Tunevall G, et al. Piperacillin-tazobactam versus imipenem-cilastatin for treatment of intra-abdominal infections. *Antimicrob Agents Chemother* 1992;36:2766–2773.
121. Solomkin JS, Reinhart HH, Dellinger EP, et al. Results of randomized trial comparing sequential i.v./oral treatment with ciprofloxacin plus metronidazole to imipenem/cilastatin for intra-abdominal infection. The Intra-Abdominal Infection Study Group. *Ann Surg* 1996;223:303–315.
122. Solomkin JS, Dellinger EP, Christou NV, et al. Results of a multicenter trial comparing imipenem/cilastatin to tobramycin/clindamycin for intra-abdominal infections. *Ann Surg* 1990;212:581–591.
123. Solomkin JS, et al. Ertapenem versus piperacillin/tazobactam in appendiceal related and other intra-abdominal abscesses [Abstract P1460]. *Clin Microbiol Infect Dis* 2001;7(suppl 1):314.
124. Ho JL, Barza M. Role of aminoglycoside antibiotics in the treatment of intra-abdominal infection. *Antimicrob Agents Chemother* 1987;31:485.
125. Brismar B, Nord CE. Monobactams and carapenems for treatment of intra-abdominal infections. *Infection* 1999;27:136–147.
126. Barie PS, Christou NV, Dellinger EP, et al. Pathogenicity of enterococcus in surgical infection. *Ann Surg* 1990;212:155–159.
127. Laroche M, Harding G. Primary and secondary peritonitis: an update. *Eur J Clin Micro Infect Dis* 1998;17:542–550.
128. Such J, Runyon BA. Spontaneous bacterial peritonitis. *Clin Infect Dis* 1998;27:669–676.
129. Yu AS, Hu KO. Management of ascites. *Clin Liver Dis* 2001;5:541–568.
130. Chang CS, Yang SS, Kao CH, et al. Small intestinal overgrowth versus antimicrobial capacity in patients with spontaneous bacterial peritonitis. *Scand J Gastroenterol* 2001;36:92–96.
131. Terg R, Cobas S, Fassio E, et al. Oral ciprofloxacin after a short course of i.v. ciprofloxacin in the treatment of spontaneous bacterial peritonitis: results of a randomized study. *J Hepatol* 2000;33:564–569.
132. Ljubicic N, Spajic D, Vrkljan MM, et al. The value of ascitic fluid polymorphonuclear cell count determination during therapy of spontaneous bacterial peritonitis. *Hepato-gastroenterology* 2000;47:1360–1363.
133. Singh N, et al. Trimethoprim-sulfamethoxazole for the prevention of spontaneous bacterial peritonitis in cirrhosis: a randomized trial. *Ann Intern Med* 1995;122: 595.
134. Bernard B, Grange JD, Khac EN, et al. Antibiotic prophylaxis for the prevention of bacterial infections in cirrhotic patients with gastrointestinal bleeding: a meta analysis. *Hepatology* 1999;29:1655–1661.
135. Rolachon A, Cordier L, Bacq Y, et al. Ciprofloxacin and long term prevention of spontaneous bacterial peritonitis: results of a prospective controlled trial. *Hepatology* 1995;22:1171–1175.
136. Peterson PK, et al. Current concepts in the management of peritonitis in patients undergoing continuous ambulatory peritoneal dialysis. *Rev Infect Dis* 1987;9:604.
137. Vas SI. Infections of continuous ambulatory peritoneal dialysis catheters. *Infect Dis Clin North Am* 1989;3:301.
138. The Ad Hoc Advisory Committee on Peritonitis Management. Peritoneal dialysis related peritonitis treatment recommendations, 1993 update. *Perit Dial Int* 1993;13:14.
139. Murray HW. Secondary peritonitis and intra-abdominal abscess. *Hosp Pract* 1990; 25:101.
140. Krisher SL, Browne A, Dibbins A, et al. Intra-abdominal abscess after laproscopic appendectomy for perforated appendix. *Arch Surg* 2001;136:438–441.
141. Memon MA, Deeik RK, Maffi TR, et al. The outcome of un-retrieved gallstones in the peritoneal cavity during laproscopic cholecystectomy. A prospective analysis. *Surg Endosc* 1999;13:848–857.

142. Tsai SC, Chao TH, Lin WY, et al. Abdominal abscesses in patients having surgery: an application of Ga-67 scintigraphic and computed graphic scanning. *Clin Nucl Med* 2001;26:761–764.
143. Garcia JC, Persky SE, Bonis PA, et al. Abscesses in Crohn's disease: outcome of medical versus surgical disease. *J Clin Gastroenterol* 2001;32:409–412.
144. vanSonnenberg E, Wittich GR, Goodacre BW, et. al. Percutaneous abscess drainage: update. *World J Surg* 2001;25:362–369.
145. Stain SC, et al. Pyogenic liver abscess: modern treatment. *Arch Surg* 1991;126:991.
146. Barnes PF, et al. A comparison of amebic and pyogenic abscess of the liver. *Medicine* 1987;66:472.
147. Alvarez Perez JA, Gonzalez JJ, Baldonero RF, et al. Clinical course, treatment, and multivariate analysis of risk factors for pyogenic liver abscess. *Am J Surg* 2001;181:177–186.
148. Alvarez JA, Gonzalez JJ, Baldonero RF, et al. Single and multiple pyogenic liver abscess: etiology, clinical course, and outcome. *Dig Surg* 2001;18:283–288.
149. Hughes MA, Petri WA Jr. Amebic liver abscess. *Infect Dis Clin North Am* 2000;14:565–582.
150. Chiu CH, Su LH, Wu TL, et al. Liver abscess caused by *Klebsiella pneumoniae* in siblings. *J Clin Microbiol* 2001;39:2351–2353.
151. Chua D, Reinhart HH, Sobel J. Liver abscess caused by *Streptococcus milleri. Rev Infect Dis* 1989;11:197.
152. Sabbaj J. Anaerobes in liver abscess. *Rev Infect Dis* 1984;6(suppl 1):152.
153. Bak SY, et al. Therapeutic percutaneous aspiration of hepatic abscesses: effectiveness in 25 patients. *AJR* 1993;160:799.
154. Hansen N, Vargish T. Pyogenic hepatic abscess: a case for open drainage. *Am Surg* 1993;59:219.
155. Chun CH et al. Splenic abscess. *Medicine* 1980;59:50.
156. Nelken N et al. Changing clinical spectrum of splenic abscess: a multicenter study and review of the literature. *Am J Surg* 1987;154:27.
157. Alonso Cohen MA et al. Splenic abscess. *World J Surg* 1990;14:513. [Reviews 227 cases from the world literature plus 7 of the authors' cases. Report from Spain.]
158. Westh H, Reines E, Skibsted L. Splenic abscess: a review of 20 cases. *Scand J Infect Dis* 1990;22:569.
159. Ho HS, Wisner DH. Splenic abscess in the intensive care unit. *Arch Surg* 1993; 128:842.
160. Hadas-Halpren I, Hiller N, Dolberg M. Percutaneous drainage of splenic abscesses: an effective and safe procedure. *Br J Radiol* 1992;65:968.
161. Altemeier WA, Alexander JW. Retroperitoneal abscess. *Arch Surg* 1961;83:512.
162. Crepps JTWelch JP. Orlando R III. Management and outcome of retroperitoneal abscesses. *Ann Surg* 1987;205:276.
163. Sacks D et al. Renal and related retroperitoneal abscess: percutaneous drainage. *Radiology* 1988;167:447.
164. Leu SY et al. Psoas abscess: changing patterns of diagnosis and etiology. *Dis Colon Rectum* 1986;29:694.
165. Bresee JS, Edwards MS. Psoas abscess in children. *Pediatr Infect Dis J* 1990;9:201.
166. Greenwald I, Abrahamson J, Cohen O. Psoas abscess: case report and review of the literature. *J Urol* 1992;147:1624.
167. Schwartz SI. Appendix. In: Schwartz SI, et al., eds. *Principles of surgery,* 6th ed. New York: McGraw-Hill, 1994:1307.
168. Bauer T, et al. Antibiotic prophylaxis in acute non-perforated appendicitis: the Danish Multicenter Study Group III. *Ann Surg* 1989;209:307.
169. Nylander WA Jr. The acute abdomen in the immunocompromised host. *Surg Clin North Am* 1988;68:457.
170. Goodgame RW. Gastrointestinal cytomegalovirus disease. *Ann Intern Med* 1993; 119:924.
171. Coyle CM, Wittner M, Kotler DP, et al. Prevalence of microsporidiosis due to *Enterocytozoon bieneusi* and *Encephalitozoon intestinalis* among patients with AIDS related diarrhea: determination by polymerase chain reaction to the midrosporidian small subunit rRNA gene. *Clin Infect Dis* 1996;23:1002–1006.

172. Enriquez FJ, Taren D, Cruz-L'opez A, et al. Prevalence of intestinal encephalitozoonosis in Mexico. *Clin Infect Dis* 1198;26:1227–1229.
173. Freeman SR, McNally PR. Diverticulitis. *Med Clin North Am* 1993;77:1149–1167.
174. Schoetz DJ. Uncomplicated diverticulitis: indications for surgery and surgical management. *Surg Clin North Am* 1993;73:965.
175. Kellum JM, Sugerman HJ. Randomized, prospective comparison of cefoxitin and gentamicin-clindamycin in the treatment of acute colonic diverticulitis. *Clin Ther* 1992;14:376.
176. Roslyn JJ, Zinner MJ. Gallbladder and extrahepatic biliary system. In: Schwartz SI, et al., eds. *Principles of surgery,* 6th ed. New York: McGraw-Hill, 1994:1367.
177. Cooperberg PI, Gibney RG. Imaging of the gallbladder. *Radiology* 1987;163:605.
178. Marton KI, Doubilet P. How to image the gallbladder in suspected cholecystitis. *Ann Intern Med* 1988;109:722.
179. Williams RA, Kourtesis G, Wilson SE. Cholecystitis and cholangitis. In: Gorbach SL, Bartlett JG, Blacklow NR, eds. *Infectious diseases.* Philadelphia: WB Saunders, 1992:736.
180. Brook I. Aerobic and anaerobic microbiology of biliary tract disease. *J Clin Microbiol* 1989;27:2373.
181. Kadaskia SC. Biliary tract emergencies: acute cholecystitis, acute cholangitis, and acute pancreatitis. *Med Clin North Am* 1993;77:1015.
182. Glenn F, Becker CG. Acute acalculous cholecystitis: an increasing entity. *Ann Surg* 1982;195:131.
183. Frazee RC, Nagorney DM, Mucha P Jr. Acute acalculous cholecystitis. *Mayo Clin Proc* 1989;64:163.
184. Hanau LH, Steigbigel NH. Cholangitis: pathogenesis, diagnosis, and treatment. *Curr Clin Top Infect Dis* 1995;15:153.
185. Huang T, Bass JA, Williams RD. The significance of biliary pressure in cholangitis. *Arch Surg* 1969;98:629.
186. Welch JP, Donaldson GA. The urgency of diagnosis and surgical treatment of acute suppurative cholangitis. *Am J Surg* 1976;131:527.
187. Jolly BT, Love JN. Emphysematous cholecystitis in an elderly woman: case report and review of the literature. *J Emerg Med* 1993;11:593.
188. Deviere J, et al. Septicemia after endoscopic retrograde cholangiopancreatography. *Endoscopy* 1990;22:72.
189. Calleja GA, Barkin JS. Acute pancreatitis. *Med Clin North Am* 1993;77:1037.
190. Steinberg W, Termer S. Acute pancreatitis. *N Engl J Med* 1994;330:1198.
191. Lee SP, Nicholls JF, Park HZ. Biliary sludge as a cause of acute pancreatitis. *N Engl J Med* 1992;326:589.
192. Frey CF. Management of necrotizing pancreatitis. *West J Med* 1993;159:675.
193. Reber HA, McFadden DW. Indications for surgery in necrotizing pancreatitis. *West J Med* 1993;159:704.
194. Buchler M, et al. Human pancreatic tissue concentrations of bactericidal antibiotics. *Gastroenterology* 1992;103:1902.
195. Bradley EL III. Antibiotics in acute pancreatitis: current and future directions. *Am J Surg* 1989;158:472.
196. Pederzoli P, et al. A randomized multicenter clinical trial of antibiotic prophylaxis of septic complications in acute necrotizing pancreatitis with imipenem. *Surg Gynecol Obstet* 1993;176:480.
197. Slavin J, Neoptolemos JP. Antibiotic prophylaxis in severe pancreatitis. What are the facts? *Langenbecks Arch Surg* 2001;386:155–159.
198. Bassi C, Mangiante G, Falconi M, et al. Prophylaxis for septic complications of acute necrotizing pancreatitis. *J Hepatobil Pancreat Surg* 2001;8:211–215.
199. Ratschko M, Fenner T, Lankisch PG. The role of antibiotic prophylaxis in acute pancreatitis. *Gastroenterol Clin North Am* 1999;28:641–659, ix–x.
200. Sharma VK, Howden CW. Prophylactic antibiotic administration reduces sepsis and mortality in acute necrotizing pancreatitis: a meta analysis. *Pancreas* 2001;22:28–31.
201. Warshaw AL, Gongliang J. Improved survival in patients with pancreatic abscess. *Ann Surg* 1985;202:408.

202. Reber HA. Pancreas. In: Schwartz SI, et al., eds. *Principles of surgery,* 6th ed. New York: McGraw-Hill, 1994:1412–1413.
203. Witt MD, Edwards JE Jr. Pancreatic abscess and infected pancreatic pseudocyst: diagnosis and treatment. *Curr Clin Top Infect Dis* 1992;12:111.
204. McClave SA, et al. Pancreatic abscess: 10-year experience at the University of South Florida. *Am J Gastroenterol* 1986;81:180.
205. Fink AS, et al. Indolent presentation of pancreatic abscess: experience with 100 cases. *Arch Surg* 1988;123:1087.
206. Altemeier WA, Alexander JW. Pancreatic abscess. *Arch Surg* 1963;87:80.
207. Mullins RJ, et al. Controversies in the management of pancreatic pseudocysts. *Am J Surg* 1988;155:165.

## 14. HEPATITIS VIRUSES

James R. Burton, Jr. and Thomas A. Shaw-Stiffel

**I. Introduction.** Hepatitis denotes an inflammation of the liver. The causes of hepatitis are varied and include viruses, bacteria, protozoa, drugs, toxins, and autoimmune disease. The clinical symptoms and course can be similar regardless of the etiology.

**A. Hepatitis viruses.** Viral hepatitis is the most common cause of chronic liver disease (Table 14.1).

1. **Hepatitis A virus (HAV),** also referred to as "infectious hepatitis."
2. **Hepatitis B virus (HBV),** also known as "serum hepatitis."
3. **Hepatitis C virus (HCV),** formerly known as "non-A, non-B hepatitis."
4. **Hepatitis D virus (HDV),** also known as the "delta agent," requires coinfection with HBV.
5. **Hepatitis E virus (HEV),** similar to HAV in many respects but with a different geographic distribution.

**B. Systemic viral illnesses with a hepatitis-like component**

1. **Epstein-Barr virus** (see Chapter 9)
2. **Cytomegalovirus** (see Chapter 9)
3. **Yellow fever virus** (see Chapter 22)
4. **Varicella-zoster virus** (see Chapter 20)
5. **Herpes simplex virus** (see Chapter 20)
6. **Miscellaneous** (e.g., rubella, rubeola, Coxsackie B virus, adenovirus, etc.)

**C. Nonviral etiologies**

1. **Infectious hepatitis** (e.g., toxoplasmosis and leptospirosis)
2. **Alcoholic hepatitis**
3. **Nonalcoholic steatohepatitis**
4. **Drug-induced hepatitis** (e.g., acetaminophen, halothane, isoniazid)
5. **Toxin-induced hepatitis** (e.g., mushrooms, phosphorus, carbon tetrachloride)
6. **Autoimmune hepatitis**

**II. Approach to viral hepatitis.** Determining the specific etiologic agent of viral hepatitis depends primarily on the patient's epidemiologic setting and clinical history, as well as the use of laboratory tests to detect specific viruses and rule out other causes.

**III. HAV**

**A. Classification and structure.** HAV is a picornavirus with a nonenveloped single-stranded RNA strand and a diameter of 27 nm. Humans are the natural hosts.

**B. Epidemiology**

1. Transmission occurs almost always via the fecal–oral route, either sporadically or in epidemics after ingestion of contaminated food, water, or milk. Uncooked shellfish (e.g., clams, mussels, and oysters) from contaminated water are a common source. Fecal shedding of HAV can last for months after resolution of symptoms, and such patients could be a source of further viral spread in the community [1].
2. HAV is found worldwide with the highest prevalence in regions with low standards of sanitation, where asymptomatic infections occur early in life. As sanitation standards improve exposure is reduced, thus increasing the risk of acquiring HAV if exposed later in life when the clinical course can be more complicated.
3. Parenteral transmission is rare. Although roughly paralleling viral levels in the stool, systemic viremia is 100- to 1,000-fold lower in magnitude [2]. Viremia is likely the source of HAV spread among illicit intravenous drug users and hemophiliacs receiving solvent-detergent inactivated factor VIII preparations.
4. Sexual transmission is not a significant problem. However, men who have sex with men, especially those with oral–anal sexual contact, are at increased risk.

**C. Pathogenesis**

1. After HAV is ingested, it first replicates within the crypt cells of the small intestine before entering the bloodstream to spread to the liver.
2. HAV then enters the hepatocyte, sheds its coat, and initiates viral replication. The resulting new viral particles are released into the bile.

Table 14.1. Review of Viral Hepatitis

| | Hepatitis A | Hepatitis B | Hepatitis C | Hepatitis D | Hepatitis E |
|---|---|---|---|---|---|
| Genome | RNA | DNA | RNA | RNA | RNA |
| Route of infection | Predominately fecal–oral | Parenteral, sexual, and perinatal | Parenteral | Parenteral (requires co-infection with HBV) | Fecal–oral |
| Endemic areas | Low standards of sanitation | SE Asia, China, sub-Saharan Africa | Worldwide | Northern S. America Mediterranean region | Middle East, India northern Africa |
| Incubation | 15–50 days (mean 30) | 1–4 mo | 2–12 weeks (mean 7) | 1–4 mo | 15–60 days (mean 40) |
| Vaccination available | Yes | Yes | No | Yes, if vaccinated against HBV | No |
| Diagnosis | Anti-HAV IgM | HepBsAg | Anti-HCV and HCV RNA by PCR | Anti-HDV in HepBsAg positive patient | Anti-HEV |
| Chronic hepatitis | No | Yes | Yes | Yes, requires HBV infection | No |
| Treatment | None needed | Interferon and Lamivudine | Interferon with/without ribavirin | High dose interferon | None needed |

3. Hepatocyte necrosis is thought to occur via cell-mediated immunity in response to viral antigens expressed by hepatocytes rather than by direct cytopathic damage [3].
4. HAV may be found in the stool for 2 weeks before the onset of jaundice and then 1 week afterward [4]. Fecal shedding of HAV reaches its height just before the onset of hepatocellular disease, at which point the patient is also maximally infectious.

**D. Clinical disease**

1. HAV results in a wide range of clinical manifestations, from subclinical infection, to overt infections with or without jaundice, to acute liver failure and death. However, most cases are self-limited.
2. The mean incubation period of 15 to 50 days (mean, 30 days) [5] is followed by the acute onset of malaise, anorexia, nausea, vomiting, abdominal pain, and fever, all of which characterize "symptomatic" disease. Symptoms can last up to a week in jaundiced patients. Cigarette smokers tend to lose interest in smoking.
3. The liver can be enlarged and tender. Serum aminotransferases (alanine aminotransferase [ALT] and aspartate aminotransferase [AST]) are elevated during the symptomatic phase followed by an elevated total bilirubin.
4. Age at acquisition of HAV is a major determinant of the severity of illness [6]. Symptomatic icteric hepatitis occurs in most infected adults but is less common in children and rare under the age of 2. Jaundice is associated with symptomatic improvement. Jaundice typically resolves after 2 weeks.
5. Fulminant HAV is relatively rare, yielding about 100 deaths each year in the United States [6]. The risk increases with advancing age, especially over the age of 40.
6. Patients with chronic hepatitis B and C who acquire acute HAV may be more likely to have an adverse outcome, including fulminant hepatitis [7,8].
7. A small proportion of patients may develop a protracted, but usually self-limited, cholestatic phase after the acute illness. Short-course corticosteroids may help [9].
8. A tiny percentage of patients experience recurrent signs and symptoms of acute HAV [9]. This is self-limited, and full recovery is invariably the case.

**E. Diagnosis**

1. The diagnosis of acute HAV is made by detecting IgM-specific antibody to the virus (anti-HAV-IgM). This antibody is present before symptom onset. It peaks during the acute phase and becomes undetectable in most cases by 6 months, except in those with relapsing hepatitis in whom it usually remains present throughout the course.
2. The presence of IgG-specific antibody to the virus (anti-HAV-IgG) indicates either prior HAV infection or vaccination against HAV. This also implies protection if exposed once again to HAV. The level of this antibody peaks during the convalescent period and remains detectable for many years.

**F. Management.** Currently, there is no specific treatment for HAV other than supportive care. Corticosteroids are often helpful for the prolonged cholestatic form of HAV. Any patient with severe symptoms and/or signs of acute HAV should be monitored closely for a prolongation of the prothrombin time and/or the onset of hepatic encephalopathy, both of which suggest acute liver failure [10]. These should prompt early transplant referral.

**G. Passive immunization**

1. Passive immunization remains the intervention of choice for postexposure prophylaxis. Antibody response after active immunization (see below) takes 2 weeks to develop fully and does not provide effective early protection.
2. Because a substantial proportion of the population has been infected with HAV, pooled lots of gamma globulin (human immunoglobulin [HIG]) contain sufficient antibody for this purpose.
3. A single dose of HIG, 0.02 mL/kg in the gluteus muscle, confers immunity that lasts up to 6 months [9]. This is recommended for those exposed (or potentially exposed) to HAV who have no prior history of HAV infection.

4. Candidates for prophylaxis include household contacts of those with acute HAV, those known to have eaten uncooked food prepared by an infected individual, and those who will be traveling to at-risk areas of the world within 2 weeks, time insufficient for active HAV immunization.
5. Once clinical symptoms of HAV infection have developed, the patient is already producing antibody, and the administration of IG is not indicated.
6. It is important to note that the simultaneous administration of active and passive immunization reduces the ultimate antibody level by 50%.

**H. Active immunization**

1. Two recombinant inactivated HAV vaccines (Havrix, GlaxoSmithKline, Research Triangle Park, NC, and VAQTA, Merck, Whitehouse Station, NJ) have been available in the United States since 1995 and 1996, respectively. Both vaccines have been shown to be safe and effective. After vaccination, the levels of protective antibody approach the levels seen after natural HAV infection. A combination hepatitis A and B vaccine (Twinrix, GlaxoSmithKline) was approved in the United States in 2001.
2. The current HAV vaccine schedule involves an initial dose followed by a booster 6 to 12 months later. The vaccines are safe in children over the age of 2 years. Their safety in pregnancy is not known.
3. The following should receive HAV vaccination: children living in areas of the United States where the rates of HAV infection are at least two times the national average (e.g., ≥20 cases per 100,000 population), persons traveling to countries with intermediate endemicity, men who have sex with men, persons with clotting disorders, persons who use illegal drugs, and personnel in HAV research laboratories [11].
4. Side effects of vaccine include injection site soreness, erythema, and induration. Systemic reactions, including fever, occur in less than 5% of subjects.
5. Patients with chronic liver disease due to HBV and HCV should also be vaccinated, because they are at risk of more severe disease if they contract HAV [7]. Seroconversion rates after two doses of the HAV vaccine are the same in these individuals as in healthy subjects [12]. However, efficacy of vaccination in patients with advanced cirrhosis and in liver transplant recipients is currently unknown.

## IV. HBV

**A. Classification and structure**

1. HBV is a DNA virus that belongs to the family of hepadnaviruses. The intact virion (or Dane particle) is a 42-nm sphere that contains the nucleocapsid, with its DNA of approximately 3,200 base pairs. HBV replicates via an RNA intermediate using viral-encoded reverse transcriptase.
2. The HBV genome consists of four open reading frames encoding for the surface envelope (pre-S/S), core (pre-core/core), polymerase, and X proteins. The S open reading frame encodes for the viral envelope protein, hepatitis B surface antigen (HBsAg), the hallmark of HBV infection. The X protein is crucial for viral life cycle *in vivo* and probably functions by interacting with multiple cellular pathways.
3. Seven genotypes of HBV (A through G) have been identified. Currently, there are insufficient data to correlate differences in clinical outcomes or responses to treatment with genotype.

**B. Epidemiology**

1. Worldwide, close to 400 million people are infected with HBV [13]. In the United States, HBV infection causes 5% to 10% of chronic liver disease and cirrhosis [14].
2. The distribution of HBV infection varies greatly throughout the world. Areas with the highest prevalence include southeast Asia, China, and sub-Saharan Africa, where approximately 10% of the population are chronic carriers [14]. Intermediate prevalence areas (3%–5%) include Mediterranean countries, Japan, Central Asia, the Middle East, Latin and South America, and indigenous population groups in the Arctic [15]. Low prevalence areas (0.1%–2%) include the United States, Canada, western Europe, Australia, and New Zealand [16].
3. The wide range of carrier rates in different parts of the world relates primarily to the individual's age at time of infection. The rate of progression to chronic

hepatitis approximates 90% for perinatally acquired infection, 20% to 50% for infection between the ages of 1 and 5 years, and less than 5% for infection acquired in adulthood [15].

4. Most infections in developed countries occur as a result of sexual activity, intravenous drug use, or occupational exposure. Less common causes include household contact, hemodialysis, and recipients of solid organs or blood products. No clear risk factors are identified in 20% to 30% of infected individuals [13].

**C. Serologic markers of HBV infection**

1. **HBsAg** is the hallmark of HBV infection. It is usually detectable 1 to 10 weeks after acute infection and 2 to 6 weeks before clinical symptoms. Patients who recover from acute infection clear HBsAg within 4 to 6 months. Persistence of HBsAg for more than 6 months implies chronic infection.
2. **Hepatitis B surface antibody (anti-HBs)** is a neutralizing antibody that confers protective immunity against HBV. Anti-HBs is found in patients who have recovered from HBV infection or responded to HBV vaccination.
3. **Hepatitis B core antigen** is the nucleocapsid that encloses the viral DNA. It is an intracellular antigen, not detected in the serum.
4. **Hepatitis B core antibody (anti-HBc).** Anti-HBc-IgM develops initially and appears within 1 month after HBsAg. Anti-HBc-IgG develops later and is found in association with anti-HBs in those who have recovered from hepatitis B or with HBsAg in chronic HBV, between the disappearance of HBsAg and the development of anti-HBs, and for many years after recovery of acute HBV. Transmission of HBV occurs via organ donors with isolated anti-HBc.
5. **Hepatitis B e antigen (HBeAg)** signifies HBV replication and infectivity. HBeAg is a peptide derived from the core gene, modified and exported from the cell. It is associated with serum HBV DNA. In the recovery phase of infection, HBeAg is cleared, ahead of HBsAg. In chronic HBV, HBeAg remains detectable for years. With seroconversion from HBeAg to anti-HBe, HBV DNA disappears and liver disease remits. Spontaneous seroconversion occurs at a rate of 5% per year in the West but much less so in the Far East [17]. During seroconversion, some develop HBeAg-negative variants due to mutations of the HBV genome. These patients have anti-HBe but have low or undetectable levels of HBeAg. Transcription of pregenomic RNA is not affected, so viral replication and liver disease persist [18]. The highest prevalence of HBeAg-negative variants is in the Mediterranean region followed by Asia, whereas they are uncommon in North America and western Europe.
6. **HBV DNA** assays used to assess HBV replication include hybridization, branched DNA, and polymerase chain reaction (PCR) assays. Each differs in its detection limits. Detection of HBV DNA may precede HBsAg. Serum HBV DNA levels determine candidacy for treatment and response to therapy in chronic HBV. HBV DNA is often associated with HBeAg. Seroconversion to anti-HBe leads to the loss of HBV DNA, although it may remain detectable by more sensitive PCR assays.

**D. Pathogenesis**

1. HBV is not cytopathic for hepatocytes. Liver injury occurs via T cells cytotoxic for hepatocytes expressing surface hepatitis B core antigen. A successful immune response occurs if all infected cells are destroyed, viral replication ceases, and anti-HBs is generated (which prevents reinfection of hepatocytes). Alternatively, immune responses may inhibit viral replication without killing infected cells and minute amounts of virus remain in hepatocytes indefinitely, even if HBsAg and HBV DNA are not detectable [19].

**E. Acute hepatitis B**

1. The incubation period is 1 to 4 months, which may be followed by anorexia, malaise, nausea and vomiting, and right upper quadrant tenderness. As these symptoms subside, jaundice ensues and lasts up to 1 to 3 months.
2. Nearly 70% of patients with acute HBV infection have anicteric hepatitis (Fig. 14.1), whereas 30% develop jaundice. Acute liver failure develops in less than 1%. [15].

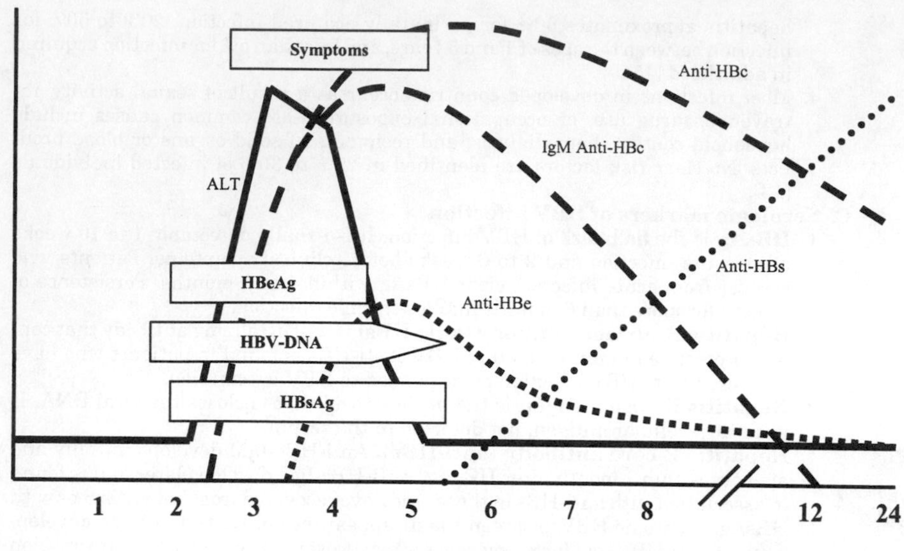


**FIG. 14.1** A typical case of acute hepatitis B. HbsAg, hepatitis B surface antigen; HBV-DNA, hepatitis B virus DNA; HbeAg, hepatitis B e antigen; ALT, alanine aminotransferase; Anti-HBe, antibody to hepatitis e antigen; Anti-HBc, antibody to hepatitis core antibody; Anti-HBs, antibody to hepatitis B surface antibody.

3. Elevations in aminotransferases to 1,000 to 2,000 IU/mL are common. Normalization occurs in 1 to 4 months, then bilirubin. Enzyme elevation for more than 6 months usually indicates chronic infection. Prothrombin time is the best prognosticator [20].

**F. Chronic hepatitis B**

1. Patients who develop chronic HBV infection usually have a mild or subclinical presentation. Others manifest fatigue and right upper quadrant discomfort. Some have exacerbations mimicking acute hepatitis. Others develop end-stage liver disease characterized by ascites, encephalopathy, and variceal bleeding.
2. A National Institutes of Health Workshop [21] defined chronic HBV as persistent HBV infection causing necroinflammatory liver disease with (a) positive HBsAg for more than 6 months, (b) serum HBV DNA levels higher than $10^5$ copies/mL or positive hepatitis B core antigen by immunostaining, (c) persistent or intermittent elevation in AST/ALT levels, and (d) a liver biopsy showing chronic hepatitis.
3. Predictors of progression to cirrhosis and hepatocellular carcinoma (HCC) include the state of the immune system, age, sex, geography, and genetics [22,23]. The overall reported incidence of HCC in surveillance studies is 0.8% to 4.1% [23].
4. Patients with inactive hepatitis B (previously a "healthy carrier") have detectable HBsAg for more than 6 months without any ongoing necroinflammatory disease. Most have lost HBeAg and developed anti-HBe, with HBV DNA levels less than $10^5$ copies/mL and a persistently normal ALT/AST. In some, disease relapses after a period of inactivity.

**G. Therapy.** The goal of treatment is to suppress HBV replication (disappearance of HBeAg and HBV DNA), thereby preventing the progression to cirrhosis and HCC.

1. **Interferon-$\alpha$(IFN-$\alpha$)** therapy was approved in 1992 for immunocompetent patients at doses of 5 to 10 million units (MIU) daily or three times a week for

16 weeks. A meta-analysis of 15 studies [24] demonstrated a sustained loss of HBV replication in those treated for at least 3 months (33% lost HBeAg vs. 12% of control subjects and 37% lost HBV DNA vs. 17% of control subjects). Eight percent lost all markers, including HBsAg, compared with 2% of control subjects. Favorable response factors included a negative human immunodeficiency virus (HIV) test, chronic active hepatitis on liver biopsy, moderately high ALT levels (>100 U/L), HBV DNA levels less than 200 pg/mL, and a history of acute hepatitis [25]. Wild-type virus (HBeAg positive) is associated with improved response rates compared with the situation with HBV variants (see section IV.C.5 above). In a 5-year follow-up of 103 patients treated with IFN-$\alpha$, survival without clinical complications was significantly prolonged in patients who cleared HBeAg [26]. IFN-$\alpha$ is also associated with a decreased incidence of HCC [27]. IFN-$\alpha$ treatment of patients with decompensated cirrhosis (ascites, variceal bleeding, encephalopathy) is contraindicated because benefit is limited, severe adverse effects are common, and, most of all, during treatment significant flares in liver enzymes are seen and this may precipitate acute decompensation and the need for urgent liver transplantation.

2. **Lamivudine** (Epivir-HBV, GlaxoSmithKline) is a nucleoside analogue that inhibits HBV reverse transcriptase, thus inhibiting HBV replication. It has negligible side effects. Treatment-naive patients or nonresponders to IFN-$\alpha$ with elevated AST/ALT and HBeAg and HBV DNA treated for 12 months were more likely to have HBeAg seroconversion (see section IV.C.5 above), sustained ALT normalization, and improvement on biopsy than placebo recipients [28–30]. Prolonging treatment to 2 years yields a further improvement in necroinflammation [31] and an increase in the sustained seroconversion rate [32]. Unlike IFN-$\alpha$, lamivudine is effective against HBV variants (see section IV.C.5 above) [33] and is safe and effective in decompensated HBV cirrhosis [34].
3. After 1 year, 15% to 30% of patients may develop **mutations in the YMDD motif** of the HBV polymerase gene [14]. Patients with this mutation have lower (but not undetectable) serum levels of HBV DNA than before treatment but improved ALT and histology, similar to patients without the YMDD mutation. Because the lamivudine-resistant mutants do not replicate as proficiently as the wild-type virus, stopping the drug results in a rapid reversion to wild-type that may be associated with a marked rise in HBV DNA and ALT levels [35].
4. **Combination of lamivudine and interferon** appears to enhance the HBeAg seroconversion rate, particularly for treatment-naive patients with moderately elevated baseline ALT levels [36]. However, this approach was not recommended at the recent National Institutes of Health Workshop on HBV [21].
5. The observations with lamivudine monotherapy suggest that combining various antivirals in a cocktail as for HIV may lead to improved response and/or less resistance. Other nucleoside analogues (e.g., adefovir, entecavir, emtricitabine) are being investigated.

**H. HBV after transplantation.** HBV recurrence after transplantation has been reduced significantly with the use of long-term high-dose intravenous hepatitis B immune globulin (HBIG). Now lamivudine added to HBIG has led to further improvements in allograft and patient survival [37]. A cost-effective alternative is low-dose intramuscular HBIG in combination with lamivudine [38].

**I. Prevention/HBV vaccine**

1. HBV vaccine prevents disease and sequelae such as HCC. It is safe and effective. The most common side effect is pain at the injection site.
2. Universal vaccination of newborns is routine in many countries, especially for infants born to HBsAg-positive mothers. Adults who should be vaccinated include health-care workers, sexual partners and family members of HBsAg-positive cases, patients with chronic liver disease, patients on hemodialysis, persons in institutions for the developmentally disabled and long-term correctional facilities, travelers staying for more than 6 months in countries with high endemic rates of HBV, and drug users.
3. Current HBV vaccines consist of HBsAg produced in yeast using recombinant DNA technology. The vaccine is given intramuscularly, usually at 0, 1, and

6 months, at a dose for adults of 10 to 20 $\mu$g and for children 2.5 to 10 $\mu$g. In 1999 the U.S. Food and Drug Administration approved an optional two-dose schedule of Recombivax HB (Merck & Co., Inc., West Point, PA) for 11 to 15 year olds. For adults, the dose of Recombivax HB is 10 $\mu$g with the second dose given 4 to 6 months later.

4. An anti-HBs titers higher than 10 IU/L is deemed protective. Maximum antibody response occurs 6 weeks after the last dose, so testing is done 1 to 2 months after completing the series, except in infants born to HBsAg-positive mothers, in whom testing should be performed at ages 9 to 15 months. In normal subjects, a favorable response occurs in 90% to 95%, but in the elderly or the immunosuppressed, response can be as low as 40% to 60% [39]. Additional doses (one to three) are recommended for nonresponders. This yields a 25% to 50% response after one additional dose and 50% to 75% after three [39].
5. Although anti-HBs titers decrease over time, the duration of protection is probably lifelong, because most responders mount an amnestic anti-HBs response upon rechallenge. Booster doses of HBV vaccine are indicated only in hemodialysis patients. Serologic testing to monitor antibody levels is not recommended.

J. **Postexposure prophylaxis** should be provided for individuals known to be anti-HBs negative, those never vaccinated, and nonresponders to prior HBV vaccination. Individuals who have been vaccinated but whose anti-HBs status is unknown should have anti-HBs testing, and if titers are less than 10 mIU/mL they should undergo prophylaxis. The Centers for Disease Control and Prevention suggests administering both a single dose of HBIG and initiating a course of HBV vaccination.

## V. HCV

A. **Classification and structure.** HCV is the only member of the genus *Hepacivirus* in the *Flaviviridae* family of viruses. It is an enveloped virus about 50 nm in diameter that contains a positive-sense single-stranded RNA genome.

B. **Epidemiology**

1. HCV was the most common blood-borne infection in the United States in the 1980's, but the incidence of HCV had declined by more than 80% to 36,000 in 1996 [40–42].
2. Some 3.9 million people (1.8%) have positive HCV antibody and 74% have detectable HCV RNA by PCR, indicating chronic infection [43,44]. In African Americans, the prevalence rate is 3.2%, compared with 1.5% for non-Hispanic whites. The highest prevalence is in men aged 30 to 49 years with large or repeated direct percutaneous exposures to blood [43].
3. After introduction of the sensitive ELISA II screening antibody in 1992, the risk for HCV infection has fallen to 0.001% per unit of blood transfused [45,46]. Another common source for HCV was the use of clotting factor concentrates before 1985. Transplantation of organs from infected donors also carried a high risk before HCV screening was initiated in the early 1990's.
4. **Intravenous drug use** now accounts for most cases of HCV transmission in the United States. For current users, the rate of HCV may be as high as 79% [40]. After 5 years of injecting, as many as 90% are infected with HCV [40].
5. **Intranasal cocaine use** ("snorting") may also serve as a route for transmission, probably due to nasal ulceration and/or bleeding and the sharing of contaminated straws [47]. However, intranasal cocaine use in the absence of intravenous drug use is relatively uncommon.
6. In contrast to HBV, **sexual transmission** is relatively infrequent. Sexual partners of patients with HCV reveal a low rate of HCV, ranging from 0 to 4.4% (mean, 1.5%) [40]. The risk of HCV transmission from men to women and from men to men is greater than that transmission from women to men, but it is still less common than that for HBV or HIV.
7. The rate of HCV infection among health-care workers is no higher than that found in the general population [40]. The risk of acquiring HCV from a needlestick injury is approximately 0.1%, but it rises to approximately 5% to 10% if the index case is confirmed to have viremia by PCR [48]. HCV transmission is particularly high in patients on hemodialysis in whom the prevalence is approximately 10% but occasionally is as high as 60% [49].

8. The rate of **vertical transmission** of HCV from mother to child is approximately 5%, but it may be 14% or more if the mother is HIV positive [40]. Elective cesarean section before membrane rupture is associated with lower HCV transmission rates compared with vaginal delivery or emergency cesarean section (0 vs. 7.4%, $p = 0.01$) [50]. The sensitivity of HCV RNA by PCR in infants is only 22% before 1 month of age, rising to 97% thereafter, which suggests that HCV infection occurs at the time of delivery [50].
9. **Nonsexual household contacts** (e.g., via razor blades, toothbrushes, or other household items) represent very low risk for HCV transmission.
10. HCV infection related to procedures (e.g., tattooing) is reported in other countries, but case studies have failed to reveal such an association in the United States [40].

**C. Pathogenesis**

1. Hepatocellular injury occurs from nonspecific immune mechanisms and a virus-specific immune response (both humoral and cellular), not from viral cytotoxicity.
2. HCV has great genetic heterogeneity. Isolates from around the world have been classified into six major genotypes. Individual isolates consist of closely related yet heterogeneous populations of viral genomes (i.e., quasi-species). This genetic diversity probably accounts for the ease with which HCV escapes the host's immune system and leads to chronic infection.

**D. Acute hepatitis C**

1. Acute hepatitis C is almost always asymptomatic and therefore rarely recognized.
2. HCV RNA typically becomes detectable in the serum by PCR about 7 to 21 days after exposure. Specific HCV antibodies appear within 20 to 150 days (mean, 50 days) [51].
3. Clinical symptoms (e.g., jaundice, fatigue, lethargy, myalgias, and right upper quadrant discomfort) occur in less than 20% of patients [41]. They occur within 2 to 12 weeks (mean, 7 weeks) after exposure [41]. Elevation in ALT is usually mild. Fulminant hepatitis is very rare. Those with clinical hepatitis are much more likely to completely clear HCV, probably due to a more vigorous immune response.

**E. Chronic hepatitis C**

1. After acute infection, approximately 15% appear to resolve infection with no detectable HCV RNA, a normal ALT, and no sequelae [52]. In the remaining 85%, chronic hepatitis develops [44]. HCV currently accounts for 40% of chronic liver disease in the United States, resulting in approximately 8,000 to 10,000 deaths each year [40]. The Centers for Disease Control and Prevention predicts that the mortality rate from HCV will triple by 2020. HCV-related end-stage liver disease is now the most common reason for liver transplantation in the United States [53].
2. The **natural history** of HCV remains a controversial issue because strategies to examine disease progression are complicated by both recall and selection bias. However, despite this it is estimated that 15% to 20% of persons who acquire HCV infection progress to end-stage liver disease (and its sequelae) during a 20- to 30-year period [54] and approximately 1% to 5% will develop HCC [40].
3. **Risk factors for more rapid disease progression** include the consumption of at least 50 g of alcohol on a daily basis, HCV acquisition after age 40, male gender, immunosuppression, and/or coinfection with HIV [55,56].
4. A key feature of chronic HCV infection is its seemingly indolent course with minimal, if any, symptoms and its discovery on routine blood studies. About 60% to 70% of patients with chronic HCV have a persistently elevated ALT. The remainder have either intermittently elevated or persistently normal ALT levels. On liver biopsy, patients with a persistently normal ALT tend to have less severe histologic findings and a lower rate of progression to cirrhosis.
5. Chronic HCV infection has been associated with numerous **extrahepatic manifestations**, the most common of which are thyroid dysfunction, porphyria cutanea tarda, Sjögren syndrome, vasculitis, and/or renal disease secondary to cryoglobulinemia and membranoproliferative glomerulonephritis.

### F. Diagnosis

1. The first step is to detect test for **antibodies to HCV** using an enzyme immunoassay. After HCV exposure, the average time to develop antibodies is approximately 8 to 9 weeks [57]. Because the symptoms of acute HCV infection usually begin at 7 weeks, a negative anti-HCV antibody does not rule out hepatitis C. HCV RNA by PCR is more helpful in high risk situations (see below).
2. The recombinant immunoblot assay is rarely used today except to confirm positive ELISA II tests during blood donation screening.
3. **HCV RNA by PCR is used to confirm viremia.** It may be qualitative (viremia present or absent) or quantitative (which is slightly less sensitive but detects viremia in the vast majority of infected individuals). PCR is useful after a needlestick injury, because this becomes positive within 6 to 8 weeks of exposure.
4. Determining **HCV genotype** does not aid in the diagnosis, but it does help decide on the duration of treatment, whenever deemed necessary (see below).

### G. Therapy

1. In the past, a biochemical response (normalization of serum aminotransferases) to treatment was the primary end point, but currently the goal of treatment is the eradication of HCV RNA from the serum (i.e., a virologic response).
2. **End-of-treatment virologic response** indicates viral clearance from the blood at the end of treatment, whereas a **sustained virologic response** (SVR) indicates the absence of virus at 6 months after the end of treatment. Of patients who achieve an SVR, 96% will have undetectable HCV RNA in the serum and no histologic progression on serial liver biopsy when followed for a mean of 4 years [58].
3. **Relapsers** achieve an end-of-treatment virologic response but subsequently redevelop viremia. **Nonresponders** fail to clear HCR RNA after completing a course of treatment. A subcategory of nonresponders initially respond with a fall in HCV RNA titer (even to undetectable levels) only to "break through" despite ongoing treatment. Their outcome is similar to other nonresponders.
4. **Predictors of response** to antiviral therapy include HCV genotypes other than type 1 or 4, pretreatment levels of HCR RNA by PCR less than 2 million copies/mL or less than 850,000 IU/mL using the new World Health Organization system, absence of bridging fibrosis or cirrhosis, age less than 40 years, and female gender [59]. HCV genotype is the most important.
5. **Monotherapy with IFN-$\alpha$,** once the mainstay of HCV treatment, is now used only when combination treatment with ribavirin is not tolerated or contraindicated. For details see previous reports [60–64].
6. **Consensus interferon alfacon-1** (Infergen, Amgen, Thousand Oaks, CA) combines the most common amino acid sequences from 11 naturally occurring IFNs. In treatment-naive patients, consensus interferon 9 $\mu$g subcutaneously three times a day leads to an SVR similar to that with standard-dose IFN-$\alpha$ monotherapy [65]. However, high-dose consensus interferon (15 $\mu$g subcutaneously three times a day for 48 weeks) enhances SVR to 13% in prior nonresponders and to 58% in relapsers after prior IFN-$\alpha$ [66].
7. Since its introduction in 1998, **ribavirin in combination with IFN- $\alpha$2b** (Rebetron, Schering-Plough, Kenilworth, NJ), so-called combination therapy, has become the gold standard. Patients must be able to tolerate the hemolysis and other side effects associated with ribavirin and have no specific contraindications to its use (see below). Ribavirin (1,000–1,200 mg orally in two divided doses a day) is an oral guanosine analogue and does not ameliorate viremia on its own, but when used in combination with IFN-$\alpha$2b it leads to a significant increase in SVR in treatment-naive patients. After 48 weeks of combination therapy SVR is 38% compared with only 13% after 48 weeks of IFN-$\alpha$2b monotherapy [59]. Recent evidence suggests that the SVR can be improved further when the dose of ribavirin is based on body weight (and at least 10.6 mg/kg/day is given) [63]. This also appears to be the case if patients take 80% of their IFN-$\alpha$2b and 80% of their ribavirin for 80% of the time (the so-called 80-80-80 rule) [64]. Combination therapy also improves SVR in relapsers (48%) and nonresponders (35%).
8. **Pegylated IFN-$\alpha$** was recently developed to overcome the rapid absorption and clearance of IFN-$\alpha$. Pegylation involves the addition of a 40-kDa branched

polyethylene glycol (PEG) polymer to IFN-$\alpha$2a (PEG-IFN-$\alpha$2a, PEGASYS, Hoffman LaRoche Laboratories, Nutley, NJ) or a 12-kDa linear PEG polymer to IFN-$\alpha$2b (PEG-IFN-$\alpha$2b, PEG-Intron, Schering-Plough). Both are dosed once weekly. In a recent pivotal trial in treatment-naive patients, PEG-IFN-$\alpha$2a 180 $\mu$g subcutaneously for 48 weeks led to an SVR of 39% compared with 19% in patients treated with INF-$\alpha$2a [67]. In compensated cirrhotics, PEG-IFN-$\alpha$2a achieved an SVR of 30% compared with 8% with standard IFN-$\alpha$2a, both given for 48 weeks [68]. In contrast, PEG-IFN-$\alpha$2b 1.5 $\mu$g/kg subcutaneously once weekly for 48 weeks led to an SVR of only 23% versus 12% with standard IFN-$\alpha$2b [69]. There is additional benefit when ribavirin is added. In a recent phase III open-label trial, patients treated with PEG-IFN-$\alpha$2b 1.5 $\mu$g/kg subcutaneously once weekly plus ribavirin 800 to 1,200 mg/day had an SVR of 54% compared with 46% with standard IFN-$\alpha$2b plus ribavirin [63].

9. **Contraindications** to the use of IFN-$\alpha$ include decompensated liver disease, severe depression or bipolar illness, autoimmune disease, active drug or alcohol use, pregnancy, and significant comorbid disease (e.g., unstable coronary artery disease, epilepsy, diabetes, or hypertension). Contraindications to the use of ribavirin include anemia (hemoglobin less than 11 g/dL), hemolysis, renal insufficiency, coronary artery disease, and cerebral vascular disease. Because of ribavirin's teratogenic risk, it is contraindicated during pregnancy. It should also not be administered to any women at risk of becoming pregnant or their male partners without advising two forms of contraception while on ribavirin and for at least 6 months after it is stopped. Serial pregnancy tests are required.

**H. HCV after liver transplantation.** HCV recurrence is almost universal, but overall graft and patient survival for the first decade at least after liver transplantation appears to be unaffected [70]. By the second decade, the prevalence of HCV-related graft failure may begin to increase. The natural history of HCV infection appears accelerated in transplant recipients as compared with immunocompetent individuals [71]. Optimal antiviral strategies for hepatitis C after transplantation have yet to be developed.

**I. Postexposure prophylaxis.** Immunoglobulin is not effective to prevent HCV [40]. Although IFN-$\alpha$ begun early in the course of HCV infection is associated with a high rate of success [72], no data exist that treatment during the acute phase after exposure is more effective than treatment begun early in the course of chronic infection.

**J. Prevention.** Currently there is no vaccine for HCV. Efforts to develop one are not without formidable challenges because of high rates of mutation in the hypervariable region of the envelope protein, slow antibody response to envelope proteins with only modest titers during primary infection, and the lack of an appropriate animal model.

## VI. HDV

**A. Classification and structure.** HDV is an unusual infectious agent (the so-called delta" agent) that requires HBsAg for its survival. Although HDV can replicate independently, HBV must be present for complete HDV virion assembly and secretion. As a result, individuals with HDV are always dually infected with HDV and HBV. The 36-nm virion consists of a 1.7-kb single-stranded RNA genome (the smallest known to infect humans), the hepatitis delta antigen (delta-Ag), and an envelope composed of lipid and HBsAg. The envelope, which is required for virion formation and infection, is the only helper function provided by HBV.

**B. Epidemiology**

1. HDV is transmitted in the same fashion as HBV.
2. About 5% of HBV carriers worldwide are infected with HDV [16]. However, the geographic distribution of HDV does not parallel that of HBV because there are three distinct genotypes with differing geographic distributions and disease severity [73]. The most widespread is genotype I, associated with a broad spectrum of chronic disease.
3. Slowly progressive liver disease appears to predominate in some HDV-endemic areas such as the Mediterranean region, where transmission occurs by inapparent permucosal, percutaneous, or intrafamilial spread.

4. Despite the high prevalence of HBV in Asia, the prevalence of HDV infection (genotype II) is generally low and is associated with milder disease. Transmission usually occurs sexually or via intravenous drug use.
5. The most severe forms of HDV infection are seen in low prevalence areas (North America and northern Europe) among intravenous drug users.
6. Outbreaks of acute HDV infection (genotype III) have been seen in northern parts of South America where the disease often has a rapidly progressive course [74].

**C. Clinical features**

1. **Acute coinfection** with HBV and HDV occurs with simultaneous exposure to both viruses. Usually, coinfection is self-limited. As the immune response clears HBsAg, HDV infection also resolves. A small number become chronically infected with both.
2. **Superinfection** develops in those infected with HBV. Because HBsAg expression is established before HDV exposure, there is a more rapid course, with high levels of HDV RNA and delta-Ag. In at least 70%, HDV becomes chronic [75]. Chronic HDV is associated with rising titers of antibodies to hepatitis D, which are not protective because the delta-Ag is an internal virus component.

**D. Diagnosis**

1. **Total HDV antibody (anti-HDV) assays** are the only commercially available tests for HDV infection in many countries. Anti-HDV-IgM levels are transient and delayed if the course of HDV is self-limited. In chronic cases, anti-HDV-IgM is long lasting, present in high titers, and correlates with the severity of disease [16]. Anti-HDV-IgG titers are high in chronic HDV infection.
2. **Serum HDV RNA** is an early sensitive marker of HDV infection in patients with acute hepatitis D. and most cases with chronic HDV infection have a positive PCR.
3. **Tissue markers of HDV infection (delta-Ag)** detected by immunohistochemical staining of liver tissue are considered the gold standard to confirm ongoing HDV.

**E. Therapy.** Current options are limited. Controlled trials [76–78] have shown that in certain groups IFN-$\alpha$ normalizes ALT, eradicates serum HDV RNA, and improves liver histology. However, high doses of IFN-$\alpha$ (5 MIU daily or 9–10 MIU three times day) for 1 to 2 years are usually needed. Most patients relapse once therapy is stopped. With lamivudine, neither HDV viremia nor liver disease activity are improved [79].

**F. Prevention** of HDV infection involves the use of vaccination against its helper virus HBV. Vaccines specifically against HDV superinfection have not been successful.

## VII. HEV

**A. Classification and structure.** HEV is a nonenveloped single-stranded RNA virus 32 nm in diameter. Viral particles were first isolated from the stool in 1983 and named HEV in 1988. Originally classified in the family *Caliciviridae* (e.g., Norwalk agent), HEV was recently found to be more similar to the rubella virus and beet necrotic yellow vein virus [80]. HEV remains unclassified at present. A number of different HEV strains have been identified, and the divergence appears to be based on geography.

**B. Epidemiology**

1. HEV is transmitted via the **fecal–oral route.** Risk factors include poor hygiene and contaminated water supplies. Person-to-person transmission accounts for few cases.
2. Unlike HAV, which has a worldwide distribution, HEV is restricted to tropical and subtropical developing countries. The highest endemic areas are the Middle East and northeast Africa, followed by India, Asia, and Mexico [81].
3. HEV causes epidemics of acute hepatitis [82,83]. In India, 90% of epidemic hepatitis is due to HEV, which follows a 10-year cycle for unknown reasons.
4. HEV mainly affects older children and adults. Serious disease seems to primarily occur in young adults from developing rather than developed countries, again for unknown reasons. In India, fewer than 5% of children under the age of 10 are seropositive [84] compared with the seropositivity rate for HAV (>90%) in the same population.

5. In the United States and northern Europe, up to 2% of the population has antibodies to HEV [85]. The prevalence of HEV antibody increases with age, and it is rarely found in those less than 30 years of age. The incidence of symptomatic disease is even lower. Cases in the United States usually have history of travel to HEV-endemic areas elsewhere in the world. Higher rates of HEV seropositivity in the United States have been reported in men who have sex with men and in intravenous drug users.
6. HEV may be zoonotic [86]. In the United States, swine and rodents infected with an attenuated strain may be the source of infection of humans. This might explain the high prevalence of antibody in certain groups who have never had symptomatic disease.
7. The greatest impact of HEV is on pregnant women, who have a high mortality rate (up to 20%–25%), especially during the second and third trimesters [87].

C. **Pathogenesis**. Like HAV, HEV enters through the gastrointestinal tract, reaching the liver via the portal vein, before being excreted in bile. Pathogenesis is poorly understood but probably involves both cytotoxic and immunologic mechanisms. The reason for the high mortality rates seen in pregnant women remains uncertain.

D. **Diagnosis.** As with HAV, acute HEV is diagnosed by the presence of the IgM class of HEV antibodies, typically present for 3 to 4 months. The IgG class is also usually detectable, and titers may rise to very high levels during the convalescence period. These IgG antibodies diminish over time and their ability to sustain immunity is unproven.

E. **Clinical features**
1. HEV infection is self-limited and does not progress to chronic liver disease.
2. The incubation period is 15 to 60 days (mean, 40 days). One to 3 weeks after exposure, HEV is detected in the blood and feces. Fecal excretion may last approximately 3 to 5 weeks.
3. Acute HEV resembles HAV, with low mortality rates except in pregnant women.

F. **Prevention and control measures**
1. In HEV-endemic regions, travelers should avoid water of unknown purity, uncooked shellfish, and fruits and vegetables not peeled by the travelers themselves.
2. Passive immunoprophylaxis with IG has been shown to be effective in controlled clinical trials [88], but commercially available lots of IG from donors collected in regions where HEV is endemic probably lack sufficient antibody to be efficacious.
3. HEV vaccines are currently under clinical evaluation.

## REFERENCES


1. Yotsuyanagi H, Koike K, Yasuda K, et al. Prolonged fecal excretion of hepatitis A virus in adult patients with hepatitis A as determined by polymerase chain reaction. *Hepatology* 1996;24:10–13.
2. Lemon SM. The natural history of hepatitis A: the potential for transmission by transfusion of blood or blood products. *Vox Sang* 1994;67[Suppl]:19–26.
3. Karayiannis P, Jowett T, Enticott M, et al. Hepatitis A virus replication in tamarins and the host immune response in relation to pathogenesis of liver cell damage. *J Med Virol* 1986;18:261–271.
4. Krugman S, Ward R, Giles JP, et al. Infectious hepatitis: detection of virus during the incubation period and in clinically inapparent infection. *N Engl J Med* 1959;261:729–734.
5. Koff RS. Hepatitis A. *Lancet* 1998;351:1643–1649.
6. Willner IR, Uhl MD, Howard SC, et al. Serious hepatitis A: an analysis of patients hospitalized during an urban epidemic in the United States. *Ann Intern Med* 1998;128:111–114.
7. Keeffe EB. Is hepatitis A more severe in patients with chronic hepatitis B and other chronic liver diseases? *Am J Gastroenterol* 1995;90:201–205.
8. Vento S, Garofano T, Renzini C, et al. Fulminant hepatitis associated with hepatitis A virus superinfection in patients with chronic hepatitis C. *N Engl J Med* 1998;338:286.
9. Koff RS. Hepatitis A. *Lancet* 1998;351:1643–1649.
10. O'Grady JG, Alexander GJM, Hayllar KM, et al. Early indicators of prognosis in fulminant hepatic failure. *Gastroenterology* 1989;97:439–445.

11. Centers for Disease Control and Prevention. Prevention of hepatitis A through active or passive immunization: recommendations of the Advisory Committee on Immunization Practices (ACIP). *MMWR Morb Mortal Wkly Rep* 1999;48:1–37.
12. Keeffe EB, Iwarson S, McMahon BJ, et al. Safety and immunogenicity of hepatitis A vaccine in patients with chronic liver disease. *Hepatology* 1998;27:881–886.
13. Lee WM. Hepatitis B virus infection. *N Engl J Med* 1997;337:1733–1745.
14. Malik AH, Lee WM. Chronic hepatitis B virus infection: treatment strategies for the next millennium. *Ann Intern Med* 2000;132:723–731.
15. Lok ASF, Chan HLY. Viral hepatitis B and D. In: O'Grady JG, Lake JR, Howdle PD, eds. *Comprehensive clinical hepatology,* 1st ed. London: Harcourt Publishers, 2000;:3.12.1–21.
16. Kane M. Global programme for control of hepatitis B infection. *Vaccine* 1995;13 [Suppl 1]:S47–S49.
17. Wong JB, Koff RS, Tinè F, et al. Cost-effectiveness of interferon $\alpha$2b treatment for hepatitis B e antigen-positive chronic hepatitis B. *Ann Intern Med* 1995;122:664–675.
18. Omata M, Ehata T, Yokouka O, et al. Mutations in the precore region of hepatitis B virus DNA in patients with fulminant and severe hepatitis. *N Engl J Med* 1991;324:1699–1704.
19. Chisar FV. Cytotoxic T cells and viral hepatitis. *J Clin Invest* 1997;99:1472–1477.
20. O'Grady JG, Alexander GJM, Hayllar KM, et al. Early indicators of prognosis in fulminant hepatic failure. *Gastroenterology* 1989;97:439–445.
21. Lok AS, Heathcote EJ, Hoofnagle JH. Management of hepatitis B: 2000—summary of a workshop. *Gastroenterology* 2001;120:1828–1853.
22. Merican I, Guan R, Amarapuka D, et al. Chronic hepatitis B virus infection in Asian countries. *J Gastroenterol Hepatol* 2000;15:1356–1361.
23. Chu CM. Natural history of chronic hepatitis B virus infection in adults with emphasis on the occurrence of cirrhosis and hepatocellular carcinoma. *J Gastroenterol Hepatol* 2000;15:E25–E30.
24. Wong DKH, Cheung AM, O'Rourke K, et al. Effect of alpha-interferon treatment in patients with hepatitis B e antigen-positive chronic hepatitis B: A meta-analysis. *Ann Intern Med* 1993;119:312–323.
25. Brook MG, Karayiannis P, Thomas HC. Which patients with chronic hepatitis B virus infection will respond to alpha-interferon therapy? A statistical analysis of predictive factors. *Hepatology* 1989;10:761–763.
26. Niederau C, Heintges T, Lange S, et al. Long-term follow-up of HBeAg–positive patients treated with interferon alfa for chronic hepatitis B. *N Engl J Med* 1996;334:1422–1427.
27. Lin SM, Sheen IS, Chien RN, et al. Long-term beneficial effect of interferon therapy in patients with chronic hepatitis B virus infection. *Hepatology* 1999;29:971–975.
28. Lai C-L, Chien R-N, Leung N, et al. A one-year trial of lamivudine for chronic hepatitis B. *N Engl J Med* 1998;339:61–68.
29. Dienstag JL, Schiff ER, Wright TL, et al. Lamivudine as initial treatment for chronic hepatitis B in the United States. *N Engl J Med* 1999;341:1256–1263.
30. Schiff E, Karayalcin S, Grimm I, et al. A placebo controlled study of lamivudine and interferon alpha-2b in patients with chronic hepatitis B who previously failed interferon therapy. *Hepatology* 1998;28:388A(abst).
31. Leung N, Wu PC, Tsang S, et al. Continued histological improvement in Chinese patients with chronic hepatitis B with 2 years lamivudine. *Hepatology* 1998;28:489A (abst).
32. Liaw YF, Lai CL, Leung NW, et al. Two-year lamivudine therapy in chronic hepatitis B infection: results of a placebo controlled multicenter study in Asia. *Gastroenterology* 1988;114:1289A(abst).
33. Tassopoulos NC, Volpes R, Pastore G, et al. Efficacy of lamivudine in patients with hepatitis B e antigen-negative/hepatitis B virus DNA-positive (precore mutant) chronic hepatitis B. *Hepatology* 1999;30;29:889–896.
34. Villeneuve J-P, Condreay LD, Willems B, et al. Lamivudine treatment for decompensated cirrhosis resulting from chronic hepatitis B. *Hepatology* 2000;31:207–210.
35. Chayama K, Suzuki Y, Kobayashi M, et al. Emergence and takeover of YMDD motif mutant hepatitis B virus during long-term lamivudine therapy and re-takeover by wild type after cessation of therapy. *Hepatology* 1998;27:1711–1716.
36. Schalm SW, Heathcote J, Cianciara J, et al. Lamivudine and alpha interferon

combination treatment of patients with chronic hepatitis B infection: a randomized trial. *Gut* 2000;46:562–568.
37. Markowitz JS, Martin P, Conrad AJ, et al. Prophylaxis against hepatitis B recurrence following liver transplantation using combination lamivudine and hepatitis B immune globulin. *Hepatology* 1998;28:585–589.
38. Yao FY, Osorio RW, Roberts JP, et al. Intramuscular hepatitis B immune globulin continued with lamivudine for prophylaxis against hepatitis B recurrence after liver transplantation. *Liver Transpl Surg* 1999;5:491–496.
39. Magolis H. Hepatitis B vaccine. Presented at the AASLD postgraduate course 2000: Update on viral hepatitis. October 27–28, 2000, Dallas, Texas.
40. Centers for Disease Control and Prevention. Recommendations for prevention and control of hepatitis C virus (HCV) infection and HCV-related chronic disease. *MMWR Morb Mortal Wkly Rep* 1998;47(RR-19):1–54.
41. Centers for Disease Control and Prevention. Public Health Service inter-agency guidelines for screening donors of blood, plasma, organs, tissues, and semen for evidence of hepatitis B and hepatitis C. *MMWR Morb Mortal Wkly Rep* 1991;40(RR-4):1–17.
42. Alter MJ. Epidemiology of hepatitis C. *Hepatology* 1997;26:62S–65S.
43. McQuillan GM, Alter MJ, Moyer LA, et al. A population based serologic study of hepatitis C virus infection in the United States. In: Rizzetto M, Purcell RH, Gerin JL, et al., eds. *Viral hepatitis and liver disease.* Turin: Edizioni Minerva Medica, 1997:267–270.
44. Alter MJ, Kruszon-Moran D, Nainan OV, et al. The prevalence of hepatitis C virus infection in the United States, 1988 through 1994. *N Engl J Med* 1999;341:556–562.
45. Donahue JG, Munoz A, Ness PM, et al. The declining risk of post-transfusion hepatitis C virus infection. *N Engl J Med* 1992;327:369–373.
46. Schreiber GB, Busch MP, Kleinman SH, et al. The risk of transfusion-transmitted viral infections. *N Engl J Med* 1996;334:1685–1690.
47. Conry-Cantilena C, VanRaden M, Gibble J, et al. Routes of infection, viremia, and liver disease in blood donors found to have hepatitis C virus infection. *N Engl J Med* 1996;334:1691–1696.
48. Alter MJ. Epidemiology of hepatitis C in the West. *Semin Liver Dis* 1995;15:5–15.
49. Tokars JI, Miller ER, Alter JM, et al. National surveillance of dialysis associated disease in the United State, 1995. *ASAIO J* 1998;44:98–107.
50. Gibb DM, Goodall RL, Dunn DT, et al. Mother-to-child transmission of hepatitis C virus: evidence for preventable peripartum transmission. *Lancet* 2000;356:904–907.
51. Orland JR, Wright TL, Cooper S. Acute hepatitis C. *Hepatology* 2001;33:321–327.
52. Shakil AO, Conry-Cantilena C, Alter HJ, et al. Volunteer blood donors with antibody to hepatitis C virus: clinical, biochemical, virologic, and histologic features. *Ann Intern Med* 1995;123:330–337.
53. Detre KM, Belle SH, Lombardero M. Liver transplantation for chronic viral hepatitis. *Viral Hepat Rev* 1997;2:219–228.
54. Seeff LB. Natural history of hepatitis C. *Ann Intern Med* 2000;132:299–300.
55. Poynard T, Bedossa P, Opolon P. Natural history of liver fibrosis progression in patients with chronic hepatitis C. *Lancet* 1997;349:825–832.
56. Benhamou Y, Bochet M, DiMartino V, et al. Liver fibrosis progression in human immunodeficiency and hepatitis C virus coinfected patients. *Hepatology* 1999;30:1054–1058.
57. Koretz RL, Brezina M, Polito AJ, et al. Non-A, non-B posttransfusion hepatitis: Comparing C and non-C hepatitis. *Hepatology* 1993;17:361–365.
58. Marcellin P, Boyer N, Gervais A, et al. Long-term histologic improvement and loss of detectable intrahepatic HCV RNA in patients with chronic hepatitis C and sustained response to interferon-alpha therapy. *Ann Intern Med* 1997;127:875–881.
59. McHutchison JG, Gordon SC, Schiff ER, et al. Interferon alfa-2b alone or in combination with ribavirin as initial treatment for chronic hepatitis C. *N Engl J Med* 1998;339:1485–1492.
60. Carithers R, Emerson SS. Therapy of hepatitis C: meta-analysis of interferon alpha-2b trials. *Hepatology* 1997;25[Suppl 1]:83S–88S.
61. Shiffman ML. Use of high-dose interferon in the treatment of chronic hepatitis C. *Semin Liver Dis* 1999;19[Suppl 1]:25–33.
62. Iino S. High dose interferon treatment in chronic hepatitis C. *Gut* 1993;34[Suppl 1]:114S–118S.

63. Mann MP, McHutchison JG, Gordon S, et al. Peg interferon alfa-2B plus ribavirin compared to interferon alfa-2B plus ribavirin for the treatment of chronic hepatitis C: 24 week treatment analysis of a multicenter, multinational phase III randomized controlled trial. Presented at the 51st annual meeting of the AASLD, October 27–31, 2000, Dallas, Texas.
64. McHutchison JG, Poynard T, Harvey J, et al. The effect of dose reduction on sustained response in patients with chronic hepatitis C receiving interferon alfa-2b in combination with ribavirin. *Hepatology* 2000;32:223A(abst).
65. Ozes ON, Reiter Z, Klein S, et al. A comparison of interferon-con1 with natural recombinant interferons-alpha: antiviral, antiproliferative, and natural killer-inducing activities. *J Interferon Res* 1992;12:55–59.
66. Heathcote EJ, Keeffe EB, Lee SS, et al. Re-treatment of chronic hepatitis C with consensus interferon. *Hepatology* 1998;27:1136–1143.
67. Zeuzem S, Feinman SV, Raseneck J, et al. Peginterferon alfa-2a in patients with chronic hepatitis C. *N Engl J Med* 2000;343:1666–1672.
68. Heathcote EJ, Shiffman ML, Cooksley WG, et al. Peginterferon alfa-2a in patients with chronic hepatitis C and cirrhosis. *N Engl J Med* 2000;343:1673–1680.
69. Trepo C, Lindsay K, Niederau C, et al. Pegylated interferon alpha-2A (PEG-Intron) monotherapy is superior to interferon alfa-2B (Intron A) for treatment of chronic hepatitis C. *J Hepatol* 2000;118:A950(abst).
70. Boker K, Dalley G, Bahr M, et al. Long-term outcome of hepatitis C virus infection after liver transplantation. *Hepatology* 1997;25:203–210.
71. Gane EJ, Portmann BC, Naoumouv NV, et al. Long-term outcome of hepatitis C infection after liver transplantation. *N Engl J Med* 1996;334:821–827.
72. Camma C, Almasio P, Craxi A. Interferon as treatment for acute hepatitis C. A meta-analysis. *Dig Dis Sci* 1996;41:1248–1255.
73. Hsu SC, Syu WJ, Ting LT, et al. Immunohistochemistry differentiation of hepatitis D virus genotypes. *Hepatology* 2000;32:1111–1116.
74. Torres JR. Hepatitis B and hepatitis delta virus infection in South America. *Gut* 1996:38[Suppl 2]:S48–S55.
75. Casey J. Hepatitis D virus. Presented at the AASLD postgraduate course 2000: Update on viral hepatitis. October 27–28, 2000, Dallas, Texas.
76. Farci P, Mandas A, Coiana A, et al. Treatment of chronic hepatitis D with interferon alfa-2a. *N Engl J Med* 1994;330:88–94.
77. DiMarco V, Giacchino R, Timitilli A, et al. Long-term interferon- treatment of children with chronic hepatitis delta: a multicenter study. *J Viral Hepat* 1996;3:123–128.
78. Battegay M, Simpson LH, Hoofnagle JH, et al. Elimination of hepatitis delta virus infection after loss of hepatitis B surface antigen in patients with chronic delta hepatitis. *J Med Virol* 1994;44:389–392.
79. Lau DT, Doo E, Park Y, et al. Lamivudine for chronic delta hepatitis. *Hepatology* 1999;30:546–549.
80. Pringle CR. Virus taxonomy—San Diego 1998. *Arch Virol* 1998;143:1449.
81. Balayan MS. Epidemiology of hepatitis E virus infection. *J Viral Hepat* 1997:4;155–165.
82. Isaacson M, Frean J, He J, et al. An outbreak of hepatitis E in Northern Namibia, 1983. *Am J Trop Med* 2000;62:619–625.
83. Skidmore SJ, Yarbough PO, Garbor KA, et al. Hepatitis E virus: the cause of waterbourne hepatitis outbreak. *J Med Virol* 1992;37:58–60.
84. Mast EE, Krawczynski K. Hepatitis E: an overview. *Annu Rev Med* 1996;47:257.
85. O'Grady J. Viral hepatitis A and E. In O'Grady JG, Lake JR, Howdle PD, eds. *Comprehensive clinical hepatology,* 1st ed. London: Harcourt Publishers, 2000;3.11.1–12.
86. Kabrane-Lazizi Y, Fine JB, Elm J, et al. Evidence for widespread infection of wild rates with hepatitis E virus in the United States. *Am J Trop Med* 1999;61:331–335.
87. Asher LV, Innis BL, Shrestha MP, et al. Virus-like particles in the liver of a patient with fulminant hepatitis and antibody to hepatitis E virus. *J Med Virol* 1990;31:229.
88. Tsarev SA, Tsareva TS, Emerson SU, et al. Successful passive and active immunization of cynomolgus monkeys against hepatitis E. *Proc Natl Acad Sci USA* 1994;91:10198.

# 15. GENITOURINARY TRACT INFECTIONS

Thomas T. Ward and Stephen R. Jones

Urinary tract infections (UTIs) are the most prevalent infection of adults for which antimicrobials are used. UTIs are most often an infection of otherwise healthy people and usually are treated on an outpatient basis. In the United States, symptoms of dysuria, urgency, or frequency result in three to four clinic visits per 100 women, and 80% or more of such episodes lead to the use of laboratory tests or to the prescription of drug therapy, or both. In addition to the inconvenience and cost posed by UTIs, infections occasionally result in protracted illness and serious disease, including gram-negative sepsis and death.

## GENERAL APPROACH TO URINARY TRACT INFECTIONS

I. **Terminology.** The term **urinary tract infection** is a general one, referring only to the presence of bacteria in the urine. More appropriate terminology should indicate the anatomic area actually involved in infection.

A. **Lower UTIs.** In women, dysuria and increased urinary frequency may be seen with cystitis, urethritis, or vaginitis. As discussed later, attention to the patient's history, with detailed characterization of dysuric symptoms, may help differentiate the site of infection.

1. **Cystitis** refers to infection of the bladder and is itself frequently called **lower UTI.** This most common site of UTI is a **superficial mucosal infection** and is much easier to eradicate than renal parenchymal infection.
2. **Urethritis,** or inflammation of the urethra, frequently is caused by sexually transmitted pathogens.
   a. **Urethritis in men** is associated with urethral discharge or dysuria, or both, but without increased frequency. This entity is discussed in detail in Chapter 16 under Urethritis.
   b. **Urethritis in women** is associated with the same symptoms as cystitis. These patients often complain of dysuria and increased frequency, but their urine cultures are sterile or show small numbers of bacteria.
3. **Prostatitis and epididymitis.** Infections of the prostate may be associated with syndromes of acute and chronic disease. Chronic bacterial prostatitis is the principal cause of recurrent cystitis in men. Complications of prostatitis such as epididymitis may uncommonly occur.

B. **Upper UTIs**

1. **Acute pyelonephritis** refers to an **inflammatory process of the renal parenchyma.** This is most often due to bacteria but occasionally may be caused by fungi. These deep tissue infections are more difficult to eradicate than cystitis.
2. **Chronic pyelonephritis** refers to a histopathologic pattern of diffuse, interstitial, inflammatory disease of the kidneys that is not specific for infection. When related to infection, it is not possible to differentiate changes of active disease from residuum of past infection. Although this term continues to be used, it has **little clinical meaning.** Relapsing infection from presumptive, silent, persistent renal parenchymal infection is better termed **subclinical pyelonephritis.**

C. **Uncomplicated versus complicated UTI**

1. **Uncomplicated UTI** generally refers to cystitis in nonpregnant young adult to middle-aged women without underlying anatomic (structural) abnormality or neurologic dysfunction. These patients represent **the largest single group with UTI.** They are characterized by the ease with which their infections respond to antimicrobial therapy. Recently, sexually active young men with acute dysuria and uncomplicated cystitis have been described (see discussion under Urinary Tract Infection in Men, below).
2. **Complicated UTI** includes those UTIs that occur at sites other than the bladder (e.g., pyelonephritis) and those in children, most men, and pregnant women, as well as UTIs associated with obstruction, foreign body (e.g., catheter), elevated postvoiding residual volume (see section II.C.3.a), renal transplant recipients,

Table 15.1. Overview of the Epidemiology of Urinary Tract Infection by Age Group

| | Females | | Males | |
|---|---|---|---|---|
| Age Group (yr) | Period Prevalence (%) | Risk Factors | Period Prevalence (%) | Risk Factors |
| <1 | 1 | Anatomic or functional urologic abnormalities | 1.0 | Anatomic or functional urologic abnormalities |
| 1–5 | 4–5 | Congenital abnormalities, vesicoureteral reflux | 0.5 | Congenital abnormalities, uncircumcised penis |
| 6–15 | 4–5 | Vesicoureteral reflux | 0.5 | None |
| 16–35 | 20 | Sexual intercourse, diaphragm use | 0.5 | Homosexuality |
| 36–65 | 35 | Gynecologic surgery, bladder prolapse | 20.0 | Prostatic hypertrophy, obstruction, catheterization, surgery |
| Over 65 | 40 | As above, plus incontinence, chronic catheterization | 35.0 | As above, plus incontinence, long-term catheterization |

From Stamm WE. Approach to the patient with urinary tract infection. In: Gorbach SL, Bartlett JG, Blacklow NR, eds. *Infectious disease.* Philadelphia: Saunders, 1992; with permission.

and surgically created ileal loop [1,2]. Some have further suggested a **"high-risk" group,** which includes a patient with immunosuppression, pregnancy, diabetes mellitus, sickle cell anemia, or UTI caused by an organism resistant to most antibiotics [2]. **Complicated UTIs** are characteristically more difficult to treat and may deserve radiographic or urologic investigation.

II. **Epidemiology and pathophysiology.** In early infancy (<3 months of age), UTIs occur more frequently in boys than in girls, but the ratio reverses thereafter; elderly men and women have about the same prevalence of infection (Table 15.1).

The normal urinary tract in men and women is bacteriologically sterile, with the exception of the distal urethra, which may be colonized with a variety of gram-positive and gram-negative bacteria.

A. **Ascending infection.** Work by Stamey [3] showed that the **ascending route of infection** (i.e., urethral organisms spreading to or invading the bladder) **is the most important** means by which the urinary tract becomes infected.

1. Microorganisms causing initial and recurrent infections in women are coliform bacteria that colonize the vaginal introitus, the urethra, and, subsequently, the bladder.
2. **In men, the prostate plays a major role in recurrent UTIs.** These infections may or may not be associated with obstruction of the urinary tract.

B. **Hematogenous infection** is much less common. UTIs secondary to bacteremia may occur but are rare.

1. **Renal abscess.** The kidney may be the site of the UTI in patients with bacteremia or endocarditis due to *Staphylococcus aureus,* as discussed under Intrarenal and Perinephric Abscess, later in this chapter.
2. **Acute pyelonephritis** can occur by the hematogenous route as a result of gram-negative bacteremia, but this is rare.

**C. Determinants of infection.** The inoculum of bacteria present, virulence of the organism, and defense mechanisms inherent in the urinary tract will determine whether infection is established [4,5].

1. **Inoculum size.** Size of the inoculum is particularly important and has been best studied in hematogenous infections. Experimental evidence has shown that delivery of large numbers of organisms to the kidney is required to initiate infection.
2. **Virulence of the organism.** The ability of bacteria to establish infection within the urinary tract varies with the individual strain. Nearly any species of bacterium or fungus can produce lower UTI. Only certain species, however, are likely to cause pyelonephritis. These include Enterobacteriaceae, *Pseudomonas* species, enterococci, and certain fungi.

   Fimbria-mediated adherence (i.e., the ability to attach to a mucosal surface) by uropathogenic *Escherichia coli* to vaginal and uroepithelial cells determines infectivity and, in some cases, the propensity to develop upper UTI. Studies have characterized several specific bacterial protein ligands and host cell carbohydrate receptor sites. Cranberry juice has been purported to prevent adherence of uropathogens to uroepithelial cells, and regular use may decrease the frequency of bacteriuria [6,7].
3. **Host defense mechanisms.** As many as one-third of patients with bacteriuria undergo spontaneous cure. Defense mechanisms are present throughout the urinary tract and contribute to resistance of the tract to infection. Some examples follow.
   a. **Complete bladder emptying** is one of the most important defense mechanisms. When residual urine volumes are high, large numbers of bacteria may remain in the urine. The ability to expel bacteria is complete when voiding is complete. This concept is important in understanding the association between urinary infection and neurologic or urologic diseases (e.g., diabetes with neurogenic bladder or obstruction) that allow bacteria to grow in the residual urine [3]. A postvoiding residual urine volume of more than 100 mL is considered severe enough urinary retention to be associated with UTI [2].
   b. **High fluid intake and frequent voiding** may also be important. These may allow for washout of bacteria and form the basis for recommendations that patients with UTI increase their fluid intake and void frequently. Theoretically, such advice seems sound, but there is no evidence that hydration improves the results of appropriate antibiotic therapy.
   c. **The vesicoureteral valve** also may provide a barrier to the spread of infection by preventing reflux of bacteria once bladder bacteriuria is established.
   d. **Length of the urethra.** The relatively long urethra is believed to protect against infection in men. The shorter female urethra probably allows entry of bacteria from urethra to bladder, and this, in part, may account for the higher frequency of UTI in women.
   e. **Vaginal flora.** Vaginal colonization with lactobacilli appears to prevent vaginal colonization and bacteriuria with *E. coli* and other uropathogens. **By altering the normal vaginal flora, contraceptive diaphragm and spermicide use, as well as postmenopausal vaginal atrophy,** increase introital colonization with Enterobacteriaceae and result in an increased likelihood of recurrent UTIs [8].
4. **Urinary tract abnormalities.** A number of urinary tract abnormalities interfere with the defense mechanisms just noted [4,5].
   a. **Obstruction** anywhere in the urinary tract increases susceptibility of the kidney to infection. The exact role of urinary stasis in obstruction-related infection, however, has not been defined. Specific types of obstruction include ureteral obstruction (ureteral calculi and congenital abnormalities such as stenosis and ureteral valves) and urethral obstruction (prostatic hypertrophy).
   b. **Vesicoureteral reflux** increases the susceptibility of the kidney to infection by providing a route for ascending infection and interfering with the normal flow of urine. Reflux can be either the cause of infection or its result. Endotoxin from gram-negative bacteria inhibits ureteral peristalsis. During acute lower

UTI in adults, reflux from bladder to ureter often is present and resolves as the acute infection resolves.

c. **Incomplete bladder emptying.** Because urine acts as a culture medium for bacterial growth, residual urine can serve as a source of infection.

d. **Foreign bodies** also serve as a nidus for infection. Renal **calculi** and **indwelling bladder catheters** are the foreign bodies implicated most frequently in UTI.

5. **Diabetes mellitus in women** appears to increase the frequency of UTI, including upper tract infections and nosocomial infections [9]. The cause of the high prevalence of UTI with upper tract involvement is speculative, and a combination of factors is probably involved, including bladder dysfunction as a result of diabetic neuropathy, structural abnormalities (e.g., cystocele, rectocele), recurrent vaginitis, and underlying vascular disease [9].

**III. Clinical manifestations.** Localization studies make it clear that clinically it is very difficult, if not impossible, to distinguish upper from lower UTIs. Urinary frequency, dysuria, lower abdominal–suprapubic discomfort, and even costovertebral angle (CVA) or flank discomfort are nonspecific and may be seen both in upper and lower UTI [5].

**A. Lower UTIs. Clinically, it is not possible to distinguish cystitis from urethritis in women; vaginitis may also cause dysuria. UTI symptoms in men should direct attention to excluding concurrent prostate disease.**

**1. Acute cystitis**

a. **Dysuria,** or burning during or just after urination, and urgency and increased frequency of urination often are associated with cystitis. Suprapubic pain, fullness, or a sensation of pressure may also be present. Gross or microscopic hematuria occurs in approximately 50% of women with acute cystitis [2] but is uncommon with other causes of dysuria. Obstructive symptoms may predominate in men. The patient may complain of CVA or flank discomfort, making these latter findings unreliable in distinguishing upper from lower UTI.

Physical examination often is unremarkable; the patient may complain only of pain on suprapubic palpation. Patients should be examined for CVA tenderness. Inspection and palpation of the external genitalia along with rectal examination should be performed in men. In women, vaginal examination may be indicated.

Ordinarily, no systemic symptoms are present in uncomplicated lower UTI. Fever generally is absent, although low-grade temperature elevations are not uncommon. In women, prior episodes of confirmed cystitis and diaphragm use suggest a diagnosis of cystitis [8].

b. **Vaginitis** also must be considered because it may present with dysuria caused by irritation of the mucosal surface by the urine stream. **Vaginitis should be suspected when patients complain of perineal, labial, or external dysuria, which may be accompanied by odor, itching, or vaginal discharge.** Patients may describe the pain on urination as being more delayed than the discomfort that often begins before or at initiation of voiding with cystitis or urethritis. If these symptoms are present, a pelvic examination should be performed and appropriate vaginal, cervical, and urethral cultures obtained. See Chapter 16 for a discussion of vulvovaginitis.

**2. Urethritis**

a. **Urethritis in women** is a very common problem. Studies have shown that as many as **one third of women presenting with symptoms of lower UTI have urethritis without cystitis.** These patients exhibit symptoms of increased frequency and dysuria, and therefore the clinical presentation is identical to that in cystitis. Patients usually are afebrile. Urinalysis demonstrates pyuria but not bacteriuria. Clues in the history that suggest a sexually transmitted cause of urethritis include suspected or proved sexually transmitted disease in a sex partner or the presence of a new or multiple sex partners.

b. **Urethritis in men** frequently is suggested by concurrent dysuria and urethral discharge. Urinalysis may demonstrate pyuria. Historic clues to sexually transmitted disease should be sought, as discussed above. Urethritis in men is discussed in Chapter 16.

3. **Prostatitis** symptoms may be those of cystitis, with dysuria, frequency, and urgency, or symptoms of bladder outlet obstruction may predominate, with hesitancy, diminished stream, nocturia, or postmicturition dribbling. Perineal or low back pain may, on occasion, be the only manifestation. Physical examination findings that help differentiate acute from chronic prostatitis are discussed in section III under Urinary Tract Infection in Men, below. Examination should include inspection and palpation for evidence of urethral discharge, penile lesions, local epididymal or testicular disease, and inguinal adenopathy [10].

**B. Upper UTIs.** Clues from the history that suggest an increased likelihood of upper UTI include a prior history of pyelonephritis or structural abnormalities of the urinary tract, UTIs in childhood, diabetes, prolonged symptoms with the current episode (7 or more days), and failure to respond to short-course therapy administered for presumed cystitis.

1. **Pyelonephritis** [11]. Some patients with **acute pyelonephritis** have characteristic findings of high fever (39.5°–40.5° [103°–105°F]), shaking chills, and lumbar pain. Many authorities argue that **fever may be the most reliable clinical finding** in differentiating between upper and lower UTI. Presence of shaking chills implies that the UTI may be complicated by bacteremia. These findings may develop rapidly over a period of a few hours or 1 to 2 days and occur with or without antecedent or concurrent symptoms of lower UTI. Nausea, vomiting, and diarrhea or constipation also may be seen. Examination often reveals CVA and flank tenderness, but this may be a nonspecific finding. Urinalysis in most patients reveals significant pyuria (at least 10 leukocytes/mm$^3$ or per high power field of the unspun sediment), but 4% to 5% of cases of pyelonephritis do not involve pyuria [12].

   Some authors have subdivided syndromes of pyelonephritis [11].

   a. **Uncomplicated pyelonephritis,** which usually refers to pyelonephritis in women, includes many episodes of acute pyelonephritis, pyelonephritis in pregnancy, and silent (subclinical) pyelonephritis.

   b. **Complicated pyelonephritis** is generally the result of structural and functional abnormalities (e.g., obstruction, including prostate hypertrophy, calculi, reflux, neurogenic bladder) and/or urologic manipulations (catheters, renal transplantation) and is seen in those with underlying disease (e.g., diabetes, immunosuppression, cystic renal disease) and the elderly.

2. **Renal abscesses** present with signs and symptoms identical to pyelonephritis and should be **considered** in the patient with upper UTI whose **fever persists beyond 48 to 72 hours despite appropriate antimicrobial therapy** [13].

**IV. Laboratory diagnosis of UTI** focuses on the determination of the presence or absence of pyuria and bacteriuria. Rapid tests for the detection of leukocytes and bacteria in urine are available. Comprehensive laboratory testing in every patient is not needed for clinical management; indiscriminate use of urine cultures results in unnecessary costs. The management of UTI, the most common infection for which adults receive antimicrobial agents, should emphasize cost-effective strategies.

**A. Microscopic examination of urine.** Laboratory diagnosis in the patient with suspected UTI should usually begin with microscopic examination for leukocytes in the urine sediment. **Pyuria still is considered a useful indicator of UTI, and its absence should suggest an alternative diagnosis.** Pyuria in the elderly may be a nonspecific finding, but its absence means that bacteriuria is unlikely (see section V.C under Urinary Tract Infection in the Elderly, below).

When a health-care provider has a long-standing relationship with a reliable patient who has recurrent uncomplicated UTIs, it is reasonable and cost-effective not to do a urinalysis (or culture) but rather to treat empirically.

1. **Pyuria.** Unspun or spun urine (2,000 rpm, for 5 minutes) can be used. The most accurate method for diagnosis is counting leukocytes in unspun urine using a chamber method [2,14], although many clinical laboratories find this a cumbersome technique. Although different levels for pyuria have been proposed, a white blood cell (WBC) count of 10 cells/mm$^3$ by the counting chamber method seems to be the best diagnostic cutoff [2]. When examining spun urine sediment, more than 10 WBC per high power field indicates pyuria.

a. The **leukocyte esterase dipstick** is used widely as a rapid alternative office test for the detection of pyuria; it is 75% to 95% sensitive in detecting pyuria associated with infection. Although not as reliable as the chamber method to define pyuria, the leukocyte esterase dipstick is an acceptable alternative [14]. (See related discussion in section C.)

b. The WBC count may vary depending on urine flow, state of hydration, previous antibiotic treatment, and method of specimen collection.

c. "Sterile pyuria" may be associated with acute urethritis, renal tuberculosis, foreign body or tumor of the urinary tract, nonbacterial infections in the genital tract [12], and a poorly understood entity called interstitial cystitis, which is typically seen in women with chronic dysuria and urgency. (The etiology and treatment of this problem remains unclear [15].)

d. **The absence of pyuria in the symptomatic patient suggests that cystitis is not the cause of dysuria,** and urethritis or vaginitis should be considered as alternative diagnoses.

2. **Bacteria** seen on microscopic examination, especially of the unspun urine, can be a useful test for the presumptive diagnosis of UTI. Generally, bacterial counts of fewer than $10^5$ colony-forming units (CFU)/mL cannot be seen microscopically in unspun urine. Falsely elevated numbers of bacteria may be noted if the specimen was improperly collected or if the specimen was allowed to stand at room temperature for long periods of time. Numbers of bacteria may be decreased by the same factors that cause low numbers of WBCs in urine.

a. **A Gram stain** of one drop of freshly voided unspun urine can be done quickly and easily. The finding of one bacterium or more in each oil-immersion field suggests the presence of at least $10^5$ CFU/mL urine. When several fields must be searched for the presence of bacteria, the quantitative counts are generally lower, ranging from approximately $10^4$ to $10^5$ CFU/mL. With experience in its use, this Gram stain technique has been shown to correlate well with the quantitative urine culture.

**Gram stains of urine are especially useful in patients with presumed urosepsis, severe pyelonephritis, and in those at risk for enterococcal UTI** (e.g., elderly men). If the Gram stain of the unspun urine shows gram-positive cocci, enterococci may be the pathogen and empiric therapy should be active against enterococci. By contrast, if the Gram stain of unspun urine reveals gram-negative bacilli, empiric therapy aimed at enterococci is not necessary.

b. **Microscopic examination of spun urine** for WBCs and bacteria can be done under high dry power. With this method, the presence of more than one bacteria on a Gram stain correlates well with more than $10^4$ bacteria/mL [16].

3. **Hematuria,** as detected by rapid dipstick methods within the office setting, occurs in approximately 50% of women with acute cystitis but is uncommon in urethritis or vaginitis. Thus, microscopic hematuria in acutely dysuric young women is a marker of cystitis.

4. The **nitrate test** is sensitive for detecting more than $10^5$ CFU/mL of Enterobacteriaceae, but it may miss cases of cystitis with lower colony counts and it will not detect enterococci and staphylococci.

B. **Urine culture.** Urine is normally a sterile body fluid. Care in urine collection for culture is important to prevent contamination from the urethra, vagina, or perineum. It is to be emphasized that obtaining a clean-catch, midstream, voided urine is cumbersome and difficult for many patients.

It has become common practice and is more cost effective in women who have uncomplicated UTIs (i.e., symptoms of cystitis and urinalysis findings of pyuria) to prescribe treatment without an initial or follow-up urine culture [17,18]. **Urine cultures still are advised in pyelonephritis, complicated UTI** (see section I.C), and **in recurrent UTI** (except in recurrent episodes of UTI that are clearly associated with sexual activity) [2]. Cultures are also suggested to help assess for asymptomatic bacteriuria in certain settings, including pregnancy, before and after urologic manipulation, and after definitive removal of a chronic indwelling Foley catheter [2].

1. **Clean-catch urine specimen.** Collection of the urine specimen should be done with care. The specimen can be split, with a portion being used for urinalysis and the rest for culture.
   a. **Female patients** can be instructed to wash their hands, straddle or squat over the toilet, and spread the labia with the nondominant hand. Then, using the dominant hand, they should swab the vulva three times, front to back, with sterile gauze pads soaked in sterile water or with a sponge soaked in a mild nonhexachlorophene soap. The first 10 mL of voided urine is the urethral specimen and is discarded, unless it is saved to help diagnose urethritis. The urine specimen collected in a sterile cup during the middle of voiding (midstream sample) is used for culture. It should be quickly processed or refrigerated [2].
   b. **Male patients** can be instructed to retract the foreskin and clean the glans penis three times using gauze pads or sponges. However, some studies have questioned the necessity of these steps in a male, when only a midstream collection is necessary [2]. (See related discussion under section III.A.1 under Urinary Tract Infection in Men, below.)
   c. **Other collections. In the very obese, acutely ill, or infirm, a single straight (in-and-out) catheterization may be performed to obtain a clean sample for urinalysis and culture.** Suprapubic aspirations also can be performed and may be particularly useful in children.
2. **Urine culture interpretation.** It is important for physicians and microbiology laboratory personnel to work together in interpreting how the bacteriologic workup of urine should be approached in the laboratory.
   a. **Clean-catch urine.** The older criterion proposed that urine counts exceeding 100,000 CFU/mL (i.e., $\geq 10^5$ bacteria/mL) were significant, and counts of 10,000 CFU/mL or less from clean-catch specimens were generally considered contaminants. Studies from Stamm [14], Stamm et al. [19,20], and Kunin [21] emphasized that approximately one-third of women with acute lower UTI have colony counts in midstream urine of between $10^2$ and $10^4$ CFU/mL. **In acutely dysuric women with confirmed pyuria, therefore, the threshold for significant bacteriuria should be $10^2$ CFU/mL or more of a single or predominant uropathogen** (e.g., *E. coli, Pseudomonas aeruginosa, Staphylococcus saprophyticus*). Low colony counts of diphtheroids, lactobacilli, *Gardnerella vaginalis,* and *Staphylococcus epidermidis* are consistent with contaminants [14].

      In men, only limited data on the significance of lower colony counts in voided urine are available; in one study comparing voided urine with bladder specimens, approximately one-third of men with bladder bacteriuria had colony counts in midstream urine of greater than $10^3$ CFU/mL but less than $10^5$ CFU/mL [22]. **In dysuric men, growth of $10^3$ CFU/mL or more of a single or predominant uropathogen should be regarded as significant for presumptive UTI.**
   b. **Multiple isolates.** Voided urine cultures revealing two or more species of bacteria with no predominant organism are seen frequently. In people with normal urinary tracts, these usually represent contaminated urine samples; therefore, the culture should be repeated, with meticulous care in the collection of the specimen.
   c. **Straight catheter and suprapubic aspiration specimens.** Colony counts are considered to be significant if greater than $10^2$ CFU/mL of a single or predominant uropathogen are cultured.
   d. **Indwelling catheter.** Culture of urine specimens obtained by indwelling catheter frequently yields multiple isolates that change rapidly over time. Identification and susceptibility testing is most commonly performed on the one or two organisms that are clearly predominant at $10^4$ CFU/mL or more.
   e. **Limitations of urine culture** [12]
      (1) **Transport time.** Delays in transport from collection of the urine specimen to processing in the laboratory can affect colony counts considerably. In general, a urine culture should be processed as soon as possible after

collection. Urine specimens may be stored at room temperature for 1 hour or in a refrigerator for up to 48 hours without appreciable changes in bacterial counts. **Storage at room temperature for 2 hours or more will result in significant increases in bacterial counts, and the results of such specimens cannot be reliably interpreted.**

(2) **Fastidious microorganisms.** Standard urine culture procedures are directed toward routine uropathogens. Unusual microorganisms should be considered in patients with unexplained pyuria or when there is suspicion of sexually transmitted disease. Mycobacteria, fungi, gonococci, chlamydiae, and viruses require special transport media or special culture techniques.

**C. Rapid diagnostic tests.** Multiple tests have become available to detect pyuria and bacteriuria more rapidly. The most reliable chemical measurement of pyuria is the leukocyte esterase dipstick test; although somewhat less sensitive than microscopic examination for leukocytes, it is a useful alternative for the detection of pyuria when urine microscopy is unavailable [23] (see section A.1.a.).

Newer bacteriuria screening tests use nephelometry, bioluminescence, or a colorimetric filtration system. They yield comparable results, and all have a sensitivity similar to the urine Gram stain; none of the tests detect fewer than $10^4$ CFU/mL. Because a urine culture is often not done in young to middle-aged women with uncomplicated UTI, the need for these rapid culture screens has diminished. For recurrent UTI or complicated UTI, a urine culture with susceptibilities is advised (see section B).

**D. Blood cultures.** As many as 30% to 40% of patients with pyelonephritis will have positive blood cultures. In general, blood cultures should be obtained in those patients with a fever and a history of rigors, as well as in patients sufficiently ill to be hospitalized, especially if prior antibiotic therapy may have selected out resistant pathogens. The need for blood cultures has been debated by some in this cost conscious era. If complex UTIs (e.g., pyelonephritis) with or without bacteremia are to be treated for 2 weeks, the need for blood cultures may be superfluous [15]. However, the availability of potent oral agents has led to the use of shorter courses of therapy in some patients with mild disease. This is an unresolved issue, and the approach needs to be individualized.

**V. Microbiologic features of UTIs.** Organisms causing UTI are derived primarily from the aerobic members of the fecal flora. In women these microorganisms colonize the perineum as a way station to the urinary tract, and in men the prostate may be colonized or subclinically infected.

**A. Bacteria.** Bacteria involved include members of the family Enterobacteriaceae: *E. coli* and *Klebsiella, Enterobacter, Serratia, Proteus,* and *Providencia* species are most frequently seen in uncomplicated UTI. Of these, *E. coli* accounts for up to 80% of all infections. *Pseudomonas* species and group D streptococci account for approximately 5% to 10% of uncomplicated infections and are associated most often with instrumentation of the urinary tract.

**Coagulase-negative staphylococci (e.g., *S. saprophyticus*) may be pathogenic more often than was previously realized.** Formerly believed to be urinary contaminants, *S. saprophyticus* have been documented in urine by suprapubic catheterization, ureteral aspiration, and renal biopsy culture. Generally, patients with UTI due to *S. saprophyticus* are young female patients aged 16 to 25 years old, have pyuria, and have symptoms of lower UTI. *S. saprophyticus* is rarely the cause of UTI in hospitalized patients unless there has been instrumentation of the genitourinary tract. The organism will be recovered on serial cultures if it is a significant pathogen. Cefixime and certain other oral cephalosporins have relatively poor *in vitro* activity against *S. saprophyticus*, yet in limited clinical studies they have appeared active.

See Table 15.2 for a list of microbial species commonly associated with UTIs.

**B. Fungi.** The presence of fungi in the urine often presents a diagnostic dilemma. For the purpose of this and later discussions, the term **fungi** will refer to yeasts such as *Candida albicans,* other *Candida* species, and *Torulopsis glabrata* (*Candida glabrata*). Fungi are isolated most frequently in diabetics, in patients with indwelling

Table 15.2. Microbial Species Most Often Associated with Specific Types of Urinary Tract Infections (UTIs)

| | Acute Uncomplicated Cystitis (%) | Acute Uncomplicated Pyelonephritis (%) | Complicated UTI (%) | Catheter-Associated UTI (%) |
|---|---|---|---|---|
| *E. coli* | 79 | 89 | 32 | 24 |
| *S. saprophyticus* | 11 | 0 | 1 | 0 |
| *Proteus* | 2 | 4 | 4 | 6 |
| *Klebsiella* | 3 | 4 | 5 | 8 |
| Enterococci | 2 | 0 | 22 | 7 |
| *Pseudomonas* | 0 | 0 | 20 | 9 |
| Mixed | 3 | 5 | 10 | 11 |
| Other | 0 | 2 | 5 | 10 |
| Yeast | 0 | 0 | 1 | 28 |
| *S. epidermidis* | 0 | 0 | 15 | 8 |

From Falagas ME, Gorbach SL. Practical guidelines: urinary tract infections. *Infect Dis Clin Pract* 1995;4:242; with permission.

bladder catheters, in those receiving antibiotics, and, occasionally, in patients who have had previous instrumentation of the urinary tract.

C. **Viruses.** Viruria occurs in a variety of systemic illnesses such as measles, mumps, and infections with herpes simplex virus, cytomegalovirus, and adenovirus. There is indirect evidence to suggest that viruses may also be responsible for certain renal lesions, including glomerulonephritis. The role of varicella-zoster virus in hemorrhagic cystitis is well documented, and adenovirus has been strongly implicated as a cause of a similar syndrome. Adenovirus type 8 has been associated with hemorrhagic cystitis in children.

D. ***Chlamydia trachomatis, Neisseria gonorrhoeae,* and herpes simplex virus.** These are the major causes of urethritis in women, an infection in which dysuria may falsely suggest a diagnosis of cystitis [19].

E. ***Trichomonas vaginalis* and *Candida* species.** These are the principal pathogens associated with vaginitis, an alternative cause of dysuria in young women that may be confused with UTI (see Chapter 16).

VI. **Indications for urologic workup.** In treating patients with UTIs, the question of when to perform a urologic evaluation often arises. The goals of radiologic imaging studies and urologic evaluation are to identify correctable anatomic abnormalities (e.g., obstruction) that may predispose to recurrent UTIs and/or prevent adequate response without urologic intervention. It is indicated when urinary lithiasis is suspected or proven and to evaluate persistent hematuria.

Although the intravenous pyelogram was commonly used in the past [24], in recent years **renal ultrasound and abdominal computed tomography (CT) have commonly replaced the intravenous pyelogram** [2,14,15]. Renal ultrasound is very useful to assess noninvasively for obstructive uropathy. CT will help identify renal abscesses.

A. **UTI in male patients.** UTIs in men are infrequent compared with their incidence in women, and bacteriuria in men may be the first sign of an anatomic or functional abnormality.

1. **In boys,** the first UTI warrants ultrasonographic evaluation of the kidneys (to detect malformation or scarring) and voiding cystography (to detect vesicoureteral reflux and urethral obstruction) [25]. See related discussion under Urinary Tract Infection in Children, below.
2. **In young men,** there has been recent recognition that uncomplicated cystitis can occur and that urologic evaluation usually is unrewarding in those who respond to a 7-day course of therapy (see Urinary Tract Infection in Men, below). In older men, persistent or recurrent bacteriuria is frequently an indication of prostatic enlargement and obstruction or of chronic prostatitis. In addition to a

physical examination of the prostate, intravenous pyelogram and cystoscopy may also be useful. For further discussion, see sections II and III under Urinary Tract Infection in Men, below.

**B. UTI in female patients.** When to initiate investigation in female patients is controversial, particularly in the highly prevalent group of middle-aged to older women with recurrent UTIs, a group who rarely exhibit anatomic or functional abnormalities.

1. Imaging studies should be performed after the first UTI in girls younger than 5 years of age, older girls with recurrent UTIs, and in any child with pyelonephritis. As in boys, renal ultrasonography and voiding cystography are indicated; however, radionuclide voiding cystography can be substituted as a screening test to detect the presence of vesicoureteral reflux. If the facilities are available, radionuclide cystography greatly reduces ovarian radiation exposure in comparison with conventional fluoroscopic voiding cystourethrography. See related discussion under Urinary Tract Infection in Children later in this chapter.
2. Most recurrent UTIs in women are exogenous reinfections rather than relapsing infections due to the same organism. Documented relapsing infections should prompt urologic evaluation to exclude a treatable anatomic defect. Postmenopausal women should be evaluated for increased postvoiding residual associated with bladder or uterine prolapse.

**C. Pyelonephritis.** Upper UTI should manifest a clinical response within 72 hours of initiation of appropriate antimicrobial therapy. If flank pain or fever persists for longer than 72 hours, ultrasonography or CT should be performed to exclude unrecognized obstruction or intrarenal or perinephric abscess. Routine radiologic imaging studies for all cases of pyelonephritis are generally unrewarding and unnecessarily expensive. Patients with a prolonged clinical course, recurrent upper UTI, or a childhood history of infection should be evaluated for anatomic or functional abnormalities.

## GENERAL MANAGEMENT PRINCIPLES OF URINARY TRACT INFECTIONS

**I. Nonspecific treatment** [26]

**A. Hydration.** Forcing fluids has long been advocated in the initial treatment of UTI. There are theoretic reasons for and against it. The benefit of hydration has never been critically documented in clinical studies; it probably is not necessary once appropriate antimicrobial treatment has been instituted.

**B. Urinary analgesics.** Such pain relievers as phenazopyridine hydrochloride (e.g., Pyridium, 200 mg orally three times a day after meals) may be useful to relieve symptoms of severe dysuria or urethral irritation but generally are necessary only for the first 24 to 48 hours of treatment if they are used at all. It is best to prescribe only a small number of tablets, for a 1- or 2-day period, because many patients mistakenly will use the drug as primary treatment and will avoid consulting a physician in the event of relapse or reinfection. It should be stressed to the patient that this drug is only adjunctive treatment and is not an antibiotic. Phenazopyridine should be avoided in pregnancy and probably in nursing mothers also.

**II. General principles of antimicrobial therapy** [26]. The choice of therapy in UTI will depend on the patient's age and gender, on whether the infection is symptomatic or asymptomatic, on the presumed site of infection (upper vs. lower), and on whether the UTI is recurrent. **Specific treatment guidelines based on these considerations are discussed in this section and are summarized in Table 15.3.** Factors such as whether the infection is community or hospital acquired and host considerations such as the presence of impaired renal function or abnormal collecting systems often influence the likely causative pathogen, the severity of illness, and the response to therapy and therefore will influence the choice of antimicrobial agent.

**A. Choice of antimicrobial agent.** Many antimicrobial agents with a broad gram-negative spectrum of activity are effective in the treatment of UTI [27]. Most UTIs are localized to the collecting system, and active urine levels are achieved after oral administration of essentially all commonly used antimicrobial agents. Bacteriostatic and bactericidal drugs are of equal efficacy. Given the availability of several drugs microbiologically active against known or suspected uropathogens, considerations in choosing empiric antimicrobial therapy are the patient's history of drug allergy, relative drug toxicities, and cost of available agents.

1. **Resistance to sulfonamides, ampicillin, and amoxicillin is now present in** 25% to 35% of *E. coli* strains causing outpatient cystitis, making these agents **no longer the standards for empiric therapy** of gram-negative UTIs [28].

   Although resistance to trimethoprim and trimethoprim-sulfamethoxazole (TMP-SMX) has been increasing nationwide, in some geographic areas it still is sufficiently uncommon that these two antimicrobial agents remain the empiric therapies of choice on the basis of cost. Resistance to nitrofurantoin and to the fluoroquinolones among *E. coli* remains below 5% in most areas. If a geographic area has a high incidence of TMP resistance to common urinary pathogens (e.g., >15%–20%), then a fluoroquinolone is a reasonable alternative (see Chapter 27).
2. **UTIs** are the **most common indication** for which antimicrobial agents are prescribed. Small increments in cost of individual therapies have the potential for large aggregate expense. Because of cost and concern with emergence of resistance, the fluoroquinolones should be reserved for UTIs in which resistance to older less expensive agents has been demonstrated or is likely. For this reason, fluoroquinolones are usually not the agents of choice for first episodes of uncomplicated cystitis (see Chapter 27).
3. With **renal functional impairment,** dosage modification is necessary for agents that are primarily renally excreted (see Chapter 27).

   UTIs in patients with **end-stage renal disease** pose a therapeutic challenge because of the lack of the usual high concentration of antimicrobial agents in the urine. In general, the penicillins and cephalosporins have little nephrotoxicity, attain adequate urine levels despite severe renal functional impairment, and may be the agents of choice in renal failure.
4. **Oral and parenteral therapies** are equally effective in the treatment of UTI provided that the patient is able to take and absorb oral medication adequately. Most patients with pyelonephritis who are ill enough to require hospitalization should be treated initially with parenteral agents until there is symptomatic improvement and fever subsides. (See section III.A under Urinary Tract Infection in Women.) Then, therapy can be completed with an oral regimen.

**B. Duration of therapy.** This primarily depends on the presumed site of infection. **For cystitis** in women, short-course therapy, usually for 3 days, is preferable to the historic 7- to 14-day therapeutic regimen because it is equally efficacious, costs less, is associated with fewer side effects, has a lower incidence of emergence of resistant gastrointestinal flora, and allows for better compliance. **The authors support the Infectious Diseases Society of America guidelines advocating 3-day regimens as more effective than single-dose therapy.** (For single-dose therapy, the best results have been observed with TMP-SMX, 320/1,600 mg, as a single dose. Single-dose therapy with drugs such as amoxicillin and the oral cephalosporins, which are excreted rapidly, has been less efficacious.) Short-course regimens of documented efficacy are shown in Table 15.3 and are discussed in section II.D.2 under Urinary Tract Infection in Women. **For pyelonephritis,** a 2-week course of antibiotics is advised [11].

Extended-duration antimicrobial therapy may be indicated for recurrent infection (as discussed later) and in pyelonephritis failing a 14-day regimen. See section III.A under Urinary Tract Infection in Women.

**III. Determinants of specific antimicrobial therapy. Asymptomatic and symptomatic, acute and recurrent, upper and lower UTIs in children, in men and women, in the elderly, and in catheterized patients are discussed separately and in detail later in this chapter.** General comments regarding several of these major determinants of therapy follow.

**A. Age and gender.** Children with UTIs and severe vesicoureteral reflux are at high risk for progressive renal scarring and eventual functional impairment. Most UTIs in women represent cystitis, which is easily treated. UTI in men is usually related

Table 15.3. Antibiotic Therapy for Adults with Symptomatic Urinary Tract Infection (UTI)

| Syndrome | Duration | Route | Medication | Dose[a] (mg) | Interval |
|---|---|---|---|---|---|
| Cystitis, females, uncomplicated[b] | 3 d | p.o. | TMP[c] | 100 | q12h |
| | | | TMP-SMX[c] | 160/800 | q12h |
| | | | Tetracycline | 500 | q6h |
| | | | Norfloxacin[d] | 400 | q12h |
| | | | Ciprofloxacin[d] | 250 | q12h |
| | | | Levofloxacin | 250 | q24 |
| | | | Cefixime | 400 | q24h |
| | | | Cefpodoxime proxetil | 100 | q12h |
| | 7 d (see text) | | Nitrofurantoin | 100 | q6h |
| | | | Amoxicillin + clavulanate | 500 | q12h |
| | 1 d | | Fosfomycin[e] | 3000 | Single dose |
| Cystitis complicated[f] | 10–14 d[g] | p.o. | Same as 3-d regimens for uncomplicated cystitis (shown above) | | |
| | | | Also: | | |
| | | | Lomefloxacin[d] | 400 | q24h |
| | | | Enoxacin[d] | 400 | q12h |
| Urethritis, female | See Chapter 16 | | | | |
| Urethritis, male | See Chapter 16 | | | | |
| Prostatitis, acute[h] | 4 wk[g,i] | p.o. | TMP[c] | 100 | q12h |
| | | | TMP-SMX[c] | 160/800 | q12h |
| | | | Ciprofloxacin[j] | 500 | q12h |
| | | | Levofloxacin[j] | 250 | q24h |
| Prostatitis, chronic[h] | 6–12 wk[g] | p.o. | TMP[c] | 100 | q12h |
| | | | TMP-SMX[c] | 160/800 | q12h |
| | | | Ciprofloxacin[j] | 500 | q12h |
| | | | Levofloxacin[j] | 250 | q24h |
| Pyelonephritis, outpatient[k] | 14 d[g] | p.o. | TMP[c] | Same as 3-d regimens for uncomplicated cystitis | |
| | | | TMP-SMX[c] | | |
| | | | Amoxicillin + clavulanate | | |
| | | | Ciprofloxacin | 500 | q12h |
| | | | Enoxacin | 400 | q12h |
| | | | Gatifloxacin | 400 | q24h |
| | | | Levofloxacin | 250 | q24h |
| Pyelonephritis, hospitalized patient[k] | 14 days[g] | i.v. and p.o.[l] | See footnote[m] | | |

[a] **See individual chapter discussions for dose modification in renal failure and details of intramuscular and intravenous regimens.**
[b] Short-course therapy (3 days) is preferable to single-dose regimens [1,27]; therefore, the 3-day regimens are emphasized. **Uncomplicated** UTI is cystitis in nonpregnant adult women (young to middle-age), without genitourinary tract structural abnormality or bladder neurologic dysfunction.
[c] Preferred antibiotic selections on the basis of cost; empiric use limited to those geographical areas where frequency of resistance is less than 20%.

(*Table Footnote Continued.*)

[d]**The fluoroquinolones are reserved for regions having a higher frequency of more resistant pathogens** (see Chapter 27). These agents should be avoided in pregnancy, nursing mothers, and adolescents younger than 17 years of age.

[e]Fosfomycin single dose therapy has comparable efficacy to 7-day nitrofurantoin therapy.

[f]See definition of uncomplicated UTI in footnote b. Other UTIs, including those in men, are, by definition, complicated.

[g]Susceptibility of pathogen to selected antibiotic must be confirmed with *in vitro* susceptibility testing.

[h]**In acute prostatitis,** symptoms included fever, acute perineal pain and discomfort, and, usually, signs of an acute lower UTI such as dysuria, frequency, and urgency. The rectal examination reveals a swollen prostate that often is exquisitely tender on palpation, and prostatic massage may precipitate bacteremia. **In chronic prostatitis,** the prostate can remain a persistent source of UTI, with recurrent episodes of UTI. Symptoms are variable, including asymptomatic bacteriuria, perineal or low back discomfort, and relapsing UTI. For further discussion, see text.

[i]Some experts prefer to treat both acute and chronic prostatitis for protracted periods of time (e.g., 4–6+ weeks) to eradicate the infection clearly.

[j]Other fluoroquinolones are potentially useful agents in this setting, but there is less experience with their use in prostatitis (see Chapter 27).

[k]The decision regarding outpatient or in-hospital treatment of acute pyelonephritis is primarily one of clinical judgment. It is influenced by the patient's clinical condition, age, underlying disease, and potential compliance. In general, older or frail patients, bacteremic patients, toxic patients, and noncompliant patients will require inpatient therapy initially [5].

[l]Change from intravenous to oral therapy when the patient has clinically improved and is afebrile at least 24–48 hours.

[m]The optimal regimen for a patient admitted with acute pyelonephritis depends on many factors. Enterococci can be in part ruled out if a Gram stain of the urine shows no gram-positive cocci.

- In patients without prior UTI and only moderate illness, cefazolin, 1 g q6–8h, is reasonable.
- In patients who are very ill or who have a history of prior UTI (therefore the potential of a resistant gram-negative infection), ampicillin-sulbactam (3 g q6–8h) with or without an aminoglycoside or ampicillin (1.5 g q4h) and an aminoglycoside (see Chapter 27) can be used, especially if enterococci are a concern. Vancomycin (see Chapter 27) can be used instead of ampicillin in the penicillin allergic patient.
- If *Pseudomonas aeruginosa* is a concern, an aminoglycoside should be used initially until culture data are available. In addition to the above regimens, it may be given with an anti-pseudomonal penicillin (e.g. piperacillin or ticarcillin) or carbapenem (e.g. imipenem or meropenem). Ceftazidime or cefepime with an aminoglycoside may be used initially when enterococci are not also a concern.
- In patients in whom enterococci is not a concern, a third-generation cephalosporin (e.g., ceftriaxone 2 g q24h) can be used.
- Intravenous TMP-SMX, fluoroquinolones, and aztreonam are options for the patient unable to receive the aforementioned regimens. Neither TMP-SMX nor aztreonam is active against enterococci.
- For activity against enterococci, ampicillin, ampicillin-sulbactam, or vancomycin is preferred. The fluoroquinolones also are active against many enterococci.

TMP, trimethoprim; SMX; sulfamethoxazole.

Adapted from Hooton TM, Stamm WB. Diagnosis and treatment of uncomplicated urinary tract infection. *Infect Dis Clin North Am* 1997;11:551; and Warren JW, Abrutyn E, Hebel JR, et al. Guidelines for antimicrobial treatment of uncomplicated acute bacterial cystitis and acute pyelonephritis in women. *Clin Infect Dis* 1999;29:745, with permission.

to prostatic enlargement or infection. Women have many more UTIs than men until approximately age 65, after which time the prevalence of bacteriuria rises with age and functional status in both men and women.

**B. Asymptomatic versus symptomatic bacteriuria.** Detection of asymptomatic bacteriuria is often the result of laboratory screening procedures because, as the term implies, such patients are indeed symptomless. Asymptomatic bacteriuria is likely to occur in patients with indwelling catheters, patients with urologic abnormalities, pregnant women, the elderly, and approximately 5% of school-aged girls.

Because of the problems of contamination of clean-catch specimens, this diagnosis should not be based on the results of a single urine culture.

**1. Criterion to establish the diagnosis of asymptomatic bacteriuria**

**a.** Two consecutive clean-catch specimens having greater than 100,000 organisms/mL, with the same organism in both specimens.

**b.** Alternatively, a single urethral catheter specimen with greater than 100 organisms/mL.

2. **Approach** to the treatment of asymptomatic bacteriuria depends on an appreciation of the prognosis of the untreated infection and the long-term results that are anticipated from therapy. The side effects and cost of therapy are of paramount importance.
   a. **Screening for asymptomatic bacteriuria in children is controversial.** Although bacteriuria can be associated with hypertension and renal insufficiency, these complications are rare as is asymptomatic bacteriuria, occurring in only 1% to 2% of children. Although there is up to a 3% prevalence of asymptomatic bacteriuria in premature infants, the difficulties in obtaining a clean urine specimen make screening neonates impractical. (See related discussion in section IV.D under Urinary Tract Infection in Children, below.)
   b. **Screening for asymptomatic bacteriuria in adults is of particular value in two situations: before urologic surgery and during pregnancy.** Postoperative infectious complications are reduced by treating bacteriuria preoperatively. The importance of routine screening during the first trimester is discussed in section 1.C under Urinary Tract Infection in Women, below.

C. **Localization of the site of infection.** It is well recognized that upper UTI (pyelonephritis) requires longer duration therapy than lower UTI (cystitis). As previously discussed, the clinical presentation may not be reliable enough to make an accurate distinction between upper and lower infection. Although several methods have been developed to help distinguish upper from lower UTI, such methods are either invasive with resultant considerable patient discomfort or are not widely available for clinical application. They are sometimes used in clinical research studies.

1. **Invasive techniques** include ureteral catheterization with direct culturing and the bladder washout technique with sequential sampling of bladder and ureteral urine. Both techniques are complex urologic and microbiologic procedures, requiring close cooperation between physicians and the clinical laboratory.
2. **The noninvasive technique** that has received most attention is the antibody-coated bacteria test [29]. The test detects antibodies against infecting bacteria that are believed to form when tissue infection (upper tract or prostatitis) is present (in contrast to cystitis). Because it is not widely available, the test has been used primarily as an epidemiologic and research tool and, to date, has not had a major role in influencing management of UTI in a given patient.
3. **In most clinical settings, therapy is based on clinical manifestations,** recognizing that most UTIs are lower tract infections. Patients with fever and flank pain are likely to have upper tract disease.

   The outcome of therapy has implications about whether upper versus lower tract infection may be present. **Relapse of infection after short-course therapy in women is associated with upper UTI.**

D. **Recurrent UTI.** Repeated episodes of UTI can be either **reinfection** (i.e., new infections with new organisms) or **relapse** (i.e., a recrudescence of a prior partially treated infection). The distinction is an important one to make because it has implications both for the type and extent of workup indicated for therapy. **Reinfections** tend to occur more than 2 weeks after completion of therapy for the initial episode and are more frequent after uncomplicated cystitis. **Relapses** tend to occur within 2 weeks after completion of therapy of complicated UTI [2].

1. **Reinfection** is more common than relapse in women; conversely, in men most recurrent infection is due to relapse. After successful therapy of a prior infection, recurrence of symptoms and evidence of **clinical infection with a new organism** (either a new bacterial species or a new serologic type of *E. coli*) indicates reinfection. In general, most reinfections occur within weeks to months of the preceding UTI.
   a. **Reinfection in women** (of childbearing age to middle age) is common. As discussed under Urinary Tract Infection in Women (see below), it is recommended that women with three or more symptomatic lower UTIs within a 6-month period should receive extended-duration (6- to 12-month) prophylactic therapy.
   b. **Reinfection in men** is a much less common cause of recurrent infection than is relapse and, as discussed under Urinary Tract Infection in Men (see below),

is most commonly related to prostatic enlargement causing partial urethral obstruction.

2. **Relapse** refers to the recurrence of symptoms and clinical infection after the cessation of treatment. Implied in this definition is that relapse involves the **same organism** or same serotype of *E. coli* that caused the initial infection. Most relapses occur shortly after the patient has completed a course of therapy (i.e., perhaps within a few days and certainly within 1 month).
   a. **Setting.** Relapse is likely to occur if there is persistent infection in the renal parenchyma or prostate gland, if the patient does not receive the proper antibiotic therapy, or if there is an underlying renal pathologic process, such as renal calculi.
   b. **Implications. Relapse often implies underlying urologic abnormality.** Therefore, **urologic evaluation is mandatory,** particularly if previous antibiotic therapy was adequate on the basis of susceptibility data.
   c. The **approach** should be directed initially at defining the underlying urologic defect, if possible. **If no correctable urologic defect is found and the patient has failed conventional 10- to 14-day therapy, one may presume there is a deeply seated tissue infection. In this group of patients, prolonged therapy (e.g., 4–8 weeks) may eradicate the infection.**
   d. **Suppressive therapy.** If a prolonged course of therapy also fails, chronic suppressive therapy may be necessary. *In vitro* susceptibility results should be used to determine the choice of chronic suppressive antibiotic therapy. The agent should be administered in full therapeutic dose. In recurrent UTI, there are limited indications for this approach. The major use is in patients with urologic abnormalities that cannot be corrected surgically. **This approach should not be taken in patients with indwelling urethral catheters.**

## URINARY TRACT INFECTION IN WOMEN

Women constitute the largest group of patients with UTI [5]. Most such UTIs represent cystitis, but the overlapping clinical symptoms of urethritis or vaginitis may cause confusion. **In most patients, short-course antibiotic therapy (3 days) may be administered empirically on the basis of symptoms along with urinalysis confirmation of pyuria, without the use of pretherapy or posttherapy urine cultures.** Recurrent UTI poses a frequent and troublesome problem.

I. **Asymptomatic bacteriuria**
   A. **Significance.** There are insufficient data regarding the long-term effects of asymptomatic bacteriuria in young or middle-aged nonpregnant women. Many patients in this group will clear their bacteriuria spontaneously and will not require treatment.
   B. **Approach. The current consensus is that this entity in the nonpregnant adult patient does not require treatment,** provided there is no urinary tract obstruction.
   C. **Pregnancy.** It is important to screen for and treat asymptomatic bacteriuria in women only during pregnancy because morbidity associated with UTI in pregnant women has been clearly demonstrated [5,30]. Asymptomatic bacteriuria occurs in about 5% of pregnant women with the most common onset between weeks 9 and 17 of pregnancy. Approximately 40% of pregnant women with asymptomatic bacteriuria will develop acute pyelonephritis in their pregnancy if not treated [2]. Pyelonephritis in the mother and low birth weight in the infant are sufficiently common complications to warrant mandatory screening for bacteriuria during gestation. Treating pregnant bacteriuric patients lowers the subsequent incidence of symptomatic UTIs by 80% to 90% [30]. Increased rates of premature labor have been seen in pregnant women with symptomatic UTI. The mechanisms for premature labor developing in patients with symptomatic infection are not completely clear but may be related, in part, to microorganism production of phospholipase $A_2$. Human term labor is believed to be initiated by amniotic and chorionic phospholipase $A_2$ [30].
      1. **All pregnant women should be screened for the presence of bacteriuria** on the first prenatal visit and again at the 28th week in women with a history

of frequent UTIs. If only a single cost-effective screening culture is done, the 16th gestational week may be an optimal time [30]. Cultures with colony counts exceeding $10^5$ bacteria warrant therapy. The significance of lower colony counts of clean-catch samples is less well defined [10].

2. **Treatment.** Because of the risk of pyelonephritis and subsequent stillbirth or prematurity, **asymptomatic bacteriuria in pregnant women should be treated. Oral antimicrobials that are safe to give during pregnancy** include amoxicillin, cephalosporins, nitrofurantoin, and sulfonamides. **(The use of sulfonamides should be avoided in the third trimester.) Recommended duration of therapy is 7 to 10 days** [30].
3. **Follow-up. Eradication of bacteriuria is the goal.** This should be confirmed with follow-up cultures at 1 and 4 weeks after therapy ends.

   If infection returns with the same bacterium, a relapsing infection from an occult source should be suspected. In this setting, a second course of antibiotics for a longer duration and an agent based on susceptibility data may be tried. If infection is present on further follow-up cultures, then a short course of antibiotics to which the bacterium is susceptible can be used to suppress the infection, followed by nitrofurantoin, 50 to 100 mg daily at bedtime, until delivery, with the hopes of suppressing recurrent infection. (For susceptible pathogens, chronic suppression with amoxicillin or a cephalosporin is also a potential regimen.) Serial urine cultures should be performed to detect the possibility of a resistant pathogen. Follow-up urine cultures should be performed after delivery, and urologic evaluation should be undertaken 3 to 6 months after delivery [30].
4. See related discussion in section V.

D. **Diabetes mellitus in women.** Although studies are limited, many experts believe that asymptomatic bacteriuria in diabetics without obvious anatomic abnormalities should be treated when detected because of the frequency of upper UTI in diabetics when bacteriuria is present [9].

II. **Lower UTI** [5,31]. Women with dysuria but without fever constitute the largest group of UTI patients and the largest group of adults for whom antimicrobials are prescribed. With such women, the **first step is to exclude vaginitis from the differential diagnosis.** Women with vaginitis usually experience dysuria as an external discomfort, and those with cystitis have a deeper and more visceral dysuria. If vaginitis is suspected, a pelvic examination should be done. Clinical and laboratory evaluation of vaginitis or cervicitis should be performed as described in Chapter 16.

A. **Cystitis.** Women with lower UTIs form a homogenous group of patients who are appropriately managed as outpatients. As a common outpatient illness, this type of UTI presents a challenge to the primary care provider. Because a UTI generally is seen more as a nuisance and an inconvenience than a harmful state, the practitioner may be lulled into unwarranted indifference and may thus not acknowledge uncommon but significant events (e.g., the presence of occult or subacute pyelonephritis with or without mechanical or neurologic dysfunction). However, with confirmation of pyuria on urinalysis, there is an opportunity for use of cost-effective antimicrobial therapy. The absence of comorbidity and the limited extent of the infection makes this bacterial infection particularly appropriate for short-course therapy, now the standard of management for lower UTI (see section D.2). The **microbial agents responsible** include *E. coli* (60%), other Enterobacteriaceae organisms (20%), and *S. saprophyticus* (10%).

B. **Urethritis.** Acute onset of dysuria along with pyuria also occurs with urethritis. Previously discussed clues about the nature of the dysuria may help distinguish cystitis from urethritis (see section III under General Approach to Urinary Tract Infections, above). Recent onset of dysuria in patients who have a new coital partner in the month before onset of symptoms and who have not had symptoms of a UTI in the preceding 2 years may signal urethritis due to a sexually transmitted infection. *C. trachomatis,* trichomoniasis, gonorrhea, and herpes simplex virus may be the etiologic agent (see Chapter 16).

**Strong consideration should be given to performing a pelvic examination in sexually active women with dysuria.**

1. Obtain a culture or Gram stain for the gonococcus.
2. If ulcerations are present, herpes simplex virus cultures should ideally be performed.
3. Testing of a first-void urine sample by nucleic acid amplification methods is at least as sensitive as culture for *C. trachomatis*; choice of the most appropriate diagnostic test will depend on local test availability and cost.

C. **Vaginitis** as a cause of dysuria should be suspected in the patient who lacks pyuria; has vaginal discharge, odor, pruritus, or dyspareunia; relates external dysuria; or has dysuria without frequency or urgency.

D. **Clinical approach to acute dysuria.** If vaginitis is excluded, the next step is to examine the urine sediment for leukocytes.

1. **Diagnostic clues**
   a. A positive leukocyte esterase test or the presence of more than 10 WBCs within a high power field of spun urine is consistent with but not diagnostic of UTI or urethritis.
   b. In the patient with acute dysuria, if pyuria is not present the probability of infection is less than 5%. The diagnosis of vaginitis should be considered in the absence of pyuria.
   c. If pyuria is present, the unspun urine should be examined carefully using a Gram stain for bacteria, and if bacteria are seen in most fields under oil immersion, it is likely that the urine contains 100,000 bacteria or more per milliliter. If bacteria are not seen, then the infection may still be bacterial with low colony counts or it may be nonbacterial.
2. **Therapy**
   a. **Most authorities advocate administering empiric short-course antibiotic therapy for uncomplicated UTI without obtaining an initial urine culture.** Indeed, treatment decisions are made and completed before culture results would be available, and this approach is supported by cost-effectiveness studies [18].
   b. **Not all antimicrobials have been shown to be effective in short-course therapy,** and only the doses and agents with proven efficacy should be used (Table 15.3). **Overall, most experts favor the 3-day regimen over the single-dose regimen** [2,15].
      (1) **Short-course (3-day) therapy is indicated for only those women with uncomplicated infections.**
      (2) **Contraindications for short-course therapy** include pregnancy, suspected upper UTI or known prior pyelonephritis, relapsing infection, recent antibiotic use or bladder instrumentation, suspected or known urinary tract structural abnormality, childhood UTIs, symptoms for longer than 7 days, recent diaphragm use [2], and inability to provide follow-up. Because of the high rate of upper UTI in **diabetic women,** many experts do not recommend 3-day regimens for acute uncomplicated UTI in diabetic women; a 7-day regimen is preferred [1,9]. Furthermore, **use of the $\beta$-lactams in 3-day regimens is less effective** than other 3-day regimens (e.g., TMP-SMX, quinolones), and therefore experts prefer 7- to 10-day courses of cephalosporins rather than use of a 3-day course, even for uncomplicated cystitis [15,26,32]. Macrodantin, likewise, is not quite as effective in 3-day regimens when compared with TMP-SMX or the quinolones [15]; a 7-day course of therapy is recommended.
3. **Indications for urine culture**
   a. **Urine culture should be obtained** in acutely dysuric women who lack pyuria, in situations when urethritis and cystitis are not clearly distinguished clinically, in patients with relapsing or frequent recurrent infections, in complicated UTIs, and in pregnant women.
   b. **In women with sterile cultures,** acute dysuria, and pyuria, chlamydial urethritis should be suspected. The sexually active woman should have a pelvic examination with appropriate urethral or cervical cultures. Empiric therapy with tetracycline, 500 mg orally every 6 hours for 7 days (or doxycycline, 100 mg orally twice daily), or azithromycin, 1 g orally as a single dose (see

Chapter 16), should be administered if not contraindicated (see Chapter 27), and test-of-cure cultures should be obtained as appropriate.

4. **Follow-up**
   a. **If symptoms resolve with short-course therapy, no follow-up culture is necessary.**
   b. If short-course therapy fails or symptoms recur, then a urine culture should be obtained.
      (1) Such patients should be suspected of having occult or subclinical pyelonephritis [2]. See section VI under General Approach to Urinary Tract Infections (above) for decisions on urologic evaluation.
      (2) Significant bacteriuria ($>10^2$ CFU/mL) should be treated with at least 14 days of antibiotics directed by susceptibility testing.
5. It is unclear how to treat dysuric patients with negative cultures and with no pyuria. Vaginitis should be excluded in all such patients. Observation and a short course of phenazopyridine hydrochloride (e.g., Pyridium) may be reasonable.

E. **Recurrent cystitis** requires that urine cultures be obtained and susceptibility tests be performed.

1. **Antibiotic therapy** directed by susceptibility test results should be administered for 7 to 14 days.
2. **Follow-up urine cultures** should be obtained at 1 and 4 weeks after the end of therapy.

## III. Upper UTI

A. **Pyelonephritis.** The syndrome of acute pyelonephritis includes dysuria and increased frequency accompanied by **fever** (temperature usually exceeds 102°F) or definite CVA tenderness; the patient may also appear septic. However, upper UTI may be difficult to distinguish from lower UTI or so-called silent (subclinical) pyelonephritis. Up to 30% of women in a primary care setting and up to 80% of indigent patients suffering from clinically apparent cystitis in emergency rooms also have silent invasive bacterial infections of renal parenchyma; this infection is indistinguishable from lower UTI because most patients have dysuria and pyuria but not back pain. (See section III.B under General Approach to Urinary Tract Infections, above.) **Women who fail short-course antibiotic therapy for presumed lower UTI should be assumed to have subclinical or occult pyelonephritis [2].** Subclinical pyelonephritis is more common in pregnant women with UTI, in patients who have had a UTI before age 12, and those who have had previous pyelonephritis or more than three UTIs in the past year. Patients with UTI and positive blood cultures have pyelonephritis with invasive tissue infection.

**Painless complicated pyelonephritis,** which in fact is a different entity than subclinical pyelonephritis, can be observed in diabetics, renal transplant patients, and alcoholics. These patients have minimal symptoms due to autonomic nervous system damage associated with underlying disease but often have severe pyelonephritis [11].

1. **Microbiologic features.** *E. coli* causes approximately 85% of all cases of community-acquired pyelonephritis. Other members of the family Enterobacteriaceae cause approximately 10%, and gram-positive bacteria such as *Streptococcus faecalis* or *S. saprophyticus* the remainder. More antibiotic-resistant gram-negative aerobes, including *P. aeruginosa,* should be anticipated in patients with hospital-acquired infection and in women who have had recurrent UTIs or who have recently failed antimicrobial therapy (Table 15.2).
2. **Principles of antibiotic therapy.** The best way to treat pyelonephritis is poorly defined in the literature, and despite initial therapy with 2 weeks of an antibiotic effective *in vitro*, approximately 20% of patients may fail this therapy (i.e., patients may have relapsing infection) [11].
   a. The relatively high failure rates reported may in part be due to the absence of sufficient levels of antibiotic in renal tissue to sterilize the infected medulla. Whether or not the antibiotic must reach inhibitory concentrations in the bloodstream and urine and renal tissue to be effective in pyelonephritis is debated, but some reviewers believe it is important for inhibitory levels to be attained in both the kidney tissue and urine of patients with pyelonephritis [11].

**b.** Laboratory studies have suggested that pyelonephritic and endotoxemic kidneys accumulate more aminoglycosides (e.g., gentamicin, tobramycin) and quinolones than $\beta$-lactams (e.g., cephalosporins). TMP-SMX penetrates renal tissue adequately [11]. Furthermore, renal tissue levels of aminoglycosides are prolonged, and their effectiveness in treating pyelonephritis is confirmed in the animal model [11].

Therefore, especially while awaiting susceptibility data, when parenteral therapy is needed for acute gram-negative bacilli pyelonephritis, **aminoglycosides are clinically effective and cost effective if not contraindicated** (see Chapter 27). Because of their prolonged tissue levels, even 48 to 72 hours of initial aminoglycoside therapy may be effective; therapy can then be narrowed based on susceptibility data [14].

**3. Outpatient versus inpatient therapy.** The decision regarding outpatient or in-hospital treatment of acute pyelonephritis is primarily one of clinical judgment. It is influenced by the patient's clinical condition, age, underlying disease, and potential for compliance. In general, patients who are older or more frail, bacteremic, toxic, or immunocompromised will require inpatient therapy initially. In mild cases in which the actual diagnosis of upper or lower UTI may be unclear, outpatient therapy is reasonable [33].

**a. Outpatient therapy.** Empiric therapy with oral antibiotics should be started as outlined in Table 15.3 pending receipt of urine culture results and susceptibility data. **Antibiotics usually are given for 2 weeks** because renal parenchymal infections are more difficult to treat than superficial bladder infections.

**b. Inpatient therapy** with empiric, parenteral, antimicrobial treatment is indicated for many patients with pyelonephritis.

**(1)** Initial antibiotic therapy should include agents that are known to be active against anticipated pathogens. Doses should be appropriate to provide sufficient drug levels within the renal parenchyma and at distant nonrenal sites, as indicated in Table 15.3. Intravenous ampicillin alone probably is inadequate. Up to 30% of organisms may be resistant, even in community-acquired infections [4].

**(2)** However, ampicillin (or vancomycin in the penicillin-allergic patient) should be used when urine Gram staining suggests the possibility of enterococcal infection (i.e., gram-positive cocci).

**(3)** Patients in whom multiple antibiotic-resistant isolates are anticipated (e.g., hospital-acquired infection) should be given agents that have broad gram-negative coverage, to include *P. aeruginosa*. Often, the most cost-effective agent is an aminoglycoside, unless contraindicated. Aztreonam, ceftazidime, cefepime, and imipenem may be used as alternatives to an aminoglycoside. See Chapter 27 for a discussion of these agents.

**(4)** Therapy should be modified to the narrowest spectrum agent possible and to a less expensive antibiotic when the results of susceptibility tests are available.

**(5)** Once the infection is well controlled with intravenous therapy, outpatient therapy with either oral or intravenous antibiotics is reasonable.

**4. Duration of therapy.** In pyelonephritis, antibiotics usually are given for a **total of 14 days** [34]. Because of the occasional difficulties in eradicating renal tissue infection in patients failing 14-day therapy, longer courses of therapy (e.g., 4–6 weeks) should be used. For the hospitalized patient, parenteral therapy usually is continued until the patient has clinically improved and is afebrile for 24 to 48 hours. Then the patient can be placed on oral antibiotics. This decision must be individualized, particularly in a patient with complications such as obstruction or bacteremia.

**5. Response to therapy.** It is important to recognize and treat the complications of acute pyelonephritis. Nearly all patients with uncomplicated acute pyelonephritis are afebrile after 3 days of effective antimicrobial therapy, and the remainder are afebrile by 4 days [13,35]. **The persistently febrile patient may have a collection of undrained pus in or around the kidney, a metastatic site**

**of infection,** or obstruction with pyonephrosis, or she may have received ineffective therapy. If fever or toxicity persists beyond 48 hours of appropriate therapy, an obstructive uropathy or renal abscess should be excluded (e.g., with renal ultrasonography). **Intrarenal and perinephric abscesses** are discussed later in this chapter. Diabetics have an increased incidence of these complications [9].

6. **Follow-up.** Approximately 48 hours after initiation of therapy, results of susceptibility testing will be available. If the organism isolated is **not** susceptible to the treatment given, treatment should be changed to the most appropriate drug.
   a. The urine should become sterile 2 or 3 days after initiation of appropriate therapy, with no bacteria noted in the urine sediment. Some authorities recommend routine culturing of the urine at 2 to 3 days to assess response to therapy. This rarely is done in outpatient settings but may be indicated in hospitalized patients, especially if there is a question of resistant organisms, if the infection is complicated by mechanical or neurologic obstruction, or if the patient is not responding clinically.
   b. Whereas antibiotic treatment may relieve or reduce the patient's symptoms, such treatment does not always result in bacteriologic cure. For this reason, follow-up after treatment is important. Recommendations of experts in the field vary with regard to the extent of follow-up, but the **minimum follow-up should be a repeat urine culture 1 to 2 weeks after completion of antimicrobial therapy** in all patients. In patients with frequent UTIs, repeat cultures at 4 to 6 weeks after treatment may be useful.
7. **Urologic evaluation** generally is indicated for any patient with relapsing pyelonephritis.

B. **Infection in patients with known urinary tract abnormalities.** In patients with known renal calculi, obstructive uropathies, or other abnormalities, antibiotic therapy may suppress infection temporarily but may not eradicate it. Treatment of these patients therefore should be directed toward correction of the underlying abnormality if this is possible.

C. **Miscellaneous.** UTIs in patients with polycystic kidney disease are difficult to treat, in part because of the poor penetration of antibiotics (e.g., aminoglycosides) into cystic fluid [36]. Infectious disease consultation is advised in these difficult cases. UTI in the setting of renal transplantation is discussed in Chapter 20.

IV. **Recurrent infections.** The healthy young woman who has had two UTIs within the last 6 months and is now presenting with her third is a candidate for long-term prophylactic therapy to prevent recurrent symptomatic bacteriuria [37].

A. The **source** of the recurrent bacteriuria is usually reinfection from the periurethral flora, or less commonly it may be the result of persistent or relapsing infection in the upper urinary tract—that is, smoldering pyelonephritis. Some women will clearly indicate sexual intercourse as a causal factor for recurrent infections [38].

B. **Prophylactic therapy.** In patients with reinfection, 6 to 12 months of continuous preventive or antibiotic therapy has been shown to decrease recurrences by 95% during the period of active treatment [39,40]. **Prophylactic therapy should be initiated only after the acute episode is bacteriologically cured.** For individuals with reinfection immediately after discontinuation of prophylactic therapy, more extended duration of prophylaxis (2 or more years) has been shown to be effective.

C. **Recommended prophylactic antibiotics** of equal efficacy include TMP-SMX, one-half regular tablet at bedtime every other night; TMP, 100 mg/day at bedtime; or nitrofurantoin, 50 or 100 mg/day at bedtime (see related discussions in Chapter 27).

D. **Alternative approaches**

1. Some prefer **patient-administered short-course therapy** at the onset of symptoms, which may be more efficacious, economical, and desirable than conventional prophylactic therapy [41]. This approach probably is justified only for the highly motivated, compliant, and well-educated patient with uncomplicated infection.

2. **Postintercourse, single-dose prophylactic therapy** can be effective inpatients who identify intercourse as a precipitating factor [38].
3. **In postmenopausal women,** topically applied intravaginal estradiol cream is a possible alternative to antimicrobial prophylaxis [42].
4. Drinking **cranberry juice** daily may reduce the frequency of UTI [6,7].

**E. Behavioral changes may be important** [15]

1. Voiding after intercourse has been suggested as a way of reducing UTI episodes related to sexual intercourse.
2. If a diaphragm and spermicide are used for contraception, an alternative method [8] may reduce the frequency of recurrent UTI.
3. Voiding when the urge to void occurs rather than delaying may help some individuals (e.g., school teachers who postpone voiding during school hours).

**F. Urologic evaluation**

1. When accurate classification is possible, women with recurrent infections characterized as **relapse** should be examined at least once for the presence of mechanical (e.g., obstruction or stones) or neurologic dysfunction of the urinary tract. The role of suppressive long-term antibiotic therapy in these patients is discussed in section III.D under General Management Principles of Urinary Tract Infections, above.
2. Women with sporadic **reinfections** that respond to short-course therapy or low-dose prophylaxis usually do not have urologic abnormalities. Therefore, invasive evaluation is not warranted.

## V. UTI in pregnancy [30]

**A.** The overall **prevalence of bacteriuria** in pregnancy ranges from 4% to 7% in most studies but is as high as 11% in socially indigent multiparas and as low as 2% in private patients [30]. Pyelonephritis in pregnancy occurs in 3% to 7% of pregnant women who have asymptomatic bacteriuria [11]. Sickle cell trait has been associated with bacteriuria also. Catheterization should be avoided in the pregnant patient because pregnancy sets the stage for the development of symptomatic infection [30].

**B. Physiologic changes with pregnancy**

1. The most impressive changes involve dilatation of the collecting system, called **hydroureters of pregnancy.** This is a normal condition in pregnancy and extends to the level of the pelvic brim. The changes are more pronounced on the right side. Dilatation begins as early as the seventh week of gestation and gradually progresses until term. Although the precise explanation for the development of hydroureters is unclear, both mechanical and hormonal factors are involved.
2. In the third trimester, the **bladder** undergoes a relative **change in position,** becoming an abdominal rather than a pelvic organ, and undergoes a progressive **decrease in tone** due to hormonal changes.
3. The net effect of these changes is to increase the risk of UTI, especially in the third trimester.
4. After delivery, in the absence of infection, the hydroureters return to normal in 66% of patients by 1 month and in most patients by 2 months [30].

**C. Therapy**

1. **Asymptomatic UTI.** See discussion in section I.C.
2. **Symptomatic UTI** deserves 7 to 10 days of antibiotic therapy based on susceptibility data. (Antibiotic use in pregnancy is discussed in Chapter 27.) Short 3-day courses are not recommended.
3. **Pyelonephritis.** Hospitalization is usually advised. Empiric therapy with a broad-spectrum cephalosporin (e.g., ceftriaxone) is appealing until culture data are available that may allow one to use a narrower spectrum cephalosporin. Aztreonam is another possible parenteral $\beta$-lactam antibiotic [2,11]. There is some concern about using aminoglycosides in pregnancy because of the potential of ototoxicity for the fetus [11] (see Chapter 27). The duration of therapy for pyelonephritis has not been well studied. After a 2-week course of an appropriate antibiotic based on susceptibility data, suppression with nitrofurantoin until delivery is rational [30] (see section I.C).

**D. Follow-up.** See related discussion in section I.C.

## URINARY TRACT INFECTION IN MEN

UTI in men [43] occurs most commonly in those with prostatic hypertrophy and partial urethral obstruction or in association with persistent infection of the prostate gland. UTIs in children and the elderly are discussed separately (see below).

I. **Asymptomatic infections.** Bacteriuria is uncommon without symptoms in the healthy man, although it is relatively common in the elderly man (see section I under Urinary Tract Infection in the Elderly, below).
   A. **Screening** for bacteriuria in asymptomatic healthy men is not suggested.
   B. **Therapy.** If bacteriuria is found by chance, it should lead to an investigation to exclude predisposing structural or functional abnormalities of the urinary tract, especially chronic prostatitis. Routine antibiotic treatment in asymptomatic men is not supported by available data. Patients should be treated before genitourinary instrumentation.

II. **Lower UTI**
   A. **It is important to recognize the concept of the relationship between lower UTI in men and prostatitis.** Prostatitis may cause symptomatic infection with or without bladder infection. Bladder infection in the man with a mechanically normal urinary system often is associated with bacterial prostatitis [44,45]. However, uncomplicated cystitis alone can also occur (see section B.1.c). Instrumentation is the most common identifiable cause of infection, but in most cases the events leading to infection are not clear. Obstruction is often coexistent with and inseparable from instrumentation.
   B. **General approach to lower UTI in men**
      1. **Clinical presentation.** The history is important.
         a. **Dysuria alone (with or without urethral discharge).** Initially, one should identify patients having dysuria alone, with or without a urethral discharge, because these patients usually have urethritis rather than a true UTI. Most men between the ages of 15 and 30 years will have either nonspecific urethritis or gonococcal urethritis. The clinical approach to this problem is discussed in Chapter 16 under Urethritis.
         b. Patients may have **dysuria, frequency, and urgency,** symptoms similar to those seen in uncomplicated UTI in women. Acute perineal pain and discomfort may occur in patients with prostatitis, as discussed in section III. **Prostatitis is particularly common in men between 40 and 45 years of age who present with a UTI.**
         c. **Uncomplicated cystitis can occur in sexually active young men with acute dysuria.** Risk factors include homosexuality with anorectal intercourse, lack of circumcision, human immunodeficiency virus infection with a CD4 lymphocyte count of less than 200 cells/$mm^3$, or a sexual partner with vaginal colonization with uropathogens [2,31]. Urethritis should be excluded and/or treated (see Chapter 16).
      2. **Diagnosis**
         a. **Examination of any urethral discharge** should be performed if possible, as discussed in Chapter 16 under Urethritis. This will usually allow one to make the distinction between nonspecific urethritis and gonococcal urethritis.
         b. **Routine urinalysis and quantitative urine culture are essential** for proper evaluation of patients with no urethral discharge but with symptoms of a UTI.
         c. **Rectal examination.** If the prostate gland is swollen, firm, and exquisitely tender, an associated acute prostatitis is likely; this entity is discussed in section III.
         d. **Prostatic localization technique.** A technique for localizing the site of UTI in men is discussed in section III.B. This technique is seldom performed at present, and the methodologic validity of testing is questionable. However, it **may be useful in the diagnosis of chronic prostatitis** and in the evaluation of men with relapsing UTI [45]. It appears to be used with diminishing frequency, even by urologists. It is **not appropriate in acute prostatitis.**

3. **Treatment**
   a. **Antimicrobial therapy**
      (1) **Urethritis alone.** The approach to and treatment of this problem is discussed in Chapter 16 under Urethritis.
      (2) **Prostatitis** therapy is discussed in section III.
      (3) **Initial therapy** in the adult man who presents with his first UTI believed to be **unrelated to a prostatic focus** is uncertain. (This may be a particular problem in the young or middle-aged man compared with the older man, who is more likely to have a prostatic focus.) A subclinical prostatic focus still is possible, as is an occult genitourinary structural problem. With **recurrent UTI,** the prostatic localization test (see section III.B) sometimes is performed to help localize the problem. It is reasonable to use TMP-SMX (which penetrates the prostate well) because of the possibility of a prostatic focus in all men with UTI. Alternatively, one may use TMP alone in the sulfa-allergic patient or a fluoroquinolone because these agents also penetrate the prostate well (see Chapter 27).
      (4) For that subgroup of sexually active young males (see section 2.c) a 7-day course of TMP-SMX, TMP, or fluoroquinolone is suggested [2] once urethritis is excluded. Failure of this regimen necessitates more careful evaluation, including consideration of a prostatic focus [2].
   b. **Urologic evaluation.** In addition to antimicrobial therapy, urologic evaluation to determine whether a urinary tract abnormality exists should be considered. It is reasonable to treat a first UTI in a man who has no history of prior genitourinary abnormalities, then watch closely, and eventually proceed with a urologic workup when and if a second UTI or relapse occurs. Cystoscopy usually is indicated in patients with recurrent infections. **In patients with a typical initial episode of cystitis or acute prostatitis responding to antibiotics, a complete urologic evaluation is not necessary.** The approach to patients with an enlarged prostate (compatible with benign prostate hypertrophy) is an evolving area, with the increased availability of medical therapy for some forms of benign prostate hypertrophy. Also, stents can be inserted in the prostatic urethra segment (instead of conventional prostatic surgery) only in carefully selected patients. Urologic consultation is therefore important [15].

III. **Bacterial prostatitis** [10,43,46] can present as either an acute or a chronic disease. It has been estimated that prostatitis constitutes approximately 25% of annual office visits for genitourinary complaints by men. Unfortunately, many aspects of prostatitis have been poorly understood, and both patients and clinicians often become confused and frustrated in dealing with this condition [10].

The common forms of prostatitis are summarized in Table 15.4. Bacterial prostatitis is associated with a UTI, positive cultures localizing the bacterial pathogen to the prostatic fluid, and excessive numbers of inflammatory cells (WBCs and macrophages containing fat) in the prostatic secretion [10,46]. **Studies suggest that nearly 90% of patients with prostatitis symptoms have nonbacterial prostatitis or prostatodynia [10,47].**

A. **Acute bacterial prostatitis** is an abrupt febrile illness. Symptoms include fever, chills, and low back and acute perineal pain and discomfort. In addition, symptoms of acute lower UTI such as dysuria, frequency, and urgency usually are present.
   1. **Diagnosis.** The signs and symptoms are sufficiently abrupt, severe, and typical that the clinician seldom has difficulty in making the diagnosis [10].
      a. **Rectal examination** often is not necessary, thereby avoiding the discomfort and potential risk of prostate massage, because symptoms and urinalysis usually support the diagnosis of acute bacterial prostatitis. If a single gentle rectal examination is performed, it reveals a swollen prostate that often is exquisitely tender on palpation.
      b. **Urinalysis** usually demonstrates pyuria and bacteriuria.
      c. **Prostatic localization studies,** as discussed later, require prostatic massage and are **unnecessary** to support the clinical diagnosis in patients with acute prostatitis. Massage may precipitate bacteremia and causes considerable patient discomfort.

Table 15.4. Clinical Features of Common Prostatitis Syndromes

| Syndrome | History of Confirmed UTI | Prostate Abnormal on Rectal Examination | Excessive WBCs in EPS | Positive Culture of EPS | Common Causative Agents | Response to Antimicrobial Treatment | Impaired Urinary Flow Rate |
|---|---|---|---|---|---|---|---|
| Acute bacterial prostatitis | Yes | Yes | Yes | Yes | Coliform bacteria | Yes | Yes |
| Chronic bacterial prostatitis | Yes | ± | Yes | Yes | Coliform bacteria | Yes | ± |
| Nonbacterial prostatitis | No | ± | Yes | No | None<br>? *Chlamydia*<br>? *Ureaplasma* | Usually no | ± |
| Prostatodynia | No | No | No | No | None | No | Yes |

UTI, urinary tract infection; WBCs, white blood cells; EPS, expressed prostatic secretions.
From Meares EM Jr. Prostatitis. *Med Clin North Am* 1991;75:497; with permission.

d. **Clean-catch urine culture.** Because acute cystitis usually is associated with acute prostatitis, **the infecting pathogen generally can be identified by routine culture of a clean-catch urine specimen.** Data suggest a clean-catch culture may not be necessary in men. Neither meatal cleansing nor mid-stream sampling generally is needed to obtain urine for culture [43].

2. **Therapy.** The inflammation of acute bacterial prostatitis allows most antibiotics to achieve high prostatic concentration, and patients generally respond rapidly to antibiotic therapy. Most infections are caused by enteric gram-negative bacilli (75%), particularly *E. coli* (25%), although gram-positive infections occur in the other 25% [10,43].

   a. **Antibiotic choice.** Currently, **TMP-SMX, or TMP alone, is the treatment of choice** for acute bacterial prostatitis because of cost and the good penetration of prostatic tissue by TMP (Table 15.3) [10,48]. TMP alone may be administered in the sulfa-allergic patient. Comparable results have been published with the fluoroquinolones, and these agents are the drugs of choice for TMP-SMX–resistant organisms or as another alternative in sulfa-allergic patients (see Chapter 27). There are few data to support the use of oral carbenicillin indanyl.

   b. **Other antibiotics.** Some patients with acute prostatitis are systemically ill and may require therapy with parenteral antibiotics initially. Ampicillin and aminoglycosides have commonly been used in combination while awaiting cultures, especially if enterococci are a concern. Broad-spectrum penicillins, cephalosporins, and aminoglycosides are effective in many patients with acute prostatitis, even though these drugs are generally not believed to penetrate the prostate well. The inflammation in acute prostatitis allows these drugs to penetrate the prostate to a greater extent in acute infections than in chronic prostatitis.

   c. **Duration of therapy.** The optimal duration of therapy is not well defined. Conventionally, treatment spans a minimum of 14 days. However, continuing therapy for prolonged durations in an attempt to treat a focus of chronic prostatitis has often been advocated [10,44]. If the antibiotic is well tolerated, we tend to treat acute infection for a 4-week course, and chronic infection for 6 to 12 weeks.

3. **Prognosis.** Most patients recover from acute prostatitis with appropriate treatment. Relapse may occur in some cases, or the prostate may remain a persistent source of infection, as discussed next.

B. **Chronic bacterial prostatitis** is a more subtle condition than acute prostatitis. Bacterial organisms in this disease are **difficult to eradicate** despite antibiotic therapy, and the prostate can remain a persistent source of UTI. The prostatic focus can repeatedly infect the bladder urine and is believed to be responsible for most relapsing lower UTIs in men. Infection usually is due to gram-negative bacilli but occasionally may be due to gram-positive organisms (e.g., enterococci). The role of other gram-positive bacteria is unclear. *S. aureus* at times may be a pathogen, but *S. epidermidis*, micrococci, and diphtheroids probably are not pathogens [10].

Infected prostate calculi that cannot be appreciated by rectal examination or simple plain-film radiographic studies may function as infected foreign bodies, explaining in part why it may be difficult to eradicate infection in chronic bacterial prostatitis.

1. **Symptoms** are highly variable, and some patients are detected because of asymptomatic bacteriuria. Many patients may not have a history of acute prostatitis. Some complain of perineal or low back discomfort. Periodic episodes of cystitis symptoms or irritative voiding dysfunction, such as urgency, frequency, nocturia, and dysuria, may occur. **The best clue to this diagnosis is that prostatitis is the most common cause of relapsing UTIs** (with the same pathogen) **in men.** Because many antibiotics penetrate the prostate poorly, the pathogen remains viable in the prostatic tissue. Some antibiotic regimens will eradicate concomitant cystitis and sterilize the patient's urine, temporarily providing relief of symptoms, but symptoms return when the antibiotic is discontinued, because the prostatic infection persists.

**2. Diagnosis**

**a. Rectal examination** reveals no characteristic findings on prostatic palpation. An enlarged or slightly boggy prostate is a nonspecific finding.

**b. Localization studies.** The historical method of diagnosis was to perform prostatic localization studies, with **careful microscopic and culture examination of the segmented urine and the prostatic fluid. Localization studies are now regarded as seldom if ever necessary;** the procedure is time-consuming, fairly expensive, and uncomfortable for patients and therefore is infrequently performed [49]. **They should not be performed in bacteriuric patients in whom the causative agent is already identified.** A justifiable alternative to performing prostatic localization studies is to treat bacteriuric men with prolonged courses of antibiotics known to penetrate the prostate. Studies may be useful in the patient who is not bacteriuric, to distinguish bacterial from nonbacterial prostatitis, to confirm a prostatic focus of infection for patients in whom prostatic surgery is contemplated because of recurrent UTI, or to help confirm the diagnosis in patients with recurrent symptoms.

The prostatic localization method requires that the patient is well hydrated and has a full bladder before starting. The glans must be cleaned as previously noted, and the foreskin must be fully retracted during the procedure. The specimens collected usually are examined microscopically and cultured immediately after collection, using methods that allow quantitation of small numbers of bacteria. **Careful microscopic examination alone can provide useful information** (see section (6)).

**(1)** The patient first voids 20 mL urine ($VB_1$) into one container.

**(2)** A midstream specimen then is obtained in a second container ($VB_2$).

**(3)** During prostatic massage, expressed prostatic secretions (EPS) are collected.

**(4)** Finally, 10 mL of urine is collected after prostatic massage ($VB_3$).

**(5) Interpretation.** Meares [10] reviewed the interpretation of this technique in detail, including illustrative cases. Briefly, if colony counts in specimen $VB_1$ exceed those in $VB_3$, the bacteria are localized to the anterior urethra. If $VB_1$ and $VB_2$ are negative or have low counts of bacteria and the EPS and $VB_3$ have larger numbers of bacteria, bacterial prostatitis must be considered. If the specimens all yield more than $10^5$ CFU/mL, interpreting the test is not possible. In this instance, the patient should be treated with a 2- to 3-day course of nitrofurantoin, which will eradicate bladder bacteriuria but will not penetrate the chronically inflamed prostate; then the four-specimen test should be repeated.

**(6) In chronic prostatitis, the prostatic fluid (EPS) should reveal more than 15 WBCs per high power field.** Culture of prostatic fluid should reveal the offending organism. Colony counts of fewer than 100,000 CFU/mL generally are seen, with counts of 1,000 CFU/mL or fewer on occasion.

**Provided that the urethral and midstream specimens show insignificant pyuria, more than 15 WBCs per high power field in the prostate expressate is diagnostic of prostatic inflammation.** The most convincing sign of prostatitis is the finding of both excessive WBCs and macrophages containing fat droplets (ovoid fat bodies) in EPS.

**3. Treatment.** Eradication of a persistent prostatic focus of infection often is difficult. Except for TMP (alone or in combination with SMX), erythromycin (for gram-positive bacteria), and the quinolones, most antibiotics useful against gram-negative bacteria diffuse poorly into the prostatic fluid. Therefore, despite prolonged 6- to 12-week courses of appropriate antibiotics, cure rates of only about 30% to 40% are reported [10], but these rates are better than those for short-course regimens.

**a. TMP-SMX or a quinolone** (Table 15.3) has been reported to be most successful for chronic prostatitis when used for prolonged periods. Therapy with TMP-SMX (one double-strength tablet twice daily) should be continued for a minimum of 6 weeks and preferably for 12 weeks. Optimal duration of therapy with the quinolones awaits further study. Ciprofloxacin (500 mg twice a day), norfloxacin (400 mg twice a day), or ofloxacin (300 mg twice a day) for 30 days has been suggested [10].

**b.** Even prolonged courses of antibiotics may be unsuccessful, particularly if there are prostatic calculi. Further urologic evaluation and partial prostatectomy may be indicated in refractory cases. Complete prostatectomy may result in incontinence or sexual impotency and therefore is contraindicated. Chronic suppressive therapy with TMP-SMX (one tablet daily) or TMP alone is appropriate in patients who continue to relapse after a 12-week course of full-dose therapy. Nitrofurantoin (100 mg/day) has been used [10]. The quinolones also are used for chronic suppression, but these agents are far more expensive than TMP or TMP-SMX (see Chapter 27).

**C. Nonbacterial prostatitis** is far **more common than chronic bacterial prostatitis.** It is defined as symptomatic prostatic inflammation with negative culture of urine and prostatic secretions. It has also been referred to as **prostatosis** [50]. Some authorities believe that prostatosis is merely bacterial prostatitis caused by small numbers of organisms. The etiology remains unclear; it is an inflammatory condition of unknown cause [10]. Systematic reviews have recently questioned the methodologic quality of historical diagnostic standards for chronic abacterial prostatitis [51].

1. **Symptoms.** Complaints are similar to those of patients with chronic bacterial prostatitis. The patient often has no prior history of a UTI.
2. **Diagnosis.** Physical examination generally is unremarkable, although some patients may complain of prostatic tenderness on palpation. **EPSs show more than 10 to 15 WBCs per high power field,** but routine urine cultures and prostatic localization cultures show no bacterial etiology.
3. **Treatment.** There is **no accepted approach** to therapy because the etiology of this disease is unknown. Empiric treatment directed toward chlamydiae, with a 2-week trial of tetracycline (500 mg four times a day), doxycycline (100 mg twice a day), or erythromycin (250–500 mg four times a day), may provide symptomatic relief, and a partial response in some patients may justify longer therapy with these agents (e.g., 4–6 weeks).

   Other antibacterial agents are neither effective nor indicated [10,52]. Sitz baths, therapy with nonsteroidal antiinflammatory agents, and, in some patients, prostatic massage also may provide symptomatic relief. Surgical intervention is not indicated. Some patients have greater relief from aspirin than from nonsteroidal antiinflammatory agents, which may aggravate the problem.

**D. Prostatodynia.** Patients with this condition have no associated UTI, noninflammatory prostatic secretions with negative cultures of EPS, and no excessive inflammatory cells in their prostatic secretions. This is a common condition [10].

1. **The typical patient** is a young to middle-aged man with irritative voiding symptoms (frequency, urgency, and nocturia) and symptoms of abnormal urinary flow (hesitancy, diminution of stream force and size, postvoid dribbling).
2. General physical and neurologic examinations are normal except that many patients have "tight" anal sphincters and tender prostates and paraprostate tissues on rectal examination [10].
3. Cystoscopic examination often suggests mild to moderate bladder neck obstruction and variable bladder trabeculation. Meares [10] believed that these patients have "spastic" dysfunction of the bladder neck and prostate urethra and therefore called this the **bladder neck–urethral spasm syndrome.**

   Smooth-muscle spasm and high prostatic urethral pressures during voiding probably lead to intraprostatic reflux of urine and an associated chemical prostatitis. $\alpha$-Blocking agents are beneficial in some patients [10,52].
4. Most men with this syndrome admit to stress and emotional tension. Whether stress is a cause or merely an effect of prostatodynia is unclear [10].

**IV. Epididymitis.** This condition is diagnosed readily by physical examination. Most infections in sexually active men are caused by *C. trachomatis* and *N. gonorrhoeae*; urethritis and prostatitis may occur concurrently [53,54]. Infection in older men is caused by the usual uropathogens, gram-negative bacilli, and, infrequently, enterococci; infection may occur as a complication of concurrent prostatitis. Etiologic agents generally are recovered from culture of the urethra, urine, or prostatic secretions; alternatively, direct aspiration of the epididymis may be required. Therapy is directed at the etiologic agent and, if present, concurrent sites of infections.

**V. Upper UTI.** The approach to pyelonephritis in the normal man does not differ from that in the normal woman. See section III under Urinary Tract Infection in Women, above.

**VI. Recurrent infections.** The **definition** of recurrent UTIs in men differs from that used for women. The defining, but arbitrary, time limit set for repeated infections in women is 6 months. For men, because UTIs are much less common and less likely to occur as a sporadic event, **two or more UTIs at any time within a 3-year period** has been used to define the syndrome [44].

**A. Predisposing factors.** The association of prostatitis and recurrent UTIs is even stronger than for sporadic lower UTIs. Unlike women, men with recurrent UTIs almost always have evidence of tissue-invasive disease. **Most men with recurrent UTIs will be found to have structural defects of the urinary tract.** In those without structural defects, most will be found to have chronic bacterial prostatitis. **Urologic evaluation is essential** in these patients.

**B. Therapy**

**1.** The ideal antimicrobial agent is one that penetrates the prostate–blood barrier. TMP and TMP-SMX are agents with an appropriate antimicrobial spectrum. The dosages given in Table 15.3 are appropriate for recurrent infection. The best chance for cure is with 6 weeks of therapy. The quinolones are other commonly used agents (see Chapter 27).

**2.** If recurrences are frequent and severe, it may be appropriate to give chronic suppressive therapy, as discussed in section III.D under General Management Principles of Urinary Tract Infections. Treatment should be with full therapeutic dosages (not the low-dose suppressive regimens used in women) in an attempt to eradicate the focus of tissue infection and, therefore, cause cessation of symptomatic episodes.

## URINARY TRACT INFECTION IN THE ELDERLY

Although many of the basic principles in the understanding and treatment of UTI in the elderly are similar to those for younger patients, several differences are noted in the elderly, and these deserve emphasis [55–63].

**I. Asymptomatic bacteriuria** is much more common in the geriatric population than in younger patients [55–58]. Among young to middle-aged women, the prevalence of bacteriuria is less than 5% and, among young to middle-aged men, less than 0.1%. By contrast at least 20% of women and 10% of men who are older than 65 years and are living at home have bacteriuria. Some, but not all, studies suggest the incidence of bacteriuria in the elderly rises with increasing age [56].

**A. Factors** [56–58]

**1.** The **place of residence** is a major factor in determining the prevalence of bacteriuria. Approximately 25% of women and 20% of men living in nursing homes or extended-care facilities have bacteriuria; even higher percentages of hospitalized elderly patients have bacteriuria.

**2. Debilitated state** (i.e., the frail elderly). The higher rates of bacteriuria are related to the more debilitated state of patients (e.g., after cerebrovascular accidents, presence of decreased functional status), perineal soiling, poor hygiene, less complete bladder emptying, and more frequent catheterization.

**B.** Serial studies show that although at one point in time an elderly patient may not have bacteriuria, at another point in time he or she will. It seems likely that most elderly persons experience episodes of asymptomatic bacteriuria at some time [56].

**C. Significance of asymptomatic bacteriuria** [56–58]

**1. Therapy** of asymptomatic bacteriuria in the elderly **to prevent renal insufficiency is not justified.** No causal relationship between uncomplicated UTI and worsening of renal function has been shown.

**2.** Therapy of asymptomatic bacteriuria is unlikely to result in improvement of incontinence when present; asymptomatic bacteriuria rarely, if ever, causes incontinence.

3. **Bacteriuria and mortality.** Although it has been suggested that the elderly with asymptomatic bacteriuria die earlier than their noninfected cohorts, randomized controlled trials have shown that therapy does not provide a permanently sterile urine and has no effect on mortality [57–63].

D. **Treatment.** In recent reviews, the authors conclude that the treatment of asymptomatic bacteriuria is best avoided because the bacteriuria cannot usually be eradicated, therapy is associated with side effects, and treatment is not cost effective [56–58].

**Available data do not support routinely treating asymptomatic bacteriuria in the frail elderly** [58,63]. Asymptomatic bacteriuria may be treated, however, before perioperative urethral catheterization or genitourinary instrumentation.

II. **Pathogenesis.** The same principles for UTI in adults apply to the elderly. A few points warrant special emphasis. Most UTIs in the elderly follow invasion of the urinary tract with bacteria by the **ascending route.** The inoculum size probably is increased by a shift of the normal vaginal flora toward coliforms, by soiling of the perineum from fecal incontinence in women, and by catheterization. Lack of estrogen effect may be important in elderly women (see section II.C under General Approach to Urinary Tract Infections). Prostatitis is a very important cause of recurrent UTI in men.

Micturition with complete emptying of the bladder often is impaired in the elderly due to prostate disease in men, bladder prolapse in women, and neurogenic bladder in either gender.

III. **Microbiologic features** [56–58]

A. ***E. coli*** is still the **most common** pathogen infecting the elderly.

B. ***S. saprophyticus*** is **uncommon** in the elderly compared with its incidence in young women.

C. Elderly men have a higher incidence of gram-positive isolates (e.g., enterococci) for unclear reasons.

D. Elderly patients have often had prior therapy for UTI or other infections and often are infected with other gram-negative bacteria (e.g., *Proteus, Klebsiella, Enterobacter, Pseudomonas* species). Frequently, these bacteria are more resistant to antibiotics than bacteria isolated from younger patients.

E. The frequency of true polymicrobial infections is unclear.

IV. **Clinical presentation.** Catheter-related infections are discussed separately later in this chapter under Cather-associated Urinary Tract Infection.

A. **Lower UTIs.** These usually are easy to recognize if patients are capable of expressing complaints of dysuria, frequency, and urgency [58].

B. **Upper UTIs.** Acute pyelonephritis in the frail elderly, like other intraabdominal processes, may present in an atypical fashion. Elderly patients may not have the classic presentation of high fever, chills, flank pain, and symptoms of lower UTI. At times, gastrointestinal (nausea or vomiting, abdominal tenderness) or respiratory symptoms may be the patients' initial complaint, even though they do not have another underlying gastrointestinal or respiratory infection. **Clinicians must always exclude UTIs in the differential diagnosis of disease in septic-appearing elderly patients.** Because of the nonspecificity of pyuria in this age group and the coexistence of asymptomatic bacteriuria with other causes of sepsis, some ambiguity will always have to be accepted. The criteria for diagnosis, however, do not differ from those described earlier (see section V).

Absence of fever in the elderly does not exclude upper UTI because elderly patients may have difficulty mounting a fever. Peripheral leukocytosis may also be absent. Bacteremia and shock are more common in the elderly with pyelonephritis than in young adults [56]. Blood cultures should be routinely obtained.

V. **Diagnosis.** In general, the same diagnostic principles that apply to younger patients apply also to the elderly, with a few noteworthy differences [56–58].

A. **Urine collection.** It may be difficult to obtain a reliable midstream clean-catch urine sample for culture in the elderly woman. A single straight-catheter sample is a reasonable approach in symptomatic patients.

B. **Significant urine culture colony counts** (midstream collections)

1. For symptomatic infections, Enterobacteriaceae in at least $10^5$ CFU/mL, and probably more than $10^2$ CFU/mL, are significant [58].
2. For asymptomatic bacteriuria, more than $10^5$ CFU/mL of the same organism in two sequential specimens are needed [58].

**C. Nonspecificity of pyuria** [58]. Unlike younger people, in the elderly the presence of pyuria does not correlate highly with bacteriuria. In a population-based study in Finland, 47% of residents had pyuria, but only half of those had bacteriuria [59]. Other studies have shown even higher rates of pyuria in elderly women.

The presence of pyuria is a poor predictor of the presence of bacteriuria, but the **absence of pyuria is a good indicator of the absence of bacteriuria.**

**D. Necessity of routine urine culture** [56–58]

1. For **elderly women** with typical symptoms of lower UTI, urine **culture at the time of first presentation is suggested but not mandatory** [57]. If pyuria is present, empiric therapy is rational; if the patient does not respond, a urine culture should be done as an aid to future antibiotic choices. However, **urine culture is recommended in the frail elderly prior to therapy for UTI** [57,58].
2. In recurrent UTI in the elderly woman, urine cultures are advisable to help guide antibiotic therapy choices.
3. **In men, routine cultures are advised** [58].

**E. Blood cultures.** Obtain blood cultures in febrile patients or in any elderly patient who may have pyelonephritis because bacteremia is relatively common in the elderly with upper urinary tract disease.

**F. Urologic evaluation.** Consider urologic evaluation in

1. **Men** to help assess for obstructive uropathy. (A residual urine volume or bladder sonogram is a useful screen.)
2. **Women** with bacteremia or pyelonephritis that does not respond well to antibiotics.

**VI. Therapy.** Asymptomatic bacteriuria should not be treated, as previously discussed.

**A. Lower UTI**

1. **Women.** Although some experts recommend that elderly women are treated initially with 3-day regimens, a more conventional 7-day regimen is favored [57,58]. Anyone who fails a 3-day regimen should be tried on a 2-week course for presumed upper UTI. Because of the drug's spectrum of activity and low toxicity, TMP alone, norfloxacin, or ciprofloxacin is favored by Baldassarre and Kaye [56]; a more recent review suggests TMP-SMX or nitrofurantoin [57]. For elderly women with recurrent UTI, a trial of local vaginal topical estrogen therapy may be beneficial by normalizing vaginal flora (see section IV.C.1 under Urinary Tract Infection in Women, above).
2. **Men** deserve at least the conventional duration of therapy (e.g., 10–14 days) and consideration of underlying structural abnormality or prostatitis, which may warrant protracted therapy, especially if recurrent infections occur [58].
3. Long-term suppressive therapy may be indicated for patients with frequently recurring symptomatic infections.

**B. Upper UTI.** Elderly patients with pyelonephritis are more likely to have bacteremia and hypotension, and hospitalization usually is indicated [56].

Although *E. coli* remains the most common bacterium, more resistant bacteria are more often found in the frail elderly. For those patients who have acquired their infection in a long- term care facility, the likelihood of a multiple antibiotic-resistant bacterium is appreciable [57,58].

A **Gram stain of the unspun urine** will help guide therapy, in part by helping to determine whether enterococci are a concern. This is more likely in men.

1. **Empiric choice of an agent.** Most frail elderly will have some degree of renal impairment, whether recognized or covert (see Chapter 27). If an aminoglycoside is used in a very ill patient, careful serum level monitoring is advised. Once susceptibility data are available, alternative safer agents may often be selected. Alternatives are indicated in Table 15.3. Careful attention to dosage modification of antibiotics for renal impairment is important (see Chapter 27).

For empiric therapy of pyelonephritis with or without urosepsis, intravenous ampicillin and gentamicin have commonly been used, especially if enterococci are suggested on the Gram stain of an unspun urine or if urine Gram staining has not been performed. If only gram-negative bacilli are seen on a Gram stain, an aminoglycoside or a third generation cephalosporin alone is a rational choice. If *P. aeruginosa* or a multiresistant gram-negative organism is a concern, an aminoglycoside can be used with another agent while awaiting culture data.

2. **Definitive therapy.** Once the bacterium is isolated, therapy can be modified based on the susceptibility data of the causative agent. Complete eradication of bacteriuria often is not a reasonable goal for the frail elderly, and in the absence of bacteremia, we sometimes use a shorter course of therapy—that is, 3 days beyond the time the patient has become afebrile if the patient has responded well to therapy. Otherwise, a routine 10- to 14-day course of therapy seems prudent [57,58].

C. **Urologic evaluation.** An evaluation for the exclusion of obstructive disease is important for men but is not cost effective for frail elderly women responding to therapy. However, in both men and women, if the patient is not clinically responding after 72 hours of appropriate antibiotic therapy, renal ultrasonography is suggested to help rule out an obstructive uropathy (see under Urinary Tract Infection in Men, above). A CT is indicated if renal abscess is a concern.

VII. **Recurrent infections.** Because they have not been studied in a focused manner, recurrent infections in the frail elderly should be managed as described in section VI under Urinary Tract Infection in Men and in section IV under Urinary Tract Infection in Women (see above).

VIII. **Foley catheter-related infections.** These are discussed separately later in this chapter under Catheter-associated Urinary Tract Infection.

## URINARY TRACT INFECTION IN CHILDREN

Neonatal UTIs are discussed in Chapter 3 under Selected Specific Infections in the Newborn. Both acute and chronic UTIs in children are relatively common. Several points deserve special emphasis [64–66].

I. **Incidence.** UTI occurs in as many as 5% of female and 1% to 2% of male children [64].

II. **Pathogenesis.** Hematogenous spread of infection to the kidney is the most common mode of infection in neonates. In older children, the ascending route of infection is most common.

A. **Obstruction with urinary stasis predisposes to UTI.** Posterior urethral valve, obstruction at the ureteropelvic junction or ureterovesical junction, and ectopic ureterocele are the main causes of anatomic obstruction in children [64].

B. **Vesicoureteral reflux is the most common underlying abnormality.** The likelihood of parenchymal scarring and renal damage is related to the severity of vesicoureteral reflux.

C. **Risk groups. Children who are at increased risk for bacteriuria or symptomatic UTI with subsequent renal damage include**

1. Premature infants discharged from neonatal intensive care units (see Chapter 3).
2. Children with systemic or immunologic diseases.
3. Children with urinary tract abnormalities, renal calculi, neurogenic bladder, voiding dysfunction, constipation, or a family history of UTI with anomalies such as reflux.
4. Girls younger than 5 years with a previous history of UTI.
5. **Uncircumcised** males [15].

III. **Etiology** is essentially the same as in adults, with at least 80% of infections due to *E. coli*. Patients with underlying structural abnormalities and recurrent infections are more likely to demonstrate other pathogens (*Klebsiella*, *Proteus*, and *Pseudomonas* species) over time.

IV. **Asymptomatic bacteriuria**

A. **Incidence.** Approximately 1% of preschool children, 1.2% to 1.8% of school-aged girls, and 0.03% of school-aged boys have asymptomatic bacteriuria [64].

**B. Diagnosis** is made when, in an asymptomatic child, cultures of two properly obtained, clean-voided, midstream urine specimens grow at least $10^5$ organisms (of one bacterial type)/mL.

**C. Implications** [64]. Asymptomatic bacteriuria in children is associated with increased risk of recurrent symptomatic infections that may result in renal scarring. Hypertension or renal insufficiency, however, is unusual.

1. **In 20% to 30% of school-aged girls with asymptomatic bacteriuria,** radiographic investigation will reveal upper tract damage, vesicoureteral reflux, or both. **Most of the kidney damage occurs before 5 years of age.**
2. Most prospective studies of school-aged girls older than 5 years with asymptomatic bacteriuria have failed to demonstrate decreased glomerular filtration rates, impaired renal growth, or progressive parenchymal damage in kidneys that are normal at the start, even if the bacteriuria is left untreated.
3. Bacteriuria in neonates and infants, and in boys beyond infancy, is associated with a high incidence of urinary tract abnormalities and necessitates prompt diagnosis and early treatment.

**D. Screening** neonates and infants for asymptomatic bacteriuria is not practical because of the difficulties of obtaining a clean urine specimen in this age group. **The only children who should definitely be screened at 6- to 12-month intervals are those at high risk for bacteriuria and subsequent renal damage** (see section II.B).

**E. Radiographic studies.** Appropriate imaging studies should be performed in boys of any age with bacteriuria, in girls younger than 5 years, and in older girls with recurrent episodes of bacteriuria. (See detailed discussion of this in section V.E.)

**F. Treatment of asymptomatic bacteriuria.** Some have argued that therapy of asymptomatic bacteriuria may eradicate organisms of low virulence and facilitate UTI with more resistant bacteria or, alternatively, may be associated with unnecessary antibiotic side effects. Although this remains a controversial area, **we agree with recent reviewers who suggest the use of antibiotic therapy in children** younger than 5 years, with underlying structural abnormalities, and who progress to symptomatic UTI. A 7- to 10-day course of therapy is suggested, and failure to respond suggests noncompliance, improper antibiotic therapy, or underlying structural defect requiring radiographic evaluation [64].

## V. Symptomatic bacteriuria

**A. Clinical manifestations.** The usual signs and symptoms of lower UTIs in adults (e.g., dysuria and frequency) often are not present, and patients may have a variety of symptoms depending on their age. Fever may not be present, and by history, examination, and routine tests, it often is difficult to distinguish upper from lower UTI in children.

1. **See Table 15.5.**

Table 15.5. Signs and Symptoms of Urinary Tract Infections in Different Age Groups

| Age | Presentation |
|---|---|
| Neonate and infant | Hypothermia, hyperthermia, failure to thrive, vomiting, diarrhea, sepsis, irritability, lethargy, jaundice, malodorous urine |
| Toddler | Abdominal pain, vomiting, diarrhea, constipation, abnormal voiding pattern, malodorous urine, fever, poor growth |
| School-aged child | Dysuria, frequency, urgency, abdominal pain, abnormal voiding pattern (including incontinence or secondary enuresis), constipation, malodorous urine, fever |
| Adolescent | Dysuria, frequency, urgency, abdominal discomfort, malodorous urine, fever |

From Sherbotic JR, Cornfeld D. Management of urinary tract infections in children. *Med Clin North Am* 1991;75:328; with permission.

2. When fever is present in a child, the diagnosis of UTI should routinely be considered [66].
3. **Dysuria, especially without bacteriuria,** when present may be attributable to other causes such as vaginitis, local perineal irritation, use of bubble baths, masturbation, and pinworm infections. At times, it may be a clue to sexual molestation [64,66].

**B. Physical examination.** A careful abdominal examination, gentle rectal examination, and inspection of the genitals are suggested [64]. Growth failure or hypertension may be present in a child with renal insufficiency.

**C. Diagnosis. A positive urine culture** that is properly obtained **is essential** for the diagnosis [64,65].

1. **Pyuria** (≥5 WBCs per high power field) may be absent in centrifuged urine sediment in 30% to 50% of children with UTI [64,66]. If pyuria is present, it is strong supportive evidence of a UTI.
2. The **leukocyte esterase** and **nitrite tests** on a urinalysis may be falsely negative or positive in 15% to 30% of childhood cases [64].
3. **Urine culture** is advised. A properly collected sample may be difficult to obtain but is essential.
   a. **For neonates,** see Chapter 3.
   b. **For infants and toddlers,** either urethral catheterization (growth of ≥1,000 CFU/mL is significant) or suprapubic bladder aspiration (any growth on culture is significant) is suggested.
      "Bagged" urine specimens frequently are contaminated and, when positive for growth, are difficult to interpret. A negative urine culture from a bagged sample is useful in ruling out a UTI [64].
   c. **For older and cooperative children,** clean-voided midstream collection for urinalysis, Gram stain, and culture is suggested. Significant colony counts have already been reviewed under Urinary Tract Infection in Men and Urinary Tract Infection in Women and in section IV.B.2 under General Approach to Urinary Tract Infections (see above).
4. **Gram stain (or unstained examination) of unspun urine under a 40-power microscope lens.** If bacteria and leukocytes are seen, UTI is likely [64,66].

**D. Antimicrobial therapy.** In general, children who appear ill or who are at significant risk of becoming seriously ill because of their age (e.g., young infants) or who have urinary tract abnormalities should be admitted to the hospital and treated aggressively.

1. **Neonates.** See Chapter 3.
2. **Infants** are at risk for serious sequelae of UTI (e.g., sepsis) and so should be treated with intravenous antibiotics. Initial therapy with intravenous ampicillin plus gentamicin or a third-generation cephalosporin alone is appropriate (Table 15.6).
   a. A repeat urine culture 48 hours after starting therapy is advised. It should be negative.
   b. Intravenous antibiotics are continued until there is clinical improvement and consistent oral intake [65]. If the patient improves rapidly, a switch may be made to oral antibiotics after 24 to 48 hours; a total course of 7 to 14 days of antibiotics (intravenous plus oral) is advised [65].
   c. Radiographic evaluation is advised, as below.
   d. A repeat urine culture 1 week after completion of therapy is suggested.
3. **Children**
   a. **Uncomplicated UTI.** Children older than 6 to 12 months of age with normal urinary tracts who are not toxic can be treated with oral outpatient regimens.
      (1) Ideally, a urine culture at 48 hours is suggested to ensure that the urine has become sterile.
      (2) A conventional 7- to 14-day course of therapy is advised [64–66] (Table 15.6). Ampicillin or amoxicillin still is commonly used in children with

Table 15.6. Suggested Antimicrobial Therapy for Urinary Tract Infections: Dosages and Alternatives

| |
|---|
| Parenteral therapy (suspected upper UTI or sepsis) |
| Neonates and infants <4–6 mo old |
| Ampicillin, 75–200 mg/kg/d divided into 4 doses |
| *plus* |
| Gentamicin, 5–7.5 mg/kg/d divided into 2–3 doses |
| Older children |
| Ampicillin, 100 mg/kg/d divided into 4 doses |
| *plus* |
| Gentamicin, 7.5 mg/kg/d divided into 3 doses |
| *or* |
| A third-generation cephalosporin alone (e.g., cefotaxime, 100–200 mg/kg/d divided into 3–4 doses) |
| Oral therapy (acute cystitis, resolving upper UTI) |
| Neonates and infants <4–6 mo old |
| Amoxicillin, 40 mg/kg/d divided into 3 doses |
| *or* |
| TMP-SMX,[a] 6–12 mg/kg/d TMP with 30–60 mg/kg/d SMX, divided into 2 doses |
| *or* |
| Cephalexin, 50 mg/kg/d divided into 3 doses |
| Older children |
| TMP-SMX, 6–12 mg/kg/d TMP with 30–60 mg/kg/d SMX, divided into 2 doses |
| *or* |
| Amoxicillin, 40 mg/kg/d divided into 3 doses |
| Prophylaxis (for recurrent infections) |
| TMP-SMX, based on 2 mg/kg/d of TMP as a single nighttime dose |
| *or* |
| Nitrofurantoin, 2 mg/kg/d as a single nighttime dose |

[a]Sulfonamide agents (e.g., TMP-SMX) should not be used in children younger than 6 weeks.
Antibiotic dosages should be adjusted for the level of renal function, and serum levels should be followed where appropriate.
UTI, urinary tract infection; TMP, trimethoprim; SMX, sulfamethoxazole.
Modified from Sherbotic JR, Cornfeld D. Management of urinary tract infections in children. *Med Clin North Am* 1991;75:335; with permission.

initial uncomplicated UTI, because resistance to *E. coli* occurs less in childhood UTI than in adult UTI.

**(3)** Single-dose regimens are not advised in children.

**(4)** The use of short-course therapy for UTI in children remains controversial. Until further data are available, 3-day regimens should be reserved only for selected patients with asymptomatic bacteriuria and girls older than 5 years with clinical findings of lower UTI, a documented normal genitourinary tract, and poor compliance (in which case a short course would be beneficial) [64].

**b. Complicated UTI.** For patients with fever, chills, CVA tenderness, or gastrointestinal upset (i.e., presumed pyelonephritis); those who have undergone recent instrumentation; or those with significant anatomic abnormalities, aggressive intravenous antibiotics are suggested [64,66].

**(1)** Empiric therapy with ampicillin and gentamicin or a third- generation cephalosporin can be started (Table 15.6). Regimens can be revised after susceptibility data are available.

**(2)** Clinical improvement with a decrease in the fever usually begins within 48 hours. If this does not occur, obstruction or a resistant pathogen should be sought [65].

(3) Intravenous therapy is continued until the patient improves clinically, with completion of treatment orally based on susceptibility studies [64,65].

(4) A follow-up urine culture is advised 1 week after therapy and, when possible, 1 to 6 weeks after therapy.

E. **Radiographic evaluation.** In children with UTI, radiographic evaluation of the urinary tract is indicated to identify vesicoureteral reflux, obstruction, or other urinary tract abnormalities. In approximately 30% to 50% of young children with their first symptomatic UTI, a structural abnormality will be found. Most commonly this is vesicoureteral reflux, which is rare in children without UTI.

1. **Indications** [64–66]

   a. **Any male or female child younger than 5 years** with asymptomatic UTI or asymptomatic bacteriuria.

   b. **Any male child** with a first episode of UTI or asymptomatic bacteriuria.

   c. **Recurrent UTI or recurrent asymptomatic bacteriuria in female children older than 5 years** who have not been previously evaluated. A sexually active adolescent girl with recurrent lower UTI does not need radiographic evaluation.

   d. **A child with his or her first UTI and a family history of urinary tract abnormalities** (e.g., reflux) or recurrent UTI and abnormal voiding pattern, poor growth, or hypertension.

   Data suggest that siblings of patients with known vesicoureteral reflux should have a screening study done for early detection of reflux, which may be found in as many as 45% of these children. This is a somewhat controversial recommendation [64].

   e. Any child with **pyelonephritis**.

2. **The choice of radiographic examinations depends on the facilities available, the skills and experience of the radiologist, and clinical findings** [64–66]. The clinician should review options and plan studies after discussion with the radiologist.

   a. **Voiding cystourethrography** will detect vesicoureteral reflux, grade the severity of reflux, and provide anatomic and functional information of the lower urinary tract.

   b. **Intravenous urogram** has been the time-honored method to evaluate upper tract abnormalities but exposes the patient to more radiation than other options. Sonography and radionuclide scintigraphy provides similar data more safely.

   c. **Renal ultrasonography** is noninvasive and free of ionizing radiation. It can reveal obstruction, renal size and contour, stones, size of the collecting system, and bladder anatomy. Upper tract infection may be associated with increases of renal volume of more than 30%. Ultrasonography provides anatomic information only, and often must be combined with a functional study.

   d. **Radionuclide scans**

   (1) **Direct radionuclide voiding cystography** will detect reflux with a 50- to 100-fold decrease in gonadal radiation exposure when compared with voiding cystourethrography, but anatomic detail is not sufficient enough to grade the severity of reflux [64]. **If this test is used as a screen and is abnormal, then a more definitive voiding cystourethrography can be done.** Periodic radionuclide cystography examinations can be performed to assess the degree of reflux over time.

   (2) **Technetium succimer (Tc-99m dimercaptosuccinic acid [DMSA])** accumulates in functional renal cortex and provides exquisite renal images. When available, **this test is preferred over intravenous urography**. It is useful in demonstrating acute pyelonephritis and evaluating focal parenchymal scarring.

   e. **A reasonable approach** for the radiographic evaluation of UTI in children is shown in Figure 15.1 [64].

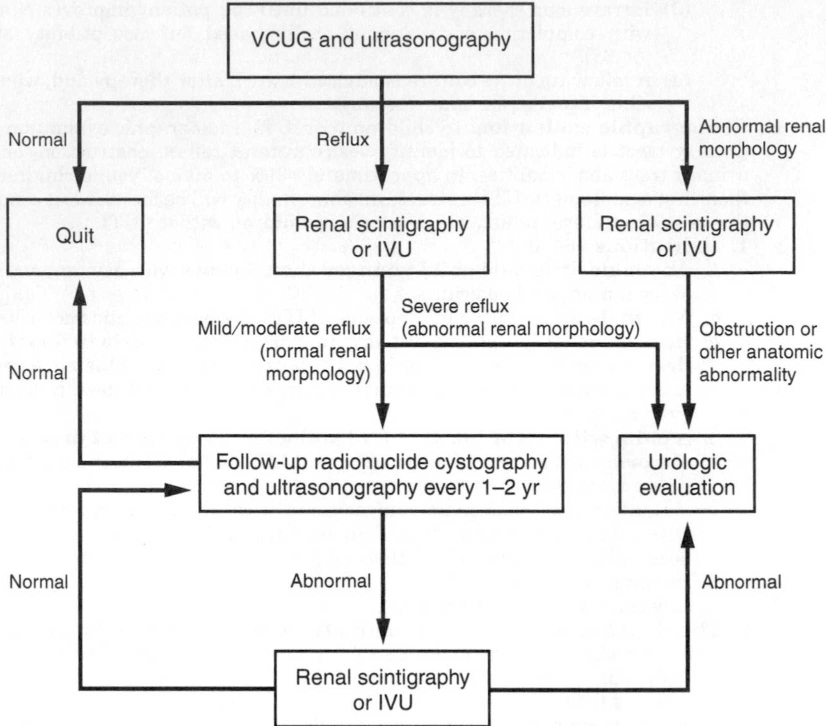


**FIG. 15.1** The protocol for radiologic evaluation of urinary tract infection in children. IVU, intravenous urography; VCUG, voiding cystourethrography. (From Zelikovic I, et al. Urinary tract infections in children: an update. *West J Med* 1992;157:558; with permission.)

**(1)** Immediate sonography can be done in the acutely ill child to exclude obstruction [64,65].

**(2)** **The optimal timing of radiographic studies.** Because transient reflux can be masked or overestimated during an acute UTI, it was previously believed that the ideal time for imaging studies was 4 to 6 weeks after antibiotic therapy. However, it is now recommended that radiographic studies should be done when infection is controlled and there is no longer evidence of bladder irritability [65]. If radiographic studies are delayed, it is prudent to continue low dose prophylactic agents until the urinary tract anatomy has been defined [65,66].

**(3)** Patients with abnormalities deserve careful evaluation by a specialist in this area.

3. **Follow-up studies. Mild to moderate reflux usually disappears with increasing age.** The goal of management of reflux is to prevent recurrent UTI and the resultant potential for renal scarring. In patients with documented reflux, repeated ultrasonography every 1 to 2 years is indicated to follow renal growth, and radionuclide cystograms should be used (e.g., every 1–2 years) serially to determine the resolution of reflux so that antimicrobial prophylaxis can be discontinued when appropriate [66].

## VI. Sequelae [64,66]

**A.** As many as 80% of children with uncomplicated UTI will have **recurrences.**

**B. Renal parenchymal infection and renal scarring are well-established complications of UTI in children.** Parenchymal scarring is found in 10% to 15% of children with UTIs. It has been estimated that nearly 10% may develop hypertension and a smaller percent renal insufficiency [64]. **The risk is especially great in infants and neonates.** To reduce the risk of renal damage, the diagnosis and therapy of UTI must be prompt. Most of the damage to the kidney caused by vesicoureteral reflux occurs in infancy and early childhood, and therefore careful workup to prevent sequelae in this age group is essential.

**C. Recurrent infections.** The approach to these patients depends on whether there is an underlying structural abnormality and on the degree of symptomatology.

1. **Patients with normal urinary tract anatomy and recurrent UTI.** Usually, three documented UTIs in a 1-year period indicate the need for prophylactic therapy. After a conventional course of antibiotics aimed at the susceptible pathogen, either TMP-SMX (10 mg/kg/day of the SMX component, given nightly or every other night) or nitrofurantoin (1–2 mg/kg/day, given nightly) is administered [64]. These agents are very effective and have few side effects. Usually prophylactic antibiotics are given for 6 to 24 months and are discontinued if the patient remains free of infection.
2. **Children with structural abnormalities,** especially vesicoureteral reflux, are best managed with continuous use of prophylactic antibiotics after the urine has been successfully sterilized with a conventional course of antibiotics. Antibiotic regimens similar to those listed in section C.1 can be used. A prophylactic antibiotic is used to prevent UTIs and possible renal damage secondary to reflux of infected urine.

   Prophylaxis often is continued for 12 to 24 months or longer while waiting for mild to moderate reflux to resolve spontaneously. Serial ultrasonography and scanning studies will help determine optimum duration of prophylactic antibiotics for patients with vesicoureteral reflux.

**VII. Surgical intervention**

**A.** Mild to moderate vesicoureteral reflux will resolve spontaneously with growth of the child in most patients [64,66].

**B.** High-grade vesicoureteral reflux, nonresolving vesicoureteral reflux, or reflux in those children unable to take prophylactic antibiotic therapy may require surgical intervention. These patients should be carefully followed by an experienced pediatric urologist and pediatric nephrologist with a special interest and expertise in these problems.

Even in patients with high-grade vesicoureteral reflux, conservative management with prophylactic antibiotics often is attempted and frequently is successful. Overall, in approximately 70% of patients with vesicoureteral reflux that is managed conservatively, the condition resolves spontaneously.

## CATHETER-ASSOCIATED URINARY TRACT INFECTION

The most common nosocomial infections are of the urinary tract, accounting for approximately 40% of all nosocomial infections [67–72]. Most patients with nosocomial UTI have had genitourinary manipulation, usually urethral catheterization (approximately 80%) or urologic manipulation (about 20%) [71]. Foley catheters are commonly used in hospitalized patients and in aged nursing home residents.

**I. Methods of catheterization and risk of UTI**

**A. Single (straight) catheterization.** After this procedure, bacteriuria develops in approximately 1% to 5% or more (up to 20%) of patients. The risk of infection is lowest in healthy outpatients and greatest in certain high risk patients such as diabetics, prepartum or postpartum patients, and especially in the elderly, debilitated, hospitalized patient [71].

**Indications** for single catheterization include (a) providing relief of temporary obstruction or inability to void; (b) obtaining urine from patients who are unable to provide a clean specimen because of weakness, debility, or other medical problems; (c) determining the amount of residual urine; and (d) conducting a urologic study of urethral anatomy.

**B. Intermittent catheterization.** This method has been helpful in avoiding long-term catheterization, **especially in young patients with spinal cord injuries** [73,74]. The technique, as originally described after World War II, was a "no-touch" technique performed by a nurse or urologic technician wearing mask, sterile gown, and gloves. Using this technique, approximately 65% of male patients and 50% of female patients were discharged from the hospital with sterile urine [73]. In recent years, a "clean" (as opposed to "sterile") technique has been taught to paraplegic patients who have been able to learn the procedure rather easily. Quadriplegics have been successfully catheterized by a caregiver using a similar technique. This has become a very useful approach for treating spinal cord-injured patients [73,74]. Intermittent catheterization might also be useful in the postoperative patient who is unable to void.

**Intermittent catheterization should not be used** in circumstances in which traumatic catheterization may be a problem, such as in obstruction of the urinary tract due to benign prostatic hypertrophy or carcinoma of the prostate. In these cases, an indwelling urethral or suprapubic catheter generally is indicated.

There is little, if any, role of prophylactic antibiotics in this setting. An attempt to use TMP-SMX in patients with spinal cord injuries demonstrated little benefit [75]; likewise, although limited published data suggest that fluoroquinolones might be effective, this is not an established practice. This approach is likely only to delay episodes of bacteriuria and pose a concern for selecting resistant pathogens.

**C. Short-term catheterization.** This may be necessary for monitoring acutely ill patients who are unable to void or who are incontinent and in whom measurement of urine output is mandatory (e.g., postoperative patients or selected patients in intensive care areas). The catheter should be removed as soon as possible to avoid increasing the risks of nosocomial UTI.

1. **Risk factors** associated with catheter-related infection [71]
   a. **Unalterable factors** that increase the risk of infection include female gender, older or debilitated patients, and patients with meatal colonization.
   b. **Potentially alterable factors,** such as duration of catheterization, catheter care techniques, type of drainage system (a closed system is preferred), and whether the patient is receiving systemic antibiotics or not affect infection rates.
2. The per-day risk of developing bacteriuria is approximately 3% to 6%, and the cumulative risk increases with duration of catheterization. Therefore, **nearly 50% of hospitalized patients catheterized for longer than 7 to 10 days develop bacteriuria** [71].

**D. Chronic catheterization.** The patient with a long-term indwelling catheter is at high risk of morbidity due to this procedure. The risk of bacteriuria increases with the duration of catheterization, at a rate of approximately 5% per day. **With protracted catheterization** (>30 days) **bacteriuria** with at least one bacterial strain **is universal,** and many patients have at least two bacterial strains [58,67].

1. **Indications for long-term bladder catheterization**
   a. Patients with atonic bladders, such as those with diabetes or other chronic neurologic disorders.
   b. Patients with obstructive uropathy preoperatively, or patients who are not surgical candidates but who have benign prostatic hypertrophy, prostatic carcinoma, and the like.
2. **Chronic catheterization should be avoided in the chronically ill incontinent patient if at all possible.** When other methods of incontinent management such as nursing care, behavioral modification, medication, special clothes, and special bed linens are not successful, there may be no alternative to long-term urethral catheterization in an attempt to prevent skin maceration and resultant decubitus ulcers. Condom catheters are an option for the incontinent male patient.

**II. Pathogenesis of catheter-associated UTI.** Bacteria can enter the urinary tract by either the periurethral or the intraluminal route [67,70,72].

**A. Periurethral or transurethral route.** This route of entry is especially important in catheterized women, probably accounting for 70% of episodes of bacteriuria. Bacteria involved in UTI emanate from the rectal flora and organisms colonize the periurethral zone. Then organisms enter the urinary tract via the external surface of the catheter in the mucous sheath between the catheter and urethral mucosa, similar to the pathogenesis of UTI in noncatheterized women [67,70,71]. This route may be less important in men.

**B. Intraluminal route.** Microorganisms can ascend through the lumen of the urinary catheter into the bladder.

1. In approximately 15% to 20% of infected patients, the infecting organism appears in the collecting bag before entry into the bladder, which occurs 24 to 48 hours later.
2. Once in the bladder, small numbers of microorganisms (e.g., 100 organisms/mL) can increase to large numbers (e.g., $>10^5$) in 24 to 48 hours.
3. **Two populations of bacteria** exist in the catheterized urinary tract.
   a. **Planktonic growth** (bacteria growing in the urine itself). Particularly adherent strains of *E. coli* (to uroepithelial cells) may be more likely to cause UTI.
   b. **Biofilm growth** (those bacteria growing on the surface of the catheter). The growth of a bacterial biofilm progresses in an orderly fashion: Bacteria attach to the catheter and initiate a biofilm form of growth in which organisms coat the catheter and secrete an extracellular matrix of bacterial glycocalyces in which they become embedded. Host urinary proteins such as Tamm-Horsfall protein and urinary salts can be incorporated into this biofilm growth, which eventually leads to encrustation of the inner surface of the catheter [66–72].
      (1) Certain bacteria (e.g., *Proteus* and *Pseudomonas* species) appear especially to contribute to biofilm growth.
      (2) In general, biofilm seen on the inner surface of the catheter is much thicker and of a different nature than that seen on the external surface [67–72].
      (3) **Implications of the biofilm** [67]
         (a) **To retard bacterial growth within the catheter biofilm, silver and silver alloy coated** catheters have been developed. Such catheters have been effective in decreasing the frequency of bacteriuria and symptomatic UTIs [68]. However, because of the greater acquisition costs, it is not clear whether routine use of silver coated catheters is cost effective [69].
         (b) **Urine cultures** obtained from the catheter may not reflect bladder bacteriuria in patients who have organisms in a biofilm on the inner surface of the catheter. Bladder urine could be sterile, but organisms from the catheter biofilm may contaminate the aspirated urine culture.
         (c) Biofilms have been demonstrated to retard the activity of antimicrobials. **Therefore, if bacteriuria is treated in a given patient, it may be prudent to replace the catheter.**
4. Breaking the connection at the junction of the catheter and drainage tube or contamination by improper manipulation of the collection bag may facilitate retrograde migration.

**C. Catheter insertion.** Only occasionally do nosocomial UTIs result from direct introduction of urethral microorganisms at the time of catheter insertion, assuming proper technique is used [71].

**III. Complications arising in use of urinary catheters.** Before using indwelling catheters in a patient, one should be thoroughly familiar with the complications associated with their use. Whenever possible, an indwelling catheter should be avoided, and when used it should be left in place for the shortest time possible.

**A. Bacteriuria.** The incidence of bacteriuria with a bladder catheter depends on the host and the method and duration of catheterization, as discussed previously [71].

1. Most episodes of bacteriuria are asymptomatic. Criteria have not been established for differentiating asymptomatic colonization of the urinary tract from symptomatic infection [67,71].
2. Pyuria accompanies most episodes of symptomatic infection, and its presence suggests host invasion rather than simple bladder colonization.

**B. Pyelonephritis.** The association between bacteriuria and subsequent pyelonephritis is well documented in both clinical and research settings.

1. The incidence of bacteriuria associated with upper tract disease has not been well defined or studied.
2. In studies using the antibody-coated bacterial test, as many as 25% of episodes of catheter-associated bacteriuria were positive, suggesting upper UTI [71]. Fever, flank pain, or other symptoms of pyelonephritis are uncommon in these patients.
3. Patients with prolonged use of catheters (>10 days) are at increased risk.

**C. Bacteremia or gram-negative sepsis.** In hospitalized patients, approximately 30% to 40% of all nosocomial gram-negative bacteremias originate from a UTI, usually catheter associated [71]. It is estimated that 30,000 deaths per year occur as a result of catheter-related sepsis due to gram-negative bacilli [71].

**D. Increased mortality.** Epidemiologic studies have related nosocomial bacteriuria to an approximate threefold relative increase in death. The exact explanation for this is not known but may involve unrecognized episodes of bacteremia [67,71].

**E. Other complications** of prolonged urinary catheterization include urinary stones, vesicoureteral reflux, and local periurethral complications such as prostatitis, prostatic abscesses, epididymitis, and scrotal abscesses. The frequency of these infections remains ill defined.

**IV. Catheter care.** Once the decision to use a catheter has been made, the following guidelines may be useful in decreasing or minimizing the risk of infection. **Catheters should be used only when absolutely necessary and then for the shortest time possible.**

**A.** For short-term use, two or three single straight catheterizations (every 6 hours) over a 24- to 72-hour period may be preferable to an indwelling catheter because of the lower risk of infection. Repeated straight catheterizations are not advisable in the patient who may be difficult to catheterize (e.g., patients with prostatic hypertrophy, prostatic cancer, or urethral strictures).

**B. Insertion** of the catheter should be **performed under aseptic conditions,** with the use of sterile gloves, sterile catheter, liquid antiseptic soap or an iodophor for perineal cleaning, and sterile water-soluble lubricating jelly for the catheter. Studies of siliconized or silver ion-coated catheters in comparison with latex catheters have given mixed results. We believe that the limited value, if any, of newer catheters does not warrant their added cost.

**C. A sterile closed drainage system** with a disposable plastic bag and connecting tubes should be used. The **junction of the catheter and drainage tube should not be disconnected** unless irrigation of an obstructed catheter is necessary, and irrigation should be done with sterile technique. Urine for culture should be aspirated from the aspiration port or distal-most portion of the catheter.

**D. Maintain adequate urine flow** at all times. Ideally, sufficient fluid to maintain a urine output of greater than 100 mL/h should be given if it is not contraindicated by the patient's clinical condition. Such a urine flow may prevent the ascent of bacteria through the collecting system.

**E. Gravity drainage** should be maintained, with the collection bag lower than the level of the bladder at all times. The bag should never touch the floor and should have a valve adequate to prevent reflux of urine into the bladder if the bag is accidentally raised above the level of the bladder. Urine in the collection bag may have very high bacterial colony counts. The downward drainage will help prevent retrograde spread of bacteria to the patient's bladder. The catheter should not be clamped except when the patient must be separate from his or her drainage bag or temporarily when a culture specimen is being collected.

**F.** Although some have suggested routine catheter change every 2 to 3 weeks [2], we concur with other experts [15] who suggest that a chronic catheter should **not be changed on a routine schedule. Indications for catheter change include** (a) malfunction or leakage; (b) obstruction of the catheter; (c) contamination of the system (e.g., breaking the connection between catheter and drainage tube); (d) concretions felt in the catheter lumen, which may precede obstruction of the catheter; (e) bacteriuria requiring antibiotic therapy as previously discussed in section II.B.3; and (f) in candiduria, catheter-change may be associated with clearing of the candiduria [15] (see Chapter 17).

**G.** To minimize the risks of cross-contamination, **a patient with an indwelling catheter should not be placed in the same room** as another patient with an indwelling catheter. Likewise, it is important that **hospital personnel wash their hands** before and after handling any portion of the collection system. Gloves should be used whenever the collection bag is handled, because the bag may be contaminated.

**H.** After the catheter has been removed, a follow-up urine culture should be done. Symptomatic or persistent bacteriuria should be treated.

**I. Urinary catheters should not be used as a matter of convenience** for the nursing staff or physician.

**J.** Cleansing the periurethral area with povidone-iodine solution or daily cleansing with soap and water are not recommended. These forms of **meatal care** may, in fact, cause meatal irritation and increase the risk for retrograde extraluminal bacterial migration. In addition, they are expensive.

**K. Additional measures** have been used. Attempts to prevent collection bag–related infection using a variety of bag antibacterial substances (e.g., hydrogen peroxide) have demonstrated no difference in the incidence of bacteriuria among patients whose bags were treated and those whose bags were not. Attempts to modify the catheter by incorporating a vent or by coating the catheter with various antibacterial substances require further study before they can be recommended for routine use.

**L. Condom catheters** are a preferred alternative in selected alert cooperative patients who can receive meticulous skin care to prevent meatal ulceration. See discussion in section VI.

**M. Chronic catheterization.** Prevention of infection is very difficult in these patients, who universally develop bacteriuria over time.

**V. Management of catheter-associated bacteriuria.** While the catheter is in place, systemic antimicrobial **treatment of asymptomatic catheter-associated bacteriuria is not recommended** [58,67,71]. Because complications of long-term catheterization are primarily infectious in nature, there is a temptation to treat all patients with catheter-associated bacteriuria; such treatment during catheterization is not helpful in eradicating infection for prolonged periods of time and serves only to select populations of organisms that are resistant to the antibiotics being used. Therefore, **while the catheter is in place, antibiotic treatment is recommended only for symptomatic infection** (i.e., bacteremia, pyelonephritis, epididymitis) [58,67,71].

**A. Short-term catheterization.** Not all patients who have been catheterized for short periods of time require a urine culture after the catheter is removed. Most patients who have bacteriuria immediately after catheter removal are asymptomatic and many patients, especially younger women, will have cleared the bacteria on repeat culture 1 to 2 weeks later. If symptomatic bacteriuria is present or if the patient is at high risk for symptomatic infection (pregnancy, diabetes, age over 65, or prolonged catheterization over 10 days), a urine culture should be obtained and appropriate antibiotic treatment based on susceptibility data should be instituted. The optimal antibiotic regimen in this setting is unclear. In one study of women, persistent bacteriuria after short-term catheterization (e.g., 4–6 days) that was asymptomatic or associated with lower UTI symptoms only was treated as effectively with single doses of TMP-SMX (320–1,600 mg) as with a 10-day course of TMP-SMX (160–800 mg twice a day) in women younger than 65 years old [76]. For older women, patients with upper tract symptoms, and males (with possible prostatic involvement), we favor conventional therapy (i.e., 10–14 days of antibiotic therapy based on susceptibility studies).

**B. Long-term catheterization.** Certain guidelines are helpful in monitoring and managing these patients.

1. **Urine cultures** in patients with chronic indwelling catheters often reveal multiple species of organisms, frequently with counts of 100,000 CFU/mL or more. These results are difficult to interpret and frequently change over short periods

of time. **Routine urine cultures are not recommended if the catheter is draining properly.**

2. **Antibiotic irrigation** of the catheter and bladder is of no advantage. Although bacteria can be suppressed, the beneficial effect is canceled by the contamination that occurs by periodically opening the collecting system.
3. **Asymptomatic bacteriuria should not routinely be treated.** This condition is very common, as was indicated previously. Because of the presence of a foreign body (i.e., the catheter), one cannot sterilize the bladder for prolonged periods of time. Unnecessary or prolonged use of antibiotics will only increase the likelihood of selecting out more resistant organisms.
4. **Systemic antibiotics should be used for catheterized patients who are febrile and ill-appearing, presumably from a UTI, with signs or symptoms suggesting a possible UTI-related bacteremia or pyelonephritis. Causes of fever other than a urinary tract source should be evaluated,** the catheter should be assessed for partial or complete obstruction, the patient should be examined for periurethral complication of urethral catheterization, and a urine culture should be aseptically obtained. **Because these are hospital-acquired infections, relatively resistant bacteria should be anticipated when selecting empiric antibiotic therapy.** Definitive antibiotic therapy should be adjusted based on susceptibility studies once they are available.
   a. **Bacteremic patients.** If bacteremia is suspected or known, broad-spectrum antibiotics are indicated while one is awaiting results of urine and blood cultures. For the hospitalized patient, enterococcal bacteremia would be uncommon and could, for all practical purposes, be excluded if an unspun urine Gram stain showed no gram-positive cocci. While awaiting cultures, an aminoglycoside, extended-spectrum penicillin or cephalosporin, or a fluoroquinolone alone could then be chosen on the basis of local antibiotic susceptibility patterns.

      These patients usually require a full 10- to 14-day course of antibiotics because of the associated bacteremia. Once culture data are available, initial empiric therapy can be tailored based on susceptibility data.
   b. **Nonbacteremic UTI.** If no bacteremia is suspected or documented, these patients should be treated with less than 10 days of antibiotics, and shorter courses (e.g., 5–7 days) are suggested [58]. This will usually sterilize the urine without selecting out more resistant bacteria. The optimal duration of therapy for a UTI in a male with a chronic catheter is not established. Prolonged therapy may only select out resistant organisms. However, a 3- to 5-day course may allow a prostatic focus to persist. While awaiting further guidelines in this setting, a 7-day course may be a reasonable compromise.

      For a patient who has just a low-grade temperature and is clinically stable, observation may be reasonable as the low-grade temperature may be transient.
   c. **Catheter change.** When antibiotics are to be given for catheter-related infections, the catheter should be changed and the urine cultured from the new catheter, as discussed in section II.B.3.
5. **Chronic antibiotic suppressive therapy is not effective** in these patients. Because the catheter acts as a foreign body, the urine of these patients cannot be sterilized for a prolonged period. Therefore, there are no data to support the use of daily TMP-SMX, quinolones, or other antibiotics in this group of patients. In addition, chronic use of methenamine and ascorbic acid is not effective in these patients. Methenamine requires 30 to 90 minutes to form formaldehyde, the active urinary suppressant. If the catheter is providing adequate drainage, the necessary "contact time" is not provided in the catheterized patient. (See methenamine discussion in Chapter 27.)
6. **Follow-up therapy.** When the catheter is discontinued, the urine should be cultured and persistent or symptomatic bacteriuria should be treated (see section V.A).

**VI. Condom catheters.** To obtain adequate urinary outputs, to maintain dryness of the patient with urinary incontinence, or to prevent soiling of an adjacent wound of the sacrum or perineum, a condom catheter system is an excellent alternative to indwelling urethral catheters in the male patient without outlet obstruction. This avoids problems associated with having a catheter within the bladder; however, bladder bacteriuria may still develop in condom-catheterized patients [77].

**A.** The **risk for bladder bacteriuria** in condom-catheterized patients is increased in uncooperative patients who frequently manipulate their condom drainage system.

**B.** Other **complications** of condom catheterization include local skin maceration, breakdown, and ulceration.

**C.** These problems should not occur if (a) constriction by the condom roller ring is avoided; (b) kinking of the collection roller ring or the collection system, which would result in urine retention, is prevented; and (c) the condom is removed once or twice daily to wash and dry the skin. Circumcision may be necessary if the prepuce is macerated and inflamed.

**D.** Physicians should be aware of the potential for bladder distention and vesicoureteral reflux in some patients with neurogenic bladders, including spine-injured patients.

## FUNGAL URINARY TRACT INFECTIONS

The presence of fungi in the urine often presents a diagnostic dilemma. *C. albicans* and other *Candida* species in the urine are seen most frequently in diabetics, in patients with indwelling bladder catheters, in patients receiving antibiotics, and occasionally in patients who have had previous instrumentation of the urinary tract.

**The presence of fungi in the urine is most often due to colonization** of the bladder and does not represent true infection. **This topic is discussed in Chapter 17.**

## INTRARENAL AND PERINEPHRIC ABSCESS

Intrarenal abscess occurs either as an uncommon consequence of ascending UTI, usually in patients with pyelonephritis and underlying obstructive urinary tract abnormalities; diabetes [9]; or hematogenous spread of bacteria from an extrarenal primary focus of infection [78]. Intrarenal abscess also may result from spontaneous infection of preexisting renal cysts. Perinephric abscess usually is the result of rupture of an intrarenal abscess into the perinephric space [78]. These are uncommon complications of UTI, and because the onset of symptoms is **characteristically insidious,** they may be overlooked as a cause of fever and flank or abdominal pain.

**I. Clinical manifestations**

**A. Setting.** Intrarenal and perinephric abscesses are most frequently associated with pyelonephritis in patients with underlying obstructive urinary tract abnormalities. Sometimes, intrarenal abscess is caused by *S. aureus*. Although one-third of patients with hematogenously derived *S. aureus* intrarenal abscesses will have no discernible primary focus of infection, most will have clinically apparent skin and soft tissue infections due to *S. aureus;* predisposing conditions are those that increase the risk for *S. aureus* bacteremia, including hemodialysis, intravenous drug abuse, and diabetes mellitus. Renal cyst infection in patients with polycystic kidney disease usually follows ascending UTI; however, on occasion, infection may be iatrogenic after cyst instrumentation.

**B. Signs and symptoms.** Intrarenal and perinephric abscesses usually present with fever, chills, and flank or abdominal pain [78]. Confusion and resultant delay in diagnosis occur when no localized signs or symptoms are present; when nausea, vomiting, or abdominal symptoms predominate; and because of the usual insidious nature of the onset of symptoms. Flank and CVA tenderness are the most common physical findings, with some patients demonstrating a tender flank or abdominal mass. Dysuria may or may not be present.

**II. Diagnosis**

**A. Signs and symptoms.** Clinical findings of fever, chills, and back pain are nonspecific and may be seen with pyelonephritis, renal and perirenal abscesses, and, occasionally, with renal tumor. An abscess or other space-occupying lesion and pyelonephritis complicated by obstruction **should be considered in the patient with UTI when fever persists beyond 48 to 72 hours despite appropriate antimicrobial therapy.**

**B. Urinalysis.** Pyuria, proteinuria, bacteriuria, or hematuria usually are present in patients whose infections originate from ascending infection; however, **in one-third**

**of patients, abscess collections will not be in communication with the collecting system and urinalysis will be normal** [78]. Patients with intrarenal abscesses due to *S. aureus* bacteremia and those with infected cysts often will have a normal urinalysis.

C. **Urine culture.** Two-thirds of patients will have urine cultures positive for aerobic gram-negative bacilli, most commonly *E. coli, Klebsiella* species, and *Proteus* species. **However, urine cultures frequently are sterile in patients with infected renal cysts.** Low colony counts ($10^2$ to $10^4$ CFU/mL) of *S. aureus* are present in one-half of patients with bacteremic intrarenal abscesses; **urine cultures positive for *S. aureus* in patients who have neither been catheterized nor treated by instrumentation should suggest an underlying *S. aureus* bacteremia** and, if clinical manifestations are present, possible secondary intrarenal abscess [78].

D. **Blood cultures.** Bacteremia is confirmed in fewer than one-third of patients [78]. Sustained *S. aureus* bacteremia suggests concurrent endocarditis (see Chapter 12).

E. **Radiographic studies. Ultrasonography and CT** are the imaging tests preferred for definite diagnosis. **Ultrasonography** can identify associated urinary obstruction, and **CT** allows precise anatomic information on the extent of extrarenal soft tissue extension. Both imaging procedures provide guidance for percutaneous aspiration and drainage. Infected intrarenal cysts may be identified by gallium scanning. Scan-guided percutaneous cyst aspiration and culture provide the definite diagnosis. Excretory urography is used less frequently today for diagnosis; abnormalities suggestive of intrarenal or perinephric abscess include decreased renal mobility, diminished renal function, calyceal abnormalities, and displacement of the kidney or ureter.

III. **Therapy**

A. **Intrarenal abscesses** often respond to antimicrobial therapy alone, and surgical intervention generally is not required. Empiric antimicrobial therapy should be directed against aerobic gram-negative bacilli and *S. aureus*. An aminoglycoside (gentamicin or tobramycin) or aztreonam in combination with a semisynthetic penicillinase-resistant penicillin (nafcillin or oxacillin) or a first-generation cephalosporin (cephalothin, cephapirin, or cefazolin) provide appropriate therapy pending the results of culture and susceptibility testing. Intravenous antibiotics are suggested in doses used for bacteremic patients, because high renal and extrarenal tissue levels of antibiotics are desirable.

Once susceptibility data are available, a conservative course of therapy of 6 to 8 weeks usually is begun; however, longer term therapy may be necessary based on the clinical response. Treatment of patients with polycystic disease is complicated by the unpredictable penetration of antibiotics into infected cysts [79], and infectious disease consultation is advised. Percutaneous drainage is indicated in a patient with a large intrarenal abscess, persistent fever, and no clinical improvement after 5 to 7 days of appropriate antimicrobial therapy. Prompt percutaneous nephrostomy drainage of obstructive lesions should be performed acutely, with delayed permanent corrective surgery.

B. **Perinephric abscesses** usually require percutaneous or open drainage, and frequently nephrectomy is necessary for definitive therapy. Along with early drainage, empiric antibiotic therapy, as stated in section A, should be instituted. Despite improved diagnostic and surgical techniques, the mortality for perinephric abscesses remains high [78]. Early urologic and infectious disease consultations are advised.

## GENITOURINARY TUBERCULOSIS

I. **Renal tuberculosis.** As in most forms of extrapulmonary tuberculosis, renal tuberculosis is the result of blood-borne dissemination from a primary focus elsewhere in the body, usually the lung but occasionally the gastrointestinal tract. The tubercle bacilli may be dormant for many years and may reactivate at a later time, with subsequent formation of caseous and cavitary necrosis of the kidney, prostate, or other genitourinary organs [80–82]. Tuberculosis is discussed in detail in Chapter 11.

**A. Clinical presentation**

1. Symptoms of dysuria, frequency, nocturia or urgency, and flank or back pain are frequently reported, but fever and constitutional symptoms generally are absent.
2. Approximately one-third of patients with renal tuberculosis have a history of tuberculosis elsewhere in the body that occurred many years previously. Sites of concurrent infection include the lung, bones, joints, other genitourinary organs, and adrenal glands.

**B.** The **tuberculin skin test** generally is positive in these patients.

**C.** The **urinalysis** frequently is abnormal, demonstrating the presence of pyuria or hematuria or both. Proteinuria also may be present. Routine bacterial cultures of urine are characteristically negative—hence, the so-called sterile pyuria that often is associated with renal tuberculosis.

**D.** Abnormal **chest roentgenograms** may be obtained in as many as 75% of such patients, most of whom have inactive pulmonary disease. Some patients have active pulmonary tuberculous infection concurrently.

**E. Special studies**

1. **Smears.** Urine smears for acid-fast bacilli may have false-positive results because of saprophytic mycobacteria present in the urine of healthy patients.
2. **PCR** is a sensitive and specific rapid diagnostic test [83]. However, it may not be widely available.
3. **Acid-fast bacilli cultures.** Three first-morning clean-catch specimens of urine are preferred over 24-hour collections, which often are contaminated samples. The urine culture will be positive in as many as 90% of patients.
4. **Intravenous pyelogram.** The radiographic appearance may support the diagnosis but is nonspecific. In addition, autonephrectomy is common in renal tuberculosis, and often there is secondary calcification.

**F. Therapy.** Extrapulmonary tuberculosis is treated in a manner similar to pulmonary tuberculosis if isoniazid and rifampin can be used for sensitive isolates, with 6 to 9 months of therapy sufficient for most patients. If isoniazid and rifampin cannot be used together, more protracted therapy (18–24 months) is indicated (see Chapter 11).

Surgery was the mainstay of treatment before the advent of antituberculous chemotherapy. At present, surgery generally is reserved for complications of renal tuberculosis, such as hemorrhage, sepsis, pain, inability to sterilize the urine, or ureteral stricture [84].

**G. Prognosis** with chemotherapy is good, with few relapses occurring in patients completing a full course of chemotherapy. Complications may result even though bacteriologic cure has been achieved. Hypertension, bacterial UTI, and ureteral obstruction may be seen.

**II. Male genital tuberculosis.** Tuberculosis of other portions of the male genitourinary tract may be present concurrently with renal tuberculosis. This suggests that infection may occur directly from the urine itself, although hematogenous spread can occur. Epididymitis is the most common form of male genital tuberculosis. A palpable painful lesion is characteristic of this disease, and the tuberculin skin test generally is positive. Diagnosis is made by biopsy and culture of the mass.

**III. Female genital tuberculosis.** Tuberculosis of the female genital tract is the result of hematogenous spread of tubercle bacilli. The **fallopian tubes** are most commonly involved. Common complaints are chronic pelvic and abdominal pain, menstrual disorders, and infertility. The tuberculin skin test generally is positive, and constitutional symptoms and fever are absent. The demonstration of tubercle bacilli is necessary for diagnosis. Endometrial curettage may reveal granulomas in half the patients with tuberculous **endometritis.** However, monthly sloughing of the endometrium in the menstruating patient may make histologic diagnosis difficult. Culdoscopy, laparoscopy, and laparotomy ultimately may be required to establish the diagnosis.

## REFERENCES

1. Preheim LC. Complicated urinary tract infections. *Am J Med* 1985;79:62.
2. Falagas ME, Gorbach SL. Practice guidelines: urinary tract infections. *Infect Dis Clin Pract* 1995;4:241.

3. Stamey TA. *Pathogenesis and treatment of urinary tract infections.* Baltimore: Williams & Wilkins, 1980.
4. Stamm WE, et al. Urinary tract infections: from pathogenesis to treatment. *J Infect Dis* 1989;159:400.
5. Kunin CM. Urinary tract infections in females. *Clin Infect Dis* 1994;18:1.
6. Avorn J, et al. Reduction of bacteriuria and pyuria after ingestion of cranberry juice. *JAMA* 1994;271:751.
7. Kontiokari T, Sundqvist K, Nuutinen M, et al. Randomised trial of cranberry-lingonberry juice and Lactobacillus GG drink for the prevention of urinary tract infections in women. *BMJ* 2001;322:1571.
8. Hooton TM, et al. *Escherichia coli* bacteriuria and contraceptive method. *JAMA* 1991;265:64–69.
9. Patterson JE, Andriole VT. Bacterial urinary tract infections in diabetes. *Infect Dis Clin North Am* 1995;9:25.
10. Meares EM, Jr. Prostatitis. *Med Clin North Am* 1991;75:405.
11. Bergeron MG. Treatment of pyelonephritis in adults. *Med Clin North Am* 1995;79:619.
12. Stamm WE. Measurement of pyuria and its relation to bacteriuria. *Am J Med* 1983;75:53.
13. Mears EM. Renal abscess. In: Gorbach SL, Bartlett JG, Blacklow NR, eds. *Infectious diseases.* Philadelphia: Saunders, 1992:805–808.
14. Stamm WE. Quantitative urine cultures in infectious disease diagnosis: use and abuse. Symposium on quantitative cultures in infectious disease diagnosis: use and abuse. 35th Interscience Conference on Antimicrobial Agents and Chemotherapy. San Francisco, California, Sept. 19, 1995.
15. Stamm WE, Warren JE. Meet the Professor Session: Urinary Tract Infection. Infectious Disease Society of America 33rd Annual Meeting. San Francisco, California, Sept. 16, 1995.
16. Jenkins RD, Fenn JP, Matson JM. Review of urine microscopy for bacteriuria. *JAMA* 1986;255:3397.
17. Komaroff AL. Urinalysis and urine culture in women with dysuria. *Ann Intern Med* 1986;104:212.
18. Stamm WE. When should we use urine cultures? *Infect Control* 1986;7:431.
19. Stamm WE, et al. Causes of acute urethral syndrome in women. *N Engl J Med* 1980;303:409.
20. Stamm WE, et al. Diagnosis of coliform infection in acutely dysuric women. *N Engl J Med* 1982;307:463.
21. Kunin CM. A reassessment of the importance of "low-count" bacteriuria in young women with acute urinary symptoms. *Ann Intern Med* 1993;119:454.
22. Lipsky BA, et al. Diagnosis of bacteriuria in men: specimen collection and culture interpretation. *J Infect Dis* 1987;155:847–854.
23. Scheer WE. The detection of leukocyte esterase activity in urine with a new reagent strip. *Am J Clin Pathol* 1987;87:86.
24. American College of Physicians. Common uses of intravenous pyelography in adults. *Ann Intern Med* 1989;111:83. [See also Mushlin AL, Thornbury JR. Intravenous pyelography: the case against its routine use. *Ann Intern Med* 1989;111:58.]
25. Belman AB. Urinary imaging in children. *Pediatr Infect Dis J* 1989;8:548.
26. Sobel JD, Kaye D. Urinary tract infections. In: Mandell GL, Bennett JE, Dolin R, eds. *Principles and practice of infectious diseases,* 5th ed. New York: Churchill Livingstone, 2000:773–805.
27. Warren JW, Abrutyn E, Hebel JR, et al. Guidelines for antimicrobial treatment of uncomplicated acute bacterial cystitis and acute pyelonephritis in women. *Clin Infect Dis* 1999;29:745.
28. Gupta K, Sahm DF, Mayfield D, et al. Antimicrobial resistance among uropathogens that cause community-acquired urinary tract infections in women: a nationwide analysis. *Clin Infect Dis* 2001;33:89.
29. Jones SR, Smith JW, Sanford JP. Localization of urinary tract infections by detection of antibody-coated bacteria in urine sediment. *N Engl J Med* 1974;290:591.
30. Andriole VT, Patterson TF. Epidemiology, natural history, and management of urinary tract infections in pregnancy. *Med Clin North Am* 1991;75:359.

31. Stamm WE, Hooton TM. Management of urinary tract infections in adults. *N Engl J Med* 1993;329:1328–1334.
32. Norrby SR. Short-term treatment of uncomplicated lower urinary tract infections in women. *Rev Infect Dis* 1990;12:458.
33. Safrin S, et al. Pyelonephritis in women: inpatient vs. outpatient treatment. *Am J Med* 1988;85:793.
34. Stamm WE, McKevitt M, Counts GW. Acute renal infection in women: treatment with trimethoprim-sulfamethoxazole or ampicillin for two or six weeks. A randomized trial. *Ann Intern Med* 1987;106:341.
35. Behr MA, Drummond R, Libman MD, et al. Fever duration in hospitalized acute pyelonephritis patients. *Am J Med* 1996;101:277–280.
36. Schwab SJ, Bander SJ, Klahr S. Renal infection in autosomal dominant polycystic kidney disease. *Am J Med* 1987;82:714.
37. Nicolle LE, Ronald AR. Recurrent urinary tract infection in adult women: diagnosis and treatment. *Infect Dis Clin North Am* 1987;1:793–806.
38. Stapleton A, et al. Postcoital antimicrobial prophylaxis for recurrent urinary tract infection: a randomized, double-blind, placebo-controlled trial. *JAMA* 1990;264:703–706.
39. Stamm WE, McKevitt M, Toberts NJ. Natural history of recurrent urinary tract infections in women. *Rev Infect Dis* 1991;13:77–84.
40. Stamm WE, et al. Antimicrobial prophylaxis of recurrent urinary tract infections. A double-blind, placebo-controlled trial. *Ann Intern Med* 1980;106:341–345.
41. Gupta K, Hooton TM, Roberts PL, et al. Patient-initiated treatment of uncomplicated recurrent urinary tract infections in young women. *Ann Intern Med* 2001;135:9–16.
42. Raz R, Stamm WE. A controlled trial of intravaginal estriol in postmenopausal women with recurrent urinary tract infections. *N Engl J Med* 1993;329:753–756.
43. Lipsky BA. Urinary tract infections in men. Epidemiology, pathophysiology, diagnosis and treatment. *Ann Intern Med* 1989;110:138–150.
44. Smith JW, et al. Recurrent urinary tract infections in men. Characteristics in response to therapy. *Ann Intern Med* 1979;91:544.
45. Meares EM Jr, Stamey TA. Bacteriologic localization patterns in bacterial prostatitis and urethritis. *Invest Urol* 1968;5:492.
46. Krieger JN, Nyberg L Jr, Nickel JC. NIH consensus definition and classification of prostatitis. *JAMA* 1999;282:236.
47. Nickel JC, Downey J, Hunter D, et al. Prevalence of prostatitis-like symptoms in a population based study using the National Institutes of Health chronic prostatitis symptom index. *J Urol* 2001;165:842.
48. Meares EM Jr. Prostatitis and related disorders. In: Walsh PC, et al., eds. *Campbell's urology,* 7th ed. Philadelphia: Saunders, 1998:615–630.
49. McNaughton Collins M, Fowler FJ Jr, Elliott DB, et al. Diagnosing and treating chronic prostatitis: do urologists use the four-glass test? *Urology* 2000;55:403.
50. Meares EM, Jr. Bacterial prostatitis versus "prostatosis." A clinical and bacteriological study. *JAMA* 1973;224:1372.
51. Collins MM, MacDonald R, Wilt TJ. Diagnosis and treatment of chronic abacterial prostatitis: a systematic review. *Ann Intern Med* 2000;133:367–381.
52. Nickel JC, Downey J, Johnston B, et al. Predictors of patient response to antibiotic therapy for the chronic prostatitis/chronic pelvic pain syndrome: a prospective multicenter clinical trial. *J Urol* 2001;165:1539.
53. Ireton RC, Berger RE. Prostatitis and epididymitis. *Urol Clin North Am* 1984;11: 83–93.
54. Berger RE, Kessler D, Holmes KK. Etiology and manifestations of epididymitis in young men: correlations with sexual orientation. *J Infect Dis* 1987;155:1341–1343.
55. Vorland LH, Carlson K, Aalen O. An epidemiological survey of urinary tract infections among outpatients in Northern Norway. *Scand J Infect Dis* 1985;17:277–283.
56. Baldassarre JS, Kaye D. Special problems of urinary tract infection in the elderly. *Med Clin North Am* 1991;75:375.
57. Nicolle LE. Urinary tract infection in long-term-care facility residents. *Clin Infect Dis* 2000;31:757–761.
58. Nicolle LE. Urinary tract infections in long-term-care facilities. *Infect Control Hosp Epidemiol* 2001;22:167–175.

59. Heinamaki P, et al. Urinary characteristics and infection in the very aged. *Gerontology* 1984;30:403.
60. Yoshikawa TT. Unique aspects of urinary tract infection in the geriatric population. *Gerontology* 1984;30:339–344.
61. Ouslander JG, Schapira M, Schnelle JF, et al. Does eradicating bacteriuria affect the severity of chronic urinary incontinence in nursing home residents? *Ann Intern Med* 1995;122:749.
62. Nicolle LE, et al. The association of bacteriuria with resident characteristics and survival in elderly institutionalized men. *Ann Intern Med* 1987;106:682–686.
63. Boscia JA, et al. Epidemiology of bacteriuria in an elderly ambulatory population. *Am J Med* 1986;80:208–214.
64. Zelikovic I, Adelman RD, Nancarrow PA. Urinary tract infections in children, an update. *West J Med* 1992;157:554–561.
65. American Academy of Pediatrics. Practice parameter: the diagnosis, treatment, and evaluation of the initial urinary tract infection in febrile infants and young children. *Pediatrics* 1999;103:843–852.
66. Carmack MA, Arvin AM. Urinary tract infections-navigating complex currents. *West J Med* 1992;157:587–588.
67. Stamm WE. Catheter-associated urinary tract infections: epidemiology, pathogenesis, and prevention. *Am J Med* 1991;91[Suppl 3B]:65–71.
68. Saint S, Elmore JG, Sullivan SD, et al. The efficacy of silver alloy-coated urinary catheters in preventing urinary tract infection: a meta-analysis. *Am J Med* 1998;105: 236.
69. Saint S, Veenstra DL, Sullivan SD, et al. The potential clinical and economic benefits of silver alloy urinary catheters in preventing urinary tract infection. *Arch Intern Med* 2000;160:2670.
70. Tambyah PA, Halvorson KT, Maki DG. A prospective study of pathogenesis of catheter-associated urinary tract infections. *Mayo Clin Proc* 1999;74:131.
71. Stamm WE. Nosocomial urinary tract infections. In: Bennett JV, Brachman PS, eds. *Hospital infections,* 4th ed. Philadelphia: Lippincott-Raven, 1998:477–485.
72. Warren JW. The catheter and urinary tract infection. *Med Clin North Am* 1991;75:481.
73. Perkash I, Giroux J. Clean intermittent catheterization in spinal cord injury patients: a follow-up study. *J Urol* 1993;149:1068.
74. Kamitsuka PF. The pathogenesis, prevention, and management of urinary tract infections in patients with spinal cord injury. *Curr Clin Top Infect Dis* 1993;13:1.
75. Gribble MJ, Putterman ML. Prophylaxis of urinary tract infection in persons with recent spinal cord injury: a prospective, randomized, double-blind, placebo controlled study of trimethoprim-sulfamethoxazole. *Am J Med* 1993;95:141.
76. Harding GKM, et al. How long should catheter-associated urinary tract infections in women be treated? A randomized controlled study. *Ann Intern Med* 1991;114:713.
77. Hirsh DD, Fainstein V, Musher DM. Do condom catheter collecting systems cause urinary tract infection? *JAMA* 1979;242:340.
78. Dembry LM, Andriole VT. Renal and perirenal abscesses. *Infect Dis Clin North Am* 1997;11:663–680.
79. Andriole V. Intrarenal and perinephric abscess. In: Hoeprich PD, Jordan MC, Arnold AR, eds. *Infectious diseases,* 5th ed. Philadelphia: Lippincott, 1994:617.
80. Simon HB, et al. Genitourinary tuberculosis: clinical features in a general hospital population. *Am J Med* 1977;63:410.
81. Garcia-Rodriguez JA, et al. Genitourinary tuberculosis in Spain: a review of 81 cases. *Clin Infect Dis* 1994;18:557.
82. Lenk S, Schroeder J. Genitourinary tuberculosis. *Curr Opin Urol* 2001;11:93–98.
83. Hemal AK, Gupta NP, Rajeev TP, et al. Polymerase chain reaction in clinically suspected genitourinary tuberculosis: comparison with intravenous urography, bladder biopsy, and urine acid fast bacilli culture. *Urology* 2000;56:570–574.
84. Carl P, Stark L. Indications for surgical management of genitourinary tuberculosis. *World J Surg* 1997;21:505–510.

# 16. SEXUALLY TRANSMITTED DISEASES AND OBSTETRIC AND GYNECOLOGIC INFECTIONS

Eric R. Houpt and Michael F. Rein

## GENERAL PRINCIPLES IN MANAGEMENT

I. **Definition.** The sexually transmitted diseases (STDs) are grouped together because sexual contact is epidemiologically significant, although it is not the only mechanism through which the diseases are acquired.

II. **Consequences**

A. Sexual partners of patients with STDs are at high risk of infection and must be evaluated. The risk of infection may be so high that such partners are treated when first evaluated, even if their infection has not yet been confirmed. This is termed **epidemiologic treatment and is a cornerstone of STD management** [1].

B. **Coprevalence**

1. **Patients with one STD are significantly likely to have others.** A patient in whom one STD has been diagnosed should be carefully evaluated for others that may be clinically silent but of much greater eventual medical consequence (e.g., human immunodeficiency virus [HIV]) [2].

2. **Patient education regarding risk reduction** is an important aspect of management.

C. **Management** of an STD **always involves dealing with more than one patient.**

1. All patients must have completed treatment before resuming unprotected sexual contact.

2. Several STDs (syphilis, gonorrhea, chancroid, lymphogranuloma venereum, acquired immunodeficiency syndrome [AIDS], and, in some states, asymptomatic HIV infection) must be reported to local health departments.

III. A careful and complete **sexual history** must be obtained from each patient.

A. The history must be taken in terms understandable to the patient. Thus, the examiner must become desensitized to using street terms (e.g., "Do you take your partner's penis into your mouth?" or "Do you give head?") rather than technical jargon (e.g., "Do you practice fellatio?").

B. **Never make assumptions regarding your patient's sexual orientation.** Obtain a sexual history in gender-neutral terms (e.g., "Have you had sex with any new partners in the past month?" rather than "Have you had sex with any new women [men] in the past month?") until the patient's sexual preferences have been defined explicitly.

IV. **A history of recent antibiotic use** is critical, because antibiotics may mask clinical features of disease without producing a cure.

## URETHRITIS

Urethritis is a common presenting syndrome. Initial evaluation requires differentiating gonococcal from nongonococcal urethritis.

I. **Epidemiology.** The major single specific etiology of acute urethritis is *Neisseria gonorrhoeae,* producing **gonococcal urethritis** (GCU). Urethritis of all other etiologies is collectively referred to as **nongonococcal urethritis** (NGU).

A. NGU is twice as common as GCU in the United States, especially among higher socioeconomic groups [3].

B. GCU is relatively more common among homosexual than heterosexual men with acute urethritis [4].

II. **Clinical features in men. GCU and NGU cannot be differentiated reliably on clinical features alone.** A significant proportion of men with GCU or NGU may be asymptomatic [5–7].

A. **Incubation period** can sometimes be assessed if the patient has had a single sexual exposure or sex with a new partner within the preceding several weeks.

1. Seventy-five percent of symptomatic men with GCU develop symptoms within 4 days and 80% to 90% within 2 weeks [7].

2. Fifty percent of symptomatic men with NGU develop symptoms within 4 days, but the incubation period ranges from 2 to 35 days [7].
3. An incubation period of less than 1 week has no differential diagnostic significance.
4. Incubation periods can be prolonged by subcurative doses of antibiotics.

**B. Urethral discharge.** Discharge is described by 75% of men with GCU but by only 11% to 33% of men with NGU [7].

1. Discharge present at the meatus without stripping suggests GCU.
2. Mucopurulent discharge (purulent flecks in a mucoid matrix) is seen in 50% of cases of NGU but also in 25% of cases of GCU.
3. A completely clear urethral discharge suggests NGU.
4. The discharge in NGU may be so slight as to be present only as a meatal bead or a crust noted when the patient first arises.

**C. Dysuria** is common in both GCU and NGU.

1. Urethral discomfort may occur at other times and be described as itching or irritation.
2. Urethral symptoms may mimic those of cystitis, particularly in women.

**D. Onset.** Symptoms usually begin fairly abruptly with GCU, whereas the onset of NGU may be less acute.

**E. Natural history.** The clinical features of acute urethritis will eventually resolve without treatment.

1. Ninety-five percent of patients with GCU will become asymptomatic within 6 months.
2. Chronic gonorrhea sometimes manifests as gleet, a thin discharge containing only small numbers of gonococci.
3. Of patients with NGU, 30% to 70% become asymptomatic over 1 to 3 months [7].

**III. Diagnosis and differential diagnosis in men**

**A. Examination of the patient.** Men should stand before the seated examiner, and the entire genital area should be examined.

1. It is preferable that the patient be examined at least 2 hours after micturition.
2. The underwear may reveal stains of discharge.
3. Erythema around the meatus may indicate urethritis, but some degree of perimeatal blush is often a normal finding.
4. If discharge is not spontaneously present, the urethra should be gently stripped by placing the gloved thumb along the ventral surface of the penis with the fingers above, applying gentle pressure, and moving the thumb forward to deliver discharge.

**B. Examination of the urethral specimen**

1. If no discharge is expressed from the meatus, urethral material must be recovered by inserting a small swab into the urethra.
   a. The patient should be warned about the brief discomfort that will result.
   b. A 1- to 2-mm calcium alginate or rayon swab on a metal shaft is inserted approximately 1.5 to 2.0 inches into the urethra and removed while the shaft is being rotated.
2. The swab is rolled across a microscope slide and then rolled across a plate of medium selective for *N. gonorrhoeae.*
3. The slide is fixed and Gram stained using standard methods.
4. The slide is examined using the oil-immersion objective (950–1,000 × X).
   a. The proximal urethra has cuboidal epithelium.
   b. The distal urethra supports a **normal bacterial flora** consisting primarily of gram-positive cocci and rods, which have no clinical significance.
   c. **Spermatozoa** sometimes are present in physiologic secretions. The heads are gram-positive and characteristically fade out toward the acrosomal cap. Gram-negative tails are sometimes observed.
   d. The diagnostic criterion of five polymorphonuclear neutrophils (PMNs) per oil-immersion field is insensitive, and 16% to 50% of men with acute urethritis will fail to show this number of PMNs in the densest portion of the slide [7]. The number of PMNs observed is reduced by recent micturition. **Even**

**the presence of a few PMNs on a urethral smear provides objective evidence of urethritis.**

e. The **complete absence of PMNs** argues against urethritis. The discomfort of symptomatic patients may persist from adequately treated urethritis or reflect psychosomatic symptoms or perhaps discomfort resulting from excessive consumption of urethral irritants such as caffeine or alcohol. Such patients are best managed with reassurance and reexamination if symptoms persist.

f. The presence of PMNs supports the diagnosis of urethritis. If, in addition, one sees characteristic **gram-negative, intracellular diplococci,** the diagnosis of gonorrhea is established. If such organisms are not observed, the patient is said to have NGU. This test is more than 95% accurate in men with symptomatic acute urethritis. The presence of extracellular organisms with the same morphology has no diagnostic significance [7,8].

5. **One cannot diagnose concurrent NGU by Gram staining in the presence of gonorrhea. Thus, one should assume that patients with gonorrhea are coinfected with nongonococcal pathogens.**

## IV. Microbiologic features in men

### A. Gonorrhea

1. *N. gonorrhoeae* is a gram-negative kidney-shaped diplococcus with flattened opposed margins. Some strains of *N. gonorrhoeae* are susceptible to the vancomycin contained in selective media and will not grow thereon. **A negative culture in the face of a positive Gram stain does not rule out GCU.**
2. **Nonculture diagnostic techniques.** Newer techniques have supplanted the culture in many clinical settings.
   a. **Ligase chain reaction** has a sensitivity of 99% and a specificity of 98% [9].
   b. **Nonamplified DNA probe** has a sensitivity of 96% and a specificity of 98% [10].
   c. Antigen detection tests are insensitive compared with culture and genetic probes.
3. **Antimicrobial susceptibility.** The gonococcus has developed resistance to antimicrobial agents by two mechanisms.
   a. **Chromosomal mutations.** are additive, and strains with relatively high resistance to many classes of antibiotics, including fluoroquinolones, are now widely observed [11–13].
   b. **Plasmids.** Gonococci bearing plasmids coding for **penicillinase production and tetracycline resistance** are prevalent in the United States [11].

### B. NGU

1. NGU is caused by any of several organisms. The cause of perhaps 20% of cases has not been identified.
2. ***Chlamydia trachomatis*** causes 15% to 50% of cases of NGU in various studies [3,4,7].
   a. The organism is an obligate intracellular parasite, which possesses both DNA and RNA; replicates by binary fission, like bacteria; and is **sensitive to a variety of antimicrobials [3,13,14].**
   b. The organism can be grown only in tissue culture, but its presence in urogenital specimens can be detected with new techniques, such as the polymerase chain reaction (PCR) and the ligase chain reaction, both of which will detect 95% of cases from urethral swabs or from urine specimens [15–17].
   c. The spectrum of diseases caused by *C. trachomatis* closely parallels that caused by *N. gonorrhoeae.* **Coinfection with these two organisms is very common and affects management strategies.**
3. ***Ureaplasma urealyticum*** causes about 15% to 30% of NGU [3,7,18,19].
   a. *Ureaplasmas* are free-living agents that can be grown in broth or on culture plates, although cultures are rarely performed in clinical practice.
   b. Some ureaplasmas are resistant to the tetracyclines and must be treated with a macrolide or a fluoroquinolone [20–22].
4. ***Mycoplasma genitalium*** is a recently characterized mycoplasma, which appears to be associated with up to 30% of NGU. Although its precise contribution

remains to be defined, it may be more strongly associated with chronic or recurrent than with acute urethritis. It is sensitive to the tetracyclines [23–26].

5. ***Trichomonas vaginalis*** usually is carried asymptomatically by men but may cause NGU that fails to respond to standard antibacterial treatment [27–29].
6. **Herpes simplex virus (HSV)** can infect the urethra and cause dysuria, which is usually far more severe than the amount of discharge would suggest [30]. The urethritis usually occurs in the setting of external lesions.
7. **Other organisms,** such as Enterobacteriaceae, adenovirus, *Neisseria meningitidis, Streptococcus pneumoniae,* microsporidia (in AIDS), and possibly *Staphylococcus saprophyticus, Haemophilus species,* and *Bacteroides* are rare causes of NGU but are not sexually transmitted [7].

## V. Treatment in men

**A. Gonorrhea.** Because of increasing resistance of *N. gonorrhoeae* to antimicrobials, the treatment for uncomplicated anogenital gonorrhea has changed. Examples of currently acceptable regimens include

1. Ceftriaxone 125 mg intramuscularly (i.m.) made up in 1% lidocaine as a single dose.
2. Ciprofloxacin, 500 mg orally as a single dose.
3. Ofloxacin, 400 mg orally as a single dose.
4. Cefixime, 400 mg orally as a single dose.
5. Cefpodoxime, 200 mg orally as a single dose.
6. Azithromycin 2 g orally as a single dose. Although this regimen will cure coincident chlamydial infection, it is very costly, and resistance is developing rapidly in several parts of the country.
7. Gatifloxacin, 400 mg orally as a single dose.

**B. Because 10% to 30% of heterosexual men and 40% to 60% of women with gonorrhea (in STD clinics) are also infected with *Chlamydia,* treatment for gonorrhea should include a second regimen effective against this organism.**

**C. NGU.** Because it is impossible to differentiate among the common etiologies of NGU, the condition is treated syndromically, including in the initial treatment regimen those drugs effective against the common causative agents. There is no advantage to extending the initial regimen beyond 7 days [31]. Examples of regimens useful in the treatment of NGU include the following:

1. Azithromycin 1 g orally provides the only single dose regimen for chlamydial infections [32,33].
2. Doxycycline 100 mg orally twice a day for 7 days.
3. Tetracycline hydrochloride 500 mg orally four times a day for 7 days.
4. Erythromycin 500 mg orally four times a day for 7 days or, if the larger dose is not tolerated, 250 mg orally four times a day for 7 days.
5. Ofloxacin 300 mg orally twice a day for 7 days. One may use equivalent (approximately half) doses of levofloxacin.
6. Minocycline 100 mg orally at bed time (qhs) for 7 days [34].

**D. The following additional regimens may be used if the infection is known to be chlamydial.** These regimens are not active against mycoplasmas.

1. Clindamycin, 450 mg orally three times a day for 10 days [35].
2. Amoxicillin 500 mg orally three times a day for 7 days [36].
3. Sulfisoxazole, 500 mg orally four times a day for 10 days. Trimethoprim-sulfamethoxazole has no greater efficacy.

**E. Epidemiologic treatment** of sexual partners of men with urethritis is essential. The practice of testing such partners for chlamydial infection and basing therapy on the result is erroneous, because NGU is very likely to be nonchlamydial [7,37].

## VI. Management of recurrent disease.

A careful sexual history regarding reexposure and adequate treatment of sexual partners is critical, because **reinfection is the most common cause of recurrence.** The pattern of recurrence of NGU can be of great value in deciding further management.

**A. Response, reexposure, recurrence.** Initial response suggests infection with a sensitive agent. Reexposure followed by recurrence strongly suggests reinfection, supports retreatment with an effective regimen, and demands careful investigation of possible sources of reinfection.

**B. Failure to respond.** Lack of response **to doxycycline** suggests infection with a tetracycline-resistant agent (see section IV.B.3–5) such as *U. urealyticum* or *T. vaginalis*.

1. The persistence of urethritis is documented by observing PMNs on a urethral smear. The absence of PMNs suggests resolution of the infectious process with a persistent pain syndrome that does not require further treatment with antimicrobials.
2. Patients with documented persistent urethritis should be empirically treated for both organisms with metronidazole, 2 g orally as a single dose, and erythromycin, azithromycin, or an appropriate fluoroquinolone.

**C. Response with relapse** in the absence of reinfection is poorly understood. Such patients are disproportionately those men who are initially culture negative for chlamydiae and ureaplasmas [22]. Appropriate treatment is not clearly defined.

1. Of such patients, 50% to 75% may respond to a 3- to 6-week course of erythromycin or a tetracycline [38,39].
2. Patients relapsing after this treatment should probably be referred for urologic evaluation [40].
3. These patients do not develop complications, and their sexual partners have no clinical evidence of infection.
4. Patients who relapse after an initial 3- to 6-week treatment course may be rendered asymptomatic with a standard regimen and then placed on long-term suppressive doses of a tetracycline [7,39]. Tetracycline hydrochloride is preferred because it is more economical, and one should use the lowest dose that keeps the patient free of symptoms, often 500 mg orally once daily. Treatment for 6 to 12 months is well tolerated and might be followed by discontinuation of the drug and reevaluation [7,39].

## VII. Urethritis in women

### A. Clinical features

1. **Women are usually unaware of urethral discharge, and urethritis presents as dysuria and frequency.**
2. Women with dysuria should be asked whether it is external or internal. Internal dysuria is associated with urethritis or cystitis, whereas external dysuria is more frequently associated with vulvovaginitis.
3. Infected women usually manifest **pyuria.**
4. If routine urine cultures are negative, affected women are said to have the **acute urethral syndrome** [41,42].

### B. Etiology

1. Some women have cystitis caused by small numbers of Enterobacteriaceae [41] or urethritis caused by Enterobacteriaceae [43].
2. Some patients have GCU or NGU [41,42], which may respond initially to standard urinary tract treatments. Recurrence of such an apparently culture-negative urinary tract infection may result from reinfection with sexually transmitted urethritis.

### C. Treatment of GCU or NGU in women is the same as treatment in men. Treatment in pregnancy involves the following [35–37]:

1. **Tetracyclines and fluoroquinolones are contraindicated.**
2. Gonorrhea can be treated with a cephalosporin or, in the setting of $\beta$-lactam allergy, with 2 g of azithromycin; the latter is followed by a test-of-cure 1 to 2 weeks later.
3. Chlamydial infection can be treated with erythromycin, azithromycin, amoxicillin, or clindamycin.

## VIII. Asymptomatic urethritis

**A.** GCU or NGU can occur without symptoms [5,6].

**B.** Asymptomatic urethritis is prevalent among the male partners of women whose gonococcal or chlamydial infections are detected on routine screening or who present with symptoms or complications [6,44]. **Asymptomatic male partners of infected women should be treated on initial presentation.**

**C.** Many men with asymptomatic urethritis have PMNs on a Gram-stained smear of a urethral specimen [5,6,44]; thus, a urethral smear should be part of the workup of asymptomatic men.

**D.** The sensitivity of the urethral smear for gonococci in asymptomatic GCU is probably only 70% [6].

**E.** Most men harboring trichomonads are asymptomatic [27].

## CERVICITIS

**I. Etiology.** Major pathogens include *N. gonorrhoeae, C. trachomatis,* and herpes simplex. However, most infected women do not have mucopurulent cervicitis (MPC) [13,45].

**A.** ***N. gonorrhoeae*** is most frequently isolated from the endocervix of infected women.

**B.** ***C. trachomatis*** can be recovered from the endocervix of 60% to 90% of the sexual partners of men with chlamydial urethritis, and cervical abnormalities, often subtle, have been observed in 80% to 90% of infected women [45–49].

**C. HSV** is isolated from the cervix in 88% of women with primary infection but from only 12% of women with recurrent herpetic infection [30,50]. **Herpetic cervicitis may be present without external lesions.**

**D.** Certain types of **human papillomavirus (HPV)** preferentially infect the cervix [51].

1. Several lines of evidence support the contention that certain types of HPV cause cervical cancer [16,18,31,33,35,39,45,51,52].
   a. Cervical cancer behaves epidemiologically as an STD [52].
   b. HPV DNA, particularly types 16 and 18, is found in more than 90% of cervical cancers [53].
   c. Prospective data indicate that acquisition of cervical HPV confers a high risk of premalignant lesions developing within 1 to 2 years [54].
   d. A molecular mechanism for malignant transformation is currently being defined [55].
2. Cervical carriage of HPV is, however, self-limited, with a median persistence of about 8 to 10 months [56–60].

**E. Other organisms** [45] that occasionally cause cervicitis include adenovirus, measles virus, cytomegalovirus, *Enterobius vermicularis,* amoebae, *Mycobacterium tuberculosis,* group B streptococci, *Neisseria meningitidis,* and actinomycetes, the last usually in association with the use of intrauterine contraceptive devices.

**II. Diagnosis.** The clinical features of specific cervical infections overlap too much to permit an accurate etiologic diagnosis without laboratory assistance [46,47]. **Multiple infections are common [48].**

**A. Clinical features.** About one-third of infected women note a discharge from the vagina that actually originates in the inflamed cervix. Inguinal adenopathy is rare unless the disease is accompanied by lesions of the external genitalia, because lymphatic drainage of the cervix involves the external iliac rather than the inguinofemoral nodes.

**B. Examination**

1. **Erythema around the cervical os may indicate infection or may merely represent cervical ectropion,** migration of endocervical epithelium over the surface of the cervix, which is symmetric about the os and is not particularly friable. It is often impossible on clinical grounds alone to differentiate ectropion from true infection. Normal cervical discharge is clear and mucoid. Purulent or mucopurulent discharge (MPC) is associated with gonococcal, chlamydial, or, less frequently, herpetic infection [46–49].
2. **Chlamydiae** have been isolated from 50% to 90% of sexually active patients with hypertrophic cervicitis. Only 19% to 32% of women with chlamydial cervical infection manifest hypertrophic cervicitis, an intensely erythematous, raised, irregular lesion that bleeds easily [45–49], and only 30% or so have a mucopurulent or purulent cervical discharge [45–49,61]. On examination, **20% to 70% of infected women have a completely normal cervix [62–65]. Therefore, physical examination never adequately excludes chlamydial or gonococcal cervicitis.**

3. **Cervicitis is seen on physical examination** in approximately 90% of women whose cervical cultures are positive for **HSV** [30,50]. Cervical discharge is usually mucoid but is occasionally mucopurulent, and in one series herpetic cervical infection caused 8% of cases of MPC [46].

C. **Laboratory tests**

1. **Microscopy**
   a. Observation of 10 to 30 PMNs per oil-immersion field in the densest portion of a Gram-stained specimen of cervical discharge correlates statistically with the presence of gonococci or chlamydiae [46,63,66–69], but the sensitivity and positive predictive value of the observation (both 25%–45% in a high risk population) are far too low for a definitive diagnosis.
   b. In the setting of MPC, a Gram stain diagnosis of gonorrhea mandates treatment for both gonococci and chlamydiae. A Gram stain negative for gonococci rules out the infection with a sensitivity of only 50%, and so such patients must still be treated for both gonococcal and nongonococcal cervicitis. **The cervical Gram stain has very limited utility in the management of MPC.**
2. **Culture and other tests**
   a. **Gonorrhea.** The standard method for detecting *N. gonorrhoeae* is culture (sensitivity approximately 90%). The organism can also be detected by DNA hybridization (sensitivity approximately 92%) and the ligase chain reaction (sensitivity approximately 97%) [70–72].
   b. ***C. trachomatis.*** Culture of the organism is an expensive and time-consuming procedure. Chlamydiae can be identified in cervical specimens using immunofluorescence microscopy (sensitivity 75%–95%), enzyme immunoassays (sensitivity 65%–95%), DNA probes (sensitivity 60%–80%), PCR (sensitivity approximately 88%) or ligase chain reaction (sensitivity approximately 93%) [15,73–75].
   c. **HSV.** The sensitivity of diagnostic tests is poorly defined, but all are relatively specific. The diagnosis may be made by observing multinucleate giant cells, often with intranuclear inclusions on Papanicolaou (Pap) smear; by recovering the virus in tissue culture; by immunofluorescent staining; or by PCR [76,77].

III. **Therapeutic approach**

A. Specifically diagnosed gonococcal or chlamydial cervicitis should be treated in the same manner as gonococcal and chlamydial urethritis.

B. Mucopurulent cervicitis in patients at risk for STD should be treated with a regimen that is effective against both *N. gonorrhoeae* and *C. trachomatis.* In a patient whose history suggests she is at very low risk for STD and in whom compliance is good, one could await the results of the screening tests.

C. **Female partners of men with NGU and male partners of women with MPC should be treated epidemiologically.**

D. **HSV.** Management of cervicitis due to HSV is identical to that of other genital herpes infections.

## PHARYNGEAL INFECTIONS AND SEXUALLY TRANSMITTED PHARYNGITIS

The oropharynx can be infected by *N. gonorrhoeae, C. trachomatis, Treponema pallidum,* HSV, or HPV.

I. **Gonococcal pharyngeal infection** [78]

A. **Epidemiology.** The major risk factor is fellatio. Cunnilingus is less likely to transmit infection, and transmission by kissing is very rare.

B. **Most infected patients are asymptomatic,** although erythematous and exudative gonococcal pharyngitis does occur.

C. The identity of *N. gonorrhoeae* on culture must be confirmed by biochemical or immunologic testing because *N. meningitidis,* will also grow on selective media and resembles gonococcus.

D. Workup for disseminated gonococcal infection should include pharyngeal cultures.

**E. Treatment**

1. Ceftriaxone, 125 to 250 mg i.m. as a single dose
2. Cefixime 400 mg orally as a single dose
3. For $\beta$-lactam–allergic patients in whom fluoroquinolones are not contraindicated: ciprofloxacin 500 mg, ofloxacin 400 mg, or levofloxacin 400 mg orally as a single dose

**II. Chlamydial pharyngeal infection**

A. *C. trachomatis* is occasionally isolated from the pharynx of the patient who practices fellatio [79].

B. Such infection is usually but not always asymptomatic.

C. Treat with those regimens effective for genital chlamydial infection.

**III. Pharyngeal herpetic infection** [30,50]

A. **Epidemiology.** In adults, this syndrome generally is associated with primary genital infection.

B. **Clinical features.** Patients usually are symptomatic, and one may see erythema or frank ulcers on the oropharynx. Fever and anterior cervical adenopathy are common.

C. **Treatment** is the same as for genital lesions.

D. Herpetic pharyngitis **may recur** and be particularly severe in immunocompromised patients, in whom extension to the esophagus is frequent.

## GENITAL LESIONS

I. **Significance.** Genital lesions present problems in differential diagnosis because of clinical overlaps in presentation. The issue is further complicated by the frequency with which different infections coexist. Ulcerative genital lesions probably predispose to the transmission of HIV infection by acting as the portal of exit or entry for the virus [2]. The morphology of genital lesions may be greatly modified in AIDS [2].

II. **Initial approach.** The initial approach to genital lesions in the sexually active patient involves taking a careful history, including the following information [80–82].

A. The **incubation period** can be assessed by inquiring about new or recent sexual contacts.

1. A very short incubation period of minutes to hours suggests trauma or an allergic reaction to a topical chemical used by a partner. Infectious diseases do not have such short incubation periods.
2. An incubation period of 2 to 5 days is seen with most cases of chancroid or HSV infection, although the mean incubation period for the latter is approximately 6 days [30,50,76,77].
3. Longer incubation periods of 1 to 3 weeks are seen with syphilis, 4 to 12 weeks with venereal warts, and approximately 4 weeks for pubic lice and scabies.
4. The incubation periods for some conditions such as molluscum contagiosum [83] and donovanosis [84] are poorly defined, but the latter may be 1 to 12 weeks.

B. A **travel history** influences the likelihood of various etiologies. Lymphogranuloma venereum is far more common in Africa and the Far East than in the United States. Donovanosis is endemic in India, New Guinea, the West Indies, and some parts of Africa and South America, but it is distinctly rare in the United States. Chancroid has become more common in the United States, particularly in major metropolitan areas.

C. **Pain** usually accompanies the lesions of herpes and chancroid. Although not classically painful, the lesions of primary syphilis cause some discomfort in up to 30% of patients [85]. Intense **pruritus** is characteristic of crabs and scabies.

D. A **history of STD in a partner** is an important clue to the differential diagnosis.

E. **Recurrence** at intervals is characteristic and highly suggestive of herpes.

F. The **morphologic features of the lesions** are key to the differential diagnosis.

G. **Recent use of antimicrobials** or other drugs may dramatically modify the morphology of lesions, and drugs may cause **fixed drug eruptions,** which are commonly limited to the genitals.

**III. Ulcerative lesions**

**A. General principles**

1. A clinical differential diagnosis of genital ulcers is the most challenging aspect of venereal dermatology [80–82].

2. Chancroid has become more common in the United States and must be considered in differential diagnosis [86].
3. Rare causes of genital ulceration include tuberculosis, amebiasis, and histoplasmosis.
4. Although the classic descriptions of lesions have high specificity, only about one-third of patients present with "classic" lesions [82].

**B. Genital herpes simplex infection**

1. **Epidemiologic considerations**
   a. Approximately 70% to 95% of genital herpes infections are caused by HSV type 2 [30]. Type 1 genital infections may result from orogenital sexual contact.
   b. Serologic studies suggest that 20% of young adults in the United States are infected with HSV type 2 [87,88].
   c. Initial infections are classified as **primary** if the patient has had no prior exposure to HSV (either type 1 or type 2); otherwise the episode is referred to as **nonprimary initial infection.** Patients with prior exposure to HSV have milder initial episodes than do those patients suffering true primary genital infection.
   d. **Approximately 70% to 90% of patients have asymptomatic initial and recurrent genital infections** [89–94]. Most infections appear to have been contracted from sexual partners who are asymptomatic shedders of virus. Because asymptomatic shedding only occurs about 3% to 7% of the time, an asymptomatically infected individual may transmit infection to a sexual partner only after years of regular contact.
   e. The rate of recurrence decreases over time [95].
   f. The rate of transmission of HSV type 2 from symptomatic to uninfected partners who have been advised not to have unprotected intercourse when the infected partner is symptomatic is approximately 10% per year [96].
2. **Clinical features. Because only about 20% of infected patients present with typical clinical features, standard clinical evaluation can never rule out genital herpes [91].**
   a. Lesions appear 2 to 20 days after exposure, but the mean incubation period is approximately 6 days. Classical lesions are initially **vesicular,** grouped, sometimes umbilicated, and surmount an erythematous base. Particularly in women, the vesicles quickly rupture to form clean, shallow, markedly painful **ulcers,** which are usually all about the same size and are not indurated. Ulcers may coalesce.
   b. Lesions are usually located on the penis or on the labia or vulva. The adult vagina is involved in only about 5% or so of cases and the cervix in nearly 90% of primary infections [30].
   c. Involvement of the urethra is common.
   d. **Regional lymphadenopathy,** usually tender, generally develops toward the end of the first week of illness.
   e. Lesions heal by **crusting** over. Primary disease often lasts 3 weeks.
   f. **Extragenital manifestations. Fever, malaise, and anorexia** are common in primary infection. A true **aseptic meningitis** without encephalitis accompanies some primary infections with HSV type 2. These manifestations are rare in recurrent disease [30].
   g. Within the first year after infection, **recurrent disease** is seen in approximately 90% of symptomatic patients with HSV type 2 genital infections but in only about 25% to 50% of those infected with HSV type 1 [94,95]. Recurrences with HSV type 2 appear four to eight times per year, whereas recurrences with HSV type 1 are, on average, nearly 10 times less frequent. The rate of recurrence varies dramatically from patient to patient. Many patients give a history of recurrences triggered by stress.
      (1) Recurrent disease may be preceded by a prodrome of itching, tingling, or burning that begins 6 to 24 hours before lesions appear [30].
      (2) Recurrences generally last 7 to 10 days and proceed through the same stages as primary disease.

3. **Direct diagnosis** can usually be made clinically in classic cases, but most cases are not classic.
   a. A **dark-field examination** may be performed **if syphilis is suspected.** Multiple chancres may be seen in almost half of patients with primary syphilis [85,97].
   b. The **Tzanck smear** is prepared by making a smear of a fresh **vesicular** lesion, which then is stained with Wright or Giemsa stain and examined for the presence of characteristic multinucleated giant cells. The sensitivity of the test is only 40% for ulcers, for which clinical differential diagnosis is more difficult [81,90].
   c. **HSV antigen detection tests,** such as direct immunofluorescence and ELISA, vary in sensitivity and specificity from about 70% to 90% [90,98].
   d. **Viral DNA** can be detected by PCR with 100% specificity and sensitivity, which is higher than any other direct technique [90,99,100].
   e. **Culture has been the gold standard for diagnosis,** but its sensitivity rapidly diminishes in recurrent disease, and it is often negative if taken from lesions that are just a few days old [91]. DNA amplification techniques are more sensitive.
4. **Serologic diagnosis** has been used in many epidemiologic studies but is of limited clinical utility.
   a. Older tests do not reliably differentiate between type 1 and type 2 virus. **Even with type-specific tests, many sexually active patients are HSV 1 antibody positive, and HSV 1 *genital* infection cannot be excluded in these patients.**
   b. An ELISA based on glycoprotein gG can differentiate between HSV types and is about 95% sensitive [101,102].
   c. A Western blot assay, also capable of differentiating among HSV types, is highly sensitive and specific but is available only from research centers [90].
   d. A new commercially available ELISA specific for HSV 2, the POCkit HSV-2 Rapid Test [103], can be performed in the clinic and becomes positive in 80% of infected patients after 4 weeks [104].
5. **Treatment. Oral antiherpetic agents** are the treatment of choice. Topical therapy is far less effective [13,105,106], and occlusive topical treatment increases the risk of maceration and delays healing. The lesions should be kept clean and dry. Valacyclovir is a prodrug of acyclovir and is therefore a more convenient but more expensive means of administration of acyclovir. Famciclovir is a prodrug of penciclovir. Various **clinically equivalent oral regimens** include the following:
   a. **Initial infection:** 7 to 10 days of oral therapy with one of the following: 400 mg acyclovir three times a day, 200 mg acyclovir five times daily, 250 mg famciclovir three times a day, or 1 g valacyclovir twice a day.
   b. **Recurrent episodes** may be treated with one of the following 5-day oral regimens: 400 mg acyclovir twice a day, 200 mg acyclovir five times per day, acyclovir 800 mg twice a day, famciclovir 125 mg twice a day, or valacyclovir 500 mg twice a day. **The effect on recurrent disease is substantially less than that observed with initial infection,** and its value depends on starting the drug early in the course of the relapse, preferably during the prodrome. In this setting, the patient should keep a supply of the drug at home so that therapy can be started immediately.
   c. **Frequently recurring disease** can be controlled with long-term **suppressive oral therapy** consisting of acyclovir 400 mg twice a day; famciclovir 250 mg twice a day; or valacyclovir 250 mg twice a day, 500 mg/day, or 1,000 mg/day [13,106–108]. After 1 year of continuous daily therapy, the drug should be discontinued and the frequency and severity of recurrences should be reassessed. Approximately 75% of patients will remain free of symptomatic recurrences. **Such suppressive therapy prevents symptomatic recurrences and reduces but does not eliminate viral shedding.** Patients should be warned that they may still be contagious.

6. **Special considerations**
   a. **Intravenous (i.v.) acyclovir** is used for serious infection, in immunocompromised patients, or when accompanying clinical problems make oral administration inadvisable. The drug is given as 5 to 10 mg/kg i.v. every 8 hours for 5 to 7 days or until clinical resolution occurs [13]. Adequate hydration reduces the risk of nephrotoxicity caused by tubular precipitation.
   b. **AIDS** patients suffer from chronic necrotizing herpetic infection, and infection may disseminate. Longer term, higher dose, or i.v. therapy may be required. Resistance has developed and should be suspected if lesions persist among patients undergoing acyclovir therapy. An alternative regimen for resistant infections is foscarnet, 40 mg/kg body weight i.v. every 8 hours until clinical resolution is obtained [13].
   c. **Pregnancy** poses problems for mother and baby, and **management remains controversial** [109]. The risk to the newborn is highest among women with their first episode of genital herpes near the time of delivery and is lower among women with recurrent herpes. The likelihood that a completely asymptomatic individual is shedding virus at the time of delivery is probably as low as 1%. Antepartum cultures are not useful, but women should be carefully examined for the presence of active lesions, which are considered by many to be an indication for cesarean section. The safety of acyclovir in pregnancy has not been completely defined, and its use should probably be restricted to treatment of initial genital herpes in this setting [13,106].

C. **Syphilis in the United States** is now at its lowest levels in the history of reporting [110].

1. **Microbiologic features.** *T. pallidum* is a spirochete 5 to 15 $\mu$m long and less than 0.5 $\mu$m wide. Living organisms are visualized by reflected light using **dark-field** microscopy. The organism can also be identified by silver staining or by direct immunofluorescence [111].
2. **Epidemiology**
   a. From 1986 to 1990, an epidemic of syphilis occurred in the United States. However, in 1991 the number of reported cases of primary and secondary syphilis declined for the first time since 1985 and has declined yearly since that time [112,113]. The reasons are uncertain but may include the use of ceftriaxone for treatment of gonorrhea, HIV prevention education with personal protection measures being followed (e.g., condom use), or HIV partner notification (which may allow for early therapy of new cases of contacts).
   b. Rates of infection remain highest in the rural South [114] and among lower socioeconomic inner-city populations. Several studies have found a strong epidemiologic association between syphilis and crack cocaine use, probably due to crack cocaine–associated changes in sexual behavior, such as sex-for-drugs prostitution [115–117].
   c. After an initial drop, syphilis has reappeared among some groups of gay men [118].
   d. Sexual transmission occurs by direct contact with a moist lesion, and transplacental transmission is the second major route of acquisition. Transfusion syphilis is no longer a problem.
3. **Clinical manifestations.** Syphilis is a chronic infection, usually latent, the course of which is punctuated by clinically apparent stages.
   a. The **incubation period** averages approximately 3 weeks but is said to range from 10 to 90 days. During this interval, infected patients have, by definition, neither clinical nor serologic evidence of disease.
   b. **Primary syphilis** consists of one or more **ulcerated lesions, called *chancres,*** which appear at the site of initial infection and multiplication by the spirochetes [85]. There are multiple lesions in many cases. Chancres usually are minimally painful or tender (compared, most dramatically, with chancroid or herpes, both of which produce tender ulcers) and are usually clean ulcerations with distinctly indurated edges. Regional **adenopathy** develops within the first week and usually consists of several discrete nodes that are relatively nontender and rubbery. Inguinal adenopathy generally is bilateral. The

cervix, proximal third of the vagina, and the glans penis are drained by deep iliac nodes, and regional lymphadenopathy is not detected on physical examination of patients infected at these sites. Although most chancres occur on the genitalia, the examiner must maintain a high index of suspicion for lesions about the mouth or anus as well. Untreated, the manifestations of primary syphilis usually resolve in 3 to 6 weeks. **Nontreponemal serologic tests for syphilis are positive in only approximately 50% of patients at the time the chancre first appears.** A nonreactive test does not rule out syphilis in such patients.

c. **Secondary syphilis.** *T. pallidum* disseminates throughout the body even before the appearance of the chancre. Approximately 3 to 6 weeks after the appearance of the chancre (indeed, often after its resolution) this dissemination manifests as a generalized rash, commonly involving the palms and soles and almost always involving the oral mucous membranes and the genitalia. The rash is highly variable, and differential diagnosis is often challenging [119,120]. **The rash generally is maculopapular, bilaterally symmetric,** and nonpruritic or minimally pruritic and is described classically as having a "sinister" coppery or boiled-ham color [121]. It may, however, be papular or, rarely, papulopustular. The rash may resemble pityriasis rosea. The dry lesions of secondary syphilis are not contagious, because they contain very few organisms. Arguing against secondary syphilis in the adult is sparing of the mouth and genitalia, a markedly pruritic eruption, or bullous lesions [121].

(1) Secondary syphilis generally begins with a nonspecific constitutional illness that commonly includes a sore throat and myalgias.
(2) Patchy alopecia is frequent.
(3) Generalized lymphadenopathy is observed in approximately 75% of patients.
(4) *Condylomata lata* are hypertrophic lesions, resembling flat warts, that occur in moist areas (e.g., around the anus) and are highly contagious.
(5) Painless shallow ulcers of the mucous membranes—**mucous patches—are highly contagious.**
(6) **Serologic tests are almost always reactive in secondary syphilis,** usually in high titer. Therefore, a negative test can be used to rule out secondary syphilis. Rarely, patients have such high levels of antibody that the nontreponemal tests are falsely negative, a so-called **prozone phenomenon.** One can avoid this by performing quantitative nontreponemal tests, in which serial dilutions of serum are examined.
(7) The manifestations of secondary syphilis resolve without treatment.
(8) Nearly 25% of patients will again develop the manifestations of secondary syphilis, termed **mucocutaneous relapse,** during the first year of infection. Such patients are again contagious to sexual partners.

d. **Latent syphilis** is clinically silent, and diagnosis can be made only on the basis of serologic tests.

e. **Late (tertiary) syphilis** eventually develops in approximately one-third of infected patients. A discussion of late syphilis is beyond the scope of this chapter, but good descriptions are available elsewhere [122]. Briefly, tertiary syphilis should be suspected in the following clinical settings:

(1) **Lymphocytic meningitis** may be a manifestation of secondary syphilis or may appear somewhat later as **meningovascular syphilis.** A cerebrovascular accident without other cause in a young person should raise suspicion. See further related discussions in Chapter 6.
(2) **Destructive lesions of skin and bones** may represent so-called **late benign syphilis.**
(3) **Dementia** may be due to **general paresis.**
(4) **Posterior column disease** may result from **tabes dorsalis.** Stabbing (lightning) pains are suggestive.
(5) Disease of the **aorta or incompetence of the aortic valve** for which other etiologies are not documented may represent **cardiovascular syphilis.**

(6) The diagnosis of late syphilis is confounded by the lack of sensitivity of the nontreponemal tests in these conditions. **A nonreactive nontreponemal test should be confirmed with a treponemal test in the workup of patients with suspected late syphilis.**

f. Approximately one-third of patients will remain seroreactive but will not develop late manifestations of syphilis. Nearly one-third remain well and become nonreactive on nontreponemal testing.

4. **Diagnosis of syphilis is undergoing a true revolution, as newer molecular techniques are applied.**

a. Syphilis can be diagnosed by identifying *T. pallidum* in lesions. The traditional method is the **dark-field examination** in which material from a lesion is examined using a microscope that sends light rays obliquely through the specimen, illuminating the organism by reflected light against a dark background. Obtaining the specimen and interpreting the test require experience and are more difficult in areas such as the mouth, where other spirochetes may be part of the normal flora. **Direct immunofluorescence** has the same sensitivity, but specimens may be sent to a central laboratory [123]. Silver staining is less sensitive and specific. PCR methods are far more sensitive and are available in a research setting [124,125]. Because syphilis is subclinical for much of its course, we have come to rely heavily on **serologic diagnosis. Potential pitfalls in serodiagnosis must be recognized** [123,124, 126].

b. **Nontreponemal tests. Screening tests for syphilis** exploit the observation that patients with syphilis develop IgG antibodies, traditionally termed **reagin,** reactive with a variety of poorly defined lipids. Classical tests include the **VDRL** (Venereal Disease Research Laboratory), **RPR** (rapid plasma reagin), **ART** (automated reagin test), and **TRUST** (toluidine red unheated serologic test), among others. An ELISA for antiphospholipid antibody, the Spirotek Reagin II, is about 95% sensitive in early syphilis [127].

(1) **Nontreponemal tests are nonspecific,** reacting in a variety of acute and chronic conditions such as acute viral illnesses, collagen vascular disease, pregnancy, i.v. drug use, old age, and leprosy. A nontreponemal test is diagnostic in the setting of a highly suggestive clinical syndrome (e.g., chancre) but cannot be used to diagnose latent syphilis without confirmation by a treponemal test.

(2) The tests **often are quantitated** and reported as the highest twofold dilution of serum eliciting a positive reaction. Titers of 1:8 or higher are unusual among false positives. The highest titers (1:128) may be seen in secondary syphilis.

(3) The tests are **relatively insensitive in primary** (except for the ELISA) **and late syphilis,** and here it may be prudent to order a treponemal test even when the nontreponemal test is nonreactive.

(4) **The titer of the test diminishes after adequate treatment of syphilis. A fourfold drop in titer is considered evidence of adequate treatment** [127–130] and should occur within 3 months of treatment of early syphilis and within 6 months of treatment of latent syphilis.

(5) **After treatment, one should follow serologic tests at 3 and 6 months and then every 6 months thereafter until titers stabilize or disappear.**

(6) The RPR converts to nonreactive within 2 years in only 72% or so of patients treated for primary syphilis and approximately 56% of patients treated for secondary syphilis [129]. The VDRL is more likely to revert to nonreactive after treatment.

(7) The failure of the nontreponemal test titer to drop fourfold requires careful follow-up but is not associated with clinical relapse within 12 months [130].

(8) A subsequent reappearance or fourfold rise in titer of nontreponemal tests is considered evidence of relapse or reinfection.

(9) **It is essential that the same nontreponemal tests are used in follow-up as were used for the original testing, because the RPR**

**can yield two- to eightfold higher titers on the same specimen than does the VDRL. Switching between tests invites confusion.**

c. **Treponemal tests.** Confirmatory tests for syphilis use *T. pallidum,* or fractions thereof, as antigen. The treponemal tests are **more specific and more sensitive** than the nontreponemal tests, **particularly in very early primary and late syphilis.** They are not quantitated but are reported as reactive or nonreactive.
   (1) The fluorescent treponemal antibody absorption test has been regarded as the most sensitive test for syphilis, but it is less sensitive than the newer DNA-based tests.
   (2) The microhemagglutination test for *T. pallidum* has been superseded by tests using particulate gelatin or latex, such as the **Serodia TP-PA** and the **PK-TP,** which are suitable as screening tests and now used extensively by blood banks [124,131–134]. They are not subject to misreading due to heterophile antibodies and are about 97% specific.
   (3) Several **treponemal ELISA tests** are now available, the most commonly used being the **Captia syphilis G test,** [132,134], which is 98% sensitive and about 100% specific. Several ELISA tests use cloned *T. pallidum* antigens and have high sensitivity and specificity [135–137].
   (4) **Western blot tests** have very high specificity and may be used in problem cases [124,138].
   (5) **Treponemal tests may be used to confirm a diagnosis of past or present treponemal infection in patients with reactive nontreponemal tests.**
   (6) **The treponemal tests remain positive for extended periods, probably for life, even after adequate treatment of syphilis in most (but not all) patients. A persistently reactive treponemal test does not indicate inadequate treatment, relapse, or reinfection [119].**
   (7) Although they are highly specific, **the treponemal tests are reactive in other treponemal diseases** (e.g., yaws, pinta, bejel) and **in some other spirochetal diseases (e.g., Lyme disease)** [139].

5. **Treatment. Penicillin remains the drug of choice for all stages of syphilis,** unless the patient is hypersensitive [13,140,141]. **All patients being treated for syphilis should be strongly advised to undergo testing for HIV antibody.**
   a. **Contact to syphilis** (epidemiologic treatment, incubating syphilis). Infection is present in 25% to 50% of the sexual partners of patients with syphilitic lesions. Syphilis may take up to 90 days to become clinically or serologically manifest. Thus, **all patients presenting as contacts to syphilis within the past 90 days (the so-called critical period) are treated with a regimen effective for early syphilis.** Patients whose exposure was more than 90 days previously may be evaluated serologically to determine whether they need treatment.
   b. **Early syphilis** (primary, secondary, and latent syphilis of <1 year's duration)
      (1) **Recommended:** benzathine penicillin G, 2.4 million units i.m., in one treatment.
      (2) **In penicillin allergy:** doxycycline, 100 mg orally twice a day for 2 weeks, **or** tetracycline, 500 mg orally four times a day for 2 weeks.
      (3) **The pregnant woman with severe penicillin allergy** ideally should be desensitized to penicillin so she can receive penicillin, because tetracyclines are contraindicated in pregnancy and erythromycin should not be used because it cannot be relied on to cure an infected fetus (see Chapter 24).
      (4) Ceftriaxone may be a suitable alternative in patients whose allergy to penicillin is not manifested by anaphylaxis [140,141]. It is not advised in pregnancy [13].

**c. Latent syphilis of unknown duration or of more than 1 year's duration, late benign syphilis, or cardiovascular syphilis**

**(1) Recommended:** benzathine penicillin G, 7.2 million units total, administered as three doses of 2.4 million units i.m., given 1 week apart for 3 consecutive weeks.

(2) Alternatively **for penicillin-allergic nonpregnant patients:** doxycycline, 100 mg orally twice a day for 4 weeks, or tetracycline, 500 mg orally four times a day for 4 weeks.

(3) Management of the **penicillin-allergic pregnant woman** is uncertain and should probably involve desensitization to penicillin.

**(4) Examination of cerebrospinal fluid is recommended in the following situations** [141]:

**(a)** Neurologic signs or symptoms;

**(b)** Treatment failure;

**(c)** Other evidence of active syphilis (e.g., aortitis, gumma, iritis);

**(d)** Nonpenicillin therapy planned;

**(e)** Concurrent HIV infection.

**d. Neurosyphilis** (see related discussion in Chapter 6)

**(1) Recommended:** aqueous crystalline penicillin G, 12 to 24 million units/day i.v. for 10 to 14 days, administered 2 to 4 million units every 4 hours or by continuous drip. In the HIV-positive patient, neurosyphilis may be particularly difficult to treat, and failures of therapy can occur despite optimal therapy with high dose i.v. aqueous penicillin [141–143].

(2) Alternatively, procaine penicillin G, 2.4 million units/day i.m., and probenecid, 500 mg orally four times a day, both for 10 to 14 days.

(3) An alternative for which data are limited: ceftriaxone, 1 g/day i.m. for 14 days [143]. This might be used in patients whose allergy to penicillin is not manifested by anaphylaxis.

**(4) It is believed by many workers that the benzathine penicillin G regimen formerly recommended for neurosyphilis is inadequate.** Because the currently recommended regimen is shorter than that recommended for late syphilis in the absence of neurosyphilis, **some experts administer one or more doses of benzathine penicillin, 2.4 million units i.m., after completion of regimen (1) or (2) [13].**

**e. The Jarisch-Herxheimer reaction** occurs 1 to 6 hours **after beginning treatment for syphilis** and is seen in approximately 50% of patients with primary syphilis and in most patients with secondary syphilis. It manifests as fever, increased rash, adenopathy, and sometimes hypotension. The mechanism is not fully defined, but it probably results from the release of treponemal antigens on lysis of the organisms. The Jarisch-Herxheimer reaction is self-limited and usually requires only treatment with antipyretics, but patients should be warned of the likelihood of its occurrence.

**f. Serologic follow-up** (see section 4.b)

**g. Syphilis in pregnancy** should be managed according to the maternal stage of syphilis. Monthly serologic follow-up is required to ensure that treatment has been effective and reinfection has not occurred. The tetracyclines are to be avoided in pregnancy [144].

**h.** The effect of **HIV infection** on the clinical course of syphilis is incompletely defined. Such patients may present with multiple and persistent chancres [2,145]. It is unclear whether HIV infection affects the serologic manifestations, the natural history, or the response to therapy in patients coinfected with *T. pallidum* [146,147]. However, many clinicians remain particularly **concerned about reports suggesting that neurosyphilis may occur more rapidly in patients with HIV** [148,149]. **Some experts recommend that cerebrospinal fluid examination be performed on all HIV-infected patients with syphilis,** regardless of clinical stage.

**D. Chancroid** is an infection with the gram-negative rod *Hemophilus ducreyi.* The incidence of chancroid has increased in the United States, and small epidemics have occurred, usually associated with prostitutes [150–152]. Chancroid is a major public health problem in the developing world, and its significance is compounded by its striking **association with HIV infection** [2,153]. **Patients should be tested for HIV at the time of diagnosis.**

1. **Clinical manifestations** [82,151,152,154]
   - **a.** The incubation period is 4 to 7 days.
   - **b.** Presents as painful ragged ulcers on the genitalia. The ulcers often are dirty or appear necrotic, are not indurated, and may vary in size. So-called **kissing lesions** of the thighs may occur by autoinoculation. Painful inguinal adenopathy occurs in more than 50% of patients, and the nodes may become fluctuant and rupture. Occasionally, one sees superinfection with mixed anaerobic organisms.
2. **Diagnosis.** The major differential diagnoses are herpes simplex genital infection and syphilis. Clinical differential diagnosis is notoriously unreliable [81,82,154].
   - **a. Dark-field examination helps to rule out syphilis.** Serology is less helpful because the diseases may coexist, and nontreponemal tests are insensitive early in primary syphilis.
   - **b. Gram staining of the lesions** may reveal chains of gram-negative streptobacilli, but the technique is insensitive and nonspecific and **is not recommended** [155].
   - **c. Culture** of the organism is definitive but difficult [155,156] and, at best, is only 80% sensitive.
   - **d. Newer tests** under development include **PCR** (sensitivity approximately 90%) and **antigen detection** (sensitivity approximately 90%) and will become the tests of choice [155–157]. Multiplex PCR can be used to diagnose simultaneous infections, which are not rare.
3. **Treatment** [158] is complicated by recent development of resistance to traditional agents.
   - **a.** Uniformly effective in the United States are (a) ciprofloxacin, 500 mg orally twice a day for 3 days; (b) ceftriaxone, 250 mg i.m. as a single dose; (c) erythromycin, 500 mg orally four times a day for 7 days; and (d) azithromycin, 1 g orally as a single dose. Trimethoprim-sulfamethoxazole should not be used [159].
   - **b.** Cure rates in other parts of the world, such as Africa, may be somewhat lower [160], and single-dose thiamphenicol, 5 g orally, appears to remain effective in South America.
   - **c.** Patients coinfected with HIV may require longer courses of therapy [2].

**E. Donovanosis (granuloma inguinale)** is **very rare in the United States,** although it is far more common in other parts of the world, including India and Latin America. Caused by an intracellular gram-negative rod, *Calymmatobacterium granulomatis,* which is related to *Klebsiella,* it manifests as **painless destructive ulcers** characterized by exuberant tissue formation and healing with scarring. Diagnosis is made by biopsy of involved tissue. Treatment with azithromycin 1 g orally weekly appears effective [161] and may replace older regimens [13,162].

## IV. Papular lesions

**A. Pearly penile papules** are regular white papules that form in one to five rows on the penile corona or in the coronal sulcus. They have no pathologic significance but sometimes precipitate a consultation.

**B. Molluscum contagiosum** is seen frequently in children, among whom it is spread by nonvenereal contact. After 2 to 8 weeks, infected adults usually develop 1- to 5-mm lesions around the genitalia, thighs, and buttocks. The infection is caused by a poxvirus that has not been cultured. The **painless papules** are easily identified clinically by their **central umbilications.** Treatment is by curettage, cryotherapy, or laser ablation. Patients should be warned to avoid squeezing the lesions and touching other areas of the body, which presents the risk of autoinoculation. Disseminated cutaneous disease, seen in AIDS [163], must be differentiated from disseminated cryptococcosis and may be treated with cidofovir [164].

**C. Venereal warts (condylomata acuminata)**

1. **Etiology.** Warts are **caused by HPV,** double-stranded DNA viruses that have not been cultured. Nearly 90 types have been identified. Types 6 and 11 cause benign genital warts, but **types 16, 18, 31, 33, and 35, among others, cause cervical cancer** [51–55]. Gestational HPV infection is associated with laryngeal lesions in vaginally delivered offspring.
2. **Natural history. Cervical HPV is self-limited in women with normal immune systems, with a median duration of about 8 to 10 months** [56–60]. Premalignant lesions often develop within 1 to 2 years of infection [54] and invasive carcinoma of the cervix within about 10 years [2].
3. **Clinical features.** The incubation period probably is approximately 4 to 6 weeks. Lesions are soft papules with irregular verrucous surfaces. They are usually located around the external genitalia or inside the urethra or vagina and on the cervix. Perianal warts in women may result from spread from a primary genital focus, but perianal warts in men strongly suggest receptive anal intercourse. Daughter lesions appear near older lesions. **Subclinical infection** is extremely important, with most infected patients having papillomavirus DNA identified in normal epithelium near visible lesions.
4. **Diagnosis of overt external lesions usually is made clinically. Warts in other locations,** including flat warts of the cervix, may require **biopsy,** which reveals characteristic koilocytosis, clear zones around the nuclei of infected cells. Subclinical infections may be suspected by swabbing the vagina, cervix, or penis [165] with 3% to 5% **acetic acid,** which turns infected areas white. This test is nonspecific and requires histologic confirmation. **DNA hybridization** kits are now commercially available and can supplement or replace standard cervical cytology [166,167].
5. **Treatment** is largely unsatisfactory and generally **controversial.** The benefit of treating subclinical infection has not been demonstrated [13]. Thus, the goal of therapy is the elimination of overt warts.
   a. **Cryotherapy** with liquid nitrogen or cryoprobe is **preferred** because of its lack of toxicity, its usefulness in pregnancy, and its destruction of warts with a single treatment.
   b. **Podofilox 0.5% solution** is applied by the patient twice daily for 3 days followed by a 4-day rest interval. The cycle may be repeated up to four times. The response rate is essentially identical to that with podophyllin, but podofilox is much more expensive [168].
   c. **Trichloroacetic acid, 80% to 90%,** can be applied carefully to warts, followed by an application of sodium bicarbonate. Treatment can be repeated at weekly intervals. This regimen is safe in pregnancy.
   d. **Podophyllin, 10% to 25% in tincture of benzoin,** is widely used. It is applied directly to the warts at weekly intervals and washed off after about 6 hours. **Absorption occurs, and so the regimen is contraindicated in pregnancy.**
   e. **Imiquimod 5% cream (Aldara),** an immunostimulator, can be applied by the patient three times weekly. The response rate is the same as with podophyllin, but it is far more costly [169].
   f. **Intralesional interferon** has been used to treat warts [170], but the technique is expensive and time consuming and is inapplicable to patients with many warts.
   g. The **relapse rate** with the treatments listed in this section approaches 75%.
   h. The cervix should not be treated before cytologic studies have ruled out malignancy.

**V. Pustular lesions (disseminated gonococcal infection).** Dissemination is reported to occur in approximately 1% to 3% of patients infected with gonococci and manifests most commonly as a rash and arthritis or tenosynovitis [171,172].

**A. Epidemiology**

1. **Deficiency in the terminal components of complement,** most frequently of C8, predisposes to disseminated gonococcal infection and disseminated meningococcal infection.

2. The organism resists killing by serum [171–173].

**B. Clinical features** [171,172)

1. Bacteremia usually manifests as **fever,** accompanied by **pustular or hemorrhagic skin lesions,** usually distributed primarily **on the distal portions of the extremities.**
   - **a.** The classic lesion is a tiny pustule, sometimes with a central eschar, surmounting a hemorrhagic base.
   - **b.** Vesicular lesions sometimes are observed.
   - **c.** Although most patients have few lesions, some have hundreds [173].
   - **d. Differential diagnosis** includes meningococcemia [173], staphylococcal endocarditis, Rocky Mountain spotted fever, or dengue.
2. **Arthritis**
   - **a.** Most patients, particularly early in their course, will have a **polyarthritis,** often accompanied by prominent tenosynovitis. Effusion usually is absent. Skin lesions are common and may continue to form.
   - **b.** Some patients present with one or very few joints manifesting effusion, a septic joint picture. Skin lesions are no longer forming at this stage.
   - **c.** Differential diagnosis includes septic arthritis of other etiologies. One must consider **Reiter syndrome,** which consists of urethritis, arthritis (usually asymmetric), dermatitis, and conjunctivitis.

**C. Diagnosis** is initially made clinically.

1. **Cultures for *N. gonorrhoeae* should be obtained for all sites used for sexual contact** (urethra, anorectum, cervix, pharynx) even if asymptomatic.
2. **Blood cultures** are positive in only approximately 40% of patients.
3. **Joint effusions should be cultured** but will be positive in only approximately 20% of cases.
4. Skin lesions are rarely positive by culture or by Gram stain. Direct fluorescent antibody staining may be useful.
5. In many patients, all cultures are negative, and diagnosis depends on clinical impression and response to therapy.

**D. Treatment** must take into account new patterns of gonococcal resistance [13].

1. **Initial therapy** should consist of **any of the following:**
   - **a.** Ceftriaxone, 1 g i.m. or i.v. every 24 hours.
   - **b.** Ceftizoxime, 1 g i.v. every 8 hours.
   - **c.** Cefotaxime, 1 g i.v. every 8 hours.
   - **d.** In $\beta$-lactam allergy, use ciprofloxacin, 500 mg orally or i.v. every 2 hours or an equivalent newer fluoroquinolone.
2. **Intravenous therapy may be discontinued 24 to 48 hours after symptoms resolve, and 1 week of total therapy may be completed with:**
   - **a.** Cefixime, 400 mg orally twice a day, or
   - **b.** Ciprofloxacin, 500 mg orally twice a day **(contraindicated in pregnancy and in children younger than 16 years).**
3. **Special considerations**
   - **a. Sexual partners** must be evaluated and treated, even if asymptomatic.
   - **b.** Patients with disseminated gonococcal infection should also be treated for chlamydial infection.
   - **c. Meningitis** or **endocarditis** rarely complicates this infection. These conditions require longer duration treatment [13,171,172].

**VI. Ectoparasites.** Infected patients should be evaluated for other STDs. Sexual partners should be treated.

**A. Pubic (crab) lice** (*Phthirus pubis*) infestation is markedly pruritic and has an incubation period of approximately 4 weeks [174,175). Signs include observation of the **lice,** 1- to 2-mm-long gray-brown organisms; **nits,** 0.5-mm brown or white ovoids attached to the hair shafts; **excreta,** tiny red dots on the skin among the hair; or rarely, **maculae ceruleae,** blue-gray macules [176]. Infestation may include the pubic and perianal, abdominal, chest, axillary, and superciliary hair.

1. Various **treatment regimens** are equally effective [13,175,177,178).
   - **a.** Permethrin (e.g., Nix) 1% creme rinse, applied to affected areas and washed off after 10 minutes.

**b.** Pyrethrins and piperonyl butoxide (e.g., RID) applied to affected areas and washed off after 10 minutes.

**c.** Lindane ($\gamma$-benzene hexachloride) (e.g., Kwell) 1% shampoo applied for 4 minutes and then washed off.

**2. Additional measures.** Clothing or bed linen contaminated within the past 48 hours should be washed before reuse. The eyelids should be carefully examined.

**3. Follow-up.** Patients should be reevaluated after 1 week if they remain symptomatic. The presence of **any lice** or the presence of **nits at the base of the hair shafts is an indication for retreatment.**

**B. Scabies** is caused by infestation with the itch mite, *Sarcoptes scabiei* [175]. After an incubation period of approximately 4 weeks, most patients develop severe pruritus of the infected areas, usually worse at night or after bathing.

**1. Diagnosis** is confirmed by **demonstrating the mite** in unexcoriated papules or burrows. The mites often are difficult to demonstrate. The female adult has a rounded body with four pairs of legs and is less than 0.5 mm long.

**a.** A hand lens is used to identify suspicious lesions. The classic linear burrows, occurring most frequently in the interdigital spaces and on the penis, are the best sites from which to take the scrapings.

**b.** With a needle or a scalpel blade, a superficial epidermal shave biopsy is performed.

**c.** The specimen is suspended in immersion oil and covered with a glass coverslip.

**d.** The mite or its products will, one hopes, be visible under the high dry lens of a light microscope.

**2. Treatment for adults**

**a. Recommended** [13,175,177–180]. **Permethrin 5% cream** applied to all areas of the body below the chin and washed off after 8 to 14 hours; **or**

**b. Lindane ($\gamma$-benzene hexachloride) 1% lotion or cream** applied to all areas of the body below the chin and washed off after 8 hours. **Application must be complete, including the interdigital spaces. Patients should be cautioned not to wash their hands after applying the medication.** Avoid in pregnant or lactating women, people with dermatitis, or in children under the age of 2.

**c. Alternatively,** one can use **crotamiton** 10%, applied to all areas of the body below the chin for two successive nights and washed off thoroughly 24 hours after the second application. This regimen appears less effective than those above [181].

**d. Ivermectin** as a single oral dose of 200 $\mu$g/kg has been used successfully in patients with standard and severe crusted scabies [182–184]. The drug has been used topically in a small number of cases [185].

**3. Additional measures**

**a.** Clothing or bed linens contaminated within the previous 48 hours should be washed before reuse.

**b.** Sexual and close household contacts should be treated.

**4. Follow-up.** Pruritus may persist for several weeks after adequate treatment. A single retreatment may be indicated if pruritus is not *improved* after 1 week.

**5. HIV-infected patients,** especially those with advanced HIV disease, may present with **atypical and severe forms** of scabies that may not respond to first-line agents [186,187]. Management may include repeated applications and should be done in consultation with a dermatologist.

## VULVOVAGINITIS

Vulvovaginitis is a common clinical syndrome and is diagnosed in more than one-fourth of women attending STD clinics (Table 16.1) [188].

**I. Differential diagnosis of vulvovaginitis**

**A. Candidiasis**

**1. Epidemiology**

Table 16.1. Typical Features of Common Vaginal Infections

| | Trichomoniasis | Candidiasis | Bacterial Vaginosis |
|---|---|---|---|
| Epidemiology | | | |
| Sexual transmission | Yes | Very rarely, if ever | Often but not always |
| Symptoms | | | |
| Relation to menses | Often postmenstrual | Often premenstrual | None |
| Vulvar irritation | Mild to marked | Mild to marked | Absent to mild |
| Dysuria | Internal and external | External | Absent |
| Odor | Sometimes | Absent | Fishy, aminelike |
| Signs | | | |
| Labial erythema | Variable | Variable | No |
| Satellite lesions | No | Yes | No |
| Vaginal tenderness | Yes | Yes | No |
| Rugal hypertrophy | Yes | Sometimes | No |
| Adnexal tenderness | Occasionally | No | No |
| Discharge | | | |
| Consistency | Frothy 25% | Sometimes curdy | Homogeneous, frothy |
| Color | Yellow-green (25%) | White | Gray, white |
| Adherent to vaginal walls | No | Yes | Yes |
| PH | Usually ≥4.7 | ≤4.5 | ≥4.7 |
| Microscopy | | | |
| Epithelial cells | Normal | Normal | Studded with coccobacilli (clue cells) |
| Polymorphonuclear neutrophils | Usually increased | Variable | Not increased |
| Bacteria | Gram-positive rods | Gram-positive rods | Gram-variable coccobacilli |
| Pathogens | Trichomonads (70%) | Yeasts or pseudohyphae (50%) | Coccobacilli and short motile rods |

**a.** Vulvovaginal candidiasis (VC) accounts for approximately one-third of the vaginitis cases seen in private practice. It is estimated that 75% of adult women suffer at least one episode of VC during their lifetimes [189].

**b.** ***Candida albicans*** is isolated from nearly 80% to 90% of cases of VC, but infection due to other species (*C. glabrata* approximately 10%, *C. tropicalis* approximately 1%–5%) is apparently increasing and is associated with higher failure and relapse rates [190–193].

**c.** Inhibition of normal bacterial flora by **broad-spectrum antibiotics** favors the growth of yeasts and predisposes to the development of VC.

**d.** **Overgrowth of yeast is favored by high estrogen levels** [194]. This may explain the observation that VC is more common in **pregnancy.** Some nonpregnant women note recurrent or increasing symptoms **preceding each menstrual period.** The prevalence of vaginal carriage of *Candida* is higher among women using **oral contraceptives** compared with those using other methods of birth control [195].

**e.** There is some evidence that tight, insulating clothing predisposes to VCiasis by increasing vulvar warmth and moisture [196].

**f.** **Patients with AIDS** often experience severe and recalcitrant disease [2,197].

**2. Clinical features**

**a. Symptoms.** Patients generally complain of **perivaginal pruritus,** often with little or no discharge. Dysuria, if noted, is likely to be vulvar rather than urethral.

**b. Physical findings.** The labia may be pale, erythematous, or excoriated. **Shallow linear fissures,** especially on the posterior portion of the introitus, are common. Tiny **satellite papules** or papulopustules just beyond the main area of erythema are helpful diagnostically. The vaginal walls may be erythematous. Candidal discharge may be thick, adherent, and curdy or thin and loose.

**3. Diagnosis**

**a.** A **wet mount** to which 10% to 20% KOH is added will reveal fungi in 50% to 70% of infected women. If negative, a presumptive diagnosis must be made on the basis of clinical features, pH, "whiff test," and microscopy negative for other pathogens.

**b.** The **vaginal pH** generally is **normal** (approximately 4.5) in women with VC, in contrast to trichomoniasis and bacterial vaginosis (BV), in which it is characteristically elevated.

**c.** The **whiff test** (see section II.B.2.b) is characteristically **negative** in VC.

**d.** The discharge usually contains relatively few PMNs.

**e.** A commercially available latex agglutination test has a limited sensitivity of approximately 60% [198].

**B. Trichomoniasis.** *Trichomonas vaginalis* is an anaerobic, flagellated, motile protozoan, approximately the size of a polymorphonuclear leukocyte.

**1. Epidemiology**

**a.** An estimated 3 million American women contract trichomoniasis every year. Its incidence has declined, possibly because of the widespread use of metronidazole for BV, but it remains common in populations at risk for other STD [199–201].

**b.** Trichomoniasis is only rarely acquired nonvenereally. Sexual partners should be treated and infected patients should be evaluated for other STD [201].

**2. Clinical features**

**a. History.** The incubation period in women is 5 to 28 days [202]. Infected women usually note **vaginal discharge and vulvovaginal soreness or irritation. Dysuria** and **dyspareunia** are common. Although up to two-thirds of infected women complain of a disagreeable **odor,** this symptom may actually be more suggestive of BV. Symptoms often begin or exacerbate during the menstrual period. **Abdominal discomfort** is described by only 5% to 12% of infected women and should prompt careful evaluation for a second process, such as pelvic inflammatory disease (PID). Approximately 10% to 50% of infected women attending STD clinics carry the organism asymptomatically.

Most men infected with *T. vaginalis* are asymptomatic [29].

**b. Physical findings**

**(1)** Examination usually reveals a copious rather loose **discharge** pooling in the posterior vaginal fornix, often yellow or green. Bubbles are observed in 10% to 33% of cases, and as many as half have a relatively thick discharge that may be confused with VC.

**(2)** There is usually **inflammation of the vaginal walls** and the exocervix. Punctate hemorrhages (colpitis macularis), including the so-called **strawberry cervix,** are observed colposcopically in 45% of infected women but in only 2% by visual inspection alone [202].

**(3)** Vaginal discharge from 90% of women with trichomoniasis has a **pH level elevated above the normal value of 4.5.**

**c. Diagnosis.** The accurate diagnosis of trichomoniasis depends on **demonstrating the organism** in genital specimens.

**(1) Trichomonads may be identified** in vaginal secretions using the **wet-mount** technique, which will detect their **characteristic movements** in nearly 60% of infected women [203]. The wet mount generally also reveals large numbers of **white blood cells,** although asymptomatic women may have very few.

(2) Direct fluorescent antibody staining [203], latex agglutination [204], and ELISA techniques [205] are more sensitive than a wet mount (80%–90%) but less sensitive than culture. More sensitive, however, are newly developed DNA probes [206] and PCR [207,208] that are becoming available.

(3) **Culture remains the most sensitive technique,** and commercially available kits have increased the ease with which the organism can be cultured [209].

(4) **Serologic testing has no current role in the evaluation of the individual patient.**

(5) The Pap smear is specific but insensitive.

**C. BV is the most common vaginal infection in the United States.** Seen primarily in sexually active women, it is characterized by a **nonirritating malodorous vaginal discharge.** Though previously called *nonspecific vaginitis* and originally attributed to infection with *Gardnerella vaginalis,* there is now considerable evidence that BV is actually a **synergistic infection** involving not only *G. vaginalis* but also certain anaerobic bacteria [210,211]. Loss of hydrogen peroxide-producing lactobacilli, possibly through the action of a recently described bacteriophage [212], probably sets the stage for this infection [210,211].

**1. Epidemiology**

**a.** BV is common in populations with a high prevalence of STDs. **The precise contribution of sexual transmission to the overall epidemiology of the condition remains controversial.**

**b.** Recurrence in the absence of sexual reexposure is well described. **It is not demonstrably necessary to treat male sexual partners** initially, but some women with frequent recurrences will benefit if sexual partners are treated well [213].

**2. Clinical features**

**a. History.** Affected women usually are sexually active and often **complain predominantly of vaginal odor.** Approximately 90% of patients also notice a **mild to moderate discharge.** If present, inflammation and perivaginal irritation are mild. Dysuria and dyspareunia are rare. Abdominal discomfort, if present, is usually mild and should prompt evaluation for coincident infections including salpingitis.

**b. Physical findings. Discharge** often is present at the introitus and is visible on the labia minora. The labia and vulva generally are not erythematous or edematous. On speculum examination, the vaginal walls are uninflamed. The vagina often contains a grayish-white, thin, homogeneous discharge manifesting **small bubbles.** This discharge differs from normal physiologic discharge in that the latter has a floccular appearance, and bubbles are absent. Because it is **relatively thin but adherent to the vaginal walls,** this discharge is often apparent only as an increased light reflex. The endocervix is unaffected by the process.

**3. Diagnosis.** BV is perhaps most easily differentiated from trichomoniasis on the basis of direct microscopic examination of vaginal discharge.

**a.** A **wet mount** of the discharge reveals **clue cells,** which are vaginal epithelial cells studded with tiny coccobacilli. **Some clue cells are seen in more than 90% of patients with BV.**

**b.** The **pH of vaginal discharge is elevated** above the normal of 4.5 in approximately 90% of cases.

**c.** A **positive whiff test** is found in nearly 70% of cases.

**d.** Bacterial flora can also be assessed on a wet-mount slide. In healthy women, the predominant morphotype is a large rod (presumably *Lactobacillus* species). In the discharge from a patient with BV, these rods have been completely supplanted by **clumps of coccobacilli.**

**e.** Discharge in BV contains **few PMNs.**

**f.** It has been suggested [214] that the clinician **look for (a) a pH greater than 4.5; (b2) homogeneous, white, adherent vaginal discharge; (c) a positive whiff test; and (d) clue cells. Finding any three of these four**

**signs strongly supports the diagnosis of BV;** the finding of clue cells is the most specific of the criteria [214].

g. Culture for *G. vaginalis* does not prove that the patient has BV or suggest a need for treatment.

4. **BV and pregnancy.** BV has been associated with adverse outcomes of pregnancy (e.g., preterm labor, preterm delivery, premature rupture of membranes, postpartum endometritis) [215]. Treatment of BV in pregnant women apparently reduces the risk of adverse pregnancy outcomes [216,217].
5. BV is **associated with an increased risk of PID** [218,219].

D. **Other vaginal conditions** to consider include vaginitis due to foreign bodies, HSV, HPV, and, much less commonly, *Mycobacterium tuberculosis,* salmonellae, actinomycetes, schistosomes, and pinworms. ***N. gonorrhoeae* and *C. trachomatis* can cause true vaginitis in prepubescent girls** [45].

E. **Noninfectious causes** of vulvovaginal complaints include genital neoplasms, chemical irritation, or focal vulvitis. Physiologic vaginal fluid can sometimes be perceived by the patient as vaginal discharge.

## II. Approach to the patient with vaginal complaints [45]

### A. Historical features

1. **Mode of onset.** An abrupt and identifiable time of onset of symptoms suggests infection. Symptoms beginning during or immediately after the menstrual period are somewhat suggestive of trichomoniasis, whereas a premenstrual onset more frequently accompanies VC.
2. **Perineal irritation.** Pruritus with a scanty or absent discharge frequently is seen in VC and is less common with trichomoniasis. Perineal discomfort is an infrequent complaint in BV. Severe episodic perineal pain sometimes preventing urination strongly suggests herpes genitalis, which affects the labia but usually spares the vagina *per se.* **Chronic discomfort, often interfering with sexual activity, should prompt consideration of focal vulvitis.**
3. **Abdominal pain.** Abdominal discomfort **is rare in uncomplicated vulvovaginitis** except for occasional cases of trichomoniasis. Women complaining of abdominal pain should be examined carefully for evidence of coincidental cystitis or PID.
4. **Medication. Use of antibiotics, corticosteroids, or oral contraceptives** predisposes to VC.
5. **New or multiple sexual contacts** increases the risk of trichomoniasis or BV.

### B. Examination of the female genitalia

1. A **complete pelvic examination** should be performed.
2. **Other bedside evaluation**
   a. After the speculum is withdrawn, the **pH of vaginal secretions** can be determined by inserting a strip of indicator paper into the material collected in the lower lip of the speculum. A normal pH of 4.5 is seen in most patients with VC, whereas a pH elevated to 5.0 or higher is associated with BV or trichomoniasis.
   b. Several drops of 10% KOH are then added to the material on the speculum. A resultant pungent, fishy, aminelike odor constitutes a positive **whiff test.** The whiff test is positive in more than 90% of patients with BV and in many patients with trichomoniasis. This test may also be evaluated on a slide that has been prepared for KOH microscopic examination.

### C. Laboratory examination

1. A **wet mount is of greatest value in the differential diagnosis of a vaginal discharge,** and the specimen may be prepared in several ways. A swab of vaginal discharge may be agitated in a tube containing approximately 0.5 mL of normal saline. One drop of the resulting suspension is put on a microscope slide, and a coverslip is applied. Alternatively, the examiner may place a drop of saline on the slide and mix in a loopful of vaginal material, after which a coverslip is applied. The slide is examined at 400 × with the substage condenser racked down and with the substage diaphragm closed. Phase-contrast microscopy is an excellent means of evaluating vaginal wet mounts.

a. **The relative numbers of epithelial cells and PMNs should be noted.** Finding more than one PMN per epithelial cell should raise the examiner's suspicion of cervical or vaginal inflammation. The relative absence of PMNs is characteristic of the discharge of BV.

b. The wet preparation should be **scanned for motile trichomonads.** Trichomonads are best recognized by their characteristic twitching motility. Trichomonad motility is improved by gently warming the preparation. Unfortunately, the wet mount is negative in approximately 30% of the women with trichomoniasis, and a negative wet mount does not rule out this infection, particularly in relatively asymptomatic women.

c. Normal squamous epithelial cells have transparent cytoplasm and small nuclei. Epithelial cells covered with tiny coccobacillary forms are **clue cells** and are associated with BV. Clue cells are best recognized by observing the edges of epithelial cells, which may be obscured by the adherent coccobacilli.

d. The **bacterial flora can be assessed** on the wet mount. Normal vaginal flora consists primarily of rods. In BV, the predominant flora is tiny coccobacilli.

e. Combining a drop of 10% or 20% **KOH** with the vaginal material on a microscope slide, applying a coverslip, and gently heating will destroy cellular elements but leave the bacteria and fungi unscathed.

2. A **Gram stain of vaginal material can be used for the diagnosis of BV** [220], but trichomonads are very difficult to identify.

## III. Treatment

### A. Candidiasis

1. **Topical therapy.** VC usually is treated with the topical application of an antifungal agent. Commercially available preparations are characterized by high patient acceptability and safety in pregnancy. The choice of an agent is based primarily on cost, the patient's preference for cream versus suppository, and the availability of agents. We prefer 3- or 7-day regimens.

a. **One 14-day regimen** is nystatin, a 100,000-unit suppository at bedtime. The cure rate exceeds 90%.

b. **Seven days of treatment with an imidazole** yields cure rates ranging from 80% to 94% [45].

(1) Miconazole 2% cream, 5 g daily at bedtime
(2) Miconazole, 100-mg vaginal suppository daily at bedtime
(3) Clotrimazole, 100-mg vaginal suppository daily at bedtime
(4) Clotrimazole 1% cream, 5 g daily at bedtime
(5) Terconazole 0.4% cream, 5 g daily at bedtime
(6) Fenticonazole 2% cream, 5 g daily at bedtime

c. **Three-day regimens.** Some reviews suggest marginally better results with 7 days of therapy [221]. Patient compliance is likely to be better [222].

(1) Miconazole, 200-mg vaginal suppository daily at bedtime
(2) Clotrimazole, 200-mg suppository daily at bedtime
(3) Butoconazole 2% cream, 5 g daily at bedtime
(4) Tioconazole 2% cream, 5 g daily at bedtime
(5) Econazole, 150-mg suppository daily at bedtime
(6) Terconazole 0.8% cream, 5 g daily at bedtime
(7) Terconazole, 80-mg suppository daily at bedtime

d. **Single-dose regimens** with large amounts of imidazoles may be preferred for the sake of convenience in the treatment of mild infections, but cure rates obtained in some of these studies have not quite matched those obtained with longer courses. Treatment in pregnancy is more often unsuccessful, and so the longer course regimens may be preferred in this setting [223].

(1) Clotrimazole, 500-mg vaginal tablet at bedtime (single dose)
(2) Tioconazole 6.5% ointment, 4.6 g at bedtime (single application)
(3) Miconazole 1200 mg suppository at bedtime (single administration)

2. **Oral therapy.** Considerable data support the value of oral imidazoles and triazoles in treating VC [45]. **Results do not appear to be substantially superior to those obtained with topical regimens, and the clinician must consider**

**carefully the need for systemic therapy for VC in view of the potential toxicities and possible teratogenicity of the drugs. Only the fluconazole single-dose regimen is approved for this use by the U.S. Food and Drug Administration.**

a. **Single-dose fluconazole,** 150-mg single oral dose, is at least as effective as intravaginal treatment of VC, and many patients may prefer the convenience of a single-dose oral regimen.

b. Other oral regimens (**not U.S. Food and Drug Administration approved)** with very limited clinical data include (a) ketoconazole, 200 mg orally twice a day for 3 to 5 days; (b) ketoconazole, 200 mg orally every day for 3 days; (c) itraconazole, 200 mg orally twice a day for 1 day; and (d) itraconazole, 200 mg orally every day for 3 days.

3. **Recurrent infection. The optimal therapy for recurrent VC has not been defined.** Several approaches have been tried with limited success in individual cases.

   a. **Replacement of lactobacillary flora by diet.** This is ineffective. Vaginal lactobacilli are not *Lactobacillus acidophilus,* women with recurrent candidiasis do not lack vaginal lactobacilli, and a double-blind trial of live versus killed yogurt failed to show any differences in recurrences [224,225].

   b. **Monthly premenstrual treatment with an antifungal.** Although this is effective, many women with somewhat less frequent symptoms prefer to use therapy only when they become symptomatic, and efficacy disappears when the regimen is discontinued [226,227].

   c. **Treatment of sexual partners.** This too is ineffective in most cases [228,229].

   d. **Elimination of a rectal focus.** This is ineffective. Note the large number of studies of the new oral regimens, which would eliminate a rectal focus but are not associated with a delay in next recurrence [229,230].

   e. **Higher dose or alternative treatment for *Candida* species other than *C. albicans*,** many of which are resistant to the imidazole/triazoles. Note that *C. glabrata* may require treatment with fluconazole 150 mg orally on days 1 and 4 or may be better treated with 7 days of a topical imidazole. Boric acid powder, 600 mg in a gelatin capsule *per vaginum* daily for 14 days, is effective against highly resistant yeasts [231,232].

   f. **Long-term, continuous, suppressive therapy for 6 months** [223,233]. This is effective for the duration of suppression and in some women for the long term. This approach may work by allowing women to become desensitized to yeast products. Regimens tested include ketoconazole 100 mg orally daily; itraconazole 50 to 100 mg orally daily; **fluconazole 150 mg orally weekly;** and clotrimazole suppositories 500 mg *per vaginum* once per week. **Because of its potential toxicity, the ketoconazole regimen is not recommended. The fluconazole regimen is the most convenient. Cost of any of these regimens is a major consideration.**

B. **Trichomoniasis.** The index case and all sex partners should be treated. Cure rates of 95% have been achieved when recommended metronidazole regimens are used [13,201].

1. The **standard treatment is metronidazole, 2 g, as a single oral dose.**
2. An **alternative regimen** is metronidazole, 250 mg orally three times a day or 500 mg orally twice a day for 7 days. **Note:** Metronidazole gel has been approved for treatment of BV but it is ineffective for trichomoniasis.
3. **Metronidazole may be used in pregnancy.**
4. **Metronidazole resistance is increasing** in prevalence. Treating metronidazole-resistant trichomoniasis usually involves the administration of high doses of metronidazole, which can be associated with toxicity [201]. Usually, retreatment with metronidazole, 500 mg twice a day for 7 days, is tried. If repeated failure occurs, the patient can be treated with a single 2-g dose of metronidazole once daily for 3 to 5 days. Patients with culture-documented infection who do not respond to these regimens and in whom reinfection has been excluded should be referred for consultation with an expert, so that susceptibility of the *T. vaginalis* to metronidazole can be determined.

C. **BV.** Successful regimens have been aimed at the anaerobic bacteria that participate in the infection. Male sexual contacts do not require therapy [13] for the initial episode. In women with recurrent episodes of BV, it would be prudent also to treat sexual contacts.

1. **Oral regimens**
   a. Metronidazole, 500 mg orally twice a day for 7 days.
   b. Metronidazole, 250 mg orally three times a day for 7 days.
   c. Clindamycin, 300 mg orally twice a day for 7 days. This regimen has the advantage of being safe in pregnancy [234].
   d. Cefadroxil, 500 mg orally twice a day for 7 days. This regimen is safe in pregnancy but is supported by very limited data [235].
2. **Topical regimens** appear to have acceptable cure rates, although data are limited.
   a. Clindamycin 2% vaginal cream, 5 g (one full applicator) vaginally at bedtime for 7 days [236–238]. **This regimen should not be used in pregnancy because it is less effective than metronidazole in preventing gestational complications** [13,239,240].
   b. Metronidazole 0.75% vaginal gel, 5 g (one full applicator) vaginally twice a day or qhs for 5 days [237,241–243].

## SEXUALLY TRANSMITTED INTESTINAL INFECTIONS

Sexually transmitted intestinal infections (e.g., due to *Salmonella* species, *Campylobacter jejuni, Shigella* species, *Cryptosporidium* species) are discussed in Chapters 13 and 18.

## OBSTETRIC/GYNECOLOGIC INFECTIONS

I. **Basic concepts**

A. The **lower genital tract** (cervix and vagina) contains a complex flora of more than 100 species of bacteria, viruses, and fungi.

B. The **upper genital tract** (uterus, fallopian tubes, ovaries, pelvic peritoneum) is normally sterile.

C. When the upper genital tract is anatomically disrupted (e.g., by STDs, surgery, or the trauma of delivery) and local defense mechanisms are impaired, the "normal flora" of the lower genital tract can ascend and cause disease [244]. **Accordingly, most gynecologic and obstetric infections are polymicrobial with these normal flora** (Table 16.2). Conversely, some **"pathogens"** are readily isolated from the healthy woman's vagina [245].

II. **Bacteria**

A. There are **$10^8$ to $10^9$ colony-forming units** of bacteria per milliliter of vaginal secretions.

B. **Anaerobes** predominate over aerobes by a ratio of approximately 10:1.

C. *Staphylococcus aureus* and *Streptococcus pyogenes* (group A streptococcus) are rarely found in normal flora; thus, their presence in the setting of toxic shock syndrome is important.

D. *Mycoplasma hominis* and *U. urealyticum* are frequently found in the vaginas of sexually active women. In the absence of illness they do not warrant therapy, but there is speculation as to their role in the development of PID.

III. **Fungi**

A. Yeasts are the only fungi of importance regularly isolated from the normal genital tract.

B. *C. albicans* is the most common species, although *C. glabrata* may be found.

IV. **Viruses**

A. **Cytomegalovirus** has been recovered in the healthy lower genital tract, particularly in highly sexually active individuals [246].

## PELVIC INFLAMMATORY DISEASE

I. **Definition. PID** refers to infection of the upper female genital tract, anywhere from the endometrium to the fallopian tubes to the ovaries to the peritoneum. **Various combinations of *C. trachomatis, N. gonorrhoeae,* and mixed bacteria of the lower genital tract are the causal organisms.**

Table 16.2. Normal Flora of the Lower Female Genital Tract

| Isolate | Approximate % of Normal Carriage |
|---|---|
| *Lactobacillus* | ~45 |
| Anaerobic gram-positive cocci | ~25 |
| *Prevotella* species | ~20 |
| *Ureaplasma urealyticum* | ~18 |
| *Gardnerella vaginalis* | ~12 |
| *Streptococcus agalactiae* (group B streptococcus) | ~11 |
| *Escherichia coli* | ~7 |
| Anaerobic gram-negative rods | ~5 |
| *Candida* species | ~5 |
| *Mycoplasma hominis* | ~3 |
| *Bacteroides fragilis* | ~3 |
| Other gram-negative rods | ~1 |

Note: The compendium of "normal flora" changes dramatically with menses, postoperatively, with tampon usage, with bacterial vaginosis, and with other sexually transmitted diseases.
From Eschenbach DA, Thwin SS, Patton DL, et al. Influence of the normal menstrual cycle on vaginal tissue, discharge, and microflora. *Clin Infect Dis* 2000;30:901–907, with permission [245].

**II. Risk factors**

- **A.** Heterosexual activity (young at first intercourse, multiple partners, recent new sexual partner, frequency of intercourse, etc.)
- **B.** Prior STD (gonorrhea, *Chlamydia,* probably BV)
- **C.** Age: incidence peaks among 15 to 24 year olds.
- **D.** Intrauterine device (IUD, especially the Dalkon shield) or no contraception greater than barrier methods or oral contraceptives
- **E.** Invasive gynecologic procedures
- **F.** Menstruating women (PID is rare during pregnancy and after menopause)

**III. Diagnosis**

- **A. Gold standards** for diagnosis are often impractical to achieve in the outpatient setting [13].
  - **1.** Endometrial biopsy showing changes consistent with PID
  - **2.** Transvaginal ultrasound showing thickened fluid-filled tubes
  - **3.** Laparoscopic evidence of PID
- **B. Clinical diagnosis**
  - **1. Symptoms** classically include fever (temperature > 101°F) and lower abdominal or adnexal tenderness.
  - **2. Examination** may reveal cervical motion tenderness or abnormal cervical discharge.
  - **3. Laboratory values** may include elevated C-reactive protein or erythrocyte sedimentation rate and cervical culture of *N. gonorrhoeae* or *C. trachomatis.*
  - **4. Clinical diagnosis is insensitive and nonspecific.** Many patients with these findings will not have true PID [247], and likewise many patients without such findings will have PID. Sole endometritis can have particularly mild symptoms [248].
  - **5. Gonococcal PID** is usually relatively acute with significant symptoms, high fever, peritoneal signs, and vaginal discharge.
  - **6. Chlamydial PID** usually displays mild to moderate symptoms (e.g., chronic pain, irregular bleeding) but severe inflammation on laparoscopy.
  - **7. Nongonococcal/nonchalmydial PID** is often marked by abscess formation.

**IV. Therapy. The Centers for Disease Control and Prevention (CDC) recommend empirical treatment for all sexually active women with lower**

**abdominal/adnexal tenderness and cervical motion tenderness on examination with no other explanation** [13].

A. **There are no large-scale trials that support one therapeutic regimen over another.**

B. All treatment regimens should be effective against **gonorrhea, chlamydia, and anaerobes,** regardless of endocervical or other cultures. The rationale is that negative endocervical cultures for *N. gonorrhoeae* and *C. trachomatis* do not preclude upper tract infection and anaerobes are likely pathogenic and therefore also should be treated [249].

C. Failure rates of 15% to 20% are documented for single drug regimens; thus, most authorities recommend **multiple-drug regimens.** These provide clinical and microbiologic cure rates of approximately 90%.

D. **Whether to hospitalize** and use i.v. therapy relies on clinical judgment, but most authorities suggest hospitalization in the following scenarios:
   1. Tubo-ovarian abscess (see below)
   2. Peritonitis (cannot rule out other abdominal processes)
   3. Pregnant patients (because of high rates of preterm labor, stillbirths, and maternal morbidity)
   4. Immunosuppressed patients (including HIV patients, who often have more severe presentations)
   5. The patient cannot tolerate oral medications
   6. Possibly in young adolescents when compliance is in question

E. The CDC recommends any of the following **parenteral** regimens:
   1. **Cefotetan** 2 g i.v. every 12h + **doxycycline** 100 mg orally every 12h
   2. **Cefoxitin** 2 g i.v. every 6 hours + **doxycycline** 100 mg orally every 12 hours
   3. **Clindamycin** 900 mg i.v. every 8 hours + **gentamicin** 2 mg/kg i.v. loading dose, then 1.5 mg/kg every 8 hours

   **Note:** Limited trials also suggest that parenteral ofloxacin + metronidazole, ampicillin/sulbactam + doxycycline, or ciprofloxacin + doxycycline + metronidazole are effective.

F. **Duration of i.v. therapy.** Most trials on inpatients have used parenteral treatment for at least 48 hours, after which the patient is switched to oral doxycycline 100 mg twice a day to complete a 14-day course.

G. **Stable patients who do not require hospitalization can be managed with outpatient therapy with any of the following regimens:**
   1. **Ofloxacin** 400 mg orally twice a day + **metronidazole** 500 mg orally twice a day for 14 days
   2. **Ceftriaxone** 250 mg i.m. × 1 + **doxycycline** 100 mg orally twice a day for 14 days
   3. **Cefoxitin** 2 g i.m. + probenecid 1 g orally once + **doxycycline** 100 mg orally twice a day for 14 days
   4. **Ceftizoxime** or cefotaxime i.m. once + **doxycycline** 100 mg orally twice a day for 14 days

   **Note:** Amoxicillin/clavulanate plus doxycycline may also be effective. There are no data on oral cephalosporins nor azithromycin (instead of doxycycline) in the treatment of PID.

H. **IUD-associated PID.** The need to remove an IUD has not been proven, but clinical response seems to be faster with removal. It is recommended for mild IUD-associated PID that oral antibiotics are started before removal to reduce the likelihood of bacteremia upon instrumentation. IUDs are also associated with *Actinomyces israelii* colonization and infection (see below).

V. **Follow-up.** All patients with PID whether given i.v. or oral therapy should have a **follow-up examination in 2 to 3 days. Male partners** who have had sexual contact with the PID patient in the preceding 60 days should be **seen and treated** empirically for both *C. trachomatis* and *N. gonorrhoeae.*

VI. **PID sequelae:**

A. Disease recurrence (approximately 43%).

B. Chronic pelvic pain (approximately 24%) [250].

C. Infertility (20%–40% in some series of PID patients).

**D.** Ectopic pregnancy (2.5%–10%) [251].

**E.** PID is also associated with premature rupture of membranes, preterm delivery, and amnionitis [252].

**VII. Prevention.** Strategies revolve around aggressive screening for chlamydial infection [250].

**VIII. Tubo-ovarian abscess**

**A. Epidemiology.** Tubo-ovarian abscess is a major complication of PID and occurs in up to one-third of hospitalized PID patients. The microbiology is generally the same as for PID.

**B. Clinical presentation. Like PID, symptoms are insensitive and nonspecific.** In a large review 89% of tubo-ovarian abscess patients had abdominal pain, 50% a history of fever/chills, 28% vaginal discharge, 26% nausea, and 21% abnormal vaginal bleeding. Fever may be present in only 60% and leukocytosis in only 70% [254].

**C. Diagnosis** requires demonstration of an inflammatory mass on imaging (usually ultrasound or computed tomography [CT]).

**D. Management**

1. **Antibiotics. Approximately 75% to 80% of tubo-ovarian abscesses respond to antibiotic therapy alone, especially when small (<7 cm)** [255].
   - **a.** The i.v. clindamycin + gentamicin regimen detailed above for PID has commonly been used.
   - **b.** In retrospective reviews, many patients receive 7 to 10 days of i.v. antibiotics before switching to oral therapy. Oral clindamycin or metronidazole is often added to the oral doxycycline to complete the 14-day PID treatment course.
2. **Surgery is required for** tubo-ovarian abscesses that rupture (approximately 3%).
3. **Surgery is usually performed for**
   - **a.** Poor response despite i.v. antibiotics
   - **b.** In the setting of an enlarging abscess
   - **c.** With bilateral tubo-ovarian abscess
   - **d.** In cases of chronic pain
4. **Unilateral adnexectomy,** often under laparoscopy, with continued antibiotics is accepted treatment (vs. total abdominal hysterectomy/bilateral salpingo-oophorectomy)[256]. Percutaneous and endovaginal ultrasound-guided **drainage** are also used.

**IX. Actinomycotic salpingitis** [257]

**A.** *Actinomyces israelii* is an anaerobic, gram-positive, branching, non–acid-fast rod.

**B. Colonization** of the lower genital tract occurs most often in the setting of IUDs (especially in long-time users) and colonization **portends an increased risk of PID.**

1. **Colonization** is usually diagnosed by Pap smears showing characteristic "sulfur granules."
2. **Colonization management.** Patients either can be followed expectantly with repeat Pap smears or treated for 10 to 14 days with oral penicillin. Rarely does the IUD need to be removed for colonization [257].

**C. Infection** ensues in a small percentage of colonized women.

1. **Clinical presentation** may be irregular vaginal bleeding or mild pelvic discomfort.
2. **Pathology** can reveal significant destruction, fibrosis, and stricturing of pelvic/retroperitoneal structures.
3. **Management.** If there is a concern of active actinomycotic endometritis/salpingitis in an IUD user, the patient should receive i.v. penicillin (plus the i.v. therapy for PID), the IUD should be removed, and surgery may be required.
4. **Note:** The tetracyclines, erythromycin, and clindamycin are also effective against *Actinomyces.*

**X. Genital tract tuberculosis**

**A.** Most common in developing countries.

**B.** Usually results from **hematogenous spread** from pulmonary infection, rarely from contiguous intraperitoneal disease or direct sexual inoculation.

C. **Clinically,** an indolent infection. Chief presentation is infertility and also vaginal bleeding or chronic pelvic pain.
D. **Diagnosis:** Hysterosalpingogram may show characteristic changes; however, endometrial or fallopian tube histology, which demonstrates granulomas, positive acid-fast stains, or positive culture of endometrial aspirates, is required.
E. **Therapy.** Antibiotics (see Chapter 27) and surgery (often TAH/BSO) if symptoms persist.

## INFECTIONS AFTER GYNECOLOGIC SURGERY OR PROCEDURES

It is helpful to realize that animal models of intraabdominal infection reveal an early and late-onset clinical pattern with **early** infection marked by **gram-negative** peritonitis with **sepsis** and **late** infection marked by **abscess** formation caused by **anaerobes.**

I. **Risk factors** for postgynecologic surgical infections
  A. Hysterectomy, especially vaginal
  B. Lower socioeconomic status
  C. Duration of surgery
  D. BV at the time of surgery
  E. Increased age

II. **Pelvic cellulitis** is the most common infection after hysterectomy.
  A. **Clinical presentation.** Fever and abdominal and pelvic pain (usually more severe on one side), typically on postoperative days 2 to 3, with parametrial tenderness on bimanual examination.
  B. **Diagnosis** is clinical. The value of obtaining cultures is controversial.
  C. **Therapy:** cefotetan, cefoxitin, ampicillin/sulbactam, ticarcillin/clavulanate. An alternate regimen is clindamycin plus gentamicin. Intravenous therapy is typically continued until the patient is afebrile for 24 to 36 hours and then stopped.

III. **Pelvic abscess.** This occurs rarely but is the most serious postoperative complication.
  A. **Epidemiology.** Risk is greatest after hysterectomy, particularly vaginal hysterectomy. There need not be preceding pelvic cellulitis. It is most common in premenopausal women.
  B. **Clinical presentation:** May present weeks after surgery (average 18 to 20 days) with high fever (usually late in the afternoon), leukocytosis, elevated erythrocyte sedimentation rate, and often a palpable mass high in the pelvis.
  C. **Diagnosis.** Ultrasound or CT to confirm presence of the mass/loculations/ relationship to bowel.
  D. **Microbiology.** Abscess pus and abscess tissue should be inoculated into anaerobic transport vials for culture. Such anaerobic cultures will be adequate for aerobes, fungi, and mycobacteria as well.
  E. **Therapy**
    1. **Antibiotic therapy alone is often successful.**
    2. Surgery should be considered because of the high mortality of abscess rupture.
    3. *Bacteroides fragilis* is most frequently isolated; thus, anaerobic coverage with **i.v. clindamycin or metronidazole** is recommended. Failure to respond to antibiotics usually attests to the need for surgical **drainage** and not antibiotic resistance.
    4. **Drainage** can be performed percutaneously or via colpotomy or laparotomy. There are numerous reports of ultrasound-guided drainage procedures. The abscess should be completely evacuated and a pigtail or equivalent catheter left in place until drainage ceases, usually 4 to 8 days.
    5. **Duration.** Intravenous antibiotics should be administered until temperature, white blood cell count, and symptoms normalize. Some clinicians treat these patients for 7 days after discharge with oral **amoxicillin/clavulanate** or **metronidazole.**
    6. **Follow-up.** Patients are often reexamined at 2 weeks.

IV. **Vaginal cuff cellulitis.** Inflammation at the vaginal cuff incision is normal after hysterectomy, but frank infection at this site is relatively rare.

**A. Clinical presentation:** Usually presents after discharge from the hospital with lower abdominal/pelvic pain, increased vaginal discharge, and low-grade fever. On bimanual examination only the superior vaginal surgical area is tender.

**B. Therapy.** Oral therapy such as amoxicillin/clavulanate is usually effective within 72 hours.

**V. Vaginal cuff abscess**

**A. Clinical presentation.** Cuff abscess generally presents acutely on postoperative days 2 to 3 with fullness in the lower abdomen, often pain with defecation, and a well-localized collection above the vaginal cuff.

**B. Management.** Therapy requires surgical drainage, which can usually be accomplished through the vagina, and i.v. antibiotics (e.g., clindamycin + gentamicin) until the patient is afebrile for 24 to 36 hours.

**VI. Osteomyelitis pubis.** A rare infection that usually results from contiguous extension after urethral suspension, radical vulvectomy, pelvic exenteration, or, rarely, hematogenous seeding.

**A. Clinical presentation.** Patients usually present approximately 8 weeks after the operation with pubic bone pain, avoidance of ambulation, and pain on abduction. Wound drainage, low fever, and elevated erythrocyte sedimentation rate and alkaline phosphatase may be present.

**B. Diagnosis.** Plain films, bone scans, CT, or magnetic resonance imaging can confirm the presence of osteomyelitis.

**C. Therapy.** Intravenous coverage for both *S. aureus* and gram-negative rods should be started **after** surgical debridement is performed. Coverage can then be narrowed based on operative cultures. Duration of therapy is 6 weeks.

## MATERNAL INFECTIONS AFTER DELIVERY

**I. Postpartum fever.** Fever (oral temperature >38.0°C) in the first 24 hours after delivery is common but usually due to breast engorgement, atelectasis, aspiration pneumonia (particularly after cesarean section), or urinary tract infection. In the setting of vaginal delivery, only approximately 20% of fevers **on** postdelivery day 1 are due to pelvic infection; in the setting of cesarean section, the percentage rises to approximately 70%. Fever **after** postdelivery day 1 is then generally due to pelvic infection. Such infections are an important cause of maternal death, accounting for between 8% and 13% of maternal deaths.

**II. Episiotomy infections**

**A. Epidemiology.** Only 0.1% to 0.3% of episiotomies become infected overall, highest for third- or fourth-degree tears (1%–2%).

**B. Risk factors:** Cigarette smoking, coagulation disorders, HPV infection.

**C. Classification**

1. **Simple episiotomy infection**
2. **Infection of the superficial fascia without necrosis**
3. **Infection of the superficial fascia with necrosis**
4. **Myonecrosis, most commonly caused by *Clostridium perfringens***

**D. Clinically presents** as a wound with red swollen edges, often with dysuria.

**E.** Management includes opening and exploration of the wound with adjunctive antibiotics for the usual vaginal flora.

**III. Postcesarean section wound infections**

**A. Epidemiology.** Incidence averages approximately 6%, with prophylactic antibiotics 2%.

**B. Risk factors:** obesity, diabetes mellitus, corticosteroid therapy, immunosuppression, or hematoma formation.

**C. Clinical presentation.** Fever on about postoperative day 4, often preceded by endometritis. Erythema and drainage are found on examination.

**D. Diagnosis.** Wound cultures are almost always positive, and the organisms are usually the same as those that cause endometritis. Hospital-acquired gram-negative pathogens may be considered, however.

**E. Therapy.** Surgical drainage and antibiotics; if fascia not intact (i.e., wound dehiscence), secondary closure.

**IV. Postpartum endometritis.** "Postpartum endometritis" technically involves not only the endometrium but also the myometrium and parametrium.

**A. Risk factors** [258]

1. Cesarean delivery
2. Poor socioeconomic status
3. Prolonged rupture of membranes
4. Prolonged labor
5. Multiple cervical examination
6. Internal fetal monitoring
7. Midforceps delivery
8. Vaginal colonization with certain organisms (group B streptococcus, *C. trachomatis, M. hominis, G. vaginalis, U. urealyticum*)
9. Chorioamnionitis

**B. Clinical presentation.** Any postpartum fever should be evaluated for endometritis. Classically entails fever on postpartum days 1 to 2 (temperature >38–39°C), chills (may suggest bacteremia), abdominal pain, fundal tenderness, parametrial tenderness, foul-smelling lochia, and leukocytosis.

**C. Microbiology.** Typically multiple organisms of the normal vaginal flora are isolated from the endometrium (approximately 2.5 on average), including

1. Anaerobes: *Peptostreptococcus, Peptococcus, Bacteroides, Clostridium.*
2. Aerobes: *Enterococcus,* group B streptococcus, *E. coli.*
3. *Gardnerella vaginalis.*
4. *M. hominis.*
5. *U. urealyticum.*
6. **Note:** The utility of endometrial cultures in routine cases is controversial, because results will not likely affect antibiotic choice.
7. An estimated 10% to 20% will have documentable bacteremia, often with group B streptococcus or *G. vaginalis.* Bacteremia does not predict the severity of illness.

**D. Special pathogens to consider**

1. *C. trachomatis:* implicated as a cause of late-onset (2–6 days postpartum), indolent, postpartum endometritis.
2. Group A streptococcus causes severe presentation with high fever, erythroderma, desquamation, and sepsis ("toxic shock") and carries a more than 55% mortality. Organisms are often associated with transmission from a caregiver, and the CDC recommends screening caregivers. Consider i.v. immunoglobulin.

**E. Therapy.** An antimicrobial regimen effective for all putative pathogens is impractical, but empirical therapy against a broad range of anaerobes and aerobes tends to be effective.

1. **After vaginal delivery:** i.v. clindamycin + gentamicin is effective in 95%.
2. If fever persists at 48 to 72 hours, most add ampicillin as enterococcus has been implicated in this setting.
3. **After cesarean section:** Many include ampicillin along with clindamycin and gentamicin.
4. $\beta$-Lactams have less of a track record, but extended-spectrum penicillins with $\beta$-lactamase inhibitors such as ampicillin/sulbactam or piperacillin/tazobactam could be considered.

**F. Duration of therapy.** Typically antibiotics are stopped after the patient is afebrile for 24 hours. Improvement should follow in 48 to 72 hours in 90%. Bacterial resistance and drug fever are extremely rare in this population, and persistence of fever after 72 hours should prompt a search for complications such as parametrial phlegmons, incisional or pelvic abscesses, infected hematomas, and septic pelvic thrombophlebitis.

**G. Prevention.** Prophylactic antibiotics decrease the postcesarean endometritis rate.

1. For routine cesarean section: cefazolin 1 g for one dose after cord-clamp
2. For cesarean section plus chorioamnionitis: clindamycin plus gentamicin (every 8 hours for three doses postoperatively)

**V. Phlegmon** is an extensive induration of the parametrium within the leaves of the broad ligament.

A. **Presentation.** Should be considered when fever persists after 72 hours despite standard antibiotic therapy. Usually unilateral, may stay limited to the base of the broad ligament or extend laterally or posteriorly.

B. **Therapy** is with i.v. antibiotics; fever may persist for more than 7 days; surgery is reserved for women in whom uterine incisional necrosis is suspected. Surgery usually requires hysterectomy and debridement is difficult.

VI. **Necrotizing fasciitis**

A. **Epidemiology.** Extremely rare but may complicate episiotomy incisions and perineal lacerations

B. **Risk factors:** diabetes mellitus, obesity, hypertension

C. **Clinically.** Symptoms usually begin at 3 to 5 days.

D. **Diagnosis.** Histopathology consistently reveals panniculitis and can help confirm the diagnosis [259].

E. **Microbiology:** polymicrobial with streptococci, coliforms, and anaerobes or monomicrobial with group A streptococci.

F. **Therapy.** Prompt wide debridement in the operating room and antibiotics, usually clindamycin plus a $\beta$-lactam. High mortality (approximately 100% without surgical treatment, 50% with aggressive excision), particularly in obstetric/gynecologic patients [260].

## INTRAPARTUM INFECTIONS

I. **Chorioamnionitis,** also known as **intraamniotic infection syndrome,** is an ascending infection of the uterus and its contents (placenta, amniotic membranes, umbilical cord) during pregnancy. It occurs in 1% to 2% of women with full-term pregnancies but increases to over 25% with the following **risk factors.**

A. **Risk factors**

1. Prolonged rupture of membranes
2. Prolonged labor with multiple vaginal examinations
3. Preterm labor
4. Meconium staining of amniotic fluid
5. Obstetric procedures (cervical cerclage, amniocentesis, cordocentesis)
6. Young age
7. Low socioeconomic class
8. Nulliparity
9. Preexisting BV

B. **Clinically:** maternal fever, tachycardia, uterine tenderness. Occasionally foul or purulent amniotic fluid. Fetal heart rate abnormalities.

C. **Diagnosis:** based largely on clinical findings, especially tachycardia. Amniotic fluid obtained in the setting of intact membranes (e.g., preterm labor unresponsive to tocolytics) that reveals a positive Gram stain, positive leukocyte esterase, or low glucose is suggestive.

D. **Microbiology.** With the rare exception of hematogenous listerial amnionitis, this ascending infection is polymicrobial with organisms similar to other gynecologic infections: anaerobes, streptococci (group B streptococcus, viridans group), *E. coli, Gardnerella, Mycoplasma,* and so on.

E. **Management** is antibiotic therapy with the understanding that delivery is required for cure. Antibiotics seek to prevent neonatal pneumonia and therefore antibiotics which target group B streptococcus and *E. coli* (such as ampicillin plus gentamicin) are common initial regimens. Antibiotics provide a better cure rate when given immediately upon diagnosis of chorioamnionitis rather then postpartum. With **cesarean delivery,** clindamycin should be added after cord clamping because 20% to 30% of these patients will fail ampicillin plus gentamicin. Cephalosporins and $\beta$-lactam/$\beta$-lactamase inhibitor combinations may also be successful.

II. **Postabortion infections**

Maternal mortality from septic abortion is a huge problem worldwide, annually accounting for over 100,000 deaths [261].

A. **Risk factors**

1. Increased gestational age

2. Method of termination (intraamniotic injection or hysterotomy higher risk than suction curettage)
3. Untreated gonorrhea or chlamydial cervicitis, possibly BV
4. IUDs

**B. Clinical.** Typical symptoms of fever, chills, tachycardia, and lower abdominal/pelvic pain develop within 4 days of the procedure. Exceptions are *S. aureus* or group A streptococcal infections, which typically present within 24 hours. Examination may reveal an enlarged uterus, foul-smelling exudate, and an open or bleeding os (indicating retained products). Septic shock occurs in 5% to 15%, usually in the setting of delayed treatment.

**C. Diagnosis.** A positive pregnancy test will rule in a recent (4–6 week) pregnancy. Gram stains of endometrial smears may be useful in fulminant cases, if gram-positive cocci, suggestive of staphylococcus or streptococci, or Gram-positive rods, suggestive of *Clostridium,* are present. Cultures should be performed. Abdominal plain films are used to exclude intraperitoneal air or (rarely) gas in the myometrium. Massive hemolysis is a clue to infection with *C. perfringens.*

**D. Microbiology.** As with PID, usually a polymicrobial infection consisting of lower genital tract flora +/− gonococci or chlamydia [261].

**E. Management:** Except for rare instances, patients should be admitted for

1. **Intravenous antibiotics**
   a. In mild to moderate infection, therapy with cefoxitin, cefotetan, or ampicillin/sulbactam can be adequate.
   b. In severe infection with septic shock, clindamycin or metronidazole + gentamicin + ampicillin has commonly been used. Depending on local methicillin-resistant *S. aureus* (MRSA) rates, vancomycin may be substituted for ampicillin. A third-generation cephalosporin + metronidazole or imipenem alone are other options. Penicillin has the largest track record for known clostridial infection.
2. **Evacuation of the uterus.** Evacuation should ideally be performed by suction curettage after adequate serum levels of antibiotics are obtained. Laparotomy is required with free intraperitoneal air, failure to respond to uterine evacuation, or myometritis and often entails hysterectomy.

## SEPTIC PELVIC THROMBOPHLEBITIS

Septic pelvic thrombophlebitis is a complication of postpartum or postoperative infections, occurring in about 0% to 2% of cases. Heparin alone is often not successful for therapy, and bacteria can be demonstrated in resected thrombi. Septic pulmonary emboli complicate up to 30% of untreated cases.

**I. Postpartum septic pelvic thrombophlebitis** can be due to superficial, deep pelvic, or ovarian vein thrombophlebitis, but **ovarian vein thrombophlebitis** is the "classic" obstetric infection. It occurs in 1 in 2,000 deliveries, most commonly in the setting of postcesarean endometritis.

**A. Clinically.** Patients can be well or ill appearing with fever, tachycardia, and lower abdominal pain. Patients classically have a "ropelike" abdominal mass on examination.

**B. Diagnosis.** Doppler ultrasonography, CT, or magnetic resonance imaging can make the diagnosis, visualizing clot extending to one or both ovarian vein plexi or the inferior vena cava (occurs in one-fourth). Blood cultures are usually negative.

**C. Therapy** consists of antibiotics against the common pelvic pathogens (third-generation cephalosporin plus clindamycin or metronidazole; clindamycin plus gentamicin) and, historically, heparin anticoagulation. A recent large study, however, showed no benefit in women treated with heparin plus antibiotics over antibiotics alone [262]. Most clinicians use a course of 7 to 10 days of both antibiotics with or without heparin.

**D. Surgery** is reserved for persistent fever or persistent pulmonary emboli to remove the associated infected area.

**II. Postoperative septic pelvic thrombophlebitis**

**A. Clinical.** Generally develops 4 to 8 days after gynecologic surgery, almost always with an operative site infection. The typical presentation is when the patient with an operative infection improves clinically on antibiotic therapy but fever persists ("**enigmatic fever**"). Physical findings are minimal.

**B. Diagnosis.** Blood cultures are positive in 35%. The diagnosis is supported by defervescence after anticoagulation with heparin.

## MATERNAL INFECTIONS DURING PREGNANCY

Though pregnancy is often considered a semi-immunosuppressed state due to maternal tolerance to the allogeneic fetal "graft," significant changes in maternal immunoglobulin, cell-mediated immunity, and polymorphonuclear cell function are difficult to demonstrate. Nonetheless, certain viral, bacterial, and protozoal infections are particularly severe in pregnancy and bear mentioning.

**I. Varicella-zoster virus**

**A. Clinical.** Varicella infection is severe in adults and probably even more severe in pregnancy. Approximately 10% of varicella-zoster virus–infected pregnant women develop **pneumonitis.**

**B. Prevention.** Varicella-zoster immune globulin can prevent or attenuate infection in nonimmune individuals upon exposure to varicella-zoster virus if administered within 96 hours. Most individuals (90%) who report never having had chickenpox are seropositive (i.e., immune) upon testing. Many authors recommend varicella-zoster immune globulin administration for all nonimmune pregnant women if exposed to chickenpox. An ideal preventive strategy would be to screen women of childbearing age for a history of varicella and administer the vaccine before pregnancy.

**II. Influenza**

**A. Clinical.** Influenza infection is common in pregnancy and **may** be associated with pregnancy complications [263].

**B. Prevention.** Vaccination against influenza is recommended by the CDC for all pregnant women after the first trimester. There is no evidence of teratogenicity.

**III. Parvovirus**

**A. Epidemiology.** Approximately 50% of pregnant women are seropositive (immune) for parvovirus; the remainder are at risk. The virus is associated with outbreaks, during which the attack rate is 20% to 30%, often asymptomatic. In infected pregnant women, the fetal loss rate is approximately 5% to 10%, due to miscarriage or hydrops fetalis. Term infants appear to develop normally [264].

**B. Management.** For women with positive IgM, ultrasound examination is indicated. If there is hydrops, fetal transfusion is recommended by some.

**IV. Rubella**

**A. Epidemiology.** Despite widespread immunization in the United States, 6% to 25% of women are susceptible.

**B. Clinically.** Maternal rubella infection is asymptomatic in about 25%; in the 75% of symptomatic infections, viremia precedes symptoms (usually a rash) by about 1 week.

**C. Management.** Given the profound teratogenicity of rubella, preconception vaccination is a priority. The use of immunoglobulin is not recommended for exposure.

**V. Cytomegalovirus**

**A. Epidemiology.** Cytomegalovirus is the most common perinatal infection, usually acquired from reactivated (not primary) infection in the mother.

**B. Clinically.** There is no evidence that pregnancy increases the risk or severity of maternal cytomegalovirus infection.

**C. Management.** Serologic screening is not recommended by the American College of Obstetrics and Gynecology, there is no effective preventive strategy, and there is no vaccine.

**VI. Group B streptococcus**

**A. Epidemiology.** Asymptomatic vaginal carriage of group B streptococcus is common, occurring in 15% to 20% of pregnant women. The organism has been implicated in preterm labor, premature rupture of membranes, chorioamnionitis, postpartum sepsis, and severe fetal/neonatal infections.

**B. Management.** Guidelines for prevention are published by the American College of Obstetrics and Gynecology, the CDC, and the Association of American Physicians using either a risk-based (treat the high-risk mother intrapartum) or screening-based (treat colonized mothers intrapartum) strategy. Implementation of either protocol diminishes group B streptococcus neonatal sepsis from 1.5 to 0.2 per 1,000.

**VII. Listeria**

**A. Epidemiology.** Infection with *L. monocytogenes* is uncommon, with approximately 2,500 infections in the United States annually, but over one-third occur in pregnant women.

**B. Clinically.** Infection in the pregnant woman may be asymptomatic or a nonspecific febrile illness. Maternal listeremia causes amnionitis/fetal infection, and neonatal mortality approaches 50%.

**C. Management.** Therapy is with ampicillin.

**VIII. Toxoplasmosis**

**A. Epidemiology.** Maternal infection occurs through ingestion of infected raw or undercooked meat, through ingestion of toxoplasma oocysts, and transplacentally. Prior infection confers immunity, so maternal infection must be primary for fetal infection. About one-third of American women have preexisting immunity, and the CDC estimates that 0.1% to 0.5% of pregnancies are complicated by acute toxoplasmosis.

**B. Clinical.** Maternal infection is usually asymptomatic but can include fatigue, muscle pains, and lymphadenopathy. Maternal infection in the first trimester leads to a severe infection in 10% of infants, whereas infection in the third trimester leads to a milder infection in 60% of infants.

**C. Management.** The American College of Obstetrics and Gynecology does not recommend routine prenatal screening except with concurrent HIV infection. For the woman with active disease (diagnosed by a rise in IgG titer or PCR), treatment is with pyrimethamine plus sulfadiazine or with spiramycin.

## MASTITIS

**I. Postpartum mastitis** may or may not be infectious. Bacteria enter through fissures and cracks in the nipple and cause infection in the setting of an inflamed breast.

**A. Clinical presentation.** Typically begins weeks to months after delivery (average 5.5 weeks) with abrupt fever, chills, and breast soreness. Usually a cellulitis is visible, classically V-shaped, extending from the nipple.

**B. Diagnosis.** Samples of breast milk may be obtained for leukocyte count and culture. Leukocyte count more than $10^6$/mL of milk **plus high bacterial counts** in milk confirms infectious mastitis. If pus can be expressed, it should be cultured and Gram stained. Blood cultures may be obtained if the patient appears systemically ill. The neonate should also be examined for evidence of infection.

**C. Microbiology.** ***S. aureus*** is the most common organism. Less common organisms include *S. epidermidis*, $\beta$-hemolytic streptococci, enterococci, and *E. coli*.

**D. Therapy.** Infectious mastitis may resolve with simple emptying of the breast, but antibiotics are recommended to prevent abscesses that otherwise develop in 11% of patients. Most patients are managed with **oral** antistaphylococcal antibiotics such as **dicloxacillin** (250–500 mg orally four times a day) or a first-generation cephalosporin such as **cephalexin** (500 mg orally four times a day). In severe cases or with systemic toxicity, i.v. **oxacillin** or **nafcillin** (1–1.5 g every 4 hours) or **cefazolin** (1 g every 8 hours) can be used. In the penicillin-allergic patient, **erythromycin, clarithromycin,** or **clindamycin** is acceptable. Adjunctive measures such as breast emptying (continued nursing is not problematic [265]) and anti-inflammatories are important.

**E. Duration of therapy** is usually 10 days.

**F. Abscess.** In the unusual scenario when an abscess develops, nursing should be interrupted. In addition to therapy with parenteral antibiotics, prompt incision and drainage should be performed.

**II. Mastitis in the nonlactating breast is uncommon.**

**A. Breast abscess** may rarely occur in premenopausal and postmenopausal women and is often polymicrobial, including anaerobes.

**Treatment** consists of surgical incision or excision, in conjunction with antimicrobial therapy based on culture results.

B. **Granulomatous mastitis** presents as firm hard masses and may mimic carcinoma. This condition has been attributed to chronic bacterial abscess, tuberculous disease, or fungi but may be idiopathic. **Diagnosis** requires biopsy and culture.

## REFERENCES


1. Handsfield HH. Principles of treatment of sexually transmitted diseases. In: Holmes KK, Sparling PF, Mårdh P-A, et al., eds. *Sexually transmitted diseases,* 3rd ed. New York: McGraw-Hill, 1999:711–721.
2. Rein MF. The interaction between HIV and the classic sexually transmitted diseases. *Curr Infect Dis Rep* 2000;2:87–95. [Also see Rottengin JA, Cameron DW, Garnett GP. A systematic review of the epidemiologic interactions between classic sexually transmitted diseases and HIV: how much is really known. *Sex Transm Dis* 2001;28:579–587.]
3. Burstein GR, Zenilman JM. Nongonococcal urethritis—a new paradigm. *Clin Infect Dis* 1999;28[Suppl 1]:S66–S73.
4. Stamm WE, Koutsky LA, Benedetti JK, et al. *Chlamydia trachomatis* urethral infections in men. Prevalence, risk factors, and clinical manifestations. *Ann Intern Med* 1984;100:47–51.
5. Swartz SL, Kraus SJ. Persistent urethral leukocytosis and asymptomatic chlamydial urethritis. *J Infect Dis* 1979;140:614–617.
6. Handsfield HH, Lipman TO, Harnisch JP, et al. Asymptomatic gonorrhea in men: diagnosis, natural course, prevalence, and significance. *N Engl J Med* 1974;290:117–123.
7. McCormack WM, Rein MF. Urethritis. In: Mandell GL, Bennett JE, Dolin R, eds. *Principles and practice of infectious diseases* 5th ed. New York: Churchill Livingstone, 2000:1208–1218.
8. Goodhart ME, Ogden J, Zaidi AA, et al. Factors affecting the performance of smear and culture tests for the detection of *Neisseria gonorrhoeae. Sex Transm Dis* 1982;9:52–55.
9. Koumans EH, Johnson RE, Knapp JS, et al. Laboratory testing for *Neisseria gonorrhoeae* by recently introduced nonculture tests: a performance review with clinical and public health considerations. *Clin Infect Dis* 1998;27:1171–1180.
10. Hale YM, Melton ME, Lewis JS, et al. Evaluation of the Pace 2 *Neisseria gonorrhoeae* assay by three public health laboratories. *J Clin Microbiol* 1993;31:451–453.
11. Fox KK, Knapp JS, Holmes KK, et al. Antimicrobial resistance in *Neisseria gonorrhoeae* in the United States 1988–1994: the emergence of decreased susceptibility to the fluoroquinolones. *J Infect Dis* 1997;175:1396–1403.
12. Thompkins JR, Zenilman JM. Quinolone resistance in *Neisseria gonorrhoeae. Curr Infect Dis Rep* 2001;3:156–161.
13. Centers for Disease Control and Prevention. 1998 Sexually transmitted disease treatment guidelines. *MMWR Morb Mortal Wkly Rep* 1997;47(RR-1):1–116.
14. Weber JT, Johnson RE. New treatments for *Chlamydia trachomatis* genital infection. *Clin Infect Dis* 1995;20[Suppl1]:S66–S71.
15. Østergaard L. Diagnosis of urogenital *Chlamydia trachomatis* infection by the use of DNA amplification. *Acta Pathol Microbiol Immunol Scand Suppl* 1999;S89:5–36.
16. Howell MR, Quinn TC, Brathwaite W, et al. Screening women for *Chlamydia trachomatis* in family planning clinics: the cost-effectiveness of DNA amplification assays. *Sex Transm Dis* 1998;25:108–117.
17. Warren R, Dwyer B, Plackett M, et al. Comparative evaluation of detection assays for *Chlamydia trachomatis. J Clin Microbiol* 1993;31:1663–1666.
18. Handsfield HH, Alexander ER, Pin Wang S, et al. Differences in the therapeutic response of chlamydia-positive and chlamydia-negative forms of nongonococcal urethritis. *J Am Vener Dis Assoc* 1976;2:5–9.
19. Bowie WR, Wang SP, Alexander ER, et al. Etiology of nongonococcal urethritis: evidence for *Chlamydia trachomatis* and *Ureaplasma urealyticum. J Clin Invest* 1977;59:735–742.
20. Stimson JB, Hale J, Bowie WR, et al. Tetracycline-resistant *Ureaplasma urealyticum:* a cause for persistent nongonococcal urethritis. *Ann Intern Med* 1981;94:192–194.

21. Magalhaes M. Persistent nongonococcal urethritis associated with a minocycline-resistant strain of *Ureaplasma urealyticum. Sex Transm Dis* 1983;10:151–152.
22. Arya OP, Pratt BC. Persistent urethritis due to *Ureaplasma urealyticum* in conjugal or stable partnerships. *Genitourin Med* 1986;62:329–332.
23. Horner P, Thomas B, Gilroy CB, et al. Role of *Mycoplasma genitalium* and *Ureaplasma urealyticum* in acute and chronic nongonococcal urethritis. *Clin Infect Dis* 2001;32:995–1003.
24. Totten PA, Schwartz MA, Sjostrom KE, et al. Association of *Mycoplasma genitalium* with nongonococcal urethritis in heterosexual men. *J Infect Dis* 2001;183:269–276.
25. Keane FE, Thomas BJ, Gilroy CB, et al. The association of *Chlamydia trachomatis* and *Mycoplasma genitalium* with non-gonococcal urethritis: observations on heterosexual men and their female partners. *Int J STD AIDS* 2000;11:435–439.
26. Maeda S-I, Tamaki M, Kojima K, et al. Association of *Mycoplasma genitalium* persistence in the urethra with recurrence of nongonococcal urethritis *Sex Transm Dis* 2001;28:472–476.
27. Krieger JN, Jenny C, Verdon M, et al. Clinical manifestations of trichomoniasis in men. *Ann Intern Med* 1993;118:844–849.
28. Borchardt KA, al-Haraci S, Maida N. Prevalence of *Trichomonas vaginalis* in a male sexually transmitted disease clinic population by interview, wet mount microscopy, and the InPouch TV test. *Genitourin Med* 1995;71:405–406.
29. Krieger JN. Trichomoniasis in men: old issues and new data. *Sex Transm Dis* 1995;22:83–96.
30. Corey L, Adams HG, Brown ZA, et al. Genital herpes simplex virus infection: clinical manifestations, course, and complications. *Ann Intern Med* 1983;98:958–972.
31. Bowie WR, Alexander ER, Stimson JB, et al. Therapy for non-gonococcal urethritis: double blind, randomized comparison of two doses and two durations of minocycline. *Ann Intern Med* 1981;95:306–311.
32. Stamm WE, Hicks CB, Martin DH, et al. Azithromycin for empirical treatment of the nongonococcal urethritis syndrome in men: a randomized double-blind study. *JAMA* 1995;274:545–549.
33. Magid D, Douglas JM Jr, Schwartz JS. Doxycycline compared with azithromycin for treating women with genital *Chlamydia trachomatis* infections: an incremental cost-effectiveness analysis. *Ann Intern Med* 1996;124:389–399.
34. Romanowski B, Talbot H, Stadnyk M, et al. Minocycline compared with doxycycline in the treatment of nongonococcal urethritis and mucopurulent cervicitis. *Ann Intern Med* 1993;199:16–22.
35. Campbell WF, Dodson MG. Clindamycin therapy for *Chlamydia trachomatis* in women. *Am J Obstet Gynecol* 1990;162:343–347.
36. Cromblehome WR, Schacter J, Grossman M, et al. Amoxicillin therapy for *Chlamydia trachomatis* infections in pregnancy. *Obstet Gynecol* 1990;75:752–756.
37. Centers for Disease Control and Prevention. Recommendations for the prevention and management of *Chlamydia trachomatis* infections, 1993. *MMWR Morb Mortal Wkly Rep* 1993;42(RR-12):1–39.
38. Wong ES, Hooton TM, Hill CC, et al. Clinical and microbiological features of persistent or recurrent nongonococcal urethritis in men. *J Infect Dis* 1988;158:1098–1101.
39. Berger RE. Recurrent nongonococcal urethritis. *JAMA* 1983;249:409.
40. Krieger JN, Hooton TM, Brust PJ, et al. Evaluation of chronic urethritis: defining the role for endoscopic procedures. *Arch Intern Med* 1988;148:703–707.
41. Stamm WE, Wagner KF, Amsel R, et al. Causes of the acute urethral syndrome in women. *N Engl J Med* 1980;303:409–415.
42. Stamm WE. Etiology and management of the acute urethral syndrome. *Sex Transm Dis* 1981;8:235–238.
43. Fihm SD, Johnson C, Stamm WE. *Escherichia coli* urethritis in women with symptoms of acute urinary tract infection. *J Infect Dis* 1988;73:196–199.
44. Kamwendo F, Johansson E, Moi H, et al. Gonorrhea, genital chlamydial infection, and nonspecific urethritis in male partners of women hospitalized and treated for acute pelvic inflammatory disease. *Sex Transm Dis* 1993;20:143–146.

45. Rein MF. Vulvovaginitis and cervicitis. In: Mandell GL, Bennett JE, Dolin R, eds. *Principles and practice of infectious diseases,* 5th ed. New York: Churchill Livingstone, 2000:1218–1235.
46. Brunham RC, Paavonen J, Stevens CE, et al. Mucopurulent cervicitis—the ignored counterpart in women of urethritis in men. *N Engl J Med* 1984;11:1–6.
47. Tait IA, Rees E, Hobson D, et al. Chlamydial infection of the cervix in contacts of men with nongonococcal urethritis. *Br J Vener Dis* 1980;56:37–45.
48. Mardh PA, Moller BR, and Paavonen J. Chlamydial infection of the female genital tract with emphasis on pelvic inflammatory disease. A review of Scandinavian studies. *Sex Transm Dis* 1981;8:140.
49. Paavonen J, Vesterinen E. *Chlamydia trachomatis* in cervicitis and urethritis in women. *Scand J Infect Dis* 1982;32[Suppl]:45–54.
50. Pazin GH. Management of oral and genital herpes simplex viral infections: diagnosis and treatment. *Disease A Month: DM* 1986;32:725–784.
51. Reid R, Greenburg M, Jenson AB, et al. Sexually transmitted papillomavirus infections. I. The anatomic distribution and pathologic grade of neoplastic lesions associated with different viral types. *Am J Obstet Gynecol* 1987;156:212–222.
52. Franco EL. Epidemiology of anogenital warts and cancer. *Obstet Gynecol Clin North Am* 1996;23:597–623.
53. Anends MJ, Buckley CH, Wells M. Aetiology, pathogenesis, and pathology of cervical neoplasia. *J Clin Pathol* 1998;51:96–103.
54. Koutsky LA, Holmes KK, Critchlow CW, et al. A cohort study of the risk of cervical intraepithelial neoplasia grade 2 or 3 in relation to papillomavirus infection. *N Engl J Med* 1992;327:1272–1278.
55. Kabbutat MHG, Vousden KH. Role of E6 and E7 oncoproteins in HPV-induced anogenital malignancies. *Semin Virol* 1996;7:295–304.
56. Ho GYF, Bierman R, Beardsly L, et al. Natural history of cervicovaginal papillomavirus infection in young women. *N Engl J Med* 1998;338:423–428.
57. Kotloff KL, Wasserman SS, Russ K, et al. Detection of genital human papillomavirus and associated cytological abnormalities among college women. *Sex Transm Dis* 1998;25:243–250.
58. Moscicki A-B, Shiboski S, Broering J, et al. The natural history of human papillomavirus infection as measured by repeated DNA testing in adolescent and young women. *J Pediatr* 1998;132:277–284.
59. Minkoff H, Feldman J, DeHovitrz J, et al. A longitudinal study of human papillomavirus carriage in human immunodeficiency virus-infected and human immunodeficiency virus-uninfected women. *Am J Obstet Gynecol* 1998;178:982–986.
60. Franco EL, Villa LL, Sobrinho JP, et al. Epidemiology of acquisition and clearance of cervical human papillomavirus infection in women from a high-risk area for cervical cancer. *J Infect Dis* 1999;180:1415–1423.
61. Wentworth BB, Bonin P, Holmes KK, et al. Isolation of viruses, bacteria and other organisms from venereal disease clinic patients: methodology and problems associated with multiple isolations. *Health Lab Sci* 1973;10:75–81.
62. Spence MR, Barbacci M, Kappus E, et al. A correlative study of Papanicolaou smear, fluorescent antibody, and culture for the diagnosis of *Chlamydia trachomatis. Obstet Gynecol* 1986;68:691–695.
63. Paavonen J, Critchlow CW, DeRouen T, et al. Etiology of cervical inflammation. *Am J Obstet Gynecol* 1986;154:556–564.
64. Harrison HR, Costin M, Meder JB, et al. Cervical *Chlamydia trachomatis* infection in university women: relationship to history, contraceptives, ectopy, and cervicitis. *Am J Obstet Gynecol* 1985;153:224–251.
65. Quinn TC, Gupta PK, Burkman RT. Detection of *Chlamydia trachomatis* cervical infections: acomparison of Papanicolaou and immunofluorescent staining with cell cultures. *Am J Obstet Gynecol* 1987;157:394–399.
66. Moscicki B, Shafer MA, Millstein SG, et al. The use and limitations of endocervical Gram stain and mucopurulent cervicitis as predictors for *Chlamydia trachomatis* in female adolescents. *Am J Obstet Gynecol* 1987;157:65–71.
67. Nugent RP, Hillier SL. Mucopurulent cervicitis as a predictor of chlamydial infection and adverse pregnancy outcome. *Sex Transm Dis* 1992;19:198–202.

68. Knud-Hansen CR, Reichart C, Pabst KM, et al. Surrogate methods to diagnose gonococcal and chlamydial cervicitis: comparison of leukocyte esterase dipstick, endocervical Gram stain, and culture. *Sex Transm Dis* 1991;18:211–216.
69. Katz BP, Caine VA, Jones RB. Diagnosis of mucopurulent cervicitis among women at risk for *Chlamydia trachomatis* infection. *Sex Transm Dis* 1989;16:103–106.
70. Dolter J, Bryant L, Janda JM. Evaluation of five rapid systems for the identification of *Neisseria gonorrhoeae. Diagn Microbiol Infect Dis* 1990;13:265–267.
71. Stary A, Ching SF, Teodorowicz L, et al. Comparison of the ligase chain reaction and culture for the diagnosis of *Neisseria gonorrhoeae* in genital and extragenital specimens. *J Clin Microbiol* 1997;35:239–242.
72. Kouomans EH, Johnson RE, Knapp JS, et al. Laboratory testing for *Neisseria gonorrhoeae* by recently introduced nonculture tests: a performance review with clinical and public health considerations. *Clin Infect Dis* 1998;27:1171–1180.
73. Howell MR, Quinn TC, Brathwaite W, et al. Screening women *for Chlamydia trachomatis* in family planning clinics: the cost-effectiveness of DNA amplification assays. *Sex Transm Dis* 1998;25:108–117.
74. Stamm WE. *Chlamydia trachomatis* infections in the adult. In: Holmes KK, Sparling PF, Märdh P-A, et al., eds. *Sexually transmitted diseases,* 3rd ed. New York: McGraw-Hill, 1999:407–422.
75. Mardh P-A. Chlamydia screening—yes, but of whom, when, by whom, and with what. *Ann N Y Acad Sci* 2000;900:286–292.
76. Cusini M, Ghislanzoni M. The importance of diagnosing genital herpes. *J Antimicr Chemother* 2001;47[Suppl T1]:9–16.
77. Marques AR, Straus SE. Herpes simplex type 2 infections—an update. *Adv Intern Med* 2000;45:175–208.
78. Wiesner PJ, Tronca E, Bonin P, et al. Clinical spectrum of pharyngeal gonococcal infections. *N Engl J Med* 1973;288:181–185.
79. Jones RB, Rabinovitch RA, Katz BP, et al. *Chlamydia trachomatis* in the pharynx and rectum of heterosexual patients at risk for genital infection. *Ann Intern Med* 1985;102:757–762.
80. Ronald A. Genital ulceration and clinical acumen. *Clin Infect Dis* 1997;25:299–300.
81. Rein MF. Genital skin and mucous membrane lesions. In: Mandell GL, Bennett JE, Dolin R, eds. *Principles and practice of infectious diseases,* 5th ed. New York: Churchill Livingstone, 2000:1201–1207.
82. DiCarlo RP, Martin DH. The clinical diagnosis of genital ulcer disease in men. *Clin Infect Dis* 1997;25:292–298.
83. Brown ST, Nalley JF, Kraus SJ. Molluscum contagiosum. *Sex Transm Dis* 1981;8:227–234.
84. Sehgal VN, Shyam-Prasad AL. Donovanosis: current concepts. *Int J Dermatol* 1986;25: 8–16.
85. Chapel TA. The variability of syphilitic chancres. *Sex Transm Dis* 1978;5:68–70.
86. DiCarlo RP, Armentor BS, Martin DH. Chancroid epidemiology in New Orleans men. *J Infect Dis* 1995;172:446–452.
87. Johnson RE, Nahmias AJ, Magder LS, et al. A seroepidemiologic survey of the prevalence of herpes simplex virus type 2 infection in the United States. *N Engl J Med.* 1989;321:7–12.
88. Flemming DT, McQuillan GM, Johnson RE, et al. Herpes simplex virus type 2 in the United States, 1976 to 1994. *N Engl J Med* 1997;337:1105–1111.
89. Wald A, Zeh J, Selke S, et al. Reactivation of genital herpes simplex virus type 2 infections in asymptomatic seropositive persons. *N Engl J Med* 2000;342:844–850.
90. Cusini M, Ghislanzoni M. The importance of diagnosing genital herpes. *J Antimicr Chemother* 2001;47[Suppl T1]:9–16.
91. Koutsky LA, Stevens CE, Holmes KK, et al. Underdiagnosis of genital herpes by current clinical and viral isolation procedures. *N Engl J Med* 1992;326:1533–1539.
92. Kulhanjian JA, Soroush V, Au DS, et al. Identification of women at unsuspected risk of primary infection with herpes simplex virus type 2 during pregnancy. *N Engl J Med* 1992;326:916–920.
93. Guinan MS, Wolinsky SM, Reichman RC. Epidemiology of genital herpes simplex virus infections. *Epidemiol Rev* 1985;7:127–146.

94. Lafferty WE, Coombs RW, Benedetti J, et al. Recurrences after oral and genital herpes simplex virus infection. Influence of the site of infection and viral type. *N Engl J Med* 1987;316:1444–1449.
95. Benedetti J, Corey L, Ashley R. Recurrence rates in genital herpes after symptomatic first episode infection. *Ann Intern Med* 1994;121:847–854.
96. Mertz GJ, Ashley R, Burke RL, et al. Double-blind, placebo-controlled trial of a herpes simplex virus type 2 glycoprotein vaccine in persons at high risk for genital herpes infection. *J Infect Dis* 1990;161:653–60.
97. Diaz-Mitoma F, Benningen G, Slutchuk M, et al. Etiology of nonvesicular genital ulcers in Winnipeg. *Sex Transm Dis* 1987;14:33–36.
98. Ashley R. Laboratory techniques in the diagnosis of herpes simplex infection. *Genitourin Med* 1993;69:174–183.
99. Marshall DS, Linfert DR, Draghi A, et al. Identification of herpes simplex virus genital infection: comparison of multiplex PCR assay and traditional viral isolation techniques. *Mod Pathol* 2001;14:152–156.
100. Lucotte G, Bathelier C, Lespiaux V, et al. Detection and genotyping of herpes simplex virus type 1 and 2 by polymerase chain reaction. *Mol Cell Probes* 1995;9:287–290.
101. Ashley RL, Wu L, Pickering JW, et al. Premarket evaluation of a commercial glycoprotein G-based enzyme immunoassay for herpes simplex virus type-specific antibodies. *J Clin Microbiol* 1998;36:294–295.
102. Prince HE, Ernst CE, Hogrefe WR. Evaluation of an enzyme immunoassay system for measuring herpes simplex (HSV) type 1-specific and HSV type 2-specific IgG antibodies. *J Clin Lab Anal* 2000;14:3–6.
103. Diagnology, Inc. P.O. Box 14643, Research Triangle Park, NC 27709. *www.diagnology.com*
104. Ashley RL, Eagelton M. Evaluation of a novel point of care test for antibodies to herpes simplex virus type 2. *Sex Transm Infect* 1998;74:228–229.
105. Corey L, et al. A trial of topical acyclovir in genital herpes simplex virus infections. *N Engl J Med* 1982;306:1313–1319.
106. Wald A. New therapies and prevention strategies for genital herpes. *Clin Infect Dis* 1999;28[Suppl 1]:S4–S13.
107. DiMitoma F, Sibbald RG, Shafran SD, et al. Oral famciclovir for the suppression of recurrent genital herpes: a randomized controlled trial. *JAMA* 1998;280:887–892.
108. Reitano M, Tyring S, Land W, et al. Valacyclovir for the suppression of recurrent genital herpes simplex virus infection: a large-scale dose range-finding study. *J Infect Dis* 1998;178:603–610.
109. Prober CG, Corey L, Brown ZA, et al. The management of pregnancies complicated by genital infections with herpes simplex virus. *Clin Infect Dis* 1992;15:1031–1038.
110. Centers for Disease Control and Prevention, Division of STD Prevention. *National Plan to Eliminate Syphilis from the United States.* October 1999.
111. Larsen SA, Hunter EF, Creighton ET. Syphilis. In: Holmes KK, et al., eds. *Sexually transmitted diseases,* 2nd ed. New York: McGraw-Hill, 1990:927–934.
112. Nakashima AK, Rolfs RT, Flock ML, et al. Epidemiology of syphilis in the United States, 1941–1993. *Sex Transm Dis* 1996;23:16–23.
113. Williams LA, Klausner JD, Whittington WLH, et al. Elimination and reintroduction of primary and secondary syphilis. *Am J Public Health* 1999;89:1093–1097.
114. St. Louis ME, Farley TA, Aral SO. Untangling the persistence of syphilis in the South. *Sex Transm Dis* 1996;23:1–4.
115. Rolfs RT, Goldberg M, Sharrar RG. Risk factors for syphilis: cocaine use and prostitution. *Am J Public Health* 1990;80:853–857.
116. Greenberg J, Schnell D, Conlon R. Behaviors of crack cocaine users and their impact on early syphilis intervention. *Sex Transm Dis* 1992;19:346–350.
117. Finelli L, Budd J, Spitalny KC. Early syphilis: relationship to sex, drugs, and changes in high-risk behavior from 1987–1990. *Sex Transm Dis* 1993;20:89–95.
118. Handsfield HH, Whittington WLH, Desmon S, et al. Resurgent bacterial sexually transmitted disease among men who have sex with men—King County, Washington, 1997–1999. *MMWR Morb Mortal Wkly Rep* 1999;48:773–777.
119. Chapel TA. The signs and symptoms of secondary syphilis. *Sex Transm Dis* 1980;7:161–164.

120. Chapel TA. Physician recognition of the signs and symptoms of secondary syphilis. *JAMA* 1981;246:250–251.
121. Stokes JH, Beerman H, Ingraham NR. *Modern clinical syphilology,* 3rd ed. Philadelphia: Saunders, 1944.
122. Swartz MN, Musher DM, Healy BP. Late syphilis. In: Holmes KK, Sparling PF, Mårdh P-A, et al., eds. *Sexually transmitted diseases,* 3rd ed. New York: McGraw-Hill, 1999:487–510.
123. Larsen SA, Steiner BM, Rudolph AH. Laboratory diagnosis and interpretation of tests for syphilis. *Clin Microbiol Rev* 1995;8:1–21.
124. Wicher K, Horowitz HW, Wicher V. Laboratory methods of diagnosis of syphilis for the beginning of the third millennium. *Microbes Infect* 1999;1:1035–1049.
125. Liu H, Rodes B, Chen CY, et al. New tests for syphilis: rational design of a PCR method for detection of *Treponema pallidum* in clinical specimens using unique regions of the DNA polymerase I gene. *J Clin Microbiol* 2001;39:1941–1946.
126. Young H. Guidelines for serologic testing for syphilis. *Sex Transm Infect* 2000;76:403–405.
127. White TJ, Fuller SA. Visuwell reagin, a nontreponemal enzyme-linked immunosorbent assay for the serodiagnosis of syphilis. *J Clin Microbiol* 1989;27:2300–2304.
128. Brown ST, Zaidi A, Larsen SA. Serological response to syphilis treatment: a new analysis of old data. *JAMA* 1985;253:1296–1299.
129. Romanowski B, Sutherland R, Fick GH, et al. Serologic response to treatment of infectious syphilis. *Ann Intern Med* 1991;114:1005–1009.
130. Rolfs RT, Joesoef MR, Hendershot EF, et al. A randomized trial of enhanced therapy for early syphilis in patients with and without human immunodeficiency virus infection. *N Engl J Med* 1997;337:307–314.
131. Orton SL, Dodd RY, Williams AE, et al. Absence of risk factors for false-positive test results in blood donors with a reactive automated treponemal test (PK-TP) for syphilis. *Transfusion* 2001;41:744–750.
132. Halling VW, Jones MF, Bestrom JE, et al. Clinical comparison of the *Treponema pallidum* CAPTIA syphilis-G enzyme immunoassay with the fluorescent treponemal antibody absorption immunoglobulin G assay for syphilis testing. *J Clin Microbiol* 1999;37:3233–3234.
133. Alberle-Grasse J, Orton SL, Notari E 4th, et al. Predictive value of past and current screening tests for syphilis in blood donors: changing from a rapid plasma reagin test to an automated specific treponemal test for screening. *Transfusion* 1999;39:206–211.
134. Pope V, Fears MB, Morrill WE, et al. Comparison of the Serodia *Treponema pallidum* particle agglutination, Captia Syphilis-G, and SpiroTek Reagin II tests with standard test techniques for diagnosis of syphilis. *J Clin Microbiol* 2000;38:2543–2545.
135. Schmidt BL, Edjlalipour M, Luger A. Comparative evaluation of nine different enzyme-linked immunosorbent assays for determination of antibodies against *Treponema pallidum* in patients with primary syphilis. *J Clin Microbiol* 2000;38:1279–1282.
136. Young H, Moyes A, Seagar L. A novel recombinant-antigen enzyme assay for serological diagnosis of syphilis. *J Clin Microbiol* 1998;36:913–917.
137. Sambri V, Marangoni A, Simone MA, et al. Evaluation of recomWell Treponema, a novel recombinant antigen-based enzyme-linked immunosorbent assay for the diagnosis of syphilis. *Clin Microbiol Infect* 2001;7:200–205.
138. Murphy FT, George R, Kubota K, et al. The use of Western blotting as the confirmatory test for syphilis in patients with rheumatic disease. *J Rheumatol* 1999;26:2448–2453.
139. Magnarelli LA, Anderson JF, Johnson RC, et al. Cross-reactivity in serological tests for Lyme disease and other spirochetal infections. *J Infect Dis* 1987;156:183–188.
140. Rolfs RT. Treatment of syphilis, 1993. *Clin Infect Dis* 1995;20[Suppl 1]:S23–S38.
141. Augenbraun MH, Rolfs RT. Treatment of syphilis 1998: nonpregnant adult. *Clin Infect Dis* 1999;28[Suppl 1]:S21–S28.
142. Musher DM, Baughin RE. Neurosyphilis in HIV-infected persons. *N Engl J Med* 1994; 331:1516.
143. Hook EW, III, Baker-Zander SA, Moskovitz BL, et al. Ceftriaxone therapy for asymptomatic neurosyphilis. *Sex Transm Dis* 1986;13:185–188.
144. Genc M, Ledger WJ. Syphilis in pregnancy. *Sex Transm Infect* 2000;76:73–79.

145. Rompalo AM, Joesoef MR, O'Donnell JA, et al. Clinical manifestations of early syphilis by HIV status and gender: results of the syphilis and HIV study. *Sex Transm Dis* 2001;28:158–165.
146. Musher DM, Hamill RJ, Baughn RE. Effect of human immunodeficiency virus (HIV) infection on the course of syphilis and on the response to treatment. *Ann Intern Med* 1990;113:872–881.
147. Gourevitch MN, Selwyn PA, Davenny K, et al. Effects of HIV infection on the serologic manifestations and response to treatment of syphilis in intravenous drug users. *Ann Intern Med* 1993;118:350–355.
148. Musher DM. Syphilis, neurosyphilis, penicillin and AIDS. *J Infect Dis* 1991;163:1201–1206.
149. Johns DR, Tierney M, Felsenstein D. Alteration in the natural history of neurosyphilis by concurrent infection with human immunodeficiency virus. *N Engl J Med* 1987;316:1569–1572.
150. Trees DL, Morse SA. Chancroid and *Haemophilus ducreyi:* an update. *Clin Microbiol Rev* 1995;8:357–375.
151. Marrazzo JM, Handsfield HH. Chancroid: new developments in an old disease. *Curr Clin Top Infect Dis* 1995;15:129–152.
152. DiCarlo RP, Armentor BS, Martin DH. Chancroid epidemiology in New Orleans men. *J Infect Dis* 1995;172:446–452.
153. Jessamine PG, Ronald AR. Chancroid and the role of genital ulcer disease in the spread of human retroviruses. *Med Clin North Am* 1990;64:1417–1431.
154. Ronald A. Genital ulceration and clinical acumen. *Clin Infect Dis* 1997;25:299–300.
155. Lewis DA. Diagnostic tests for chancroid. *Sex Transm Infect* 2000;76:137–141.
156. Morse SA, Trees DL, Htun Y, et al. Comparison of clinical diagnosis and standard laboratory and molecular methods for the diagnosis of genital ulcer disease in Lesotho: association with human immunodeficiency virus infection. *J Infect Dis* 1997;175:583–589.
157. Totten PA, Kuypers JM, Checn CY, et al. Etiology of genital ulcer disease in Dakar, Senegal, and comparison of PCR and serologic assays for detection of *Hemophilus ducreyi. J Clin Microbiol* 2000;38:268–273.
158. Schmid GP. Treatment of chancroid, 1997. *Clin Infect Dis* 1999;28[Suppl 1]:S14–S20.
159. D'Souza P, Pandhi RK, Khanna N, et al. A comparative study of therapeutic response of patients with clinical chancroid to ciprofloxacin, erythromycin, and cotrimoxazole. *Sex Transm Dis* 1998;25:293–295.
160. Malonza IM, Tyndall MW, Ndinya-Achola JO, et al. A randomized, double-blind, placebo-controlled trial of single-dose ciprofloxacin versus erythromycin for the treatment of chancroid in Nairobi, Kenya. *J Infect Dis* 1999;180:1886–1893.
161. Bowden FJ, Mein J, Plunkett C, et al. Pilot study of azithromycin in the treatment of genital donovanosis. *Genitourin Med* 1996;72:17–19.
162. Anonymous. National guideline for the management of donovanosis (granuloma inguinale). *Sex Transm Infect* 1999;75[Suppl 1]:S38–S39.
163. Schwartz JJ, Myskowski PL. Molluscum contagiosum in patients with human immunodeficiency virus infection. *J Am Acad Dermatol* 1992;27:583–588.
164. Meadows KP, Tyring SK, Paviz AT, et al. Resolution of recalcitrant molluscum contagiosum virus lesions in human immunodeficiency virus-infected patients treated with cidofovir. *Arch Dermatol* 1997;133:987–990.
165. Schultz RE, Skelton HG. Value of acetic acid screening for flat genital condylomata in men. *J Urol* 1988;139:777–779.
166. Clavel C, Masure M, Bory JP, et al. Human papillomavirus testing in primary screening for the detection of high-grade cervical lesions: a study of 7932 women. *Br J Cancer* 2001;84:1616–1623.
167. Denny L, Kuhn L, Risi L, et al. Two stage cervical cancer screening: an alternative for resource-poor settings. *Am J Obstet Gynecol* 2000;183:383–388.
168. Medical Letter. Podofilox for genital warts. *Med Lett Drugs Ther* 1991;33:117–118.
169. Beutner KR, Spraunce SL, Hougham AJ, et al. Treatment of genital warts with an immune-response modifier (imiquimod). *J Am Acad Dermatol* 1998;38:230–239.

170. Eron LJ, Judson F, Tucker S, et al. Interferon therapy for condylomata acuminata. *N Engl J Med* 1986;315:1059–1064.
171. Eisenstein BI, Masi AT. Disseminated gonococcal infections (DGI) and gonococcal arthritis (GCA). 1. Bacteriology, epidemiology, host factors, pathogen factors, and pathology. 2. Clinical manifestations, diagnosis, complications, treatment, and prevention. *Semin Arthr Rheum* 1981;10:155–172.
172. O'Brien JP, Goldenberg DL, Rice PA, et al. Disseminated gonococcal infection: a prospective analysis of 49 patients and a review of pathophysiology and immune mechanisms. *Medicine (Baltimore)* 1983;62:395–406.
173. Rompalo AM, Hook EW 3rd, Roberts PL, et al. The acute arthritis-dermatitis syndrome: The changing importance of *Neisseria gonorrhoeae* and *Neisseria meningitidis. Arch Intern Med* 1987;147:281–283.
174. Chapel TA, Katta T, Kusmar T, et al. Pediculosis pubis in a clinic for sexually transmitted diseases. *Sex Transm Dis* 1979;6:257–260.
175. Chosidow O. Scabies and pediculosis. *Lancet* 2000;355:819–826.
176. Miller RA. Maculae ceruleae. *Int J Dermatol* 1986;25:383–384.
177. Brown S, Becher J, Brady W. Treatment of ectoparasitic infections: review of the English-language literature, 1982–1992. *Clin Infect Dis* 1995;20[Suppl1]:S104–S109.
178. Anonymous. National guideline for the management of *Phthirus pubis* infestation. *Sex Transm Infect* 1999;75[Suppl 1]:S78–S79.
179. Anonymous. National guideline for the management of scabies. *Sex Transm Infect* 1999;75[Suppl 1]:S76–S77.
180. Meinking TL, Taplin D. Safety of permethrin vs lindane for the treatment of scabies. *Arch Dermatol* 1996;132:959–962.
181. Taplin D, Meinking TL, Chen JA, et al. Comparison of crotamiton 10% cream (Eurax) and permethrin 5% cream (Elemite) for the treatment of scabies in children. *Pediatric Dermatol* 1990;7:67–73.
182. Meinking TL, Taplin D, Hermida JL, et al. The treatment of scabies with ivermectin. *N Engl J Med* 1995;333:26–30.
183. Usha V, Gopalakrishnan Nari TV. A comparative study of oral ivermectin and topical permethrin cream in the treatment of scabies. *J Am Acad Dermatol* 2000;42:236–240.
184. Elmogy M, Fayed H, Marzok H, et al. Oral ivermectin in the treatment of scabies. *Int J Dermatol* 1999;38:926–928.
185. Victoria J, Trujillo R. Topical ivermectin: a new successful treatment for scabies. *Pediatric Dermatol* 2001;18:63–65.
186. Funkhauser ME, Ross A. Management of scabies in patients with human immunodeficiency virus disease. *Arch Dermatol* 1993;129:911–913.
187. Corbett EL, Crossley I, Holton J, et al. Crusted ("Norwegian") scabies in a specialist HIV unit: successful use of ivermectin and failure to prevent nosocomial transmission. *Genitourin Med* 1996;72:115–117.
188. Centers for Disease Control and Prevention. Nonreported sexually transmitted diseases. *MMWR Morb Mortal Wkly Rev* 1979;28:61.
189. Sobel JD. Epidemiology and pathogenesis of recurrent vulvovaginal candidiasis. *Am J Obstet Gynecol* 1985;152:924–935.
190. Spinillo A, Capuzzo E, Gulminetti R, et al. Prevalence of and risk factors for fungal vaginitis caused by non-albicans species. *Am J Obstet Gynecol* 1997;176:138–141.
191. Redondo-Lopez V, Lynch M, Schmitt CA, et al. *Torulopsis glabrata* vaginitis: clinical aspects and susceptibility to antifungal agents. *Obstet Gynecol* 1990;76:651–655.
192. Geiger AM, Foxman B, Sobel JD. Chronic vulvovaginal candidiasis: characteristics of women with *Candida albicans, C. glabrata* and no candida. *Genitourin Med* 1995;75:304–307.
193. Sobel JD, Chaim W. Treatment of *Torulopsis glabrata* vaginitis: a retrospective review of boric acid therapy. *Clin Infect Dis* 1997;24:649–652.
194. Larsen B. Vaginal flora in health and disease. *Clin Obstet Gynecol* 1993;36:107–121.
195. Sobel JD. Pathogenesis and treatment of recurrent vulvovaginal candidiasis. *Clin Infect Dis* 1992;14[Suppl 1]:5148–5153.
196. Heidrich FE, Berg AO, Bergman JJ. Clothing factors and vaginitis. *J Fam Pract* 1984;19:491–494.

197. Imam N, Carpenter CCJ, Mayer KH, et al. Hierarchical pattern of mucosal *Candida* infections with HIV seropositive women. *Am J Med* 1990;89:142–146.
198. Reed BD, Pierson CL. Evaluation of a latex agglutination test for identification of *Candida* species in vaginal discharge. *J Am Board Fam Pract* 1992;5:375–380.
199. Pastorek JG II, Cotch MF, Martin DH, et al. Clinical and microbiological correlates of vaginal trichomoniasis during pregnancy. *Clin Infect Dis* 1996;23:1075–1080.
200. Sorvillo F, Kovacs A, Kerndt P, et al. Risk factors for trichomoniasis among women with human immunodeficiency virus (HIV) infection at a public clinic in Los Angeles County, California: implications for HIV prevention. *Am J Trop Med Hyg* 1998;58:495–500.
201. Rein MF. *Trichomonas vaginalis.* In: Mandell GL, Bennett JE, Dolin R, eds. *Principles and practice of infectious diseases,* 5th ed. New York: Churchill Livingstone,2000:2894–2898.
202. Wolner-Hanssen P, Krieger JN, Stevens CE, et al. Clinical manifestations of vaginal trichomoniasis. *JAMA* 1989;264:571–576.
203. Krieger JN, Tam MR, Stevens CE, et al. Diagnosis of trichomoniasis: comparison of conventional wet mount examination with cytologic studies, cultures, and monoclonal antibody straining of direct specimens. *JAMA* 1988;259:1223–1227.
204. Carney JA, Unadkat P, Yule A, et al. A new rapid agglutination test for the diagnosis of *Trichomonas vaginalis* infection. *J Clin Pathol* 1988;41:806–808.
205. Yule A, Gellan MC, Oriel JD, et al. Detection *of Trichomonas vaginalis* antigen in women by enzymc immunoassay. *J Clin Pathol* 1987;40:566–568.
206. DeMeo LR, Draper DL, McGregor JA, et al. Evaluation of a deoxyribonucleic acid probe for the detection of *Trichomonas vaginalis* in vaginal secretions. *Am J Obstet Gynecol* 1996;174:1339–1342.
207. Heine RP, Wiesenfeld HC, Sweet RL. Polymerase chain reaction analysis of distal vaginal specimens: a less invasive strategy for detection of *Trichomonas vaginalis. Clin Infect Dis* 1997;24:985–987.
208. Shaio MF, Lin PR, Liu JY. Colorimetric one-tube nested PCR for detection of *Trichomonas vaginalis* in vaginal discharge. *J Clin Microbiol* 1997;35:132–138.
209. Levi MH, Torres J, Pina C, et al. Comparison of the InPouch TV culture system and Diamond's modified medium for detection of *Trichomonas vaginalis. J Clin Microbiol* 1997;35:3308–3310.
210. Thorsen P, Jensen IP, Jeune B, et al. Few microorganisms associated with bacterial vaginosis may constitute the pathologic core: a population-based microbiologic study among 3596 pregnant women. *Am J Obstet Gynecol* 1998;178:580–587.
211. Hawes SE, Hillier SL, Benedetti J, et al. Hydrogen peroxide-producing lactobacilli and acquisition of vaginal infections. *J Infect Dis* 1996;174:1058–1063.
212. Blackwell AL. Vaginal bacterial phaginosis? *Sex Transm Infect* 1999;75:352–353.
213. Hay PE. Recurrent bacterial vaginosis. *Curr Infect Dis Rep* 2000;2:506–511.
214. Thomason JL, Gelbart SM, Anderson RJ, et al. Statistical evaluation *of* diagnostic criteria for bacterial vaginosis. *Am J Obstet Gynecol* 1990;102:155–160.
215. Goldenberg RL, Iams JD, Mercer BM, et al. The preterm prediction study: the value of new *vs* standard risk factors in predicting early and all spontaneous preterm births. NICHD MFMU Network. *Am J Public Health* 1998;88:233–238.
216. Morales WJ, Schorr S, Albritton J, et al. Effect of metronidazole in patients with preterm birth in preceding pregnancy and bacterial vaginosis: a placebo-controlled, double-blind study. *Am J Obstet Gynecol* 1994;171:345–347.
217. McDonald HM, O'Loughlin JA, Vigneswaran R, et al. Impact of metronidazole therapy on preterm birth in women with bacterial vaginosis flora (*Gardnerella vaginalis*): a randomized, placebo controlled trial. *Br J Obstet Gynaecol* 1997;104:1391–1397.
218. Peipert JF, Mantagno AB, Cooper AS, et al. Bacterial vaginosis as a risk factor for upper genital tract infection. *Am J Obstet Gynecol* 1997;177:1184–1187.
219. Sweet RL. Role of bacterial vaginosis in pelvic inflammatory disease. *Clin Infect Dis* 1995;20[Suppl 2]:S271–S275.
220. Schwebke JR, Hillier SL, Sobel JD, et al. Validity of the vaginal gram stain for the diagnosis of bacterial vaginosis. *Obstet Gynecol* 1996;88:573–576.
221. Weisberg M. Treatment of vaginal candidiasis in pregnant women. *Clin Therap* 1986;8:563–567.

222. Nixon SA. Vulvovaginitis: the role of patient compliance in treatment success. *Am J Obstet Gynecol* 1991;165:1207–1209.
223. Reef SE, Levine WC, McNeil MM, et al. Treatment options for vulvovaginal candidiasis, 1993. *Clin Infect Dis* 1995;20[Suppl 1]:S80–S90.
224. Sobel JD, Chaim W. Vaginal microbiology of women with recurrent vulvovaginal candidiasis. *J Clin Microbiol* 1996;34:2497–2502.
225. Shalev E, Battino S, Weiner E, et al. Ingestion of yogurt containing *Lactobacillus acidophilus* compared with pasteurized yogurt as prophylaxis for recurrent candidal vaginitis and bacterial vaginosis. *Arch Fam Med* 1996;5:593–596.
226. Fong IW. The value of prophylactic (monthly) clotrimazole versus empiric self-treatment in recurrent vaginal candidiasis. *Genitourin Med* 1994;70:124–126.
227. Spinillo A, Colonna L, Piazzi G, et al. Managing recurrent vulvovaginal candidiasis: intermittent prevention with itraconazole. *J Reprod Med* 1997;42:83–87.
228. Fong IW. The value of treating sexual partners of women with recurrent vaginal candidiasis with ketoconazole. *Genitourin Med* 1992;68:174–176.
229. Spinillo A, Carrata L, Pizzoli G. Recurrent vulvovaginal candidiasis: results of a cohort study of sexual transmission and intestinal reservoir. *J Reprod Med* 1992;37:343–347.
230. Sobel JD, Faro S, Force RW. Vulvovaginal candidiasis: epidemiologic, diagnostic, and therapeutic considerations. *Am J Obstet Gynecol* 1996;178:203–211.
231. Sobel JD, Chaim W. Treatment of *Torulopsis glabrata* vaginitis: a retrospective review of boric acid therapy. *Clin Infect Dis* 1997;24:649–652.
232. Van Slyke KK, Michel VP, Rein MF. Boric acid powder treatment of vulvovaginal candidiasis. *Am J Obstet Gynecol* 1981;141:145–148.
233. Fidel PJ Jr, Sobel JD. Immunopathogenesis of recurrent vulvovaginal candidiasis. *Clin Microbiol Rev* 1996;9:335–348.
234. Greaves WL, Chungafung J, Morris B, et al. Clindamycin versus metronidazole in the treatment of bacterial vaginosis. *Obstet Gynecol* 1988;72:799–802.
235. Wathne B, Hovelius B, Holst E. Cefadroxil as an alternative to metronidazole in the treatment of bacterial vaginosis. *Scand J Infect Dis* 1989;21:585–586.
236. Mikamo H, Kawazoe K, Izumi K, et al. Comparative study on vaginal or oral treatment of bacterial vaginosis. *Chemotherapy* 1997;43:60–68.
237. Ferris DG, Litaker MS, Woodward L, et al. Treatment of bacterial vaginosis: a comparison of oral metronidazole, metronidazole vaginal gel, and clindamycin vaginal cream. *J Fam Pract* 1995;41:443–449.
238. Mikamo H, Kawazoe K, Izumi K, et al. Bacteriological epidemiology and treatment of bacterial vaginosis. *Chemotherapy* 1996;42:78–84.
239. McGregor JA, French JL, Jones W, et al. Bacterial vaginosis is associated with prematurity and vaginal fluid mucinase and sialidase: results of a controlled trial of topical clindamycin cream. *Am J Obstet Gynecol* 1994;171:1048–1060.
240. Joesoef MR, Hillier SL, Wiknjosastro G, et al. Intravaginal clindamycin treatment for bacterial vaginosis: effects on preterm delivery and low birth weight. *Am J Obstet Gynecol* 1995;173:1527–1531.
241. Galask RP, Bowdler N. Open label evaluation of 0.75% metronidazole gel in the treatment of bacterial vaginosis. Annual Meeting of the Infectious Disease Society for Obstetrics and Gynecology, August 6–8, 1992, San Diego.
242. McGregor JA, Livengood C III, French JI, et al. Intravaginal metronidazole gel (0.75%) for bacterial vaginosis: results of a double-blinded, randomized, placebo-controlled trial. Annual Meeting of the Infectious Disease Society for Obstetrics and Gynecology, August 6–8, 1992, San Diego.
243. Hillier SL, Lipinski C, Briselden AM, et al. Efficacy of intravaginal 0.75% metronidazole gel for the treatment of bacterial vaginosis. *Obstet Gynecol* 1993;81:963–967.
244. Larsen B. Vaginal flora in health and disease. *Clin Obstet Gynecol* 1993;36:107–121.
245. Eschenbach DA, Thwin SS, Patton DL, et al. Influence of the normal menstrual cycle on vaginal tissue, discharge, and microflora. *Clin Infect Dis* 2000;30:901–907.
246. Chandler SH, Holmes KK, Wentworth BB, et al. The epidemiology of cytomegaloviral infection in women attending a sexually transmitted disease clinic. *J Infect Dis* 1985;152:597–605.

247. Jacobson L, Westrom L. Objectivized diagnosis of acute pelvic inflammatory disease. Diagnostic and prognostic value of routine laparoscopy. *Am J Obstet Gynecol* 1969;105:1088–1098.
248. Paavonen J, Aine R, Teisala K, et al. Comparison of endometrial biopsy and peritoneal fluid cytologic testing with laparoscopy in the diagnosis of acute pelvic inflammatory disease. *Am J Obstet Gynecol* 1985;151:645–650.
249. Walker CK, Workowski KA, Washington AE, et al. Anaerobes in pelvic inflammatory disease: implications for the Centers for Disease Control and Prevention's guidelines for treatment of sexually transmitted diseases. *Clin Infect Dis* 1999;28[Suppl 1]:S29–S36.
250. Safrin S, Schachter J, Dahrouge D, et al. Long-term sequelae of acute pelvic inflammatory disease. A retrospective cohort study. *Am J Obstet Gynecol* 1992;166:1300–1305.
251. Westrom L. Effect of acute pelvic inflammatory disease on fertility. *Am J Obstet Gynecol* 1975;121:707–713.
252. Toth M, Witkin SS, Ledger W, et al. The role of infection in the etiology of preterm birth. *Obstet Gynecol* 1988;71:723–726.
253. Scholes D, Stergachis A, Heidrich FE, et al. Prevention of pelvic inflammatory disease by screening for cervical chlamydial infection. *N Engl J Med* 1996;334:1362–1366.
254. Landers DV, Sweet RL. Tubo-ovarian abscess: contemporary approach to management. *Rev Infect Dis* 1983;5:876–884.
255. Reed SD, Landers DV, Sweet RL. Antibiotic treatment of tuboovarian abscess: comparison of broad-spectrum $\beta$-lactam agents versus clindamycin-containing regimens. *Am J Obstet Gynecol* 1991;164:1556–1561; discussion 1561–1562.
256. Wiesenfeld HC, Sweet RL. Progress in the management of tuboovarian abscesses. *Clin Obstet Gynecol* 1993;36:433–444.
257. Lippes J. Pelvic actinomycosis: a review and preliminary look at prevalence. *Am J Obstet Gynecol* 1999;180:265–269.
258. Chaim W, Bashiri A, Bar-David J, et al. Prevalence and clinical significance of postpartum endometritis and wound infection. *Infect Dis Obstet Gynecol* 2000;8:77–82.
259. Schorge JO, Granter SR, Lerner LH, et al. Postpartum and vulvar necrotizing fasciitis. Early clinical diagnosis and histopathologic correlation. *J Reprod Med* 1998;43:586–590.
260. Nolan TE, King LA, Smith RP, et al. Necrotizing surgical infection and necrotizing fasciitis in obstetric and gynecologic patients. *South Med J* 1993;86:1363–1367.
261. Stubblefield PG, Grimes DA. Septic abortion. *N Engl J Med* 1994;331:310–314.
262. Brown CE, Stettler RW, Twickler D, et al. Puerperal septic pelvic thrombophlebitis: incidence and response to heparin therapy. *Am J Obstet Gynecol* 1999;181:143–148.
263. Irving WL, James DK, Stephenson T, et al. Influenza virus infection in the second and third trimesters of pregnancy: a clinical and seroepidemiological study. *Br J Obstet Gynaecol* 2000;107:1282–1289.
264. Rodis JF, Rodner C, Hansen AA, et al. Long-term outcome of children following maternal human parvovirus B19 infection. *Obstet Gynecol* 1998;91:125–128.
265. Niebyl JR, Spence MR, Parmley TH. Sporadic (nonepidemic) puerperal mastitis. *J Reprod Med* 1978;20:97–100.

# 17. INFECTIONS DUE TO FUNGI, *ACTINOMYCES,* AND *NOCARDIA*

Harold M. Henderson and Stanley W. Chapman

An organized approach to fungal infections is outlined in this chapter, which is divided into sections that describe each mycosis. The epidemiologic settings, host status, skin tests, and serologic information associated with the major fungal diseases are listed in Table 17.1 and should assist the reader in narrowing down the diagnostic possibilities in a given patient. The decision to initiate systemic antifungal chemotherapy may be difficult, and infectious disease consultation is strongly recommended to help determine the indications for the potentially toxic antifungal agents and to assist in their administration. Actinomycosis and nocardiosis are caused by organisms that are no longer classified as fungi. They are discussed separately at the end of this chapter.

## CANDIDIASIS

***Candida* species are normal inhabitants of mucocutaneous body surfaces** and commonly cause superficial skin disease and vaginitis. Under certain circumstances, they may **cause invasive disease if alterations in host defenses occur.** The incidence of *Candida* infections has increased markedly with the widespread use of antibiotics and immunosuppressive therapy, increased numbers of patients in critical care settings, and infection with human immunodeficiency virus (HIV) [1].

**I. Growth and identification characteristics. Many *Candida* species cause infection in humans,** including *C. tropicalis, C. krusei, C. parapsilosis,* and *C. glabrata,* **but the most common cause of clinical infection is *C. albicans.*** *Candida* species are yeasts and can be cultured easily on blood agar and Sabouraud dextrose agar in 24 to 48 hours. Presumptive identification of *C. albicans* can be made in 2 to 3 hours by a positive germ tube test (i.e., characteristic morphologic change seen on incubation of the yeast colony in serum). Definite species identification requires an additional 2 to 8 days.

**II. Epidemiologic and host factors.** *Candida* species are found worldwide and are normal commensals of humans.

**A. Colonization.** *Candida* is commonly cultured from the female genital tract, gastrointestinal (GI) tract, diseased skin, and from the urine of patients with indwelling Foley catheters. Colonization is more prevalent in hospitalized patients than in healthy individuals and is promoted by antibiotics that suppress normal bacterial growth.

**B. Host defense.** Intact skin, phagocytic cells such as neutrophils and monocytes, and the cell-mediated immune system are all important components of the host's resistance to infection by *Candida* species. **Alterations in host defenses** may lead to a change in the organism's normal commensal status, with subsequent tissue invasion and clinical disease. These alterations may be naturally occurring as in the cases of **diabetes mellitus** and **acquired immunodeficiency syndrome (AIDS).** More often, **iatrogenic factors** predispose to invasive candidiasis. The use of broad-spectrum antibiotics and corticosteroids, mucosal damage from instrumentation or chemotherapeutic agents, or a breach in the integrity of the skin by intravenous catheters or pressure-monitoring devices increases the risk of invasive disease.

**III. Clinical aspects**

**A. Cutaneous infections.** *Candida* commonly causes infection in warm moist areas of the skin such as the axillary, inguinal, and intergluteal regions. Perineal infection with involvement of the perianal area, thighs, scrotum, and penis (balanitis) is common. Diaper rash in infants often is caused by *Candida,* and angular cheilitis at the corners of the mouth may be caused by the organism as well. Each of these conditions is characterized by **erythematous papules or macules that may be confluent and are very pruritic.** Infection tends to be more extensive in the presence of immunosuppression. The diagnosis can be made by wet-mount examination of scrapings from the infected area with 10% to 20% KOH. *Candida* may also cause nail infection in the forms of paronychia or onychomycosis. Persons who frequently immerse their hands in water or wear occlusive gloves are particularly susceptible,

Table 17.1. Summary of Major Fungal Infections

| Fungus | Epidemiologic Features | Major Clinical Entities | Host/Setting | Skin Test | Immunologic Test | Value of Immunologic Studies |
|---|---|---|---|---|---|---|
| *Candida* | Worldwide | Cervical; vaginal | Normal; antibiotic use | Not helpful | | |
| | | Oropharyngeal | Normal; antibiotic use; steroid inhalers; immunocompromised | | | |
| | | Gastrointestinal; disseminated; isolated fungemia | Antibiotic use; i.v. catheters; immunocompromised; diabetes mellitus; extensive burns | | Precipitating antibody<br>Agglutinating antibody<br>Antigens<br>PCR | Not helpful (false-positive and false-negative results) |
| | | Endocarditis | Recent cardiac surgery; i.v. catheters; heroin addicts | | | |
| *Histoplasma* | Midwestern and southeastern U.S.[a]<br>Avian feces exposure | Acute pulmonary | Normal | Usually positive in endemic area; can cause false-positive *Histoplasma* serologic result | Complement fixation | More than 90% positive; some falsely positive |
| | | | | | Immunodiffusion | |
| | | | | | M band | 70%–80% positive |
| | | | | | H band | 10%–20% positive in active infection |
| | | Chronic cavitary | Chronic obstructive pulmonary disease | Not useful | Complement fixation | Majority positive[b] |
| | | Progressive disseminated | Immunocompromised; elderly; probably infants | Not useful | Complement fixation | Majority positive |
| | | | | | Antigen-EIA | Serum 80% positive<br>Urine >90% positive |

(*Continued*)

Table 17.1. (*Continued*)

| Fungus | Epidemiologic Features | Major Clinical Entities | Host/Setting | Skin Test | Immunologic Test | Value of Immunologic Studies |
|---|---|---|---|---|---|---|
| *Cryptococcus* | Worldwide | Pulmonary | Normal; immunocompromised | Not useful | Latex agglutination (antigen) | Some positive; false-positive results with rheumatoid factor |
| | | CNS | Normal; immunocompromised | | Latex agglutination | Sensitive and specific |
| *Coccidioides* | Southwestern U.S. | Acute pneumonitis | Normal | 95% positive[c]; can cause false-positive *Histoplasma* serologic results | Precipitins | 75% positive; disappears after 4–6 weeks |
| | | | | | Complement fixation | >50% positive; develops after 4–12 weeks |
| | | Chronic cavitary | Normal | Minority positive[c] | Precipitins | Usually negative |
| | | | | | Complement fixation | 50%–60% positive |
| | | Pulmonary nodule | Normal | Not useful[d] | Precipitins | Usually negative |
| | | | | | Complement fixation | Minority positive |
| | | Disseminated | Immunocompromised; Filipinos, Mexicans, blacks, pregnant women | Not useful | Precipitins | Usually negative |
| | | | | | Complement fixation | 80%–95% positive; 75%–95% positive in CSF if meningeal infection |

| | | | | | | |
|---|---|---|---|---|---|---|
| *Aspergillus* | Worldwide | Allergic broncho-pulmonary aspergillosis | Asthma | 99% positive; false-positive results occur | Precipitating antibody (precipitins) | 70% or more positive; false-positive results occur |
| | | | | | Serum IgE | Markedly elevated |
| | | Aspergilloma | Prior pulmonary cavity | Minority positive | Precipitins | 90%–100% positive |
| | | Invasive aspergillosis | Immunocompromised; rare in normal host | Insufficient data | Precipitins antibody | Not helpful |
| *Blastomyces* | Southeastern and midwestern U.S. soil contact | Acute pneumonitis; chronic (lungs, 75%; skin, bone, genitourinary tract) | Normal | Not available | Complement fixation | Not helpful |
| | | | | | Immuno-diffusion | Variable; up to 70%–80% in cases of disseminated disease |
| *Mucorales (Zygomycetes)* | Worldwide | Rhinocerebral; pulmonary | Diabetes in poor control; immunocompromised | Not available | Not available | |
| | | Disseminated | Immunocompromised; extensive burns | | | |
| | | Gastrointestinal | Young children with malnutrition or colitis | | | |
| *Sporothrix* | Worldwide: soil; sphagnum moss; rose and berry bushes | Cutaneous lymphatic | Normal | Not available | Agglutinating antibody | 90% positive |
| | | Pneumonitis | Normal; alcoholics | | Agglutinating antibody | |
| | | Disseminated | Normal; immuno-compromised; alcoholics | | | |

[a] May also occur in many cities in the United States. See text. Cultures necessary for diagnosis.
[b] Tissue histopathologic examination or if recent conversion from negative to positive reactivity is shown
[c] Helpful diagnostically.
[d] Does not differentiate between active disease and past infection.
i.v., intravenous; PCR, polymerase chain reaction; EIA, enzyme immunoassay; CNS, central nervous system; CSF, cerebrospinal fluid.

and diabetics have a higher incidence of paronychia than does the general population. Therapy with topical agents such as nystatin or miconazole creams are usually very effective for cutaneous infection in the normal host. Onychomycosis and more extensive cutaneous disease in the immunocompromised host requires treatment with an oral azole, such as fluconazole or itraconazole. Itraconazole 200 mg twice daily for 1 week repeated monthly for 3 to 4 months is recommended for onychomycosis [2].

**B. Mucosal infections**

1. **Oral candidiasis.** Thrush may occasionally occur in normal hosts such as neonates and denture wearers but is **most common in persons with** recent antibiotic treatment, inhaled or systemic steroid use, other immunosuppressive therapy, cancer, and AIDS [3]. The lesions most often appear as raised white plaques on the tongue and other oral mucosal surfaces. Oral candidiasis may also present with an atrophic appearance or as angular cheilitis. The diagnosis may be made by examining scrapings under light microscopy, which reveals masses of yeasts and pseudohyphae.
2. **Esophageal candidiasis.** Esophagitis generally **occurs in immunocompromised patients,** particularly patients with hematologic malignancy or AIDS. **Dysphagia and retrosternal pain with swallowing** are the most common symptoms. Oral candidiasis is often but not always present. Many clinicians initiate empiric therapy for esophageal candidiasis in high-risk patients who have typical symptoms in the presence of thrush [4]. Definitive diagnosis requires endoscopy.
3. **Nonesophageal involvement of the GI tract** by *Candida* is diagnosed most commonly in cancer patients [5]. The stomach is the organ most often involved. *Candida* may cause significant gastritis, invade ulcer beds, and cause superficial ulcerations in the small and large intestine. Disseminated candidiasis frequently is present in these settings.
4. **Vulvovaginal candidiasis** (see Chapter 16).
5. **Therapy**
   a. **Oral candidiasis** may be treated initially with either **nystatin** oral suspension 5 mL four times a day or **clotrimazole** troches four times a day for 7 to 10 days. Oral azoles are also effective; fluconazole 100 mg daily for 7 to 14 days was more effective than topical therapy in some studies. Oropharyngeal candidiasis that does not respond to fluconazole may be treated with itraconazole solution 200 mg/day [4,6].
   b. **Esophagitis.** Systemic therapy is required for esophageal candidiasis. Fluconazole 100 to 200 mg/day is highly effective and is a reasonable first choice. Esophageal disease refractory to fluconazole can be treated with itraconazole oral solution 200 mg/day or amphotericin B intravenously (i.v.) [4,6,7].

   Recurrence of oral and/or esophageal candidiasis is common in immunosuppressed hosts, particularly patients with HIV infection. Chronic suppressive therapy with fluconazole is effective at preventing recurrences but unfortunately is associated with the emergence of resistance [8,9]. It is therefore recommended that suppressive therapy is used only in the setting of very frequent severe recurrences [4] (see Chapter 18).

**C. Chronic mucocutaneous candidiasis.** This group of disorders is typified by persistent and recurrent *Candida* infections of the skin, nails, and mucous membranes [10]. Chronic mucocutaneous candidiasis may occur in young children or adults and is associated with large disfiguring cutaneous lesions. Disseminated candidiasis usually is not seen, but other infections with bacteria or dermatophytes may occur. Endocrinopathies, such as Addison disease, hypothyroidism, or hypoparathyroidism, are present in some patients. Various immune defects have been documented in patients with chronic mucocutaneous candidiasis, but the most consistent finding is that of abnormal T-lymphocyte function, as shown by anergy to delayed hypersensitivity testing. Treatment of chronic mucocutaneous candidiasis centers around therapy for the individual *Candida* infections. The **oral azoles** are the drugs of choice, and chronic suppressive therapy for many years has proven safe and successful.

**D. Disseminated candidiasis.** Once a rare disease, **disseminated candidiasis has become a very important nosocomial infection** because of the increased numbers of susceptible hosts. *Candida* species are now the fourth most common cause of bloodstream infections in hospitalized patients in the United States [11]. The clinical spectrum ranges from widespread involvement of multiple organs in a severely ill patient to isolated candidemia in a minimally symptomatic patient. Most cases are caused by *C. albicans,* but disseminated candidiasis caused by non-*albicans* species is becoming more common [12].

1. **Risk factors.** Several risk factors have been identified in patients with disseminated candidiasis: recent **abdominal surgery, neutropenia, broad-spectrum antibiotics, indwelling intravenous catheters, peripheral alimentation, cancer chemotherapy, immunosuppressive therapy in transplant recipients, and colonization with *Candida* species** [12–14]. In addition, recent evidence suggests the acquisition of candidal infection from hospital environmental sources [15,16]. Multiple risk factors are often present simultaneously in an individual patient.
2. **Manifestations.** Dissemination may present as **fever of unclear etiology or as the sepsis syndrome** with chills, spiking fevers, hypotension, and prostration. Multiple organs are usually involved with the formation of diffuse microabscesses. **Dissemination to brain, lungs, liver, and spleen** reflects a major and often preterminal breakdown in host defense. Spread to any organ may occur in this setting, but **infections of the eye and skin** are particularly important, because they may provide important diagnostic clues.
   a. **Macronodular skin lesions** represent embolic foci but are seen in only some patients. They are 0.5 to 1.0 cm in diameter, pink or red, and single or multiple and generalized. **Punch biopsy** may reveal the fungi on histopathologic study and culture. *Candida* may also produce lesions that resemble ecthyma gangrenosum or purpura fulminans.
   b. **Endophthalmitis** [17] occurs in approximately 20% to 50% or more of disseminated candidiasis patients and correlates closely with multiple visceral organ involvement. Endophthalmitis may cause blurry vision, scotomas, or ocular pain, but extensive disease may be present without symptoms. Endophthalmitis is a clinical diagnosis made in the proper setting and at times requires **serial funduscopic examinations,** which reveal white, cotton-like, circumscribed exudates with filamentous borders in the chorioretina extending into the vitreous. A **good ophthalmologic examination is an important part of the evaluation** of a patient with risk factors for disseminated disease.
3. **Diagnosis is problematic.** The definitive diagnosis of disseminated candidiasis can be made only by histopathologic demonstration of the organism invading tissue or by the isolation of *Candida* species from normally sterile body sites such as blood. Positive blood cultures are the most common way to make the diagnosis, but unfortunately blood cultures are negative in many patients with disseminated infection, and the rate of premortem diagnosis is only 10% to 40%. Thus, a **presumptive clinical diagnosis based on the presence of typical signs and symptoms in a high-risk patient is often the basis for initiating antifungal therapy,** because time is of the essence if the underlying disease is severe. The most important diagnostic technique in a high-risk patient is a thorough daily physical examination.
   a. **Serologic tests** to detect *Candida* antibodies or antigens such as arabinotol or enolase as an aide to diagnosis have been reviewed extensively elsewhere [18,19]. Current serologic tests lack sensitivity for the diagnosis of invasive candidiasis and cannot reliably differentiate colonization and invasive disease. As noted by Edwards [1], the decision to initiate antifungal therapy in a patient with suspected disseminated candidiasis should not be made on the basis of serologic test results alone, but in the context of a **comprehensive evaluation of a high-risk patient.** Because of their limitations, serologic tests have not become widely used in clinical practice as of this writing.
   b. **Colonization often precedes dissemination.** Positive cultures of urine, sputum, or stool are common in patients with disseminated disease. Isolation of *Candida* species from these specimens has some predictive value but

is not diagnostic. Only a small proportion of patients who are colonized by *C. albicans* develop invasive disease due to this organism [20]. The **isolation of *C. tropicalis* from an immunocompromised patient, however, has been shown to be more predictive of disseminated disease** [21].

**c. Polymerase chain reaction** assays using universal fungal primers, multicopy gene targets, and species specific probes are currently being developed for the early diagnosis of invasive fungal infections, including candidiasis. The sensitivity, specificity, and predictive value of these polymerase chain reaction-based assays need to be established in prospective clinical trials and correlated with clinical outcome [21a].

**4. Therapy.** Systemic candidal infection must be treated with systemic antifungal chemotherapy. The most effective currently available systemic antifungal agents for the treatment of invasive candidal infections are amphotericin and fluconazole. The choice of therapy is dependent on the clinical status of the patient and knowledge of the particular infecting *Candida* species.

**a. Amphotericin B** (0.5–0.7 mg/kg/day) has broad activity against various *Candida* species and has traditionally been the drug of choice in treating patients with disseminated disease, but recent comparative studies have shown that therapy with **fluconazole** provides comparable efficacy with less toxicity [22–24]. Most experts now recommend **initiating treatment with fluconazole 400 to 800 mg/day** in patients infected with an unknown *Candida* species who are clinically stable and have not recently been treated with azoles [4,25]. Because of concern for the presence of azole-resistant *Candida* species, **amphotericin B is recommended for patients recently treated with fluconazole** [25]. For patients who are clinically unstable (hypotension, rapidly worsening condition, multiorgan failure), high-dose amphotericin B 0.7 to 1.5 mg/kg/day is recommended as initial therapy.

Disseminated infection with ***C. albicans, C. parapsilosis,* or *C. tropicalis*** may be treated with either fluconazole or amphotericin B at usual doses, because these species are generally broadly susceptible to both azoles and amphotericin in most clinical settings. ***C. krusei* strains are resistant to fluconazole** and should be treated with amphotericin B. Most experts also recommend amphotericin B as treatment for infections due to ***C. glabrata,*** although high-dose fluconazole (800 mg/day) has been suggested [4]. **Many strains of *C. lusitaniae* are resistant to amphotericin B,** and fluconazole 400 to 800 mg daily is recommended as therapy for infections with this species. Infectious disease consultation is advised.

**b. Lipid-based preparations of amphotericin B** may be used in patients who are intolerant or refractory to amphotericin B deoxycholate or are at high risk for nephrotoxicity due to amphotericin B. Three lipid formulations are currently available: amphotericin B lipid complex (ABLC, Abelcet), amphotericin B colloidal dispersion (ABCD, Amphotec), and liposomal amphotericin B (L-AMB, Ambisome). Doses of 3 to 5 mg/kg/day are recommended [26]. For further discussion of amphotericin lipid formulations, see section **II** under Antifungal Chemotherapy later in this chapter.

**c. Flucytosine.** Flucytosine may be used for selected patients in combination with amphotericin B or fluconazole for its synergistic effect against *Candida* species. Candidates for dual therapy include those patients with endocarditis, meningitis, and endophthalmitis. Patients whose blood cultures remain positive after therapy with amphotericin or fluconazole is started may also be candidates for combination therapy. Bone marrow suppression may be a complication of flucytosine therapy. The recommended flucytosine dose is 25 mg/kg every 6 hours, but this should be adjusted in the presence of renal insufficiency [25].

**d. New therapeutic options are on the horizon** for the treatment of invasive candidiasis.

**(1) Caspofungin (Cancidas)** is the first commercially available echinocandin. This new class of antifungal agents interferes with fungal cell wall synthesis and, as the case with caspofungin, is fungicidal against *Candida* species [27,28]. The results of initial clinical trials using caspofungin for the treatment of candidal infections appear to be promising. See section **V** under Antifungal Chemotherapy later in this chapter.

(2) **Voriconazole** is a new triazole recently approved. Voriconazole has excellent *in vitro* activity against *Candida* species and has proven efficacious in several animal models of candidal infection [29]. Large-scale clinical trials are currently ongoing to study the effectiveness of voriconazole in the treatment of invasive candidiasis in neutropenic and non-neutropenic patients. See section **IV.E.** under Antifungal Chemotherapy later in this chapter for further discussion.

**e.** The presence of intravascular catheters is a risk factor for the development of disseminated candidiasis, and data indicate that **all intravenous lines should be changed** as soon as candidemia is detected, if possible [30].

**f.** The recommended duration of therapy is 2 weeks after the last positive blood culture for *Candida* and resolution of signs and symptoms of disseminated infection [4].

(1) **Isolated catheter-related candidemia.** Candidemia frequently occurs in patients with indwelling catheters but in whom signs of disseminated disease are minimal or absent. Several reports have documented late complications of disseminated candidiasis in such patients who did not receive antifungal chemotherapy, particularly immunocompromised patients but also normal hosts. Most authorities recommend **removal of the catheter and a course of antifungal chemotherapy** in patients in this setting [25,30]. The principles of therapy are as outlined for disseminated candidiasis (see section **D.4**).

**E. Empiric therapy for suspected disseminated candidiasis** is considered most commonly in two situations:

1. **Neutropenic patients,** after chemotherapy, with persisting fever despite treatment with antibiotics. The approach to these patients is discussed in section **I.H** under Antifungal Chemotherapy, below.
2. **Critically ill intensive care unit patients.** In febrile patients who lack an obvious focal infection and have risk factors for disseminated candidiasis (e.g., broad-spectrum antibiotics, hyperalimentation, surgery, *Candida* colonization of multiple sites), empiric antifungal therapy with fluconazole or amphotericin B may be warranted.

**F. Specific deep organ infections**

1. **Hepatosplenic candidiasis** is seen typically in patients with acute leukemia and prolonged leukopenia that has resolved [31]. This condition is characterized by widespread microscopic and macroscopic abscesses in the liver, spleen, kidney, and lungs.

**a. Manifestations** include persistent fevers, abdominal pain, hepatosplenomegaly, increased alkaline phosphatase levels, and leukocytosis.

**b. Diagnosis.** Computed tomography (CT), magnetic resonance imaging (MRI), and ultrasonography reveal multiple hepatosplenic (and occasionally renal) filling defects and/or abscesses. **CT is the most specific diagnostic tool.** The lesions are hypodense, and ring enhancement often is seen. Definitive diagnosis requires biopsy with culture and histopathologic examination or, if possible, aspiration of one or more of these abscesses in an attempt to identify the infecting organism.

**c. Treatment requires long-term antifungal therapy.** Fluconazole 400 to 800 mg/day for months is recommended by most experts [4]. Some authorities would initiate therapy with a short course of amphotericin B followed by a prolonged course of fluconazole. Therapy should be continued until radiographic resolution of all lesions has occurred. Infectious disease consultation is advised.

2. **Candidal endocarditis** is particularly **common in heroin addicts,** in patients with prolonged intravenous catheterization, and after recent cardiac surgery [32]. Most cases are caused by *C. albicans.* Addicts have a predilection for tricuspid involvement (see Chapter 12).

a. **Manifestations** are similar to those of bacterial endocarditis, except for a propensity toward large valvular vegetations. Many patients suffer **major embolic episodes** with occlusion of medium-size arteries (brain, extremities, lungs, mesentery). Invasion of the myocardium may occur and generally is irreversible.

b. **Diagnosis. Although early diagnosis is crucial** in preventing significant morbidity or death, **only 50% of patients have positive blood cultures** (up to 75% are positive in prosthetic valve endocarditis), and fever and leukocytosis may be absent. **Clinical clues strongly suggestive of the diagnosis** include the presence of endophthalmitis, major embolic episodes, or large vegetations demonstrated by echocardiography. Biopsy of skin lesions may be diagnostic.

c. **Therapy** combines early surgical intervention with amphotericin B (0.5–0.8 mg/kg/day). Prolonged intravenous therapy and careful follow-up are vital because relapse is common (see also Chapter 12).

d. **Prognosis** has been poor, especially in patients treated with medical therapy alone. Successful therapy is being described with increasing frequency, however, due mostly to earlier diagnosis and surgical intervention. With amphotericin B and surgical therapy, 50% of patients may survive.

3. **Genitourinary infection. Candiduria is common in hospitalized patients,** especially in an intensive care setting. **Risk factors include diabetes, broad-spectrum antibiotics, indwelling urinary catheters, and immunosuppressive therapy.** The most commonly involved species is *C. albicans.*

a. **Colonization versus infection.** There are no established criteria that reliably distinguish urinary colonization with *Candida* species from invasive infection, although the absence of pyuria makes invasive infection less likely [33]. Urinary colonization is asymptomatic and usually associated with an indwelling urinary catheter and may not require antifungal therapy. **Invasive disease is more likely in the presence of risk factors** such as neutropenia and immunosuppression and does require antifungal therapy.

b. **Manifestations.** Lower tract infection (cystitis) is usually asymptomatic, but symptoms when present include dysuria, hematuria, and frequency. Upper tract infection presents with typical signs and symptoms of bacterial pyelonephritis: fever, elevated white count, and costovertebral angle tenderness. **The presence of granular casts with hyphal elements** on urinalysis indicates involvement of the renal parenchyma. Hematogenous spread is the most common route resulting in renal infection, but urinary obstruction may on occasion lead to upper tract candidiasis via ascending infection.

c. **Therapy. Asymptomatic candiduria does not generally require antifungal therapy** [4,25]. Most patients with asymptomatic candiduria do not have invasive disease, and antifungal therapy does not necessarily result in long-term eradication of *Candida* species. **Catheter removal alone** resulted in eradication of candiduria in 41% of patients in a recent study and can be generally recommended if possible [33,34].

**Symptomatic patients and those with risk factors for invasive disease—renal transplant recipients, neutropenic patients, or patients about to undergo a genitourinary tract procedure—should be treated with antifungal therapy. Fluconazole 200 mg/day** is recommended [4,25]. **Amphotericin B** is an alternative and may be given either i.v. or as a bladder irrigation 50 to 200 $\mu$g/mL for 3 to 5 days [4,35]. Catheters and other urinary tract instruments should be removed if possible. **Persistence of candiduria in an immunocompromised host** despite antifungal therapy should prompt abdominal CT or ultrasound to rule out focal renal abscess or fungus ball.

4. **Central nervous system (CNS) infection** is usually a complication of disseminated disease in critically ill adults or neonates. Most cases have occurred in the setting of immune suppression, trauma, neurosurgery, and, more recently, AIDS [36,37]. The diagnosis is generally made on the basis of isolation of *Candida* species from cerebrospinal fluid (CSF). Therapy with amphotericin B and

flucytosine is recommended [4]. Shunts, if present, should be removed if possible. The role of fluconazole in therapy of CNS infection is unknown. Infectious disease consultation is advised. See related discussion in Chapter 6.

5. **Pulmonary infection** is usually secondary to hematogenous dissemination and results in fever and cough. Although positive sputum cultures are common in hospitalized patients, this usually represents colonization. Definitive diagnosis relies on biopsy, with demonstration of tissue invasion. Primary *Candida* pneumonia is rare except in the compromised host, and even in this setting it is uncommon [38].
6. **Peritonitis** caused by *Candida* species is generally a complication of peritoneal dialysis or GI surgery [39,40]. Dissemination is uncommon in patients undergoing chronic ambulatory peritoneal dialysis but may occur in association with bowel surgery. All patients with candidal peritonitis should be treated with either amphotericin B or fluconazole, and in chronic ambulatory peritoneal dialysis patients the dialysis catheter should be removed [4]. See additional discussion in Chapter 13.
7. **Musculoskeletal infection** with *Candida* species is another complication of disseminated disease. Arthritis may be acute or chronic and presents in a fashion similar to bacterial arthritis [41]. Bone disease usually involves the vertebral spine in adults or the long bones in children [42]. Diagnosis requires aspiration of the infected area. Treatment of osteomyelitis generally requires initial surgical debridement combined with systemic antifungal therapy. Both amphotericin B and fluconazole have been used successfully, and some experts recommend an initial 2 to 3 weeks of amphotericin B followed by a prolonged course of fluconazole [4]. Joint drainage combined with a lengthy course of systemic antifungal therapy is indicated in the management of candidal arthritis.
8. **Ocular infection** due to hematogenous dissemination of *Candida* was discussed in section **D.2.b.** Exogenous infection after trauma or surgery may also occur. Systemic therapy with fluconazole or amphotericin B with or without flucytosine is indicated [4]. The role of vitrectomy is unclear. Infectious disease and ophthalmologic consultation is recommended.
9. **Septic thrombophlebitis** of the peripheral or great vessels may occur in association with intravenous catheters. Fever, signs of sepsis, and persistent candidemia are characteristic of peripheral thrombophlebitis caused by *Candida* species. If suppuration is found with a peripheral phlebitis, the vein should be excised and antifungal therapy initiated. Septic thrombophlebitis of the great vessels has been treated successfully with amphotericin B [43].

## HISTOPLASMOSIS

***Histoplasma capsulatum*** is a dimorphous fungus that causes histoplasmosis, the most common systemic fungal infection in the United States. Inhalation of the infectious spores of *H. capsulatum* usually results in asymptomatic infection. Symptomatic pulmonary disease may occur in the normal host, and the organism may occasionally produce chronic progressive pulmonary infection or disseminated disease in some patients. *H. capsulatum* **is an important opportunistic pathogen in the immunocompromised host, especially persons infected with HIV** [44].

I. **Growth and identification characteristics.** *H. capsulatum* can be grown on routine fungal culture media, although growth is augmented on enriched agar such as brain-heart infusion. The mycelial phase requires 10 to 21 days to grow at room temperature and can be identified in the laboratory by characteristic large tuberculate spores. Conversion to the yeast phase at 37°C requires another 7 to 14 days. Biopsied tissue specimens should be stained and cultured; Gomori methenamine silver and periodic acid–Schiff preparations may reveal characteristic small intracellular yeasts. The organism may also be detected by Wright stain of sputum or blood.

II. **Epidemiologic features**

A. **Endemic areas.** Although histoplasmosis occurs throughout the world, **the disease is endemic in the central United States, particularly in the Ohio and**

**Mississippi River valleys.** In areas of Tennessee and Kentucky, more than 90% of the adult population has been infected with *H. capsulatum,* as manifested by positive skin test reactions. As far east as Maryland and Virginia, 85% of those tested have been exposed.

**B. Sources of infection.** *H. capsulatum* is found in nature in the soil. The organism grows particularly well in soil contaminated with excreta of birds (e.g., starlings, chickens, and blackbirds) and bats. Persons involved in cleaning chicken houses or blackbird roosts and in exploring caves are at risk for heavy exposures, and these conditions provide the setting for epidemic outbreaks [45]. Histoplasmosis may also be seen in urban residents. Foci of *H. capsulatum* spores may be present in open fields, parks, or old buildings, and an outbreak of acute pulmonary histoplasmosis may result if these foci are disturbed by construction or demolition [46,47].

**III. Pathogenesis**

**A. Agent. Infection occurs via inhalation of airborne spores.** The spores are deposited in pulmonary alveoli, where conversion to the yeast form and phagocytosis by macrophages occur. Infected macrophages spread through lymphatic channels to regional lymph nodes, followed by hematogenous spread to organs of the reticuloendothelial system, liver, spleen, and bone marrow.

**B. In the normal host,** cell-mediated immunity develops within 7 to 21 days of primary exposure [44]. T lymphocytes secrete cytokines that activate macrophages to kill intracellular yeasts, eventually resulting in caseating or noncaseating granulomas at infected sites. This response controls the infection. The granulomas become calcified with time, resulting in the characteristic Gohn complex and splenic calcifications commonly seen on roentgenography.

**C. In some persons, effective cellular immunity never develops.** The infection is not contained, and **disseminated histoplasmosis occurs.** Persons at greatest risk for disseminated disease include the elderly and very young children and immunosuppressed patients, such as those with leukemia or lymphoma, transplant recipients, and patients receiving corticosteroids. **Persons with AIDS are at very high risk for developing disseminated histoplasmosis.**

**IV. Clinical presentation, diagnosis, and therapy**

**A. Acute pulmonary histoplasmosis**

**1. Manifestations**

**a. In the normal host, infection after a mild inhalational exposure is usually subclinical and asymptomatic.** Uncommonly, mild exposure results in symptomatic illness, usually in children or infants. Rarely, pulmonary infection may result in disseminated disease.

**b. Infection after a heavy inhalational exposure** to spores may cause symptomatic disease, referred to as **acute pulmonary histoplasmosis** [45–47].

**(1) Acute illness in those without prior exposure** often presents with an **influenza-like picture** (chills, fever, malaise, headache, myalgias, nonproductive cough, and chest pain) after an incubation period of 10 to 18 days. Erythema nodosum, erythema multiforme, and migrating polyarthritis have been described in this setting. The **chest x-ray** generally reveals bilateral, patchy, nodular infiltrates with hilar or mediastinal adenopathy. Pleural effusion is uncommon. Symptoms in most patients resolve within 2 to 3 weeks.

**(2) Acute disease in a previously exposed individual** follows a slightly different pattern. Symptoms are similar but milder in degree and occur after a shorter incubation period (3–7 days). The chest roentgenogram may be different in that nodules are fine and miliary and there is no adenopathy, pleural involvement, or late calcification.

**2. Diagnosis**

**a. Subclinical infections** are diagnosed retrospectively by skin test conversion or by characteristic x-ray patterns of calcification.

**b. Acute symptomatic pulmonary histoplasmosis** can be diagnosed by culture and examination of sputum in no more than 10% of patients. Additional diagnostic aids include the following:

(1) **The chest x-ray** may be suggestive, as noted previously.

(2) **Skin tests** generally are not useful to diagnose acute infection because most individuals in endemic areas will react due to prior exposure.

(3) **Complement fixation tests** detect antibodies to either yeast or mycelial antigens. If either or both tests are performed, more than 90% of patients with acute disease will have titers of 1:8 or greater, and 70% will have titers of at least 1:32 [48]. Titers of 1:8 to 1:16 are suspect because false-positive results in healthy persons often fall into this range, particularly in endemic regions. False-positive results, generally titers of 1:8 or 1:16, are also seen in 20% to 40% of persons with other fungal or granulomatous diseases. A complement fixation titer of at least 1:32, or a fourfold rise in titer, in conjunction with a compatible clinical syndrome is strongly suggestive of acute pulmonary histoplasmosis.

The **immunodiffusion test** for precipitins to the H and M antigens is more specific than complement fixation but is not very sensitive. Antibodies may be undetectable for more than 3 weeks after exposure, and the immunodiffusion and complement fixation tests often are negative if performed early in the course of infection.

(4) **Antigen test.** The polysaccharide antigen of *H. capsulatum* may be detected in the urine or serum in up to 20% of patients with acute pulmonary infection [49].

3. **Therapy.** Most normal hosts have benign self-limited infection and require no therapy. Treatment with itraconazole 200 mg daily for 6 to 12 weeks is recommended for patients whose symptoms persist for more than 2 to 4 weeks [50]. Amphotericin B 0.5 to 0.7 mg/kg/day should be used initially in patients who have respiratory failure and require ventilatory support. Infectious disease consultation is advised.

B. **Progressive disseminated histoplasmosis** [51,52] is uncommon, occurring in approximately 1 of 2,000 to 5,000 acute infections and generally in an immunocompromised host (e.g., AIDS, transplant recipients). On occasion, it has been reported in an otherwise healthy adult. Disseminated disease may occur soon after an acute exposure or years later, after the patient has left an endemic region and subsequently developed immunosuppression. **Infection with HIV should be excluded in patients with disseminated disease** who have no apparent predisposing condition.

1. **Clinical manifestations** may vary from very severe illness (usually seen in infants and patients with AIDS) to more chronic disease, extending over months to years [52].
   a. **Systemic symptoms** of fever, chills, malaise, anorexia, and weight loss are common. Symptoms that follow an acute inhalational exposure and last more than 3 weeks may indicate systemic involvement.
   b. **Hepatosplenomegaly** and abnormal liver tests are common and may be striking in infants.
   c. **Mucosal ulcerations** occur in 35% to 40% of patients throughout the GI tract, especially the ileum, causing anorexia, nausea, abdominal pain, diarrhea, frank bleeding, or perforation. **Oropharyngeal, nasal, labial, gingival, and laryngeal ulcers** provide excellent biopsy sites for diagnosis.
   d. **The adrenal glands** are frequently infected and adrenal insufficiency can occur early or even years after initial infection. The incidence of clinically significant adrenal insufficiency is unclear.
   e. **Chest x-rays** may be normal or show interstitial or nodular infiltrates.
   f. **Anemia and leukopenia** are common, especially in patients with severe disease.
   g. **Uncommon manifestations** include meningitis, skin lesions (papules, nodules, or ulcers), endocarditis, and lytic bone lesions.
   h. **Patients with AIDS and disseminated histoplasmosis** frequently have severe disease and may present with shock, adult respiratory distress syndrome, disseminated intravascular coagulopathy, and CNS involvement [51,52].

2. **Diagnosis**
   a. **Complement fixation tests** are positive in 50% to 70% of patients but should be interpreted with caution, as previously discussed (see section **A.2.b.(3)**).
   b. **Antigen detection.** *H. capsulatum* polysaccharide antigen may be detected in the blood of more than 50% and in the urine of more than 90% of patients with disseminated histoplasmosis [48]. **Serial antigen measurements are helpful in following treatment response** because the antigen disappears with treatment and reappears with relapse.
   c. **Cultures of bone marrow** are positive in more than 75% of patients with disseminated disease, and **blood cultures** are positive in 40% to 70% of cases [51,52]. The lysis-centrifugation technique improves the yield from blood cultures and is particularly useful in AIDS patients. The organism can be isolated from **sputum and urine** cultures in more than half of the patients.
   d. **Special stains.** Demonstration of organisms by methenamine silver stain from specimens such as bone marrow or sputum provides a diagnosis within 24 to 48 hours in many patients. A Wright stain of the peripheral blood may reveal organisms within leukocytes in patients with severe disease. Biopsy specimens may also be obtained from oral lesions, the liver, and lymph nodes.
3. **Therapy. Antifungal therapy is clearly indicated in all cases of progressive disseminated histoplasmosis.**
   a. **In the immunocompromised HIV-negative patient** with symptoms severe enough to require hospitalization, amphotericin B 0.7 to 1.0 mg/kg/day is recommended [50,52]. A total dose of 30 to 35 mg/kg should be given to adults. Alternatively, amphotericin may be discontinued when symptoms have resolved and antifungal therapy may be completed with itraconazole, 200 to 400 mg daily for 6 months [52,53]. Itraconazole alone may be used at the indicated dose in patients with mild disease not requiring hospitalization.
   b. **Patients with AIDS** who have CNS involvement or immediately life-threatening disease should receive an **induction course of amphotericin B.** Induction therapy may be completed with itraconazole 200 mg twice daily for 8 to 12 weeks after resolution of symptoms [50,53,54]. AIDS patients with mild to moderate disease may be treated with **itraconazole** 300 mg twice daily for 3 days and then 200 mg twice daily for 8 to 12 weeks as induction therapy [50,53,54]. To prevent relapse, all AIDS patients should be placed on **maintenance** therapy with itraconazole (200–400 mg/day) indefinitely after resolution of the acute illness [55]. Itraconazole prophylaxis (200 mg daily) to prevent disseminated histoplasmosis may be considered for AIDS patients with CD4 counts less than 100/mm$^3$ who live in an area with a high incidence of histoplasmosis [56,57].
   c. **In immunocompetent HIV-negative patients,** itraconazole, 200 mg/day for 6 months, is well tolerated and very effective [50,53]. Fluconazole 400 to 800 mg daily and ketoconazole 200 to 400 mg daily are alternatives for patients who do not tolerate itraconazole [50,58]. Patients with severe disease or involvement of the CNS should be treated with amphotericin B. Infectious disease consultation is advised.
4. **Prognosis.** Without treatment, mortality is approximately 90%. In HIV-negative patients, treatment with amphotericin B decreases the mortality rate to 7% to 15%. The prognosis in AIDS patients is related to the severity of the histoplasmosis on presentation. Most relapses occur within 1 year of treatment.

C. **Chronic pulmonary histoplasmosis** [59] occurs in the setting of preexisting chronic lung disease. It manifests initially as a lingering segmental interstitial pneumonitis. Approximately 10% to 20% of cases progress to chronic cavitary disease.
1. **Early noncavitary pneumonitis**
   a. **Manifestations.** Malaise, fever, cough, and pleuritic pain are common, but some patients may be asymptomatic. Chest x-ray shows an interstitial infiltrate occurring typically in the apical-posterior area of the lung. The infiltrate disappears in 2 to 3 months, and the infarct-like necrotic areas become larger, leading to contraction and volume loss.

**b. Diagnosis.** Sputum cultures are positive in about one-third of cases.

**c. Therapy.** Early pneumonitis episodes usually are self-limited and generally follow a benign course but may result in the destruction of significant amounts of lung tissue, thereby exacerbating any existing respiratory insufficiency. In some patients, large air spaces, or bullae, become infected, and this progresses to chronic cavitary disease. When patients show evidence of clinical progression and/or progressive pulmonary infiltrates, treatment should be initiated as outlined for cavitary histoplasmosis (see section **2.c**).

**2. Cavitary infection**

**a. Manifestations.** Cough and sputum production are prominent and are usually accompanied by weight loss, low-grade fever, and easy fatigability. Hemoptysis is common, and in general there is an acceleration of the manifestations of the underlying chronic lung disease. **Chest x-ray** reveals cavitation, usually immediately adjacent to a pneumonic lesion and at the extreme apex. If inflammation subsides, cavitary walls often remain thin, but active infection leads to wall thickening. Continuing infection is probable if wall thickness exceeds 2 mm.

**b. Diagnosis**

**(1) Definitive bacteriologic diagnosis** by culture or Wright stain of sputum may be achieved in 35% to 60% of patients, but positive cultures do not necessarily indicate active disease or threat of relapse.

**(2) The chest x-ray** affords a better index of disease activity than do microbiologic data.

**(3) Complement fixation tests** are positive in 75% of patients but should be interpreted with caution.

**c. Therapy.** Many cases, especially those with thin-walled lesions (<2 mm), may regress spontaneously. Such cases can therefore be managed with an initial period of observation. Without treatment, 30% to 40% of thin-walled cavities persist and enlarge, and progressive pulmonary insufficiency results. If cavitation progresses and clinical improvement does not occur, antifungal therapy is indicated [50,53]. Oral therapy with itraconazole (200–400 mg/day) or ketoconazole (400 mg/day) for 6 months or more yields response rates of 65% to 80% [50,53], which compare favorably with results seen with amphotericin B. The indications for surgical resection are not well defined, and underlying lung disease often precludes a surgical approach. Infectious disease consultation is advised.

**D. Uncommon manifestations of histoplasmosis**

**1. Histoplasmomas** may form during the healing phase of a primary lung infection. These asymptomatic lesions may appear as solitary pulmonary nodules (1–4 cm in diameter) that have central calcification. **No antifungal therapy is indicated.**

**2. Mediastinal fibrosis** is the term used to describe a very thick (> 1 cm) fibrotic capsule in the mediastinal perihilar region, with actual invasion or compression of adjacent structures [60]. The process tends to be slowly but relentlessly progressive, and no therapeutic approach has proven to be reliably effective.

**3. Mediastinal granuloma** refers to large caseous lymph nodes that mat together and become encapsulated after primary infection. These may occasionally result in symptoms due to compression of adjacent structures in the mediastinum [60]. Treatment with amphotericin B 0.7 to 1.0 mg/kg/day or itraconazole 200 to 400 mg daily may be beneficial [50].

## CRYPTOCOCCOSIS

*Cryptococcus neoformans* is a saprophytic fungus that may cause disease in normal hosts as well as in the immunosuppressed. Meningitis and pulmonary infection are the most common manifestations, and *C. neoformans* is a common cause of meningoencephalitis in AIDS patients [61].

**I. Growth and identification characteristics.** Clinical cryptococcal isolates are encapsulated yeast and often are identifiable on India ink and Wright stain. Visualization in clinical specimens may yield an early presumptive diagnosis. Standard culture techniques are used. Media used for isolation should not contain cycloheximide because it inhibits growth of the organism. Growth generally occurs in 3 to 7 days, with identification in 3 to 4 days. Occasionally growth is slower, however, and incubation should be continued for 4 to 6 weeks before the culture is discarded as negative.

**II. Epidemiologic features and host factors.** *C. neoformans* is an ubiquitous fungus that is found worldwide in avian feces, particularly pigeon droppings. It has also been found in soil, certain fruits, contaminated milk, and food products [62]. Disease generally occurs after inhalation of the organism. **Many patients have no demonstrable underlying immune defect.** Patients who are immunocompromised, however, especially those with defective cell-mediated immunity, are prone to more serious infections, with rapid progression and dissemination. **Patients at highest risk for severe disease** include those with AIDS and lymphoma or leukemia, transplant recipients, and those receiving corticosteroids [61,63].

**III. Pulmonary involvement** [64,65]. The respiratory tract is presumed to be the primary portal of entry of *C. neoformans.* Pulmonary cryptococcosis is probably the **most common form of the disease,** although it is diagnosed less often than meningoencephalitis because it is **usually transient and often subclinical.**

**A. Clinical presentation.** Pulmonary infection usually results in few sequelae, and **many patients are asymptomatic.** If a patient inhales a large inoculum of organisms or if host defenses are compromised systemically or locally (because of a chronic respiratory disorder), the occurrence of symptomatic pulmonary disease is more likely. Clinically significant illness typically manifests as a subacute process with dull chest pain, cough with scant sputum production, and dyspnea. Low-grade fever and weight loss may occur with illness of longer duration.

**B. Diagnosis.** The manifestations of cryptococcal infection are nonspecific, and diagnosis depends on a high index of suspicion. **Patients who are immunocompromised are especially at risk.** Because of the lack of a vigorous inflammatory response, the routine indices of infection, such as leukocytosis and sedimentation rate elevations, may be absent.

1. **Sputum cultures** will isolate the organism in only 10% to 30% of patients with invasive disease. Because saprophytic colonization of the respiratory tract may result in a positive sputum culture, definitive diagnosis often requires open lung or bronchoscopic biopsy and **demonstration of tissue invasion.** Characteristic yeasts are readily seen with methenamine silver, periodic acid–Schiff, or Mayer mucicarmine stains.
2. **Chest x-ray findings are variable** and may range from solitary nodules in asymptomatic individuals to focal or lobar infiltrates with symptomatic infection. Patients may present with diffuse interstitial infiltrates and the adult respiratory distress syndrome. Cavitation and pleural effusion are uncommon.
3. **In all patients suspected or proven to have pulmonary cryptococcosis, the spinal fluid and blood should also be cultured** for *C. neoformans,* and the cryptococcal antigen test should be performed on CSF and serum to rule out disseminated disease [61].

**C. Therapy.** Pulmonary cryptococcosis does not need to be treated in every patient.

1. **A 2- to 4-month period of observation without therapy is acceptable in a normal host if** the following conditions are met: (a) Extrapulmonary lesions are absent; (b) cultures of blood, CSF, and urine are negative; (c) cryptococcal antigen is negative in the CSF and the serum titer is absent, low, stable, or falling; and (d) pulmonary lesions are small, few, stable, or regressing.
2. **Antifungal therapy should be instituted if** (a) the radiographic picture worsens, (b) increasing ventilatory impairment is evident, (c) dissemination is evident, or (d) the patient is immunocompromised. **Patients who are immunosuppressed need antifungal therapy because the risk of dissemination is high** [63,64]. Fluconazole 200 to 400 mg daily for 3 to 12 months may be used in immunocompetent hosts with mild to moderate symptoms [65,66]. Amphotericin B 0.5 to 0.7 mg/kg/day is recommended for severe disease in the normal host and in the case of fluconazole treatment failure. In immunosuppressed patients with pulmonary disease, initial therapy with amphotericin B 0.7 to 1.0 mg/kg/day for

2 weeks followed by fluconazole 400 to 800 mg daily for 8 to 10 weeks and then fluconazole 200 mg daily for 6 to 12 months has been suggested [66]. Infectious disease consultation is recommended.

IV **Disseminated disease.** Blood-borne cryptococcal yeast may disseminate from the lung to any organ but has a **predilection for the CNS.** Skin and bone involvement may also occur. All patients with disseminated disease require antifungal therapy.

A. **CNS.** Meningoencephalitis is the most common clinical manifestation of infection with *C. neoformans.* Most persons with cryptococcal CNS infection are immunocompromised. **See related discussion in Chapters 6 and 18.**

1. **The clinical manifestations** of cryptococcal meningitis are highly variable. Patients may present with acute symptoms of only a few days' duration, particularly if they are very immunosuppressed (e.g., HIV-infected persons). Conversely, others may have subtle symptoms for weeks or months before the diagnosis is made. The most common signs and symptoms include headache, fever, nuchal rigidity (often absent), cranial nerve palsies, impaired memory and judgment, lethargy, obtundation, and coma [67].

2. **Diagnosis**

a. **CSF**

(1) **Standard tests.** Of symptomatic patients, 90% demonstrate some abnormality of the CSF—increased opening pressure, elevated protein, decreased glucose, or a lymphocytic pleocytosis—although on occasion the CSF may be normal. Normal or only slightly abnormal CSF parameters are common in AIDS patients, and greater reliance should be placed on more specific tests [67].

(2) **India ink stains.** Cryptococcal yeast may be demonstrated on India ink stain in at least 50% of non-AIDS patients with CNS involvement and in more than 70% of AIDS patients. False-positive results may occur, however, if yeasts are confused with artifact or lymphocytes. Organisms may also be seen on Gram stain of the CSF.

(3) **Definitive diagnosis** generally requires isolation of the organism in culture of the CSF. Centrifuged sediments from large volumes of CSF (4–8 mL) should be used.

b. **Cryptococcal polysaccharide antigen** may be detected by the latex agglutination slide test. **The cryptococcal antigen test is particularly useful for making a presumptive diagnosis of cryptococcal meningitis,** with virtually all patients demonstrating titers of 1:8 or higher in the CSF. The test is more than 90% sensitive and specific for cryptococcal infection when performed properly. Rarely, false-positive results may occur in the presence of rheumatoid factor or the opportunistic fungus *Trichosporon beigelii.* Cryptococcal antigen may also be detected in serum and urine. **The serum antigen test is usually positive in persons with AIDS and cryptococcal meningitis and is therefore a useful screening test in this cohort of patients.**

3. **Therapy. Cryptococcal meningoencephalitis is an absolute indication for systemic antifungal chemotherapy.**

a. **In patients with AIDS** and cryptococcal meningitis the primary goal of treatment is to **gain control of the acute illness** and then continue therapy with an easily tolerated agent that will **suppress continuing cryptococcal infection** and allow patients to maintain their functional status. An aggressive **induction course** of **amphotericin B** (0.7 mg/kg/day) with **flucytosine** (25 mg/kg every 6 hours) for the initial 2 to 3 weeks is recommended by most experts [66,68]. Amphotericin effects more rapid sterilization of the CSF than does fluconazole. If induction therapy is successful, consolidation therapy with fluconazole 400 mg daily for 8 weeks may then be administered. Infectious disease consultation is suggested.

b. **Maintenance therapy** in AIDS patients is critical to prevent the otherwise inevitable relapse. When consolidation therapy has been completed, patients should receive **fluconazole** 200 mg/day indefinitely. This is both a highly effective and well-tolerated maintenance regimen. Fluconazole is preferred over itraconazole for maintenance [69].

c. **HIV-negative immunocompetent patients** may be treated successfully with the traditional combination of amphotericin B 0.3 mg/kg/day and flucytosine 25 to 37.5 mg orally every 6 hours for 4 to 6 weeks [70]. However, given the relative toxicity and inconvenience of this regimen, many experts advocate an induction course of amphotericin B 0.5 to 1.0 mg/kg/day with flucytosine 25 mg/kg every 6 hours for 2 weeks followed by fluconazole 400 mg daily for another 8 to 10 weeks [66]. Lumbar puncture should be repeated to document CSF sterilization.

d. **HIV-negative immunosuppressed patients** (e.g., transplant recipients) require prolonged therapy. Amphotericin B 0.7 to 1.0 mg/kg/day for 2 weeks followed by fluconazole 400 to 800 mg daily for 8 to 10 weeks and then fluconazole 200 mg daily for 6 to 12 weeks has been recommended [71].

e. **Elevated intracranial pressure** is common in patients with cryptococcal meningitis and is associated with increased morbidity and mortality [72]. Treatment options include lumbar puncture repeated daily or the placement of a lumbar drain ar a ventriculoperitoneal shunt [72,73]. Infectious disease consult is recommended.

f. **See additional discussion in Chapter 6.**

**B. Non-CNS extrapulmonary disease**

1. **Skin.** Nearly 10% to 15% of patients with disseminated disease have skin involvement, which occurs most frequently on the face and scalp. Although rare reports suggest the occurrence of primary skin cryptococcosis, essentially **all patients with cryptococcal skin lesions should be considered to have disseminated disease.** Cryptococcal skin involvement should be suspected in any immunosuppressed patient with erythematous papules, pustules, warts with a molluscum contagiosum-like appearance, subcutaneous nodules, or ulceration. Mucosal lesions are uncommon. Skin biopsy with fungal stains and cultures may be diagnostic.
2. **Bone.** Approximately 5% of patients with disseminated disease manifest osseus lesions. The prominences of long bones, cranial bones, and vertebrae are involved most commonly. Radiographs reveal round lytic areas without sclerosis. Biopsy with culture is necessary for diagnosis.
3. Spread to most organs has been documented at postmortem examination in patients with disseminated disease. **Detection of cryptococcal organisms in any organ always mandates a search for the presence of cryptococcal infection elsewhere in the body.** Patients infected with HIV may have a syndrome of disseminated cryptococcal infection without specific organ localization. These patients have fever, chills, myalgias, lethargy, and a positive serum cryptococcal antigen.
4. **The therapeutic approach** to patients with non-CNS extrapulmonary cryptococcosis should be similar to that described above for CNS disease [66]. Prolonged treatment may be required.

## COCCIDIOIDOMYCOSIS

*Coccidioides immitis* is a highly infectious fungus that frequently causes pulmonary infection in endemic areas of the United States. **Although most disease caused by this organism is benign and self-limited, infection may occasionally result in chronic pulmonary or skin disease, meningitis, or disseminated illness [74,75].**

I. **Growth and identification characteristics.** Routine culture methods are used, with presumptive identification in 2 to 5 days. The fungus grows readily on most culture media. **All culture plates should be handled with extreme care, because they are highly infectious to laboratory personnel. Direct human-to-human transmission is not known to occur, however.** *C. immitis* spherules may be identified in sputum, drainage material, or infected tissue. It is doubly refractile and thick walled, measures 20 to 80 mm, and is typically seen in several stages of development. Several preparations may be used to identify spherules, including potassium hydroxide, hematoxylin and eosin, methenamine silver, and periodic acid–Schiff stain.

**II. Epidemiologic features.** Coccidioidomycosis is endemic in the southwestern United States, Mexico, and parts of Central and South America. Cases may be seen outside endemic areas in persons who have traveled through these regions or as reactivation of infection acquired years earlier by a former resident of an endemic area. Because **infection is caused by inhalation of airborne arthrospores,** outbreaks may occur in dry weather in association with fresh diggings, newly plowed ground, and dust storms.

**III. Clinical aspects**

**A. Acute pulmonary coccidioidomycosis.** Most persons with primary infection by *C. immitis* **have an acute self-limited infection in the lungs.**

**1. Subclinical or asymptomatic illness** occurs in approximately 60% of patients. Prior infection in these persons can be detected only by skin testing.

**2. Symptomatic illness.** Forty percent of patients develop flulike symptoms after an incubation period of 7 to 28 days (average, 10–16 days).

**a. Signs and symptoms.** Fever, malaise, dry cough, shortness of breath, night sweats, anorexia, and pleuritic chest pain are common. Within the first few days of the onset of symptoms, a fine, generalized, erythematous maculopapular rash, sometimes urticarial in appearance, develops in 10% to 40% of patients. Peripheral eosinophilia may be present. The development of cutaneous hypersensitivity may be manifest as erythema nodosum or erythema multiforme, which occurs in fewer than 25% of infected individuals. This finding often is accompanied by arthralgias and, in association with pneumonitis, constitutes the classic picture of so-called valley fever.

**b. Roentgenographic findings.** The most common radiologic manifestation of acute coccidioidal pneumonitis is a segmental pneumonia, seen in approximately 50% of cases. Minimal infiltrates occur in nearly 30%, whereas hilar adenopathy and pleural effusion, sometimes massive, are seen in approximately 20%. In addition, solitary or multiple nodules, thin- or thick-walled cavities, and mediastinal lymphadenopathy may occur. Chest x-ray abnormalities usually resolve in 1 to 3 weeks.

**3. Diagnosis**

**a. Sputum.** Approximately 40% to 70% of primary infections will yield positive cultures [76]. A positive sputum culture is virtually diagnostic of pulmonary coccidioidomycosis, because this organism rarely colonizes the oropharynx.

**b. Skin tests** cannot differentiate between acute and remote infection and often are negative in persons with disseminated disease. They are, therefore, primarily useful only in epidemiologic evaluations.

**c. Serologic tests often are diagnostic** in primary coccidioidomycosis. **Serum precipitins,** as detected by tube precipitin, immunodiffusion, or latex agglutination testing, are IgM antibodies that are demonstrable in more than 75% of patients within 3 weeks of the onset of symptoms. Precipitins usually cannot be detected after 4 weeks. **Complement fixation detects IgG antibodies,** which appear more slowly but persist longer than IgM precipitins. More than 50% of patients will have a positive complement fixation titer, usually less than 1:32 by 3 months after the occurrence of clinical disease. More than 90% of patients with symptomatic acute pulmonary disease will have detectable antibodies by either precipitin testing or complement fixation [74,75]. Rising or persistently high complement fixation titers are a poor prognostic sign, whereas decreasing titers indicate improvement.

**4. Treatment. In many patients with acute coccidioidomycosis, the disease resolves within 6 to 8 weeks without specific therapy.** However, systemic **antifungal therapy should be considered in the following settings:** debilitation, pregnancy, immunosuppression, racial groups predisposed to disseminated disease (see section **C**), rising or persistently high (>1:16) complement fixation titers, progressive pulmonary disease, and persistent symptoms for more than 2 weeks [74]. For uncomplicated acute pulmonary coccidioidomycosis, most experts recommend itraconazole 200 mg twice daily or fluconazole 400 to 800 mg daily for 3 to 6 months [74,77]. If diffuse infiltrates are present, therapy with amphotericin B is recommended until significant clinical improvement has occurred, followed by oral azole therapy for at least 1 year.

B. **Other pulmonary manifestations** may occur.

1. **Chronic pulmonary coccidioidomycosis.** In some patients, symptoms of the acute pneumonia may persist for months or years. These patients have low-grade fever, weight loss, and cough. Serum complement fixation titers are positive, and sputum cultures often grow *C. immitis.* Therapy with itraconazole or fluconazole for at least 1 year is recommended [77].
2. **Solitary pulmonary nodules** due to *C. immitis* are common in endemic areas. In the absence of symptoms or immunosuppression no antifungal therapy is indicated.
3. **Cavitary disease** may be seen after acute primary infection and usually resolves spontaneously, but persistent cavitation sometimes occurs. Patients may be asymptomatic or have hemoptysis and low-grade fever. Sputum cultures often are positive. The course of persistent coccidioidal cavities is unpredictable, but most will resolve spontaneously over a period of 1 to 2 years. In a few patients, complications such as hemoptysis or rapid expansion with involvement of the adjacent lung may require some combination of azole drug therapy and surgery [77].

C. **Disseminated coccidioidomycosis.** Fewer than 1% of infected individuals will develop disseminated (extrapulmonary) infection. This complication **most often occurs in immunocompromised hosts such as transplant recipients, patients with hematologic malignancies, or those receiving immunosuppressive chemotherapy** [74]. **AIDS patients are at increased risk for disseminated disease,** although focal pulmonary disease may also be seen [78,79]. Dissemination appears to be more common during pregnancy, particularly in the third trimester. In addition, persons of non-white ethnic groups (e.g., Filipino, Hispanic, African American) more commonly have disseminated disease than do whites. Dissemination may occur within a few weeks of the primary infection or years later, after reactivation of quiescent disease.

1. **Osteoarticular disease.** More than one-third of patients with disseminated disease have **involvement of the bones or joints** [74]. The bones most commonly affected are the skull and vertebrae and the bones of the hands and feet. **Lytic lesions** are typical and frequently involve the overlying soft tissue, producing abscesses or draining sinuses. Articular lesions usually are limited to a single joint, generally the knee or ankle.
2. **Cutaneous disease.** The skin is commonly involved in patients with disseminated coccidioidomycosis. The lesions may vary in appearance from pustules or plaques to verrucous wart-like growths. Rarely, skin lesions may result from the direct inoculation of *C. immitis.*
3. **Meningitis.** CNS involvement by *C. immitis* usually is subtle and nonspecific and generally occurs within several months of the primary infection. Headache, fever, and weight loss are common symptoms [80]. Examination of the CSF typically reveals a mononuclear pleocytosis with an elevated protein. Peripheral blood eosinophilia has been noted (see also Chapter 6).
4. **Other less common manifestations** of dissemination include involvement of the genitourinary tract in the form of prostatitis or epididymitis. Coccidioidal peritonitis and lymphadenitis have been described, and, rarely, the eyes may be involved. **Miliary disease,** as manifested by diffuse reticular infiltrates on chest x-ray, is a common presentation **in AIDS patients** [78] (see Chapter 18).
5. **Diagnosis.** Definitive diagnosis requires **histopathologic evidence and/or culture of the organism** from infected tissue or fluid. Positive blood or urine cultures are uncommon. CSF cultures are positive in approximately one-third of patients with meningitis. **Elevated complement fixation titers** are the rule in disseminated coccidioidomycosis. Most patients have serum titers of 1:32 or higher [74,75]. The exception to this generalization is meningitis, in which serum titers tend to be much lower. Complement-fixing antibodies are **detectable in the spinal fluid** in more than 75% of patients with meningitis. Complement fixation titers show considerable variation between laboratories. The reporting laboratory's experience with these assays should thus be borne in mind when assessing the significance of a particular result.

6. **Therapy. Systemic antifungal therapy is indicated in all forms of disseminated disease.**
   a. **Treatment of nonmeningeal forms of disseminated disease** is usually initiated with an oral azole, generally **itraconazole or fluconazole 400 mg daily.** Duration of treatment should be at least 1 year and for 6 months beyond the point at which the disease has become inactive. **Amphotericin B 0.5 to 0.7 mg/kg/day** may be used as an alternative, especially for severe disease with rapidly progressive lesions [74,75].
   b. **Oral fluconazole 400 to 800 mg daily** is now recommended by most experts as the **preferred treatment for coccidioidal meningitis** [81]. Response rates with fluconazole are comparable with those seen with intrathecal amphotericin B with much less toxicity. Itraconazole 400 to 800 mg daily has also been used successfully. Relapse rates are unfortunately quite high, and an indefinite duration of treatment is indicated [82]. Infectious disease consultation is recommended. **See further discussion in Chapter 6.**

## ASPERGILLOSIS

***Aspergillus*** species are common contaminants in the bacteriology laboratory, and the relationship of a positive culture to clinical disease must always be questioned. However, *Aspergillus* may cause a variety of illnesses, from **hypersensitivity pneumonitis to disseminated overwhelming infection in immunosuppressed patients.**

I. **Growth and identification characteristics.** *Aspergillus* species are easily grown on routine fungal culture media, with identification possible within 48 to 72 hours. The species most frequently associated with human infections are *A. fumigatus* and *A. flavus.* Although a positive culture may suggest a causative relationship in the setting of a typical clinical syndrome, it may also represent benign colonization. **Definitive diagnosis of *Aspergillus* infection depends on demonstration of the organism invading tissue.** Staining with periodic acid–Schiff and methenamine silver permits ready identification of *Aspergillus* organisms in clinical specimens by visualization of their acutely branching septate hyphae.

II. **Epidemiologic features.** *Aspergillus* species are ubiquitous soil saprophytes that are found in all parts of the world. *Aspergillus* frequently is cultured in hospital wards from unfiltered outside air circulating through open windows. Aspergillosis usually is acquired through the inhalation of airborne conidia by a susceptible host.

III. **Clinical aspects.** Infection with *Aspergillus* species may result in one of several forms of a broad range of illnesses known as aspergillosis.
   A. **Tracheobronchial colonization.** *Aspergillus* may colonize ectatic bronchi or cavities in the lungs of patients with chronic pulmonary disease without invasion of the surrounding pulmonary parenchyma, and therefore the organism may be isolated in the absence of associated clinical illness. In these instances, allergic or invasive aspergillosis is not present. In most cases no specific therapy is required. Sometimes, however, slowly progressive pulmonary infiltrates develop in some patients, and treatment is required.
   B. **Allergic aspergillosis** may involve either the alveoli (extrinsic allergic alveolitis) or the airways (allergic bronchopulmonary aspergillosis [ABPA]).
      1. **Extrinsic allergic alveolitis is a hypersensitivity pneumonitis** that occurs in nonatopic individuals who are repeatedly exposed to conidia of *Aspergillus,* as in farmers who work in close proximity to moldy grain. Cough, dyspnea, fever, chills, and malaise typically develop 4 to 8 hours after exposure. Repeated attacks can lead to granulomatous disease and pulmonary fibrosis.
      2. **ABPA** results from a **hypersensitivity reaction of the airways** to *Aspergillus* fungal antigens present in the bronchial tree [83]. The pathophysiology of this disorder is complex and only partially understood. The immediate hypersensitivity (type I) reaction is believed to be IgE-mediated, probably accounting for the bronchospastic symptoms that are so characteristic of this disorder. A type III reaction (mediated by immune complexes) is most likely responsible for the roentgenographic features and more destructive changes of the bronchi [84].

a. **Manifestations. ABPA is characterized by symptoms of bronchospasm,** particularly episodic wheezing and dyspnea. Cough that produces mucopurulent sputum, low-grade fever, peripheral eosinophilia, and pulmonary infiltrates are common. Pleuritic chest pain and hemoptysis may also be seen. The illness may be mild and without sequelae, but recurrent episodes frequently result in progression to bronchiectasis and pulmonary fibrosis.

b. **Diagnosis.** ABPA is highly likely in a patient if several diagnostic criteria are present [84].
   (1) Patients will have a history of episodic asthma.
   (2) Peripheral blood **eosinophilia** is a nearly universal feature.
   (3) The **skin test** with *Aspergillus* antigenic extract usually is positive but is nonspecific, because it may be positive in patients who do not have ABPA.
   (4) **Serum precipitating antibodies** to *Aspergillus* antigens are present in 70% to 100% of cases.
   (5) **Total serum IgE** levels are markedly elevated. Both total IgE and IgE specific for *Aspergillus* antigens are increased in active ABPA and decrease with remissions.
   (6) **Chest x-rays** show a wide variety of abnormalities from small, patchy, **fleeting infiltrates** (commonly in the upper lobes) to lobar consolidation, atelectasis, or cavitation. Most patients eventually develop central bronchiectasis.
   (7) **Sputum cultures** often are positive for *A. fumigatus* and are suggestive but not diagnostic.

c. **Differential diagnosis. Tuberculosis** may be suggested by the upper lobe infiltrates or cavitation. **Cystic fibrosis** has features in common with ABPA, and this disorder must be excluded before treatment with steroids is begun. **Carcinoma of the lung and eosinophilic pneumonia or bronchiectasis** of other etiologies are additional considerations [83].

d. **Therapy** is determined by the severity and frequency of attacks. Mild disease may not require specific treatment.
   (1) **Corticosteroids are the mainstay of therapy for ABPA.** During acute exacerbations, large daily doses of prednisone (0.5–1.0 mg/kg) have been recommended until the chest x-ray has cleared, followed by alternate-day therapy at 0.5 mg/kg. This is continued for 3 to 6 months and then gradually tapered [83]. Aggressive treatment of early episodes may halt or delay progression to the final fibrotic stage.
   (2) **Bronchodilators** and **physiotherapy** with postural drainage may help prevent mucous plugging.
   (3) **Serial chest x-rays and monitoring of IgE levels** are helpful in guiding corticosteroid therapy and detecting exacerbations.
   (4) **Preventive aspects.** Patients should avoid locations (e.g., compost heaps and grain silos) and activities (e.g., smoking marijuana) in which exposure to *Aspergillus* spores is likely.
   (5) A recent randomized study demonstrated an **additional benefit of itraconazole 200 mg twice daily for 16 weeks** to that of steroids in patients with ABPA [85], so itraconazole can now be recommended as a steroid-sparing agent [86].

C. **Aspergillomas** ("fungus balls") generally represent **secondary saprophytic colonization of preexisting pulmonary cavities,** most commonly in patients with a history of chronic lung disease such as tuberculosis, sarcoidosis, or emphysema [87,88]. Aspergillomas may occur as a late consequence of invasive aspergillosis and have been described, on occasion, in patients with ABPA. Aspergillomas are masses of tangled hyphal elements, fibrin, and mucus.

1. **Manifestations. Hemoptysis** is the most common symptom associated with aspergilloma, occurring in 55% to 85% of cases. Hemoptysis may vary from blood-streaked sputum to active bleeding that requires urgent surgical resection. Chronic cough is not uncommon. **Many patients are asymptomatic.**
2. **Diagnosis** can be established by a typical radiologic picture, sputum culture, and serologic tests.

a. **Chest x-rays or CTs usually** show the characteristic intracavitary mass partially surrounded by a crescent of air.
b. **Sputum cultures** are positive in one-half to two-thirds of patients.
c. **Serum precipitins** are present in more than 90% of cases and are suggestive of the diagnosis when accompanied by the characteristic x-ray appearance.

3. **Therapy and prognosis.** The natural history of aspergilloma is variable, and therapy must be individualized based on symptoms and underlying pulmonary status. A conservative approach is prudent, with observation alone indicated for asymptomatic patients and those with mild infrequent hemoptysis. Spontaneous disappearance or lysis of aspergillomas has been reported in 7% to 10% of cases. Surgical resection is indicated for patients with severe hemoptysis [89]. A beneficial role of antifungal therapy has not been demonstrated definitively [86].

D. **Invasive aspergillosis.** ***Aspergillus* is a common opportunistic pathogen in the compromised host and occasionally occurs in those whose immunocompromise is not obvious.** Cancer patients with prolonged neutropenia from cytotoxic chemotherapy are particularly prone to infection. Patients receiving high-dose corticosteroids or other immunosuppressive agents or those with chronic granulomatous disease of childhood are also at increased risk [90]. Invasive aspergillosis occurs in AIDS patients, especially those patients who are leukopenic and on multiple antibiotics (azithromycin, trimethoprim-sulfamethoxazole) [91,92].

1. **Manifestations**

a. **Pulmonary involvement** is by far the most common manifestation of invasive aspergillosis [90]. The lungs typically manifest a necrotizing bronchopneumonia, ranging from small areas of infiltrate to intensive bilateral hemorrhagic infarction. The most common presentation is that of **unremitting fever and a new pulmonary infiltrate despite broad-spectrum antibiotic therapy in an immunosuppressed patient.** Dyspnea and nonproductive cough are common. Hemoptysis is uncommon. Chest x-ray may reveal patchy bronchopneumonia, nodular densities, consolidation, or cavitation. In immunocompromised patients, invasive pulmonary aspergillosis (IPA) generally is acute and evolves over days to weeks. Less commonly, patients with normal or only mild abnormalities of their immune systems may develop a more chronic slowly progressive form of IPA [93].

b. **Extrapulmonary dissemination** is found at autopsy in many patients with IPA [90].

(1) **Involvement of the CNS** may occur after either hematogenous dissemination or direct extension of invasive disease in the sinuses and results in infarction or abscess. The CSF may show a pleocytosis and increased protein content, but **cultures of CSF usually are negative.**

(2) **Necrotizing skin ulcers,** usually on the extremities, may occur secondary to hematogenous dissemination or after direct inoculation from an environmental source.

(3) **Osteomyelitis** due to *Aspergillus* typically involves a rib or the vertebral column and is most common in the immunosuppressed patient.

c. **Rapidly invasive infections of the paranasal sinuses** may occur in immunocompromised hosts and may extend into the orbit or cranial vault. A chronic form of invasive *Aspergillus* sinusitis typically occurs in normal hosts [90].

2. **Diagnosis of invasive aspergillosis. Definitive diagnosis requires the demonstration of tissue invasion** seen on a biopsy specimen or a positive culture from tissue obtained by an invasive procedure such as transbronchial biopsy. These patients often are severely ill, however, and invasive procedures may be associated with a high morbidity. **Noninvasive tests in the presence of an appropriate clinical syndrome may suggest the diagnosis.** For example, **pulmonary invasive disease is probable** in patients with chest radiographs that show new nodules or new cavities in the context of neutropenia, cytotoxic chemotherapy, or chronic corticosteroid therapy **and** sputum cultures or bronchoalveolar lavage washings or brush cultures for *Aspergillus* species or

cytologic examination on bronchoalveolar lavage that reveals characteristic septate hyphae.

a. **Sputum and nasal cultures** are positive in some patients with invasive aspergillosis, and the organisms can sometimes be isolated from these sites in the absence of invasive disease. **In the high-risk patient, isolation of *Aspergillus* from sputum, bronchoalveolar lavage fluid, or bronchial washings is strongly suggestive of invasive aspergillosis [94,95].**

b. **Serologic studies.** The standard *Aspergillus* precipitin assay, usually elevated in ABPA, rarely is elevated in patients with invasive disease and in general is not helpful.

c. **Blood cultures** usually are negative.

d. **Lung biopsy usually is necessary for definitive diagnosis of IPA,** because parenchymal invasion of lung tissue must be demonstrated to confirm the diagnosis. Most investigators recommend open lung biopsy to ensure adequate tissue for histopathologic evaluation. The transbronchial biopsy approach has also been used. Unfortunately, lung biopsy cannot be performed safely in many patients at high risk for invasive aspergillosis. Therefore, **if the suspicion for IPA is very high, based on the clinical syndrome and positive sputum or nasal cultures, empiric antifungal therapy may be indicated.** Infectious disease consultation is advised.

e. **Biopsy and culture of extrapulmonary lesions** will provide the diagnosis in patients with invasive disease outside the lungs.

3. **Therapy.** Invasive aspergillosis is often a fulminating illness that results in death. With early therapy, many patients have survived [96]. Prognosis is highly dependent on the course of the underlying disease. Infectious disease consultation is advised.

a. **Amphotericin B has traditionally been standard treatment.** Most clinicians prescribe high daily doses (0.8–1.0 mg/kg/day). Doses as high as 1.5 mg/kg/day have been given to patients who respond poorly. The optimal duration of therapy has not been defined and should be individualized based on the severity of illness and the degree of immunosuppression. Lipid preparations of amphotericin may be preferred in patients with renal dysfunction or in those receiving other nephrotoxic agents [86,97].

b. Studies of **itraconazole** in the treatment of invasive aspergillosis have demonstrated similar response rates to those of amphotericin B [98,99]. **Therapy with itraconazole 300 mg twice daily for 4 days and then 200 mg twice daily** is an alternative to amphotericin B for selected patients not receiving other agents that may interact with itraconazole [86].

c. An initial course of treatment with intravenous itraconazole or amphotericin B until disease stabilization or regression has occurred followed by prolonged oral therapy with itraconazole has been suggested by some clinicians [86].

d. **Caspofungin** is the first of the new echinocandin class of antifungal agents and was recently approved by the U.S. Food and Drug Administration (FDA) for the treatment of invasive aspergillosis (70 mg i.v. on day 1, then 50 mg i.v. daily) in patients who have failed or have been intolerant to amphotericin and/or itraconazole. It has not been studied as initial therapy [100].

e. **Voriconazole,** is a newly approved triazole that has been used in open-labeled studies of invasive aspergillosis. Complete or partial response rates of 50% or greater have been reported for patients treated with voriconazole who have been intolerant to or failed other therapies for invasive aspergillosis [86]. Other investigational triazoles such as posaconazole also exhibit excellent activity against *Aspergillus* species [101].

f. **Combination therapy.** Because of the high mortality rates of invasive aspergillosis treated with single antifungals, a variety of combination therapies using amphotericin B with azoles, flucytosine, or rifampin has been evaluated both *in vitro* and in animal models. A combination of caspofungin and itraconazole has been used successfully in the treatment of invasive aspergillosis in a small number of patients [102]. The combination of caspofungin with newer azoles, such as voriconazole and posaconazole, appears to be promising.

   g. **Reduction of corticosteroids or cytotoxic chemotherapy,** if possible, appears to improve prognosis.
   h. **Surgical resection** may be useful in selected patients with focal lesions.
4. **Prognosis** is improved with early diagnosis and aggressive therapy, remission of the underlying disease, and reversal of chemotherapy-induced bone marrow suppression. **Resolution of neutropenia is particularly important** if a favorable response to therapy is to be seen.
5. **Future chemotherapy if the patient survives.** Patients who have survived a prior episode of invasive aspergillosis are at risk for reactivation of invasive disease during subsequent myelosuppression with repeat courses of chemotherapy. Some studies suggest at least a 50% rate of reactivation during chemotherapy in patients who have recovered from prior invasive aspergillosis. **Prophylactic amphotericin B (1 mg/kg/day) beginning at least 48 hours before chemotherapy** and continuing until the time of granulocyte recovery to prevent relapse of invasive disease in patients undergoing repeat chemotherapy has been recommended [103].

E. **Rare manifestations of aspergillosis**
   1. ***Aspergillus* endocarditis** mimics *Candida* endocarditis in that it occurs most commonly on prosthetic heart valves and is associated with large vegetations that embolize to medium-sized vessels. **Diagnosis is difficult because blood cultures are rarely positive.** Early valve replacement is essential if cure is to be achieved.
   2. **Allergic *Aspergillus* sinusitis** is a recently recognized form of sinusitis that occurs primarily in young atopic persons [104]. Nasal polyps and mucoid material containing eosinophils and fungal hyphae are found commonly. Optimal therapy requires corticosteroids and surgical debridement.

## BLASTOMYCOSIS

***Blastomyces dermatitidis*** is a dimorphous fungus that causes the acute and chronic illness blastomycosis. Infection with *B. dermatitidis* occurs via the lungs and then may be followed by hematogenous dissemination. Pulmonary disease is most common, followed by disease of skin, bone, and genitourinary tract. **Widely disseminated disease is most common in immunocompromised hosts, especially those with AIDS.**

I. **Growth and identification characteristics.** *B. dermatitidis* mycelial colonies are usually visible 1 to 2 weeks after clinical specimens are incubated at 30°C. Conversion to the yeast phase at 37°C is necessary for definitive diagnosis and usually occurs within another 10 days of culture. Microscopic examination of sputum, pus, or drainage from skin lesions is a rapid method for presumptive diagnosis of blastomycosis. When seen in a wet preparation or after digestion with KOH, the **characteristic yeast forms** are as spherical cells with a diameter of 8 to 15 $\mu$m, have a highly refractile thick cell wall, are multinucleate, and reproduce by a single broad-based bud. These same characteristics allow identification of the organism in histopathologic specimens with the use of special stains such as periodic acid–Schiff, Gomori methenamine silver, Papanicolaou, and Giemsa stains.

II. **Epidemiologic and host characteristics.** Infection caused by *B. dermatitidis* has been reported only occasionally outside of North America. Most patients reside in the southeastern and south central states, especially those bordering the Mississippi and Ohio River valleys, and the midwestern states and Canadian provinces that border the Great Lakes [105–107]. Isolates from the environment indicate that ***B. dermatitidis* exists in nature in warm moist soil that is rich in organic material,** usually decaying vegetation [108,109]. When these microfoci are disturbed, either during work or recreational activities, the aerosolized spores (conidia) are inhaled into the lungs. Disease at other body sites is the result of dissemination from this initial pulmonary infection. Primary cutaneous disease, however, has been reported after dog bite and after accidental inoculation injury. A rare case of vaginal infection transmitted sexually from a man with genitourinary blastomycosis has been described [105].

*B. dermatitidis* is a primary pathogen that causes disease primarily in normal hosts. Virulence is probably mediated to some extent by the rapid conversion of conidia to the yeast form after inhalation into the lung. The yeast form is more resistant to phagocytosis and killing by leukocytes. Additionally, the elegant work of Klein and coworkers [110–114] has clearly documented a 120-kDa protein antigen on the cell wall surface, designated WI-1, which is not only a major immunodominant epitope for humoral and cellular immunity but also is an important virulence factor for *B. dermatitidis.*

**III. Clinical manifestations.** Blastomycosis is a systemic disease with both pulmonary and extrapulmonary manifestations. Pulmonary disease may be acute or chronic. Extrapulmonary disease occurs most commonly during the chronic form of illness.

**A. Acute blastomycosis** often is unrecognized and is characterized by **pneumonitis** that occurs after a median incubation time of 30 to 45 days. Analysis of point source outbreaks indicate that only 50% or so of infected individuals become symptomatic [108,109].

1. **Symptomatic patients** usually have an influenza-like syndrome with fever, chills, arthralgias, myalgias, cough, fatigue, and pleuritic chest pain. The symptoms may be mild or severe. Spontaneous resolution of disease is well recognized, and the duration of illness in these cases is generally less than 4 weeks [115].
2. **Chest roentgenograms** usually show lobar or segmental consolidation. Small pleural effusions are seen occasionally. Hilar adenopathy usually does not occur [116].

**B. Chronic blastomycosis** is indolent in onset and follows a widely variable course. Recent clinical experience indicates that extrapulmonary disease occurs in only approximately one-fourth of patients with blastomycosis [117]. Infection has been documented in almost every body organ, but skin, bone, and genitourinary sites of disease are most common [105,106].

1. **Pulmonary manifestations.** Most patients have signs and symptoms of a **chronic pneumonia that mimics tuberculosis.** The most frequent symptoms are cough, sputum production, hemoptysis, pleuritic chest pain, and weight loss. Fever tends to be low grade. The chest roentgenogram is nonspecific, with a wide variety of findings [116]. Lobar or segmental alveolar infiltrates, especially of the upper lobes are most common. These infiltrates may progress to cavitation. Masslike infiltrates that mimic lung cancer occur nearly as often as alveolar infiltrates. Other radiologic findings include solitary cavities, lung nodules, and fibronodular infiltrates, with or without cavities. Pleural thickening and small pleural effusions occur, whereas large pleural effusions are uncommon. Miliary disease and diffuse pneumonitis, often associated with respiratory failure, are occasionally reported and are associated with a high mortality.
2. **Skin lesions are the most common form of extrapulmonary blastomycosis.** Skin disease usually occurs in conjunction with pulmonary disease but may occur alone. Skin lesions tend to occur on exposed parts of the body. The characteristic lesion begins as a small papule or pustule that gradually enlarges over a period of weeks or months, becoming elevated, verrucous, and crusted (Color Plate 4.6). Outer borders are well demarcated and indurated. Older lesions commonly exhibit central healing and scarring at the same time that the outer border of the lesion is active and advancing. Removal of the crust reveals a granulomatous base with numerous small abscesses exuding purulent material. Less frequently, the lesion may begin as a small pustule that ulcerates. These ulcerative lesions bleed easily. Subcutaneous abscesses that sometimes drain spontaneously are seen in a minority of patients. **The organism easily is seen and is cultured from pus aspirated from these abscesses.**
3. **Bone infection** has been reported in 10% to 50% of patients. Lesions are osteolytic and often painless. The long bones, vertebrae, and ribs are most commonly involved. Some patients present with a contiguous soft tissue abscess or draining sinus. Contiguous spread to joints may cause a pyarthrosis. **Diagnosis is made by biopsy** of the involved bone or aspiration of the contiguous soft tissue abscess.
4. **Genitourinary disease** has been noted in 10% to 30% of patients. The prostate and epididymis are most commonly involved. The kidney usually is spared.

Patients may note a painful swelling of the testis or epididymis, a perineal ache, or symptoms of urinary obstruction. The prostate may be tender and enlarged. Cultures of urine or prostatic secretions obtained after massage frequently are positive.

5. **CNS disease** is reported in fewer than 5% of cases. However, CNS complications of blastomycosis are more common in AIDS patients, noted in 40% of patients with blastomycosis and AIDS in one series [118]. Abscesses are most common and present as mass lesions. Meningitis is usually a late complication and is frequently associated with multiorgan disease.
6. **Other sites** of disease are reported less frequently and include the lymph nodes, spleen, larynx, esophagus, thyroid, pituitary, and heart.

C. **Infections in the compromised host.** Blastomycosis in the immunocompromised host is more severe and more often disseminated and is associated with greater mortality than in immunocompetent patients [118,119]. As noted in the preceding section, CNS infection is especially common in AIDS patients. Death rates of 30% to 40% are reported despite treatment with amphotericin B.

IV. **Diagnosis.** Definitive diagnosis is **established by culture.** A presumptive diagnosis can be made by visualizing the distinctive yeast forms in clinical specimens and is often sufficient to initiate antifungal therapy. Serologic studies must be interpreted with caution because of their high false-positive and false-negative rates.

A. **Culture.** Clinical specimens should be cultured on Sabouraud or more enriched agar. Sputum, pus from soft tissue abscesses, scrapings from skin lesions, and prostatic secretions may all be cultured successfully.

B. **Direct examination of clinical specimens**

1. **Wet preparation.** Sputum, scrapings from skin lesions, pus, or pleural fluid should be examined microscopically as a fresh wet preparation. The use of 10% KOH to digest cellular debris may facilitate seeing the organism. Occasionally, multiple specimens must be collected before the organism can be seen on smear. Bronchoscopy is helpful in patients who are unable to produce sputum. Visualization of the yeast form on cytology preparations is facilitated by Papanicolaou stain.
2. **Histopathology.** The typical inflammatory response is characterized by pyogranulomas. Yeast forms usually are not seen with hematoxylin and eosin stains but may be demonstrated with special stains, as noted earlier in section **I.**

C. **Skin tests.** No skin test reagent is currently available for the diagnosis of blastomycosis in patients with suspected disease.

D. **Serologic tests** for the diagnosis of blastomycosis are complicated by their **lack of sensitivity and specificity** [120]. Thus, negative tests should never be used to rule out disease. Neither should an isolated positive test prompt antifungal therapy. Rather, **a positive result should stimulate the clinician to search diligently for evidence of disease.**

1. **Complement fixation** tests are neither sensitive nor specific. Fewer than 50% of patients with blastomycosis will develop a positive test, and cross-reactions with *H. capsulatum* and *C. immitis* are common.
2. **Immunodiffusion tests.** The detection of precipitating antibodies is highly specific for blastomycosis, but sensitivity is variable. Positive results have been reported in up to 80% of patients with blastomycosis. However, lower rates of positivity (33%) have been reported in patients with localized disease [120]. Positive results are most frequently noted in patients with symptoms lasting 50 days or longer. Thus, immunodiffusion is **not helpful in acute disease.**
3. **Radioimmunoassays and enzyme immunoassays** that are highly sensitive have been developed [121]. False-positive results, however, are well documented. An enzyme immunoassay is now commercially available and may prove useful for initial screening of specimens. Positive results should be confirmed with the more specific immunodiffusion test.
4. **Recent advances** in the characterization of the yeast antigens of *B. dermatitidis* may facilitate the development of more reliable serologic tests. A novel 120-kDa surface protein, designated as WI-1, has been described by Klein and Jones [110].

Preliminary results using this antigen in a radioimmunoassay appear promising, but currently this test is investigational [121].

**V. Therapy.** Although amphotericin B was previously considered the primary drug for treating all clinical forms of blastomycosis, recent studies have proven that either ketoconazole or itraconazole is an effective alternative for the treatment of immunocompetent patients with mild to moderate disease. Neither azole is indicated for patients with CNS disease.

**A. Acute blastomycosis. Some patients may not require therapy.** Because the acute form may be a benign self-limited illness, it has been suggested that patients with acute blastomycosis should be followed, without specific chemotherapy but with prolonged observation [115]. However, illness progresses in some patients to chronic infection with significant morbidity. Because there are no known clinical characteristics that predict which patients are susceptible to chronic involvement, some authorities recommend that all patients with acute blastomycosis receive chemotherapy. **The indication for antifungal therapy in this group remains controversial,** and infectious disease consultation is advised.

**B. Chronic blastomycosis**

1. **Amphotericin B** is the **drug of choice for patients with life-threatening disease,** patients who are **immunocompromised, and** patients **with CNS disease [122].** A total dose of at least 1.5 g is recommended. For selected patients treated initially with amphotericin B who are immunocompetent and who do not have CNS disease, an azole may be substituted for amphotericin B after clinical improvement is noted. Cure rates of greater than 90% are reported in immunocompetent patients who complete a full treatment course of amphotericin B, and relapse rates are less than 5%. Relapse is more frequently reported in immunocompromised patients, especially those with AIDS. Maintenance therapy with an oral azole has thus been advocated after successful primary therapy of blastomycosis in AIDS patients [118].
2. **Ketoconazole.** Two clinical trials have documented cure rates of approximately 80% for patients treated with a daily dose of 400 mg ketoconazole [123,124]. For patients who do not respond satisfactorily, the dose may be increased in 200-mg increments to a maximum of 800 mg/day. At least 6 months of treatment is recommended.
3. **Itraconazole** is highly effective against *B. dermatitidis* both *in vivo* and *in vitro.* At doses of 200 to 400 mg/day, itraconazole was effective in 90% to 95% of patients with blastomycosis [53,122]. Because efficacy rates were similar at both doses, the initial recommended daily dose of itraconazole is 200 mg. For patients who fail this initial therapy, the dose may be increased in 100-mg increments to a maximum daily dose of 400 mg. Itraconazole generally has fewer side effects than ketoconazole and is the preferred agent for the treatment of blastomycosis at the authors' medical center.
4. **Fluconazole** has been studied in only a limited number of patients. In studies using daily doses of 400 to 800 mg, a successful outcome was noted in 80% of a cohort of 39 patients [125,126]. These results indicate that fluconazole and ketoconazole are essentially equivalent when administered at equivalent doses of more than 400 mg/day. Adverse events are less common with fluconazole. Fluconazole penetrates well into the CNS and therefore may have a role in the treatment of blastomycotic meningitis and cerebral abscesses in patients who are intolerant to amphotericin B.
5. **Surgery** has a limited role in the treatment of blastomycosis.
6. **Special patient populations**
   a. **Pediatric blastomycosis.** Blastomycosis is reported less commonly in children. However, the clinical spectrum of disease and therapeutic and treatment considerations are similar to adults. That is, children with life-threatening or CNS disease should be treated with amphotericin B. Children with mild to moderate disease without CNS involvement have been successfully treated with itraconazole daily dose of 5 to 7 mg/kg/day.
   b. **Pregnancy.** Amphotericin B is the drug of choice for the treatment of blastomycosis in pregnant women.

7. **Prognosis.** Most patients (≥90%) with chronic blastomycosis are cured with therapy. Mortality is greatest in patients with AIDS and those with respiratory failure or CNS disease.

## MUCORMYCOSIS

**Mucormycosis** (or *zygomycosis*) is the term for infection caused by fungi of the order Mucorales. A number of families of this order are associated with disease, but the Mucoraceae (which include the genera *Absidia, Mucor, Rhizomucor,* and *Rhizopus*) are the most common [127]. **Mucoraceae may produce severe disease in susceptible individuals, notably patients with diabetes and leukemia.** Mixed infections with other fungi and with bacteria are common.

I. **Growth and identification characteristics.** The Mucorales are cultured on routine fungal media, and growth is abundant in 24 to 72 hours. A saline preparation will reveal broad nonseptate hyphae with right-angle branching. **The laboratory should be alerted when mucormycosis is a diagnostic possibility.** Microscopic examination of smears and histopathologic evaluation of scrapings and biopsy material often reveal the diagnosis when cultures are negative. The organisms stain readily with periodic acid–Schiff, methenamine silver, and routine hematoxylin and eosin stains.

II. **Epidemiologic and host characteristics.** The **organisms that cause mucormycosis are ubiquitous** molds commonly found in the soil and on decaying organic debris. They are infrequent contaminants in the laboratory. Occasionally, Mucorales species have been isolated from sputum or sinus specimens in the absence of invasive disease. There is **no evidence for person-to-person transmission. Certain conditions predispose** to tissue invasion by these normally saprophytic fungi, including **diabetes mellitus, leukemia, lymphoma, corticosteroid therapy, severe malnutrition, organ transplantation, extensive burns, and uremia.** Several cases of mucormycosis have been reported in dialysis patients who were being treated with the chelating agent **deferoxamine [128].**

III. **Clinical aspects.** Mucormycosis is usually an acute fulminant infection characterized pathologically by the **invasion of major blood vessels, with resultant ischemia and infarction of adjacent tissue.**

   A. **Rhinocerebral mucormycosis** most commonly manifests in the setting of **poorly controlled diabetes, especially with ketoacidosis.** The causative organism in most cases is *Rhizopus arrhizus.* The organisms invade through the palate or the mucous membranes of the nose or paranasal sinuses. Subsequently, invasion through the ethmoids may occur, with direct extension into the orbital region and the frontal lobes of the brain. Progression of disease is usually rapid, although it may become indolent if ketoacidosis resolves.

      1. **Clinical manifestations.** Local symptoms of sinusitis and palatal or orbital cellulitis may be present. **The nasal septum may be ulcerated, necrotic, or even perforated, and dark bloody nasal discharge commonly results.** The nasal turbinate bones often are black and necrotic. Soft periorbital or perinasal swelling may progress to induration and discoloration. **Neurologic sequelae** evolve after a few days and usually are rapidly progressive. Ptosis, proptosis, and dilatation or fixation of the pupil may occur. Drainage of **black** pus from the eyes sometimes is seen. Progressive neurologic deficits ensue, with ophthalmoplegia, blindness, cranial nerve involvement, and, finally, contralateral hemiplegia due to thrombosis of the internal carotid artery. Progressive lethargy develops despite control of the diabetes, and coma follows.

      2. **Diagnosis** requires a **high degree of suspicion** to permit early therapy.

         a. **A tissue biopsy or wet preparation** of the necrotic areas may demonstrate the characteristic nonseptate hyphae. This is the **best rapid diagnostic procedure** because cultures require 1 to 3 days and are often negative.

         b. **The CSF** usually shows nonspecific findings with a mononuclear pleocytosis and slight elevation of protein. CSF cultures typically are negative.

         c. **Radiologic examination** may demonstrate sinusitis or findings suggestive of osteomyelitis. CT or MRI may be useful to demonstrate tissue or bone destruction, cerebritis, or retro-orbital disease. Arteriograms may reveal filling defects, narrowing, occlusions, and infarction.

3. **Therapy. Because of the rapidity with which this disease progresses, prompt and aggressive therapy is essential** [127]. Surgical and infectious disease consultations are advised.
   a. **Treatment directed toward reversing the underlying condition** (e.g., diabetic ketoacidosis) or decreasing immunosuppressive therapy is necessary.
   b. **Amphotericin B is the only truly effective agent.** The dosage should be rapidly advanced to 1 to 1.5 mg/kg/day. If there is a favorable clinical response, an alternate-day regimen can be adopted. A total dosage of 2 to 3 g given over 2 to 3 months usually is required, depending on the clinical course and control of the underlying disease. A lipid formulation of amphotericin may be used in the presence of renal dysfunction. Cases have occurred where lipid formulations at doses as high as 16 mg/kg/day have been used and succeeded when amphotericin appeared to be failing.
   c. **Surgical debridement.** Extensive surgical extirpation or debridement of devitalized tissue and adequate drainage of sinuses and abscesses are essential elements in controlling infection.
4. **Prognosis.** With aggressive combined chemotherapy and surgery, the mortality is approximately 50%. Survivors often have significant neurologic deficits. Rapid diagnosis and treatment may improve prognosis.

B. **Pulmonary mucormycosis** may occur after inhalation of fungal spores or from hematogenous or lymphatic spread during dissemination. Most patients have hematologic malignancy, severe neutropenia, or are transplant recipients, and most have received steroids.

1. **Manifestations.** Fever is common with **pulmonary infiltration or cavitation that progresses despite antibiotic therapy.** Occasionally, subacute cases occur in diabetics, with progression over weeks to months.
2. **Diagnosis.** The diagnosis of pulmonary mucormycosis requires **histopathologic evidence of pulmonary invasion.** Cultures of respiratory secretions are usually negative. The chest x-ray is nonspecific.
3. **Therapy.** Most patients in whom pulmonary mucormycosis is diagnosed have had advanced disease with extensive tissue destruction, and results of treatment have been disappointing. Early diagnosis, reversal of the underlying disease, and high-dose amphotericin B may improve the prognosis. Surgical resection of pulmonary lesions may be beneficial in selected patients.

C. **Gastrointestinal mucormycosis** has been diagnosed primarily in patients with severe malnutrition or in transplant recipients [129]. Any part of the GI tract may be involved, but the stomach and large bowel are the most common sites of infection. Abdominal pain and bloody diarrhea are typical, and signs of peritonitis may ensue if the intestinal wall is perforated. The disease is usually acute and rapidly fatal. **Diagnosis requires biopsy of involved tissue.** A combination of surgical resection and antifungal chemotherapy with amphotericin B is indicated as treatment.

D. **Cutaneous mucormycosis.** Involvement of the skin with the Mucorales may be primary (after direct inoculation of organisms during minor trauma) or secondary (after dissemination from another site) [130]. Extensive involvement of burn wounds may result in disseminated disease. **Diagnosis depends on** the demonstration of **tissue invasion in biopsy specimens.** For patients with primary localized cutaneous disease, surgical debridement may be adequate for cure. However, in patients with evidence of disease distant to the cutaneous site of infection or invasion of hyphal forms into the subcutaneous tissue, systemic therapy with amphotericin B is required.

E. **Disseminated mucormycosis** usually occurs in debilitated patients with hematologic malignancies [131]. Dissemination is most often from the lungs or GI tract and may involve any part of the body. Multiple areas of infarction and abscess formation are common. Cutaneous lesions that resemble ecthyma gangrenosum have been described. The clinical course is acute and rapidly progressive. Biopsy of involved tissue is required to make the diagnosis. Intensive therapy with amphotericin B is indicated, but the outcome is generally poor.

## SPOROTRICHOSIS

*Sporothrix schenckii* is a saprophytic fungus found widely in nature. Infection due to *S. schenckii* generally is limited to the skin and regional lymphatics, although systemic and disseminated disease occasionally occur.

I. **Growth and identification characteristics.** *S. schenckii* is a dimorphous fungus. The mycelial phase can be grown and identified on routine culture media in 3 to 5 days. Conversion to the yeast phase is desirable for definitive diagnosis. **Isolation of *S. schenckii* in the laboratory usually indicates infection,** because it is not a normal commensal of humans.

II. **Epidemiologic features.** *S. schenckii* is found worldwide. The organism is found in the soil and on rose and barberry bushes, sphagnum moss, tree bark, and other vegetation. **Infection usually occurs after inoculation injury after contact with thorny plants** [132].

III. **Clinical aspects.** Sporotrichosis can be divided into cutaneous and extracutaneous infection.

A. **Cutaneous disease** accounts for 75% to 80% of cases of sporotrichosis. Transmission to humans typically occurs through a break in the skin, often after minor or unrecognized injuries. Cutaneous sporotrichosis is therefore an **occupational disease** of gardeners, farmers, horticulturists, nursery workers, and florists.

1. **Manifestations.** The fungus usually gains entry in the fingers or hands, where a **small papule or raised, erythematous, subcutaneous nodule develops.** The lesion may be evident at any time from 1 week to 6 months after inoculation. Spread to regional lymphatics results in **progression of secondary nodules** up the arm, which often ulcerate and drain but do not produce significant pain or disability. Localized cutaneous infection without lymphatic spread is less common; these lesions may be nodular, crusted, or fungating and may occur anywhere at a site of trauma. Lesions may wax and wane for months or years.

2. **Diagnosis.** Although the clinical appearance may be very suggestive of sporotrichosis, other infectious diseases may cause identical lesions, including nontuberculous mycobacterial infection, nocardiosis, blastomycosis, and leishmaniasis [132]. **Culture of drainage or aspirated material** should reveal the causative organism and **is diagnostic.** Histopathologic examination of punch biopsy specimens reveals granulomatous lesions with fungal cells confined to the dermis. The fungal cells may be surrounded by an aggregation of material that stains with periodic acid–Schiff, the so-called asteroid body.

3. **Therapy**

a. **Oral potassium iodide** remains an effective inexpensive treatment for cutaneous and lymphatic sporotrichosis. However, it is associated with frequent allergic reactions and GI intolerance.

(1) **Mode of administration.** Saturated potassium iodide solution is given orally in doses of 3 to 4 mL (maximum) every 8 hours, beginning with 1 mL per dose and gradually increasing the dose while monitoring for toxicity. Some advise putting the drug in root beer to disguise the taste. Treatment is continued until 1 month after the skin lesions disappear.

(2) **Toxicity.** Nausea, vomiting, parotid swelling, iodism (acne) or other skin lesions, coryza, sneezing, eyelid swelling, and depression generally respond to discontinuing the drug for a few days and restarting it at a lower dosage.

(3) Application of local heat to the lesions may also be helpful.

b. **Treatment with itraconazole** results in response rates of greater than 90% [133,134]. Itraconazole 200 mg daily for 3 to 6 months is well tolerated and more convenient than potassium iodide and can now be recommended as the **treatment of choice** [135].

B. **Extracutaneous disease** represents approximately 20% of cases of sporotrichosis. Therapy with potassium iodide is ineffective in all forms of extracutaneous disease. Treatment with itraconazole or amphotericin B is required.

1. **Pulmonary sporotrichosis is uncommon.** It may be a primary infection after inhalation of *S. schenckii* spores or may occur secondary to dissemination

[136]. Many patients have a history of chronic obstructive pulmonary disease, diabetes, alcohol abuse, or some other chronic medical condition. Symptoms include the insidious onset of cough, sputum production, malaise, weight loss, and fever. **Chest x-rays** generally reveal parenchymal infiltration progressing to cavitation, and hilar adenopathy may be marked. Infection is usually indolent but progressive. **Diagnosis depends on isolation of the fungus from sputum, bronchial washings, or lung tissue. Amphotericin B** is recommended for life-threatening disease. Mild to moderate disease may be treated with **itraconazole 200 mg twice daily** [135,137].

2. **Osteoarticular sporotrichosis** is an extremely indolent infection that primarily involves the joints and bones. Involvement of a single joint is typical. Cutaneous disease usually is absent. Most patients have pain, effusion, and decreased mobility of the affected joint. Cultures of joint fluid are frequently negative, and synovial biopsy may be required for diagnosis. **Itraconazole 200 mg twice daily** is effective and recommended for most patients [135]. Amphotericin B may be used in cases of itraconazole treatment failure.
3. **Disseminated sporotrichosis is rare,** usually occurring in an immunosuppressed host. Involvement of multiple sites, including the skin, lungs, joints, bones, and CNS, has been reported. Risk factors for dissemination include alcoholism, diabetes, chronic obstructive pulmonary disease, and AIDS [138]. Clinical manifestations depend primarily on the organ systems involved. **Skin lesions,** often ulcerative, are found in most patients. Lymphatic spread generally is not seen due to hematogenous dissemination. **Multifocal joint involvement** is common, in contrast to the normally unifocal osteoarticular disease. Nodular pulmonary lesions are present in 10% to 20% of patients. **Meningitis** is a rare manifestation of infection with *S. schenckii.*
   a. The **diagnosis** may be suspected on the basis of the characteristic skin and joint lesions. **Culture of the fungus** from an infected lesion generally is not difficult, although multiple cultures occasionally are required. Recovery of the organism from blood cultures has been reported. Repeated culture of the CSF often is necessary to isolate the organism in patients with meningitis, and serologic tests of serum and CSF may be useful [139].
   b. **Amphotericin B** is the preferred therapeutic agent for disseminated sporotrichosis, including meningitis. Itraconazole may have a role as maintenance therapy in patients with AIDS after initial treatment with amphotericin [132]. Infectious disease consultation is advised.

## MISCELLANEOUS FUNGAL INFECTIONS

I. **Paracoccidioidomycosis** is a systemic infection caused by the dimorphous fungus *Paracoccidioides brasiliensis* [140]. The **disease is endemic in Latin America, particularly Brazil,** and is diagnosed only rarely in North America. Pulmonary infection is the most common manifestation, but involvement of the mucous membranes, skin, and lymph nodes after dissemination occurs frequently. **Itraconazole** is the drug of choice for treatment.

II. **Mycetoma** (Madura foot) is a localized noncontagious infection involving cutaneous tissue, fascia, and bone [141]. The disease is reported most frequently in patients who live in tropical or temperate zones. Mycetoma may be caused by either aerobic actinomycetes or various species of fungi and generally occurs after the traumatic implantation of the organisms into the subcutaneous tissue of a healthy host. Most cases involve the foot or hand and progress very slowly over months to years. Combined surgical–medical treatment is the best therapeutic approach for mycetoma caused by fungi.

III. **Dematiaceous fungi** are a group of darkly pigmented organisms that cause infections termed *phaeohyphomycoses.* These infections occur most frequently in immunocompromised hosts and manifest clinically as subcutaneous, sinus, or cerebral infection [142]. Surgical resection of localized lesions is crucial for diagnosis and treatment, but the prognosis is usually poor.

IV. ***Penicillium marneffei*** is a dimorphic fungus endemic in southeast Asia that causes disseminated infection with papular skin lesions in persons with AIDS [143, 144]. Disseminated penicilliosis may be **treated effectively with amphotericin B**

**followed by itraconazole** 200 mg twice daily for 10 weeks and then 200 mg daily as maintenance therapy to prevent relapse [145].

V. **Emerging opportunistic fungal infections.** Many fungal species that formerly were considered nonpathogenic or only rarely were associated with invasive disease are now causing increasingly common infections in immunosuppressed hosts. *Trichosporon* and *Malassezia* species are common causes of superficial dermatologic infections but may cause disseminated disease in immunocompromised or debilitated patients [146,147]. *Fusarium* species cause disseminated infection primarily in patients with hematologic malignancies or severe burns [148]. *Pseudallescheria boydii* is an agent of mycetoma and may cause more deep-seated infections such as pneumonia or disseminated disease in the immunocompromised host [149]. There is no standard well-defined antifungal treatment for most of these infections, and infectious disease consultation is suggested.

## ANTIFUNGAL CHEMOTHERAPY

The agents currently available for the systemic therapy of mycotic infections are presented in Table 17.2. The decision regarding whether to initiate systemic antifungal chemotherapy must be based in part on consideration of the toxicity of these drugs (Table 17.3). **Infectious disease consultation is recommended** to help determine the indications for therapy and to assist in administration of the drugs. The following general guidelines provide an introduction to systemic antifungal chemotherapy.

I. **Amphotericin B (Fungizone)** has been the most reliable agent against most of the invasive fungal pathogens [150,151].
   A. **Mode of action.** Amphotericin binds to ergosterol, the primary sterol in the membrane of susceptible fungi, resulting in the opening of pores in the membrane and leakage of cellular constituents followed by cell death [152].

Table 17.2. Systemic Antifungal Agents

| Class | Route | Daily Dose | Action |
|---|---|---|---|
| Polyenes | | | |
| Amphotericin B deoxycholate | i.v. | 0.5–1.0 mg/kg | Membrane: binds to fungal sterols |
| Lipid formulations | i.v. | 3.0–6.0 mg/kg | |
| Azoles | | | |
| Ketoconazole | p.o. | 200–400 mg | Membrane: interferes with ergosterol synthesis |
| Fluconazole | p.o., i.v. | 400–800 mg | |
| Itraconazole | p.o., i.v. | 200–400 mg | |
| Voriconazole | p.o., i.v. | 200–400 mg | |
| Allylamines | | | |
| Terbinafine | p.o. | 250 mg | Membrane: interferes with ergosterol synthesis |
| Echinocandins | | | |
| Caspofungin | i.v. | 50–70 mg | Cell wall: glucan synthesis inhibitor |
| Nucleic acid analogues | | | |
| 5-Fluorocytosine | p.o. | 100–150 mg/kg | Nuclear: interferes with DNA and RNA synthesis |
| Griseofluvin | p.o. | 500 mg | Nuclear: interferes with microtubules |
| Iodides | | | |
| SSKI | p.o. | Titrate 5–40 drops t.i.d. | Unknown |

SSKI, saturated solution of potassium iodide.

Table 17.3. Principal Adverse Effects of Antifungal Agents

| Amphotericin B | Flucytosine | Ketoconazole | Fluconazole | Itraconazole | Voriconazole | Terbinafine | Caspofungin |
|---|---|---|---|---|---|---|---|
| Fever, chills, nausea, vomiting<br>Nephrotoxicity<br>Thrombophlebitis at site of administration<br>Anemia<br>Electrolyte imbalance ($K^+$ $Mg^{2+}$)<br>Pulmonary deterioration (rare) | Suppression of bone marrow<br>Nausea, vomiting<br>Diarrhea<br>Increased hepatic enzymes<br>Rash | Gastrointestinal distress<br>Rash, pruritus<br>Transiently increased hepatic enzymes<br>Severe hepatotoxicity (rare)<br>Alopecia<br>Decreased synthesis of testosterone leading to diminished libido, impotence, and gynecomastia<br>Menstrual irregularities<br>Decreased synthesis of cortisol | Gastrointestinal distress (less than with ketoconazole)<br>Rash<br>Headache<br>Transiently increased hepatic enzymes<br>Severe hepato-toxicity (?)<br>Chapped lips<br>Dry skin<br>Alopecia | Gastrointestinal distress (less than with ketoconazole)<br>Rash<br>Pruritus<br>Headache<br>Dizziness<br>Transiently increased hepatic enzymes<br>Severe hepato-toxicity (?)<br>Possible impotence and gynecomastia<br>Syndrome of mineralocorticoid excess<br>Congestive heart failure | Visual disturbances<br>Rashes<br>Photosensitivity<br>Severe dermatologic reactions (rare)<br>Infusion-related anaphylactoid reaction<br>Transiently elevated hepatic enzymes<br>Severe hepato-toxicity (?) | Gastrointestinal<br>Headaches<br>Dysgeusia<br>Rash<br>Pruritus<br>Urticaria<br>Severe cutaneous reaction (rare)<br>Increased hepatic enzymes<br>Severe hepato-toxicity (?) | Nausea, vomiting<br>Fever<br>Rash<br>Histamine reactions with infusion<br>Phlebitis at administration site |

Adapted from Patel R. Antifungal agents. Part I. Amphotericin B preparations and flucytosine. *Mayo Clin Proc* 1998;73:1205–1225; and Terrell CL. Antifungal agents. Part II. The azoles. *Mayo Clin Proc* 1999;74:78–100, with permission.

**B. The pharmacokinetics** of amphotericin B **are poorly understood.** Amphotericin B is poorly absorbed from the GI tract. Systemic infections must be treated intravenously. No metabolism of the drug has been identified, and elimination occurs slowly via the biliary tract.

**C. Distribution.** The highest concentrations of amphotericin B are achieved in the liver, spleen, lung, and kidneys [153]. Distribution into spinal fluid, parotid gland fluid, aqueous humor, urine, and hemodialysis solutions is poor. Plasma levels do not predict treatment success.

**D. Dosage and administration. The method of calculating the dose of amphotericin B remains controversial.** Many experts maintain that duration of therapy is the best predictor of therapeutic success and advocate, for example, low doses daily for 6 to 12 weeks. Other experts advocate administration of high daily doses, if tolerated, until a specific total **dose is achieved. There is no consensus as to the optimal regimen, total dose, or total duration of therapy.** General guidelines are available, however, and depend on the clinical response, site of infection, identity of the fungus, and the patient's tolerance of the drug [150,151].

1. **Some authorities suggest an initial test dose** of 1 mg i.v. over 30 minutes to 1 hour because rarely patients experience an idiosyncratic reaction of hypotension or an anaphylaxis-like reaction. The necessity of this test dose has been questioned [154] because it delays therapeutic doses. We do not routinely use a test dose.
2. **Several dosage regimens** are used. The dose may be gradually increased daily (by increments of 5–10 mg/day), or full-dose intravenous administration (e.g., 0.5 mg/kg/day) may begin immediately. **In seriously ill patients we prefer this latter approach.** The dose may be increased to as much as 0.7 to 1.0 mg/kg/day, although some prefer not to exceed a maximum daily dose of 50 mg.
3. **The daily dose is typically infused over 4 to 6 hours;** we prefer 4-hour infusion. Some authors believe a more rapid infusion of 1 to 2 hours may decrease the incidence or intensity of side effects (e.g., fever, chills, nausea, and vomiting). Studies suggest that more rapid infusions in patients with normal renal function are as well tolerated as the traditional 6-hour infusion [155]. Amphotericin B binds to some degree to cholesterol of mammalian cells, causing release of intracellular potassium, potentially resulting in severe hyperkalemia, especially in patients with renal failure. Therefore, **rapid infusion rates should not be used in patients with renal insufficiency** [156]. Arrhythmias have additionally occurred during amphotericin B administration, and rapid infusion rates should thus not be used in patients with cardiovascular disease [156]. In general, **we favor a 4-hour infusion for most patients.**
4. **Alternate-day or thrice-weekly regimens** may be used to minimize side effects. Thrice-weekly therapy facilitates outpatient or home administration. The usual maximum individual dose in these regimens is 50 to 80 mg.
5. If serum creatinine rises to exceed 2.5 to 3.0 mg/dL or blood urea nitrogen exceeds 40 mg/mL, many experts suggest lowering the dose, discontinuing the drug until renal function improves, or switching to alternate-day therapy. However, diminishing renal function does not affect the rate of elimination. Although amphotericin B is nephrotoxic, it does not accumulate in renal failure. Dosage adjustments are made to minimize toxicity, but hemodialysis patients usually receive full doses.
6. **Intrathecal** or intraventricular amphotericin B may be indicated for coccidioidal meningitis and in some refractory cases of cryptococcal meningitis [157]. Administration is technically complicated, and neurosurgical and infectious disease consultations are suggested.

**E. Toxicity**

1. **Fever and rigors** during infusion are common in the first week of therapy and usually diminish thereafter. Fever and chills may be the result of amphotericin B-induced release of interleukin-1 and tumor necrosis factor from mononuclear cells [158,159], which leads to a secondary release of prostaglandin $E_2$. Because they alter the hypothalamic set point of the brain, prostaglandins have been implicated as a cause of fever and rigors. **Some physicians premedicate**

**patients with** a standard dose of acetaminophen (e.g., 650 mg orally for adults), diphenhydramine hydrochloride (Benadryl) (e.g., 25–50 mg i.v./orally for adults), and meperidine (e.g., 25–50 mg i.v. in adults) approximately 30 minutes before the infusion of amphotericin B. Because 25% of patients who have not received premedication fail to experience an adverse event with amphotericin B infusion, **we do not advocate the routine pretreatment regimens. However, if adverse reactions occur, use of pretreatment regimens in subsequent infusions of amphotericin B is advised [160]. If the patient has additional chills during the infusion, the dose of meperidine may be repeated at 3-hour intervals.** This routine decreases the incidence of fever and rigors in many patients. **Ibuprofen** (a single dose of 10 mg/kg up to a maximum dose of 600 mg) **is also useful as premedication** [159]. Because protracted use of this agent should be associated with nephrotoxicity, ibuprofen may be helpful for the initial 1 to 2 weeks of therapy while tolerance to side effects is developing. Simultaneous administration of hydrocortisone, 25 to 50 mg i.v., may be effective when fever is particularly troublesome. Corticosteroids alone for pretreatment are not advised.

2. **Anorexia, nausea, and vomiting** are common but usually diminish as therapy progresses. Pretreatment with antiemetics may be helpful.
3. **Nephrotoxicity is the major dose limiting factor** in amphotericin administration [160]. Early toxicity is dose dependent, whereas later toxicity is related to the total dose. Renal function returns to nearly normal in most patients several months after therapy is stopped, but irreversible renal failure occurs. Renal function should be monitored at least every other day during the early stages of therapy. In the stable patient who is receiving intravenous amphotericin B at home or in an outpatient setting, serum creatinine (and potassium levels) should be monitored at least 2 to 3 times per week. Other renal abnormalities such as cylindruria and mild renal tubular acidosis are not used as guides to dosage but may be predictors of renal dysfunction.

   **The incidence of renal failure may be reduced if a saline infusion is given before each dose** or if a high salt intake is maintained [161]. In patients who can tolerate the sodium load, we often give 500 mL to1 L of normal saline over 1 to 2 hours before amphotericin B administration.
4. **Anemia** develops in more than 75% of patients, due to the inhibition of erythropoietin production and direct bone marrow suppression [162]. Leukopenia and thrombocytopenia are rare.
5. **Hypokalemia** from a renal tubular defect develops in 25% of patients and may require potassium supplementation. **Serum potassium levels should be monitored serially. Hypomagnesemia** may also occur.
6. **Infusion-related phlebitis** is common. Limiting the concentration of amphotericin to no more than 0.1 mg/mL reduces the incidence of phlebitis. The simultaneous infusion of heparin may also help to ameliorate phlebitis [160].
7. **Serious pulmonary reactions** with acute dyspnea, hypoxemia, and interstitial infiltrates on chest films have been described in patients receiving combined amphotericin B and leukocyte transfusions [163]. Therefore, it is advised that the interval between the infusion of amphotericin B and the leukocyte infusion is as long as possible.
8. **A preprinted order sheet,** including the saline load and premedications described in section **E.1, and preprinted flow sheet** are used by some institutions to monitor the daily and cumulative doses of amphotericin B, serum creatinine, and other therapies.

F. **Pregnancy.** Amphotericin B has been used during pregnancy for the treatment of systemic fungal infections, without any adverse effects on fetal development.

G. **Combination chemotherapy.** Addition of flucytosine may be synergistic, especially for cryptococcal infection in non-AIDS patients. Preliminary studies reporting the enhanced efficacy of amphotericin B in combination with other agents are encouraging but have been only studied in animal models of infection.

H. **Empiric amphotericin B therapy in the persistently febrile granulocytopenic patient.** The source of fever in neutropenic patients often defies careful physical and laboratory examination (including multiple cultures), and fever frequently persists despite broad-spectrum antibiotic therapy. Because the early diagnosis of disseminated fungal infection (e.g., candidemia) is very difficult, the empiric addition of a systemic antifungal agent is a consideration. Typically, if fever persists beyond 5 to 7 days despite negative blood cultures and broad-spectrum antibiotic therapy, empiric amphotericin B (commonly 0.5 mg/kg/day) often is started and continued until the leukopenia resolves [164]. Empiric amphotericin B sometimes is initiated even more rapidly (within hours) in the hospitalized leukopenic patient who has been stable for several days on broad-spectrum antibiotics and then becomes febrile and acutely ill. In addition to reculturing and broadening antibiotic therapy if indicated, empiric amphotericin B may be added for a possible disseminated fungal infection. The role of fluconazole as a substitute for amphotericin B in febrile neutropenic patients has been established in large prospective trials [4,22–24]. See discussion under Candidiasis, section **III.D.4.a. Infectious disease consultation is advisable in this setting.**

**I. Cost** (Table 17.4)

**II. Lipid formulations of amphotericin B.** With conventional amphotericin B, dosage is often limited by adverse effects. Targeted drug delivery systems using liposome technology has made it possible to give more amphotericin and to attain much higher drug level concentrations in some organs without any increase in systemic toxicity. Three lipid preparations are currently commercially available (26,165,166) (Table 17.4).

**A. Mechanisms for improved therapeutic index**

**1.** The mechanisms by which lipid formulations may enhance efficacy with a reduction in toxicity is unknown. However, the following is postulated:

**a.** Lipid-associated amphotericin B may be targeted preferentially to organs rich in macrophages that are commonly the site of fungal infection (i.e., liver, spleen, lungs).

**b.** The rapid uptake in tissue macrophages may spare the kidneys from the higher dose that is seen with the amphotericin B deoxycholate administration.

**c.** There may also be the selective transfer of amphotericin B from the donor lipid to the fungal cell membrane.

Table 17.4. Comparative Cost of Common Antifungal Agents

| Agent | Route | Typical Daily Dose | Approximate Daily Cost |
|---|---|---|---|
| Amphotericin B | | | |
| Deoxycholate | i.v. | 50 mg | $ 23.28 |
| Lipid preparations | | | |
| Abelcet | i.v. | 5 mg/kg/day[a] | $ 920.00 |
| Ambisome | i.v. | 3 mg/kg/day | $ 942.00 |
| | | 6 mg/kg/day | $1,413.00 |
| Amphotec | i.v. | 4 mg/kg/day | $ 559.98 |
| Flucytosine | p.o. | 100 mg/kg/day | $ 112.40 |
| Ketoconazole | p.o. | 200 mg | $ 2.78 |
| | | 400 mg | $ 5.96 |
| Fluconazole | p.o. | 400 mg | $ 26.49 |
| | i.v. | 400 mg | $ 191.29 |
| Itraconazole | p.o. | 200 mg | $ 15.56 |
| | i.v. | 200 mg | $ 184.97 |
| Voriconazole | i.v. | 400 mg | $ N/A |
| | p.o. | 400 mg | $ N/A |
| Terbinafine | p.o. | 250 mg | $ 8.68 |
| Caspofungin | i.v. | 50 mg | $ 360.00 |

[a] All mg/kg doses were calculated for a 70-kg adult with normal renal function.
From 2002 *Drug topics red book*. New Jersey: 2000. Thomson Medical Economics, with permission.

**d.** *In vitro* data indicate that lipid preparations of amphotericin B do not elicit the release of pyrogenic cytokines to the same degree as amphotericin B deoxycholate. For further discussion on these proposed mechanisms, see the recent review by Slain [26].

**B. Pharmacokinetics.** Pharmacokinetic studies have been limited with lipid-based amphotericin B products. Further, no single clinical pharmacokinetic study has systematically compared the three commercially available lipid-based products with deoxycholate amphotericin B. Although these lipid formulations alter amphotericin B pharmacokinetics, it is uncertain if and how these changes affect clinical efficacy or toxicity. A compilation of pharmacokinetic studies with the lipid-based amphotericin B formulations is presented in a comprehensive review by Slain [26].

**C. Clinical indications and dosage.** These preparations are given i.v. once daily.

1. **Ampotericin B lipid complex** (Abelcet, ABLC) is approved for the treatment of invasive fungal infections in patients intolerant or refractory to amphotericin B [167]. The recommended dose is 5 mg/kg.
2. **Lipsomal amphotericin** (Ambisome, L-AMB) is approved for the empiric therapy of presumed fungal infections in febrile neutropenic patients [168]. It is also approved for the treatment of patients with serious fungal infections who are refractory to or intolerant to amphotericin B deoxycholate. Recommended daily dose is 3 to 5 mg/kg.
3. **Amphotericin B colloidal dispersion** (Amphotec, ABCD) is approved only for the treatment of invasive aspergillosis in patients who fail treatment with or are intolerant to amphotericin B. The recommended daily dose is 3 to 4 mg/kg [169].

**D. Clinical efficacy and toxicity**

1. Although there is paucity of large, prospective, randomized trials, the cumulative data indicate that all the lipid formulations of amphotericin B have significantly less renal toxicity than amphotericin B deoxycholate. Infusion-related toxicity is still seen with lipid preparations but appears mildest with Ambisome. Abelcet and Amphotec appear to have a similar infusion-related toxicity and are intermediate between AmBisome and amphotericin deoxycholate.
2. The lipid formulations appear to be equally or more effective compared with treatment with amphotericin B deoxycholate. The ability to give higher dosages with less nephrotoxicity may take advantage of the drug's concentration-dependent pharmacodynamic effects.
3. Because of the high mortality of invasive aspergillosis and mucormycosis in the compromised host, it is our practice to initiate treatment with a liposomal AMB at the highest dose for these patients.
4. Because of their high costs, the lipid-based formulations should be reserved as an alternative therapy for patients who fail treatment with other antifungal agents, cannot tolerate deoxycholate amphotericin B, or are at great risk of developing renal failure if given amphotericin B.

**III. Flucytosine (5-fluorocytosine, Ancobon)** is an effective antifungal drug, but because drug resistance develops it rarely is used alone. It is active against *C. neoformans*, *Candida* species, and *Torulopsis* species in particular.

**A. Mode of action.** Flucytosine is converted within susceptible fungal cells to 5-fluorouracil and 5-fluor-2-deoxyuredylic acid, which inhibit the function of **RNA and DNA,** respectively, and result in subsequent cell death [170].

**B. Distribution** is excellent into all body water spaces, **particularly the CSF, where 60% to 80% of the serum drug level is achieved.**

**C. Elimination.** Approximately 90% of the drug is excreted unchanged in the urine, and so **reduced renal function will lead to accumulation of the drug.** In contrast, reduced hepatic function does not alter drug excretion. Protein binding is negligible, and flucytosine is removed by hemodialysis and peritoneal dialysis.

**D. Mode of administration and dosage.** This oral agent is well absorbed (>90%) from the GI tract. Only oral capsules (250 and 500 mg) are available.

1. Patients with normal renal function usually receive 12.5 to 37.5 mg/kg orally every 6 hours (i.e., 50–150 mg/kg/day). Most infectious disease consultants recommended a maximum daily dose of 100 mg/day.

Table 17.5. Recommended Dosages of Flucytosine in Patients with Renal Insufficiency

| Creatinine Clearance (mL/min) | Dosage (mg/kg) | Interval (h) | Total Daily Dose (mg/kg) |
|---|---|---|---|
| >40 | 25 | 6 | 100 |
| 20–40 | 25 | 12 | 50 |
| <20 | 25 | 24 | 25 |
| <10 | [a] | [a] | [a] |
| Hemodialysis | 25 | After each hemodialysis | — |

[a] Avoid or adjust use to maintain peak serum level between 40 and 60 μg/mL. See text discussion.
From Patel R. Antifungal agents. Amphotericin B preparations and flucytosine. *Mayo Clin Proc* 1998;73: 1205–1225, with permission.

2. **Dosage is reduced in the presence of renal impairment. The dose should be regulated by monitoring serum levels,**which should be maintained at less than 100 μg/mL (preferably 40–60 μg/mL). Stamm et al. [171] published a nomogram to guide therapy. Also, see dose reductions in Table 17.5.

E. **Toxicity is** noted most often in patients with blood concentrations exceeding 100 μg/mL.
   1. **Hepatic abnormalities** (e.g., elevation in transaminases) are seen in approximately 5% to 7% of patients and are generally asymptomatic and reversible. Fatal hepatic necrosis has been reported, and so weekly liver function panels are suggested.
   2. **Leukopenia and thrombocytopenia are potentially lethal complications** [171] and occur more commonly in those with previous bone marrow damage. In initial reports, many **AIDS patients** who receive flucytosine along with amphotericin B for the treatment of cryptococcal meningitis were reported to develop significant bone marrow suppression. Therefore, flucytosine use was advised with caution in AIDS patients; amphotericin B is often used alone in the treatment of HIV-related cryptococcal meningitis. Additional clinical studies, however, have determined that the combination of flucytosine and amphotericin B result in significant improvement in outcome without excess toxicity in the treatment of AIDS-associated cryptococcal meningitis as compared with amphotericin B alone [68]. Flucytosine has also been used successfully in combination with fluconazole to treat cryptococcal meningitis in patients with AIDS [172,173].
   3. **GI intolerance** usually is limited to mild diarrhea, but in severe cases patients have had copious diarrhea, anorexia, nausea, vomiting, and abdominal pain.
   4. **Teratogenic effects.** Flucytosine has been shown to be teratogenic in animals and therefore should be avoided during pregnancy unless the potential benefit is greater than the potential risk to the fetus.
   5. **Nursing mothers.** It is not known whether flucytosine is excreted in breast milk. Mothers should be advised to discontinue nursing if flucytosine is administered.

F. **Combination chemotherapy.** Although many isolates of *Candida* and *Cryptococcus* are sensitive to flucytosine, **the rapid emergence of drug resistance precludes the use of the drug as a single agent in serious infections.** The combination of flucytosine with amphotericin B has an additive or synergistic effect, both *in vitro* and *in vivo,* against *Candida* and *Cryptococcus.* The additive effects may not only offer increased efficacy but may also allow amphotericin B to be given in lower doses, thus decreasing the toxicity of this agent. **Unfortunately, amphotericin B may increase the toxicity of flucytosine by impairing its renal excretion. Therefore, serum concentrations of flucytosine must ideally be monitored in patients who are taking this combination** and the dosage lowered or the drug stopped if flucytosine accumulates. This combination is frequently recommended for cryptococcal meningitis [66,68] and, occasionally, for systemic candidiasis.

G. **Cost** (Table 17.4)

**IV. Azoles.** The azoles are safe and effective alternatives to amphotericin B for the treatment of many of the systemic mycoses [174]. They are also useful in the management of superficial mycoses recalcitrant to topical therapy. The azoles are chemically classified by the number of nitrogen atoms in their five-membered azole rings as either imidazoles (miconazole and ketoconazole) or triazoles (itraconazole or fluconazole). **All the azoles exert their fungistatic activity by the same mechanism:** inhibition of the biosynthesis of ergosterol, the main sterol in the fungal cell membrane, via interference with the cytochrome P450-dependent fungal enzyme C-14 lanosterol demethylase. This results in altered membrane permeability with inhibition of cell growth and replication. **Unfortunately, the azoles may also interact with mammalian enzymes that are dependent on the cytochrome P450 system, and this interaction may induce major toxicities and drug interactions.** The triazoles, as compared with the imidazoles, have much greater affinity for fungal rather than mammalian cytochrome P450 enzymes and, in general, have less toxicity and fewer drug interactions.

**A. Miconazole (Monistat)** is an imidazole that is available only in the United States as a topical preparation. See Chapter 16 for its topical uses. Its **usage as a systemic antifungal agent was limited by its toxicity and by the development of more effective and less toxic systemic azoles.**

**B. Ketoconazole (Nizoral),** an oral imidazole, was the first azole to prove clinically useful as a systemic antifungal drug.

1. **Antifungal activity.** Ketoconazole is active against clinical isolates of *Candida, C. immitis, H. capsulatum, B. dermatitidis,* and *Paracoccidioides brasiliensis.*
2. **Pharmacokinetics.** Only an **oral** preparation is available. Ketoconazole is well absorbed if there is enough gastric acidity. The administration of antacids, proton pump inhibitors, or $H_2$-blocking agents reduces absorption. Other situations that reduce gastric acid secretion (and that may reduce absorption) include aging, gastric surgery, and AIDS gastropathy. **Because of the uncertainty of absorption in these settings, many clinicians may prefer to use fluconazole** when appropriate. Sucralfate does not affect absorption.

   The drug is extensively degraded *in vivo,* and very little active drug is excreted by either the renal or biliary pathway. Therefore, **the dose does not have to be changed in renal failure.** Whether dosage should be adjusted in hepatic failure is unknown. Isoniazid, phenytoin, and rifampin increase the metabolism of ketoconazole, and concurrent use of these drugs may result in treatment failure. Ketoconazole does not penetrate well into the CSF.
3. **Clinical uses [175]**
   - a. **Chronic mucocutaneous candidiasis.** Ketoconazole has been very effective in treating this uncommon disease [10]. Chronic maintenance therapy over many years has been effective and well tolerated.
   - b. **Dermatophyte infections.** Ketoconazole is indicated for the treatment of severe or recalcitrant cutaneous dermatophyte infections that have not responded to topical therapy or oral griseofulvin or for patients who are unable to take griseofulvin. It has also been used with success in onychomycosis due to *Trichophyton* species, *Microsporum* species, and *Epidermophyton floccosum.*
   - c. **Oral thrush and candidal esophagitis.** These conditions in **AIDS** patients and others often respond well to ketoconazole. Treatment failure may result from the concomitant use of antacids, proton pump inhibitors, or $H_2$-receptor antagonists because an acid gastric pH is necessary for adequate absorption. Patients with AIDS frequently have gastric hypochlorhydria, which impairs ketoconazole absorption and may result in clinical failure.
   - d. **Systemic fungal infections.** Ketoconazole may be used for the treatment of a variety of systemic fungal infections in immunocompetent patients who do not have life-threatening or CNS disease, including **histoplasmosis, blastomycosis, coccidioidomycosis,** and **paracoccidioidomycosis.** (Itraconazole due to enhanced efficacy and less toxicity has supplemented the use of ketoconazole in most clinical situations.) Infectious disease consultation is recommended.

e. **Miscellaneous**
   (1) **Vaginal candidiasis.** The therapy of vaginal candidiasis is discussed elsewhere (see Chapter 16). Ketoconazole is not indicated in the routine management of this problem.
   (2) **Prophylaxis of fungal infections in neutropenic patients with ketoconazole is not advised.**
   (3) ***Candida balanitis*** often responds well to a 7- to 10-day course of ketoconazole.

4. **Dosage.** Ketoconazole is available in a scored 200-mg tablet.
   a. **Adults.** The usual starting dose for superficial candidal or dermatophyte infections is 200 mg/day. Higher doses (400–800 mg/day) are used in the treatment of histoplasmosis, blastomycosis, and coccidioidomycosis [50,122]. In a patient with candidal esophagitis and AIDS, 400 mg/day may be necessary. **Achlorhydria or concurrent administration of agents that decrease gastric acidity** (e.g., antacids, anticholinergics, proton pump inhibitors, or $H_2$ blockers) **decreases the absorption of ketoconazole.** Administering ketoconazole with cola or another liquid with an acid pH (e.g., orange juice) may improve its absorption. In such circumstances, however, fluconazole, which does not require an acid pH for absorption, is preferable.
   b. **Children.** In small numbers of children older than 2 years, ketoconazole in a single daily dose of 3.3 to 6.6 mg/kg has been used successfully (see the package insert). The potential benefits should outweigh the risks before using ketoconazole in children.
   c. **The duration of treatment** must be individualized depending on the presence of associated diseases and response to therapy. Usually only 1 or 2 weeks of treatment are necessary for the management of superficial *Candida* infections. A minimum treatment period of 6 months is recommended for the systemic mycoses [50,122].
   d. **In renal failure** dose modification is not necessary. Ketoconazole is not substantially removed by hemodialysis or peritoneal dialysis.
   e. **In hepatic insufficiency** no dose adjustment is necessary for mild to moderate hepatic insufficiency. In patients with severe liver failure, ketoconazole should be avoided or the dose reduced and serum levels monitored if no alternative agent is available.
   f. **Cost** (Table 17.4)

5. **Contraindications or drug interactions**
   a. **Pregnancy. Ketoconazole** is teratogenic in the rat model and should be avoided in pregnancy.
   b. **Nursing mothers** who must receive ketoconazole should not breast-feed for the duration of treatment.
   c. **Drug interactions**
      (1) Ketoconazole increases the blood levels of **cyclosporine, digoxin, and phenytoin.** Serum levels of these drugs should be carefully monitored.
      (2) **The coadministration of ketoconazole with terfenadine or astemizole is contraindicated.** When ketoconazole is administered with either of these antihistamines, it may prolong the QT interval, sometimes causing life-threatening ventricular arrhythmias [175,176]. A similar interaction has been described in patients receiving **cisapride (Propulsid)** for upper gastrointestinal motility problems.
      (3) **Isoniazid, rifampin, and phenytoin** increase the metabolism of ketoconazole. These drugs should not be used concomitantly. Monitoring serum ketoconazole levels may be helpful.
      (4) **The anticoagulant effect of coumadin** may be enhanced by ketoconazole. The patient's prothrombin time should be followed closely.
      (5) Ketoconazole may potentiate the hypoglycemic effect of some oral **hypoglycemic agents.**

6. **Adverse effects.** In general, ketoconazole is well tolerated (Table 17.3) [175,177].

a. **Nausea** is the most common side effect. It can be reduced when ketoconazole is taken with food or at bedtime. Abdominal pain may occur.

b. **Pruritus and skin rashes** are not uncommon. **Anaphylaxis** after the first dose has been reported rarely.

c. **Hepatotoxicity** due to hepatocellular damage **may occur,** and rare fatalities damage have been reported. Liver damage usually is reversible when the drug is discontinued. **Liver function tests should be obtained before starting therapy and at frequent intervals during drug administration,** especially in patients on prolonged therapy or those receiving other potentially hepatotoxic agents. Transient minor liver function test elevations often occur during ketoconazole therapy. The drug should be discontinued if elevated levels of transaminases persist or are three to five times greater than normal.

d. **Miscellaneous.** Gynecomastia in men, rashes, dizziness, constipation, and diarrhea have occurred. Temporary suppression of serum testosterone levels and of adrenal cortisol production in response to adrenocorticotropic hormone has been described. Rarely, adrenal crisis has been reported in the setting of high-dose ketoconazole therapy [178]. Oligospermia may occur at high daily doses, especially if the dosage exceeds 400 mg/day. Loss of libido and loss of potency also have been reported [179].

C. **Fluconazole (Diflucan)** is a bis-triazole antifungal that was released in 1990. Fluconazole is indicated for the treatment of candidal infections and for initial treatment (of selected patients) and prevention of cryptococcal meningitis in AIDS patients. It is available in both an intravenous and an oral preparation.

1. **Pharmacokinetics**

a. **Absorption** from the GI tract is **excellent,** with oral bioavailability exceeding 90% [179–181]. Serum levels are similar after oral and intravenous administration. **Gastric acid is not required for absorption.** Absorption is not reduced by concomitant use of $H_2$ blockers on antacids.

b. There is little metabolism of fluconazole, and renal excretion accounts for approximately 80% of its elimination as unchanged drug. Therefore, **dosage reduction is necessary in patients with renal failure.**

c. **Urine concentrations of fluconazole are high.** Thus, it may be an effective agent in urinary tract candidiasis [181].

d. Fluconazole has **excellent penetration into the CSF,** with levels reaching 60% to 80% of serum levels.

e. Fluconazole diffuses well into sputum, saliva, skin, and the vitreous and aqueous humor of the eye. Pharmacokinetics are similar in healthy young adults and in the elderly [180].

2. **Clinical uses**

a. Fluconazole has proven useful for **cryptococcal meningitis in AIDS patients** as both initial therapy and maintenance therapy. Amphotericin B, however, is preferred as initial therapy in those patients who are seriously ill or confused or who have other poor prognostic findings. In these patients, fluconazole may be substituted for amphotericin B once the patient has clinically stabilized and the CSF parameters have improved (see Cryptococcosis, above, and Chapters 6 and 18). For maintenance therapy of AIDS patients, oral fluconazole (200–400 mg/day) is the treatment of choice.

b. Fluconazole is effective in the treatment of **oropharyngeal and esophageal** candidiasis in immunocompromised hosts [6,179].

c. Fluconazole is not recommended for the routine management of **vaginal candidiasis.** However, it may be helpful in selected patients who fail topical therapy or who have frequent recurrences (see Chapter 16).

d. The use of fluconazole for patients with **candidemia and systemic candidiasis** has been controversial. However, recent studies indicate that fluconazole has equivalent efficacy to amphotericin B for treating these syndromes in patients with and without neutropenia. See section **III.D** under Candidiasis, above.

e. Fluconazole has also been used successfully to prevent candidiasis in patients undergoing bone marrow transplantation. Unfortunately, an increased rate of infections due to fluconazole-resistant *C. krusei* was noted in these studies [182,183]. Many AIDS patients receive fluconazole either continuously or intermittently over long periods of time. Concomitant with its widespread use (over 15 million patients since 1988), there have been **increasing reports of fluconazole resistance.** This topic has been reviewed elsewhere [184].

f. The role of fluconazole in the treatment of coccidioidomycosis, histoplasmosis, blastomycosis, and sporotrichosis is currently under investigation. Initial studies indicate that fluconazole will be a useful agent in treating coccidioidal meningitis.

g. **Hepatosplenic candidiasis** has responded to fluconazole (see section **III.F.1** under Candidiasis, above).

3. **Dosages.** Because fluconazole is well absorbed after oral therapy, **the daily doses for oral and intravenous therapy are the same.** Intravenous administration is preferred when GI motility is impaired or nasogastric suction is used. Tablets are available in 50, 100, or 200 mg. A suspension is also available.

a. **For oropharyngeal candidiasis,** 200 mg on the first day followed by 100 mg once daily is continued until infection has subsided. Most patients respond in a few days, and treatment for longer than 1 week usually is not necessary. Frequent relapses of disease are noted in AIDS patients, and maintenance therapy has proven helpful in these instances. We found a dose of 100 mg once weekly is effective in preventing relapse in most of our patients [7].

b. **For esophageal candidiasis,** 200 mg on the first day followed by 100 mg once daily is routinely suggested. Higher doses (up to 400 mg/day) may be necessary. Patients should be treated for a minimum of 2 weeks.

c. **Systemic candidiasis or candidemia.** Two recent randomized trials indicate that non-neutropenic patients treated with fluconazole, 400 mg/day, have similar outcomes to those treated with amphotericin B [22,23]. However, some non-*albicans* species, such as *C. krusei,* are resistant to fluconazole, and amphotericin B should be used in individuals infected with these organisms.

d. **For cryptococcal meningitis**

(1) **For suppression of relapse** in patients with AIDS, 200 mg once daily is suggested [67–69].

(2) **For primary therapy of cryptococcal meningitis** in patients with AIDS, after an initial 400 mg on the first day, 200 to 400 mg once daily may be effective in selected low-risk patients [65]. However, most experts recommend an initial course of amphotericin, followed by fluconazole once the patient has clinically stabilized and the CSF parameters have improved. Infectious disease consultation is advised in this setting. See section **IV.A.3** under Cryptococcosis, above.

(3) The role of fluconazole in the treatment of cryptococcal meningitis in HIV-negative individuals is yet to be defined.

e. **Dosage needs to be reduced in patients with renal failure.** After the initial loading dose, the following dose reductions are suggested: For a creatinine clearance in excess of 50 mL/min, give the normal dose; if the clearance is 21 to 50 mL/min, give 50% of the usual dose; if the clearance is 11 to 20 mL/min, give 25% of the usual dose. In patients on regular hemodialysis, give the usual dose once after each dialysis treatment.

f. **Intravenous fluconazole** is used in patients who cannot take the oral, less expensive, route, as in patients who have nausea and vomiting, are taking nothing by mouth, and so on. Otherwise, there is no advantage of the intravenous preparation, which provides serum concentrations similar to the oral preparation. For dosages see section **3.**

g. **Pregnancy.** The package insert notes that there are no adequate and well-controlled studies in pregnant women; this agent should be used in pregnancy only if the potential benefit justifies the possible risk to the fetus.

   h. **Nursing.** The package insert notes that fluconazole is excreted in human milk at concentrations similar to plasma. Therefore, the use of fluconazole in nursing mothers is not recommended.

4. **Side effects.** Fluconazole has been well tolerated, with reports of toxicity most frequent in AIDS patients (Table 17.2) [179,180].
   a. **Rash** occurs in fewer than 5% of recipients.
   b. **Nausea and vomiting** occur in 2% to 10% of recipients. Nausea is less frequent with fluconazole than with ketoconazole.
   c. **Stevens-Johnson syndrome** and **hepatotoxicity** are reported rarely. Transient elevations of liver function tests are relatively common in AIDS patients.
   d. Fluconazole affects adrenal steroid synthesis much less than does ketoconazole. Endocrine side effects, including impotence, gynecomastia, and menstrual disturbances, are reported less frequently.
5. **Drug interactions.** Drug interactions are less frequent and less pronounced as compared with ketoconazole. When another agent is administered with fluconazole, the following drug interactions may occur.
   a. **Rifampin** decreases serum concentrations of fluconazole.
   b. The hypoglycemic effects of oral agents, especially **tolbutamide,** may be enhanced.
   c. **Warfarin, phenytoin, rifabutin, and cyclosporine** levels are variably increased, especially with higher doses of fluconazole [185]. Monitoring the prothrombin time or serum drug levels is important in patients receiving fluconazole.
   d. **The potential interaction between fluconazole and terfenadine or astemizole has not been adequately studied. Until these data are available, it seems prudent to avoid these combinations.** Fluconazole may interact with **cisapride** (Propulsid), and these two agents should not be used together.
6. **Cost.** Fluconazole is expensive (Table 17.4).

D. **Itraconazole (Sporanox)** is a triazole that was originally released as an oral agent for the systemic treatment of fungal infections. It has subsequently been formulated with a $\beta$-cyclodextrin as an oral suspension and intravenous agent [186–188]. It is approved for primary therapy of histoplasmosis and blastomycosis. Recent approval has been obtained for the treatment of invasive aspergillosis.

1. **Pharmacokinetics**
   a. **Absorption of the capsules** while fasting is only 30% to 40%. **Bioavailability** is significantly **enhanced by food,** and it is recommended that the drug be taken with meals. Absorption is also enhanced by the presence of gastric acid and is reduced by antacids [187].
   b. **The oral suspension** is better absorbed on an empty stomach and is less dependent on acid for absorption.
   c. Itraconazole is **highly protein bound** (99.8%), and there is little or no CSF penetration.
   d. The drug is lipophilic, and **tissue levels exceed serum concentrations.** The drug can be detected in tissue, including the skin and nails, for longer periods of time than in serum after the drug has been discontinued.
   e. Extensive hepatic metabolism occurs, but one of the major metabolites has antifungal activity. Less than 1% of active drug is excreted in the urine.
   f. Renal failure, hemodialysis, and peritoneal dialysis do not alter serum levels or metabolism of itraconazole when given as capsules or suspensions. Note, however, that the $\beta$-cyclodextrin present in the intravenous preparation is excreted by the kidneys [188].
2. **Clinical uses**
   a. Itraconazole currently is approved for the treatment of **histoplasmosis** and **blastomycosis** [50,122] and as an alternative agent in aspergillosis [96]. See individual discussions of these topics earlier in this chapter.
   b. Itraconazole has a broad range of *in vitro* antifungal activity, including *Candida* species, *C. immitis, S. schenckii, C. neoformans,* and *Aspergillus* species.

c. Itraconazole has proven helpful in the management of selected patients with chronic skin and nail infections due to dermatophyte fungi. The role of itraconazole for onychomycosis was recently reviewed; doses of 200 mg once a day, with a meal, for 3 months are suggested [189,190].

3. **Dosage.** Itraconazole is available in 100 mg capsules, which **should be taken with meals.** An oral suspension is also available and has enhanced bioavailability. The availability of an intravenous preparation has proven useful in patients unable to tolerate oral medications. Doses above 200 mg/day should be given in divided doses.
   a. **Histoplasmosis and blastomycosis.** In a recent prospective trial, patients treated with 200 mg/day had a similar outcome to those treated with 400 mg/day. Thus, the initial recommended daily dose of itraconazole is 200 mg. Patients whose disease progresses on therapy should have their dose increased in 100-mg increments to a maximum daily dose of 400 mg. A minimum of 6 months' therapy is recommended, but the successful treatment of histoplasmosis frequently requires treatment for 1 year or longer [50,122].
   b. **Aspergillosis.** Itraconazole was later approved for use in the treatment of pulmonary and extrapulmonary aspergillosis in patients who are intolerant of or refractory to amphotericin B therapy. A loading dose of 200 mg three times day should be given for the first 3 days (in severe infection) and then 200 to 400 mg/day is suggested. Itraconazole has also been used for the treatment of ABPA and mycetomas [85,86].
   c. Although not FDA approved for **sporotrichosis,** initial studies indicate that itraconazole is an effective alternative to potassium iodide in this setting. For cutaneous or lymphocutaneous disease, the usual dose is 200 mg/day for 3 to 6 months. Higher doses (200 mg twice daily) are used for osseous or articular disease and pulmonary disease [133,135]. Therapy for 1 or 2 years may be required in extracutaneous disease. Infectious disease consultation is recommended.
   d. **Pediatric use.** The safety and efficacy of itraconazole in children has not been established.
   e. **Renal failure.** Dosage adjustments of the capsules and suspension are not necessary in renal failure. Neither hemodialysis nor peritoneal dialysis alters serum levels of itraconazole. The $\beta$-cyclodextrin contained in the intravenous formulation is cleared by the kidneys. As such, dose should be adjusted in patients with renal insufficiency. It is recommended that intravenous itraconazole should not be used in patients with a creatinine clearance of less than 30 mL per minute.
   f. **Hepatic dysfunction.** Whether dosage adjustment is necessary in patients with hepatic dysfunction is unclear. Plasma concentrations should be monitored in patients with severe hepatic insufficiency.

4. **Toxicity.** Itraconazole is generally well tolerated in the currently recommended doses of 200 to 400 mg/day. Toxicity is reported more frequently at doses of 600 mg or higher.
   a. **Nausea and vomiting** are seen in approximately 10% of patients but usually do not necessitate discontinuation of therapy. Giving the dose with the evening meal or dividing the daily dosage into two equal doses may be helpful.
   b. **Liver function abnormalities** are mild and transient; symptomatic hepatitis is rare.
   c. Less common side effects include **pruritus, skin rash, headache, hypertension, hypokalemia, pedal edema, and congestive heart failure.**
   d. **Impotence,** usually reversible, has been reported despite normal testosterone levels.
   e. At doses of less than 600 mg/day, itraconazole has little or no effect on adrenal cortisol production.

5. **Drug interactions** have been well documented between itraconazole and a variety of other medications. Compared with ketoconazole, it is not as potent an inhibitor of liver microsomal enzymes.

a. **Antacids, and possibly proton pump inhibitors and $H_2$-receptor antagonists,** will decrease peak serum levels and so should be avoided if possible.
b. **Rifampin and phenytoin** will induce the metabolism of itraconazole and **result in decreased serum levels.** The dosage of itraconazole may need to be increased in patients failing therapy when these agents are used concurrently. Some suggest that concurrent use of rifampin, phenytoin, carbamazepine, and phenobarbital should be avoided in patients receiving itraconazole for life-threatening infection (e.g., invasive aspergillosis) [86].
c. **The coadministration of itraconazole and terfenadine, or astemizole, is contraindicated. A prolonged QT interval and life-threatening ventricular arrhythmias have been reported** [191]. A similar potential interaction has been noted for **cisapride** (Propulsid).
d. Itraconazole will raise the levels of **cyclosporine, digoxin, and phenytoin** when coadministered with these agents. Levels should be monitored.
e. The anticoagulant effect of **warfarin** may be increased by itraconazole.
f. The hypoglycemic effect of **oral sulfonylurea drugs,** especially tolbutamide, may be enhanced when coadministered with itraconazole.

6. **Pregnancy.** Itraconazole is teratogenic in rats and should not be given during pregnancy unless benefits outweigh potential risks. The drug is secreted in breast milk and should not be administered to nursing mothers.
7. **Cost.** Itraconazole is an expensive agent (Table 17.4).

E. **Voriconazole** is a new triazole antifungal agent recently approved for the treatment of invasive aspergillosis. In addition, it has also been approved for the treatment of serious fungal infections caused by *Scedosporium apiospermum* (the asexual form of *Pseudallescheria boydii*) and *Fusarium* species in patients intolerant or refractory to other therapies. Voriconazole also has good activity *in vitro* against many other pathogenic fungi, including *Candida* species, *Cryptococcus* species, and *Dermatophyte* species [192–194]. Voriconazole can be administered either orally or parenterally and has a favorable adverse events profile. The most commonly reported adverse effects are visual disturbances and elevation in liver function tests.

1. **Pharmacokinetics** [195,196]. Voriconazole is available for both oral and intravenous administration and has a wide tissue distribution, including the CNS. The drug is hepatically metabolized with the renal excretion of metabolites and exhibits nonlinear pharmacokinetics.
   a. **The oral tablets contain 50 or 200 mg of voriconazole.** The bioavailability of these tablets is approximately 96% in humans, and peak concentrations occur within 2 hours after an oral dose. Other pharmacokinetic properties of voriconazole are similar after intravenous and oral administration.
   b. **The intravenous formulation contains a sulfobutyl ether $\beta$-cyclodextrin.** This cyclodextrin is not excreted by the kidneys and thus may accumulate in patients with renal failure. Dosage adjustment is necessary for patients with renal failure.
   c. Approximately 58% of voriconazole in the blood is protein bound.
   d. The distribution of voriconazole is rapid and extensive; the volume of distribution is 4.6 L/mg. Concentrations have been measured in the CSF between 30% and 68% of simultaneous serum concentrations.
   e. **Voriconazole is metabolized in the liver** by the cytochrome P450 enzyme system. The pharmacokinetics of voriconazole are nonlinear due to saturation of its metabolism. A dosage adjustment is necessary in patients with hepatic insufficiency.
   f. Peak plasma concentrations approach steady-state levels in the first 24 hours of dosing if a loading dose is administered.
2. **Clinical usage**
   a. Voriconazole is approved for the treatment of invasive aspergillosis, both as primary or salvage therapy. **As primary therapy for invasive aspergillosis,** a satisfactory response rate of 53% was reported for voriconazole as compared with 32% in amphotericin B-treated patients. In the combined clinical

data on salvage therapy (no comparator group), an overall favorable response rate of 44% was noted. (Data submitted to FDA and cited in the product insert.)

   **b.** Although the cohort of patients treated was small, voriconazole has been shown to be effective against *Scedosporium apiospermum* and *Fusarium* species, with favorable response rates reported of 63% and 43%, respectively. (Data submitted to FDA and cited in the product insert.)

   **c.** Potential future uses of voriconazole include the treatment of invasive candidiasis, candidemia, and as an alternative to amphotericin for the treatment of febrile neutropenic patients [197].

**3. Dosage.** A loading dose should be given on day 1 to achieve plasma concentrations close to steady state. A loading dose of 6 mg/kg every 12 hours for two doses is recommended.

   **a. Maintenance dose.** The maintenance dose is 4 mg/kg every 12 hours. If patients are started on intravenous therapy, they should be switched to tablets once they can tolerate oral medications. When administered orally, for patients who weigh more than 40 kg the recommended maintenance dose is 200 mg every 12 hours. For smaller adults weighing less than 40 kg, 100 mg every 12 hours is recommended.

   **b. A dosage adjustment is necessary in patients with hepatic insufficiency.** It is recommended that the standard loading dose is a given but the maintenance dose reduced by 50% in patients with mild to moderate hepatic disease (Child-Pugh class A or B). Voriconazole has not been studied in patients with severe hepatic cirrhosis (Child-Pugh class C).

   **c. Use of patients with renal failure.** The pharmacokinetics of oral voriconazole is not significantly effected by renal insufficiency and no dosage adjustment is necessary for oral therapy. In contrast, the sulfobutyl ether $\beta$-cyclodextrin in the intravenous formulation will accumulate in patients with moderate or severe renal insufficiency (e.g., 50 mL/min). Voriconazole is hemodialyzed, but the sulfobutyl ether $\beta$-cyclodextrin is not.

**4. Toxicity. The most commonly reported side effects include visual disturbances, dermatologic reactions, and elevations in liver function tests. (Data on file with manufacturer.)**

   **a.** Visual disturbances have been reported in approximately 30% of patients enrolled in clinical trials. The mechanism of action of the visual disturbances is unknown but is most likely due to direct effects on the retina and appears to be associated with higher plasma concentrations and doses. The visual disturbances reported to date have generally been mild and transient. Discontinuation of the drug due to visual changes has been rare. Visual hallucinations that are distinct from other visual perception changes also may occur in up to 4% of patients [197].

   **b.** Dermatologic reactions are reported in approximately 6% of voriconazole-treated patients. For those exposed to the sun, significant sun sensitivity develops. Most of the reactions are mild, although serious cutaneous reactions have been reported.

   **c.** Clinically significant transaminase elevations were noted in approximately 13.4% of patients treated in prerelease clinical trials. Most abnormal liver function tests resolved during treatment with or without a dosage adjustment. Liver function tests should be monitored at the start of and routinely during the course of voriconazole treatment.

**5. Drug interactions.** Voriconazole is hepatically metabolized. Drugs cleared by the cytochrome P450 system have been investigated for potential interactions with voriconazole.

   **a. Voriconazole has been shown to significantly increase the serum levels of the following agents to such a degree that concurrent use is contraindicated: sirolimus, terfenadine, astemizole, cisapride, pimozide, quinidine, and the ergot alkaloids.**

   **b.** The coadministration of voriconazole with cyclosporine, tacrolimus, warfarin, statins, benzodiazepines, calcium channel blockers, sulfonylureas, and the vinca alkaloids will result in increased activity of these drugs. Although not contraindicated, careful monitoring or dosing adjustment of these drugs is required.

**c.** Some drugs when given concurrently will result in significant reduction in voriconazole serum/tissue levels and may adversely effect clinical outcome. These include rifampicin, rifabutin, and phenytoin. Increasing the voriconazole dose in patients receiving these agents is suggested. Avoiding the use of these agents in patients with life-threatening infections seems more prudent.

**d.** Although not well studied, carbamazepine and long-acting barbiturates are also likely to decrease plasma voriconazole concentrations.

**e.** Little or no significant interactions have been noted between voriconazole and cimetidine, ranitidine, digoxin, macrolide antibiotics, or indinavir.

**6. Voriconazole is Pregnancy Category D and should not be used in pregnant women.**

**7. Pediatric experience is limited but promising [198], and the safety of voriconazole in children has not been adequately established.**

**V. Echinocandins** are a new class of antifungal drugs that inhibit the synthesis of B-(1,3)-d-glucan, an integral component of the fungal cell wall. Caspofungin acetate (Cancidas) is the first glucan synthesis inhibitor commercially available [100]. Caspofungin acetate is currently indicated only for the treatment of invasive aspergillosis in patients refractory or intolerant to other therapies. Because of its excellent *in vitro* and *in vivo* activity against isolates of *Candida* species (including non-*albicans Candida*), caspofungin will assume a prominent role in the treatment of patients with invasive candidiasis and candidemia. **Caspofungin has little or no activity *in vitro* or *in vivo* against *Cryptococcus neoformans* or *Mucor* species.**

**A. Pharmacokinetics of caspofungin**

**1. Caspofungin acetate** is only available as an intravenous formulation.

**2. Caspofungin** is extensively bound to albumin (approximately 97%).

**3. Caspofungin** is slowly metabolized by hydroxylation and *N*-acetylation. Thus, dosing adjustments are necessary in patients with liver failure.

**4. Dosing in patients with renal failure.** No dosage adjustment is necessary for patients with renal insufficiency. Caspofungin is not dialyzed, and supplemental dosing after hemodialysis is not necessary.

**B. Clinical uses**

**1.** Caspofungin is currently indicated only for the treatment of invasive aspergillosis in patients refractory or intolerant to other therapies, including amphotericin B, lipid formulations of amphotericin B, or itraconazole. Studies using caspofungin as initial therapy for invasive aspergillosis have not been completed. Although this is the only approved use, observations in disseminated candidiasis and refractory candida esophagitis in AIDS suggest that approval for these uses will occur very soon.

**2.** Caspofungin exhibits good *in vitro* activity against *Aspergillous fumigatus, Aspergillus flavis,* and *Aspergillus tereus.*

**3.** Sixty-nine patients were enrolled in an open-label noncomparative study of caspofungin in patients with invasive aspergillosis intolerant or refractory to other therapies. Sixty-three patients met entry criteria and had outcome data. Overall, 41% (26 of 63) receiving at least one dose of caspofungin had a favorable response. For those patients who received greater than 7 days of therapy, 50% had a favorable response. The favorable response rate for patients intolerant to previous therapy was 70% as compared with 36% of those who failed previous therapy.

**4. Combination therapy with caspofungin and itraconazole** has been used successfully in the treatment of patients with invasive aspergillosis who have failed monotherapy. We believe that combination therapy may be especially important in patients with prolonged immunosuppression.

**C. Dosage**

**1.** For the treatment of invasive aspergillosis a single 70-mg intravenous dose is given on day 1 followed by 50 mg/day thereafter. Limited safety data indicate that a 70-mg daily dose is also well tolerated. Doses above 70 mg/day are currently undergoing evaluation but have not been adequately studied for either safety or efficacy.

2. No dosage adjustments are needed in patients with renal failure.
3. **Dosing in patients with hepatic insufficiency.** No dosage adjustments are needed for patients with mild hepatic insufficiency (Child-Pugh class A). For patients with moderate hepatic insufficiency (Child-Pugh class B) the daily dose (after the initial 70-mg loading dose) should be reduced to 35 mg. There is no clinical experience in treating patients with severe hepatic insufficiency as defined by Child-Pugh class C.

**D. Toxicity.** Caspofungin is generally well tolerated in the currently recommended doses of 50 to 70 mg/day.

1. **Histamine-mediated symptoms** during infusion have been reported. Symptoms include rash, facial swelling, pruritus, and the sensation of warmth. Anaphylaxis has also been rarely reported.
2. Other reported adverse effects include fever, rash, nausea, vomiting, and phlebitis at the injection site.
3. Elevations in hepatic transaminases have also been reported especially when caspofungin and cyclosporine are given concurrently.

**E. Drug interactions.** Caspofungin is not an inhibitor of any of the enzymes in the cytochrome P450 system. Additionally, caspofungin does not appear to induce the CYP 3A4 metabolism of other drugs.

1. Although caspofungin is not metabolized by the hepatic cytochrome system, its concurrent use with other drugs that broadly activate hepatic enzyme systems may accelerate the metabolism of caspofungin. This may have an adverse effect on clinical outcome. Thus, increasing the dose of caspofungin is warranted when administered with efavirenz (Sustiva), nelfinavir (Viracept), phenytoin, dexamethasone, rifampin, and carbamazepine.
2. Serum levels of tacrolimus are reduced by approximately 25% when caspofungin is coadministered.

**F. Special considerations**

1. Caspofungin is **Pregnancy Category C** and should only be used in pregnant women if the potential benefits of therapy justifies the potential risk to the fetus.
2. Safety in pediatric patients has not been adequately established.

**VI. Allylamines.** The allylamines exert their antifungal activity by inhibition of the fungal squalene epoxidase. Inhibition of this enzyme not only decreases ergosterol synthesis but also results in the accumulation of squalene, which is toxic to the fungus and is responsible for the fungicidal action seen with this class of agents [199]. The first of these compounds available for systemic use is terbinafine (Lamisil). Terbinafine is the most active antifungal agent *in vitro* against the dermatophyte fungi. Hence, its primary use is for treatment of onychomycosis of the toenails or fingernails due to the dermatophytes (tinea unguium).

**A. Pharmacokinetics [199]**

1. Terbinafine is well absorbed from the GI tract (>70%) with a peak plasma concentration occurring within 2 hours after an oral dose.
2. Terbinafine is greater than 99% bound to plasma proteins.
3. The drug is also lipophilic and keratophilic, which results in a depot effect in the skin and nails. A terminal elimination half-life of 200 to 400 hours has been reported and represents the slow elimination of terbinafine from skin and adipose tissue.
4. Before excretion, terbinafine is extensively metabolized in the liver. Most metabolites (70%–80%) are excreted in the urine.

**B. Clinical indications and dosage [199].** Terbinafine tablets are currently indicated only for treatment of onychomycosis of the toenails or fingernails. Antifungal activity has been established *in vitro* against other fungi, including *S. schenkii* and *C. albicans.* Clinical efficacy in treating lymphocutaneous sporotrichosis has also been documented, but this usage is not currently FDA approved.

1. **Onychomycosis [190,199,200]**
   a. **Fingernails.** A dose of 250 mg/day given over 6 weeks is currently recommended for onychomycosis of the fingernails. Clinical and mycologic cure rates are reported in up to 60% of patients.
   b. **Toenails.** For treatment of toenail infections, the same daily dose is extended for 12 weeks. Clinical and mycologic cure rates of 38% to 59% have been reported.
   c. **Relapse** of infection (especially of toenails) after apparent successful therapy is significant and remains problematic.
   d. **Alternative treatment regimens that take advantage of the high concentrations achieved in the nails and skin (depot effect) have been developed.** In these "pulse therapy" protocols, 500 mg of terbinafine is given daily for 1 week for 4 successive months for toenail infections and 3 months for fingernail infections. Cure rates for patients treated with terbinafine pulse therapy was similar for that reported in patients treated with daily terbinafine or pulse with itraconazole.
2. **Sporotrichosis.** Terbinafine has also shown clinical efficacy in the treatment of lymphocutaneous sporotrichosis. In open-label studies, terbinafine in a daily dose of 250 to 500 mg had a favorable clinical response [135].

C. **Toxicity.** In general, terbinafine has been well tolerated. The most frequently reported toxicities are as follows [199]:
   1. GI symptoms (nausea, abdominal pain, diarrhea) are most common and are dose dependent.
   2. Skin reactions, headache, and dysgeusia are also uncommonly reported.
   3. Elevated hepatic transaminases are also reported. Rare cases of liver failure, some leading to death or transplantation, have been reported. Thus, liver function studies should be monitored regularly.

D. **Drug interactions.** Terbinafine is metabolized in the liver by the cytochrome P450 enzyme system. However, it has only moderate affinity for these enzymes and has less drug interaction than noted for the azoles.
   1. Terbinafine does not effect the clearance of digoxin, warfarin, or terfenadine.
   2. Terbinafine does increase clearance of cyclosporine by approximately 15% and monitoring drug levels is prudent.
   3. Rifampin increases the clearance of terbinafine by 100%, and this combination of drugs should be avoided.
   4. Cimetidine decreases the clearance of terbinafine by approximately one-third.

E. **Special considerations.**
   1. **Terbinafine is Pregnancy Category B** and should not be initiated during pregnancy.
   2. The safety and efficacy of terbinafine has not been established in pediatric patients.

VII. **Other agents**

A. **Potassium iodide** has long been an effective agent for the treatment of the cutaneous-lymphatic form of sporotrichosis. See the discussion in section **III** under Sporotrichosis.

B. **Griseofulvin** is produced by a species of *Penicillium.* It exerts its fungicidal activity by inhibiting fungal mitosis, most likely due to the polymerization of cell microtubules and disruption of the mitotic spindle [201]. Griseofulvin is active against the dermatophytes (*Trichophyton, Epidermophyton,* and *Microsporum* species) that cause ringworm of the skin, hair, and nails. It has no clinically significant activity against *Candida* species or any other pathogenic fungi.
   1. **Mode of administration.** Griseofulvin is sold in a microsize form in capsules (125 and 250 mg), in an ultramicrosize form in tablets (165 and 330 mg), and as a pediatric suspension (125 mg/5 mL) [201].
      a. The **usual adult dose** is 500 mg/day of the microsize preparation or 330 mg of the ultramicrosize preparation given as a single daily dose. In severe or more recalcitrant cases of disease, these doses may be doubled.
      b. The duration of therapy varies depending on the site of infection and clinical response. For skin infections, treatment courses of 4 to 8 weeks usually

are curative. Nail infections are more difficult to treat and usually require a minimum of 4 months for fingernails and 6 months for toenails.

2. **Toxicity and drug interactions.** Griseofulvin is **generally well tolerated.** Headache is common but usually resolves during the first week of therapy. A variety of skin reactions has been reported and may necessitate stopping the drug. Occasionally nausea, vomiting, a bad taste in the mouth, paresthesias of the hands and feet, insomnia, confusion, or dizziness may occur. Reversible granulocytopenia and hepatotoxicity have been reported. Patients on high-dose or prolonged therapy should have blood count and liver tests followed on a routine basis.

## ACTINOMYCOSIS

*Actinomyces* species are gram-positive **filamentous bacteria** that once were classified as fungi. These organisms cause subacute and chronic granulomatous inflammations that closely resemble true fungal infections.

I. **Growth and identification characteristics.** Clinical actinomycosis is almost always caused by *Actinomyces israelii* [202]. *Actinomyces* can be grown on routine culture media with augmentation using brain–heart infusion. The **primarily anaerobic character of *Actinomyces* requires rapid transport of abscess material to the laboratory or direct inoculation into an anaerobic container.** Mature colonies may be present after 3 to 7 days of incubation. In some cases, however, growth may take up to 21 days. Prior antibiotic use may dramatically decrease culture yields. We recommend notifying the laboratory to hold all cultures for at least 21 days when the diagnosis of actinomycosis is suspected. *A. israelii* is seen on Gram stains of exudates or tissue sections as pleomorphic, beaded, branching gram-positive rods. Infection with *Actinomyces* may result in the formation of yellow, white, gray, or brown macroscopic particles called **sulfur granules,** which represent conglomerate masses of organisms.

II. **Epidemiologic features.** *Actinomyces* is worldwide in distribution and is a common saprophyte of the oral cavity, pharynx, and intestines. Therefore, **simple recovery of the organism from culture does not necessarily establish the presence of infection.**

III. **Pathogenesis.** The normal commensal status of *Actinomyces* is altered when the organism gains entrance to deeper tissues through a break in intact mucous membranes. Once it enters a microaerophilic or anaerobic atmosphere, *Actinomyces* produces a subacute or chronic granulomatous infection with a tendency to cause externally draining sinuses.

IV. **Clinical syndromes.** Actinomycosis most commonly involves the cervicofacial, thoracic, or abdominal regions and on occasion the CNS.

   A. **Cervicofacial actinomycosis** commonly occurs one to several weeks after dental extraction or minor trauma to the oral mucous membrane or in association with poor oral hygiene.

      1. **Manifestations.** The patient usually has a bluish swollen lesion at the angle of the mandible or in the neck. The lesion may enlarge slowly and may be painless or may progress rapidly and cause considerable pain. A visible sinus tract or fistula may be present. Sulfur granules may be seen in the exudate. Nonspecific symptoms of fever, weight loss, chills, and trismus may occur. Infection spreads without regard to fascial tissue planes and may involve the salivary and lacrimal glands, mandible, orbit, or paranasal sinuses.

      2. **Diagnosis.** Definitive diagnosis is made by culture of the organism from biopsy specimens or exudate. Pus should be collected by aspiration from closed lesions, transferred to an anaerobic environment quickly, and examined for the presence of sulfur granules. X-rays may reveal bony changes ranging from a minor subperiosteal reaction to overt lytic destruction.

   B. **Thoracic actinomycosis** may result from oropharyngeal aspiration of the organism, direct extension from the neck into the mediastinum, or spread from the abdominal cavity. Severe periodontal disease is commonly present.

      1. **Manifestations.** Nonproductive cough, low-grade fever, and weight loss are common, gradually progressing to mucopurulent sputum production, occasional

hemoptysis, and pleuritic chest pain. **Local chest wall spread may involve pleura and ribs and may produce externally draining cutaneous sinuses.** Extension of a pulmonary lesion through the thoracic wall may occur. Infection may extend to the pericardium, heart, and thoracic vertebrae or through the diaphragm, producing subphrenic or subhepatic abscesses. Hematogenous dissemination may result in spread to other organs, particularly the skin. Chest x-rays may show mass lesions, dense infiltrates, cavities, or pleural disease. **Draining sinus tracts through the chest wall are particularly suggestive of actinomycosis.**

2. **Diagnosis.** Because *A. israelii* may colonize the upper respiratory tract, **definitive diagnosis requires isolation of the organism from a resected specimen,** growth in culture from an **empyema** cavity, **or recovery from a draining sinus.**

C. **Abdominal infection** occurs most frequently after appendectomy, appendiceal abscess, or traumatic perforation of the bowel and represents 20% to 50% of all cases of actinomycosis [203].

1. **Manifestations.** Infection occurs most commonly in the ileocecal area and produces abdominal discomfort, fever, and a palpable mass. The process may localize or spread directly into the peritoneal cavity, abdominal wall, or pelvis. The course is usually subacute to chronic. Sinuses may appear in the abdominal wall. Extension to the urinary tract, pelvic organs, or vertebral bodies may occur. Anorectal involvement may result from secondary extension or may arise primarily through a break in an anal crypt. Pelvic actinomycosis may occur in women in association with an intrauterine device.
2. **Diagnosis** is by culture of specimens at the time of exploratory laparotomy, unless draining sinuses are present in the abdominal wall. Culture isolation may be frequently lacking, and diagnosis is made on the basis of sulfur granules on histopathology along with the characteristic clinical syndrome.

D. **Involvement of the CNS** is usually in the form of brain abscess and generally results from hematogenous spread of primary infection from the lung or abdomen [202]. Diagnosis requires culture of the organism from a biopsy specimen.

V. **Therapy. Penicillin** remains the drug of choice for actinomycosis [203]. Prolonged treatment with large doses is required to ensure adequate penetration into areas of fibrosis. Intravenous aqueous penicillin G (10–20 million units/day) for 4 to 6 weeks, followed by oral penicillin for 6 to 12 months, is suggested. Some recommend probenecid along with oral penicillin. Tetracyclines may be used in the nonpregnant penicillin-allergic patient. Other alternative agents include erythromycin and clindamycin. Surgical drainage of abscesses and excision of sinus tracts are important aspects of treatment. Infectious disease consultation is advised.

## NOCARDIOSIS

Nocardiosis is a localized or disseminated disease most commonly caused by *Nocardia asteroides* and less often by *Nocardia brasiliensis* and *Nocardia caviae. Nocardia* species are gaining increased recognition as **opportunistic pathogens, although they also cause illness in normal hosts.** Although originally believed to be fungi, *Nocardia* are now classified as higher order **bacteria** and are related to the *Actinomyces.*

I. **Growth and identification characteristics.** *Nocardia* species are gram-positive, aerobic, **weakly acid-fast bacilli** and are readily isolated on routine bacterial, fungal, and mycobacterial media. Colonies usually appear within 4 days but in some instances may require 2 to 4 weeks of culture. *Nocardia* can be difficult to isolate by culture, particularly because of overgrowth by nonpathogenic colonizers. **If nocardiosis is suspected clinically, the bacteriology laboratory should be informed and cultures should be kept longer than usual.** Gram-stained preparations reveal delicately branching, gram-positive, beaded filaments. With a modified Ziehl-Neelsen or Kinyoun stain, *Nocardia* organisms are weakly acid-fast, a characteristic that helps to distinguish them from *Actinomyces.* **However, the histologic appearance of *Nocardia* is not unique, and culture is necessary for definitive diagnosis.**

**II. Epidemiologic and host factors.** *Nocardia* species are soil saprophytes with worldwide distribution. *N. brasiliensis* most often causes primary cutaneous disease. Infection with *N. asteroides* most frequently occurs after inhalation of the organism into the lungs of predisposed individuals. The organism is an **opportunistic invader** in the setting of compromised host defenses; patients with leukemia, lymphoma, solid tumors, AIDS, dysgammaglobulinemia, collagen vascular disease, and chronic granulomatous disease and individuals on steroids or immunosuppression for organ transplantation are especially susceptible. In addition, prior pulmonary disease, including chronic obstructive lung disease and pulmonary alveolar proteinosis, are risk factors. Nevertheless, **approximately 15% of patients with nocardiosis have no underlying disorder** [204,205].

**III. Clinical aspects.** Although a few cases of skin or subcutaneous disease may occur by primary inoculation, clinical infection usually begins in the lungs, with 75% of patients exhibiting a primary pneumonitis. Secondary dissemination occurs by hematogenous spread and is almost always due to *N. asteroides.*

**A. Pulmonary and systemic nocardiosis** usually follows a subacute to chronic course, spanning weeks to months. Fulminant disease may occur in severely immunosuppressed patients. Pulmonary disease may be much more common than previously reported. Sputum cultures obtained for *Legionella pneumophila* in perplexing pneumonia often yield *Nocardia.*

1. **Manifestations.** Constitutional symptoms of fever, night sweats, malaise, anorexia, and weight loss are reported in most cases. Leukocytosis is not consistently present.
   a. **Pulmonary findings.** Cough may be dry but usually is productive of thick mucopurulent sputum. Hemoptysis and pleuritic chest pain also are reported. **Chest roentgenograms** are variable and **nonspecific.** Localized infiltrates, often in the upper lobes, are common. Single or multiple nodules, cavities, diffuse infiltrates, consolidation, abscesses, large masses, and pleural effusions have all been reported.
   b. CNS involvement has been noted in approximately 25% of patients. This is usually in the form of a **brain abscess,** and the diagnosis may be suspected on the basis of CT or MRI. Meningitis has been reported. Decreased mental status, unsteadiness, headaches, nausea and vomiting, seizures, or focal neurologic deficits may occur. (CSF does not reveal *Nocardia* on smear or culture, and brain biopsy may be necessary.)
   c. **Skin and subcutaneous abscesses** are present in approximately 10% of patients.
   d. **Pleural and chest wall invasion** from a contiguous pneumonic infection occurs in 10% of cases. Patients may complain of pleuritic pain or may manifest sinus tracts. Pleural effusions may become infected, with the development of empyema.
   e. **Metastatic infection** to virtually every organ has been documented.
2. **Diagnosis. Nocardiosis should be considered in any chronic pneumonia that persists despite conventional antimicrobial therapy. The combination of pulmonary and CNS or skin infection in a compromised host is particularly suggestive.**
   a. **Sputum or pulmonary specimens.** Positive sputum cultures are diagnostic, but false-negative results are common. Invasive procedures such as thoracentesis, transtracheal aspiration, lung aspiration, or lung biopsy may be necessary.
   b. **Blood cultures** are rarely positive.
   c. **Smears and culture material** obtained from skin lesions, sinus tracts, and tissue biopsy specimens are important sources. Histologic examination is suggestive but not diagnostic.
   d. **Skin and serologic tests are not available.**
3. **Therapy.** Sulfonamide-based regimens have proven to be the most effective treatment for nocardiosis. Infectious disease consultation is advised.
   a. **Trimethoprim-sulfamethoxazole** is considered to be the treatment of choice for nocardiosis [205–207]. This rationale is supported by the *in vitro*

synergy, the excellent tissue levels achieved (including the CNS), and their excellent bioavailability when given orally. Sulfa levels in serum should be monitored to achieve concentrations of 12 to 15 mg/dL [207].

b. **Sulfonamides** as single agents are also very effective against *Nocardia*. For example, sulfadiazine, 8 to 12 g/day, can be used (see Chapter 27). The dosage should be monitored to achieve peak serum concentrations of approximately 15 mg/dL.

c. **Other regimens** may be necessary if the organisms are resistant or if patients are intolerant to sulfa drugs. Susceptibility testing is difficult and ideally should be performed at reference laboratories. **Minocycline, doxycycline, and amoxicillin-clavulanate** have been effective. Many *Nocardia* strains are susceptible to **amikacin,** and this drug may be added to a sulfa regimen or an alternative regimen [208]. **Imipenem** may be another alternative agent.

d. The duration of therapy is not well defined, but **most authorities recommend a prolonged course of treatment.** For minor infections and in immunocompetent hosts, therapy is given for at least 2 to 3 months. For severe infections or in immunosuppressed individuals, therapy for up to 1 year is recommended. Some experts suggest maintenance therapy to prevent relapse in transplant recipients or in patients continuing on immunosuppressive therapy [205,206].

e. **Surgical drainage and excision** should be performed on abscesses, if possible.

4. **Prognosis.** Mortality varies with the site of disease and the severity of the patient's underlying immunosuppression. Survival definitely is improved if therapy is initiated early and before hematogenous seeding occurs. Individuals with CNS infection have the highest mortality, approximately 40%. Mortality in patients with isolated pulmonary disease ranges between 10% and 29%, the higher rate being reported in transplant recipients and other immunocompromised patients [204,205].

B. *N. asteroides* **is a rare laboratory contaminant,** and **isolation from sputum usually indicates active disease.** However, positive sputum cultures have been found in asymptomatic patients, individuals with mild upper respiratory tract infections, and some persons with bronchitis. In patients with malignancies or immunosuppressive disorders, the isolation of *Nocardia* from clinical specimens should prompt the initiation of therapy. On the other hand, in immunocompetent individuals a positive culture for *Nocardia* should stimulate further investigation but may not mandate therapy if solid evidence of invasive disease cannot be found. Infectious disease consultation is advised.

## REFERENCES

1. Edwards JE. *Candida* species. In: Mandell GL, Bennett JE, Dolin R, eds. *Principles and practice of infectious diseases,* 5th ed. Philadelphia: Churchill Livingstone, 2000:2656.
2. De Doncker P, et al. Pulse therapy with one-week itraconazole monthly for three or four months in the treatment of onychomycosis. *Cutis* 1995;56:180.
3. Fotos PG, Vincent SD, Hellstein JW. Oral candidosis: clinical, historical, and therapeutic features of 100 cases. *Oral Surg Oral Med Oral Pathol* 1992;74:41.
4. Rex JH, et al. Practice guidelines for the treatment of candidiasis. *Clin Infect Dis* 2000;30:662.
5. Eras P, Goldstein MJ, Sherlock P. *Candida* infection of the gastrointestinal tract. *Medicine* 1972;51:367.
6. Darouiche RO. Oropharyngeal and esophageal candidiasis in immunosuppressed patients: treatment issues. *Clin Infect Dis* 1998;26:259.
7. Lopez-Dupla M, et al. Clinical, endoscopic, immunologic, and therapeutic aspects of oropharyngeal and esophageal candidiasis in HIV-infected patients: a survey of 114 cases. *Am J Gastroenterol* 1992;87:1771.
8. Fichtenbaum CJ, Powderley WG. Refractory mucosal candidiasis in patients with human immunodeficiency virus infection. *Clin Infect Dis* 1998;26:556.
9. Sobel JD, et al. The evaluation of *Candida* species and fluconazole susceptibility among

oral and vaginal isolates recovered from human immunodeficiency virus-seropositive and at-risk HIV-seronegative women. *J Infect Dis* 2001;183:286.
10. Kirkpatrick CH. Chronic mucocutaneous candidiasis. *J Am Acad Dermatol* 1994; 31:S14.
11. Pfaller MA, et al. National surveillance of nosocomial bloodstream infection due to *Candida albicans*: frequency of occurrence and antifungal susceptibility in the SCOPE program. *Diagn Microbiol Infect Dis* 1998;31:327.
12. Wenzel RP. Nosocomial candidemia: risk factors and attributable mortality. *Clin Infect Dis* 1995;20:1531.
13. Blumberg HM, et al. Risk factors for candidal bloodstream infections in surgical intensive care unit patients: the NEMIS prospective multicenter study. *Clin Infect Dis* 2001;33:177.
14. Fraser VJ, et al. Candidemia in a tertiary care hospital: epidemiology, risk factors, and predictors of mortality. *Clin Infect Dis* 1992;15:414.
15. Vasquez JA, et al. Nosocomial acquisition of *Candida albicans*: an epidemiologic study. *J Infect Dis* 1993;168:195.
16. Pertowski CA, et al. Nosocomial outbreak of *Candida albicans* sternal wound infections following cardiac surgery traced to a scrub nurse. *J Infect Dis* 1995;172:817.
17. Edwards JE Jr, et al. Ocular manifestations of *Candida* septicemia: review of 76 cases of hematogenous *Candida* endophthalmitis. *Medicine* 1974;53:47.
18. Reiss E, Morrison CJ. Nonculture methods for diagnosis of disseminated candidiasis. *Clin Microbiol Rev* 1993;6:311.
19. Verweij PE, et al. Current trends in the detection of antigenemia, metabolites and cell wall markers for the diagnosis and therapeutic monitoring of fungal infections. *Med Mycol* 1998;36[Suppl 1]:146.
20. Sandford GR, et al. The value of fungal surveillance cultures as predictors of systemic fungal infections. *J Infect Dis* 1980;142:503.
21. Marina NW, et al. *Candida tropicalis* and *Candida albicans* fungemia in children with leukemia. *Cancer* 1991;68:594.
21a. Reiss E, Tanaka K, Bruker G, et al. Molecular diagnosis and epidemiology of fungal infections. *Med Mycol* 1998;36:249–257.
22. Rex JH, et al. A randomized trial of fluconazole vs. amphotericin B for the treatment of candidemia in patients without neutropenia. *N Engl J Med* 1994;331:1325.
23. Anaissie EJ, et al. Management of invasive candidal infections: results of a prospective, randomized, multicenter study of fluconazole versus amphotericin B and review of the literature. *Clin Infect Dis* 1996;23:964.
24. Phillips P, et al. Multicenter randomized trial of fluconazole versus amphotericin B for treatment of candidemia in non-neutropenic patients. *Eur J Clin Microbiol Infect Dis* 1997;16:337.
25. Edwards JE, et al. International conference for the development of a consensus on the management and prevention of severe candidal infections. *Clin Infect Dis* 1997;25:43.
26. Slain D. Lipid-based amphotericin B for the treatment of fungal infections. *Pharmacotherapy* 1999;19:306.
27. Pfaller MA, Jones RN, Doern GV, et al. International surveillance of blood stream infections due to *Candida* species in the European SENTRY program: species distribution and antifungal susceptibility including the investigational triazole and echinocandin agents. *Diagn Microbiol Infect Dis* 1999;35:19–25.
28. Abruzzo GK, Flattery AM, Gill CJ, et al. Evaluation of the echinocandin antifungal MK-0991 (L-743,872): efficacies in mouse models of disseminated aspergillosis, candidiasis, and cryptococcosis. *Amtimicrob Agents Chemother* 1997;41:2333–2338.
29. Marco F, Pfaller MA, Messer S, et al. *In vitro* activities of voriconazole (UK-109,496) and four other antifungal agents against 394 clinical isolates of *Candida* spp. *Antimicrob Agents Chemother* 1998;42:161–163.
30. Rex JH, et al. Intravascular catheter exchange and duration of candidemia. *Clin Infect Dis* 1995;21:994.
31. Thaler M, et al. Hepatic candidiasis in cancer patients: the evolving picture of the syndrome. *Ann Intern Med* 1988;108:88.
32. Melgar GR, et al. Fungal prosthetic valve endocarditis in 16 patients. An 11-year experience in a tertiary care hospital. *Medicine* 1997;76:94.

33. Lundstrom T, Sobel J. Nosocomial candiduria: a review. *Clin Infect Dis* 2001;32:1602.
34. Sobel JD, et al. Candiduria: a randomized, double-blind study of treatment with fluconazole and placebo. *Clin Infect Dis* 2000;30:19.
35. Fan-Havard P, et al. Oral fluconazole versus amphotericin B bladder irrigation for treatment of candidal funguria. *Clin Infect Dis* 1995;21:960.
36. McCullers JA, et al. Candidal meningitis in children with cancer. *Clin Infect Dis* 2000;31:451.
37. Casodo JL, et al. Candidal meningitis in HIV-infected patients: analysis of 14 cases. *Clin Infect Dis* 1997;25:673.
38. Haron E, et al. Primary *Candida* pneumonia. Experience at a large cancer center and review of the literature. *Medicine* 1993;72:137.
39. Alden SM, et al. Abdominal candidiasis in surgical patients. *Am Surg* 1989;55:45.
40. Goldie SJ, et al. Fungal peritonitis in a large chronic peritoneal dialysis population: a report of 55 episodes. *Am J Kidney Dis* 1996;28:86.
41. Hansen BL, Anderson K. Fungal arthritis. *Scand J Rheumatol* 1995;24:248.
42. Hendrickx L, et al. Candidal vertebral osteomyelitis: report of 6 patients, and a review. *Clin Infect Dis* 2001;32:527.
43. Benoit D, et al. Management of candidal thrombophlebitis of the central veins: case report and review. *Clin Infect Dis* 1998;26:393.
44. Deepe GS. *Histoplasma capsulatum*. In: Mandell GL, Bennett JE, Dolin R, eds. *Principles and practice of infectious diseases,* 5th ed. Philadelphia: Churchill Livingstone, 2000:2718.
45. Goodwin RA Jr, Loyd JE, Des Prez RM. Histoplasmosis in normal hosts. *Medicine* 1981;60:231.
46. Wheat LJ, et al. A large urban outbreak of histoplasmosis: clinical features. *Ann Intern Med* 1981;94:331.
47. Stobierski MJ, et al. Outbreak of histoplasmosis among employees in a paper factory–Michigan, 1993. *J Clin Microbiol* 1996;34:1220.
48. Wheat LJ, et al. The diagnostic laboratory tests for histoplasmosis. Analysis of experience in a large urban outbreak. *Ann Intern Med* 1982;97:680.
49. Wheat LJ, Kohler RB, Tewari RP. Diagnosis of disseminated histoplasmosis by detection of *Histoplasma capsulatum* antigen in serum and urine specimens. *N Engl J Med* 1986;314:83.
50. Wheat J, et al. Practice guidelines for the management of patients with histoplasmosis. *Clin Infect Dis* 2000;30:688.
51. Goodwin RA Jr, et al. Disseminated histoplasmosis: clinical and pathologic correlations. *Medicine* 1980;59:1.
52. Wheat LJ, et al. Disseminated histoplasmosis in the acquired immunodeficiency syndrome: clinical findings, diagnosis, treatment and review of the literature. *Medicine* 1990;69:361.
53. Dismukes WE, et al. Itraconazole therapy for blastomycosis and histoplasmosis. *Am J Med* 1993;93:489–497.
54. Wheat LJ, et al. Itraconazole treatment of disseminated histoplasmosis in patients with acquired immunodeficiency syndrome. *Am J Med* 1995;98:336.
55. Wheat LJ, et al. Prevention of relapse of histoplasmosis with itraconazole in patients with the acquired immunodeficiency syndrome. *Ann Intern Med* 1993;118:610.
56. McKinsey DS, et al. Itraconazole prophylaxis for fungal infections in patients with advanced immunodeficiency virus infection: randomized, placebo-controlled, double-blind study. *Clin Infect Dis* 1999;28:1049.
57. Hajjeh RA, et al. Multicenter case-control study of risk factors for histoplasmosis in human immunodeficiency virus-infected persons. *Clin Infect Dis* 2001;32:1215.
58. McKinsey DS, et al. Fluconazole therapy for histoplasmosis. *Clin Infect Dis* 1996;23:996.
59. Goodwin RA, et al. Chronic pulmonary histoplasmosis. *Medicine* 1976;55:413–452.
60. Loyd JL, et al. Mediastinal fibrosis complicating histoplasmosis. *Medicine* 1988;67:295.
61. Mitchell TG, Perfect JR. Cryptococcosis in the era of AIDS—100 years after the discovery of *Cryptococcus neoformans*. *Clin Microbiol Rev* 1995;8:515.

62. Kerkering TM, Duma RJ, Shadomy S. The evolution of pulmonary cryptococcosis. *Ann Intern Med* 1981;94:611.
63. Sugar A, et al. Cryptococcal disease in patients with the acquired immunodeficiency syndrome. *Ann Intern Med* 1986;104:234.
64. Cameron ML, et al. Manifestations of pulmonary cryptococcosis in patients with acquired immunodeficiency syndrome. *Rev Infect Dis* 1991;13:64.
65. Nunez M, Peacock JE, Chin R Jr. Pulmonary cryptococcosis in the immunocompetent host. *Chest* 2000;118:527.
66. Saag MS, et al. Practice guidelines for the management of cryptococcal disease. *Clin Infect Dis* 2000;30:710.
67. Dismukes WE. Cryptococcal meningitis in patients with AIDS. *J Infect Dis* 1988; 157:624.
68. Van der Horst CM, et al. Treatment of cryptococcal meningitis associated with the acquired immunodeficiency syndrome. *N Engl J Med* 1997;337:15.
69. Saag MS, et al. A comparison of itraconazole versus fluconazole as maintenance therapy for AIDS-associated cryptococcal meningitis. *Clin Infect Dis* 1999;28:291.
70. Bennett JE, et al. A comparison of amphotericin B alone and combined with flucytosine in the treatment of cryptococcal meningitis. *N Engl J Med* 1979;301:126.
71. Dismukes WE, et al. Treatment of cryptococcal meningitis with combination amphotericin B and flucytosine for four as compared with six weeks. *N Engl J Med* 1987;317:334.
72. Denning DW, et al. Elevated cerebrospinal fluid pressures in patients with cryptococcal meningitis and the acquired immunodeficiency syndrome. *Am J Med* 1991;91: 267.
73. Park MK, Hospenthal DR, Bennett JE. Treatment of hydrocephalus secondary to cryptococcal meningitis by use of shunting. *Clin Infect Dis* 1999;28:629.
74. Galgiani J. *Coccidioides immitis.* In: Mandell GL, Bennett JE, Dolin R, eds. *Principles and practice of infectious diseases,* 5th ed. Philadelphia: Churchill Livingstone, 2000:27–46.
75. Stevens DA. Coccdioidomycosis. *N Engl J Med* 1995;332:1077.
76. Bayer AS. Fungal pneumonias: pulmonary coccidioidal syndromes. I. Primary and progressive coccidioidal pneumonias—diagnostic, therapeutic, and prognostic considerations. *Chest* 1981;79:575.
77. Galgiani JN, et al. Comparison of oral fluconazole and itraconazole for progressive, nonmeningeal coccidioidomycosis. *Ann Intern Med* 2000;133:676.
78. Fish DG, et al. Coccidioidomycosis during human immunodeficiency virus infection. A review of 77 patients. *Medicine* 1990;69:384.
79. Singh RS, et al. Coccidioidomycosis in patients infected with human immunodeficiency virus: review of 91 cases at a single institution. *Clin Infect Dis* 1996;23:563.
80. Bouza E, et al. Coccidioidal meningitis. *Medicine* 1981;60:139.
81. Galgiani JN, et al. Fluconazole therapy for coccidioidal meningitis. *Ann Intern Med* 1993;119:28.
82. Dewsnup DH, et al. Is it ever safe to stop azole therapy for *Coccidioides immitis* meningitis? *Ann Intern Med* 1996;124:305.
83. Glimp RA. Fungal pneumonias. III. Allergic bronchopulmonary aspergillosis. *Chest* 1981;80:85.
84. Rosenberg M, et al. Clinical and immunologic criteria for the diagnosis of allergic bronchopulmonary aspergillosis. *Ann Intern Med* 1977;86:405.
85. Stevens DA, et al. A randomized trial of itraconazole in allergic bronchopulmonary aspergillosis. *N Engl J Med* 2000;342:756.
86. Stevens DA, et al. Practice guidelines for diseases caused by *Aspergillus. Clin Infect Dis* 2000;30:696.
87. Tomlinson JR, Sahn SA. Aspergilloma in sarcoid and tuberculosis. *Chest* 1987;92:505.
88. Addrizzo-Harris D, Harkin McGuinness G, et al. Pulmonary aspergillomas and AIDS. A comparison of HIV-infected and HIV-negative individuals. *Chest* 1997;111: 612.
89. Babasti G, Massetti M, Chapelier A, et al. Surgical treatment of pulmonary aspergilloma: current outcome. *J Thorac Cardiovasc Surg* 2000;199:906.
90. Denning DW. Invasion aspergillosis. *Clin Infect Dis* 1998;26:781.

91. Lortholary O, et al. Invasive aspergillosis in patients with acquired immunodeficiency syndrome: report of 33 cases. *Am J Med* 1993;95:177.
92. Holding KJ, et al. Aspergillosis among people infected with human immunodeficiency virus: incidence and survival. *Clin Infect Dis* 2000;31:1253.
93. Binder RE, et al. Chronic necrotizing aspergillosis: a discrete clinical entity. *Medicine* 1982;61:109.
94. Perfect JR, Cox GM, Lee JY, et al. The impact of culture isolation of aspergillus species: a hospital-based survey of aspergillosis. *Clin Infect Dis* 2001;33:1824–1833.
95. Horvatch JA, Dummer S. The use of respiratory-tract cultures in the diagnosis of invasive pulmonary aspergillosis. *Am J Med* 1996;100:171.
96. Denning DW, Stevens DA. Antifungal and surgical treatment of invasive aspergillosis: review of 2,121 published cases. *Rev Infect Dis* 1990;12:1147.
97. White MH, et al. Amphotericin B colloidal dispersion vs. amphotericin B as therapy for invasive aspergillosis. *Clin Infect Dis* 1997;24:635.
98. Denning DW, et al. NIAID Mycoses Study Group multicenter trial of oral itraconazole therapy of invasive aspergillosis. *Am J Med* 1996;100:171.
99. Stevens DA, Lee JY. Analysis of compassionate use itraconazole therapy for invasive aspergillosis by the NIAID Mycoses Study Group criteria. *Arch Intern Med* 1997; 157:1857.
100. Medical Letter. Caspofungin (Cancidas) for aspergillosis. *Med Lett Drugs Ther* 2001; 43:58.
101. Andriole VT. Current and future antifungal therapy: new targets for antifungal agents. *J Antimicrob Chemother* 1999;44:151.
102. Rubin MA, Carroll KC, Cahill BC, et al. Caspofungin in combination with itraconazole for the treatment of invasive aspergillosis in humans. *Clin Infect Dis* 2002;34:1158–1159.
103. Karp JE, Burch PA, Merz WG. An approach to intensive antileukemia therapy in patients with previous invasive aspergillosis. *Am J Med* 1988;85:203.
104. DeShazo RD, Chapin K, Swain RE. Fungal sinusitis. *N Engl J Med* 1997;337:254.
105. Chapman SW. *Blastomyces dermatitidis.* In: Mandell GL, Bennett JE, Dolin R, eds. *Principles and practice of infectious diseases,* 5th ed. Philadelphia: Churchill Livingstone, 2000:2733.
106. Bradsher RW. Blastomycosis. *Infect Dis Clin North Am* 1988;2:877–898.
107. Al-Dorry Y. DiSalvo AF, eds. *Blastomycosis.* New York: Plenum, 1992.
108. Klein BS, et al. Isolation of *Blastomyces dermatitidis* in soil associated with a large outbreak of blastomycosis in Wisconsin. *N Engl J Med* 1986;314:529.
109. Klein BS, et al. Two outbreaks of blastomycosis along river banks in Wisconsin are described. Isolation of *B. dermatitidis* from river bank soil and evidence of transmission along waterways is obtained. *Am Rev Respir Dis* 1987;136:1333.
110. Klein BS, Jones JM. Isolation, purification, and radiolabeling of a novel 120-kd surface protein on *Blastomyces dermatitidis* yeasts to detect antibody in infected patients. *J Clin Invest* 1990;85:152.
111. Klein BS, Sondel PM, Jones JM. WI-1 a novel 120-kilodalton surface protein on *Blastomyces dermatitidis* yeast cells, is a target antigen of cell-mediated immunity in human blastomycosis. *Infect Immun* 1992;60:4291.
112. Klein BS, Chaturvedi S, Hogan LH, et al. Altered expression of surface protein WI-1 in genetically related strains of *Blastomyces dermatitidis* that differ in virulence regulates recognition of yeast by human macrophages. *Infect Immun* 1994;62:3536.
113. Bradhorst TT, Wuthrich M, Warner T, et al. Targeted gene disruption reveals an adhesin indispensable for pathogenicity of *Blastomyces dermatitidis*. *J Exp Med* 1999; 189:1207.
114. Hogan LH, Klein BS. Altered expression of surface a-1,3-glucan in genetically related strains of *Blastomyces dermatitidis* that differ in virulence. *Infect Immun* 1994; 62:3543.
115. Sarosi GA, Davies SF, Phillips JR. Self-limited blastomycosis: a report of 39 cases. *Semin Respir Infect* 1986;1:40.
116. Brown LR, et al. Roentgenologic features of pulmonary blastomycosis. *Mayo Clin Proc* 1991;66:29.

117. Chapman SW, Lin AC, Hendricks KA, et al. Endemic blastomycosis in Mississippi: epidemiological and clinical studies. *Semin Respir Infect* 1997;12:219–228.
118. Pappas PG, et al. Blastomycosis in patients with acquired immunodeficiency syndrome. *Ann Intern Med* 1992;116:847.
119. Pappas PG, et al. Blastomycosis in immunocompromised patients. *Medicine* 1993;72:311.
120. Turner S, Kaufman L. Immunodiagnosis of blastomycosis. *Semin Respir Infect* 1986;1:22.
121. Klein BS, et al. Comparison of enzyme immunoassay, immunodiffusion and complement fixation tests in detecting antibody in human serum to the A antigen of *B. dermatitidis. Am Rev Respir Dis* 1986;133:144.
122. Chapman SW, Bradsher RW Jr, Campbell GD Jr, et al. Practice guidelines for the management of patients with blastomycosis. *Clin Infect Dis* 2000;30:679.
123. Bradsher RW, Rice DC, Abernathy RS. Ketoconazole therapy for endemic Blastomycosis. *Ann Intern Med* 1985;103:872.
124. National Institute of Allergy and Infectious Diseases Study Group. Treatment of blastomycosis and histoplasmosis with ketoconazole: results of a prospective randomized trial. *Ann Intern Med* 1985;103:861–872.
125. Pappas PG, Bradshaer RW, Chapman SW, et al. Treatment of blastomycosis with fluconazole: a pilot study. *Clin Infect Dis* 1995;20:267.
126. Pappas PG, Bradsher RW, Kayffman CA, et al. Treatment if blastomycosis with higher dose fluconazole. *Clin Infect Dis* 1997;25:200.
127. Sugar AM. Agents of mucormycosis and related species. In: Mandell GL, Bennett JE, Dolin R, eds. *Principles and practice of infectious diseases,* 5th ed. Philadelphia: Churchill Livingstone, 2000:26–85.
128. Boelaert JR, Fenves AZ, Coburn JW. Deferoxamine therapy and mucormycosis in dialysis patients: report of an international registry. *Am J Kidney Dis* 1991;18:660.
129. Singh N, et al. Invasive gastrointestinal zygomycosis in a liver transplant recipient: case report and review of zygomycosis in solid-organ transplant recipients. *Clin Infect Dis* 1995;20:617.
130. Adam RD, et al. Mucormycosis: emerging prominence of cutaneous infections. *Clin Infect Dis* 1994;19:67.
131. Ingram CW, et al. Disseminated zygomycosis: report of four cases and review. *Rev Infect Dis* 1989;11:741.
132. Kauffman CA. Sporotrichosis. *Clin Infect Dis* 1999;29:231.
133. Restrepo A, et al. Itraconazole therapy in lymphangitic and cutaneous sporotrichosis. *Arch Dermatol* 1986;122:413.
134. Sharkey-Mathis PK, et al. Treatment of sporotrichosis with itraconazole. *Am J Med* 1993;95:279.
135. Kauffman CA, Hajjeh R, Chapman SW. Practice guidelines for the management of patients with sporotrichosis. *Clin Infect Dis* 2000;30:684.
136. Pluss JL, Opal SM. Pulmonary sporotrichosis: review of treatment and outcome. *Medicine* 1986;65:143.
137. Winn RE, et al. Systemic sporotrichosis treated with itraconazole. *Clin Infect Dis* 1993;17:210.
138. Heller HM, Fuhrer J. Disseminated sporotrichosis in patients with AIDS: case report and review of the literature. *AIDS* 1991;5:1243.
139. Scott EX, et al. Serologic studies in the diagnosis and management of meningitis due to *Sporothrix schenckii. N Engl J Med* 1987;317:935.
140. Brummer E, Castaneda E, Restrepo A. Paracoccidioidomycosis: an update. *Clin Microbiol Rev* 1993;6:89.
141. Mahgoub ES. Agents of mycetoma. In: Mandell GL, Bennett JE, Dolin R, eds. *Principles and practice of infectious diseases,* 5th ed. Philadelphia: Churchill Livingstone, 2000:2702.
142. Rossman SNB, Cernoch PL, Davis JR. Dematiaceous fungi are an evolving cause of human disease. *Clin Infect Dis* 1996;22:73.
143. Duong TA. Infection due to *Penicillium marneffei*, an emerging pathogen: review of 155 reported cases. *Clin Infect Dis* 1996;23:125.

144. Sirisanthana T, et al. Amphotericin B and itraconazole for treatment of disseminated *Penicillium marneffei* infection in human immunodeficiency virus-infected patients. *N Engl J Med* 1998;339:1739.
145. Supparatpinyo K, et al. A controlled trial of itraconazole to prevent relapse of *Penicillium marneffei* infection in patients infected with the human immunodeficiency virus. *N Engl J Med* 1998;339:1739.
146. Fridkin SK, Jarvis WR. Epidemiology of nosocomial fungal infections. *Clin Microbiol Rev* 1996;9:499.
147. Barber GR, et al. Catheter-related *Malassezia furfur* fungemia in immunocompromised patients. *Am J Med* 1993;95:365.
148. Boutati EI, Anaissie EJ. *Fusarium*, a significant emerging pathogen in patients with a hematologic malignancy: ten years' experience at a cancer center and implications for management. *Blood* 1997;90:999.
149. Travis LB, Roberts GD, Wilson WR. Clinical significance of *Pseudallescheria boydii:* a review of ten years' experience. *Mayo Clin Proc* 1985;60:531.
150. Gallis HA, Drew RH, Pickard WW. Amphotericin B: 30 years of clinical experience. *Rev Infect Dis* 1990;12:308.
151. Peacock JE Jr, Herrington DA, Cruz JM. Amphotericin B: past, present, and future. *Infect Dis Clin Pract* 1993;2:81.
152. Brajtburg J, et al. Amphotericin B: current understanding of mechanisms of action. *Antimicrob Agents Chemother* 1990;34:183.
153. Christiansen KJ, et al. Distribution and activity of amphotericin B in humans. *J Infect Dis* 1985;152:1037.
154. Goodwin SD, et al. Pretreatment regimens for adverse events related to infusion of amphotericin B. *Clin Infect Dis* 1995;20:755.
155. Cruz JM, et al. Rapid intravenous infusion of amphotericin B: a pilot study. *Am J Med* 1992;93:123.
156. Drutz DJ. Rapid infusion of amphotericin B: is it safe, effective and wise? *Am J Med* 1992;93:119.
157. Polsky B, et al. Intraventricular therapy of cryptococcal meningitis via a subcutaneous reservoir. *Am J Med* 1986;81:24.
158. Cleary JD, Chapman SW, Nolan RL. Pharmacologic modulation of interleukin-1 expression by amphotericin B-stimulated human mononuclear cells. *Antimicrob Agents Chemother* 1992;36:977.
159. Gigliotti F, et al. Induction of prostaglandin synthesis as the mechanism for the chills and fever produced by infusing amphotericin B. *J Infect Dis* 1987;156:784.
160. Clements JS Jr, Peacock JE Jr. Amphotericin B revisited: reassessment of toxicity. *Am J Med* 1990;88:22–27.
161. Branch RA. Prevention of amphotericin B-induced renal impairment: a review on the use of sodium supplementation. *Arch Intern Med* 1988;148:2389–2394.
162. Lin AC, et al. Amphotericin B blunts erythropoietin response to anemia. *J Infect Dis* 1990;161:348.
163. Wright DA, et al. Lethal pulmonary reactions associated with combined use of amphotericin B and leukocyte transfusions. *N Engl J Med* 1981;304:1185.
164. Hughes WT, et al. Guidelines for the use of antimicrobial agents in neutropenic patients with unexplained fever. *J Infect Dis* 1990;161:381.
165. Wong-Beringer A, Jacobs RA, Guglielmo BJ. Lipid formulations of amphotericin B: clinical efficacy and toxicities. *Clin Infect Dis* 1998;27:603.
166. Hiemenz JW, Walsh TJ. Lipid formulations of amphotericin B: recent progress and future directions. *Clin Infect Dis* 1996;22:S133.
167. Walsh TJ, Hiemenz JW, Seibel NL, et al. Amphotericin B lipid complex for invasive fungal infections: analysis of safety and efficacy in 556 cases. *Clin Infect Dis* 1998;26:1383.
168. Walsh TJ, Finberg RW, Arndt C, et al. Liposomal amphotericin B for empirical therapy in patients with persistent fever and neutropenia. National Institute of Allergy and Infectious Diseases Mycoses Study Group. *N Engl J Med* 1999;340:764.
169. White MH, Anaissie EJ, Kusne S, et al. Amphotericin B colloidal dispersion vs. amphotericin B as therapy for invasive aspergillosis. *Clin Infect Dis* 1997;24:635.

170. Francis P, Walsh TJ. Evolving role of flucytosine in immunocompromised patients: new insights into safety, pharmacokinetics, and antifungal therapy. *Clin Infect Dis* 1992;15:1003.
171. Stamm AM, et al. Toxicity of amphotericin B plus flucytosine in 194 patients with cryptococcal meningitis. *Am J Med* 1987;83:236.
172. Larsen RA, Leal MAE Chan LS. Fluconazole compared with amphotericin B plus flucytosine for the treatment of cryptococcal meningitis in AIDS: a randomized trial. *Ann Intern Med* 1990;113:183.
173. Mayanja-Kizza H, Oishi K, Mitaral S, et al. Combination therapy with fluconazole and flucytosine for cryptococcal meningitis in Ugandan patients with AIDS. *Clin Infect Dis* 1998;26:1362.
174. Como JA, Dismukes WE. Oral azole drugs as systemic antifungal therapy. *N Engl J Med* 1994;330:263.
175. Medical Letter. Ketoconazole (Nizoral), a new antifungal agent. *Med Lett Drugs Ther* 1981;23:85.
176. Honig PK, et al. Terfenadine-ketoconazole interaction: pharmacokinetic and electrocardiographic consequences. *JAMA* 1993;269:1513.
177. Symoens J, et al. An evaluation of two years of clinical experience with ketoconazole. *Rev Infect Dis* 1980;2:674.
178. Khosia S, et al. Adrenal crisis in the setting of high-dose ketoconazole therapy. *Arch Intern Med* 1989;149:802.
179. Medical Letter. Drugs for treatment of deep fungal infections. *Med Lett Drugs Ther* 1994;36:16.
180. Bennett JG. Overview of the symposium on fluconazole: a novel advance in the therapy for systemic fungal infections. *Rev Infect Dis* 1990;12[Suppl 3]:S263.
181. Brammer KW, Farrow PR, Faulkner JK. Pharmacokinetics and tissue penetration of fluconazole in humans. *Rev Infect Dis* 1990;12[Suppl 3]:5318.
182. Wingard JR, et al. Increase in *Candida krusei* infection among patients with bone marrow transplantation and neutropenia treated prophylactically with fluconazole. *N Engl J Med* 1991;325:1274.
183. Goodman JL, et al. A controlled trial of fluconazole to prevent fungal infections in patients undergoing bone marrow transplantation. *N Engl J Med* 1992;376:845.
184. Rex JH, et al. Minireview: resistance of *Candida* species to fluconazole. *Antimicrob Agents Chemother* 1995;39:1.
185. Trapnell CB, et al. Increased plasma rifabutin levels with concomitant fluconazole therapy in HIV-infected patients. *Ann Intern Med* 1996;124:573.
186. Grant SM, Clissold SP. Itraconazole: a review of its pharmacodynamic and pharmacokinetic properties, and therapeutic use in superficial and systemic mycoses. *Drugs* 1989;37:310.
187. Cleary JD, Taylor JW, Chapman SW. Itraconazole in antifungal therapy. *Ann Pharmacother* 1992;26:502.
188. Slain D, Rogers PD, Chapman SW, et al. Intravenous itraconazole: a formulary focus. *Ann Pharmacother* 2001;35:720–729.
189. Medical Letter. Itraconazole for onychomycosis. *Med Lett. Drug Ther* 1996;38:5.
190. De Backer M, De Vroey C, Lesaffre E, et al. Twelve weeks of continuous oral therapy for toenail onychomycosis caused by dermatophytes: a double-blind comparative trial of terbinafine 250 mg/day versus itraconazole 200 mg/day. *J Am Acad Dermatol* 1998;38:S57.
191. Crane JK, Shih H. Syncope and cardiac arrhythmia due to an interaction between itraconazole and terfenadine. *Am J Med* 1993;95:445.
192. Wildfeuer A, Seidl HP, Paule I, et al. In vitro evaluation of voriconazole against clinical isolates of yeasts, moulds and dermatophytes in comparison with itraconazole, ketocconazole, amphotericin B and griseofulvin. *Mycoses* 1998;41:309–319.
193. McGinnis MR, Pasarell L, Sutton DA, et al. In vitro activity of voriconazole against selected fungi. *Med Mycol* 1998;36:239–242.
194. Espinel-Ingroff A. In vitro fungicidal activities of voriconazole, itraconazole, and amphotericin B against opportunistic monillaceous and dematiaceous fungi. *J Clin Microbiol* 2001;39:954–959.

195. Jezequel SG, Clark M, Cole S. UK-109,496 a novel, wide-spectrum triazole derivative for the treatment of fungal infections: pre-clinical pharmacokinetics. Program and Abstracts of the 35th Interscience Conference on Antimicrobial Agents and Chemotherapy, San Francisco, CA, 1995. Abstract F76, p. 126. American Society for Microbiology, Washington, DC.
196. Patterson BE, Coates PE. UK-109,496 a novel, wide-spectrum triazole derivative for the treatment of fungal infections: pharmacokinetics in man. In Program and Abstracts of the 35th Interscience Conference on Antimicrobial Agents and Chemotherapy, San Francisco, CA, 1995. Abstract F78, p. 126. American Society for Microbiology, Washington, DC.
197. Walsh TJ, Pappas P, Winston DJ, et al. Voriconazole compared with liposomal amphotericin B for empirical antifungal therapy in patients with neutropenia and persistent fever. *N Engl J Med* 2002;346:225–234.
198. Walsh TJ, Lutsar I, Driscoll T, et al. Voriconazole in the treatment of aspergillosis, scedosporiosis, and other invasive fungal infections in children. *Pediatr Infect Dis J* 2002;21:240–248.
199. Abdel-Rahman SM, Nahata MC. Oral terbinafine: a new antifungal agent. *Ann Pharmacother* 1997;31:445.
200. Angello JT, Voytovich RM, Jan SA. A cost/efficacy analysis of oral antifungals indicated for the treatment of onychomycosis: griseofulvin, itraconazole, and terbinafine. *Am J Manag Care* 1997;3:443.
201. Araujo OE, Flowers FP, King MM. Griseofulvin: a new look at an old drug. *DICP* 1990;24:851.
202. Weese WC, Smith IM. A study of 57 cases of actinomycosis over a 36-year period. *Arch Intern Med* 1975;135:1562.
203. Smego RA, Foglia G. Actinomycosis. *Clin Infect Dis* 1998;26:1255.
204. Berkey P, Bodey GP. Nocardial infection in patients with neoplastic disease. *Rev Infect Dis* 1989;11:407.
205. Wilson JP, et al. Nocardial infection in renal transplant patients. *Medicine* 1989;68:38.
206. Chapman SW, Wilson JP. Nocardiosis in transplant recipients. *Semin Respir Med* 1990;5:74.
207. Wallace RJ, et al. Use of trimethoprim-sulfamethoxazole for treatment of infections due to *Nocardia. Rev Infect Dis* 1982;4:315.
208. Gombert ME. Susceptibility of *Nocardia asteroides* to various antibiotics, including newer beta-lactams, trimethoprim-sulfamethoxazole, amikacin and N-formidoyl thienamycin. *Antimicrob Agents Chemother* 1982;21:1101.

# 18. OPPORTUNISTIC INFECTIONS IN HIV DISEASE

Jin S. Suh and Kent A. Sepkowitz

This chapter focuses on current diagnostic and treatment modalities against opportunistic infection, updates of preventive strategies, and the changing spectrum of disease associated with immune reconstitution. The U.S. Public Health Service/Infectious Diseases Society of America (USPHS/IDSA) guidelines for preventing opportunistic infections have been published in *Morbidity and Mortality Weekly Reports* [1] and *Clinical Infectious Diseases* [2]; updated information is available as a "living document" on the AIDS Treatment Information Service (ATIS) website at *www.hivatis.org.* A comprehensive review of the pathophysiology and treatment of acquired immunodeficiency syndrome (AIDS), and of its complications, is beyond the scope of this chapter. The reader is directed to excellent reference sources that are both practical and useful for keeping up with progress in this disease [3–5]. Antiretroviral therapy is reviewed in Chapter 19.

## I. HIV in the HAART era

**A. Introduction.** Since the recognition of the first cases of AIDS in 1981, there have been an estimated 21.8 million deaths worldwide from the devastating human immunodeficiency virus (HIV) pandemic. UNAIDS and the World Health Organization (WHO) estimated that the number of people living with HIV or AIDS at the end of the year 2001 was 40 million, including 5 million who became infected within the preceding year. The virus has spread to all of the continents of the world. The bulk of the epidemic resides in sub-Saharan Africa, where some epicenters report an adult prevalence rate as high as 33% [6]. HIV continues to be spread by sexual contact, by exposure to infected blood or blood products, and by transmission from mother to child.

There has been much progress toward understanding the pathogenesis, clinical presentation, treatment, and prevention of HIV [7]. **The hallmark of infection is immune suppression, making patients susceptible to opportunistic infections (OIs)** [8]. The **CD4 cell count remains the single most important predictor of risk for OIs.** Although the measurement of HIV viral load has led to a greater understanding of the natural history of HIV as well as therapeutic monitoring, no useful scale of viral load exists to determine when patients are at risk for developing specific OIs. It is clear that prevention and treatment of OIs remain priorities in reducing the morbidity and mortality associated with HIV/AIDS. The introduction of **highly active antiretroviral therapy (HAART) has exerted a profound effect on the epidemiology, natural history, clinical manifestations, and responses to treatment of OIs** [9–11]. HAART is defined as at least three medications with activity against HIV, including either a protease inhibitor or a non-nucleoside reverse transcriptase inhibitor.

**B. Effects of HAART on opportunistic infections and mortality.** The incidence of nearly all AIDS-defining opportunistic infections decreased significantly in the United States between 1992 and 1998 [12]. Decreases in the most common OIs, including *Pneumocystis carinii* pneumonia (PCP), esophageal candidiasis, and disseminated *Mycobacterium avium* complex (MAC), were most pronounced during this period when HAART was introduced (Fig. 18.1). The incidence of major OIs in eight U.S. cities declined from 21.9/100 person-years in 1994 to 3.7/100 person-years by mid-1997 [13]. Mortality declined from 29.4/100 person-years in 1995 to 8.8/100 person-years in 1997 [14], after remaining constant during 1994 and 1995. Several reports have described reductions in mortality and in the rate of hospitalization of HIV-infected patients [15,16]. There were reductions in mortality regardless of sex, race, age, and risk factors for transmission of HIV [13,14,17]. Overall mortality nationally has declined an estimated 21% or a rate of 4.6 deaths per 100,000 in 1998, the lowest rate since 1987. HIV mortality has declined more than 70% since 1995 (Fig. 18.2).

**C. Prophylaxis for OIs.** The success of HAART in reducing the incidence of AIDS-related OIs has led to a reassessment of the role of prophylaxis against these

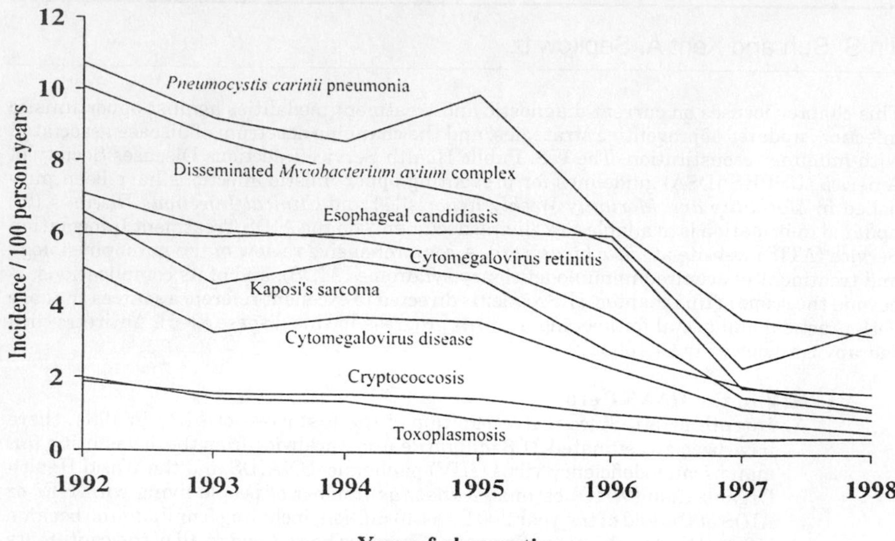


**FIG. 18.1** Trends for opportunistic infections in HIV-infected adults and adolescents, Adult and Adolescent Spectrum of Disease Project, 1992–1998. (Reprinted from Kaplan JE, Hanson D, Dworkin MS, et al. Epidemiology of human immunodeficiency virus–associated opportunistic infection in the United States in the era of highly active antiretroviral therapy. *Clin Infect Dis* 2000;30(suppl):2–15, with permission.)

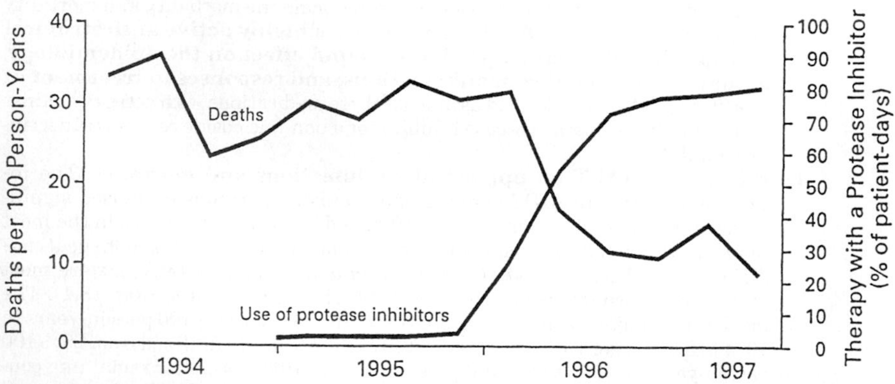


**FIG. 18.2** Mortality and frequency of use of combination antiretroviral therapy including a protease inhibitor among HIV-infected patients with fewer than 100 CD4$^+$ cells/mm$^3$, according to calendar quarter, from January 1994 through June 1997. (Reprinted from Palella FJ, Delaney KM, Moorman AC, et al. Declining morbidity and mortality among patients with advanced human immunodeficiency virus infection. *N Engl J Med* 1998;338:853–860, with permission.)

infections [18–20]. Previously, prophylaxis was continued based on the lowest, or nadir, CD4 cell count [21]. This was based on a concern that recovery of the immune system was incomplete, and patients who lost specific immunity would not regain it even as the CD4 cell count rose. There are now sufficient data to recommend that for patients who have CD4 T-lymphocyte count responses, primary or secondary prophylaxis for some OIs can be discontinued. Consequently, in 2001 the USPHS/IDSA amended their prophylaxis guidelines to include prophylaxis discontinuation [1].

**D.** The declining rates of morbidity and mortality, as well as improvement in quality of life, have been well documented among HIV-infected individuals who have access to diagnostic monitoring and potent combinations of antiretroviral drugs. But despite the encouraging trends in incidence of OIs, **patients are still dying from HIV and associated OIs. This is most notable in** yet undiagnosed patients not receiving antiretroviral therapy, patients who cannot adhere to regimens, and those who fail therapy. These three groups pose an important challenge in management, especially because the best treatment for many OIs may be effective antiretroviral therapy. Thus, the treatment of OIs may depend heavily on the effectiveness and tolerability of future antiretroviral regimens.

**II. Immune reconstitution**

**A. Phases of immune reconstitution with HAART.** It is important to keep in mind that antiretroviral medications, in general, have no intrinsic antimicrobial effect; therefore, **the change in rates of opportunistic infections are mostly a consequence of improvements in immune function,** usually accompanied by viral suppression and an elevation in CD4 cell count. Several previously untreatable opportunistic infections have responded to HAART, presumably due to immune system recovery, including progressive multifocal leukoencephalopathy (PML), cytomegalovirus (CMV), and AIDS-associated microsporidiosis and cryptosporidiosis. Immune restoration from HAART can be divided into two distinct phases. The initial increase of CD4 cell count after initiation of HAART, which is observed within the first 8 weeks, is believed to be due to the release of trapped memory cells from lymphoid tissues to the blood. There is a minimal increase in these cells as time progresses. Decreased risk of OIs has been demonstrated in this early period [22]. Later, there is a slower, more modest increase in naive cells that have matured in the thymus and extrathymic sites. During this period, both CD4-naive cells and CD8-naive cells tend to increase while memory CD4 cells stabilize or increase modestly and memory CD8 cells tend to decrease [23]. Naive cells respond to newly encountered antigens, and memory cells are capable of rapid responses to previously encountered antigens. It is not clear whether and for how long immune reconstitution persists after the loss of viral suppression. It is also not known whether immune recovery is more effective with earlier antiretroviral intervention [22]. However, it is abundantly clear that the increase in CD4 cell count is associated with clinical evidence of recovery of the immune system.

**B. Immune reconstitution syndromes.** Paradoxically, some patients who have virologic and immunologic responses to HAART develop inflammation at sites of preexistent or subclinical infection by opportunistic pathogens. These episodes of unexpected exacerbation of disease while on appropriate therapy have been seen within the first 3 months on HAART as the immune response against the specific pathogens is restored.

1. **MAC lymphadenitis** has been described in patients with localized disease who develop **fever and painful generalized adenopathy,** associated with initiation of HAART. This has been linked to the restoration of mycobacteria-specific cell-mediated immune responses. Patients may appear systemically ill with severe abdominal pain, malaise, and leukocytosis. Mediastinal or mesenteric adenopathy with associated endobronchial lesions, pulmonary infiltrates, and inflammatory skin lesions have been reported [24,25]. Biopsies

of involved lymph nodes may demonstrate granulomatous inflammation. Adenopathy may persist for months despite appropriate therapy. Corticosteroids have been used once other possibilities, including lymphoma, have been ruled out.

2. **Paradoxic reactions with tuberculosis** (TB) have been reported in 36% of patients receiving concomitant therapy for both HIV and TB [26]. Manifestations include fever, intrathoracic and cervical lymphadenopathy, and worsening pulmonary infiltrates. Treatment involves the use of antiinflammatory agents, including corticosteroids or pentoxyfylline, along with continuation of antitubercular therapy. Corticosteroid-responsive cerebral tuberculoma and relapsing corticosteroid-dependent focal cerebritis also have been reported [27], giving support to the assumption that these exacerbations are distinct from TB treatment failure due to resistance or noncompliance.
3. **CMV vitritis** has occurred in patients with and without retinitis who begin HAART. This appears related to the restoration of T-cell responses against CMV antigens. Vitreal inflammation may occur even though retinitis, if present, undergoes remission. This is usually associated with macular edema and epiretinal membrane formation; retinal detachment also can occur [28]. One study reported an annual incidence of CMV vitritis at 83 cases per 100 person-years [29]. It is not possible to predict which patients are at risk for a relapse of CMV retinitis or vitritis, although use of markers for anti-CMV T-cell response is under investigation. Antiinflammatory therapy should be considered for patients with evidence of vitreal inflammation.
4. **Hepatitis C virus (HCV)–or hepatitis B virus–related hepatitis** has been reported in patients being treated with HAART [30–32]. It may be asymptomatic or present with nausea, abdominal pain, and jaundice. Abnormalities in liver function test results may resolve with discontinuation of HAART. This syndrome must be distinguished from medication-related hepatotoxity, although the clinical symptoms are similar.
5. **Other syndromes** of immune reconstitution recently described include **herpes zoster** [33,34], and **inflammatory folliculitis** [35]. According to one study, the incidence of herpes zoster associated with HAART was estimated at 9 episodes per 100 patient-years. Case patients were more likely than controls to manifest an increase in CD8 cell count immediately before clinical disease appeared.
6. **Strategies for the prevention of immune reconstitution syndromes** are poorly defined at present. Withdrawal of effective antiretroviral therapy most often is inappropriate. Options include continuation of HAART with the addition of antimicrobial therapy to suppress the OI, and antiinflammatory agents for symptoms of pain or organ dysfunction. Discontinuation of HAART, even temporarily, should be reserved as a last resort. Prospective studies using measurement of pathogen-specific immune response are needed to distinguish immune reconstitution syndromes from new OIs, treatment failures, or adverse effect of antiretroviral drugs, which currently pose a diagnostic challenge.

III. **Prevention of opportunistic infections.** Whenever possible, preventing an OI is preferred to treating an active infection. **Guidelines for preventing OIs in persons infected with HIV** were first published in the summer of 1995 following a year-long effort by federal authorities, professional societies, researchers, clinicians, community groups, and HIV-infected persons, with comments invited from the general public [21]. Because important new data concerning the prevention of opportunistic diseases have emerged since 1995, they were revised in 1999 and 2001. **The guidelines are posted on the Internet as a "living document" where the latest update is available [1]. Health-care providers actively involved in the care of HIV-infected patients are encouraged to review this excellent source material.** The guidelines provide background information and recommendations on those behavioral changes, drug regimens, and immunizations that are most likely to be beneficial, safe, feasible, and cost effective (Tables 18.1–18.13). The most recent version discusses 19 OIs or groups of OIs, including human herpesvirus 8 (HHV-8) and HCV, two pathogens not previously considered, and provide criteria for discontinuing prophylaxis [1].

Recommendations in the tables designated "A" are supported by evidence that is both statistically and clinically persuasive; the measures designated are strongly recommended, should always be offered, and are considered standard of care. Those designated "B" are recommended for consideration; such measures should be generally offered, but their use should involve some discussion of the "pros and cons" between the provider and patient. Those designated "C" are considered optional, those designated "D" generally should not be offered, and those designated "E" are contraindicated [1]. Recommendations are further rated as I (evidence from at least one properly reported controlled trial), II (evidence from at least one well-designed clinical trial without randomization, or case-controlled studies), or III (evidence from opinions of respected authorities based on clinical experience, from descriptive studies, or from expert communities) [1].

A. **For prophylaxis for OIs** in adults and adolescents, see Tables 18.1 and 18.2. For prophylaxis for OIs in infants and children, see Tables 18.3 and 18.4.
B. **For criteria for discontinuing and restarting prophylaxis** for adults and adolescents whose CD4 counts increased because of HAART, see Table 18.5.
C. **For suggestions to help patients avoid OIs,** see Table 18.6.
D. **For important drug interactions,** see Tables 18.7 through 18.9.
E. **For adverse effects of commonly used drugs to prevent OIs,** see Table 18.10.
F. **For recommended dosing in renal insufficiency** of commonly used drugs to treat or prevent OIs, see Table 18.11.
G. **For a summary of the costs of various prophylactic regimens,** see Table 18.12.
H. **For recommended immunizations in HIV-infected children,** see Table 18.13.

IV. ***Pneumocystis carinii* pneumonia.** In the pre-AIDS era, PCP was seen uncommonly in patients with impaired cellular immunity: premature, debilitated infants; children with primary immunodeficiency states, particularly severe combined immunodeficiency; and patients receiving immunosuppressive drugs for cancer or organ transplantation. During this period, *P. carinii* was misidentified as a protozoan due to its morphology, failure to grow on fungal media, and its response to drugs used to treat protozoan infections. Molecular analysis of its ribosomal RNA and mitochondrial DNA revealed that it is phylogenetically related to the ascomycetes yeast, and thus is now classified as a fungus.

A. **Epidemiology.** Reports of PCP in previously healthy men heralded the onset of the AIDS epidemic [36,37]. In the following two decades, PCP gained notoriety as the most common opportunistic infection associated with HIV and the most common infection among persons who died with AIDS. **The best predictor of PCP occurrence in HIV-infected patients is the CD4 lymphocyte blood count.** The majority of AIDS patients have CD4 cell counts in the range of 50 to 70/mm$^3$ at the time of their first episode of PCP, and more than 90% of episodes occur when counts are below 200/mm$^3$ [38]. Clinical manifestations including a history of thrush, herpes zoster, unexplained fever, and weight loss are correlated with an increased risk independent of the CD4 cell count.

Even in the HAART era, PCP continues to be the most common complication of HIV infection. According to the Centers for Disease Control and Prevention (CDC) Surveillance Report, from 1992 through 1997, PCP was the most common AIDS-defining OI, accounting for 36% of AIDS index cases, the most common incident AIDS-defining OI (87.9 cases per 1,000 person-years), and the most common OI among persons who had died of AIDS (53%) [17]. Although the incidence of PCP declined from 108 cases per 1,000 person-years in 1992 to 46 cases per 1,000 person-years in 1997, largely attributed to widespread prophylaxis and HAART, the absolute rates of these infections were still high.

*(Text continues on p. 663.)*

Table 18.1. Prophylaxis to Prevent First Episode of Opportunistic Disease in Adults and Adolescents Infected with Human Immunodeficiency Virus

| | Preventive Regimens | | |
|---|---|---|---|
| Pathogen | Indication | First Choice | Alternatives |
| Strongly recommended as standard of care | | | |
| *Pneumocystis carinii*[a] | CD4$^+$ count <200/$\mu$L or oropharyngeal candidiasis | TMP-SMX 1 DS orally daily (AI)<br>TMP-SMX 1 SS orally daily (AI) | Dapsone 50 mg orally b.i.d. or 100 mg orally daily (BI); dapsone 50 mg orally daily plus pyrimethamine 50 mg orally weekly plus leucovorin 25 mg orally weekly (BI); dapsone 200 mg orally plus pyrimethamine 75 mg orally plus leucovorin 25 mg orally weekly (BI); aerosolized pentamidine 300 mg monthly via Respirgard II nebulizer (BI); atovaquone 1,500 mg orally daily (BI); TMP-SMX 1 DS orally t.i.w. (BI) |
| *Mycobacterium tuberculosis* | | | |
| Isoniazid-sensitive[b] | TST reaction $\geq$5 mm or prior positive TST result without treatment or contact with case of active tuberculosis regardless of TST result (BIII) | Isoniazid 300 mg orally plus pyridoxine 50 mg orally daily for 9 mo (AII), or isoniazid 900 mg orally plus pyridoxine 100 mg orally b.i.w. for 9 mo (BII) | Rifampin 600 mg orally daily (BIII) for 4 mo or rifabutin 300 mg orally daily (CIII) for 4 mo<br>Pyrazinamide 15–20 mg/kg orally daily for 2 mo plus either rifampin 600 mg orally daily (BI) for 2 mo rifabutin 300 mg orally daily (CIII) for 2 mo |
| Isoniazid-resistant | Same as above; high probability of exposure to isoniazid-resistant tuberculosis | Rifampin 600 mg orally (AIII) or rifabutin 300 mg orally (BIII) daily for 4 mo | Pyrazinamide 15–20 mg/kg orally daily plus either rifampin 600 mg orally (BI) or rifabutin 300 mg orally (CIII) daily for 2 mo |

| | | | |
|---|---|---|---|
| Multidrug (isoniazid and rifampin)-resistant | Same as above; high probability of exposure to multidrug-resistant tuberculosis | Choice of drugs requires consultation with public health authorities. Depends on susceptibility of isolate from source patient. | — |
| *Toxoplasma gondii*[c] | IgG antibody to *Toxoplasma* and CD4$^+$ count $<100/\mu$L | TMP-SMX 1 DS orally daily (AII) | TMP-SMX 1 SS orally daily (BIII); dapsone 50 mg orally daily plus pyrimethamine 50 mg orally weekly plus leucovorin 25 mg orally weekly (BI); dapsone 200 mg orally plus pyrimethamine 75 mg orally plus leucovorin 25 mg orally weekly (BI); atovaquone 1,500 mg orally daily with or without pyrimethamine 25 mg orally daily plus leucovorin 10 mg orally daily (CIII) |
| *Mycobacterium avium* complex[d] | CD4$^+$ count $<50/\mu$L | Azithromycin, 1,200 mg orally weekly (AI) or clarithromycin[d] 500 mg orally b.i.d. (AI) | Rifabutin 300 mg orally daily (BI); azithromycin 1,200 mg orally weekly plus rifabutin 300 mg orally daily (CI) |
| Varicella zoster virus (VZV) | Significant exposure to chickenpox or shingles for patients who have no history of either condition or, if available, negative antibody to VZV | Varicella zoster immune globulin 5 vials (1.25 mL each) i.m., administered $\leq$96 h after exposure, ideally within 48 h (AIII) | |
| Generally recommended | | | |
| *Streptococcus pneumoniae*[e] | CD4$^+$ count $\geq 200/\mu$L | 23 valent polysaccharide vaccine, 0.5 mL i.m. (BII) | None |
| Hepatitis B virus[f,g] | All susceptible (anti-HBc–negative) patients | Hepatitis B vaccine: 3 doses (BII) | None |

*(Continued)*

Table 18.1. (*Continued*)

| Pathogen | Preventive Regimens | | |
|---|---|---|---|
| | Indication | First Choice | Alternatives |
| Influenza virus[f,h] | All patients (annually, before influenza season) | Inactivated trivalent influenza virus vaccine: one annual dose (0.5 mL) i.m. (BIII) | Oseltamivir 75 mg orally daily (influenza A or B) (CIII); rimantadine 100 mg orally b.i.d. (CIII), or amantadine 100 mg orally b.i.d. (CIII) (influenza A only) |
| Hepatitis A virus[f,g] | All susceptible (anti-HAV–negative) patients at increased risk for HAV infection (e.g., illicit drug users, men who have sex with men, hemophiliacs) or with chronic liver disease, including chronic hepatitis B or hepatitis C | Hepatitis A vaccine: two doses (BIII) | None |
| **Evidence for efficacy but not routinely indicated** | | | |
| Bacteria | Neutropenia | Granulocyte colony-stimulating factor 5–10 $\mu$g/kg s.c. daily for 2–4 wk or granulocyte-macrophage colony-stimulating factor 250 $\mu g/m^2$ s.c. for 2–4 wk (CII) | None |
| *Cryptococcus neoformans* | $CD4^+$ count <50/$\mu$L | Fluconazole 100–200 mg orally daily (CI) | Itraconazole capsule, 200 mg orally daily (CIII) |
| *Histoplasma capsulatum*[i] | $CD4^+$ count <100/$\mu$L, endemic geographic area | Itraconazole capsule 200 mg orally daily (CI) | None |
| Cytomegalovirus (CMV)[j] | $CD4^+$ count <50/$\mu$L and CMV antibody positivity | Oral ganciclovir 1g orally t.i.d. (CI) | None |

Information included in these guidelines might not represent U.S. Food and Drug Administration (FDA) approval or approved labeling for the particular products or indications in question. Specifically, the terms "safe" and "effective" might not be synonymous with the FDA-defined legal standards for product approval. The Respirgard II nebulizer is manufactured by Marquest, Englewood, Colorado. Letters and roman numerals in parentheses after regimens indicate the strength of the recommendation and the quality of evidence supporting it. Anti-HBc, antibody to hepatitis B core antigen; b.i.w., twice a week; DS, double-strength tablet; HAART, highly active antiretroviral therapy; HAV, hepatitis A virus; HIV, human immunodeficiency virus; i.m., intramuscular; i.v., intravenous; SS, single-strength table; t.i.w., three times a week; TMP-SMX, trimethoprim-sulfamethoxazole; s.c., subcutaneous; TST, tuberculin skin test.

[a]Prophylaxis should also be considered for persons with a CD4+ percentage of <14%, for persons with a history of an AIDS-defining illness, and possibly for those with CD4+ counts >200 but <250 cells/μL. TMP-SMX also reduces the frequency of toxoplasmosis and some bacterial infections. Patients receiving dapsone should be tested for glucose-6 phosphate dehydrogenase deficiency. A dosage of 50 mg daily is probably less effective than 100 mg daily. The efficacy of parenteral pentamidine (e.g., 4 mg/kg/mo) is uncertain. Fansidar (sulfadoxine-pyrimethamine) is rarely used because of severe hypersensitivity reactions. Patients who are being administered therapy for toxoplasmosis with sulfadiazine-pyrimethamine are protected against *Pneumocystis carinii* pneumonia (PCP) and do not need additional prophylaxis against PCP.

[b]Directly observed therapy is recommended for isoniazid, e.g., 900 mg b.i.w.; isoniazid regimens should include pyridoxine to prevent peripheral neuropathy. If rifampin or rifabutin are administered concurrently with protease inhibitors or non-nucleoside reverse transcriptase inhibitors, careful consideration should be given to potential pharmacokinetic interactions. There have been reports of fatal and severe liver injury associated with the treatment of latent TB infection in HIV-uninfected persons treated with the 2-month regimen of daily rifampin and pyrazinamide; therefore, it may be prudent to use regimens that do not contain pyrazinamide in HIV-infected persons whose completion of treatment can be assured. (Centers for Disease Control and Prevention. Update: fatal and severe liver injuries associated with rifampin and pyrazinamide for latent tuberculosis infection and revisions in American Thoracic Society/CDC recommendations, United States 2001. *MMWR* 2001;50:733.) Exposure to multidrug-resistant tuberculosis might require prophylaxis with two drugs; consult public health authorities. Possible regimens include pyrazinamide plus either ethambutol or a fluoroquinolone.

[c]Protection against toxoplasmosis is provided by TMP-SMX, dapsone plus pyrimethamine, and possibly by atovaquone. Atovaquone may be used with or without pyrimethamine. Pyrimethamine alone probably provides little, if any, protection.

[d]During pregnancy, azithromycin is preferred over clarithromycin because of demonstrated teratogenicity in animals with clarithromycin.

[e]Vaccination may be offered to persons who have a CD4+ T-lymphocyte count of <200 cells/μL, although the efficacy is likely to be diminished. Revaccination 5 years after the first dose or sooner if the initial immunization was given when the CD4+ count was <200 cells/μL and the CD4+ count has increased to >200 cells/μL on HAART is considered optional. Some authorities are concerned that immunizations might stimulate the replication of HIV.

[f]Although data demonstrating clinical benefit of these vaccines in HIV-infected persons are not available, it is logical to assume that those patients who develop antibody responses will derive some protection. Some authorities are concerned that immunizations might stimulate HIV replication, although for influenza vaccination, a large observational study of HIV-infected persons in clinical care showed no adverse effect of this vaccine, including multiple doses, on patient survival (J. Ward, CDC, personal communication). Also, this concern may be less relevant in the setting of HAART. However, because of the theoretical concern that increases in HIV plasma RNA following vaccination during pregnancy might increase the risk of perinatal transmission of HIV, providers may wish to defer vaccination for such patients until after HAART is initiated.

[g]Hepatitis B vaccine has been recommended for all children and adolescents and for all adults with risk factors for hepatitis B virus. For persons requiring vaccination against both hepatitis A and hepatitis B, a combination vaccine is now available. For additional information regarding vaccination against hepatitis A and B, see CDC. Hepatitis B virus: a comprehensive strategy for eliminating transmission in the United States through universal childhood vaccination. Recommendations of the Advisory Committee on Immunization Practices (ACIP). *MMWR* 1991;40(RR-13):1.

[h]Oseltamivir is appropriate during outbreaks of either influenza A or influenza B. Rimantadine or amantadine are appropriate during outbreaks of influenza A (although neither rimantadine nor amantadine is recommended during pregnancy). Dosage reduction for antiviral chemoprophylaxis against influenza might be indicated for decreased renal or hepatic function, and for persons with seizure disorders. Physicians should consult the drug package inserts and the annual CDC influenza guidelines for more specific information about adverse effects and dosage adjustments. For additional information about vaccination, antiviral chemoprophylaxis and therapy against influenza, see CDC. Prevention and control of influenza: recommendations of the Advisory Committee on Immunization Practices (ACIP). *MMWR* 2001;50(RR-4):1.

[i]In a few unusual occupational or other circumstances, prophylaxis should be considered; consult a specialist.

[j]Acyclovir is not protective against cytomegalovirus (CMV). Valacyclovir is not recommended because of an unexplained trend toward increased mortality observed in persons with AIDS who were being administered this drug for prevention of CMV disease.

From Masur H, Kaplan JE, Holmes KK, and the USPHS/IDSA Prevention of Opportunistic Infections Working Group. 2001 USPHS/IDSA guidelines for the prevention of opportunistic infections in persons infected with human immunodeficiency virus, pages 38–41. Posted November 28, 2001 as a "living document" at *www.hivatis.org/trtgdlns.html#Opportunistic*.

Table 18.2. Prophylaxis to Prevent Recurrence of Opportunistic Disease in Adults (after Chemotherapy for Acute Disease) in Adults and Adolescents Infected with Human Immunodeficiency Virus

| | Preventive Regimens | | |
|---|---|---|---|
| Pathogen | Indication | First Choice | Alternatives |
| Recommended as standard of care | | | |
| *Pneumocystis carinii* | Prior *P. carinii* pneumonia | TMP-SMX 1 DS orally daily (AI); TMP-SMX 1 SS orally daily (AI) | Dapsone 50 mg orally b.i.d. or 100 mg orally daily (BI); dapsone 50 mg orally daily plus pyrimethamine 50 mg orally weekly plus leucovorin 25 mg orally weekly (BI); dapsone 200 mg orally plus pyrimethamine 75 mg orally plus leucovorin 25 mg orally weekly (BI); aerosolized pentamidine 300 mg monthly via Respirgard II nebulizer (BI); atovaquone 1,500 mg orally daily (BI); TMP-SMX 1 DS orally t.i.w. (CI) |
| *Toxoplasma gondii*[a] | Prior toxoplasmic encephalitis | Sulfadiazine 500–1,000 mg orally q.i.d. plus pyrimethamine 25–50 mg orally daily plus leucovorin 10–25 mg orally daily (AI) | Clindamycin 300–450 mg orally every 6–8 h plus pyrimethamine 25–50 mg orally daily plus leucovorin 10–25 mg orally daily (BI); atovaquone 750 mg orally every 6–12 h with or without pyrimethamine 25 mg orally daily plus leucovorin 10 mg orally daily (CIII) |
| *Mycobacterium avium* complex[b] | Documented disseminated disease | Clarithromycin[b] 500 mg orally b.i.d. (AI) plus ethambutol 15 mg/kg orally daily (AII); with or without rifabutin 300 mg orally daily (CI) | Azithromycin 500 mg orally daily (AII) plus ethambutol 15 mg/kg orally daily (AII), with or without rifabutin 300 mg orally daily (CI) |
| Cytomegalovirus | Prior end-organ disease | Ganciclovir 5–6 mg/kg/day i.v. 5–7 days/wk or 1,000 mg orally t.i.d. (AI); or foscarnet 90–120 mg/kg i.v. daily (AI); or (for retinitis) ganciclovir sustained-release implant every 6–9 mo plus ganciclovir 1.0–1.5 g orally t.i.d. (AI) | Cidofovir 5 mg/kg i.v. q.o.w. with probenecid 2 orally 3 h before the dose followed by 1 g orally 2 h after the dose, and 1 g orally 8 h after the dose (total of 4 g) (AI). Fomivirsen 1 vial (330 $\mu$g) injected into the vitreous, then repeated every 2–4 wk (AI); valganciclovir 900 mg orally daily (BI) |

| | | | |
|---|---|---|---|
| *Cryptococcus neoformans* | Documented disease | Fluconazole 200 mg orally daily (AI) | Amphotericin B 0.6–1.0 mg/kg i.v. 1–3 times/wk (AI); itraconazole 200 mg capsule orally daily (BI) |
| *Histoplasma capsulatum* | Documented disease | Itraconazole capsule 200 mg orally b.i.d. (AI) | Amphotericin B 1.0 mg/kg i.v. weekly (AI) |
| *Coccidioides immitis* | Documented disease | Fluconazole 400 mg orally daily (AII) | Amphotericin B 1.0 mg/kg i.v. weekly (AI); itraconazole 200 mg capsule orally b.i.d. (AII) |
| *Salmonella* species, (nontyphi)[c] | Bacteremia | Ciprofloxacin 500 mg orally b.i.d. for several months (BII) | Antibiotic chemoprophylaxis with another active agent (CIII) |
| Recommended only if subsequent episodes are frequent or severe | | | |
| Herpes simplex virus | Frequent/severe recurrences | Acyclovir 200 mg orally t.i.d. or 400 mg orally b.i.d. (AI)<br>Famciclovir 250 mg orally b.i.d. (AI) | Valacyclovir 500 mg orally b.i.d (CIII) |
| *Candida* (oropharyngeal or vaginal) | Frequent/severe recurrences | Fluconazole 100–200 mg orally daily (CI) | Itraconazole solution 200 mg orally daily (CI) |
| *Candida* (esophageal) | Frequent/severe recurrences | Fluconazole 100–200 mg orally daily (BI) | Itraconazole solution 200 mg orally daily (BI) |

Information included in these guidelines might not represent U.S. Food and Drug Administration (FDA) approval or approved labeling for the particular products or indications in question. Specifically, the terms "safe" and "effective" might not be synonymous with the FDA-defined legal standards for product approval. The Respirgard II nebulizer is manufactured by Marquest, Englewood, Colorado. Letters and roman numerals in parentheses after regimens indicate the strength of the recommendation and the quality of evidence supporting it.

b.i.d., twice a day; DS, double-strength tablet; i.v., intravenous; q.o.w., every other week; SS, single-strength tablet; t.i.d., three times a day; t.i.w., three times a week; TMP-SMX, trimethoprim-sulfamethoxazole.

[a] Pyrimethamine-sulfadiazine confers protection against *Pneumocystis carinii* pneumonia (PCP) as well as toxoplasmosis; clindamycin-pyrimethamine does not offer protection against PCP.

[b] Many multiple-drug regimens are poorly tolerated. Drug interactions (e.g., those seen with clarithromycin and rifabutin) can be problematic; rifabutin has been associated with uveitis, especially when administered at daily doses of >300 mg or concurrently with fluconazole or clarithromycin. During pregnancy, azithromycin is recommended instead of clarithromycin because clarithromycin is teratogenic in animals.

[c] Efficacy for eradication of *Salmonella* has been demonstrated only for ciprofloxacin.

From Masur H, Kaplan JE, Holmes KK, and the USPHS/IDSA Prevention of Opportunistic Infections Working Group. 2001 USPHS/IDSA guidelines for the prevention of opportunistic infections in persons infected with human immunodeficiency virus, pages 42–43. Posted November 28, 2001 as a "living document" at *www.hivatis.org/trtgdlns.html#Opportunistic*.

Table 18.3. Prophylaxis to Prevent First Episode of Opportunistic Disease in Infants and Children Infected with Human Immunodeficiency Virus

| Pathogen | Indication | Preventive Regimens | |
|---|---|---|---|
| | | First Choice | Alternatives |
| Strongly recommended as standard of care | | | |
| *Pneumocystis carinii*[a] | HIV-infected or HIV-indeterminate, infants aged 1–12 mo; HIV-infected children aged 1–5 yr with $CD4^+$ count $<500/\mu L$ or $CD4^+$ percentage $<15\%$; HIV-infected children aged 6–12 yr with $CD4^+$ count $<200/\mu L$ or $CD4^+$ percentage $<15\%$ | TMP-SM, 150/750 $mg/m^2$/day in 2 divided doses orally t.i.w. on consecutive days (AII) Acceptable alternative dosage schedules (AII): Single dose orally t.i.w. on consecutive days; or 2 divided doses orally daily; or 2 divided doses orally t.i.w. on alternate days | Dapsone (children aged $\geq 1$ mo) 2 mg/kg (max 100 mg) orally daily or 4 mg/kg (max 200 mg) orally weekly (CII); aerosolized pentamidine (children aged $\geq 5$ yr) 300 mg monthly via Respirgard II nebulizer (CIII); atovaquone (children aged 1–3 mo and $>24$ mo, 30 mg/kg orally daily; children aged 4–24 mo, 45 mg/kg orally daily) (CII) |
| *Mycobacterium tuberculosis*[b] | | | |
| Isoniazid-sensitive | TST reaction $\geq 5$ mm or prior positive TST result without treatment, or contact with any case of active tuberculosis regardless of TST result | Isoniazid 10–15 mg/kg (max 300 mg) orally daily for 9 mo (AII) or 20–30 mg/kg (max 900 mg) orally b.i.w. for 9 mo (BII) | Rifampin 10–20 mg/kg (max 600 mg) orally daily for 4–6 mo (BIII) |
| Isoniazid-resistant | Same as above; high probability of exposure to isoniazid-resistant tuberculosis | Rifampin 10–20 mg/kg (max 600 mg) orally daily for 4–6 mo (BIII) | Uncertain |
| Multidrug (isoniazid and rifampin)-resistant | Same as above; high probability of exposure to multidrug-resistant tuberculosis | Choice of drugs requires consultation with public health authorities and depends on susceptibility of isolate from source patient | |
| *Mycobacterium avium* complex[b] | For children aged $\geq 6$ yr, $CD4^+$ count $<50/\mu L$; aged 2–6 yr $CD4^+$ count $<75/\mu L$; aged 1–2 yr, $CD4^+$ count $<500/\mu L$; aged $<1$ yr, $CD4^+$ count $<750/\mu L$ | Clarithromycin 7.5 mg/kg (max 500 mg) orally b.i.d. (AII), or azithromycin 20 mg/kg (max 1,200 mg) orally weekly (AII) | Azithromycin, 5 mg/kg (max 250 mg) orally daily (AII); children aged $\geq 6$ yr, rifabutin 300 mg orally daily (BI) |

| | | | |
|---|---|---|---|
| Varicella zoster virus[c] | Significant exposure to varicella or shingles with no history of chickenpox or shingles | VZIG 1 vial (1.25 mL)/10 kg (max 5 vials) i.m., administered ≤96 h after exposure, ideally within 48 h (AII) | None |
| Vaccine-preventable pathogens[d] | HIV exposure/infection | Routine immunizations (see Table 18.13) | None |
| **Generally recommended** | | | |
| *Toxoplasma gondii*[e] | IgG antibody to *Toxoplasma* and severe immunosuppression | TMP-SMX 150/750 mg/m$^2$/day in 2 divided doses orally daily (BIII) | Dapsone (children aged ≥1 mo), 2 mg/kg or 15 mg/m$^2$ (max 25 mg) orally daily plus pyrimethamine 1 mg/kg orally daily plus leucovorin 5 mg orally every 3 days (BIII)<br>Atovaquone (aged 1–3 mo and >24 mo, 30 mg/kg orally daily; aged 14–24 mo, 45 mg/kg orally daily) (CIII) |
| Varicella zoster virus | HIV-infected children who are asymptomatic and not immunosuppressed | Varicella zoster vaccine (see vaccine-preventable pathogens section of this table) (BII) | None |
| Influenza virus | All patients (annually, before influenza season) | Inactivated split trivalent influenza vaccine (see vaccine-preventable section of this table) (BIII) | Oseltamivir (during outbreaks of influenza A or B) for children ≥13 years, 75 mg orally daily (CIII); rimantadine or amantadine (during outbreaks of influenza A) aged 1–9 yr, 5 mg/kg in 2 divided doses (max 150 mg/day) orally daily; aged ≥10 yr, use adult doses (CIII) |
| **Not recommended for most children; indicated for use only in unusual circumstances** | | | |
| Invasive bacterial infections[f] | Hypogammaglobulinemia (i.e., IgG <400 mg/dL) | IVIG (400 mg/kg every 2–4 wk) (AI) | None |
| *Cryptococcus neoformans* | Severe immunosuppression | Fluconazole 3–6 mg/kg orally daily (CII) | Itraconazole 2–5 mg/kg orally every 12–24 h (CII |

(*Continued*)

Table 18.3. (*Continued*)

| Pathogen | Indication | Preventive Regimens: First Choice | Preventive Regimens: Alternatives |
|---|---|---|---|
| *Histoplasma capsulatum* | Severe immunosuppression, endemic geographic area | Itraconazole 2–5 mg/kg orally every 12–24 h (CIII) | None |
| Cytomegalovirus (CMV)[g] | CMV antibody positivity and severe immunosuppression | Oral ganciclovir 30 mg/kg t.i.d. (CII) | None |

Information included in these guidelines might not represent U.S. Food and Drug Administration (FDA) approval or approved labeling for the particular products or indications in question. Specifically, the terms "safe" and "effective" might not be synonymous with the FDA-defined legal standards for product approval. The Respirgard II nebulizer is manufactured by Marquest, Englewood, Colorado. Letters and roman numerals in parentheses after regimens indicate the strength of the recommendation and the quality of the evidence supporting it.

b.i.w., twice a week; i.m., intramuscular; IVIG, intravenous immune globulin; t.i.d., three times a day; t.i.w., three times a week; TMP-SMX, trimethoprim-sulfamethoxazole; VZIG, varicella zoster immune globulin.

[a]Daily TMP-SMX reduces the frequency of some bacterial infections. TMP-SMX, dapsone-pyrimethamine, and possibly atovaquone (with or without pyrimethamine) appear to protect against toxoplasmosis, although data have not been prospectively collected. When compared with weekly dapsone, daily dapsone is associated with lower incidence of *Pneumocystis carinii* pneumonia (PCP) but higher hematologic toxicity and mortality (McIntosh K, Cooper E, Xu J, et al. Toxicity and efficacy of daily vs. weekly dapsone for prevention of *Pneumocystis carini* pneumonia in children infected with HIV. *Pediatr Infect Dis J* 1999;18:432–439).

The efficacy of parenteral pentamidine (e.g., 4 mg/kg every 2–4 wk) is controversial. Patients receiving therapy for toxoplasmosis with sulfadiazine-pyrimethamine are protected against PCP and do not need TMP-SMX.

[b]Significant drug interactions can occur between rifamycins (rifampin and rifabutin) and protease inhibitors and nonnucleoside reverse transcriptase inhibitors. Consult a specialist.

[c]Children routinely being administered IVIG should receive VZIG if the last dose of IVIG was administered >21 days before exposure.

[d]HIV-infected and HIV-exposed children should be immunized according to the childhood immunization schedule in Table 18.13, which has been adapted from the January–December 2001 schedule recommended for immunocompetent children by the Advisory Committee on Immunization Practices, the American Academy of Pediatrics, and the American Academy of Family Physicians. This schedule differs from that for immunocompetent children in that both the conjugate pneumococcal vaccine (PCV-7) and the pneumococcal polysaccharide vaccine (PPV-23) are recommended (BII), and vaccination against influenza (BIII) should be offered. MMR should not be administered to severely immunocompromised children (DIII). Vaccination against varicella is indicated only for asymptomatic nonimmunosuppressed children (BII). Once an HIV-exposed child is determined not to be HIV infected, the schedule for immunocompetent children applies.

[e]Protection against toxoplasmosis is provided by the preferred antipneumocystis regimens and possibly by atovaquone. Atovaquone may be used with or without pyrimethamine. Pyrimethamine alone probably provides little, if any, protection.

[f]Respiratory syncytial virus (RSV) IVIG (750 mg/kg), not monoclonal RSV antibody, may be substituted for IVIG during the RSV season to provide broad antiinfective protection, if this product is available.

[g]Oral ganciclovir and perhaps valganciclovir results in reduced CMV shedding in CMV-infected children. Acyclovir is not protective against CMV.

From Masur H, Kaplan JE, Holmes KK, and the USPHS/IDSA Prevention of Opportunistic Infections Working Group. 2001 USPHS/IDSA guidelines for the prevention of opportunistic infections in persons infected with human immunodeficiency virus, pages 55–57. Posted November 28, 2001 as a "living document" at *www.hivatis.org/trtgdlns.html#Opportunistic.*

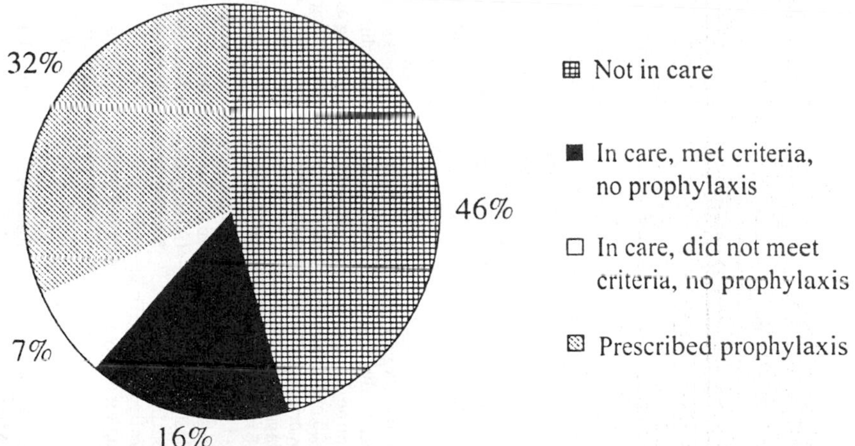


**FIG. 18.3** Reasons why persons developed *Pneumocystis carinii* pneumonia, from the Adult and Adolescent Spectrum of Disease Project, 1996–1998 (N = 1,837). (Reprinted from Kaplan JE, Hanson D, Dworkin MS, et al. Epidemiology of human immunodeficiency virus–associated opportunistic infection in the United States in the era of highly active antiretroviral therapy. *Clin Infect Dis* 2000;30(suppl):2–15; with permission.)

PCP still occurs, particularly among individuals who are unaware of their HIV seropositivity or adhere poorly to prophylaxis, or those with poor access to adequate health care (Fig. 18.3). Even with appropriate prophylaxis, PCP is one of the most common serious opportunistic infections among HIV-infected persons, because prophylaxis failure may occur. Thus, PCP continues to be a substantial cause of morbidity and mortality during the HAART era.

**B. Clinical manifestations**

1. **Symptoms** are often present for weeks and are accompanied by weight loss and malaise. Slowly worsening exertional dyspnea, nonproductive cough, fever, and hypoxemia are common. Some patients may have pleuritic chest pain, but rigors, chills, and hectic fevers are uncommon. **Results of the lung examination** are usually normal, although fine bibasilar inspiratory rales may occasionally be heard. Tachypnea and tachycardia may be present, depending on the severity of illness. Findings that reflect the degree of CD4 depletion also may be noted, including thrush.
2. **Laboratory findings** often include an elevated serum lactate dehydrogenase (LDH) level, although this abnormality is neither sensitive nor specific for PCP. Some studies have suggested a strong correlation between the degree of LDH elevation and survival [39,40]. **The best indicator of prognosis is the alveolar-arterial gradient at the time that specific therapy is initiated.**
3. **Chest radiographs** classically reveal a diffuse bilateral, interstitial, and then alveolointerstitial infiltrate progressing from perihilar to peripheral regions. Pneumatoceles are associated with more prolonged, indolent disease. Apical disease, often confused with TB, has been associated with use of aerosol pentamidine prophylaxis [41]. Pleural effusions and intrathoracic adenopathy are rare, whereas spontaneous pneumothorax is more common, in PCP. Normal chest radiographs have been reported in the range of 0% to 40% [4], particularly early in the process.
4. **Extrapulmonary disease** is rarely encountered in patients receiving systemic chemoprophylaxis. Reported sites of disseminated *P. carinii* infection include the lymph nodes, liver, spleen, bone marrow, intestine, peritoneum, adrenal gland, pancreas, skin, eye, ear, and meninges [42,43]. Most case

(*Text continues on p. 673.*)

**Table 18.4. Prophylaxis to Prevent Recurrence of Opportunistic Disease (after Chemotherapy for Acute Disease) in HIV-infected Infants and Children**

| | | Preventive Regimens | |
|---|---|---|---|
| Pathogen | Indication | First Choice | Alternatives |
| Recommended for life as standard of care | | | |
| *Pneumocystis carinii* | Prior *P. carinii* pneumonia | TMP-SMX 150/750 mg/$m^2$/day in 2 divided doses orally t.i.w. on consecutive days (AII) Acceptable alternative schedules for same dosage (AII): single dose orally t.i.w. on consecutive days; 2 divided doses orally daily; 2 divided doses orally t.i.w. on alternate days | Dapsone (children aged ≥1 mo) 2 mg/kg (max 100 mg) orally daily or 4 mg/kg (max 200 mg) orally weekly (CII); aerosolized pentamidine (children aged ≥5 yr) 300 mg monthly via Respirgard II nebulizer (CIII); atovaquone (aged 1–3 mo and >24 mo, 30 mg/kg orally daily; aged 4–24 mo, 45 mg/kg orally daily) (CII) |
| *Toxoplasma gondii*[a] | Prior toxoplasmic encephalitis | Sulfadiazine 85–120 mg/kg/day in 2–4 divided doses orally daily plus pyrimethamine 1 mg/kg or 15 mg/$m^2$ (max 25 mg) orally daily plus leucovorin 5 mg orally every 3 days (AI) | Clindamycin 20–30 mg/kg/day in 4 divided doses orally plus pyrimethamine 1 mg/kg orally daily plus leucovorin 5 mg orally every 3 days (BI) |
| *Mycobacterium avium* complex[b] | Prior disease | Clarithromycin 7.5 mg/kg (max 500 mg) orally b.i.d. (AII) plus ethambutol 15 mg/kg (max 900 mg) orally daily (AII), with or without rifabutin 5 mg/kg (max 300 mg) orally daily (CII) | Azithromycin 5 mg/kg (max 250 mg) orally daily (AII) plus ethambutol 15 mg/kg (max 900 mg) orally daily (AII), with or without rifabutin 5 mg/kg (max 300 mg) orally daily (CII) |
| *Cryptococcus neoformans* | Documented disease | Fluconazole 3–6 mg/kg orally daily (AII) | Amphotericin B 0.5–1.0 mg/kg i.v. 1–3 times/week (AI); itraconazole 2–5 mg/kg orally every 12–24 h (BII) |
| *Histoplasma capsulatum* | Documented disease | Itraconazole 2–5 mg/kg orally every 12–48 h (AIII) | Amphotericin B 1.0 mg/kg i.v. weekly (AIII) |

| | | | |
|---|---|---|---|
| *Coccidioides immitis* | Documented disease | Fluconazole 6 mg/kg orally daily (AII) | Amphotericin B 1.0 mg/kg i.v. weekly (AIII); itraconazole 2–5 mg/kg orally every 12–48 h (AIII) |
| Cytomegalovirus | Prior end-organ disease | Ganciclovir 5 mg/kg i.v. daily; or foscarnet 90–120 mg/kg i.v. daily (AI) | (For retinitis) ganciclovir sustained-release implant every 6–9 mo plus ganciclovir 30 mg/kg orally t.i.d. (BIII) |
| *Salmonella* species (nontyphi)[c] | Bacteremia | TMP-SMX 150/750 mg/$m^2$ in 2 divided doses orally daily for several months (CIII) | Antibiotic chemoprophylaxis with another active agent (CIII) |
| Recommended only if subsequent episodes are frequent or severe | | | |
| Invasive bacterial infections[d] | >2 infections in 1-yr period | TMP-SMX 150/750 mg/$m^2$ in 2 divided doses orally daily (BI); or IVIG 400 mg/kg every 2–4 wk (BI) | Antibiotic chemoprophylaxis with another active agent (BIII) |
| Herpes simplex virus | Frequent/severe recurrences | Acyclovir 80 mg/kg/day in 3–4 divided doses orally (AII) | |
| *Candida* (oropharyngeal) | Frequent/severe recurrences | Fluconazole 3–6 mg/kg orally daily (CIII) | |
| *Candida* (esophageal) | Frequent/severe recurrences | Fluconazole 3–6 mg/kg orally daily (BIII) | Itraconazole solution 5 mg/kg orally daily (CIII) |

Information included in these guidelines might not represent U.S. Food and Drug Administration (FDA) approval or approved labeling for the particular products or indications in question. Specifically, the terms "safe" and "effective" might not be synonymous with the FDA-defined legal standards for product approval. The Respirgard II nebulizer is manufactured by Marquest, Englewood, Colorado. Letters and roman numerals in parentheses after regimens indicate the strength of the recommendation and the quality of evidence supporting it. i.v., intravenous; IVIG, intravenous immune globulin; t.i.d., three times a day; t.i.w., three times a week; TMP-SMX, trimethoprim-sulfamethoxazole.

[a]Only pyrimethamine plus sulfadiazine confers protection against *Pneumocystis carinii* pneumonia as well as toxoplasmosis. Although the clindamycin plus pyrimethamine regimen is recommended in adults, it has not been tested in children. However, these drugs are safe and are used for other infections.

[b]Significant drug interactions might occur between rifabutin and protease inhibitors and non-nucleoside reverse transcriptase inhibitors. Consult an expert.

[c]Drug should be determined by susceptibilities of the organism isolated. Alternatives to TMP-SMX include ampicillin, chloramphenicol, or ciprofloxacin. However, ciprofloxacin is not approved for use in persons aged <18 years; therefore, it should be used in children with caution and only if no alternatives exist.

[d]Antimicrobial prophylaxis should be chosen based on the microorganism and antibiotic sensitivities. TMP-SMX, if used, should be administered daily. Providers should be cautious about using antibiotics solely for this purpose because of the potential for development of drug-resistant microorganisms. IVIG might not provide additional benefit to children receiving daily TMP-SMX but may be considered for children who have recurrent bacterial infections despite TMP-SMX prophylaxis. Choice of antibiotic prophylaxis vs. IVIG should also involve consideration of adherence, ease of intravenous access, and cost. If IVIG is used, respiratory syncytial virus (RSV) IVIG (750 mg/kg), not monoclonal RSV antibody, may be substituted for IVIG during the RSV season to provide broad antiinfective protection, if this product is available.

From Masur H, Kaplan JE, Holmes KK, and the USPHS/IDSA Prevention of Opportunistic Infections Working Group. 2001 USPHS/IDSA guidelines for the prevention of opportunistic infections in persons infected with human immunodeficiency virus, pages 58–59. Posted November 28, 2001 as a "living document" at *www.hivatis.org/trtgdlns.html#Opportunistic.*

Table 18.5. Criteria for Starting, Discontinuing, and Restarting Opportunistic Infection Prophylaxis for Adults with Human Immunodeficiency Virus Infection

| Opportunistic Illness | Criteria for Initiating Primary Prophylaxis | Criteria for Discontinuing Primary Prophylaxis | Criteria for Restarting Primary Prophylaxis | Criteria for Initiating Secondary Prophylaxis | Criteria for Discontinuing Secondary Prophylaxis | Criteria for Restarting Secondary Prophylaxis |
|---|---|---|---|---|---|---|
| *Pneumocystis carinii* pneumonia | $CD4^+$ <200 cells/$\mu$L or oropharyngeal candidiasis (AI) | $CD4^+$ >200 cells/$\mu$L for ≥3 months (AI) | $CD4^+$ <200 cells/$\mu$L (AIII) | Prior *Pneumocystis carinii* pneumonia (AI) | $CD4^+$ >200 cells/$\mu$L for ≥3 months (BII) | $CD4^+$ <200 cells/$\mu$L (AIII) |
| Toxoplasmosis | IgG antibody to toxoplasma and $CD4^+$ <100 cells/$\mu$L (AI) | $CD4^+$ >200 cells/$\mu$L for ≥3 months (AI) | $CD4^+$ <100–200 cells/$\mu$L (AIII) | Prior toxoplasmic encephalitis (AI) | $CD4^+$ >200 cells/$\mu$L sustained (e.g., ≥6 mo) and completed initial therapy and asymptomatic for toxoplasmosis (CIII) | $CD4^+$ <200 cells/$\mu$L (AIII) |
| Disseminated *Mycobacterium avium* complex (MAC) | $CD4^+$ <50 cells/$\mu$L (AI) | $CD4^+$ >100 cells/$\mu$L for ≥3 months (AI) | $CD4^+$ <50–100 cells/$\mu$L (AIII) | Documented disseminated disease (AII) | $CD4^+$ >100 cells/$\mu$L sustained (e.g., ≥6 months) and completed 12 mo of MAC therapy and asymptomatic for MAC (CIII) | $CD4^+$ <100 cells/$\mu$L (AIII) |

| | | | | | | |
|---|---|---|---|---|---|---|
| Cryptococcosis | None | Not applicable | Not applicable | Documented disease (AI) | CD4$^+$ >100–200 cells/$\mu$L sustained (e.g., ≥6 mo) and completed initial therapy and asymptomatic for cryptococcosis (CIII) | CD4$^+$ <100–200 cells/$\mu$L (AIII) |
| Histoplasmosis | None | Not applicable | Not applicable | Documented disease (AI) | No criteria recommended for stopping | Not applicable |
| Coccidioidomycosis | None | Not applicable | Not applicable | Documented disease (AI) | No criteria recommended for stopping | Not applicable |
| Cytomegalovirus retinitis | None | Not applicable | Not applicable | Documented end-organ disease (AI) | CD4$^+$ >100–150 cells/$\mu$L sustained (e.g., ≥6 mo) and no evidence of active disease and regular ophthalmic examination (BII) | CD4$^+$ <100–150 cells/$\mu$L (AIII) |

From Masur H, Kaplan JE, Holmes KK, and the USPHS/IDSA Prevention of Opportunistic Infections Working Group. 2001 USPHS/IDSA guidelines for the prevention of opportunistic infections in persons infected with human immunodeficiency virus, page 60. Posted November 28, 2001 as a "living document" at *www.hivatis.org/trtgdlns.html#Opportunistic.*

Table 18.6. Recommendations to Help Patients Avoid Exposure to or Infection with Opportunistic Pathogens

Sexual exposures

Patients should use a latex condom during every act of sexual intercourse to reduce the risk for acquiring cytomegalovirus, herpes simplex virus, and human papillomavirus, as well as other sexually transmitted pathogens (AII). Condom use also will, theoretically, reduce the risk for acquiring human herpesvirus 8, as well as superinfection with an HIV strain that has become resistant to antiretroviral drugs (BIII) and will prevent transmission of HIV and other sexually transmitted pathogens to others (AII). Data regarding the use and efficacy of female condoms are incomplete, but these devices should be considered as a risk-reduction strategy (BIII).

Patients should avoid sexual practices that might result in oral exposure to feces (e.g., oral-anal contact) to reduce the risk for intestinal infections (e.g., cryptosporidiosis, shigellosis, campylobacteriosis, amebiasis, giardiasis, and hepatitis A) (BIII). Latex condom use alone may not reduce the risk of acquiring these fecal-orally transmitted pathogens, especially those that have low infectious doses. Persons wishing to reduce their risk of exposure might consider using dental dams or similar barrier methods for oral-anal and oral-genital contact, changing condoms after anal intercourse, and wearing latex gloves during digital-anal contact. Frequently washing hands and genitals with warm soapy water during and after activities which may bring these body parts in contact with feces may further reduce risk of illness (CIII).

Hepatitis B immunization is recommended for all susceptible (anti-HBc–negative) HIV-infected patients (BII).

Hepatitis A immunization is recommended for all susceptible men who have sex with men, as well as others at risk for infection with hepatitis A virus (BIII).

Injection drug use exposures

Injection drug use is a complex behavior that puts HIV-infected persons at risk for hepatitis B virus and hepatitis C virus infection, other possibly drug-resistant strains of HIV, and other blood-borne pathogens. Providers should assess the individual's readiness to change this practice and encourage efforts to provide education and support directed at recovery. Patients should be counseled to stop using injection drugs (AIII) and to enter and complete substance-abuse treatment, including relapse prevention programs (AIII).

If they are continuing to inject drugs, patients should be advised (BIII):

- to never reuse or share syringes, needles, water, or drug preparation equipment; if, nonetheless, injection equipment that has been used by other persons is shared, to first clean the equipment with bleach and water (U.S. Public Health Service. HIV prevention bulletin: medical advice for persons who inject illicit drugs. May 8, 1997. Rockville, MD: CDC, 1997)
- to use only sterile syringes obtained from reliable source (e.g., pharmacies or syringe exchange programs)
- to use sterile (e.g., boiled) water to prepare drugs; if not possible, to use clean water from a reliable source (e.g., fresh tap water); to use a new or disinfected container ("cooker") and a new filter ("cotton") to prepare drugs
- to clean the injection site with a new alcohol swab before injection
- to safely dispose of syringes after one use

All susceptible injection drug users should be immunized against hepatitis B (BII) and hepatitis A (BIII).

Environmental and occupational exposures

Certain activities or types of employment might increase the risk for exposure to tuberculosis (BIII). These include volunteer work or employment in health-care facilities, correctional institutions, and shelters for the homeless, as well as other settings identified as high risk by local health authorities. Decisions about whether to continue with such activities should be made in conjunction with the health-care provider and should be based on such factors as the patient's specific duties in the workplace, the prevalence of tuberculosis in the community, and the degree to which precautions designed to prevent the transmission of tuberculosis are taken in the

Table 18.6. (*Continued*)

workplace (BIII). These decisions will affect the frequency with which the patient should be screened for tuberculosis.

Child care providers and parents of children in child care are at increased risk for acquiring CMV infection, cryptosporidiosis, and other infections (e.g., hepatitis A and giardiasis) from children. The risk for acquiring infection can be diminished by good hygienic practices, such as hand washing after fecal contact (e.g., during diaper changing) and after contact with urine or saliva (AII). All children in child-care facilities also are at increased risk for acquiring these same infections; parents and other caretakers of HIV-infected children should be advised of this risk (BIII).

Occupations involving contact with animals (e.g., veterinary work and employment in pet stores, farms, or slaughterhouses) might pose a risk for cryptosporidiosis, toxoplasmosis, salmonellosis, campylobacteriosis, or *Bartonella* infection. However, the available data are insufficient to justify a recommendation against work in such settings.

Contact with young farm animals, especially animals with diarrhea, should be avoided to reduce the risk for cryptosporidiosis (BII).

Hand washing after gardening or other contact with soil might reduce the risk for cryptosporidiosis and toxoplasmosis (BIII).

In areas endemic for histoplasmosis, patients should avoid activities known to be associated with increased risk (e.g., creating dust when working with surface soil; cleaning chicken coops that are heavily contaminated with compost droppings; disturbing soil beneath bird-roosting sites; cleaning, remodeling, or demolishing old buildings; and cave exploring) (CIII).

In areas endemic for coccidioidomycosis, when possible, patients should avoid activities associated with increased risk, including those involving extensive exposure to disturbed native soil (e.g., at building excavation sites or during dust storms) (CIII).

Pet-related exposures

Health-care providers should advise HIV-infected persons of the potential risk posed by pet ownership. However, they should be sensitive to the possible psychologic benefits of pet ownership and should not routinely advise HIV-infected persons to part with their pets (DIII). Specifically, providers should advise HIV-infected persons of the following precautions.

*General*

Veterinary care should be sought when a pet develops diarrheal illness. If possible, HIV-infected persons should avoid contact with animals that have diarrhea (BIII). A fecal sample should be obtained from animals with diarrhea and examined for *Cryptosporidium*, *Salmonella*, and *Campylobacter*.

When obtaining a new pet, HIV-infected patients should avoid animals aged <6 months (or <1 year for cats; see Cats section, which follows), especially those with diarrhea (BIII). Because the hygienic and sanitary conditions in pet-breeding facilities, pet stores, and animal shelters are highly variable, the patient should be cautious when obtaining a pet from these sources. Stray animals should be avoided. Animals aged <6 months, especially those with diarrhea, should be examined by a veterinarian for *Cryptosporidium*, *Salmonella*, and *Campylobacter* (BIII).

Patients should wash their hands after handling pets (especially before eating) and avoid contact with pets' feces to reduce the risk for cryptosporidiosis, salmonellosis, and campylobacteriosis (BIII). Hand washing for HIV-infected children should be supervised.

*Cats*

Patients should be aware that cat ownership increases their risk for toxoplasmosis and *Bartonella* infection, as well as enteric infections (CIII). Those who elect to obtain a cat should adopt or purchase an animal that is aged >1 year and in good health to reduce the risk for cryptosporidiosis, *Bartonella* infection, salmonellosis, and campylobacteriosis (BII).

Litter boxes should be cleaned daily, preferably by an HIV-negative, nonpregnant person; if the HIV-infected patient performs this task, he or she should wash hands thoroughly afterward to reduce the risk for toxoplasmosis (BIII).

*Continued*

Table 18.6. (*Continued*)

To reduce the risk for toxoplasmoisis, HIV-infected patients should keeps cats indoors, not allow them to hunt, and not feed them raw or undercooked meat (BIII).

Although declawing is not generally advised, patients should avoid activities that might result in cat scratches or bites to reduce the risk for *Bartonella* infection (BII). Patients should also wash sites of cat scratches or bites promptly (CIII) and should not allow cats to lick the patients' open cuts or wounds.

Care of cats should include flea control to reduce risk for *Bartonella* infection (CIII).

Testing cats for toxoplasmosis (EII) or *Bartonella* infection (DII) is not recommended.

*Birds*

Screening healthy birds for *Cryptococcus neoformans, Mycobacterium avium*, or *Histoplasma capsulatum* is not recommended (DIII).

*Other*

Contact with reptiles (e.g., snakes, lizards, iguana, and turtles) as well as chicks and ducklings should be avoided to reduce the risk for salmonellosis (BIII).

Gloves should be used during the cleaning of aquariums to reduce the risk for infection with *Mycobacterium marinum* (BIII).

Contact with exotic pets (e.g., nonhuman primates) should be avoided (CIII).

Food- and water-related exposures

Raw or undercooked eggs (including foods that might contain raw eggs [e.g., some preparations of hollandaise sauce, Caesar and certain other salad dressings, some mayonnaises, uncooked cookie and cake batter, eggnog]); raw or undercooked poultry, meat, and seafood (especially raw shellfish); unpasteurized dairy products; unpasteurized fruit juice; and raw seed sprouts (e.g., alfalfa sprouts, mung bean sprouts) should not be eaten. Poultry and meat are safest when adequate cooking is confirmed with a thermometer (internal temperature of 180°F for poultry and 165°F for red meats). If a thermometer is not used, the risk for illness is decreased by consuming poultry and meat that have no trace of pink. Color change of the meat (e.g., absence of pink) does not always correlate with internal temperature. Produce should be washed thoroughly before being eaten (BIII).

Cross-contamination of foods should be avoided. Uncooked meats should not be allowed to come in contact with other foods; hands, cutting boards, counters, knives, and other utensils should be washed thoroughly after contact with uncooked food (BIII).

Although the incidence of listeriosis is low, it is a serious disease that occurs frequently among HIV-infected persons who are severely immunosuppressed. An immunosuppressed HIV-infected person who wishes to reduce the risk of acquiring listeriosis as much as possible may choose to do the following:

Avoid soft cheeses (e.g., feta, Brie, Camembert, blue-veined, and Mexican-style cheese such as queso fresco). Hard cheeses, processed cheeses, cream cheese (including slices and spreads), cottage cheese, or yogurt need not be avoided.

Cook leftover foods or ready-to-eat foods (e.g., hot dogs) until steaming hot before eating.

Avoid foods from delicatessen counters (e.g., prepared salads, meats, cheeses) or heat/reheat these foods until steaming before eating.

Avoid refrigerated pates and other meat spreads, or heat/reheat these foods until steaming if eaten. Canned or shelf-stable pate and meat spreads need not be avoided.

Avoid raw or unpasteurized milk (including goat's milk) or milk products, or foods that contain unpasteurized milk or milk products (CIII).

Patients should not drink water directly from lakes or rivers because of the risk for cryptosporidiosis and giardiasis (AIII). Water-borne infection also might result from swallowing water during recreational activities. Patients should avoid swimming in water that is likely to be contaminated with human or animal waste and should avoid swallowing water during swimming (BII).

During outbreaks or in other situations in which a community "boil water advisory" is issued, boiling water for 1 minute will eliminate the risk for acquiring cryptosporidiosis (AI). Using submicron, personal-use water filters (home/office types) and/or drinking bottled water might also reduce risk (CIII). Current data are inadequate to support a recommendation that all HIV-infected persons boil or otherwise avoid drinking tap

Table 18.6. (*Continued*)

water in nonoutbreak settings. However, persons who wish to take independent action to reduce their risk from water-borne cryptosporidiosis may choose to take precautions similar to those recommended during outbreaks. Such decisions are best made in conjunction with a health-care provider. Persons who opt for a personal-use filter or bottled water should be aware of the complexities involved in selecting the appropriate products, the lack of enforceable standards for destruction or removal of oocysts, the cost of the products, and the difficulty of using these products consistently. Patients taking precautions to avoid acquiring cryptosporidiosis from drinking water should be advised that ice made from contaminated water also can be a source of infection (BII). Such persons should be aware that fountain beverages served in restaurants, bars, theaters, and other public places might also pose a risk, because these beverages, as well as the ice they might contain, are made from tap water. Nationally distributed brands of bottled or canned carbonated soft drinks are safe to drink.

Commercially packaged noncarbonated soft drinks and fruit juices that do not require refrigeration until after they are opened (i.e., those that can be stored unrefrigerated on grocery shelves) also are safe. Nationally distributed brands of frozen fruit juice concentrate are safe if they are reconstituted by the user with water from a safe source. Fruit juices that must be kept refrigerated from the time they are processed to the time of consumption might be either fresh (unpasteurized) or heat-treated (pasteurized); only juices labeled as pasteurized should be considered free of risk from *Cryptosporidium*. Other pasteurized beverages and beers are also considered safe to drink (BII). No data are available concerning survival of *Cryptosporidium* oocytes in wine.

Travel-related exposures

Travel, particularly to developing countries, might result in significant risks for the exposure of HIV-infected persons to oppotunistic pathogens, especially for patients who are severely immunosuppressed. Consultation with health-care providers or with experts in travel medicine will help patients plan itineraries (BIII).

During travel to developing countries, HIV-infected persons are at even higher risk for food-borne and water-borne infections than they are in the United States. Foods and beverages—particularly raw fruits and vegetables, raw or undercooked seafood or meat, tap water, ice made with tap water, unpasteurized milk and dairy products, and items purchased from street vendors—might be contaminated (AII). Items that are generally safe include steaming hot foods, fruits that are peeled by the traveler, bottled (especially carbonated) beverages, hot coffee or tea, beer, wine, and water brought to a rolling boil for 1 minute (AII). Treating water with iodine or chlorine might not be as effective as boiling but can be used, perhaps in conjunction with filtration, when boiling is not practical (BIII).

Water-borne infections might result from swallowing water during recreational activities. To reduce the risk for cryptosporidiosis and giardiasis, patients should avoid swallowing water during swimming and should not swim in water that might be contaminated (e.g., with sewage or animal waste) (BII).

Antimicrobial prophylaxis for traveler's diarrhea is not recommended routinely for HIV-infected persons traveling to developing countries (DIII). Such preventive therapy can have adverse effects and can promote the emergence of drug-resistant organisms. Nonetheless, several studies (none involving an HIV-infected population) have shown that prophylaxis can reduce the risk for diarrhea among travelers (CDC. *Health information for international travel, 1999–2000*. Atlanta, GA: U.S. Department of Health and Human Services, 1999:202). Under selected circumstances (e.g., those in which the risk for infection is very high and the period of travel brief), the provider and patient may weigh the potential risks and benefits and decide that antibiotic prophylaxis is warranted (CIII). For those persons to whom prophylaxis is offered, fluoroquinolones (e.g., ciprofloxacin [500 mg daily]) can be considered (CIII), although fluoroquinolones should not be given to children or pregnant women. Trimethoprim-sulfamethoxazole (TMP-SMX) (one double-strength tablet daily) also has been shown

*Continued*

Table 18.6. (*Continued*)

to be effective, but resistance to this drug is now common in tropical areas. Persons already taking TMP-SMX for prophylaxis against *Pneumocystis carinii* pneumonia (PCP) might gain some protection against traveler's diarrhea. For HIV-infected persons who are not already taking TMP-SMX, health-care providers should be cautious in prescribing this agent for prophylaxis of diarrhea because of the high rates of adverse reactions and the possible need for the agent for other purposes (e.g., PCP prophylaxis) in the future.

All HIV-infected travelers to developing countries should carry a sufficient supply of an antimicrobial agent to be taken empirically should diarrhea develop (BIII). One appropriate regimen is 500 mg of ciprofloxacin twice a day for 3–7 days. Alternative antibiotics (e.g., TMP-SMX) should be considered as empirical therapy for use by children and pregnant women (CIII). Travelers should consult a physician if their diarrhea is severe and does not respond to empirical therapy, if their stools contain blood, if fever is accompanied by shaking chills, or if dehydration develops. Antiperistaltic agents (e.g., diphenoxylate and loperamide) are used for the treatment of diarrhea; however, they should not be used by patients with high fever or with blood in the stool, and their use should be discontinued if symptoms persist beyond 48 hours (AII). Antiperistaltic agents are not recommended for children (DIII).

Travelers should be advised about other preventive measures appropriate for anticipated exposures (e.g., chemoprophylaxis for malaria, protection against arthropod vectors, treatment with immune globulin, and vaccination) (AII). They should avoid direct contact of the skin with soil or sand (e.g., by wearing shoes and protective clothing and using towels on beaches) in areas where fecal contamination of soil is likely (BIII).

In general, live-virus vaccines should be avoided (EII). One exception is measles vaccine, which is recommended for nonimmune persons. However, measles vaccine is not recommended for persons who are severely immunosuppressed (DIII); immune globulin should be considered for measles-susceptible, severely immunosuppressed persons who are anticipating travel to measles-endemic countries (BIII). Another exception is varicella vaccine, which may be administered to asymptomatic nonimmunosuppressed children (BII). Inactivated (killed) poliovirus vaccine should be used instead of oral (live) poliovirus vaccine, which is contraindicated for HIV-infected persons. Persons at risk for exposure to typhoid fever should be administered an inactivated parenteral typhoid vaccine instead of the live attenuated oral preparation. Yellow fever vaccine is a live-virus vaccine with uncertain safety and efficacy in HIV-infected persons. Travelers with asymptomatic HIV infection who cannot avoid potential exposure to yellow fever should be offered the choice of vaccination. If travel to a zone with yellow fever is necessary and vaccination is not administered, patients should be advised of the risk, instructed in methods for avoiding the bites of vector mosquitoes, and provided with a vaccination waiver letter.

In general, killed and recombinant vaccines (e.g., diphtheria-tetanus, rabies, hepatitis A, hepatitis B, Japanese encephalitis vaccines) should be used for HIV-infected persons just as they would be used for non–HIV-infected persons anticipating travel (BIII). Preparation for travel should include a review and updating of routine vaccinations, including diphtheria-tetanus for adults and all routine immunizations for children. The currently available cholera vaccine is not recommended for persons following a usual tourist itinerary, even if travel includes countries reporting cases of cholera (DII).

Travelers should be informed about other area-specific risks and instructed in ways to reduce those risks (BIII). Geographically focal infections that pose a high risk to HIV-infected persons include visceral leishmaniasis (a protozoan infection transmitted by the sandfly) and several fungal infections (e.g., *Penicillium marneffei* infection, coccidioidomycosis, and histoplasmosis). Many tropical and developing areas have high rates of tuberculosis.

From Masur H, Kaplan JE, Holmes KK, and the USPHS/IDSA Prevention of Opportunistic Infections Working Group. 2001 USPHS/IDSA guidelines for the prevention of opportunistic infections in persons infected with human immunodeficiency virus, pages 61–65. Posted November 28, 2001 as a "living document" at *www.hivatis.org/trtgdlns.html#Opportunistic.*

Table 18.7. Effects of Food on Drugs Used to Prevent Opportunistic Infections

| Drug | Food Effect | Recommendation |
|---|---|---|
| Atovaquone | Bioavailability increased up to threefold with high-fat meal | Administer with food |
| GCV (capsules) | High-fat meal results in 22% (GCV) or 30% (VGCV) increase in AUC | High-fat meal may increase toxicity of VGCV |
| Itraconazole | Grapefruit juice results in 30% decrease in AUC | Avoid concurrent grapefruit juice |
| Itraconazole (capsules) | Significant increase in bioavailability when taken with a full meal | Administer with food |
| Itraconazole (solution) | 31% increase in AUC when taken under fasting conditions | Take without food if possible |

GCV, ganciclovir; VGCV, valganciclovir; AUC, area under the curve.
From Masur H, Kaplan JE, Holmes KK, and the USPHS/IDSA Prevention of Opportunistic Infections Working Group. 2001 USPHS/IDSA guidelines for the prevention of opportunistic infections in persons infected with human immunodeficiency virus, page 44. Posted November 28, 2001 as a "living document" at *www.hivatis.org/trtgdlns.html#Opportunistic.*

reports associate extrapulmonary disease with the use of aerosol pentamidine [44].

C. **Diagnosis.** Patients who present with an illness suggestive of PCP should undergo chest radiography. If the chest film is supportive, then attempts should be made to confirm the diagnosis by identification of *P. carinii* on microscopic examination with Gomori **methenamine silver stain** or **toluidine blue O.** If the chest film is negative but PCP is still suspected, further studies are indicated to help support the diagnosis prior to treatment.

1. **Sputum.** Expectorated sputum is rarely suitable for microscopic evaluation. Similarly, purulent sputum, even when induced, may be inadequate for examination due to the presence of cellular debris and artifact. Sensitivity of the induced sputum examination greatly depends on the quality of the sampling and the experience of the laboratory, and has ranged from 30% to 90% [45,46].
2. **Bronchoscopy with bronchoalveolar lavage (BAL) is the diagnostic procedure of choice for obtaining adequate pulmonary secretions.** A negative BAL for *P. carinii* should strongly suggest an alternative diagnosis. Transbronchial biopsy or open lung biopsy usually are not necessary to diagnose PCP in AIDS patients.
3. **Other tests.** Gallium citrate scanning is highly sensitive (90%) but nonspecific (50%) for PCP [47,48]; it is seldom used due to the high cost and time delay for results (3 days). Likewise, high-resolution computed tomography (CT) showing ground glass infiltrates and pulmonary function testing are nonspecific and do not provide an etiologic diagnosis. Polymerase chain reaction (PCR) tests to detect *P. carinii* DNA has yielded positive results in patients without pneumonia. Refinements in the methodology may make this sensitive assay appropriate for routine clinical use in the future [49].
4. **Empiric treatment without attempts to confirm a diagnosis is not generally recommended.** However, this may be appropriate in patients with mild illness who are clinically stable and not hypoxic; have clinical, laboratory, and radiographic support for PCP; and are at low risk for other OIs or conditions that may mimic PCP. It also may be used for individuals who do not have prompt access to diagnostic facilities.

Table 18.8. Effects of Medications on Drugs Used to Prevent Opportunistic Infections

| Affected Drug | Interacting Drug(s) | Mechanism/Effect | Recommendation |
|---|---|---|---|
| **Atovaquone** | Rifampin | Induction of metabolism/ decreased drug levels | Concentrations might not be therapeutic; avoid combination or increase atovaquone dose. |
| **Atovaquone** | Lopinavir-ritonavir | Potential for induction of metabolism/ decreased drug levels | Concentrations may not be therapeutic; may require increased atovaquone dose, but data insufficient to make specific recommendation. |
| **Clarithromycin** | Efavirenz | Induction of metabolism/decrease in clarithromycin AUC by 39%, increase in AUC of 14-OH clarithromycin by 34% | Clarithromycin efficacy uncertain. |
| **Clarithromycin** | Ritonavir | Inhibition of metabolism/increased clarithromycin drug levels by 77% | Dose adjustment of clarithromycin necessary only if renal dysfunction is present. For CrCl <60 mL/min, reduce clarithromycin dose by 50%; for CrCl <30 mL/min, reduce dose by 75%. |
| **Clarithromycin** | Lopinavir-ritonavir | Inhibition of metabolism/increased clarithromycin drug levels | Dose adjustment of clarithromycin necessary only if renal dysfunction is present. For CrCl <60 mL/min, reduce clarithromycin dose by 50%; for CrCl <30 mL/min, reduce dose by 75%. |
| **Clarithromycin** | Nevirapine | Induction of metabolism/decrease in clarithromycin AUC by 35%, increase in AUC of 14-OH clarithromycin by 27% | Efficacy of MAC prophylaxis may be decreased; monitor closely. |
| **Ketoconazole** | Lopinavir-ritonavir | Inhibition of metabolism/increased ketoconazole AUC | Use with caution at ketoconazole doses>200 mg/day |

(*Continued*)

Table 18.8. (*Continued*)

| Affected Drug | Interacting Drug(s) | Mechanism/Effect | Recommendation |
|---|---|---|---|
| Ketoconazole | Antacids, didanosine (but not didanosine EC), buffered products, $H_2$ blockers, proton pump inhibitors | Increase in gastric pH that impairs absorption of ketoconazole | Avoid use of ketoconazole with pH-raising agents or use alternative antifungal drug. |
| Quinolone antibiotics (ciprofloxacin, levofloxacin, gatifloxacin, moxifloxacin) | Didanosine (but not didanosine EC), antacids, iron products, calcium products, sucralfate (cation preparations) | Chelation results in marked decrease in quinolone drug levels | Administer cation preparation at least 2 h after quinolone. |
| Rifabutin | Fluconazole | Inhibition of metabolism/marked increase in rifabutin drug levels | Monitor for rifabutin toxicities such as uveitis, nausea, neutropenia. |
| Rifabutin | Efavirenz | Induction of metabolism/ significant decrease in rifabutin AUC | Increase rifabutin dose to 450–600 mg daily or 600 mg twice weekly.[a] |
| Rifabutin | Ritonavir, lopinavir-ritonavir, ritonavir-saquinavir | Inhibition of metabolism/marked increase in rifabutin drug levels | Decrease rifabutin to 150 mg every other day or three times per week. |
| Rifabutin | Indinavir, nelfinavir, amprenavir | Inhibition of metabolism/marked increase in rifabutin drug levels | Decrease rifabutin to 150 mg daily or 300 mg three times per week. |

AUC, area under the curve; MAC, *Mycobacterium avium* complex; $H_2$, histamine; CrCl, creatinine clearance.
[a] Appropriate dose of efavirenz is uncertain if a protease inhibitor is used with efavirenz plus rifabutin.
From Masur H, Kaplan JE, Holmes KK, and the USPHS/IDSA Prevention of Opportunistic Infections Working Group. 2001 USPHS/IDSA guidelines for the prevention of opportunistic infections in persons infected with human immunodeficiency virus, pages 45–46. Posted November 28, 2001 as a "living document" at *www.hivatis.org/trtgdlns.html#Opportunistic.*

5. **A firm diagnosis must be established in patients on prophylaxis** who present with a clinical picture that is suggestive of PCP. Patients on oral prophylaxis who develop PCP have the same manifestations as described above. However, systemic PCP prophylaxis is quite effective, and many other conditions (including infections) may yield the same clinical picture.
6. **A diagnosis must be established for the pulmonary process, and other OIs should be sought in hypoxic patients given corticosteroids** (see below). This is because the degree of immunosuppression that predisposes to PCP is also a risk for other OIs that may be the true pulmonary diagnosis, or a mixed infection may be present, and the corticosteroids may exacerbate these other infections.

Table 18.9. Effects of Opportunistic Infection Medications on Antiinfective Drugs Commonly Administered to Persons Infected with Human Immunodeficiency Virus

| Affected Drug | Interacting Drug(s) | Mechanism/Effect | Recommendation |
|---|---|---|---|
| Amprenavir, delavirdine, indinavir, lopinavir-ritonavir, nelfinavir, saquinavir | Rifampin | Induction of metabolism/marked decrease in protease inhibitor or delavirdine drug levels | Avoid concomitant use. |
| Efavirenz, ritonavir, ritonavir-saquinavir, nevirapine | Rifampin | Induction of metabolism/decrease in protease or nevirapine levels | Combinations could possibly be used but limited clinical experience. Consider efavirenz 800 mg daily when used with rifampin. |
| Delavirdine | Rifabutin | Induction of metabolism/50%–60% decrease in delavirdine levels | Avoid concomitant use. |
| Indinavir, nelfinavir, amprenavir[a] | Rifabutin | Induction of metabolism/50% decrease in protease inhibitor levels | Consider increase in indinavir dose to 1,000 mg q8h; If indinavir is the sole protease inhibitor, decrease rifabutin dose to 150 mg daily. |
| Ritonavir, ritonavir-saquinavir, lopinavir-ritonavir | Rifabutin | Induction of metabolism of ritonavir | No dosage change for protease inhibitors. Consider rifabutin 150 mg q.o.d. or three times per week. |
| Efavirenz | Rifabutin | Potential for decreased efavirenz levels | No dosage change necessary for efavirenz; adjust rifabutin dose to 450–600 mg daily or 600 mg twice weekly. |
| Saquinavir | Rifabutin | Potential for decreased saquinavir levels | Limited data |
| Didanosine (ddI) | Ganciclovir (oral) | Increased ddI AUC by approximately 100% | Clinical significance unknown; monitor for ddI-related adverse effects. |

q 8h, every 8 hours; q.o.d., every other day; AUC, area under the curve.

[a] Little data are available for use of rifamycin drugs with ritonavir-boosting protease inhibitor regimens except for ritonavir-saquinavir and ritonavir-lopinavir. Therefore, concomitant use of rifamycins with these regimens must be approached cautiously.

From Masur H, Kaplan JE, Holmes KK, and the USPHS/IDSA Prevention of Opportunistic Infections Working Group. 2001 USPHS/IDSA guidelines for the prevention of opportunistic infections in persons infected with human immunodeficiency virus, page 47. Posted November 28, 2001 as a "living document" at *www.hivatis.org/trtgdlns.html#Opportunistic.*

Table 18.10. Adverse Effects of Drugs Used in the Prevention of Opportunistic Infections

| | |
|---|---|
| Bone marrow suppression | Cidofovir, dapsone, ganciclovir, pyrimethamine, rifabutin, sulfadiazine, TMP-SMX |
| Diarrhea | Atovaquone, clindamycin |
| Hepatotoxicity | Clarithromycin, fluconazole, isoniazid, itraconazole, ketoconazole, pyrazinamide, rifabutin, rifampin, TMP-SMX |
| Nephrotoxicity | Amphotericin B, cidofovir, foscarnet, pentamidine, high-dose acyclovir |
| Ocular effects | Cidofovir, ethambutol, rifabutin |
| Pancreatitis | Pentamidine, TMP-SMX |
| Peripheral neuropathy | Isoniazid |
| Neurotoxicity | Acyclovir (high-dose), quinolones |
| Skin rash | Atovaquone, dapsone, pyrimethamine, sulfadiazine, TMP-SMX, ribavirin |

TMP-SMX, trimethoprim-sulfamethoxazole.
From Masur H, Kaplan JE, Holmes KK, and the USPHS/IDSA Prevention of Opportunistic Infections Working Group. 2001 USPHS/IDSA guidelines for the prevention of opportunistic infections in persons infected with human immunodeficiency virus, page 48. Posted November 28, 2001 as a "living document" at *www.hivatis.org/trtgdlns.html#Opportunistic.*

**D. Treatment.** Even with proper therapy, **response is gradual:** respiratory rate, dyspnea, and arterial-alveolar gradient improve within 4 to 8 days. Several options are available:

1. **Trimethoprim** (15–20 mg/kg/day) and **sulfamethoxazole** (75 mg/kg/day) (**cotrimoxazole**) orally or intravenously (i.v.) in three to four divided doses for at least 21 days **is always the drug regimen of choice** unless the patient has a history of life-threatening intolerance. No other agent has demonstrated higher efficacy for PCP. Cotrimoxazole is well absorbed orally and can be used for outpatient therapy for mild disease (room air partial pressure of oxygen [$Po_2$] of >80 mm Hg) in patients with no major gastrointestinal dysfunction. Side effects include rash, fever, pruritis, digestive disturbances, cytopenias, and hyperkalemia, most of which are easily managed. Life-threatening reactions such as Stevens-Johnson syndrome are rare. Recent reports have documented mutations in the dihydropteroate synthase gene leading to sulfonamide resistance in some human isolates [50,51]. The frequency and clinical significance of these and other mutations are currently being studied, and they could have an obvious negative impact on the efficacy of prophylaxis.
2. **Trimethoprim** (15 mg/kg/day in three divided doses) **plus dapsone** (100 mg orally once daily) for 21 days has efficacy that is comparable with trimethoprim-sulfamethoxazole and may be somewhat better tolerated but less convenient because they are taken at different times. Side effects include rash, methemoglobinemia, hemolytic anemia, and neutropenia. It is rarely necessary to screen for **G6PD deficiency** prior to dapsone therapy unless there is a strong suspicion of deficiency, as might be the case for those of Mediterranean ancestry. A history of life-threatening trimethoprim-sulfamethoxazole intolerance should preclude the use of dapsone plus trimethoprim.
3. **Intravenous pentamidine** (4 mg/kg once daily) for 21 days is about as effective as trimethoprim-sulfamethoxazole. Pentamidine was the first drug successfully used in patients who did not have AIDS. Adverse reactions can be life threatening, such as hypotension, hypoglycemia, renal insufficiency, and various cardiac arrhythmias, including torsades de pointes. Other side effects include pancreatitis and diabetes. In addition, patients often feel ill during therapy, with an abnormal taste in their mouth and a loss of appetite. This agent should be restricted to patients with severe disease who cannot tolerate or fail to respond to cotrimoxazole or trimethoprim-dapsone.

*(Text continues on p. 681.)*

Table 18.11. Dosing of Drugs for Primary Prevention or Maintenance Therapy for Opportunistic Infections in Renal Insufficiency

| Drug | Normal Dose | Renal Dysfunction | | |
|---|---|---|---|---|
| **Acyclovir** | 200 mg 5 times/day to 800 mg b.i.d. | Regimen | CrCl (mL/min/1.73m²) | Adjusted Dose |
| | | 200 mg orally t.i.d. | <10 | 200 mg q12h |
| | | 400 mg orally q12h | <10 | 200 mg q12h |
| | | Hemodialysis | | Additional dose after each dialysis |
| **Cidofovir** | 5 mg/kg i.v. every other week (with probenecid and hydration) | Reduce from 5 mg/kg to 3 mg/kg for an increase in serum creatinine of 0.3–0.4 mg/dL above baseline. Discontinue for an increase in creatinine ≥0.5 mg/dL above baseline or development of 3+ proteinuria. Not recommended for patients with baseline serum creatinine >1.5 mg/dL, CrCl ≤55 mL/min, or ≥2+ proteinuria | | |
| **Ciprofloxacin** | 500 mg orally q12h | CrCl (mL/min/1.73m²) | | Dose |
| | | 30–50 mg/dL | | 250–500 mg q12h |
| | | <30 | | 250–500 mg q18h |
| | | Hemodialysis | | 250–500 mg after dialysis |
| **Clarithromycin** | 500 mg b.i.d. | Reduce dose by one-half or double interval if creatinine clearance <30 mL/min | | |
| **Famciclovir** | 250–500 mg q12h | CrCl | | Dose |
| | | 20–39 (mL/min/1.73$\mu^2$) | | 125–250 mg q12h |
| | | <20 | | 125–250 mg q24h |
| | | Hemodialysis | | 125 mg after each dialysis |
| **Fluconazole** | 50–400 mg/day | CrCl | | Dose |
| | | <50 (mL/min/1.73$\mu^2$) | | Half dose |
| | | (not on dialysis) dialysis | | Full dose after dialysis |
| **Foscarnet** | 90–120 mg/kg/day | | Maintenance | |
| | | CrCl (mL/min/kg) | Low Dose | High Dose |
| | | >1.4 | 90 mg q12h | 120 mg q24h |
| | | 1.0–1.4 | 70 mg q24h | 90 mg q24h |
| | | 0.8–1.0 | 50 mg q24h | 65 mg q24h |
| | | 0.6–0.8 | 80 mg q48h | 104 mg q48h |
| | | 0.5–0.6 | 60 mg q48h | 80 mg q48h |
| | | 0.4–0.5 | 50 mg q48h | 65 mg q48h |
| | | <0.4 | Not recommended | Not recommended |

| | | | | |
|---|---|---|---|---|
| **Ganciclovir** | Oral: | CrCl (mL/min) | i.v. Dose (mg/kg) | Capsules |
| | 1 g t.i.d. (capsules) | 50–69 | 2.5 q24h | 1,500 mg daily or 500 mg t.i.d. |
| | i.v.: | 25–49 | 1.25 q24h | 1,000 mg daily or 500 mg b.i.d. |
| | 5 or 6 mg/kg/day | 10–24 | 0.625 q24h | 500 mg daily |
| | for 5 days/wk (i.v.) | <10 | 0.625 t.i.w. after dialysis | 500 mg t.i.w. after dialysis |
| **Levofloxacin** | 250–500 mg/day | CrCl (mL/min) | | Dose |
| | | 50–80 | | 500 mg LD, then 250 mg q24h |
| | | <50 | | 500 mg LD, then 250 mg q48h |
| **TMP/SMX** | | CrCl (mL/min) | | Dose |
| | 1 DS daily | 15–30 | | Half dose |
| | 1 DS t.i.w. | <15 | | Half dose[a] or use alternative agent |
| | 1 SS daily | | | |
| **Valacyclovir** | 500 mg to 1 g q24h | CrCl(mL/min/1.73 m$^2$) | | Dose |
| | | <30 | | 500 mg every 24–48 h |
| **Valganciclovir** | 900 mg/day | CrCl | | Dose |
| | | 40–59 | | 450 mg daily |
| | | 25–39 | | 450 mg daily |
| | | 10–24 | | 450 mg twice weekly |
| | | <10 | | Not recommended |
| | | Dialysis | | Not recommended |

b.i.d., twice daily; CrCl, creatinine clearance; DS, double-strength tablet; i.v., intravenous; LD, loading dose; q12h, every 12 hours; SS, single-strength tablet; t.i.d., three times daily; t.i.w., three times a week; TMP-SMX, trimethoprim-sulfamethoxazole.

[a]For hemodialysis, give after each dialysis.

From Masur H, Kaplan JE, Holmes KK, and the USPHS/IDSA Prevention of Opportunistic Infections Working Group. 2001 USPHS/IDSA guidelines for the prevention of opportunistic infections in persons infected with human immunodeficiency virus, pages 49–50. Posted November 28, 2001 as a "living document" at *www.hivatis.org/trtgdlns.html#Opportunistic.*

Table 18.12. Wholesale Acquisition Costs of Agents Recommended for the Prevention of Opportunistic Infections in Adults Infected with Human Immunodeficiency Virus

| Opportunistic Pathogen | Drug/Vaccine | Dose | Annual Cost per Patient |
|---|---|---|---|
| *Pneumocystis carinii* | Trimethoprim sulfamethoxazole | 160/800 mg daily | $135 |
| | Dapsone | 100 mg daily | $72 |
| | Aerosolized pentamidine | 300 mg monthly | $1,185 |
| | Atovaquone | 1,500 mg daily | $11,627 |
| *Mycobacterium avium* complex | Clarithromycin | 500 mg b.i.d. | $2,843 |
| | Azithromycin | 1,200 mg weekly | $3,862 |
| | Rifabutin | 300 mg daily | $3,352 |
| Cytomegalovirus | Ganciclovir (oral) | 1,000 mg t.i.d. | $17,794 |
| | Ganciclovir implant[a] | | $5,000 |
| | Ganciclovir (i.v.) | 5 mg/kg daily | $13,093 |
| | Foscarnet (i.v.) | 90–120 mg/kg daily | $27,770–37,027 |
| | Cidofovir (i.v.) | 375 mg q.o.w. | $20,904 |
| | Fomivirsen (intravitreal) | 1 vial every 4 wk | $12,000 |
| | Valganciclovir | 900 mg daily | $21,582 |
| *Mycobacterium tuberculosis* | Isoniazid[b] | 300 mg daily | $23 (9 months) |
| | Rifampin | 600 mg daily | $294 (2 months) |
| | Pyrazinamide | 1,500 mg daily | $194 (2 months) |
| Fungi | Fluconazole | 200 mg daily | $4,603 |
| | Itraconazole capsules | 200 mg daily | $5,340 |
| | Itraconazole solution | 200 mg daily | $5,673 |
| | Ketoconazole | 200 mg daily | $1,230 |
| Herpes simplex virus | Acyclovir | 400 mg b.i.d. | $1,384 |
| | Famciclovir | 500 mg b.i.d. | $5,311 |
| | Valacyclovir | 500 mg b.i.d. | $2,538 |
| *Toxoplasma gondii* | Pyrimethamine | 50 mg weekly | $49 |
| | Leucovorin | 25 mg weekly | $988 |
| | Sulfadiazine | 500 mg q.i.d. | $1,490 |
| *Streptococcus pneumoniae* | 23-valent pneumococcal vaccine | 0.5 mL i.m. once | $13 |
| Influenza virus | Inactivated trivalent influenza vaccine | 0.5 mL i.m. once | $3 |
| Hepatitis A virus | Hepatitis A vaccine | 1.0 mL i.m. twice | $124 |
| Hepatitis B virus | Recombinant hepatitis B | 10–20 $\mu$g i.m. three times | $70 |
| Bacterial infections | G-CSF | 300 $\mu$g t.i.w. | $29,406 |
| Varicella zoster virus | VZIG | 5 vials (6.25 mL) | $562 |

b.i.d., twice daily; G-CSF, granulocyte colony-stimulating factor; i.v., intravenous; i.m., intramuscular; q.o.w., every other week; t.i.d., three times daily; t.i.w., three times a week; VZIG, varicella zoster immune globulin.

[a]Implant generally lasts 6–9 months.

[b]Cost for 9 months of therapy.

From Medical Economics. Drug topics red book. Montvale, New Jersey: Medical Economics Inc., 2000; and Masur H, Kaplan JE, Holmes KK, and the USPHS/IDSA Prevention of Opportunistic Infections Working Group. 2001 USPHS/IDSA guidelines for the prevention of opportunistic infections in persons infected with human immunodeficiency virus, page 51. Posted November 28, 2001 as a "living document" at *www.hivatis.org/trtgdlns.html#Opportunistic.*

4. **Clindamycin** (600 mg i.v. every 8 hours or 300–450 mg orally every 6 hours) **plus primaquine** (30 mg orally daily) for 21 days is an alternative for mild PCP, although efficacy also has been shown in moderate and severe disease. Side effects include rash, methemoglobinemia, hemolysis, elevated serum transaminase, and digestive disturbances. This is an attractive alternative for oral therapy.
5. **Atovaquone** (750 mg suspension orally twice daily) for 21 days is a second-line alternative for mild to moderate PCP. It should be administered with food to maximize absorption (Table 18.7). A micronized formulation has been developed that might have better oral bioavailability. It is not available in a parenteral form. The primary toxicity is skin rash.
6. **Trimetrexate** (45 mg/m$^2$ i.v. daily) **plus folinic acid** (leucovorin; 20 mg/m$^2$ orally or i.v. every 6 hours) is effective when used alone or in combination with a sulfonamide. Leucovorin is needed to rescue the inhibition of dihydrofolate reductase in human cells, thus preventing cytopenia, its major adverse event. Higher relapse rates have been reported when compared to therapy with cotrimoxazole.
7. **Adjunctive corticosteroids** have been shown to be beneficial for improving oxygenation, reducing the risk of fibrosis, decreasing the need for mechanical ventilation, and reducing the case fatality rate [52]. Tapering doses of corticosteroids are recommended in patients with severe disease ($Po_2$ <70 mm Hg or A-a gradient >35 mm Hg): prednisone 40 mg orally twice daily on days 1 through 5, followed by prednisone 40 mg/day orally on days 6 through 10, then prednisone 20 mg/day orally on days 11 through 21 for those older than 13 years of age. In patients with preexisting severe immune dysfunction, corticosteroids must be given with extreme caution, because reactivation of other latent coinfections such as mycobacteria and herpes infections may occur.

E. **Prevention** (Tables 18.1–18.5). All patients with a CD4 count of less than 200/mm$^3$, CD4 percentage less than 14%, clinical manifestations from HIV (see section **A**), or another AIDS-defining condition should receive chemoprophylaxis to prevent a first episode of PCP (primary prophylaxis). All patients should receive prophylaxis following a course of treatment for PCP (secondary prophylaxis). Primary and secondary prophylaxis can be safely discontinued after the CD4 cell count has increased to at least 200/mm$^3$ for more than 3 months in response to HAART [53–58]. Prophylaxis should resume if any indication cited above recurs. Decisions about discontinuing prophylaxis should be individualized in patients whose episode of PCP occurred at a CD4 count or greater than 200/mm$^3$. The following are accepted regimens for prophylaxis in adults (Tables 18.1 and 18.2); see Tables 18.3 and 18.4 for dosing recommendations in children.

1. **Trimethoprim-sulfamethoxazole (cotrimoxazole)** orally (one double-strength [DS] or single-strength [SS] tablet daily) **is the agent of choice.** Alternatively, one DS tablet three times weekly may be used. Daily cotrimoxazole also protects against toxoplasmosis and some bacterial infections.
2. **Dapsone** 100 mg orally daily is an acceptable alternative; 50 mg daily may be less effective. Dapsone (50 mg daily) plus pyrimethamine (50 mg orally weekly) plus leucovorin (25 mg orally weekly), or dapsone (200 mg weekly) plus pyrimethamine (75 mg weekly) plus leucovorin (25 mg weekly) may be used and also offers protection against toxoplasmosis (dapsone alone does not).
3. **Atovaquone** 1,500 mg orally daily is as effective as dapsone and probably protects against toxoplasmosis, but is more expensive.
4. **Aerosolized pentamidine** 300 mg monthly delivered by the Respirgard II nebulizer (Marquest, Englewood, CO) does not offer systemic protection, and has been associated with extrapulmonary disease or apical relapses.

V. **Candidiasis** is the most common fungal condition seen in HIV-positive persons. Progression of HIV infection to AIDS is associated with development of oropharyngeal candidiasis [59]. Candidial infections are estimated to occur at some time

Table 18.13. Recommended Immunization Schedule for Human Immunodeficiency Virus–Infected Children

| Vaccine | Age: Birth | 1 mo | 2 mos | 4 mos | 6 mos | 12 mos | 15 mos | 18 mos | 24 mos | 4–6 yrs | 11–12 yrs | 14–16 yrs |
|---|---|---|---|---|---|---|---|---|---|---|---|---|
| Recommendations for these vaccines are the same as those for immunocompetent children. | | | | | | | | | | | | |
| Hepatitis B[1] | Hep B #1 | | | | | | | | | | | |
| | | Hep B #2 | | | Hep B #3 | | | | | | Hep B | |
| Diphtheria and Tetanus toxoids, Pertussis[2] | | | DTaP | DTaP | DTaP | | DTaP | | | DTaP | Td | |
| Haemophilus influenzae type b[3] | | | Hib | Hib | Hib | Hib | | | | | | |
| Inactivated Polio[4] | | | IPV | IPV | IPV | | | | | IPV | | |
| Hepatitis A[5] | | | | | | | | | Hep A in selected areas | | | |
| Recommendations for these vaccines differ from those for immunocompetent children. | | | | | | | | | | | | |
| Pneumococcus[6] | | | PCV | PCV | PCV | PCV | | | PPV23 | PPV23 (age 5-7 yrs) | | |
| Measles, Mumps, Rubella[7] | Do not give to severely immuno-suppressed (Category 3) **children** | | | | | MMR | | | | MMR | MMR | |
| Varicella[8] | Give only to asymptomatic non-immunosuppressed (category 1) children. Contraindicated in all other HIV infected children. | | | | | Var | Var | | | | Var | |
| **Influenza**[9] | | | | | A dose is recommended every year | | | | | | | |

Legend:

- Open box: Range of recommended ages for vaccination.
- Oval: Vaccines to be given if previously recommended doses were missed or were given earlier than the recommended minimum age.
- Shaded box: Recommended in selected states and/or regions.

This schedule indicates the recommended ages for routine administration of currently licensed childhood vaccines as of November 1, 2000, for children through age 18 years. Additional vaccines may be licensed and recommended during the year. Licensed combination vaccines may be used whenever any components of the combination are indicated and the vaccine's other components are not contraindicated. Providers should consult the manufacturer's package inserts for detailed recommendations.

[1]Infants born to hepatitis B surface antigen (HBsAg)-negative mothers should receive the first dose of hepatitis B vaccine (Hep B) at birth and no later than age 2 months. The second dose should be administered at least 1 month after the first dose. The third dose should be administered at least 4 months after the first dose and at least 2 months after the second dose, but not before age 6 months. Infants born to HBsAg-positive mothers should receive Hep B and 0.5 mL hepatitis B immune globulin (HBIG) within 12 hours of birth at separate sites. The second dose is recommended at age 1–2 months and the third dose at age 6 months. Infants born to mothers whose HBsAg status is unknown should receive Hep B within 12 hours of birth. Maternal blood should be drawn at delivery to determine the mother's HBsAg status; if the HBsAg test result is positive, the infant should receive HBIG as soon as possible (no later than age 1 week). All children and adolescents (through age 18 years) who have not been immunized against hepatitis B should begin the series during any visit. Providers should make special efforts to immunize children who were born in or whose parents were born in areas of the world where hepatitis B virus infection is moderately or highly endemic.

in the course of HIV disease in 90% to 95% of patients [60]. *Candida albicans* causes most disease; however, other species, including *C. tropicalis, C. krusei,* and *C. dubliniensis,* also have been reported, although much less frequently [60]. *C. glabrata* and *C. parapsilosis* tend to occur in patients with advanced disease and previous exposure to antifungals [61]. Chronic courses of azole therapy (e.g., in prophylaxis) may result in selection of azole-resistant species.

A. **Clinical presentation** is generally limited to oral, vaginal, or esophageal mucosa. Systemic disease is extremely rare and should not be included in the differential diagnosis of unexplained fever.

   1. Symptoms of **oropharyngeal candidiasis** include burning, pain, and altered taste sensation, although many patients are asymptomatic. Pseudomembranous candidiasis or "thrush" appears as removable white plaques on any oral mucosal surface. The erythematous form is seen as smooth red patches and is often missed on routine examination. Candidiasis also can cause angular cheilitis producing erythema, cracks, and fissures at the corner of the mouth.
   2. **Vaginal candidiasis** presents as a creamy white vaginal discharge and often is the first evidence of immune dysfunction in women [62]. Recurrent infection is common, and chronic suppressive therapy may be necessary (see Chapter 16).

---

(*Table Footnote Continued.*) [2]The fourth dose of diphtheria and tetanus toxoids and acellular pertussis vaccine (DTaP) may be administered as early as age 12 months, provided 6 months have elapsed since the third dose and the child is unlikely to return at age 15–18 months. Tetanus and diphtheria toxoids (Td) are recommended at age 11–12 years if at least 5 years have elapsed since the last dose of diphtheria and tetanus toxoids and pertussis vaccine (DTP), DTaP, or diphtheria and tetanus toxoids (DT). Subsequent routine Td boosters are recommended every 10 years.

[3]Three *Haemophilus influenzae* type b (Hib) conjugate vaccines are licensed for infant use. If Hib conjugate vaccine (PRP-OMP) (PedvaxHIB or ComVax [Merck]) is administered at ages 2 and 4 months, a dose at age 6 months is not required. Because clinical studies in infants have demonstrated that using some combination products may induce a lower immune response to the Hib vaccine component, DTaP/Hib combination products should not be used for primary immunization in infants at ages 2, 4, or 6 months unless approved by the U.S. Food and Drug Administration for these ages.

[4]An all-inactivated poliovirus vaccine (IPV) schedule is recommended for routine childhood polio vaccination in the United States. All children should receive four doses of IPV at age 2 months, age 4 months, between ages 6 and 18 months, and between ages 4 and 6 years. Oral poliovirus vaccine should not be administered to HIV-infected persons or their household contacts.

[5]Hepatitis A vaccine (Hep A) is recommended for use in selected states or regions, and for certain high-risk groups such as those with hepatitis B or hepatitis C infection. Information is available from local public health authorities.

[6]The heptavalent pneumococcal conjugate vaccine (PCV) is recommended for all children age 2–59 months with HIV. Children 2 years and older should also receive the 23 valent pneumococcal polysaccharide vaccine; a single revaccination with the 23 valent vaccine should be offered to children after 3–5 years. Refer to the Advisory Committee on Immunization Practices recommendations on dosing intervals for children starting the vaccination schedule after 2 months of age. (See Chapter 11)

[7]MMR should not be administered to severely immunocompromised (category 3) children. HIV-infected children without severe immunosuppression would routinely receive their first dose of MMR as soon as possible after reaching their first birthday. Consideration should be given to administering the second dose of MMR as soon as 1 month (i.e., a minimum of 28 days) after the first dose rather than waiting until school entry.

[8]Varicella zoster virus vaccine should be given only to asymptomatic, nonimmunosuppressed children. Eligible children should receive two doses of vaccine with at least a 3-month interval between doses. The first dose may be given as early as 12 months of age.

[9]Inactivated split influenza virus vaccine should be administered to all HIV-infected children $\geq$6 months of age each year. For children aged 6 months to <9 years who are receiving influenza vaccine for the first time, two doses given $\geq$1 month apart are recommended. For specific recommendations, see CDC. Prevention and control of influenza: recommendations of the Advisory Committee on Immunization Practices (ACIP). *MMWR* 2001;50(RR-4):l.

From Masur H, Kaplan JE, Holmes KK, and the USPHS/IDSA Prevention of Opportunistic Infections Working Group. 2001 USPHS/IDSA guidelines for the prevention of opportunistic infections in persons infected with human immunodeficiency virus, pages 53–54. Posted November 28, 2001 as a "living document" at *www.hivatis.org/trtgdlns.html#Opportunistic.*

3. **Esophageal candidiasis** may present with severe dysphagia or odynophagia in patients with or without evidence of oral infection. At endoscopy, exudate, ulcers, and deep erosions are seen lining the esophagus [63].

**B. Diagnosis** of oral or vaginal disease often is made on clinical appearance alone. In patients who fail to respond to standard therapy, KOH preparation and fungal cultures are indicated. Esophageal disease is diagnosed by endoscopic examination and culture, although response to empiric antifungal therapy is often used.

**C. Treatment.**

1. **Localized oral** or **vulvovaginal candidiasis** responds well to topical therapy.
   - **a. Clotrimazole** oral troches 10 mg five times per day, or **nystatin** oral pastilles (200,000 units) or oral suspension (500,000 units/5 mL) five times per day may be used for oral disease.
   - **b.** Over-the-counter clotrimazole or miconazole may be used for vaginitis. Fluconazole 150 mg as a single oral dose is also effective.
   - **c.** For patients who do not respond to standard therapy or who also have esophageal disease, the oral azole compounds (fluconazole, itraconazole) are effective.
   - **d. Prevention.** Chronic suppression may be needed for frequent recurrences, but otherwise prophylaxis is not recommended [1]. Fluconazole is superior to clotrimazole in preventing relapses of thrush (Tables 18.2 and 18.4 for drug choices and dosing recommendations in adults and children, respectively); 200 mg thrice weekly for oral and once weekly for vaginal candidiasis have been used. Azoles should be avoided during pregnancy.
2. **Treatment of esophageal candidiasis** requires systemic therapy. Drug resistance, particularly azole-resistant candidiasis, is increasingly common [64]. Some patients respond to increased doses of the drug, and some respond to a switch from one azole to another (e.g., fluconazole to itraconazole). However, low-dose therapy with i.v. amphotericin B is required for many. In pregnancy, azoles should be avoided if possible. The role of the new i.v. **echinocandins,** which may be as effective but less toxic than amphotericin B, has yet to be determined [65,66].
   - **a. Fluconazole** (100–200 mg/day, oral or i.v., in adults) for 14 to 21 days is preferred; up to 800 mg/day may be successful despite *in vitro* resistance. Maintenance suppressive therapy may be necessary in cases of recurrent esophagitis. Direct comparative trials also have demonstrated superiority versus ketoconazole [67]. Side effects include nausea and skin rash, but generally it is well tolerated.
   - **b. Itraconazole** tablets or oral suspension (100 mg twice daily in adults) is equally effective. It requires gastric acid for absorption, and should be taken 1 hour before or 2 hours after antacids; the liquid formulation shows better absorption (serum levels can be followed). Adverse reactions include gastrointestinal upset, rash, and hepatic dysfunction. Concurrent use with cisapride, quinidine, triazolam, and possibly other drugs metabolized by cytochrome P450 3A4 is not recommended. Itraconazole may increase levels of protease inhibitors (e.g., ritonavir, indinavir, saquinavir). Inducers of cytochrome P450 3A4 isoenzymes, such as nevirapine, will decrease itraconazole levels (see Chapters 19 and 27).
   - **c. Ketoconazole** 200 mg/day orally is effective, but an increase in gastric pH impairs absorption. Adverse reactions include rash and hepatotoxicity. Ketoconazole suppresses the hepatic cytochrome p450 system; drug interactions are similar to those with itraconazole.
   - **d. Amphotericin B** 0.3 mg/kg/day i.v. for 7 days (or 100 mg oral suspension four times daily if available) may be used for disease refractory to other agents. Lipid amphotericins may be better tolerated, but their use is limited by high costs.
   - **e. Prevention.** Frequent recurrences require chronic suppression, but primary prophylaxis is not recommended. Fluconazole or itraconazole

solution is effective for most patients (Tables 18.2 and 18.4). Maintenance with oral azoles often can be resumed after i.v. amphotericin B therapy for esophagitis exacerbations, although some patients must be maintained on once- or twice-weekly i.v. amphotericin B.

**VI. *Mycobacterium tuberculosis.*** TB continues to be a devastating disease worldwide (see also Chapter 11). It is estimated to cause 3 million deaths annually [68]. **HIV infection is by far the most important predisposing factor for the development of TB.** Experts believe that TB accounted for 30% of the 5.0 million AIDS-related deaths in the year 2000 [69]. The risk for a patient with AIDS developing TB is 170 times higher than that for a nonimmunosuppressed person. The risk for death in HIV-infected patients with TB was reported to be twice that in HIV-infected patients without TB, independent of CD4 cell count [70].

**A. Epidemiology.** In 2000, a total of 16,377 new TB cases were reported in the United States [71], and approximately 25% to 30% were HIV coinfected. The groups with the greatest increases in rates of TB, specifically black and Hispanic men 25 to 40 years of age, are also the groups with the highest rates of HIV infection, demonstrating how closely intertwined these two epidemics have become [72]. Anonymous HIV testing of serum from TB clinics demonstrated that as many as 40% of all TB patients are HIV infected [73]. This number may be even higher in certain urban areas. In addition, TB is unique among AIDS-related OIs because it is contagious to otherwise healthy persons. This, combined with several nosocomial outbreaks affecting both patients and staff [74], has led to extensive reconsideration of hospital infection control efforts [75]. Finally, resistant TB has been increasing, especially in urban areas [76,77], and is particularly difficult to treat in the HIV-infected patient.

**B. Clinical presentation** depends largely on the overall immune status of the patient [78]. Patients with high CD4 cell counts (>200–300/mm$^3$), generally will have classic TB, with apical cavitary lung disease, respiratory symptoms, fevers, and weight loss. As immunity wanes, presentations become less specific, and diagnosis becomes more difficult as atypical chest radiographic features and extrapulmonary TB are encountered. The most common extrapulmonary manifestations are asymmetric lymphadenopathy, pericarditis, pleurisy, bone disease, and skin lesions. Fever, weight loss, and fatigue may be the only symptoms with disseminated TB, mimicking lymphoma, CMV disease, AIDS wasting syndrome, MAC, and other illnesses [70]. Hilar or mediastinal adenopathy may be the primary chest radiographic abnormality. In addition, pulmonary TB may show lobar and interstitial infiltrates resembling primary TB, and 10% to 20% may have normal radiographs [78]. Thus, HIV-induced immunosuppression may result in unusual presentations and delay the diagnosis.

**Concurrent HIV and TB** interact in several other ways: (a) HIV-infected persons latently infected with TB develop reactivation TB at a rate of 8% to 10% per year, rather than 5% to 10% per lifetime [73]; (b) HIV-infected persons exposed to an infectious index case develop acute TB at a rate as high as 40% over 6 to 12 months rather than 2% to 5% over 2 years in normal hosts [78]; (c) TB may accelerate the progression of HIV infection by activating expression of HIV from macrophages [70]; and (d) immune reconstitution syndromes may occur (see section **II**).

**C. Diagnosis** requires culturing *M. tuberculosis* from appropriate specimens. The sputum smear for acid-fast bacilli is approximately 50% sensitive in HIV-infected persons, a rate similar to that among HIV-negative persons [79]. Cultures using a radiometric system (BACTEC) may speed the diagnosis. Because the initial acid-fast smear cannot distinguish *M. tuberculosis* from MAC, culture with identification and susceptibility tests must be routinely performed. Direct tests of nucleic acid amplification for rapid diagnosis are available. Newer procedures using enzyme immunoassay (EIA) may make serologic testing for *M. tuberculosis* possible in the future (see Chapter 11).

**D. Treatment** guidelines of the CDC and the American Thoracic Society state that the minimal duration of therapy is 6 months for drug-susceptible TB in patients coinfected with HIV. If clinical or bacteriologic response is slow, they recommend extending treatment for a total of 9 months, or for 4 months after cultures become negative [72].

1. **Initial therapy** should consist of standard daily isoniazid (INH) 300 mg orally daily, rifampin 600 mg orally daily, pyrazinamide 20 to 35 mg/kg orally daily, and ethambutol 15 to 25 mg/kg orally daily (see Chapter 11).
2. **Considerations for patients on HAART.** Important **drug interactions** occur between the rifamycins and protease inhibitors and other commonly used agents (Tables 18.8 and 18.9). Rifampin induces the activity of cytochrome P450 CYP3A, which lowers the concentration of protease inhibitors and non-nucleoside reverse transcriptase inhibitors, resulting in incomplete viral suppression [80]. Most experts, however, advise against withholding antiretroviral therapy until completion of TB therapy. **Three principles for treatment of TB in HIV-infected patients have been emphasized:**
   - **a.** Antiretroviral therapy should be administered when indicated.
   - **b.** A short-course regimen (6–9 months, depending on the regimen) should be administered as directly observed therapy to enhance compliance.
   - **c.** Rifabutin at a lower dose (150 mg) is preferred over rifampin because of significant drug interactions of rifampin with protease inhibitors and non-nucleoside reverse transcriptase inhibitors (Tables 18.8 and 18.9).
3. **Patients with CD4 counts of less than 100/mm$^3$** should receive daily therapy for the first 2 months, and no less often than three times weekly during the remainder of treatment. This will minimize the risk of rifampin or rifabutin resistance developing on less frequent intermittent regimens [81].
4. **Sputum cultures and smears** should be checked monthly to document clearing of infection. If they remain positive after 3 months of therapy, resistance, noncompliance, drug interactions, and impaired absorption should be considered.
5. Persistence of fever for more than 2 to 4 weeks in a patient receiving standard four-drug regimen suggests **multidrug-resistant TB** (MDR TB). If susceptibility results are pending, treatment options should be guided by prior drug exposure, history of exposure to a case of MDR TB, and susceptibility patterns in the community [76,82]. Drug fever and a second infection should also be considered.

**E. Chemoprophylaxis** (Tables 18.1 and 18.3) with INH (300 mg orally daily) for 9 months should be administered to any HIV-infected patient with a tuberculin skin test induration that is at least 5 mm in diameter, once active TB has been ruled out. Chemoprophylaxis also should be initiated regardless of the tuberculin skin test result in patients with a history of positive results who were not adequately treated, a close contact with infectious TB, or a chest radiograph that is consistent with previous untreated TB. Recent studies have shown that the results of anergy testing are not reproducible and that INH prophylaxis does not reduce the incidence of TB in HIV-infected patients with anergy [83]. Therefore, **anergy testing is no longer recommended** in this population (see also Chapter 11).

**VII. *Mycobacterium avium* complex** disease has been much less common since the widespread use of HAART. Despite declining incidence, the relative frequency of MAC infection compared with other OIs has not changed. MAC disease continues to be the most common systemic bacterial infection in AIDS and is responsible for significant morbidity.

**A. Epidemiology.** According to the CDC's Adult and Adolescent Spectrum of Disease (ASD) Project, the incidence of MAC declined 39.9% per year between 1996 and 1998, compared with 4.7% per year between 1992 and 1995 [17]. The HIV Outpatient Study reported similar decreases in incidence rates in eight U.S. cities [13]. The prevalence of disseminated MAC for patients with CD4 cell counts of less than 100/mm$^3$ is approximately 10% [83]; at autopsy, prior to HAART and routine use of prophylaxis, the rate was approximately 50% [84].

**B. Clinical presentation** of disseminated MAC includes fever, night sweats, severe weight loss, and, less often, diarrhea. High "spiking" temperatures and a toxic appearance may be seen. Hepatosplenomegaly may be present, but the examination often is quite nonspecific and unrevealing. Common laboratory abnormalities include anemia, neutropenia, and elevated alkaline phosphatase. Immune reactivation lymphadenitis may occur soon after the initiation of HAART (see section **II**).

**C. Diagnosis** depends on culturing the organism from blood or bone marrow. The utility of cultures from other sites, including lymph node and liver, is less well established. Isolation of organisms from respiratory secretions, stool, or urine does not establish the presence of disseminated infection. Blood cultures using special media (i.e., BACTEC or Dupont Isolator systems) yield the highest results. Whereas a single positive blood culture is diagnostic, a negative culture does not rule out disseminated infection because patients can have low levels of mycobacteremia [85]. Specific DNA probes for MAC can rapidly differentiate MAC from other mycobacteria when there is sufficient growth in culture.

**D. Treatment** of MAC continues to improve. Active drugs include the macrolides (azithromycin and clarithromycin), the rifamycins (rifabutin and rifampin), ciprofloxacin, ethambutol, and amikacin [86–88]. Therapy initially should include a macrolide and ethambutol. A third agent, such as a rifamycin or ciprofloxacin, can either be included in the initial regimen or added if there is a slow response. The addition of amikacin as a fourth agent may be needed in some patients who fail to respond or who relapse [89]. In very ill patients, some experts recommend a multidrug regimen (e.g., clarithromycin, ethambutol, arifamycin, and amikacin) to rapidly diminish the bacteremia. Once the patient clinically responds, at least two oral agents (e.g., ethambutol and clarithromycin) may be substituted to simplify an outpatient regimen. Clofazimine is not recommended due to an association with increased mortality. Susceptibility testing is not routinely performed unless the likelihood of drug resistance is high, as in the case of a patient developing mycobacteremia while receiving macrolide therapy.

**E. Prophylaxis** (Tables 18.1–18.5) for MAC disease is recommended for patients with CD4 cell counts of less than 50/mm$^3$. Patients with a prior history of opportunistic infections, or colonization with MAC in the respiratory or gastrointestinal tract, should also be considered for chemoprophylaxis. It is essential to rule out MAC bacteremia and active TB. Clarithromycin (500 mg orally twice daily) or azithromycin (1,200 mg once per week) is more effective than rifabutin and with fewer potential drug interactions [90–92]. In one comparative trial, clarithromycin was superior to azithromycin in time to clearing MAC bacteremia [86]. Preliminary data suggest that low-dose clarithromycin (500 mg orally daily) may be effective [93]. Azithromycin is preferred in pregnancy because clarithromycin has been teratogenic in animals. Recent studies support the **discontinuation of primary prophylaxis** in patients who respond to HAART with sustained increases in CD4 cell counts to **greater than 100/mm$^3$ for 3 to 6 months** (Table 18.5) [1,94]. There are only limited data to recommend discontinuation of secondary prophylaxis, although this may be considered for adult patients on HAART with CD4 counts of greater than 100/mm$^3$ for at least 6 months (Table 18.5) [1,95]. Children should be given lifelong prophylaxis [1].

## VIII. Other mycobacteria

**A. *Mycobacterium kansasii*** is the second most common nontuberculous mycobacterial infection in patients with AIDS [96,97]. Most often disease is localized to the lungs, but the organism also can cause extrapulmonary infection.

1. **Clinical presentation** resembles that of TB and includes fever, cough, and dyspnea. Chest radiographic appearance includes either upper lobe or diffuse infiltrates.
2. **Diagnosis** is made by culture. *M. kansasii* is always considered pathogenic. Of note, *M. kansasii* is not transmitted person to person, so respiratory isolation is not required.

3. **Treatment** recommendations include high-dose INH (600 mg/day), rifampin (600 mg/day), and ethambutol (15–25 mg/kg/day), even though most strains are resistant to INH. Clarithromycin (500 mg orally twice daily) can be substituted for rifampin for patients on protease inhibitors or with rifampin resistance. *M. kansasii* is intrinsically resistant to pyrazinamide. Other antimycobacterial agents, including erythromycin, ciprofloxacin, and streptomycin, have been used with some success [97]. Infectious disease or pulmonary consultation is advised.

B. ***Mycobacterium haemophilum*** is a rare mycobacterium that causes disease in immunosuppressed patients with and without HIV [98].

1. **Clinical presentation** most often includes involvement of skin, bone, or joints. Lung involvement also has been described and is associated with a high mortality rate [99].
2. **Diagnosis** is made by special culture of specimens plated on chocolate heme-enriched agar and incubated at 30°C.
3. **Treatment** has not been standardized but should include a macrolide, rifampin, or rifabutin, and probably at least one other agent from among ciprofloxacin, ethambutol, and amikacin [99,100]. Duration of therapy is not known, but usually extends 12 to 24 months. Infectious disease consultation is advised.

C. **Many other mycobacteria,** including *M. xenopi, M. simiae, M. scrofulaceum, M. malmoense, M. genavense, M. gordonae, M. fortuitum, M. chelonei,* and *M. marinarum,* also have been recovered [101–103]. In the future, additional mycobacterial strains undoubtedly will be associated with disease in persons with advanced AIDS due both to improvements in mycobacteriology and to prolonged survival. Distinguishing colonization from invasive disease will remain difficult. Treatment regimens for many unusual mycobacterial infections are not standardized, but often include a macrolide, ethambutol, and either a rifamycin or quinolone. More severe infections should be treated with amikacin or streptomycin as well. Infectious disease consultation is advised.

IX. **Cytomegalovirus** disease has declined with the availability of more potent HIV therapies. Prior to HAART, CMV was diagnosed in up to 40% of AIDS patients [104], and at autopsy more than 90% had documented CMV infection [105]. **Virtually all patients with disease due to CMV have CD4 counts below 100/mm$^3$** [106]. CMV syndromes still occur during the early months of HAART (presumably before immunorestoration), in those who fail or are intolerant of HAART, and in patients with limited medical care. The shedding of CMV as detected by culture does not necessarily indicate invasive disease. Clinical presentation, histopathologic findings, and viral culture all must be considered in the diagnosis. CMV is often cultured in blood and urine specimens, and detected histopathologically at autopsy. However, the positive predictive values of CMV viremia (35%) and viruria (28%) for the development of end-organ disease were poor in one study [107].

A. **Chorioretinitis** is now seldom the presenting manifestation but occurs when the CD4 count is less than 50/mm$^3$ [108]. It remains the most common intraocular infection in patients with AIDS, accounting for at least 90% of HIV-related infectious retinopathies [109]. Symptoms include decreasing visual acuity, the presence of so-called floaters, and visual field defects. Blindness will result if CMV is left untreated [110].

1. **Diagnosis** is made by **ophthalmologic examination.** Typical findings include creamy or yellow-white granular areas with perivascular exudates and hemorrhages. These lesions are found initially in the periphery of the fundus but can progress to involve the macula and optic disk [110]. Recently, molecular diagnostic testing has been utilized to predict and detect CMV disease. Antigenemia testing and nucleic acid amplification testing have been used to identify at-risk patients and predict CMV end-organ disease, but their value for this purpose has not been established. Following serial antigen results is a means of assessing viral response to treatment [111].
2. **Therapy.** Drugs currently available that act to inhibit viral DNA polymerase are **ganciclovir (and valganciclovir), foscarnet,** and **cidofovir.**

Induction therapy includes 2 weeks or more of high-dose drug. At times, ganciclovir and foscarnet are given together to control relapsed or rapidly advancing disease (ocular or extraocular). When retinitis is stable, patients are placed on lifelong maintenance therapy until there is evidence of immune recovery (discussed below).

a. **Ganciclovir** has an initial response rate of 80% to 90%; however, 30% of patients relapse within 1 year [112]. Side effects include myelosuppression, particularly neutropenia. The induction dose is 5 mg/kg i.v. every 12 hours for 14 to 21 days or until there is an adequate clinical response; the maintenance dose is 5 mg/kg/day i.v. or 1.0 g every 8 hours orally. Oral ganciclovir, despite its low bioavailability of 8%, at a dose of 1,000 mg three times a day, is nearly equivalent to i.v. ganciclovir in preventing progression and preserving vision, particularly if the initial CMV retinitis was not sight threatening. Oral ganciclovir alone is not approved for initial treatment.

b. **Foscarnet** is only available for i.v. use. A comparison trial with ganciclovir found no difference in the frequency and rate of retinitis progression. Although foscarnet was not as well tolerated as ganciclovir, it offered survival advantage, perhaps secondary to its direct antiretroviral activity [106]. Side effects include renal impairment, periuretheral ulceration, paresthesia, seizures, and other central nervous system (CNS) symptoms. The induction dose is 60 mg/kg every 8 hours or 90 mg/kg every 12 hours; the maintenance dose is 90 to 120 mg/kg/day.

c. **Cidofovir** plus probenicid (2 g orally 3 hours before each dose, 1 g orally 2 and 8 hours postdose) to limit nephrotoxicity may be effective in patients who fail or are intolerant of ganciclovir or foscarnet [113]. Its long half-life permits administration every 2 weeks during maintenance therapy. No oral form is available. The induction dose is 5 mg/kg i.v. weekly; the maintenance dose is 5 mg/kg i.v. every other week.

d. **An intraocular ganciclovir release device** (every 6 months) **plus oral ganciclovir or valganciclovir** is preferred by some clinicians, especially for immediately sight-threatening infection. This is superior to i.v. ganciclovir in time to relapse, but there is increased risk of involvement of the other eye and extraocular disease [114].

e. **Valganciclovir,** the first oral drug for CMV induction therapy (900 mg orally twice daily), is a prodrug of ganciclovir that is well absorbed from the gastrointestinal tract conferring greater bioavailability; absorption is increased, and the potential for toxicity enhanced, if taken with high-fat meals (Table 18.7). Efficacy is comparable with i.v. ganciclovir without the risk of catheter-related complications; side effects are similar to those of ganciclovir [115,116]. The maintenance dose is 900 mg daily.

f. **Alternative therapy** includes **intraocular injections** of foscarnet 1.2 to 2.4 mg in 0.1 mL or ganciclovir 2,000 $\mu$g in 0.05 to 0.1 mL. Fomivirsen (330 $\mu$g by intravitreal injection at days 1 and 15, then monthly) is a new antisense compound [117]. Any local therapy should be accompanied by systemic anti-CMV therapy such as oral ganciclovir or valganciclovir [118].

3. **Prophylaxis (Tables 18.1–18.5).** Current data suggest that long-term ganciclovir prophylaxis can be safely discontinued in adults after resolution of lesions, if the CD4 cell count has been above 100 to 150/mm$^3$ for at least 6 months, if the lesions are not sight threatening, and if regular follow-up with an ophthalmologist can be assured (Table 18.5) [1,109,119,120]. There are insufficient data about the safety of this approach in children. Discontinuation of secondary prophylaxis for extraocular CMV disease is not supported by the current literature.

B. **CMV colitis** previously developed in 5% to 10% of AIDS patients but is now uncommon. Symptoms are nonspecific and may include diarrhea, weight loss, abdominal pain and cramping, anorexia, and fever [121].

1. **Diagnosis** is made by endoscopic biopsy. Endoscopy reveals mucosal ulceration and submucosal hemorrhage. Biopsy shows the pathognomonic "owl eye" inclusions in tissue, or demonstrates CMV antigens (e.g., by immunohistochemical staining).
2. **Therapy** with ganciclovir and foscarnet is variably effective. Some studies have shown improvement of symptoms and the appearance of the colon, as well as decreased incidence of extracolonic CMV infection. However, not all patients respond, and the optimal dose and length of treatment are not well defined. One approach is to treat patients for 2 weeks and follow them clinically off therapy.

**C. CMV pneumonitis** is a major concern in bone marrow transplantation, but seldom is seen in AIDS. CMV is often isolated in respiratory specimens, yet treatment of other pathogens alone usually results in clinical improvement [122]. True CMV pneumonitis is seen in fewer than 10% of patients who undergo evaluation of pulmonary infiltrates of unknown etiology [123]. **Symptoms** include worsening shortness of breath, dyspnea on exertion, and dry cough. Chest radiographs may show diffuse infiltrates similar to those seen in PCP.

1. **Diagnosis** is established by finding pathognomonic intranuclear inclusion bodies (owl eyes) in biopsy samples. The diagnosis is suggested in patients with positive CMV cultures, no other recovered pathogens, and response to appropriate therapy.
2. **Therapy** is with ganciclovir at routine doses. Unlike bone marrow transplant patients, there is no proven benefit to concurrent i.v. immunoglobulins. Maintenance therapy should be considered for responders.

**D. CMV esophagitis** is less common than that caused by *C. albicans.* Symptoms include odynophagia, dysphagia, or vague dyspepsia [124]. Diagnosis is made by endoscopic biopsy. Ganciclovir is effective for treatment. Maintenance therapy is not used unless symptoms recur.

**E. CMV encephalitis** usually is diagnosed postmortem [125]. Symptoms are varied and include cognitive deficits, personality changes, increased somnolence, and focal neurologic signs [126]. Diagnosis often is confused with progressive AIDS dementia. Antiviral treatment has not been shown to be effective, although combination therapy with ganciclovir and foscarnet is often recommended.

**F. CMV ventriculoencephalitis** is a late infection with acute onset often associated with cranial nerve palsies. Patients may either have no history of CMV disease [127] or are already on therapy for CMV [125]. Spinal fluid analysis shows pleocytosis, usually with lymphocytes but sometimes with polymorphonuclear leukocytes, marked increase in protein, and low glucose [127]. Magnetic resonance imaging (MRI) may reveal a characteristic periventricular ringlike enhancement [125]. Viral culture of the cerebrospinal fluid (CSF) is not always positive; CMV DNA can often be detected in CSF using PCR. Therapy with ganciclovir or foscarnet may ameliorate symptoms if given early, but response is unpredictable and most cases progress [128].

**G. CMV polyradiculitis** may cause radicular pain, progressive Guillain-Barré–like ascending paralysis, and urinary retention [129]. The CSF may have a pleocytosis with a predominance of neutrophils (unusual for viral infection), elevated protein, and low glucose [130]. Diagnosis is made by viral culture of CSF; PCR also may be useful [131]. Therapy with ganciclovir has resulted in improvement of symptoms in some patients [132]. Some experts give ganciclovir concurrently with foscarnet.

**H. CMV involvement of the adrenal glands** is seen at autopsy in up to 50% of patients [133]. However, adrenal insufficiency is less common, and the correlation between adrenal infection and clinical adrenal dysfunction is incomplete. Adrenal insufficiency should be considered in all patients with CMV and symptoms consistent with Addison disease (e.g., electrolyte abnormalities, unexplained hypotension, fever, and fatigue). Diagnosis is confirmed by **cosyntropin stimulation test.** Dramatic improvement may be seen with steroid replacement therapy.

**X. Toxoplasmosis.** *Toxoplasma gondii* is the most common cause of focal encephalitis in AIDS patients [134]. Disease is usually due to recrudescence of latent infection; therefore, all patients with antibodies to *T. gondii* are at risk. Seroprevalence varies among geographic locations. In the United States, 20% to 40% of the general population has evidence of past infection [135]. Approximately 25% to 40% of seropositive patients with AIDS will develop disease unless given prophylaxis [136]. The risk of reactivation infection increases with a decreasing CD4 cell count, especially when the CD4 count falls below 100/mm$^3$. In the United States, toxoplasmic encephalitis (TE) has been reported in 1% to 5% of patients with AIDS. TE in AIDS patients is associated with a mortality rate of 70% by 12 months after diagnosis [137]. Effective prophylaxis and potent combination antiretroviral regimens have resulted in a marked decrease in the incidence of this disease [136,138].

**A. Clinical presentation** ranges from focal neurologic findings to generalized symptoms, including weakness, confusion, seizures, and coma. Constitutional symptoms such as fever and malaise are variable, but meningismus is rare. The CSF may show a mononuclear pleocytosis and elevated protein, or may be normal. **Disseminated toxoplasmosis,** involving heart, lung, colon, skeletal muscles, and other organs, has been described [139]. Septic shock also has been seen, with presentation of prolonged fever, dyspnea, thrombocytopenia, and high lactate dehydrogenase levels [140].

**B. Serologic tests** for antitoxoplasma antibodies are highly reliable but not specific for active disease. Almost all patients with toxoplasmosis have immunoglobulin G (IgG) antibody. From a practical standpoint, a patient with CNS symptoms and a recent negative test result for toxoplasma IgG antibody is unlikely to have TE. Seronegative toxoplasmosis is rare, accounting for only 0% to 3% of cases [135,141]; however, one study reported a seronegative rate of 22% [141]. The level of antibody is not predictive of likelihood of reactivation or severity of disease.

**C. Radiographic evaluation** reveals single or multiple CNS lesions with ring or nodular enhancement. Lesions are most frequently found in the basal ganglia or corticomedullary junction [142]. The MRI scan is the best imaging technique and may detect lesions not seen by CT scanning [143]. The presence of edema, a mass effect, and hemorrhage may help to distinguish TE from CNS lymphoma. Thallium 201 single-photon emission computed tomography (SPECT) scans may distinguish between these two entities because a negative scan is unlikely to represent lymphoma [144], although their value has recently been questioned [145]. Positron emission tomography is useful but is not as widely available [146].

**D. Diagnosis** is definitive when *T. gondii* tachyzoites are seen on brain biopsy; however, this can be difficult because the organism may be difficult to find and histopathologic changes may resemble other infections [147]. Most often, a presumptive diagnosis is made based on positive serology, typical radiographic findings, and response to specific therapy.

**E. Polymerase chain reaction** can detect *T. gondii* DNA in brain tissue, CSF, BAL fluid, sputum, and blood in patients with AIDS [148,149]. The sensitivity of PCR in CSF has been between 11% and 77%, and the specificity is almost 100% [150,151]. PCR is widely available and should be used when the diagnosis is in question.

**F. Differential diagnosis.** The main diagnosis of exclusion is CNS lymphoma. All patients with characteristic lesions on CT or MRI and positive serology for *T. gondii* should be treated empirically for toxoplasmosis. In patients with single lesions, the predictive value for TE is less. CNS lymphoma is four times more likely to present with a single lesion than multiple lesions [143]. Patients with CNS lymphoma often have Epstein-Barr virus (EBV) detected on PCR of CSF. However, toxoplasma antibody–positive patients with a single lesion also should receive empiric treatment for TE. Response to empiric treatment is the most practical means of making the diagnosis. Half of patients with toxoplasmosis will clinically respond by day 3 and 90% by day 14 [134], and radiographically within 2 weeks. For responders, a repeat scan in 1 month is reasonable. For those who do not respond by day 14 or do not have a positive serology, brain biopsy should be considered. **Corticosteroids** will result in radiologic improvement with either lymphoma or toxoplasmosis and should not be given unless the diagnosis is already secured.

**G. Treatment** is based on combination chemotherapy, with most agents acting to block folic acid metabolism.

1. **Standard regimens** include **pyrimethamine** (100–200 mg loading dose, then 50–100 mg orally daily) plus **folinic acid** (10 mg orally daily) plus either **sulfadiazine** (1–1.5 g orally every 6 hours) or **clindamycin** 900 mg i.v. every 6 hours or 450 to 600 mg orally every 6 hours for at least 6 weeks.
2. **Alternatives** include pyrimethamine plus folinic acid plus either **azithromycin** (1,200–1,500 mg orally daily) or **clarithromycin** (1 g orally twice daily) or **atovaquone** (750 mg orally with food four times daily). These combinations are clearly inferior and should therefore be reserved for patients with true intolerance to standard regimens.
3. **Corticosteroids** (**decadron** 4 mg orally or i.v. every 6 hours) are used for significant edema/mass effect.

**H. Prevention** (Tables 18.1–18.6). Patients seronegative for *T. gondii* antibodies should be educated about appropriate precautions to avoid exposure, for example, while working with soil or in considering cat ownership (Table 18.6).

1. **Primary prophylaxis** (Tables 18.1 and 18.3) is used for patients with positive IgG antibody and a CD4 count of less than 100/mm$^3$. **Trimethoprim-sulfamethoxazole,** 1 DS or SS tablet orally daily is the agent of choice. **Dapsone** 50 mg orally daily plus **pyrimethamine** 50 mg orally weekly plus folinic acid 25 mg orally weekly is an alternative. Both regimens also prevent PCP. See Table 18.3 for pediatric dosing recommendations. Primary prophylaxis may be discontinued in adults if HAART raises the CD4 count to more than 200/mm$^3$ for at least 3 months (Table 18.5).
2. **Secondary prophylaxis** (Tables 18.2 and 18.4), or suppressive therapy, should be given following treatment for toxoplasmosis; 80% relapse after discontinuation of therapy. **Pyrimethamine** 25 to 50 mg orally daily plus **folinic acid** 10 to 25 mg orally daily plus **sulfadiazine** 500 to 1,000 mg orally four times daily is preferred. Alternatives include **clindamycin** 300 to 450 mg orally every 6 hours plus **pyrimethamine** 25 to 50 mg orally daily plus **folinic acid** 10 mg orally daily (which does not protect against PCP), or **atovaquone** 750 mg orally two to four times daily with or without pyrimethamine plus folinic acid. See Table 18.4 for pediatric dosing recommendations. Discontinuation of secondary prophylaxis in adults may be considered if HAART raises the CD4 count to greater than 200/mm$^3$ for at least 6 months (Table 18.5).
3. **Other considerations.** The safety of discontinuing prophylaxis in children has not been evaluated and is not recommended [1]. Pyrimethamine should be used only with caution in pregnancy because of potential teratogenicity.

**XI. Cryptococcosis.** *Cryptococcus neoformans* most often causes meningitis or disseminated disease. Six percent to 10% of patients with AIDS will develop cryptococcosis. It is the most common systemic fungal infection and third most common CNS disorder (behind toxoplasmosis and lymphoma) in HIV-infected patients. The incidence of cryptococcosis has decreased due to more widespread use of azoles and potent antiretroviral therapy.

**A. Presentation.** Cryptococcal meningitis is usually an indolent disease (see Chapter 6). Symptoms, including headache, fever, and malaise [152] typically are present for weeks prior to diagnosis. The headache often is worse with sneezing or coughing. Lethargy, mental status changes, and forgetfulness are common. Classic meningismus and focal neurologic signs are uncommon, occurring less than 10% of the time. Pulmonary symptoms with an abnormal chest radiograph may be seen. Prostatitis occurs and the prostate may serve as a nidus for subsequent recurrence [153]. Other sites of involvement include the joints, pericardium, myocardium, mediastinum, skin, and oral cavity. CSF often reveals a poor inflammatory response; protein and glucose levels may be normal, with little pleocytosis. Poor prognostic factors include impaired mental status at presentation [154], fewer than 20 white blood cells (WBCs) per $mm^3$ in CSF, elevated opening pressure (>200 mm $H_2O$), and a CSF cryptococcal antigen titer greater than 1:1,024 [155].

**B. Diagnosis.** Isolation of *C. neoformans* from blood, CSF, or other specimens is the standard for diagnosis. However, the latex agglutination test for cryptococcal polysaccharide antigen is highly sensitive and specific. In one large study of patients with culture-proven meningitis, 98% tested positive for a serum antigen and 91% for a CSF antigen, whereas CSF India ink stains tested positive in 74% [156]. In general, a serum titer of greater than 1:4 should be repeated and a full evaluation considered; a titer of greater than 1:32 is considered diagnostic. All patients with a positive serum antigen titer should undergo a spinal tap. Routine screening with the serum cryptococcal antigen test is not recommended.

**C. Therapy** for cryptococcosis in AIDS patients is lifelong (see Chapters 6 and 17). The treatment of choice is **amphotericin B** (0.7–1.0 mg/kg/day i.v.) **with concurrent flucytosine** (25 mg/kg orally every 6 hours) **for 14 days, followed by fluconazole** 400 mg daily **to complete an 8- to 10-week course. Suppression with fluconazole** 200 mg daily is then recommended. Pregnancy should be avoided during chronic fluconazole therapy because of potential teratogenicity. Weekly amphotericin B produces a higher relapse rate than fluconazole, but amphotericin is an alternative (0.6–1.0 mg/kg one to three times weekly). Itraconazole (200 mg/day) is not as effective as fluconazole for suppressive therapy [157]. Increased intracranial pressure greater than 250 mm $H_2O$ requires urgent CSF drainage. In the absence of obstructive hydrocephalus, serial lumbar punctures are recommended for increased intracranial pressure. In addition, corticosteroids may ameliorate the sequelae of increased intracranial pressure. If cerebral edema occurs, high-dose steroids may offer temporary benefits. Long-term use, however, is discouraged because it may interfere with the effectiveness of antifungal therapy.

**D. Prevention** (Tables 18.1–18.5). Studies to support the use of primary prophylaxis for cryptococcosis are limited. Although cryptococcal meningitis decreased with either fluconazole or itraconazole prophylaxis, no survival benefit was noted. Due to concerns regarding development of antifungal resistance, especially in *Candida* species, the relative infrequency of cryptococcal disease, the possibility of drug interactions, and costs, USPHS/IDSA guidelines do not endorse routine primary prophylaxis [158]. Discontinuation of suppressive therapy (secondary prophylaxis) may be considered if HAART raises the CD4 count to greater than 100 to 200/$mm^3$ for at least 6 months (Table 18.5); this is not recommended in children [1].

**XII. Histoplasmosis** occurs in at least 5% of HIV-infected patients residing within endemic regions (central and south central) of the United States, and it often is their first OI (>70%). Nearly all cases are disseminated at the time of diagnosis. In these regions, histoplasmosis has been the second or third most common opportunistic disease [159]. Dissemination may result either from primary or reactivation *H. capsulatum* infection.

**A. Clinical presentation** includes fever and weight loss in greater than 95% of patients, and at least 50% have pulmonary complaints. Examination is often notable for hepatosplenomegaly, lymphadenopathy, and, rarely, skin lesions [160]. The chest radiograph may show streaky infiltrates but can be normal in 50%. An **elevated LDH** level, often over 1,000 U/L, may be a clue to diagnosis. The median CD4 cell count at the time of diagnosis is 50/$mm^3$. Disseminated disease can cause a sepsis-like syndrome characterized by hypotension, respiratory and liver failure, and disseminated intravascular coagulopathy. On rare occasions, histoplasmosis may cause retinitis, prostatitis, pericarditis, pancreatitis, or colitis [161,162].

**B. Diagnosis** of active disease is made by isolation of *H. capsulatum* from appropriate sites, including blood, bone marrow, lung tissue, or lymph node. Sensitivity is approximately 90% for blood and bone marrow cultures, and slightly less for respiratory specimens. Isolates are confirmed using a DNA probe for specific ribosomal DNA. **Detection of polysaccharide antigen is the mainstay of rapid diagnosis.** In one series of HIV-positive patients, it had a sensitivity of greater than 90% in urine and approximately 75% in blood [163]. Monitoring antigen levels is much more sensitive than serology for detecting early relapse [164]. The complement fixation test does not distinguish past and active disease, and is less sensitive in HIV-infected patients [164]. Following the LDH level is also a sensitive means of detecting early relapse, and is used with serial urine antigen tests.

**C. Therapy with amphotericin B** until there is definite clinical improvement (usually 0.7–1.0 mg/kg for 7–14 days; some clinicians suggest giving 10–15 mg/kg total cumulative dose) **is followed by itraconazole** (200 mg orally twice daily) for 12 weeks. **Liquid formulation itraconazole is preferred** due to improved absorption and fewer drug interactions. Interactions of itraconazole preparations with food are listed in Table 18.7. Failures of this approach were seen in patients who were severely ill at diagnosis [160]. Oral itraconazole can be used alone for mild nonmeningeal, nonsepticemic cases (200 mg three times daily for 3 days, then 200 mg twice daily for 12 weeks total). **Lifetime maintenance therapy is required** to prevent relapse (Tables 18.2, 18.4, and 18.5) [160]. Although weekly or biweekly amphotericin B (1 mg/kg) decreases relapse rates from 80% to 10%–15%, itraconazole (200 mg orally once or twice daily in adults) is equally effective, more convenient, and better tolerated [165]. **Fluconazole** has less *in vitro* activity for *H. capsulatum* and is inferior for both initial and maintenance therapy [166,167]. See Table 18.4 for pediatric doses.

**D. Prevention.** Routine primary prophylaxis is not recommended, although some clinicians argue that patients with low CD4 counts living in endemic areas would benefit. Concern for developing resistant organisms is the major argument against this practice. Further study is necessary before this controversial issue can be resolved. Secondary prophylaxis has been discussed above.

**XIII. Coccidioidomycosis** is endemic to areas of the southwestern United States (see Chapter 17). Rates and severity of illness are higher in HIV-infected persons [168]. The majority of these patients have CD4 counts of less than 250/mm$^3$. Primary antifungal prophylaxis is not recommended.

**A. Presentation** depends on the immunologic status of the patient. Patients with relatively normal immune function have either subclinical illness or lower respiratory symptoms [169]. For patients with CD4 cell counts of less than 250/mm$^3$, pneumonia and meningitis are more common. Illness may resemble PCP, with fever, dyspnea, nonproductive cough, and a chest radiograph with diffuse nodular infiltrates [168,169]. Coccidioidal meningitis presents with headache, fever, and lethargy. The CSF may have more than 50 WBCs per mm$^3$ (predominantly lymphocytes) with low glucose and high protein. In addition, the disease may present as a fever of unknown origin with diffuse lymphadenopathy and pancytopenia.

**B. Diagnosis.** Results of coccidioidal **serologic tests are positive in approximately 90%** of HIV-positive patients. **Titers reflect the activity of infection and therefore can be used to monitor response to therapy.** Antibody detection tests include the tube precipitins method, complement fixation, latex agglutination, immunodiffusion, and EIA. Skin testing for delayed-type hypersensitivity to coccidioidal antigens has a limited diagnostic role because of anergy and a positive test result indicates only prior infection. **Definitive diagnosis is made from clinical specimens by culture of the organism or identification of coccidioidal spherules on histopathologic examination,** using stains such as methenamine silver or Papanicolaou. Although it is difficult to culture the organism from CSF, the presence of complement-fixing antibodies suggests the diagnosis of meningitis. Laboratory personnel need to take appropriate precautions when coccidioidiomycosis is suspected.

**C. Treatment** of disseminated disease is with **amphotericin B** (1 mg/kg/day) for a total dose of as much as 2.5 g. The oral azoles including **itraconazole** (200 mg twice daily) and **fluconazole** (400 mg/day) also have been used with success as initial therapy [170,171]. Although meningitis has been treated with i.v. and intrathecal amphotericin B, currently oral fluconazole (400–800 mg/day) is often used initially. Lifelong maintenance therapy with oral azoles (400 mg/day in adults) is recommended to prevent relapse (Tables 18.2, 18.4, and 18.5) [172]. Studies are under way to evaluate optimal regimens for both induction and maintenance therapy.

**XIV. Blastomycosis** is endemic to areas of the midwestern and south central United States. It rarely causes disease in HIV-infected persons even in endemic regions [173]. Most patients have had a prior opportunistic infection and CD4 cell counts of less than 200/mm$^3$.

- **A. Presentation.** Pulmonary or disseminated disease may be seen. Unlike normal hosts, in whom skin, bone, and prostate involvement is common, HIV-positive persons with disseminated disease frequently have infection in the CNS (meningitis or blastomycoma), liver, spleen, and bone marrow [174].
- **B. Diagnosis** by growth in culture may require 2 to 4 weeks. **Microscopic examination** of sputum, BAL fluid, and other tissue specimens should be used to rapidly detect the characteristic organism (see Chapter 17). Serologic tests lack sensitivity and specificity.
- **C. Treatment.** Patients should receive amphotericin B until they are stable (usually 10–20 mg/kg total dose) followed by lifelong maintenance therapy with itraconazole [173,175].

**XV. Penicilliosis.** *Penicillium marneffei* is a dimorphic fungus endemic in Southeast Asia, especially Vietnam, Thailand, and parts of southern China. Although rare in the United States, it is the third most common opportunistic infection in HIV-infected patients in Northern Thailand. Most reported cases in the United States occur in individuals who have traveled to endemic regions [176]. The actual route of human infection with this organism is unknown. *P. marneffei* infection is serious and potentially fatal without therapy. Travelers to endemic regions should be informed of the risk for acquiring this infection (Table 18.6).

- **A. Clinical presentation** may be similar to that of disseminated histoplasmosis. Fever is the most common symptom, along with anemia and weight loss. Respiratory complaints occur in approximately half of cases. The majority of patients with disseminated disease present with cutaneous involvement characterized by multiple papular lesions. Disseminated infection usually occurs in advanced HIV infection (CD4 cells <50/mm$^3$).
- **B. Diagnosis** is made by direct microscopy or culture of blood, skin lesions, lymph nodes, and bone marrow [176].
- **C. Treatment.** Amphotericin B (0.6 mg/kg/day) for 2 weeks followed by oral itraconazole (200 mg twice daily) for 10 weeks is regarded as standard therapy [177]. As with other endemic mycoses, relapse is common; therefore, chronic suppressive therapy with itraconazole (200 mg/day) is recommended [177]. Although ketoconazole is active *in vitro,* it is less effective than itraconazole both for treatment and prevention [178].

**XVI. Herpes simplex virus (HSV) types 1 and 2 commonly cause mucocutaneous disease** in HIV-infected persons; 95% of homosexual men with AIDS have antibodies to HSV [179,180], as do up to 77% of the HIV-infected population in general [181]. Reactivation occurs frequently, resulting in chronic lesions in patients with AIDS. Direct contact with oral (HSV-1) or genital (HSV-2) secretions is the primary mode of transmission.

- **A. Clinical manifestations** may vary from typical grouped vesicles with an erythematous base, to chronic, nonhealing ulcers or indistinct erosions; they most frequently involve the orolabial, genital, and anorectal regions. Disseminated disease, which occurs rarely in AIDS patients, may involve the esophagus, lung, liver, and adrenal glands. CNS infection is rare but life threatening (see Chapter 6). Fever and weight loss are common with gastrointestinal involvement [181].
- **B. Diagnosis** is usually suggested by the clinical appearance. Techniques for diagnosis include cytologic preparations for multinucleated giant cells (e.g., Tzanck test), fluorescein-conjugated monoclonal antibody staining of scrapings from lesions, viral culture, and PCR assays for HSV DNA [182].

C. **Therapy.** Oral **acyclovir** (200 mg five times daily or 400 mg three times daily, up to 800 mg five times daily) for 7 to 10 days **is the treatment of choice for an initial mucocutaneous outbreak.** Bioavailability of oral acyclovir is approximately 10% to 20%. Topical acyclovir is not highly effective in patients with HIV infection and should not be used. **Famciclovir** (250 mg orally three times daily) **or valacyclovir** (1.0 g orally twice daily) given for 7 to 10 days is equally effective. Both have excellent bioavailability after oral administration. **Severe mucocutaneous disease may require i.v. acyclovir** (5 mg/kg every 8 hours). **Esophagitis or other visceral disease also is treated with i.v. acyclovir** (10 mg/kg every 8 hours for up to 21 days). **Recurrent mucocutaneous lesions** are treated with acyclovir (400 mg three times daily), famciclovir (125 mg twice daily), or valacyclovir (500 mg twice daily) orally for 5 days. **Suppressive therapy** (Tables 18.2 and 18.4) is recommended for frequent recurrent infections or relapses [183,184]. Many patients are controlled with acyclovir 400 to 800 mg/day in divided doses, famciclovir 125 to 250 mg orally twice daily, or valacyclovir 500 mg orally twice daily or 1 g orally daily. Dosages should be individualized to the patient's response. Acyclovir is the agent of choice for children (Table 18.4).

**Acyclovir-resistant HSV infection** is increasingly common, particularly in those with an extensive prior history of acyclovir use. **Foscarnet** (40–60 mg/kg/day i.v.) is the treatment of choice despite its potential toxicity and added costs [185].

XVII. **Varicella-zoster virus (VZV)** is a common pathogen that causes an array of clinical syndromes, ranging from chickenpox and shingles, to disseminated skin involvement and visceral disease, to postinfectious vasculitis. Because shingles may be the first evidence of HIV infection, many experts recommend HIV testing for any young to middle-aged individual presenting with shingles [186].

A. **Clinical features.** The typical rash associated with **primary VZV (chickenpox)** appears 10 to 21 days after exposure/infection. Lesions evolve over 1 to 3 days to form vesicles, pustules, and various stages of crusting. Early cases with few vesicles or multidermatomal cases may be more difficult to diagnose clinically. In such cases, confirmatory viral culture is recommended. A Tzanck preparation from scrapings from the base of lesions may reveal multinucleated giants cells but is not specific for VZV. Fluorescein-conjugated monoclonal antibody staining is specific and more rapid than viral culture [187].

The unique unilateral dermatomal distribution of clustered vesicles allows clinical diagnosis of most cases of **shingles (herpes zoster).** Herpes zoster in the immunocompromised patient is often more severe. HIV-positive patients (regardless of the CD4 cell count) have a higher incidence of dermatomal zoster and are at increased risk for disseminated disease compared with age-matched immunocompetent hosts [186]. **Involvement of the ophthalmic division of the trigeminal nerve (V1), herpes zoster ophthalmicus,** causes anterior uveitis and corneal scarring with visual loss.

B. **Other syndromes.** Varicella-zoster virus rarely has been recovered from retinal tissue in patients with sudden blindness due to **acute retinal necrosis** [188]. Most cases appear to be postinflammatory in nature. **Varicella encephalitis,** a subacute encephalitis characterized by slowly progressive dementia and confusion that involves the white matter preferentially, also may be seen. Granulomatous vasculitis causing contralateral stroke syndrome is a rare CNS complication of herpes zoster ophthalmicus [189].

C. **Treatment of VZV** requires higher doses of antivirals than that used for HSV.

1. **Dermatomal zoster** may be treated orally, although patients with advanced disease or uncertain absorption are best treated intravenously until stable. The standard i.v. acyclovir dose for adults and children under 1 year of age is 10 mg/kg every 8 hours (500 mg/$m^2$ every 8 hours in children between 1 and 2 years of age) for 7–10 days. Oral dosages in adults with uncomplicated cases are acyclovir 800 mg five times daily, valacyclovir 1.0 g three times daily, or famciclovir 500 mg three times daily.

2. **Chickenpox, disseminated zoster, multidermatomal zoster, or involvement of V1 should be treated with i.v. acyclovir** until stable.
3. **Acyclovir-resistant VZV infection** has been reported. The vesicles in this syndrome often are atypical, with a more necrotic base and larger, more leathery appearance. Foscarnet is the antiviral agent of choice for infection with acyclovir-resistant VZV [185].
4. The best therapy for **retinal necrosis** is not known. There is no apparent response to either steroids or antiviral therapy, although antiviral therapy is often tried. Ophthalmologic consultation is recommended.
5. **Aspirin should not be given to children** with varicella to reduce the risk for Reye syndrome.

**D. Prevention.** HIV-infected children and adults known to be susceptible to VZV are candidates for varicella-zoster immune globulin within 96 hours of an exposure. There are no data to support the use of postexposure acyclovir. Asymptomatic children in CDC class I (CD4 counts $\geq$25%) may be considered for varicella vaccination (Table 18.13). (See also Chapter 23.)

**XVIII. Human herpesvirus 8 and Kaposi sarcoma (KS).** KS is the most common neoplasm in AIDS. Early in the AIDS epidemic, a 20,000-fold increased rate of KS was noted among homosexual men [190]. Promiscuity and oral-fecal contact were identified as risk factors, suggesting the presence of an infectious etiology [191,192]. In 1994, HHV-8 was detected in biopsy samples of KS tissues from a patient with AIDS [191,193]. Abundant data now support the assertion that **HHV-8 infection is etiologically related to KS** [191,194]. It also is linked to the development of B-cell body cavity lymphomas and Castleman disease.

**A. Epidemiology.** HHV-8 infection appears restricted to the human population. About 30% to 40% of homosexual men with HIV are seropositive for HHV-8 [192]. Although all infections result from human-to-human transmission, the exact modes of transmission have not been defined. HHV-8 most often is acquired through sexual contact or body fluids, and is not readily transmitted by blood, although injection drug use is a risk. Moreover, the mechanisms by which HHV-8 infection induce KS remain incompletely understood. A 10- to 30-fold decreased incidence of KS has been reported since the introduction of HAART in 1996 [195,196]. Despite declining frequencies, KS was present in 20.5% of U.S. patients who died from AIDS in 1997 [17].

Before the AIDS epidemic, KS was recognized as a rare, indolent dermal tumor usually found on the lower extremities of elderly white men of Mediterranean or Eastern European origin. KS also was known to occur occasionally in renal transplant patients in whom lesions often regressed when immunosuppressive agents were discontinued.

**B. KS in AIDS patients** is usually aggressive. It is a multicentric tumor that initially presents as purplish nodules on the skin or mucous membranes. Patients with high CD4 cell counts (>300–400/mm$^3$) may develop limited cutaneous lesions. In the early stage, lesions are irregular, reddish blue or purple to violaceous, nonblanching macules. The macules may become papular or nodular, or coalesce to form large patches, plaques, and fusiform or ovoid tumors. Individual lesions are usually asymptomatic, although pain, itching, and burning can be noted [197]. Lesions commonly are less than 1 cm in diameter. KS frequently spreads to lymph nodes and visceral organs and can be seen in any organ. In advanced disease, lymph node involvement may result in edema, particularly of the legs and scrotum. More than half of patients with cutaneous KS have oral involvement. Oral lesions are especially common on the hard palate and gingival margins and often are asymptomatic. Immunosuppression is an important risk factor for KS, although it may occur in persons with CD4 cell counts of greater than 500/mm$^3$. Remission of cutaneous and pulmonary disease has been noted in patients receiving HAART.

**C. Diagnosis of KS** is confirmed by biopsy, which shows vascular proliferation. Any patient with presumed KS should have a biopsy, because other conditions, such as bacillary angiomatosis, may mimic the disease.

**D. Therapy for KS** can be local or systemic. Local therapies include surgical excision, cryotherapy, laser, intralesional injections, and radiation therapy. Recombinant interferon-$\alpha$ (IFN-$\alpha$) therapy has been used for extensive cutaneous lesions [198–200]. In life-threatening situations, where KS lesions may obstruct vital structures such as the bronchus, bowel, or biliary tract, either radiation or chemotherapy may be necessary. Systemic treatments involve various combinations of vinblastine, etoposide, bleomycin, and doxorubicin. Paclitaxel (taxol) is generally well tolerated and is the treatment of choice for refractory KS [201]. **Lesions may regress in response to HAART** [202].

**E. Prevention.** There is currently no recommended drug regimen for preventing HHV-8 infection. Thus, HIV-infected patients should avoid sexual and injection drug use exposures to HHV-8 (Table 18.6). However, there is evidence that some antiherpesvirus drugs (i.e., ganciclovir, foscarnet, and cidofovir) may inhibit HHV-8 replication. In addition, the incidence of KS has decreased since the advent of potent antiretroviral therapy.

**XIX. Progressive multifocal leukoencephalopathy** is a demyelinating disease caused by **JC virus,** a polyomavirus that infects the oligodendrocytes. Pre-HAART, approximately 4% of AIDS patients developed PML [203], which typically progressed to death within months from diagnosis.

**A. Clinical presentation** varies from diffuse encephalopathy to focal deficits such as ataxia, hemiparesis, or speech difficulties. Symptoms tend to progress rapidly over several months, although rare patients have a waxing and waning course extending for years. Unlike global dementia of AIDS, the cognitive deficit of PML often progresses rapidly and can occur with other focal neurologic deficits. The typical finding is progressive dementia concurrent with a stroke syndrome.

**B. Definitive diagnosis** must be made by brain biopsy, which shows focal myelin loss with bizarre astrocytes and other changes. Suggestive CT findings include multiple nonenhancing lesions scattered throughout the white matter without mass effect. MRI shows lesions as hypodense in T1 images and hyperdense in T2 images [204]. **PCR detection of JC virus** has a diagnostic sensitivity of 70% to 80% and a specificity of virtually 100% [205] and is increasingly used in place of brain biopsy. The value of markers for JC-specific cellular and humoral immune responses, including VP-1, the major capsid protein of JCV, are being studied [206].

**C. There is no proven treatment** for PML. Prednisone, acyclovir, vidarabine, HLA-matched platelets, amantadine, IFN-$\alpha$, and cytarabine have not resulted in consistent improvement [207]. One study demonstrated clearance of JC virus DNA in five of six patients treated with HAART for 35 to 365 days [206]. Cytarabine did not affect survival [207,208]. Response to cidofovir has been disappointing; in a recent pilot study, cidofovir did not prolong PML survival beyond what has been reported without treatment [209]. Cidofovir added to HAART, however, has been associated with improved survival due to more effective control of JC virus replication [210]. **Improvement with HAART has been reported** and this is the treatment of choice [211,212].

**XX. Cryptosporidiosis** was considered a rare and insignificant protozoan infection prior to the AIDS epidemic. *Cryptosporidium parvum,* the parasite that causes human cryptosporidiosis, is now known to be ubiquitous. It is recognized as one of the most common enteric pathogens in humans and domesticated animals worldwide. Transmission is primarily by the fecal-oral route; numerous U.S. waterborne outbreaks in normal hosts have heightened awareness of this parasite's threat to public health [213]. Person-to-person transmission and animal-to-person transmission also have been described. The prevalence of cryptosporidiosis in HIV-infected patients was estimated to be 10% to 15% prior to the advent of HAART [214]. According to the CDC, the incidence of chronic cryptosporidiosis has decreased from 16.4 per 1,000 person-years in 1992 to 3.7 cases per 1,000 person-years in 1997 [17]. This decline is consistent with the decreasing rates of other OIs [215].

**A. Clinical presentation** varies depending on host immune status. Whereas immunocompetent patients have a transient illness, patients with AIDS have a spectrum of disease ranging from asymptomatic carriage to fulminant, persistent, cholera-like diarrhea [214]. *Cryptosporidium* causes diarrhea, nausea, vomiting, abdominal pain, and weight loss; fever is uncommon. Biliary tract involvement occurs in at least 15% of AIDS patients and results in severe right upper quadrant pain with protracted nausea and vomiting. Laboratory studies reveal an elevated alkaline phosphatase level, and ultrasonography demonstrates gallbladder wall thickening and dilated bile ducts [216,217]. CMV and microsporidia cause similar signs and symptoms, and often are concomitant pathogens.

**B. Diagnosis** is made by modified acid-fast stain of stool or other tissue specimens. Biopsy of the small intestine may be less sensitive than stool examination owing to focal intestinal involvement and the absence of inflammatory changes to guide the endoscopist. Immunofluorescent antibody assays and enzyme linked immunosorbent assays (ELISAs) are available; ELISA sensitivities range from 66% to 100% and specificities from 93% to 100% [218]. Serologic detection is primarily used as an investigational tool because antibody persistence limits its utility in diagnosis of acute infection. PCR assays have not undergone large clinical trials.

**C. Treatment.** There is no reliable palliative or curative therapy for cryptosporidiosis in immunodeficient hosts. There are numerous reports of limited success with the nonabsorbable aminoglycoside paromomycin, but its unpredictable activity and limitations in preventing extraintestinal spread have dampened enthusiasm. A recent controlled trial showed that 3 to 6 weeks of paromomycin was no more effective than placebo for treatment of symptomatic cryptosporidial enteritis in HIV-infected patients [219]. Lactose-free azithromycin was found to have some promise in a placebo-controlled trial, but further studies are needed. Other tested agents with marginal results include spiramycin, diclazuril, roxithromycin, allicin, and immunomodulatory therapies such as bovine colostral immunoglobulins and hyperimmune egg yolks [220–222]. Responses are usually transient or incomplete; therefore, symptomatic therapy with loperamide, opioids, and somatostatin analogues may be necessary. Restoration of immune function with HAART appears to be the most effective intervention, resulting in significant clinical, microbiologic, and histologic improvements [223].

**D. Prevention.** Patients with CD4 cell counts of less than 200/mm$^3$ should be educated about measures to reduce the risk for acquiring cryptosporidiosis (Table 18.6). **Chemoprophylaxis is not available,** although patients taking clarithromycin or rifabutin for MAC may have less cryptosporidiosis [1].

**XXI. Microsporidiosis.** *Microsporidium* species are pathogens of animals, but only since 1985 have they been recognized as an AIDS-associated infection [224,225]. At least 11 species are known to cause human disease, and serious illness is restricted to persons with abnormal immunity. In AIDS patients with chronic diarrhea, the prevalence of microsporidiosis has ranged from 4% to 50% [224] prior to HAART. Similar to cryptosporidiosis, the prevalence of microsporidiosis has dropped off dramatically with the use of HAART [17].

**A. Clinical presentation.** Over 90% of intestinal microsporidiosis is caused by *Enterocytozoon bieneusi.* Chronic diarrhea, anorexia, and weight loss are the most common manifestations [224]. *E. bieneusi* also has been associated with cholangitis and cholecystitis in AIDS patients. *Encephalitozoon hellem* appears to disseminate to lungs and kidneys and often spares the intestine [225]. *Septata intestinalis* involves the intestine but also causes disseminated disease [226]. *Pleistophora* and *Nosema* are rare in HIV-infected patients.

**B. Diagnosis** is by stool examination using special stains, including modifications of Weber chromotrope-based stains and other chemofluorescent agents. Such tests may be available only at reference laboratories or hospitals with a special interest in this diagnosis. Transmission electron microscopic examination of a small-bowel biopsy specimen is often used to confirm the diagnosis of microsporidiosis and to determine the genus and species. The specificity of serologic tests for antibodies to microsporidia is unknown, and their clinical utility is unclear.

C. **Treatment.** There is no effective therapy, but anecdotal reports suggest that albendazole (400 mg every 12 hours) for 2 to 4 weeks may be useful for certain microsporidial species. There are case reports of patients treated with azithromycin, metronidazole, atovaquone, furazolidone, and various other antibiotics [227]. Eradication of the parasite was reported with fumagilin, but follow-up found frequent relapses [228]. Although HAART is promising, its potential role in preventing microsporidiosis is unclear [223].

D. **Prevention** involves the same precautions as for cryptosporidiosis (Table 18.6). There is no effective chemoprophylaxis [1].

**XXII. Isosporiasis.** *Isospora belli* is an acid-fast coccidian protozoan that causes a clinical syndrome indistinguishable from cryptosporidiosis. Infection follows ingestion of food and water contaminated with human feces. Humans are the only known reservoir. Isosporiasis accounts for less than 1% of AIDS-defining illness in the United States [17], with higher prevalence in developing regions. Thus, precautions during overseas travel are indicated (Table 18.6). Profuse watery diarrhea, anorexia, malaise, and weight loss are common clinical findings. Atypical presentations include acalculous cholecystitis and reactive arthritis [229]. Isospora can be eradicated with trimethoprim-sulfamethoxazole therapy (one DS tablet four times daily for 10 days). Alternatively, pyrimethamine (75 mg daily) plus folinic acid (10 mg daily) may be successful. Because of a high relapse rate (up to 50% within 6–8 weeks), chronic suppression with trimethoprim-sulfamethoxazole (1 DS tablet three times per week) or pyrimethamine (25 mg/day) plus folinic acid (5 mg/day) is recommended.

**XXIII. Cyclosporiasis.** Infection caused by *Cyclospora cayetanensis,* an acid-fast coccidian, occurs worldwide but is relatively rare among AIDS patients in the United States [230,231]. The parasite is transmitted by the fecal-oral route, and likely acquired through contaminated water or food. Direct person-to-person transmission is unlikely because excreted oocytes require time outside the host to sporulate and become infective [232]. Clinical presentation is similar to cryptosporidiosis, microsporidiosis, or isosporiasis. Diagnosis requires identification of oocytes in the stool; *Cyclospora* (8 $\mu$m) is about twice the size of *Cryptosporidium* (4 $\mu$m). Repeat stool examinations may be necessary because the parasite is excreted intermittently and in low numbers. Tests for *Cyclospora* species, *Isospora* species, *Cryptosporidium* species, and *Microsporidia* should be requested specifically, in addition to routine stool ova and parasites, to ensure that specific methods to detect these organisms are applied. The only treatment is trimethoprim-sulfamethoxazole (1 DS tablet four times daily) for 10 days followed by one DS tablet three times a week indefinitely [231].

**XXIV. Syphilis** and HIV infection are uniquely associated. Epidemiologic studies have shown that a history of sexually transmitted diseases is associated with increased risk of HIV infection, and genital ulcerations caused by *Treponema pallidum* may facilitate HIV transmission [233–235]. In fact, recent *in vitro* studies have shown induction of HIV-1 gene expression in human monocytes by this spirochete [236]. HIV infection may alter the clinical course of syphilis, especially latent and tertiary disease [237–239]. Annual syphilis screening should be performed in HIV-infected patients due to high rates of coinfection [5,240].

A. **Clinical presentation** varies depending on the stage of HIV infection. Most HIV-infected patients with early syphilis have clinical manifestations comparable with those of primary and secondary lesions observed in HIV-uninfected persons [241]. A higher incidence of neurosyphilis may be seen, which may develop rapidly. Some case reports indicate that syphilis in HIV-infected patients can present with atypical lesions and in aggressive forms; the frequency of these atypical presentations, however, is unknown [238]. (See Chapters 6 and 16.)

B. **Diagnosis.** Serologic tests, patient history, clinical examination, and darkfield examination of tissue are all used. Serology remains a cornerstone of diagnosis.

1. **Venereal Disease Research Laboratory (VDRL)** test and the **rapid plasma reagin** test are nontreponemal screening tests. Up to 6% of HIV-infected patients have biologic false-positive test results [242].

False-negative results also occur, but are rare. The fluorescent **treponemal antibody-absorption test** and the **microhemagglutination *T. pallidum*** treponemal test detect antibodies directed against *T. pallidum* antigens. Treponemal tests are used to confirm reactive nontreponemal tests. Therefore, a negative test result does not always rule out current or previous infection. Once positive, treponemal test results usually stay positive for life, although some studies indicate that HIV-positive patients appear more likely to serorevert to negative following therapy [243]. In addition, microhemagglutinating antibody may be lost with progression of HIV disease.

2. **Dark-field examination** with biopsy of lesions may be useful when serologic tests are nonreactive but clinical suspicion remains high. Dark-field examination is the only means of practical, direct diagnosis.
3. **Lumbar puncture** is recommended for all patients with latent syphilis regardless of the apparent duration of infection [240]. CSF evaluation is also indicated for any HIV patient with unexplained behavioral changes or neurologic abnormalities. Diagnosis of **neurosyphilis** is made by a positive CSF serology, high protein level, or pleocytosis; however, there are many false-negative results [244].

C. **Treatment** with penicillin is recommended by the CDC whenever possible for all stages of syphilis in HIV-infected patients [240]. Furthermore, there are no proven alternatives to penicillin for treatment of congenital syphilis, neurosyphilis, or syphilis in pregnancy. Penicillin desensitization is recommended for these situations.

1. **Benzathine penicillin G** (2.4 million units intramuscularly) is recommended for primary or secondary syphilis in patients who have no evidence of neurosyphilis. A total of 7.2 million units (2.4 million units intramuscularly weekly for 3 weeks) is advised for treatment of non-neurologic latent syphilis regardless of apparent duration of infection.
2. **Follow-up nontreponemal serologies** should be obtained at 3, 6, 9, and 12 months. In HIV-positive patients, a slower decrease in serologic response may be seen, but clinical failures are rare [245,246]; reinfection is more common than relapse. However, even after proper therapy some patients have stable or increasing serologic titers. Therefore, careful long-term follow-up is essential, and repeated courses of penicillin may be needed [244]. Optimal therapy in this setting is not clear, and some experts advocate higher doses of penicillin for primary and secondary syphilis in the HIV-positive patient (see Chapter 16). Infectious disease consultation is suggested for complicated or puzzling cases.
3. **Treatment of neurosyphilis** is with high-dose i.v. penicillin G (3–4 million units every 4 hours) for 10 to 14 days. Penicillin-sensitive patients should be desensitized.

D. **Prevention.** Patients should be counseled on means to reduce the risk for sexually transmitted diseases (Table 18.6).

XXV. **Hepatitis C virus** infects approximately 4 million people in the United States, of whom an estimated 10,000 die each year [247,248]. HCV is a major pathogen in HIV-infected patients, reflecting shared epidemiologic risk factors. HCV is transmitted chiefly by percutaneous exposure to blood through injection drug use in the United States. Sexual transmission occurs less commonly. All HIV-infected patients should be screened for HCV because approximately 30% to 50% (about 240,000 persons in the United States) are coinfected [249,250]. Children born to coinfected mothers also should be screened for HCV. HIV is an important cofactor for HCV disease progression. Moreover, coinfected individuals have poorer responses to HAART compared with HIV-positive matched controls [251]. The majority of these patients will develop chronic hepatitis; others may progress to cirrhosis, hepatic decompensation, and hepatocellular carcinoma [252]. Awareness of HCV status is also important so that liver function abnormalities can be properly evaluated during HAART. Hepatotoxicity may be more common in persons with chronic HCV; some clinicians may be reluctant to use certain antiretroviral medications for fear of inducing severe hepatic damage. However, current data do not support withholding antiretroviral therapy in patients with concomitant HCV infection. Immune reconstitution hepatitis is also possible (see section **II.B.4**). Overall morbidity and mortality related to HCV among HIV-infected persons are substantial [247] (see also Chapter 14).

**A. Clinical presentation.** Most patients with chronic HCV are asymptomatic and unaware of their infection. Patients may complain of lethargy, inability to concentrate, or abdominal pain. Jaundice, encephalopathy, ascites, splenomegaly, or gastrointestinal bleeds secondary to portal hypertension indicate decompensated cirrhosis. Laboratory findings may include hypoalbuminemia, thrombocytopenia, coagulopathy, and elevated hepatic transaminases. **Extrahepatic manifestations** include mixed cryoglobulinemia, membranous proliferative glomerulonephritis, and porphyria cutanea tarda. Hepatocellular carcinoma should be suspected in patients with sudden decompensation in previously stable chronic liver disease and elevated $\alpha$-fetoprotein (see Chapters 13 and 14).

**B. Diagnosis** is made by detection of antibody to HCV in blood by EIA. EIA-positive patients should undergo confirmation testing with recombinant immunoblot assay or reverse transcriptase PCR for HCV RNA. Acute HCV, however, cannot be reliably diagnosed by antibody tests because of a prolonged window period. If clinical suspicion remains high despite negative HCV antibody test results, HCV RNA is useful. However, unlike HIV viral load, the HCV RNA quantitative level is not closely associated with outcome or overall prognosis. Similarly, the magnitude of alanine aminotransferase elevation or other abnormality in liver biochemistry does not correlate well with disease outcome or histologic changes. Liver biopsy provides information about degree of inflammation and the stage of fibrosis. A recent prospective study revealed that the combination of several basic serum markers ($\alpha_2$-macroglobulin, haptoglobin, $\gamma$-globulin, apolipoprotein $A_1$, $\gamma$-glutamyltranspeptidase, and total bilirubin) may have predictive value similar to liver biopsy in determining significant fibrosis [253].

**C. Treatment.** Despite advancements in treatment, the data regarding safety and efficacy in HIV-coinfected persons is limited. The majority of trials with IFN for chronic hepatitis C have excluded patients with HIV coinfection.

1. **Interferon-$\alpha$** was the first licensed treatment for HCV, but its mechanisms of action in viral hepatitis remain uncertain. About 15% to 20% of patients achieve a long-term or sustained virologic response with IFN monotherapy. A standard dosing regimen is 3 million units three times weekly for 6 months. Adverse events commonly associated with IFN therapy include self-limited, dose-dependent, flulike illness with mild fever, chills, headache, lethargy, arthralgias, and myalgias. Other important side effects include depression, irritability, anorexia, rash, and alopecia. Patients need to be warned about potential adverse events. Results of therapy in HIV-coinfected patients have been limited and mostly disappointing. In one prospective, controlled trial, a response rate of 38% was noted in coinfected patients compared with 47% in HIV-negative patients [254]. However, a sustained virologic response was diminished in both groups. Given the low sustained response rate, use of monotherapy has been abandoned in favor of combination therapy with ribavirin.
2. **Ribavirin** is an oral nucleoside analogue that is active *in vitro* against many RNA and DNA viruses. The precise mechanism of action of ribavirin in chronic hepatitis C is not well understood. The major toxic effect of ribavirin appears to be reversible, dose-dependent hemolytic anemia.
3. **Combination therapy with IFN-$\alpha$ and ribavirin,** which is approved by the U.S. Food and Drug Administration, is more effective than IFN alone [255]. Used together, sustained response rates increase to approximately 50%. Combination therapy in smaller series with HIV-infected patients is encouraging; larger controlled trials are currently under way.
4. **Pegylated IFN-$\alpha$** (PEG-IFN) is approved by the U.S. Food and Drug Administration, and is easier to administer because of a longer half-life [256]. Polyethylene glycol (PEG), an inert polymer, is covalently bonded to

standard IFN, resulting in delayed recognition as a foreign substance by the immune system, thus prolonging the half-life of PEG-IFN to approximately 54 hours compared with 8 hours for routine IFN-$\alpha$. PEG-IFN administered once weekly with daily ribavirin is now the treatment of choice in HIV-negative patients. Prospective multicenter trials comparing PEG-IFN alone, PEG-IFN plus ribavirin, and IFN plus ribavirin in HIV-infected populations are in progress.

5. Susceptible patients should be **vaccinated against hepatitis A and B** (see Table 18.13 for recommended childhood immunizations).
6. **Alcohol** consumption should be limited.

**D. Hepatotoxicity due to antiretroviral medications.** Zidovudine may be the most potentially hepatotoxic drug in the nucleoside analogue class. Among protease inhibitors, indinavir and ritonavir are hepatotoxic, and nelfinavir and saquinavir are much less so. Nevirapine and other non-nucleoside reverse transcriptase inhibitors are also potentially hepatotoxic [251] (see Chapter 19).

**E. Prevention.** Patients should be counseled on how to limit their risk for acquiring hepatitis C [1], and offered referral for substance abuse treatment when appropriate (Table 18.6). Risks from body piercing and tattooing, sharing needles, sharing dental equipment and razors, and sexual practices should be reviewed.

**XXVI. Bacillary angiomatosis (BA)** is a disease caused by small gram-negative organisms of the genus *Bartonella* (formerly *Rochalimaea*), specifically *B. henselae* and *B. quintana.* These vascular proliferative lesions can form in many different organs, including skin, bone, brain parenchyma, lymph nodes, bone marrow, and the gastrointestinal and respiratory tracts. Most patients with BA are significantly immunocompromised. In one study of 42 patients with BA, the median CD4 count was 21 cells/mm$^3$. Disseminated infection may be more common in immunosuppressed patients with a history of cat contact or homelessness.

**A. Clinical presentation** depends on the organ system involved.

1. **Cutaneous lesions** are raised erythematous areas that bleed when traumatized. They also can appear as a cellulitic plaque, which often overlies osteolytic lesions. They can occur singly or multiply and can occur in any location. These lesions are indolent and may be present for as long as 1 year before diagnosis is made. Most often they are confused with KS.
2. **Osseous BA,** often seen with cutaneous lesions, causes pain and radiologically lytic lesions. Bones most often affected include the tibia, fibula, and radius.
3. **Hepatic BA (peliosis hepatis)** is characterized histopathologically by cystic spaces of varying size filled with blood [257,258]. Patients present with abdominal pain, fever, and high alkaline phosphatase. CT demonstrates heterogeneity in the liver. Lesions are also seen in the spleen [259].
4. **Other manifestations** without vascular proliferation include necrotizing lymphadenitis, cat-scratch disease–type necrotizing infection, and bacteremias. Endocarditis has been reported in HIV-infected patients in the absence of cutaneous involvement.

**B. Diagnosis** is made by tissue biopsy and demonstration of the organisms by **Warthin-Starry stain.** Histopathologic evaluation demonstrates vascular proliferation that can be mistaken for KS, angiosarcoma, or pyogenic granuloma. The organism has been cultured from blood, but specimens need to be incubated at 35°C for 3 weeks. Use of the Isolator lysis centrifugation system may increase the yield of blood cultures, which should be incubated at least 14 days. Isolation of *Bartonella* species directly from cutaneous BA lesions is difficult because of the organism's fastidious growth characteristics. Indirect immunofluorescence assay to detect antibodies to *B. henselae* are useful for diagnosis of both acute disease and relapse [260]. PCR detection techniques remain experimental and are not routinely available.

**C. Treatment.** Clarithromycin (500 mg orally twice daily), azithromycin (250 mg orally daily), and fluoroquinolones are first-line therapy, although cures also have been reported with doxycycline, trimethoprim-sulfamethoxazole, and minocycline [261]. Despite *in vitro* susceptibility, penicillins and first-generation cephalosporins have no activity against *Bartonella.* Cutaneous lesions are treated for 8 to 12 weeks, and osseous and liver lesions are treated for at least 3 months [259]. However, the optimal duration of therapy is unknown. Rifampin may have a role when added to either erythromycin or doxycycline for severely ill patients. There have been numerous reports of relapse of *Bartonella* infection in immunocompromised patients. If relapse occurs in the HIV-infected patient, lifelong maintenance therapy with erythromycin or doxycycline is recommended.

**D. Prevention.** Patients should be counseled on the potential risks of cat ownership, and how to limit their exposure to this organism (Table 18.6). There is no known chemoprophylaxis for *Bartonella,* although the widespread use of macrolides for prophylaxis against MAC may decrease the incidence of BA. Secondary prophylaxis is not generally indicated unless there is relapse or reinfection.

**XXVII. Salmonellosis,** particularly bacteremias, is seen in higher frequency in HIV-infected patients and often presents without intestinal symptoms [262]. Nontyphoid *Salmonella* species, especially *S. enteritidis* and *S. typhimurium,* are isolated most often. Travelers' diarrhea may be a severe illness that is more resistant to therapy in HIV-infected patients [263]. One study found an increased risk of salmonellosis among HIV-positive persons who were residents of the Northeast, had a history of injection drug use, or were African American or Hispanic [264]. The incidence of *Salmonella* bacteremia has declined with the use of trimethoprim-sulfamethoxazole prophylaxis and antiretroviral therapy [265].

**A. The clinical course** in patients with AIDS is more severe than in normal hosts (see Chapter 13). Rates of bacteremia are increased, fever may persist for 1 to 2 weeks, and relapse rates are higher. Bacteremic relapse may be secondary to hidden foci of infection. Other sites of involvement include the prostate, heart, CNS, joints, parotids, and bones.

**B. Diagnosis** is made by bacterial culture of blood, stool, or urine. Other localized infections are diagnosed by culture of the appropriate anatomic site.

**C. Treatment** with ampicillin, quinolones, third-generation cephalosporins, or trimethoprim-sulfamethoxazole is effective. Therapy should extend for at least 7 to 10 days after defervescence. Some experts place all patients with salmonellosis on **chronic suppressive therapy** (Tables 18.2 and 18.4) [1]; others give suppressive therapy only to those with recurrent disease. Oral ciprofloxacin 500 mg twice daily in adults is recommended for susceptible isolates, although amoxicillin and trimethoprim-sulfamethoxazole are equally effective for chronic suppression (Table 18.2). Trimethoprim-sulfamethoxazole is the drug of choice for suppression in children (Table 18.4) [1]. Fluoroquinolones should not be used in children or during pregnancy (see Chapter 27).

**D. Prevention.** Steps to avoid acquisition of *Salmonella* should be reviewed with patients, including animal exposures, safe food handling, and during travel (Table 18.6). Household contacts with salmonellosis should be checked for chronic carriage of the organism to limit the risk for reinfection [1].

**XXVIII. AIDS-associated bacterial pneumonia.** Pulmonary infections cause significant morbidity and mortality in HIV-infected patients. Recurrent bacterial pneumonia as an AIDS-defining disease is defined as two or more episodes of bacterial pneumonia within 1 year, regardless of CD4 cell count [266,267]. Although the incidence of bacterial pneumonia has declined with widespread use of PCP and MAC prophylaxis [268], the rate of recurrent pneumonia was still approximately 20.2 cases per 1,000 person-years from 1992 to 1997 [17]. In contrast to PCP, bacterial pneumonia can occur at any CD4 cell level.

**A. Etiology.** *Streptococcus pneumoniae* is the most commonly identified cause. Pneumococcal bacteremia occurs at an approximately 100-fold greater rate in the HIV population [269,270]. Injection drug use is an independent risk factor for both bacterial pneumonia and pneumococcal bacteremia. Other pathogens causing bacterial pneumonia in HIV-infected patients include *Staphyloccocus aureus, Haemophilus influenzae,* and gram-negative organisms, most notably *Klebsiella* and *Pseudomonas* [271–273]. Patients with low CD4 cell counts have higher rates of *Pseudomonas aeruginosa* pneumonia, which is usually indolent, resembling infection in patients with cystic fibrosis, and may be recurrent [274,275]. Risk factors include CD4 cell counts of less than 50/mm$^3$, neutropenia, bronchiectasis, and corticosteroid therapy.

**B. Clinical presentation.** Bacterial pneumonia may be more severe when associated with HIV disease. Symptoms usually occur with abrupt onset and include fever, productive cough, dyspnea, and acute pleuritic chest pain. This is usually distinct from PCP, which typically is indolent and associated with dry cough and infrequent chest pain, but symptom overlap occurs. Thus, diagnosis should not be based only on clinical findings.

**C. Diagnosis** is based on radiographic findings and appropriate laboratory tests, including blood cultures and sputum Gram stains plus culture. A lobar infiltrate generally suggests bacterial pneumonia, but radiographic findings alone will not identify the cause. Blood cultures should be obtained in all patients. HIV patients with pneumonia have higher rates of bacteremia compared with HIV-negative individuals [276]. It is essential to identify the pathogen to appropriately treat the pneumonia and improve outcome. Invasive procedures such as bronchoscopy may be necessary, particularly in patients with poor response to therapy or when PCP is suspected (see Chapter 11).

**D. Empiric treatment** is warranted in order to improve the outcome (see Chapter 11). Selection of agents should be based on local patterns of drug resistance. Once the pathogen has been identified, appropriate adjustments in therapy should be made (see Chapter 11) [277].

**E. Prevention** (Tables 18.1, 18.3, and 18.13). Protection against *Streptococcus pneumoniae* is best achieved with pneumococcal vaccine (see also Chapter 11). However, efficacy is blunted by diminished antibody responses in patients with CD4 cell counts of less than 200/mm$^3$. *H. influenzae* type B vaccine is not generally recommended for adults because most infections involve nontypeable strains. Children should receive these vaccines according to current recommendations (Table 18.13) [1]. Trimethoprim-sulfamethoxazole used for PCP prophylaxis has coverage against several pathogens responsible for bacterial pneumonia (*Streptococcus, Haemophilus, Staphylococcus, Pseudomonas,* and *Klebsiella*). However, indiscriminate use, when not indicated for PCP prophylaxis, may lead to development of resistant organisms. Antibiotic prophylaxis or i.v. gamma globulin is not recommended to prevent bacterial pneumonia except in children with recurrent sinopulmonary or other serious bacterial infections (Tables 18.3 and 18.4) [1]. Annual influenza vaccine (Tables 18.1, 18.3, and 18.13) may help to prevent some bacterial pneumonias.

**XXIX. Malignancies associated with AIDS.** The association between certain malignancies and HIV infection was recognized early in the AIDS epidemic when **KS** was noted in homosexual men at a 20,000-fold increased rate compared with the pre-AIDS era [190]. Increased incidence of other cancers such as **squamous cell neoplasia,** particularly cervical and anal intraepithelial neoplasia (CIN, AIN), **non-Hodgkin lymphoma, Hodgkin disease,** and **primary CNS lymphoma** also has been well documented [278–280]. A correlation with viral coinfections exists with several of these malignancies. HHV-8 or KS herpesvirus promotes the development of KS, although the exact mechanism is not defined (see section **XVIII**). Moreover, certain types of **human papilloma virus** are associated with more advanced CIN lesions (CIN II and CIN III) and are found in the majority of cases of invasive carcinoma [281]. The presence of EBV has been reported in approximately 40% of systemic HIV-associated lymphomas and in a majority of primary CNS lymphomas [282].

Some AIDS-related malignancies have declined in frequency in the HAART era similar to other opportunistic infections. According to data from the ASD project, reductions were noted for KS and CNS lymphoma as a result of antiretroviral combinations, presumably by slowing the progression of HIV disease and delaying the onset of severe immunosuppression [283]. Lymphomas other than primary CNS lymphoma have not changed dramatically despite the widespread use of HAART. Similarly, available but limited data indicate no significant impact of HAART on

CIN or AIN. Although the presentation of malignancy in patients infected with HIV is often different from that seen in immunocompetent hosts, patients with controlled HIV and moderate CD4 counts generally are capable of tolerating full-dose chemotherapy and radiotherapy.

## REFERENCES


1. 1999 USPHS/IDSA guidelines for the prevention of opportunistic infections in persons infected with human immunodeficiency virus: United States Public Health Service (USPHS) and the Infectious Diseases Society of America (IDSA). *MMWR* 1999;48:1–66. Updated November 28, 2001 as a "living document" at *www.hivatis.org/trtgdlns.html#Opportunistic,* and in print as Guidelines for preventing opportunistic infections among HIV-infected persons–2002. *MMWR* 2002;51:(RR-8):1–52.
2. Masur H, Holmes KK, Kaplan JE. Introduction to the 1999 USPHS/IDSA guidelines for the prevention of opportunistic infections in persons infected with human immunodeficiency virus. *Clin Infect Dis* 2000;30(suppl):1–4.
3. Streicher HZ, Reitz MS, Gallo RC. Human immunodeficiency viruses. In: Mandell GL, Bennett JE, Dolin R, eds. *Principles and practice of infectious diseases,* 5th ed. Philadelphia: Churchill Livingstone, 2000:1874–1887.
4. Sande MA, Volberding PA. *The medical management of AIDS.* Philadelphia: WB Saunders, 1999.
5. Bartlett JG, Gallant JE. *2001–2002 Medical management of HIV infection.* Baltimore: Johns Hopkins University, 2001.
6. UNAIDS report on the global HIV/AIDS epidemic. Joint United Nations Programme on HIV/AIDS and World Health Organization (WHO), December 2001.
7. Sepkowitz KA. AIDS—the first 20 years. *N Engl J Med* 2001;344:1764–1772.
8. Armstrong D. Treatment of opportunistic infections. *Clin Infect Dis* 1993;16:1–7.
9. Murphy EL, Collier AC, Kalish LA, et al. Highly active antiretroviral therapy decreases mortality and morbidity in patients with advanced disease. *Ann Intern Med* 2001;135:17–26.
10. Sepkowitz KA. Effect of HAART on natural history of AIDS-related opportunistic disorders. *Lancet* 1998;351:228–230.
11. Sepkowitz KA, Armstrong D. Treatment of opportunistic infections in AIDS. *Lancet* 1995;346:588–589.
12. Kaplan JE, Masur H, Holmes KK, et al. An overview of the 1999 US Public Health Service/Infectious Diseases Society of America guidelines for preventing opportunistic infections in human immunodeficiency virus–infected persons. *Clin Infect Dis* 2000;30(suppl):15–28.
13. Palella FJ, Delaney KM, Moorman AC, et al. Declining morbidity and mortality among patients with advanced human immunodeficiency virus infection. *N Engl J Med* 1998;338:853–860.
14. Hogg RS, Shaughnessy MV, Gataric N, et al. Decline in deaths from AIDS due to new antiretrovirals. *Lancet* 1997;349:1294.
15. Detels R, Munoz A, Macfarlane G, et al. Effectiveness of potent antiretroviral therapy on time to AIDS and death in men with known HIV duration. *JAMA* 1998;280:1497–1503.
16. Selik RM. Trends in fatal infectious diseases among persons dying of HIV infection in the era of HAART. Paper presented at the 7th CROI, San Francisco, CA, 2000.
17. Jones JL, Hanson DL, Dworkin MS, et al. Surveillance for AIDS-defining opportunistic illnesses, 1992–1997. *MMWR* 1999;48:1–22.
18. Currier JS. Discontinuing prophylaxis for opportunistic infection: guiding principles. *Clin Infect Dis* 2000;30(suppl):66–71.
19. Kovacs JA, Masur H. Prophylaxis against opportunistic infections in patients with human immunodeficiency virus infection. *N Engl J Med* 2000;342:1416–1429.
20. Powderly WG. Prophylaxis for opportunistic infections in an era of effective antiretroviral therapy. *Clin Infect Dis* 2000;31:597–601.
21. 1995 USPHS/IDSA guidelines for the prevention of opportunistic infections in persons infected with human immunodeficiency virus: United States Public Health

Service (USPHS) and the Infectious Diseases Society of America (IDSA). *MMWR* 1995;44:1–34.

22. Ledergerber B, Egger M, Erard V, et al. AIDS-related opportunistic illnesses occurring after initiation of potent antiretroviral therapy. *JAMA* 1999;282:2220–2226.
23. Lederman MM, Valdez H. Immune restoration with antiretroviral therapies. *JAMA* 2000;284:223–228.
24. Powderly WG, Landay A, Lederman MM. Recovery of the immune system with antiretroviral therapy: the end of opportunism? *JAMA* 1998;280:72–77.
25. Race EM, Adelson-Mitty J, Kriegel GR, et al. Focal mycobacterial lymphadenitis following initiation of protease-inhibitor therapy in patients with advanced HIV-1 disease. *Lancet* 1998;351:252–255.
26. Narita M, Ashkin D, Hollender ES, et al. Paradoxical worsening of tuberculosis following antiretroviral therapy in patients with AIDS. *Am J Respir Crit Care Med* 1998;158:157–161.
27. Afghani B, Lieberman JM. Paradoxical enlargement or development of intracranial tuberculomas during therapy. *Clin Infect Dis* 1994;19:1092–1099.
28. Johnson SC, Benson CA, Johnson DW, et al. Recurrences of cytomegalovirus retinitis in a human immunodeficiency virus-infected patient, despite potent antiretroviral therapy and apparent immune reconstitution. *Clin Infect Dis* 2001;32:815–819.
29. Karavellas MP, Plummer DJ, MacDonald JC, et al. Incidence of immune recovery vitritis in cytomegalovirus retinitis following institution of successful highly active antiretroviral therapy. *J Infect Dis* 1999;179:697–700.
30. John M, Flexman J, French M. Hepatitis C virus–associated hepatitis following treatment of HIV-infected patients with HIV protease inhibitors: an "immune restoration disease"? *AIDS* 1998;12:2289–2293.
31. Mastroianni CM, Trinchieri V, Santopadre P, et al. Acute clinical hepatitis in an HIV-seropositive hepatitis B carrier receiving protease inhibitor therapy. *AIDS* 1998;12: 1939–1940.
32. Carr A, Cooper DA. Restoration of immunity to chronic hepatitis B infection in HIV-infected patient on protease inhibitors. *Lancet* 1997;349:995–996.
33. Domingo P, Torres OH, Ris J, et al. Herpes zoster as an immune reconstitution disease after initiation of combination antiretroviral therapy in patients with human immunodeficiency virus type-1 infection. *Am J Med* 2001;110:605–609.
34. Martinez E, Gatell JM, Moran T, et al. High incidence of herpes zoster in patients with AIDS soon after therapy with protease inhibitors. *Clin Infect Dis* 1998;27:1510–1513.
35. Bouscaret F, Maubec E, Matheron S, et al. Immune recovery inflammatory folliculitis. *AIDS* 2000;14:617–618.
36. Pneumocystis pneumonia—Los Angeles. *MMWR* 1981;30:250–252.
37. Gottlieb MS, et al. *Pneumocystis carinii* pneumonia and mucosal candidiasis in previously healthy homosexual men: evidence of a new acquired cellular immunodeficiency. *N Engl J Med* 1981;305:1425–1431.
38. Kovacs JA, Masur H. Prophylaxis for *Pneumocystis carinii* pneumonia in patients with human immunodeficiency virus. *Clin Infect Dis* 1992;14:1005.
39. Garay SM, Greene J. Prognostic indicators in the initial presentation of *Pneumocystis carinii* pneumonia. *Chest* 1989;95:769.
40. Kagawa FT, Kirsch CM, Yenokida GG, et al. Serum lactate dehydrogenase activity in patients with AIDS and *Pneumocystis carinii* pneumonia: an adjunct to diagnosis. *Chest* 1988;94:1031.
41. Chaffey MH, Klein JS, Gamsu G, et al. Radiographic distribution of *Pneumocystis carinii* pneumonia in patients with AIDS treated with prophylactic inhaled pentamidine. *Radiology* 1990;175:715.
42. Telzak EE, Cote RJ, Gold JW, et al. Extrapulmonary *Pneumocystis carinii* infections. *Rev Infect Dis* 1990;12:380–386.
43. Northfelt DW, Clement MJ, Safrin S. Extrapulmonary pneumocystosis: clinical features in human immunodeficiency virus infection. *Medicine* 1990;69:392–398.
44. Noskin GA, Murphy RL. Extrapulmonary infection with *Pneumocystis carinii* in patients receiving aerosolized pentamidine. *Rev Infect Dis* 1991;13:525.
45. O'Brien RF, Quinn JL, Miyahara BT, et al. Diagnosis of *Pneumocystis carinii* pneumonia by induced sputum in a city with moderate incidence of AIDS. *Chest* 1989;95:136.

46. Bigby TD, Margolskee D, Curtis JL, et al. The usefulness of induced sputum in the diagnosis of *Pneumocystis carinii* pneumonia in patients with acquired immunodeficiency syndrome. *Am Rev Respir Dis* 1986;133:515.
47. Moser E, Tatsch K, Kirsch CM, et al. Value of 67gallium scintigraphy in primary diagnosis and follow-up of opportunistic pneumonia in patients with AIDS. *Lung* 1990;168:692–703.
48. Kramer EL, Sanger JJ, Garay SM, et al. Gallium-67 scans of the chest in patients with acquired immunodeficiency syndrome. *J Nucl Med* 1987;28:1107–1114.
49. Larsen HH, Masur H, Kovacs JA, et al. Development and evaluation of a quantitative, touch-down, real-time PCR assay for diagnosing *Pneumocystis carinii* pneumonia. *J Clin Microbiol* 2002;40:490–494.
50. Mei Q, Gurunathan S, Masur H, et al. Failure of co-trimoxazole in *Pneumocystis carinii* infection and the mutations in dihydropterase synthase gene. *Lancet* 1998;351:1631–1632.
51. Helweg-Larsen J, Benfield TL, Eugen-Olsen J, et al. Effects of mutations in *Pneumocystis carinii* dihydropteroate synthase gene on outcome of AIDS-associated *P. carinii* pneumonia. *Lancet* 1999;354:1347–1351.
52. Masur H, Meier P, McCutchan JA, et al. Consenus statement on the use of corticosteroids as adjunctive therapy for pneumocystic pneumonia in acquired immunodeficiency syndrome. *N Engl J Med* 1990;323:1500–1504.
53. Furrer H, Egger M, Opravil M, et al. Discontinuation of prophylaxis for *Pneumocystis carinii* pneumonia in HIV-1 infected adults treated with combination antiretroviral therapy. *N Engl J Med* 1999;340:1301–1306.
54. Ledergerber B, Mocroft A, Reiss P, et al. Discontinuation of secondary prophylaxis against *Pneumocystis carinii* pneumonia in patients with HIV infection who have a response to antiretroviral therapy. *N Engl J Med* 2001;344:168–174.
55. Lopez Bernaldo de Quiros J, Miro JM, Pena JM, et al. A randomized trial of the discontinuation of primary and secondary prophylaxis against *Pneumocystis carinii* pneumonia after highly active antiretroviral therapy in patients with HIV infection. *N Engl J Med* 2001;344:159–167.
56. Schneider MME, Borleffs JCC, Stolk RP, et al. Discontinuation of prophylaxis for *Pneumocystis carinii* pneumonia in HIV-1 infected patients treated with highly active antiretroviral therapy. *Lancet* 1999;353:210–213.
57. Weverling GJ, Mocroft A, Ledergerber B, et al. Discontinuation of *Pneumocystis carinii* pneumonia prophylaxis after start of highly active antiretroviral therapy in HIV-1 infection. *Lancet* 1999;353:1293–1298.
58. Yangco BG, Von Bargen JC, Moorman AC, et al. Discontinuation of chemoprophylaxis against *Pneumocystis carinii* pneumonia in patients with HIV infection. HIV Outpatient Study (HOPS) Investigators. *Ann Intern Med* 2000;132:201–205.
59. Wilcox CM. Esophageal disease in the acquired immunodeficiency syndrome: etiology, diagnosis, and management. *Am J Med* 1992;92:412–421.
60. Coleman DC, Sullivan DJ, Bennett DE. Candidiasis: the emergence of a novel species, *Candida dubliniensis. AIDS* 1997;11:557–567.
61. Vasquez JA, Peng G, Sobel JD, et al. Evolution of antifungal susceptibility among *Candida* species isolates recovered from human immunodeficiency virus–infected women receiving fluconazole prophylaxis. *Clin Infect Dis* 2001;33:1069–1075.
62. Iman W. Hierarchical pattern of mucosal *Candida* infections in HIV seropositive women. *Am J Med* 1990;89:142–146.
63. Darouiche RO. Oropharyngeal and esophageal candidiasis in immunocompromised patients: treatment issues. *Clin Infect Dis* 1998;26:259–274.
64. Fichtenbaum CJ, Powderly WG. Refractory mucosal candidiasis in patients with human immunodeficiency virus infection. *Clin Infect Dis* 1998;26:556–565.
65. Dodds ES, Drew RH, Perfect JR. Antifungal pharmacodynamics: review of the literature and clinical applications. *Pharmacotherapy* 2000;20:1335–1355.
66. Onishi J, Meinz M, Thompson J, et al. Discovery of novel antifungal (1,3)-beta-D-glucan synthase inhibitors. *Antimicrob Agents Chemother* 2000;44:368–377.
67. Laine L, Dretler RH, Conteas CN, et al. Fluconazole compared with ketoconazole for the treatment of *Candida* esophagitis in AIDS. A randomized trail. *Ann Intern Med* 1992;117:655–660.

68. Zumla A, Malon P, Henderson J, et al. Impact of HIV infection on tuberculosis. *Postgrad Med J* 200;76:259–268.
69. Small PM, Fujiwara PI. Management of tuberculosis in the United States. *N Engl J Med* 2001;345:189–200.
70. Whalen C, Horsburgh CR, Hom D, et al. Accelerated course of human immunodeficiency virus infection after tuberculosis. *Am J Respir Crit Care Med* 1995;151:129–135.
71. Surveillance reports: the reported tuberculosis in the United States, 2000. Division of Tuberculosis Elimination, National Center for HIV, STD and TB Prevention, CDC website: *www.cdc.gov/nchstp/tb/surv/surv2000.*
72. Centers for Disease Control and Prevention. Prevention and treatment of tuberculosis among patients infected with human immunodeficiency virus: principles of therapy and revised recommendations. *MMWR* 1998;47:1–58.
73. Havlir DV, Barnes PE. Tuberculosis in patients with human immunodeficiency virus infection *N Engl J Med* 1999;340:367–373.
74. Sepkowitz KA, Telzak EE, Recalde S, et al. Tuberculosis susceptibility trends in New York City, 1987–1991. *Clin Infect Dis* 1994;18:755–759.
75. Sepkowitz KA. Tuberculosis and the health care worker: a historical perspective. *Ann Intern Med* 1994;120:71–79.
76. Bloch AB et al. Nationwide survey of drug-resistant tuberculosis in the United States. *JAMA* 1994;271:665–671.
77. Iseman MD. Treatment of multi-drug resistant tuberculosis. *N Engl J Med* 1993; 329:784–791.
78. Fitzgerald JM, Grzybowski S, Allen EA. The impact of human immunodeficiency virus infection on tuberculosis and its control. *Chest* 1991;100:1991–2000.
79. Finch D, Beaty CD. The utility of a single sputum specimen in the diagnosis of tuberculosis; comparison between HIV-infected and non–HIV-infected patients. *Chest* 1997;111:1174–1179.
80. Burman WJ, Gallicano K, Peloquin C. Therapeutic implications of drug interactions in the treatment of human immunodeficiency virus-related tuberculosis. *Clin Infect Dis* 1999;28:419–430.
81. Centers for Disease Control and Prevention. Acquired rifamycin resistance in persons with advanced HIV disease being treated for active tuberculosis with intermittent rifamycin-based regimens. *MMWR* 2002;51:214–215.
82. Gordin FM, Nelson ET, Matts JP, et al. The impact of human immunodeficiency virus infection on drug resistant tuberculosis. *Am J Respir Crit Care Med* 1996;154:1478–1483.
83. Benson CA, Ellner JJ. *Mycobacterium avium* complex infection and AIDS: advances in theory and practice. *Clin Infect Dis* 1993;17:7–20.
84. Havlir DV, Dube MP, Sattler FR, et al. Prophylaxis against disseminated *Mycobacterium avium* complex with weekly azithromycin, daily rifabutin, or both. *N Engl J Med* 1996;335:392.
85. Gordin FM, Cohn DL, Sullam PM, et al. Early manifestations of disseminated *Mycobacterium avium* complex disease: a prospective evaluation. *J Infect Dis* 1997;176:126–132.
86. Ward TT, Rimland D, Kauffman C, et al. Randomized open-label trial of azithromycin plus ethambutol vs. clarithromycin plus ethambutol as therapy for *Mycobacterium avium* complex bacteremia in patients with human immunodeficiency virus infection. *Clin Infect Dis* 1998;27:1278–1285.
87. May T, Brel F, Beuscart C, et al. Comparison of combination therapy regimens for treatment of human immunodeficiency virus–infected patients with disseminated bacteremia due to *Mycobacterium avium. Clin Infect Dis* 1997;25:621–629.
88. Benson CA. Treatment of disseminated disease due to the *Mycobacterium avium* complex in patients with AIDS. *Clin Infect Dis* 1994;18(suppl):237–242.
89. Chiu J, Nussbaum J, Bozzette S, et al. Treatment of disseminated *Mycobacterium avium* complex infection in AIDS with amikacin, ethambutol, rifampin, and ciprofloxacin. *Ann Intern Med* 1990;113:358.
90. Benson CA, Williams PL, Cohn DL, et al. Clarithromycin or rifabutin alone or in combination for primary prophylaxis of *Mycobacterium avium* compex disease in

patients with AIDS: a randomized, double-blind, placebo-controlled trial. *J Infect Dis* 2000;181:1289–1297.
91. Chassion RE, Benson CA, Dube MP, et al. Clarithromycin therapy for bacteremic *Mycobacterium avium* complex disease. A randomized, double-blind, dose-ranging study in patients with AIDS. *Ann Intern Med* 1994;121:905–911.
92. Nightingale SD, Cameron DW, Gordin FM, et al. Two controlled trials of rifabutin prophylaxis *Mycobacterium avium* complex infection in AIDS. *N Engl J Med* 1993;329:828–833.
93. Hewitt RG, Papandonatos GD, Shelton MJ, et al. Prevention of disseminated *Mycobacterium avium* complex infection with reduced dose clarithromycin in patients with advanced HIV disease. *AIDS* 1999;13:1367–1372.
94. El-Sadr WM, Burman W, Grant L, et al. Discontinuation of prophylaxis against *Mycobacterium avium* complex disease in HIV-infected patients who have a response to antiretroviral therapy. *N Engl J Med* 2000;342:1085–1092.
95. Shafran SD, Gill MJ, Lajonde RG, et al. Successful discontinuation of MAC therapy following effective HAART [Abstract 547]. Presented at the 8th Conference on Retroviruses and Opportunistic Infections, February 4–8, 2001, Chicago, Illinois.
96. Levine B, Chaisson RE. *Mycobacterium kansasii*: a cause of treatable pulmonary disease associated with advanced human immunodeficiency virus infection. *Ann Intern Med* 1991;114:861–868.
97. Bamberger DM, Driks MR, Gupta MR, et al. *Mycobacterium kansasii* among patients infected with human immunodeficiency virus in Kansas City. *Clin Infect Dis* 1994;18:395–400.
98. Strauss WL, Ostroff SM, Jernigan DB, et al. Clinical and epidemiologic characteristics of *Mycobacterium haemophilum,* an emerging pathogen in immunocompromised patients. *Ann Intern Med* 1994;120:118–125.
99. Dever LL, et al. Varied presentations and responses to treatment of infections caused by *Mycobacterium haemophilum* in patients with AIDS. *Clin Infect Dis* 1992;14:1195–2000.
100. Bernard EM, Edwards FF, Kiehn TE, et al. Activities of antimicrobial agents against clinical isolates of *Mycobacterium haemophilum*. *Antimicrob Agents Chemother* 1993;37:2323.
101. Piersimoni C, Tortoli E, de Lalla F, et al. Isolation of *Mycobacterium celatum* from patients infected with human immunodeficiency virus. *Clin Infect Dis* 1997;24:144.
102. Pechere M, Opravil M, Wald A, et al. Clinical and epidemiologic features of infection with *Mycobacterium genavense. Arch Intern Med* 1995;155:400.
103. Bottger EC, Teske A, Kirschner P, et al. Disseminated *Mycobacterium genavense* infection in patients with AIDS. *Lancet* 1992;340:76.
104. Jacobsen MA, Mills J. Serious cytomegalovirus disease in the acquired immunodeficiency syndrome. *Ann Intern Med* 1988;108:58.
105. Reichert CM, et al. Autopsy pathology in the acquired immune deficiency syndrome. *Am J Pathol* 1983;12:357.
106. Palestine AG, Polis MA, DeSmet MD, et al. A randomized, controlled trial of foscarnet in the treatment of cytomegalovirus retinitis in patients with AIDS. *Ann Intern Med* 1991;115:665–673.
107. Zurlo JJ, O'Neill D, Polis MA, et al. Lack of clinical utility of cytomegalovirus blood and urine cultures in patients with HIV infection. *Ann Intern Med* 1993;118:12–17.
108. Back MC, et al. 9-(1,3-Dihydroxy-2-propoxymethyl) guanine for cytomegalovirus infections in patients with immunodeficiency syndrome. *Ann Intern Med* 1985;103:381–382.
109. Whitcup SM, Fortin E, Linblad AS, et al. Discontinuation of anticytomegalovirus therapy in patients with HIV infection and cytomegalovirus retinitis. *JAMA* 1999;282:1633–1637.
110. Bloom JN, Palestine AG. The diagnosis of cytomegalovirus retinitis. *Ann Intern Med* 1988;109:963.
111. Bowen EF, Sabin CA, Wilson P, et al. Cytomegalovirus (CMV) viremia detected by polymerase chain reaction identifies a group of HIV-positive patients at high risk for CMV disease. *AIDS* 1997;11:889–893.

112. Jacobsen MA. Treatment of cytomegalovirus retinitis in patients with acquired immunodeficiency syndrome. *N Engl J Med* 1997;337:105–114.
113. Lalezari JP, Staag RJ, Kuppermann BD, et al. Intravenous cidofovir for peripheral cytomegalovirus retinitis in patients with AIDS—a randomized controlled trial. *Ann Intern Med* 1997;126:257–263.
114. Musch DC, Martin DF, Gordon JF, et al. The Ganciclovir Implant Study Group. Treatment of cytomegalovirus retinitis with a sustained-release ganciclovir implant. *N Engl J Med* 1997;337:83–90.
115. Curran M, Noble S. Valganciclovir. *Drugs* 2001;61:1145–1150.
116. Martin DF, Sierra-Madero J, Walmsley S, et al. A controlled trial of valganciclovir as induction therapy for cytomegalovirus retinitis. *N Engl J Med* 2002;346:1119–1126.
117. Piascik P. Fomivirsen sodium approved to treat CMV retinitis. *J Am Pharm Assoc* 1999;39:84–85.
118. Whitley RJ, Jacobsen MA. Friedberg DN, et al. Guidelines for the treatment of cytomegalovirus diseases in patients with AIDS in the era of potent antiretroviral therapy. *Arch Intern Med* 1998;158:957.
119. MacDonald JC, Torriani FJ, Morse LS, et al. Lack of reactivation of cytomegalovirus (CMV) retinitis after stopping CMV maintenance therapy in AIDS patients with sustained elevation in CD4$^{+}$cells in response to highly active antiretroviral therapy. *J Infect Dis* 1998;177:1182–1187.
120. Jacobson MA, Zegans M, Pavan PR, et al. Cytomegalovirus retinitis after initiation of highly active antiretroviral therapy. *Lancet* 1997;349:1443–1445.
121. Goodgame RW. Gastrointestinal cytomegalovirus disease. *Ann Intern Med* 1993; 119:924–935.
122. Rodriquez-Barradas MC, Stool E, Musher DM, et al. Diagnosing and treating cytomegalovirus pneumonia in patients with AIDS. *Clin Infect Dis* 1996;23:76–81.
123. Miles PR, Baughman RP, Lindeneman CC. Cytomegalovirus in the bronchoalveolar lavage fluid of patients with AIDS. *Chest* 1990;97:1072.
124. Wilcox CM, Staub RF, Schwartz DA. Cytomegalovirus esophagitis in AIDS: a prospective evaluation of clinical responses to ganciclovir therapy, relapse rate, and long-term outcome. *Am J Med* 1995;98:169–176.
125. Berman SM, Kim RC. The development of cytomegalovirus encephalitis in AIDS patients receiving ganciclovir. *Am J Med* 1994;96:415–419.
126. McCutchan JA. Clinical aspects of cytomegalovirus infections of the nervous system in patients with AIDS. *Clin Infect Dis* 1995;21(suppl):196–201.
127. Kalayjian RC, Cohen ML, Bonomo RA, et al. Cytomegalovirus ventriculoencephalitis in AIDS. A syndrome with distinct clinical and pathologic features. *Medicine* 1993;72:67–77.
128. Price TA, Digioia RA, Simon GL. Ganciclovir treatment of cytomegalovirus ventriculitis in a patient infected with human immunodeficiency virus. *Clin Infect Dis* 1992;15(4):606–608.
129. Kim YS, Hollander H. Polyradiculopathy due to CMV: report of two cases in which improvement occurred after prolonged therapy and review of the literature. *Clin Infect Dis* 1993;17:32–37.
130. DeGans J, et al. Predominance of polymorphonuclear leukocytes in cerebrospinal fluid of AIDS patients with cytomegalovirus polyradiculomyelitis. *J AIDS* 1990;12:1155–1158.
131. Wolf OG, Spector SA. Diagnosis of human CMV central nervous system disease in AIDS patients by DNA amplification from cerebrospinal fluid. *J Infect Dis* 1992;166:1412–1415.
132. Fuller GN, et al. Ganciclovir for lumbosacral polyradiculopathy in AIDS. *Lancet* 1990;335:48–49.
133. Bricaire F, et al. Adrenal cortical lesions and AIDS. *Lancet* 1988;1:881.
134. Luft BJ, Hafner R, Korzun AH, et al. Toxoplasmic encephalitis in patients with the acquired immunodeficiency syndrome. *N Engl J Med* 1993;329:995–1000.
135. Luft BJ, Remington JS. Toxoplasmic encephalitis. *J Infect Dis* 1988;157:1.
136. Carr A, Tindall B, Brew BJ, et al. Low-dose trimethoprim-sulfamethoxazole prophylaxis for toxoplasmic encephalitis in patients with AIDS. *Ann Intern Med* 1992;117:106–111.

137. Oksenhendler E, Charreau I, Tournerie C, et al. *Toxoplasma gondii* infection in advanced HIV infection. *AIDS* 1994;8:483–437.
138. Jacobson MA, Besch CL, Child C, et al. Primary prophylaxis for toxoplasmic encephalitis in patients with advanced HIV disease: results of a randomized trial. *J Infect Dis* 1994;169:384–394.
139. Rabaud C, May T, Amiel C, et al. Extracerebral toxoplasmosis in patients infected with HIV. *Medicine* 1994;73:306.
140. Lucet JC, Bailly MP, Bedos JP, et al. Septic shock due to toxoplasmosis in patients infected with human immunodeficiency virus. *Chest* 1993;104:1054.
141. Derouin F, Thylliez P, Garin YJF. Value and limitations of toxoplasmosis serology in HIV patients. *Pathol Biol* 1991;39:255–259.
142. Elkin CM, Leon E, Grenell SL, et al. Intracranial lesions in acquired immunodeficiency syndrome: radiologic (CT) features. *JAMA* 1985;253:393.
143. Kupfer MC, Zee CS, Colletti PM, et al. MRI evaluations of AIDS-related encephalopathy: toxoplasmosis vs. lymphoma. *MRI* 1990;8:51.
144. Ruiz A, Ganz WI, Post MJ, et al. Use of thallium-201 brain SPECT to differentiate cerebral lymphoma from toxoplasma encephalitis in AIDS patients. *Am J Neuroradiol* 1994;15:1885–1894.
145. Licho R, Litofsky NS, Senitko M, et al. Inaccuracy of Tl-201 brain SPECT in distinguishing cerebral infections from lymphoma in patients with AIDS. *Clin Nucl Med* 2002;27:81–86.
146. Pierce MA, Johnson MD, Maciunas RJ, et al. Evaluating contrast-enhancing brain lesions in patients with AIDS by using positron emission tomography. *Ann Intern Med* 1995;123:594–598.
147. Tirard V, Niel G, Rosenheim M, et al. Diagnosis of toxoplasmosis in patients with AIDS by isolation of the parasite from the blood. *N Engl J Med* 1991;324:634.
148. Cristina N, Pelloux H, Goulhot C, et al. Detection of *Toxoplasma gondii* in AIDS patients by polymerase chain reaction. *Infection* 1993;21:150–153.
149. Parmly S, Goebel F, Remington J. Detection of *Toxoplasmic gondii* in cerebrospinal fluid from AIDS patients by polymerase chain reaction. *J Clin Microbiol* 1992;30:3000–3002.
150. Burg JL, Grover CM, Pouletty P, et al. Direct and sensitive detection of a pathogenic protozoan, *Toxoplasma gondii* by polymerase chain reaction. *J Clin Microbiol* 1989; 27:1787.
151. Dupouy-Camet J, Lavareda de Souza S, Maslo C, et al. Detection of *Toxoplasma gondii* in venous blood from AIDS patients by polymerase chain reaction. *J Clin Microbiol* 1993;31:1866.
152. Dismukes WE. Cryptococcal meningitis in patients with AIDS. *J Infect Dis* 1988; 157:624.
153. Powderly WG. Cryptococcal meningitis and AIDS. *Clin Infect Dis* 1993;17:837–842.
154. Saag MS, Powderly WG, Cloud GA, et al. Comparison of amphotericin B with fluconazole in the treatment of acute AIDS-associated cryptococcal meningitis. *N Engl J Med* 1992;326:83–89.
155. Powderly WG, Cloud GA, Dismukes WE, et al. Value of serum and cerebrospinal fluid cryptococcal antigen measurement in the management of AIDS-associated cryptococcal meningitis. *Clin Infect Dis* 1994;18:789–792.
156. Chuck SL, Sande MA. Infections with Cryptococcal neoformans in the acquired immunodeficiency syndrome. *N Engl J Med* 1989;321:794–799.
157. Saag MS, Cloud GA, Graybil JR, et al. A comparison of itraconazole versus fluconazole as maintenance therapy for AIDS-associated cryptococcal meningitis. *Clin Infect Dis* 1999;28:291–296.
158. Saag MS, Graybill RJ, Larsen RA, et al. Practice guidelines for the management of cryptococcal disease. Infectious Diseases Society of America. *Clin Infect Dis* 2000;30:710–718.
159. Hajjeh RA, Pappas PG, Henderson H, et al. Multicenter case-control study of risk factors for histoplasmosis in human immunodeficiency virus–infected persons. *Clin Infect Dis* 2001;32:1215–1220.
160. Wheat LJ, Connolly-Stringfield PA, Baker RL, et al. Disseminated histoplasmosis in

the acquired immune deficiency syndrome: clinical findings, diagnosis and treatment, and review of the literature. *Medicine* 1990;69:361–373.

161. Wheat LJ, Chetchotisakd P, Williams B, et al. Factors associated with severe manifestations of histoplasmosis in AIDS. *Clin Infect Dis* 2000;30:877–881.
162. Suh KN, Anekthananon T, Mariuz PR. Gastrointestinal histoplasmosis in patients with AIDS: case report and review. *Clin Infect Dis* 2001;32:483–491.
163. Wheat LJ, Connolly-Stringfield PA, Kohler RB, et al. *Histoplasma capsulatum* polysaccharide antigen detection in diagnosis and management of disseminated histoplasmosis in patients with acquired immunodeficiency syndrome. *Am J Med* 1989;87:360–400.
164. Wheat LJ, Connolly-Stringfield PA, Blair R, et al. Histoplasmosis relapse in patients with AIDS: detection using *Histoplasma capsulatum* variety capsulatum antigen levels. *Ann Intern Med* 1991;115:936–941.
165. Mocherla S, Wheat LJ. Treatment of histoplasmosis. *Semin Respir Infect* 2001;16: 141–148.
166. Wheat LJ, Connolly P, Smedema M, et al. Emergence of resistance to fluconazole as a cause of failure during treatment of histoplasmosis in patients with acquired immunodeficiency disease syndrome. *Clin Infect Dis* 2001;33:1910–1913.
167. McKinsey DS, Kaufmann CA, Pappas et al. Fluconazole therapy for histoplasmosis. *Clin Infect Dis* 1996;23:996–1001.
168. Bronnimann DA, Adam RD, Galgiani JN, et al. Coccidioidomycosis in the acquired immunodeficiency syndrome. *Ann Intern Med* 1987;106:372–379.
169. Fish DG, Ampel NM, Galgiani JN, et al. Coccidioidomycosis during HIV infection: a review of 77 patients. *Medicine* 1990;69:384–391.
170. Tucker RM, Galgiani JN, Denning DW, et al. Treatment of coccidioidal meningitis with fluconazole. *Rev Infect Dis* 1990;12(suppl):380–389.
171. Galgiani JN, Catanazaro A, Cloud GA, et al. Comparison of oral fluconazole and itraconazole for progressive, nonmeningeal coccidioidomycosis. A randomized, double-blind trial. Mycoses Study Group. *Ann Intern Med* 2000;133:676–686.
172. Galgiani JN, Ampel NM, Catanazaro A, et al. Practice guideline for the treatment of coccidioidomycosis. Infectious Diseases Society of America. *Clin Infect Dis* 2000;30:658–661.
173. Pappas PG, Pottage JC, Powderly WG, et al. Blastomycosis in patients with the acquired immunodeficiency syndrome. *Ann Intern Med* 1992;116:847–853.
174. Tan G, Kaufman L, Peterson EM, et al. Disseminated atypical blastomycosis in two patients with AIDS. *Clin Infect Dis* 1993;16:107–111.
175. Chapman SW, Bradsher RW Jr, Campbell GD, et al. Practice guidelines for the management of patients with blastomycosis. Infectious Diseases Society of America. *Clin Infect Dis* 2000;30:679–683.
176. Kok I, Veenstra J, Rietra PJ, et al. Disseminated *Penicillium marneffei* infection as an imported disease in HIV-1 infected patients: description of two cases and a review of the literature. *Neth J Med* 1994;44:18–22.
177. Sirisanthana T, Supparatpinyo K, Perriens J, et al. Amphotericin B and itraconazole for treatment of disseminated *Penicillium marneffei* infection in human immunodeficiency virus-infected patients. *Clin Infect Dis* 1998;26:1107 1110.
178. Supparatpinyo K, Perriens, Nelson KE, et al. A controlled trial of itraconazole to prevent relapse of *Penicillium marneffei* infection in patients infected with human immunodeficiency virus. *N Engl J Med* 1998;339:1739–1743.
179. Rogers MF, Morens DM, Stewart JA, et al. National case control study of Kaposi's sarcoma and *Pneumocystis carinii* pneumonia in homosexual men. Part 2. Laboratory results. *Ann Intern Med* 1983;99:151–158.
180. Whitley RJ, Kimberlin DW, Roizman B. Herpes simplex viruses. *Clin Infect Dis* 1998;26:541–555.
181. Stewart JA, Reef SE, Pellet PE, et al. Herpesvirus infections in persons infected with human immunodeficiency virus. *Clin Infect Dis* 1995;21(suppl 1):114–120.
182. Cinque P, Vago L, Marenzi R, et al. Herpes simplex virus infections of the central nervous system in human immunodeficiency virus–infected patients: clinical management

by polymerase chain reaction assay of cerebrospinal fluid. *Clin Infect Dis* 1998;27:303–309.
183. Douglas JM, Critchlow C, Benedetti J, et al. Double blind study of oral acyclovir for suppression of recurrences of genital herpes simplex virus infection. *N Engl J Med* 1984;310:1551.
184. Mertz GJ, Loveless MO, Levin MJ, et al. Oral famciclovir for suppression of recurrent genital herpes simplex virus infection in women: a multicenter, double-blind, placebo-controlled trial. *Arch Intern Med* 1997;157:343.
185. Safrin S, Berger TG, Gilson I, et al. Foscarnet therapy in five patients with AIDS and acyclovir-resistant varicella-zoster virus infection. *Ann Intern Med* 1991;115:19–21.
186. Friedman-Kien AE, Lafleur FL, Gendler E, et al. Herpes zoster: a possible early clinical sign for development of acquired immunodeficiency syndrome in high risk individuals. *J Am Acad Dermato* 1986;14:1023.
187. Murphy ME, Polsky B. Viral infection. In: Armstrong D, Cohen J, eds. *Infectious diseases* London: Harcourt, 1999:5.11.1–5.11.8.
188. Forster DJ, Dugel PU, Frangieh GT, et al. Rapidly progressive outer retinal retinal necrosis in the acquired immunodeficiency syndrome (AIDS). *Am J Ophthalmol* 1990;110:341–348.
189. Nogueira RG, Sheen VL. Images in clinical medicine. Herpes zoster ophthalmicus followed by contralateral hemiparesis. *N Engl J Med* 2002;346:1127.
190. Rutherford GW, Schwarcz SK, Lemp GF, et al. The epidemiology of AIDS-related Kaposi's sarcoma in San Francisco. *J Infect Dis* 1989;159:569.
191. Moore PS, Chang Y. Detection of herpes-virus like DNA sequences in Kaposi's sarcoma in patients with and without AIDS. *N Engl J Med* 1995;332:1181–1185.
192. Beral V, Peterman TA, Berkelman RL, et al. Kaposi's sarcoma among persons with AIDS: a sexually transmitted infection? *Lancet* 1990;1:123.
193. Chang Y, Cesarman E, Pessin MS, et al. Identification of herpesvirus-like DNA sequences in AIDS-associated Kaposi's sarcoma. *Science* 1995;266:1865.
194. Depond W, Said J, Tasaka T, et al. Kaposi's sarcoma-associated herpesvirus and human herpesvirus 8 (KSHV/HHV8)-associated lymphoma of the bowel. *Am J Surg Pathol* 1997;2:719–724.
195. Gnann JW, Pellett PE, Jaffe HW. Human herpesvirus 8 and Kaposi's sarcoma in persons infected with human immunodeficiency virus. *Clin Infect Dis* 2000;30(suppl):72–76.
196. Jones J, Hansen D, Dworkin M, et al. Effect of antiretroviral therapy on recent trends in selected cancers among HIV-infected persons. *J AIDS* 1999;21(suppl):11–17.
197. Koh HK, Davis BE. Dermatologic manifestations. In: Libman H, Witzburg RA, eds. *HIV infection: a primary care manual,* 3rd ed. Boston: Little, Brown, 1996:107–122.
198. Volberding PA, Mitsuyasu RT, Golando JP, et al. Treatment of Kaposi's sarcoma with interferon alpha-2 (Intron A). *Cancer* 1987;59:620.
199. Krown SE, Gold JWM, Niedzwiecki D, et al. Interferon-alpha with zidovudine: safety, tolerance, and clinical and virologic effects in patients with Kaposi's sarcoma associated with the acquired immunodeficiency syndrome (AIDS). *Ann Intern Med* 1990;112:812.
200. Kovacs JA, Deyton L, Davey R, et al. Combined zidovudine and interferon-alpha therapy in patients Kaposi's sarcoma and the acquired immunodeficiency syndrome (AIDS). *Ann Intern Med* 1989;111:280.
201. Saville MW, Lietzau J, Pluda JM, et al. Activity of paclitaxel (taxol) as therapy for HIV-associated Kaposi's sarcoma. *Lancet* 1995;346:26.
202. Martinelli C, Zazzi M, Ambu S, et al. Complete regression of AIDS-related Kaposi's sarcoma associated with undetectable human herpes-virus-8 sequences during anti-protease therapy. *AIDS* 1998;12:1717–1719.
203. Price RW, Worley JM. Neurological complications of HIV-1 infections and AIDS. In: Broder S, Merigan Jr TC, Bolognesi D, eds. *Textbook of AIDS medicine* Baltimore: Williams & Wilkins, 1994:494–495.
204. Berger JR, Kaszovitz B, Post MJ, et al. Progressive multifocal leukoencephalopathy associated with human immunodeficiency virus infection. A review of the literature with a report of sixteen cases. *Ann Intern Med* 1987;107:78–87.

205. Cinque P, Scarpellini P, Vago L, et al. Diagnosis of central nervous system complications in HIV-1-infected patients: cerebrospinal fluid analysis by the polymerase chain reaction [Review]. *Acquired Immunodeficiency Syndrome* 1997;11:1–17.
206. Giudici B, Vaz B, Bossolasco S, et al. Highly active antiretroviral therapy and progressive multifocal leukoencephalopathy: effects on cerebrospinal fluid markers of JC virus replication and immune response. *Clin Infect Dis* 2000;30:95–99.
207. Hall CD, Dafni U, Simpson D, Clifford D, et al. Failure of cytarabine in progressive multifocal leukoencephalopathy associated with human immunodeficiency virus infection. *N Engl J Med* 1998;338:1345–1351.
208. Enting RH, Portegies P. Cytarabine and highly active antiretroviral therapy in HIV-related progressive multifocal leukoencephalopathy. *J Neurol* 2000;247:134–138.
209. Marra CM, Rajicic N, Barker DE, et al. Prospective pilot study of cidofovir for HIV-associated progressive multifocal leukoencephalopathy [Abstract 596]. Presented at the 8th Conference on Retroviruses and Opportunistic Infections, February 4–8, 2001.
210. De Luca A, Giancola ML, Ammassari A, et al. Cidofovir added to HAART improves virological and clinical outcome in AIDS-associated progressive multifocal leukoencephalopathy. *Acquired Immunodeficiency Syndrome* 2000;14:F117–F121.
211. Clifford DB, Yiannoutsos C, Glicksman M, et al. HAART improves prognosis in HIV-associated progressive multifocal leukoencephalopathy. *Neurology* 1999;52:623–625.
212. Greenlee JE. Progressive multifocal leukoencephalopathy—progress made and lessons relearned. *N Engl J Med* 1998;338:1378–1380.
213. Soave R, Armstrong D. Cryptosporidium and cryptosporidiosis. *Rev Infect Dis* 1986;8:1012–1023.
214. Mannheimer SB, Soave R. Protozoal infections in patients with AIDS. *Infect Dis Clin North Am* 1994;8:483–498.
215. Ives NJ, Gazzard BG, Easterbrook PJ. The changing pattern of AIDS-defining illnesses with the introduction of highly active antiretroviral therapy (HAART) in a London clinic. *J Infection* 2001;42:134–139.
216. Peterson C. Cryptosporidiosis in patients infected with the human immunodficiency virus. *Clin Infect Dis* 1992;15:903–909.
217. Margulis SJ, Honig CL, Soave R, et al. Biliary obstruction in the acquired imunodeficiency syndrome. *Ann Intern Med* 1986;105:207.
218. Ungar BLP. Enzyme-linked immunoassay for detection of *Cryptosporidium* antigens in fecal specimens. *J Clin Microbiol* 1990;28:2491–2495.
219. Hewitt RG, Yiannoutsos CT, Higgs ES, et al. Paromomycin: no more effective than placebo for treatment of cryptosporidiosis in patients with advanced human immunodeficiency virus infection. *Clin Infect Dis* 2000;31:1084–1092.
220. Holmberg SD, Moorman AC, Von Bargen JC, et al. Possible effectiveness of clarithromycin and rifabutin for cryptosporidiosis chemoprophylaxis in HIV disease. HIV Outpatient Study (HOPS) Investigators. *JAMA* 1998;279:384–386.
221. Giacometti A, Cirioni O, Scalise G. *In-vitro* activity of macrolides alone and in combination with artemisin, atovaquone, dapsone, minocycline or pyrimethamine against *Cryptosporidium parvum*. *J Antimicrob Chemother* 1996;38:399–408.
222. Nord J, Ma P, DiJohn D, et al. Treatment with bovine hyperimmune colostrum of cryptosporidial diarrhea in AIDS patients. *AIDS* 1990;4:581–584.
223. Carr A, Marriott D, Field A, et al. Treatment of HIV-1 associated microsporidiosis and cryptosporidiosis with combination antiretroviral therapy. *Lancet* 1998;351:256–261.
224. Asmuth DM, DeGirolami PC, Federman M, et al. Clinical features of microsporidiosis in patients with acquired immunodeficiency syndrome. *Clin Infect Dis* 1994;18:819–825.
225. Orenstein JM, Dieterich DT, Kotler DP. Systemic dissemination by a newly recognized microsporidia species in AIDS. *Acquired Immunodeficiency Syndrome* 1992;6:1143–1150.
226. Molina JM, Oksenhendler E, Beauvais B, et al. Disseminated microsporidiosis due to *Septata intestinalis* in patients with AIDS. Clinical features and response to albendazole therapy. *J Infect Dis* 1995;171:245–249.
227. Anwar-Bruni DM, Hogan SE, Schwartz DA, et al. Atovaquone is effective treatment for the symptoms of gastrointestinal microsporidiosis in HIV-1 infected patients. *Acquired Immunodeficiency Syndrome* 1996;10:619–624.

228. Molina JM, Goguel J, Sarfati C, et al. Potential efficacy of fumagilin in intestinal microsporidiosis due to *Enterocytozoon bieneusi* in patients with HIV infection: results of a drug screening study. *AIDS* 1997;11:1603–1610.
229. Benator DA, French AL, Beaudet LM, et al. *Isospora belli* infection associated with acalculus cholecystitis in a patient with AIDS. *Ann Intern Med* 1994;121:663–664.
230. Ortega YR, Sterling CR, Gilman RH, et al. *Cyclospora* species—a new protozoan pathogen of humans. *N Engl J Med* 1993;328:1308–1312.
231. Pape JW, Verdier RI, Boncy M, et al. Cyclospora infection in adults infected with HIV. *Ann Intern Med* 1994;121:654–657.
232. Taylor AD, Davis LJ, Soave R. *Cyclospora*—review. *Curr Clin Top Infect Dis* 1997;17: 256–268.
233. Darrow WW, Echenberg DF, Jaffe HW, et al. Risk factors for human immunodeficiency virus infections in homosexual men. *Am J Public Health* 1987;77:479–483.
234. Telzak EE, Chiasson MA, Berier PJ, et al. HIV-1 seroconversion in patients with and without genital ulcers. *Ann Intern Med* 1993;119:1181–1186.
235. Greenblatt RM, Lukehart SA, Plummer FA, et al. Genital ulceration as a risk factor for human immunodeficiency virus infection. *Acquired Immunodeficiency Syndrome* 1988;2:47–50.
236. Theus SA, Harrich DA, Gaynor R, et al. *Treponema pallidum,* lipoproteins, and synthetic lipoprotein analogues induce human immunodeficiency virus type I gene expression in monocytes via NF-$\kappa$B activation. *J Infect Dis* 1998;177:941–950.
237. Johns DR, Tierney M, Felenstein D. Alteration in the natural history of neurosyphilis by concurrent infection with human immunodeficiency virus infection. *N Engl J Med* 1987;316:1569–1572.
238. Hutchinson CM, Hook EW III, Shephard M, et al. Altered clinical presentation of early syphilis in patients with human immunodeficiency virus infection. *Ann Intern Med* 1994;121:94–100.
239. Tomberlin MG, Holtom PD, Owens JL, et al. Evaluation of neurosyphilis in human immunodeficiency virus–infected individuals. *Clin Infect Dis* 1994;18:288–294.
240. Centers for Disease Control and Prevention. 1998 guidelines for treatment of sexually transmitted diseases. *MMWR* 1998;47:1–116.
241. Collis TK, Celum CL. The clinical manifestations and treatment of sexually transmitted diseases in human immunodeficiency virus–positive men. *Clin Infect Dis* 2001;32:611–622.
242. Hicks CB, Benson PM, Lupton GP, et al. Seronegative secondary syphilis in a patient infected with the human immunodeficiency virus with Kaposi's sarcoma: a diagnostic dilemma. *Ann Intern Med* 1987;107:492–495.
243. Janier M, Chasting C, Spindler E, et al. A prospective study of the influence of HIV status on the seroconversion of serological tests for syphilis. *Dermatology* 1999;198:362–369.
244. Malone JL, Wallace MR, Hendrick BB, et al. Syphilis and neurosyphilis in a human immunodeficiency virus type-1 seropositive population: evidence for frequent serologic relapse after therapy. *Am J Med* 1995;99:55–63.
245. Telzak EE, Greenberg MS, Harrison J, et al. Syphilis treatment response in HIV-infected individuals. *AIDS* 1991;5:591–598.
246. Rolfs RT, Joesoef R, Hendershot EF, et al. A randomized trial of enhanced therapy for early syphilis in patients with and without human immunodeficiency virus. *N Engl J Med* 1997;337:307–314.
247. Monga HK, Rodriguez-Barradas MC, Breaux K, et al. Hepatitis C virus infection–related morbidity and mortality among patients with human immunodeficiency virus infection. *Clin Infect Dis* 2001;33:240–247.
248. Centers for Disease Control and Prevention. Recommendations for prevention and control of hepatitis C virus (HCV) infection and HCV-related chronic disease. *MMWR* 1998;47:1–39.
249. Sulkowski MS, Mast EE, Seeff LB, et al. Hepatitis C virus infection as an opportunistic disease in persons infected with human immunodeficiency virus. *Clin Infect Dis* 2000;30(suppl):77–84.

250. Poles MA, Dieterich D. Hepatitis C virus/human immunodeficiency virus coinfection: clinical management issues. *Clin Infect Dis* 2000;31:154–161.
251. Sulkowski MS, Thomas DL, Chaisson RE, et al. Hepatotoxicity associated with antiretroviral therapy in adults with HIV and the role of hepatitis B or C infection. *JAMA* 2000;283:74–80.
252. Horvath J, Raffanti SP. Clinical aspects of the interactions between human immunodeficiency virus and the hepatotropic viruses. *Clin Infect Dis* 1994;18:339–347.
253. Imbert-Bismut F, Ratziu V, Pieroni L, et al. Biochemical markers of liver fibrosis in patients with hepatitis C virus infection: a prospective study. *Lancet* 2001;357:1069–1075.
254. Soriano V, Gracia-Samaniego J, Bravo R, et al. Efficacy and safety of interferon-$\alpha$ treatment for chronic hepatitis C in HIV-infected patients. *J Infect Dis* 1995;31:9–13.
255. Reichard O, Norkrans G, Fryden A, et al. Randomized, double-blind, placebo-controlled trial of interferon $\alpha$2b with and without ribavirin for chronic hepatitis C. *Lancet* 1998;351:83–87.
256. Emilie D, Burgard M, Lascoux-Combe C, et al. Early control of HIV replication in primary HIV-1 infection treated with antiretroviral drugs and pegylated IFN alpha: results from the Primoferon A (ANRS 086) Study. *AIDS* 2001;15:1435–1437.
257. Mohle-Boetani JC, Koehler JE, Berger TG, et al. Bacillary angiomatosis and bacillary peliosis in patients infected with human immunodeficiency virus: clinical characteristics in a case-control study. *Clin Infect Dis* 1996;22:794–800.
258. Perkocha LA, Geaghan SM, Yen TSB, et al. Clinical and pathologic features of bacillary peliosis hepatis in association with human immunodeficiency virus infection. *N Engl J Med* 1990;323:1581–1586.
259. Koehler JE, Tappero JW. Bacillary angiomatosis and bacillary peliosis in patients infected with human immunodeficiency virus. *Clin Infect Dis* 1993;17:612–624.
260. Spach DH, Koehler JE. *Bartonella*-associated infections. *Infect Dis Clin North Am* 1998;12:137–155.
261. Guerra LG, Neira CJ, Boman D, et al. Rapid response of AIDS-related bacillary angiomatosis to azithromycin. *Clin Infect Dis* 1993;17:264–266.
262. Gruenewald R, Blum S, Chan J. Relationship between human imunodeficiency virus infection and salmonellosis in 20- to 59-year-old residents of New York City. *Clin Infect Dis* 1994;18:358–363.
263. Matila L. Clinical features and duration of traveler's diarrhea in relation to its etiology. *Clin Infect Dis* 1994;19:728–734.
264. Levine WC, Buehler JW, Bean NH, et al. Epidemiology of nontyphoidal *Salmonella* bacteremia during the human immunodeficiency virus epidemic. *J Infect Dis* 1991;164:81–87.
265. Celem CL, Chaisson RE, Rutherford GW, et al. Incidence of salmonellosis in patients with AIDS. *J Infect Dis* 1987;156:998–1001.
266. Sanders A. HIV-associated bacterial pneumonia. *AIDS Reader* 1999;9:580–583.
267. Hirschtick RE, Glassroth J, Jordan MC, et al. Bacterial pneumonia in persons infected with the human immunodeficiency virus. *N Engl J Med* 1995;333:845–851.
268. Currier J, Williams P, Feinberg J, et al. Impact of prophylaxis for *Mycobacterium avium* complex on bacterial infections in patients with advanced human immunodeficiency virus disease. *Clin Infect Dis* 2001;32:1615–1622.
269. Mundy LM, Auwaeter PC, Oldach D, et al. Community-acquired pneumonia: impact of immune status. *Am J Respir Crit Care* 1995;152:1309–1315.
270. Janoff EN, Breiman RF, Daley CL, et al. Pneumococcal disease during HIV infection. Epidemiologic, clinical, and immunologic perspectives. *Ann Intern Med* 1992;117:314–324.
271. Tumbarello M, Tacconelli E, de Gaetano DK, et al. HIV-associated bacterial pneumonia in the era of highly active antiretroviral therapy. *J AIDS Hum Retrovirol* 1999;20:208–209.
272. Wallace JM, Hansen NI, Lavange L, et al. Respiratory disease trends in the pulmonary complications of HIV infections study cohort. *Am J Respir Crit Care Med* 1997;155:72–80.
273. Munoz P, Miranda ME, Llancaqueo A, et al. *Haemophilus* species bacteremia in adults. *Arch Intern Med* 1997;157:1869–1873.

274. Kielhofner M, Atmar RL, Hamill RJ, et al. Life-threatening *Pseudomonas aeruginosa* infections in patients with human immunodeficiency virus. *Clin Infect Dis* 1992;14:403–411.
275. Mitchell DM, Miller RF. New developments in the pulmonary diseases affecting HIV infected individuals. *Thorax* 1995;50:294–302.
276. Polsky B, Gold JW, Whimbey E, et al. Bacterial pneumonia in patients with the acquired imunodeficiency syndrome. *Ann Intern Med* 1986;104:38–41.
277. Bartlett JG, Breiman RF, Mandell LA, et al. Guidelines from the Infectious Disease Society of America. Community-acquired pneumonia in adults: guidelines for management. *Clin Infect Dis* 1998;26:811–838.
278. Ellerbrock TV, Chiasson MA, Bush TJ, et al. Incidence of cervical squamous intraepithelial lesions in HIV-infected women. *JAMA* 2000;283:1031–1037.
279. Goedert J, Cote T, Virgo P, et al. Spectrum of AIDS-associated malignant disorders. *Lancet* 1998;351:1833–1839.
280. Kaplan LD, Abrams DI, Feigal E, et al. AIDS-associated non-Hodgkin's lymphoma in San Francisco. *JAMA* 1989;261:719–724.
281. Manos MM, Kinney WK, Hurley LB, et al. Identifying women with cervical neoplasia: using human papillomavirus DNA testing for equivocal Papanicolaou results. *JAMA* 1999;281:1605–1610.
282. MacMahon EM, Glass JD, Hayward SD, et al. Epstein-Barr virus in AIDS-related primary central nervous system lymphoma. *Lancet* 1991;338:969–973.
283. Jones J, Hansen D, Dworkin M, et al. Effect of antiretroviral therapy on recent trends in selected cancers among HIV-infected persons. *J AIDS* 1999;21(suppl):11–17.

# 19. ANTIRETROVIRAL THERAPY: THERAPEUTIC AGENTS, DOSING, PHARMACOKINETICS, AND THEIR USE

Amneris E. Luque, Susan E. Cohn, Geoffrey A. Weinberg, and Peter R. Mariuz

**I. Introduction and background.** The advent of potent combination antiretroviral therapy (ARVT) in 1996, also referred to as highly active antiretroviral therapy (HAART), has revolutionized the treatment of human immunodeficiency virus (HIV) infection. The time to progression from HIV infection to acquired immunodeficiency syndrome (AIDS) has been delayed. Dramatic decrease in AIDS mortality and morbidity from opportunistic infections and certain malignancies (e.g., Kaposi sarcoma) has occurred [1–3]. The attendant increase in CD4 cell counts and return of pathogen-specific lymphoproliferative responses (immune reconstitution) [4] has permitted the discontinuation of primary prophylaxis for *Pneumocystis carinii* pneumonia (PCP) and for disseminated *Mycobacterium avium* complex infection (MAC). Accumulating evidence suggests that secondary prophylaxis of CMV retinitis [5], PCP [6], MAC [7], toxoplasmosis [8], and cryptococcosis [9] also can be discontinued. However, up to 62% of patients fail HAART therapy [10,11]. Furthermore, none of the current HAART regimens eradicates HIV even after continued use for up to 3 years [12]. In fact, a recent review suggests that eradication would require complete suppression of viral replication for decades [13], and thus is not a realistic goal at the present time. This finding—coupled with concerns about the complexity of drug regimens, drug interactions, the adverse effects of long-term ARVT, and antiretroviral resistance—has recently led to changes in the guidelines on initiation of therapy in asymptomatic HIV infection.

**II. The virus**

**A. Life cycle.** Understanding the life cycle (Fig. 19.1) and pathogenesis of HIV helps explain the mechanism of action of antiretroviral agents, the rationale for therapy, antiretroviral resistance, and future therapeutic targets.

**B. Virus structure**

1. **HIV, an enveloped RNA virus,** belongs to the lentivirus genus of retroviruses.
2. **The HIV genome** contains three primary genes: *gag, pol,* and *env.* These genes encode for the major structural proteins (*gag*), enzymatic proteins (*pol*), and envelope (*env*). Five other genes (*tat, nef, rev, vpu,* and *vif*) regulate expression of proteins, assembly, and release of virus from infected cells.
3. **Steps in synthesis**
   a. **HIV binds** via surface glycoprotein 120 (gp120) to CD4 receptors (on lymphocytes, macrophages, and dendritic cells). Cells without CD4 receptors are infected by another mechanism.
   b. **Fusion** with the host cell plasma occurs by the interaction of the HIV fusion protein (gp41) and a coreceptor on the host cell membrane. This is chemokine receptor 5 (CCR5) on macrophages or CXCR4 on lymphocytes. This is followed by nucleocapsid penetration of the cell membrane followed by release of the viral genome (two single strands of RNA) into the cytoplasm.
   c. **Reverse transcription** of HIV RNA to DNA requires viral reverse transcriptase (RT), which is an RNA-dependent DNA polymerase. RT generates a first-strand copy of proviral DNA. After viral ribonuclease H partially degrades the original RNA template, RT controls the synthesis of second-strand DNA.
   d. **Mechanism of resistance.** Because of the low fidelity of RT, which lacks the error-correcting mechanisms seen in eukaryotic and prokaryotic polymerases, and the high degree of guanine-to-adenine nucleotide hypermutation in HIV (a characteristic of all lentiviruses) [14], mutations are frequent. A high mutation rate coupled with the extraordinarily large daily production of virions ensures that resistance may occur easily, particularly under pressure of therapy. A single mutation in RT confers resistance to lamivudine (3TC), which occurs by 1 week with 3TC monotherapy [15].
   e. **Comparative mechanisms of action of antiretroviral agents.** The nucleoside reverse transcriptase inhibitors (NRTIs) and non-nucleoside reverse

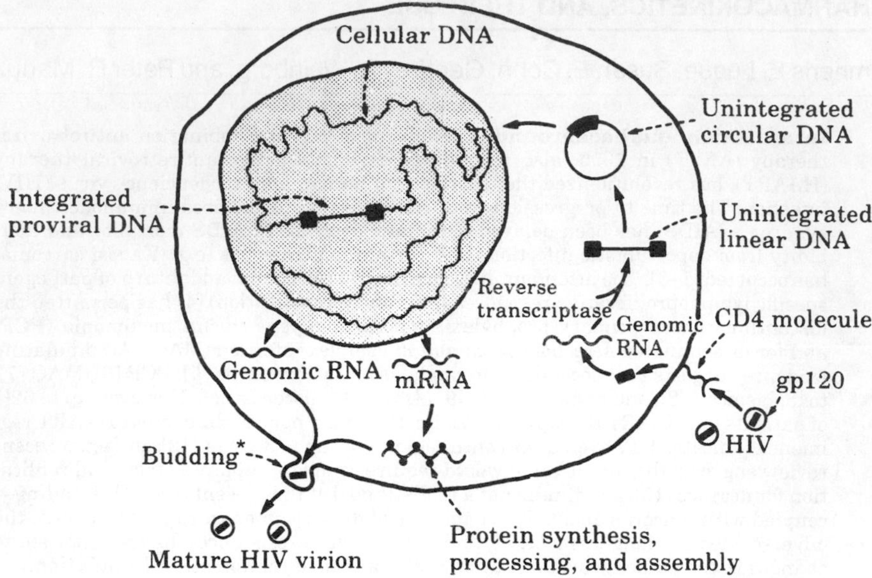


**FIG. 19.1** The life cycle of human immunodeficiency virus (HIV). *Immature viral particles bud. (Reprinted from Fauci AS. The human immunodeficiency virus: infectivity and mechanisms of pathogenesis. *Science* 1988;239:619, with permission.)

transcriptase inhibitors (NNRTIs) block the function of RT by different mechanisms. Proviral DNA transported to the host cell nucleus is inserted into the host genome by viral integrase. Subsequent viral replication depends on the coordinated activity of both cellular and viral factors (HIV regulatory proteins tat, rev, and nef) that activate and regulate HIV transcription. Viral DNA is translated to genomic and messenger RNA, and production of virion structural and enzymatic proteins occurs. At the cell membrane HIV RNA is incorporated into capsids that bud from the cell surface, taking up viral envelope glycoproteins. An HIV protease mediates final viral maturation by cleaving first itself, then other viral proteins (RT, integrase, capsid, matrix, and nucleocapsid proteins) from a precursor polyprotein. This maturation step, blocked by protease inhibitors (PIs), is essential for viral release and infectivity. Currently available antiretroviral agents inhibit two essential steps in the HIV life cycle: reverse transcription and protease activity. Other potential targets include inhibition of fusion, integrase, and regulatory proteins (see section VII on investigational drugs), and binding to CD4 receptors. In addition, methods of improving specific anti-HIV immunity are being investigated.

**III. Pathogenesis of HIV infection**

**A. CD4 cell changes.** With continuous HIV replication in $CD4^+$ T cells, their numbers gradually decline (50–75 per year). This eventually leads to AIDS [16]. The mean time from HIV infection to AIDS is 8 to 10 years. Twenty percent of patients develop AIDS in less than 5 years. Less than 5% remain asymptomatic with normal immune function for more than 10 years [17].

**B. Virus changes.** Billions of virions are produced and destroyed every day [18] in a dynamic equilibrium between production in lymphoid tissues and clearance by the immune system. The HIV 1 RNA level in plasma (viral load) [19] predicts disease progression. This can be measured using branched-chain DNA signal amplification (bDNA assay) or reverse transcriptase polymerase chain reaction (RT-PCR). The assays used should be constant because HIV RNA values by RT-PCR are about twice those of bDNA assay.

**C. Viral load and CD4 cell interaction.** HIV replication and its associated CD4 cell destruction are assessed by measuring HIV viral load. CD4 cell counts independently predict disease progression and give an estimate of HIV induced immune destruction. Viral load and CD4 cell count measurements are best used together to assess the risk of disease progression. When the CD4 cell count was over 750/mL and the HIV-1 RNA level was less than or equal to 1,500 copies/mL (by RT-PCR), 1.7% developed AIDS within 6 years. When the CD4 cell count was less than or equal to 200/mL and the HIV-1 RNA level was over 60,000 copies/mL, 97.9% develop AIDS in 6 years [20]. Viral load and CD4 cell counts from several studies have been used to generate guidelines for the U.S. Department of Health and Human Services and the International AIDS Society (IAS)-USA [21,22] for when to initiate ARVT (Table 19.1). It is extremely useful to review this information

Table 19.1. Risk of Progression to AIDS-Defining Illness in a Cohort of Homosexual Men Predicted by Baseline CD4$^{+}$ T-Cell Count and Viral Load

| Plasma Viral Load (Copies/mL)[a] | | | % AIDS (AIDS-Defining Complication)[b] | | |
|---|---|---|---|---|---|
| bDNA | RT-PCR | n | 3 Years | 6 Years | 9 Years |
| CD4 Count ≤ 200 | | | | | |
| ≤500 | <1,500 | 0[c] | — | — | — |
| 501–3,000 | 1,501–7,000 | 3[c] | — | — | — |
| 3,001–10,000 | 7,001–20,000 | 7 | 14.3 | 28.6 | 64.3 |
| 10,001–30,000 | 20,001–55,000 | 20 | 50.0 | 75.0 | 90.0 |
| >30,000 | >55,000 | 70 | 85.5 | 97.9 | 100.0 |
| CD4 Count 201–350[d] | | | | | |
| ≤500 | ≤1,500 | 3[c] | — | — | — |
| 501–3,000 | 1,501–7,000 | 27 | 0 | 20.0 | 32.2 |
| 3,001–10,000 | 7,001–20,000 | 44 | 6.9 | 44.4 | 66.2 |
| 10,001–30,000 | 20,001–55,000 | 53 | 36.4 | 72.2 | 84.5 |
| >30,000 | >55,000 | 104 | 64.4 | 89.3 | 92.9 |
| CD4 Count >350 | | | | | |
| ≤500 | ≤1,500 | 119 | 1.7 | 5.5 | 12.7 |
| 501–3,000 | 1,501–7,000 | 227 | 2.2 | 16.4 | 30.0 |
| 3,001–10,000 | 7,001–20,000 | 342 | 6.8 | 30.1 | 53.5 |
| 10,001–30,000 | 20,001–55,000 | 323 | 14.8 | 51.2 | 73.5 |
| >30,000 | >55,000 | 262 | 39.6 | 71.8 | 85.0 |

RT-PCR, reverse transcriptase polymerase chain reaction.

[a]MACS numbers reflect plasma HIV RNA values obtained by version 2.0 bDNA testing. RT-PCR values are consistently 2- to 2.5-fold higher than first-generation bDNA values, as indicated. It should be noted that the current generation bDNA assay (3.0) gives similar HIV-1 RNA values as RT-PCR except at the lower end of the linear range (<1,500 copies/mL).

[b]In this study AIDS was defined according to the 1987 CDC definition and does not include asymptomatic individuals with CD4$^{+}$ T-cell counts of <200 mm$^3$.

[c]Too few subjects were in the category to provide a reliable estimate of AIDS risk.

[d]A recent evaluation of data from the MACS cohort by of 231 individuals with CD4$^{+}$ T-cell counts of >200 and <350 cells/mm$^3$ demonstrated that of 40 (17%) individuals with plasma HIV RNA <10,000 copies/mL, none progressed to AIDS by 3 years (Alvaro Muñoz, personal communication). Of 28 individuals (29%) with plasma viremia of 10,000–20,000 copies/mL, 4% and 11% progressed to AIDS at 2 and 3 years, respectively. Plasma HIV RNA was calculated as RT-PCR values from measured bDNA values.

Data are from the Multi-Center AIDS Cohort Study (MACS) as reported by Alvaro Muñoz, Ph.D. (personal communication.) Reprinted from the Report of the NIH panel to define principles of therapy of HIV infection and guidelines for the use of antiretroviral agents in HIV-infected adults and adolescents. *MMWR* 1998; with permission.

with patients when discussing the rationale and indications for antiretroviral treatment.

**D. Effect of HAART on viral load and CD4 cell count.** HAART is a combination drug regimen that reduces plasma HIV RNA viral load to an undetectable level (<50 copies/mL) in treatment-naive patients. This leads to biphasic increases in CD4 cell counts [23] with associated clinical benefits, delayed disease progression, and decreased morbidity and mortality from HIV infection. The initial response is an increase in memory $CD4^+$ cells that may reflect release of trapped memory cells from lymphoid tissues. The second phase, usually seen after 6 months, is made up of new naive $CD4^+$ cells [23]. Plasma HIV-1 RNA viral load and CD4 cell counts are used to decide when to begin therapy, to monitor the efficacy of therapy, and as end points in clinical trials.

**IV. Historical milestones in ARVT.** In 1987 in placebo-controlled trials, zidovudine (or azidothymidine, or AZT) was shown to improve survival and decrease disease progression to AIDS [24]. In less advanced HIV, AZT decreased disease progression, but there was no survival advantage [25]. In clinical trials of dual NRTI therapy versus AZT alone, combination therapy provided improved and more durable clinical and survival benefits. In 1997, combination therapy with a PI and two NRTIs was shown to be superior to dual NRTI therapy [26]. More recently, two NRTIs with one NNRTI have been compared with regimens containing a PI and two NRTIs [27]. Results from all of these trials indicate that resistance to antiretroviral agents eventually leads to therapeutic failure. The most effective way to avoid the emergence of antiretroviral resistant HIV-1 is to achieve maximum suppression of HIV replication.

**V. Pharmacology of individual antiretroviral agents.** Currently available antiretroviral agents can be grouped according to the site and mode of action as NRTIs, nucleotide reverse transcriptase inhibitors, NNRTIs, and PIs.

**A. Nucleoside reverse transcriptase inhibitors.** The available NRTIs are listed in Table 19.2.

1. **Description. NRTIs** are synthetic nucleoside analogue prodrugs. AZT and stavudine (d4T), for example, are analogues of thymidine. NRTIs must be phosphorylated to the active 5′-triphosphate form by intracellular enzymes (kinases, nucleotidases). Certain NRTIs (AZT, d4T) are primarily active against proliferating HIV-infected cells [28]. Others, such as didanosine (2′,3′-dideoxyinosine, or ddI) and zalcitabine (dideoxycytidine, or ddC), are active even in HIV-infected resting cells. This is dependent on the growth phase during which the cellular kinases that metabolize NRTIs to the 5′-triphosphate form are most active [29].
2. **Mechanism of action.** NRTIs competitively bind to HIV-RT in place of the natural nucleotide. They lack the 3′-hydroxyl group on the ribose sugar needed for the 5′–3′ linkages essential for DNA synthesis and thus cause chain termination [30]. High intracellular levels of AZT monophosphate may impair HIV-1 RNAse H activity [31].
3. **NRTI class-related toxicity. Lactic acidosis/hepatic steatosis** is a rare, frequently fatal complication associated with the use of AZT, ddI, d4T as monotherapy and combinations of AZT/ddC or 3TC with other NRTIs [32]. It is seen more commonly in obese women, typically after several months of therapy.

Table 19.2. Nucleoside Reverse Transcriptase Inhibitors

| |
|---|
| Zidovudine (AZT, ZDV, Retrovir) |
| Didanosine (ddI, Videx) |
| Zalcitabine (ddC, HIVID) |
| Stavudine (d4T, Zerit) |
| Lamivudine (3TC, Epivir) |
| Abacavir (ABC, Ziagen) |
| Combivir (AZT+3TC) |
| Trizivir (AZT+3TC+Abacavir) |

Symptoms include nausea, vomiting, early satiety, abdominal bloating and pain, malaise, fatigue, dyspnea, occasionally fever, and right upper quadrant pain. Laboratory tests show anion gap acidosis, decreased bicarbonate, elevated lactic acid, and mild to moderate elevations of transaminases. Ultrasonography or abdominal computed tomography (CT) shows hepatomegaly and hepatic steatosis. Histopathology shows microvesicular, macrovesicular, or mixed steatosis, and electron microscopy (EM) shows abnormal mitochondria. NRTIs inhibit (to different degrees) mitochondrial DNA polymerase gamma, which is responsible for mitochondrial DNA synthesis [33]. Mitochondrial dysfunction leads to increased lactic acid production and acidosis [34]. Asymptomatic lactic acidemia (or lactemia), an increase in venous lactate levels in the absence of abnormal arterial pH, also has been described [35,36]. Coexistent riboflavin deficiency also may play a role. The incidence of lactemia increases over time in patients treated with NRTIs [37]. Whether this leads to lactic acidosis/hepatic steatosis is not certain. Fatal cases have occurred in pregnant patients taking ddI and d4T. **This combination should therefore be avoided. Treatment** with AZT (or other NRTIs) should be discontinued. There is no known effective therapy. Anecdotal reports suggest riboflavin 50 mg orally daily, or L-carnitine alone or in combinations with complex vitamin B may be effective [38,39] because some patients have riboflavin deficiency. The use of mechanical ventilation, thiamine supplements, and bicarbonate infusions have not been effective. Currently there are no recommendations to screen for this entity (by measuring lactate levels) in NRTI-treated patients. **Lactic acidosis/hepatic steatosis** should be suspected in any patient taking NRTIs with an unexplained decrease in serum bicarbonate level, increased anion gap, or elevated hepatic transaminases, particularly if associated with fatigue, nausea, abdominal pain, or bloating. Dyspnea without other pulmonary findings on physical examination and chest radiography is a late manifestation, consistent with respiratory compensation for metabolic acidosis.

**4. Zidovudine**

**a. Formulations:** 300-mg tablets, 100-mg capsules, syrup 10-mg/mL, and intravenous (i.v.) infusion 10 mg/mL.

**b. Dosage**

**(1)** Adults may be given 300 mg orally twice daily or 200 mg three times daily, taken without regard to meals.

**(2)** Children over age 12 may be given the adult dosage; or 180 mg/m$^2$ of body surface area (BSA) per dose three times daily (which approximates the adult dosage). For children under age 13, 160 mg/m$^2$ BSA/dose is given three times daily [40].

**(3)** Newborns are given 2 mg/kg/dose orally every 6 hours for 6 weeks as part of a tripartite regimen to prevent vertical transmission of HIV (see section **VIII.C.1–3**). The suggested dose for premature newborns (28–33 weeks' gestation) is 1.5 mg/kg/dose orally or i.v. every 12 hours for the first 2 weeks of life, then 2 mg/kg/dose orally or i.v. every 8 hours for the next 8 weeks [40,41].

**c. *In vitro* activity.** AZT is active against HIV-1 and HIV-2. *In vitro,* AZT is active predominantly against HIV-infected proliferating cells [28].

**d. Pharmacology** [42]

**(1) Absorption.** Bioavailability is 65% to 70%. Protein binding ranges from 18% to 38%.

**(2) Half-life** in plasma is 1 hour. Active 5′-triphosphate has an intracellular half-life of 3 to 4 hours, allowing twice-daily dosing. Plasma and intracellular 5′-triphosphate levels do not correlate [43].

**(3) Tissue distribution.** AZT is widely distributed to most tissues and fluids [42], including breast milk and semen. AZT crosses the placenta.

**(4) Cerebrospinal fluid (CSF).** AZT crosses into CSF, yielding 60% of serum levels (CSF:plasma ratio = 0.3:1 to 1.35:1) [44].

**(5) Metabolism and elimination.** Liver conjugates to an inactive glucuronide, which is rapidly excreted in the urine; less than 20% is found unchanged in the urine. Renal clearance is greater than creatinine clearance, indicating both glomerular filtration and tubular secretion.

**(6) Dose modifications.** In **hepatic disease,** clearance of AZT is reduced by 70% in patients with cirrhosis [45], resulting in two- to threefold increases in peak plasma levels and half-life. In the setting of severe hepatic dysfunction, a reduced dose of 100 mg orally every 8 hours seems appropriate [42]. In **renal disease,** the half-lives of AZT and its glucuronide increase. Dose adjustments [46] should be instituted as follows: in the setting of glomerular filtration rate (GFR) of more than 10 mL/min, no change; GFR of less than than 10 mL/min, 100 mg orally every 8 hours. For patients on hemodialysis, the dose should be the same as that in the setting of GFR of less than 10 mL/min. For patients on continuous ambulatory peritoneal dialysis (CAPD), the dose should be the same as that in the setting of GFR of less than 10 mL/min. Patients with continuous arterial venous diafiltration (CAVH) should be given 100 mg orally every 8 hours.

**(7) Drug interactions.** Myelosuppressive drugs (e.g., ganciclovir) may increase marrow toxicity, particularly granulocytopenia [47]. Other drugs to be used with caution include trimethoprim-sulfamethoxazole, sulfadiazine, pyrimethamine, dapsone, flucytosine, adriamycin, vinblastine, vincristine, hydroxyurea, interferon, and amphotericin B. Contrary to findings in early studies, acetaminophen has no effect on the metabolism of AZT [42]. These drugs can be given concomitantly. There is antagonism (competition for phosphorylation to the active moiety) between AZT and d4T [48,49]. These drugs should not be used together. Ribavirin inhibits phosphorylation of AZT. AZT plus ddI, ddC, $\alpha$-interferon, or foscarnet are synergistic against HIV-1. Probenecid increases AZT serum levels and half-life by inhibiting renal secretion and hepatic glucuronidation.

**e. Pregnancy category C**

**f. Adverse effects**

**(1) Subjective adverse effects.** Headache, gastrointestinal (GI) upset, altered taste, insomnia, fatigue, myalgia, and malaise occur early and usually subside with continued therapy. The currently used dosage of 600 mg/day of AZT is better tolerated and less toxic than the initial regimens (1,200–1,500 mg/day).

**(2) Hematologic toxicity** is related to the dose and duration, degree of marrow reserve, and stage of disease. The mechanism is likely multifactorial and may be related to inhibition of DNA synthesis both in marrow progenitor cells and in mitochondria [29,42]. **Anemia** may occur within 4 weeks, but the greatest risk is in months 3 through 8. Two percent of asymptomatic HIV-infected patients taking 600 mg/day [50] and up to 29% of AIDS patients taking 600 to 1,500 mg/day develop anemia (Retrovir package insert). Anemia usually resolves several weeks after discontinuation of AZT. **Macrocytosis** occurs in over 90% of AZT recipients but does not correlate with development of anemia and is not associated with abnormal vitamin $B_{12}$ or folate levels. Marrow may be normal or show hypoplasia or aplasia if severe anemia is present [51]. Pure red cell aplasia also has been described [52]. **Neutropenia** occurs in 8% of asymptomatic patients with HIV infection versus 37% of patients with AIDS. **Thrombocytopenia** rarely occurs [51]. AZT is the preferred treatment for HIV-1–associated thrombocytopenia. The effect is dose related; 2.5- and 4.9-fold increases in platelets over baseline with 600 and 1,200 mg/day, respectively [42]. If severe anemia (hemoglobin $<8.0$ g/dL) or neutropenia develops ($<750$ cells/mm$^3$), the clinician should switch to another agent rather than using colony-stimulating factors or transfusions.

**(3) Myopathy** is uncommon. Long-term ($>6$ months) high-dose ($>1,200$ mg/day) therapy with AZT has been associated with symptomatic myopathy in 6% to 18% of patients [42,53–55]. Manifestations include myalgia and diffuse symmetrical weakness of hip or shoulder girdle muscles, resulting in difficulty climbing stairs or arising from a squatting position or a chair. Serum creatinine kinase (CK) is usually elevated. Electromyography shows fibrillation potentials, positive sharp waves, and complex repetitive discharges. Histology shows mitochondrial abnormalities on Gomori trichrome staining (ragged red fibers) and EM, as well as inflammatory infiltrates of the endomysium consisting of $CD8^+$ lymphocytes and macrophages [53]. Discontinuation of AZT leads to gradual resolution of weakness over 6 to 8 weeks in 70% to 100% of patients [42]. Myalgia and serum CK improve more quickly. Patients not responding to discontinuation of AZT respond to steroid treatment [53]. AZT myopathy has become rare with the 600 mg/day dosage.

(4) **Hepatitis.** Reversible liver function abnormalities occasionally occur within 2 to 4 weeks.

(5) **Hepatic steatosis/lactic acidosis. See pharmacology of NRTIs in section V.A.3 above.**

(6) **Dermatologic.** AZT causes hyperpigmentation of skin and nails. Melanonychia occurs in 40%. The incidence in blacks is 81% versus white, 20%, and Hispanic, 31% [42].

(7) **Children.** AZT is generally well tolerated in children, with its major toxicities similar to those in adults: commonly macrocytic anemia and neutropenia, rarely myopathy, and very rarely lactic acidosis. Cardiomyopathy has occurred in children on AZT but it is more likely due to the effects of HIV itself [56–58].

5. **Didanosine** (Videx, Videx EC) is a purine nucleoside analogue of inosine. It is triphosphorylated by host kinases intracellularly to the active moiety 2′,3′-dideoxyadenosine 5′-triphosphate (ddATP). Unlike AZT, ddI is more active in resting cells [59].

a. **Formulations.** Chewable/dispersible tablets containing buffers are available in 25, 50, 100, 150, and 200 mg; buffered powder packets in 100, 167, and 250 mg; pediatric powder for solution (reconstituted with sterile water and antacid buffers) 10 mg/mL; enteric coated capsules (Videx EC, without buffer) in 125, 200, 250, and 400 mg. Advantages compared with buffered tablets are lack of buffer-related side effects and drug interactions, as well as better palatability.

b. **Dosage**

(1) **Adults**

(a) For adults weighing at least 60 kg, either 200 mg (buffered tablets) orally twice daily or 250 mg (buffered powder) orally twice daily is preferred. An alternative is 400 mg (buffered tablets) orally daily.

(b) For adults weighing no more than 60 kg, either 125 mg (buffered tablets) orally twice daily or 167 mg (buffered powder) orally twice daily is preferred. An alternative is 250 mg (buffered powder) orally daily.

(c) Videx EC has the following advantages relative to buffered tablets/powder: lack of buffer-related side effects and drug interactions, and better convenience and palatability. For adults weighing at least 60 kg, 400 mg orally daily is preferred. For adults weighing no more than 60 kg, 250 mg orally daily is preferred.

(d) All buffered forms are to be taken half an hour before or 2 hours after a meal.

(2) **Children.** Children over 13 years of age may use the adult dose of ddI formulations. Children under 13 years of age should be given 90 mg/m$^2$ BSA/dose orally every 12 hours of either the buffered tablets, powder, or pediatric solution (dose range 90–150 mg/m$^2$ BSA/dose orally every 12 hours). When using tablets, at least two should be given to ensure adequate buffering (e.g., two 50-mg tablets are preferred to one 100-mg tablet when delivering a 100-mg dose) [40].

c. ***In vitro*** activity. ddI inhibits HIV-1(including AZT-resistant strains) [30]. It is also active against HIV-2.

**d. Pharmacology.**

**(1)** Rapidly **absorbed** bioavailability varies widely depending on formulation of ddI, gastric pH, and presence of food (mean bioavailability 30%); ddI is very acid labile; therefore, oral formulations contain buffering agents (except Videx EC). The chewable tablet is 20% to 25% more bioavailable than powder. Food reduces absorption by 50% or more [60] (presumably by gastric acidity). It should be taken on an empty stomach 1 hour before or 2 hours after a meal.

**(2) Half-life.** The active triphosphate (ddATP) has an intracellular half-life of 8 to 24 hours [61].

**(3) Tissue distribution.** Less than 5% protein bound, ddI crosses the placenta and undergoes placental metabolism with only 15% to 50% of the drug reaching the fetal circulation (significantly lower than AZT). ddI penetration into the CNS is also lower than AZT. CSF levels are 20% of serum levels after an i.v. dose [61] (CSF:plasma ratios are 0.16:1 to 0.19:1).

**(4) Metabolism and elimination.** ddI is metabolized to hypoxanthine (major metabolite) and uric acid. Thirty percent to 50% of an administered dose is excreted unchanged by glomerular filtration and tubular secretion [61]. Approximately 20% of a dose is cleared by 4 to 6 hours of hemodialysis.

**(5) Dose modification.** In renal disease the half-life increases (Table 19.3).

**e. Drug interactions:** Concurrent use of ddC and ddI is contraindicated. Drugs that increase risk of pancreatitis (d4T, hydroxyurea, ethyl alcohol [EtOH], pentamidine, azathioprine) or that cause peripheral neuropathy, (isoniazid [INH], ethambutol, ethionamide, chloramphenicol, thalidomide, metronidazole, nitrofurantoin, vincristine, cisplatin, gold, phenytoin [62]), should be used with caution or avoided. Ganciclovir and valganciclovir increase plasma ddI concentrations (57.7% with i.v. ganciclovir). Patients should be monitored for risk of ddI toxicity [63]. If the buffered formulations of ddI are used, drugs requiring gastric acidity for optimal absorption (itraconazole, ketoconazole, dapsone, indinavir [IDV], ritonavir [RTV], delavirdine [DLV]) should be given 1 to 2 hours before or after ddI. The divalent cations in the buffer chelate quinolones and tetracyclines [64].

**f. Pregnancy category B**

**g. Adverse effects**

**(1) Pancreatitis** can occur 3 to 5 months after starting ddI. The mechanism is unknown. It is sometimes fatal and is dose related (25% of patients receiving 10–12 mg/kg/day [65] vs. <10% with current doses [66]). Perhaps discontinuation of therapy with asymptomatic hyperamylasemia accounts for the low incidence of pancreatitis in some studies [66,67]. Risk is higher with a history of pancreatitis or alcohol abuse, or in the presence of hypertriglyceridemia, AIDS, or obesity, or with the concomitant use of d4T, hydroxyurea, and pentamidine [65,68]. It presents with the typical signs and symptoms. DdI should be discontinued and

Table 19.3. Dose[a] (in mg) Adjustments of ddI per GFR, Weight, and Formulation

| GFR (mL/min) | >60 | >59 | >59 | 30–59 | 30–59 | 10–29 | 10–29 | <10 | <10 |
|---|---|---|---|---|---|---|---|---|---|
| kg | Any | >60 | <60 | >60 | <60 | >60 | <60 | >60 | <60 |
| Buffered tablet | Usual dose | | | 200 | 150 | 150 | 100 | 100* | 75 |
| Videx EC | | 400 | 250 | 200 | 125 | 125 | 125 | 125 | [b] |

GFR, glomerular filtration rate.

[a] An extra dose should be given postdialysis. In the setting of continuous ambulatory peritoneal dialysis or continuous arterial venous diafiltration, the dose given should be the same as when GFR is <10 mL/min. In the setting of hepatic disease, the need for a change in dose is unknown. The patient should be monitored for evidence of ddI toxicity.

[b] An alternative formulation should be used.

pancreatitis usually resolves. Recurrence can occur in patients rechallenged [69]. Routine monitoring of enzymes during therapy is not recommended. Asymptomatic elevations of amylase and lipase (up to two times the upper limit of normal [ULN]) are common in HIV-infected patients [70]. In one study 39% of ddI patients developed asymptomatic increases in pancreatic enzymes, yet none developed pancreatitis during a mean follow-up of 8 months [65].

**(2) Peripheral neuropathy.** DdI can cause distal symmetric polyneuropathy. The incidence (5%–15%) varies by dose and duration of therapy, by the prevalence of underlying HIV-associated distal symmetric sensory neuropathy, by the presence of AIDS, and according to different criteria used to define neuropathy in various studies [71–73]. With the currently used dose, neuropathy is uncommon, the incidence being similar to that among patients treated with AZT (600 mg/day) [66,73]. It usually occurs after 2 to 7 months of treatment [69], with numbness, tingling, burning, or aching pain over the soles of the feet [69,72]. Over time, lancinating pain of the lower extremities follows, and if ddI is continued, the hands and upper extremities become involved. Initially pain occurs only when ambulating, but eventually becomes continuous. In more advanced cases, pain can interfere with sleep and routine daily activities [69]. Initially, examination and nerve conduction studies are usually unremarkable, but eventually sensory loss appears (vibratory sense, pinprick, and temperature) in a stocking-glove distribution, Achilles reflex is decreased, and nerve conduction studies show an axonal neuropathy. In severe cases mild weakness may be found. Symptoms gradually resolve or substantially improve in most patients 4 to 8 weeks after stopping ddI. In some patients, symptoms worsen for up to 6 weeks (coasting) and then gradually improve. Patients with AIDS or severe neuropathy may not fully recover. Patients with AIDS or HIV neuropathy (or other causes of neuropathy) or those taking ddI with d4T or taking d4T and hydroxyurea are at higher risk of developing ddI-associated neuropathy [74]. It has been suggested, but not proven, that ddI (and d4T and ddC) cause neuropathy by inhibiting mitochondrial DNA synthesis [33,75,76]. Treatment is helped by early recognition, and discontinuation of ddI is most important because this gives a better chance of full recovery. Physicians should make patients aware of the coasting phenomenon [72,77] noted above. Although some patients tolerate rechallenge with a lower dose of ddI, the use of subinhibitory doses of antiretroviral agents cannot be advocated. No specific therapy exists.

**(3) Hepatitis.** Asymptomatic elevations of liver function test (LFT) results (more than five times normal) may occur in up to 9% of patients [66]. Fulminant hepatitis occurs rarely [78].

**(4) Lactic acidosis/hepatic steatosis.** ddI can cause lactic acidosis/hepatic steatosis (see section **V.A.3**).

**(5) Miscellaneous effects.** Because GI upset and diarrhea are relatively common with the powdered form, Videx EC is preferred. Hyperuricemia is rare with the current dose [66]. Sodium and magnesium in the powder and buffered tablets may be a concern in patients with decreased renal function or on low-sodium diets.

**(6) Children.** Pancreatitis, although reported, is less commonly observed in children than in adults, although it tends to occur in children with other risk factors, including previous pancreatitis or use of other medications such as d4T or pentamidine. Peripheral sensory neuropathy may occur as in adults. Children given ddI develop asymptomatic peripheral retinal depigmentation, which appears to reverse with discontinuation of the agent. It occurs in fewer than 5% of courses [40]. Lactic acidosis occurs rarely as in adults.

**6. Zalcitabine** (HIVID) is a dideoxynucleoside analogue of cytidine. It requires triphosphorylation by cellular kinases to convert to the active 5′-triphosphate.

This takes place most efficiently in resting cells (in contrast to AZT) (DdC package insert).

a. **Formulations** : 0.375- and 0.75-mg tablets
b. **Dosage**
   (1) **Adults.** Adults weighing at least 30 kg should receive 0.75 mg orally three times daily; those under 30 kg should receive 0.375 mg orally three times daily.
   (2) **Children.** Children at least 13 years of age may be given the adult dosage; those under 13 should be given 0.01 mg/kg/dose orally every 8 hours [40].
c. ***In vitro* activity:** HIV-1 (including AZT-resistant strains), HIV-2, hepatitis B [79]
d. **Pharmacology** [79a]
   (1) **Absorption.** ddC is 70% to 90% bioavailable. Administration with food decreases the rate and extent of absorption. However, the clinical relevance of this is not known.
   (2) **Half-life.** The plasma elimination half-life is 1 to 3 hours [79a].
   (3) **Tissue distribution.** ddC is not highly protein bound. CSF concentration is 20% of plasma i.v. levels (less than that of AZT) (CSF:plasma ratio is 0.14:1 to 0.20:1) [79a]. ddC diffuses across the placenta (50%).
   (4) **Metabolism and elimination.** ddC does not undergo hepatic metabolism. Sixty-two percent of an oral dose is excreted both by filtration and secretion unchanged in urine. Dideoxyuridine is the major metabolite. It is not known whether ddC is dialyzed by any method. Dosage modifications for renal disease are as follows: patients with a GFR of 10 to 40 mL/min should receive 0.75 mg orally every 12 hours; those with a GFR of less than 10 mL/min should receive 0.75 mg orally every 24 hours.
   (5) **Drug interactions.** ddC should not be coadministered with ddI or d4T because of increased risk for neurotoxicity. Other drugs that cause neuropathy (see discussion of ddI, section V.5) should be administered with caution.
e. **Pregnancy category C**
f. **Adverse effects**
   (1) **Peripheral neuropathy** occurs in 5% to 18% of patients and is dose related [80–83]. Neuropathy due to ddC is more common than that related to ddI [81,83] (see discussion of ddI, section V.5, for features). Patients with AIDS, diabetes mellitus, EtOH abuse, low baseline vitamin $B_{12}$ levels, and a history of peripheral neuropathy are at higher risk for developing neurotoxicity [84,85]. ddC should be discontinued when symptoms occur. Although some patients can tolerate rechallenge with a lower dose, the use of subinhibitory doses of ddC cannot be recommended.
   (2) **Oral and esophageal ulcers.** Stomatitis (ulcers of the buccal mucosa, pharynx, tongue, and soft palate) occurs in 2.6% to 8% of patients [82,83]. Esophageal ulcerations also occur [86].
   (3) **Rash.** Transient erythematous maculopapular rash on the extremities and trunk, associated with fever, malaise, and stomatitis, may occur, usually during the first 30 days of therapy [79a]. In a phase I trial, 70% developed rash [79a], although in larger trials, the incidence of rash was not noted [82,83].
   (4) **Pancreatitis** occurred in 0.5% to 3% of patients in large trials [81–83] but less frequently than with ddI and ddC (0.5% vs. 1%–2%) [81,83].
   (5) **Lactic acidosis.** Hepatic steatosis has been described with ddC (see discussion of AZT, section V.4, for details).
   (6) **Hepatitis.** Elevations of LFT results were reported in 6% of patients on ddC monotherapy [82] and in 7.1% of subjects receiving AZT and ddC [83].
   (7) **Children.** Peripheral neuropathy, stomatitis, and lactic acidosis occur as in adults.

7. **Stavudine (Zerit)** is a nucleoside analogue of thymidine.
   a. **Formulations:** 15-, 20-, 30-, and 40-mg capsules and 1 mg/mL oral solution.
   b. **Dosage**
      (1) **Adults.** Adults weighing at least 60 kg should receive 40 mg orally twice daily; those weighing less than 60 kg should receive 30 mg orally twice daily. It may be taken without regard to meals.
      (2) **Children.** Children at least 13 years of age or weighing over 30 kg may be given the adult weight-based dosage; those under 13 should be given 1 mg/kg/dose orally twice daily [40]. Use of either the oral solution or opening the capsules and sprinkling the medication onto a spoonful of food facilitates administration of medication to children.
   c. ***In vitro* activity.** d4T is active against HIV-1 and HIV-2, especially in proliferating cells [29].
   d. **Pharmacology** [87]
      (1) **Absorption.** Bioavailability is 70%. It is not protein bound.
      (2) **Half-life.** The intracellular half-life of the triphosphate form is 3.5 hours, similar to that of AZT [88]. The 3.5-hour half-life allows twice-daily dosing.
      (3) **Tissue distribution.** CSF levels are 30% to 55% of those found in plasma (similar to those for AZT). d4T crosses the placenta by simple diffusion, with tissue levels lower than those achieved with AZT (approximately 75%). This is consistent with d4T being less lipophilic than AZT [29].
      (4) **Metabolism and elimination.** d4T is excreted by renal and nonrenal routes. Forty percent of a dose is excreted, unchanged in urine by both glomerular filtration and tubular secretion. The remaining portion is metabolized to thymine, which may then be used in pyrimidine-based salvage pathways [89].
      (5) **Dose modifications.** Dose adjustment for renal failure is necessary (Table 19.4).
      (6) **Hemodialysis.** Patients weighing at least 60 kg should receive 20 mg orally every 24 hours; those weighing less than 60 kg should be given 15 mg orally every 24 hours. The dose should be given after dialysis and at the same time on nondialysis days.
      (7) **Drug interactions.** d4T should not be used with AZT [79a,88] (see discussion of AZT, section V.4) or ddC. Drugs that cause peripheral neuropathy should be used with caution or avoided when possible and include vincristine, nitrofurantoin, ethambutol, INH, ethionamide, gold, phenytoin, thalidomide, dapsone, chloramphenicol, cisplatinum, ethanol, colchicine, and metronidazole. The risk for peripheral neuropathy is higher when d4T is used in combination with ddI, and with ddI plus hydroxyurea.

Table 19.4. Adjustment of Stavudine (Zerit) in Patients with Varying Degrees of Renal Function

| | Recommended Stavudine Dose by Patient Weight | |
|---|---|---|
| Creatinine Clearance (mL/min) | >60 kg | <60 kg |
| >50 | 40 mg q12h | 30 mg q12h |
| 26–50 | 20 mg q12h | 15 mg q12h |
| 10–25 | 20 mg q24h | 15 mg q24h |

q12h, every 12 hours.
There are insufficient data to recommend a dose for patients with a creatinine clearance of <10 mL/min or for patients undergoing dialysis.
Reprinted from *Physicians' Desk Reference*, 50th ed. Montvale, NJ: Medical Economics Data, 1996:732; with permission.

Patients should be monitored closely for signs and symptoms of neurotoxicity. Ribavirin *in vitro* interferes with the phosphorylation of d4T [49]. The clinical relevance of this is not known.

**e. Pregnancy category C**

**f. Adverse effects**

**(1) Peripheral neuropathy.** The incidence is similar to that seen with ddI and ddC. The risk is dose related. One-year incidence rates were 6% and 37% for dosages of 0.1 and 2.0 mg/kg/day, respectively [90]. With the currently recommended dosing (1 mg/kg/day), neuropathy develops in 12% of patients [91]. As with ddI and ddC, neurotoxicity occurs more commonly in patients with AIDS (25% 1-year rate vs. 10% among HIV-infected asymptomatic patients) [91]. Upon discontinuation, neuropathy completely resolved within 4 to 57 days (median 17 days) in 63% [91]. The risk is significantly increased when d4T is given in combination with ddI or with ddI plus hydroxyurea [74].

**(2) Hepatic steatosis/lactic acidosis** occurs in those receiving d4T (see section V.A.3). Asymptomatic elevations of liver enzymes (greater than five times the ULN) occurred in 12/100 person-years versus 10/100 person-years with AZT [91].

**(3) Pancreatitis.** There is no clear association between d4T use and an increased risk for pancreatitis [91].

**(4) Children.** d4T is generally well tolerated by children, with similar rates of toxicity as observed in adults. However, peripheral neuropathy is uncommon, and lactic acidosis is rare [40].

**8. Lamivudine (Epivir)** is a pyrimidine nucleoside analogue of cytosine. It must be triphosphorylated to the active moiety (3TC-triphosphate).

**a. Formulations** include 150-mg tablets and 10 mg/mL oral solution. In combination with AZT it is available as Combivir (150 mg 3TC and 300 mg AZT). In combination with AZT and abacavir (ABC) it is available as Trizivir (150 mg 3TC + 300 mg AZT + 300 mg ABC).

**b. Dosage**

**(1) Adults.** Adults should be given 150 mg every 12 hours. As Combivir, adults should receive one tablet orally twice daily; As Trizivir, they should receive one tablet orally twice daily (administered without regard to food).

**(2) Children.** Children at least 13 years of age may be given the adult dosage; those under 13 should be given 4 mg/kg/dose orally twice daily up to a maximum of 150 mg orally twice daily; those under 1 month of age should be given 2 mg/kg/dose orally twice daily. For children and adolescents one may use Combivir or Trizivir tablets or half-tablets to approximate weight-based doses.

**c. *In vitro* activity.** 3TC is active against HIV-1 (including AZT-resistant strains) and HIV-2 in acutely infected cells [92]. It is also active against hepatitis B virus.

**d. Pharmacology** [93]

**(1) Absorption.** Bioavailability is 82%. It can be taken without regard to meals.

**(2) Half-life.** The intracellular half-life of the active moiety is 10.5 to 15.5 hours.

**(3) Tissue distribution.** Protein binding varies from 20% to 30%. CSF penetration is 4% to 8% of serum concentration (CSF:plasma ratio of 0.06:1). These levels exceed the 50% inhibitory concentration ($IC_{50}$) of HIV-1 and are clinically relevant. 3TC diffuses freely across the placenta and is secreted into breast milk [93].

**(4) Metabolism and elimination.** Approximately 70% of an oral dose is eliminated via renal mechanisms as unchanged drug. About 5% is metabolized to an inactive trans-sulfoxide metabolite.

**(5) Dose modification.** 3TC doses need adjustment in **renal insufficiency** (Table 19.5). Patients undergoing hemodialysis should receive 25 to

Table 19.5. Adjustment of Lamivudine (Epivir) in Patients with Varying Degrees of Renal Function

| Creatinine Clearance (mL/min) | Dosage of Lamivudine |
|---|---|
| ≥50 | 150 mg twice daily |
| 30–49 | 150 mg/day |
| 15–29 | 150 mg first dose, then 100 mg/day |
| 5–14 | 150 mg first dose, then 50 mg/day |
| <5 | 50 mg first dose, then 25 mg/day |

There are insufficient data to recommend a dosage of lamivudine in patients undergoing hemodialysis.
From Epivir (Lamivudine). Package insert, November 1995.

50 mg orally daily and should receive a supplemental dose after dialysis. For patients on CAPD, the dose should be the same as that in the setting of GFR of 5–14 mL/min. For patients with CAVH, the dose should be the same as that in the setting of GFR of 15–29 mL/min. In the presence of **hepatic dysfunction,** the 3TC dose is unaltered (see Table 19.5).

(6) **Drug interactions.** Clinically relevant adverse drug interactions have not been reported.

e. **Pregnancy category C**

f. **Adverse effects**

(1) **Adults.** 3TC is well tolerated. No dose-related toxicities occurred in large phase I/II studies [94,95]. The most common complaints were headache, fatigue, GI upset, and insomnia. These were mild and transitory. In a trial of AZT versus 3TC plus AZT there was no additional toxicity versus AZT alone, and the adverse effects in both arms were felt to be secondary to AZT [96,97].

(2) **Children.** 3TC is very well tolerated. Uncommonly, pancreatitis, peripheral neuropathy, or lactic acidosis occurs. The rare precipitous decrease in hemoglobin following institution of combined AZT/3TC therapy reported in adults [98] has been seen by us in one older adolescent and one newborn of a mother receiving AZT/3TC [99].

9. **Abacavir (Ziagen)** is a 2′-deoxynucleoside analogue of guanosine that is triphosphorylated by a unique set of enzymes to the active, carboxylic guanosine triphosphate.

a. **Formulations** include 300-mg tablets and 20 mg/mL oral suspension. In combination with AZT and 3TC it is available as Trizivir (300 mg AZT + 150 mg 3TC + 300 mg ABC).

b. **Dosage**

(1) **Adults.** Adults should be given 300 mg orally twice daily. As Trizivir, they should be given one tablet orally twice daily, which may be taken without regard to food.

(2) **Children.** Children at least 13 years of age may be given the adult dosage; those under 13 should be given 8 mg/kg/dose orally twice daily up to a maximum of 300 mg orally twice daily.

c. ***In vitro* activity.** ABC is active against HIV-1 and HIV-2, including AZT-resistant strains.

d. **Pharmacology** [100,101]

(1) **Absorption.** Bioavailability is 80%. Approximately 50% is protein bound.

(2) **Half-life.** The intracellular half-life of the active moiety is 3.3 hours, which allows dosing every 12 hours.

(3) **Tissue distribution.** CSF penetration data are scant. In three patients, ABC 200 mg every 8 hours yielded a CSF level that was 18% of plasma

level, 1.5 to 2 hours postdose. The mean ABC CSF concentration was twice the established $IC_{50}$ against clinical isolates of HIV [102]. Using different doses of ABC, the average CSF:plasma concentration ratio was 0.42:1 [103]. Animal data suggest that CSF penetration is similar to that for AZT [100]. In an *ex vivo* human placental model, ABC crosses the placenta [104].

(4) **Metabolism and elimination.** ABC is metabolized to inactive 5′-carboxylated and 5′-glucuronide compounds. The major excretion is renal. Less than 2% is found unchanged in urine [105].

(5) **Dose modifications.** None for patients with renal insufficiency.

(6) **Drug interactions.** ETOH can increase ABC levels [105].

e. **Pregnancy category C**

f. **Adverse effects.** In placebo-controlled studies the most common adverse effects have been mild and reversible and include nausea, abdominal pain, vomiting, headache, fatigue, and malaise [101,103,106]. There was a trend toward increased frequency of nausea and headache at higher doses [101,106]. At 300 mg twice daily, 45% had nausea, 40% headache, and 40% fatigue over 12 weeks. It was not specified if these adverse effects were solely from ABC [106]. Ten percent of patients on higher doses stopped taking the drug owing to adverse events (nausea, dizziness, photophobia, and palpitations or hypersensitivity syndrome) considered secondary to ABC.

(1) **Hepatic steatosis/lactic acidosis** (see section **V.A.3**). ABC (relative to the other NRTIs) is a weak inhibitor of mitochondrial DNA polymerase gamma [107]. However, hepatic steatosis/lactic acidosis occurs when using ABC in combination with other NRTIs. Asymptomatic elevations of LFT results have not been reported [106].

(2) **Hypersensitivity reaction.** This is a serious and potentially fatal adverse effect reported in 3% of patients [97,106,108]. Onset occurred at a mean of 11 days (range 1–28 days) [108]. **Manifestations initially** include malaise and fever, accompanied by nausea (with or without vomiting) and progression with additional dosing. An urticarial or maculopapular or generalized erythematous rash was present at onset or developed 1 to 3 days after constitutional symptoms began. Rash may be a dominant sign or an incidental finding. Some may have cough. ABC hypersensitivity can be difficult to distinguish from a viral respiratory syndrome [109,110]. Although influenza is less likely to cause GI symptoms, it can be difficult to distinguish these entities on clinical grounds alone [109]. Laboratory value abnormalities may include neutropenia, elevated LFT results, and increased creatinine phosphokinase (CPK). No risk factors have been identified, but there may be a genetic predisposition with certain HLA types [111,112]. The pathogenesis is not known, and there is no specific therapy. Upon discontinuation of ABC, symptoms resolve rapidly (1–2 days). Rechallenge is associated with rapid (within hours) reoccurrence of more severe symptoms, and deaths have been reported [109,111]. Patients should never be rechallenged with ABC.

(3) **Children.** Toxicities, similar to those occurring in adults include the uncommon (3%–5%) hypersensitivity reaction and the rare lactic acidosis and hepatic steatosis syndromes.

B. **Non-nucleoside reverse transcriptase inhibitors** are listed in Table 19.6.

1. **Mechanism of action** [113,114]. NNRTIs are a structurally diverse group of drugs that do not require intracellular processing (phosphorylation, etc.) to

Table 19.6. Non-nucleoside Reverse Transcriptase Inhibitors

| |
|---|
| Nevirapine (NVP, Viramune) |
| Efavirenz (EFV, Sustiva) |
| Delavirdine (DLV, Rescriptor) |

exert their activity. Thus, unlike NRTIs, they are active in many different cell lines (resting and active, T-lymphocytes and macrophages). They bind to a site on RT distinct from NRTIs, and they are neither DNA chain terminators nor competitive inhibitors of RT. Nucleotide binding is not altered in the presence of NNRTIs. NNRTIs probably slow the rate of the chemical reaction catalyzed by RT [12]. The activity of NNRTIs is highly specific for HIV-1 RT, leaving human DNA polymerase unaffected.

**2. Nevirapine (NVP, Viramune)**, is a dipyridodiazepinone NNRTI.

**a. Formulations** include 200-mg tablets and 10 mg/mL syrup.

**b. Dosage**

**(1) Adults.** Initial dosage is 200 mg orally daily for 14 days then 200 mg orally every 12 hours. This decreases the frequency of rash (see section on adverse effects below) and compensates for autoinduction of hepatic metabolism. If a rash occurs during days 1 to 14, the second daily dose should not be added until the rash has resolved. Some clinicians suggest an even slower dose escalation (100 mg daily for 7 days then increasing by 100 mg/day for the next 7 days and so forth until the 400 mg daily dose is reached) and considering giving prednisone 50 mg every other day for the first 2 weeks. Evaluation in a small group of subjects suggested that this approach is safe [115].

**(2) Children.** Plasma clearance of NVP by children is greater than by adults, especially in children under 9 years of age. Similar to adults, however, are the increase in clearance of NVP by children of all ages after the first 2 weeks of use and the apparent decrease in rash if a stepwise increase in dose is instituted. The majority of pediatric clinical trials used a dose of 120 to 200 mg/m$^2$ BSA orally once daily (maximum dose 200 mg) for 14 days, followed by a full dose of 120 to 200 mg/m$^2$ BSA orally every 12 hours if no rash had occurred. It should be noted that the U.S. Food and Drug Administration (FDA) recently licensed an alternative pediatric regimen of 7 mg/kg orally every 12 hours for children under 8 years of age and 4 mg/kg for children at least 8 years of age. Again, one begins with once-daily dosing for 14 days and then increases to twice-daily dosing up to a maximum at any age of 200 mg orally twice daily. The alternative regimen is designed by pharmacokinetic modeling to achieve similar plasma concentrations as dosing of 150 mg/m$^2$ BSA orally twice daily, but results in an abrupt 43% decrease in dose size after the 8th birthday rather than the more gradual change when BSA-based dosing is used. Some clinicians (including us) prefer to use the BSA-based dosing regimens studied in clinical trials [40]. Neonatal dosing is being studied in clinical trials.

**c. *In vitro* activity.** NVP is active only against HIV-1, including NRTI- and PI-resistant strains. NVP-resistant HIV-1 is frequently resistant to all NRTIs.

**d. Pharmacology**

**(1) Absorption.** Bioavailability is greater than 90% [116] without regard to meals or buffering agents.

**(2) Half-life.** Plasma half-life is 25 to 30 hours at steady state [116]; therefore, studies of once-daily dosing are under way.

**(3) Tissue distribution.** NVP is 60% protein bound, nonionized at physiologic pH, lipophilic, and widely distributed in human tissues. It crosses the placenta completely [117] and is secreted in breast milk [118]. CSF concentrations are 45% of plasma levels [119]. Semen levels are 60% of plasma levels [120].

**(4) Metabolism and elimination.** NVP is extensively metabolized to several hydroxylated inactive metabolites by hepatic cytochrome P-450 (primarily CYP3A). The metabolites are excreted in urine (<3% of an oral dose is excreted unchanged). NVP is an inducer of cytochrome P-450 enzymes that metabolize many other drugs (see following section on drug interactions). NVP dose must be increased after 14 days because of autoinduction of NVP's own hepatic metabolism (see section on dosing) [116].

(5) **Dose modifications.** Few data about dosage adjustments for hepatic or renal disease are available. Standard doses should be used with caution.

(6) **Drug interactions.** NVP induces the CYP3A4 group isoenzymes of hepatic cytochrome P-450, reaching maximum induction 4 weeks after starting therapy. Therefore, certain drugs require dose modification. NVP substantially lowers levels of **methadone and other opiates.** This may precipitate withdrawal beginning on days 4 to 10 of NVP administration [121]. In one study [121], some patients required a mean dose increase of 16%. Used in conjunction with **IDV or lopinavir (LPV) plus RTV,** NVP lowers levels of both IDV and LPV, requiring a dose increase (see respective PI section (6)).

(7) **Drugs to avoid with NVP.** With ketoconazole, NVP levels are decreased by more than 60%; with oral contraceptives, ethinyl estradiol levels are decreased by 20% (alternative or additional contraceptive methods should be used); and with rifampin, NVP levels are decreased by 37%. St. John's wort (hypericum perforatum) also decreases NVP levels. Drug interactions with lipid lowering agents or anticonvulsants are unknown.

e. **Pregnancy category C**

f. **Adverse effects**

(1) **Rash** occurs in up to 22% of patients, sometimes leading to discontinuation [122–124]. Onset is usually within the first 4 to 6 weeks. Risk factors include ETOH use, concomitant hepatitis C infection, and Chinese ancestry [125]. The rash is erythematous maculopapular in nature; occasionally pruritus involves the face, trunk, and extremities. Palms and soles may be spared. It is usually mild and self-limited. Extensive skin involvement associated with fever, constitutional symptoms, and occasionally oral ulcers has been described in 4% to 32% of patients [122]. Stevens-Johnson syndrome with fatalities was reported in less than 1% to 7.6% of patients [123,126,127]. The mechanism of the rash is uncertain.

(a) **Treatment.** Mild rash (no systemic symptoms/signs or mucosal lesions) can be treated with antihistamines while patients continue NVP. Severe rash or signs and symptoms suggestive of Stevens-Johnson syndrome (confluent, painful, edematous rash; mucosal membrane and conjunctiva blisters or ulcers; and fever, malaise, and myalgia) require immediate discontinuation of NVP. Patients should not be rechallenged with NVP. Corticosteroids given in conjunction with the lead-in dose (200 mg orally daily) of NVP may decrease the incidence of rash [115], although this is not routine practice.

(b) **NNRTI dermatologic cross-reactions.** The molecular structures of the NNRTIs are unrelated; thus, the risk for developing a rash when given another NNRTI would not be expected. However, studies to evaluate this are limited. Two patients with severe hypersensitivity reactions to NVP tolerated efavirenz (EFV) in addition to a tapering dose of prednisone over 11 days [128]. Protection by steroids may have played a role. Other investigators have reported one of six patients with an NVP-associated rash previously also developed a rash when given EFV [129]. However, these investigators concluded that EFV is safe in patients with known hypersensitivity reactions to NVP.

(2) **Hepatitis.** In phase I/II studies, 10% of subjects had isolated elevation of $\gamma$-glutamyl transpeptidase that was five times normal [125,130,131]. However, some of these patients had baseline elevations of the enzyme. Hepatitis occurred in less than 2% of patients in controlled trials [125,130,131], although jaundice and elevated LFT results, with fever,

malaise, anorexia, nausea, and a rash occurring within 2 to 4 weeks of starting NVP, have been reported [125,132]. Clinical manifestations and LFT results resolved within 8 weeks of therapy cessation. Twelve cases of hepatotoxicity (two life threatening) were reported in non–HIV-infected health-care workers given an NVP containing an antiretroviral regimen for postexposure prophylaxis [133,134]. NVP is not recommended for postexposure prophylaxis [134]. Thus far, no serious toxicity has been reported among mother-infant pairs using single-dose NVP for the prevention of perinatal HIV transmission [133,134].

(3) **Miscellaneous.** In phase I/II studies, mild somnolence, headache, and nausea were occasionally observed that did not require discontinuation of NVP [116].

(4) **Children.** The incidence of skin rash, Stevens-Johnson syndrome, hepatotoxicity, and drug interactions is similar in children and adults.

3. **Efavirenz (Sustiva)** is a 1,4-dihydro-2H-3,1-benzoxazin-2-one NNRTI.

a. **Formulations** include 50-, 100-, and 200-mg capsules and 600-mg tablets.

b. **Dosage**

(1) **Adults.** Adults may be given 600 mg orally once daily, usually prior to bedtime to reduce the CNS side effects. Patients should avoid taking it after a high-fat meal, which can cause EFV levels to increase markedly (>50%).

(2) **Children.** Children at least 13 years of age may be given the adult dosage (600 mg orally daily). Children under 13 should be given EFV based on their body weight (BW) once daily. The dose is as follows: BW 10 to 14 kg, 200 mg; 15 to 19 kg, 250 mg; 20 to 24 kg, 300 mg; 25 to 32 kg, 350 mg; 33 to 40 kg, 400 mg; over 40 kg, 600 mg. Capsule contents may be sprinkled on food. The somewhat bitter taste can be masked with grape jelly or chocolate syrup.

c. ***In vitro* activity.** EFV is active against HIV-1, including NRTI- and PI-resistant strains. It requires no intracellular metabolism to become activated.

d. **Pharmacology** [135,136]

(1) **Absorption.** Bioavailability is 45%, but meals high in fat increase bioavailability by 50% (see section on dose below). EFV is 99.5% to 99.75% protein bound.

(2) **Half-life** in plasma is more than 24 hours, allowing once-daily dosing.

(3) **Tissue distribution.** EFV crosses the blood–brain barrier, and CSF ratios are 0.26 to 1.19 of corresponding plasma levels. These levels are over the $IC_{95}$ for wild-type HIV-1 [135] and were clinically relevant in one small study [137]. EFV crosses the placenta, and malformations have been observed in fetuses of EFV-treated monkeys.

(4) **Metabolism and elimination.** EFV is metabolized primarily by hepatic cytochrome P-450 and by CYP3A4 and CYP2B6 isoenzymes to inactive hydroxylated metabolites. Fourteen percent to 34% of an oral dose is excreted in the urine as glucuronide metabolites, 16% to 61% in feces as unchanged drug. Less than 1% of a dose is excreted unchanged in urine.

(5) **Dose modification.** None is required for hepatic or renal disease.

(6) **Drug interactions.** EFV is both an inducer and inhibitor of CYP3A4 isoenzymes. *In vitro* EFV also inhibits isoenzymes CYP2C9 and CYP2C19, leading to alteration of metabolism of other drugs. Similarly, EFV plasma levels may be lower if drugs that induce CYP3A4 are used in conjunction. **Drugs that should be avoided** include saquinavir (SQV) (but SQV and RTV combination therapy can be used with EFV); clarithromycin (EVF levels decrease by 40%); and astemizole, terfenadine, midazolam, triazolam, and ergot derivatives. **Drugs that require dose adjustments** include IDV (increase dose to 1g every 8 hours), amprenavir (APV; increase dose to 1,200 mg every 8 hours), LPV/RTV (Kaletra; increase dose to 4 teaspoons every 12 hours); and methadone (increase

dose to achieve effect). For phenobarbital, phenytoin, and carbamazepine, the anticonvulsant levels should be monitored and doses adjusted. When used with warfarin, the anticoagulation effect should be monitored closely. EFV decreases rifabutin levels by 35%, so the dose should be increased to 450 to 600 mg/day. Levels of rifampin are not affected, but EFV levels decrease by 25%; the clinical implications are not clear. Estradiol levels increase by 37%. The clinical significance is not known. Because the effect of EFV on other oral contraceptives is not known, a reliable method of barrier contraception is recommended in addition to oral agents.

e. **Pregnancy category C** (similar to other antiretroviral agents). However, EFV should not be used during the first trimester because fetal malformations have been described in monkeys. Women of childbearing age should be informed of this and contraceptive protection should be ensured.

f. **Adverse effects**

(1) **Central nervous system** effects occur after the first dose. Manifestations include insomnia, dizziness, abnormal dreaming, impaired concentration, and mood changes in 58% to 73% of patients taking EFV in combination with other antiretroviral agents versus 27% for controls [138,139]. No severe reactions were reported. Median duration of symptoms was 19 to 22 days, but they may persist for several weeks. Less than 2% of patients discontinued EFV because of CNS side effects. **Psychiatric side effects,** including hallucinations, changes in personality, depression, anxiety, and marked cognitive dysfunction, have been described. The cause of CNS effects is not known.

(2) **Dermatologic.** Rash was reported in 10% to 34% of patients [27], usually occurring in the second week. It is maculopapular in nature, self-limited, and requires no therapy, or a brief course of oral antihistamines. Mean duration of rash is 14 days, and it usually does not lead to discontinuation of EFV [27]. Stevens-Johnson syndrome has rarely been reported [140].

(3) **Laboratory values.** Occasionally both high-density lipoprotein (HDL) and low-density lipoprotein (LDL) cholesterol are increased [140].

(4) **Children.** CNS manifestations of EFV are similar to those in adults but less common, whereas skin rash is more common [40]. Drug interactions are similar to those in adults.

4. **Delavirdine (Rescriptor).** DLV is a bisheteroarylpiperazine NNRTI.

a. **Formulations** include 100- and 200-mg tablets. The 100-mg tablets only may be dispersed in water (see package insert for instructions).

b. **Dosage**

(1) **Adults.** Adults should be given 400 mg every 8 hours without regard to meals. Buffering agents (ddI) or antacids should be given at least 1 hour apart from DLV (see section below on drug interactions). Twice-daily dosing (600 mg every 12 hours) is being studied.

(2) **Children.** Adolescents are given the same dose as adults. Few data are available to guide dosage for children under 13.

c. ***In vitro* activity.** DLV is active only against HIV-1, including NRTI- and PI-resistant strains. It does not require any intracellular metabolism to become active.

d. **Pharmacology** [141–143]

(1) **Absorption.** Bioavailability is 85%, and peak plasma concentrations occur in 1 to 2 hours. DLV is a weak base, with poor solubility at pH above 3.0. Therefore, the rate and extent of absorption is affected by hypochlorhydria of any cause or by drugs that decrease gastric acidity. DLV levels are significantly decreased (by 40%–45%) in patients with hypo- or achlorhydria compared to subjects with normal gastric acidity, even when DLV is given concomitantly with an acidic beverage. DLV is 98% protein bound, primarily to albumin.

(2) **Half-life** is 2.35 to 4.12 hours, necessitating dosing every 8 hours.

(3) **Tissue distribution.** Given extensive protein binding, CSF penetration is only 0.4% of plasma concentration; 2% of the serum concentration has been reported in semen. DLV is teratogenic in rats and is excreted in milk. No studies have been done in pregnant women.

(4) **Metabolism and elimination.** DLV is extensively biotransformed to several inactive metabolites by hepatic CYP3A pathways primarily and to a lesser extent CYP2D6. Five percent appears unchanged in urine, and the metabolites are excreted in the feces (51%) and urine (44%). DLV reversibly inhibits the activity of CYP3A and CYP2C9, common metabolic pathways for other drugs (see drug interactions).

(5) **Dose modifications.**

(a) **Renal disease.** Less than 5% of DLV is excreted intact in urine; no dose adjustment is needed.

(b) **Hepatic disease.** The pharmacokinetics of DLV in patients with hepatic impairment have not been studied. Given that DLV undergoes extensive hepatic metabolism, it should be used with caution in patients with liver disease.

(6) **Drug interactions.** DLV inhibits hepatic CYP3A microsomal enzymes. Elevated levels of drugs metabolized by this pathway may occur and result in serious side effects.

Drugs that should not be coadministered include astemizole, terfenadine, alprazolam, midazolam, triazolam, rifampin, rifabutin, nifedipine, cisapride, sildenafil, quinidine, warfarin, ergot derivatives, clarithromycin, dapsone, simvastatin, and lovastatin. Levels of IDV, SQV, RTV, and APV are increased. Doses need to be adjusted (see section (6) on individual PI). **Drugs that induce CYP3A** can result in significant decreases in DLV serum levels and should not be coadministered: rifampin, rifabutin, phenytoin, phenobarbital, and carbamazepine. **Drugs that increase gastric pH** can lower DLV bioavailability; antacids or buffered ddI should be administered at least 1 hour before or after DLV. Chronic histamine receptor antagonists are not recommended. Data are unavailable regarding the use of DLV with methadone or oral contraceptive agents.

e. **Pregnancy category C**

f. **Adverse effects** [142]

(1) **Dermatologic.** An erythematous maculopapular rash, which may be pruritic, becomes confluent and is occasionally associated with fever. It occurs in up to 44% of subjects, typically 7 to 15 days (range 2–18) following the initiation of therapy. It may be dose related and is observed more frequently in patients with CD4 cell counts of less than 200/mL [144]. Over 90% of patients were able to continue therapy despite rash [142,144]. Upon discontinuation of DLV, rash resolved in 3 to 5 days. Severe or life-threatening rash (Stevens-Johnson syndrome) has been reported rarely (1 case among the first 1,000 patients given DLV). Rash resulted in discontinuation of DLV therapy in fewer than 5% of patients [142].

(2) **Miscellaneous adverse effects.** Headache and nausea occasionally occur.

(3) **Laboratory values.** No significant LFT or hematologic abnormalities have occurred [142–144].

(4) **Children.** Rash, headache, nausea, and drug interactions are similar to those observed in adults.

C. **Nucleotide reverse transcriptase inhibition**

1. **Tenofovir (disoproxil fumarate, TDF)** is the first drug of this class approved for treatment of HIV-1 infection. The nucleotide analogues (e.g., tenofovir itself) have poor oral bioavailability and low cellular penetration (because of highly polar phosphate moieties). These disadvantages have been circumvented by the attachment of labile lipophilic groups to mask the polarity of the phosphate moieties. This allows passive diffusion across cellular membranes. Nucleotide

analogues are thus given as prodrugs (e.g., TDF) that require further intracellular processing to become pharmacologically active.

a. **Formulation** is 300-mg tablets.

b. **Dosage**
   (1) **Adults.** Adults may be given 300 mg once daily.
   (2) **Children.** As of spring 2002, there are no published clinical trials providing data for TDF pediatric dosing. Older adolescents could presumably use the adult dose.

c. **Mechanism of action** [145,146]. TDF is a prodrug of the acyclic adenosine analogue tenofovir. It requires intracellular phosphorylation to become active. In its diphosphorylated form it competes with deoxyadenine triphosphate for uptake by RT (competitive inhibition) and also functions as a chain terminator. It is active in both resting and activated cells [146].

d. ***In vitro* activity.** TDF is active against HIV-1 (including strains with mutations that confer resistance to most NRTIs), HIV-2, and simian immunodeficiency virus [147].

e. **Pharmacology**
   (1) **Absorption.** Oral bioavailability is estimated to be 25% in the fasting state. Bioavailability is improved when TDF is administered with food (particularly a high-fat meal).
   (2) **Half-life** in serum is 12 to 15 hours; intracellular half-life is 10 to 50 hours, allowing once-daily dosing.
   (3) **Tissue distribution.** Only 7.2% of TDF is protein bound. No information is available on CSF penetration, or to what degree TDF crosses the placenta.
   (4) **Metabolism and elimination.** TDF is not metabolized by cytochrome P-450 enzymes. When multiple (300 mg/day) oral doses are given with food, 22% to 42% is found as unchanged drug in urine. TDF is eliminated by glomerular filtration and active tubular secretion.
   (5) **Dose modification**
      (a) **Hepatic disease.** TDF is not metabolized by liver enzymes.
      (b) **Renal disease** has not been evaluated. The kidneys primarily eliminate TDV. Other drugs may compete with TDV for elimination by this route. TDF should not be given if the rate of creatinine clearance is less than 60 mL/min.
   (6) **Drug interactions.** TDF increases (by an unknown mechanism) serum levels of ddI by 44% to 60% in various fasting and fed states [148]. Patients using these drugs concomitantly should be monitored for ddI-related adverse effects [149]. Drugs that compete for active tubular secretion or reduce renal function may increase TDF levels or serum concentrations of other drugs eliminated by the kidneys. Examples include acyclovir, valacyclovir, cidofovir, ganciclovir, and valganciclovir [149].

f. **Pregnancy category B**

g. **Adverse effects.** In a phase I/II trial of 49 patients receiving TDF, the only grade III and i.v. adverse events were laboratory value abnormalities: 5 subjects had CK elevations, 2 greater than four times the ULN. All of the CK elevations were associated with recent exercise [146]. Two of five subjects with increased CK had concurrent elevations in aspartate aminotransferase (AST) or alanine aminotransferase (ALT) (greater than five times the ULN), suggestive of a skeletal muscle etiology. In larger placebo-controlled trials of TDF in patients receiving other antiretroviral agents, GI events (nausea 11%, vomiting 5%, abdominal pain 3%) were the most common adverse effects. These were observed with similar frequency in placebo recipients. Discontinuation of TDF because of GI complaints was rare. Laboratory value abnormalities were no more common in TDF than in placebo recipients [150].
   (1) **Lactic acidosis/hepatic steatosis.** TDF has much less effect on mitochondrial DNA polymerase gamma than the NRTIs, and no cases have been reported [145,149].
   (2) **Children.** As of spring 2002, there are no data available.

Table 19.7. Currently Available Protease Inhibitors

| |
|---|
| Saquinavir |
| Ritonavir |
| Indinavir |
| Nelfinavir |
| Amprenavir |
| Lopinavir |

**D. Protease inhibitors. The currently available PIs are listed in Table 19.7.**

1. **Mechanism of action.** Structural protein components of the viral core and the viral replicative enzymes (RT, integrase, and protease) are synthesized as polyproteins. These must be cleaved, by viral protease, to produce mature infectious virions. PIs mimic the peptide cleavage site of HIV protease. By competitive inhibition, they prevent HIV protease–mediated processing of viral polyproteins. Immature, defective viral particles are produced [151–153], preventing further rounds of infection. PIs do not require any intracellular metabolism to become active and are effective in latently infected cells. The PIs alter the pharmacokinetics of other drugs by inhibiting or inducing hepatic cytochrome P-450. All PIs inhibit cytochrome P-450 enzymes. RTV is the most potent, SQV is the least potent, and IDV and nelfinavir (NFV) are in between [154]. PIs have low affinity for human aspartyl endopeptidases.
2. **PI class-related adverse effects** include lipid abnormalities, insulin resistance and diabetes mellitus, lypodystrophy syndrome, gynecomastia, osteonecrosis, and abnormal bleeding in patients with hemophilia or von Willebrand disease.
3. **Saquinavir** [155] **(Fortovase [soft-gelatin capsule], Invirase [hard-gelatin capsule])**
   a. **Formulations** include 20-mg soft-gelatin capsule (Fortovase; SQV- SGC) and 200-mg hard-gel capsule (Invirase).
   b. **Dosage**
      (1) **Adults.** Fortovase is preferred: 1,200 mg every 8 hours, 400 mg every 12 hours if given with RTV 400 mg every 12 hours. Invirase has poor bioavailability and should be used only in combination with RTV and only if Fortovase is unavailable.
      (2) **Children.** Few data are available on pediatric dosing guidelines for either SQV hard-gelatin or soft-gelatin capsules. Older adolescents could be given the adult dosage of SQV-SGC 1,200 mg orally every 8 hours. No liquid preparation makes SQV impractical for treatment of younger children.
   c. ***In vitro* activity.** SQV is active against HIV-1 and HIV-2, including NRTI- and NNRTI-resistant strains.
   d. **Pharmacology** [155–157]
      (1) **Absorption.** Invirase is poorly absorbed, and SQV undergoes extensive first-pass hepatic metabolism. Both contribute to the low bioavailability of Invirase (4%). Although the absolute bioavailability of SQV-SGC has not been assessed, it is estimated to be three to four times that of Invirase. Absorption is markedly increased when SQV is taken with meals (particularly fatty foods). This has been attributed (in part) to better solubilization created by increased gastric pH.
      (2) **Half-life** is 1 to 2 hours, which necessitates dosing every 8 hours.
      (3) **Tissue distribution.** SQV is highly protein bound (97%) and appears to penetrate poorly into semen (<5%) and CSF (<1% concurrent plasma levels) [155,157–160]. It is not known if SQV is excreted in breast milk. Placental transfer of SQV is expected to be very low (<5% of plasma concentrations) based on the high level of protein binding. An *ex vivo* placental transfer model in animals confirms this [161,162].

(4) **Metabolism and elimination.** SQV undergoes rapid and extensive first-pass hepatic and intestinal metabolism, primarily (50%) by CYP3A4 isoenzymes. Several inactive mono- and dihydroxylated compounds are the end result. Biliary is the major route of elimination (88% of SQV is excreted in feces); 1% is found in urine as unchanged drug [157].

(5) **Dose modification.** SQV has not been studied. **Renal disease** should not affect SQV pharmacokinetics. Given the extensive hepatic metabolism, this drug should be used with caution in patients with **hepatic disease.**

(6) **Drug interactions** [154]. Drugs contraindicated for concurrent use because SQV increases their serum levels include **antihistamines,** terfenadine, astemizole, **GI motility agents** (e.g., cisapride), **sedatives/hypnotics** (e.g., triazolam, midazolam, St. John's wort), **lipid-lowering agents** (e.g., simvastatin, lovastatin), and ergot derivatives. Rifampin and rifabutin are contraindicated for concurrent use because they significantly decrease SQV levels. EFV is contraindicated for concurrent use because SQV decreases its serum levels. Sildenafil requires dose modification when used with SQV (25 mg/48 hours). Drugs that increase SQV levels include RTV, IDV, NFV, DLV, ketoconazole, and clarithromycin. Low-dose RTV with SQV allows twice-daily dosing (see section on dosing). Drugs that may decrease SQV levels and should be avoided if possible include anticonvulsants, phenobarbital, carbamazepine, phenytoin (monitor levels), **corticosteroids** (e.g., dexamethasone), and garlic supplements.

e. **Pregnancy category B**

f. **Adverse effects** [154,157]

(1) **Gastrointestinal.** The most frequent side effects with both formulations are diarrhea, nausea, and abdominal pain (5%–10% and 10%–20% of patients, respectively). Most side effects were described as mild.

(2) **Laboratory value abnormalities.** CPK (6%), ALT (3%), and AST (4%) elevations have been observed.

(3) **Children.** Clinical studies, all of which enrolled only small numbers of children given SQV-SGC with NFV, revealed no unexpected adverse effects beyond those seen in adults. Further studies are needed.

4. **Ritonavir (Norvir)**

a. **Formulations** include 100-mg soft-gelatin capsules and 80 mg/mL elixir (unpalatable).

b. **Dosage**

(1) **Adults.** Adults may be given 600 mg every 12 hours. To improve tolerability (GI upset), the following dose escalation regimen is recommended: 300 mg every 12 hours on day 1, then increased by 100 mg every 12 hours at 2- to 3-day intervals.

(2) **Children.** Adolescents at least 13 years of age may be given the adult dosage of 600 mg orally twice daily. Administration should begin with 300 mg twice daily and the dose increased stepwise by 100 mg orally twice daily every 1 to 3 days to achieve the full dose by 1 to 2 weeks. **Children under 13** should be given 350 to 400 mg/m$^2$ BSA orally twice daily, with a similar stepwise increase in dose starting at 250 mg/m$^2$ BSA orally twice daily to achieve full dose by 1 to 2 weeks. Infant and newborn dosing is under study. RTV as a pharmacologic enhancer is given at a dosage of 200 to 400 mg orally twice daily along with another PI used in adolescents and adults.

c. ***In vitro* activity.** RTV is active against HIV-1 and HIV-2, including NRTI- and NNRTI-resistant strains.

d. **Pharmacology** [154,163]

(1) **Absorption.** Bioavailability is 66% to 75%. Food affects the rate and extent of absorption to a moderate degree depending on dose and formulation of RTV (overall absorption of caplets increases with food but is less pronounced when liquid formulation is used).

(2) **Half-life** is 3 to 5 hours.

(3) **Tissue distribution.** RTV is 98% to 99% protein bound; CSF concentrations are only 1% of concomitant plasma levels. RTV is highly protein bound, so placental transfer and secretion in breast milk is likely to be minimal. An *in vitro* model confirms negligible placental transfer [164]. In a small study, levels in semen were less than 5% of plasma concentrations [160].

(4) **Metabolism and elimination.** RTV is metabolized by hepatic CYP3A microsome enzymes and to a lesser degree by CYP2D6 enzymes. Eighty-five percent of an RTV dose is excreted in stool (34% as unchanged drug), and 11% is excreted in urine, of which 3.5% is unchanged [163].

(5) **Dose modifications.** No studies have been conducted in patients with renal or hepatic disease. RTV **renal clearance is negligible,** so doses do not have to be adjusted. Given the extensive hepatic metabolism of RTV, **caution** should be exercised when using RTV in patients **with liver disease.**

(6) **Drug interactions** [166,170]. RTV is a potent inhibitor of CYP3A and CYP2D6. It slows metabolism of drugs by these isoenzymes, leading to potentially life-threatening toxicities. For drugs that should not be coadministered with RTV, see Table 19.8.

RTV increases the levels of several other PIs, such as IDV, SQV, APV, and LPV. Small doses of RTV allow less frequent dosing of the other PIs (boosting) when used in combination (see section IX.C.4.b). RTV can decrease the plasma concentrations of methadone (dose increase may be necessary), ethinyl estradiol (dose should be increased or alternative contraceptive measures used), theophylline (levels should be monitored and dose increased if required), warfarin (international normalized ratio should be monitored), phenytoin, divalproex, lamotrigine (levels should be monitored), and atovaquone. RTV decreases meperidine concentrations, but levels of an active metabolite (norperidine) are increased. Long-term use of meperidine is not recommended. Rifampin, rifabutin, and St. John's wort should not be used with RTV because they significantly decrease RTV levels. Plasma levels of rifabutin or its metabolites may be concomitantly increased, leading to dose alteration of rifabutin to 150 mg daily.

Many other drugs that may have increased plasma concentrations when coadministered with RTV (Table 19.9) should be used with caution. When possible, their levels should be monitored. Patients must be followed closely for adverse effects, and reduced doses may be needed.

e. **Pregnancy category B**

Table 19.8. Drugs that Should Not Be Coadministered with Ritonavir

| Drug Class | Drugs | Possible Effects |
|---|---|---|
| Antihistamines | Astemizole, terfenadine | Cardiac arrhythmias |
| Antiarrhythmics | Amiodarone, quinidine flecainide, encainide, propafenonis, bepridil | Cardiac arrhythmias |
| Sedative/hypnotic | Triazolam, midazolam | Prolonged or increased sedation, respiratory depression |
| Antimigraine | Dihydroergotamine, ergotamine | Peripheral vasospasm, ischemia of the extremities |
| GI motility agent | Cisapride | Cardiac arrhythmias |
| Neuroleptic | Pimozide | Increased or prolonged sedation, respiratory depression |
| Lipid-lowering agents | Simvastatin, lovastatin, atorvastatin, cerivistatin | ?Increased risk of myopathy and rhabdomyolysis |

Table 19.9. Drugs for which Ritonavir Increases the Plasma Concentrations

| Drug Class | Drugs |
|---|---|
| Antiarrhythmics | Lidocaine, mexilitine, disopyramide |
| Calcium channel blockers | Diltiazem, verapamil, nifedipine |
| β-blockers | Metoprolol, timolol |
| Anticonvulsants | Carbamazepine, clonazepam, ethosuximide (monitor levels) |
| Antidepressants | Desipramine (monitor levels), bupropion, SSRIs, tricyclics, nefazodone |
| Neuroleptics | Perphenazine, risperidone, thioridazine |
| Sedatives/hypnotics | Diazepam, flurazepam, estazolam, zolpidem, chlorazepate |
| Antiemetics | Dronabinol |
| Antiparasitics | Quinine |
| Stimulants | Methamphetemines |
| Steroids | Dexamethasone, prednisone |
| Immunosuppressants | Cyclosporine, tacrolimus (monitor levels) |
| Analgesics | Propoxyphene, tramadol |
| Antibiotics | Clarithromycin (dose needs to be adjusted in presence of renal failure) |
| Antifungals | Ketoconazole (doses >200 mg/day not recommended) |
| Other | Sildenafil (dose should not exceed 25 mg in 48 hours) |

Ritonavir formulations contain alcohol and can produce disulfiram-like reactions when given with metronidazole or disulfiram.

f. **Adverse effects.** In placebo-controlled studies, GI toxicity, nausea (25%), diarrhea (18%–46%), vomiting (15%), headache (27%), fatigue (15%), and circumoral paresthesia (7%–15%) were common. Seventeen percent of patients withdrew, mostly during the initiation of therapy. Adverse effects are related to RTV concentration. Dose escalation (see section on dosing) may reduce the incidence [165].

(1) **Hepatitis.** Significant asymptomatic increases (>200% of ALT, AST, γ-glutamyl transferase) were seen in 4% to 6% of patients receiving the highest doses of RTV (500–600 mg twice daily) versus placebo [166,167]. In another placebo-controlled study, only elevations of GGT were noted more frequently (24%) in RTV-treated subjects [168]. Hepatitis occurs more frequently with RTV (vs. other PIs), particularly in patients coinfected with hepatitis C or B [169].

(2) **Lipid abnormalities** include insulin resistance, fat redistribution, osteonecrosis, and increased bleeding with hemophilia (see section on class-related adverse reactions).

5. **Indinavir (Crixivan)**

a. **Formulations** include 200- and 400-mg capsules.

b. **Dosage**

(1) **Adults.** Adults may be given 800 mg every 8 hours on an empty stomach (1 hour before or 2 hours after a meal) or with a light nonfat meal (e.g., cornflakes with skim milk or toast and jelly). To avoid IDV-associated nephrolithiasis (see section below on adverse effects), patients should drink 48 ounces of fluid daily. Twice-daily dosing can be achieved when 800 mg of IDV is boosted with 100 mg of RTV.

(2) **Children.** Adolescents at least 13 years of age may be given an adult dosage of 800 mg orally every 8 hours. In children under 13, limited clinical trial data suggest that 350 to 500 mg/m$^2$ BSA orally every 8 hours may be used. No information is available for newborn dosing. No liquid formulation is available for children [40].

c. ***In vitro* activity.** IDV is active against HIV-1 and HIV-2, including NRTI- and NNRTI-resistant strains.

**d. Pharmacology** [154,171]

(1) **Absorption is reduced by food.** Bioavailability is 65% in the fasting state or with a light meal. A full or fatty meal decreases absorption by more than 70%. If IDV is boosted with RTV, food has no effect on absorption.

(2) **Half-life** is 1.8 hours.

(3) **Tissue distribution.** IDV is the least protein bound of the PIs (60% vs. 90%–99%). CSF penetration is low (CSF:plasma ratio is 0.004:1 to 2.28:1) but exceeds that of other PIs. CSF levels are generally greater than the $IC_{95}$ of IDV-sensitive strains [172]. Both CSF and semen concentrations of IDV are greatly enhanced by RTV administered at a dose of 100 mg every 12 hours [173]. Human placental transfer studies are lacking, but IDV crosses the placenta in animals (indinavir sulfate).

(4) **Metabolism and elimination.** Most IDV is excreted in bile as metabolites (64%) and unchanged drug (19%). IDV is metabolized by hepatic glucuronidation and cytochrome P-450 enzymes, mainly the CYP3A4 isoform. Unchanged drug (9%) and metabolites (10%) are excreted in urine.

(5) **Dose modifications**

(a) **Hepatic disease.** The half-life of IDV is prolonged in cirrhosis and mild to moderate hepatic insufficiency. With liver disease, 600 mg every 8 hours is recommended (indinavir sulfate).

(b) **Renal disease.** Limited data are available. Because less than 20% of IDV is excreted in urine, substantial dosage reductions are not necessary [174,175]. However, because IDV is nephrotoxic, another PI should be considered in the presence of renal disease or there must be close monitoring.

(6) **Drug interactions.** Like other PIs, IDV interacts with drugs that induce or inhibit hepatic cytochrome P-450. **Contraindicated drugs for concomitant use** are listed in Table 19.10.

(a) **Drugs that decrease IDV levels** include rifabutin (dose should be decreased to 150 mg/day and IDV increased to 1 g every 8 hours), NVP (IDV should be increased to 1 g every 8 hours), and EFV (IDV should be increased to 1 g every 8 hours). Depending on the specific concentration of flavenoids, grapefruit juice may decrease IDV levels by 25% by inducing intestinal cytochrome P-450 metabolism (coadministration should be avoided). Buffered ddI should be administered either 2 hours before or after IDV, or the Videx EC formulation used. Anticonvulsants (e.g., phenobarbital, phenytoin, carbamazepine) can decrease PI levels (levels of anticonvulsant should be monitored; when possible, alternative anticonvulsants should be used).

(b) **Drugs that increase IDV levels.** When using RTV (see section D.4.d.(6)), ketoconazole, or itraconazole, the IDV dose should be decreased to 600 mg every 8 hours. Limited data are available

Table 19.10. Drugs Contraindicated for Concomitant Use with Indinavir

| Drug Class | Drugs |
|---|---|
| Antihistamines | Astemizole, terfenadine |
| Gastric motility agents | Cisapride |
| Sedatives/hypnotics | Triazolam, midazolam |
| Antidepressants | St. John's wort |
| Migraine therapy | Ergotamines |
| Lipid-lowering agents | Lovastatin, simvastatin |

on using boosted IDV plus NFV in twice-daily dosing. IDV increases serum levels of norethindrone and ethinyl estradiol (no dose changes needed), as well as sildenafil (not to exceed 25 mg/48 hours), trimethoprim, and clarithromycin.

e. **Pregnancy category C**

f. **Adverse effects** (see class-related side effects in section **VI.A–E**).

(1) **Renal toxicity.** IDV is poorly soluble in water at pH greater than 4. Several consequences have been described, including nephrolithiasis with frank renal colic, flank or back pain without evidence of IDV stones, obstructive uropathy with acute renal failure from stones, sludge, dysuria or urgency (often mistaken for infectious urethritis) associated with crystalluria, crystal-induced tubulointerstitial nephritis (with pyuria and eosinophiluria), and asymptomatic crystalluria or pyuria [176–178]. **Nephrolithiasis** is the most serious side effect of IDV, with an incidence of 3% to 15% [178]. However, in one 3-year follow-up study of 33 patients, the incidence was 39% [179]. Most patients have no prior risk factors for nephrolithiasis. Most cases occur after 5 to 7 months of treatment but have manifested within 1 week of starting IDV [176]. Risk factors for IDV stones include inadequate fluid intake, urinary pH greater than 6, elevated plasma levels of IDV, living in a warmer climate, and possibly hepatitis C coinfection [32]. The clinical presentation is similar to that of standard renal colic. IDV stones are usually radiolucent. Ultrasonography or CT may reveal stones, hydronephrosis, or ureteral obstruction. Light microscopy reveals rectangular plate-like forms with irregular borders, sheafs of densely packed crystals, and rosette or starburst forms [176]. **Crystalluria** occurred in 20% of 142 asymptomatic patients on standard-dose (2,400 mg/day) IDV [32,177]. The clinical presentation is similar to that of nephrolithiasis. Urinalysis shows hematuria, pyuria, proteinuria, and crystalluria. Clinical manifestations similar to nephrolithiasis can be caused by IDV sludge without discrete stone formulation [176]. CT scans reveal bilateral renal parenchymal defects. Hydronephrosis also may be present. Symptomatic crystalluria occurred in 8% of patients taking IDV [177]. Symptoms consisted of dysuria and urgency or symptoms similar to nephrolithiasis without stones. **Treatment** for any of these complications consists of i.v. fluid administration and pain control. Antiretroviral agents should be temporarily discontinued and renal function monitored. Up to 55% of patients respond to conservative therapy. In five patients with biopsy-proven tubulointerstitial disease, elevated serum creatinine and leukocyturia resolved after discontinuation of IDV [174]. In crystalluria and pyuria, drug can be continued and fluids given, but if they do not resolve, IDV should be discontinued.

Most patients can resume IDV therapy, but there may be recurrence. IDV should not be restarted with persistent renal insufficiency or tubulointerstitial disease (increasing blood urea nitrogen or creatinine, or pyuria). IDV stones, asymptomatic crystalluria, and pyuria are **preventable** by increasing daily fluids [177].

(2) **Gastrointestinal.** Nausea and vomiting occur in 10% to 12% of patients [154,177]. They usually improve or resolve with continued therapy and are rarely a reason to discontinue therapy [180,181]. Asymptomatic hyperbilirubinemia (predominantly indirect bilirubin) occurs in 1% to 15% of patients [154,177]. This is not an indication for discontinuation [177]. Severe cases of hyperbilirubinurea (greater than five times the ULN) occurred in 5.2% of 116 patients taking IDV in the presence of hepatitis C or B coinfection [169]. Overall, this degree of elevation occurs in greater than 10% of patients [154,177]. Clinically significant hepatitis rarely occurs in patients not coinfected with hepatitis C or B, alcoholic patients, or those using other hepatotoxic medications.

(3) **Dermatologic** effects include dry skin, dry lips, hair loss (scalp and extremities), paronychia, and cheilitis, secondary to its effect on retinoid metabolism [177]. Hair regrowth occurred (as did regression of other skin changes) when a different PI or an NNRTI was substituted [182].

(4) **Children.** Nephrolithiasis, crystalluria, and hematuria occur in children as they do in adults in about 10% to 15% of patients. These adverse effects occur slightly more often in children due to the difficulty in assuring adequate fluid intake. Hyperbilirubinemia is seen in 10% of children receiving IDV, similar to the rate in adults. This effect has restricted the use of IDV in newborns, who tolerate hyperbilirubinemia poorly.

**6. Nelfinavir (Viracept)**

a. **Formulations** include 250-mg tablets and 50 mg/g oral powder.

b. **Dosage**

(1) **Adults.** Adults may be given 750 mg every 8 hours or 1,250 mg every 12 hours, preferably with food.

(2) **Children.** Adolescents at least 13 years of age may be given the adult dosage, 750 mg orally every 8 hours or 1,250 mg orally every 12 hours. For children 2 to 13, 20 to 30 mg/kg/dose has been approved by the FDA, but this dose is being reassessed in clinical trials. Some clinicians use 30 to 45 mg/kg/dose orally every 8 hours to improve serum concentrations of NFV. Limited data support NFV dosing of children 6 to 13 years of age at 55 mg/kg/dose orally every 12 hours. Although the oral powder was developed for administration to young children in food or liquid, it requires a large amount of powder to deliver the desired dosage and is consequently poorly palatable. Most parents find it far easier to dissolve the tablets in a small volume of liquid; the tablets disperse readily enough that a few children might prefer dissolving them in their mouths. For those who do not like the taste, chocolate syrup or peanut butter disguises NFV very well.

c. ***In vitro* activity.** NFV and several of its metabolites are active against HIV-1 and HIV-2, including NRTI- and NNRTI-resistant strains [183,184].

d. **Pharmacology**

(1) **Absorption.** NFV has good oral bioavailability, which is markedly improved in the fed state [185]. Bioavailability is 70% to 80%.

(2) **Half-life** is 3.5 to 5 hours. Coupled with relatively slow absorption, this allows twice-daily dosing.

(3) **Tissue distribution.** NFV is highly protein bound (>98%) primarily to $\alpha_1$-acid glycoprotein. In animal models, organ distribution is extensive, but not into CSF [186].

(4) **Metabolism and elimination.** NFV is metabolized by the hepatic cytochrome P-450 enzyme system. At least four different cytochrome P-450 enzymes are involved (CYP3A4, CYP2C9, CYP2CI9, and CYP2D6). Several metabolites have antiretroviral activity. Eighty-seven percent is eliminated via the biliary tract into stool. Of this, 78% is oxidative metabolites, 22% unchanged NFV; 1% to 2% is excreted mostly as unchanged drug in urine.

(5) **Dose modifications**

(a) **Renal disease.** No dose modification is required [174].

(b) **Hepatic disease.** The pharmacokinetics of NFV in this setting have not been studied. Given its extensive hepatic metabolism, NFV should be used with caution in liver disease.

(6) **Drug interactions.** NFV inhibits cytochrome P-450, primarily CYP3A. **Drugs contraindicated for concurrent use include** astemizole, terfenadine, midazolam, triazolam, cisapride, ergot derivatives, St. John's wort, simvastatin, lovastatin, rifampin, amiodarone, and quinidine.

(a) **Drugs that require dose modification.** Ethinyl estradiol serum levels decrease by 47% (an alternative birth control method should be used). Sildenafil levels increase up to 11-fold (dosage should not exceed 25 mg/48 hours). Methadone levels decrease by 30% to 50%, and should be monitored for signs of opiate withdrawal. Rifabutin levels increase 200%, whereas NFV levels decrease by 30%; 150 mg/day rifabutin should be used. Tacrolimus and cyclosporine levels may be increased (drug levels should be monitored).

(b) **Others.** Carbamazepine, phenobarbital, and phenytoin may significantly decrease NFV levels. A different anticonvulsant should be considered. DLV levels decrease by 40%, NFV levels increase, and a greater than 20% incidence of neutropenia occurs (this combination should be used with caution).

e. **Pregnancy category B**

f. **Adverse effects** (see class-related side effects in section **VI.A–E**).

(1) **Gastrointestinal.** Mild to moderate diarrhea, greatest at initiation of NFV, is most common (20%–25% of patients), leading to discontinuation in less than 2% [183,187]. The mechanism is unknown. In many patients diarrhea resolves over time with continued NFV use [188]. Treatment of diarrhea [188] has included use of the following agents: oat bran, psyllium, loperamide, calcium, diphenoxylate/atropine, SP-303, and pancreatic enzymes. Nausea or elevated LFT results have been observed in fewer than 10% of patients [154,183,187]. Many of these have coinfection with hepatitis B or C [189].

(2) **Children.** NFV is relatively well tolerated by children, even at high doses. The most common adverse events are diarrhea, flatulence, abdominal pain, and, less commonly, rash.

7. **Amprenavir (Agenerase)** [190] is the only PI that is a sulfonamide.

a. **Formulations** include 50- and 150-mg soft-gelatin capsules and 15 mg/mL oral solution. The oral solution and the capsules contain large amounts of propylene glycol (550 mg/mL), which is used to achieve adequate solubility of APV. Because of the potential risk for propylene glycol toxicity, the oral solution is contraindicated in pregnant women, children under 4 years of age, patients with hepatic or renal dysfunction, or those taking metronidazole or disulfiram; APV capsules should be substituted. In addition, both the capsule and the oral form of Agenerase contain a high concentration of vitamin E. There is sufficient concentration that the vitamin E intake exceeds the daily requirement by 50 to 100 times. The consequences of this are unknown, but the patient should avoid taking any additional vitamin E supplement.

b. **Dosage**

(1) **Adults.** Adults may be given 1,200 mg (eight 150-mg caps) every 12 hours without regard to meals (although high-fat food should be avoided).

(2) **Children.** Adolescents at least 13 years of age (and >50 kg BW) should be given 1,200 mg orally twice daily; children 4 to 12 years of age and greater than 12 but less than 50 kg BW should be given 20 mg/kg/dose orally twice daily up to a maximum of 2,400 mg per day. APV is not recommended for children under 4 years of age because of the propylene glycol content, vitamin E content, and paucity of data concerning dosing. The drug in the liquid preparation is less bioavailable than the capsule. When used, the dose of the liquid should be 14% greater than the capsule dose, or 22.5 mg/kg/dose of liquid orally twice daily up to a maximum of 2,800 mg.

c. ***In vitro* activity.** APV is active against HIV-1 and HIV-2, including HIV-1 strains resistant to NRTIs, NNRTIs, and some PIs.

d. **Pharmacology** [190]

(1) **Absorption.** APV is well absorbed, but the absolute bioavailability has not been established. Absorption is reduced by food. This is significant only with high-fat meals, however.

(2) **Half-life** is 7 to 11 hours, which allows twice-daily dosing.

(3) **Tissue distribution.** APV is 90% protein bound (mostly $\alpha_1$-acid glycoprotein). CSF penetration is presumed to be limited by extensive protein binding and P-glycoprotein–mediated efflux. Placental levels and penetration into breast milk has not been studied. HIV-1 RNA levels in semen

decreased significantly in 14 of 19 men on APV monotherapy [190] (APV levels not measured).

**(4) Metabolism and elimination.** APV is primarily metabolized by hepatic CYP3A4. Most of an administered dose is found as metabolites in stool. There is minimal (<3% unchanged APV) renal excretion

**(5) Dose modification.**

**(a) Renal disease.** No dose modifications are necessary. The oral solution should not be used.

**(b) Hepatic disease.** Only APV capsules should be used, and caution should be exercised in patients with moderate or severe hepatic impairment. With a Child-Pugh score of 5 to 8, the dose should be decreased to 450 mg every 12 hours, and to 300 mg every 12 hours for a Child-Pugh score of 9 to 12 [191].

**(6) Drug interactions** [190, 192]. **Drugs contraindicated for concomitant use** include astemizole, terfenadine, cisapride, ergot derivatives, St. John's wort, midazolam, triazolam, pimozide, lovastatin, simvastatin, and rifampin. **Drugs that should be used with caution, require dose adjustments, or require monitoring of serum level** include amiodarone, lidocaine, quinidine, amitriptyline, nortriptyline, desipramine, imipramine, and warfarin. For sildenafil, dosage should not exceed 25 mg/48 hours. **Drugs that lower APV levels** include phenobarbital, carbamazepine, and phenytoin, and **concomitant use should be avoided.** The dose of rifabutin should be decreased to 150 mg daily. **Clinically important APV interactions occur with the following antiretroviral agents:** EFV decreases APV levels by 36% (EFV levels increase by 15%), so APV dosing should be increased to three times daily. RTV increases APV levels by more than 300%. Using RTV (100–200 mg twice daily) to boost APV is currently recommended (see section on dosing). APV may lower serum levels of oral contraceptives, so an alternative method of birth control should be used.

**e. Pregnancy category C**

**f. Adverse effects** (see class-related side effects in section **VI.A–E**).

**(1) Dermatologic.** A maculopapular rash, variably pruritic (mild to moderate severity leading to maximum 3% discontinuation), occurs in 28% of patients, usually during the first few weeks of therapy [179,190]. One percent of patients developed Stevens-Johnson syndrome. The higher incidence of rash compared with other PIs has been attributed to its sulfa moiety. However, patients with known allergy to sulfa drugs may take APV [179]. Therapy can be continued in patients with mild rash not associated with pruritus or systemic symptoms [179]. Antihistamines can be used for pruritus. APV should be discontinued, and rechallenge should not be attempted in patients with rash associated with fever, vomiting, chills, and severe pruritus or mucous membrane involvement.

**(2) Gastrointestinal.** GI adverse effects (mild to severe) led to discontinuation in 11% of patients and included nausea (38%–73%), vomiting (20%–23%), and diarrhea (33%–56%) [192]. Giving APV immediately after meals ameliorates nausea. Antidiarrheal therapies may be useful.

**(3) CNS.** Perioral dysesthesias (26%–30%), headache (7%–44%), and depression and mood changes (4%–15%) rarely lead to discontinuation. Headache, usually self- limited, responds to analgesics. No data are available on therapy for APV-related psychiatric adverse effects or dysesthesias.

**(4) Laboratory value abnormalities** [190]. Grade 3 (more than five times the ULN) elevations in AST (3.1%), ALT (2.8%), and bilirubin (0.6%) are infrequent. Hypertriglyceridemia is also infrequent (3.9%).

**(5) Children.** Nausea, vomiting, diarrhea, and rash (including Stevens-Johnson syndrome) are the most common side effects and similar to those in adults. As noted above, APV is a sulfonamide that may cause hypersensitivity reactions in the sulfonamide-allergic patient. The recommended daily allowance for vitamin E in children is 10 IU/day; that for adolescents and adults is 30 IU/day. APV oral solution, at the recommended doses noted above, contains 138 IU/kg/day up to 8,757 IU/day maximum. APV capsules contain up to 1,744 IU/day of vitamin E. Vitamin E toxicity has been associated with necrotizing enterocolitis in infants, and with coagulopathy, creatinuria, and decreased wound healing in adults. Therefore, patients taking APV should be cautioned not to take supplemental vitamin E. Propylene glycol may cause hyperosmolalitiy, lactic acidosis, seizures, and respiratory depression in infants. Children under 4 years of age should not be given APV oral solution.

8. **Lopinavir (Kaletra [LPV + RTV])** [193] is the first pharmacologically enhanced PI.
   a. **Formulations.** Each capsule contains 133 mg of LPV and 33 mg of RTV. Oral solution contains 80 mg LPV and 20 mg RTV per milliliter. Oral administration of LPV alone produces only transient, low levels in plasma (2). Coadministration with RTV (which inhibits hepatic metabolism of LPV) increases LPV plasma levels over 100-fold. The combination of LPV/RTV is active against HIV-1 and HIV-2, including NRTI- and NNRTI-resistant strains [194].
   b. **Dosage**
      (1) **Adults.** Adults may be given three capsules (400 mg LPV/100 mg RTV) every 12 hours with food.
      (2) **Children.** Adolescents at least 13 years of age may be given the adult dose of 400 mg LPV/100 mg RTV (three capsules or 5 mL elixir) orally twice daily. For children 6 months to 12 years of age, LPV dosage is based on weight. Children 7 to 14 kg BW should be given 12 mg/kg/dose orally twice daily; 15 to 40 kg BW, 10 mg/kg/dose orally twice daily. Dosage of LPV must be increased for children receiving concurrent NVP or EFV (see section below on drug interactions). The suggested adolescent dose is 533 mg (four capsules every 12 hours). Children 7 to 14 kg BW should be given 13 mg/kg/dose orally twice daily. Children 15 to 40 kg BW should be given 11 mg/kg/dose orally twice daily. LPV is best absorbed with food.
   c. **Pharmacology** [193]
      (1) **Absorption.** The absolute bioavailability of LPV/RTV has not been established in humans. Plasma levels are increased when administered with food and should be given with meals to enhance bioavailability and minimize pharmacokinetic variability.
      (2) **Half-life** is 5.8 hours.
      (3) **Tissue distribution.** LPV is 98% to 99% protein bound to $\alpha_1$-acid glycoproteins and albumin. There are no human data on the levels achieved in CSF or semen, or on placental transfer.
      (4) **Metabolism and elimination.** LPV is rapidly metabolized by hepatic CYP3A4. The major metabolites are less active against HIV-1 than LPV [193,195]. Most LPV is excreted in stool as unchanged drug (19%), and metabolites with less than 3% excreted unchanged in urine.
      (5) **Dose modification.** No dose adjustments would be expected in **renal failure.** This was confirmed in one patient receiving LPV/RTV while on hemodialysis [196]. With regard to **hepatic disease,** although not specifically studied, LPV is extensively metabolized in the liver, and concentrations may be increased in the presence of liver disease. LPV/RTV should be used with caution.
      (6) **Drug interactions.** LPV/RTV use is contraindicated with drugs that are extensively metabolized by CYP3A or CYP2D6 enzymes and for which elevated plasma levels are associated with serious or life-threatening effects (Table 19.11). **Several drugs increase the metabolism of LPV/RTV leading to subtherapeutic levels,** including anticonvulsants (e.g., carbamazepine, phenytoin, phenobarbital), rifampin, and St. John's wort. Concomitant use with rifampin and St. John's wort is contraindicated.

Table 19.11. Drugs Contraindicated for Use with Lopinavir/Ritonavir

| Drug Class | Drugs |
|---|---|
| Antiarrhythmics | Flecainide, propafenone |
| Antihistamines | Astemizole, terfenadine |
| Ergot derivatives | Ergotamine, dihydroergotamine, ergonovine, methylergonovine |
| Gastric motility agents | Cisapride |
| Neuroleptics | Pimozide |
| Sedatives/hypnotics | Midazolam, triazolam |
| Lipid-lowering agents | Lovastatin, simvastatin |

**When used concomitantly with LPV/RTV, several drugs require dose adjustments, level monitoring, or close clinical monitoring. Levels of the following drugs are increased when used with LPV/RTV:** sildenafil (should be used with caution, and the dose reduced [25 mg every 48 hours]), dihydropyridine calcium channel blockers (e.g., nifedipine, felodipine, nicardipine), antiarrhythmics (e.g., amiodarone, lidocaine [systemic use], quinidine, depredil], rifabutin and its metabolites (which are increased, so dose should be reduced to 150 mg three times per week and the patient monitored for uveitis), lipid-lowering agents (e.g., atorvastatin, cerivastatin, of which the lowest possible dose should be used, or an alternative agent considered [pravastatin]), immunosuppressants (e.g., cyclosporine, tacrolimus, rapamycin; levels should be monitored), clarithromycin (dose adjustment is necessary for patients with decreased renal function [among those with creatinine clearance of 30–60 mL/min, and the dose should be reduced by 50%; <30 mL/min, reduced by 75%]), and ketoconazole and itraconazole (doses of >200 mg/day are not recommended).

**Levels of the following drugs are decreased when used with LPV/RTV:** methadone (patient should be monitored for withdrawal symptoms, and methadone dose may need to be increased), ethinyl estradiol (an additional or alternative contraceptive method is recommended), and atovaquone (clinical significance is not known; dose may need to be increased).

**Drugs that significantly lower LPV levels** include EFV and NVP. The dose of LPV/RTV should be increased to 4 capsules every 12 hours. **Drugs that increase LPV/RTV levels** include DLV (appropriate dose for either drug is not known when these are coadministered). LPV/RTV can increase the levels of other PIs (appropriate doses for combination therapy with other PIs are unknown). LPV/RTV oral elixir contains alcohol, and when used with disulfiram/metronidazole, disulfiram-like reactions may occur.

**d. Pregnancy category C**

**e. Adverse effects** [193,197] (see class-related side effects in section **VI.A–E**).

**(1) Gastrointestinal.** In two large prospective double-blind randomized trials involving over 700 therapy-naive patients, moderate diarrhea (more than three loose stools/day) occurred in 17% to 25% of patients, nausea in 9%, abnormal stools (fewer than three loose stools/day) in 6% to 19%, and vomiting in less than 5%.

**(2) Others.** Headache and asthenia were reported in 6% to 13% of patients.

**(3) Laboratory value abnormalities.** LFT elevations (more than five times the ULN) developed in 14% of subjects on the currently recommended dose. Some had coinfection with hepatitis B or C. Hepatitis B surface antigen or hepatitis C virus antibody at baseline was associated with an eightfold increased relative risk of developing a grade III/IV AST or ALT elevation on LPV/RTV.

(4) **Children.** The most common adverse effects associated with LPV in children are diarrhea, asthenia, and elevation of triglycerides and cholesterol, similar to that occurring in adults. LPV/RTV elixir is somewhat more palatable than RTV elixir.

**VI. Protease inhibitor class–related adverse effects**

**A. Glucose intolerance** occurs with all currently available PIs, with the possible exception of APV [198]. The prevalence of abnormal glucose metabolism in PI-treated patients varies widely. Two percent to 25% had hyperglycemia, 16% to 35% had glucose intolerance, and 4% to 9% had frank diabetes mellitus (type II) [32]. Significant elevation in fasting plasma glucose occurs by 4 weeks [198,199]. PIs cause abnormal insulin secretion and peripheral insulin resistance in both HIV-1–and non HIV-1–infected patients [152,200].

**B. Weight.** Patients in whom this occurs are often overweight. Inhibition of the insulin-responsive glucose transporter GLUT-4 [201] is the proposed mechanism. Blood glucose should be monitored at 3-month intervals, especially with a history of impaired glucose tolerance or risk factors for type II diabetes. Insulin doses may require adjustment. Given the similarities between PI-associated hyperglycemia and type II diabetes, dietary modifications, exercise, and weight loss for obese patients should be attempted. No large studies are available to guide the selection of specific oral hypoglycemic agents. Metformin is associated with lactic acidosis (also a complication of NRTI use), particularly in renal insufficiency. Some patients require insulin therapy. Improvement in insulin resistance and normalization of blood sugars occur over months after PIs are discontinued (switched to an NNRTI) [136,202,203].

**C. Hyperlipidemia.** Untreated HIV-1 infection and particularly AIDS are associated with hypertriglyceridemia and decreased LDL and HDL and cholesterol [204]. Triglyceride levels correlate with elevated $\alpha$-interferon levels (the host response to HIV-1 infection). Both triglyceride and interferon levels decrease with antiretroviral treatment. By contrast, fasting triglycerides, and total and LDL cholesterol increase significantly after a mean of 7 months of PI therapy, whereas HDL levels do not change [199]. These lipid abnormalities may occur in the absence of significant weight gain or lipodystrophy [199]. Patients treated with PIs for 3 to 36 months have a prevalence of hypertriglyceridemia of 50% to 78% and hypercholesterolemia of 26% to 83% [32]. For many patients, the PI-associated increase in LDL is a correction of the prior HIV infection–associated decrease in LDL. However, some patients will have significant elevations of triglycerides and cholesterol that require therapy. Of the HMG CoA reductase inhibitors (statins), only pravastatin is not metabolized by hepatic CYP3A4 enzymes. Levels of the other statins may increase significantly when coadministered with PIs (see section on individual PIs). If dietary restrictions, weight loss, and pharmacotherapy are not effective, changing the PI to another agent (NNRTI) is an option [205].

**D. Lipodystrophy syndrome** (i.e., fat redistribution syndrome) refers to three body habitus changes discernible in some patients: lipoatrophy, lipohypertrophy, or a combination of the two. Changes occur with either stable or increased total body weight (as opposed to HIV-associated wasting syndrome). Lipodystrophy syndrome is usually accompanied by hyperlipidemia and insulin resistance [206,207]. The onset is often insidious. It is not clear if lipodystrophy is dose related, and it has been reported in patients receiving PI therapy for acute HIV-1 infection and for post-exposure prophylaxis [206]. It also has been reported in antiretroviral-naive patients and some receiving non–PI-containing regimens [32]. NRTI use (particularly Zerit) correlates with lipoatrophy [208]. Unfortunately, at present no definition of lipodystrophy syndrome exists. Most studies have not been prospective, nor have standardized methods to measure changes in adipose tissue always been used. Thus, reports on the prevalence of lipodystrophy syndrome vary widely (1.8%–71%). Efforts are under way to develop standardized criteria and methods. Dyslipidemia associated with insulin resistance and central (truncal/abdominal) adiposity has raised concern about associated cardiovascular disease [209]. Case reports of coronary artery disease in young patients on HAART have been described [206], as has endothelial dysfunction [210]. The etiology of lipodystrophy remains unknown [211]. There is no known effective therapy at the present time [212]. Switching the PI to another agent has not been effective in reversing lipodystrophy (particularly fat wasting) [207]. Possible therapeutic approaches were recently reviewed [212]. Physical signs are first observed 1 to 7 months after starting therapy.

1. **Lipoatrophy** (fat wasting) is usually manifested as loss of subcutaneous fat in the face or limbs and buttocks. Loss of buccal adipose tissue resulting in hollow cheeks, sunken eyeballs and a cachectic appearance occurs. There may be symmetric loss of subcutaneous fat of the upper or lower extremities and buttocks (particularly in women), resulting in thinning of the limbs and development of prominent veins. Muscle mass and strength in wasted areas is not affected.
2. **Lipohypertrophy** (fat accumulation) manifests as fat deposition in the abdomen in both the subcutaneous and visceral areas (manifested as increased abdominal girth), dorsocervical region (buffalo hump), breasts (sometimes accompanied by pain), face, neck, and salivary glands. Increased abdominal girth is occasionally accompanied by GI symptoms (distention, fullness, bloating). Serum prolactin levels, 24-hour urinary free-cortisol concentrations, plasma cortisol levels, testosterone, $\beta$-human chorionic gonadotropin, dehydroepiandrostene, follicle-stimulating hormone, luteinizing hormone, results of thyroid function tests, and response to dexamethasone suppression are normal. Alcoholism does not seem to be a factor. CT, magnetic resonance imaging, and dual-energy x-ray absorptiometry reveal intraabdominal fat accumulation (particularly of visceral abdominal adipose tissue) and loss of adipose tissue in lipoatrophic areas but no organomegaly or ascites. Mammograms are unrevealing. At least some of the body habitus changes (particularly lipoatrophy and increased abdominal girth) may be due to the normal aging process [213].
3. **Abnormal bleeding.** Increased rates of spontaneous bleeding in PI-treated patients with hemophilia or von Willebrand disease occurs [214,215]. Bleeding occurs in both usual and unusual (e.g., finger joint) sites. Hematuria and mucous membrane bleeding is common. It is more resistant to treatment with factor concentrates, although some patients are able to tolerate continued PI therapy without further episodes [214]. The mechanism of the bleeding tendency is unknown.

**E. Bone disease.** The incidence of avascular necrosis (AVN) may be increasing in HIV [216], but there is no evidence that AVN or decreased bone density is associated with PI use [217].

## VII. Investigational drugs for HIV infection

The goal of this summary is not to detail all drugs now under consideration for trials against HIV. However, a few comments may help the reader become aware of some of the new agents or new combinations now undergoing clinical investigation [218].

### A. New formulations of existing medications

1. Sustained-release versions (e.g., of AZT and D4T) to allow for less frequent dosing.
2. Higher dose versions of medications or prodrug formulations to reduce total pill burden (e.g., EFV 600 mg, SQV [Invirase] 800 mg for use with RTV, and FOS-APV, a prodrug of APV [219]).

### B. Nucleosides

1. **Emtricitabine-FTC.** Emtricitabine (2′,3′-dideoxy-5-fluoro-3′-thiacytidine, or FTC) is a fluorinated NRTI that has potent *in vivo* antiretroviral activity. It is remarkably similar to 3TC, but its pharmacokinetic profile allows once-daily dosing. It was compared with 3TC, combined either with d4T or with an NNRTI, in a randomized blinded study in 468 treatment-naive subjects [220]. The activity and toxicities of the two regimens were comparable. Unfortunately, the M184V resistance mutation, occurring in patients failing a 3TC-containing regimen, confers cross-resistance to emtricitabine. Its long-term toxicity profile needs further evaluation.
2. **Diaminopurine dioxolane (DAPD).** DAPD (B-D-2,6-diaminopurine dioxolane) is a purine nucleoside analogue metabolized to dioxolane guanosine

(DXG), which has potent *in vitro* activity against wild-type and AZT-resistant and 3TC-resistant HIV-1 variants, including those containing the multi-NRTI resistance insert at codon 69. It is well tolerated and shows antiretroviral activity in both naive and treatment-experienced patients, although the antiretroviral activity of DAPD is diminished in patients with prior NRTI experience.

3. **ACH-126,443** is an L-nucleoside analogue RTI with 10- to 20-fold greater anti-HIV activity than 3TC, a half-life of longer than 24 hours, and little apparent mitochondrial toxicity. It maintained activity *in vitro* against virus with the known NRTI-resistance mutations, including M4lL, M184V, T215Y, Q151M, and 69S [221]. Clinical studies will soon be under way.
4. **(−)dOTC** The thiacytidine derivative dOTC (2′-deoxy-3′-oxa-4′-thiocytidine) is a racemic mixture similar in structure to 3TC, but with *in vitro* activity against AZT- and 3TC-resistant strains. The negative enantiomer (−)dTC, which maintains antiretroviral activity but has little *in vitro* toxicity, has been selected for further development.

**C. Non-nucleoside reverse transcriptase inhibitors**

1. **TMC120** (R147681) is a diaminopyrimidine that retains *in vitro* activity against virus resistant to current NNRTIs [222]. In a 7-day study in naive patients, TMC120 demonstrated potent dose-dependent activity, the highest dose 100 mg twice daily, achieving a 30-fold reduction in plasma HIV-1 RNA levels [223]. Mild somnolence was the most common side effect. Studies are in development.

**D. Protease inhibitors**

1. **Tipranavir** is the first nonpeptidomimetic PI, and has potent *in vitro* activity against HIV-1 resistant to current PIs. In a panel of 105 isolates with at least 10-fold resistance to three or more PIs, only 10 had a greater than fourfold increase in the $IC_{50}$ for tipranavir, compared with wild-type virus, and only two had a greater than 10-fold increase [224]. Development has been delayed by problems in producing a formulation that offers both adequate bioavailability and an acceptable pill burden. However, when combined with RTV, twice-daily dosing is feasible. Studies in PI-experienced patients are needed to determine if *in vitro* promise of tipranavir translates into clinical utility [225].
2. **Atazanavir** (BMS-232632), a novel azapeptide PI, is highly potent *in vitro,* with *in vitro* activity against most HIV-1 strains that are resistant to 1, 2, or 3 currently available PIs, including NFV, SQV, RTV, and APV. If the virus tested is resistant to four current PIs, greater than sixfold decreases in susceptibility to atazanavir is observed. All viruses resistant to all five current PIs were resistant [226]. Mutations emerging during *in vitro* passage are different from those seen with other PIs, suggesting that cross-resistance to current agents may be limited. This observation remains to be confirmed *in vivo* [226]. Pharmacokinetic studies support once-daily dosing without RTV boosting [227]. Of particular interest, atazanavir appears to be less likely to induce the lipid abnormalities and provoke insulin resistance compared with current PIs. It has little effect on triglyceride levels. Increased bilirubin and jaundice have been reported with atazanavir that was not associated with major alterations in liver enzymes and resolves after the drug is discontinued. Also, cardiac arrhythmias may be more frequent during atazanavir therapy. Clinical studies are under way.

**E. Inhibitors of HIV-I fusion and entry**

1. **T20-pentafuside.** Work is currently under way to develop medications that inhibit the binding of the HIV envelope protein gp120 to the CD4 molecule on the cell surface or the binding of the viral envelope to chemokine coreceptors (e.g., CXCR4 and CCR5). These are still in early development. Some progress has been made with inhibition of fusion between virus and cell, thus preventing HIV entry into the host cell. These would be used in conjunction with the RT and PI inhibitors. T-20 is a 36–amino acid peptide that corresponds to the HR-2 sequence of the viral envelope protein gp41. For successful fusion to occur, the HR-1 and HR-2 regions of gp41 must form a hairpin structure. However, T-20 binds to HR1 near the fusion domain, preventing interactions with the HR-2 region and fusion of the virus and cell membranes. T-20 must be administered parenterally, but has significant short-term antiretroviral activity when given

by means of i.v. infusion or twice-daily subcutaneous injection [228]. T-20 was generally well tolerated, but some patients developed subcutaneous skin nodules that in some cases evolved into subcutaneous abscesses. They were slow to resolve. Because resistance has developed during T-20 monotherapy, this agent should ideally be used in conjunction with several other agents [229].

2. **T-1249.** Development of a second more potent fusion inhibitor is under way. A 39–amino acid peptide, it retains activity against HIV variants that are resistant to T-20 [230] and has significant antiretroviral activity. Adverse events were uncommon. No cases of subcutaneous skin abscesses were seen. T-1249 elimination kinetics allows once-daily dosing.

**F. Other experimental drugs**

1. **Interleukin-2 (IL-2).** HIV-1 infection is associated with decreased production of IL-2. Replacement of IL-2 has been viewed as a possible form of immunotherapy [231,232]. Recombinant IL-2 therapy is combined with potent ARVT. Although IL-2 is known to upregulate the production of HIV-1 *in vitro* and may increase viral load, the rate of CD4 cell destruction, and theoretically worsen clinical progression, in clinical trials, high-dose intermittent IL-2 has resulted in impressive increases in peripheral CD4 cell counts. The impact of these changes on long-term clinical outcome is unknown. In addition, lower doses of IL-2 are associated with a sustained increase in natural killer (NK) cell function and interferon-$\gamma$ production, both of which could be beneficial. For now, IL-2 use in HIV should be restricted to experimental protocols.
2. **Mycophenolate mofetil** (MMF, CellCept) is used in solid organ transplantation. After oral adsorption, it is hydrolyzed to mycophenolic acid (MPA), the active metabolite. MPA is a potent inhibitor of inosine monophosphate dehydrogenase (IMPDH), and thus inhibits the *de novo* synthesis of guanosine nucleotide synthesis [233]. *In vitro,* MPA increases the activity of ABC, ddI, and TDF against wild-type and multinucleoside RT inhibitor-resistant HIV. A clinical trial is planned to assess the safety, tolerability, and antiretroviral activity of combining MMF with DAPD to provide a potent salvage antiretroviral regimen.

## VIII. HIV in pregnant women

**A. Transmission of HIV to the baby during pregnancy.** The rate of perinatal HIV transmission in the absence of ARVT is approximately 25%. Transmission can occur during the course of pregnancy, during labor and delivery, or postpartum through breast-feeding. Two-thirds to three-fourths of transmissions occur during or close to the intrapartum period, particularly in non–breast-feeding populations [234,235]. Perinatal transmission is multifactorial, and influenced by viral, immune, and clinical factors in both the mother and infant (Table 19.12) [236,237]. Maternal plasma viral load is the strongest predictor of transmitting HIV perinatally. Although the risk is low with undetectable plasma viral load, transmission has occurred at all maternal plasma viral loads [238]. Perinatal transmission also appears to be more common with advanced HIV disease (CD4 cell counts of $<$200/mL), with acute maternal seroconversion, and vaginal delivery. Other obstetric factors thought to be associated with increased perinatal HIV-1 transmission include chorioamnionitis, placenta previa, and invasive interventions such as scalp monitoring, chorionic villus sampling, amniocentesis, cord blood sampling, and placental biopsy [239,240].

**B. Antiretroviral use in pregnancy**

1. **Introduction.** Antiretroviral therapy should be offered to pregnant women with HIV infection. To prevent perinatal transmission, AZT chemoprophylaxis should be incorporated into the antiretroviral regimen when possible [241]. The use of ARVT by pregnant women to treat HIV infection, to reduce perinatal transmission, or for both purposes should be accompanied by a discussion of the known and unknown short- and long-term benefits and risks of such therapy for infected women and their infants [242,242a]. Because information on the use of ARVT in pregnancy is rapidly evolving, we strongly recommend reviewing the U.S. Public Health Service Guidelines, which are updated regularly at *hivatis.org/trtgdlns.html,* link perinatal.

Table 19.12. Potential Factors Influencing Mother-to-Child Transmission of HIV

| |
|---|
| Maternal factors |
| Advanced HIV disease as measured by |
| Clinical staging |
| Low CD4 count |
| Higher viral loads |
| p24 antigenemia |
| Primary HIV infection |
| Viral phenotype: syncytium-inducing |
| Viral genotype: resistant HIV mutant strains |
| Coinfection with other sexually transmitted diseases |
| Vitamin A deficiency |
| First born twins |
| Obstetrical events |
| Vaginal delivery |
| Invasive procedures/fetal monitoring during labor |
| Prolonged premature rupture of membranes (>4 h) |
| Older maternal age |
| Cigarette smoking and illicit drug use during pregnancy |
| Breast-feeding |
| Unprotected sexual intercourse with multiple partners |
| Lack of antiretroviral use |
| Fetal/placental factors |
| Chorioamnionitis |
| Prematurity |
| Low birth weight |
| Labor/birth canal factors |
| Cervicovaginal viral load |
| Local HIV-specific immune response |
| Maternal-fetal transfusion of blood |
| Immune factors |
| Humoral |
| Neutralizing antibody |
| Antibody-dependent cellular cytotoxicity |
| gp 120 V3 loop antibody |
| MCH concordance |
| Other |
| Cell-mediated |
| Cytotoxic T-lymphocytes |
| CD8 suppression |
| Mucosal immunity |

Data from Bryson YJ. Perinatal HIV-1 transmission: recent advances and therapeutic interventions. *AIDS* 1996;10(suppl 3)33–42; and Mofenson LM. Mother-child HIV-1 transmission: timing and determinants. *Obstet Gynecol Clin North Am* 1997;24:759–784.

2. **Nucleoside reverse transcriptase inhibitors**
   a. **Zidovudine** was the first agent studied. It reduced perinatal transmission by 67.5% [243,244]. Women with more than 200 CD4 cells/mL received 100 mg oral AZT five times a day initiated between 14 and 34 weeks' gestation and continued throughout pregnancy. When labor commenced, a 2 mg/kg loading dose was given over 1 hour, followed by an i.v. infusion of 1 mg/kg/h that was continued until delivery. Newborn infants received AZT syrup, 2 mg/kg every 6 hours, for 6 weeks after delivery. Perinatal transmission was reduced to 8.3% in 205 women who received AZT versus 25.5% in 204 not on ARVT ($p = 0.00006$) [244]. In August 1994, the U.S. Public Health Service task force issued recommendations for the use of AZT for reduction of

perinatal HIV-1 transmission [245]. This was followed in July 1995 by recommendations for universal prenatal HIV-1 counseling and HIV-1 testing with informed consent for all pregnant women in the United States [246]. Rate of transmission is dependent on when AZT prophylaxis was begun. If begun prenatally, the rate was 6.1%; when begun intrapartum, the rate was 10.0%; when begun within 48 hours of life, the rate was 9.3%; and when begun on day 3 of life or later, the rate was 18.4% [247]. Without AZT prophylaxis, the rate of transmission was 26.6% [247]. The AZT regimen was well tolerated, and the only toxicity observed more frequently in the treatment group was a lower hemoglobin concentration in neonates that was not clinically significant. Hemoglobin levels in the AZT infants were equivalent to the untreated group by week 12. Because the long-term effects are unknown, all exposed children, regardless of HIV status, should receive careful long-term follow-up [248]. The mechanism of reduction in transmission is unknown. The effect of AZT on maternal HIV viral load is insufficient to explain fully its efficacy, especially when given to pregnant women with extensive prior AZT experience [249,250]. Whatever the explanation, the use of AZT by HIV-infected pregnant women in the United States and Europe has resulted in marked declines in perinatal transmission rates, typically as low as 3% to 4%. Because of its complexity and cost, this extended prenatal or postnatal AZT regimen unfortunately has not been used in most developing countries.

**b. Other NRTIs.** All of the NRTIs are classified as FDA pregnancy category C, except for ddI, which is classified as category B [241]. Only AZT, 3TC, and ddI pharmacokinetics have been evaluated in clinical trials [251,252]. The pharmacokinetics of 3TC are not altered by pregnancy, so no dose modification is indicated. In the newborn, the dose is decreased because of reduced clearance in infants 1 week of age. The oral pharmacokinetics of ddI antepartum are not different postpartum, nor are they different from the published mean values for pregnant and nonpregnant women. No dose adjustment is necessary for oral ddI [252].

**Mitochondrial toxicity of NRTIs** may be of particular concern for pregnant women and infants with *in utero* exposure to nucleoside analogue drugs. Pregnancy may mimic some of the early symptoms of lactic acidosis/hepatic steatosis syndrome. It is unclear if pregnancy is a risk factor for lactic acidosis/hepatic steatosis syndrome, which may have a female preponderance and has similarities to the syndrome of acute fatty liver of pregnancy. The triad of hemolysis, elevated LFT results, and a low platelet count (HELLP syndrome), which rarely occurs during the third trimester, is a concern. The frequency of HELLP syndrome in HIV is not known. Pregnant women receiving NRTIs should have hepatic enzymes and electrolytes assessed more frequently during the last trimester (every 4–6 weeks) of pregnancy, and any new suggestive symptoms should be evaluated thoroughly. Additionally, because of several cases of maternal mortality secondary to lactic acidosis from prolonged use of the combination of d4T and ddI, this antiretroviral combination should be used during pregnancy with caution and generally only when other NRTI combinations cannot be used. Thus far, severe or fatal mitochondrial disease in infants exposed to NRTIs is rare [241].

**3. NNRTIs (pregnancy category C).** The safety and pharmacokinetics of **NVP** have been evaluated. A single 200-mg dose at labor onset and a single 2 mg/kg dose to the infant 48 to 72 hours after birth were well tolerated, and no adverse effects occurred in women or infants. NVP pharmacokinetics in pregnant women are similar, although somewhat more variable, than in nonpregnant adults. The half-life and elimination were prolonged in the infants. A single 200-mg dose of NVP was sufficient to maintain serum antiviral activity for the first week of life [241]. One needs to be aware that severe, life-threatening, and, in some cases, fatal hepatotoxicity (fulminant, cholestatic hepatitis and hepatic failure), have occurred in HIV-infected patients receiving NVP with other antiretroviral agents. This has occurred in a small number of individuals receiving NVP with other antiviral agents for postexposure prophylaxis of nosocomial or sexual HIV exposure. **DLV and EFV** have not been studied in pregnant women. DLV at high doses is known to be teratogenic in rodents. Of seven women who inadvertently became pregnant while enrolled in DLV trials, three had ectopic pregnancies, three had healthy infants, and one delivered a premature infant with a muscular ventricular septal defect [241]. EFV studies have been performed on pregnant monkeys that were given human doses. Of 13 monkey infants, one had a cleft palate, one microphthalmia, and another anencephaly and anophthalmia [253]. Long-term and transplacental animal carcinogenicity studies are not available for these three non-nucleosides. Until additional data are available, EFV and DLV should be given to pregnant women only if the benefits outweigh the potential risks.

4. **Protease inhibitors** cause insulin resistance. Pregnancy is a risk factor for hyperglycemia. It is unknown whether PIs increase this risk. Pregnant women should be aware of the risk of hyperglycemia and informed how to recognize the early symptoms and thus seek medical care if such symptoms develop. Blood glucose levels should be monitored. No data are available regarding drug dosage, safety, and tolerance of any of the PIs in pregnant women or in neonates. Phase I studies of IDV, RTV, NFV, and SQV in combination with AZT and 3TC in pregnant HIV-infected women and their infants are currently under way in the United States. APV and LPV/RTV (Kaletra) have not yet been studied. IDV is associated with hyperbilirubinemia, which may be a concern in neonates. Preliminary data suggest that serum levels of IDV, NFV, and SQV in pregnant women may be lower than in nonpregnant women. PIs are highly protein bound, and it is likely that minimal placental transfer occurs. RTV, NFV, and SQV are classified as pregnancy category B, and IDV, APV, and LPV are classified as pregnancy category C.
5. **Other antiretroviral agents.** Hydroxyurea should be avoided because of significant anomalies occurring in multiple animal species exposed to this drug, and because of the uncertain role of hydroxyurea in HIV. TDF, a nucleotide RTI, is classified as pregnancy category B, but no data are available on its use in pregnant women or neonates [242].

**C. Management of pregnant HIV-infected women**

1. **Evaluation of the pregnant HIV-infected woman.** In evaluating the patient's history, the clinician should assess factors that enhance perinatal transmission: past sexually transmitted diseases, drug and alcohol use, tobacco use, sexual activity, and lack of condom use [254,254a]. Addressing these practices may reduce perinatal transmission risk nonpharmacologically. A pelvic examination may reveal ongoing conditions that warrant therapy. CD4/CD8 subsets and viral load should be done at least every trimester. Some clinicians suggest HIV genotyping to help guide optimal ARVT. Pregnant women should be treated with an antiretroviral regimen that suppresses HIV replication to fewer than 50 copies/mL.
2. **Antiretroviral therapy.** Despite the lack of controlled clinical trials for most antiretroviral agents in pregnancy, current guidelines indicate that ARVT in pregnant women should generally be the same as for nonpregnant adults. Pregnancy is not a reason to defer therapy. However, the physician should assess whether clear fetal or maternal contraindications exist. Further research is needed of combination ARVT in pregnancy before it can be stated to be without risk to the woman or the fetus. Standard combination antiretroviral regimens for treatment of HIV infection should be discussed with and offered to all pregnant women with HIV infection regardless of viral load. However, some women may wish to restrict exposure of their fetus to antiretroviral drugs during pregnancy but still wish to reduce the risk of transmitting HIV to their infant. For those women, antiretroviral prophylaxis provides benefit in preventing perinatal transmission even for RNA levels of less than 1,000 copies/mL. In a meta-analysis of women with fewer than 1,000 copies/mL HIV-1 RNA at or near delivery, the rate of transmission was only 1.0% if the women received antenatal ARVT (primarily AZT alone) compared with 9.8% among those who received no antenatal therapy [238,241]. Furthermore, although the time-limited use of

AZT alone during pregnancy for chemoprophylaxis of perinatal transmission is controversial because of the potential for resistance development, for women with HIV-1 RNA levels of 1,000 copies/mL, induced resistance is unlikely to occur. This is because there is limited viral replication existing in the patient and the exposure is brief. The development of AZT resistance was unusual among the population of antiretroviral-naive women with CD4 cell counts of greater than 200/mL who participated in Pediatric AIDS Clinical Trials Group Protocol 076 [241,255]. This combination of observations implies that the use of prophylaxis is reasonable for all pregnant women with HIV infection regardless of antenatal HIV RNA level.

3. **Timing of antiretroviral therapy in pregnancy.** After discussion with her health-care provider about the known and unknown benefits and risks of therapy, the pregnant woman should decide whether to use antiretroviral medication in pregnancy. Because the risk of teratogenicity is greatest during the first trimester, many providers advocate waiting until the end of the first trimester before starting new medications. The clinical, immunologic, and virologic status of the mother must be weighed against the potential effect of antiretroviral agents on the fetus. Pregnant women already receiving ARVT may choose either to continue therapy or temporarily discontinue it until 14 weeks' gestational age [241]. If therapy is discontinued, all drugs should be stopped and reintroduced simultaneously to avoid the development of antiretroviral drug resistance. However, discontinuing antiretroviral medications may result in a surge in the viral load that may have an impact on HIV transmission and the subsequent ability to obtain virologic control.
4. **Treatment and prophylaxis of opportunistic infections.** Treatment and prophylaxis of opportunistic infections during pregnancy should follow the guidelines for nonpregnant women [256]. As with antiretroviral medications, the potential benefits must be weighed against their potential risks. Pneumococcal, hepatitis B, and influenza vaccines may be given during pregnancy if indicated. Live vaccines such as rubella, measles, mumps, and varicella are contraindicated during pregnancy and labor, and during the early postpartum period.
5. **Perinatal transmission and mode of delivery.** Recent studies suggest that cesarean section (C-section) performed before the onset of labor and rupture of membranes significantly reduces the risk for perinatal HIV transmission by 55% to 60% [251,257]. These studies were performed in populations not receiving HAART with PIs or NNRTIs. Whether C-section confers protection to patients on HAART or with undetectable plasma viral loads is not known. Furthermore, for HIV-positive women, C-section may be associated with increased risk for postoperative endometritis and other postoperative morbidity, especially in women with advanced HIV disease [258]. Although the morbidity from C-section was low in the prospective randomized trial, postpartum fever was significantly more frequent than in the women who underwent vaginal delivery (6.7% vs. 1.1%, $p = 0.002$) [257]. HIV-infected women should be informed about these study results, and the decision about method of delivery should be individualized. It is possible that C-section plays the most important role in preventing transmission to the newborn in those women with a high viral load that are not receiving prenatal ARVT.
6. **Timing of scheduled cesarean section and intrapartum antiretroviral medications.** Elective C-section delivery should be performed at 38 weeks of gestation. Amniocentesis should be avoided [259]. This contrasts with recommendations for women not infected with HIV. In that setting, unless amniocentesis is performed, one waits until 39 completed weeks, or the onset of labor, to reduce the chance of complications in the neonate. Cesarean delivery at 38 compared with 39 weeks entails a small but definite increased risk of development of infant respiratory distress requiring mechanical ventilation. This increased risk must be balanced against the potential risk for labor or membrane rupture by waiting until 39 weeks. Women should be informed of the risk/benefit ratio to themselves and their infants in choosing the timing and mode of delivery [241].

Table 19.13. Factors that Influence Adherence to Antiretroviral Therapy

| Negative Predictors of Adherence | Positive Predictors of Adherence |
|---|---|
| Active drug or alcohol use | Good understanding of the benefits of antiretroviral therapy |
| Regimen complexity and side effects | Regimen ease of administration, tolerability |
| Depression or other psychiatric illness | Good relationship with provider |
| | Social support |

For a scheduled cesarean delivery, i.v. the patient should begin receiving AZT 3 hours before surgery, using standard dosing [241]. Other antiretroviral medications taken during pregnancy should not be interrupted, regardless of route of delivery. Because maternal infectious morbidity is potentially increased, clinicians may opt to give perioperative antimicrobial prophylaxis. However, there are no controlled data supporting this approach [241].

7. **Breast-feeding.** The U.S. Public Health Service recommends that all HIV-infected women completely refrain from breast-feeding to avoid postnatal transmission of HIV-1 to their infants, whether or not they are being treated [241]. These guidelines should be ignored only in developing countries without access to clean water and infant formula [260]. Passage of antiretroviral drugs into milk has been evaluated for only a few antiretroviral drugs. NVP, AZT, and 3TC have been detected in breast milk, and ddI, ddC, d4T, ABC, DLV, EFV, TDF, IDV, RTV, SQV, NFV, lopinavir, and APV have been detected in the milk of rats [242]. Whether ARVT prevents postnatal transmission of HIV-1 through breast milk and whether the drug containing milk is toxic to the infant are both unknown.

**IX. Therapeutic management in HIV infection.** The goals of ARVT are to maximally suppress viral replication (<50 copies/mL) and to preserve or restore immune system function.

**A. Initiating therapy in chronic or established HIV infection** (Tables 19.13 and 19.14). The optimal time to initiate ARVT in asymptomatic HIV-infected patients is unknown. Initiation of ARVT at CD4 cell counts of greater than 350/mL has been associated with a higher rate of AIDS-free survival at 2 years. Suppression of HIV RNA is easier to achieve and maintain at higher CD4 cell counts and lower levels

Table 19.14. Initiation of Antiretroviral Therapy

| | $CD4^+$ T-cell Count | Plasma HIV-1 RNA | Recommendation |
|---|---|---|---|
| Symptomatic | Any value | Any value | Treatment |
| Asymptomatic, AIDS | <200/mm$^3$ | Any value | Treatment |
| Asymptomatic | >200/mm$^3$ but <350/mm$^3$ | Any value | Treatment should be offered |
| Asymptomatic | >350/mm$^3$ | >55,000 (RT-PCR) | Some clinicians recommend therapy because the risk of developing AIDS in 3yr if untreated is >30% |
| Asymptomatic | >350/mm$^3$ | <55,000 (RT-PCR) | Many clinicians would defer therapy because the risk of developing AIDS in 3yr is <15% |

RT-PCR, reverse transcriptase polymerase chain reaction.
Adapted from the U.S. Department of Health and Human Services and Henry J. Kaiser Family Foundation. Guidelines for the use of antiretroviral Agents in HIV-infected adults and adolescents, August 2001.

of plasma viral load [261,262]. However, no clinical outcome data are currently available, and no comparative trials of immediate versus delayed treatment have been conducted in asymptomatic HIV-infected patients with CD4 cell counts of greater than 350/mL to support this approach.

1. **Factors that favor early initiation of ARVT in asymptomatic individuals:**
   May be more effective in immune reconstitution.
   May elicit HIV-specific immune responses that contribute to the effectiveness of ARVT.
   May suppress viral reservoirs to a greater degree than more advanced HIV disease.
   May be important in prevention of HIV transmission.
   May tolerate medications less well in more advanced disease stages.
2. **Arguments against early initiation of ARVT:**
   Longer exposure to antiretroviral agents and the inherent risk of short- and long-term side effects.
   Higher cost.
   ARVT can elicit immune reconstitution even in advanced disease.
   Delays exposure to antiretroviral agents and their side effects.
   No clear survival benefit from early therapy.
3. **Adherence. The decision of when to initiate therapy** depends largely on an individual patient's ability to adhere to therapy, which is crucial for long-term therapeutic success. Patients need to be aware that ARVT is life long, that strict adherence is required for success, and that there are inherent costs, inconveniences of side effects, and impact on quality of life. When choosing therapy, the comparative pill burden, dosing frequency, food requirements, convenience, toxicity, and potential for drug interactions between regimens need to be considered. Thus, ARVT can be individualized. The aid of an adherence counselor is valuable in preparing the patient for all of the above.
   a. **Factors that influence adherence to ARVT**
   b. **Other patient factors.** Patient race, gender, disease stage, and history of substance abuse as well as the physician assessment of patient adherence do not predict adherence.

**B. Other considerations regarding initiation of therapy**

1. **Resistance factors.** Concern about the long-term complications of ARVT and about the resistance development has dictated a more conservative approach to initiation of treatment.
2. **Symptoms or disease.** There is unanimous agreement to initiate therapy in all HIV-infected patients who have symptomatic HIV-infection or AIDS.
3. **Viral load.** Patients with high plasma viral loads (>100,000 copies/mL) are at a higher risk for disease progression and death (see Table 19.1).
4. **Lymphocyte markers.** In general, patients with CD4 counts of less than 350 cells/$\mu$L should be offered therapy. The short-term risk of the development of AIDS in 3 to 6 years, at all levels of plasma HIV RNA (see Table 19.1), is substantial for patients with CD4 cell counts of less than 350/mL. Waiting to initiate therapy when CD4 cell counts are below 200/mL has been associated with shorter survival [263].

**C. Selecting the initial regimen for the patient naive to ARVT** (Table 19.15). The initial antiretroviral regimen used offers the best chance for therapeutic success [264]. That regimen must be carefully chosen to achieve this goal. Rational sequencing of antiretroviral drugs is also necessary to preserve future therapeutic options.

1. **NRTIs, NNRTIs, and PIs.** Randomized clinical trials indicate that either two NRTIs in combination with a PI or two NRTIs and an NNRTI are effective.
   a. **Viral suppression** is achieved in various tissue reservoirs, including the genital tract and CSF with either regimen.
   b. **Sequence treatment.** Both regimens spare a class of antiretroviral drugs for future use. However, the PI-based regimen involves a greater pill burden and more potential for drug-drug interactions, and may be more

Table 19.15. Recommended Antiretroviral Agents for Initial Treatment of Established HIV Infection

| Column A | Column B |
|---|---|
| Strongly recommended | |
| Efavirenz | Didanosine + lamivudine |
| Indinavir | Stavudine + didanosine |
| Nelfinavir | Stavudine + lamivudine |
| Lopinavir/ritonavir | Zidovudine + didanosine |
| Saquinavir + ritonavir | Zidovudine + lamivudine |
| Recommended as alternatives | |
| Abacavir | Zidovudine + zalcitabine |
| Amprenavir | |
| Delavirdine | |
| Nelfinavir + saquinavir sgc | |
| Nevirapine | |
| Ritonavir | |
| Saquinavir sgc | |
| Not recommended: should not be offered | |
| Saquinavir hgc | Stavudine + zidovudine |
| | Zalcitabine + didanosine |
| | Zalcitabine + lamivudine |
| | Zalcitabine + stavudine |

Adapted from the U.S. Department of Health and Human Services and Henry J. Kaiser Family Foundation. Guidelines for the use of antiretroviral agents in HIV-infected adults and adolescents, August 2001.

demanding for adherence. An NNRTI-based regimen is easier to use and has fewer potential drug-drug interactions. Conversely, resistance to NNRTI confers cross-resistance to the entire class, limiting the future use of another NNRTI, whereas multiple mutations are required for PI resistance.

2. **Specific factors to consider**
   a. **Viral load** is an essential parameter to consider when initiating ARVT. A greater virologic response was achieved in ARVT-naive patients on a PI-based regimen when using LPV/RTV than when using NFV [265]. Preliminary data from another trial suggests that a higher proportion of ARVT-naive patients with baseline viral loads above 100,000 copies/mL achieved better virologic suppression when receiving LPV/RTV and two NRTIs versus NFV plus two NRTIs [266].
   b. **Resistance.** To avoid the development of resistance, all three selected antiretroviral agents must be started simultaneously [267].
   c. **RTV boost.** Although no trial has been conducted to prove the benefit of the inhibitory effect of RTV on the cytochrome P-450 system, it has been used to enhance the pharmacokinetics of other PIs. This boosting results in higher plasma levels and prolonged half-life of the boosted PI, allowing a reduction in the number of pills and daily doses used (see section on PI dosing).
3. **Regimens.** Two agents from column B and one agent from column A in Table 19.15 are used
   a. **Nucleoside combinations** listed as strongly recommended (column B in Table 19.15) have similar potency and are usually chosen based on their adverse effect profile, ease of administration, and patient preference.
   b. **Once-daily dosing.** At present, among the NRTIs only ddI is recommended. A daily dose of 3TC (300 mg/day) has yielded good results, but trials are lacking.

c. **Regimens to avoid or for special attention.** The combination of AZT and d4T are antagonistic and should not be used [268]. The combination of either ddC and ddI, ddC and 3TC, or ddC and d4T may have overlapping and additive toxicity and are not recommended.

4. **Specific classes**

a. **Among the PIs, SQV** in the hard-gelatin capsule formulation (SQV-HGC) has poor bioavailability and is not recommended unless boosted with RTV. It is associated with inferior virologic and clinical outcome compared with other PIs when used as the only PI [269,270]. Using SQV soft-gelatin capsules (SQV-SGC) has improved bioavailability but requires a high pill burden. The addition of RTV allows a decrease in the number of pills and twice-daily administration. This combination (SQV-SGC/RTV) has been shown to be comparable with IDV or RTV alone [271]. Once a day administration of SQV-SGC (1,600 mg) together with RTV (100 mg) has shown a favorable pharmacologic profile in normal volunteers [272]. Preliminary information in HIV-infected patients appears promising.

b. **RTV,** although potent, when used at full dose (600 mg twice daily) causes frequent and severe side effects. It interferes with the metabolism of numerous drugs through the cytochrome P-450 system. Currently its use is limited to boosting other PIs.

c. **IDV** has a short half-life, requiring dosing three times daily and food restriction for better absorption. When administered every 8 hours, in combination with two nucleosides, it is effective [181,273] even in advanced HIV disease with previous exposure to AZT (45% of patients with CD4 cell counts of <50/mL achieved HIV RNA counts of <50 copies/mL at 24 weeks) [274]. The addition of RTV (100 mg twice daily) inhibits IDV metabolism, resulting in an increased area under the curve (AUC) and trough levels [275,276]. When IDV is used (800 mg twice daily), it is boosted with RTV (100 mg twice daily). This combination eliminates the food restriction requirement, but the risk for nephrolithiasis may be higher [277]. The daily fluid intake requirements (see section D.5.b) cannot be waived.

d. **NFV** can be dosed twice daily, and resistance to this PI does not necessarily confer cross-resistance to other PIs. This makes salvage therapy possible with another PI-containing regimen. However as noted in section **2.a** above, NFV may be inferior to LPV/RTV in viral suppression.

e. **APV** (1,200 mg daily or 600 mg twice daily) boosted with RTV (100 mg daily or 100 mg twice daily) yields an increase in the AUC and trough levels that are similar to those achieved with the current recommended dose of 1,200 mg orally twice daily [278]. The use of APV boosted with RTV allows the use of fewer APV capsules, although the pill burden remains significant.

f. **Summary of PIs.** Only a few comparative trials have been done to compare PIs. One large multicenter trial did not find any differences in the percentage of patients with an HIV-1 RNA level of less than 20 copies/mL at 72 weeks between RTV, IDV, or SQV/RTV combination therapy. Only half of the patients achieved viral loads of fewer than 20 copies/mL [271]. Comparative trials among PI-based regimens that include the newer PIs are lacking, except for preliminary information as noted in section **2.a** above.

5. **Combinations of NRTIs and NNRTIs.** Two NRTIs and an NNRTI (either NVP or EFV) have shown good efficacy with durable viral suppression achievable even in subjects with high (>100,000 copies/mL) viral loads. EFV and NVP have a convenient dosing schedule with few pills and therefore have gained wide acceptance as first-line regimens. Care should be exercised to prevent failure with these regimens because resistance to one NNRTI usually confers complete cross-resistance to the entire class. DLV requires dosing three times daily and is seldom used in ARVT-naive patients. However, DLV increases the levels of PIs and may have a role in PI boosting in salvage regimens where both an NNRTI and PI are used (see section B.3.d.(6)).

6. **Comparisons between regimens.** Prospective and retrospective studies comparing PI-based regimens (RTV/SQV or IDV every 8 hours) to NNRTI (EFV)-based regimens have shown that the latter are associated with better virologic response rates regardless of baseline viral load [27,279].
7. **Alternative regimens.** Three NRTIs with ABC as one of the agents for ARVT-naive patients has generated great interest given its ease of administration. AZT, 3TC, and ABC are marketed in combination in one pill (Trizivir) given twice daily. This regimen had similar virologic response rates when compared with IDV plus two NRTIs, particularly in patients with baseline HIV RNA levels of less than 100,000 copies/mL. For patients with HIV RNA levels of greater than 100,000 copies/mL, a three-NRTI combination may not be as potent as the standard PI- or NNRTI-based regimens [280,281] and is not currently recommended for routine use in these patients.

**D. Monitoring ARVT**

1. **Monitoring response to therapy.** Reviewing the details of the ARVT regimen after instituting therapy should be routine practice. This is always useful in disclosing any misunderstandings regarding dosing or food requirements that could lead to failure. Prompt corrective actions may reestablish the regimen's success early on.
2. **Plasma HIV-1 RNA analysis** should be performed 4 to 8 weeks after starting therapy. A decline of at least 1 log is a satisfactory response. The ultimate goal of therapy (HIV RNA <50 copies/mL) is usually achieved within 6 months. HIV-1 RNA should then be repeated every 3 months to monitor efficacy. Significant declines in HIV-1 RNA at 8 weeks predict the achievement (at 6 months) of HIV-1 RNA levels of less than 50 copies/mL [282]. Once the HIV-1 RNA level has been less than 50 copies/mL, episodic levels of greater than 50 copies/mL but less than 200 copies/mL, or "blips," may occur. In a retrospective analysis of 241 patients receiving triple-combination therapy for 4.5 years who achieved viral suppression, blips occurred in 40%. There was no association between these blips and virologic failure [283]. These blips do not warrant changes in therapy.
3. **Lymphocyte markers** should be measured every 3 months or when clinically indicated in all patients receiving ARVT. A significant increase in CD4 cell counts (>160/mL) at week 48 after initiation of HAART is seen in most patients [284]. There is considerable variation in the degree and timing of the response. The absence of an increase in CD4 cell count does not indicate ARVT failure if the viral load has declined appropriately. Greater median maximum CD4 cell count changes are seen with PI-based regimens, younger patients, and higher baseline CD4 cell counts [285,286].
4. **Other laboratory and clinical parameters** are monitored depending on the side effect profile of the different antiretroviral agents, potential for drug interactions, and the patient's specific comorbid conditions (e.g., hepatitis C, seizure disorders, renal insufficiency).
5. **Poor response.** Failure of ARVT is defined as the inability to achieve an undetectable plasma HIV RNA level within 4 to 6 months of starting therapy, or a less than 0.5 to 0.75 $\log_{10}$ reduction in plasma HIV RNA by 4 weeks after starting therapy or less than 1 $\log_{10}$ reduction by 8 weeks. If an adequate virologic response is not obtained or is suboptimal, adherence and possible drug-drug interactions needs to be assessed.
6. **Resistance development.** Reappearance of virus after initial suppression to undetectable levels or a reproducible significant increase (threefold or greater) from the plasma HIV RNA nadir that is not attributable to intercurrent infection, vaccination, or problems inherent to the test suggests the development of resistance.
7. **Causes of ARVT failure:**
   Development of resistance (most common cause)
   Drug-drug interactions
   Use of a suboptimal regimen
   Poor absorption leading to inadequate ARV levels

**E. Salvage therapy.** The choice of ARVT after use of an initial regimen (salvage therapy) should be based on a careful review of past antiretroviral treatment, adherence to the current regimen and the use of resistance testing. Currently there are two types of tests available to assess HIV resistance.

1. **Genotype testing** detects drug resistance mutations by either sequencing relevant genes (RT and protease) or by using probes to detect selected mutations. Assessment of viral genotype involves comparison of the relevant genetic region of the test sample with a consensus wild-type sequence. The results report any amino acid substitutions at the codons tested. The interpretation of genotypic tests remains complex. Assays may vary in their performance at different codons, and their reliability may vary between laboratories. ARVT selection based on genotype results in concert with expert advice has been linked to a better outcome [287–289]. Because wild-type virus usually outgrows resistant virus, resistance testing should be performed while the patient is on antiretroviral medications or within 2 weeks of their discontinuation [290]. Some laboratories report the results of genotype testing accompanied by a virtual phenotype report. Phenotype testing is performed with viral strains of similar genotype resistance pattern to the patient's viral strain. The influence of this interpretation on clinical outcome has not been definitively established but is commonly used in practice. Viruses resistant to newer antiretroviral medications have not been studied long enough to establish genotype resistance patterns, and the patient's genotypic pattern may be difficult to match with the existing ones in the database. In addition, some mutations can increase drug susceptibility.
2. **Phenotype testing** uses cells infected with a fixed amount of the patient's virus. This is intuitively an excellent approach to the study of clinical resistance. Unfortunately the only study conducted to compare both genotype and phenotype testing to standard of care failed to show an effect on the clinical outcome and warrants further study [291].

**F. Therapeutic drug monitoring (TDM).** Factors other than poor adherence to ARVT or viral resistance may be responsible for suboptimal response or failure. These include inadequate drug levels caused by differing levels of phosphorylation to the active moiety (NRTIs), membrane efflux pumps (described for PIs and NNRTIs) that extrude ARVs from cells, differing ability to absorb and metabolize drugs, as well as drug-drug interactions. These factors may help explain inter- and intrasubject drug level variability. A significant correlation between *in vivo* antiviral activity and plasma drug concentrations has been demonstrated for PIs [292]. The PI plasma levels are inversely correlated with plasma HIV RNA levels [293]. PIs seem to be the best candidate for TDM because their AUC and trough levels appear to predict their efficacy. TDM may become, along with resistance testing, instrumental in optimizing ARVT. The use of the inhibitory quotient (IQ = the trough concentration of a drug in plasma divided by the *in vitro* $IC_{50}$) is being studied in clinical trials to assess its role in clinical management.

**G. Laboratory monitoring of potential side effects of antiretroviral medications**

1. **Bone marrow suppression** is caused by AZT, a widely used agent. A baseline complete blood count and differential are repeated at least every 3 months or when clinically indicated. A different NRTI can be substituted if anemia occurs. Erythropoietin for patients with inappropriately low erythropoietin levels is an option for patients with fewer ARV alternatives, but requires parenteral administration and constitutes an additional expense. Neutropenia is managed by changing AZT to another NRTI, or by administering parenteral granulocyte colony-stimulating factor. Substitution of the ARV is the preferred choice.
2. **Hepatitis.** Retrospective data were compiled from 10,611 HIV-infected patients with baseline LFT results showing less than grade 1 toxicity enrolled in 21 AIDS Clinical Trials Group (ACTG) studies including all drug classes between 1991 and 2000. An overall rate of hepatotoxicity of 9% was noted [294]. The development of grade 3 to 4 toxicity led to permanent discontinuation of ARVT in 23%. Most of these patients developed toxicity after 24 weeks, but in some it occurred quite early. PIs, particularly RTV, were associated with the highest

rate of hepatotoxicity, but those on NRTI regimens were more likely to die or to discontinue therapy. Among NNRTIs, DLV was associated with the lowest rate and NVP had the highest rate of hepatotoxicity and permanent discontinuation of therapy and the only hepatic-related death in this class. Overall, 2.5% of deaths were related to hepatotoxicity. Elevated LFT results are seen more frequently in patients coinfected with hepatitis B or C receiving ARVT. It is difficult to know the exact etiology of the liver damage.

3. **LFTs should be conducted** at baseline and every 3 months in stable patients. They should also be repeated when ARVT changes occur and whenever clinically indicated. More frequent monitoring of LFT results (every 4–6 weeks) is indicated in patients with underlying liver disease. Given the potential for fatal hepatotoxicity with NVP, transaminases should be monitored during the first 12 weeks of therapy. NVP should be discontinued if moderate to severe abnormalities (greater than three times the ULN) develop (NVP package insert) [125].
4. **Hyperglycemia** (see section VI.A). Blood glucose levels should be monitored every 3 months or when clinically indicated. The management of diabetes in HIV-infected patients is the same as in non–HIV-infected patients.
5. **Development of dyslipidemias** (see section VI.C–D). A baseline fasting serum lipid profile should be obtained before initiating ARVT that includes a PI or an NNRTI. The lipid profile should be repeated in 3 to 6 months [295]. Baseline screening for cardiovascular risks and factors that exacerbate dyslipidemia is indicated and should be repeated at least yearly thereafter unless abnormalities are detected or other risk factors for dyslipidemia are present.
6. **Management of dyslipidemias.** Clinical studies to determine the most appropriate treatment for dyslipidemia are ongoing. Meanwhile, initiating treatment according to the NECP guidelines appears reasonable (see section on PI drug-drug interactions with lipid-lowering agents). Preliminary data suggest that switching the PI to NVP (in patients naive to NNRTI) or to ABC may be useful in controlling dyslipidemia, but switching to EFV has yielded inconsistent results.
7. **Lactic acidosis** (see section V.A.3). Currently there are no specific recommendations for laboratory monitoring for lactic acidosis in patients without symptoms (see section on NRTI class-related adverse effects). Risk factors for lactic acidosis include treatment with NRTI, African-American ethnicity, obesity, hepatitis C, and female gender.
8. **Pancreatitis** (see section V.A.5.g.(1)). Unless symptoms of pancreatitis develop, monitoring amylase and lipase levels is not routinely recommended. Risk factors include a history of pancreatitis, use of ddI, d4T, or ddC, CD4 cell count below 50/mL, alcohol use, obesity, hypertriglyceridemia, gallstones, or use of medications that can cause pancreatitis. When pancreatitis occurs, all medications should be held until resolution is complete. A different antiretroviral agent should be substituted for the agent felt to be the cause of the pancreatitis. Hyperamylasemia of nonpancreatic origin may occur in HIV-infected patients. A serum lipase should be obtained in this setting. Patients with asymptomatic elevations of serum amylase and lipase levels (up to three times the ULN) should be monitored clinically without a change in therapy.
9. **Neuropathy** (see section V.A.5.g.(2)). Glucose level, vitamin $B_{12}$ level, and thyroid function tests should be obtained in HIV-infected patients presenting with signs and symptoms of neuropathy. Electrophysiologic studies may not be necessary for the diagnosis of typical distal symmetric polyneuropathy but may be useful in diagnosing other neuropathies. Analgesics should be offered in a stepwise fashion. Supplementation with antidepressants or antiseizure medications might be useful. If alternative non-neurotoxic antiretroviral agents are available, they should be substituted.
10. **Myopathy** (see section V.A.4.f.(3)). When myopathy is suspected, muscle enzymes should be measured and muscle biopsy performed. Antiretroviral

agents should be discontinued until symptoms and laboratory value abnormalities resolve.

11. **Bone disorders** (see section VI.E). Osteopenia and avascular necrosis usually involving weight-bearing joints occur in HIV-infected patients receiving ARVT. No definitive association with a particular class of antiretroviral agent has been confirmed. Currently there are no specific recommendations for monitoring of these disorders.
12. **Fat redistribution syndrome** (see section on PI class-related toxicities). A definition of fat redistribution syndrome has yet to be established. This term describes a variety of changes in subcutaneous and visceral fat, most commonly loss of subcutaneous fat on the face and legs, and dorsocervical fat deposition (buffalo hump) and increase in visceral fat. Fat redistribution does not require a specific intervention unless cosmetically disturbing to the patient. Changing ARVT has not proven successful, but large trials have not been conducted; growth hormone has yielded unimpressive results. Glitazone did not demonstrate a significant effect on fat redistribution in a small placebo-controlled trial. Fat redistribution syndrome may coincide with dyslipidemia and hyperglycemia. There are no recommended laboratory tests to monitor for fat redistribution syndrome.

**H. Changing therapy.** Antiretroviral therapy may need to be changed for several reasons: toxicity, treatment failure, convenience, or drug interactions.

1. **Toxicity** (see section on individual agent adverse effects). If a side effect can be attributed to a particular antiretroviral agent with certainty (e.g., anemia from AZT or nephrolithiasis with IDV), and maximal viral suppression has been achieved, the antiretroviral agent may be substituted (see Table 19.15). If the adverse effect requires holding the antiretroviral agent (e.g., pancreatitis), all antiretroviral medications should be held. A new regimen with a different side effect profile should be used once the adverse event has resolved.
2. **Treatment failure** is the inability to obtain a significant decrease in viral load or development of an increase in viral load above 200 copies/mL after achieving viral suppression (<50 copies/mL). In general, agents to which the patient has not been exposed offer the best opportunity for further suppression. Cross-resistance among antiretroviral medications may make it difficult to achieve this goal. A better outcome can be expected when past history of ARVT use is obtained, resistance testing is employed, and expert opinion is used in concert to guide the selection of ARVT for salvage therapy. At least two clinical trails have demonstrated the short-term benefit of genotypic and phenotypic resistance testing to guide the selection of salvage therapy. There are scant data supporting the longer term benefit of resistance testing. Some recent yet unpublished trials have failed to show the benefit of resistance testing [291]. The contrasting results of these trials may be due to many factors, including poorly defined thresholds for resistance, difference in the number of new drugs given, or different past histories of antiretroviral agents used. Nonetheless, many clinicians consider resistance testing the standard of care in this setting at the present time.
3. **Cross-resistance** among the NRTIs has emerged as one of the most important issues related to sequencing therapy. Mutations at RT codons 41, 67, 70, 210, and 215 (referred to as thymidine analogue mutations [TAMs] or nucleoside analogue mutations [NAMs]) cause cross-resistance among the NRTIs. 3TC, when used in regimens that are not suppressive, produces rapid development of resistance conferred by a single point mutation at codon 184 that confers complete 3TC resistance but increases susceptibility to AZT and the nucleotide analogue TDF. The accumulation of increasing numbers of TAMs is associated with increased phenotypic resistance to all of the NRTIs. Resistance mutations with the use of NNRTI often confer cross-resistance to all NNRTIs. Consistently, the K103 mutation of RT that can be selected by EFV, NVP, or DLV confers resistance to all three NNRTIs. The RT mutation Y 181C, selected by NVP, does not exclude the subsequent use of EFV.
4. **Resistance to the PIs** usually requires the development of three or more specific mutations on the protease-encoding gene. SQV's primary mutations include

G48V and L90M. The latter is a secondary mutation for all the other PIs and may confer cross-resistance to all PIs except APV. IDV's primary mutations include M46I/L and V82A/F/T. The latter mutation confers cross-resistance to RTV. NFV has a unique resistance pattern, with D30N selected in two-thirds of patients. This mutation does not compromise the activity of other PIs. Some clinicians therefore prefer to use NFV as the initial PI. However, approximately one-third of individuals who fail NFV develop L90 M, which as noted causes broad PI cross-resistance. APV also has a unique resistance pattern, with I50V as the primary mutation. Thus far this has not been identified as conferring cross-resistance to other PIs. Early failures on APV can be managed successfully by switching to other PI-containing regimens. LPV appears to have a high genetic barrier to the development of resistance compared with other PIs. Perhaps a larger number of mutations must accumulate for resistance to be detected.

5. **Convenience.** European and North American trials support making changes to simplify therapy (fewer pills, less frequent dosing). This should be done only when maximal viral suppression has been achieved. Switching a patient from a less convenient PI inhibitor–based regimen to an NNRTI-based regimen is safely done as long as adherence continues.

**I. Therapy for acute or primary HIV-1 infection.** Treatment of acute or primary HIV infection can dramatically suppress HIV-1 RNA and preserve HIV-1–specific immune responses. Several uncontrolled studies have documented normalization of $CD4^+$ and $CD8^+$ lymphocyte subsets as well as virologic suppression. Furthermore, preservation of HIV specific CD4 cell lymphoproliferative responses and stabilization of the T-cell receptor repertoire have been observed (see following section on structured treatment interruptions). Combination ARVT is recommended for acute HIV infection.

**J. Virus characteristics.** The virus is relatively uniform genetically and typically of a non–syncytium-inducing phenotype. Moreover, infection may not be fully established in all tissues until some time after exposure [296]. These features may render the infection easier to control. Clinical trials with potent antiretroviral medications are under way to determine the feasibility of intense time-limited treatment for acute HIV infection.

**K. Structured or supervised treatment interruptions (STIs).** With effective HAART, HIV-specific cell-mediated immunity may actually be decreased because the immune system is not exposed to HIV antigens. In theory, during STI when HAART is stopped, HIV antigen is once again provided by the rebound in viral replication. This may stimulate HIV-specific T-helper and cytotoxic T-lymphocyte responses.

1. **Acute HIV infection.** STI may be useful in acute, primary HIV infection. Small pilot studies of individuals with HIV infection of less than 180 days, who had achieved good virologic control with HAART, showed increases in median cytotoxic T-lymphocyte responses after STI. A similar response was achieved in other subjects after a second round of STI. Sixty percent achieved viral suppression after STI in the absence of further HAART. Larger studies are obviously needed to clarify the role of STI in acute or recent HIV infection.
2. **Chronic HIV infection.** Several small nonrandomized, uncontrolled studies of STI, using different durations of drug cessation, have yielded conflicting results. However, in all of these studies treatment interruption was followed in the majority of patients by an increase in viremia. The time to viral rebound after discontinuation of HAART varied from as early as 2 to 3 days to as late as 3 weeks. In one study, rebound viremia exceeded pretreatment levels by 27-fold [297]. Upon reinitiation of HAART, although viral suppression was observed, reduction in viral load was delayed by up to 2 months compared with the initial virologic response. Other features of concern include the inconsistent increase in CD4 cell count, the inconsistent HIV-1–specific T-cell helper response to p24 antigen (recovery in only 2 of 12 patients in one study), and inconsistent lymphocyte proliferative response to HIV-1 p24 antigen in only 4 of 22 patients [298]. Fortunately, no mutations associated with resistance developed.

3. **Modified STI.** A small preliminary study using shorter cycles of therapy (7 days) [299] showed no rebound in viremia.
4. **STI summary.** It is not clear which patients with chronic HIV infection are most likely to benefit. Whether STI leads to lasting enhancement of the immunologic response to HIV remains to be firmly established, and further data are needed before its use is adopted. Treatment interruptions, especially in chronic HIV infection, can be potentially dangerous, leading to dramatic increases in HIV viral load and precipitous declines in CD4 cell counts.

**X. Use of antiretroviral agents in children**

**A. Introduction.** The pathogenesis of HIV infection and the general principles of ARVT in infants, children, and adolescents are similar to those in adults but there are unique considerations. In addition, the dramatic decline in rates of maternal-infant transmission of HIV when ARVT is given to pregnant women (see section VIII) has resulted in far fewer HIV-infected infants in the United States. This has limited the available number of ARVT-naive subjects for performance of clinical trials. Thus, health-care providers for HIV-infected infants, children, and adolescents should seek consultation with, or refer such patients to, a pediatric HIV specialist. Ideally, these children should be treated in a center with access to pediatric clinical trials [40,235]. Pediatric guidelines for ARVT use are available at *www.hivatis.org*, and information on pediatric clinical trials is available at *www.hivactis.org*.

**B. Differences between adult and pediatric HIV infection that may impact use of ARVT**

1. **Paucity of pediatric clinical trials data.** Decisions about use of ARVT in children are complex and may rely on assumptions based on adult data only. This is because infants and children make up only 1% to 2% of the HIV-infected population in the United States, and traditional pharmaceutical research practices use testing of compounds in adults before children.
2. **Pediatric acquisition of HIV.** Nearly all infants and children in the United States, and in much of the world, have acquired HIV vertically from their mothers. Thus, infection occurs during the development of the immune system, at a time when the thymus is active and $CD4^+$ lymphocytes circulate in the blood in great numbers. Clinical and immunologic manifestations of pediatric HIV, therefore, differ from those of adults [235]. For example, immunologic compromise in children is associated with $CD4^+$ lymphocyte counts that would be in the normal range in adults. Thus, starting points for ARVT differ in children [40,235].
3. **Virologic parameters.** Children tend to have a greater "set point" of plasma RNA copy numbers. This may be because of the establishment of infection in the developmentally immature immune system at a time when high numbers of $CD4^+$ lymphocytes are circulating in the blood. Thus, a 2 log reduction of 500,000 copies/mL yields a posttherapy viral load of 5,000 copies/mL. Five thousand copies would be considered a failure in adults, but may be tolerated in such children.
4. **Pharmacokinetic parameters.** Plasma clearance of many drugs is increased in children relative to adults. Clearance also may change during puberty. Current guidelines suggest that adolescents in early puberty (Tanner stages I–II) be given pediatric dosage of antiretroviral agents, whereas those in late puberty (Tanner V) should be dosed using adult schedules [40]. Clinical trials are assessing proper dosing, especially for PIs, in midpuberty.
5. **Pediatric formulations.** Not all antiretroviral agents have been licensed for use in children, nor do all have palatable liquids available for use in children who may not be able to swallow large pills.
6. **Adherence issues in children and adolescents.** Because essentially all children and many adolescents require supervision of ARVT administration, there is a necessarily different dynamic of working with a family unit rather than a single patient. Issues affecting adherence include willingness of a child to take a drug. There are also feelings of guilt in mothers who transmitted the virus. This may affect the interaction between caregiver and receiver. There is the complexity of the need to administer the drug in the fasting or fed state when

the infected infant is fed so often. There is the unwillingness to disclose the fact of HIV infection status to young children, their school officials, or other family members, creating a situation where doses are missed frequently. Adolescents may have additional issues revolving around denial and fear of HIV infection, distrust of the medical establishment, unstructured and chaotic lifestyle, and lack of familial and social support [40].

C. **ARVT regimens for HIV-infected children.** Despite the difficulties posed by the lack of clinical trial data, and differences between adult and pediatric HIV infection mentioned previously, all antiretroviral agents approved for use in adults may be used in children when indicated, irrespective of labeling notations. Continually updated pediatric guidelines are published electronically along with adult guidelines by U.S. Public Health Service task forces. These are available at *www.hivatis.org*. In general, the most strongly recommended ARV regimen for children is two NRTIs plus one PI. Generally the PI is NFV or RTV. For older children who can swallow capsules, two NRTIs plus EFV is an increasingly used alternative initial therapy. Other combinations include NVP plus two NRTIs or even ABC/AZT/3TC. The consultation of a pediatric HIV specialist should be sought because the field is rapidly changing.

## REFERENCES

1. Palella FJ, Delaney KM, Moorman AC, et al. Declining morbidity and mortality among patients with advanced human immunodeficiency virus infection. HIV Outpatient Study Investigators. *N Engl J Med* 1998;338:853–860.
2. Mocroft A, et al. AIDS across Europe, 1994–98: the EuroSIDA study. *Lancet* 2000;356:291–296.
3. Hogg RS, et al. Improved survival among HIV-infected patients after initiation of triple-drug antiretroviral regimens. *CMAJ* 1999;160:659–665.
4. Powderly WG, Landay A, Lederman MM. Recovery of the immune system with antiretroviral therapy: the end of opportunism? *JAMA* 1998;280:72–77.
5. U.S. Public Health Service/Infectious Diseases Society of America. 1999 Guidelines for the prevention of opportunistic infections in persons infected with human immunodeficiency virus. *MMWR* 1999;48:1–59,61–66.
6. Ledergerber B, et al. Discontinuation of secondary prophylaxis against *Pneumocystis carinii* pneumonia in patients with HIV infection who have a response to antiretroviral therapy. Eight European Study Groups. *N Engl J Med* 2001;344:168–174.
7. Aberg JA, Yajko DM, Jacobson MA. Eradication of AIDS-related disseminated *Mycobacterium avium* complex infection after 12 months of antimycobacterial therapy combined with highly active antiretroviral therapy. *J Infect Dis* 1998;178:1446–1449.
8. Soriano V, et al. Discontinuation of secondary prophylaxis for opportunistic infections in HIV-infected patients receiving highly active antiretroviral therapy. *AIDS* 2000;14:383–386.
9. Martinez E, et al. Discontinuation of secondary prophylaxis for cryptococcal meningitis in HIV-infected patients responding to highly active antiretroviral therapy. *AIDS* 2000;14:2615–2617.
10. Bartlett J, Demasi R, Quinn J, et al. Meta-analysis of efficacy of triple combination therapy in antiretroviral-naive HIV-1 infected adults. January 30–February 2 [Abstract 519]. Presented at the 7th Conference on Retroviruses and Opportunistic Infections, San Francisco, CA, 2000.
11. Lucas GM, Chaisson RE, Moore RD. Highly active antiretroviral therapy in a large urban clinic: risk factors for virologic failure and adverse drug reactions. *Ann Intern Med* 1999;131:81–87.
12. Zhang L, et al. Quantifying residual HIV-1 replication in patients receiving combination antiretroviral therapy. *N Engl J Med* 1999;340:1605–1613.
13. Pomerantz RJ. Reservoirs of human immunodeficiency virus type 1: the main obstacles to viral eradication. *Clin Infect Dis* 2002;34:91–97.
14. Balzarini J, et al. Exploitation of the low fidelity of human immunodeficiency virus type 1 (HIV-1) reverse transcriptase and the nucleotide composition bias in the HIV-1 genome to alter the drug resistance development of HIV. *J Virol* 2001;75:5772–5777.

15. Schuurman R, et al. Rapid changes in human immunodeficiency virus type 1 RNA load and appearance of drug-resistant virus populations in persons treated with lamivudine (3TC). *J Infect Dis* 1995;171:1411–1419.
16. Lyles RH, et al. Natural history of human immunodeficiency virus type 1 viremia after seroconversion and proximal to AIDS in a large cohort of homosexual men. Multicenter AIDS Cohort Study. *J Infect Dis* 2000;181:872–880.
17. Vergis EN, Mellors JW. Natural history of HIV-1 infection. *Infect Dis Clin North Am* 2000;14:809–825, v–vi.
18. Ho DD, et al. Rapid turnover of plasma virions and CD4 lymphocytes in HIV-1 infection. *Nature* 1995;373:123–126.
19. Mellors JW, et al. Quantitation of HIV-1 RNA in plasma predicts outcome after seroconversion. *Ann Intern Med* 1995;122:573–579.
20. Mellors JW, et al. Plasma viral load and CD4$^{+}$ lymphocytes as prognostic markers of HIV-1 infection. *Ann Intern Med* 1997;126:946–954.
21. Centers for Disease Control and Prevention. Report of the NIH panel to define principles of therapy of HIV infection and guidelines for the use of antiretroviral agents in HIV-infected adults and adolescents. *MMWR* 1998;47:3.
22. Carpenter CC, et al. Antiretroviral therapy in adults: updated recommendations of the International AIDS Society—USA Panel. *JAMA* 2000;283:381–390.
23. Evans TG, et al. Highly active antiretroviral therapy results in a decrease in CD8$^{+}$ T cell activation and preferential reconstitution of the peripheral CD4$^{+}$ T cell population with memory rather than naive cells. *Antiviral Res* 1998;39:163–173.
24. Fischl M, Richman DD, Grieco MH, et al. The efficacy of azidothymidine (AZT) in the treatment of patients with AIDS and AIDS-related complex: a double blind, placebo-controlled trial. *N Engl J Med* 1987;317:185–190.
25. Fischl M, Richman DD, Hansen J, et al. The safety and efficacy of zidovudine (AZT) in the treatment of subjects with mildly symptomatic human immunodeficiency virus type 1 (HIV) infection: a double-blind, placebo-controlled trial. *Ann Intern Med* 1990;12:727–732.
26. Hammer S, Katzenstein DA, Hughes MD, et al. A trial comparing nucleoside monotherapy with combination therapy in HIV-infected adults with CD4 cell counts from 200 to 500 per cubic millimeter. *N Engl J Med* 1996;335:1081–1090.
27. Staszewski S, et al. Efavirenz plus zidovudine and lamivudine, efavirenz plus indinavir, and indinavir plus zidovudine and lamivudine in the treatment of HIV-1 infection in adults. Study 006 Team. *N Engl J Med* 1999;341:1865–1873.
28. Pincus SH, Wehrly K. AZT demonstrates anti-HIV-1 activity in persistently infected cell lines: implications for combination chemotherapy and immunotherapy. *J Infect Dis* 1990;162:1233–1238.
29. Sommadossi JP. Comparison of metabolism and *in vitro* antiviral activity of stavudine versus other 2′,3′-dideoxynucleoside analogues. *J Infect Dis* 1995;171(suppl 2):88–92.
30. St. Clair MH, et al. 3′-Azido-3′-deoxythymidine triphosphate as an inhibitor and substrate of purified human immunodeficiency virus reverse transcriptase. *Antimicrob Agents Chemother* 1987;31:1972–1977.
31. Tan CK, et al. Inhibition of the RNase H activity of HIV reverse transcriptase by azidothymidylate. *Biochemistry* 1991;30:4831–4835.
32. Stenzel MS, Carpenter CC. The management of the clinical complications of antiretroviral therapy. *Infect Dis Clin North Am* 2000;14:851–878.
33. Chen CH, Vazquez-Padua M, Cheng YC. Effect of anti-human immunodeficiency virus nucleoside analogs on mitochondrial DNA and its implication for delayed toxicity. *Mol Pharmacol* 1991;39:625–628.
34. Stacpoole PW. Lactic acidosis and other mitochondrial disorders. *Metabolism* 1997;46:306–321.
35. Boubaker K, et al. Hyperlactatemia and antiretroviral therapy: the Swiss HIV Cohort Study. *Clin Infect Dis* 2001;33:1931–1937.
36. Lonergan JT, et al. Hyperlactatemia and hepatic abnormalities in 10 human immunodeficiency virus–infected patients receiving nucleoside analogue combination regimens. *Clin Infect Dis* 2000;31:162–166.
37. John M, et al. Chronic hyperlactatemia in HIV-infected patients taking antiretroviral therapy. *AIDS* 2001;15:717–723.

38. Fouty B, Frerman F, Reves R. Riboflavin to treat nucleoside analogue-induced lactic acidosis. *Lancet* 1998;352:291–292.
39. Brinkman K, et al. Treatment of nucleoside reverse transcriptase inhibitor–induced lactic acidosis. *AIDS* 2000;14:2801–2802.
40. Working Group on Antiretroviral Therapy and Medical Management of HIV-infected children. Guidelines for the use of antiretroviral agents in pediatric HIV infection. Available at *www.hivatis.org.* Version of December 14, 2000.
41. Perinatal HIV Guidelines Working Group. Recommendations for use of antiretroviral drugs in pregnant HIV-1–infected women for maternal health and interventions to reduce perinatal HIV-1 transmission in the United States. Available at *www.hivatis.org.* Version of February 4, 2002.
42. McLeod GX, Hammer SM. Zidovudine: five years later. *Ann Intern Med* 1992;117:487–501.
43. Rodman JH, et al. A systemic and cellular model for zidovudine plasma concentrations and intracellular phosphorylation in patients. *J Infect Dis* 1996;174:490–499.
44. Klecker RW, et al. Plasma and cerebrospinal fluid pharmacokinetics of 3′-azido-3′-deoxythymidine: a novel pyrimidine analog with potential application for the treatment of patients with AIDS and related diseases. *Clin Pharmacol Ther* 1987;41:407–412.
45. Taburet AM, et al. Pharmacokinetics of zidovudine in patients with liver cirrhosis. *Clin Pharmacol Ther* 1990;47:731–739.
46. Aronoff G, Bennett W, Berns JS, et al. *Drug prescribing in renal failure: dosing guidelines for adults,* 4th ed. Philadelphia: American College of Physicians, 1999.
47. Jacobson MA, et al. Prolonged pancytopenia due to combined ganciclovir and zidovudine therapy. *J Infect Dis* 1988;158:489–490.
48. National Institutes of Health. Important information on the combination of zidovudine (ZDV) and stavudine (d4T) in ZDV-experienced patients [NIH press release]. Bethesda, MD: National Institutes of Health, 1996.
49. Back D, Haworth S, Hoggard P, et al. Drug interactions with d4T phosphorylation *in vitro* [Abstract MO.B.1194]. Presented at the XIth International Conference on AIDS, Vancouver, Canada, 1996.
50. Koch MA, et al. Toxic effects of zidovudine in asymptomatic human immunodeficiency virus–infected individuals with $CD4^+$ cell counts of $0.50 \times 10^9$/L or less. Detailed and updated results from protocol 019 of the AIDS Clinical Trials Group. *Arch Intern Med* 1992;152:2286–2292.
51. Richman DD, et al. The toxicity of azidothymidine (AZT) in the treatment of patients with AIDS and AIDS-related complex. A double-blind, placebo-controlled trial. *N Engl J Med* 1987;317:192–197.
52. Cohen H, et al. Reversible zidovudine-induced pure red-cell aplasia. *AIDS* 1989;3:177–178.
53. Dalakas MC, et al. Mitochondrial myopathy caused by long-term zidovudine therapy. *N Engl J Med* 1990;322:1098–1105.
54. Lange DJ. AAEM minimonograph #41: neuromuscular diseases associated with HIV-1 infection. *Muscle Nerve* 1994;17:16–16.
55. Mhiri C, et al. Zidovudine myopathy: a distinctive disorder associated with mitochondrial dysfunction. *Ann Neurol* 1991;29:606–614.
56. Lipshultz SE, et al. Cardiac structure and function in children with human immunodeficiency virus infection treated with zidovudine. *N Engl J Med* 1992;327:1260–1265.
57. Lipshultz SE, et al. Absence of cardiac toxicity of zidovudine in infants. Pediatric Pulmonary and Cardiac Complications of Vertically Transmitted HIV Infection Study Group. *N Engl J Med* 2000;343:759–766.
58. Domenski M, Sloas MM, Fallmann DE, et al. Effect of zidovudine and didanosine treatment on heart function in children infected with human immunodeficiency virus. *J Pediatr* 1995;127:131–146.
59. Gao WY, et al. Divergent anti-human immunodeficiency virus activity and anabolic phosphorylation of 2′,3′-dideoxynucleoside analogs in resting and activated human cells. *J Biol Chem* 1994;269:12633–12638.

60. Hartman NR, et al. Pharmacokinetics of 2′,3′-dideoxyinosine in patients with severe human immunodeficiency infection. II. The effects of different oral formulations and the presence of other medications. *Clin Pharmacol Ther* 1991;50:278–285.
61. Shelton MJ, O'Donnell AM, Morse GD. Didanosine. *Ann Pharmacother* 1992;26:660–670.
62. Yarchoan R, et al. The National Cancer Institute phase I study of 2′,3′-dideoxyinosine administration in adults with AIDS or AIDS-related complex: analysis of activity and toxicity profiles. *Rev Infect Dis* 12(suppl 5):522–533.
63. Trapnell C, Cimoch P, Gaines K, et al. Altered didanosine pharmacokinetics with concomitant oral ganciclovir [Abstract 193]. Presented at the 95th Annual Meeting of the American Society of Clinical Pharmacology and Therapeutics, 1994.
64. Sahai J. Avoiding the ciprofloxacin-didanosine interaction. *Ann Intern Med* 1995; 123:394–395.
65. Maxson CJ, Greenfield SM, Turner JL. Acute pancreatitis as a common complication of 2′,3′-dideoxyinosine therapy in the acquired immunodeficiency syndrome. *Am J Gastroenterol* 1992;87:708–713.
66. Kahn JO, et al. A controlled trial comparing continued zidovudine with didanosine in human immunodeficiency virus infection. The NIAID AIDS Clinical Trials Group. *N Engl J Med* 1992;327:581–587.
67. Floridia M, et al. A randomized trial (ISS 902) of didanosine versus zidovudine in previously untreated patients with mildly symptomatic human immunodeficiency virus infection. *J Infect Dis* 1997;175:255–264.
68. Grasela TH, et al. Analysis of potential risk factors associated with the development of pancreatitis in phase I patients with AIDS or AIDS-related complex receiving didanosine. *J Infect Dis* 1994;169:1250–1255.
69. Lambert JS, et al. 2′,3′-dideoxyinosine (ddI) in patients with the acquired immunodeficiency syndrome or AIDS-related complex. A phase I trial. *N Engl J Med* 1990;322:1333–1340.
70. Argiris A, et al. Abnormalities of serum amylase and lipase in HIV-positive patients. *Am J Gastroenterol* 1999;94:1248–1252.
71. Simpson DM, Tagliati M. Nucleoside analogue–associated peripheral neuropathy in human immunodeficiency virus infection. *J AIDS Hum Retrovir* 1995;9:153–161.
72. Schaumberg H, Berger AR, Thomas PK. In: Plum F, ed. Disorders of peripheral nerves. Philadelphia: FA Davis, 1992:257–273.
73. Kelleher T, Cross A, Dunkle L. Relation of peripheral neuropathy to HIV treatment in four randomized clinical trials including didanosine. *Clin Ther* 1999;21:1182–1192.
74. Moore RD, et al. Incidence of neuropathy in HIV-infected patients on monotherapy versus those on combination therapy with didanosine, stavudine and hydroxyurea. *AIDS* 2000;14:273–278.
75. Cui L, et al. Effect of nucleoside analogs on neurite regeneration and mitochondrial DNA synthesis in PC-12 cells. *J Pharmacol Exp Ther* 1997;280:1228–1234.
76. Lewis W, Dalakas MC. Mitochondrial toxicity of antiviral drugs. *Nature Med* 1995; 1:417–422.
77. Kieburtz K, et al. A randomized trial of amitriptyline and mexiletine for painful neuropathy in HIV infection. AIDS Clinical Trial Group 242 Protocol Team. *Neurology* 1998;51:1682–1688.
78. Lai KK, et al. Fulminant hepatic failure associated with 2′,3′-dideoxyinosine (ddI). *Ann Intern Med* 1991;115:283–284.
79. Larder BA, Darby G. Richman DD. HIV with reduced sensitivity to zidovudine (AZT) isolated during prolonged therapy. *Science* 1989;243:1731–1734.
79a. Shelton MJ, O'Donnell AM, Morse GD. Zalcitabine. *Ann Pharmacother* 1993;27:480.
80. Merigan TSG, Bozzette S, et al. and the ddC study group of the AIDS Clinical Trials Group. Circulating p24 antigen levels and responses to dideoxycytidine in human immunodeficiency virus (HIV) infections. *Ann Intern Med* 1998;110:189.
81. Saravolatz LD, et al. Zidovudine alone or in combination with didanosine or zalcitabine in HIV-infected patients with the acquired immunodeficiency syndrome or fewer than 200 CD4 cells per cubic millimeter. Investigators for the Terry Beirn Community Programs for Clinical Research on AIDS. *N Engl J Med* 1996;335:1099–1106.

82. Fischl MA, et al. Combination and monotherapy with zidovudine and zalcitabine in patients with advanced HIV disease. The NIAID AIDS Clinical Trials Group. *Ann Intern Med* 1995;122:24–32.
83. Delta Coordinating Committee. Delta: a randomised double-blind controlled trial comparing combinations of zidovudine plus didanosine or zalcitabine with zidovudine alone in HIV-infected individuals. *Lancet* 1996;348:283–291.
84. Fichtenbaum CJ, Clifford DB, Powderly WG. Risk factors for dideoxynucleoside-induced toxic neuropathy in patients with the human immunodeficiency virus infection. *J AIDS Hum Retrovir* 1995;10:169–174.
85. Berger AR, et al. 2′,3′-dideoxycytidine (ddC) toxic neuropathy: a study of 52 patients. *Neurology* 1993;43:358–362.
86. Indorf AS, Pegram PS. Esophageal ulceration related to zalcitabine (ddC). *Ann Intern Med* 1992;117:133–134.
87. Dudley MN, et al. Pharmacokinetics of stavudine in patients with AIDS or AIDS-related complex. *J Infect Dis* 1992;166:480–485.
88. Ho HT, Hitchcock MJ. Cellular pharmacology of 2′,3′-dideoxy-2′,3′-didehydrothymidine, a nucleoside analog active against human immunodeficiency virus. *Antimicrob Agents Chemother* 1989;33:844–849.
89. Cretton EM, et al. *In vitro* and *in vivo* disposition and metabolism of 3′-deoxy-2′,3′-didehydrothymidine. *Antimicrob Agents Chemother* 1993;37:1816–1825.
90. Petersen EA, et al. Dose-related activity of stavudine in patients infected with human immunodeficiency virus. *J Infect Dis* 1995;171(suppl 2):131–139.
91. Spruance SL, et al. Clinical efficacy of monotherapy with stavudine compared with zidovudine in HIV-infected, zidovudine-experienced patients. A randomized, double-blind, controlled trial. Bristol-Myers Squibb Stavudine/019 Study Group. *Ann Intern Med* 1997;126:355–363.
92. Coates JA, et al. (−)-2′-deoxy-3′-thiacytidine is a potent, highly selective inhibitor of human immunodeficiency virus type 1 and type 2 replication *in vitro. Antimicrob Agents Chemother* 1992;36:733–739.
93. Johnson MA, et al. Clinical pharmacokinetics of lamivudine. *Clin Pharmacokinet* 1999;36:41–66.
94. van Leeuwen R, et al. Evaluation of safety and efficacy of 3TC (lamivudine) in patients with asymptomatic or mildly symptomatic human immunodeficiency virus infection: a phase I/II study. *J Infect Dis* 1995;171:1166–1171.
95. Pluda JM, et al. A phase I/II study of 2′-deoxy-3′-thiacytidine (lamivudine) in patients with advanced human immunodeficiency virus infection. *J Infect Dis* 1995;171:1438–1447.
96. Eron JJ, et al. Treatment with lamivudine, zidovudine, or both in HIV-positive patients with 200 to 500 CD4$^+$ cells per cubic millimeter. North American HIV Working Party. *N Engl J Med* 1995;333:1662–1669.
97. Staszewski S, et al. A dose-ranging study to evaluate the safety and efficacy of abacavir alone or in combination with zidovudine and lamivudine in antiretroviral treatment-naive subjects. *AIDS* 1998;12:197–202.
98. Tseng A, et al. Precipitous declines in hemoglobin levels associated with combination zidovudine and lamivudine therapy. *Clin Infect Dis* 1998;27:908–909.
99. Watson WJ, Stevens TP, Weinberg GA. Profound anemia in a newborn infant of a mother receiving antiretroviral therapy. *Pediatr Infect Dis J* 1998;17:435–436.
100. Foster RH, Faulds D. Abacavir. *Drugs* 1998;55:729–736; discussion 737–738.
101. Kumar PN, et al. Safety and pharmacokinetics of abacavir (1592U89) following oral administration of escalating single doses in human immunodeficiency virus type 1-infected adults. *Antimicrob Agents Chemother* 1999;43:603–608.
102. Rajitch J, Jarret J, White HR, et al. Central nervous system penetration of the antiretroviral abacavir (1592) in human and animal models [Abstract 636]. Presented at the 5th Conference on Retroviruses and Opportunistic Infections, Chicago, IL, 1998.
103. McDowell JA, et al. Multiple-dose pharmacokinetics and pharmacodynamics of abacavir alone and in combination with zidovudine in human immunodeficiency virus–infected adults. *Antimicrob Agents Chemother* 2000;44:2061–2067.
104. Bawdon RE. The *ex vivo* human placental transfer of the anti-HIV nucleoside inhibitor

abacavir and the protease inhibitor amprenavir. *Infect Dis Obstet Gynecol* 1998;6:244–246.

105. McDowell JA, et al. Pharmacokinetics of [$^{14}$C] abacavir, a human immunodeficiency virus type 1 (HIV-1) reverse transcriptase inhibitor, administered in a single oral dose to HIV-1–infected adults; a mass balance study. Antimicrob Agents Chemother 1999;43:2855–2861.
106. Saag MS, et al. Antiretroviral effect and safety of abacavir alone and in combination with zidovudine in HIV-infected adults. Abacavir Phase 2 Clinical Team. *AIDS* 1998;12:203–209.
107. Kakuda TN. Pharmacology of nucleoside and nucleotide reverse transcriptase inhibitor-induced mitochondrial toxicity. *Clin Ther* 2000;22:685–708.
108. Glaxo-Wellcome. Letter to clinicians regarding abacavir hypersensitivity syndrome, 1997.
109. Keisel P, Andrews C, Yazdani B, et al. Comparison of symptoms of influenza A infection with abacavir-associated hypersensitivity reaction [Abstract 622]. Presented at the 8th Conference on Retroviruses and Opportunistic Infections, Chicago, IL, 2001.
110. Hetherington S, Steel H, Kafon S, et al. Safety and tolerance of abacavir (1592, ABC) alone and in combination therapy for HIV-1 infection [Abstract 12353]. Presented at the 12th World AIDS Conference, Geneva, Switzerland, 1998.
111. Hewitt RG. Abacavir hypersensitivity reaction. *Clin Infect Dis* 2002;34:1137–1142.
112. Mallal S, et al. Association between presence of HLA-B*5701, HLA-DR7, and HLA-DQ3 and hypersensitivity to HIV-1 reverse transcriptase inhibitor abacavir. *Lancet* 2002;359:722–773.
113. de Clercq E. Antiviral therapy for human immunodeficiency virus infections. *Clin Microbiol Rev* 1995;8:200–239.
114. Spence RA, et al. Mechanism of inhibition of HIV-1 reverse transcriptase by nonnucleoside inhibitors. *Science* 1995;267:988–993.
115. Barreiro P, et al. Prevention of nevirapine-associated exanthema using slow dose escalation and/or corticosteroids. *AIDS* 2000;14:2153–2157.
116. Cheeseman SH, Hattox SE, McLaughlin MM, et al. Pharmacokinetics of nevirapine: initial single-rising-dose study in humans. *Antimicrob Agents Chemother* 1993;37:178–182.
117. Mirochnick M. Antiretroviral pharmacology in pregnant women and their newborns. *Ann NY Acad Sci* 2000;918:287–297.
118. Musoke P, et al. A phase I/II study of the safety and pharmacokinetics of nevirapine in HIV-1-infected pregnant Ugandan women and their neonates (HIVNET 006). *AIDS* 1999;13:479–486.
119. Beach JW. Chemotherapeutic agents for human immunodeficiency virus infection: mechanism of action, pharmacokinetics, metabolism, and adverse reactions. *Clin Ther* 1998;20:2–25; discussion 1.
120. Taylor S, et al. Concentrations of nevirapine, lamivudine and stavudine in semen of HIV-1–infected men. *AIDS* 2000;14:1979–1984.
121. Clarke SM, et al. Pharmacokinetic interactions of nevirapine and methadone and guidelines for use of nevirapine to treat injection drug users. *Clin Infect Dis* 2001;33:1595–1597.
122. Carr A, et al. A controlled trial of nevirapine plus zidovudine versus zidovudine alone in p24 antigenaemic HIV-infected patients. The Dutch-Italian-Australian Nevirapine Study Group. *AIDS* 1996;10:635–641.
123. d'Aquila RT, et al. Nevirapine, zidovudine, and didanosine compared with zidovudine and didanosine in patients with HIV-1 infection. A randomized, double-blind, placebo-controlled trial. National Institute of Allergy and Infectious Diseases AIDS Clinical Trials Group Protocol 241 Investigators. *Ann Intern Med* 1996;124:1019–1030.
124. Montaner JS, et al. A randomized, double-blind trial comparing combinations of nevirapine, didanosine, and zidovudine for HIV-infected patients: the INCAS Trial. Italy, The Netherlands, Canada and Australia Study. *JAMA* 1998;279:930–937.
125. Prakash M, et al. Jaundice and hepatocellular damage associated with nevirapine therapy. *Am J Gastroenterol* 2001;96:1571–1574.
126. Viramune (Mevirapine) Product Monograph (package insert), Roxanne Laboratories. 1998.

127. Warren KJ, et al. Nevirapine-associated Stevens-Johnson syndrome. *Lancet* 1998; 351:567.
128. Podzamczer D, et al. Efavirenz associated with corticosteroids in patients with previous severe hypersensitivity reaction due to nevirapine. *AIDS* 2000;14:331–332.
129. Soriano V, et al. Is there cross-toxicity between nevirapine and efavirenz in subjects developing rash? *AIDS* 2000;14:1672–1673.
130. Cheeseman SH, Havlir D, McLaughlin MM, et al. Phase I/II evaluation of nevirapine alone and in combination with zidovudine for infection with human immunodeficiency virus. *J AIDS Hum Retrovirol* 1995;8:141–151.
131. Havlir D, et al. High-dose nevirapine: safety, pharmacokinetics, and antiviral effect in patients with human immunodeficiency virus infection. *J Infect Dis* 1995;171:537--545.
132. Cattelan AM, et al. Severe hepatic failure related to nevirapine treatment. *Clin Infect Dis* 1999;29:455–456.
133. Boxwell D, Haverkos H, Kukich S, et al. Serious adverse events attributed to nevirapine regimens for postexposure prophylaxis after HIV exposures worldwide, 1997–2000. *MMWR* 2001;49:1153–1156.
134. Centers for Disease Control and Prevention. Updated U.S. Public Health Service guidelines for the management of occupational exposures to HBC, HCV, and HIV and recommendations for post-exposure prophylaxis. *MMWR* 2001;50:51.
135. Adkins JC, Noble S. Efavirenz. *Drugs* 1998;56:1055–1064; discussion 1065–1066.
136. Molina JM, et al. Once-daily combination therapy with emtricitabine, didanosine, and efavirenz in human immunodeficiency virus–infected patients. *J Infect Dis* 2000;182:599–602.
137. Tashima KT, et al. Cerebrospinal fluid human immunodeficiency virus type 1 (HIV-1) suppression and efavirenz drug concentrations in HIV-1–infected patients receiving combination therapy. *J Infect Dis* 1999;180:862–864.
138. Morales-Ramirez J, Tashima K, Hardy D, et al. A phase II multicenter randomized, open-label study to compare the antiretroviral activity and tolerability of efavirenz (EFV) + indinavir (IDV), versus EFV + zidovudine (ZDV) + lamivudine (3TC), versus IDV + 3TC + ZDV at >36 weeks [DMP266-006] [Abstract 394]. Presented at the 38th Interscience Conference on Antimicrobial Agents and Chemotherapy, San Diego, CA, 1993.
139. Lang JP, et al. [Apropos of atypical melancholia with Sustiva (efavirenz)]. *Encephale* 2001;27;290:293.
140. Moyle G. The emerging roles of non-nucleoside reverse transcriptase inhibitors in antiretroviral therapy. *Drugs* 2001;61:19–26.
141. Tran JQ, Gerber JG, Kerr BM. Delavirdine: clinical pharmacokinetics and drug interactions. *Clin Pharmacokinet* 2001;40:207–226.
142. Scott LJ, Perry CM. Delavirdine: a review of its use in HIV infection. *Drugs* 2000;60:1411–1444.
143. Davey RT, Bhat N, Yoder C, et al. HIV-1 and T cell dynamics after interruption of highly active antiretroviral therapy (HAART) in patients with a history of sustained viral suppression. Proc Natl Acad Sci USA 1999;96:15109–15114.
144. Para MF, Meehan P, Holden-Wiltse J, et al. ACTG 260: a randomized, phase I-II, dose-ranging trial of the anti-human immunodeficiency virus activity of delavirdine monotherapy. The AIDS Clinical Trials Group Protocol 260 Team. *Antimicrob Agents Chemother* 1999;43:1373–1378.
145. Squires KE. An introduction to nucleoside and nucleotide analogues. *Antiviral Ther* 2001;6(suppl 3):1–14.
146. Barditch-Crovo P, et al. Phase I/II trial of the pharmacokinetics, safety, and antiretroviral activity of tenofovir disoproxil fumarate in human immunodeficiency virus–infected adults. *Antimicrob Agents Chemother* 2001;45:2733–2739.
147. Srinivas RV, Fridland A. Antiviral activities of 9-R-2-phosphonomethoxypropyl adenine (PMPA) and bis(isopropyloxymethylcarbonyl)PMPA against various drug-resistant human immunodeficiency virus strains. *Antimicrob Agents Chemother* 1998;42:1484–1487.
148. Bristol Myers Squibb. Bristol Myers letter to health professionals, May 7, 2002.
149. Gilead S. Viread product information.

150. Schooley R, Myers R, Ruane P, et al. Tenofovir disoproxil fumarate (TDF) for the treatment of antiretroviral experienced patients. A double-blind placebo-controlled study [Abstract 692]. Presented at the 40th Interscience Conference on Antimicrobial Agents and Chemotherapy, Toronto, Ontario, Canada, September 17–20, 2000.
151. Paterson DL, et al. Adherence to protease inhibitor therapy and outcomes in patients with HIV infection. *Ann Intern Med* 2000;133:21–30.
152. Noor MA, et al. Metabolic effects of indinavir in healthy HIV-seronegative men. *AIDS* 2001;15:11–18.
153. Winslow DL, Otto MJ. HIV protease inhibitors. *AIDS* 1995;9(suppl A):183–192.
154. Flexner C. HIV-protease inhibitors. *N Engl J Med* 1998;338:1281–1292.
155. Montaner J, Saag M, Schwarts R. Pharmacokinetic and safety evaluations of a once daily regimen of saquinavir soft gel capsule (SQV) in HIV infected antiretroviral naive patients. Presented at Frontiers in Drug Development for Antiretroviral Therapy (DART), Puerto Rico, 2000.
156. Figgitt DP, Plosker GL. Saquinavir soft-gel capsule: an updated review of its use in the management of HIV infection. *Drugs* 2000;60:481–516.
157. Perry CM, Noble S. Saquinavir soft-gel capsule formulation. A review of its use in patients with HIV infection. *Drugs* 1998;55:461–486.
158. Kravcik S, et al. Cerebrospinal fluid HIV RNA and drug levels with combination ritonavir and saquinavir. *J AIDS* 1999;21:371–375.
159. Gisolf EH, et al. Cerebrospinal fluid HIV-1 RNA during treatment with ritonavir/saquinavir or ritonavir/saquinavir/stavudine. *AIDS* 2000;14:1583–1589.
160. Kashuba AD, et al. Antiretroviral-drug concentrations in semen: implications for sexual transmission of human immunodeficiency virus type 1. *Antimicrob Agents Chemother* 1999;43:1817–1826.
161. Forestier F, et al. Maternal-fetal transfer of saquinavir studied in the *ex vivo* placental perfusion model. *Am J Obstet Gynecol* 2001;185:178–181.
162. Fortovase™ (Saquinavir) soft gelatin capsules prescribing information, 2000.
163. Lea AP, Faulds D. Ritonavir. *Drugs* 1996;52:541–546; discussion 547–548.
164. Casey BM, Bawdon RE. Placental transfer of ritonavir with zidovudine in the *ex vivo* placental perfusion model. *Am J Obstet Gynecol* 1998;179(part 1):758–761.
165. Gatti G, et al. The relationship between ritonavir plasma levels and side-effects: implications for therapeutic drug monitoring. *AIDS* 1999;13:2083–2089.
166. Norvir (ritonavir) capsules and oral solution prescribing information, 1996.
167. Markowitz M, et al. A preliminary study of ritonavir, an inhibitor of HIV-1 protease, to treat HIV-1 infection. *N Engl J Med* 1995;333:1534–1539.
168. Danner SA, et al. A short-term study of the safety, pharmacokinetics, and efficacy of ritonavir, an inhibitor of HIV-1 protease. European-Australian Collaborative Ritonavir Study Group. *N Engl J Med* 1995;333:1528–1533.
169. Sulkowski MS., et al. Hepatotoxicity associated with antiretroviral therapy in adults infected with human immunodeficiency virus and the role of hepatitis C or B virus infection. *JAMA* 2000;283:74–80.
170. Piscitelli SC, Gallicano KD. Interactions among drugs for HIV and opportunistic infections. *N Engl J Med* 2001;344:984–996.
171. Barry M, et al. Protease inhibitors in patients with HIV disease. Clinically important pharmacokinetic considerations. *Clin Pharmacokinet* 1997;32:194–209.
172. Letendre SL, et al. Indinavir population pharmacokinetics in plasma and cerebrospinal fluid. The HIV Neurobehavioral Research Center Group. Antimicrob Agents Chemother 2000;44:2173–2175.
173. van Praag RM, et al. Enhanced penetration of indinavir in cerebrospinal fluid and semen after the addition of low-dose ritonavir. *AIDS* 2000;14:1187–1194.
174. Jayasekara D, et al. Antiviral therapy for HIV patients with renal insufficiency. *J AIDS* 1999;21:384–395.
175. Guardiola JM, et al. Indinavir pharmacokinetics in haemodialysis-dependent end-stage renal failure. *AIDS* 1998;12:1395.
176. Kopp JB, et al. Crystalluria and urinary tract abnormalities associated with indinavir. *Ann Intern Med* 1997;127:119–125.
177. Moyle G, Gazzard B. Current knowledge and future prospects for the use of HIV protease inhibitors. *Drugs* 1996;51:701–712.

178. Perazella MA, Kashgarian M, Cooney E. Indinavir nephropathy in an AIDS patient with renal insufficiency and pyuria. *Clin Nephrol* 1998;50:194–196.
179. Max B, Sherer R. Management of the adverse effects of antiretroviral therapy and medication adherence. *Clin Infect Dis* 2000;30(suppl 2):96–116.
180. Gulick RM, et al. Treatment with indinavir, zidovudine, and lamivudine in adults with human immunodeficiency virus infection and prior antiretroviral therapy. *N Engl J Med* 1997;337:734–739.
181. Hammer SM, et al. A controlled trial of two nucleoside analogues plus indinavir in persons with human immunodeficiency virus infection and CD4 cell counts of 200 per cubic millimeter or less. AIDS Clinical Trials Group 320 Study Team. *N Engl J Med* 1997;337:725–733.
182. Bouscarat F, Prevot MH, Matheron S. Alopecia associated with indinavir therapy. *N Engl J Med* 1999;341:618.
183. Bardsley-Elliot A, Plosker GL. Nelfinavir: an update on its use in HIV infection. *Drugs* 2000;59:581–620.
184. Zhang KE, et al. Circulating metabolites of the human immunodeficiency virus protease inhibitor nelfinavir in humans: structural identification, levels in plasma, and antiviral activities. *Antimicrob Agents Chemother* 2001;45:1086–1093.
185. Quart B, Chapman SK, Peterkin J, et al. Phase I safety, tolerance, pharmacokinetics, and food effect studies of AG1343: a novel HIV protease inhibitor. Presented at the 2nd National Conference on Human Retroviruses, Washington, D.C., January 29–February 2, 1995.
186. Aweeka F, et al. Failure to detect nelfinavir in the cerebrospinal fluid of HIV-1–infected patients with and without AIDS dementia complex. *J AIDS* 1999;20:39–43.
187. Tebas P, Powderly WG. Nelfinavir mesylate. *Expert Opin Pharmacother* 2000;1:1429–1440.
188. Sherman DS, Fish DN. Management of protease inhibitor–associated diarrhea. *Clin Infect Dis* 2000;30:908–914.
189. Markowitz M, et al. A preliminary evaluation of nelfinavir mesylate, an inhibitor of human immunodeficiency virus (HIV)-1 protease, to treat HIV infection. *J Infect Dis* 1998;177:1533–1540.
190. Noble S, Goa KL. Amprenavir: a review of its clinical potential in patients with HIV infection. *Drugs* 2000;60:1383–1410.
191. Veronese L, Rautureau J, Sadler BM, et al. A study to compare the pharmacokinetics of a single, oral, 100 mg dose of amprenavir in healthy volunteers and patients with cirrhosis. Presented at the 39th Interscience Conference on Antimicrobial Agents and Chemotherapy, San Francisco, CA, September 26–29, 1999.
192. Amprenavir (agenerase) capsules [package insert], 1999.
193. Hurst M, Faulds D. Lopinavir. *Drugs* 2000;60:1371–1379; discussion 1380–1381.
194. Sham HL, et al. ABT-378, a highly potent inhibitor of the human immunodeficiency virus protease. *Antimicrob Agents Chemother* 1998;42:3218–3224.
195. Kumar GN, et al. *In vitro* metabolism of the HIV-1 protease inhibitor ABT-378: species comparison and metabolite identification. *Drug Metab Disposition* 1999;27:86–91.
196. Izzedine H, et al. Pharmacokinetic of nevirapine in haemodialysis. *Nephrol Dial Transplant* 2001;16:192–193.
197. Murphy RL, et al. ABT-378/ritonavir plus stavudine and lamivudine for the treatment of antiretroviral-naive adults with HIV-1 infection: 48-week results. *AIDS* 2001;15:1–9.
198. Dube MP, et al. Protease inhibitor–associated hyperglycaemia. *Lancet* 1997;350:713–714.
199. Mulligan K, et al. Hyperlipidemia and insulin resistance are induced by protease inhibitors independent of changes in body composition in patients with HIV infection. *J AIDS* 2000;23:35–43.
200. Mariuz P, Woerle HF, Meyer C, et al. Protease inhibitors cause insulin resistance and impair beta cell function: a model to study the pathogenesis of type 2 diabetes [Abstract 783]. Presented at the 37th Meeting of the European Association for the Study of Diabetes, Glasgow, UK, 2001.
201. Hruz PW, Murata H, Mueckler M. Adverse metabolic consequences of HIV protease

inhibitor therapy: the search for a central mechanism. *Am J Physiol Endocrinol Metab* 2001;280:549–553.

202. Botella JI, et al. Complete resolution of protease inhibitor induced diabetes mellitus. *Clin Endocrinal (Oxf)* 2000;52:241–243.
203. Domingo P, et al. Switching to nevirapine decreases insulin levels but does not improve subcutaneous adipocyte apoptosis in patients with highly active antiretroviral therapy–associated lipodystrophy. *J Infect Dis* 2001;184:1197–1201.
204. Grunfeld C, et al. Lipids, lipoproteins, triglyceride clearance, and cytokines in human immunodeficiency virus infection and the acquired immunodeficiency syndrome. *J Clin Endocrinol Metab* 1992;74:1045–1052.
205. Martinez E, et al. Impact of switching from human immunodeficiency virus type 1 protease inhibitors to efavirenz in successfully treated adults with lipodystrophy. *Clin Infect Dis* 2000;31:1266–1273.
206. Graham NM. Metabolic disorders among HIV-infected patients treated with protease inhibitors: a review. *J AIDS* 2000;25(suppl 1):4–11.
207. John M, Nolan D, Mallal S. Antiretroviral therapy and the lipodystrophy syndrome. *AIDS* 2001;6:9–20.
208. Chene G, et al. Role of long-term nucleoside-analogue therapy in lipodystrophy and metabolic disorders in human immunodeficiency virus–infected patients. *Clin Infect Dis* 2002;34:649–657.
209. Hadigan C, et al. Metabolic abnormalities and cardiovascular disease risk factors in adults with human immunodeficiency virus infection and lipodystrophy. *Clin Infect Dis* 2001;32:130–139.
210. Stein JH, et al. Use of human immunodeficiency virus-1 protease inhibitors is associated with atherogenic lipoprotein changes and endothelial dysfunction. *Circulation* 2001;104:257–262.
211. Nolan D, John M, Mallal S. Antiretroviral therapy and the lipodystrophy syndrome, part 2: concepts in aetiopathogenesis. *Antiviral Ther* 2001;6:145–160.
212. Wanke CA, et al. Clinical evaluation and management of metabolic and morphologic abnormalities associated with human immunodeficiency virus. *Clin Infect Dis* 2002;34:248–259.
213. Kingsley L, Smit E, Riddler S, et al. Prevalence of lipodystrophy and metabolic abnormalities in the multicenter AIDS cohort study (MICS) [Abstract 538]. Presented at the 8th Conference on Retroviruses and Opportunistic Infections, Chicago, IL, 2001.
214. Wild J. Protease inhibitor therapy and bleeding. *Haemophilia* 2000;6:487–490.
215. Hollmig KA, Beck SB, Doll DC. Severe bleeding complications in HIV-positive haemophiliac patients treated with protease inhibitors. *Eur J Med Res* 2001;6:112–114.
216. Kernly J, Chaisson RE, Moore RD. Increasing incidence of avascular necrosis of the hip in HIV-infected patients [Abstract 637]. Presented at the 8th Conference on Retroviruses and Opportunistic Infections, Chicago, IL, 2001.
217. Masur H. Metabolic complications in HIV disease: lactemia and bone disease. *Top HIV Med* 2001;9:1–8.
218. de Clercq E. New developments in anti-HIV chemotherapy. *Curr Med Chem* 2001; 8:1543–1572.
219. Wood R, Arestetr K, Pollard R, et al. GW433908, a novel prodrug of the HIV protease inhibitor (PI) amprenavir (APV): safety, efficacy, and pharmacokinetics (PK) (APV20001) [Abstract 333]. Presented at the 8th Conference on Retroviruses and Opportunistic Infections, Chicago, IL, 2001.
220. Van der Horst C, Sanne I, Wakeford C, et al. Two randomize, controlled, equivalence trials of emtricitabine (FTC) to lamivudine (3TC) [Abstract 18]. Presented at the 8th Conference on Retroviruses and Opportunistic Infections, Chicago, IL, 2001.
221. Dunkle L, Oshana SC, Cheng Y-C, et al. ACH-126,443: a new nucleoside analog with potent activity against wild-type and resistant HIV-1 and a promising pharmacokinetic and mitochondrial safety profile [Abstract 303]. Presented at the 8th Conference on Retroviruses and Opportunistic Infections, Chicago, IL, 2001.
222. De Bethune M, Andries K, Ludovici D, et al. TMC120(r147681), a next-generation NNRTI, has potent *in vitro* activity against NNRTI-resistant HIV variants [Abstract

304]. Presented at the 8th Conference on Retroviruses and Opportunistic Infections, Chicago, IL, 2001.
223. Gruzdev B, Horban A, Boron-Kaezmarska A, et al. TMC120 a new non-nucleoside reverse transcriptase inhibitor, is a potent antiretroviral in treatment naive HIV-1 infected subjects [Abstract 13]. Presented at the 8th Conference on Retroviruses and Opportunistic Infections, Chicago, IL, 2001.
224. Larder BA, et al. Tipranavir inhibits broadly protease inhibitor–resistant HIV-1 clinical samples. *AIDS* 2000;14:1943–1948.
225. Eron J, Murphy RL. New agents for anti-HIV therapy. HIV-AIDS Annual Update 2001. Incorporated in proceeding of the 11th annual Clinical Care Options for HIV symposium article 1418646 http://www.medscape.com.
226. Gong YF, et al. *In vitro* resistance profile of the human immunodeficiency virus type 1 protease inhibitor BMS-232632. *Antimicrob Agents Chemother* 2000;44:2319–2326.
227. O'Mara E, Mummaneni V, Randall D, et al. BMS-232632: a summary of multiple dose pharmacokinetic, food effect and drug interaction studies in healthy subjects [Abstract 504]. Presented at the 7th Conference on Retroviruses and Opportunistic Infections, San Francisco, CA, 2000.
228. Lalezari J, Eron J, Carlson M, et al. Safety, pharmacokinetics, and antiviral activity of T-20 as a single agent in heavily pre-treated patients [Abstract LB13]. Presented at the 6th Conference on Retroviruses and Opportunistic Infections, Chicago, IL, 1999.
229. Lalezari J, Drucker J, Demasi R, et al. A controlled phase II trial assessing three doses of T-20 in combination with abacavir, amprenavir, low dose ritonavir and efavirenz in non-nucleoside naive protease inhibitor experienced HIV-1 infected adults [Abstract LB5]. Presented at the 8th Conference on Retroviruses and Opportunistic Infections, Chicago, IL, 2001.
230. Lambert D, Zhou J, Medinas R, et al. T1249 a second generation hybrid synthetic peptide inhibitor of i.v.: isolates from T20-treated patients are sensitive to T1249. *Antiviral Ther* 1999;4(Suppl 1); 8 abst 10.
231. Durier C, Emilie D, Estaquier J, et al. Effect of subcutaneous IL-2 combined with HAART on immunological restoration in HIV-infected patients [Abstract 345]. Presented at the 8th Conference on Retroviruses and Opportunistic Infections, Chicago, IL, 2001.
232. Hardy G, Imamil N, Sullivan A, et al. Immunomodulation of chronic HIV-1 infection: impact of HAART, interleukin-2 and/or an inactivated gp120-depleted HIV-1 immunogen (REMUNE) [Abstract 349]. Presented at the 8th Conference on Retroviruses and Opportunistic Infections, Chicago, IL, 2001.
233. Coull J, Betts M, Turner D, et al. A pilot study of the use of mycophenolate mofetil (MMF) as a component of therapy for multidrug resistant HIV-1. *J AIDS* 2001;26:423–434.
234. Mofenson LM, et al. Risk factors for perinatal transmission of human immunodeficiency virus type 1 in women treated with zidovudine. Pediatric AIDS Clinical Trials Group Study 185 Team. *N Engl J Med* 1999;341:385–393.
235. Weinberg GA. Pediatric human immunodeficiency virus (HIV) infection. In: Mandell G, Bennett JE, Dolin R, eds. *Principles and practice of infectious diseases,* 5th ed. Philadelphia: WB Saunders, 2000:1467–1479.
236. Bryson YJ. Perinatal HIV-1 transmission: recent advances and therapeutic interventions. *AIDS* 1996;10(suppl 3):33–42.
237. Mofenson LM. Mother-child HIV-1 transmission: timing and determinants. *Obstet Gynecol Clin North Am* 1997;24:759–784.
238. Ioannidis J, Abrams EJ, Ammann A, et al. Perinatal transmission of human immunodeficiency virus type 1 by pregnant women with RNA virus loads <1000 copies/mL. *J Infect Dis* 2001;183:539–545.
239. Landesman SH, et al. Obstetrical factors and the transmission of human immunodeficiency virus type 1 from mother to child. The Women and Infants Transmission Study. *N Engl J Med* 1996;334:1617–1623.
240. Zorrilla CD. Obstetric factors and mother-to-infant transmission of HIV-1. *Infect Dis Clin North Am* 1997;11:109–118.
241. U.S. Public Health Service. Public Health Service Task Force recommendations for the use of antiretroviral drugs in pregnant HIV-1 infected women for maternal health and

interventions to reduce perinatal HIV-1 transmission in the United Stated. Updated February 4, 2002 (updates available at HIV/AIDS Treatment Information Service website *www.hivatis.org.*)

242. U.S. Public Health Service. Safety and toxicity of individual antiretroviral agents in pregnancy—updated May 23, 2002 (updates available at *www.hivatis.org.*)

242a. Tuomala RE, Shapiro DE, Mofenson LM, et al. Antiretroviral therapy during pregnancy and the risk of an adverse outcome. *N Engl J Med* 2002;346:1863–1870.

243. Connor EM, et al. Reduction of maternal-infant transmission of human immunodeficiency virus type 1 with zidovudine treatment. Pediatric AIDS Clinical Trials Group Protocol 076 Study Group. *N Engl J Med* 1994;331:1173–1180.

244. Cooper E, Nugent RP, Diaz C, et al. After AIDS clinical trial 076: the changing pattern of zidovudine use during pregnancy, and the subsequent reduction in the vertical transmission of human immunodeficiency virus in a cohort of infected women and their infants. Women and Infants Transmission Study Group. *J Infect Dis* 1996;174:1207–1211.

245. Centers of Disease Control and Prevention. Recommendations of the US Public Health Service Task Force on the use of zidovudine to reduce perinatal transmission of human immunodeficiency virus. *MMWR* 1994;43:1–20.

246. Centers for Disease Control and Prevention. US Public Health Service recommendations for human immunodeficiency virus counseling and voluntary testing for pregnant women. *MMWR* 1995;44:1–14.

247. Wade NA, et al. Abbreviated regimens of zidovudine prophylaxis and perinatal transmission of the human immunodeficiency virus. *N Engl J Med* 1998;339:1409–1414.

248. Khalsa AM, Currier J. Women and HIV. A review of current epidemiology, gynecologic manifestations, and perinatal transmission. *Primary Care Clin Office Pract* 1997;24:617–641.

249. Sperling RS, et al. Maternal viral load, zidovudine treatment, and the risk of transmission of human immunodeficiency virus type 1 from mother to infant. Pediatric AIDS Clinical Trials Group Protocol 076 Study Group. *N Engl J Med* 1996;335:1621–1629.

250. Aleixo LF, Goodenow MM, Sleasman JW. Zidovudine administered to women infected with human immunodeficiency virus type 1 and to their neonates reduces pediatric infection independent of an effect on levels of maternal virus. *J Pediatr* 1997;130:906–914.

251. International Perinatal HIV Group. The mode of delivery and the risk of vertical transmission of human immunodeficiency virus type 1. A meta-analysis of 15 prospective cohort studies. *N Engl J Med* 1999;340:977–987.

252. Wang Y, et al. Pharmacokinetics of didanosine in antepartum and postpartum human immunodeficiency virus–infected pregnant women and their neonates: an AIDS clinical trials group study. *J Infect Dis* 1999;180:1536–1541.

253. National Institute of Allergy and Infectious Disease/National Institutes of Health. Safety information of DMP-266, 1998.

254. Anderson J. A guide to the clinical care of women with HIV. Rockville, MD: U.S. Dept. of Health and Human Services, 2001.

254a. Watts DH. Management of human immunodeficiency virus infection in pregnancy. *N Engl J Med* 2002;346:1879–1891.

255. Eastman PS, et al. Maternal viral genotypic zidovudine resistance and infrequent failure of zidovudine therapy to prevent perinatal transmission of human immunodeficiency virus type 1 in Pediatric AIDS Clinical Trials Group Protocol 076. *J Infect Dis* 1998;177:557–564.

256. U.S. Public Health Service/Infectious Diseases Society of America (USPHS/IDSA). 2001 Guidelines for the prevention of opportunistic infections in persons infected with human immunodeficiency virus. USPHS/IDSA Prevention of Opportunistic Infections Working Group. Available at *www.cdc./gov/hiv/pubs/guidelines.htm#treatment.*

257. Anonymous. Elective caesarean-section versus vaginal delivery in prevention of vertical transmission: a randomized clinical trial. The European Mode of Delivery Collaboration. *Lancet* 1999;353:1035–1039.

258. Urbani G, de Vries MM, Cronje HS, et al. Complications associated with cesarean section in HIV-infected patients. *Int J Gynaecol Obstet* 2001;74:9–15.

259. American College of Obstetricians and Gynecologists Committee Opinion. Scheduled cesarean delivery and the prevention of vertical transmission of HIV infection. Number 234, May 2000.
260. Weinberg G. The dilemma of postnatal mother-to-child transmission of HIV: to breastfeed or not? *Birth* 2000;27:199–205.
261. Kaplan J, et al. Early initiation of combination therapy (ART): does it affect clinical outcome? [Abstract LbPeB7051]. Presented at the 13th International AIDS Conference, Durban, South Africa, 2001.
262. Opravil M, Ledergerber B, Furrer H, et al. Clinical benefit of early initiation of HAART in patients with asymptomatic HIV and CD4 counts >350 cells/mm$^3$ [Abstract LB-6]. Presented at the 8th Conference on Retrovirus and Opportunistic Infections, Chicago, IL, 2001.
263. Egger M, et al. Prognosis of HIV-1 infected drug naive patients starting potent antiretroviral therapy: multicohort analysis of 12,040 patients. Presented at the 41st ICAAC. Chicago, IL, 2001, abst LB-18:14.
264. Deeks SG. Determinants of virological response to antiretroviral therapy: implications for long-term strategies. *Clin Infect Dis* 2000;30(suppl 2):177–184.
265. Johnson M, Beall G, Badley A, et al. ABT-378/ritonavir (ABT-378/rit) versus nelfinavir in antiretroviral naive subjects: week 48 comparison in a phase III blinded randomized clinical trial [Abstract PL6.5]. *AIDS* 2000;14(suppl 4):7.
266. King M, Bernstein B, Kempf D, et al. Comparison of time to achieve HIV RNA <400 copies/mL and <50 copies/mL in a phase III, blinded randomized clinical trial of ABT 378/r vs. NFV in ARV-naive patients [Abstract 329]. Presented at the 8th Conference on Retrovirus and Opportunistic Infections, Chicago, IL, February 2–4, 2001.
267. Gulick RM, et al. Simultaneous vs sequential initiation of therapy with indinavir, zidovudine, and lamivudine for HIV-1 infection: 100-week follow-up. *JAMA* 1998;280:35–41.
268. Havlir DV, et al. *In vivo* antagonism with zidovudine plus stavudine combination therapy. *J Infect Dis* 2000;182:321–325.
269. Kirk O, Mocroft A, Pradier C, et al. Clinical outcome among HIV-infected patients starting saquinavir hard gel compared to ritonavir or indinavir. *AIDS* 2001;15:999–1008.
270. d'Arminio Monforte ATL, Adorni F, et al. Clinical outcome and predictive factors of failure of highly active antiretroviral therapy in antiretroviral-experienced patients in advanced stages of HIV-1 infection. *AIDS* 1998;12:1631–1637.
271. Katzenstein TL, et al. The Danish Protease Inhibitor Study: a randomized study comparing the virological efficacy of 3 protease inhibitor-containing regimens for the treatment of human immunodeficiency virus type 1 infection. *J Infect Dis* 2000;182:744–750.
272. Kilby JM, et al. Safety and pharmacokinetics of once-daily regimens of soft-gel capsule saquinavir plus minidose ritonavir in human immunodeficiency virus–negative adults. *Antimicrob Agents Chemother* 2000;44:2672–2678.
273. Gulick RM, et al. 3-year suppression of HIV viremia with indinavir, zidovudine, and lamivudine. *Ann Intern Med* 2000;133:35–39.
274. Hirsch M, et al. A randomized, controlled trial of indinavir, zidovudine, and lamivudine in adults with advanced human immunodeficiency virus type 1 infection and prior antiretroviral therapy. *J Infect Dis* 1999;180:659–665.
275. van Heeswijk R, Veldkamp AI, Hoetelmans RM, et al. The steady-state plasma pharmacokinetics of indinavir alone and in combination with a low dose of ritonavir in twice daily dosing regimens in HIV-1 infected individuals. *AIDS* 1999;13:95–99.
276. Burger D, Hugen PW, Aarnoutse RE, et al. A retrospective cohort-based survey of patients using twice-daily indinavir + ritonavir combination: pharmacokinetics, safety and efficacy. *J AIDS* 2001;26:218–224.
277. Voigt E. Presented at the 1st IAS Conference on HIV Pathogenesis and Treatment. Buenos Aires, Argentina, 2001.
278. Sadler B, Piliero PJ, Preston SL, et al. Pharmacokinetics and safety of amprenavir and ritonavir following multiple dose, co-administration to healthy volunteers. *AIDS* 2001;15:1009–1018.

279. Lucas GM, Chaisson R, Moore RL. Comparison of initial combination antiretroviral therapy with a single protease inhibitor, ritonavir and saquinavir, or efavirenz [Abstract 686]. Presented at the 39th Meeting of the Infectious Diseases Society of America, San Francisco, CA.
280. U.S. Department of Health and Human Services. Guidelines for the use of antiretroviral agents in HIV-infected adults and adolescents. Washington, DC: February, 2001.
281. Vibhagool A, et al. Poster 063. Presented at the 1st IAS Conference on HIV Pathogenesis and Treatment. Buenos Aires, Argentina, 2001.
282. Demeter LM, et al. Predictors of virologic and clinical outcomes in HIV-1–infected patients receiving concurrent treatment with indinavir, zidovudine, and lamivudine. AIDS Clinical Trials Group Protocol 320. *Ann Intern Med* 2001;135:954–964.
283. Havlir D, Bassett R, Levitan D, et al. Prevalence and predictive value of intermittent viremia with combination HIV therapy. *JAMA* 2001;286:171–179.
284. Connick E, et al. Immune reconstitution in the first year of potent antiretroviral therapy and its relationship to virologic response. *J Infect Dis* 2000;181:358–363.
285. Viard J, Mocroft A, Chiesi A, et al. Influence of age on CD4 cell recovery in human immunodeficiency virus-infected patients receiving highly active antiretroviral therapy: evidence from the EuroSIDA study. *J Infect Dis* 2001;183:1290–2004.
286. Kaufman G, Block M, Finlayson R, et al. The extent of HIV-1 related immunodeficiency and age predict the longterm CD4 lymphocyte response to antiretroviral therapy. *AIDS* 2002;16:359–367.
287. Brosgart CL, et al. Clinical experience and choice of drug therapy for human immunodeficiency virus disease. *Clin Infect Dis* 1999;28:14–22.
288. Kitahata MM, et al. Physicians' experience with the acquired immunodeficiency syndrome as a factor in patients' survival. *N Engl J Med* 1996;334:701–706.
289. Stone VE, et al. The relation between hospital experience and mortality for patients with AIDS. *JAMA* 1992;268:2655–2661.
290. Devereux HL, et al. Rapid decline in detectability of HIV-1 drug resistance mutations after stopping therapy. *AIDS* 1999;13:123–127.
291. Meynard J, Vray M, et al. Presented at the 1st IAS Conference on HIV pathogenesis and treatment (ANRS 088). Buenos Aires, Argentina, 2001.
292. Burger DM, et al. Low plasma concentrations of indinavir are related to virological treatment failure in HIV-1–infected patients on indinavir-containing triple therapy. *Antiviral Ther* 1998;3:215–220.
293. Durant J, Clevenbergh P, Garraffo R, et al. Importance of protease inhibitor plasma levels in HIV-infected patients treated with genotypic-guided therapy: pharmacological data from the Viradapt Study. *AIDS* 2000;14:1333–1339.
294. Servoss JC, Sherman KE, Robbins G, et al. Hepatotoxicity in the U.S. Adults AIDS Clinical Trial Group. *Gastroenterology* 2001;120(suppl 1):54.
295. Dube MP, Sprecher D, Henry WK, et al. Preliminary guidelines for the evaluation and management of dyslipidemia in adults infected with human immunodeficiency virus and receiving antiretroviral therapy: recommendations of the Adult AIDS Clinical Trial Group cardiovascular disease focus group. *Clin Infect Dis* 2000;31(5):1216–1224.
296. Pantaleo G, Cohen OJ, Schacker T, et al. Evolutionary pattern of human immunodeficiency virus (HIV) replication and distribution in lymph nodes following primary infection: implications for antiviral therapy. *Nature Med* 1998;4:341–345.
297. de Jong MD, et al. Overshoot of HIV-1 viraemia after early discontinuation of antiretroviral treatment. *AIDS* 1997;11:79–84.
298. Haslett PA, et al. Strong human immunodeficiency virus (HIV)-specific $CD4^+$ T cell responses in a cohort of chronically infected patients are associated with interruptions in anti-HIV chemotherapy. *J Infect Dis* 2000;181:1264–1272.
299. Fauci AS. Host factors in the pathogenesis of HIV disease: implications for therapeutic strategies [Abstract S16]. Presented at the 8th Conference on Retroviruses and Opportunistic Infections, Chicago, IL, 2001.

# 20. INFECTIONS IN TRANSPLANTATION

Sally H. Houston and John T. Sinnott

Transplantation patients have dramatically increased in numbers over the past 40 years. In 2000, approximately 45,000 bone marrow transplants were performed worldwide, and in the United States, 4,954 liver, 2,198 cardiac, 13,372 kidney, 956 lung, 48 heart-lung, and 435 pancreas transplants were performed. As of November 2001, there were 78,802 individuals awaiting organs. One-third of patients waiting for a heart or liver die before an organ becomes available.

The immunosuppressive regimens yield continual risk for infection. This chapter and references to other chapters will orient the reader to the fundamental causes of infection.

## BASIC PRINCIPLES

**I. Donor selection** is the responsibility of a trained procurement team. Because cadavers are a major source of tissue for all but bone marrow recipients, infection with human immunodeficiency virus (HIV) must be ruled out [1]. In general, hearts and kidneys are harvested from donors under 50 years of age, and livers are harvested from donors 2 months to 65 years of age [2], with exceptions made on a case-by-case basis. For solid organs, organ size and ABO compatibility but not human lymphocyte antigen (HLA) compatibility are considered. For bone marrow transplantation (BMT), HLA typing is very important [1].

- **A. General contraindications** for organ donation include systemic malignancy or active infections [1]. Covert bacteremia should be excluded by history and blood cultures.
- **B. Infectious disease considerations are paramount in this setting. The donor should be screened for** syphilis, hepatitis B (HBV) and C viruses (HCV), HIV-1, HIV-2, human T-lymphotropic virus type I (HTLV-I), Epstein-Barr virus (EBV), *Toxoplasma gondii,* and cytomegalovirus (CMV) antibody [3]. These tests guide transfusion and prophylactic strategies after transplantation [4].

**II. Recipient selection.** Every indication that the recipient will be compliant is crucial. Findings of the presence of varicella-zoster virus (VZV), HIV-1, and HIV-2, HTLV-I, syphilis, toxoplasma, HBV, HCV, EBV, herpes simplex virus (HSV), and CMV antibody guide management. A purified protein derivative (PPD) test (see Chapter 11) should be performed. Patients from developing countries and those from the rural southern United States should have three stool specimens screened for *Strongyloides* cysts. Carriers should be treated with thiabendazole or ivermectin [5]. Transplantation in HIV-positive recipients has been reviewed [6]. Recommendations are to restrict renal transplantation to those with a $CD_4$ count of greater than 200, and to restrict hepatic grafts to those with a $CD_4$ count of greater than 100 and an undetectable viral load for at least 3 months on a stable antiretroviral regimen.

**Contraindications include** recent hemorrhage, active infection, or malignancy [1]. Pretransplantation bacteremia or pneumonia is associated with a poor outcome.

- **A. Kidney recipients** should have disease in which recurrence in the allograft is unlikely. Contraindications include comorbid disease that limits life expectancy to less than 2 years.
- **B. Heart recipients** usually have irreversible vascular, valvular, or idiopathic cardiomyopathy. Contraindications include irreversible pulmonary hypertension, recent pulmonary infarction, and severe peripheral vascular disease [1].
- **C. Liver recipients** must have end-stage cirrhosis, Budd-Chiari syndrome, or primary hepatocellular carcinoma. Children receive transplants for congenital cirrhosis, primary biliary atresia, and metabolic defects such as $\alpha_1$-antitrypsin deficiency, tyrosinemia, and glycogen storage disease types I and IV. Contraindications include the extrahepatic complications of cholangiocarcinoma or advanced cardiopulmonary disease. Relative contraindications include patient age over 55 years, portal vein thrombosis, hepatitis B e antigen (HBeAg) seropositivity, active alcohol abuse, or prior hepatobiliary or portocaval surgery [7].
- **D. Bone marrow recipients.** See later in this chapter, under Bone Marrow Transplantation.

III. **Immunosuppressive therapy.** The ultimate goal of immunosuppression is, after engraftment, to induce tolerance [1]. Most regimens use a combination of agents. Customarily, a daily maintenance regimen is established. Pulse therapy (corticosteroids or antilymphocyte globulin [ALG]) is used for episodes of rejection. Infection and neoplasia [8] occur as a consequence of immune suppression. In cardiac transplantations, about 30% of infections occur after therapy for rejection [9].

A. **Cyclosporine,** a cyclic polypeptide, inhibits interleukin-2 (IL-2) production, thereby suppressing CD4 proliferation and activation of cytotoxic T cells. Because IL-3 is not inhibited by cyclosporine, the suppressor T-cell population increases, and the ratio of suppressor to cytotoxic cells is increased. Cyclosporine does not lyse effector cells, so it **is more useful for prophylaxis.** Infectious complications are reduced because lower dosages of steroids can be used. Cyclosporine is metabolized in the liver, and its effects are dose dependent [8]. Optimum trough levels vary depending on the type of organ transplanted, time interval since transplantation, and level of rejection.

1. **Side effects** include nephrotoxicity, hepatotoxicity, hypertension, hirsutism, tremor, gingival hyperplasia, and tumorigenesis. Nephrotoxicity may be potentiated by high-dose trimethoprim-sulfamethoxazole (TMP-SMX) aminoglycosides, vancomycin, erythromycin, amphotericin B, acyclovir (ACV), and ganciclovir (GCV) [10]. Although most patients tolerate prolonged therapy, with long-term cyclosporine use, the kidney is subject to renal vasoconstriction and possible hypertension or nephrotoxicity [11].
2. Monitoring levels is important. **Ketoconazole and erythromycin increase cyclosporine levels** and side effects, whereas rifampin, isoniazid (INH), and TMP-SMX lower levels, increasing the risk for rejection [10]. Drugs stimulating cytochrome P450 activity will result in more rapid metabolism and lower levels of cyclosporine. Idiosyncratic interactions such as renal failure after single doses of aminoglycosides, amphotericin B, or fluoroquinolones may occur. St. John's wort decreases cyclosporine levels [12].

B. **Tacrolimus** (Prograf; **previously called FK506**) was approved in 1994 for primary prevention of rejection in patients receiving liver transplants. The drug also has been used as rescue therapy for graft rejection unresponsive to other immunosuppressive drugs. Tacrolimus is a bacteria-derived macrolide unrelated to cyclosporine but with similar activity [13]. It interferes with cytotoxic T-cell proliferation and production of IL-1 and -2, interferon-$\gamma$ (IFN-$\gamma$), and IL-2 receptors. It is approximately 10 times more active than cyclosporine, and reduces the incidence of acute rejection and steroid-resistant rejection. Adverse effects and drug interactions are similar to those seen with cyclosporine, although there is an increased risk for glucose intolerance associated with tacrolimus [14].

C. **Corticosteroids** interfere with production of IL-1 through IL-5, IFN-$\gamma$, and immunoglobulin secretion. Acute inflammatory responses are blunted. They predispose to side effects, especially infection. Leukocytosis occurs, but rarely with a white blood cell count of greater than 20,000/mm$^3$ without an underlying infection. Osteoporosis, aseptic hip necrosis, glucose intolerance, cataracts, and hypercholesterolemia often complicate long-term therapy [8,10]. **Modern immunosuppression involves attempting to use a dose that balances** rejection and side effects.

D. **Azathioprine,** a purine analogue, interrupts DNA synthesis, thereby suppressing T-cell proliferation. It is used in rejection prophylaxis. Dose-related side effects include leukopenia, thrombocytopenia, macrocytic anemia, pancreatitis, hepatotoxicity, tumorigenesis, and infection [10]. Azathioprine does not interact with antibiotics but enhances hematologic toxicity [8]. Used with allopurinol, doses should be reduced.

E. **Mycophenolate mofetil** (MMF; Cellcept was approved in 1995 for oral use and is superior to azathioprine in preventing organ rejection in renal transplants) [15]. Similar to azathioprine, MMF blocks T- and B-cell proliferation by stopping production of guanine nucleotides needed for DNA synthesis. Proliferation of fibroblasts, endothelial cells, arterial smooth muscle cells, and B-cell production of antibodies is diminished. Side effects include leukopenia and gastrointestinal problems.

F. **Sirolimus,** also a macrolide, is 27 times more potent than tacrolimus and is used in combination with calcineurin inhibitors to prevent rejection. It inhibits T- and B-cell proliferation by interfering with cytokine signals after cytokine attachment to the cell receptor [16]. Doses of calcineurin inhibitors and steroids can be reduced when sirolimus is part of the regimen. Drug interactions are similar to those seen with calcineurin inhibitors. Side effects include elevated cholesterol and triglyceride levels, hypertension, thrombocytopenia, anemia, and leukopenia. The effects of hypercholesterolemia and hypertriglyceridemia seem to be offset by reduction of graft vasculopathy [17].

G. **Antilymphocyte globulins, antithymocyte globulins (ATGs), and OKT3 murine monoclonal antibody** are biologic preparations that lyse host immunocytes. They are effective for both prophylaxis and treatment of rejection. Potential side effects include fever, serum sickness, aseptic meningitis, pulmonary edema, and diarrhea, which may be confused with symptoms of infection or rejection. Concurrent administration of corticosteroids, acetaminophen, and diphenhydramine palliates the side effects of fever and rigors [8]. Rabbit ATG is better tolerated than others and is more effective than horse-derived ATG. All reactivate CMV; however, rabbit ATG is less likely to cause disease [18].

H. **Interleukin-2 inhibitors.** Monoclonal antibodies block T-cell receptors for IL-2, thus inhibiting the signal for T-cell proliferation. They decrease rejection and permit withdrawal of steroids. The incidence of infusion side effects or infection is low [19,20].

I. **Radiation therapy** is used routinely for BMT preparation. Total lymphoid irradiation has been used to treat chronic stubborn rejection in heart recipients [21].

IV. **Problems resembling infection in solid organ transplantation**

A. **Although the patient may feel well, with signs of rejection seen only on biopsy, rejection mimics infection.** Fever, myalgias or arthralgias, and leukocytosis occur. **In any febrile episodes, rejection is considered, but after cultures antibiotics should be initiated.**

B. **Medications** can cause fever. Azathioprine or cyclosporine hepatotoxicity should be considered in posttransplantation hepatitis. Usually fever due to OKT3 occurs early in therapy.

V. **Clinical signs of infection on immunosuppressive therapy may be obscure.** The impaired inflammatory response results in a paucity of signs. The insidious onset and possible rapid progression of infection warrant a prompt and thorough evaluation. This includes a complete history and physical examination, with attention to the skin and oropharynx. A complete blood count (CBC), chest radiography, urinalysis, and blood cultures are indicated. Initiation of empiric broad-spectrum antibiotics is reasonable pending the outcome of studies.

VI. **CMV** is the most important cause of transplant-associated infection. Three clinical syndromes occur between 1 and 6 months posttransplantation. **Primary infection,** the most serious, develops in seronegative recipients of grafts or blood products from a CMV-seropositive donor. **Reactivation** of latent virus occurs. **Reinfection** develops because donor or blood product virus is transmitted into the "immune" recipient [22].

A. **Illness** The proportion of a syndrome group that becomes ill is highest in primary infection. In all groups illness presents as fever and malaise. Some, especially with primary disease, progress to pneumonitis, encephalitis, hepatitis, and other organ involvement. **Graft dysfunction may ensue** [23–26].

B. **Laboratory studies usually show a leukopenia and mild increase in liver enzymes.**

C. **Viral studies.** Antigenemia assays or polymerase chain reaction (PCR) of peripheral blood are early indicators of CMV active infection that predicts disease [27–29].

D. **CMV exerts effects in addition to clinical infectious syndromes** [23,30,31].

1. CMV enhances net immunosuppression by causing leukopenia and depressing cell-mediated immunity and alveolar macrophage function. This may result in opportunistic infections with *Pneumocystis, Nocardia,* and *Listeria* species [23,30].

2. CMV mediates allograft injury (and possibly rejection), accelerates atherosclerosis in hearts, and increases the incidence of bronchiolitis obliterans in lung transplants [22,23,28,29].
3. Malignancy may be induced [23].

**VII. Strategy to prevent infection** in solid organ transplantation and BMT

A. **Surgical prophylaxis pretransplantation** [6,32]

1. In renal transplantation, cefazolin with or without aminoglycoside is used. The use of prophylactic **TMP-SMX daily for 6 months after renal transplantation has been shown to reduce urinary tract infections** (UTIs) in patients free of anatomic abnormalities [33,34].
2. Heart transplantation. Cefuroxime or cefepime may be given for 24 to 48 hours.
3. Liver transplantation. Selective bowel decontamination for gram-negative organisms and fungi must be undertaken at least 7 days pretransplantation [34], and concurrent fungal prophylaxis with clotrimazole or nystatin should be administered. Cefepime and/or piperacillin/tazobactam is started pretransplantation and continued for 5 days postoperatively. Fluconazole is used in patients with prolonged intubation or operative time, in those undergoing surgical reexploration, in those who require multiple blood products, and in those on perioperative antibiotics or dialysis [35].
4. Lung and heart-lung recipients should receive prophylaxis with activity against *Pseudomonas aeruginosa*. Regimens are then adjusted based on results of donor sputum/endotracheal cultures and recipient sputum/lavage cultures [32,34,36].
5. BMT patients often receive oral ciprofloxacin at the onset of neutropenia and oral acyclovir 400 to 600 mg/day for 6 months for HSV prophylaxis [37,38]. Decreased levels of immunoglobulin reported posttransplantation have been associated with a greater incidence of infections. Data to recommend administration of intravenous immunoglobulin (IVIG) posttransplantation is lacking [39].

B. **CMV prevention.** Oral GCV or valacyclovir given for 90 days after kidney transplantation prevents CMV disease [40,41]. CMV-negative recipients of CMV-negative grafts must receive CMV-negative blood products or, if not available, leukocyte poor blood products (equivalent to CMV-negative products) [42]. Cases of serious and refractory hypotension during transfusion of blood products through in-line filters have been reported [43]. **Cytomegalovirus immunoglobulin (CMVIG)** has high titers of antibody against CMV and is more effective than IVIG for prevention of CMV disease in renal [44], liver [45], and lung grafts that are CMV mismatches [46]. CMVIG has the additional benefit of decreasing the risk for other opportunistic infections [45].

C. **Opportunistic infection prophylaxis**

1. **Isoniazid** is used in patients with positive PPD test results, but side effects may outweigh benefits. It is indicated for patients with a history of active tuberculosis (TB), a positive PPD test result and nonwhite background, malnourishment, an abnormal chest radiograph, or with other immune-compromising conditions (i.e., diabetes mellitus, achlorhydria) [33].
2. **TMP/SMX** protects against *Pneumocystis, Listeria,* and *Nocardia* infections [33,47]. **Other infection prevention measures pretransplantation** also should be considered.
3. **Dental and other procedures [47].** Heart transplant recipients should receive prophylaxis when undergoing dental, gastrointestinal, or genital urinary procedures [37]. Liver transplant patients should receive antibiotic prophylaxis prior to liver biopsy or cholangiography. See Chapter 27B.
4. **Infection control.** Health care workers must adhere to strict hand washing practices. Recipients must not be exposed to other patients or to visitors with upper respiratory infection, chicken pox, or tuberculosis.
5. **Hot water decontamination** and filtering air may be necessary if *Legionella* or *Aspergillus* outbreaks occur.
6. **Environmental pathogens.** Avoid contact with zoonotic vectors such as birds (chlamydia), cats (toxoplasmosis), and fresh flowers. For the first six months posttransplantation, the patient should wear a mask when going into public. Airplane travel should be avoided, especially to areas where sanitation is

inadequate. Infectious diseases consultation should be sought for travel after that time.

7. **Pretransplant vaccination** against pneumococci [48] once and influenza seasonally is recommended. If not current, inactivated vaccination against tetanus, *Haemophilus infuenza type B (HiB),* and poliovirus, as well as the live mumps, measles, and rubella (MMR) vaccination should be given. Seronegative recipients to the respective viruses should receive hepatitis A, hepatitis B and varicella vaccines. Meningococcal vaccine should be provided to college-age recipients. In BMT, vaccination of the donor may be helpful.
8. **Posttransplant vaccination.** In BMT, inactivated vaccines: that for influenza starting at 6 months, and those for diphtheria-tetanus-acellular pertussis (DTaP), *Pneumococcus* diphtheria-tetanus (DT), tetanus-diphtheria (Td), HiB, hepatitis B, and inactivated polio vaccine after 12 months. The live MMR vaccine should be given 24 months later [49].
9. **In the transplant unit,** fresh fruits and vegetables should be washed and all meats must be thoroughly cooked [34]. Intravenous lines and Foley catheters should be meticulously maintained and discontinued promptly. Patients should be mobilized as soon as possible. Masks are indicated for patients transported through construction areas [34] and for health-care workers with respiratory infections.
10. **Varicella prophylaxis.** Patients who are seronegative to varicella and exposed to chicken pox or to zoster, require varicella-zoster immune globulin (VZIG). See related discussion in Chapter 26.

## INFECTIONS IN RENAL TRANSPLANTATION

**During the first month after transplantation, the patient is most likely to experience a nosocomial infection, whereas the second interval (at 1–6 months) is marked by a predominance of opportunistic infections. After 6 months, if immunosuppression is reduced, the major risk is community-acquired infections.** (Fig. 20.1). Infectious disease problems of the diabetic transplant recipient have recently been reviewed [50].

**The clinical presentation of infection or rejection is similar and sometimes can be resolved only by biopsy of the transplanted kidney.** Renal transplant patients differ from other transplant recipients in that in the face of overwhelming infection, immunosuppression may be discontinued and dialysis used as an alternative therapy.

I. **Immediate posttransplantation period (first month).** Nosocomial infections with or without fever occur particularly during the immediate posttransplantation period. Because the net immunosuppression is still low, opportunistic infections occur only rarely in this interval, and their presence should prompt consideration of environmental exposure [33].

A. **Nosocomial infections,** including intravenous (i.v.) catheters, lung, wound, and urinary tract sites. These infections are frequent sources of fever. [33]. Other hospital-acquired infections include sinusitis, prostatitis, and disseminated *Candida* infections.

1. **Specific syndromes of the early posttransplantation period**

a. **Intravenous line infections** are common at both central and peripheral sites. If blood cultures are positive, i.v. lines discontinued in a febrile transplant patient should be quantitatively cultured. See Chapter 2 for a discussion of catheter-related sepsis.

b. **Pneumonia may be difficult to distinguish from postoperative atelectasis, adult respiratory distress syndrome, hemorrhage, congestive heart failure, or emboli.** Pneumonia in this period is a complex nosocomial process, and the reader is referred to Chapter 11 for further discussion. Empiric therapy should be based on the clinical setting, sputum Gram stain results, and local susceptibility patterns. If Gram stain does not suggest *Staphylococcus* or yeast, use piperacillin-tazobactam or a third- or fourth-generation cephalosporin as initial therapy. Nephrotoxic antibiotics and

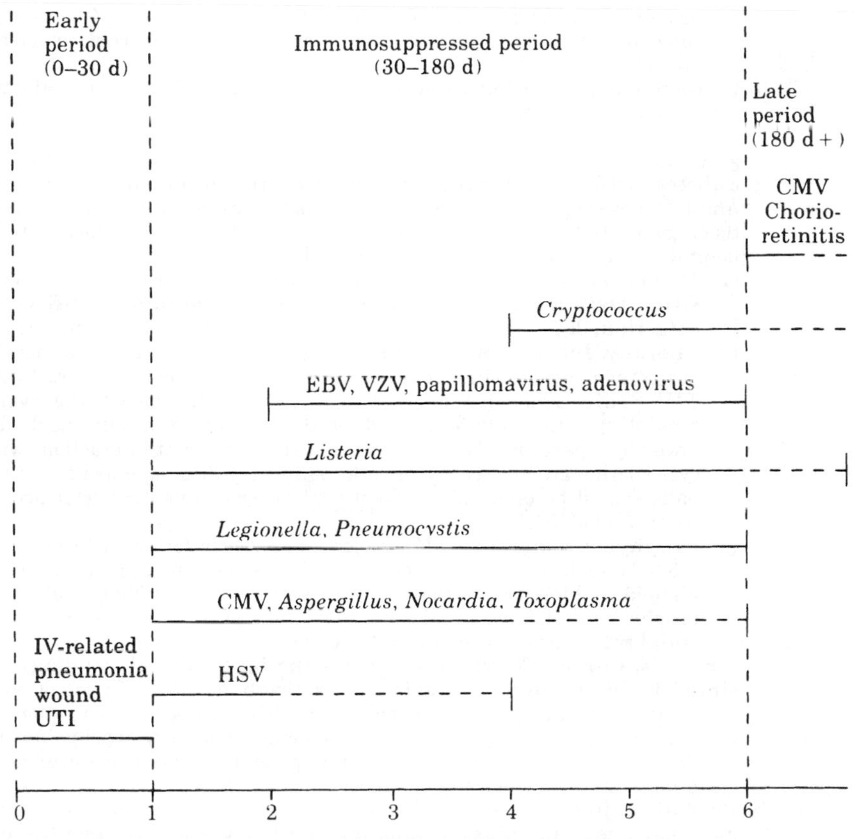


**FIG. 20.1** Infection timetable. CMV, cytomegalovirus; EBV, Epstein-Barr virus; VZV, varicella-zoster virus; HSV, herpes simplex virus; UTI, urinary tract infection. (Modified from Rubin RH, et al. Infection in the renal transplant recipient. *Am J Med* 1981;70:405; with permission.)

antibiotics that interact with immunosuppressive agents should be avoided (see section **III.A.1**).

**c. Wound infection** caused by staphylococci or gram-negative organisms is linked to technical complications that result in urine leaks from anastomoses, wound hematomas, or lymphoceles [51]. The use of systemic antibiotics and improved surgical techniques has decreased the incidence to 1% [51]. **However,** incisional pain, erythema, and fever are either mild or absent. **A high index of suspicion is necessary for early diagnosis.**

**(1)** A Gram stain and culture should be performed on any wound drainage, and blood cultures should be obtained. A CBC and a urinalysis with culture are indicated.

**(2)** Computed tomography (CT) of the transplanted kidney will show changes of infection. Aspiration of perirenal fluid for Gram stain and culture should be performed. Management may require surgical drainage and antibiotics. Empiric *Pseudomonas* coverage until Gram stain or culture results are available is indicated. In early studies, 75% of deep infections required a nephrectomy to prevent anatomic disruption and for cure [51].

d. **Urinary tract infections.** Due to surgical handling, for the first 90 days the urinary tract is a prime site of infection [51]. An infected allograft is a source of upper tract infection or sepsis. Infection due to hospital-acquired gram-negative rods or *Candida* species usually originates with an indwelling catheter. Graft loss due to *Candida* pyelonephritis has been reported [52]. Another cause of graft failure is BK virus, a polyomavirus. Hemorrhagic cystitis or interstitial nephritis with possible graft failure occur. Cidofovir may be helpful [53]. A mild febrile episode may be the only finding.
   (1) **Diagnosis.** With bacteria, urinalysis reveals white blood cells and casts. **Gram stain** results of urine **will often guide therapy. In BK virus infection,** decoy cells present on urine cytology or PCR is diagnostic.
   (2) **Therapy. Intravenous therapy is used** for these early (4–6 months posttransplantation) intrarenal processes then therapy is completed with TMP-SMX or a quinolone for 4 to 6 weeks [54]. Candiduria, whether symptomatic or not, should be treated for 10 days with oral antifungals followed by repeat urinalysis and culture [54]. Significant interactions with cyclosporine are not seen. Search for surgically drainable foci or fungus balls should be undertaken. Treatment of asymptomatic bacteriuria is controversial [54,55].
   (3) **Prophylaxis** with TMP-SMX yields significantly fewer bacterial UTIs [56]. Those at high risk for recurrence (diabetics, patients on cyclophosphamide or high-dose steroids, or those with recurrent UTIs) should have prophylaxis indefinitely [56]. Antifungal prophylaxis is not indicated [57].

2. **Nosocomial infections less commonly seen**
   a. **Sinusitis. Coronal head CT scans are the best methods to diagnose sinusitis related to nasogastric or nasotracheal tubes.** Oxymetazoline 0.5% and removal of the tube on the affected side may be sufficient therapy. Optimal management may require antral puncture or surgery. Febrile sinusitis should be treated with antibiotics such as piperacillin-tazobactam to cover gram-negative organisms and anaerobes.
   b. **Prostatitis** from the Foley catheter may manifest as pus around the indwelling catheter. Rectal examination reveals a boggy, tender prostate. Culture of expressed prostatic secretions may identify the pathogens. TMP-SMX is a reasonable empiric choice. Quinolones are an alternative in the sulfa-sensitive patient. Patients receiving quinolones and cyclosporine should be monitored for nephrotoxicity.
   c. **Disseminated fungal infections** occur from line sepsis, especially in association with prolonged antibiotic use [33]. New lipid formulations of amphotericin B are less nephrotoxic than standard amphotericin B. The latter may cause increased serum creatinine levels in 50% to 100% of patients [58,59]. At doses ranging from 1 to 4 mg/kg/day, liposomal amphotericin B concentrations are greater than the inhibitory concentrations of most fungal organisms [60]. Among the three formulations, liposomal amphotericin B has the best toxicity profile (61) and a clinical response in invasive aspergillosis of 61% [61a]. Caspofungin (Cancidas) shows promise for treatment of *Candida* or *Aspergillus* infections. Elevation of liver function tests (LFTs) occur if cyclosporine but not tacrolimus is used. Approval by the U.S. Food and Drug Administration of voriconazole, which is active against filamentous and dimorphic fungi and *Candida* species, is expected early in 2002. It does interfere with cytochrome P450.

B. **Reactivation of latent infection**
   1. **CMV** often reactivates and may produce a self-limited febrile illness with malaise and neutropenia. See section **VI** under Basic Principles.
   2. **Preexisting tuberculous** disease can disseminate, resulting in miliary disease.
   3. ***Strongyloides stercoralis*** infestation may evolve into a hyperinfection syndrome with pulmonary infiltrates and polymicrobial bacteremia. Mortality

approaches 70% [6]. Treatment employs thiabendazole or ivermectin [6]. Screening of stool (five samples), sputum, and duodenal aspirate will identify larvae in 91% of these patients.

C. **Allograft-derived infections.** Pyelonephritis, occasionally developing immediately after transplantation, results from the graft having been seeded prior to being harvested [62]. Donors who have been in the intensive care unit for more than 1 week pose the greatest risk. Graft contamination during preservation may be more common than donor infection. Culture of perfusate identifies this potential source of infection. Kidney recipients with a culture-positive perfusate should receive 7 to 14 days of i.v. antibiotics. CMV, EBV, TB, hepatitis, syphilis, *Strongyloides, Candida,* and HIV have all been transmitted by renal allografts [63].

II. **Immunosuppressive period (1–6 months).** This is the interval of maximum immunosuppression. Both primary and reactivated CMV infection add to the immunosuppression. The combination of these factors predisposes both to infection and to tumorigenesis [29,30]. **Infections may present in an unusual fashion and may be caused by exotic and unexpected pathogens.**

A. **Pulmonary infections mandate a rapid diagnostic approach.** Diagnosis within 5 days yields 80% versus 35% survival if diagnosis is delayed [64].

1. **Clinical approach** to pulmonary infections

a. **A history and physical examination** should be performed, with particular attention to mode of onset; travel; serostatus of the donor and recipient with respect to CMV, EBV, HSV, and VZV; animal contacts; exposure to ill persons; compliance with prophylactic regimens; vaccination history; and receipt of blood products. The immunosuppression regimen should be reviewed, including pulse immunotherapy for rejection. Recall that CMV predisposes to other complications [23,29,30].

b. **Expectorated or induced sputum (using inhalation of 10% glycerin plus 10% NaCl for 10 minutes)** is obtained for Gram and regular and modified acid-fast stains, as well as routine, acid-fast, and *Legionella* culture. Because atypical pneumonia and opportunistic processes present with a dry cough, sputum induction improves identification of mycobacteria and fungi as well as *Pneumocystis* species. Cultures should be held for 2 weeks to detect *Nocardia* or *Legionella.* A Papanicolaou smear should be performed to search for *Strongyloides.*

c. Blood cultures, arterial blood gases, and serial chest radiography are appropriate. **Samples for serum analysis of cryptococcal antigen should be obtained, and urinalysis should be performed to look for *Legionella* urinary antigen.**

d. **Imaging studies** must be carefully interpreted. Chest x-ray patterns do not correlate with a specific etiology. Radiographs are abnormal in only 56% of cases of pneumonia; CT scans are often helpful when the chest radiograph is nondiagnostic.

e. **Bronchoscopy** should be performed if diagnosis is uncertain within **24 to 48 hours,** or earlier if the clinical course mandates. Quantitative cultures obtained by protected brush, bronchoalveolar lavage, and biopsy are helpful. With a protected brush, $10^3$ bacteria/mL suggests infection [65]. If these studies are unrevealing, open lung biopsy is indicated [66].

f. **Transthoracic needle aspiration** of discrete peripheral lesions or infiltrates can be attempted, especially if the lesions are cavitary. Limited tissue is a drawback when attempting to diagnose a process that may be multietiologic (see Chapter 11).

g. **Initial empiric therapy** should be initiated immediately after bronchoscopy (or immediately after specimen collection if bronchoscopy is not performed initially) and should be based on clinical setting and results of Gram staining. Coverage for resistant gram-negative organisms with a third- or fourth-generation cephalosporin and a second-generation quinolone is reasonable. For dosing, see Chapter 27F and G. Macrolides including azithromycin should be avoided in patients on calineurin inhibitors.

Table 20.1. Immunocompromised Protocol: Studies Done on Biopsy Samples of Lung Tissue or Bronchoalveolar Lavage Washings

| |
|---|
| Gram stain and bacterial culture |
| Fungal culture |
| Acid-fast bacilli smear and culture |
| *Nocardia* smear and culture |
| *Legionella* smear and culture |
| Respiratory viral culture |
| Cytomegalovirus smear and culture |
| Smears for herpes simplex virus and adenovirus and, in the proper season, influenza virus, respiratory syncytial virus, and parainfluenza virus |
| Cytology |
| Gomori methenamine silver stain for *Pneumocystis carinii* pneumonia |

Empiric therapeutic doses of TMP-SMX can be initiated if the patient has not received prophylaxis for *Pneumocystis* (see Chapter 18). Cyclosporine levels should be followed closely when TMP-SMX is used. Sputum for acid-fast bacilli (AFB) smear and culture postbronchoscopy have an increased yield of mycobacteria after the procedure [67].

2. **The laboratory approach** is complex (see also Chapters 11 and 25). Bronchoscopy and open-lung biopsy specimens must be handled meticulously (Table 20.1).
   a. **The protected brush technique** is used to differentiate upper airway colonization from lower infection. A quantity of greater than $10^3$ organisms suggests that the organism is the cause of the infection [68].
   b. **Bronchoalveolar lavage** fluid should be stained for *Pneumocystis* species, fungi, and AFB. Direct fluorescent antibody testing of smears is useful for detecting *Legionella* species and viruses such as CMV, herpes simplex adenovirus, and, in the appropriate season influenza, parainfluenza, or respiratory syncytial virus (RSV). Bronchoalveolar lavage can be used to detect organisms in 69% of cases [65].
   c. **Biopsy tissue is** stained with hematoxylin and eosin and examined for viral inclusions and granulomas. Tissue should be cultured for viruses and *Mycobacterium tuberculosis* and stained by the immunoperoxidase technique for toxoplasma (see Chapter 25).
   d. **Open lung biopsy** is relatively safe and should not be delayed in the critically ill patient. It is especially useful in diffuse infiltrates. Lung tissue should be studied as in section **c.**

B. **Dermal infections** present a diagnostic challenge. **Biopsy of the lesion is usually necessary for accurate diagnosis.** Lesions should be evaluated promptly. They may be a *forme fruste* of disseminated infection, and early systemic therapy can be successful [69].

1. **Skin infections** may be similar to those seen in immunocompetent individuals.
   a. **Cellulitis due to staphylococci or streptococci** is commonly observed because of skin fragility from chronic corticosteroids. Ampicillin-sulbactam, an antistaphylococcal penicillin, or clindamycin for penicillin-allergic individuals, should be used. A portal of entry such as dermatophyte infection should be sought.
   b. **Cellulitis caused by unusual pathogens.** Gram-negative bacteria, cryptococci, or *Candida,* may be clinically indistinguishable from pyogenic cellulitis. **Biopsy with culture is indicated when response to standard therapy is lacking** [33].
2. **Skin infections producing localized or mild infections.**
   a. **Herpes simplex viruses.** The severity of HSV infection is governed by the type and intensity of immunosuppressive therapy. Lympholytic preparations (OKT3, ALG) are major promoters of HSV infection. Approximately one-half

of kidney recipients experience reactivation of cutaneous lesions within 30 to 60 days after transplantation [33]. With lympholytic therapy, these infections may develop earlier.

(1) **Herpes labialis** usually is caused by HSV type 1 and is exacerbated by the presence of endotracheal and nasogastric tubes. It may progress to involve the oral and esophageal mucosa and may mimic *Candida* esophagitis radiographically. The lesions often become superinfected with *Candida* [69]. Acyclovir is effective [47].

(2) **Anogenital lesions due to HSV type 2 are less common.** Lesions after transplantation may be typical vesicles or less characteristic ulcers. A Tzanck preparation is helpful diagnostically, as are viral cultures. There is a potential for secondary infection with gastrointestinal flora and subsequent bacteremia. Oral acyclovir is effective.

(3) **Cutaneous dissemination of HSV,** (Kaposi varicelliform eruption), presents with crops of vesicles arising in separate sites. This is due to autoinoculation. It usually involves areas of prior trauma (e.g., burns). Treatment is i.v. acyclovir.

b. **Varicella-zoster virus.**

(1) **Reactivation of latent VZV** occurs in a dermatomal distribution in 10% of renal transplant recipients; dissemination is a rare event. Immunosuppression need not be changed. Acyclovir enhances healing and decreases acute pain. With normal renal function, 10 mg/kg every 8 hours is indicated. Patients should be isolated until lesions crust [47].

(2) **Primary VZV infection** (chickenpox) is uncommon because of immunity. When it occurs, hepatitis, pneumonitis, central nervous system (CNS) infection, and disseminated intravascular coagulation can result. **Prophylaxis with VZIG is imperative for seronegative patients exposed to VZV.** VZIG will prolong the incubation period (see Chapter 26). If lesions occur, acyclovir 10 mg/kg i.v. every 8 hours, should be initiated promptly (assuming normal renal function) [33].

c. **Papillomavirus,** the cause of warts, affects 40% of renal transplant patients and occasionally develops into extensive or disfiguring lesions [33]. Furthermore, malignant transformation of warts can occur. Initial therapy is reduction of immunosuppression followed by cryosurgery. Dermatologic consultation is suggested.

3. **Primary skin infections caused by opportunistic organisms usually are diagnosed by biopsy with histologic examination and routine, fungal, and mycobacterial cultures.**

a. **Localized infections** with atypical mycobacteria, fungi, and algae occur.

b. **Systemic spread** can follow cutaneous infection with *Candida* and the zygomycetes. The lung and gastrointestinal tract are the usual portals of entry for *Aspergillus* and *Candida* organisms, respectively. The zygomycetes have been introduced by trauma from dressings or i.v. line placement.

4. **Disseminated skin infection may originate from a noncutaneous source,** heralding a systemic infection that requires systemic therapy. *Nocardia, Cryptococcus,* and *Candida* are noted for this. In 25% of patients with cryptococcosis, dermal lesions appear weeks to months prior to CNS disease. Disseminated candidal infections present with skin lesions in 15% of patients [33]. *Nocardia* is noted for the concurrence of dermal and lung lesions.

C. **Central nervous system infections**

1. **Meningoencephalitis and brain abscess** are the most frequent CNS infections and present in a subacute fashion. Causative organisms include *Aspergillus, Toxoplasma, Nocardia,* and viruses. **See related discussions in Chapter 6.**

a. ***Aspergillus*** infection is common in the first 1 to 2 months posttransplantation [69a]. It usually originates from a pulmonary focus (83%–90%). Mental status changes vary between those that rapidly progress to obtundation and death or focal neurologic findings occur. **The diagnosis should be suspected if sinus or pulmonary aspergillosis is present. Magnetic resonance imaging (MRI) is more sensitive than CT.** Lesions are multifocal at the gray and white junction [69a,70]. Lipid complex amphotericin B is the drug of choice. Fatality rates approach 100% [71].

b. ***Toxoplasma gondii*** is uncommon. The initial presentation is altered mental status in 45% and seizures in 35%; MRI demonstrates single- or multiple-ring–enhancing lesions in periventricular areas [71]. A stereotactic biopsy is useful for diagnosis. Sulfisoxazole and pyrimethamine are the agents of choice [72]. Clindamycin may be substituted for the sulfonamide in the sulfa-allergic patient (see Chapter 18).

c. **Nocardiosis.** See section **II.A.2** under Infections in Heart Transplantation.

2. **Meningitis** is another common presentation of CNS infection during this period. Patients may complain of headache, lethargy, or fever, or may demonstrate meningismus. The organism responsible for **acute meningitis usually is *Listeria*, whereas *Cryptococcus* and *Coccidioides* present in a subacute fashion.** Meningitis often occurs after treatment for rejection, regardless of the time that has elapsed since transplantation [70].

a. ***Cryptococcus*** causes a basilar meningitis with increased intracranial pressure and the risk for deafness and blindness. CT findings are often normal. Infection usually occurs more than 3 months posttransplantation and presents with headache (80%) and fever (60%). Cerebrospinal fluid (CSF) crytpococcal antigen is obtained, which is positive in 100% of cases; whereas culture is positive in only 90%. Opening pressure should be measured. Fluconazole or lipid complex amphotericin B and flucytosine are the drugs of choice [73,74] for the transplant recipient in whom interactions with cyclosporine are a primary concern. Repeated lumbar puncture to lower pressure is indicated if initial pressure is elevated.

b. ***Listeria*** occurs late after transplantation. It presents as brain stem encephalitis with cranial nerve palsies or pontomedullary signs [75]. CSF Gram stain is always negative. Treatment is ampicillin plus an aminoglycoside. TMP-SMX is used in penicillin-allergic patients.

c. ***Coccidioides immitis.*** Fluconazole or itraconazole are effective, but amphotericin B—systemically or, in refractory cases, intrathecally—remains the standard of care [76–78]. If possible, immunosuppression should be decreased.

d. **Rhinocerebral phycomycoses** due to *Mucor* and *Rhizopus* are encountered only rarely in renal transplant recipients, even during the height of immunosuppression. Physical examination reveals periorbital swelling, cranial nerve palsies, and necrosis of the nasal turbinates. Biopsy with histologic examination demonstrating hyphal elements is diagnostic. Lipid complex amphotericin B is adjunctive to extensive surgical resection.

D. **Urinary tract infections** in this period parallel those seen in the immediate posttransplantation period (see section **I.A.1.d**).

E. **Gastrointestinal complaints in the renal transplant recipient warrant aggressive diagnostic evaluation, because the severity of illness can be masked by immunosuppression.** See related discussions in Chapter 13.

1. **Viral infections are common.**

a. Stomatitis or esophagitis usually is caused by concurrent HSV and *Candida* infections. In stomatitis, the diagnosis is made clinically, but esophagitis requires endoscopy with biopsy and culture. Acyclovir is effective for HSV esophagitis. Oral or i.v. fluconazole is used for candidal esophagitis [77].

b. **Gastrointestinal ulceration** and bleeding may be caused by CMV. Diagnosis requires endoscopy with biopsy and viral culture. GCV is the drug of choice [79]. *Helicobacter pylori* and rarely invasive fungal disease may be etiologic.

2. **Bacterial infections are seen less often.**

a. **Acute gastroenteritis** is caused by pathogens that occur in immunocompetent patients.

b. **Hemorrhagic diarrhea** can be seen with *M. tuberculosis* infection, CMV, pseudomembranous colitis, posttransplantation lymphoproliferative disorder, diverticulitis, or *Campylobacter* or *Salmonella* infection (see section **III.E**).

c. **Intraabdominal abscess.** Chronic steroid therapy leads to perforation at any weak area in the bowel. Perforation is followed by abscess formation. Diagnosis can be made via ultrasonography or CT.

3. **Diverticulitis** caused by chronic constipation is seen in patients given long-term phosphate-binding antacids. It should be suspected with abdominal pain or change in bowel habits. Diverticulosis before transplantation predisposes a patient to diverticulitis. Classic signs of peritonitis frequently are absent in the immunosuppressed patient. Surgical evaluation, CT scanning, or a water-soluble contrast enema may be helpful (see Chapter 13).
4. **Cholecystitis** may be calculous or acalculous. In the latter, dehydration is a contributing factor. **Corticosteroids can mask the manifestations of cholecystitis** [69].

F. **Fever of uncertain origin.** A search for hepatic, neurologic, and gastrointestinal disease is indicated, and a low threshold for biopsy of the involved organ with routine AFB smear, viral culture, and histology is necessary. Human parvovirus B19 infections following transplantation may cause fever of unknown origin, myalgias, and refractory anemia [80]. IVIG may be helpful. **However, in this period fever often is caused by CMV** (see section **VI** under Basic Principles). Neutropenia accompanying CMV infection may necessitate decreasing the dose of MMF or azathioprine. In our experience, CMV infection contributes profoundly to the net immunosuppressive effect. A CMV-infected patient should be observed for the development of other opportunistic infections or malignancies.

III. **The late period (>6 months posttransplantation)** is **characterized by community-acquired infections** in patients who are successfully grafted. Patients chronically infected with CMV and hepatitis viruses and those with ongoing rejection remain at risk for opportunistic disease.

A. **Late pulmonary infections**

1. ***M. tuberculosis*** **and atypical mycobacterial infections** may exhibit unusual presentations. A history of exposure or a reactive PPD test result may be difficult to obtain. Accordingly, a **high index of suspicion** must be maintained when late pulmonary infiltrates develop. Acid-fast stains of sputum may be negative, and bronchoscopy may be necessary to obtain adequate specimens. Optimal treatment for highly susceptible *M. tuberculosis* and atypical mycobacteriosis is controversial. Although 9 months of INH and rifampin may be sufficient, the immunocompromised patient may require an additional 9 months of therapy [47,67] (see Chapter 11).

   Greater controversy surrounds the treatment of multiply resistant TB. Consideration of this possibility must be made when evaluating individuals exposed to TB. Resistant and atypical mycobacterial infections require individualized therapy based on the results of susceptibility testing. Infectious disease consultation is suggested (see Chapter 11). Lung resection is an alternative in patients with localized pulmonary involvement caused by atypical mycobacteria [47].
2. **Fungal infection** with *Histoplasma, Coccidioides,* and *Cryptococcus* species can present without obvious pulmonary involvement. Histoplasmosis and coccidioidomycosis generally are encountered in endemic areas, whereas cryptococcosis occurs throughout the United States. The clinician should alert the laboratory when sputum is submitted. Positive culture should be assumed to represent invasive disease. For treatment of cryptococcosis, fluconazole is used. Histoplasmosis and blastomycosis respond to itraconazole, which exhibits 90% efficacy [78] (see Chapter 17). The clinician should be alert to interactions with the calcineurin inhibitors.
3. **Pneumococcal and *H. influenzae*** pretransplantation vaccination is important. See section **VII.C.6–7** under Basic Principles. Influenza vaccine should be administered annually posttransplantation. Renal transplant recipients have a reduced antibody response to vaccine, but vaccine does not compromise graft function [81].

B. **Dermal infections.** See section **II.B.**

C. **Central nervous system infection** is more likely if the patient has continued rejection or persistent viral infection. See section **II.C.** In the patient requiring low-dose immunosuppression, routine bacterial pathogens and cryptococci should be suspected.

D. **Urinary tract infections.** During this period, these usually are benign, and the incidence of such infections is decreased by prophylactic use of TMP-SMX. **Low-dose quinolones** are effective and relatively safe in the transplant patient. Bacteremic pyelonephritis suggests anatomic abnormality and warrants urologic evaluation [33].

E. **Gastrointestinal infections**

1. **Chronic hepatitis caused by HBV,** with or without hepatitis delta virus (HDV) and HCV infection, is a leading cause of morbidity and mortality in patients with functioning renal allografts who survive 10 years [82]. Donor and recipient serologies for HBV must be analyzed carefully prior to transplantation. Hepatitis surface antigen (HBsAg)-positive or anti–hepatitis core antibody (HBcAb) IgM-positive donors pose a high risk for transmission of HBV. Anti-HBcAb IgG-positive or HBsAb-positive grafts are unlikely to transmit HBV to kidney recipients. Pretransplantation immunization and posttransplantation prophylaxis may allow use of seropositive grafts [83]. Hepatocellular injury is cytopathic in HBV and primarily immune mediated in HCV. IFN is a difficult drug to use in transplant recipients because it has an immunostimulatory effect [84]. A recent study by Pereira et al. showed that liver disease was increased in recipients of HCV-positive organs but the rate of graft loss or mortality during a 3.5-year follow-up period [85] was similar. In a more recent study, HCV-positive recipients of renal allografts had an increased incidence of membranoproliferative glomerulonephritis compared with HCV-negative recipients, and HCV positivity was a predictor of graft loss [86]. Interestingly, HCV exerts an immunomodulating effect during the first year. Allograft survival is significantly greater in these patients. The infection rate is also greater in the first year. Boletis et al. established that liver biopsy, not simply transaminase level, is required to determine the severity of disease, prognosis, and response to treatment [87]. Cirrhosis may ensue.

2. ***Salmonella* infections** may result in metastatic infection or bowel perforation. **Any patient with *Salmonella* gastroenteritis should always be treated** (see Chapter 13).

F. **Eye infection.** Visual field defects are a common manifestation of CMV retinitis. However, this occurs rarely in transplant recipients. The patient may be asymptomatic and the clinical course evolves over weeks. GCV 5 mg/kg every 12 hours for 2 weeks will halt disease progression, but patients may relapse (see Chapter 18). Toxoplasmosis presents similarly but is very uncommon. Ophthalmologic consultation is imperative (see Chapter 27).

G. **Epstein-Barr virus** is associated with a spectrum of B-cell lymphoproliferative diseases that infrequently develop following kidney transplantation. These have recently been reviewed [88].

## INFECTIONS IN HEART TRANSPLANTATION

Problems in cardiac transplantation parallel those in renal transplantation. However, prevention of rejection is the top priority in heart transplant recipients, because retransplantation is risky and expensive. The 1-year survival rate for repeat cardiac transplantation is approximately 55% [89]. Therefore, aggressive immunosuppression must be enforced, but this increases the incidence and severity of infection. Patients who receive transplants for ischemic disease tend to experience more infections than those who receive transplants for other reasons, but this may be related to their greater mean age [90]. Infection in heart transplant recipients has been reviewed [91].

I. **Immediate posttransplantation period (first month).** The infectious complications encountered during this period are the same as those in renal transplant recipients, with the exception of surgical wound infections.

A. **Nosocomial infections** are a common cause of fever in this time period.

1. **Intravenous catheter** infections should be managed as for renal transplant recipients. The avoidance of bacteremia is paramount because of the vascular anastomoses (see Chapter 2). Lines should be removed as soon as feasible, and pacer wires should be removed promptly.

2. Refer to section **I.A** under Infections in Renal Transplantation and Chapter 11 for the presentation, diagnosis, and treatment of **pneumonia.** A recent review of pneumonia found rates of 21.1 per 100 heart recipients—75% occurred in the first 2 months. Sixty percent were caused by opportunistic organisms, 25% were nosocomial pathogens, and 15% were community-acquired pathogens. Bronchoscopy was 95% sensitive for diagnosis [92]. Influenza vaccination is safe after heart transplantation and induces adequate antibody responses in most patients [93]. *Pneumocystis carinii* pneumonia (PCP) prophylaxis should be given for 1 year posttransplantation and reinstituted following treatment of rejection [32].
3. **Surgical wound** infections are uncommon, but potential progression into the mediastinum makes this a grave complication. Needle aspirate or bone biopsy is important [94]. Diagnosis is made by results of Gram staining and culture. Responsible organisms include coagulase-positive and -negative staphylococci, as well as by *Enterobacter, Serratia,* and *Pseudomonas* species. Sternotomy infections require debridement and systemic antibiotics.
4. **Urinary tract** infections are less common than in renal transplant recipients and are managed as would be any nosocomial UTI. Prophylaxis with TMP-SMX for PCP also reduces the incidence of UTIs (see Chapter 15).
5. **Pleural effusions** might occur postoperatively. In an asymptomatic patient, these may be observed, but if infection is suspected, a diagnostic thoracentesis is indicated.

B. **Reactivation of prior infection can occur.** Refer to section **I.B** under Infections in Renal Transplantation. With respect to HBV, some investigators suggest that transplantation of HBV-positive carriers is safe given that lamivudine controls viral replication posttransplantation [95]. Despite the finding that survival posttransplantation was not impacted by HBV status pretransplantation, others caution against transplantation in this setting. Liver biopsy pretransplantation may be helpful. Fagiuoli's group found that HBV and HCV behaved more aggressively after cardiac transplantation [96].

C. **Various infections may be transmitted by allograft.**

1. **Transplantation of a *Toxoplasma*-**seropositive heart into a seronegative patient poses a 25% to 50% risk for disseminated toxoplasmosis, with a high risk for mortality [97]. A 6-month course of TMP-SMX or pyrimethamine and folinic acid prophylaxis should be initiated [34,97,98].
2. The risk for **CMV** disease is higher in heart than in kidney recipients. Prophylaxis involves short-term i.v. GCV, then 3 months oral GCV [32,99]. Prophylaxis including immunoglobulin seems to be more effective than use of either agent alone [100]. Alternatively, preemptive approaches have become popular. Various regimens have been identified. One is to start i.v. GCV when ATG/ALG is given for rejection. Addition of oral GCV for 3 months after rejection therapy nullifies the risk for CMV disease [101]. Many centers use quantitative PCR or pp65 antigenemia assays to determine when to give preemptive i.v. GCV [102–107]. Advantages of preemptive approaches include avoidance of drug toxicity and reduction in CMV resistance because fewer patients receive GCV [107]. Furthermore, prophylactic GCV prevents induction of CMV-specific T-cell responses, allowing for late-onset CMV disease after prophylaxis is stopped [103], whereas preemptive therapy allows this T-cell response to occur. Hibberd showed a 52% reduction of CMV disease if GCV was used with ALG [108].
3. **HCV**-positive donors are a possibility for critically ill heart patients. However, the risk for HCV transmission approaches 80%. Consequences of HCV remain to be seen [109].
4. **HBV.** Some programs use hearts from donors positive for HBsAg or HBcAb if the recipient has natural immunity to HBV or has been successfully immunized [110].

II. **Immunosuppressive period (1–6 months).** As in renal transplantation, this is the time of maximum immunosuppression. Opportunistic infections surpass nosocomial infections as the most common causes of fever. Infections are similar but often more severe than in renal transplants. *Legionella* and *Nocardia* are more common in heart transplant recipients. With TMP-SMX prophylaxis, the incidence of *Nocardia* has diminished.

A. **Pulmonary infections** constitute the most commonly encountered infectious process [111] and are similar to those encountered in renal transplant patients (see section **II.A** under Infections in Renal Transplantation) [112].

1. **Legionellosis** is more common in some centers. (See related discussion in Chapter 11.)

   a. **Legionellosis usually presents as a patchy, interstitial pneumonia** that progresses to an alveolar infiltrate. Any appearance is possible; cavitation has been described [33].

   b. ***Legionella* is difficult to isolate from sputum.** Bronchoscopy with culture may be necessary [113]. An indirect fluorescent antibody study is available, but an increase in titer may be delayed. A single titer of 1:256 or greater is presumptive evidence, whereas paired sera reflecting a fourfold increase are diagnostic. Eighty percent of cases of *Legionella* are caused by serogroup 1. Urinary antigen detection tests, which detect only serogroup 1, have good sensitivity and specificity. Histologic examination usually reveals a bronchopneumonia.

   c. **Treatment.** A second-generation quinolone should be started empirically because of the difficulty in confirming the diagnosis and given for 21 days. Late relapse can occur. Rifampin 600 mg orally twice daily may be added in severe or refractory cases [113]. Azithromycin is generally avoided when patients are on tacrolimus or cyclosporine. Clarithromycin has significant interactions with calcineurin inhibitors.

2. **Nocardiosis is seen in heart transplant recipients [114].**

   a. *Nocardia* infections have decreased with use of TMP-SMX prophylaxis for PCP. Most patients have symptomatic lung disease. Although radiographic findings are variable, **the concurrence of skin lesions and a pulmonary infiltrate strongly suggests nocardiosis or cryptococcosis.** See related discussion in Chapter 17.

   b. Sputum cultures have a yield of only 30%. **Diagnosis often requires invasive procedures** to obtain tissue for culture and histologic examination. As in renal transplants, about 30% of open-lung biopsy specimens yield a previously unexpected diagnosis [66]. In sputum or lung tissue, acid-fast, gram-positive, filamentous bacteria suggest nocardiosis. All patients with nocardiosis should undergo brain MRI to exclude intracranial disease.

   c. **The drug of choice** is a sulfonamide (e.g., sulfadiazine 2 g orally every 6 hours or TMP-SMX 2 double-strength tablets orally three times daily) for 3 to 6 months (see Chapters 17 and 27L). Serum levels ideally should be monitored, with peak levels adjusted to 12 to 15 mg/dL. Sulfadiazine may crystallize in the renal tubules, resulting in acute renal failure. To prevent this outcome, sodium bicarbonate (or sodium citrate and citric acid [Bicitra]) should be used to maintain the urine pH at greater than 7. In patients allergic to sulfonamides, various combinations of amikacin, minocycline, ceftriaxone, and imipenem have been used with success. Duration of therapy has not been well defined. Infectious disease consultation is advised.

B. **Dermal infections.** See section **II.B** under Infections in Renal Transplantation.

C. **Central nervous system infections.** See section **II.C** as above.

D. **Urinary tract infections.** See section **II.D** under Infections in Renal Transplantation.

E. **Gastrointestinal infections.** See section **II.E** under Infections in Renal Transplantation.

F. **Posttransplantation lymphoproliferative disorders** (PTLDs).

1. **Etiology and pathogenesis.** Most PTLDs are of B-lymphocyte origin and are often the result of primary EBV infection [115]. **Early diagnosis is essential, because the syndrome may be reversible in the early stages, but** progresses to malignancy if diagnosis is delayed. Those at risk for developing PTLD include a seronegative recipient (10% of the population [116]) of a seropositive graft; patients receiving ALG therapy [116], cyclosporine, or tacrolimus; recipients of nonrenal grafts; and patients with other infections, particularly CMV [117]. Clinical presentation may mimic CMV, with fever, malaise, leukopenia, adenopathy, or splenomegaly. Involvement of the GI tract, lungs, CNS, or the graft itself is

typical [116,118]. A spectrum may occur after transplantation. EBV-associated disease occurs early posttransplantation (≤1 year). Several histopathologic patterns have been described. Posttransplantation infectious mononucleosis and plasma cell hyperplasias are distinct forms of PTLD. EBV-associated polymorphic lymphomas, polymorphic B-cell hyperplasia, and lymphomatous PTLD characterize true PTLDs [115]. Adults are more likely to have EBV-negative non-Hodgkin lymphomas after transplantation and are most often EBV-seropositive men over 45 years of age. Retransplantation is another risk factor for EBV-negative non-Hodgkin lymphomas [119]. Lesions are monomorphic and respond poorly to conventional antineoplastic therapies [120].

2. **Diagnosis.** Semiquantitative PCR has been developed to monitor for PTLD. It appears that this assay is better for ruling out PTLD than confirming the diagnosis [121].
3. **Treatment** is relatively ineffective. Initially it involves minimizing immunosuppression. Because high EBV viral loads may be immunosuppressive, the risk for rejection with this reduction is minimal. Because CMV may serve as a cofactor, treatment with GCV and CMVIG may be helpful [115]. Localized symptomatic lesions may be removed surgically; radiation and chemotherapy are reserved for systemic involvement and failure to respond to initial treatment. Monoclonal anti-CD 20, 21, and 24 B-cell antibodies are efficacious against PTLD lesions that contain the targeted cell marker [122].

G. **Fever of uncertain origin.** See section **II.F** under Infections in Renal Transplantation.

III. **Late period (>6 months).** The infectious problems encountered in this period are similar to those described in section **III** under Infections in Renal Transplantation.

## INFECTIONS IN LIVER TRANSPLANTATION

Infection, the most important determinant of morbidity and mortality in orthotopic liver transplantation (OLT) [123–126], is difficult to **diagnose because of the similarities between infection and rejection.** Bacterial infections tend to occur during treatment of rejection episodes, and devitalized liver tissue is a haven for bacteria. Infections or their treatment may contribute to hepatic dysfunction. Furthermore, liver histology may be altered by infection. The differentiation between rejection and infection is difficult [127].

I. **Infection or not infection—that is the question.**

A. **Rejection** may be acute or chronic.

1. **Acute rejection** crisis is the most common cause of graft dysfunction and typically occurs on approximately the fifth day after transplantation.
   a. **Symptoms and signs** of malaise, anorexia, abdominal discomfort, fever, increased organ size, or clear bile are present in rejection [128].
   b. **Laboratory studies** should assess for rapidly rising hepatic values, especially bilirubin and prothrombin time. **Liver biopsy is the best diagnostic tool** for evaluating rejection but is dangerous because of preexisting coagulopathy or neovascularization of the implanted liver [128].
   c. **Radionuclide scans** (dimethyl iminodiacetic acid [HIDA]) shows decreased uptake and excretion not only in rejection but also in ischemic, obstructive, viral, drug, and septic complications. Ultrasonography undertaken with HIDA scan can be used to distinguish between tumor, biloma, abscess, and hepatic infarction.
   d. **Treatment** of acute rejection requires pulse immunosuppression, which can potentiate infectious complications. **The prognosis** of rejection is guarded; children fare better than adults. Acute rejection leads to 20% of all posttransplantation deaths in OLT [128].
2. **Chronic rejection** targeting the intrahepatic ducts is an ongoing process and may eventuate in a "vanishing bile duct syndrome" at any time [128].
   a. **Jaundice,** which reflects the obliteration of bile ducts during the rejection process, is the hallmark of chronic rejection, whereas increasing aspartate aminotransferase (AST) and alanine aminotransferase (ALT) values are less specific.

b. **Treatment** of vanishing bile duct syndrome has been disappointing. In approximately 20% of such recipients, retransplantation is required; survival averages 50% [129].

B. **Hepatic dysfunction** can occur with viral or bacterial infection. CMV that is established by liver biopsy, or by other diagnostic approaches is most common [130]. Less commonly, bacteremia, an intraabdominal abscess, or pneumonia can produce hyperbilirubinemia, usually in association with an elevated alkaline phosphatase and minimally elevated transaminases [128]. This is referred to as cholestatic jaundice. Hepatotoxic drugs and technical problems such as biliary leak or stricture, bleeding, or hepatic artery thrombosis may simulate infection or rejection.

II. **Infection complicates liver transplantation in 80% of recipients.** Many will have polymicrobial infection or multiple episodes of infection. Mortality varies between 20% and 30%. Risk factors include length of surgery, multiple blood products, Roux-en-Y anastomosis, CMV infection, and prior abdominal surgery [123–126]. In OLT, the timing of specific infections is less predictable because the graft is an "immunologic" organ. **All patients with fever of unclear origin should undergo CT or ultrasonography to rule out abscess or ductal dilatation. Additionally, because the biliary tree is colonized, antibiotic prophylaxis is essential before biopsy or cholangiogram and should be continued for 48 hours** [32].

A. **Immediate posttransplant period (first month). Rejection and infection, the latter involving the peribiliary liver tissue, and the biliary and vascular anastomoses, mark this period.** The greater infection rates in liver transplantation can be directly attributed to the technical complexity of the surgery. **Procedure-related infections** increase with the duration of surgery and the number of prior operations [125]. They occur at vascular or enterobiliary anastomoses. Thrombocytopenia is a marker of risk for early infections and increased mortality [131]. **Organisms** are similar to those in renal transplants, although in some centers vancomycin-resistant *Enterococcus faecium* is a significant problem. Selective bowel decontamination seems to lower the incidence of infections [132, 133].

1. **Hepatic artery anastomoses can become infected** or undergo thrombosis, especially in children, during the first posttransplantation week. This results in peribiliary duct necrosis with secondary abscess formation. Bacteremias have arisen from hepatic or portal vein thrombosis as well. The clinical onset often is heralded by an isolated episode of fever. Alternatively patients may present with ascites or an increase in liver function tests [128].
2. **Biliary anastomoses** may leak, become obstructed, or become infected by the adjacent gastrointestinal flora. The normal flora will not cause clinical infection unless leaks or an obstruction is present. The manifestations are variable and may include cholangitis, liver abscess, or bacteremia [128]. Postoperative ileus may lead to increased pressure on biliary anastomoses, with subsequent biliary leak and infection.
3. **Invasive candidiasis** arising from the upper small bowel can occur in up to 44% of patients [134]. Risk factors include hemodialysis, perioperative antibiotics, multiple blood products, prolonged mechanical ventilation, and need for surgical reexploration. These patients should receive prophylactic fluconazole. Use of amphotericin B should be entertained for patients who are intubated for long periods of time. Clotrimazole (10-mg troche) or nystatin suspension (10 mL orally four times daily) often is given to reduce colonization [35].

B. **Infection after 30 days** more typically mirrors the processes seen in patients receiving heart or kidney transplants. Mortality is lower than in patients who develop infectious complications during the immediate posttransplantation period [33]. However, the infections are more diverse and reflect prolonged immunosuppression.

1. **Nosocomial infections** can occur in any hospitalized transplant patient. See section **I.A** under Infections in Renal Transplantation.
2. **Opportunistic infections** are seen in this period and decrease only when immunosuppression is decreased. See section **II.A–F.**

   a. **CMV infection** causes mild persistent hepatic dysfunction and can be distinguished from rejection only by biopsy with **histology and viral culture.**

CMV prophylaxis after liver transplantation consists of two approaches. A short course of i.v. GCV (until bowel function returns) followed by 90 days of oral VGCV lowers the risk for CMV disease even in donor-positive/recipient-negative patients [29]. Oral GCV has proved effective in recipients of anti-lymphocyte therapy [135]. Preemptive therapy (based on quantitative pp65 antigenemia or PCR assays) consisting of 14 to 21 days of i.v. GCV has established efficacy for prevention of CMV disease [29]. A cost-effectiveness study by Das found that universal prophylaxis consisting of 100 days of oral GCV was the most cost-effective strategy [136]. See section **VI** under Basic Principles and section **II** under Infections in Renal Transplantation.

**b. Human herpesvirus 6 (HHV-6) is** a member of the herpesvirus family. Most studies have examined liver transplant recipients. Seroprevalence rates in adults are greater than 90% [137]. Although this is a controversial area, infections have been reported in 30% to 50% of solid organ recipients [137a]. Based on positive CSF PCR results, HHV-6 has been linked with mental status changes and fever (as high as 40°C). However 50% of normal children have a positive CSF PCR result. There is general agreement that HHV-6 causes fever and a rash and possibly thrombocytopenia, leukopenia, and anemia. Infections have peak incidence at 4 weeks. Like other herpesviruses, it is postulated that HHV-6 diminishes cell-mediated function, perhaps elevating the risk for CMV, invasive fungal disease, and mortality [137b]. Calcineurin inhibitors have been associated with an immunosuppression-induced leukoencephalopathy, which may mimic those allegedly related to HHV-6 [138]. MRI demonstrates subcortical white matter lesions in posterior cortical hemispheres. Because both the development and the time of onset of immunosuppression-induced seizures is similar, the exact role of HHV-6 is uncertain.

**c. Hepatitis B** can significantly affect graft survival. There is a high rate of recurrence (83%–100%) of HBV following OLT [139], with progression to chronic active hepatitis by 9 to 12 months, and cirrhosis 2 to 3 years posttransplantation. HBV leads to increased levels of IFN-$\gamma$ and tumor necrosis factor-$\alpha$ (TNF-$\alpha$), along with upregulation of TNF-$\alpha$ receptor expression by hepatocytes with subsequent graft injury. Prophylaxis against HBV infections is useful. Regimens of i.v. or intramuscular HBIG reduce recurrence of HBV to less than or equal to 20% [140]. Lamivudine or famciclovir have been given posttransplantation [141], but lamivudine has better activity than famciclovir. Both are more effective in the setting of HBeAg-positive patients, higher ALT levels pretreatment, and HDV coinfection. About 5% of patients have breakthrough elevated HBV DNA levels after initial viral suppression [141]. Despite the emergence of resistance, ongoing lamivudine results in a less aggressive disease course. HBV-positive liver recipients have more infectious complications and probably a greater risk for hepatic neoplasm if HBV recurs [128].

**d. Hepatitis C.** The implications of HCV infection in liver transplantation are unclear. The rate of recurrence of HCV after transplantation is 42% to 88%. Approximately 10% of patients will die or have graft failure due to recurrent HCV. However, 5-year graft survival rates in HCV-positive liver transplant recipients are similar to those for HCV-negative recipients [142]. HCV genotype 1B, high cumulative doses of corticosteroids, and steroid-resistant rejection result in elevated HCV viral loads [142]. Pegylated IFN with or without ribavirin should be considered, before the serum bilirubin exceeds 3 mg/dL, in those who demonstrate histologic recurrence of HCV. Rejection risk is not increased [143]. If IFN three times weekly is not tolerated, benefit may accrue from low-dose daily IFN.

**C. In the late period (>6 months),** opportunistic infections diminish in frequency. The transition from opportunistic infection to community-acquired infection is less clear in the liver transplant recipient. TB presents a particularly difficult problem because of hepatotoxicity from standard antituberculous drugs. Meyers et al. reported on regimens of 2 months of induction followed by continued treatment with ethambutol and ofloxacin for 9 months in patients who developed TB posttransplantation. Six of seven patients treated with this protocol were alive and free of TB at the end of follow-up [144].

## INFECTIONS IN LUNG TRANSPLANTATION (A UNIQUE AND FREQUENTLY ENCOUNTERED SET OF PROBLEMS)

I. **Outcome.** Survival rates after lung transplantation are 74% the first year, 65% the second year, and 47% at 5 years. Infectious complications account for 50% of deaths, and two thirds involve the respiratory tract [145]. The cumulative incidence of bacterial pneumonia during the first year after lung transplantation is 70%.

II. **Pathophysiology.** Sinus surgery to decrease colonization pretransplantation is controversial. As a result of the procedure, the graft is denervated, resulting in a diminished cough reflex and disrupted mucociliary clearance. Environmental exposure further escalates the risk for pneumonia. [145]. The bronchial anastomosis is subject to ischemic/infection that may lead to dehiscence or stenosis.

III. **Etiology**

A. Common pathogens include *Pseudomonas* species, other gram-negative organisms, *Staphylococcus aureus*, and *Enterococcus* species. Colonizing organisms found pretransplantation, especially in cystic fibrosis (CF) patients, produce postoperative infections. CF patients benefit from double lung transplantation to lower the risk for graft pneumonia. Colonization by *Aspergillus* species leads to invasive disease in 13% to 26% and is consistently fatal [146]. Risk for invasive aspergillosis peaks in the first 6 months posttransplantation, but 30% occur more than 6 months out.

B. CMV incidence is increased after lung transplantation. Risks include size of the organ and amount of lymphoid tissue in the graft. CMV disease occurs in 90% to 100% of donor-positive/recipient-negative patients and in 60% of donor-positive/recipient-positive patients [147]. CMV has been linked to obliterative bronchiolitis, which leads to progressive deterioration in lung function [145,147].

C. PTLD occurs more frequently after lung transplantation than for other solid organs. The risk approaches 30% [148] and most often affects the graft. Bronchoscopic lung biopsy (BLB) is an important diagnostic technique and is also useful for diagnosis of infectious complications. BLB specimens are less reliable for detecting graft rejection. Blood loss in excess of 100 mL is the leading complication.

IV. **Prevention and treatment.** Special considerations after lung transplantation address prevention of invasive fungal infections, multiply resistant bacteria, CMV, viral respiratory pathogens, HSV, and EBV-associated PTLD. For fungus, some centers use a combination of antifungal agents, including lipid complex amphotericin B or itraconazole and inhaled amphotericin B to achieve higher local tissue levels [149]. Lifelong PCP prophylaxis is recommended by some clinicians; at a minimum it should be reinstated with antirejection treatment. TB may occur either due to reactivation, to posttransplantation exposure, or to transmission from the donor. INH prophylaxis is safe and effective [144]. Prophylaxis against HSV with acyclovir or valacyclovir for 3 months posttransplantation is given because HSV pneumonia may be severe. For CMV there may be a benefit to adding CMVIG to GCV.

**Infections in pancreatic transplantation will not be reviewed here.**

## BONE MARROW TRANSPLANTATION

Bone marrow transplantation differs significantly from solid organ transplantation. In BMT patients, HLA typing is closely observed; the immunosuppression is profound; and graft-versus-host disease (GVHD) occurs frequently. Most marrow recipients have undergone therapy for leukemia and have received at least one round, and often several rounds, of antibiotics. Other differences are the absence of a surgical wound and the presence of an initial period of complete immunosuppression lasting approximately 30 days. Absolute leukopenia and the absence of cell-mediated immunity make predictions of infectious agents difficult.

I. **Basic principles. Allogeneic transplantation is distinctly different from reinfusion of autologous marrow/stem cells. Immunosuppression posttransplanta-**

**tion is not done, and GVHD does not occur in the latter group, only the pretransplantation conditioning.**

**A. Donor and recipient selection and preparation before BMT**

1. **The marrow donor** is ideally an HLA-identical sibling. Twenty-five percent of siblings are HLA identical. Use of partially matched family member marrow and matched, unrelated donor marrow is increasing. It is preferable that the donor and recipient be matched at the HLA-A, -B, and -DR locus, and their mixed lymphocyte cultures must have mutual nonreactivity. Donors should be screened for syphilis, CMV, HSV, HIV, HCV, VZV, EBV, and HBV. Cardiac and pulmonary status should be evaluated if anesthesia will be used for marrow harvest.
2. **Recipient selection.** BMT is used to treat leukemia, lymphoma, multiple myeloma, severe combined immunodeficiency, aplastic anemia, sickle cell disease, and enzyme deficiencies. Common to these disorders is an immunologic deficiency that predisposes to infection even prior to marrow irradiation and immunosuppression therapy. Research into BMT for solid organ tumors is ongoing.
3. **Immunosuppressive therapy.** Before BMT, patients receive a regimen that ablates existing disease and allows donor marrow engraftment, combining chemotherapy with total body irradiation for those with malignancy. Potential regimens include methotrexate (MTX), cyclosporine, ATG, and corticosteroids. Donor marrow is pretreated with monoclonal antibody or lectins to remove T cells in an attempt to prevent GVHD [150].

**B. Measures to prevent infection**

1. **Protective environment.** Patient hygiene and fastidious handwashing by staff and visitors is essential. Allogeneic recipients should be housed in rooms that have at least 12 air exchanges per hour. Use of portable high-efficiency particulate air filters is recommended [151]. If available, laminar air flow rooms are useful, but patients find them uncomfortable for prolonged periods of time [49].
2. **Antimicrobial prophylaxis.** In the early posttransplantation period, before fever develops, many centers use ciprofloxacin prophylaxis. Later, one TMP-SMX double-strength tablet daily is useful for chronic GVHD because of the high incidence of bacterial infections. This also decreases the frequency of PCP [151], toxoplasmosis, and nocardiosis. IVIG may be indicated in patients who are hypogammaglobulinemic to prevent upper and lower respiratory tract infections [151]. Prophylactic fluconazole 400 mg/day orally reduces the incidence of superficial and systemic fungal infections in allogeneic and high-risk autologous BMT patients if they are likely to have prolonged neutropenia [152]; itraconazole prophylaxis has been effective as well [153].
3. **CMV prophylaxis** with CMVIG is considered for seropositive marrow into a seronegative recipient. However, the risk for CMV disease is greatest in the seropositive recipient. Options for CMV prevention include i.v. GCV from engraftment to day 100 posttransplantation or preemptive i.v. GCV triggered by a positive CMV antigenemia or PCR assay result. If the CMV pairing is donor positive/recipient negative, preemptive therapy coupled with leukocyte-poor blood products is preferred for BMT recipients because the risk for CMV disease is low [49].

**II. Infections in BMT** have been recently reviewed [154].

**A. The early period (0–21 days)** is characterized by an **absolute neutrophil count (ANC) of less than 100, lymphopenia,** and mucositis. Fever, which usually is the only sign of infection, is the hallmark and almost invariably complicates the early neutropenic period. Noninfectious fever—from transfusion, embolism, deep hemorrhage, or drugs—may occur. Central venous and Foley catheters contribute to the breakdown of normal anatomic barriers. Both increase the chance for bacteremia [49]. HSV infection occurs at this time [155].

1. **Blood cultures must be obtained. In the febrile patient, bacteremia** occurs in 20% to 30% of patients. Patients appear septic. Organisms include Enterobacteriaceae, coagulase-negative staphylococci, and viridans streptococci [156]. Empiric $\beta$-lactam antibiotic (e.g., piperacillin, cefepime, or imipenem) with or without an aminoglycoside is administered (see Chapter 2). With the increasing incidence of gram-positive infections, two options exist. Many authorities hold vancomycin until gram-positive organisms are isolated [156a]. Others initiate therapy with

vancomycin and stop it if blood cultures are negative. Antibiotics are continued until the ANC increases to 500/mm$^3$, unless infection is proven, then duration should follow standard practice. Treatment may be abbreviated in the febrile clinically stable patient after 1 week, when the ANC is greater than 200/mm$^3$ and cultures remain negative. For indwelling catheter infections, see Chapter 2.

2. ***Candida* infections** are considered if fever persists or recurs while the patient is on antibiotic treatment. The incidence is related to the duration of neutropenia [152]. Febrile patients should undergo urine, blood, and sputum cultures, biopsy of skin lesions, and retinal examination for lesions. A course of antifungal therapy is warranted even with negative cultures [35,157]. As noted above, these individuals are on prophylactic oral fluconazole. Therefore, for allogeneic transplant patients on nephrotoxic immunosuppressive agents, lipid complex amphotericin B is the agent used [35]. In auto-BMT recipients with a serum creatinine level of at least 2.0 mg/dL, 50% will require hemodialysis; if amphotericin is initiated and creatinine increases, early switch to lipid complex amphotericin B is reasonable. **Molds such as *Aspergillus*** that are resistant to fluconazole present as sinusitis and lung nodules or abscess and are difficult to treat. Although initially they may look very well, the rate of mortality is high in patients with *Aspergillus.* Radiographic imaging of the chest and sinuses may demonstrate otherwise occult fungal infections. The treatment regimen for *Aspergillus* is not settled. Some clinicians administer liposomal amphotericin up to 15 mg/kg.
3. **Orolabial HSV reactivation** occurs in 75% of seropositive patients and progresses to esophagitis or pneumonia [151,158]. Oral acyclovir is used for prophylaxis and in i.v. preparation for treatment.

B. **The middle period (21–100 days) often** is characterized by continued granulocytopenia from graft failure or rejection. Bacterial and fungal infection remain important. With successful engraftment and the gradual return of immune function, **the main obstacle is acute GVHD.** This presents with rash, diarrhea, and hepatic dysfunction, and is believed to result from proliferation of donor T-lymphocytes reacting to host tissue antigens. In parallel, viruses and protozoa become important causes of infection.

1. **Interstitial pneumonia. The second major risk to the patient during this period is interstitial pneumonia** [159], which is seen in 40% to 60% of patients. The mortality rate exceeds 50% [159]. Fever, increased respiratory rate, and nonproductive cough occurring approximately 45 days after BMT are characteristic. CMV is found in one-half of the cases. Pretransplantation lung function is a predictor of interstitial pneumonia due to CMV. HHV-6 infections may cause interstitial pneumonia in BMT recipients (137a). The incidence of PCP is declining with the use of prophylactic TMP-SMX. Uncommonly, *Aspergillus*, adenovirus, HSV, parainfluenza, adenovirus, RSV, and *Chlamydia* are causative agents. RSV is associated with a high mortality rate [160]. Thirty percent to 45% of cases are idiopathic [159]. **Idiopathic interstitial pneumonia** [161–163] has a similar presentation, but no infectious etiology can be demonstrated. Pulmonary fibrosis may be immune mediated. Risk factors include preconditioning irradiation and chemotherapy, MTX to control GVHD, age greater than 20 years, and a low pretransplantation Karnovsky score [161]. Treatment is supportive. Superinfection is a frequent complication. The mortality rate approaches 60% [161].
   a. **Diagnosis.** Hypoxemia and infiltrates characterize interstitial pneumonia. If bronchoscopy with lavage and biopsy is nondiagnostic and the patient has not improved after 24 to 48 hours of appropriate antibiotics, open lung biopsy should be performed.
   b. **Treatment. Until biopsy results are known, a broad-spectrum $\beta$-lactam with an aminoglycoside is recommended** [151]. GCV in combination with CMV immunoglobulin is used for CMV pneumonitis [162].
2. **Dermal infections** are associated with acute GVHD or with indwelling catheters.
   a. **Acute GVHD** with its generalized maculopapular skin rash can evolve into bullae, ulcers, and epidermolysis. The rash mimics maculopapular drug eruption. Histologic confirmation is necessary. Corticosteroids, MTX, ATG, and

cyclosporine have been used for treatment. HHV-6 infections and GVHD are interrelated. Both cause increase in cytokines with subsequent reactivation of HHV-6 or induction of GVHD.

b. **Skin infections are often associated with an indwelling catheter** (see Chapter 4).

3. **Central nervous system infections can** present as meningitis or as subtle changes in mental status (see Chapter 6).
4. **Urinary tract infections** (see Chapter 15).
5. **Gastrointestinal tract infections.** Nausea, vomiting, and anorexia during the first 2 weeks after BMT are usually side effects of chemoradiotherapy or of drugs. Between days 15 and 60, acute GVHD, HSV infections, and drug toxicity are possibilities.
   a. **Diarrhea** is common in this period. Chemoradiotherapy sequelae are diagnosed by biopsy and treated supportively. Drug toxicity is excluded by discontinuation or substitution of medications. Chemotherapeutic agents and antimicrobials may cause *Clostridium difficile* colitis (see Chapter 13). Patients developing acute GVHD present with nausea and vomiting and have hemoccult-positive, watery stools with a high protein content. CT scans or sonograms showing edematous intestine, or mucosal biopsies of duodenum or colon may aid in the diagnosis. Enteroviruses, rotavirus, and especially adenovirus may mimic or be associated with GVHD. The same may be said for fungi, parasites, and bacteria. Stool should be cultured for viruses and enteric pathogens and examined for ova and parasites. Endoscopic biopsy with viral culture is indicated if CMV or HSV is suspected or if the diagnosis remains unclear.
   b. **Mucositis or acute GVHD often causes gastrointestinal bleeding**, but other causes include CMV, EBV-induced PTLD, peptic ulcer, and Mallory-Weiss tears.
   c. **Esophagitis** caused by chemoradiotherapy occurs early in the posttransplantation period and usually is self-limited. Because viruses, fungi, or bacteria may cause disease singly or in combination [164], diagnosis requires biopsy. Stricture formation may be a late sequela.
   d. **Abdominal pain. Early-onset** abdominal pain may be caused by **chemoradiotherapy or venoocclusive disease.** Right upper quadrant pain, ascites, and fluid retention can be seen with the latter. Such disease involves the terminal hepatic venules and sublobular veins, with necrosis of hepatocytes leading to fibrosis and obstruction of sinusoidal blood flow. No intervention has altered the disease course, which carries a mortality rate of 30% [164].

      **Later, acute GVHD and infectious enteritis** are common causes of abdominal pain and may occur together. Bacterial invasion and inflammation of the bowel wall characterize typhlitis or neutropenic enterocolitis that presents with right lower quadrant pain, vomiting, fever, and diarrhea. *Clostridium septicum* may be cultured from blood, although other anaerobes, gram-negative organisms, or yeast may be involved. Sepsis syndrome and edema of the colonic mucosa on CT scanning further suggest this diagnosis. Supportive therapy with appropriate antibiotic treatment is indicated; surgical resection is a consideration while waiting for the neutropenia to resolve [164].
6. **Disseminated CMV infection.** GVHD predisposes to symptomatic disease. Approximately 50% of cases are caused by reactivation, but other CMV infections are acquired from the donor or from CMV-seropositive blood products. The nonspecific presentation may include fever, neutropenia, or organ dysfunction. Many patients are asymptomatic [49]. One-fifth or so of CMV infections culminate in pneumonia, with a mortality rate of 50% to 60% [153,165]. Diagnosis requires biopsy of the involved organ and CMV cultures of blood and urine. Alternatively, PCR or pp65 antigenemia assays may be helpful. Avoidance of seropositive marrow donors, use of filtered blood products, and early preemptive therapy based on quantitative PCR or pp65 antigen can prevent most disease [35]. Treatment of visceral disease comprises GCV with CMVIG [162].
7. **Line-related bacteremias.** The patient's immunosuppressed state, the presence of GVHD, and indwelling venous catheters all contribute to the development

of *Candida, Staphylococcus epidermidis,* or *Corynebacterium* species sepsis (see Chapter 2).

**C. The late period (>100 days)** is associated with fewer infections because most i.v. lines have been removed, fewer immunosuppressive agents are used, and the immune system has progressively recovered. **Chronic GVHD** occurs in 30% to 50% of patients. It may follow acute GVHD or arise *de novo* [164]. It may be focal and mild, or it may be generalized, resembling autoimmune disease with scleroderma-like skin lesions, hepatitis, malabsorption, and sicca syndrome. Chronic GVHD leads to an increased risk for infection owing to interruption of skin and mucosal barriers, delayed recovery of cell-mediated and humoral immunity, and functional asplenia.

1. **Pulmonary infections.** The entire respiratory tract is susceptible to infection because chronic GVHD leads to IgA deficiency and sicca syndrome. *Streptococcus pneumoniae* predominates, whereas fungi, CMV, and PCP are less common. TMP-SMX is used for bacterial and PCP prophylaxis.
2. **Dermal infections.** VZV occurs in 30% of all patients and 45% of patients with chronic GVHD. Both primary and reactivation disease are encountered. Bacterial superinfection, scarring, postherpetic neuralgia, and trigeminal zoster occur. Visceral involvement is life threatening, affecting pelvic and abdominal organs, the lungs, the oral and genital mucous membranes, and the CNS. Patients with cutaneous or visceral VZV should be isolated and treated with i.v. acyclovir. VZIG is indicated for primary exposure to prevent or ameliorate illness. See discussions in Chapters 4 and 26.
3. **Disseminated infections.** Pneumococcal sepsis is seen, as are bacteremias with *H. influenzae, Neisseria meningitidis, S. aureus,* and gram-negative aerobes. A $\beta$-lactam and aminoglycoside should be used empirically when these bacteremic syndromes are suspected. TMP-SMX prophylaxis is effective in decreasing the incidence of bacteremia.

## REFERENCES

1. Perlroth MG. The role of organ transplantation in medical therapy. In: Rubenstein E, Federman DD, eds. *Scientific American medicine.* New York: Scientific American, 1989, CTM V, 1–16.
2. Symposium on Liver Transplantation. The Department of Continuing Education in Health Sciences, UCLA Extension and the Liver Transplant Program, Department of Surgery, School of Medicine, University of California, Los Angeles, 1986.
3. Schaffner A. Pretransplant evaluation for infections in donors and recipients of solid organs. *Clin Infect Dis* 2001;33(suppl 1):9–14.
4. Keating MR, Wilhelm MP, Walker RC. Strategies for prevention of infection after cardiac transplantation. *Mayo Clin Proc* 1992;67:676–684.
5. Kuo PC, Stock PG. Transplantation in the HIV+ patient. *Am J Transplant* 2001; 1:13–17.
6. Avery RK, Ljungman P. Prophylactic measures in the solid-organ recipient before transplantation. *Clin Infect Dis* 2001;33(suppl 1):15–21.
7. Busuttil RW (moderator). Liver transplantation today. *Ann Intern Med* 1986;104:377–389.
8. Council on Scientific Affairs. Introduction to the management of immunosuppression. *JAMA* 1987;257:1781.
9. Grossi P, et al. Infections in heart transplant recipients: the experience of the Italian Heart Transplantation Program. *J Heart Lung Transplant* 1992;11:847–866.
10. McGoon MD, Franz RP. Techniques of immunosuppression after cardiac transplantation. *Mayo Clin Proc* 1992;67:586–595.
11. Burke JF Jr, et al. Long-term efficacy and safety of cyclosporine in renal-transplant recipients. *N Engl J Med* 1994;331:358.
12. Barone GW, Gurley BJ, Ketel BL, et al. Herbal supplements: a potential for drug interactions in transplant recipients. *Transplantation* 2001;71:239–241.
13. Medical Letter. Tacrolimus (FK506) for organ transplants. *Med Lett Drugs Ther* 1994;36:82.

14. Knoll GA, Bell R. Tacrolimus versus cyclosporin for immunosuppression in renal transplantation: meta-analysis of randomized trials. *Br Med J* 1999;318:1104–1107.
15. Sollinger HW, for The U.S. Renal Transplant Mycophenolate Mofetil Study Group. Mycophenolate mofetil for the prevention of acute rejection in primary cadaveric renal allograft recipients. *Transplantation* 1995;60:215–232.
16. Kelly P, Gruber S, Behbod F, et al. Sirolimus, a new, potent immunosuppressive agent. *Pharmacotherapy* 1997;17:1148–1156.
17. Cao W, Mohacsi P, Shorthouse R, et al. Effects of rapamycin on growth factor–stimulated vascular smooth muscle cell DNA synthesis. Inhibition of basic fibroblast growth factor and platelet-derived growth factor action and antagonism of rapamycin by FK506. *Transplantation* 1995;59:390–395.
18. Brennan DC, Flavin K, Lowell JA, et al. A randomized, double-blinded comparison of *Thymoglobulin* versus *Atgam* for induction immunosuppressive therapy in adult renal transplant recipients. *Transplantation* 1999;67:1011–1018.
19. Onrust SV, Wiseman LR. Basiliximab. *Drugs* 1999;57:207–213.
20. Nashan B, Light S, Hardie IR, et al. Reduction of acute renal allograft rejection by daclizumab: Daclizumab Double Therapy Study Group. *Transplantation* 1999;67:110–115.
21. Bourge RC, et al. Total lymphoid irradiation in cardiac transplantation: Is there a prolonged effect on allograft rejection? *J Heart Lung Transplant* 1993;12(suppl 86):2.
22. Smyth RL, et al. Infection and reactivation with cytomegalovirus strains in lung transplant recipients. *Transplantation* 1991;52:480–481.
23. Paya CV. Indirect effects of CMV in the solid organ transplant patient. *Transplant Infect Dis* 1999;1(suppl):8–12.
24. Koskinen P, Krogerus LA, Nieminen MS, et al. Quantification of cytomegalovirus infection-associated histologic findings in endomyocardial biopsies of heart allografts. *J Heart Lung Transplant* 1993;12:343–354.
25. Valantine HA, Gao S-Z, Santosh G, et al. Impact of prophylactic immediate posttransplant ganciclovir on development of transplant atherosclerosis. A post-hoc analysis of a randomized, placebo-controlled study. *Circulation* 1999;100:61–66.
26. Rubin RH. Discussion and consensus points. *Transplant Infect Dis* 1999;1:40–41.
27. Camargo LF, Uip DE, Simpson AA, et al. Comparison between antigenemia and a quantitative-competitive polymerase chain reaction for the diagnosis of cytomegalovirus infection after heart transplantation. *Transplantation* 2001;71:412–417.
28. Barber L, Egan JJ, Lomax J, et al. A prospective study of a quantitative PCR ELISA assay for the diagnosis of CMV pneumonia in lung and heart-transplant recipients. *J Heart Lung Transplant* 2000;19:771–780.
29. van der Bij W, Speich R. Management of cytomegalovirus infection and disease after solid-organ transplantation. *Clin Infect Dis* 2001;33(suppl 1):32–37.
30. Rubin RH. Importance of CMV in the transplant population. *Transplant Infect Dis* 1999;(suppl 1):3–7.
31. Valantine HA. Role of CMV in transplant coronary artery disease and survival after heart transplantation. *Transplant Infect Dis* 1999;(suppl 1):25–30.
32. Villacian JS, Paya CV. Prevention of infections in solid organ transplant recipients. *Transplant Infect Dis* 1999;1:50–64.
33. Rubin RH. Infection in the organ transplant recipient. In: Rubin RH, Young LS, eds. *Clinical approach to infection in the compromised host,* 3rd ed. New York: Plenum, 1994.
34. Soave R. Prophylaxis strategies for solid-organ transplantation. *Clin Infect Dis* 2001;33(suppl 1):26–31.
35. Sepkowitz K. Infectious challenges in solid organ and bone marrow transplant recipients. 40th Interscience Conference Antimicrobial Agents and Chemotherapy, Day 1—September 17, 2000. Retrieved July 6, 2001, from Medscape.com. *www.medscape.com/medscape/cno/2001/ICAAC/Story.cfm?story_id=1641.*
36. Corris PA. Prophylaxis post-transplant. The role of monitoring surveillance bronchoscopy and antimicrobials. *Clin Chest Med* 1997;18:311–318.
37. Kirk JL, et al. Analysis of early infectious complications after autologous bone marrow transplantation. *Cancer* 1988;62:2445–2450.

38. Taylor CE, et al. Virus infections in bone marrow transplant recipients: a three-year prospective study. *J Clin Pathol* 1990;43:633–637.
39. Corales R, Chua J, Mawhorter S, et al. Significant post-transplant hypogammaglobulinemia in six heart transplant recipients: an emerging clinical phenomenon? *Transplant Infect Dis* 2000;2:133–139.
40. Lowance D, Neumayer HH, Legendre CM, et al. Valacyclovir for the prevention of cytomegalovirus disease after renal transplantation. International Valacyclovir Cytomegalovirus Prophylaxis Transplantation Study Group. *N Engl J Med* 1999;13:1462–1470.
41. Kletzmayr J, Kreuzwieser E, Watkins-Riedel T, et al. Long-term oral ganciclovir prophylaxis for prevention of cytomegalovirus infection and disease in cytomegalovirus high-risk renal transplant recipients. *Transplantation* 2000;27:1174–1180.
42. Strauss RG. Leukocyte-reduction to prevent transfusion-transmitted cytomegalovirus infections. *Pediatr Transplant* 1999;3(suppl 1):19–22.
43. Lavee J, Yoav P. Hypotensive reactions associated with transfusion of bedside leukocyte-reduction filtered blood products in heart transplanted patients. *J Heart Lung Transplant* 2001;20:759–761.
44. Tsevat J, et al. Which renal transplant patients should receive cytomegalovirus immune globulin? *Transplantation* 1991;52:259–265.
45. Snydman DR, Werner BG, Dougherty NN, et al. Cytomegalovirus immune globulin prophylaxis in liver transplantation. A randomized, double blind, placebo-controlled trial. The Boston Center for Liver Transplantation CMVIG Study Group. *Ann Intern Med* 1993;10:984–991.
46. Avery RK. Special considerations regarding CMV in lung transplantation. *Transplant Infect Dis* 1999;(suppl 1):13–18.
47. Peterson PK, Anderson RC. Infection in renal transplant recipients. *Am J Med* 1986;81(suppl 1A):2.
48. Amber JI, et al. Increased risk of pneumococcal infections in cardiac transplant recipients. *Transplantation* 1990;49:122–125.
49. Guidelines for preventing opportunistic infections among hematopoietic stem cell transplant recipients. *MMWR* 2000;49:1–128.
50. Tolkoff-Rubin NE, Rubin RH. The infectious disease problems of the diabetic renal transplant recipient. *Infect Dis Clin North Am* 1995;9:117.
51. Cuvelier R, Pirson Y, Alexandre G. Late urinary tract infection after transplantation: prevalence, predisposition and morbidity. *Nephron* 1985;40:76.
52. Martinez-Marcos F, Cisneros J, Gentil M, et al. Prospective study of renal transplant infections in 50 consecutive patients. *Eur J Clin Microbiol Infect Dis* 1994;13:1023–1028.
53. Gonzalez-Fraile MI, Canizo C, Caballero D, et al. Cidofovir treatment of human polyomavirus-associated acute haemorrhagic cystitis. *Transplant Infect Dis* 2001; 3:44–46.
54. Munoz P. Management of urinary tract infections and lymphocele in renal transplant recipients. *Clin Infect Dis* 2001;33(suppl 1):53–57.
55. Snydman DR. Posttransplant microbiological surveillance. *Clin Infect Dis* 2001; 33(suppl 1):22–25.
56. Fox BC, Sollinger HW, Belzer FO, et al. A prospective, randomized, double-blind study of trimethoprim-sulfamethoxazole for prophylaxis of infection in renal transplantation: clinical efficacy, absorption of trimethoprim-sulfamethoxazole, effects on the microflora, and the cost-benefit of prophylaxis. *Am J Med* 1990;89:255–274.
57. Anonymous. Chemoprophylaxis for candidosis and aspergillosis in neutropenia and transplantation: a review and recommendations. Working Party of the British Society for Antimicrobial Chemotherapy. *J Antimicrob Chemother* 1993;32:5–21.
58. White MH, Bowden RA, Sandler ES, et al. Randomised, double blind clinical trial of amphotericin B colloidal dispersion vs. amphotericin B in the empirical treatment of fever and neutropenia. *Clin Infect Dis* 1998;27:296–302.
59. White M, Anaissie EJ, Kusne S, et al. Amphotericin B colloidal dispersion vs. amphotericin B as therapy for invasive aspergillosis. *Clin Infect Dis* 1997;24:635–642.
60. Ellis M. Amphotericin B preparations: a maximum tolerated dose in severe invasive fungal infections? *Transplant Infect Dis* 2000;2:51–61.

61. Wingard JR, White MH, Anaissie E, et al. A randomized double-blind comparative trial evaluating the safety of liposomal amphotericin B versus amphotericin lipid complex in the empiric treatment of febrile neutropenia L Amph/ABLC Collaborative Study Group. *Clin Infect Dis* 2000;31:1155–1163.

61a. Mills W, Chopra R, Linch DC, et al. Liposomal amphotericin B in the treatment of fungal infections in neutropenic patients: a single center experience of 133 episodes in 116 patients. *Br J Haematol* 1994;86:754–760.

62. Bijnen AB, et al. Infections after transplant of a contaminated kidney. *Scand J Urol Nephrol Suppl* 1985;92:49.

63. Gottesdiener KM. Transplanted infections: donor-to-host transmission with allograft. *Ann Intern Med* 1989;110:1001–1016.

64. Ramsey PG, et al. The renal transplant patient with fever and pulmonary infiltrates: etiology, clinical manifestations and management. *Medicine (Baltimore)* 1980;59:296.

65. Reichenberger F, Dickenmann M, Binet I, et al. Diagnostic yield of bronchoalveolar lavage following renal transplantation. *Transplant Infect Dis* 2001;3:2–7.

66. Toledo-Pereya LH, et al. The benefit of open lung biopsy in patients with previous non-diagnostic transbronchial lung biopsy; a guide to appropriate therapy. *Chest* 1980;77:647.

67. Bass JB. Chairman, Subcommittee of the Scientific Assembly on Microbiology, Tuberculosis and Pulmonary Infections. American Thoracic Society—diagnostic standards and classification of tuberculosis. *Am Rev Respir Dis* 1990;142:725–735.

68. Winterbauer RH, et al. The use of quantitative cultures and antibody coating of bacteria to diagnose bacterial pneumonia by fiberoptic bronchoscopy. *Am Rev Respir Dis* 1983;128:98.

69. Auchincloss H, Rubin RH. Clinical management of the critically ill renal transplant patient. In: Parillo JE, Masur H, eds. *The critically ill immunosuppressed patient.* Rockville, MD: Aspen, 1987:347–376.

69a. Selby R, Ramirez CB, Singh R, et al. Brain abscess in solid organ transplant recipients receiving cyclosporine-based immunosuppression. *Arch Sur* 1997;132:304.

70. Aksamit AJ. Central nervous system. In: Bowden RA, Ljungman P, Paya CV, eds. *Transplant infections.* Philadelphia: Lippincott-Raven, 1998:133–151.

71. Singh N, Husain S. Infections of the central nervous system in transplant recipients. *Transplant Infect Dis* 2000;2:101–111.

72. Britt RH, Enzmann DR, Remington JS. Intracranial infection in cardiac transplant recipients. *Ann Neurol* 1981;9:107.

73. Paya CV. Fungal infections in solid-organ transplantation. *Clin Infect Dis* 1993; 16:677–688.

74. Dismukes WE. Management of cryptococcosis. *Clin Infect Dis* 1993;17(suppl 2):507–512.

75. Armstrong RW, Fung PC. Brain stem encephalitis (rhomboencephalitis) due to *Listeria monocytogenes:* case report and review. *Clin Infect Dis* 1993;16:702.

76. Meyer RD. Current role of therapy with amphotericin B. *Clin Infect Dis* 1992; 15(suppl):154–160.

77. Bodey GP. Azole antifungal agents. *Clin Infect Dis* 14(suppl):161–169.

78. Graybill JR. Future directions of antifungal chemotherapy. *Clin Infect Dis* 1992; 14(suppl):170–181.

79. Sinnott JT, Cullison JP, Rogers K. Treatment of CMV gastrointestinal ulceration in a heart transplant patient. *J Heart Transplant* 1987;6:186.

80. Pamidi S, Friedman K, Kampalath B, et al. Human parvovirus B19 infection presenting as persistent anemia in renal transplant recipients. *Transplantation* 2000;69:2666–2669.

81. Sanchez-Fructuoso AI, Prats D, Naranjo P, et al. Influenza virus immunization effectivity in kidney transplant patients subjected to two different triple-drug therapy immunosuppression protocols: mycophenolate versus azathioprine. *Transplantation* 2000;69:436–439.

82. Chan PC, Lok AS, Cheng IK, Chan MK. The impact of donor and recipient hepatitis B surface antigen status on liver disease and survival in renal transplant recipients. *Transplantation* 1992;53:128–131.

83. Chung RT, Feng S. Delmonico FL. Approach to the management of allograft recipients following the detection of hepatitis B virus in the prospective organ donor. *Am J Transplant* 2001;1:185–191.
84. Rostaing L, et al. Treatment of chronic hepatitis C with recombinant interferon alpha in kidney transplant recipients. *Transplantation* 1995;59:1426.
85. Pereira BJ, et al. A controlled study of hepatitis C transmission by organ transplantation. *Lancet* 1995;345:484.
86. Cruzado JM, Carrera M, Torras J, et al. Hepatitis C virus infection and *de novo* glomerular lesions in renal allografts. *Am J Transplant* 2001;1:171–178.
87. Boletis J, et al. Liver biopsy is essential in anti-HCV (+) renal transplant patients irrespective of liver function tests and serology for HCV. *Transplant Proc* 1995;27: 945.
88. Hanto DW. Classification of Epstein-Barr virus–associated posttransplant lymphoproliferative diseases: implications for understanding their pathogenesis and developing rational treatment strategies. *Annu Rev Med* 1995;46:381.
89. Ensley RD, et al. Predictors of survival after repeat heart transplantation. *J Heart Lung Transplant* 1992;11:5142–5158.
90. Cooper DKC, et al. Infectious complications after heart transplantation. *Thorax* 1983;38:822.
91. Petri WA Jr. Infections in heart transplant recipients. *Clin Infect Dis* 1994;18:141.
92. Cisneros JM, Munoz P, Torre-Cisneros J, et al. Pneumonia after heart transplantation: a multi-institutional study. Spanish Transplantation Infection Study Group. *Clin Infect Dis* 1998;27:324–331.
93. Fraund S, Wagner D, Pethig K, et al. Influenza vaccination in heart transplant recipients. *J Heart Lung Transplant* 1999;18:220–225.
94. Bernabeu-Wittel M, Cisneros JM, Rodriguez-Hernandez MJ, et al. Suppurative mediastinitis after heart transplantation: early diagnosis with CT-guided needle aspiration. *J Heart Lung Transplant* 2000;19:512–514.
95. Ko WJ, Chou NK, Hsu RB, et al. Hepatitis B virus infection in heart transplant recipients in a hepatitis B endemic area. *J Heart Lung Transplant* 2001;20:865–875.
96. Fagiuoli S, Minniti F, Pevere S, et al. HBV and HCV infections in heart transplant recipients. *J Heart Lung Transplant* 2001;20:718–724.
97. Montoya JG, Giraldo LF, Efron B, et al. Infectious complications among 620 consecutive heart transplant patients at Stanford University Medical Center. *Clin Infect Dis* 2001;33:629–640.
98. Wreghitt TG, Gray JJ, Pavel P, et al. Efficacy of pyrimethamine for the prevention of donor acquired *Toxoplasma gondii* in heart and heart-lung transplant patients. *Transplant Int* 1992;5:197–200.
99. Rubin RH, Kemmerly SA, Conti D, et al. Prevention of primary cytomegalovirus disease in organ transplant recipients with oral ganciclovir or oral acyclovir prophylaxis. *Transplant Infect Dis* 2000;2:112–117.
100. Valantine HA, Luikart H, Doyle R. Impact of cytomegalovirus hyperimmune globulin on outcome after cardiothoracic transplantation. *Transplantation* 2001;72:1647–1652.
101. Turgeon N, Fishman JA, Basgoz N, et al. Effect of oral acyclovir or ganciclovir after preemptive i.v. ganciclovir therapy to prevent CMV disease in CMV seropositive renal and liver transplant patients receiving antilymphocyte antibody therapy. *Transplantation* 1998;66:1780–1786.
102. Kunzle N, Petignat C, Francioli P, et al. Preemptive treatment approach to cytomegalovirus (CMV) infection in solid organ transplant patients: relationship between compliance with the guidelines and prevention of CMV morbidity. *Transplant Infect Dis* 2000;2:118–126.
103. Boeckh M, Gooley TA, Myerson D, et al. Cytomegalovirus pp65 antigenemia-guided early treatment with ganciclovir versus ganciclovir at engraftment after allogeneic marrow transplantation: a randomized double-blind trial. *Blood* 1996;88:4063–4071.
104. Singh N, Yu VL, Mieles L, et al. High-dose acyclovir compared with short-course preemptive ganciclovir therapy to prevent cytomegalovirus disease in liver transplant recipients: a randomized trial. *Ann Intern Med* 1994;120:375–381.

105. Koehler M, St. George K, Ehrlich GD, et al. Prevention of CMV disease in allogeneic BMT recipients by cytomegalovirus antigenemia-guided preemptive ganciclovir therapy. *J Pediatr Hematol Oncol* 1997;19:43–47.
106. Paniagua MJ, Crespo-Leiro MG, Rodriguez JA, et al. Preemptive and prophylactic ganciclovir therapy for CMV infection in heart transplant patients. *Transplant Proc* 1999;31:2528–2529.
107. Singh N. Preemptive therapy versus universal prophylaxis with ganciclovir for cytomegalovirus in solid organ transplant recipients. *Clin Infect Dis* 2001;32:742–751.
108. Hibberd P, et al. Preemptive ganciclovir therapy to prevent cytomegalovirus disease in cytomegalovirus antibody-positive renal transplant recipients. *Ann Intern Med* 1995;123:18.
109. Pfau PR, Rho R, DeNofrio D, et al. Hepatitis C transmission and infection by orthotopic heart transplantation. *J Heart Lung Transplant* 2000;19:350–354.
110. Ko WJ, Chou N-K, Hsu R-B, et al. Hepatitis B virus infection in heart transplant recipients in a hepatitis B endemic area. *J Heart Lung Transplant* 2001;20:865–875.
111. Hofflin JM, et al. Infectious complications in heart transplant recipients receiving cyclosporine and corticosteroids. *Ann Intern Med* 1987;106:209.
112. Rubin RH, et al. Infection in the renal transplant recipient. *Am J Med* 1981;70:405.
113. Saravolatz LD, et al. The compromised host and Legionnaires' disease. *Ann Intern Med* 1979;90:533–537.
114. Kramer MR, Marshall SE, Starnes VA, et al. Infectious complications in heart–lung transplantations. Analysis of 200 episodes. *Arch Int Med* 1993;153(17):2010–2016.
115. Green M. Management of Epstein-Barr virus–induced post-transplant lymphoproliferative disease in recipients of solid organ transplantation. *Am J Transplant* 2001;1:103–108.
116. Straus SE (moderator). Epstein-Barr virus infections: biology, pathogenesis, and management. *Ann Intern Med* 1993;118:45.
117. Preiksaitis JK, Keay S. Diagnosis and management of posttransplant lymphoproliferative disorder in solid-organ transplant recipients. *Clin Infect Dis* 2001;33(suppl 1): 38–46.
118. Chen J, et al. Management of lymphoproliferative disorders after cardiac transplantation. *Ann Thorac Surg* 1993;56:527–538.
119. Swerdlow AJ, Higgins CD, Hunt BJ, et al. Risk of lymphoid neoplasia after cardiothoracic transplantation. A cohort study of the relation to Epstein-Barr virus. *Transplantation* 2000;69:897–904.
120. Dotti G, Fiocchi R, Motta T, et al. A. Epstein-Barr virus–negative lymphoproliferate disorders in long-term survivors after heart, kidney, and liver transplant. *Transplantation* 2000;69:827–833.
121. Allen U, Hebert D, Petric M, et al. Utility of semiquantitative polymerase chain reaction for Epstein-Barr virus to measure virus load in pediatric organ transplant recipients with and without posttransplant lymphoproliferative disease. *Clin Infect Dis* 2001;33:145–150.
122. Milpied N, Vassuer B, Parquet N, et al. Humanized anti-CD20 monoclonal antibody (rituximab) in post transplant lymphoproliferative disorder: a retrospective analysis on 32 patients. *Ann Oncol* 2000;11(suppl 1):113–116.
123. Winston DJ, Emmanouilide C, Busuttil RW. Infections in liver transplant recipients. *Clin Infect Dis* 1995;21:1077–1091.
124. Paya CV, Wiesner RH, Herman PE, et al. Risk factors for cytomegalovirus and severe bacterial infections following liver transplantation: a prospective multivariate time-dependent analysis. *J. Hepatol.* 1993;18:185–195.
125. Martin M, Kusne S, Alessiani M, et al. Infections after liver transplantation: risk factors and prevention. *Transplant Proc* 1991;23:1929–1930.
126. Hadley S, Samore MH, Lewis WD, et al. Major infectious complications after orthotopic liver transplantation and comparison of outcomes in patients receiving cyclosporine of FK-506 as primary immunosuppression. *Transplantation* 1995;59:851–859.
127. Colonna JO, et al. Infectious complications in liver transplantation. *Arch Surg* 1988;123:360.
128. Busuttil MD. Liver transplantation today. *Ann Intern Med* 1986;104:372.

129. Wiesner RH, et al. Hepatic allograft rejection: new developments in terminology, diagnosis, prevention, and treatment. *Mayo Clin Proc* 1993;68:69–79.
130. Kanj SS, et al. Cytomegalovirus infection following liver transplantation: review of the literature. *Clin Infect Dis* 1996;22:537.
131. Chang FY, Singh N, Gayowski T, et al. Thrombocytopenia in liver transplant recipients: predictors, impact on fungal infections, and role of endogenous thrombopoietin. *Transplantation* 2000;69:70–75.
132. Badger IL, Crosby HA, Kong KL, et al. Is selective bowel decontamination of the digestive tract beneficial in liver transplant patients? Interim results of a prospective, randomized trial. *Transplant Proc* 1991;23:1460–1461.
133. Smith SD, Jackson RJ, Hannakan CJ, et al. Selective decontamination in pediatric liver transplants: a randomized prospective study. *Transplantation* 1993;55:1306–1309.
134. Wajszczuk CP, et al. Fungal infections in liver transplant recipients. *Transplantation* 1985;40:347.
135. Rubin RH, Kemmerly SA, Conti D, et al. Prevention of primary cytomegalovirus disease in organ transplant recipients with oral ganciclovir and oral acyclovir prophylaxis. *Transplant Infect Dis* 2000;2:112–117.
136. Das A. Cost-effectiveness of different strategies of cytomegalovirus prophylaxis in orthotopic liver transplant recipients. *Hepatology* 2000;31:311–317.
137. Okuno T, Takahashi K, Balachandra K, et al. Seroepidemiology of human herpesvirus 6 infection in normal children and adults. *J Clin Microbiol* 1981;27:651–653.
137a. Rogers J, Rohal S, Carrigan DR, et al. Human herpesvirus-6 in liver transplant recipients: role in pathogenesis of fungal infections, neurologic complications, and outcome. *Transplantation* 2000;69:2566–2573.
138. Singh N, Bonham A, Fukui M. Immunosuppressive associated leukoencephalopathy in organ transplant recipients. *Transplantation* 2000;69:467–472.
139. Marinos G, Rossol S, Carucci P, et al. Immunopathogenesis of hepatitis B virus recurrence after liver transplantation. *Transplantation* 2000;69:559–568.
140. Terrault NA, Zhou S, Combs C, et al. Prophylaxis in liver transplant recipients using a fixed dosing schedule of hepatitis B immunoglobulin. *Hepatology* 1996;24:1327–1333.
141. Rayes N, Seehofer D, Hopf U, et al. Comparison of famciclovir and lamivudine in the long-term treatment of hepatitis B infection after liver transplantation. *Transplantation* 2001;71:96–101.
142. Charlton M, Seaberg E, Wiesner R, et al. Predictors of patient and graft survival following liver transplantation for hepatitis C. *Hepatology* 1998;28:823–830.
143. Charlton M. Hepatitis C infection in liver transplantation. *Am J Transplant* 2001;1:197–203.
144. Meyers BR, Papanicolaou GA, Sheiner P, et al. Tuberculosis in orthotopic liver transplant patients: increased toxicity of recommended agents; cure of disseminated infection with nonconventional regimens. *Transplantation* 2000;69:64–69.
145. Speich R, van der Bij W. Epidemiology and management of infections after lung transplantation. *Clin Infect Dis* 2001;33(suppl 1):58–65.
146. Westney GE, Kesten S, De Hoyos A, et al. Aspergillus infection in single and double lung transplant recipients. *Transplantation* 1996;61:915–919.
147. Boehler K, Kesten S, Weder W, et al. Bronchiolitis obliterans after lung transplantation. *Chest* 1998;114:1411–1426.
148. Cohen AH, Sweet SC, Mendeloff E, et al. High incidence of posttransplant lymphoproliferative disease in pediatric patients with cystic fibrosis. *Am J Respir Crit Care* 2000;161:1252–1255.
149. Palmer SM, Perfect JR, Howell DN, et al. Candidal anastomotic infection in lung transplant recipients: successful treatment with a combination of systemic and inhaled antifungal agents. *J Heart Lung Transplant* 1998;17:1029–1033.
150. Martin PJ, et al. A clinical trial of *in-vitro* depletion of T-cells in donor marrow for prevention of acute graft-versus-host disease. *Transplant Proc* 1985;17:486.
151. Bowden RA, Myers JD. Infection complicating bone marrow transplantation. In: Rubin RH, Young LS, eds. *Clinical approach to infection in the compromised host,* 3rd ed. New York: Plenum, 1994.

152. Slavin MA, Osborne B, Adams R, et al. Efficacy and safety of fluconazole for fungal infections after marrow transplant: a prospective, randomized, double-blind study. *J Infect Dis* 1995;171:1545–1552.
153. Menichetti F, Del Favero A, Martino P. GINEMA infection program. Itraconazole oral solution as prophylaxis for fungal infections in neutropenic patients with haematological malignancies: a randomized, placebo-controlled, double-blind, multicenter trial. *Clin Infect Dis* 1999;28:250–255.
154. Sable CA, Donowitz GR. Infections in bone marrow transplant recipients. *Clin Infect Dis* 1994;18:273.
155. Saral R, et al. Acyclovir prophylaxis of herpes simplex virus infections. A randomized double blind, controlled trial in bone marrow recipients. *N Engl J Med* 1981;305:63.
156. Valteau D, et al. Streptococcal septicaemia following autologous bone marrow transplantation in children treated with high-dose chemotherapy. *Bone Marrow Transplant* 1991;7:415–419.
156a. Feld R. Vancomycin as part of initial empirical antibiotic therapy for febrile neutropenia in patients with cancer: pros and cons. *Clin Infect Dis* 1999;29:503–507.
157. EORTC Cooperative Group. Empiric antifungal therapy in febrile granulocytopenic patients. *Am J Med* 1989;86:668.
158. Ramsay PG, et al. Herpes simplex pneumonia: clinical, virological and pathological features in twenty patients. *Ann Intern Med* 1984;100:823.
159. Hertz MI, et al. Respiratory syncytial virus-induced acute lung injury in adult patients with bone marrow transplants: a clinical approach and review of the literature. *Medicine (Baltimore)* 1989;68:269–281.
160. Crawford SW, Hackman RC. Clinical course of idiopathic pneumonia after bone marrow transplantation. *Am Rev Respir Dis* 1993;147:1393–1400.
161. Weiner RS, et al. Risk factors for interstitial pneumonia following bone marrow transplantation for severe aplastic anaemia. *Br J Haematol* 1989;71:535–543.
162. Reed EC, et al. Treatment of cytomegalovirus pneumonia with ganciclovir and intravenous cytomegalovirus immunoglobulin in patients with bone marrow transplants. *Ann Intern Med* 1988;109:783.
163. Meyers JD, et al. Biology of interstitial pneumonia after marrow transplant. In: Gale RP, ed. *Recent advances in bone marrow transplantation.* New York: Alan R. Liss, 1983:405–423.
164. Wolford JL, McDonald GB. A problem-oriented approach to intestinal and liver disease after marrow transplant. *J Gastroenterol* 1988;10:419.
165. Donowitz GR. Infections in bone marrow transplant recipients. In: Mandell GL, Bennett JE, Dolin R, eds. *Principles and practice of infectious diseases,* update 12. New York: Churchill Livingstone, 1992.

# 21. ZOONOSES (INCLUDING LYME DISEASE)

Candace L. Mitchell and J. Thomas Cross, Jr.

## ZOONOSES

Although Virchow coined the phrase "zoonosis," zoonoses have been identified for over 4,000 years. The Eshunni Code of Mesopotamia (before 2300 B.C.) stated that the owner of a vicious dog who had bitten a man causing his death should be fined. This was likely the first description of rabies. In 1959, the World Health Organization convened a committee of experts and **defined zoonosis as "Those diseases and infections naturally transmitted between animals and man."** Today we know that over 200 different zoonoses are transmitted from animals to humans. A single chapter is inadequate to provide the depth necessary to explore each of the many zoonoses encountered in the United States and their widely varying geographic and vector-dependent features. We have selected a few zoonoses and the animals associated with them for a brief review. Lyme disease, which is the most common vector-borne infection in the United States today, is discussed in greater detail.

**I. Factors influencing acquisition of zoonoses.** The probability of zoonotic disease transmission from animals to humans is influenced by many factors: length of time the animal is infective, length of the incubation period in animals, stability of the organism in the environment, available modes of transmission, virulence of the organism for humans, density of infected animals in a community, and community control of wild rodents and insects.

**A. Human contacts with animals.** Domesticated animals are an important part of almost all cultures, including in the United States (Table 21.1). However, many opportunities exist for contact with other animals and disease vectors. **Thus, a thorough exposure and travel history is essential in evaluating patients for a suspected zoonosis.** This identifies the likely animals and vectors encountered, which in turn suggests the most likely possible infections (Tables 21.2 to 21.12).

1. **Pets.** In the United States, it is estimated that 55% of households have a dog or cat. Additionally, 15% to 20% have pet birds. Common pets in the United States are listed in Table 21.1. Their presence in the household should always be sought in the history.
2. **Farm animals** are also frequent in rural households, including those that are not working farms.
3. **Outdoor exposure.** Many people venture into the wilderness for recreation or build houses in undeveloped settings. Others spend their time gardening or similar outdoor activity nearer to the home. This increases the likelihood of exposure to specific animals or vectors for zoonoses. For example, a person camping in Connecticut in the summer is much more likely to be exposed to Lyme disease than is a person camping in southern Louisiana. International travel adds the possibility of more exotic diseases.

**B. Animal and vector contact with humans.** Climate and habitat changes may increase animal and vector populations, permitting their encroachment into residential areas and increasing the chances for disease transmission.

**C. Combinations of human and animal/vector factors** are usually present to influence the transmission of animal-borne infections to humans. For example, the return of forests in the northeast enabled population expansion of the white-tailed deer and white-footed mouse, important hosts in the life cycle of *Ixodes* ticks. Suburban living near forested areas and outdoors activities brought more susceptible people into contact with the tick and contributed to the risk for Lyme disease. Other influences on these complex interactions include natural cycles of food sources for animal reservoirs (such as acorns) and choice of landscaping [1,2].

**D. Routes of transmission.** Zoonoses can be transmitted by any of the following routes:

1. **Direct or indirect contact** with animals (e.g., their feces, urine, saliva, blood, milk, and bedding).
2. **Biting insects.**

Table 21.1. Common Household Pets in the United States

| |
|---|
| Dogs |
| Cats |
| Birds |
| Rodents |
| Hamsters |
| Gerbils |
| Mice |
| Rats |
| Squirrels |
| Reptiles |
| Snakes |
| Iguanas |
| Turtles |
| Fish |
| Monkeys |
| Miniature pigs, goats |
| Ferrets |
| Rabbits |

3. **Inhalation** of airborne contaminated secretions.
4. **Ingestion** of contaminated foods or drinks.
5. **Xenotransplantation** refers to the transfer of animal tissue into humans. This new and developing field is regulated in the United States because of the theoretical risks for transferring animal viruses or other agents into human recipients. Resulting infections have been called "xenoses" or "xenozoonoses" [3]. The risks of cross-species infection have been underscored by the recent demonstration of replication-competent baboon cytomegalovirus in blood from a patient who had received a baboon liver 4 weeks earlier [4] and the propensity of retroviruses to infect varying species [3]. As xenotransplantation becomes more common, surveillance must be maintained for the emergence of new infectious diseases.
6. Interestingly, humans can also transmit infection to animals (e.g., *C. jejuni* spread from owner to dog).

## II. Infections acquired from cats (Table 21.2)

### A. Cat bites [5]

**1. Microbiology**

a. ***Pasteurella multocida*** is a small, nonmotile, polymorphic, gram-negative bacillus. It inhabits the oral cavity and upper respiratory tract of many

Table 21.2. Diseases Associated with Cats

| |
|---|
| Anthrax |
| Campylobacteriosis |
| Cat scratch disease (*Bartonella henselae*) |
| Cryptosporidiosis |
| Pasteurellosis |
| Plague |
| Q fever |
| Rabies |
| Rat bite fever |
| Salmonellosis |
| Toxoplasmosis |
| Tularemia |

animals besides cats (rabbits, rodents, dogs, mice, and birds). Cats and dogs are frequently healthy carriers. This organism has been cultured from 75% of cat bites.

   b. **Other aerobes commonly involved** include *Streptococci, Staphylococci, Moraxella,* and *Neisseria*. **Common anaerobes** include *Fusobacterium, Bacteroides, Porphyromonas,* and *Prevotella. Erysipelothrix rhusiopathiae* has been isolated from cat bites on occasion [3].

2. **Clinical manifestations.** Most bites and scratches lead to local inflammation around the site and can be complicated by abscess formation and/or systemic symptoms. Patients usually present with a wound infection from bites and scratches (Color Plate 4.11). Occasionally, cat bites can lead to meningitis, endocarditis, septic arthritis, and septic shock [6].

3. **Treatment.** Cat bites in general require treatment at the time of the bite because 80% will become infected. **Amoxicillin/clavulanate or doxycycline** is recommended for treatment [7]. It should be noted that *P. multocida* is resistant to dicloxacillin, cephalexin, and clindamycin.

**B. Cat scratches**

1. **Cat scratch disease** was described more than 50 years ago [8]. The causative organism has been identified as ***Bartonella henselae*** (formerly *Rochalimaea*) [9,10]. More than 40,000 cases are diagnosed in the United States annually, with more than 2,000 hospitalizations [10,11]. Most reported cases occur in males under the age of 20 with a peak incidence in the fall and winter [12]. More than 90% of patients have a history of some type of contact with cats, and 57% to 83% have a history of a cat scratch. Highest risk seems to occur with kittens younger than 12 months of age and being exposed to a kitten with fleas.

   a. **The cardinal clinical manifestation is tender regional lymphadenopathy.** Because adenopathy usually appears 1 to 2 weeks after a cat scratch or bite, the **primary inoculation papule or pustule** proximal to the nodes may have subsided or be overlooked. Malaise and other systemic symptoms are common, but significant fever is infrequent. Long-standing nodes may suppurate, but these are the minority. Adenopathy is self-limited, slowly subsiding over several months. Parinaud oculoglandular syndrome occurs with infection of the conjunctiva and ipsilateral preauricular nodes. Other less common manifestations include encephalitis, meningitis, myelitis, hepatic or splenic infection, and osteomyelitis.

   b. **Diagnosis** can be made on clinical grounds for patients with a typical presentation and history of recent cat scratch. Testing for serum antibodies to *B. henselae* is helpful. Biopsy of involved nodes reveals a characteristic granulomatous reaction that is not diagnostic. Organisms can be visualized by Warthin-Starry stain or similar silver impregnation methods. Polymerase chain reaction (PCR) on tissue is sensitive and specific but not readily available. Skin testing is not useful.

   c. **Treatment** of cat scratch disease with most antimicrobials has been ineffective. However, azithromycin in a small (29 patients) prospective, randomized, double-blind, placebo-controlled trial showed 80% reduction in node size in 7 of 14 azithromycin-treated patients during the first 30 days of infection [13]. After 30 days, there was no difference between placebo and azithromycin.

2. **Other syndromes caused by *B. henselae*** include fever of unknown origin and encephalitis in children [10,14]. In patients with acquired immunodeficiency syndrome (AIDS), *B. henselae* from cats has been shown to produce bacillary angiomatosis and hepatic and splenic peliosis; it also frequently causes fever of unknown origin in human immunodeficiency virus-infected patients (see Chapter 18).

3. Occasionally other agents are associated with cat scratches and fleas (Table 21.2). These include tularemia, plague [15], *Capnocytophaga canimorsus* septicemia [16], and the newly recognized gram-negative organism Centers for Disease Control and Prevention (CDC) group NO-1 [17].

**C. Toxoplasmosis (*Toxoplasma gondii*)**

**1.** Cats are the definitive host for the protozoan parasite *T. gondii*. Toxoplasmosis is of particular concern in immunocompromised patients and in pregnant women.

**a. Congenital toxoplasmosis** is the "T" in TORCH infections. *T. gondii* may infect the unborn child by transplacental passage during initial maternal infection. If a mother seroconverts during pregnancy there is a 50% probability that the infant will be infected at the time of delivery; however, only about 10% have clinical manifestations of disease. Clinical presentation in newborns can include chorioretinitis, meningitis, microcephaly, and cerebral calcifications. Additionally, petechiae, hepatosplenomegaly, jaundice, various rashes, and pneumonitis are commonly seen. Diagnosis can be difficult and relies on serologic assays (see Chapter 3).

**b. Toxoplasmosis in immunocompetent hosts** is usually asymptomatic. When clinically apparent the most common manifestation is cervical adenopathy, although other nodes may also be involved. Many patients also have systemic symptoms, and the illness may mimic mononucleosis (see Chapter 9).

**Ocular toxoplasmosis** may cause symptomatic progressive chorioretinitis. Most cases represent congenitally acquired infection, and both eyes may be affected. Acquired toxoplasmosis may also result in retinal involvement; this may occur during acute infection or from later progression. Thus, ocular toxoplasmosis may present at any age (see Chapter 7).

**c. Toxoplasmosis in immunocompromised hosts** is a potentially life-threatening illness. This may result from newly acquired infection or from reactivation of latent infection. Patients with AIDS and others with impaired cell-mediated immunity (e.g., bone marrow or solid organ transplantation) are at greatest risk. Although encephalitis is the most commonly recognized syndrome, other sites of involvement may result in pneumonia, retinitis, myocarditis, and hepatitis. Seronegative immunocompromised patients should take precautions to avoid acquiring toxoplasmosis (see Chapters 6 and 18).

**D. Cat organisms not infectious to humans include** tapeworms, feline giardia, feline immunodeficiency virus, feline infectious peritonitis, and feline leukemia virus.

**III. Infections associated with dogs (Table 21.3).** Dogs may transmit the same organisms as cats. In fact, a case of meningitis due to *Pasteurella* occurred in a woman who kissed her dog frequently.

Table 21.3. Diseases Associated with Dogs

| |
|---|
| Anthrax |
| Blastomycosis |
| Brucellosis |
| Campylobacteriosis |
| *Capnocytophaga* infection |
| Cryptosporidiosis |
| Giardiasis |
| Leptospirosis |
| Lyme borrelliosis |
| Mite infestation |
| Pasteurellosis |
| Rabies |
| Rat bite fever |
| Rocky Mountain spotted fever |
| Salmonellosis |
| Strongyloidiasis |
| Tularemia |
| Yersiniosis |

A. **Rabies** is the most deadly of the diseases that can be transmitted from animals to humans. In the United States the largest concern for this organism occurs in areas where humans infringe on the habitat of infected wild animals, especially raccoons.

1. **The virus** that causes rabies belongs in the genus *Lyssavirus* of the family Rhabdoviridae [18] and causes an acute almost invariably fatal disease. In the United States, wildlife rabies most frequently involves skunks, raccoons, and bats. Only about 5% to 10% of cases occur in domesticated animals each year. Transmission occurs in virus-laden saliva by bite, scratch, or abrasion. Rabid dogs can shed virus for 5 to 7 days before symptoms occur. Aerosol transmission has occurred in laboratory workers, as well as in caves where bats roost.
2. **Animal rabies.** The clinical course in dogs can be divided into three phases: the prodromal, the excitative, and the paralytic. In any animal, the first sign is a change in behavior, which can be indistinguishable from an injury, foreign body in the mouth, poisoning, or an early infectious disease. Temperature change is usually not significant. Animals usually stop eating and drinking and may seek solitude. After the prodromal period of 1 to 3 days, animals either show signs of paralysis or become vicious. The disease progresses rapidly after paralysis develops and death occurs within 10 days of the first signs of infection. Bats flying in daytime are probably rabid.
3. **Human rabies.** Cases in the United States rarely have a history of an animal bite, although this is much more common in other parts of the world. Pain appears at the site of the bite, followed by paresthesias. The skin is sensitive to changes of temperature, especially wind or air-conditioning currents. Attempts at drinking cause extremely painful laryngeal spasm, so that the patient refuses to drink (hydrophobia). Large amounts of thick tenacious saliva are present. The patient is restless and behaves in an unusual manner. Muscle spasm, laryngospasm, and extreme excitability are present. Seizures are common.
4. **Diagnosis** in animals can be established by viral isolation from body fluid or tissue or fluorescent antibody staining of tissues, including cornea, frozen skin, and brain. Human diagnosis premortem is usually made by PCR or staining for viral antigen in saliva, skin, brain, or cornea. Nuchal skin biopsy and saliva offer better yields than do corneal specimens.
5. **Treatment** is usually supportive and the disease is invariably fatal in humans.
6. **Prevention [19].** Prophylaxis is essential because there is no treatment for clinical rabies. Nonetheless, each year in the United States many more persons than necessary receive postexposure rabies prophylaxis.
   a. **Preexposure prophylaxis** with vaccine is indicated for veterinarians, animal handlers, and persons with potential exposure to rabies (e.g., spelunkers). Booster doses are indicated when antibody levels fall.
   b. **Postexposure prophylaxis** is given after a careful consideration of the animal and the exposure. In the United States rabies is almost never transmitted by adequately vaccinated dogs or cats, squirrels, lagomorphs, and small rodents, including gerbils and hamsters. If a biting dog, cat, or ferret is healthy and available, prophylaxis may be withheld while the animal is observed for 10 days. Prophylaxis should be started at the first sign of a rabies-compatible illness, and the animal should be killed for testing. **Animals such as skunks, foxes, raccoons, coyotes, and bats should be regarded as rabid** unless captured and proven otherwise. Local authorities should be consulted to review the current epidemiology of rabies in the animal species under scrutiny, including dogs and cats that are unavailable for observation or testing.

      **The circumstances of the incident should be thoroughly elucidated.** Unprovoked attacks are an indication of increased risk. The details of the exposure must be ascertained, including whether a bite occurred and if there was saliva exposure to cuts, broken skin, or mucous membranes (see also Chapters 4 and 23).
      (1) **The wound should be cleaned** with soap and water or a virucidal preparation (e.g., povidone-iodine).
      (2) **Rabies immune globulin, 20 IU/kg,** should be infiltrated around the wound to the fullest possible extent. Any remaining rabies immune

globulin should be given intramuscularly at a site distant from vaccine. Previously vaccinated individuals do not need rabies immune globulin.

(3) **Rabies vaccine** (any of the available preparations) should be given. It is administered intramuscularly in the deltoid on days 0, 3, 7, 14, and 28; previously vaccinated individuals only need injections on days 0 and 3. Small children may be given vaccine in the thigh (see Chapter 23).

**B. Leptospirosis**

1. **Animal sources.** Dogs, rats, mice, guinea pigs, gerbils, rabbits, hamsters, and reptiles can transmit *Leptospira* to humans. It has been noted that 40% of stray dogs may be seropositive for this organism. Rodents are the only major animal species that can shed leptospires throughout their lifespan without clinical evidence of disease. Active shedding by lab animals can go unnoticed until personnel handling the animals become ill.
2. **Transmission.** The organism is most often transmitted to humans by the urine of the reservoir host and may survive in water for prolonged periods. Handling affected animals, contaminating hands or abrasions with urine, or aerosol exposure during cage cleaning are among the most common routes of acquisition. Many infections are reported in those after bathing or swimming in infected waters or with infected pets. The organism may also enter through minor skin abrasions and the conjunctiva. Outdoor activities, including athletic events, are important risk factors [20].
3. **Animal disease.** In cattle, fever and anorexia occur with rapid decline in milk yield and atypical mastitis. Pregnant cows abort with retention of placenta. In dogs and cats, gastroenteritis, jaundice, and nephritis may occur.
4. **Human disease.** This ranges from inapparent infection (most) to severe illness and death. Although leptospirosis is classically a biphasic illness, signs and symptoms are frequently continuous and not biphasic. Initially, weakness, headache, myalgias, chills, and fever occur. This is accompanied by leukocytosis, painful orchitis, conjunctival suffusion, and nonspecific rash. Improvement generally occurs within a week, but fever and myalgias may recur if the patient has a biphasic illness. It is during this phase that aseptic meningitis may be present (see Chapter 6). Icteric leptospirosis (Weil syndrome) is the most severe form of the disease, characterized by impaired renal and hepatic function, abnormal mental status, pulmonary infiltrates, hypotension, and a 5% to 10% mortality rate.
5. **Diagnosis.** The organism may be identified by darkfield examination of the patient's blood or urine, but this requires expert interpretation. Culture of blood, urine, and cerebrospinal fluid (CSF) should be attempted but is difficult and requires several weeks. Cultures are usually only positive in the blood and central nervous system (CNS) in the first week of infection and in the urine later in disease. Antibody testing may provide a retrospective diagnosis. PCR testing is not widely available.
6. **Treatment.** The value of treatment in mild cases is controversial, but antibiotics should be given to patients with more severe illness. Penicillin G (1.5 million units qid) or ampicillin can be used intravenously for moderate or severe disease, and amoxicillin or doxycycline may be used orally for mild disease.
7. **Prevention** involves several steps. Vaccination in cattle, swine, and dogs is important to eliminate domestic reservoirs. Risky activities should be avoided, particularly swimming in or drinking from potentially contaminated water. Animal workers should wear boots and gloves. Rodent control is also important. Weekly doxycycline has been used for those who cannot avoid prolonged potential exposures [20].

**IV. Diseases associated with other animals (Tables 21.4 to 21.12)**

**A. Salmonellosis.** For many years, infections with *Salmonella* species have been a problem in the United States. Animals commonly associated with this infection included chickens and turtles, but the recent popularity of iguanas has resulted in these animals as a commonly reported source. This has been especially important in pediatric cases (see Chapter 13).

**B. Plague** is an acute febrile illness caused by the gram-negative bacillus *Yersinia pestis*. Human infection results from the bites of infected rodent fleas. The incubation

Table 21.4. Diseases Associated with Amphibians, Iguanas, Snakes, and Turtles

| |
|---|
| *Aeromonas* infection |
| *Campylobacter* infection |
| *Edwardsiella* infection |
| *Mycobacterium ulcerans* infection |
| *Ophionyssus* infestation |
| Pentastomiasis |
| Q fever |
| Salmonellosis |
| Sparganosis |

Table 21.5. Diseases Associated with Cattle, Horses, Sheep, and Goats

| |
|---|
| *Actinobacillus* infection |
| *Actinomyces* infection |
| Anthrax |
| Brucellosis |
| Campylobacteriosis |
| *Chlamydia psittaci* infection |
| Cowpox |
| Crytposporidiosis |
| *Escherichia coli* 0157:H7 infection |
| Giardiasis |
| Leptospirosis |
| *Mycobacterium bovis* infection |
| Orf virus infection |
| Q fever |
| Rabies |
| Salmonellosis |
| Variant Creutzfeldt-Jakob disease (mad cow disease) |
| Yersiniosis |

Table 21.6. Diseases Associated with Pigs

| |
|---|
| Anthrax |
| Ascariasis |
| Botulism |
| Brucellosis |
| Cryptosporidiosis |
| *Entamoeba* infection |
| *Erysipelothrix* infection |
| Leptospirosis |
| *Pasteurella* infection |
| Rabies |
| Sarcosporidiosis |
| $\beta$-Hemolytic *Streptococcus* infection |
| Swine influenza virus infection |
| *Yersinia enterocolitica* infection |

Table 21.7. Diseases Associated with Bats

| |
|---|
| Histoplasmosis |
| Lyssavirus infection |
| Mokola virus infection |
| Rabies |

Table 21.8. Diseases Associated with Rabbits and Hares

| |
|---|
| Brucellosis |
| *Microsporum canis* infection |
| Q fever |
| Tularemia |
| *Yersinia pestis* infection (plague) |

Table 21.9. Diseases Associated with Birds

| |
|---|
| Campylobacteriosis |
| Histoplasmosis |
| Newcastle disease virus infection |
| Psittacosis |
| Salmonellosis |
| *Streptococcus pyogenes* infection |
| *Yersinia pseudotuberculosis* infection |

Table 21.10. Diseases Associated with Rodents

| |
|---|
| Campylobacteriosis |
| Endemic (murine) typhus |
| Hantavirus infection |
| *Hymenolepis diminuta* infection |
| Lassa fever |
| Leptospirosis |
| Listeriosis |
| Lymphocytic choriomeningitis virus infection |
| Rabies |
| Rat bite fever |
| Rat mite infestation |
| Relapsing fever |
| Rickettsialpox |
| Venezuelan hemorrhagic fever |
| *Yersinia pestis* infection (plague) |

Table 21.11. Diseases Acquired from Fish

| |
|---|
| Anisakiasis |
| Botulism |
| Capillariasis |
| *Clonorchiasis sinensis* infection |
| Diocytophymatid larval nematode infection |
| Diphyllobothriasis |
| *Erysipelothrix* infection |
| Gnathostomiasis |
| Intestinal fluke infection |
| *Mycobacterium marinum* infection |
| *Nanophyetus salmincola* infection |
| Opisthorchiasis |
| Salmonellosis |
| *Vibrio* infection |

period is usually 2 to 8 days. The clinical course can be rapidly fatal without prompt therapy. In the United States, plague is generally confined to the southwestern United States with ground squirrels, prairie dogs, and wood rats being the common reservoirs. Classic bubonic plague occurs with sudden onset of fever, chills, and headache followed quickly by a localized lymphadenitis known as a bubo. See Chapters 4 and 11 for a further discussion of plague.

**C. Brucellosis (undulant fever)**

1. **Epidemiology.** Most cases in the United States are due to occupational exposure to *Brucella abortus* from cattle; veterinarians, farmers, and abattoir workers are at greatest risk. Those affected are mainly men, and occasionally laboratory and technical personnel are infected. However, in Texas and Florida the ingestion of unpasteurized dairy products infected with *Brucella melitensis* (from goats, sheep, and camels) occurs in adults and children of both sexes. *B. melitensis* produces a more severe clinical pattern and can produce a chronic form. *B. suis* is found in swine, and *B. canis* is found in dogs.
2. **Clinical manifestations.** Acute infection presents with high fever, malaise, headache, sweats, and arthralgias. In many cases, constipation, back pain, and weight loss are found. Weight loss of 20 pounds in 2 months is not uncommon. Localization of infection may occur at any time in the illness and is heralded by symptoms and signs in that organ system. Hepatic enlargement may indicate granulomatous hepatitis or abscess, and splenomegaly may be seen. Hematologic manifestations include various forms of cytopenias. Articular complaints are seen with reactive arthritis and septic arthritis. Vertebral osteomyelitis may also occur. CNS findings may indicate neurobrucellosis. Renal and cardiac involvement are possible.

   A subacute form occurs more commonly in endemic areas of the world (known as Malta fever). The chronic form occurs after a year of illness and usually requires bone marrow biopsy to diagnose.
3. **Diagnosis** is usually made by routine agglutination assays to detect antibodies to *Brucella*. However, *B. canis* does not react in the standard assay, and must be requested from the CDC. Blood or bone marrow cultures are helpful but must be incubated for at least 2 weeks. The laboratory should be notified when brucellosis is suspected to correctly process cultures.
4. **Treatment** is difficult because of the intracellular nature of the infection. In adults oral doxycycline 100 mg twice daily for 45 days plus streptomycin 1 g intramuscularly daily for 2 weeks or doxycycline 100 mg twice daily plus oral rifampin 600 mg daily for 45 days are recommended. In children under the age of 8, a combination of oral rifampin 15 to 20 mg/kg once daily for 4 weeks plus gentamicin for 5 to 10 days is effective.
5. **Prevention** is by control of animal infections and proper food safety measures.

Table 21.12. Diseases Acquired from Exotic Animals

| |
|---|
| Armadillos |
| Leprosy |
| Bears |
| Trichinosis |
| Camels |
| Brucellosis |
| *Camploybacter* infection |
| Plague |
| Salmonellosis |
| Elephants |
| Anthrax |
| *Mycobacterium tuberculosis* infection |
| Salmonellosis |
| Vaccinia |
| Marsupials |
| Leptospirosis |
| *Pasturella* infection |
| Q fever |
| Salmonellosis |
| *Sarcoptes scabei* infestation |
| Tinea |
| Monkeys and other nonhuman primates |
| *Bertiella* infection |
| *Campylobacter* infection |
| *Entamoeba* infection |
| Hepatitis A |
| *Herpesvirus simiae* infection |
| Leprosy |
| Measles |
| Monkeypox |
| *Mycobacterium bovis* infection |
| *Mycobacterium tuberculosis* infection |
| Salmonellosis |
| Shigellosis |
| Simian immunodeficiency virus infection |
| Tularemia |
| Raccoons |
| *Baylisascaris* infection |
| *Edwardsiella* infection |
| Rabies |
| Salmonellosis |
| Seals, sea lions, and walruses |
| Influenza A |
| Trichinosis |
| Weasels, otters, badgers, skunks |
| Bovine tuberculosis |
| Rabies |
| Whales, dolphins, porpoises |
| *Mycobacterium marinum* infection |

**D. Psittacosis.** *Chlamydia psittaci* has a wide range of host species, including birds, humans, and lower mammals. The systemic illness associated with *C. psittaci* has been termed "psittacosis" because of its association with parrots and other psittacine birds. The term "ornithosis" is likely more appropriate because of the wide range of birds that harbor this organism.

1. **Epidemiology.** Those at greatest risk include workers in aviaries, poultry abattoirs, zoos, pet shops, and veterinary offices. Poultry breeders are at significant risk and account for most outbreaks. It must be noted that birds can be healthy appearing yet transmit the disease.
2. **Clinical manifestations.** *C. psittaci* is inhaled in aerosol form and travels to the alveoli. It disseminates to regional lymph nodes and the reticuloendothelial system. Classically it presents as an atypical pneumonia (see Chapter 11), although it may also manifest as fever of unknown origin (see Chapter 1). Endocarditis, rash, panniculitis, and a pseudotyphoid presentation can occur. Incubation periods range from 5 to 21 days. In about 20% of cases no exposure to birds is found. Most patients present with fever, sweats, and minimally productive cough. Headache may be prominent and can be helpful in the setting of pneumonitis. Diarrhea and myalgias are also common. Splenomegaly and hepatomegaly may be found. Chest radiography usually shows a lobar infiltrate, but any pattern is possible.
3. **Diagnosis** is based on serologic confirmation. A fourfold rise in complement fixation antibody titer, or a random titer greater than 1:32, supports the diagnosis in a patient with a compatible illness. Because the complement fixation test detects cross-reacting antibodies with other *Chlamydia,* the serum microimmunofluorescence assay may be used to detect specific antibodies.
4. **Therapy.** The antibiotic of choice is usually a tetracycline, and patients usually improve within the first few days. Most use doxycycline 100 mg twice daily for 14 to 21 days. In endocarditis, courses up to 6 weeks of a tetracycline are recommended and valve replacement is almost invariably necessary. The newer agent azithromycin has been shown to be effective at a dose of 10 mg/kg of body weight for 7 days.

**E. Tularemia**

1. **Epidemiology.** *Francisella tularensis* is a gram-negative coccobacillus that causes the disease tularemia. Sources of the organism include over 100 species of wild animals (most commonly rabbits, hares, squirrels, and deer), some domestic animals (rabbits, cats, dogs, and cattle), and arthropods (particularly ticks, deerflies, and mosquitoes). In the United States, rabbits and ticks are the major sources for infection. People at risk are those with occupational or recreational exposure to infected animals or their habitat. The incubation period is usually 1 to 21 days, with most cases occurring 3 to 5 days after exposure.
2. **Clinical manifestations.** Tularemia can occur in six distinct forms. The most common is the ulceroglandular syndrome characterized by a primary painful maculopapular skin lesion at the site of entry (see Chapter 4). Illness usually begins acutely or subacutely with nonspecific symptoms that include fevers, myalgias, and malaise. There is subsequent ulceration and slow healing of the skin lesion (Color Plates 4.10 and 4.25), with associated painful and acutely inflamed lymph nodes that may drain spontaneously.

   The other forms of tularemia are glandular (where no skin or mucous membrane lesion is present), oculoglandular (severe conjunctivitis and preauricular lymph node involvement), oropharyngeal (severe exudative pharyngitis), typhoidal (high fever, hepatosplenomegaly), and pneumonic (see Chapter 11).
3. **Diagnosis** is most often established by serologic assays (see Chapter 11). A fourfold rise in tube agglutinin titer frequently is found after the second week of illness. An isolated titer of 1:160 or greater, or a microagglutination titer of 1:128 or greater, is consistent with recent or past infection.
4. The **treatment** of choice has been streptomycin. However, with recent shortages of the drug, gentamicin has become the recommended agent. Duration of therapy is usually 6 to 10 days. Tetracyclines may be used but have a higher relapse rate and are usually reserved for less severe infections.

### F. Ehrlichiosis

1. **Epidemiology** [21]. There are two distinct forms of ehrlichiosis infection in the United States. The human monocytic form (HME) occurs in persons from the southeastern and south central United States. HME is caused by *Ehrlichia chaffeensis* and is transmitted by the Lone Star tick (*Amblyomma americanum*). Most cases of human granulocytic ehrlichiosis (HGE) have been reported from Wisconsin, Minnesota, Connecticut, and New York, but cases have been reported in many states, particularly those on the west coast. Most cases of HGE are due to *Ehrlichia phagocytophila* [22]. HGE is transmitted by the *Ixodes scapularis* tick, which also is the vector of *Borrelia burgdorferi* (the agent of Lyme disease). The principal reservoirs for the agents of human ehrlichiosis remain to be identified, although white-tailed deer and white-footed mice may be infected naturally with *E. chaffeensis* and *E. phagocytophila*. Patients with *Ehrlichia* are characteristically older than those with Rocky Mountain spotted fever, and age-specific incidences are highest in persons older than 40 years of age. Most infections occur between April and September; peak occurrence is in May through July. Coinfections with other tick-borne diseases, including babesiosis and Lyme disease, are reported [23]. The incubation period typically is 7 to 14 days after a tick bite. The canine species *E. ewingii* may occasionally cause human infections, including in patients with AIDS [24].
2. **Clinical manifestations.** The two disease forms have different causes but similar presentations [25,26]. Both are acute, systemic, febrile illnesses that are similar to Rocky Mountain spotted fever except more frequently have leukopenia, anemia, and hepatitis. Ehrlichiosis presents with rash less frequently than Rocky Mountain spotted fever. The febrile illness often is accompanied by headache, chills, malaise, myalgias, arthralgias, nausea, and vomiting. If rash does occur, it typically develops 1 week after onset of illness and occurs in only 50% of reported cases of HME and fewer than 10% of those with HGE. Diarrhea, abdominal pain, and change in mental status occur on occasion. Reported complications of both forms include pulmonary infiltrates, bone marrow hypoplasia, respiratory failure, encephalopathy, meningitis, disseminated intravascular coagulation, and renal failure; although both may cause severe infections, mortality has been higher with HME. Anemia, hyponatremia, leukopenia, thrombocytopenia, elevated liver enzyme concentrations, and CSF abnormalities are common. Both diseases typically last 1 to 2 weeks, and recovery generally proceeds without sequelae. However, neurologic complications have been reported in some children. Additionally, fatal and asymptomatic infections are reported.
3. **Diagnosis.** The CDC defines a confirmed case of ehrlichiosis as one with a fourfold or greater rise in indirect immunofluorescent assay antibody titer between acute and convalescent samples (ideally collected 3–6 weeks apart), or PCR amplification of ehrlichial DNA from a clinical sample, or detection of intraleukocytoplasmic *Ehrlichia* microcolonies (morulae) and a single immunofluorescent assay titer of more than 64. A probable case is defined as a single immunofluorescent assay titer of more than 64 or the presence of morulae within infected leukocytes. Tests for HME and HGE must be requested separately because they are designed to detect the different specific causative agents.
4. **Treatment.** Doxycycline is the drug of choice for treatment. The recommended dosage of doxycycline is 100 mg intravenously or orally twice daily for adults and 3 to 4 mg/kg/day in two divided doses for children (to a maximum of the adult dose). For children younger than 8 years of age, the recommendations are to use doxycycline as the risk of serious disease is much greater than the risk of teeth or bone abnormalities for the short course of therapy. Treatment is continued for 3 days after defervescence and a minimum total course of 5 to 7 days. Severe or complicated disease may require longer treatment courses. It is prudent to start presumptive therapy with doxycycline for patients with clinical evidence of disease and no other identified cause.
5. **Prevention.** Specific measures should focus on limiting exposure to ticks. No data exist on the use of prophylactic antibiotics after tick bite for this infection.

**G. Babesiosis** [27]

1. **Epidemiology** [28]. The primary reservoir for *Babesia microti* is the white-footed mouse (*Peromyscus leucopus*), and the primary vector is the tick *Ixodes scapularis*. This tick can also transmit Lyme disease and human granulocytic ehrlichiosis. Humans acquire infection from the bites of infected ticks, although recently lice and fleas have also been implicated as vectors. The white-tailed deer (*Odocoileus virginianus*) is the important host for the tick but is not a reservoir for *B. microti*. An increase in the deer population in the last few decades is thought to be a major factor in the spread of *I. scapularis* and the infections they transmit. Rare cases have been reported from blood transfusions. Transplacental and perinatal transmission of babesiosis have also been reported. Most cases have been reported in the northeast, midwest, and west coast of the United States. Most cases occur in the summer or fall. In endemic areas, asymptomatic infections are common. The incubation period ranges from 1 to 9 weeks.
2. **Clinical manifestations** [29]. Many clinical features are similar to those of malaria. Patients with babesiosis present with gradual onset of malaise, anorexia, and fatigue. This is followed by fever, with temperatures as high as 40°C, and one or more of the following symptoms: chills, sweats, myalgias, arthralgias, nausea, and vomiting. Less common findings are emotional lability and depression, hyperesthesia, headache, sore throat, abdominal pain, conjunctival injection, photophobia, weight loss, and nonproductive cough. Physical examination usually has minimal findings often consisting only of fever, but mild splenomegaly and hepatomegaly have been reported. The illness can last for a few weeks to several months with a prolonged recovery taking up to 18 months. Severe illness is most likely in people older than 40 years of age, those with asplenia, and in the immunocompromised (including human immunodeficiency virus infection). Splenectomized persons are particularly at risk for death and severe infection.
3. **Diagnosis.** Microscopic identification of the organism on Giemsa- or Wright-stained thick and thin blood smears establishes the diagnosis. Multiple thick and thin smears may be required. Serologic tests are available from the CDC but require 2 to 4 weeks to become positive; thus, examination of blood smears should always be done.
4. **Therapy** is generally reserved for those with moderate or severe disease. Most with a mild clinical course are undiagnosed and recover without specific therapy. The combination of clindamycin (adult dose of 1.2 g twice daily intravenously or 600 mg three times daily orally) and oral quinine (adult dose of 650 mg three times a day) for 7 days or atovaquone (adult dose of 750 mg orally every 12 hours) and azithromycin (adult dose of 500 mg orally on day 1 and then 250 mg/day) for 7 days are the current regimens of choice [30]. Exchange transfusions have been successful in asplenic patients with life-threatening disease and should be considered in severely ill patients with a high parasitemia.
5. **Prevention.** Specific recommendations concern prevention of tick bites.

**H. *Baylisascaris procyonis* infection** is an under-appreciated emerging infection [31]. It also has the potential to be used as an agent of bioterrorism because it is quite hardy, the infectious inoculum is small, illness is severe, and there is no vaccine or effective therapy [31].

1. **Epidemiology.** The infectious roundworm of raccoons, *B. procyonis,* is an increasingly recognized human pathogen. The host raccoon, *Procyon lotor,* is widespread in its distribution, with human infections being documented in California, Massachusetts, New York, Michigan, Illinois, Pennsylvania, and Germany. Greater than 90% of juvenile raccoons are parasitized and can excrete up to 45,000,000 eggs per day in stool. Latrines where raccoons communally defecate have been found in close proximity to playgrounds and neighborhoods, raising concern over potential infection of children at play. Pica is an important risk factor for infection, with infants being especially at risk due to their propensity for oral exploration of their surroundings.
2. **Clinical manifestations.** Humans are dead-end hosts, and disease represents worm migration through tissues. The complete clinical spectrum of disease and the frequency of asymptomatic infections currently are not known. **Eosinophilic**

**meningoencephalitis** has been the most commonly recognized presentation, but retinitis and eosinophilic cardiac pseudotumor have also been described [31]. Severe neurologic and/or ocular sequelae occur early after larval invasion.

3. **Diagnosis.** This infection should be considered when meningoencephalitis, diffuse unilateral subacute neuroretinitis, or cardiac pseudotumor occurs in patients with a history of pica and raccoon exposure, especially in the setting of **blood and CNS eosinophilia.** Imaging studies reveal diffuse white matter disease. Definitive diagnosis requires observation of larval forms in the tissues. However, biopsy may not contain larvae or they may be misidentified due to the rarity of the infection. Several reported cases of diffuse unilateral subacute neuroretinitis have been associated with tissue larval parasites. Serologic testing is performed in research settings, but no serologic test is commercially available.
4. **Treatment** consists of supportive care only. Several antihelminthic agents have been tried in human infections without efficacy. All reported human cases either died or sustained severe neurologic and/or ocular sequelae [31].
5. **Prevention.** Infants and developmentally challenged adults must be observed closely for pica behaviors. Ownership of raccoons as pets should be discouraged unless the animals are routinely evaluated for the presence of intestinal parasites. A public awareness program informing communities about the risks of interaction with raccoon feces is important (discouraging feeding wild raccoons and explaining the hazards of not securing pet food), especially in neighborhoods where large numbers of raccoons share human habitat. Routine screening of children or adults is not recommended.

## LYME DISEASE

The manifestations of Lyme disease have been well described since early in the 1900's. Various worldwide clinical presentations have been recognized as "erythema chronicum migrans," "Bannwarth syndrome," and "acrodermatitis chronica atrophicans" [32]. In 1975, children in Lyme, Connecticut experienced an outbreak of oligoarticular arthritis resulting in increased investigations for an etiology [33]. Yale researchers were able to link the neurologic sequelae with the erythema migrans (EM) rash and an antecedent tick bite as a syndrome named for the town in which it appeared. In 1982, a spirochete isolated from the midgut of the *Ixodes* tick was implicated as the causative agent of Lyme disease [33–35]. This spirochete, ***Borrelia burgdorferi,*** is now established as the definitive etiologic agent and occurs in at least three groups (together referred to as *B. burgdorferi sensu lato*). Although present in many parts of the world, the focus of this discussion is on Lyme disease in the United States, which is caused by *B. burgdorferi sensu stricto*.

I. **Epidemiology.** Lyme disease is the most common vector-borne illness in the United States with more than 15,000 cases each year. Most cases occur in children and in middle-aged adults, although all ages can be affected and there is no sex predilection.

A. **Endemic regions.** The most important historical information to obtain when considering Lyme disease is whether a patient lives in or has visited an endemic area. In the absence of a classic presentation, if no endemic exposure history is elicited the diagnosis of Lyme disease is significantly more difficult [36]. **In the United States there are three endemic areas:** the Northeast (New York, New Jersey, Massachusetts, Rhode Island, Connecticut, Pennsylvania, Virginia), the Midwest (Wisconsin, Minnesota), and the Pacific Coast (Oregon, California) [37].

B. **Vectors.** Four species of *Ixodes* ticks serve as *B. burgdorferi* vectors, including *I. scapularis* (Northeast and Midwest), *Ixodes pacificus* (Pacific Coast), *Ixodes ricinum* (Europe), and *Ixodes persulcatus* (Asia) [38,39]. Human risk is predicated on the regional density of ticks and the percentage of their parasitism by spirochetes [40,41]. The ticks begin as larvae and enter adulthood after evolution through a nymphal stage, which is the period of their life cycle when most infections are transmitted. The animal reservoirs available to nymphal ticks are determinants of overall tick parasitism and thus are indirectly responsible for the prevalence of human disease. In the Northeast and Midwest, nymphal ticks feed on white-footed mice, a thriving reservoir for *B. burgdorferi*. In contrast, in the Pacific region, *I. pacificus* ticks feed on lizards, a poor spirochete reservoir, and to a much lesser extent the dusky-footed woodrat. Only those *Ixodes* ticks in the Pacific region that feed on the woodrat carry enough spirochetes to cause human infection; hence, the prevalence of Lyme disease in California and Oregon is less than that observed in the Northeast and Midwest [42–44]. Nymphal ticks reside on tips of tall grasses in the summer months, which helps account for the abundance of clinical cases in the summer and early fall [36]. White-tailed deer are hosts to adult ticks and are critical to completing the tick life cycle.

**II. Pathogenesis**

**A. Transmission and incubation period.** *B. burgdorferi* adapts to the midgut of its tick host, traverses to the tick salivary glands, and is transmitted during the blood meal. Dissemination occurs to the skin and hematogenously to many other sites including the joints, heart, and CNS. The small *Ixodes* ticks must be attached for longer than 24 hours before sufficient transfer of spirochetes occurs to cause disease. The incubation period for cutaneous lesions is generally between 7 and 14 days and ranges from 3 to 32 days after the initial bite [45]. However, in many patients there is no history of a specific tick bite in the region of the skin lesion because ticks that are noticed are removed before they can efficiently transmit the organism.

**B. Outer surface proteins** of *B. burgdorferi* are its major virulence factor, and they promote attachment to mammalian cells [37]. Organism binding to cellular and extracellular matrix components contributes to its tissue tropism. Spirochete tissue spread is accomplished in part through binding of host plasminogen and urokinase-type plasminogen activator to its surface. Plasmin is then activated and acts as a protease, which facilitates tissue invasion [46]. The spirochetes secrete no toxins and require the host to provide all elements of nutritional support [47]. They are capable of remaining viable in host tissues for prolonged periods of time in the absence of treatment.

**C. The host immune response** is slow to develop and results in a broad range of specific antibodies. In murine models there is a genetic determination of susceptibility and the host immune response in controlling early spirochete dissemination. *B. burgdorferi* is a potent stimulus for pro-inflammatory mediator production, and histology of lesions is marked by mononuclear cell infiltrates with some degree of vascular damage. In cases of chronic arthritis, joint destruction is ascribed to an ongoing inflammatory response that may continue despite antibiotic sterilization of the joint.

**III. Clinical manifestations.** The uninterrupted **disease evolves through three phases:** early localized disease; early disseminated disease to the skin, nervous system, heart, and joints; and late disease [37,48]. **It is most important to understand that not all phases may be clinically recognized and that overlap can exist among these phases.** Thus, late manifestations may occur without any preceding signs or symptoms of infection, and patients with late neurologic disease may have EM lesions or chronic arthritis.

**A. Early localized disease** begins when the tick regurgitates or salivates sufficient spirochetes into the bite, with subsequent local inflammation occurring at the site. As the spirochetes move centrifugally within the skin away from the bite, they create the classic rash of **EM** (Color Plate 4.4) [36,49]. EM lesions are flat with partial central clearing and usually have a bright red outer border and a target center; variations exist with some lesions being homogenous and losing the target center, and others having vesicular centers [37]. In fact, these "atypical" EM lesions may be more common than the classic target appearance [50].

The bite of the Lone Star tick (*A. americanum*) has been associated with an EM-like illness in the southeastern United States, called southern tick-associated rash illness or STARI [51,52]. Such patients have had no evidence by culture or serology of *B. burgdorferi* infection. *Borrelia lonestari,* an uncultured spirochete found in *A. americanum* ticks, is a likely cause for this syndrome [52].

**B. Early disseminated disease** occurs within weeks or months of infection and is marked by systemic illness with **fever, headaches, myalgias, arthralgias, and/or lymphadenopathy.** It also may involve the **skin, CNS, or heart.**

1. During this phase 50% of patients experience **new EM lesions,** which are often multiple and in new sites [36].
2. **Acute neuroborreliosis** develops in 15% of untreated patients and results from spirochetes invading the CNS during early dissemination; it usually presents weeks or months after infection. Lymphocytic meningitis (see Chapter 6), encephalitis, cranial nerve involvement, radiculopathies, mononeuritis multiplex, cerebellar ataxia, and myelitis may occur [37,53,54]. **Bell palsy** may be an isolated manifestation of early disseminated disease, or it may occur with other neurologic findings in late disease [55]. It is a common manifestation, occurring in 50% of those with meningitis, and may be bilateral. However, because isolated cranial nerve VII palsy is caused more commonly by herpes infection in nonendemic areas, it is not considered a *sina qua non* of Lyme disease [56]. Case reports detail *B. burgdorferi*-infected children who developed optic nerve damage secondary to nerve inflammation or increased intracranial pressure resulting in blindness. Pseudotumor cerebri is another rare CNS phenomenon observed in children secondary to Lyme disease [57].
3. **Lyme carditis** develops in 5% of untreated patients [37]. The median time to presentation of cardiac involvement is 5 weeks after acute infection. Common symptoms include dyspnea, syncope, dizziness, and palpitations [58]. **The most common abnormality is atrioventricular block,** and a PR interval longer than 300 ms predicts an increased risk of complete heart block [59]. Myocarditis occurs less frequently, and valvular disease has not been reported [36].

**C. Late disease**

1. **Arthritis** occurs in 60% of untreated patients months after the initial infection and is the most common form of late disease. It manifests **primarily in the large joints (especially the knees),** causing recurrent asymmetric monoarticular or oligoarticular arthritis [58]. Joints have significant swelling and warmth but minimal erythema, and joint erosions can occur, leading to significant disability. Baker cysts are seen frequently and result in further debilitation secondary to swelling and pain [60]. Joint fluid contains various numbers of leukocytes that are mostly neutrophils. Synovial biopsy reveals hypertrophy, vascular proliferation, and a mononuclear cell infiltrate. Untreated patients often have recurrent attacks and are considered to have chronic Lyme arthritis if these continue for 1 year or longer. Ten percent of cases develop chronic arthritis despite adequate antimicrobial therapy, especially in those patients with HLA-DRB1*0401 or related alleles [61], suggesting an autoimmune pathogenesis. Fatigue may be prominent in many patients with chronic arthritis and is episodic with periods of wellness between attacks [60,62,63].
2. **Chronic neurologic syndromes** develop in as many as 5% of untreated patients and may become apparent many years after the original infection [37]. "Lyme encephalopathy" is characterized by subtle cognitive deficits in adults [64,65], and children may experience mood swings, decreased concentration, and declining school performance. Focal CNS lesions may occur characterized by a chronic axonal polyneuropathy, spinal radicular pain, or distal paresthesias [54,66]. In the European species of *Borrelia,* vestibular and optic neuritis have been observed in combination with cognitive impairment [54].
3. Violaceous skin lesions that become sclerotic or atrophic over time are acrodermatitis chronica atrophicans and are found in Europe and Asia as a result of *Borrelia afzelii* infection [37].

**D. Lyme disease during pregnancy.** The clinical manifestations of Lyme disease in pregnant women are the same as in nonpregnant patients. Despite a few case reports of fetal transmission of *B. burgdorferi,* prospective studies have failed to identify documented cases of congenital infection or an adverse effect on pregnancy outcome [48,67].

**E.** "Chronic Lyme disease" and "post-Lyme disease syndrome" are terms that have been applied to heterogeneous groups of patients with myalgias, arthralgias, neurocognitive impairment, or fatigue that persists after adequate antibiotic treatment [37,68,69]. Recently the validity of these terms has been questioned because there is little evidence to support them as specific diagnoses [68,69]. **Fatigue alone,**

**without any other convincing evidence of Lyme disease, should not be considered Lyme disease.**

**IV. Diagnosis.** To reduce over-diagnosis and unnecessary treatment, the CDC developed a case definition for Lyme disease that requires the classic EM rash or another characteristic clinical manifestation with positive laboratory evidence of *B. burgdorferi* infection [70]. When evaluating patients for possible Lyme disease, routine laboratory studies (liver function tests, erythrocyte sedimentation rate, etc.) generally are not helpful.

**A. Culture** of *B. burgdorferi* from blood, synovial aspirate, or CSF is difficult [58]. Spirochetes can be grown from the leading edge of the lesions in 50% of EM cases when cultured on Barbour-Stoenner-Kelly medium [71]. A positive culture is diagnostic of Lyme disease.

**B. PCR** evaluation of blood, CSF, and urine for evidence of the organism has been unhelpful in reliably establishing the diagnosis because of low sensitivities. Although rarely positive on culture, 85% of synovial fluid or synovial biopsy specimens are PCR positive for *B. burgdorferi* DNA. However, joints with chronic erosive arthritis that persists after adequate treatment usually are PCR negative. Thus, PCR on joint specimens may be used for initial diagnosis of Lyme arthritis [72] and also to determine whether retreatment with antibiotics may be helpful for chronic arthritis [72–75].

**C. Lumbar puncture** in early localized disease is unremarkable, but in early dissemination and late disease it often reveals a CSF mononuclear cell pleocytosis associated with an elevated protein and normal glucose [76]. Patients with acute neuroborreliosis often have an elevated CSF- to-serum *B. burgdorferi* antibody ratio (>1) using an antibody-capture immunoassay, but this test is reliable only at specialized institutions [77]. Previously, single photon emission computed tomography was used to assist in evaluation of CNS Lyme disease, but its reliability has been questioned. With peripheral nerve involvement nerve conduction velocities are often abnormal [37].

**D. Electrocardiograms** in patients with Lyme carditis reveal varying degrees of atrioventricular block. As mentioned above, PR intervals greater than 300 mses predict progression to complete heart block.

**E. Current serologic testing for Lyme disease is neither sensitive nor specific,** with frequent false-positive and false-negative results in the detection of both IgM and IgG antibodies [78]. They also remain positive for prolonged periods, so they do not necessarily represent active infection. Because other studies are not usually diagnostic or readily available, diagnosis often rests on these difficult to interpret serologies. As a result, the American College of Physicians and the CDC recommend carefully applying a two-step approach to serodiagnosis [70,79–81]. Patients with a pretest probability of Lyme disease between 20% and 80% should initially undergo enzyme-linked immunosorbent assay (ELISA) testing of acute and convalescent sera. Intermediate ELISA test results require Western blot confirmation. To reduce the variability that exists among laboratories, the Western blot results should be interpreted according to the criteria established by the CDC [70]. Patients with *Treponema pallidum* infections can have false-positive ELISA results, as can patients with infectious mononucleosis or polyclonal B-cell activation from other causes [82].

1. **In early localized disease when EM lesions are seen, serology is not indicated** for diagnosis because many patients will not have made antiborrelial antibodies yet, and the pretest probability is above 80% [67,80,81].
2. Often the most challenging patients are those who complain of arthralgias, myalgias, headache, palpitation, or fatigue and who have an endemic exposure history. **These symptoms alone are not enough to warrant Lyme disease serologic testing** because such patients have a low pretest probability of having Lyme disease [80,81]. Persons with these symptoms from nonendemic regions have an even lower probability of having Lyme disease. **Patients appropriate for Lyme disease serologic testing should have objective joint, cardiac, and/or neurologic findings** either on the physical exam, electrocardiogram, synovial fluid aspirate or biopsy, nerve conduction studies, CSF analysis, or neuropsychological testing.
3. **Serologic tests should not be used for screening** of otherwise healthy individuals with a history of tick exposure.

Table 21.13. Treatment of Lyme Disease

| Stage of Disease | Antibiotic Choices[a] |
|---|---|
| Early infection (local or disseminated) | |
| Adults | Doxycycline, 100 mg orally twice daily for 14–21 days |
| | Amoxicillin, 500 mg orally three times daily for 14–21 days |
| Doxycycline or amoxicillin allergy | Cefuroxime axetil, 500 mg orally twice daily for 14–21 days |
| | Erythromycin, 250 mg orally 4 times a day for 14–21 days |
| Children | Amoxicillin, 250 mg orally 3 times per day or 50 mg/kg of body weight/day in 3 divided doses for 14–21 days |
| Penicillin allergy | Cefuroxime axetil, 125 mg orally twice daily or 30 mg/kg per day in 2 divided doses for 14–21 days |
| | Erythromycin, 250 mg orally 3 times per day or 30 mg/kg/day in 3 divided doses for 14–21 days |
| Neurologic abnormalities (early or late) | |
| Adults | Ceftriaxone, 2 g i.v. once daily for 14–28 days |
| | Cefotaxime, 2 g i.v. every 8 hours for 14–28 days |
| | Penicillin G, 3.3 million units i.v. every 4 hours (20 million units/day) for 14–28 days |
| Ceftriaxone or penicillin allergy | Doxycycline, 100 mg orally 3 times per day for 30 days |
| Facial palsy alone | Oral regimens may be adequate |
| Children | Ceftriaxone, 75–100 mg/kg/day (maximum, 2 g) i.v. once daily for 14–28 days |
| | Cefotaxime 150 mg/kg/day in 3 or 4 divided doses (maximum, 6 g) i.v. once daily for 14–28 days |
| | Penicillin G, 200,000–400,000 units/kg/day in 6 divided doses for 14–28 days |
| Arthritis (intermittent or chronic) | Oral regimens listed above for 30–60 days or i.v. regimens listed above for 14–28 days |
| Cardiac abnormalities | |
| First-degree atrioventricular block | Oral regimens listed above for 14–21 days |
| High-grade atrioventricular block (PR > 0.3 s) | i.v. regimens listed above and cardiac monitoring (treatment may be finished orally after the patient has been stabilized) |
| Pregnant women | Standard therapy for manifestation of illness; avoid doxycycline |

[a]Alternatives are in order of acceptability, with the drug of choice listed first in each category.
Modified from Steere AC. Lyme disease. *N Engl J Med* 2001;345:122, with permission.

**F.** There are no useful tests to detect *B. burgdorferi* antigens at present. In particular, a marketed urine Lyme antigen detection test is unreliable and is not recommended [83].

**V. Evidence-based treatment recommendations from the Infectious Diseases Society of America [37,69] are presented in Table 21.13.** It is important to recognize and accurately diagnose Lyme disease because the manifestations are reversible with appropriate treatment most of the time. The fear of a missed diagnosis coupled with pressure from the media and patients often results in significant over-diagnosis and treatment. This can be avoided by incorporating an endemic exposure history and an understanding of the clinical manifestations of Lyme disease, with the appropriate use of laboratory diagnostic tests (see section **IV**). This benefits patients and physicians alike by decreasing unnecessary medical expenditures and reducing the anxiety fostered by abnormal test results.

**A. Early localized and early disseminated disease. Oral therapy is appropriate for** EM, isolated cranial nerve palsy, and cardiac involvement limited to first- or second-degree heart block. **Doxycycline** is the drug of choice for patients older than 8 years of age because it also is effective against HGE, a common coinfecting agent (see section **IV.F** under Zoonoses). Alternatives are listed in Table 21.13. Macrolides should be reserved for those who cannot tolerate doxycycline, amoxicillin, or cefuroxime. More than 90% of patients with early localized disease have satisfactory outcomes after the recommended treatment regimens [37].

1. **Acute neuroborreliosis** resolves over several weeks with treatment [37]. Intravenous therapy for meningitis and radiculopathy remains the standard of care in the United States (Table 21.13).
2. In Lyme **carditis,** patients with prolonged PR intervals should be monitored for complete heart block, with placement of a temporary pacer when appropriate. Patients with third-degree block should be hospitalized and treated with intravenous ceftriaxone (Table 21.13). Patients with PR intervals great than 300 ms are also best managed initially with hospital monitoring and intravenous treatment [37]. Permanent pacing is rarely required.

**B. Late disease**

1. **Arthritis** may be treated orally or intravenously (Table 21.13) and usually resolves over several months. Oral therapy is preferred for patients without CNS disease because it is easier, less costly, and has fewer adverse effects [69]. Patients with arthritis and concomitant CNS disease should be treated intravenously. Recurrent arthritis after an initial course of appropriate therapy should be retreated with either another oral 4-week course or with 2 to 4 weeks of intravenous ceftriaxone [69]. Unfortunately, some patients will have persistent synovitis even after such therapy. It is in this select population where *Borrelia*-specific PCR synovial aspirate testing is helpful in distinguishing active infection with spirochetes versus persistent immune destruction of the joint [37]. Patients with negative PCR tests are treated symptomatically with nonsteroidals, and some eventually may require arthroscopic synovectomy.
2. **Chronic neuroborreliosis** improves slowly over months after therapy, and the response may be incomplete. Repeat treatment should not be undertaken without objective evidence of relapse, which is uncommon after 28 days of intravenous ceftriaxone [37,69].

**C. Pregnant women** should be diagnosed and treated conventionally according to the recommendations in Table 21.13. However, because maternal-to-fetal transmission of *Borrelia* is rare, the risk of doxycycline to the fetus obligates use of an alternative treatment [69].

**D. Failure to respond to recommended treatment.** There are several possibilities to explain the persistence of symptoms after appropriate treatment for Lyme disease.

1. Patients with early disease who remain symptomatic should be evaluated for possible coinfections with HGE and babesiosis (see sections **IV.F** and **IV.G** under Zoonoses) [23]. Inadequate dosing and incomplete adherence, particularly to oral therapy, also should be considered. As discussed above, late disease responds slowly to treatment, whereas early disease responds more quickly. Patients with late disease should be observed for further improvement or objective evidence of relapse before retreatment. In addition, symptoms may not be due to Lyme disease or concomitant infection but another illness such as fibromyalgia or chronic fatigue syndrome.
2. Prolonged antibiotic therapy for persistent nonspecific symptoms (musculoskeletal, cognitive, or neuropathic) is of no benefit and should not be used [84].

## VI. Prevention

A. **Avoiding exposure to ticks, using protective clothing and tick repellants, and regularly checking for and quickly removing attached ticks** are the best methods to avoid Lyme disease transmission. When traveling to endemic areas, care should be taken to avoid tick-infested environments. If possible, light-colored clothing (so ticks are easily recognizable), long pants, and long-sleeved shirts should be worn. Patients should be instructed to remain on paths away from brush and to consider the use of tick repellants. Unfortunately, spraying city lawns for ticks has not been shown to be effective in reducing infections.

B. **Prophylaxis after tick bites**

1. A single 200-mg dose of doxycycline within 72 hours of an *I. scapularis* tick bite is effective in preventing Lyme disease [85]. However, if the tick has been removed promptly, no prophylaxis is necessary nor is it recommended in nonendemic areas. Even in endemic areas, the frequency of Lyme disease after tick bite with no prophylaxis is only about 1% [85]. Furthermore, many patients experience repeated tick bites, and doxycycline should not be used in children younger than 8 years of age. Thus, this approach may be best suited for those older children and adults in endemic areas with only an occasional tick bite.
2. Anyone in an endemic area who removes an attached tick should seek medical care for febrile illnesses and skin lesions that occur within the next 30 days [69].
3. Persons treated for EM are considered susceptible to reinfection, but those who develop Lyme arthritis are usually resistant to reinfection [37].

C. **Vaccination.** The previously available recombinant OspA Lyme vaccine was withdrawn from the market by its manufacturer in February 2002. Although there was unsubstantiated controversy about its safety [86], particularly with the need for regular booster doses, the manufacturer cited economic concerns for this decision because there was waning use of the vaccine.

## REFERENCES


1. Fish D. Environmental risk and prevention of Lyme disease. *Am J Med* 1995;98 [Suppl 4A]:2S–9S.
2. Jones CG, Ostfeld RS, Richard MP, et al. Chain reactions linking acorns to gypsy moth outbreaks and Lyme disease risk. *Science* 1998;279:1023–1026.
3. Chapman LE, Folks TM, Salomon DR, et al. Xenotransplantation and xenogeneic infections. *N Engl J Med* 1995;333:1498–1501.
4. Michaels MG, Jenkins FJ, St. George K, et al. Detection of infectious baboon cytomegalovirus after baboon-to-human liver xenotransplantation. *J Virol* 2001;75:2825–2828.
5. Talan DA, Citron DM, Abrahamian FM, et al. Bacteriologic analysis of infected dog and cat bites. Emergency Medicine Animal Bite Infection Study Group. *N Engl J Med* 1999;340:85–92.
6. Feder HM Jr, Shanley JD, Barbera JA. Review of 59 patients hospitalized with animal bites. *Pediatr Infect Dis J* 1987;6:24–28.
7. Goldstein EJC, Citron DM. Comparative activities of cefuroxime, amoxicillin-clavulanic acid, ciprofloxacin, enoxacin, and ofloxacin against aerobic and anaerobic bacteria isolated from bite wounds. *Antimicrob Agents Chemother* 1988;32:1143–1148.
8. Debre R, Lamy M, Jammet M-L, et al. La maladie des griffes de chat. *Bull Mem Soc Med Hop Paris* 1950;66:76–79.
9. Regnery RL, Olson JG, Perkins BA, et al. Serological response to *Rochalimaea henselae* antigen in suspected cat-scratch disease. *Lancet* 1992;339:1443–1445.
10. Zangwill KM, Hamilton DH, Perkins BA, et al. Cat scratch disease in Connecticut—epidemiology, risk factors, and evaluation of a new diagnostic test. *N Engl J Med* 1993;329:8–13.
11. Tompkins LS. Of cats, humans, and Bartonella. *N Engl J Med* 1997;337:1915–1917.
12. Carithers HA. Cat-scratch disease: an overview based on a study of 1,200 patients. *Am J Dis Child* 1985;139:1124–1133.

13. Bass JW, Freitas BC, Freitas AD, et al. Prospective randomized double blind placebo-controlled evaluation of azithromycin for treatment of cat-scratch disease. *Pediatr Infect Dis J* 1998;17:447–452.
14. Jacobs R, Schutze G. *Bartonella henselae* as a cause of prolonged fever and fever of unknown origin in children. *Clin Infect Dis* 1998;26:80–84.
15. Doll JM, Zeitz PS, Ettestad P, et al. Cat-transmitted fatal pneumonic plague in a person who travelled from Colorado to Arizona. *Am J Trop Med Hyg* 1994;51:109–114.
16. Mahrer S, Raik E. *Capnocytophaga canimorsus* septicemia associated with cat scratch. *Pathology* 1992;24:194–196.
17. Hollis DG, Moss CW, Daneshvar MI, et al. Characterization of Centers for Disease Control group NO-1, a fastidious, nonoxidative, gram-negative organism associated with dog and cat bites. *J Clin Microbiol* 1993;31:746–768.
18. Wunner WH, Peters D. *Family Rhabdoviradae.* In: Franchi RIB, et al. *Classification and nomenclature of viruses: fifth report of the International Committee on taxonomy of Viruses. Arichl Virol Suppl 2.* New York: Springer-Verlag, 1991:250–262.
19. Human rabies prevention—United States, 1999. Recommendations of the Advisory Committee on Immunization Practices (ACIP). *MMWR Recomm Rep* 1999;48(RR-1):1–21.
20. Haake DA, Dundoo M, Cader R, et al. Leptospirosis, water sports, and chemoprophylaxis. *Clin Infect Dis* 2002;34:e40–e43.
21. Bakken JS, Dumler JS. Human granulocytic ehrlichiosis. *Clin Infect Dis* 2000;31:554–560.
22. Dumler JS. Is human granulocytic ehrlichiosis a new Lyme disease? Review and comparison of clinical, laboratory, epidemiological, and some biological features. *Clin Infect Dis* 1997;25[Suppl 1]:S43–S47.
23. Krause PJ, McKay K, Thompson CA, et al. Disease-specific diagnosis of coinfecting tick-borne zoonoses: babesiosis, human granulocytic ehrlichiosis, and Lyme disease. *Clin Infect Dis* 2002;34:1184–1191.
24. Paddock CD, Folk SM, Shore GM, et al. Infections with *Ehrlichia chaffeensis* and *Ehrlichia ewingii* in persons coinfected with human immunodeficiency virus. *Clin Infect Dis* 2001;33:1586–1594.
25. Eng TR, Harkess JR, Fishbein DB, et al. Epidemiologic, clinical, and laboratory findings of human ehrlichiosis in the United States, 1988. *JAMA* 1990;264:2251–2258.
26. Bakken JS, Krueth J, Wilson-Nordskog C, et al. Clinical and laboratory characteristics of human granulocytic ehrlichiosis. *JAMA* 1996;275:199–205.
27. Hatcher JC, Greenberg PD, Antique J, et al. Severe babesiosis in Long Island: review of 34 cases and their complications. *Clin Infect Dis* 2001;32:1117–1125.
28. Meldrum SC, Birkhead GS, White DJ, et al. Human babesiosis in New York State: an epidemiological description of 136 cases. *Clin Infect Dis* 1992;15:1019–1023.
29. Boustani MR, Gelfand JA. Babesiosis. *Clin Infect Dis* 1996;22:611–615.
30. Krause PJ, Lepore T, Sikard UC, et al. Atovaquone and azithromycin for the treatment of babesiosis. *N Engl J Med* 2000;343:1454–1458.
31. Sorvillo F, Ash LR, Berlin OG, et al. Baylisascaris procyonis: an emerging helminthic zoonosis. *Emerg Infect Dis* 2002;8:355–359.
32. Afzelius A. Verhandlungen der dermatologischen Gesellschaft zu Stockholm. *Arch Dermatol Syph* 1910;101:405–406.
33. Steere AC, et al. Lyme arthritis: An epidemic of oligoarticular arthritis in children and adults in three Connecticut communities. *Arthritis Rheum* 1977;20:7–17.
34. Burgdorfer W. The discovery of Lyme disease spirochete and its relation to tick vectors. *Yale J Biol Med* 1984;57:515.
35. Burgdorfer W. The discovery of the Lyme disease spirochete. In: Stanek G, et al., eds. *Proceedings of the Second International Symposium on Lyme Disease and Related Disorders*, Vienna, 1985. New York: Verlag, 1987.
36. Weil HFC, Frank WA, Rahn DW. Lyme disease (tickborn borreliosis). In: Reese RE, ed. *A practical approach to infectious disease*, 4th ed. Boston: Little, Brown & Company, 1996:878–902.
37. Steere AC. Lyme disease. *N Engl J Med* 2001;345:115–125.
38. Steere AC, Malawista . SE cases of Lyme disease in the United States: locations correlated with distribution of *Ixodes dammini. Ann Intern Med* 1979;91:730–733.

39. Weber K, et al. European erythema migrans disease and related disorders. *Yale J Biol Med* 1984;57:465–471.
40. Schulze TL, et al. Comparison of rates of infection by the lyme disease spirochete in selected populations of *Ixodes dammini* and *Amblyomma americanum*. In Stanek G, et al., eds. *Proceedings of the Second International Symposium on Lyme Disease and Related Disorders,* Vienna, 1985. New York: Verlag, 1987:507–513.
41. Lane RS, Lavoie PE. Lyme borreliosis in California: acarological, clinical, and epidemiological studies. *Ann NY Acad Sci* 1988;539:192–203.
42. Ciesielski CA, et al. The geographical distribution of Lyme disease in the United States. *Ann NY Acad Sci* 1988;539:283–288.
43. Spach DH, et al. Tick-borne diseases in the United States. *N Engl J Med* 1993;329:936–947.
44. Spielman A, Levine JF, Wilson ML. Vectorial capacity of North American *Ixodes* ticks. *Yale J Biol Med* 1984;57:507–513.
45. Piesman J, et al. Duration of tick attachment and *Borrelia burgdorferi* transmission. *J Clin Microbiol* 1987;25:557–558.
46. Coleman JL, Gebbia JA, Piesman J, et al. Plasminogen is required for efficient dissemination of *B. burgdorferi* in ticks and for enhancement of spirochetemia in mice. *Cell* 1997;89:1111–1119.
47. Fraser CM, Casjens S, Huang WM, et al. Genomic sequence of a Lyme disease spirochete, *Borrelia burgdorferi*. *Nature* 1997;390:580–586.
48. Shapiro ED,Gerber MA. Lyme disease. *Clin Infect Dis* 2000;31:533–542.
49. Benach JL, et al. Adult *Ixodes dammini* on rabbits: a hypothesis for the development and transmission of *Borrelia burgdorferi*. *J Infect Dis* 1987;155:1300–1306.
50. Smith RP, Schoen RT, Rahn DW, et al. Clinical characteristics and treatment outcome of early Lyme disease in patients with microbiologically confirmed erythema migrans. *Ann Intern Med* 2002;136:421–428.
51. Burkot TR, Mullen GR, Anderson R, et al. *Borrelia lonestari* DNA in adult *Amblyomma americanum* ticks, Alabama. *Emerg Infect Dis* 2001;7:471–473.
52. James AM, Liveris D, Wormser GP, et al. *Borrelia lonestari* infection after a bite by an *Amblyomma americanum* tick. *J Infect Dis* 2001;183:1810–1814.
53. Coyle PK, Goodman JL, Krupp LB, et al. *Lyme disease: continuum: lifelong learning in neurology*. Vol. 5. Philadelphia: Lippincott Williams & Wilkins, 1999.
54. Oschmann P, Dorndorf W, Hornig C, et al. Stages and syndromes of neuroborreliosis. *J Neurol* 1998;245:262–272.
55. Halperin JJ, et al. Nervous system abnormalities in Lyme disease. *Ann NY Acad Sci* 1988;539:24–34.
56. Murakami S, et al. Bell palsy and herpes simplex virus: identification of viral DNA in endoneurial fluid and muscle. *Ann Intern Med* 1996;124:27.
57. Rothermel H, Hedges TR III, Steere AC. Optic neuropathy in children with Lyme disease. *Pediatrics* 2001;108:477–481.
58. Steere AC. Lyme disease. *N Engl J Med* 1989;321:586–596.
59. Steere AC, et al. Lyme carditis: cardiac abnormalities of Lyme disease. *Ann Intern Med* 1980;93:8–16.
60. Duffy J. Lyme disease. *Infect Dis Clin North Am* 1987;1:511.
61. Steere AC Baxter-Lowe LA. Association of chronic, treatment-resistant Lyme arthritis with rheumatoid arthritis (RA) alleles. *Arthritis Rheum* 1998;41[Suppl]:S81(abstr).
62. Steere AC, Schoen RT, Taylor E. The clinical evolution of Lyme arthritis. *Ann Intern Med* 1987;107:725–731.
63. Pachner AR. Spirochetal diseases of the nervous system. *Neurol Clin* 1986;4:207–222.
64. Logigian EL, Kaplan RF, Steere AC. Chronic neurologic manifestations of Lyme disease. *N Engl J Med* 1990;323:1438–1444.
65. Halperin JJ, Luft BJ, Anand AK, et al. Lyme neuroborreliosis: central nervous system manifestations. *Neurology* 1989;39:753–759.
66. Logigian EL, Steere AC. Clinical and electrophysiologic findings in chronic neuropathy of Lyme disease. *Neurology* 1992;42:303–311.
67. Steere AC. *Borrelia burgdorferi* (Lyme disease, Lyme borreliosis). In Mandell BL, Bennett JE, Dolin R, eds. *Principles and practice of infectious diseases,* 5th ed. New York: Churchill Livingstone, 2000:2504–2518.

68. Sigal LH. Misconceptions about Lyme disease: confusions hiding behind ill-chosen terminology. *Ann Intern Med* 2002;136:413–419.
69. Wormser GP, Nadelman RB, Dattwyler RJ, et al. Practice guidelines for the treatment of Lyme disease. *Clin Infect Dis* 2000;31[Suppl]:S1–S14.
70. Case definitions for public health surveillance. *MMWR Morb Mortal Wkly Rep* 1990;39:(RR-13):1–43.
71. Berger BW, Johnson RC, Kodner C, et al. Cultivation of *Borrelia burgdorferi* from erythema migrans lesions and perilesional skin. *J Clin Microbiol* 1992;30:359–361.
72. Nocton JJ, Dressler F, Rutledge BJ, et al. Detection of *Borrelia burgdorferi* DNA by polymerase chain reaction in synovial fluid from patients with Lyme arthritis. *N Engl J Med* 1994;330:229–234.
73. Steere AC, Duray PH, Butcher EC. Spirochetal antigens and lymphoid cell surface markers in Lyme synovitis: comparison with rheumatoid synovium and tonsillar lymphoid tissue. *Arthritis Rheum* 1988;31:487–495.
74. Carlson D, Hernandez J, Bloom BJ, et al. Lack of *Borrelia burgdorferi* DNA in synovial samples in patients with antibiotic treatment-resistant Lyme arthritis. *Arthritis Rheum* 1999;42:2705–2709.
75. Rahn D. Lyme disease—where's the bug. *N Engl J Med* 1994;330:282–283.
76. Luft BJ, Dattwyler RJ. Lyme borreliosis. *Curr Clin Top Infect Dis* 1989;10:56–81.
77. Steere AC, Berardi VP, Weeks KE, et al. Evaluation of the intrathecal antibody response to *Borrelia burgdorferi* as a diagnostic test for Lyme neuroborreliosis. *J Infect Dis* 1990;161:1203–1209.
78. Dattwyler R, et al. Seronegative Lyme disease. *N Engl J Med* 1988;319:1441–1446.
79. Recommendations for test performance and interpretation from the Second National Conference on Serologic Diagnosis of Lyme Disease. *MMWR Morb Mortal Wkly Rep* 1995;44:590–591.
80. Guidelines for laboratory evaluation in the diagnosis of Lyme disease. American College of Physicians. *Ann Intern Med* 1997;127:1106–1108.
81. Tugwell P, Dennis DT, Weinstein A, et al. Laboratory evaluation in the diagnosis of Lyme disease. *Ann Intern Med* 1997;127:1109–1123.
82. Grodzicki R, Steere AC. Comparison of immunoblotting and indirect enzyme-linked immunosorbent assay using different antigen preparations for diagnosing early Lyme disease. *J Infect Dis* 1988;157:790–797.
83. Klempner MS, Schmid C, Hu L, et al. Intralaboratory reliability of serologic and urine testing for Lyme disease. *Am J Med* 2001;110:217–219.
84. Klempner MS, Hu LT, Evans J, et al. Two controlled trials of antibiotic treatment in patients with persistent symptoms and a history of Lyme disease. *N Engl J Med* 2001;345:85–92.
85. Nadelman RB, Nowakowski J, Fish D, et al. Prophylaxis with single-dose doxycycline for the prevention of Lyme disease after an *Ixodes scapularis* tick bite. *N Engl J Med* 2001;345:79–84.
86. Rahn DW. Lyme vaccine: issues and controversies. *Infect Dis Clin North Am* 2001; 15:171–187.

# 22. HEALTH ADVICE FOR INTERNATIONAL TRAVEL

David R. Hill and Richard D. Pearson

International travel, including visits to the developing world for business, vacation, study, or missionary and service activities, is a major pursuit of Americans. These travelers are often exposed to bacterial, viral, and parasitic diseases that range from traveler's diarrhea to life-threatening infection with *Plasmodium falciparum.* Complex itineraries and changing patterns of disease and international health requirements make the providing of advice on prevention and immunizations for the traveler a challenging task [1]. Whenever possible, pretravel care should be provided by an expert in the field. Many hospitals and schools of medicine in the United States have specialized travel clinics or units of tropical medicine that can render expert travel advice [2].

Travel medicine should provide preventive advice, immunizations, and medications for disease prevention or self-treatment based on an individual's itinerary and health status. To do this, an assessment of the potential health risks confronting the traveler must be developed by determining their itinerary (including whether rural sites will be visited), planned activities, duration of stay, and medical and immunization histories. This information, as well as the plan of care, should be recorded in a **permanent medical record.** There are multiple sources of information, both printed and on-line, to aid the provider of travel care in decision making (see Appendix).

## VACCINATIONS

**I. General considerations**

**A. Types of vaccinations for the traveler.** Vaccinations can be divided into those that are routinely recommended for children and adults, whether or not they are traveling; those that are required by countries for entry; and those that are recommended because of potential exposure in the country of destination (Table 22.1).

1. **Routine vaccinations. The pretravel visit is an excellent time to update routinely recommended vaccines.** Immunizations are discussed in the *Guide for Adult Immunization* [3], in *Health Information for International Travel* [4], in the pediatric *Red Book* [5], in section **II** of Chapter 23, and in recent reviews [6,7].
2. **Required vaccinations—the International Certificate of Vaccination.** The only vaccine currently required under World Health Organization (WHO) regulations for travel between countries is yellow fever vaccine. Nevertheless, some countries may still ask for evidence of cholera vaccination. This is discussed in more detail in section **III.** A list of the vaccine requirements by country is published by the Centers for Disease Control and Prevention (CDC) in *Health Information for International Travel* [4]. **According to international health regulations, yellow fever vaccination must be recorded in the document "International Certificate of Vaccination"** [8] **and validated** by a stamp issued by state health departments. No vaccinations are required for returning U.S. residents entering the United States. **Smallpox vaccination is not required by any country** (see section **III**) [9].
3. **Recommended vaccinations.** Travelers and physicians frequently confuse the distinction between **required** and **recommended** vaccines. In reality, only yellow fever may be required. Some vaccines are recommended because infection could be acquired in the country of destination. Examples include epidemic meningococcal disease, which is limited to certain areas of the world, and typhoid fever, which is present throughout developing regions but is a risk to travelers only if they encounter poor food and water sanitation. In addition to vaccination, many diseases transmitted by fecal contamination of the food and water supply can be prevented by care in selecting foods and liquids. Vaccination should never be considered a substitute for practicing preventive measures. **Exposure to foods and liquids in areas of poor sanitation (as may occur in rural areas and small villages) for more than 2 to 3 weeks may be a reasonable criterion for administering vaccines for protection against enteric pathogens (e.g., typhoid)** (see section **IV**). Unfortunately, data are not always available on the

Table 22.1. Vaccinations to Consider for Travel to the Developing World

| Vaccine | Type, Route, and Dose[a] | Schedule[a] | Indications[a] | Precautions and Contraindications[b] | Side Effects[b] |
|---|---|---|---|---|---|
| **Toxoids** | | | | | |
| Tetanus-diphtheria (Td) | Adsorbed toxoids<br>i.m. (0.5 mL) | Primary: 3 doses; first 2, 4–8 wk apart; 3rd dose after 6–12 mo<br>Booster: every 10 yr; single dose after age 50 | All adults | First trimester of pregnancy<br>Hypersensitivity or neurologic reaction to previous doses<br>Severe local reaction | Local reactions; occasional fever and systemic symptoms<br>Arthus-like reactions in persons with mutiple previous boosters<br>Rare—systemic allergy |
| **Inactivated bacteria vaccines** | | | | | |
| *Streptococcus pneumoniae* | Polysaccharide–23 serotypes<br>s.c. or i.m. (0.5 mL)<br>See text for conjugate pneumococcal vaccine | Primary: single dose<br>Booster: high-risk patients after 5 yr | Persons ≥5 yr at increased risk of pneumococcal disease and its complications<br>Healthy adults ≥65 yr | Safety in pregnancy is unknown<br>Previous pneumococcal vaccination (relative) | Approximately 50% of patients have mild erythema and pain at injection site<br>Systemic reaction in <1% of patients<br>Arthus-like reaction with booster doses |
| *Neisseria meningitidis* | Polysaccharide containing four serotypes (A, C, Y, W–135)<br>s.c. (0.5 mL) | Primary: single dose<br>Booster: not officially recommended; may be given after 3 to 5 yr in adults and after 2 to 3 yr in children vaccinated at 2 to 4 yr of age | Travelers to areas with epidemic meningococcal disease (see text)<br>Asplenia or certain complement-deficiency states | Safety in pregnancy is unknown | Infrequent, mild local reactions |
| Typhoid | Polysaccharide Vi antigen<br>i.m. (0.5 mL) | Primary: single dose for age ≥2 years<br>Booster: every 2 yr | Risk of exposure to typhoid fever (see text) | Safety in pregnancy is unknown<br>Hypersensitivity to vaccine components | Local pain and induration—10–20%<br>Systemic reaction in <5% |
| **Attenuated live bacterial vaccine** | | | | | |
| Typhoid | Attenuated Ty21a mutant of *Salmonella typhi*<br>Oral | Primary: 1 capsule every other day for 4 doses<br>Booster: every 5 yr | Risk of exposure to typhoid fever in persons ≥6 yr (see text) | Safety in pregnancy is unknown<br>Immunocompromised host[c]<br>Persons with acute febrile or gastrointestinal illness<br>Persons taking antibiotics<br>If taking mefloquine, separate doses by 24 h<br>Refrigerate capsules | Infrequent gastrointestinal upset or rash |

| | | | | | |
|---|---|---|---|---|---|
| **Attenuated live virus vaccines** | | | | | |
| Measles | Attenuated live virus (available in monovalent form or combined with rubella [MR] ± mumps [MMR]) s.c. (0.5 mL) | Primary: 2 doses; 1st at 12–15 mo, 2nd at 4–6 yr<br>For adults, 2 doses separated by at least 1 mo<br>Booster: none | Persons born after 1956 who have not had documented measles or received 2 doses of live vaccine | Pregnancy<br>Immunocompromised host[c] (asymptomatic HIV-infected persons can be considered for vaccination; see text)<br>History of anaphylaxis to eggs or neomycin<br>Administration of immune globulin within 5 mo | Temperature of ≥39.4°C, 5–21 days after vaccination in 5–15%<br>Transient rash in 5%<br>Of persons previously immunized with killed vaccine (1963–1967), 4–55% have a local reaction |
| Mumps | Attenuated live virus s.c. (0.5 mL) | Primary: 1 dose (usually given as part of MMR vaccine)<br>Booster: none | Persons born after 1956 who have not had documented mumps or mumps vaccine | Pregnancy<br>Immunocompromised host[c]<br>History of anaphylaxis to eggs or neomycin<br>Administration of immune globulin within 5 mo | Mild allergic reactions uncommon<br>Rare parotitis |
| Rubella | Attenuated live virus s.c. (0.5 mL) | Primary: 1 dose (often given as part of MR or MMR)<br>Booster: none | All persons, particularly women of childbearing age, without documented illness or live vaccine on or after first birthday | Pregnancy<br>Immunocompromised host[c]<br>History of anaphylaxis to neomycin<br>Administration of immune globulin within 5 mo | Up to [illegible]0% of postpubertal women have joint pains, transient arthralgias, beginning 3–25 days after vaccination, persisting 1–11 days<br>Frank arthritis in <2% |
| Varicella vaccine | Attenuated live virus s.c. (0.5 mL) | Primary: 1 dose, children 12 mo to 12 yr; >12 yr, 2 doses at a 4–8 wk interval | Persons ≥12 mo who have not had varicella | Pregnancy<br>Immunocompromised host[c]<br>Potential for rare transmission of vaccine virus to susceptible hosts<br>Administration of immune globulin within 5 mo | Local pain and induration ≈20%<br>Fever ≈15%<br>Localized or systemic varicella rash ≈6% |
| Yellow fever | Attenuated live virus s.c. (0.5 mL) | Primary: single dose 10 days to 10 yr before travel<br>Booster: every 10 yr | As required by individual countries | Avoid in pregnant women, unless high-risk travel<br>Infants <9 mo (see text)<br>Immunocompromised host[c]<br>Hypersensitivity to eggs | Mild headache, myalgia, fever 5–10 days after vaccination in 2–5%<br>Rare immediate hypersensitivity<br>Rare severe multiorgan system failure (see text) |

(*Continued*)

Table 22.1. (*Continued*)

| Vaccine | Type, Route, and Dose[a] | Schedule[a] | Indications[a] | Precautions and Contraindications[b] | Side Effects[b] |
|---|---|---|---|---|---|
| **Inactivated virus vaccines** | | | | | |
| Hepatitis A (Havrix and Vaqta) | Inactivated virus<br>i.m. (adult and pediatric formulations) | Primary: 2 doses, 2nd dose after 6 to 18 mo provides long-term (perhaps 10–20 yr) protection<br>Booster: not currently recommended | Travel to developing countries<br>Children residing in endemic regions of the United States [44]<br>Some persons may benefit from prevaccine hepatitis A serology (see text) | Safety in pregnancy is unknown | Local reactions with pain and tenderness <20%<br>Occasional fever, <5% |
| Hepatitis B (Recombivax and Engerix) | Recombinant-hepatitis B surface antigen<br>i.m. (adult and pediatric formulations) | Primary: 3 doses at 0, 1 and 6 mo; can accelerate vaccination (see text)<br>Booster: not routinely recommended | Health-care workers in contact with blood<br>Persons residing in areas of intermediate to high endemicity for hepatitis B<br>Others at risk for contact with blood, body fluids, or blood-contaminated medical or dental instruments | Pregnancy is not a contraindication in high-risk persons<br>Hypersensitivity to vaccine components | Mild local reaction in 10–20%<br>Occasional systemic symptoms of fever, headache, fatigue, and nausea |
| Hepatitis A and B antigens combined | Inactivated virus (A) plus recombinant hepatitis B surface antigen<br>i.m. (1.0 mL) | Primary: 3 doses at 0, 1 and 6 mo | Travelers $\geq$18 yr at risk for both hepatitis A and B (see text)<br>Give at least 2 doses of vaccine prior to departure to provide protection against hepatitis A | Safety in pregnancy is unknown<br>Hypersensitivity to vaccine components | Local reactions in $\approx$35%<br>Systemic symptoms of headache and fatigue, similar to single antigen preparations |
| Poliomyelitis | Killed poliomyelitis virus, trivalent<br>s.c. or i.m. (0.5 mL) | Primary: 3 doses, first 2 at a 4- to 8-wk interval; 3rd dose 6–12 mo after 2nd<br>Booster: one adult, lifetime dose with travel to endemic regions | Only formulation of polio vaccine used in U.S.<br>Travel to polio-endemic countries: complete primary series or receive one booster in adult lifetime | Safety in pregnancy is unknown<br>Anaphylactic reactions to streptomycin or neomycin | Mild local reactions |

| | | | | | |
|---|---|---|---|---|---|
| Influenza | Inactivated whole and split influenza A and B virus<br>i.m. (0.5 mL) | Annual vaccination with current vaccine | Persons ≥6 mo with high-risk conditions (see text)<br>Healthy persons ≥50 yr<br>Medical care personnel, others<br>Travelers at risk (see text) | First trimester of pregnancy is a relative contraindication<br>Anaphylaxis to eggs | Mild local reactions in < one-third<br>Occasional systemic reaction of malaise, myalgia, beginning 6–12 h after vaccination and lasting 1–2 days<br>Rare allergic reaction |
| Japanese B encephalitis | Inactivated virus<br>s.c. (1.0 mL) | Primary: 3 doses at days 0, 7, and 30<br>Booster: 1 dose at 3 yr interval; however, duration of protection is not known | Travelers to area of risk with rural exposure or prolonged residence (see text) | Pregnancy<br>Allergy to mice or rodents<br>History of anaphylaxis or urticaria | Local mild reactions lasting 1–3 days (20%)<br>Systemic reactions of fever, myalgia, headache, or gastrointestinal upset (10%)<br>Allergic reactions of urticaria, rash angioedema, or respiratory distress (0.1–10/1,000)<br>Rare sudden death or encephalomyelitis |
| Rabies (Imovax and RabAvert) | Inactivated virus grown in human diploid cells (HDCV) or purified chick embryo cells (PCEC)<br>i.m. (1.0 mL) | Preexposure: 3 doses at days 0, 7, and 21 or 28<br>Booster: depends on risk category and is based on serologic testing (see text) | Itineraries and activities which place the traveler at risk for rabies; dogs are primary threat in developing regions | Allergy to previous doses<br>May be given in pregnancy if indicated | ≈30% have local reactions<br>≈20% have mild systemic reactions: headache, nausea, aches, dizziness<br>Occasional (6%) immune reactions with booster doses of HDCV occurring 2–21 days after vaccination |
| **Passive prophylaxis** | | | | | |
| Immunoglobulin | Fractionated immunoglobulins (primarily IgG)<br>i.m. | Travel of <3 mo duration: 0.02 mL/kg<br>Travel >3 mo: 0.06 mL/kg every 4–6 mo | For prevention of hepatitis A<br>Some travelers may benefit from pretravel hepatitis A antibody testing (see text) | Should not be given <3 wk after or 5 mo before measles mumps, rubella, or varicella vaccines | Local discomfort<br>Rare systemic allergy |

[a]Manufacturer's full prescribing information should be consulted, because vaccines, doses, and schedules may differ between countries. Doses given are generally for adults; pediatric doses may vary.
[b]Only major precautions, contraindications, and side effects listed.
[c]Persons immunocompromised because of immunodeficiency diseases, leukemia, lymphoma, generalized malignancy, or HIV/AIDS, or who are immunosuppressed from therapy with corticosteroids, alkylating agents, antimetabolites, or radiation.

precise risk of most infectious diseases by geographic area, and the benefit-to-risk ratio of specific immunizations must be estimated by the physician [4,10].

**B. Vaccine administration pointers**

1. **Simultaneous administration of vaccines** is reviewed in detail in Chapter 23. Although most viral and bacterial vaccines, whether attenuated, live, or killed, can be administered simultaneously at different sites, cumulative side effects may preclude this, and the traveler should return for a subsequent visit if there is time before departure. **Attenuated live viral vaccines, which are not given simultaneously, should be separated by 1 month.**
2. **Live viral vaccines generally should not be given to** pregnant women, to patients who are immunocompromised, or to persons with a febrile illness (for exceptions, see discussion of individual vaccines).
3. **Immunoglobulin should not be given less than 5 months before or less than 2 weeks after measles, mumps, or rubella vaccine and not less than 3 weeks after varicella vaccine** because the passive transfer of antibodies may interfere with the immune response (see Chapter 23). These restrictions do not apply to yellow fever vaccine or inactivated viral vaccines.
4. **An individual's risk factors for infection with human immunodeficiency virus (HIV) should be determined before administering vaccines.** Although immunization of otherwise healthy HIV-infected persons is considered safe for most vaccines, progressive infection with live attenuated viruses or bacteria is a possibility [11]. The safety, immunogenicity, and efficacy of any vaccine should be matched with the risk of disease acquisition by the HIV-positive traveler. There is improved immunogenicity if CD4 counts are more than 200 cells/mm; and this CD4 count, plus clinical status and viral load, may be a reasonable yardstick for safely administering live viral vaccines [12,13].
5. **Documentation.** Before the administration of any vaccine, the full prescribing information provided by the manufacturer should be consulted. The date, dose, site, manufacturer, and lot number of each vaccine should be recorded in permanent records. Adverse reactions in the United States should be reported to the Vaccine Adverse Event Reporting System (800-822-7967) and in Canada to the Division of Immunization in Canada (613-957-1340). Vaccine Adverse Event Reporting System reporting forms can be down-loaded from *www.fda.gov/cber/vaers/vaers.htm* for the United States and from *www.hc-sc.gc.ca/hpb/lcdc/bid/di/vaae_e.html* for Canada (see Chapter 23).

**II. Routine vaccinations for travelers.** A summary is provided in this section. More detailed discussion may be found in Chapter 23.

**A. Tetanus-diphtheria toxoids.** Many adults in the United States are not adequately protected against tetanus and diphtheria. This is particularly true for persons older than 50 years in whom most cases of tetanus occur [14]; these persons may also lack protective antibodies against diphtheria [15]. Outbreaks of diphtheria have occurred in areas where vaccine coverage is lacking or protection has waned, and travelers to these regions (e.g., some countries in Africa, Asia, and Eastern Europe) should ensure immunity to diphtheria [16]. Each traveler should have completed the primary series of vaccination against tetanus-diphtheria and should have received boosters with the combined toxoids at 10-year intervals. **For routine immunization, persons 50 years of age and older should receive only one booster. Some travelers may benefit from a booster at a 5-year interval,** because a tetanus-prone wound requires neither tetanus immunoglobulin (given only to persons who have not received the primary series) nor a tetanus booster if a person has been boosted within 5 years [17]. It is usually easier and safer to be immunized before travel than to try to obtain a booster in a developing area where sterility of needles and storage conditions are less certain (see Chapter 4).

**B. Pneumococcal vaccine.** There are two pneumococcal polysaccharide vaccines available: a seven-valent conjugate vaccine (PCV7) for routine immunization of all children 2 to 23 months of age [18] and a 23-valent polysaccharide vaccine (PPV23) for use in children 5 years and older and adults [19]. The conjugate vaccine can also be considered for high risk and other children 24 to 59 months of age according to CDC guidelines: children 2 to 4 years of age (who would receive PCV7) and those

5 years of age and older (who would receive PPV23) who are at increased risk of severe pneumococcal disease, including persons with impairment of the cardiorespiratory, hepatic, or renal systems; diabetes mellitus; anatomic or functional asplenia; sickle cell disease; chronic alcoholism; HIV infection; and healthy persons 65 years of age and older [18,19]. In adults, the vaccine is given as a one-time dose, but high-risk individuals may be revaccinated after 5 or more years. See further discussion in Chapters 11 and 23.

**C. Measles.** Travelers may have substantial exposure to measles overseas, particularly if they visit countries in the African and eastern Mediterranean regions [20]. Currently, almost 70% of measles cases in the United States are imported or linked to imported cases [21]. To achieve immunity to measles, all children should receive two doses of measles vaccine, the first at 12 to 15 months of age and the second upon entry to elementary school (ages 4 to 6 years) [22]. Persons born before 1957 are usually immune secondary to natural infection. Those born in 1957 or later who have never had measles infection or received vaccine should receive two doses of a measles-containing vaccine separated by an interval of at least 1 month. Travelers born in 1957 or later who have not had two doses of a live attenuated measles vaccine, with the second dose after 1980, should also be given one or two doses of vaccine depending on their vaccination status. Serologic testing can be helpful in assessing immunity against measles and rubella.

Children traveling to high-risk areas where they are likely to be exposed at a young age can be vaccinated between 6 and 12 months with single-antigen (monovalent) measles vaccine. They should be reimmunized at 15 months with the measles-mumps-rubella vaccine. Vaccination of children younger than 2 years is reviewed elsewhere (see Chapter 23).

Measles vaccine may be carefully considered for HIV-infected individuals if they are asymptomatic with low or undetectable HIV levels and a CD4 in the normal range [22]. For further discussion of measles vaccinations, see Chapter 23.

**D. Rubella and mumps.** Women of childbearing age who are not immune to rubella should be considered for immunization. Most adults probably were infected naturally with mumps virus and are immune; however, if an adult is susceptible to mumps vaccination may be considered. If immunity to more than one virus is lacking, combined measles-mumps-rubella vaccine can be given. There are no increased side effects if a person receives a vaccine virus to which he or she is immune (see Chapter 23).

**E. Influenza.** The composition of influenza vaccine is determined annually and includes the viral subtypes projected to cause disease in the United States during the winter influenza season [23]. Vaccination is recommended for adults with chronic disorders of the cardiovascular or pulmonary system (including asthma); persons with other chronic medical conditions (e.g., diabetes mellitus, renal disease, hemoglobinopathies, and immunosuppression); nursing home and long-term-care residents; children aged 6 months to 18 years who are on chronic aspirin therapy; pregnant women in their second and third trimesters; healthy persons 50 years of age and older; and persons who provide health care in hospitals, custodial facilities, or in the home. Vaccination may also be considered for healthy persons traveling during influenza season. Influenza viruses active in the developing world may or may not be included in the vaccine in the United States.

Influenza vaccine should be given to travelers leaving the United States at any time of the year when destined for the tropics or between April and September when destined for the southern hemisphere. Outbreaks can occur in summer months in northern climates when travelers congregate from throughout the world [24]. High-risk travelers who are unable to receive vaccine may want to carry amantadine or rimantadine for self-treatment of influenza A or one of the new neuraminidase inhibitors, zanamivir or oseltamivir, for treatment of either influenza A or B [24]. Because of potential side effects and medication contraindications, self-treatment should be carefully reviewed with the traveler (see Chapter 10).

**F. *Haemophilus influenzae* type b.** Implementation of childhood vaccination with conjugate *Haemophilus* b vaccines has resulted in a greater than 95% decrement of illness with this organism [25]. All children beginning at age 2 months should be vaccinated [26] (see Chapters 6 and 23).

## III. Required vaccinations

**A. Yellow fever.** Countries that require yellow fever vaccine are listed in *Health Information for International Travel* [4]. Because of its requirement for cold storage and its viability for only 60 minutes after reconstitution, **the vaccine is given only in approved yellow fever vaccination centers,** which may be identified by calling state or local health departments. Persons who are traveling or living in areas **infected** with yellow fever and persons who visit rural areas in countries in the **endemic** zone for yellow fever should receive vaccine. Vaccine should be administered and recorded at least 10 days before travel. Worldwide, yellow fever cases have increased. Infection has spread to urban areas in South America [27,28], and fatal cases of yellow fever have occurred in short-term visitors to infected areas [29].

**Infected areas** are those where yellow fever cases are occurring; these lie primarily in equatorial South America and approximately 15 degrees on either side of the equator in Africa. They are listed in the *Summary of Health Information for International Travel,* which is published every 2 weeks by the CDC [30] and may be found on-line at the CDC travel website (*www.cdc.gov/travel/bluesheet.htm*). Zones **endemic** for yellow fever are areas in Africa and South America where yellow fever could occur. Some countries, particularly those in Asia, that are not in the endemic zones require immunization of persons who enter their country from an area in which yellow fever is occurring. Requirements for each country are clearly stated in *Health Information for International Travel* [4].

Recently, several cases of multiple organ system failure, some of them fatal, have occurred in persons receiving yellow fever vaccine [31]. A CDC analysis of U.S. persons with serious reactions to this vaccine indicated an increased risk for the elderly (particularly those 75 years of age and older) [32]. The CDC and Immunization Practices Advisory Committee have made no changes to the recommendations for yellow fever vaccine. However, before administering vaccine, the travel health professional should be sure that it is indicated for the traveler.

**It is best not to vaccinate HIV-infected travelers with yellow fever vaccine unless they are asymptomatic, have undetectable viral loads and high CD4 counts, and are traveling to yellow fever-infected areas.** Otherwise, they should avoid travel to infected areas. If they have to travel and yellow fever vaccine is required, they should carry with them a letter of medical exemption to vaccination, and they should adhere meticulously to mosquito avoidance measures. Whole-cell inactivated cholera vaccine (no longer available in the United States) given within 3 weeks of yellow fever vaccination may reduce antibody responses to both vaccines. Yellow fever vaccine may be given simultaneously with immunoglobulin.

**B. Cholera.** Production of the whole-cell inactivated cholera vaccine (the only cholera vaccine that was available in the United States) ceased in 2000. Discontinuation may have been prompted by the vaccine's limited efficacy (around 50%) for only a short duration (3–6 months) and uncomfortable side effects [33]. More importantly, use of this vaccine was extremely limited because of the negligible risk of cholera for international travelers [34,35]. This low level of risk prevails despite increased cholera infection in Latin America and a new serotype of cholera, *Vibrio cholerae* O139, which is circulating in Asian countries [36].

Two oral vaccines are marketed in countries other than the United States [37]. One is live-attenuated and uses a recombinant toxin-deleted strain of *V. cholerae,* CVD HgR 103 (Mutachol, Berna). The second is inactivated, combining whole *V. cholerae* O1 cells with recombinant B subunit of cholera toxin (Dukoral, SBL Vaccine AB). Although these vaccines are generally well tolerated and more effective (60%–80% protective efficacy) than the parenteral vaccine, they are still not recommended because of low risk [38].

Cholera immunization is no longer required for international travel, which further decreases the need for vaccination. Although no country requires vaccination for entry, some local authorities may still request documentation. In these circumstances, the traveler can try to obtain vaccine outside of the United States or may carry a letter of contraindication to vaccine. To avoid infection, travelers should exercise care in food and water consumption.

C. **Smallpox. The requirement for smallpox vaccination for international travel was discontinued in 1982** after the worldwide eradication of smallpox [9]. Stocks of the vaccinia virus vaccine have been maintained by several countries and used for vaccination of laboratory workers. With the threat of bioterrorist attacks using smallpox virus [39], there has been renewed interest in protecting a larger segment of the population and having vaccine available for use in control of an outbreak [40]. There are no recommendations for vaccine use for travel, but this is an area that should be closely monitored.

IV. **Recommended vaccinations for travelers because of risk**

A. **Hepatitis prophylaxis**

1. **Hepatitis A.** Hepatitis A virus (HAV), endemic throughout much of the developing world, is the most common vaccine-preventable illness in travelers and causes the most time lost from work in returned travelers [41]. The risk for HAV in unprotected travelers varies from 1 to 10 per 1,000 travelers for a 2- to 3-week stay and includes persons on first-class tours [41–43]. Therefore, most travelers should receive protection [44]. See related discussion in Chapters 14 and 23.

   a. **Hepatitis A vaccine.** There are two inactivated vaccines available in the United States (Havrix, GlaxoSmithKline, and Vaqta, Merck) that are highly immunogenic, protective, and cost effective [44,45]. After a single intramuscular dose in either adults or children, protective antibodies develop in 14 to 28 days and protection should last for at least a year. A dose at 6 to 18 months will likely provide protection for as long as 10 to 20 years, and perhaps for a lifetime. The manufacturers recommend administering vaccine 2 to 4 weeks before travel to allow development of a protective immune response. Indirect information, however, indicates that vaccination may be protective immediately before exposure or within the first several days after exposure [46,47]. If necessary, either Vaqta or Havrix may be administered to boost a primary dose with the other vaccine [48]. When inactivated vaccines were first released, use was often restricted to long-term (≥6 months) or frequent (three or more trips) travelers; however, these vaccines are becoming the products of choice.

   b. **Immunoglobulin,** a sterile preparation of antibodies (primarily IgG) with high titers against HAV, is available **for immediate passive protection against infection.** It may be used for children under 2 years of age in whom inactivated vaccines are not approved by the U.S. Food and Drug Administration (FDA). Immunoglobulin provides protection for 2 to 6 months, depending on the dose administered (Table 23.1) [49]. Problems with production of immunoglobulin for intramuscular use have led to intermittent shortages of the product.

   c. **Pretravel hepatitis A antibody testing may be considered for frequent visitors to the developing world or those with a higher likelihood of having had infection in the past,** such as persons older than 50 (30%–75% will be seropositive, depending on the population studied [44,50]), those born in or with prolonged residence in developing regions, and those with a history of hepatitis [51]. The cost effectiveness of this testing depends on the prevalence of hepatitis A antibody, the cost of screening, and the cost of vaccine [52]. Anti-HAV (IgG)-positive travelers do not need either immunoglobulin or inactivated vaccine.

2. **Hepatitis B.** Vaccination against hepatitis B virus (HBV) is routine for children and adolescents in the United States [26]. Travelers at risk are those who will be in contact with blood or body fluid secretions (e.g., physicians, nurses, other health-care workers, and laboratory technicians) and those likely to have sexual exposure [4]. Travelers who will live in countries with intermediate (2%–7%) or high prevalence (>8%) of hepatitis B surface antigenemia (such as parts of southeast Asia, Sub-Saharan Africa, and the interior Amazon basin) should also consider vaccination (Fig. 22.1).

   HBV vaccine (Engerix, GlaxoSmithKline, and Recombivax, Merck) is administered at 0, 1, and 6 months. Dosage varies between the two licensed products. Adolescents 11 to 15 years of age require only two doses of either vaccine (10 $\mu$g

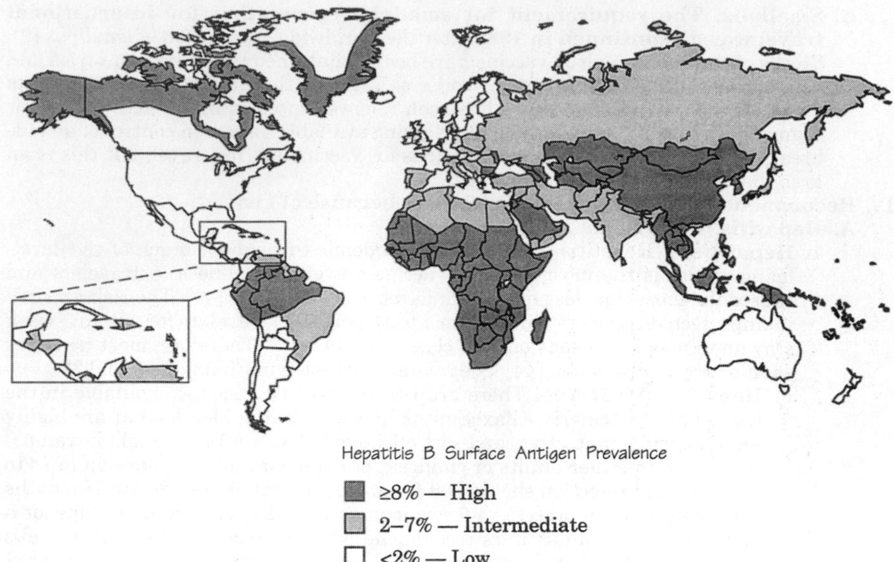


**FIG. 22.1** World prevalence of hepatitis B surface antigen. (From Centers for Disease Control and Prevention. *Health information for international travel, 2001–2002.* Atlanta, GA: U.S. Department of Health and Human Services, 2001, with permission.)

dose) at 0 and 6 months. To achieve more rapid immunity for travelers, the dosing intervals of Engerix (20 $\mu$g) may be shortened to 0, 1, and 2 months with a 6- to 12-month booster [53]. Further acceleration may be achieved by giving Engerix at 0, 7, and 21 days, which will produce seroprotective titers in 65% of recipients at 28 days [54]; this regimen is not FDA approved.

Intramuscular injections of hepatitis vaccine should be given in the deltoid. **Persons immunized against hepatitis B will also be protected against delta hepatitis** because this incomplete virus requires actively replicating hepatitis B for survival (see Chapters 14 and 23).

3. **Combination vaccination against HAV and HBV.** Twinrix (GlaxoSmithKline, released in 2001) combines both HAV and HBV antigens and is approved for persons 18 years of age and older [55]. Indications for use are the same as those for HAV and HBV. Because the vaccine has a lower dose of HAV antigen (720 ELISA Units) compared with either of the two single-antigen HAV vaccines, seroconversion to HAV may be delayed; **two doses of vaccine should be administered before travel to ensure protection.**
4. **Hepatitis C.** There is no vaccine against hepatitis C. Persons may decrease their risk of infection by avoiding exposure to blood products, blood-contaminated needles or dental instruments, and unprotected sexual contact.
5. **Hepatitis E** is recognized throughout much of the developing world [56]. An analysis of clinically apparent cases of hepatitis E in travelers indicated that most cases occurred after travel to the Indian subcontinent and in persons who were traveling for longer than 1 month [57]. Subclinical seroconversion may occur [58]. Water that has been fecally contaminated, often after heavy rains in areas with inadequate sewage disposal, is the most likely source of infection in endemic cases [59]. The overall risk for travelers appears to be less than that for hepatitis A. Pregnant women are at a relatively high risk of mortality. There is no evidence that immunoglobulin will prevent hepatitis E [60] and so proper preparation of food and purification of water needs should emphasized (see Chapter 14).

**B. Typhoid.** Typhoid immunization is indicated before traveling to areas endemic for typhoid fever where fecally contaminated food and water are likely to be ingested. Importation accounted for 72% of the 2,445 cases of typhoid in the United States from 1985 to 1994 [61]. Although most cases of typhoid originated in Mexico, travel to the Indian subcontinent presented the highest risk: 1.1 to 4.1 cases of typhoid fever occurred per 10,000 travelers, which was 18 times higher than travel to other destinations. Another reason to consider vaccination is that *Salmonella typhi* acquired internationally is frequently multidrug resistant [62].

1. **Live oral vaccine** (Vivotif Berna, Swiss Serum and Vaccine Institute). This attenuated live vaccine uses the Ty21a mutant of *S. typhi*. In a meta-analysis of typhoid vaccines, three doses of this vaccine provided a 3-year protective efficacy of 51% (95% confidence interval, 35%–63%) [63]. In the United States, four doses of vaccine are administered, which could lead to improved efficacy. The traveler takes one enteric-coated capsule with a cool to warm drink (<37°C) 1 hour before a meal every other day for a total of four capsules, beginning at least 2 weeks before departure. Although capsules should be refrigerated, they usually retain potency if left at room temperature (20–25°C) for a few days. The availability of this vaccine has been limited in the United States in recent years.

   **The safety of this vaccine in HIV-infected persons is not known. It should not be given to persons taking antimicrobials, nor should mefloquine be given simultaneously** because of the potential of killing the attenuated bacteria. Administration of mefloquine and vaccine should be separated by at least 24 hours; antibiotics can be commenced 48 hours after completing the vaccine series.
2. **Typhoid Vi polysaccharide vaccine,** which consists of purified Vi capsular polysaccharide of *S. typhi,* is given in a single intramuscular dose and should provide approximately 50% to 70% protection for 2 to 3 years [64,65]. It can be administered to persons 2 years of age or older and should be given at least 2 weeks before travel. The vaccine may be the product of choice when compliance with oral dosing and refrigeration of the Ty21a vaccine are concerns and for children aged 2 to 6 years of age. An experimental conjugate Vi antigen vaccine has demonstrated superior protective efficacy in children 2 to 6 years of age [66].
3. **Parenteral whole-cell vaccine.** Although this vaccine was as effective as the oral and Vi polysaccharide typhoid vaccines, it was often poorly tolerated, and production in the United States was discontinued in 2000. It could be given to persons 6 months of age and older. Because children under 2 years of age can no longer be vaccinated against typhoid, their parents or guardians must ensure that they ingest only safe foods and liquids during travel.

**C. Meningococcal disease.** Most international travelers are at low risk for acquiring meningococcal bacteremia or meningitis. Several areas of the world, however, have epidemic or endemic meningococcal disease, and because the consequences of meningococcal infection are severe, vaccination may be warranted [67] (Fig. 22.2). **It is required that religious pilgrims traveling to Saudi Arabia to attend the annual hajj receive vaccine. Long-term visitors to the meningitis belt in Sub-Saharan Africa should be vaccinated. Short-term visitors to this region who travel from December through June and who will have contact with local people should also consider vaccine** [4]. Although the serotype A is usually associated with epidemic disease, in the years 2000 and 2001 serotype W-135 affected hundreds of pilgrims to Saudi Arabia, who sometimes carried this serotype type back to their country of origin [68]. The meningococcal polysaccharide vaccine in the United States is polyvalent for groups A, C, Y, and W-135. Because of variable efficacy of the current vaccine in children under the age of 5 years, conjugate vaccines against *Neisseria meningitis* group C have been developed and used in England and Canada [69].

The risk of meningococcal disease is slightly greater among freshman college students who live in dormitories [70]. Therefore, the Advisory Committee on Immunization Practices has recommended that this group of students is informed of the risk and that protection (against serotypes A, C, Y, and W-135) is available by vaccination

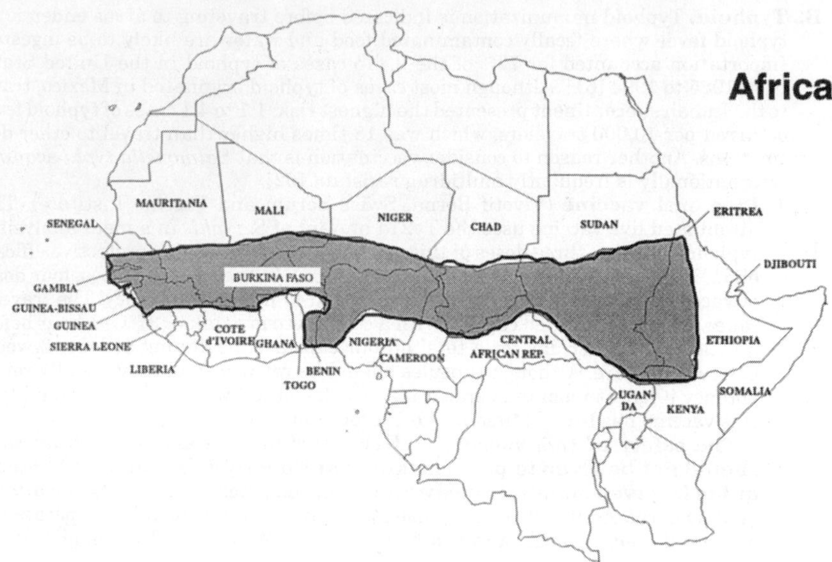


**FIG. 22.2** Areas in Sub-Saharan Africa with epidemic meningococcal disease. (From Centers for Disease Control and Prevention. *Health information for international travel, 2001–2002.* Atlanta, GA: U.S. Department of Health and Human Services, 2001, with permission.)

[71]. Other students may also consider vaccination to reduce this small risk of disease. See Chapters 6 and 23 for further discussion.

**D. Poliomyelitis.** Worldwide, much progress has been made in the elimination of poliomyelitis [72]. The Western Hemisphere was declared polio free in September 1994 and the Western Pacific in October 2000 [73]. Most of the world's polio cases occur in Africa (central and western), particularly in countries with conflict, and in the Indian subcontinent [72]. Despite the progress in control of polio, it remains important to maintain high vaccine coverage. This was illustrated recently in Haiti, the Dominican Republic, and the Philippines where cases of vaccine-strain paralytic disease occurred in unvaccinated or incompletely vaccinated persons [74].

The risk to the international traveler is extremely low [75]. In a study of paralytic poliomyelitis in the United States from 1980 through 1998, there were only six cases imported and only one after 1986 [76,77]. Nevertheless, travelers to endemic areas who are exposed to poor food and water sanitation should be immunized.

In January 2000 the CDC and the American Academy of Pediatrics initiated a change from oral poliovirus vaccine (Sabin; live attenuated, trivalent vaccine [OPV]) to inactivated polio vaccine (IPV) for routine childhood immunization [77]. This was undertaken because of the rare risk of paralytic disease in recipients and contacts of recipients of OPV; all cases of indigenous paralytic poliomyelitis in the United States since 1980 have been associated with the OPV vaccine.

1. **Primary vaccination of persons of all ages should be accomplished with inactivated poliomyelitis vaccine.** At least two doses of IPV should be given before travel; however, if time is lacking (<4 weeks before departure), a single dose of IPV can be given.
2. **It is recommended that persons who have completed a primary series receive one adult (generally those age 18 and older) lifetime booster if traveling to an area of risk.**
3. **See Chapter 23 for further discussion.**

**E. Japanese B encephalitis.** Japanese B encephalitis is a mosquito-borne encephalitis prevalent in many areas of the Indian subcontinent and Asia (Fig. 22.3). It has an

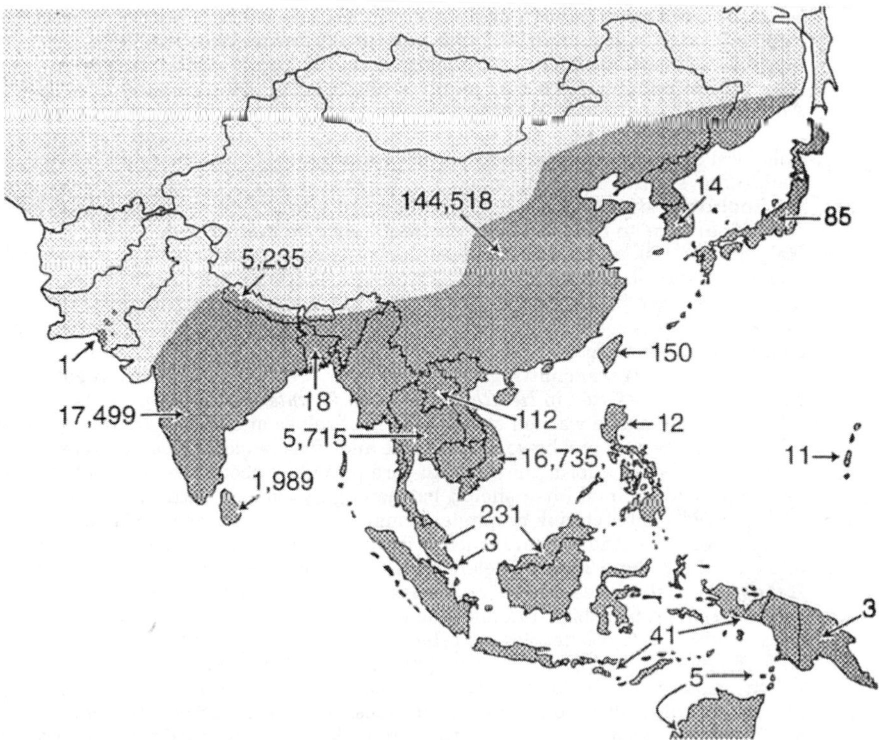


**FIG. 22.3** Reported Japanese encephalitis cases by endemic countries and regions of Southeast Asia where viral transmission is proven or suspected, 1986–1996. (From Tsai TF, Chang G-JJ, Yu YX. Japanese encephalitis vaccines. In: Plotkin SA, Orenstein WA, eds. *Vaccines.* Philadelphia: W.B. Saunders, 1999:672–710, with permission.)

inapparent-to-apparent case ratio of 50 to 500:1. Among patients with symptomatic disease; however, the fatality rate is approximately 20%, and there is high morbidity in survivors [78]. Disease occurs primarily in young children and adults older than 65 years of age. Seasons and areas of risk are delineated in *Health Information for International Travel* [4], and this guide should be consulted in determining the risk to travelers. Based on the number of cases in expatriate travelers and military personnel, the risk appears to be fewer than one case per 1 million travelers [79]. If risk is based on endemic populations, however, it could be as high as one case per 5,000 to 20,000.

Vaccination against Japanese B encephalitis should be considered for travelers with prolonged residence in endemic areas during transmission seasons or short-term travelers who will engage in high-risk activities such as fieldwork, camping, or bicycling. Transmission is most likely to occur in rural areas where there is rice farming (a breeding site for the *Culex* mosquito vector) in proximity to pig farming (the principal amplifying host for the virus). Most travelers to endemic countries will not need vaccination because their travel is short term and they typically visit only urban and major tourist destinations. All travelers should practice personal protection against the *Culex* mosquito, particularly during the dusk to dawn hours.

Japanese B encephalitis vaccine in the United States is an inactivated mouse brain-derived vaccine (Biken) distributed by Aventis Pasteur. **This vaccine may**

**be associated with severe systemic allergic reactions that occur with an approximate frequency of 0.1 to 5 per 1,000 administrations** [79–83]. Severe reactions have included urticaria, anaphylaxis, and cardiovascular collapse and can occur within minutes of vaccine administration to several days after vaccination. **An allergic history may be associated with an increased risk of adverse reactions and should be a relative contraindication to receiving vaccine** [82]. Mild local and systemic reactions occur with a frequency of 10% to 20%. **Vaccine recipients should be monitored for 60 minutes after immunization, and the final dose should preferably be completed not sooner than 10 days before departure so that untoward effects may be monitored.**

**F. Rabies.** The risk of acquiring rabies during travel is very low; there were only 10 cases in travelers from 1975 to 1984 [84]. Potential exposures (e.g., dog bites), however, may not be uncommon. Most cases in travelers and most transmission of rabies overseas is secondary to the bite of a rabid dog [85]; canine rabies is highly endemic throughout many areas of the world. Other animal species, including bats, are also capable of transmitting the rabies virus. Countries that have reported no cases of rabies are listed in *Health Information for International Travel* [4].

Travelers should be warned about the risk of rabies and if they are exposed how to treat a bite wound and how to access safe and effective postexposure rabies treatment. They should inform their health-care providers about the exposure as soon as possible. All animal bites should be thoroughly cleaned with copious amounts of water and soap. Tetanus prophylaxis may be needed if the traveler has not received a booster within 5 years, and antibiotics should be given to treat a potential bite wound infection. Then travelers should seek **postexposure** rabies treatment. If they have had no preexposure prophylaxis, postexposure treatment will consist of rabies vaccine **plus** rabies immune globulin [86]. If they have received preexposure prophylaxis, only a booster dose of rabies vaccine is necessary. See Chapters 4 and 23 for further discussion of bite wound management and rabies prophylaxis.

**Preexposure** prophylaxis is recommended based on the individual's itinerary, planned activities, duration of travel, and access to safe postexposure biologics. There are two rabies vaccines available in the United States: the purified chick embryo cell vaccine (RabAvert, Chiron) and the human diploid cell vaccine (Imovax, Aventis Pasteur). These are both administered intramuscularly in the deltoid of adults or the quadriceps of small children; the intradermal formulation of human diploid cell vaccine has been discontinued. Preexposure immunization consists of three doses of vaccine given over 21 or 28 days (Table 22.1). Routine serologic testing after preexposure immunization is not necessary unless the recipient is believed to be at risk for a diminished immune response. Intramuscular administration of vaccine overcomes the interference of immunogenicity that occurred when chloroquine (and possibly mefloquine) was administered with intradermal human diploid cell vaccine.

**Preexposure prophylaxis has the advantage of providing protection when there is an inapparent exposure to rabies** (such as may occur with small children who do not report a bite) **and when postexposure therapy is delayed. It also eliminates the need for rabies immune globulin** in the event of an exposure. This product is difficult to obtain in many countries [87] and may be manufactured from nonhuman sources that have variable purity. Equine rabies immune globulin has been used safely in many countries. **Preexposure prophylaxis does not eliminate the need for additional doses of rabies vaccine** [86]. Travelers who receive postexposure treatment overseas should be evaluated by health-care providers on return and serologic testing should be done to ensure that they developed immunity from their treatment.

**G. Plague.** The plague vaccine is not required by any country. Because of uncertain efficacy and very low risk of disease, production of the vaccine was terminated in 1999. Approximately 2,500 cases of plague are reported annually from 10 to 15 countries (including the United States) [88]. Nearly 80% of the world's plague comes from Africa. Travelers who will reside in plague endemic areas should avoid rodents and use precautions against fleas. For unavoidable exposure, adults can be given tetracycline (500 mg four times a day) or doxycycline (100 mg twice daily) chemoprophylaxis and children can be given sulfonamides [89]. The efficacy of this measure, however, has not been established.

**H. Tuberculosis prevention.** Tuberculosis exposure in the developing world usually occurs as a result of prolonged contact with respiratory droplets from infected persons in a closed setting. The risk during travel was recently defined in Dutch travelers visiting tuberculosis endemic regions for at least 3 months [90]. Travelers were bacille balié de Calmette-Guerin naive and were screened by pre- and posttravel tuberculin skin testing. The incidence of infection (based on 656 travelers) was 3.5 cases per 1,000 person-months, the incidence of disease was 0.6 cases per 1,000 person-months, and the incidence of infection in health-care workers was 7.9 cases per 1,000 person-months. These risks approach that for the most common vaccine-preventable diseases. For travelers with exposure, particularly long-term travelers and health-care workers, pretravel and posttravel (2 months after return) tuberculin skin testing is indicated. This approach is preferable to administration of the bacille balié de Calmette-Guerin vaccine [91]. For children who will have unavoidable exposure to tuberculosis and for whom other preventive measures such as prophylactic isoniazid cannot be used, bacille balié de Calmette-Guerin vaccine may be considered.

## ADVICE ON DISEASE PREVENTION OTHER THAN BY VACCINATION

**I. Traveler's diarrhea**

**A. Clinical findings. Traveler's diarrhea affects 20% to 50% of visitors to developing regions** in Latin America, Africa, and portions of Asia [92–95]. The risk is intermediate in some of the Caribbean islands and in Eastern Europe. Disease is transmitted through fecally contaminated food or liquids.

1. **Etiology.** The causative agent is identified in fewer than three-fourths of cases. Enterotoxigenic *Escherichia coli* is most common, accounting for approximately 50% of cases in which the etiology is determined [94,96]. *Shigella, Salmonella* species, *Campylobacter,* and enteroaggregative *E. coli* are seen in 10% to 30% of cases [97]. *Vibrio* species, *Aeromonas,* and *Plesiomonas* species are less frequent. Norwalk-like agents and rotavirus are implicated in approximately 20% of cases. *Giardia lamblia* is the most common parasite that causes diarrhea in travelers (approximately 5% of cases) [98]. Symptoms may appear after the traveler has returned to the United States and often persist for more than 2 weeks. *Cryptosporidium parvum* and *Cyclospora cayetanensis* are also seen, with *Entamoeba histolytica* and *Isospora belli* reported infrequently [99]. Most cases of parasitic diarrhea occur in long-term travelers [99,100].
2. **Clinical manifestations.** Traveler's diarrhea usually occurs during the first week of travel. Diarrhea and abdominal cramps are associated with nausea and malaise. Temperature exceeding 38°C occurs in only 10% to 20% of patients and vomiting in fewer than 15%. Bloody dysenteric stools are unusual (2%–10%). The duration of traveler's diarrhea, even in persons who are not treated, is 3 to 4 days, with 60% of patients recovering within 48 hours.

**B. Prevention**

1. **Routine precautions. The best precaution against traveler's diarrhea is careful choice of food and drink.** It is particularly important to exercise this precaution when traveling with infants or small children because the consequences of diarrhea at this age may be considerable. Travelers should ingest only commercially bottled or carbonated beverages (bottled carbonated water, soda, and beer), wine, heated drinks (coffee, tea, boiled water), thoroughly cooked foods and meats served piping hot (particularly seafood and shellfish), and fruits that the traveler can peel. Unpasteurized dairy products, tap water, ice cubes, food from street vendors, salads, and fresh ground-grown leafy greens and vegetables should be avoided. Even persons who exercise these precautions may not always avoid diarrhea.

   The most reliable way to purify drinking water is to bring it to a boil; boiling for an additional few minutes may be necessary at high altitude [101]. If used properly, halogens (iodine or chlorine preparations) will kill viruses and bacteria.

Chlorine preparations are more affected by water temperature, pH, and turbidity. Protozoa cysts, particularly *Cryptosporidium* and *Cyclospora,* will not be killed by halogenation [102]. Small-volume water filters of an "absolute" size no more than 1 $\mu$m remove bacteria and protozoa cysts.

2. **Antiperistaltic agents.** These should not be used for preventing traveler's diarrhea.
3. **Prophylactic bismuth subsalicylate.** The prophylactic use of bismuth subsalicylate liquid (Pepto-Bismol, 2 oz four times a day) or tablets (two tablets four times a day) can reduce by approximately 60% the incidence of diarrhea in travelers [103]. Persons taking salicylate-containing compounds may develop salicylate toxicity if bismuth subsalicylate is taken concurrently. **Patients who are allergic to salicylates or who are taking anticoagulants should not take Pepto-Bismol.**
4. **Prophylactic antibiotics.** Several antibacterials (trimethoprim, 160 mg, and sulfamethoxazole, 800 mg, 1 tablet daily; trimethoprim, 200 mg/day; doxycycline, 100 mg/day; norfloxacin, 400 mg/day; ciprofloxacin, 500 mg/day) can decrease the incidence of diarrhea to 5% to 15% for the short-term (<3 weeks) traveler [93]. However, **prophylactic antibiotics may cause serious allergic reactions in a small number of persons** (e.g., Stevens-Johnson syndrome with sulfonamides) or adverse effects in others (e.g., photosensitivity and vaginal yeast infections with doxycycline and antibiotic-associated colitis with any antibiotic) and may contribute to the development of resistance to enteric flora. **Therefore, prophylactic antibiotics to prevent this usually mild illness are not recommended for most healthy travelers** [104]. For the short-term traveler who is on a very important trip or who has a medical condition that would be adversely affected by diarrhea, antimicrobial prophylaxis may be considered after potential risks are weighed.

**C. Treatment**

1. **Fluid replacement and diet. The most important management principle is to replace fluids and electrolytes lost in diarrheal stools** (Table 22.2) [4,105,106]. This may be the only treatment necessary for many adults and children because the diarrheal illness is often self-limited and of short duration. Oral rehydration must include glucose, sodium, potassium, chloride, and free water. Except in extreme cases, this may be accomplished in adults and older children by ingesting fruit juices, caffeine-free soft drinks, broth, and bouillon. These may be supplemented with salted crackers, rice, or toast. **Dairy products should be avoided initially** because lactose intolerance may be present.

   Breast-fed infants should continue nursing. Bottle-fed children should also continue with lactose-free formulas. For oral rehydration, packets that contain glucose and salts at the appropriate concentrations after addition of purified water are available in most developing countries and in the United States (Table 22.2). Some formulas are rice based. Those who travel with infants and small children should consider carrying these packets. Children who experience persistent vomiting, bloody diarrhea, or high fever should receive immediate medical attention.
2. **Antimotility agents.** Drugs such as loperamide (Imodium) or diphenoxylate hydrochloride with atropine sulfate (Lomotil) relieve cramping and help to control diarrhea, allowing patients to participate in planned activities [107]. Loperamide is available over the counter and appears to be better tolerated than diphenoxylate-atropine, particularly in the elderly. It is favored by most physicians who advise travelers.

   Antimotility agents may predispose to complications in patients with invasive or inflammatory enterocolitis. Therefore, **they should not be used when temperature exceeds 38.5°C or when blood appears in the stool** [93]. **They should not be taken by children younger than 2 years of age.** Liquid bismuth subsalicylate has proven effective for treatment for mild diarrhea [108]. Experience with this agent in children is limited [109], and it could potentially lead to salicylate toxicity if not used properly [110]. **If symptoms persist beyond 48 hours after any of these agents are initiated, administration should be discontinued and medical attention sought.**

Table 22.2. Treatment of Traveler's Diarrhea[a]

| Agent | Dose |
|---|---|
| Oral hydration[b] | |
| Homemade solution | |
| Potable water | 1 L |
| Table salt | 1/2 teaspoon |
| Baking soda | 1/2 teaspoon |
| Table sugar (sucrose)[c] | 2–3 tablespoons |
| World Health Organization composition[d] | |
| Sodium chloride | 3.5 g/L |
| Glucose | 20.0 g/L |
| Sodium citrate | 2.9 g/L |
| Potassium chloride | 1.5 g/L |
| Bismuth subsalicylate | 1 oz q 1/2 h × 8 doses, or 2 tabs q 1/2 h × 8 doses |
| Loperamide (2 mg)[e] | 2 capsules with 1st diarrheal stool, then 1 with each subsequent loose stool, not to exceed 8 capsules/day |
| Antibiotics | |
| Quinolones[f] | |
| Ciprofloxacin, 500 mg | Single dose—750 mg; 3-day therapy—500 mg b.i.d. |
| Norfloxacin, 400 mg | Single dose—800 mg; 3-day therapy—400 mg b.i.d. |
| Ofloxacin | Single dose—400 mg; 3-day therapy—300 mg b.i.d. |
| Levofloxacin, 500 mg | Single dose—500 mg; 3-day therapy—500 mg b.i.d. |
| Azithromycin[g] | Single dose—1,000 mg; 3-day therapy—500 mg b.i.d. |
| Trimethoprim, 160 mg, and sulfamethoxazole, 800 mg[h] | 1 tablet b.i.d. |
| Doxycycline, 100 mg[h] | 1 tablet b.i.d. |

[a]Travelers who have a temperature of more than 38.5°C, severe cramping, and blood or mucus in their stools should seek prompt medical attention if symptoms do not promptly resolve.
[b]Rice-based products may also be used. Commercial preparations may be purchased from: Jianas Brothers Packaging Company, Kansas City, MO (816 421-2880); or Cera Products, Inc., 1041 Waterfowl Terrace, Columbia, MD 21044 (301 490-4941).
[c]Honey or karo syrup (2 tbsp) may be substituted for sugar.
[d]The WHO composition is sodium (90 mEq/L), potassium (20 mEq/L), chloride (80 mEq/L), citrate (30 mEq/L), glucose (20 g/L).
Sucrose (table sugar), 40 g/L, may be substituted for glucose.
Sodium bicarbonate, 2.5 g/L, may be substituted for sodium citrate.
[e]Avoid taking loperamide if there is fever >38°C and blood or mucus in the stools.
[f]Treatment of enteric infections is not an approved indication for norfloxacin. Quinolones are contraindicated in pregnancy and for children under the age of 18 years. May be safe for short-term use in the pediatric age group.
[g]Not FDA approved for treatment of travelers' diarrhea.
[h]There may be resistance to trimethoprim-sulfamethoxazole and doxycycline by enteric organisms.

3. **Antibiotic therapy.** Patients with mild to moderate traveler's diarrhea can be treated with a single dose or a short course (3 days) of one of several antibiotics [111]. Trimethoprim, trimethoprim-sulfamethoxazole [112], and doxycycline were studied initially; however, widespread resistance of enteric organisms has made these choices less effective [113]. Most experts recommend that travelers carry a quinolone antibiotic: norfloxacin, ciprofloxacin, ofloxacin, or levofloxacin (Table 22.2) [111]. *Campylobacter* species is becoming resistant to quinolones, especially in Asia; in these cases, azithromycin may be effective [114]. New agents that have not yet been approved for use in the United States may prove valuable [115].

Single-dose therapy for traveler's diarrhea has not been extensively studied but is likely to be effective [116]. A single dose may be initiated; if diarrhea does not resolve after this, treatment may be continued for up to 3 days. Although combining an antibiotic with loperamide for mild to moderate diarrhea has also been shown to effect prompt improvement of symptoms [117,118], this approach has not been found consistently effective in all regions of the world and in all etiologies of diarrhea [95,119]. It is a reasonable approach as long as the traveler is not experiencing severe cramping, fever at least 38.5°C, or bloody stools.

Patients with high fever or bloody diarrhea should seek medical evaluation. If medical attention is not available, empiric antibiotic therapy can be initiated.

**II. Malaria.** Malaria is a febrile flu-like illness caused by one of four species of malaria parasites: *Plasmodium falciparum, P. vivax, P. ovale,* or *P. malariae.* From 1993 through 1998, 85% of malaria cases imported to the United States were caused by *P. falciparum* or *P. vivax* [120]. *P. falciparum* is the species that causes the most severe illness and nearly all cases of fatal malaria [4,121]. It is widely resistant to chloroquine phosphate, and in rural and forested border areas of Thailand it is resistant to other antimalarials (Fig. 22.4). From 1995 through 1998, 83% of imported cases of falciparum malaria cases originated in Sub-Saharan Africa [120].

Exposure to malaria depends on the itinerary and duration of a trip, time of year, and prevalence of *Plasmodium* species. The overall risk of acquiring malaria ranges from 0.8 cases to 24 cases per thousand travelers [122,123] and varies greatly between and within countries, the type of travel, and whether or not chemoprophylaxis was taken (Fig. 22.4). Country-specific prevention guidelines are published by the CDC in *Health Information for International Travel* [4] and by the WHO [124]. The United Kingdom and Canada also publish their own guidelines [125,126].

Prevention of malaria requires a multifaceted approach that emphasizes protection against mosquitoes, safe and effective chemoprophylaxis, and plans for medical care if

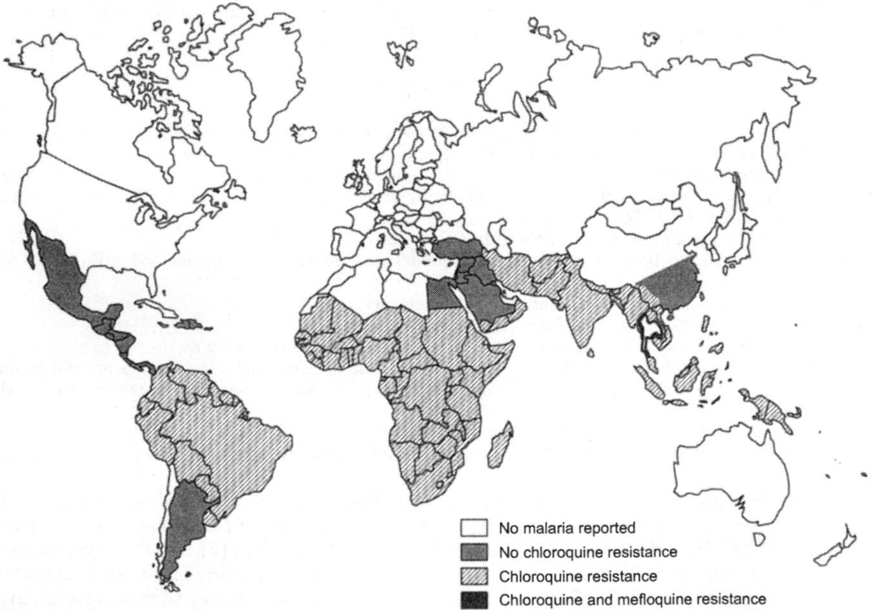


**FIG. 22.4** Distribution of malaria and chloroquine-resistant *Plasmodium falciparum.* For use only as a visual aid. Refer to up-to-date resources for actual distribution. (From Committee to Advise on Tropical Medicine and Travel (CATMAT). Canadian recommendations for the prevention and treatment of malaria among international travelers. *Can Commun Dis Rep* 2000;26[Suppl 2]:1–42, with permission.)

malaria occurs [127]. **All travelers should be informed that no prophylactic regimen is 100% effective and that malaria can develop several months or longer after returning to the United States.** Travelers must be advised to seek prompt medical attention for any acute febrile illness that might be malaria and to inform their physician of their exposure. **Patient compliance with medication and physician prescribing of correct antimalarials** are key. In the United States from 1992 to 2001 75% of United States civilians with malaria had taken either no prophylaxis or inappropriate chemoprophylaxis [128]; in Canada, similar findings have been reported [129].

**A. Mosquito avoidance.** The first step in malaria prevention is avoidance of the female *Anopheles* mosquito, which typically feeds from dusk until dawn. Travelers should wear long-sleeved, light-weight, loose-fitting, protective clothing; avoid the use of perfumes; use mosquito repellents; and sleep under netting or in well-screened rooms.

Mosquito repellents that contain diethyltoluamide (DEET) in a concentration of 15% to 35% offer best protection [127,130]. With new extended-duration formulations of DEET that may provide protection for 4 to 12 hours, there is no need for highly concentrated preparations. DEET is safe to use on children, but guidelines should be followed carefully to avoid any of the exceedingly rare neurologic complications [130]. **DEET-containing products should be applied sparingly only on exposed skin or clothing.** They should not be inhaled, ingested, or applied to mucous membranes, the eyes, or irritated skin; they should be washed off after coming indoors [4]. If a suspected reaction to a repellent occurs, treated skin should be washed and medical attention promptly sought.

Mosquito coils, sprays, and vaporizing mats may be used in enclosed areas to decrease the mosquito population. **Clothing and netting may be sprayed or dipped in the insecticide permethrin.** Permethrin remains adherent to fabric through several washings and provides weeks of protection against mosquitoes [131].

**B. Prophylactic drugs. Current recommendations for antimalarial drugs and their dosing should always be consulted** because chemoprophylactic regimens are reviewed on an ongoing basis as to efficacy and safety [4,124]. Table 22.3 lists antimalarial drugs and their recommended adult and pediatric doses.

1. **For travel to areas with chloroquine-sensitive malaria.** Currently, only the Dominican Republic, Haiti, Central America west and north of the Panama Canal, Mexico, Argentina, Egypt, most countries in the Middle East, and some areas of China have *P. falciparum* strains that are still sensitive to chloroquine. For travel to these areas, chloroquine phosphate remains the drug of choice. It can prevent clinical illness due to the erythrocytic stages of sensitive strains of *P. falciparum* and all other *Plasmodium* species. No agent, including chloroquine, will prevent mosquito bites or kill sporozoites. Occasional cases of chloroquine-resistant *P. vivax* have been reported from Indonesia and Papua [132].

   Chloroquine is taken weekly as a single oral dose, beginning 1 to 2 weeks before travel and each week thereafter in the malarious zone and for 4 weeks after leaving the endemic area. Taking the drug after meals can help to reduce any minor gastrointestinal distress. Chloroquine has been reported to exacerbate psoriasis. High doses of chloroquine [133] or hydroxychloroquine [134] taken on a daily basis for treatment of inflammatory conditions have rarely been associated with retinopathy (three cases per 1,500 users). Persons who take chloroquine at a daily dose of less than 250 mg or less than 3.0 mg/kg should have ophthalmologic screening at 6-month intervals [135]. Chloroquine should be stored in child-proof containers to prevent a risk of life-threatening toxicity with accidental ingestion or overdose of the drug in children.

2. **Travel to areas where chloroquine resistance occurs.** There are three choices for prevention of chloroquine-resistant *P. falciparum*: mefloquine (Lariam, Roche), atovaquone-proguanil (Malarone, GlaxoSmithKline), and doxycycline.

   a. **Mefloquine** is highly effective against both chloroquine-resistant and sulfadoxine-pyrimethamine-resistant *P. falciparum* infections [136–138].

Table 22.3. Drugs Used in the Prophylaxis of Malaria

| Drug | Adult Dose | Pediatric Dose |
|---|---|---|
| Chloroquine phosphate (Aralen) | 300 mg base (500 mg salt) orally, once per wk, beginning 1 wk before travel and continuing for 4 wk after travel | 5 mg/kg base (8.3 mg/kg salt), orally, once per week (not to exceed adult dose of 300 mg base) |
| Mefloquine (Lariam) | 250 mg (salt) orally, once per wk, beginning 1 wk before travel and continuing for 4 wk after travel | <15 kg: 5 mg salt/kg/wk<br>15–19 kg: 1/4 tab/wk<br>20–30 kg: 1/2 tab/wk<br>31–45 kg: 3/4 tab/wk<br>>45 kg: 1 tab/wk |
| Atovaquone/proguanil (A/P) (Malarone) | 250 mg A/100 mg P | 62.5 mg A/25 mg P |
| | 1 tablet daily, beginning 2 days before travel and continuing for 7 days after travel | 11–20 kg: 1 tablet daily<br>21–30 kg: 2 tablets daily<br>31–40 kg: 3 tablets daily<br>>40 kg: adult dosing |
| Doxycycline | 100 mg orally, 1 tablet daily, beginning 2 days before travel and continuing for 7 days after travel | >8 yr old: 2 mg/kg orally, once per day (not to exceed adult dose of 100 mg) |
| Hydroxychloroquine sulfate (Plaquenil) | 310 mg base (400 mg salt) orally once per wk | 5 mg/kg base (6.5 mg/kg salt) orally, once per wk (not to exceed adult dose of 310 mg base) |
| Proguanil | 200 mg/d orally, in combination with weekly chloroquine | <2 yr old: 50 mg/d<br>2–6 yrs old: 100 mg/d<br>7–10 yrs old: 150 mg/d<br>>10 yrs old: 200 mg/d |
| Primaquine | 15 mg base (26.3 mg salt) orally, once per day, for 14 days | 0.3 mg/kg base (0.5 mg/kg salt) orally, once per day |

Adapted from Centers for Disease Control and Prevention. *Health information for international travel, 2001-2002.* 2001, Atlanta, GA: U.S. Department of Health and Human Services.

*P. falciparum* resistance to mefloquine (and to chloroquine) occurs in rural forested areas of Thailand that border Cambodia and Myanmar (formerly Burma) [139].

**(1) Dosage.** Mefloquine is taken weekly as a single dose, beginning 1 to 2 weeks before travel and continuing weekly during exposure and for 4 weeks after leaving endemic areas. Some authorities recommend a loading dose (250 mg daily for 3 days) of mefloquine to rapidly achieve protective levels and to assess the potential for side effects [126,129]; however, this measure is not recommended by the CDC or WHO.

**(2) Side effects.** Although mefloquine is well tolerated by most persons, concern about potential neuropsychiatric side effects has adversely affected patient acceptance of the drug and physician willingness to prescribe it.

Several studies have reviewed adverse events [138,140,141]. With prophylactic doses, minor side effects of gastrointestinal disturbance and mild neuropsychiatric events occur in 5% to 30% of users. Neuropsychiatric events include sleep disturbance, vivid dreams, dizziness, mood changes, and concentration defects. Approximately 40% of these adverse reactions occur after the first dose and 78% after the third dose [142,143]. Rarely, a serious adverse event such as psychosis or convulsions will occur during prophylaxis (about one case per 13,000 users) [144,145]. Neuropsychiatric events occur more frequently with treatment doses.

**(3) Contraindications to the use of mefloquine.**

**(a)** Travelers with known hypersensitivity to mefloquine.

**(b)** Travelers with history of seizures or psychiatric disorder.

**(c)** Travelers with underlying cardiac conduction abnormalities, but not those on beta-blockers (e.g., for hypertension) if they have normal rhythms.

**(d)** Although not approved during pregnancy, mefloquine given during the last two trimesters has not been associated with adverse fetal outcomes [146–148]. Limited information also suggests safety during the first trimester. **Therefore, if exposure to chloroquine-resistant falciparum malaria is unavoidable, mefloquine may be considered** [4].

**b. Atovaquone/Proguanil (Malarone)** is a fixed combination agent approved in the United States in 2000 for the prevention and treatment of *P. falciparum* malaria in both children and adults [149–151]. It has demonstrated excellent efficacy in treatment of both chloroquine-resistant and multidrug-resistant falciparum malaria in semi-immune hosts living in endemic regions of Asia, Africa, and South America [152,153]. It has also been highly effective in prophylaxis of falciparum malaria in semi-immune hosts [154].

Two recent studies have demonstrated safety and efficacy in preventing falciparum malaria in nonimmune travelers [155,156]. It has the advantage of causal prophylaxis (kills developing exoerythrocytic phase organisms) that allows discontinuation of the drug soon after leaving the malarious area [157]. This characteristic makes it a good choice for travelers with a short period of exposure to malaria. Although there are only limited data as to its efficacy in prevention and killing of nonfalciparum malaria parasites, it is presumed to be effective against these species. It does not kill the hypnozoites of *P. vivax* or *P. ovale.*

**(1) Dosage.** Malarone is taken daily, beginning 1 to 2 days before exposure, continued daily during exposure, and continued for 7 days after leaving the malarious area (Table 22.3).

**(2) Side effects.** Malarone is well tolerated; some may experience gastrointestinal upset, headache, or rash. Absorption is enhanced by ingestion with fatty foods. Its safety during pregnancy is not known, and it should not be used in these circumstances, unless other options are not available.

**c. Doxycycline** is effective against chloroquine-resistant and multidrug-resistant falciparum malaria [158,159]. It is taken daily, beginning 1 to 2 days before departure and continued daily during travel in the endemic areas and for 4 weeks after the traveler leaves the malarious area (Table 22.3). Doxycycline is contraindicated in pregnancy and in children younger than 8 years of age. Potential problems with doxycycline include difficulty in complying with a medication taken daily for 4 weeks after return, gastrointestinal upset, photosensitivity dermatitis, vaginal candidiasis, antibiotic-associated colitis, and esophageal ulceration if the pill is not completely swallowed [160]. Use of a sunscreen may decrease the risk of photosensitivity.

**d. Other medications. Proguanil,** a dihydrofolate reductase inhibitor, has been combined with chloroquine (200 mg daily) to provide coverage for chloroquine-resistant *P. falciparum* in areas of low prevalence (e.g., in India and South America) [124,125]. This approach is not endorsed by CDC, however, because of its inferior efficacy and deaths due to malaria in persons on this regimen and the difficulty in acquiring and adhering to proguanil because it is not available in the United States [128].

**Primaquine** has been studied for prevention of malaria [150,161]. It has causal prophylaxis against all species of malaria and, like Malarone, may be discontinued soon after departing the malarious area. There is limited experience with this drug for prevention, and it is not FDA approved for this use; it may also cause hemolysis in glucose-6-phosphate dehydrogenase (G6PD)–deficient individuals. **The G6PD status of anyone receiving primaquine should be checked.**

3. **Self-treatment for malaria.** Travelers who choose not to take chemoprophylaxis or who desire to carry medication in the event of acquiring malaria despite chemoprophylaxis may carry self-treatment medications. Although malaria self-diagnosis kits are available in some countries outside of the United States, they are often not used reliably by the traveler [162]. Thus, if the traveler develops a febrile illness that could be malaria, the first step is to seek medical care. If medical care cannot be obtained within 24 hours, then self-treatment can be considered. **Two options are Fansidar (sulfadoxine/pyrimethamine) or Malarone, the latter is probably best.** Fansidar may not be effective in areas of sulfonamide resistance (southeast Asia, the Amazon River basin, and parts of East Africa) and has been associated with life-threatening severe cutaneous reactions in persons allergic to sulfonamides. Even if self-treatment is taken, travelers should still seek medical evaluation. Halofantrine should not be used for self-treatment because of the risk of sudden cardiac death in persons with cardiac conduction abnormalities [163]. Mefloquine used for self-treatment may also be associated with serious adverse events, including seizures and hallucinations.
4. **Prolonged exposure to malaria in areas intensely endemic for *P. vivax* or *P. ovale* may warrant terminal malaria prophylaxis with primaquine phosphate** to eradicate persistent hepatic forms of these species. Missionaries, Peace Corps volunteers, or refugee camp workers with prolonged exposure and returning travelers who were treated for malaria while abroad are at greatest risk for infection with these parasites. A G6PD level should be checked before prescribing this drug. Primaquine is **contraindicated during pregnancy** because the G6PD status of the fetus cannot be easily ascertained. Primaquine is not necessary for most travelers.
5. **Malaria information.** Detailed recommendations for the prevention of malaria may be obtained 24 hours a day by calling the CDC travel information system (888-232-3228) or by accessing the CDC Travel Health webpage (*www.cdc.gov/travel*).

**III. Other diseases**

**A. Dengue fever.** Dengue fever is a mosquito-borne arboviral illness characterized by the sudden onset of fever, headaches, severe myalgias and arthralgias (break bone fever), abdominal discomfort, rash, and mild liver enzyme abnormalities. The rash appears 3 to 5 days after onset of fever and may spread from the torso to the extremities and face. Dengue fever has been a long-standing problem in the Far East, and during the last 10 years it has also spread throughout the Caribbean and Latin America [164,165]. Outbreaks tend to be focal and urban. Although dengue can progress to a fatal hemorrhagic shock syndrome (more likely in persons with prior dengue infection of a different serotype), most cases in travelers are self-limited. In recent years, 20 to 50 cases of confirmed dengue have occurred in U.S. travelers [165]. **Travelers should avoid the mosquito vectors (*Aedes* species), which tend to bite during the day, by using the personal protection measures discussed for malaria. No vaccine is available.**

**B. Schistosomiasis.** Acute schistosomiasis (Katayama fever), sometimes associated with severe neurologic sequelae, may occur in travelers [166,167]. **Travelers may be exposed to the parasite in fresh water of endemic areas of the Caribbean, South America, Africa, or Asia. Travelers should avoid swimming, wading, or bathing in fresh water unless it is chlorinated.** In some areas, the local opinion may be that the body of fresh water is free of risk (such as Lake Malawi), but cases of schistosomiasis have occurred in those situations [168]. Swimming in salt water or bathing in fresh water that has been heated to 50°C for 5 minutes or that has stood more than 48 hours is safe. Praziquantel is effective treatment for schistosomiasis caused by all *Schistosoma* species

**C. Sexually transmitted diseases.** Removed from societal restraints, some travelers are more likely to engage in casual sexual activity and place themselves at risk for HIV and other sexually transmitted diseases [169]. It has been estimated that 5% or more of short-term travelers have casual sexual encounters and use condoms in fewer than half of them [170]. Among long-term male expatriates living in Sub-Saharan Africa, high-risk sexual activity approached 30% [171]. Drug-resistant isolates of *Neisseria gonorrhoeae* are prevalent in many areas, especially southeast Asia and Africa, and hepatitis B, syphilis, herpes simplex, and venereal diseases uncommon in the United States (chancroid, lymphogranuloma venereum, and granuloma inguinale) occur (see Chapter 16). Of these only hepatitis B is preventable by immunization.

The rapid spread of HIV infection throughout the world poses a major risk for transmission via the sexual route. Seroprevalence of HIV in urban female sex workers varies but has been reported to be as high as 80% in some areas of Africa [172]. **Although the risk of transmission of HIV can be decreased by the use of condoms, diaphragms, and spermicides, the safest course for the traveler is abstinence.** Additionally, condoms manufactured outside the United States may not be reliably protective. The presence of other sexually transmitted diseases and genital lesions can enhance the risk of transmission of HIV and should be an absolute indication for abstinence.

## OTHER CONSIDERATIONS FOR THE TRAVELER

**I. Jet lag.** Travel across multiple time zones is associated with disruption of the normal circadian rhythm. For many travelers this results in adverse subjective and physiologic responses during the first days after arrival. A number of approaches to restore the circadian rhythm have been suggested. Exposure to bright light after arrival facilitates adaptation. Although dietary measures have been proposed, they have not been rigorously evaluated. Short- to intermediate-acting benzodiazepines and the nonbenzodiazepine pyrazolopyrimidines can help to maintain sleep after arrival in the new time zone. These agents should be started at the lowest effective dose, and their duration of action should be matched with the time available for sleep. They should not be used during air travel because they can lead to confusion and disorientation. The hormone melatonin is naturally produced during sleep. Exogenous administration of melatonin has been proposed as a means to reestablish the circadian rhythm, but recent studies have failed to demonstrate a significant effect in travelers [173,174].

**II. Deep venous thrombosis.** Long-distance travel, particularly by air, has been associated with an increased risk of deep venous thrombosis [175]. This syndrome has been called "economy class syndrome" and may occur in as many as 5% of long-haul (10–15 hours) travelers who have increased cardiovascular risk factors [176]. A smaller percent will experience pulmonary embolism (approximately 1–2 cases per million flights longer than 5,000 km) [177]. Maintaining hydration, exercise, and wearing below the knee support stockings may help to decrease risk [176].

**III. Motion sickness.** There are several agents for motion sickness. For short-term use, over-the-counter preparations of diphenhydramine (Benadryl) (especially for children) or meclizine may be effective. Travelers should be aware of the potential sedating effects of these agents. For longer trips, such as cruises, a sustained-release transdermal preparation of scopolamine (Transderm-Scop) may be preferred. The package insert instructions should be carefully followed and, after the disk is applied, the hands should be thoroughly washed to remove any scopolamine. For severe nausea, Phenergan pills (25 mg for adults) or suppositories may be used.

**IV. Sun protection.** Travelers should avoid excessive exposure to the sun to prevent heat exhaustion and sunburn. Sunburn is caused by the effects of both ultraviolet B and ultraviolet A radiation [178]. Most sunscreens offer protection against both types of radiation. Sunscreens should be applied in sufficient quantities to cover skin and may need repeat application if there is prolonged exposure or if they are washed off during swimming. Sunscreens with a sun protection factor of at least 15 should be used. Products that are water insoluble may be longer lasting.

**V. Skin care.** Skin problems are a major health issue for the traveler [179,180]. Insect bites, sunburn, dermatophyte infections, and cellulitis all can occur. Many dermatophytoses are made worse by warm and humid tropical conditions. Therefore, skin should be kept as clean and dry as possible, especially in skinfold areas. A topical antifungal preparation should be carried. Arthropod infections such as scabies and lice can be avoided by carefully washing hands and clothes. Persons should refrain from scratching insect bites to avoid pyoderma and cellulitis. Shoes or sandals should be worn at all times to prevent penetration by various nematodes.

**VI. High-altitude illness.** Acute mountain sickness, characterized by headache, nausea, vomiting, insomnia, and lassitude, affects up to 25% of persons who rapidly ascend to altitudes of 2,500 m and an even higher percent of those who exceed altitudes of 3,000 m [181]. Acute mountain sickness occasionally progresses to the potentially fatal syndromes of high-altitude pulmonary edema or cerebral edema. Acclimatization is the best method to prevent acute mountain sickness [181]. Acclimatization can be achieved by spending a few days at an intermediate altitude (1,500–2,200 m) and then gradually ascending to higher altitudes each day, with a return to sleeping at an elevation no more than 300 to 500 m higher than the night before.

Acetazolamide (Diamox) is a carbonic anhydrase inhibitor that may help travelers who ascend rapidly from low elevations. It hastens acclimatization but does not necessarily prevent acute mountain sickness. Acetazolamide is usually taken 24 to 48 hours before and for the first several days during the ascent. Various doses have been used ranging from 125 mg to 250 mg twice daily [181]. Acetazolamide is a diuretic and can cause circumoral and peripheral paresthesias; it is contraindicated in the sulfonamide-allergic patient. Descent and supplementary oxygen are the treatments of choice for mountain sickness. A descent of as little as 500 to 1,000 m can result in resolution of symptoms. Some large expeditions carry portable hyperbaric chambers to simulate descent until affected persons can be moved to lower elevations. When descent is not possible, dexamethasone or acetazolamide can be used for the treatment of acute mountain sickness [181]. Dexamethasone is not recommended for prophylaxis [182], because it only suppresses symptoms but does not enhance acclimatization. Travelers planning trips to altitudes above 3,500 m should seek expert advice.

**VII. Personal safety.** Although many travelers consider only the risk of exotic tropical diseases, more deaths in North Americans overseas are in fact attributable to accidents, injuries, and homicides than to infectious diseases [183,184]. Travelers should try to use safe public and private transport to avoid accidents and injuries and avoid swimming and diving in unfamiliar waters. Travelers may decrease the risk of personal assault by dressing conservatively and avoiding sites and activities that might be targeted by terrorist groups. Travelers should refuse to carry a package from one country to another, even if someone they have befriended (e.g., a personal guide) asks them to carry it; bombs, illicit drugs, or other illegal items may be hidden in the package. The U.S. State Department (888-407-4747 or *travel.state.gov/*) provides callers with updated travel advisory or visa information, along with safety tips and the names, addresses, and telephone numbers of Foreign Service locations.

**VIII. The HIV-infected traveler. Travelers infected with HIV face special challenges** [12,185]. Preventive measures [186], issues of vaccine safety and efficacy, prevalence of infectious agents overseas, health-care access, and the requirement by some countries for HIV testing prior to obtaining an entry visa (requirements may be accessed at *travel.state.gov/HIVtestingreqs.html*) all must be considered. Depending on the degree of immunosuppression, vaccines may be ineffective or unsafe. In general, live vaccines should be avoided. In addition, travel to developing countries may carry with it the risk of exposure to opportunistic pathogens such as *Salmonella* species, *Cryptosporidium parvum, Isospora belli, Cyclospora* species, *Mycobacterium tuberculosis,* and *Leishmania* species.

**IX. Travelers who have chronic lung or cardiovascular diseases, are pregnant, or are traveling with infants and young children.** Some travelers travel with medical conditions or chronic illnesses [187]. Cardiovascular disease is the most common cause of death among older travelers abroad [184]. Patients with severe chronic lung disease should undergo pulmonary function testing with arterial blood gases to determine whether they need supplemental oxygen during air flight [187,188]. Travelers requiring oxygen should contact their carriers 48 to 72 hours before travel and have a prescription from their physician that indicates diagnosis and liter flow rate.

Insulin-dependent diabetics should discuss with their physician the proper adjustment of insulin and diet schedules for time zone changes. Pregnant travelers should consider the potential health risks to self and fetus by air flight, exposure to malaria, and receipt of vaccinations and prophylactic medicines [189]. All travelers with preexistent medical conditions need to be cautioned about the effects of changes in diet, jet lag, altitude, and climate. They should carry on their persons each medication in a labeled bottle as well as copies of their prescriptions. Special considerations also pertain to those traveling with infants and children [190].

X. **Avoidance of blood-borne pathogens (HIV, hepatitis C, etc.).** The safety and screening of the blood supply may be questionable. Previously used needles or intravenous administration sets, dental equipment, and tattooing and other skin-piercing instruments should be avoided to decrease the risk of HIV, hepatitis B, and hepatitis C. Hepatitis B is preventable by immunization. Travelers who visit areas without access to safe medical care may be supplied with kits containing gloves, alcohol swabs, needles, and syringes. Some have also considered obtaining blood donations if needed from fellow travelers or members of the expatriate community who have tested negative for HIV and hepatitis and who have no risk factors to suggest the likelihood of these pathogens.

XI. **Plans for emergency medical help.** Emergency medical care may be needed during travel. There are several travel health insurance companies that will help the traveler access emergency care, pay for that care, and arrange for air evacuation if medically indicated (*travel.state.gov/medical.html*). These companies may also provide baggage and trip cancellation protection. The availability of medical care in remote areas may be ascertained by inquiring at U.S. consulates or embassies or by visiting mission hospitals, which often are staffed by expatriates.

## THE RETURNED TRAVELER

Fortunately, for most travelers serious illness is unusual, but some return with symptoms or develop them later. The experience of a group of nearly 800 returned U.S. travelers indicated the most common conditions were **diarrhea (13%), upper respiratory tract infections (10%), skin rash (3%), and fever (2%)** [180]. **Febrile illness warrants immediate attention because it may be due to malaria or another potentially life-threatening pathogen.**

When formulating a differential diagnosis, the health-care provider should consider the geographic location(s) visited, the traveler's activities, the frequency of specific diseases in the region(s), the incubation periods of potential pathogens, and the vaccines and other prophylactic measures that were used [191]. Many common bacterial and viral infections have short incubation periods and will develop abroad or within the first week or two of return. Diseases with longer incubation periods, such as giardiasis and amebiasis, viral hepatitis, malaria, and tuberculosis, may present weeks to months after a traveler's return. Travelers should be informed that an illness presenting after their return could be related to travel and requires medical evaluation. Persons who were ill during their trip or who lived for a prolonged period in a developing region should be evaluated after return [192,193].

The following presents an overview of common conditions in returned travelers. More detailed discussions and information about pathogens endemic to specific geographic regions should be consulted.

I. **Traveler's diarrhea.** Traveler's diarrhea is the most common illness among travelers and can begin abroad or after return [194]. Patients should be examined and stools tested for blood, fecal leukocytes, and fecal lactoferrin. Stool culture for enteropathogens is indicated if these screening tests are positive or if the patient presents with tenesmus, fever, or gross blood in the stool. Examination of stool for ova and parasites is typically reserved for those with persistent diarrhea lasting for 10 days to 2 weeks or longer or for those who have resided for a prolonged period in regions of poor sanitation. See related discussion earlier in this chapter, Table 22.2, and Chapter 13.

A. **Noninflammatory diarrhea.** The most frequently identified cause of traveler's diarrhea is enterotoxigenic *E. coli*. Enteroaggregative *E. coli* has recently been shown to be important pathogen. Fecal leukocytes and blood are absent with both, and the temperature is normal or only mildly elevated. Oral hydration with a mixture of water, glucose, buffer, and electrolytes is the most appropriate therapy and is often all that is necessary. Antibiotics and antimotility agents can shorten the duration of symptoms. Although uncommon among North American travelers, *V. cholerae* may present as rapidly dehydrating diarrhea that requires fluid and electrolyte replacement.

**B. Bacterial dysentery.** The presence of fever higher than 38°C, bloody stools, or tenesmus suggests inflammatory enterocolitis caused by bacterial pathogens such as *Shigella* species, *Campylobacter jejuni, Salmonella* species, *Yersinia enterocolitica,* or enteroinvasive *E. coli.* **Fecal leukocytes or lactoferrin are usually present in the stool.** Hydration is important, and treatment with an antibiotic, such as one of the fluoroquinolones in adults, frequently is administered pending the results of stool culture. Azithromycin can be used in children. It has also been used for travelers to areas in which *C. jejuni* is prevalent and possibly resistant to fluoroquinolones, such as Asia. Loperamide and other antimotility agents should not be used in travelers with inflammatory enterocolitis. (See related discussions in Chapter 13.) Enterohemorrhagic *E. coli,* such as O157:H7, are generally not seen among travelers, but the development of bloody diarrhea without fever raises this possibility. Neither antibiotics nor antimotility agents should be used in that setting, particularly in children [195].

**C. Amebic colitis.** Although not common among travelers, amebic colitis is a consideration in those presenting with dysentery. Gross or occult blood is typically found in the stool, but fecal leukocytes may be pyknotic or absent. Cysts or trophozoites of *E. histolytica* may be identified on stool examination: they are morphologically indistinguishable from those of *Entamoeba dispar,* a nonpathogen. The diagnosis of invasive amebiasis can be confirmed by identifying *E. histolytica* antigen in the stool, but not all commercial kits can differentiate between *E. histolytica* and *E. dispar* [196]. Metronidazole eradicates tissue trophozoites but should be followed with a luminal agent, such as paromomycin or iodoquinol, to eradicate cysts. Loperamide and other antimotility agents are contraindicated.

**D. Prolonged diarrhea.** Noninflammatory diarrhea lasting more than 10 days to 2 weeks raises the possibility of giardiasis, cryptosporidiosis, and other protozoan infections in addition to amebiasis. Stools should be examined for ova and parasites and stained for acid-fast organisms. Three stools, properly examined, will usually yield the diagnosis. Antigen testing for *Giardia* and *Cryptosporidium* is more sensitive than ova and parasite examination. Occasionally, empiric therapy for giardiasis is warranted after other etiologies have been excluded. Metronidazole is currently the drug of choice for giardiasis [197]. Trimethoprim-sulfamethoxazole is effective for cyclosporiasis [198]. There is currently no curative therapy for cryptosporidiosis, and illness in the immunocompetent host is self-limited (see Chapter 13).

**II. Upper respiratory tract infections.** Upper respiratory tract infections are the second most common illness among travelers. Although not carefully studied, **most are presumed to be viral in etiology.** They are managed symptomatically. Influenza should be considered in returned travelers with fever, myalgia, headache, coryza, and cough. Penicillin-resistant *S. pneumoniae* may be a problem and should be considered in those presenting with pneumonia. *Legionella* pneumonia has been acquired by travelers staying at resort hotels and taking journeys on cruise ships. It is related to water systems and whirlpool spas (see Chapters 8 and 11) [199].

**III. Dermatitis.** Travelers may suffer sun-related skin injuries, insect bites, drug reactions, or cutaneous infections due to bacteria *Staphylococcus aureus* and *Streptococcus pyogenes,* fungi, parasites, or other pathogens [179]. Cutaneous larva migrans follows skin contact with sand or soil contaminated with animal feces containing dog or cat hookworms (*Ancylostoma braziliensis*) or other nematodes. Furuncular myiasis may be confused with a staphylococcal furuncle. A small round breathing hole in the center of the lesion above the maggot is helpful in the diagnosis. Tungiasis is found on the feet and toenails. Cutaneous leishmaniasis presents as a chronic, nodular, or ulcerative skin lesion(s) that is not usually painful [200].

Systemic diseases can also present with cutaneous manifestations. The combination of rash and fever may indicate a potentially life-threatening disease and warrants immediate evaluation as discussed below. The differential diagnosis of rash in the returned traveler is extensive and is reviewed in detail elsewhere [179,201]. The risk of insect bites and vector-borne diseases can be reduced by the application of repellents to skin and clothing, the presence of window screens, and use of insecticide-impregnated bed nets.

**IV. Fever.** Fever in the returning traveler may be due to a life-threatening infection and is an indication for immediate evaluation. The differential diagnosis is broad and includes the following considerations [202].

**A. Malaria. Malaria is the first consideration in a traveler returning from Africa or other malaria-endemic areas who develops fever.** The mortality of *P. falciparum* malaria among nonimmune Americans is 2% or less; death usually occurs in persons who have not taken any prophylaxis or have taken incorrect chemoprophylaxis and have experienced a delayed or missed diagnosis [120,121]. Symptoms of malaria can begin as early as a week after infection, but they may be delayed for months and occasionally years. Eighty-nine percent of *P. falciparum* cases occur in the first month after return, but 29% of *P. vivax* cases occur after more than 6 months [120]. Compliance with antimalarial chemoprophylaxis does not exclude the diagnosis.

1. **The symptoms** of malaria often are often systemic and nonspecific: fever, malaise, myalgia, and anorexia. They may be focal: headache, confusion, obtundation, seizures, chest pain, abdominal pain, diarrhea, or respiratory distress. Although a tertian (every 48 hours) or quartan (every 72 hours) pattern of fever points to the diagnosis of malaria, most nonimmune travelers have **hectic fever patterns** when evaluated. Splenomegaly may be present, but there are **no pathognomonic physical findings.**
2. **The diagnosis** of malaria is confirmed by identifying parasites in thick or thin blood smears; however, parasites may sometimes be sparse and therefore missed. **If no other diagnosis is apparent in a toxic-appearing febrile traveler, empiric treatment for malaria should be initiated.**
3. **Therapy** (Table 22.4) for chloroquine-resistant *P. falciparum* in persons who can safely be given **oral therapy** is quinine sulfate plus doxycycline, or if the presentation is uncomplicated, atovaquone/proguanil (Malarone) may be given [151,203,204]. Mefloquine can also be used but is frequently associated with side effects. Persons returning from areas with chloroquine-sensitive *P. falciparum* can be treated with chloroquine phosphate. In the United States, **parenteral quinidine gluconate should be given to patients with severe *P. falciparum* infection (and severe infection with other species)** who cannot take medications orally [203,205]. Quinidine may not always be readily available for use, and hospitals should consider maintaining a supply or having a protocol for access of the drug [206].

   *P. vivax* or *P. ovale* infections are treated orally with chloroquine. Quinine or mefloquine is used in areas where chloroquine-resistant *P. vivax* is prevalent (such as Indonesia and Papua). Treatment of *P. vivax* and *P. ovale* includes a terminal course of primaquine to eradicate hypnozoites in the liver. G6PD levels should be determined before using primaquine. Primaquine is contraindicated in pregnant women. Infectious disease consultation is advised for returning travelers with malaria. Other supportive measures are also required [205].

**B. Typhoid fever.** *S. typhi* is endemic throughout developing areas. In the United States 72% of cases of typhoid are international importations; highest risk destinations are the Indian subcontinent, Central and South America, the Philippines, Haiti, and Africa [61]. A progressive increase in fever over a period of days, malaise, headache, abdominal symptoms, a pulse-temperature deficit, Rose spots, and eventually hypotension suggest the diagnosis. Many *S. typhi* isolates are tetracycline, ampicillin, and sulfonamide resistant, so therapy with a quinolone or advanced spectrum cephalosporin is advisable (see Chapter 13).

**C. Other bacterial infections.** In addition to pneumonia, skin infections, and typhoid fever, a number of other bacteria can produce febrile syndromes in travelers.

Table 22.4. Treatment of Malaria[a]

| Drug | Adult Dose | Pediatric Dose |
| --- | --- | --- |
| ***P. vivax, P. ovale, P. malariae,* and chloroquine-susceptible *P. falciparum*** | | |
| Chloroquine | 600 mg base (1,000 mg chloroquine phosphate) p.o. initially, followed by an additional 300 mg base (500 mg salt) 6 h later, and again at 24 and 48 h | 10 mg base/kg p.o. initially (not to exceed 600 mg base) followed by an additional 5 mg base/kg 6 h later and at 24 and 48 h (total dose of 25 mg base/kg over 3 days) |
| **Chloroquine-resistant *P. falciparum*** | | |
| **Oral regimens** | | |
| Quinine sulfate plus | 650 mg q8h × 3–7 days | 25 mg/kg/day in 3 divided doses × 3–7 days |
| Doxycycline[b] | 100 mg b.i.d. × 7 days | 2 mg/kg/day (max. 100 mg) × 7 days |
| *or* | | |
| Quinine sulfate plus pyrimethamine-sulfadoxine (Fansidar) | Single dose of 3 tabs on the last day of quinine treatment | 1–3 yr: 0.5 tablet<br>4–8 yr: 1 tablet<br>9–14 yr: 2 tablets |
| *or* | | |
| Quinine sulfate plus clindamycin[b] | 900 mg t.i.d. × 3–5 days | 20–40 mg/kg/day in 3 divided doses × 3–5 days |
| *or* | | |
| Atovaquone/proguanil (Malarone) | 4 adult tabs (each 250 mg/100 mg) daily for 3 days | 11–20 kg: 1 adult tablet (each 250 mg/100 mg) daily × 3 days<br>21–30 kg: 2 adult tabs daily for 3 days<br>31–40 kg: 3 adult tabs daily for 3 days<br>>40 kg: 4 adult tabs daily for 3 days |
| *or* | | |
| Mefloquine[c] | 1,250 mg p.o. as a single dose | 25 mg/kg p.o. as a single dose |

| | | |
|---|---|---|
| **Parenteral regimes** (i.v.) (all species) | | |
| Quinidine gluconate[d] | 10 mg (salt)/kg loading dose (max 600 mg) in normal saline infused slowly over 1–2 h, followed by continuous infusion of 0.02 mg/kg/min until patient is able to begin oral treatment | Same as adult dose |
| Quinine dihydrochloride[d,e] | 20 mg (salt)/kg loading dose in 5% dextrose over 4 hr, followed by 10 mg/kg over 2–4 h q8h (max 1,800 mg/day) until patient is able to begin oral treatment | Same as adult dose |
| **Prevention of relapse due to *P. vivax* or *P. ovale*** | | |
| Primaquine phosphate[f] | 15 mg base (26.3 mg phosphate salt) per day p.o. × 14 days *or* 45 mg base (79 mg salt) per wk × 8 wk | 0.3 mg base (0.5 mg salt) per kg/day × 14 days |

[a]For help in managing patients with malaria, the CDC may be contacted at (770) 488-7788 (M–F, 8 a.m.–4:30 p.m. eastern standard time) or after hours at (404) 639-2888.
[b]Doxycycline and clindamycin are typically begun after 2–3 days of treatment with quinine to ensure that side effects from quinine are not confused with those of doxycycline or clindamycin. Doxycycline should not be given to children <8 yr or pregnant women.
[c]At this dosage, severe side effects such as nausea, vomiting, diarrhea, dizziness, psychosis, and seizures may occur. Medical Letter suggests giving adult single dose as 750 mg followed 12 h later by 500 mg (see ref. below).
[d]Continuous cardiac (EKG), blood pressure, and glucose monitoring is recommended. Parenteral quinidine may not be readily available and hospitals may need to contact their distributor, or Eli Lilly Company ([800] 821-0538) for the drug.
[e]Quinine dihydrochloride is not available in the United States.
[f]G-6-PD testing should be done prior to prescribing primaquine phosphate.
*Note:* For a related reference see Medical Letter. Drugs for parasitic infections. *Med Lett Drug Ther* 2000;1–12.
http://www.medletter.com/html_files/publicreading.htm#Parasitic
Modified from Pearson RD, Weller PF Thielman, et al. Chemotherapy of tropical infectious diseases. In: Guerrant RL, Walker DH, Weller PF, eds. *Essentials of tropical infectious diseases.* New York: Churchill Livingstone, 2001:613–637.

Leptospirosis is a risk for travelers with rural exposure to water in swamps and rivers. Brucellosis, tularemia, plague, and anthrax are rare in travelers but are potentially life-threatening [202].

D. **Rickettsial diseases.** Typhus, tick-typhus, and other rickettsial diseases may be acquired during travel [207]. Most are associated with a rash and, in some cases, an eschar at the site of inoculation, but the rash may develop relatively late in the course of infection. If a rickettsial disease is suspected, empiric therapy with doxycycline should be initiated.

E. **Viral infections**

1. **Arthropod-borne viruses.** Dengue, yellow fever, and other arthropod-borne viruses are endemic in tropical areas. **Yellow fever** poses a risk in equatorial Latin America and Sub-Saharan Africa. Fortunately, cases of yellow fever are rare among travelers due to the high degree of efficacy of the vaccine [29]. **Dengue,** in contrast, remains a risk, and there is no effective form of immunoprophylaxis [164,165]. The incubation period is short (maximum of 7–9 days), so a disease that begins more than a week after a traveler leaves the tropics is not likely to be dengue (see section **III.A** under Advice on Disease Prevention other than by Vaccination, above).
2. **Hepatitis A, B, C, D, and E.** Fever, nausea, vomiting, fatigue, malaise, and jaundice suggest the possibility of viral hepatitis. If the liver enzymes are elevated, serologic studies are indicated to make a specific diagnosis (see Chapter 14).
3. **Measles, rubella, and varicella.** The common childhood viral exanthemas must be considered in travelers with fever and rash. Measles has been acquired by young adult U.S. travelers who failed to develop immunity after a single childhood immunization. Rubella, mumps, and chickenpox may also be acquired abroad.
4. **Viral hemorrhagic fevers.** Fortunately, viral hemorrhagic fevers, such as Ebola or Marburg hemorrhagic fever, Lassa fever, Argentine or Bolivian hemorrhagic fever, Rift Valley fever, and Crimean-Congo hemorrhagic fever are rare in travelers. They must be considered in those with unexplained fever, prostration, multiorgan system involvement, and evidence of coagulopathy [208]. Barrier nursing techniques are essential in preventing the spread of these viruses to health-care workers. If a returning traveler has a syndrome suggestive of viral hemorrhagic fever, expert help should be sought, including consultation with the CDC [209].
5. **Other viral diseases.** Many other viruses can produce febrile diseases in returned travelers. Clinicians should consider infections endemic to the United States, such as Epstein-Barr virus and HIV, as well as viral infections that may be unique to areas visited.

F. **Parasitic disease other than malaria.** A number of parasitic diseases such as visceral leishmaniasis, Katayama fever (acute schistosomiasis), and Chagas disease must be considered in the differential diagnosis of fever in travelers who have had potential exposure in endemic area, but they are rare [202].

G. **Noninfectious diseases.** Drug fever should be considered in travelers who are taking antibiotics or other medications. Deep venous thrombosis with or without pulmonary emboli can occur in persons who have been seated for long periods of time.

V. **Eosinophilia.** The finding of eosinophilia (>500 total eosinophils) in a returned traveler suggests the possibility of a helminthic infection [210,211]. However, many persons will have increased eosinophil counts secondary to drug allergy or atopic conditions, so these conditions should be ruled out before extensive investigations are performed for parasites. **Worms that have an extensive tissue phase are the most common helminths that cause eosinophilia.** These include *Strongyloides stercoralis,* recent infestation with hookworms, *Schistosoma* species, visceral larva migrans (*Toxocara* species), *Trichinella spiralis,* and filaria. Appropriate studies can include three stools for ova and parasites, blood smears for filaria, serology, and skin or tissue biopsies. It may be necessary to repeat testing after 3 to 6 months because of the prolonged prepatent period of many helminths (such as hookworm) before production of ova or worms become clinically manifest. Eosinophilia is not observed in malaria and most other protozoan diseases.

## APPENDIX

### *Suggested Readings, Resources, and Websites for Health-Care Providers Who Advise Travelers*

I. **Centers for Disease Control and Prevention.** *Health information for international travel, 2001–2002.* Atlanta, GA: U.S. Department of Health and Human Services, 2001.

This publication is for sale by the Public Health Foundation (877-252-1200, or online ordering at *bookstore.phf.org*). It may be downloaded as a pdf file at the CDC travel website (*www.cdc.gov/travel/reference.htm*). It lists countries that require yellow fever vaccine, provides the epidemiology of malaria in endemic countries and recommends chemoprophylactic regimens, and discusses diseases (including detailed recommendations on vaccine-preventable disease) that present risks to travelers. **This is an essential reference for advising travelers.**

II. **Centers for Disease Control and Prevention website:** *www.cdc.gov/travel/*

This website provides the information found in *Health Information for International Travel, 2001–2002,* including health recommendations based on destination and reports of recent infectious disease outbreaks around the world. **It is revised frequently. This is an essential source to access when advising travelers.**

III. **Centers for Disease Control and Prevention.** ***Summary of health information for international travel***. Atlanta: U.S. Department of Health and Human Services, Public Health Service. *www.cdc.gov/travel/blusheet.htm*

Known as the **blue sheet,** this biweekly publication lists countries and areas within those countries (for yellow fever) that are reporting yellow fever, cholera, and plague. This publication is used in conjunction with *Health Information for International Travel* to determine whether yellow fever vaccine should be given.

IV. ***International Certificate of Vaccination*** (PHS-731). Superintendent of Documents, U.S. Public Health Service. Washington, DC: U.S. Government Printing Office.

This booklet is used to record required immunizations (currently only yellow fever), other immunizations, and personal medical history. Yellow fever vaccine must be validated by a stamp issued by state health departments.

V. ***Morbidity and Mortality Weekly Report (MMWR)*** *www.cdc.gov/mmwr/*

This CDC publication periodically reports official changes in vaccination requirements and disease outbreaks and is another source of information. Individual subscriptions are available by writing Massachusetts Medical Society, P.O. Box 9120, Waltham, MA 02454-9120.

VI. **World Health Organization.** *International Travel and Health. Vaccination Requirements and Health Advice.* Geneva: World Health Organization, 2001. *www.who.org*

The World Health Organization's version of *Health Information for International Travel.* Available from WHO Distribution and Sales, Geneva. (41 22) 791-2476, e-mail: publications@who.ch.

VII. **Other resources.** A number of excellent textbooks and reviews of travel and tropical medicine exist [10,212–214]. The *Journal of Travel Medicine* is devoted to issues pertinent to travelers (Decker Periodicals, 800-568-7281, *www.istm.org/jtm.html*). Several Internet and computer-based resources are available for travel medicine practitioners that provide ready access to information on outbreaks of travel-related disease and information on the likelihood of acquiring diseases in specific locations. These are reviewed by Keystone et al. [215].

## REFERENCES

1. Ryan ET, Kain KC. Health advice and immunizations for travelers. *N Engl J Med* 2000;342:1716–1725.
2. Hill DR. Travel clinics in the United States and Canada. In: DuPont HL, Steffen R, eds. *Textbook of travel medicine and health*. Hamilton, Ontario: B.C. Decker, 2001:52–57.
3. American College of Physicians. *Guide for adult immunization*, 3rd ed. Philadelphia: American College of Physicians, 1994.
4. Centers for Disease Control and Prevention. *Health information for international travel, 2001–2002*. Atlanta, GA: U.S. Department of Health and Human Services, 2001.
5. American Academy of Pediatrics. *2000 Red Book: report of the Committee on Infectious Diseases*. Elk Grove Village, IL: American Academy of Pediatrics, 2000.

6. Peter G, Gardner P. Standards for immunization practice for vaccines in children and adults. *Infect Dis Clin North Am* 2001;15:9–19.
7. Gardner P, Peter G. Recommended schedules for routine immunization of children and adults. *Infect Dis Clin North Am* 2001;15:1–8.
8. Superintendent of Documents USPHS. *International certificates of vaccination (PHS-731).* Washington, DC: U.S. Government Printing Office.
9. Centers for Disease Control and Prevention. Vaccinia (Smallpox) vaccine: recommendations of the Advisory Committee on Immunization Practices (ACIP), 2001. *MMWR Morb Mortal Wkly Rep* 2001;50(No. RR-10):1–25.
10. Wilson ME. *A world guide to infections. Diseases, distribution, diagnosis.* Oxford: Oxford University Press, 1991.
11. Angel JB, Walpita P, Lerch RA, et al. Vaccine-associated measles pneumonitis in an adult with AIDS. *Ann Intern Med* 1998;129:104–106.
12. Castelli F, Patroni A. The human immunodeficiency virus-infected traveler. *Clin Infect Dis* 2000;31:1403–1408.
13. Rousseau MC, Moreau J, Delmont J. Vaccination and HIV: a review of the literature. *Vaccine* 1999;18:825–831.
14. Singleton JA, Greby SM, Wooten KG, et al. Influenza, pneumococcal, and tetanus toxoid vaccination of adults—United States, 1993–1997. *MMWR Morb Mortal Wkly Rep* 2000;49(No. SS-9):39–62.
15. Karzon DT, Edwards KM. Diphtheria outbreaks in immunized populations. *N Engl J Med* 1988;318:41–43.
16. Centers for Disease Control and Prevention. Update on the supply of tetanus and diphtheria toxoids and of diphtheria and tetanus toxoids and acellular pertussis vaccine. *MMWR Morb Mortal Wkly Rep* 2001;50:189–190.
17. Centers for Disease Control. Diphtheria, tetanus, and pertussis: recommendations for vaccine use and other preventive measures. Recommendations of the Immunization Practices Advisory Committee (ACIP). *MMWR Morb Mortal Wkly Rep* 1991;40(RR-10): 1–28.
18. Centers for Disease Control and Prevention. Preventing pneumococcal disease among infants and young children: recommendations of the Advisory Committee on Immunization Practices (ACIP). *MMWR Morb Mortal Wkly Rep* 2000;49(No. RR-9):1–35.
19. Centers for Disease Control and Prevention. Prevention of pneumococcal disease. Recommendation of the Advisory Committee on Immunization Practices. *MMWR Morb Mortal Wkly Rep* 1997;46(No. RR-8):1–24.
20. Centers for Disease Control and Prevention. Global measles control and regional elimination, 1998–1999. *MMWR Morb Mortal Wkly Rep* 1999;48:1124–1130.
21. Centers for Disease Control and Prevention. Measles—United States, 1999. *MMWR Morb Mortal Wkly Rep* 2000;49:557–560.
22. Centers for Disease Control and Prevention. Measles, mumps, and rubella—vaccine use and strategies for elimination of measles, rubella, and congenital rubella syndrome and control of mumps: recommendation of the Advisory Committee on Immunization Practices (ACIP). *MMWR Morb Mortal Wkly Rep* 1998;47(No. RR-8):1–57.
23. Centers for Disease Control and Prevention. Prevention and control of influenza: recommendations of the Advisory Committee on Immunization Practices (ACIP). *MMWR Morb Mortal Wkly Rep* 2001;50(No. RR-4):1–44.
24. Centers for Disease Control and Prevention. Outbreak of influenza A infection among travelers—Alaska and the Yukon Territory, May-June 1999. *MMWR Morb Mortal Wkly Rep* 1999;48:545–546, 555.
25. Centers for Disease Control and Prevention. Impact of vaccines universally recommended for children—United States, 1990–1998. *MMWR Morb Mortal Wkly Rep* 1999;48:243–248.
26. Centers for Disease Control and Prevention. Recommended childhood immunization schedule—United States, 2001. *MMWR Morb Mortal Wkly Rep* 2001;50:7–10, 19.
27. Robertson SE, Hull BP, Tomori O, et al. Yellow fever. A decade of reemergence. *JAMA* 1996;276:1157–1162.
28. Van der Stuyft P, Gianella A, Pirard M, et al. Urbanisation of yellow fever in Santa Cruz, Bolivia. *Lancet* 1999;353:1558–1562.

29. Centers for Disease Control and Prevention. Fatal yellow fever in a traveler returning from Venezuela, 1999. *MMWR Morb Mortal Wkly Rep* 2000;49:303–305.
30. Centers for Disease Control and Prevention. *Summary of health information for international travel*. HHS publication no. 396. Atlanta, GA: U.S. Department of Health and Human Services, 2001.
31. Centers for Disease Control and Prevention. Fever, jaundice, and multiple organ system failure associated with 17D-derived yellow fever vaccination, 1996–2001. *MMWR Morb Mortal Wkly Rep* 2001;50:643–645.
32. Martin M, Weld LH, Tsai TF, et al. Advanced age a risk factor for illness temporally associated with yellow fever vaccination. *Emerg Infect Dis* 2001;7:945–951.
33. Sack DA, Cadoz M. Cholera vaccines. In: Plotkin SA, Orenstein WA, eds. *Vaccines*. Philadelphia: W.B. Saunders, 1999:639–649.
34. MacPherson DW, Tonkin M. Cholera vaccination: a decision analysis. *Can Med Assoc J* 1992;146:1947–1952.
35. Mahon BE, Mintz ED, Greene KD, et al. Reported cholera in the United States, 1992–1994. *JAMA* 1996;276:307–312.
36. World Health Organization. Cholera, 2000. *Wkly Epidemiol Rec* 2001;76:233–240.
37. Ryan ET, Calderwood SR. Cholera vaccines. *Clin Infect Dis* 2000;31:561–565.
38. An Advisory Committee Statement (ACS). Committee to Advise on Tropical Medicine and Travel (CATMAT). Statement on oral cholera vaccine. *Can Commun Dis Rep* 1998;24:1–4.
39. Henderson DA, Inglesby TV, Bartlett JG, et al. Smallpox as a biological weapon. Medical and public health management. *JAMA* 1999;281:2127–2137.
40. Medical Letter. Drugs and vaccines against biological weapons. *Med Lett Drugs Therap* 2001;43:87–89.
41. Steffen R, Rickenbach M, Wilhelm U, et al. Health problems after travel to developing countries. *J Infect Dis* 1987;156:84–91.
42. Steffen R, Kane MA, Shapiro CN, et al. Epidemiology and prevention of hepatitis A in travelers. *JAMA* 1994;272:885–889.
43. Wolfe MS. Hepatitis A and the American traveler. *J Infect Dis* 1995;171[Suppl 1]:S29–S32.
44. Centers for Disease Control and Prevention. Prevention of hepatitis A through active or passive immunization: recommendations of the Advisory Committee on Immunization Practices (ACIP). *MMWR Morb Mortal Wkly Rep* 1999;48(No. RR-12):1–37.
45. Behrens RH, Roberts JA. Is travel prophylaxis worthwhile? Economic appraisal of prophylactic measures against malaria, hepatitis A, and typhoid in travellers. *Br Med J* 1994;309:918–922.
46. Werzberger A, Mensch B, Kuter B, et al. A controlled trial of a formalin-inactivated hepatitis A vaccine in healthy children. *N Engl J Med* 1992;327:453–457.
47. Sagliocca L, Amoroso P, Stroffolini T, et al. Efficacy of hepatitis A vaccine in prevention of secondary hepatitis A infection: a randomized trial. *Lancet* 1999;353:1136–1139.
48. Bryan JP, Henry CH, Hoffman AG, et al. Randomized, cross-over, controlled comparison of two inactivated hepatitis A vaccines. *Vaccine* 2000;19:743–750.
49. Lerman Y, Shohat T, Ashkenazi S, et al. Efficacy of different doses of immune serum globulin in the prevention of hepatitis A: a three-year prospective study. *Clin Infect Dis* 1993;17:411–414.
50. Schwartz E, Raveh D. The prevalence of hepatitis A antibodies among Israeli travellers and the economic feasibility of screening before vaccination. *Int J Epidemiol* 1998;27:118–120.
51. Parry JV, Perry KR, Mortimer PP, et al. Rational programme for screening travellers for antibodies to hepatitis A virus. *Lancet* 1988;1:1447–1449.
52. Bryan JP, Nelson M. Testing for antibody to hepatitis A to decrease the cost of hepatitis A prophylaxis with immune globulin or hepatitis A vaccines. *Arch Intern Med* 1994;154:663–668.
53. Marsano LS, Greenberg RN, Kirkpatrick RB, et al. Comparison of a rapid hepatitis B immunization schedule to the standard for adults. *Am J Gastroenterol* 1996;91:111–115.

54. Bock HL, Löscher T, Scheiermann N, et al. Accelerated schedule for hepatitis B immunization. *J Travel Med* 1995;2:213–217.
55. Medical Letter. Twinrix: a combination hepatitis A and B vaccine. *Med Lett Drugs Therap* 2001;43:67–68.
56. Skidmore SJ. Tropical aspects of viral hepatitis. Hepatitis E. *Trans R Soc Trop Med Hyg* 1997;91:125–126.
57. Schwartz E, Piper Jenks N, Van Damme P, et al. Hepatitis E virus infection in travelers. *Clin Infect Dis* 1999;29:1312–1314.
58. Ooi WW, Gawoski JM, Yarbbough PO, et al. Hepatitis E seroconversion in United States travelers abroad. *Am J Trop Med Hyg* 1999;61:822–824.
59. Mast EE, Krawczynski K. Hepatitis E: an overview. *Annu Rev Med* 1996;47:257–266.
60. Centers for Disease Control and Prevention. Hepatitis E among U.S. travelers, 1989–1992. *MMWR Morb Mortal Wkly Rep* 1993;42:1–4.
61. Mermin JH, Townes JM, Gerber M, et al. Typhoid fever in the United States, 1985–1994. Changing risks of international travel and increasing antimicrobial resistance. *Arch Intern Med* 1998;158:633–638.
62. Ackers M-L, Puhr ND, Tauxe RV, et al. Laboratory-based surveillance of *Salmonella* serotype typhi infections in the United States. Antimicrobial resistance on the rise. *JAMA* 2000;283:2668–2673.
63. Engels EA, Falagas ME, Lau J, et al. Typhoid fever vaccines: a meta-analysis of studies on efficacy and toxicity. *Br Med J* 1998;316:110–115.
64. Klugman KP, Gilbertson IT, Koornhof HJ, et al. Protective effect of Vi capsular polysaccharide vaccine against typhoid fever. *Lancet* 1987;2:1165–1169.
65. Acharya IL, Lowe CU, Thapa R, et al. Prevention of typhoid fever in Nepal with the Vi capsular polysaccharide of *Salmonella typhi*. A preliminary report. *N Engl J Med* 1987;317:1101–1104.
66. Lin FY, Ho VA, Khiem HB, et al. The efficacy of a *Salmonella typhi* Vi conjugate vaccine in two- to five-year-old children. *N Engl J Med* 2001;344:1263–1269.
67. Greenwood B. Meningococcal meningitis in Africa. *Trans R Soc Trop Med Hyg* 1999;93: 341–353.
68. Centers for Disease Control and Prevention. Update: assessment of risk of meningococcal disease associated with the Hajj 2001. *MMWR Morb Mortal Wkly Rep* 2001;50:221–222.
69. MacLennan J. Meningococcal group C conjugate vaccines. *Arch Dis Child* 2001;84:383–386.
70. Bruce MG, Rosenstein NE, Capparella JM, et al. Risk factors for meningococcal disease in college students. *JAMA* 2001;286:688–693.
71. Centers for Disease Control and Prevention. Prevention and control of meningococcal disease and meningococcal disease and college students: recommendations of the Advisory Committee on Immunization Practices (ACIP). *MMWR Morb Mortal Wkly Rep* 2000;49(No. RR-7):1–20.
72. Centers for Disease Control and Prevention. Progress toward global poliomyelitis eradication, 2000. *MMWR Morb Mortal Wkly Rep* 2001;50:320–322, 331.
73. Centers for Disease Control and Prevention. Certification of poliomyelitis eradication—Western Pacific region, October 2000. *MMWR Morb Mortal Wkly Rep* 2001;50:1–3.
74. Centers for Disease Control and Prevention. Update: outbreak of poliomyelitis—Dominican Republic and Haiti, 2000–2001. *MMWR Morb Mortal Wkly Rep* 2001;50: 855–856.
75. Kubli D, Steffen R, Schär M. Importation of poliomyelitis to industrialised nations between 1975 and 1984: evaluation and conclusions for vaccination recommendations. *Br J Med* 1987;295:169–171.
76. Strebel PM, Sutter RW, Cochi SL, et al. Epidemiology of poliomyelitis in the United States one decade after the last reported case of indigenous wild virus-associated disease. *Clin Infect Dis* 1992;14:568–579.
77. Centers for Disease Control and Prevention. Poliomyelitis prevention in the United States: Updated recommendations of the Advisory Committee on Immunization Practices (ACIP). *MMWR Morb Mortal Wkly Rep* 2000;49(No. RR-5):1–22.
78. Tsai TF, Chang G-JJ, Yu YX. Japanese encephalitis vaccines. In: Plotkin SA, Orenstein WA, eds. *Vaccines*. Philadelphia: W.B. Saunders, 1999:672–710.

79. Centers for Disease Control and Prevention. Inactivated Japanese encephalitis virus vaccine. Recommendations of the advisory committee on immunization practices (ACIP). *MMWR Morb Mortal Wkly Rep* 1993;42(No. RR-1):1–15.
80. Ruff TA, Eisen D, Fuller A, et al. Adverse reactions to Japanese encephalitis vaccine. *Lancet* 1991;338:881–882.
81. Plesner AM, Ronne T. Allergic mucocutaneous reactions to Japanese encephalitis vaccine. *Vaccine* 1997;15:1239–1243.
82. Berg SW, Mitchell BS, Hanson RK, et al. Systemic reactions in U.S. Marine Corps personnel who received Japanese encephalitis vaccine. *Clin Infect Dis* 1997;24:265–266.
83. Takahashi H, Pool V, Tsai TF, et al. Adverse events after Japanese encephalitis vaccination: review of post-marketing surveillance data from Japan and the United States. The VAERS Working Group. *Vaccine* 2000;18:2963–2969.
84. Centers for Disease Control. Human rabies acquired outside the United States. *MMWR Morb Mortal Wkly Rep* 1985;34:235–236.
85. Case Records of the Massachusetts General Hospital. Case 21—1998. *N Engl J Med* 1998;339:105–112.
86. Centers for Disease Control and Prevention. Human rabies prevention—United States, 1999: recommendations of the Advisory Committee on Immunization Practices (ACIP). *MMWR Morb Mortal Wkly Rep* 1999;48 (No. RR-1):1–21.
87. Kositprapa C, Wimalratna O, Chomchey P, et al. Problems with rabies postexposure management: a survey of 499 public hospitals in Thailand. *J Travel Med* 1998;5:30–32.
88. World Health Organization. Human plague in 1998 and 1999. *Wkly Epidemiol Rec* 2000;75:338–343.
89. Centers for Disease Control and Prevention. Prevention of plague: recommendations of the Advisory Committee on Immunization Practices (ACIP). *MMWR Morb Mortal Wkly Rep* 1996;45(No. RR-14):1–15.
90. Cobelens FGJ, van Deutekom H, Draayer-Jansen IWE, et al. Risk of infection with *Mycobacterium tuberculosis* in travellers to areas of high tuberculosis endemicity. *Lancet* 2000;356:461–465.
91. Brewer TF, Colditz GA. Bacille Calmette-Guérin vaccination for the prevention of tuberculosis in health care workers. *Clin Infect Dis* 1995;20:136–142.
92. Steffen R, Van der Linde F, Gyr K, et al. Epidemiology of diarrhea in travelers. *JAMA* 1983;249:1176–1180.
93. DuPont HL, Ericsson CD. Prevention and treatment of travelers' diarrhea. *N Engl J Med* 1993;328:1821–1827.
94. von Sonnenburg F, Tornieporth N, Waiyaki P, et al. Risk and aetiology of diarrhea at various tourist destinations [Letter]. *Lancet* 2000;356:133–134.
95. Hill DR. Occurrence and self-treatment of diarrhea in a large cohort of Americans traveling to developing countries. *Am J Trop Med Hyg* 2000;62:585–589.
96. DuPont HL, Khan FM. Travelers' diarrhea: epidemiology, microbiology, prevention, and therapy. *J Travel Med* 1994;1:84–93.
97. Adachi JA, Jiang ZD, Mathewson JJ, et al. Enteroaggregative *Escherichia coli* as a major etiologic agent in travelers' diarrhea in 3 regions of the world. *Clin Infect Dis* 2001;32:1706–1709.
98. Reinthaler FF, Feierl G, Stunzner D, et al.. Diarrhea in returning Austrian tourists: epidemiology, etiology, and cost-analysis. *J Travel Med* 1998;5:65–72.
99. Okhuysen PC. Travelers' diarrhea due to intestinal protozoa. *Clin Infect Dis* 2001;33:110–114.
100. Herwaldt BL, de Arroyave KR, Wahlquist SP, et al. Multiyear prospective study of intestinal parasitism in a cohort of Peace Corps volunteers in Guatemala. *J Clin Microbiol* 2001;39:34–42.
101. Backer H. Water disinfection for international and wilderness travelers. *Clin Infect Dis* 2002;34:355–364.
102. Juranek DD. Cryptosporidiosis: sources of infection and guidelines for prevention. *Clin Infect Dis* 1995;21[Suppl 1]:S57–S61.
103. DuPont HL, Ericsson CD, Johnson PC, et al. Prevention of travelers' diarrhea by the tablet formulation of bismuth subsalicylate. *JAMA* 1987;257:1347–1350.

104. Gorbach SL, Edelman R, eds. Travelers' diarrhea: National Institutes of Health Consensus Conference. *Rev Infect Dis* 1986;8[Suppl 2]:S227–S233.
105. Centers for Disease Control and Prevention. The management of acute diarrhea in children: oral rehydration, maintenance, and nutritional therapy. *MMWR Morb Mortal Wkly Rep* 1992;41(No. RR-16):1–20.
106. Guerrant RL, Van Gilder T, Steiner TS, et al. Practice guidelines for the management of infectious diarrhea. *Clin Infect Dis* 2001;32:331–350.
107. Johnson PC, Ericsson CD, DuPont HL, et al. Comparison of loperamide with bismuth subsalicylate for the treatment of acute travelers' diarrhea. *JAMA* 1986;255:757–760.
108. DuPont HL. Bismuth subsalicylate in the treatment and prevention of diarrheal disease. *Drug Intell Clin Pharm* 1987;21:687–693.
109. Figueroa-Quintanilla D, Salazar-Lindo E, Sack RB, et al. A controlled trial of bismuth subsalicylate in infants with acute watery diarrheal disease. *N Engl J Med* 1993;328:1653–1658.
110. Barry M. Medical considerations for international travel with infants and older children. *Infect Dis Clin North Am* 1992;6:389–404.
111. Adachi JA, Ostrosky-Zeichner L, DuPont HL, et al. Empirical antimicrobial therapy for travelers; diarrhea. *Clin Infect Dis* 2000;31:1079–1083.
112. DuPont HL, Reves RR, Galindo E, et al. Treatment of travelers' diarrhea with trimethoprim/sulfamethoxazole and with trimethoprim alone. *N Engl J Med* 1982;307:841–844.
113. Gomi H, Jiang ZD, Adachi JA, et al. In vitro antimicrobial susceptibility testing of bacterial enteropathogens causing travelers' diarrhea in four geographic regions. *Antimicrob Agents Chemother* 2001;45:212–216.
114. Kuschner RA, Trofa AF, Thomas RJ, et al. Use of azithromycin for the treatment of *Campylobacter* enteritis in travelers to Thailand, an area where ciprofloxacin resistance is prevalent. *Clin Infect Dis* 1995;21:536–541.
115. DuPont HL, Jiang ZD, Ericsson CD, et al. Rifaximin versus ciprofloxacin for the treatment of traveler's diarrhea: a randomized, double-blind clinical trial. *Clin Infect Dis* 2001;33:1807–1815.
116. Salam I, Katelaris P, Leigh-Smith S, et al. Randomised trial of single-dose ciprofloxacin for travellers' diarrhoea. *Lancet* 1994;344:1537–1539.
117. Ericsson CD, DuPont HL, Mathewson J, et al. Treatment of travelers' diarrhea with sulfamethoxazole and trimethoprim and loperamide. *JAMA* 1990;263:257–261.
118. Ericsson CD, DuPont HL, Mathewson JJ. Single dose ofloxacin plus loperamide compared with single dose or three days of ofloxacin in the treatment of traveler's diarrhea. *J Travel Med* 1997;4:3–7.
119. Petruccelli BP, Murphy GS, Sanchez JL, et al. Treatment of traveler's diarrhea with ciprofloxacin and loperamide. *J Infect Dis* 1992;165:557–560.
120. Holtz TH, Kachur SP, MacArthur JR, et al. Malaria surveillance—United States, 1998. *Morb Mortal Wkly Rev* 2001;50(SS-5):1–18.
121. Kain KC, MacPherson DW, Kelton T, et al. Malaria deaths in visitors to Canada and in Canadian travellers: a case series. *Can Med Assoc J* 2001;164:654–659.
122. Lobel HO, Phillips-Howard PA, Brandling-Bennett AD, et al. Malaria incidence and prevention among European and North American travellers to Kenya. *Bull World Health Org* 1990;68:209–215.
123. Steffen R, Heusser R, Mächler R, et al. Malaria chemoprophylaxis among European tourists in tropical Africa: use, adverse reactions, and efficacy. *Bull World Health Org* 1990;68:313–322.
124. World Health Organization. *International travel and health. Vaccination requirements and health advice*. Geneva: World Health Organization, 2001.
125. Bradley DJ, Bannister B. on behalf of the Advisory Committee on Malaria Prevention for UK Travellers. Guidelines for the prevention of malaria in travellers from the United Kingdom for 2001. *Commun Dis Public Health* 2001;4:84–101.
126. Committee to Advise on Tropical Medicine and Travel (CATMAT). Canadian recommendations for the prevention and treatment of malaria among international travelers. *Can Commun Dis Rep* 2000;26[Suppl 2]:1–42.
127. Croft A. Malaria: prevention in travellers. *Br J Med* 2000;321:154–160.

128. Centers for Disease Control and Prevention. Malaria deaths following inappropriate malaria chemoprophylaxis—United States, 2001. *Morb Mortal Wkly Rev* 2001;50:597–599.
129. Kain KC, Keystone JS. Malaria in travelers. Epidemiology, disease, and prevention. *Infect Dis Clin North Am* 1998;12:267–284.
130. Fradin MS. Mosquitoes and mosquito repellents: a clinician's guide. *Ann Intern Med* 1998;128:931–940.
131. Medical Letter. Insect repellents. *Med Lett Drugs Therap* 1989;31:45–47.
132. Baird JK, Nalim MFS, Basri H, et al. Survey of resistance to chloroquine by *Plasmodium vivax* in Indonesia. *Trans R Soc Trop Med Hyg* 1996;90:409–411.
133. Easterbrook M. Ocular effects and safety of antimalarial agents. *Am J Med* 1988;85 [Suppl 4A]:23–29.
134. Levy GD, Munz SJ, Paschal J, et al. Incidence of hydroxychloroquine retinopathy in 1,207 patients in a large multicenter outpatient practice. *Arthritis Rheum* 1997;40: 1482–1486.
135. Easterbrook M, Bernstein H. Ophthalmological monitoring of patients taking antimalarials: preferred practice patterns. *J Rheumatol* 1997;24:1390–1392.
136. Lobel HO, Miani M, Eng T, et al. Long-term malaria prophylaxis with weekly mefloquine. *Lancet* 1993;341:848–851.
137. Steffen R, Fuchs E, Schildknecht J, et al. Mefloquine compared with other malaria chemoprophylactic regimens in tourists visiting East Africa. *Lancet* 1993;341:1299–1303.
138. Croft A, Garner P. Mefloquine to prevent malaria: a systematic review of trials. *Br J Med* 1997;315:1412–1416.
139. Fontanet AL, Johnston BD, Walker AM, et al. High prevalence of mefloquine-resistant falciparum in eastern Thailand. *Bull World Health Org* 1993;71:377–383.
140. Lobel HO, Kozarsky PE. Update on prevention of malaria for travelers. *JAMA* 1997; 278:1767–1771.
141. Schlagenhauf P. Mefloquine for malaria chemoprophylaxis 1992–1998: a review. *J Travel Med* 1999;6:122–133.
142. Stürchler D, Handschin J, Kaiser D, et al. Neuropsychiatric side effects of mefloquine [Letter]. *N Engl J Med* 1990;322:1752–1753.
143. World Health Organization. Review of central nervous system adverse events related to the antimalatial drug, mefloquine (1985–1990). Report: WHO/MAL/91.1063. Geneva, Switzerland: World Health Organization, 1991:1–21.
144. Weinke T, Trautmann M, Held T, et al. Neuropsychiatric side effects after the use of mefloquine. *Am J Trop Med Hyg* 1991;45:86–91.
145. Bem JL, Kerr L, Stürchler D. Mefloquine prophylaxis: an overview of spontaneous reports of severe psychiatric reactions and convulsions. *J Trop Med Hyg* 1992;95:167–179.
146. Nosten F, ter Kuile F, Maelankiri L, et al. Mefloquine prophylaxis prevents malaria during pregnancy: a double-blind, placebo-controlled study. *J Infect Dis* 1994;169:595–603.
147. Smoak BL, Writer JV, Keep LW, et al. The effects of inadvertent exposure to mefloquine chemoprophylaxis on pregnancy outcomes and infants of US Army servicewomen. *J Infect Dis* 1997;176:831–833.
148. Vanhauwere B, Maradit H, Kerr L. Post-marketing surveillance of prophylactic mefloquine (Lariam®) use in pregnancy. *Am J Trop Med Hyg* 1998;58:17–21.
149. Medical Letter. Atovaquone/proguanil (Malarone) for malaria. *Med Lett Drugs Therap* 2000;42:109–111.
150. Shanks GD, Kain KC, Keystone JS. Malaria chemoprophylaxis in the age of drug resistance. II. Drugs that may be available in the future. *Clin Infect Dis* 2001;33:381–385.
151. Pearson RD. Atovaquone/proguanil for the treatment and prevention of malaria. *Curr Infect Dis Rep* 2001;3:68–76.
152. Kremsner PG, Looareesuwan S, Chulay JD. Atovaquone and proguanil hydrochloride for treatment of malaria. *J Travel Med* 1999;6[Suppl 1]:S18–S20.
153. Looareesuwan S, Chulay JD, Canfield CJ, et al. Malarone(tm) (atovaquone and proguanil hydrochloride): a review of its clinical development for treatment of malaria. *Am J Trop Med Hyg* 1999;60:533–541.

154. Shanks GD, Kremsner PG, Sukwa TY, et al. Atovaquone and proguanil hydrochloride for prophylaxis of malaria. *J Travel Med* 1999;6[Suppl 1]:S21–S27.
155. Hogh B, Clarke PD, Camus D, et al. Atovaquone-proguanil versus chloroquine-proguanil for malaria prophylaxis in non-immune travellers: a randomised, double-blind study. *Lancet* 2000;356:1888–1894.
156. Overbosch D, Schilthuis H, Bienzle U, et al. Atovaquone-proguanil versus mefloquine for malaria prophylaxis in nonimmune travelers: results from a randomized, double-blind study. *Clin Infect Dis* 2001;33:1015–1021.
157. Berman JD, Nielsen R, Chulay JD, et al. Causal prophylactic efficacy of atovaquone-proguanil (Malarone) in a human challenge model. *Trans R Soc Trop Med Hyg* 2001; 95:429–432.
158. Ohrt C, Richie TL, Widjaja H, et al. Mefloquine compared with doxycycline for the prophylaxis of malaria in Indonesian soldiers. A randomized, double-blind, placebo-controlled trial. *Ann Intern Med* 1997;126:963–972.
159. Andersen SL, Oloo AJ, Gordon DM, et al. Successful double-blinded, randomized, placebo-controlled field trial of azithromycin and doxycycline as prophylaxis for malaria in western Kenya. *Clin Infect Dis* 1998;26:146–150.
160. Morris TJ, Davis TP. Doxycycline-induced esophageal ulceration in the U.S. Military service. *Mil Med* 2000;165:316–319.
161. Baird JK, Lacy MD, Basri H, et al. Randomized, parallel placebo-controlled trial of primaquine for malaria prophylaxis in Papua, Indonesia. *Clin Infect Dis* 2001;33:1990–1997.
162. Jelinek T, Grobusch MP. Nothdurft HD. Use of dipstick tests for the rapid diagnosis of malaria in nonimmune travelers. *J Travel Med* 2000;7:175–179.
163. Centers for Disease Control and Prevention. Sudden death in a traveler following halofantrine administration—Togo, 2000. *MMWR Morb Mortal Wkly Rep* 2001;50:169–170, 179.
164. Jelinek T. Dengue fever in international travelers. *Clin Infect Dis* 2000;31:144–147.
165. Centers for Disease Control and Prevention. Imported dengue—United States, 1997 and 1998. *MMWR Morb Mortal Wkly Rep* 2000;49:248–253.
166. Centers for Disease Control. Acute schistosomiasis in U.S. travelers returning from Africa. *MMWR Morb Mortal Wkly Rep* 1990;39:141–142, 147–148.
167. Lucey DR, Maguire JH. Schistosomiasis. *Infect Dis Clin North Am* 1993;7:635–653.
168. Cetron MS, Chitsulo L, Sullivan JJ, et al. Schistosomiasis in Lake Malawi. *Lancet* 1996;348:1274–1278.
169. Matteelli A, Carosi G. Sexually transmitted diseases in travelers. *Clin Infect Dis* 2001; 32:1063–1067.
170. Carter S, Horn K, Hart G, et al. The sexual behaviour of international travellers at two Glasgow GUM clinics. *Int J STD AIDS* 1997;8:336–338.
171. Houweling H, Coutinho RA. Risk of HIV infection among Dutch expatriates in sub-Saharan Africa. *Int J STD AIDS* 1991;2:252–257.
172. Joint United Nations Programme on HIV/AIDS (UNAIDS) and World Health Organization (WHO). *AIDS epidemic update 2001.* Geneva, Switzerland: UNAIDS, December, 2001.
173. Spitzer RL, Terman M, Williams JB, et al. Jet lag: clinical features, validation of a new syndrome-specific scale, and lack of response to melatonin in a randomized, double-blind trial. *Am J Psychiatry* 1999;156:1392–1396.
174. Edwards BJ, Atkinson G, Waterhouse J, et al. Use of melatonin in recovery from jet-lag following an eastward flight across 10 time-zones. *Ergonomics* 2000;43:1501–1513.
175. Ferrari E, Chevallier T, Chapelier A, et al. Travel as a risk factor for venous thromboembolic disease: a case-control study. *Chest* 1999;115:440–444.
176. Belcaro G, Geroulakos G, Nicolaides AN, et al. Venous thromboembolism from air travel: the LONFLIT study. *Angiology* 2001;52:369–374.
177. Lapostolle F, Surget V, Borron SW, et al. Severe pulmonary embolism associated with air travel. *N Engl J Med* 2001;345:779–783.
178. Medical Letter. Sunscreens: are they safe and effective? *Med Lett Drugs Therap* 1999; 41:43–44.
179. Caumes E, Carrière J, Guermonprez G, et al. Dermatoses associated with travel to

tropical countries: a prospective study of the diagnosis and management of 269 patients presenting to a tropical disease unit. *Clin Infect Dis* 1995;20:542–548.

180. Hill DR. Health problems in a large cohort of Americans traveling to developing countries. *J Travel Med* 2000;7:259–266.
181. Hackett PH, Roach RC. High-altitude illness. *N Engl J Med* 2001;345:107–114.
182. White AP. High-altitude illness. *N Engl J Med* 2001;345:1280.
183. Baker TD, Hargarten SW, Guptill KS. The uncounted dead—American civilians dying overseas. *Public Health Rep* 1992;107:155–159.
184. MacPherson DW, Guerillot F, Streiner DL, et al. Death and dying abroad: the Canadian experience. *J Travel Med* 2000;7:227–233.
185. Karp CL. Preparation of the HIV-infected traveler to the tropics. *Curr Infect Dis Rep* 2001;3:50–58.
186. Kovacs JA, Masur H. Prophylaxis against opportunistic infections in patients with human immunodeficiency virus infections. *N Engl J Med* 2000;342:1416–1429.
187. Mileno MD, Bia FJ. The compromised traveler. *Infect Dis Clin North Am* 1998;12:369–412.
188. Gong H. Advising patients with pulmonary diseases on air travel [Editorial]. *Ann Intern Med* 1989;111:349–351.
189. Samuel BU, Barry M. The pregnant traveler. *Infect Dis Clin North Am* 1998;12:325–354.
190. Fischer PR. Travel with infants and children. *Infect Dis Clin North Am* 1998;12:355–368.
191. Hill DR. Evaluation of the returned traveler. *Yale J Biol Med* 1992;65:343–356.
192. MacLean JD, Libman M. Screening returning travelers. *Infect Dis Clin North Am* 1998;12:431–443.
193. Brouwer ML, Tolboom JJM, Hardeman JHJ. Routine screening of children returning home from the tropics: retrospective study. *Br J Med* 1999;318:568–569.
194. Cheng AC, Thielman NM. Update on travelers' diarrhea. *Curr Infect Dis Rep* 2002;4:70–77.
195. Wong CS, Jelacic S, Habeeb RL, et al. The risk of the hemolytic-uremic syndrome after antibiotic treatment of *Escherichia coli* O157:H7 infections. *N Engl J Med* 2000;342:1930–1936.
196. Petri WA, Jr , Singh U, Ravdin JI. Enteric amebiasis. In: Guerrant RL, Walker DH, Weller PF, eds. *Tropical infectious diseases. Principles, pathogens, & practice*. Philadelphia: Churchill Livingstone, 1999:685–702.
197. Gardner TB, Hill DR. Treatment of giardiasis. *Clin Microbiol Rev* 2001;14:114–128.
198. Herwaldt BL. *Cyclospora cayetanensis*: a review, focusing on the outbreaks of cyclosporiasis in the 1990s. *Clin Infect Dis* 2000;31:1040–1057.
199. Castellani Pastoris M, Monaco RL, Goldini P, et al. Legionnaires' disease on a cruise ship linked to the water system: clinical and public health implications. *Clin Infect Dis* 1999;28:33–38.
200. Herwaldt BL, Stokes SL, Juranek DD. American cutaneous leishmaniasis in U.S. travelers. *Ann Intern Med* 1993;118:779–784.
201. Kain KC. Skin lesions in returned travelers. *Med Clin North Am* 1999;83:1077–1102.
202. Wilson ME, Pearson RD. Fever and systemic symptoms. In: Guerrant RL, Walker DH, Weller PF, eds. *Tropical infectious diseases. Principles, pathogens, & practice*. Philadelphia: Churchill Livingstone, 1999:1381–1399.
203. Medical Letter. Drugs for parasitic infections. The medical letter handbook of antimicrobial therapy, 16th ed. 2002;120–143. (This article and other useful articles for advising international travelers are available on the Internet: *www.medletter.com/-html_files/publicreading.htm#Parasitic.*)
204. Labbe AC, Loutfy MR, Kain KC. Recent advances in the prophylaxis and treatment of malaria. *Curr Infect Dis Rep* 2001;3:68–76.
205. World Health Organization. Severe falciparum malaria. *Trans R Soc Trop Med Hyg* 2000;94[Suppl 1]:S1–S90.
206. Centers for Disease Control and Prevention. Availability and use of parenteral quinidine gluconate for severe or complicated malaria. *Morb Mortal Wkly Rev* 2000;49:1138–1140.

207. Raoult D, Fournier PE, Fenollar F, et al. *Rickettsia africae,* a tick-borne pathogen in travelers to sub-Saharan Africa. *N Engl J Med* 2001;344:1504–1510.
208. Peters CJ, Zaik SR. Overview of viral hemorrhagic fevers. In: Guerrant RL, Walker DH, Weller PF, eds. *Tropical infectious diseases. Principles, pathogens, & practice*. Philadelphia: Churchill Livingstone, 1999:1182–1190.
209. Centers for Disease Control and Prevention. Update: management of patients with suspected viral hemorrhagic fever—United States. *Morb Mortal Wkly Rev* 1995;44:475–479.
210. Moore TA, Nutman TB. Eosinophilia in the returning traveler. *Infect Dis Clin North Am* 1998;12:503–522.
211. Wilson ME, Weller PF. Eosinophilia. In: Guerrant RL, Walker DH, Weller PF, eds. *Tropical infectious diseases. Principles, pathogens, & practice*. Philadelphia: Churchill Livingstone, 1999:1400–1419.
212. Guerrant RL, Walker DH, Weller PF, eds. *Tropical infectious diseases. Principles, pathogens, & practice.* Philadelphia: Churchill Livingstone, 1999.
213. Strickland GT, ed. *Hunter's tropical medicine and emerging infectious diseases,* 8th ed. Philadelphia: W.B. Saunders, 2000.
214. DuPont HL, Steffen R, ed. *Textbook of travel medicine and health,* 2nd ed. Hamilton, Ontario: B.C. Decker, 2001.
215. Keystone JS, Kozarsky PE, Freedman DO. Internet and computer-based resources for travel medicine practitioners. *Clin Infect Dis* 2001;32:757–765.

# 23. IMMUNIZATIONS

Paul J. Edelson

Prophylactic immunization is an essential part of primary care at all ages [1,2]. Although childhood immunization remains the primary control strategy for most preventable diseases, major programs for adult immunization have been developed and vaccination recommendations have now been formulated to address the needs of specialized subgroups. New vaccines, adoption of the National Childhood Vaccine Injury Act [3], and changing epidemiologic patterns of disease have affected our practice responsibilities for immunization of both child and adult patients. New approaches have already led to significant improvement in the seroprevalence levels for varicella and hepatitis B in preschoolers [4]. Immunization levels for adults, however, are still inadequate [5]. Recommendations for modern approaches to immunization programs have been published [6–8]. There are a number of reliable sources for current immunization recommendations: reports of the U.S. Advisory Committee on Immunization Practices (ACIP) of the U.S. Public Health Service are published in ***Morbidity and Mortality Weekly Reports,*** issued by the Centers for Disease Control and Prevention (CDC). This valuable publication, available via the CDC Internet site, is regularly extracted in the *Journal of the American Medical Association.* Specific ACIP recommendations are also available from the CDC National Immunization Program Office and many state health departments. A convenient source of current ACIP recommendations, as well as other immunization resources, is the Immunization Action Coalition's website (***www.immunize.org/adultrules***). Similar recommendations of the Canadian expert group are published in the *Canadian Medical Association Journal.* Recommendations of other expert panels are collected in the *Report of the Committee on Infectious Diseases* (the so-called Red Book) [9] for infants and children and in the *Guide to Adult Immunization* (the so-called Green Book) [10] for adults. Excellent summaries of current recommendations for immunization of the adult patient in general have been published [11,12]. Recommendations for specific groups of adults are provided below (see section **VI**). Recent authoritative surveys of the entire field are also available [13–16]. These recommendations are appropriate for use only in the United States because epidemiologic circumstances and vaccines may differ in other countries. Advice regarding immunization for travel abroad can be found in Chapter 22.

**I. General principles [16]**

**A. Immunobiologics.** This term refers to all biological materials involved in the artificial production of a specific immune state, including the following.

1. **Vaccine.** A suspension of live (usually attenuated) or killed microbial organisms, or portions of them, that can be used to induce immunity and prevent infectious disease when injected, inhaled, or ingested. Vaccines may have differing levels of purity. A list of currently licensed vaccines for general use is provided in Table 23.1.
2. **Toxoid.** A modified microbial toxin that still retains its antigenic specificity and can be used to stimulate immunity to the relevant toxin.
3. **Immune globulin (IG)** is prepared from large plasma pools by ethanol fractionation (the Cohn method) and was previously designated *immune serum globulin* or *gamma globulin.* It **contains specified amounts of antibody against measles, diphtheria, and poliovirus type 1.** In addition, IG contains **variable amounts of antibody against hepatitis A and B viruses, varicella virus, respiratory syncytial viruses,** and possibly some non-A, non-B hepatitis viruses. IG is not specifically designated as safe for intravenous use and **should be used only intramuscularly.** IG has never been associated with the transmission of human immunodeficiency virus (HIV), although some lots prepared before 1985 have passively transferred transient HIV seropositivity. Although the Cohn procedure has been shown to inactivate HIV, since 1985 all IG used in the United States must be prepared from HIV-seronegative blood.
4. **Intravenous immune globulin (IVIG).** A fraction of blood plasma is prepared from a large donor pool, similar to that used for IG, but treated for **intravenous**

Table 23.1. Major Types of Vaccines

| |
|---|
| Live attenuated virus |
| Measles |
| Mumps |
| Parainfluenza virus[a] |
| Poliovirus (oral) |
| Respiratory syncytial virus[a] |
| Rubella |
| Varicella |
| Yellow fever |
| Live attenuated bacteria |
| Bacillus Calmette-Guérin (BCG) |
| Tularemia |
| Typhoid (oral) |
| Inactivated virus |
| Hepatitis A |
| Hepatitis B |
| Human papillomavirus[a] |
| Influenza |
| Poliovirus (subcutaneous) |
| Rabies |
| Inactivated bacteria |
| Anthrax |
| Cholera |
| Diphtheria (toxoid) |
| Gonococcus[a] |
| *Haemophilus influenzae* type b (polysaccharide-protein conjugate) |
| Lyme disease |
| Meningococcus (polysaccharide) |
| Pertussis (acellular) |
| Pertussis (inactivated whole bacteria) |
| Plague |
| Pneumococcus (polysaccharide) |
| Pneumococcus (polysaccharide-protein conjugate) |
| Tetanus (toxoid) |
| Typhoid (subcutaneous) |
| Inactivated rickettsiae |
| Q fever (*Coxiella burnetii*) |

[a]Under development.

**administration.** Its use is generally similar to that of IG, but larger amounts can be administered than via the intramuscular route.

5. **Specific IG.** Special preparations of IGs containing high-titered antibody to specific infectious agents. They are prepared from plasma pools obtained from immunized donors or from individuals recovering from recent disease or by laboratory techniques that produce monoclonal antibodies of animal or human type, including so-called humanized animal antibodies. Human IGs are much less likely to provoke serious hypersensitivity reactions than are IGs derived from animals, which they have generally replaced. Like IG, these preparations are for **intramuscular** injection only unless specifically labeled for intravenous use. Specific IGs currently available for clinical use include hepatitis B IG, varicella-zoster IG, rabies IG, tetanus IG, and vaccinia IG. Recommendations for the use of both specific and pooled IGs have been published [17]. Adverse effects of the administration of IGs have also been reviewed [18].

6. **Antitoxin.** Antibody prepared in animals that provide passive immunity to specific microbial toxins, such as diphtheria or botulinum antitoxin.

B. **Active immunization** involves the use of immunogens, such as live attenuated virus, inactivated virus, isolated viral proteins, bacterial components, or inactivated toxins (toxoids), to stimulate a protective antibody or cell-mediated immune response, or both (Table 23.1).

1. **Live attenuated virus vaccines** generally stimulate greater and more durable immunity than do inactivated virus vaccines. The live attenuated vaccines, however, have greater inherent risks and are not appropriate for use in all individuals.
   a. **Live attenuated preparations include measles, mumps, rubella, oral poliovirus, varicella, and yellow fever vaccines.**
   b. **Limitations.** Except under special circumstances, **live attenuated vaccines should not be administered to patients with** congenital or acquired immunodeficiency; leukemia, lymphoma, or generalized malignancy; or to patients receiving immunosuppressive therapy or, in certain cases, to members of their households, because these attenuated agents may cause disease in the impaired host or may be spread after administration in immunocompromised individuals to susceptible hosts. In addition, because these agents present a theoretic risk to the developing fetus, live attenuated virus vaccines are not generally recommended for use in pregnant women or those likely to become pregnant within 3 months after immunization. For special recommendations concerning the use of live attenuated measles or trivalent measles-mumps-rubella (MMR) vaccine in children with HIV infection see section **III.A.4.h.**
2. **Inactivated virus or purified viral components** are used to produce **influenza** and **hepatitis B** vaccines. Because an inactivated virus is used, the limitations in section **1.b** may not apply to these vaccines. For example, if poliomyelitis immunization is indicated for immunosuppressed patients, their household contacts, or other close contacts, the (enhanced) inactivated poliovirus vaccine (e-IPV) can safely replace the live attenuated vaccine, as discussed in section **III.D.3.**
3. **Inactivated bacterial vaccines** include the currently available **pertussis, typhoid** (parenteral), and **cholera** vaccines. Bacterial-component immunogens may not produce lifelong immunity and may therefore require booster doses at appropriate intervals to ensure adequate and long-lasting protection.
4. **Toxoids. Diphtheria** and **tetanus** vaccines are inactivated toxins, referred to as toxoids.

C. **Passive immunization** is produced by the administration of **IG, IVIG, or specific IG.** All these preparations contain specific protective antibodies derived from human plasma.

1. This form of immunization **provides immediate protection** but is of very limited duration and is most useful for time-limited prophylaxis. It may be given up to 3 weeks before or up to 72 hours after specific disease exposure. For the clinical use of specific human IGs, refer to the following:
   a. **Varicella-zoster virus:** see Chapter 4 under Mucocutaneous Vesicles
   b. **Tetanus:** see Chapter 4 under Tetanus
   c. **Rabies:** see Chapter 4 under Bite Wounds and Rabies Prevention
   d. **Hepatitis B:** see section **IV.A**
2. **Animal-derived IGs. Except for treatment of snake and spider bites or in the treatment of diphtheria, animal sera are no longer recommended for human use.** In the past, tetanus and rabies antisera were derived from immunized animals. These were far more likely than human products to cause serum sickness or anaphylaxis.

D. **Passive and active immunizations** are sometimes combined to provide both immediate protection (with preformed antibody) and sustained protection (antigenic stimulation of host immune response). As a rule, each agent is injected at a separate site.

1. For postexposure **rabies** prophylaxis, for example, human rabies IG (passive) is combined with human diploid cell rabies vaccine (active).
2. For postexposure **tetanus** prophylaxis in the previously nonimmunized individual, human tetanus IG (passive) is combined with tetanus toxoid (active). Note, however, that in this situation **only the alum-precipitated or adsorbed toxoid, and not the fluid toxoid, should be used** (see section **V.E**).
3. Similar active-passive immunization is used in the prophylaxis of neonates born to mothers who are hepatitis B carriers (see section **IV.A**).
4. **Immunoglobulin should never be administered to modify the normal and expected reaction to a live attenuated virus vaccine,** as was previously done with the Edmonston-strain measles vaccine.

**E. Simultaneous administration of vaccines.** Studies have shown that it is safe and, in most instances, effective to administer multiple vaccines simultaneously [16]. This is often more convenient for individuals who require a number of different immunizations. When several vaccines are being administered at the same time, the vaccines should not be combined in the same syringe or administered at the same site. **Only prepackaged combination vaccines should be administered at a single site.** However, the antibody **response of both cholera and yellow fever vaccines may be decreased if given simultaneously** or within a short time of each other. If possible, cholera and yellow fever vaccinations should be separated by at least 3 weeks (see Chapter 22).

1. **Live attenuated virus vaccines** were previously administered 1 month apart, but studies have shown that simultaneous administration of some live virus vaccines (e.g., MMR) is just as effective as single injections and does not result in higher rates of adverse reactions.
2. **Inactivated vaccines** can be administered simultaneously at separate sites. When vaccines commonly associated with local or systemic side effects (e.g., cholera, parenteral typhoid, or plague) are given simultaneously, side effects could be accentuated. For patients with a history of a reaction to one or more vaccines, it is prudent to administer each on a separate occasion.
3. **An inactivated and a live attenuated vaccine** can be given simultaneously.
4. **Inactivated bacterial and viral vaccines** can be given simultaneously. An example is the simultaneous administration of influenza and pneumococcal vaccines.

**F. Contraindications and adverse reactions** [19]. The manufacturer's guidelines and recommendations, as contained in the U.S. Food and Drug Administration approved package insert, should be followed carefully.

1. **Hypersensitivity reactions**
   a. **Some vaccine antigens, particularly measles, mumps, influenza, and yellow fever, are derived from embryonated chicken eggs or embryonic chick cells.** In general, **if patients can eat a whole egg, these vaccines can be safely administered.** Protocols have been developed for immunization of the highly egg-allergic patient [20].
   b. **Anaphylactic antibiotic reactions.** Some vaccines contain trace amounts of antibiotics. In patients with a history of anaphylactic reactions to specific antibiotics, the current package insert should be carefully reviewed to ascertain whether the antibiotic of concern is in the vaccine. If the vaccine does contain the antibiotic, the vaccine should be avoided. No current vaccines contain penicillin or penicillin derivatives. The history of a minor local contact dermatitis from prior neomycin use is not a contraindication to any vaccine containing neomycin.
2. **Altered immunity.** Live attenuated virus vaccines may cause serious disease in some immunocompromised individuals. In general, these vaccines should not be used in such patients. Measles vaccine, however, has been recommended for use in certain individuals infected with HIV (see section **III.A.4.h**). **Live attenuated poliovirus vaccines should not be administered to any household member of an immunocompromised person** (see section **VI.F**).
3. **Severe febrile illness.** Minor illness, such as a mild upper respiratory infection, should not preclude immunization. Vaccination of patients with severe

febrile illnesses should be deferred so that side effects of the vaccine do not complicate the existing illness and so that symptoms of the illness are not incorrectly ascribed to the vaccine.

4. **Pregnancy.** Because **live attenuated virus vaccines pose a theoretic risk to the developing fetus**, these vaccines generally should not be given to a pregnant woman or to a woman likely to become pregnant within 3 months of immunization. Concerns and risks of immunization during pregnancy are further addressed in section **VI.B.**
5. **Recent administration of IG.** Passively acquired antibody (e.g., IG) **may interfere with the response to live attenuated virus vaccines. Administration of such vaccines should be individualized based on specific recommendations** [16].
   a. **Oral polio vaccine (OPV), yellow fever, and oral typhoid vaccine (Ty21a)** vaccines may be administered without regard to the administration of immune or specific globulins.
   b. Although it has previously been stated that MMR or any of its component vaccines may be administered as early as 6 weeks to 3 months after a dose of IG, high-titer IGs or IGs administered in large doses may interfere with measles immunization even beyond 3 months and can also inhibit the response to rubella vaccine. Effects on mumps or varicella response are unknown, but standard preparations do contain antibody to each of these agents. Blood products, except *washed* packed red cells, also contain significant amounts of antibody; precautions regarding immunization should apply to recipients of blood products. In general, live antigen vaccines, other than those in section **a,** should be delayed proportionately to the dose of antibody previously administered. When possible, IG should be delayed at least 2 weeks after the administration of live antigen vaccines.
   c. Most bacterial or inactivated viral vaccines may be administered with IG for specific postexposure prophylaxis (see section **I.D**).

## II. Immunization schedules

### A. Pediatric immunization schedules.

**A. Pediatric immunization schedules.** The details of these schedules are published in the serial editions of the **Red Book** [10] **and updated reports** of the Committee on Infectious Diseases in Pediatrics, and in recommendations made by the ACIP as published in *Morbidity and Mortality Weekly Reports.* Schedules are typically updated and issued twice yearly.

A working group of federal and state experts, medical specialty organizations, and vaccine manufacturers has promulgated a **single scientifically valid immunization program, summarized in Table 23.2.** This was intended in part to help resolve variations in prior recommendations. Important recommendations of the working group include the following:

1. The third dose of OPV should be administered routinely at 6 months of age; vaccination at as late as 18 months remains an acceptable alternative.
2. The first dose of MMR vaccine is suggested at 12 to 15 months of age. The second dose of MMR can be administered at either 4 to 6 or 11 to 12 years of age.
3. Universal hepatitis B vaccination of infants was recommended in 1991.
   a. For infants whose mothers are hepatitis B surface antigen (HBsAg) negative, routine hepatitis B vaccination series should begin at birth, with the second dose administered at 2 months of age (see acceptable ranges in Table 23.2). The third dose should be administered at 6 to 18 months.
   b. For infants of HBsAg-positive mothers, the infant should receive the first dose of vaccine at birth (along with hepatitis B immune globulin [HBIG]), the second dose at 1 month of age, and the third dose at 6 months (see related discussion in Chapter 3).
4. The schedule for diphtheria-tetanus-pertussis (DTP) vaccination in force for several years is still recommended (Table 23.2).

**B. Adult immunizations.** The indications for adult immunizations are reviewed in the discussions of individual vaccines below (see sections **III–V**) and in Table 23.3 and in related discussion in Chapter 22. False contraindications sometimes applied to various vaccines have been reviewed by the CDC [19]. Regarding a hypothesized

Table 23.2. Recommended Childhood Immunization Schedule[a]—United States

| Vaccine | Age: Birth | 1 mo | 2 mo | 4 mo | 6 mo | 12 mo | 15 mo | 18 mo | 4–6 yr | 11–12 yr | 14–16 yr |
|---|---|---|---|---|---|---|---|---|---|---|---|
| Hepatitis B[b] | Hep B-1 | | | | | | | | | | |
| | | Hep B-2 | | | Hep B-3 | | | | | Hep B[c] | |
| Diphtheria and tetanus toxoids and pertussis vaccine[d] | | | DTP | DTP | DTP | DTP (DTaP at ≥15 mo) | | | DTP or DTaP | Td | |
| *Haemophilus influenza type* b[e] | | | Hib | Hib | Hib | **Hib** | | | | | |
| Poliovirus[f] | | | OPV | OPV | **OPV** | | | | OPV | | |
| Measles-mumps-rubella[g] | | | | | | MMR | | | MMR | or MMR | |
| Varicella zoster virus[h] | | | | | | Var | | | | Var[i] | |

**Note:** Boxed information indicates range of acceptable ages for vaccination.

[a]Vaccines are listed under the routinely recommended ages. Recommendations of the ACIP are generally updated every 6 months.

[b]**Infants born to hepatitis B surface antigen (HBsAg)-negative mothers** should receive 2.5 μg of Recombivax HB (Merck) or 10 μg of Engerix-B (SmithKline Beecham). The second dose should be administered ≥1 month after the first dose. **Infants born to HBsAg-positive mothers** should receive 0.5 mL hepatitis B immune globulin (HBIG) within 12 h of birth and either 5 μg of Recombivax HB or 10 μg of Engerix-B at a separate site. The second dose is recommended at age 1–2 months and the third dose at age 6 months. **Infants born to mothers whose HBsAg status is unknown** should receive either 5 μg of Recombivax HB or 10 μg of Engerix-B within 12 hours of birth. The second dose of vaccine is recommended at age 1 month and the third dose at age 6 months.

[c]Adolescents who have not received three doses of hepatitis B vaccine should initiate or complete the series at age 11–12 years. The second dose should be administered at least 1 month after the first dose, and the third dose should be administered at least 4 months after the first dose and at least 2 months after the second dose.

[d]The fourth dose of diphtheria and tetanus toxoids and pertussis vaccine (DTP) may be administered at age 12 months, if at least 6 months have elapsed since the third dose of DTP. Diphtheria and tetanus toxoids and acellular pertussis vaccine (DTaP) is licensed for the fourth and/or fifth dose(s) for children aged ≥15 months and may be preferred for these doses in this age group. Tetanus and diphtheria toxoids, adsorbed, for adult use (Td) is recommended at age 11–12 years if at least 5 years have elapsed since the last dose of DTP DTaP, or diphtheria and tetanus toxoids, absorbed, for pediatric use (DT).

[e]Three *Haemophilus influenzae* type b (Hib) conjugate vaccines are licensed for infant use. If PedvaxHIB (Merck) *Haemophilus* b conjugate vaccine (meningococcal protein conjugate) (PRP-OMP) is administered at ages 2 and 4 months, a dose at 6 months is not required. After completing the primary series, any Hib conjugate vaccine may be used as a booster.

[f]Oral poliovirus vaccine (OPV) is recommended for routine infant vaccination. Inactivated poliovirus vaccine (IPV) is recommended for persons or household contacts of persons—with a congenital or acquired immune deficiency disease or an altered immune status resulting from disease or immunosuppressive therapy, and is an acceptable alternative for other persons. The primary three-dose series for IPV should be given with a minimum interval of 4 weeks between the first and second doses and 6 months between the second and third doses.

[g]The second dose of measles-mumps-rubella vaccine (MMR) is routinely recommended at age 4–6 years or at age 11–12 years but may be administered at any visit provided at least 1 month has elapsed since receipt of the first dose.

[h]Varicella-zoster virus vaccine (Var) can be administered to susceptible children any time after age 12 months.

[i]"Catch-up" vaccination (see also footnote c). Unvaccinated children who lack a reliable history of chickenpox should be vaccinated at age 11–12 years.

Modified from Advisory Committee on Immunization Practices, American Academy of Pediatrics, and American Academy of Family Physicians. *MMWR Morb Mortal Wkly Rev* 1996; 44:942–943.

Table 23.3. Vaccines to Be Considered for Adult Patient Groups[a]

| Patient Group | Major Vaccines[b] | Other Considerations[c] |
|---|---|---|
| Healthy adults | | |
| Adolescents and young adults | Td, MMR up to date, hepatitis B, meningococcal vaccine, completion of childhood immunizations | Varicella (see text) |
| 25–64 yr | Td, rubella (women only), polio | Varicella (see text) |
| 65 yr and older | Td, influenza, pneumococcal | |
| Pregnant women | MMR is contraindicated; test for rubella antibody and hepatitis B surface antigen | |
| Those in environmental situations | | |
| Nursing home residents | Influenza, pneumococcal | Tuberculin test |
| Institutionalized mentally retarded | Hepatitis B | Hepatitis A |
| Prison inmates | Hepatitis B, rubella | Hepatitis A |
| Homeless persons | Review all vaccines; consider pneumococcal vaccine | Tuberculin test |
| Occupational groups | | |
| College students | MMR; consider hepatitis B, polio, influenza | |
| Health-care workers | Hepatitis B, influenza, MMR | Varicella |
| Essential community services | Influenza | |
| Daycare center personnel | MMR, polio, influenza | Hepatitis A, hepatitis B |
| Laboratory personnel | Hepatitis B | Consider individually |
| Veterinarians, animal handlers, rural workers, and other field personnel | Rabies | Plague, anthrax |
| Immigrants and refugees | Review all vaccines, test for hepatitis B surface antigen | Tuberculin test |
| Those with life-style risks | | |
| Homosexual and bisexual men | Hepatitis B, hepatitis A | |
| Intravenous drug abusers | Hepatitis B, Td, hepatitis A | |
| Prostitutes, persons with multiple sexual partners or sexually transmitted diseases | Hepatitis B | Hepatitis A (see Chapter 14) |
| Accident victims | | |
| Wounds | Td | TIG |
| Animal bites | Td | Rabies vaccine, RIG |
| Snake and spider bites | Td | Specific antivenins |
| Immunocompromised | | |
| HIV infection and AIDS | Pneumococcal conjugate, hepatitis B | IG (measles), VZIG, measles, varicella |
| Splenic disorders | Pneumococcal conjugate, influenza | *Haemophilus influenzae* type b, meningococcal |
| Diabetes | Pneumococcal, influenza | |
| Renal failure and dialysis | Pneumococcal, influenza, hepatitis B | |

(*Continued*)

Table 23.3. (*Continued*)

| Patient Group | Major Vaccines[b] | Other Considerations[c] |
|---|---|---|
| Alcoholism, cirrhosis | Pneumococcal, influenza | Hepatitis B vaccine |
| Organ transplant recipients, immunosuppressive therapy | Pneumococcal, influenza | *Haemophilus influenzae* type b, meningococcal |
| Those with malignant diseases | Consider individually | |
| International travel groups | Review Td, MMR, polio; consider influenza, pneumococcal, hepatitis B | Yellow fever, IG or hepatitis A, meningococcal, typhoid, cholera, rabies, Japanese encephalitis, antimalarial prophylaxis (see Chapter 22) |

[a]See text for specific details on indications, administration, adverse reactions, precautions, contraindications, and special considerations for each vaccine, toxoid, and immunoglobulin preparation. Also see reference 10.
[b]Major vaccines include combined tetanus and diphtheria (Td) toxoids; measles-mumps-rubella (MMR) vaccine; oral polio vaccine and enhanced-potency inactivated polio vaccine; influenza vaccine; pneumococcal vaccine; and hepatitis B vaccine.
[c]Other considerations include immunoglobulin (IG), tetanus immunoglobulin (TIG), rabies immunoglobulin (RIG), varicella-zoster immunoglobulin (VZIG), and intravenous immunoglobulin (IVIG).
Modified from ACP Task Force on Adult Immunization and Infectious Diseases Society of America. *Guide to adult immunization,* 3rd ed. Philadelphia: American College of Physicians, 1994. See also Gardner P, et al. Adult immunizations. *Ann Intern Med* 1996;124:35–40.

association between vaccines and **multiple sclerosis,** two recent studies have concluded that routine immunizations, including influenza vaccine, have no effect on the risk of short-term relapse [21] and offer no support for a relationship between hepatitis B immunization and the disease [22].

**C. Requirements of the National Childhood Vaccine Injury Act of 1988.** This act, which provides for certain indemnifications for vaccine-related injuries, imposes specific record-keeping and reporting obligations on individuals who administer vaccines. Requirements of most relevance to adult vaccinees apply to the administration of tetanus and diphtheria toxoids, tetanus toxoid, and both OPV and IPV. As of March 21, 1988, **physicians and others providing these vaccines are required to maintain immunization records specifying for each recipient** the date of administration; manufacturer and lot number of the vaccine; and the name, address, and title of the person administering the vaccine. In addition, the law specifies a list of reportable events occurring within specified times after vaccine administration and the names of authorities to whom reports must be made. (Additional details are presented in Appendices 9 and 10 of the Green Book [11].)

**III. Live attenuated virus vaccines**

**A. Measles (rubeola)** [22] can be a severe disease, with pulmonary, gastrointestinal, and neurologic complications. Encephalitis occurs in approximately 1 of every 1,000 reported cases, and survivors may suffer permanent neurologic impairment or mental retardation. Death occurs in 1 to 2 of every 1,000 cases. Measles during pregnancy increases the risks of spontaneous abortion, premature labor, and low birth weight. Birth defects have been reported in infants exposed to measles virus in their first trimester, but the defects comprise no definable pattern of malformation and measles has not been confirmed as the cause of any of these malformations. Because maternal fever in the first trimester may itself be embryopathic, it is possible that the abnormalities are not the result of a specific malformation syndrome but rather represent a nonspecific result of maternal fever. Subacute sclerosing panencephalitis is also considered to be a rare but devastating complication of natural infection with measles virus. In countries where there is a significant degree of infantile and early childhood malnutrition or in the setting of large numbers of displaced persons or forced population migrations, measles is a significant cause of childhood deaths. Before measles vaccine became available in 1963, more than 400,000 measles cases were reported annually in the United States, and it is estimated that only 10% of cases were reported. Since then, reported cases (including imported cases representing overseas exposures) have fallen by 100- to 1,000-fold, and a national goal of measles eradication has been set by the U.S. Public Health Service. There has also been a striking decline in the incidence of subacute sclerosing panencephalitis.

**The currently available measles vaccine, the measles eradication program,** and recommendations for measles outbreak control **have been reviewed by the CDC** [23].

1. **Measles elimination efforts in the United States.** The adoption in 1993 of a national program to eliminate measles from the United States, involving the use of a two-dose regimen of immunizations, has markedly improved immunization rates, particularly in preschoolers, adolescents, and young adults. The transmission of indigenous measles appears to have been interrupted for the first time in this country. Further progress in eliminating measles will depend on the continuing effort to immunize all children between 12 and 15 months of age and to ensure that all children receive a second dose of vaccine before they enter school, as well as cooperating with other national governments to eliminate measles abroad.
   a. **Preschoolers**
      (1) **Continued compliance** with recommended measles vaccination programs for young children is essential.
      (2) **Two-dose measles vaccine schedule.** To reduce the number of primary vaccine failure-related cases of measles, the ACIP recommends a routine two-dose measles vaccine schedule. The initial dose is administered at 12 to 15 months of age, whereas the second dose is recommended at school entry (4–6 years of age). The second dose may be administered at any visit after the first birthday, until age 12, provided at least 1 month has elapsed since receipt of the first dose. Children can be vaccinated initially as early as 6 to 9 months of age in an actual outbreak of measles and then reimmunized at 12 months and boosted before beginning school (Table 23.2). MMR is recommended for both doses.
   b. **Young adults** (high school and college age). Many educational institutions have already adopted requirements intended to prevent measles outbreaks among individuals who may have been immunized before their first birthdays or received vaccine before 1980 or who for other reasons were among the 2% of persons estimated to be primary vaccine failures. In such people, a second dose of vaccine is generally successful. State-mandated prematriculation immunization guidelines for measles has been effective in reducing the incidence of measles outbreaks in colleges [24,25].
      (1) Evidence of measles immunity (i.e., prior diagnosis by a physician or laboratory evidence) must be provided by matriculating students born in or after 1957.
      (2) Documentation of two doses of live measles vaccine, with the second dose after 1980, must be provided. If this has not been done already, a dose of measles vaccine should be given before school begins to ensure adequate immunity.
      (3) In an outbreak of measles, all persons at risk (e.g., students attending schools where measles has occurred who have not been adequately vaccinated) should be vaccinated (see sections **1 and 2**).
      (4) **Although MMR has been considered appropriate for revaccinating college-age students,** because of the increased incidence of

Table 23.4. Current Recommendations for Measles Vaccination

| Routine Childhood Schedule, United States | |
|---|---|
| Primary immunization | Two doses[a,b]<br>First dose at 12–15 mo<br>Second dose at 4–6 yr (entry to kindergarten or first grade)[d] |
| Colleges and other educational institutions after high school | Documentation of receipt of two doses of measles vaccine after the first birthday[b] or other evidence of measles immunity[c] |
| Medical personnel beginning employment | Documentation of receipt of two doses of measles vaccine after the first birthday[b] or other evidence of measles immunity |

[a]Both doses should preferably be given as combined measles-mumps-rubella vaccine (MMR).
[b]No less than 1 month apart. If there is no documentation of any dose of vaccine, vaccine should be given at the time of school entry or employment and no less than 1 month later.
[c]A county with more than five cases among preschool-aged children during each of the last 5 years, a county with a recent outbreak among unvaccinated preschool-aged children, or a county with a large inner-city urban population. These recommendations may be applied to an entire county or to identified risk areas within a county.
[d]Some areas may elect to administer the second dose at an older age or to multiple age groups.

arthritic reactions seen in young adults after revaccination with rubella vaccine, **it may be prudent to revaccinate with measles vaccine alone if rubella immune status is not a concern** (see section **5** and Table 23.4). Arthritis and arthralgias are known adverse effects of rubella vaccine in nonimmune vaccinees. They occur in approximately 12% to 20% of adults and 0% to 3% of children and have an intermediate incidence in adolescents. Neither MMR nor measles vaccine is recommended in pregnancy.

2. **Vaccine.** The current live attenuated measles vaccine, prepared in chick embryo cell cultures, is less reactogenic than its predecessor, the Edmonston B strain. In addition, stabilizers added in 1980 seem to have improved the storage characteristics of the vaccine. The current vaccine produces a mild or inapparent noncommunicable infection, with antibody developing in over 95% of susceptible recipients vaccinated at 15 months of age or older. Both monovalent (measles only) and combination (i.e., measles and rubella and MMR) forms of the vaccine are available.
3. **Persons can be considered immune to measles if one of the following conditions is met:**
   a. **Born before 1957.** These individuals are likely to have been infected naturally and are considered immune.
   b. **Documentation of physician-diagnosed measles.** A clinical case definition includes a generalized maculopapular rash of 3 days' duration or longer (often appearing first at the hairline, forehead, and behind the ears and upper neck, then spreading downward to involve the face and neck and then the trunk and upper extremities); fever of at least 101°F orally; **and** cough, coryza, or conjunctivitis. A *confirmed* case has seropositivity or meets the preceding definition and is epidemiologically linked to a known case or outbreak of measles. A *suspected* case meets the preceding definition (but rash can be of less than 3 days' duration) but has no serologic confirmation or epidemiologic link. Serologic confirmation involves either a positive IgM test or a fourfold rise from acute to convalescent specimens in complement fixation testing without a history of recent vaccination.
   c. **Documented laboratory evidence of measles immunity.** The enzyme immunoassay and enzyme-linked immunosorbent assay (ELISA) currently used for measles immunity are more sensitive than the hemagglutination

inhibition test, which was the former standard. Demonstration of antibody by any of these tests is sufficient to document immunity. All new cases suspected of being measles should be confirmed by laboratory testing. Routine serologic screening to determine measles immunity is not recommended, except possibly for health-care workers. (See section **10** and Chapter 26 on employee health.)

d. **Adequate immunization with live measles vaccine at or after 15 months of age.** The maximal rate of seroconversion after measles vaccine occurs at 15 months of age or later. An adequate two-dose measles vaccination schedule in children or a booster dose in young adults is advised (see section **2**).

e. **During an outbreak,** proof of immunity is documentation of receipt of two doses of measles vaccine or MMR, both administered after the individual's first birthday and after 1980 and not administered with IG unless the Edmonston strain is known to have been used.

4. **Persons needing measles vaccine** (Table 23.4)

a. **Susceptible children older than 15 months, adolescents, and adults** should be vaccinated if there are no contraindications. Also, persons who did not receive two doses of the measles vaccine after their first birthday should be vaccinated (see section **2**).

b. **Those vaccinated with live measles virus before 12 months of age** should be identified and revaccinated.

c. **Those immunized with the inactivated (killed) measles vaccine in use from 1963 to 1967** (or to 1969 in Canada) are at risk for developing **atypical measles** when exposed to natural infection. This disease may have significant morbidity in adults and has been reviewed in detail elsewhere [26]. Patients may have conjunctivitis and a characteristic erythematous maculopapular rash progressing to vesicular, petechial, or purpuric lesions. The rash initially involves the palms and soles, with subsequent spread to the proximal extremities and trunk, sparing the face. Pulmonary involvement with significant hypoxemia is common. Although recipients of the killed vaccine may have an increased risk of adverse reaction when revaccinated with the live vaccine, these risks are minor compared with the severity of atypical measles developing after infection with wild-type virus.

d. **Young adults** (secondary school or college age) **who have not had measles vaccine since 1980** require revaccination (see section **2**).

e. **Persons who received IG at the time of measles vaccination** should be revaccinated. Although immunization with the Edmonston B strain vaccine probably was effective even when administered with IG, the use of IG with other vaccines, including the current one, could render the dose ineffective. All individuals in whom IG was used in combination with a vaccine other than the Edmonston B strain or in whom the vaccine type is not known should be reimmunized.

f. **Susceptible persons exposed to measles** may benefit from vaccination if the vaccine is given within 72 hours of measles exposure.

g. **Travelers to high-risk areas** may require vaccination. Measles continues to be endemic throughout many parts of Asia, Africa, and Central and South America. Nonimmune visitors run the risk of acquiring measles and of exposing others on their return. **Travelers born after 1956 who are planning trips to these areas should have their measles immune status reviewed** (see section **2**). Although serologic screening is not routinely recommended, it may be useful in evaluating prospective travelers. If the traveler has prior immunity, there is no evidence of enhanced risk from receiving the live attenuated measles vaccine. For infants traveling to measles-endemic areas, vaccination is recommended as early as 6 months of age, with a second measles immunization at age 15 months and a third dose at school entry. For further discussion see Chapter 22.

h. **Persons with HIV infection** may be at special risk for measles complications. Because of several reports of severe or fatal cases of measles in children with HIV infection [27], it has been recommended that measles vaccine is administered to all such children, regardless of the stage of their HIV disease. However, newer draft recommendations of the CDC advise that MMR not be given to severely immunosuppressed (category 3) children [27].

5. **The dosage** is the same for children and adults: a subcutaneous dose of properly stored vaccine in the 0.5-ml volume recommended by the manufacturer. The trivalent MMR form is the vaccine of choice for routine childhood immunization. **IG should not be administered with the measles vaccine or, ideally, sooner than 3 months before measles vaccine or 2 weeks after** (see Chapter 22).
6. **Precautions and contraindications**
   a. **Pregnancy.** Live measles vaccine should not be administered to women who are pregnant. Also, women should avoid becoming pregnant for 3 months after vaccination. Although there is no clinical experience of harm to the developing fetus, there is a theoretic risk of such harm. Pregnant women exposed to natural measles infection may wish to consider the use of IG within 6 days of the exposure.
   b. **Allergies.** Because the live attenuated virus vaccine is prepared in chick embryo cells, patients with a history of **egg allergy** associated with anaphylactic reaction should be vaccinated only with extreme caution. Herman et al. [20] devised a protocol for immunizing such individuals. There is no evidence that persons with other allergies to chicken or to feathers are at increased risk of reaction to the vaccine.

      The vaccine contains trace amounts of **neomycin.** Therefore, persons who have experienced anaphylactic reactions to topical or systemic neomycin also should not receive this vaccine. See related discussion in section **I. F.**
   c. **Febrile illness, recent use of IG, and states of altered immunity** are discussed in section **I.F.**
7. **Side effects.** The currently available measles vaccine is a further attenuated preparation of the Enders-Edmonston virus. It causes fewer adverse reactions than the Edmonston B or other vaccine strains and has an excellent safety record. Side effects include **fever** (beginning approximately the sixth day after inoculation and lasting up to 5 days) in 5% to 15% of recipients, **transient rashes** in approximately 5% of recipients, and **encephalitis** occurring approximately once in every million doses administered. It is estimated that severe illness or death is more than 1,000 times more likely to occur in a person who acquires the disease naturally than in one who becomes ill as a result of vaccination. **There is no association of autism with the receipt of MMR vaccine [28].**
8. **Revaccination.** Two doses of vaccine are recommended for full immunity. No additional doses are recommended for persons already immune. There is, however, no evidence that revaccination of an immune individual carries an enhanced risk.
9. **IG is effective in preventing or modifying measles in a susceptible normal host exposed within the preceding 6 days.** The dose used is 0.25 ml/kg intramuscularly, with a maximum dose of 15 ml. **The common intramuscular IG preparation should never be administered intravenously.** IG may be particularly indicated for susceptible household contacts of measles patients, especially contacts younger than 1 year, or for susceptible pregnant women. If not contraindicated, live attenuated virus vaccine should be administered again after the child's first birthday. Whether IG is protective in patients with impaired immunity is unclear. A report from CDC details experience using IG in exposed patients with HIV infection [27].
10. **Nosocomial measles** can occur, and inadequately vaccinated medical personnel are sometimes the vectors [29].

B. **Mumps** is principally a disease of school-aged children, but approximately 15% of cases occur in adolescents or adults. It is usually self-limited without long-term sequelae, but deafness, which may be profound, is a rare complication. Although orchitis may occur in up to 20% of cases in postpubertal male patients, sterility is very rare. Naturally acquired mumps infection, including the estimated 30% of cases that occur subclinically, confers durable immunity [30]. There is no evidence that mumps during pregnancy causes congenital malformations. In recent years, there has been an increased occurrence of mumps in susceptible adolescents and young adults, with several outbreaks in high schools, colleges, and occupational settings. This is due to the relative underimmunization of children born between 1967 and 1977, when the mumps vaccine was not used routinely.

1. Mumps live virus vaccine, introduced in 1967, produces a subclinical noncommunicable infection with very few side effects. The live attenuated vaccine is prepared from chick embryo cell cultures and induces antibodies in more than 95% of recipients. Studies over the 35 years since the vaccine was introduced have shown that vaccine-stimulated immunity is long lasting, but its precise duration is unclear. Mumps vaccine is available in both a monovalent form (mumps only) and in combination (e.g., measles, mumps, and rubella). The MMR vaccine is the vaccine of choice for routine administration and should be used in all situations where there are no contraindications and recipients are also likely to be susceptible to measles or rubella [23]. There is no evidence that persons who have previously had mumps or received mumps vaccine are at any increased risk of local or systemic reactions to live mumps vaccine.
2. **Persons can be considered immune to mumps** if one of the following conditions is met:
   a. **Born before 1957.** Those born before 1957 are likely to have been infected naturally.
   b. **Documentation of physician-diagnosed mumps.**
   c. **Documented laboratory evidence of mumps immunity.** Reliable serologic studies (neutralization, complement fixation, ELISA, or radial hemolysis antibody tests) are not readily available. The mumps skin test does not predict immunity reliably. Routine susceptibility testing before vaccination is unnecessary. Persons who are immune from prior infection or immunization are not at an increased risk for reaction if they receive live mumps virus vaccine.
   d. **Documentation of adequate immunization** with live mumps virus vaccine when 12 months old or older.
3. **Vaccination is indicated for any susceptible person older than 12 months.** Susceptible children, adolescents, and adults should be vaccinated against mumps unless vaccination is contraindicated. Mumps vaccine is of particular value for children approaching puberty, especially adolescent and young adult men who have not had mumps and have not previously been immunized. It should be recognized, however, that the most serious consequence of mumps infection—deafness—may occur in either gender and at any age.
4. **Dosage.** Two doses of vaccine in the volume specified by the manufacturer should be administered subcutaneously. It should not be administered to infants younger than 12 months because persisting maternal antibodies may interfere with seroconversion.
5. **Side effects.** The mumps vaccine is very well tolerated. Rarely, parotitis and allergic reactions (transient rashes and pruritus) have been reported. Very infrequently, febrile seizures or encephalitis occurring within 30 days of immunization have been reported, but an etiologic relationship between these events and prior vaccination has not been established.
6. **Precautions and contraindications**
   a. **Pregnancy.** The precautions in pregnancy are the same as for measles (see section **III.A.6.a**).
   b. **Allergies.** The vaccine is produced in chick embryo culture (see discussion in section **I.F**). Because vaccines contain traces of **neomycin,** the vaccine should be avoided if the patient has a history of anaphylaxis to neomycin. A history of contact dermatitis to neomycin is not a contraindication to receiving mumps vaccine.

c. **Prior IG administration and immunodeficiency** (see section **I.F**). An exception to these general recommendations relates to children infected with HIV. All HIV-infected children who are not severely immunosuppressed (those in class 3) should receive MMR at 15 months of age (see section **III.A.4.h**). For other groups see section **4.h** above.

d. **Febrile illness** (see section **I.F.3**).

7. **International travel** (see Chapter 22).
8. **Mumps control** measures are reviewed elsewhere [30].
9. **Nosocomial mumps** can occur rarely and is, at least in part, preventable [30].

C. **Rubella** is a common childhood disease with nonspecific signs and symptoms, including postauricular and suboccipital adenopathy, low-grade fever, and a transient erythematous rash [31]. **Because of the nonspecific nature of this infection, a history of rubella illness is not a reliable indicator of immunity. Assessment of immune status is based on the presence of demonstrable antibody.**

1. **Background. The goal of rubella immunization is unique: the prevention of the congenital rubella syndrome** rather than prevention of rubella infections per se. The most important consequences of rubella are fetal anomalies resulting from rubella infection early in pregnancy, particularly early in the first trimester (see Chapter 3). School and infant vaccination programs have reduced the overall incidence of rubella in the United States more than 1,000-fold, but cases continue to occur among nonimmunized adolescents and young adults. **Outbreaks have been reported from schools, colleges, the military, office buildings, prisons, hospitals,** and other institutions in which large numbers of young adults live or work. Therefore, a combined approach to vaccinating both infants and susceptible adolescents and young adults has been recommended.
2. **Live rubella vaccine** is prepared in human diploid cell culture. Since 1979, the available vaccine has been based on the RA 27/3 virus strain. With a single dose, approximately 95% of recipients develop antibody that provides lifelong protection.
3. **Susceptibility status** is determined by serologic studies. Hemagglutination inhibition antibody usually is used to screen for rubella immunity. Other screening tests include passive hemagglutination, hemolysis in gel, and ELISA tests. **Any detectable titer,** whether from natural infection or immunization and no matter how low, **protects against subsequent viremic infection** (i.e., the type of infection that may affect the fetus). The ACIP suggests that revaccination of persons with low levels of rubella hemagglutination inhibition antibody is unnecessary. Rather, attention should be directed toward vaccinating the truly susceptible population.

   Routinely performing serologic tests in all women of childbearing age to determine susceptibility is expensive and has been ineffective in some areas. Therefore, the ACIP recommends that rubella vaccination should be given, without prior serologic testing, to all women who are not pregnant, who have been counseled to avoid pregnancy for the subsequent 3 months, and who have no history of vaccination [31].
4. **Indications for vaccination**
   a. **All children older than 12 months.** These individuals should be vaccinated to protect against rubella and to prevent spread of the virus to susceptible women.
   b. **Susceptible** prepubertal, adolescent, and adult **women of childbearing age.**
   c. **Susceptible hospital employees. Both male and female employees should be vaccinated because any infected employee may transmit rubella to pregnant patients.**
   d. **All susceptible military recruits, applicants to educational and training institutions, and prisoners.**
5. **Risks to the pregnant patient.** Because of the theoretic risk of this live virus vaccine to the fetus, women of childbearing age should receive this vaccine only

if they are not pregnant and are counseled to avoid pregnancy for 3 months after vaccination. However, all available data indicate that teratogenicity from live rubella vaccines has not occurred. The CDC has followed more than 200 known rubella-susceptible pregnant women who were vaccinated within 3 months before or 3 months after conception [32]. None of the babies had malformations consistent with congenital rubella infection. Therefore, the ACIP states that inadvertent rubella vaccination just before or in early pregnancy should not be a reason to recommend routine interruption of pregnancy. Vaccinating susceptible children whose mother or other household member is pregnant poses no risk to the pregnant woman.

6. **Side effects** include occasional rash and lymphadenopathy in children. Arthralgia of the small joints may occur in up to 40% of those vaccinated, but frank arthritis occurs in fewer than 1%. These symptoms are more common in adults and usually occur 7 to 21 days after immunization and persist for 1 to 3 days. The risk of these reactions is no greater if persons already immune are vaccinated.
7. **Contraindications**
   a. **Pregnancy** (see section **5**). As of April 1989, the CDC discontinued accepting new enrollees into the Vaccine in Pregnancy registry. However, any suspected case of congenital rubella syndrome, whether presumed to be due to wild-type or vaccine virus infection, should continue to be reported through state and local health departments.
   b. **Immunocompromised hosts.** Because live attenuated vaccine strains may cause disease in immunocompromised patients, such patients **should not receive this live virus vaccine** (see section **I.F.2**).
   c. **Severe allergy to neomycin.** This vaccine contains trace amounts of neomycin; persons who have experienced anaphylactic reactions to neomycin should not receive rubella vaccine.

D. **Poliomyelitis** has been nearly eliminated in the United States since the introduction of poliovirus vaccines in 1955 because of the widespread use of live attenuated OPV first developed by Sabin. However, with the licensure of an e-IPV, the ACIP now recommends the use of inactivated vaccine, either alone or followed by subsequent oral doses [33], as the principal primary immunization strategy. **The routine immunization of persons over the age of 18 years is not recommended, even if they have never been fully immunized.** When polio immunization is appropriate in the adult, e-IPV is recommended. In addition to a greater reliance on IPV, the number of doses necessary for primary immunization has also been modified (see section **2**).

1. **Indications for vaccination.** Routine primary immunization of adults (generally those 18 years old or older) in the United States is not necessary. Most adults are immune because of prior immunization or prior wild-type poliovirus infection. In addition, the cessation of circulation of wild-type virus in the 1960s and the small number of cases of poliomyelitis that currently occur in this country make the risk of exposure to wild-type virus very small. **Major emphasis on primary poliovirus vaccinations in the United States is aimed at children.** Certain adults at special risk are also candidates for primary or booster vaccination (see section **4**).
2. The IPV has been used extensively since 1955 and is given subcutaneously. The original inactivated vaccine has been superseded by a new enhanced-potency vaccine released in March 1988 [34,35]. Primary vaccination of children with three doses of the **e-IPV** resulted in immunity to all three poliovirus types in more than 99% of recipients, and early results of long-term follow-up studies suggest that the durability of immunity following e-IPV will be excellent [36].
   a. **Indications.** In the United States, e-IPV has been used routinely **to vaccinate immunodeficient patients and their household contacts and adults requiring primary immunization.** This vaccine can also be used as a booster dose in adults planning international travel to developing countries (see Chapter 22). In addition, **e-IPV is now the recommended vaccine for the routine primary immunization of healthy infants and children.**

b. **Risks and side effects.** No paralytic reactions to IPV have occurred with recent preparations. In 1955, a cluster of poliomyelitis cases occurred after use of an IPV preparation containing live poliovirus that had escaped inactivation.
c. **Allergic history.** This preparation contains trace amounts of streptomycin and neomycin; **individuals with a history of anaphylactic reactions to systemic or topical streptomycin or neomycin should not receive this vaccine.**
d. **Administration.** Primary vaccination consists of three doses given subcutaneously in the volume recommended by the manufacturer. The first two doses are given at a 4- to 8-week interval, and the third dose should follow the second in 6 to 12 months. Most commonly, the first dose is administered at 2 months of age, the second at 4 months, and the third at 12 to 18 months. All children who received all three primary doses of vaccine before 4 years of age should receive a fourth dose before or at school entry. A fourth dose is not necessary if the third dose is received after the fourth birthday.

3. **OPV.** Available since 1963, this **live attenuated (Sabin) vaccine,** containing all three poliovirus strains, provides long-lasting immunity in over 95% of recipients after a three-dose primary immunization sequence.
a. **Indications. For primary immunization of normal infants and young children,** e-IPV is now the preferred vaccine for routine immunization in the United States. Full immunization may be accomplished with e-IPV or, as an interim strategy, with two doses of e-IPV followed by two doses of OPV. Although it carries the highest risk for vaccine-associated cases of paralytic polio, immunization can also be accomplished solely with OPV. Because OPV interferes with the subsequent infection of the pharynx and gastrointestinal tract by wild-type virus, it may be the vaccine of choice for vaccination campaigns undertaken to control an ongoing polio epidemic.
b. **Risks and contraindications of live attenuated poliovirus vaccines.** OPV has rarely been associated with the development of paralytic poliomyelitis in a vaccine recipient or close contact (1 in approximately 3.2 million doses distributed). This risk is increased in immunocompromised individuals (e.g., those with a primary immunodeficiency [see section **I.F**] or who are receiving immunosuppressive agents) and in adults.
(1) **Only e-IPV should be used in immunocompromised hosts or for household contacts of such patients.** If OPV is inadvertently administered to a household contact of an immunodeficient individual, close contact between the two should be avoided for approximately 1 month after vaccination. The family member and the immunosuppressed individual in particular must be carefully counseled to avoid exposure to fecal–oral contamination, essentially by practicing good personal hygiene (i.e., enteric precautions).
(2) **Healthy adults requiring primary vaccination may also be at increased risk of vaccine-associated paralysis after OPV. Thus, for primary immunization at all ages and for all health statuses, the inactivated form of the poliovirus vaccine (e-IPV) should be used.**
(3) **Pregnancy.** Because there is a theoretic risk to the fetus, vaccination of pregnant women should be avoided. In special circumstances, however, if the risk of exposure to natural infection is substantial and immediate protection is needed (e.g., for the young pregnant woman traveling to a country with endemic poliomyelitis), the risk of poliovirus exposure outweighs the theoretic risk of the vaccine. Either OPV or IPV may be used, although IPV might be preferred on theoretical grounds.
(4) Although the risk of vaccine-associated paralysis is extremely rare with OPV (an estimated one case in 5.5 million doses of vaccine in healthy adults), recipients should be informed of this risk.

4. **Vaccination of adults.** Routine vaccination of those older than 18 years of age is not indicated (see section **1**).
   a. **These adults are at special risk and warrant vaccination:**
      (1) **Travelers** to areas of countries where poliomyelitis is endemic or epidemic (see Chapter 22);
      (2) **Laboratory workers** handling specimens that may contain poliovirus;
      (3) **Medical workers** in close contact with patients who may be excreting poliovirus, including those who administer live virus vaccine;
      (4) **Members of communities or specific population groups** with a high prevalence of natural disease, such as Amish and Hutterite communities.
   b. **Regimens.** A full series of IPV is generally recommended for adults without prior primary vaccination. For details of vaccination schedules, see section **2.d.** For adults who have completed primary immunization with OPV, a booster OPV dose (or e-IPV) may be given. If adults have completed the primary series with IPV, either e-IPV or OPV may be used for the booster dose. In general, e-IPV is preferred for all uses in adults.

E. **Varicella.** Live attenuated varicella vaccine (Varivax, Merck, West Point, PA) has been used routinely in the United States since 1995, but experience in this country predates that in studies of children who are immunocompromised [36] and in healthy children [37] and adults [38]. The vaccine has been generally well tolerated in all groups, although mild chickenpox developed in 7% of healthy children and up to one-third of children who had received chemotherapy [39]. In the latter group, children with rash may transmit the virus. In immunocompromised children, a significant number of vaccinees subsequently developed natural infection, although no severe cases were reported. The risk of varicella-zoster infection after vaccine appears to be comparable with that reported by Lawrence et al. [40] or lower than that after natural infection.

In addition to its routine use in infants 12 months of age or older who have not had varicella [41], the vaccine has also been recommended for use in susceptible adolescents and young adults [42] to prevent the serious complications of adult varicella [43] and varicella during pregnancy [44]. Adult immunization may also be useful in controlling disease in hospitals [45].

Before introduction of the vaccine, nearly 100% of persons brought up in the continental United States were varicella immune. Although serious or life-threatening complications occurred at a very low rate, given the large numbers of infected individuals the incidence of serious varicella infections was striking. It is estimated that varicella accounted for about 9,300 hospital admissions annually, and in 1973 through 1979 there were 106 deaths due to varicella [46]. Complications are generally more severe in people 15 years of age or older; pregnant women are particularly susceptible to severe complications themselves and to the occurrence of the congenital varicella syndrome in their fetuses. Two other syndromes have been particularly associated with clinical varicella in childhood: **Reye syndrome** and **severe invasive group A streptococcal disease.**

1. **Recommendations for vaccine use** have been reviewed in detail elsewhere [47].
   a. **Ages 12 to 18 months.** One subcutaneous dose is recommended for universal immunization for all healthy children who lack a reliable history of varicella.
   b. **Ages 18 months to 13 years.** One dose is recommended for children who have not been immunized previously and who lack a reliable history of varicella infection.
   c. **Healthy adolescents and young adults.** Healthy adolescents older than 13 years who have not been immunized previously and have no history of varicella infection should be immunized by administration of two doses of vaccine 4 to 8 weeks apart. **A two-dose regimen is necessary for adults because of their diminished responsiveness to the vaccine** [38]. One recent report suggests that higher serum titers of antibody are

achieved when the second dose is given at an 8-week rather than a 4-week interval.

**d. Adults.** In healthy individuals older than 18 years who have no history of varicella, **performing serologic tests** before vaccination **is optional** but can be cost effective in that 71% to 93% of adults born in the continental United States who have no history of varicella nevertheless are immune to infection. Persons who grew up in tropical regions, such as the Caribbean, and who have no history of clinical disease appear less likely to be varicella immune. **For adults with negative serology** for varicella, vaccine should be considered in the following:

**(1)** Health-care workers.

**(2)** Susceptible family and/or close contacts of immunocompromised hosts.

**(3)** Those adults whose occupations place them at risk for exposure (e.g., teachers and day-care workers).

**(4)** Persons living in conditions where spread of varicella infection is likely. including college students, military personnel, and inmates of correctional facilities.

**(5)** Nonpregnant women of childbearing age who anticipate future pregnancies.

**(6)** Persons planning routine international travel (e.g., non–health-care providers), particularly if they anticipate close personal contact with local populations.

**(7)** The use of varicella vaccine has been proposed in older Americans to improve their levels of specific cell-mediated immunity and in this way to control their increased risk for zoster attacks. No recommendations currently exist for using the vaccine in this way, but a recent review by Raeder and Hayney [48] examined this issue and relevant studies.

**(8)** Other persons may also consider immunization following discussion with their personal physicians.

**e.** Use of the varicella vaccine for **postexposure prophylaxis** is not currently recommended because no data using the currently licensed vaccine in this situation are available. However, in two controlled studies using an earlier vaccine formulation, protective efficacy of more than 90% was demonstrated when immunization was accomplished within 72 hours of exposure.

**2. Contraindications and cautions** [47]

**a.** Varicella vaccine **should not be given to immunodeficient patients** or to patients who have received **high doses of systemic corticosteroids** (>2 mg/kg/day of prednisone or equivalent) for at least the 2 preceding weeks. Testing for antibody should be done at 6 weeks postvaccination; children who have not seroconverted should be reimmunized. Children receiving higher doses of steroids can be vaccinated if they have not received steroids for 3 months, as is recommended for all live virus vaccines, but 1 month is probably sufficient. Some experts recommend withholding steroids for 2 to 3 weeks after immunization. The vaccine is probably safe for children using only inhaled steroids (see section **e**).

Vaccine is not generally recommended for persons with HIV infection, but a draft of more recent CDC recommendations for persons with HIV infections does recommend varicella vaccine for asymptomatic nonimmunosuppressed children (**category 1**) [47].

**b.** Varicella should not be administered to **pregnant women** because the possible effects on fetal development are unknown. When postpubertal females are immunized, pregnancy should be avoided for 1 month after immunization.

**c.** Varicella vaccine should not be administered to individuals who have had an **anaphylactic reaction to neomycin** because trace amounts of neomycin are in the vaccine. A contact dermatitis history to neomycin is not a contraindication.

**d.** The vaccine manufacturer recommends that **salicylates are not administered for 6 weeks** after the varicella vaccine has been given because of the association between Reye syndrome, natural varicella, and salicylates.

**e.** Under special circumstances, vaccine may be appropriate under a special protocol in patients with acute lymphocytic leukemia in remission at least 1 year (see reference 47 for details).

**f. Households with potential immunocompromised contacts.** ACIP advises that there is no need to withhold varicella vaccine from persons living in the same household with immunocompromised individuals. Transmission of vaccine type varicella-zoster virus from healthy individuals has been infrequently (if at all) documented. Thus, even in families with immunocompromised individuals, including those with HIV infection, no special precautions are recommended after vaccination of healthy children (and presumably adults) who do not develop a rash. Vaccinees who develop a rash (up to 7%–8% of recipients) should avoid contact with immunocompromised susceptible hosts for the duration of the rash. If contact inadvertently occurs, the use of varicella-zoster immunoglobulin is not currently recommended. Transmission is rare, and if disease develops, it is mild and presumably treatable with acyclovir.

**3.** Doses are given subcutaneously. The **cost** of the varicella vaccine to physicians is $39 per dose; the cost of serum antibody testing to varicella is about $70 but will vary depending on the laboratory used.

**F. Rabies.** See Chapter 4 under Bite Wounds and Rabies Prevention, and Chapter 22, section IV under Vaccinations.

**G. Yellow fever** (see Chapter 22)

**IV. Inactivated virus vaccines**

**A. Hepatitis B**

**1. Hepatitis B vaccine** [49]. All hepatitis B virus (HBV) vaccines currently available in the United States are recombinant DNA derived. Heptavax, a human plasma-derived vaccine, is no longer produced in the United States.

**a. Vaccines** currently available are as follows:

**(1)** Recombivax HB (Merck) is produced by common baker's yeast into which a plasmid containing the gene for HBsAg has been inserted. Heptavax B and Recombivax are equally effective, and approximately 90% of healthy adults will develop protective antibody.

**(2)** Engerix-B (SmithKline Beecham) is a recombinant DNA derived vaccine. Studies show it is as effective as the Recombivax HB vaccine.

**(3)** Twinrix is a combination hepatitis A and B vaccine [50]. Seroresponses are excellent after at least two doses; after a single dose, protection against hepatitis B may be limited. The vaccine is approved for use in children.

**b. Dosages of vaccines.** Hepatitis B vaccines are packaged to contain 10 to 40 $\mu$g HBsAg protein/ml. The currently recommended dosage schedules are shown in Table 23.5. Primary vaccination consists of three intramuscular doses, with the second and third doses given at 1 and 6 months after the first, respectively. For more rapid protection, an accelerated regimen has been effective [51] for certain high-risk groups (e.g., those with needlestick exposures, certain travelers, infants born of infected mothers) with standard doses of Engerix-B given at 0, 1, 2, and 12 months. Other accelerated regimens have undergone preliminary investigation and may be useful in some international travelers [52]. If routine dose schedules are interrupted, alternative dose regimens are available [49].

**c. Antibody response.** Antibody response is higher when the HBV vaccine is given in the arm (deltoid muscle) than in the buttock (gluteal muscle). Therefore, the arm should be used as the site of injection in adults (unless it may jeopardize shunt access in the hemodialysis patient). For infants born to mothers who are HBV carriers, the preferred site for vaccination remains the anterolateral thigh.

Table 23.5. Recommended Doses and Schedules of Currently Licensed Hepatitis B Vaccines

| Group | Recombivax HB[a] Dose | | Engerix-B[a,b] Dose | |
|---|---|---|---|---|
| | μg | mL | μg | mL |
| Infants of HBV-carrier mothers | 5 | 0.5 | 10 | 0.5 |
| Other infants and children <11 yr | 2.5 | 0.25 | 10 | 0.5 |
| Children and adolescents 11–19 yr | 5 | 0.5 | 20 | 1.0 |
| Adults >19 yr | 10 | 1.0 | 20 | 1.0 |
| Dialysis patients and other immunocompromised persons | 40 | 1.0[c] | 40 | 2.0[d,e] |

[a] Usual schedule: three doses at 0, 1, and 6 months.
[b] Alternative schedule: four doses at 0, 1, 2, and 12 months.
[c] Special formulation for dialysis patients.
[d] Two 1.0 mL doses given at different sites.
[e] Four-dose schedule recommended at 0, 1, 2, and 6 months.
Centers for Disease Control. Hepatitis B virus. Recommendations of the Immunization Practices Advisory Committee. *MMWR Morb Mortal Wkly Rep* 1991;40(RR-13):5.

2. **Preexposure HBV immunization** is now recommended for routine use in all newborn infants in the United States [53]. The total hospital cost of the three adult doses of vaccine in the United States is approximately $55 to $65. Currently, 90.3% of children from 19 to 36 months of age have received a full series of three injections [4]. Preexposure HBV vaccine **also is recommended for** the following groups:
   a. **Persons with occupational risk.** Hepatitis B is a major infectious risk for health-care workers and public-safety workers. Any workers who may be exposed to percutaneous or permucosal contacts with blood or blood products should be immunized. Other workers may also need immunization, based on their occupational responsibilities. Because health-care workers may be exposed to significant risks while still in training, immunization is recommended while workers are still students.
   b. **Clients and staff of institutions for the developmentally disabled.** The risks for hepatitis B transmission include not only blood exposures but also bites and contact with skin lesions or other infective secretions. **Susceptible clients and staff** who work directly with clients who are hepatitis B carriers in residential settings should be immunized. **Clients discharged to community programs** should be tested for HBsAg to allow for planning to prevent transmission to others. **Staff of nonresidential day-care facilities** working with persons who are hepatitis B carriers have a risk of infection comparable with that of health-care workers and therefore should also be immunized. **Clients in such programs** have a lower risk of infection, but immunization may be considered for them as well. Immunization of **classroom contacts of HBV carriers** is strongly encouraged if the carrier displays aggressive behavior or has other medical problems that increase risk of exposure to blood or serous secretions.
   c. **Hemodialysis patients.** Hepatitis B vaccination is recommended for all susceptible hemodialysis patients, even though seroconversion rates are lower than for healthy persons. Immunization early in the course of renal disease may be more effective than waiting until renal function has deteriorated to require dialysis.
   d. **Sexually active homosexual men.** Sexually active homosexual men should be immunized regardless of age or duration of homosexual activity. Persons who are HIV positive should be tested for an anti-HBs response and counseled accordingly.

e. **Users of nonmedical injectable drugs.** All susceptible persons who engage in drug injection should be immunized as early in their use of drugs as possible.
f. **Recipients of certain blood products.** Persons with clotting disorders who require transfusion of clotting factor concentrates should be immunized at the time their disorder is first identified. Those who have already received multiple transfusions of these products should be screened for antibody before immunization.
g. **Household and sexual contacts of HBV carriers.** Household contacts are at high risk; sexual contacts are at the greatest risk for infection. When HBV carriers are identified through routine screening programs, they should be notified of their status. All household and sexual contacts should be tested and susceptibles should be immunized.
h. **Adoptees from countries where HBV is highly endemic.** Orphans or unaccompanied minors from countries of high or intermediate endemicity for HBV should be screened for HBsAg. Those who are seronegative should be immunized, and those who are seropositive should be presumed carriers; members of their adopting households should be immunized.
i. **Populations in which HBV is highly endemic.** Certain U.S. populations, including Alaskan Natives and Pacific Islanders, are highly likely to be or to have been infected during childhood. They should have universal HBV immunization in childhood. "Catch up" immunization schedules should be considered if resources permit.
j. **Refugees and immigrants** from areas of high HBV endemicity, particularly Africa, East Asia, and the Pacific Islands, should be screened for HBsAg at the time of resettlement in the United States. Even if no HBV carriers are identified, consideration should be given to immunization of susceptibles below age 7 because of the high rates of interfamilial spread of HBV infection in this group. All infants born to women who are from areas of high endemicity should be immunized as part of the program of universal newborn HBV immunization.
k. **Inmates of long-term correctional institutions.** Prison environments may be favorable settings for HBV transmission because of injection drug use or male homosexual behavior. In addition, this setting represents an opportunity to immunize injection drug users. The ACIP recommends that prison officials consider screening and immunization programs for inmates with histories of high-risk behavior.
l. **Sexually active heterosexuals.** Risk for HBV increases with the number of sexual partners. Persons recently diagnosed with a sexually transmitted disease other than HBV, sex workers, and persons who have a history of sexual activity with multiple partners in the preceding 6 months should be immunized.
m. **Other contacts of HBV carriers.** Persons in casual contact with known or possible HBV carriers in settings such as schools or offices are at minimal risk of infection and do not require immunization on these grounds alone. Transmission of HBV in child-care centers has been documented only rarely. Unless special behavioral (aggressive behavior) or medical (such as dermatologic conditions) are present, contacts of carriers do not require immunization.
n. **International travelers.** Recommendations for HBV prophylaxis for international travelers can be found in Chapter 22.

3. **Responses to hepatitis B vaccine**
   a. **Booster doses** of vaccine are not routinely recommended nor is routine serologic testing to assess antibody levels. However, previously vaccinated persons who experience percutaneous or needle exposure to HBsAg-positive blood should be tested for antibody level. If the antibody level is lower than 10 mIU/ml, two booster doses at 1-month intervals may be useful. Hemodialysis patients should be tested semiannually and may require booster doses. At least one expert group has recommended that all immunocompromised

patients should be regularly tested for anti-HBs antibodies and that they be revaccinated when the titer falls below 10 mIU/ml [54].

**b. Nonresponders.** Why some adults do not respond to the conventional hepatitis B immunization series is only partially understood. Older age, smoking, and obesity seem to be related to decreased responsiveness to hepatitis B vaccine. Determination of whether real differences exist between antibody response to the two currently available vaccines awaits further prospective studies. The optimal approach to the nonresponder is unclear [55]. Giving two booster doses at 1-month intervals appears to result in an adequate response in only a minority of recipients (see section **b**). Other innovative protocols have been suggested for nonresponders [56].

**4. Postexposure prophylaxis** of HBV infection should be exercised in the following situations: accidental percutaneous or permucosal exposure to HBsAg-positive blood, sexual exposure to an HBsAg-positive person, or perinatal exposure of an infant born to an HBsAg-positive mother (see Chapter 3 for details). Recent recommendations include the use of both HBIG (single dose) and the HBV vaccine in persons known or suspected to be negative for anti-HBs. This affords an immediate passive immunity combined with long-lasting active immunization. The cost of combined therapy is lower compared with that of previous recommendations, which called for two HBIG immunizations at a total hospital cost of approximately $300 to $350 for an average-sized adult. In addition, HBIG alone is only approximately 75% effective.

For details of postexposure prophylaxis, see Table 23.6 and the ACIP recommendations. If HBIG is not immediately available, IG should be used. The latter contains low-level anti-HBs and, although not as efficacious as HBIG, is probably better than no therapy.

**5. Prevaccination serologic screening** for susceptibility. Carriers of HBV and persons having antibody from previous infection do not need to be vaccinated. Serologic screening to detect such individuals before vaccination may or may not be cost effective in a given setting. An approach to the variables involved in screening are discussed elsewhere [57]. The vaccine is well tolerated in carriers or those with protective antibody so that these patients are not at excess risk of side effects if they receive the vaccine in the absence of screening.

**B.** IPV is discussed in section **III.D.**

**C.** Influenza (see Chapter 10)

**D.** Rabies. See Chapter 4 under Bite Wounds and Rabies Prevention and Chapter 22, section **IV** under Vaccinations.

**V. Bacterial vaccines.** Certain of these vaccines are discussed elsewhere. Only recent developments in vaccines and vaccine regimens are discussed here.

**A. Pneumococcal vaccine** (see Chapter 11). In case-control studies the pneumococcal vaccine has shown efficacies from 56% to 81%. CDC surveillance studies have reinforced this conclusion, with a 57% overall protective efficacy against invasive disease due to serotypes included in the vaccine in persons aged 6 years and over. Specialized studies of high-risk populations, including diabetics and persons with coronary vascular disease, congestive heart failure, chronic pulmonary disease, or anatomic asplenia, have shown similar efficacy [58]. Efficacy of 75% has been shown for persons 65 years or older. Despite these data and the evidence of risk provided by outbreaks of nosocomial pneumococcal disease among unimmunized residents of nursing homes [59], the principal limit on the effectiveness of the polyvalent pneumococcal polysaccharide vaccine currently available in the United States continues to be the limited use of the vaccine in high-risk individuals, with only 10% of older Americans having been immunized.

Recently, a protein conjugated pneumococcal polysaccharide vaccine has been approved for use in children under age 2 [60]. Such a vaccine might also be useful for groups of adults who have a poorer than optimal response to the unconjugated vaccine, for example, persons with sickle cell anemia or those receiving immunosuppressive chemotherapy. Because the conjugate vaccine includes only eight serotypes, use of the 23-valent pneumococcal polysaccharide vaccine is preferable in those older children and adults in whom it can be used.

Table 23.6. Recommendations for Postexposure Prophylaxis for Hepatitis B Virus

| | HBIG | | Vaccine | |
|---|---|---|---|---|
| Agent Exposure | Dose | Recommended Timing | Dose | Recommended Timing |
| Perinatal[a] | 0.5 mL i.m. | Within 12 h of birth | 0.5 mL i.m.[b] | Within 12 h of birth |
| Percutaneous | 0.06 mL/kg i.m. | Single dose within 12 h *or*[c] | 1.0 mL i.m.[b] | Start vaccination series as soon as possible after exposure[b] |
| | 0.06 mL/kg i.m. | Within 24 h; repeat at 1 mo | | |
| Sexual | 0.06 mL/kg i.m. | Single dose within 14 days of sexual contact | Vaccine is recommended for sexually active homosexual men and for regular sexual contacts of chronic hepatitis virus carriers | |
| Household contact | | | | |
| Chronic carrier | — | — | — | Start vaccination series as soon as possible[b] |
| Acute case | None, unless known exposure | | None unless known exposure | |
| Known exposure | 0.06 mL/kg i.m. | Single dose within 14 days of exposure | Vaccine is recommended if household case becomes chronic carrier | |
| In primary caregiver—infant <12 mo | 0.5 mL i.m. | As soon as possible | 0.5 mL[b] | Start vaccination series as soon as possible[b] |

[a]For further discussion, see Chapter 3.

[b]For vaccine doses and time intervals, see Table 23.5. The first dose can be given the same time as the HBIG dose but at a separate site.

[c]For those who choose not to receive hepatitis B vaccine.

HBIG, hepatitis B immunoglobulin.

Adapted from Centers for Disease Control. Hepatitis B virus. Recommendations of the Immunization Practices Advisory Committee. *MMWR Morb Mortal Wkly Rep* 1991; 40(RR-13):6.

**B. Meningococcal vaccine** (see Chapter 6 under Prophylaxis of Meningitis and Chapter 22). This polysaccharide vaccine [61] is protective against serogroups A, C, W135, and Y after a single dose. The need for booster doses is unknown. It does not protect against serogroup B infections. Travelers to areas with epidemic or endemic meningococcal disease should be vaccinated (see Chapter 22). Adolescents in group living conditions, including college residents, armed forces recruits, and inmates of institutions for the developmentally disabled and correctional institutions, should be considered for meningococcal immunization. Like *Haemophilus influenzae* polysaccharide vaccine, children less than 2 years of age respond poorly to the meningococcal vaccine. Protein conjugate vaccines are under development.

**C. Typhoid** (see Chapter 22)

**D. Plague** (see section **VII.D** and Chapter 22)

**E. Diphtheria, tetanus, and pertussis.** Universal childhood immunization has reduced the prevalence of tetanus and diphtheria to extremely low levels. Pertussis persists, although at a much reduced level, because of adult carriage with transmission to infants not yet fully immunized. In this section, we discuss only those aspects of these diseases relevant to the care of adult patients. The recommendations for DTP immunization in the United States have been comprehensively reviewed [62,63].

1. Diphtheria remains a potentially serious, although rare, disease in the United States, with fatalities in approximately 5% to 10% of respiratory cases. Most cases, in both adults and children, occur in nonimmunized or inadequately immunized individuals. However, waning immunity many years after primary vaccination may also contribute to some adult outbreaks [64]. Although adequate immunization is believed to protect for at least 10 years, recent serosurveys in the United States suggest that many adults may not have protective levels of antibodies [5]. Cutaneous diphtheria has occurred principally among certain groups of Native Americans and indigent adults. Localized epidemics have been reported in the latter group.

2. **Tetanus** incidence in the United States has declined dramatically with the routine use of tetanus toxoid in childhood. Though vaccine-induced immunity may not be lifelong, it is extremely durable. Currently, the fewer than 100 annual cases of tetanus that do occur in this country involve elderly people who never received primary immunization [65]. Tetanus control, therefore, depends most on universal primary vaccination; however, waning immunity is thought to explain the very low seroprevalence seen in persons over 65. Thus, the control strategy also includes reimmunizations every 10 years and appropriate use of toxoid and human hyperimmune anti-tetanus globulin in accident and emergency rooms. A significant number of emergency room patients are overtreated or, worse, undertreated for tetanus-prone injuries [66]. See related discussion in Chapter 4 under Tetanus.

3. **Pertussis** is caused by toxigenic strains of the gram-positive rod *Bordetella pertussis.* Its precise incidence is unclear. The disease is highly communicable, with attack rates of more than 90% reported in susceptible household contacts. Most reported illness occurs in children younger than 1 year, with classic lower respiratory symptoms. In adults, who actually represent most symptomatic cases in this country [67], the disease may manifest merely as a modest upper respiratory or catarrhal illness, but such persons can serve as unrecognized reservoirs and disseminators of infection [67,68]. This circumstance may increase the difficulty of providing effective secondary prophylaxis for susceptible contacts.

4. **Vaccines**

   a. **Diphtheria toxoid** is prepared by formaldehyde treatment of purified diphtheria toxin. The concentration of diphtheria toxoid in preparations for adult use (designated d) is lower than that in pediatric formulations (designated D) to reduce the incidence of adverse reactions, which are considered to be related to both dose and age.

   b. **Tetanus toxoid** is likewise prepared by formaldehyde inactivation of purified tetanus toxin. It is available in fluid and aluminum salt-adsorbed forms.

The adsorbed toxoid induces more persistent antitoxin titers and is strongly recommended for routine use.

c. **Pertussis vaccine** has been comprehensively reviewed [62], as have the newer acellular vaccines [69,70]. Until recently, all pertussis vaccine used in the United States was a suspension of inactivated *B. pertussis* bacteria. The use of whole killed organisms in this vaccine probably accounted for its higher rate of adverse side effects. Three combination vaccines, containing an acellular pertussis vaccine (DTaP), are now approved for use in the United States for routine primary immunization in children under 6 years of age [69]. Although the acellular vaccine may appear especially attractive for immunization or boosting of adults [70,71], at the time of this report there is no official recommendation for its use in adults. The combined DTaP would have to be reformulated with a lower dose of diphtheria toxoid for use in adults.

5. **Preparations and dosages.** Simultaneous immunization against diphtheria, pertussis, and tetanus during infancy and childhood has been routine in the United States since the late 1940's.
   a. For infants and children younger than 7 years, diphtheria toxoid, tetanus toxoid, and the acellular pertussis vaccine adsorbed (DTaP) and diphtheria and tetanus toxoids adsorbed (DT) are most commonly used. Dose schedules are reviewed elsewhere [69].
   b. For persons 7 years old or older, tetanus and diphtheria toxoids adsorbed (Td) is recommended. This product contains a smaller amount of diphtheria antigen (as indicated by the lowercase "d") for use in older children and adults. Tetanus toxoid should be given with adult-dose diphtheria toxoid every 10 years as part of routine primary medical care. If a dose is given sooner as part of wound management, the next booster is not needed for 10 years thereafter. The use of tetanus toxoid in wound management is discussed in Chapter 4. Some travelers may benefit from a booster at 5-year intervals because a tetanus-prone wound does not require tetanus IG or a booster if a person has been boosted within 5 years (see Chapter 22).
   c. Single-antigen products are available (i.e., acellular pertussis vaccine adsorbed [aP], tetanus toxoid adsorbed [T], and diphtheria toxoid adsorbed [D]) when combined preparations are not appropriate. For example, pertussis vaccine has been used in hospital personnel to help control a pertussis outbreak [68].
6. **Side effects and adverse reactions**
   a. DTP administration is commonly associated with **local reactions** such as erythema, induration, and tenderness. These usually are self-limited and require no therapy. Fever beginning several hours after administration is also common and may persist for up to 2 days. Mild somnolence, vomiting, irritability, or malaise can occur, especially with pertussis containing vaccines. Rarely, severe **systemic reactions** such as generalized urticaria, anaphylaxis, or neurologic complications may occur after administration of DTP or, to a lesser extent, after DTaP (see section **c**).
   b. **Arthus-type hypersensitivity** reactions, characterized by severe local reactions 2 to 8 hours after an injection, may be seen in persons receiving a number of booster injections at too-frequent intervals, as may happen with tetanus.
   c. **Pertussis.** Severe reactions occasionally occur after pertussis vaccine injection in infants [19]. However, large studies indicated no evidence of a causal relationship between pertussis vaccine and permanent neurologic illness [72]. The incidence of major adverse reactions is low (below 1 in 1,000 for any symptom and 100–1,000 times less frequent for the most serious reactions). In many cases, the occurrence of major reactions may be merely coincidental with the recent immunization rather than attributable to it. Sudden infant death syndrome is not more likely to occur after a DTP immunization [73,74]. The incidence of all adverse reactions seems decreased when acellular pertussis vaccine is used.

**d.** Use of multiple reduced-dose regimens. Some physicians have suggested using reduced doses of pertussis or other vaccines in a multidose regimen to reduce the risk of an adverse reaction. There is no rationale for doing this, because vaccine reactions do not appear to be dose related. In addition, the efficacy of such idiosyncratic dosing schedules is unknown, and children receiving such vaccines would be considered nonimmune for the purpose of school entrance requirements.

**7. Precautions and contraindications**

**a.** If any of the severe reactions that may be seen with DTaP has occurred, the immunizations should be completed with DT. If a serious anaphylactic reaction has occurred, further doses of DTaP should be deferred until it is clear whether the reaction was due to the tetanus toxoid component. If it was, desensitization by an allergist may be appropriate to allow completion of the immunization series with tetanus toxoid alone. Although the presence of an evolving neurologic disorder contraindicates the use of pertussis vaccine until neurologic status stabilizes, a personal or family history of seizures is not an indication to withhold pertussis vaccine. A CDC statement on contraindications to the use of pertussis vaccine has been distributed [71].

**b.** The main contraindication to the use of tetanus or diphtheria toxoids is a history of neurologic or systemic hypersensitivity reaction after a previous dose. Local side effects alone do not preclude further use. When an Arthus-like local reaction occurs after frequent tetanus toxoid doses (e.g., with frequent immunizations such as every 2 or 3 years), further routine or emergency booster doses of Td should not be given more frequently than every 10 years.

**c.** Immunosuppressive therapies may reduce the efficacy of these vaccines. When possible, routine vaccination should be deferred while patients are receiving such therapy or for 3 months thereafter (see also section **VI.F**).

**F. *H. influenzae* b** polysaccharide conjugate vaccine [75]. Four conjugate vaccines have been licensed for use in the United States: a PRP-diphtheria toxoid conjugate (**PRP-D**), a meningococcal protein conjugate (**PRP-OMP**), a mutant diphtheria protein conjugate (**HbOC**), and a tetanus toxoid conjugate (**PRP-T**). Combination vaccines composed of Hib conjugate vaccine and DtaP (TriHIBit) or OTP (Tetramane) have also been developed. Hepatitis B (Recombivax, 5 $\mu$g) and Hib (PRP-OMP) have also been combined (Comvax, Merck), and this vaccine is licensed for use at 2, 4, and 12 to 15 months.

Excellent antibody responses in infants less than 2 years old have been achieved with multidose regimens of all the conjugate vaccines except PRP-D, which is used only at 15 months of age or older. Routine immunization of all children beginning at 2 months of age is recommended. (See Table 23.2 for recommended childhood immunization schedule.) Older children with increased rates of serious Hib disease (e.g., asplenic patients, sickle cell patients, or immunosuppressed individuals) should also be considered for immunization. Rates of both meningitic and nonmeningitic childhood Hib disease have decreased by 90% since the approval of the conjugate vaccine for routine immunization of infants [76]. (See Chapter 6 for further discussion on Hib vaccine for the prevention of meningitis.)

Hib vaccines do not affect infection rates with nonencapsulated (nontypeable) strains. These organisms commonly colonize the respiratory tract and cause pneumonia in persons with chronic pulmonary disease or older Americans but rarely cause bacteremic disease. Encapsulated *H. influenzae* infections are rare in adults, and as such there appears to be little indication for the use of Hib as an adult vaccine.

**VI. Immunization considerations for special risk groups.** Specific immunization recommendations have been formulated for certain groups with recognized special risks.

**A. Older Americans.** Immunization recommendations for the elderly are well addressed elsewhere [77,78]. Recommendations for pneumococcal and influenza vaccine are discussed above (see section **V.A** and Chapter 10, respectively). Only approximately 22% of the elderly receive influenza vaccine each year, and only 10%

have received pneumococcal vaccine [79]. A survey of the attitudes and practices of the elderly concerning pneumococcal and influenza vaccines emphasizes that the most important factor in determining immunization status of the elderly is the recommendation of the individual's physician.

**B. Pregnant women.** Immunization of the pregnant woman has been reviewed [80]. In general, immunization during pregnancy should be avoided. Although there is little evidence that currently available live virus vaccines can harm the developing fetus, the theoretic risk exists, making it prudent to avoid such exposures. Inactivated vaccines do not carry this same risk, but it has been suggested that maternal fever may be a risk factor for certain congenital abnormalities, so these vaccines should also be avoided. When necessary, it is possible to administer OPV to pregnant women (see section **III.D.3.b**). Influenza vaccination during pregnancy is discussed in Chapter 10.

**C. College students.** These young adults are at special risk for epidemic illness spread by the respiratory route; outbreaks of measles, rubella, and influenza have repeatedly been reported on college campuses [81]. Since May 1983, the American College Health Association has encouraged institutions to adopt a recommended preadmission immunization policy [82], but serious gaps in immunization among college students persist. Special recommendations for measles and hepatitis B vaccine have also been published for this population.

**D. Prison populations.** As noted above (see section **IV.A.2.k**), HBV infection is a significant risk for persons in long-term incarceration, and HBV vaccine may play an important role in reducing the risks of transmission. Rubella outbreaks in prisons in several different parts of the country [83] have emphasized the need for immunization programs for young adults in prison [84]. Such outbreaks also represent occupational risks for prison staff.

**E. Homeless persons.** The fragmentary, episodic, and disorganized medical care that many of the homeless receive leaves a large group of individuals susceptible to a variety of vaccine-preventable diseases for which new immunization strategies may be required [85]. Homeless adults have been the targets of a diphtheria epidemic [86] and a cluster outbreak of pneumococcal pneumonia [87]. Homeless adolescents may be at high risk for HBV infection [88].

**F. Immunosuppressed individuals.** Immunization of the immunocompromised individual has been reviewed [89–91]. Immunization in this population is problematic for two reasons. Live virus vaccines generally are contraindicated because of their potential for causing disease, whereas many inactivated or component vaccines may not be as effective in this population. However, certain exceptions to these general rules should be noted. Because of reports of severe and even fatal measles occurring in children who were HIV infected, it has been recommended that both symptomatic and asymptomatic HIV-infected children be immunized with the measles vaccine [27]. Children who are HIV infected and who have a measles exposure, regardless of their immunization status, should also receive IG prophylaxis. Pneumococcal vaccination appears to be cost effective in adults with HIV, although routine influenza immunization may be more problematic [92].

The use of bacterial polysaccharide vaccines has been an important issue in Hodgkin disease patients who have previously undergone staging splenectomy. In these individuals, the risk of pneumococcal or *Haemophilus* sepsis is appreciably elevated. Studies of the responses of such individuals show that, although vaccine immunogenicity and durability of the antibody response may be poorer in such persons, protective levels can be achieved in some [93]. Immunization efficacy is not influenced by the scheduling of splenectomy, but better responses are achieved when chemotherapy can be delayed 3 weeks after vaccine administration [93].

**G. Additional special vaccinee categories.** Special studies and recommendations have been made for alcoholics [94], persons with rheumatologic disease [95], persons receiving hemodialysis [96], postsplenectomy patients [97], patients who have undergone bone marrow transplantation [98], and persons infected with HIV [99,100]. Recommendations have also been reviewed for health-care workers [101,102] (see Chapter 26).

**VII. Vaccines for use in the military and special occupational groups**

**A. Anthrax,** the disease caused by *Bacillus anthracis*, has historically been a disease of persons whose occupations brought them into frequent and close contact with animal hides and hair of hooved animals. Laboratory-derived cases in personnel working with the organism have also been reported. Three clinical forms of disease are recognized: cutaneous, gastrointestinal, and inhalation, the latter being the most lethal (i.e., mortality rates in excess of 80% are reported in untreated cases). *B. anthracis* has the ability to form spores that are highly resistant to most environmental conditions and hence may survive for decades. When inhaled into the lungs of humans, the spores may then germinate and result in inhalation anthrax. These properties have resulted in *B. anthracis* becoming the prototypical organism for development as a biological warfare agent. It is identified by the CDC as a high priority category A, agent for bioterrorism [103]. Since the tragic events of September 11, 2001, the role of *B. anthracis* as a weapon for domestic and international terrorism has been highlighted [104]. The most up-to-date information related to anthrax and other biological weapons may be obtained on the Internet from the CDC (*www.bt.cdc.gov*) and Johns Hopkins University (*www.hopkins-biodefense.org/mdex.html*).

A vaccine against anthrax was previously available from the state-owned Michigan Biologics Products Institute. This company was bought by Bioport and remains the only manufacturer of anthrax vaccine, almost exclusively for the Department of Defense. Despite production problems, over 700,000 military personnel have received anthrax vaccine since 1998.

The anthrax vaccine is a noninfectious culture filtrate of an attenuated strain of *B. anthracis* that is adsorbed to an aluminum hydroxide adjuvant. Protective antigen that is present in the filtrate vaccine is thought to generate antibodies that prevent the disease. The schedule for administration is 0, 2, and 4 weeks and again at 6, 12, and 18 months. Annual booster doses are necessary to maintain immunity. Efficacy of this new vaccine has only been demonstrated in animal challenge studies. Despite controversy, the frequency and severity of adverse events related to anthrax vaccine do not exceed those of other routinely used vaccines. Most people experience local injection site reactions (e.g., redness, swelling, soreness, itching). In addition to primary prevention, the anthrax vaccine has also been proposed for use in combination with antibiotics for postexposure prophylaxis [104,105].

**B. Lyme disease vaccine** (LYMErix, GlaxoSmithKline) is a recombinant outer surface lyproprotein (OspA) of *Borrelia burgdorferi* that is combined with an adjuvant [107]. Vaccination involves three intramuscular injections (30 $\mu$g) given on day 0 and at 1 month and 12 months. Although efficacious, Lyme vaccine is recommended only for individuals who work, live, or travel to areas of unusually high incidence of Lyme disease (i.e., hyperendemic areas). Local injection site pain is the most frequent adverse event, although other serious vaccine reactions have been reported by the manufacturer, including musculoskeletal, neurologic, and hypersensitivity reactions.

**C. Q fever.** An investigational inactivated vaccine is available for use in animal handlers working with sheep and in laboratory workers exposed to *Coxiella burnetii.* It is available through the U.S. Army Medical Research Institute of Infectious Diseases, Fort Detrick, Maryland.

**D. Tularemia.** A live attenuated vaccine is available from the CDC for use in individuals whose work regularly brings them into contact with wild mammals or vectors in tularemia-endemic areas.

**E. Plague.** Plague vaccine is used rarely except in laboratory or field personnel who are working with *Yersinia pestis* or in certain workers (e.g., Peace Corps volunteers and agricultural advisers) who reside in rural areas where enzootic or epidemic plague exists and where avoidance of rodents and fleas is impossible. Detailed indications and recommendations for the use of this vaccine have been reviewed [106].

**F. Rabies vaccine.** See Chapter 4 under Bite Wounds and Rabies Prevention.

**VIII.** Vaccines are currently in *de novo* development for gonorrhea, malaria, and respiratory syncytial virus, and improved vaccines also are being developed for cholera and typhoid. An adenovirus vaccine is approved for use in the military.

**IX. Vaccine use in developing countries.** This topic is beyond the scope of this chapter. However, it has been reviewed in an international symposium [108] and updated [109].

## ACKNOWLEDGMENT

Supported in part by a grant from the National Institutes of Health, HD-01312, and funds from the Lasden Family Foundation.

## REFERENCES

1. LaForce FM. Immunizations, immunoprophylaxis, and chemoprophylaxis to prevent selected infections. US Preventive Services Task Force. *JAMA* 1987;257:2464–2470.
2. Williams WW, Hickson MA, Kane MA, et al. Medicine and public issues. Immunization policies and vaccine coverage among adults: the risk for missed opportunities. *Ann Intern Med* 1988;108:616–625.
3. Centers for Disease Control and Prevention. Current trends. National Childhood Vaccine Injury Act: requirements for permanent vaccination records and for reporting of selected events after vaccination. *MMWR Morb Mortal Wkly Rep* 1988;37:197–200.
4. Centers for Disease Control and Prevention. National, state and urban area vaccination coverage levels among children aged 19–35 months—United States, 2000. *MMWR Morb Mortal Wkly Rep* 2001;50:637–641.
5. Centers for Disease Control and Prevention. Influenza, pneumococcal, and tetanus toxoid vaccination of adults—United States, 1993–1997. *MMWR Morb Mortal Wkly Rep* 2000;49(SS09):39–62.
6. Centers for Disease Control and Prevention. Successful strategies in adult immunization. *MMWR Morb Mortal Wkly Rep* 1991;40:700–703.
7. Peter G, Gardner P. Standards for immunization practice for vaccines for children and adults. *Infect Dis Clin North Am* 2001;15:9–19.
8. Fingar AR, Francis BJ. Adult immunization. American College of Preventive Medicine Practice policy statement. *Am J Prevent Med* 1998;14:156–158.
9. *Report of the Committee on Infectious Diseases,* 23rd ed. Evanston, IL: American Academy of Pediatrics, 1994.
10. ACP Task Force on Adult Immunization and Infectious Diseases Society of America. *Guide to adult immunization,* 3rd ed. Philadelphia: American College of Physicians, 1994.
11. Centers for Disease Control and Prevention. Update on adult immunization. *MMWR Morb Mortal Wkly Rep* 1991;40(RR-12):1–94.
12. Gardner P, Eickhoff T, Poland GA, et al. Adult immunizations. *Ann Intern Med* 1996;124:35–40.
13. Ryan ET. Immunization. In: Goroll AH, Mulley AG Jr, eds. *Primary care medicine,* 4th ed. Philadelphia: Lippincott Williams & Wilkins, 2000:21–36.
14. Orenstein WA, et al. Immunization. In: Mandell GL, Bennett JE, Dolin E, eds. *Mandell, Douglas, and Bennett's principles and practice of infectious diseases,* 5th ed. Philadelphia: Churchill Livingstone, 2000:3207–3234.
15. Plotkin SA, Orenstein WA, eds. *Vaccines,* 3rd ed. Philadelphia: W.B. Saunders, 1999.
16. Centers for Disease Control and Prevention. General recommendations on immunization. *MMWR Morb Mortal Wkly Rep* 1994;43(RR-1):1–38.
17. NIH Consensus Conference. Intravenous immunoglobulin. Prevention and treatment of disease. *JAMA* 1990;264:3189–3193.
18. Ratko TA, Burnett DA, Foulke GE, et al. Recommendations for off-label use of intravenously administered immunoglobulin preparations. *JAMA* 1995;273:1865–1870.
19. Centers for Disease Control and Prevention. Update: vaccine side effects, adverse reactions, contraindications, and precautions. *MMWR Morb Mortal Wkly Rep* 1996;45(RR-12):1–35.
20. Herman JJ, Radin R, Schneiderman R, et al. Allergic reactions to measles (rubeola) vaccine in patients hypersensitive to egg protein. *J Pediatr* 1983;102:196–199.
21. Confavreux C, Suissa S, Saddier P, et al. Vaccinations and the risk of relapse in multiple sclerosis. *N Engl J Med* 2001;344:319–326.
22. Ascherio A, Zhang SM, Herman MA, et al. Hepatitis B vaccination and the risk of multiple sclerosis. *N Engl J Med* 2001;344:327–332.

23. Centers for Disease Control and Prevention. Measles, mumps, and rubella. *MMWR Morb Mortal Wkly Rep* 1998;47(RR-8):1–57.
24. Kelley PW, Petruccelli BP, Stehr-Green P, et al. The susceptibility of young adult Americans to vaccine-preventable infections. A national serosurvey of US Army recruits. *JAMA* 1991;266:2724–2729.
25. Baughman AL, Williams WW, Atkinson WL, et al. The impact of college prematriculation immunization requirements on risk for measles outbreaks. *JAMA* 1994;272:1127–1132.
26. Martin DB. Atypical measles in adolescents and young adults. *Ann Intern Med* 1979;90:877–881.
27. Centers for Disease Control and Prevention. Epidemiologic notes and reports: measles in HIV-infected children. *MMWR Morb Mortal Wkly Rep* 1988;37:183–186.
28. Stratton K, et al. *Immunization safety review: measles, mumps, and rubella vaccines and autism.* Washington, DC: National Academy Press, 2001.
29. Centers for Disease Control and Prevention. Immunization of health-care workers. *MMWR Morb Mortal Wkly Rep* 1997;46(RR-18):1–42.
30. Centers for Disease Control and Prevention. Mumps prevention. *MMWR Morb Mortal Wkly Rep* 1989;38:388–392, 397–400.
31. Centers for Disease Control and Prevention. Rubella prevention. *MMWR Morb Mortal Wkly Rep* 1990;33(RR-15):1–18.
32. Centers for Disease Control and Prevention. Rubella vaccination during pregnancy—United States, 1971–1988. *MMWR Morb Mortal Wkly Rep* 1989;38:289–293.
33. Centers for Disease Control and Prevention. Poliomyelitis prevention in the United States: introduction of a sequential vaccination schedule of inactivated poliovirus vaccine followed by oral poliovirus vaccine. *MMWR Morb Mortal Wkly Rep* 1997;46(RR-3):1–25.
34. Centers for Disease Control and Prevention. Poliomyelitis prevention: enhanced-potency inactivated poliomyelitis vaccine-supplementary statement. *MMWR Morb Mortal Wkly Rep* 1987;36:795–798.
35. Bernier RH. Improved inactivated poliovirus vaccine: an update. *Pediatr Infect Dis* 1986;5:289.
36. Brunell PA, Shehab Z, Geiser C, et al. Administration of live varicella vaccine to children with leukemia. *Lancet* 1982;2:1069.
37. Weibel R, Neff BJ, Kuter BJ, et al. Live attenuated varicella virus vaccine: efficacy trial in healthy children. *N Engl J Med* 1984;310:1409–1415.
38. Gershon AA, Steinberg SP, LaRussa P, et al. Immunization of healthy adults with live attenuated varicella vaccine. *J Infect Dis* 1988;158:132–137.
39. Gershon AA, Steinberg SP, Gelb L, et al. Live attenuated varicella vaccine. Efficacy for children with leukemia in remission. *JAMA* 1984;252:355–362.
40. Lawrence R, Gershon AA, Holzman R, et al. The risk of zoster after varicella vaccination in children with leukemia. *N Engl J Med* 1988;318:543–548.
41. Vazquez M, LaRussa PS, Gershon AA, et al. The effectiveness of the varicella vaccine in clinical practice. *N Engl J Med* 2001;344:955–960.
42. Lieu TA, Finkler LJ, Sorel ME, et al. Cost-effectiveness of varicella serotesting versus presumptive vaccination of school-age children and adolescents. *Pediatrics* 1995;95:632–638.
43. Gogos CA, Bassaris HP, Vagenakis AG. Varicella pneumonia in adults: a review of pulmonary manifestations, risk factors and treatment. *Respiration* 1992;59:339.
44. Enders G, Miller E, Cradock-Watson J, et al. Consequences of varicella and herpes zoster in pregnancy: prospective study of 1739 cases. *Lancet* 1994;344:950–951.
45. Lewis DA, Jenks P, Gent AE, et al. Varicella-zoster vaccination for health care workers. *Lancet* 1994;343:1362–1363.
46. Centers for Disease Control and Prevention. Varicella-related deaths among adults—United States, 1997. *MMWR Morb Mortal Wkly Rep* 1997;46:409–412.
47. Centers for Disease Control and Prevention. Prevention of varicella. *MMWR Morb Mortal Wkly Rep* 1996;(RR-11):1–36.
48. Raeder CK, Hayney MS. Immunology of varicella immunization in the elderly. *Ann Pharmacother* 2001;34:228–234.

49. Centers for Disease Control and Prevention. Protection against viral hepatitis. *MMWR Morb Mortal Wkly Rep* 1990;39(RR-2):1–26.
50. Medical Letter. Twinrix: a combination Hepatitis A and B vaccine. *Med Lett* 2001;43: 67–68.
51. Safary A, et al. An accelerated dosing schedule of hepatitis B vaccination for those needing rapid protection (abstract 197). Presented at the Twenty-Ninth Interscience Conference on Antimicrobial Agents and Chemotherapy, Houston, September 18, 1989.
52. Marchou B, Excler JL, Bourderioux C, et al. A 3-week hepatitis B vaccination schedule provides rapid and persistent protective immunity: a multicenter, randomized trial comparing accelerated and classic vaccination schedules. *J Infect Dis* 1995;172:258–260.
53. Centers for Disease Control and Prevention. Hepatitis B virus: a comprehensive strategy for eliminating transmission in the United States through universal childhood vaccination. *MMWR Morb Mortal Wkly Rep* 1991;40(RR-13):1–19.
54. European Consensus Group on Hepatitis B Immunity. Are booster immunisations needed for lifelong Hepatitis B immunity? *Lancet* 2000;355:561–565.
55. Margolis HS, Presson AC. Host factors related to poor immunogenicity of hepatitis B vaccine in adults: another reason to immunize early. *JAMA* 1993;270:2971–2972.
56. Alimonos K, Nafziger AN, Murray J, et al. Prediction of response to hepatitis B vaccine in health care workers: whose titers of antibody to hepatitis B surface antigen should be determined after a three-dose series, and what are the implications in terms of cost-effectiveness? *Clin Infect Dis* 1998;26:566–571.
57. Stevens CE, Taylor PE. Hepatitis B vaccine: issues, recommendations, and new developments. *Semin Liver Dis* 1986;6:23–27.
58. Centers for Disease Control and Prevention. Prevention of pneumococcal disease. *MMWR Morb Mortal Wkly Rep* 1997;46(RR-8):1–24.
59. Nuorti JP, Butler JC, Crutcher JM, et al. An outbreak of multidrug-resistant pneumococcal pneumonia and bacteremia among unvaccinated nursing home residents. *N Engl J Med* 1998;338:1861–1868.
60. Centers for Disease Control and Prevention. Vaccine information statement (Interim): pneumococcal conjugate vaccine. July 18, 2000.
61. Centers for Disease Control and Prevention. Control and prevention of meningococcal disease. *MMWR Morb Mortal Wkly Rep* 1997;46(RR-5):1–21.
62. Centers for Disease Control and Prevention. Diphtheria, tetanus, and pertussis: recommendations for vaccine use and other preventive measures. *MMWR Morb Mortal Wkly Rep* 1991;40(RR-10):1–28.
63. Edwards KM. Diphtheria, tetanus, and pertussis immunizations in adults. *Infect Dis Clin North Am* 1990;4:85–103.
64. Karzon DT, Edwards KM. Diphtheria outbreaks in immunized populations. *N Engl J Med* 1988;318:41–43.
65. Centers for Disease Control and Prevention. Tetanus—United States, 1985–1986. *MMWR Morb Mortal Wkly Rep* 1987;36:477–481.
66. Brand DA, Acampora D, Gottlieb LD, et al. Adequacy of anti-tetanus prophylaxis in six hospital emergency rooms. *N Engl J Med* 1983;309:636–640.
67. Nelson JD. The changing epidemiology of pertussis in young infants: the role of adults as reservoirs of infection. *Am J Dis Child* 1978;132:371–373.
68. Linnemann CC Jr, Ramundo N, Perlstein PH, et al. Use of pertussis vaccine in an epidemic involving hospital staff. *Lancet* 1975;2:540–543.
69. Centers for Disease Control and Prevention. Pertussis vaccination: use of acellular pertussis vaccines among infants and young children. *MMWR Morb Mortal Wkly Rep* 1997;46(RR-7):1–25.
70. Keitel WA. Cellular and acellular pertussis vaccine in adults. *Clin Infect Dis* 1999;28[Suppl 2]:S118–S123.
71. Edwards KM, Decker MD, Graham BS, et al. Adult immunization with acellular pertussis vaccine. *JAMA* 1993;269:53–56.
72. Pertussis immunization and the central nervous system. Ad Hoc Committee for the Child Neurology Society Consensus Statement on Pertussis Immunization and the Central Nervous System. *Ann Neurol* 1991;29:458–460.

73. Hoffmann HJ, Hunter JC, Damus K, et al. Diphtheria-tetanus-pertussis immunization and sudden infant death: results of the National Institute of Child Health and Human Development Cooperative Epidemiological Study of Sudden Infant Death Syndrome Risk Factors. *Pediatrics* 1987;79:598–611.
74. Walker AM, Jick H, Perera DR, et al. Diphtheria-tetanus-pertussis immunization and sudden infant death syndrome. *Am J Public Health* 1987;77:945–951.
75. Centers for Disease Control and Prevention. *Haemophilus* b conjugate vaccines for prevention of *Haemophilus influenzae* type b disease among infants and children two months of age and older. *MMWR Morb Mortal Wkly Rep* 1991;40(RR-1):1–6.
76. Madore DV. Impact of immunization on *Haemophilus influenzae* type b disease. *Infect Agents Dis* 1996;5:8–20.
77. Gleich GS. Health maintenance and prevention in the elderly. *Prim Care Clin Office Pract* 1995;22:697–711.
78. Harward MP. Preventive health for the elderly. Role of vaccination. *J FL Med Assoc* 1992;79:687–689.
79. Current trends. Adult immunization—knowledge, attitudes, and practices: DeKalb and Fulton counties, Georgia, 1988. *MMWR Morb Mortal Wkly Rep* 1988;37:657–661.
80. Immunization during pregnancy (ACOG Technical Bulletin no. 160, October 1991). *Int J Gynaecol Obstet* 1993;40:69–79.
81. Centers for Disease Control and Prevention. Immunization of adolescents. *MMWR Morb Mortal Wkly Rep* 1996;45(RR-13):1–16.
82. Schaff EA, Hedberg VA. Preventive health care for teenagers and young adults. *Primary Care* 1995;22:637–652.
83. Centers for Disease Control and Prevention. Rubella outbreaks in prisons—New York City, West Virginia, California. *MMWR Morb Mortal Wkly Rep* 1985;34:615.
84. Krupp LB, Gelberg EA, Wormser GP, et al. Prisoners as medical patients. *Am J Public Health* 1987;77:859–860.
85. Brickner PW, Scanlan BC, Conanan B, et al. Medicine and public issues: homeless persons and health care. *Ann Intern Med* 1986;104:405–409.
86. Pedersen AH, Spearman J, Tronca E, et al. Diphtheria on Skid Road, Seattle, WA, 1972–1975. *Public Health Reports* 1977;92:336.
87. Mercat A, Nguyen J, Dautzenberg B. An outbreak of pneumococcal pneumonia in two men's shelters. *Chest* 1991;99:147.
88. Wang EE, King S, Goldberg E, et al. Hepatitis B and human immunodeficiency virus infection in street youths in Toronto, Canada. *Pediatr Infect Dis J* 1991;10:130.
89. Hibbard PL, Rubin RH. Approach to immunization in the immunosuppressed host. *Infect Dis Clin North Am* 1990;4:123–142.
90. Sixbey JW. Routine immunizations and the immunosuppressed child. *Adv Pediatr Infect Dis* 1987;2:79–114.
91. Centers for Disease Control. Use of vaccines and immune globulins in persons with altered immunocompetence. *MMWR Morb Mortal Wkly Rep* 1993;42(RR-4):1–18.
92. Rose DN, Schechter CB, Sacks HS. Influenza and pneumococcal vaccination of HIV-infected patients: a policy analysis. *Am J Med* 1993;94:160.
93. Siber GR, Gorham C, Martin P, et al. Antibody response to pretreatment immunization and post-treatment boosting with bacterial polysaccharide vaccines in patients with Hodgkin's disease. *Ann Intern Med* 1986;194:467–475.
94. McMahon BJ, Wainwright K, Bulkow L, et al. Response to hepatitis B vaccine in Alaska natives with chronic alcoholism compared with non-alcoholic control subjects. *Am J Med* 1990;88:460–464.
95. Turner-Stokes L, Isenberg DA. Immunisation of patients with rheumatoid arthritis and systemic lupus erythematosus. *Ann Rheum Dis* 1988;47:529–531.
96. Schwebke J, Mujais S. Vaccination in hemodialysis patients. *Int J Artif Organs* 1989;12:481–484.
97. Konradsen HB, Nielsen JL, Pedersen FK, et al. Antibody persistence in splenectomized adults after pneumococcal vaccination. *Scand J Infect Dis* 1990;22:725–727.
98. Ljungman P, Duraj V, Magnius L. Response to immunization against polio after allogeneic marrow transplantation. *Bone Marrow Transplant* 1991;7:89–93.
99. U.S. Public Health Service and Infectious Diseases Society of America. 1999

USPHS/IDSA Guidelines for the Prevention of Opportunistic Infections in Persons Infected with Human Immunodeficiency Virus. *MMWR Morb Mortal Wkly Rep* 1999;48(RR-10):1–59, 61–66.

100. Centers for Disease Control and Prevention. Notice to readers: draft of Guidelines for the Prevention of Opportunistic Infections (OIs) in Persons Infected with Human Immunodeficiency Virus. *MMWR Morb Mortal Wkly Rep* 2001;50:687.
101. Centers for Disease Control and Prevention. Immunization of health-care workers. *MMWR Morb Mortal Wkly Rep* 1997;46(RR-18):1–42.
102. Weber DJ, Rutala WA, Weigle K, et al. Selection and use of vaccines for healthcare workers. *Infect Control Hosp Epidemiol* 1997;18:682–687.
103. Block SM. The growing threat of biological weapons. *Am Sci* 2001;89:28–37.
104. Swartz MN. Recognition and management of anthrax—an update. *N Engl J Med* 2001;345:1621–1626.
105. Brookmeyer R, Blades N. Prevention of inhalation anthrax in the U.S. outbreak. *Science* 2002;295:1861.
106. Centers for Disease Control and Prevention. Prevention of plague. *MMWR Morb Mortal Wkly Rep* 1996;45(RR-14):1–15.
107. Rahm DW. Lyme vaccination: issues and controversies. *Infect Dis Clin North Am* 2001;15:171–187.
108. Bart KJ, Hinman AR, Jordan WS Jr. International symposium on vaccine development and utilization. *Rev Infect Dis* 1989;11[Suppl 3]:5491–5667.
109. Hall AJ, Greenwood BM, Whittle H. Modern vaccines. Practices in developing countries. *Lancet* 1990;335:774–777.

# 24. ALLERGY TO β-LACTAMS AND OTHER SELECTED ANTIBIOTICS

Stephen F. Kemp and Richard D. deShazo

## GENERAL PRINCIPLES OF ADVERSE DRUG REACTIONS

**I. Epidemiology.** Adverse drug reactions (ADRs) are frequent consequences of medical treatment. Estimates of fatalities in the United States due to ADRs range from 75,000 to 106,000 fatalities per year [1]. Statistics vary, however, depending on the reporting mechanism. One study found a marked disparity between national public-use databases of U.S. death certificates and the U.S. Food and Drug Administration's (FDA's) postmarketing surveillance system (MEDWatch) [2]. A critique of reports and their interpretation has been published elsewhere [3]. Clinical trials may not detect many of the serious ADRs prior to approval of a given drug [4,5]. For proper management, allergic reactions must be distinguished from other reactions.

Allergic and other immunologic drug reactions probably cause 6% to 10% of ADRs [6]. Reports suggest that the risk of an allergic reaction for most drugs is 1% to 3% [7]. Antibiotics, especially β-lactam antibiotics, are the most common cause of allergic drug reactions. Antibiotics are also the most common class of drug associated with prescribing errors. A study over 9 years in a teaching hospital determined that antibiotics were associated with 34% of prescribing errors, at least twice the incidence of any other drug class [8]. Overdose accounted for 33.5% as compared with underdose in 26.3% of instances. Allergic drug reactions accounted for 22.3%.

**II. Immunopathogenic mechanisms**

**A.** Gell and Coombs first classified four types of hypersensitivity (immunopathologic) reactions [9]:

1. Type I. Immediate hypersensitivity reactions are immunoglobulin E (IgE) dependent. Clinical examples include urticarial and anaphylaxis.
2. Type II. Cytotoxic reactions are IgG or IgM dependent. Clinical examples include Coombs-positive hemolytic anemia.
3. Type III. Immune complex disease is mediated by antigen–antibody complexes (IgM or IgG). Serum sickness is an example of this type of drug reaction.
4. Type IV. Delayed or cell-mediated hypersensitivity reactions are T-lymphocyte dependent. Contact dermatitis is a clinical example of this type of drug reaction.

**B.** Sell has proposed an alternate classification system based on seven immunopathologic mechanisms with both protective and destructive functions [10]:

1. Type 1 mechanisms are immune-mediated inactivation/activation reactions of biologically active molecules.
2. Type 2 are antibody-mediated cytotoxic or cytolytic reactions.
3. Type 3 are immune complex reactions.
4. Type 4 are allergic reactions.
5. Type 5 are T-lymphocyte–mediated cytotoxicity reactions.
6. Type 6 are delayed hypersensitivity reactions.
7. Type 7 are granulomatous reactions.

In this classification, one or more mechanisms may be active in an immunopathologic reaction (e.g., ADR) for a given individual.

**III. Classification.** Some clinicians consider the terminology used in discussions of ADR to be a "tower of Babel" [3]. A useful classification separates ADRs into two categories: types A and B [11]. **Type A reactions** are common and predictable reactions that may occur in any patient. **Type B reactions** are uncommon and unpredictable reactions that occur only in particularly susceptible patients (Table 24.1). At least 80% of ADRs are type A reactions, which are often dose dependent and reflect known pharmacologic actions of the drug.

**A. Allergic** or **hypersensitivity reactions** are type B reactions, which occur in small numbers of patients and require previous exposure to the same or a chemically related drug. They develop rapidly after reexposure and produce clinical syndromes commonly associated with immunologic reactions. Higher molecular weight drugs

Table 24.1. Classification of Adverse Drug Reactions

Type A

- Overdosage or toxicity: an exaggerated but characteristic effect from an excessive dose
- Side effects: excessive expressions of known pharmacologic effects that can occur at recommended dosages of a drug
- Drug interactions: can occur when a patient takes two or more medications
- Teratogens: capable of producing developmental defects in a fetus whose mother takes these drugs

Type B

- Intolerance: an undesirable pharmacologic outcome that occurs at a subtherapeutic dosage
- Idiosyncratic reaction: an uncharacteristic response to the administration of a drug that is usually due to a hereditary enzyme deficiency
- Allergic or hypersensitivity reactions: occur in small numbers of patients, require previous exposure to the same or a chemically related drug, develop rapidly after reexposure, and produce clinical syndromes commonly associated with immunologic reactions

Adapted from Rawlins MD, Thompson W. Mechanisms of adverse drug reactions. In: Davies DM, ed. *Textbook of adverse drug reactions.* New York: Oxford University Press, 1991:18–45, with permission.

(e.g., antisera) are more likely to produce immunologic reactions directly, whereas lower molecular weight drugs (e.g., penicillin) are haptens that must combine with carrier proteins before they can elicit reactions [12].

IV. **Risk factors.** Both drug and patient factors may increase the risk of ADRs.

A. Drug factors include the class of drug, variations in drug metabolism, and drug exposure (dose, frequency, duration, and route of administration). Patient factors include age, gender, genetic and constitutional factors, prior exposure to medications, and concurrent illnesses and medications or other biologic agents. These risk factors are reviewed in greater detail elsewhere [13].

B. Some risk factors assume particular significance for antibiotic administration. The route, dose, duration, and frequency of drug administration can influence the risk of drug allergy.

1. Sensitization may occur by any route of drug administration, but the oral route generally presents the least risk.
2. Parenterally administered medications, including $\beta$-lactam antibiotics, are more likely to cause anaphylaxis than those administered orally [14].
3. Single prophylactic doses of any antibiotic are less likely to sensitize than is high-dose, prolonged parenteral therapy.
4. Frequent courses of antibiotic therapy are more likely to result in allergic reactions than courses of therapy separated by several years, which may explain why patients with cystic fibrosis appear particularly susceptible to drug reactions [15].
5. Children of parents who are allergic to an antibiotic have been reported to be 15 times more likely to develop allergic reactions to antibiotics [16].
6. Hospitalized patients with a history of drug allergy are nine times more likely to report a history of drug allergy among their first-degree relatives [17].
7. Although atopy (the hereditary predisposition to develop allergic rhinitis, allergic asthma, or allergic dermatitis) does not affect the incidence of ADRs, it may predispose to more severe reactions [18].

C. Some patients appear to be at risk for allergic reactions to multiple drugs. The multiple drug allergy syndrome, reported to occur primarily with antimicrobial agents, may reflect a general tendency to respond immunologically to haptens rather than to react to specific classes of drugs [19,20]. Some investigators have challenged its existence [21].

**D.** Concurrent disease and therapy also may influence the risk for ADRs.

1. Viral infections may increase the frequency of cutaneous drug reactions (see section **I.C** under Common Clinical Patterns of adverse Reactions to Antibiotics below).
2. Patients with systemic lupus erythematosus may have an increased incidence of allergic drug reactions, but it is unclear whether this is related to the underlying immunologic abnormality or to more frequent exposure to drugs [22,23].

## COMMON CLINICAL PATTERNS OF ADVERSE REACTIONS TO ANTIBIOTICS

**I. Cutaneous reactions**

**A. Acute urticaria and angioedema** are common manifestations of antibiotic allergy [24]. The lesions usually appear shortly after beginning drug therapy and resolve rapidly when the drug is discontinued.

1. Acute urticaria should be considered a manifestation of anaphylaxis. Anaphylaxis is an acute, life-threatening immunologic reaction that consists of diffuse erythema, pruritus, urticaria, angioedema, bronchospasm, laryngeal edema, hyperperistalsis, hypotension, or cardiac arrhythmias, alone or in combination. Anaphylaxis usually develops rapidly, often within 5 to 30 minutes after drug administration [25].
2. Acute urticaria after an antibiotic should be treated as an anaphylactic reaction with epinephrine lest the reaction progress to full-blown anaphylaxis.

**B. Chronic urticaria** (hives persisting for 6 weeks or longer) occasionally occurs despite discontinuation of treatment with a drug to which a patient is allergic.

**C. Maculopapular or morbilliform eruptions,** overall, are the most common drug-induced cutaneous reactions.

1. These eruptions are symmetric, often confluent erythematous macules and papules that typically spare the palms and soles. They originate on the extremities of ambulatory patients or overlie pressure areas of bedridden patients.
2. Beta-lactam antibiotics and sulfonamides are common causes of antibiotic-associated maculopapular eruptions. These eruptions occur more frequently with ampicillin (approximately 10%) than with other penicillins (approximately 2%) and develop in 50% to 80% of patients with Epstein-Barr virus (including infectious mononucleosis) or cytomegalovirus infections, chronic lymphocytic leukemia, or hyperuricemia, and in patients taking allopurinol concomitantly [7].
3. Maculopapular eruptions are also common in patients with viral infections, especially those with human immunodeficiency virus (HIV) infection who receive trimethoprim-sulfamethoxazole (TMP-SMX), ampicillin, or other drugs.
4. These eruptions usually develop within 1 week of initiating the offending drug and follow a variable course. The eruptions may subside spontaneously with continued use of the responsible drug and do not always recur on repeat exposure. However, the reactions may occasionally progress to generalized erythroderma or exfoliative dermatitis. Therefore, a prudent approach to morbilliform drug reactions is to discontinue treatment with the culprit drug and to avoid subsequent administration if possible.

**D. Erythema multiforme/Stevens-Johnson syndrome.** Erythema multiforme is an erythematous, polymorphic eruption that may be caused by drugs in 10% to 20% of cases. Antibiotics, especially sulfonamides, are frequently implicated. Skin manifestations include target lesions, maculopapular rashes, urticaria, and vesicles. Lesions are typically symmetric and have a predilection for the extremities [26].

1. In the most severe form of erythema multiforme, Stevens-Johnson syndrome, 90% of patients have mucosal lesions and 85% have conjunctival lesions; epidermal loss involves 10% or less of body surface area. Approximately 50% of cases of Stevens-Johnson syndrome are associated with drugs, and readministration of a responsible drug produces recurrence.
2. Sulfonamides, anticonvulsants, nonsteroidal antiinflammatory drugs, and allopurinol account for two-thirds of these reactions.

3. Fever and influenza-like symptoms often precede the mucocutaneous lesions by 1 to 3 days.
4. Visceral involvement is associated with a poor prognosis, but the mortality rate is generally less than 5% [24].
5. Although treatment is supportive, some investigators recommend the early use of systemic corticosteroids [27]. Corticosteroids may prevent visceral involvement and decrease both the duration and severity of clinical findings [28–30]. However, corticosteroid use in Stevens-Johnson syndrome remains controversial.
6. **Readministration of any medication clearly implicated in Stevens-Johnson syndrome is contraindicated.**

E. **Toxic epidermal necrolysis (TEN).** TEN is an acute illness characterized by fever, epidermal loss exceeding 30% of body surface area, and visceral involvement with an associated mortality rate of 30% to 40% [31]. More than 80% of TEN cases are induced by the same medications that produce Stevens-Johnson syndrome [24].
1. As with Stevens-Johnson syndrome, readministration of the offending drug produces recurrence.
2. It is often difficult clinically to distinguish TEN from Stevens-Johnson syndrome without skin biopsy. For instance, both conditions produce conjunctival lesions in 85% of patients [24].
3. Treatment is supportive and corticosteroids are not advocated.
4. Intravenous immune globulin may be helpful for some patients [32].

F. **Histopathology of cutaneous antibiotic reactions**
1. T cells are the predominant cells that comprise the inflammatory infiltrate of skin in antibiotic-induced bullous and morbilliform reactions [33,34]. Cells isolated from biopsy samples of these reactions are capable of *in vitro* proliferation after stimulation with the culprit drug [33,35–37]. Several investigators have concluded that these reactions reflect lymphocyte-mediated delayed hypersensitivity because they are often associated with positive results obtained with the patch test or leukocyte transformation test (LTT), or delayed positive results (i.e., >6 hours postadministration) with the intracutaneous test [38–41].

II. **Serum sickness–like reactions**

A. Serum sickness–like reactions to antibiotics are indistinguishable from the serum sickness due to heterologous serum.
1. The serum sickness–like reaction is a syndrome characterized by fever, malaise, and an urticarial or morbilliform rash, which is often preceded by pruritus and erythema. Arthralgias or arthritis (mainly large joints), lymphadenopathy, abdominal pain (possibly with emesis or melena), nephritis, neuropathy, or vasculitis (cutaneous or systemic) may occur in some cases.
2. Serum sickness–like reactions result from immune complex (IgG) tissue deposition and may develop 6 to 21 days after drug administration, but they can occur within 12 to 48 hours in individuals who have previously been sensitized to the medication or serum.
3. Cutaneous vasculitis, also known as hypersensitivity vasculitis, is usually manifested by palpable purpura, and is most evident on the lower extremities of ambulatory individuals or on the buttocks or sacral region of bedridden patients. Purpuric lesions reflect the leakage of erythrocytes into the skin from inflamed postcapillary venules.
4. Serum sickness–like reactions associated with $\beta$-lactam antibiotics appear to be more common with cefaclor. The incidence with cefaclor is low, ranging from 0.024% in controlled clinical trials to 0.5% in published reports [42].
5. Cefaclor-induced serum sickness-like reactions are more common in children taking the oral suspension and have a predilection for the winter months [42,43].
6. No circulating immune complexes have been identified. Kearns et al. have suggested that unique hepatic biotransformation of the parent drug to reactive intermediates capable of lymphocyte activation may cause serum sickness–like reactions attributed to cefaclor [44].

III. **Drug fever.** Drug fever may occur with any drug, including antibiotics, and its mechanism is unknown. Eosinophilia, leukocytosis, elevated erythrocyte sedimentation rate, and rash may occur in patients with drug fever. Because drug fever almost always resolves within 48 to 72 hours of discontinuing treatment with the culprit drug, the most useful diagnostic test is the discontinuation of the suspect drug [45].

**IV. Other organ system patterns of ADRs**

**A. Hepatitis.** Drug-induced allergic hepatitis may be accompanied by fever, rash, lymphadenopathy, hemolysis, and eosinophilia.

**1.** Hepatitis begins after several weeks of drug treatment and recurs rapidly on reexposure. Histologic patterns of liver injury may include hepatocellular necrosis, cholestasis, or both.

**2.** More than 150 drugs have been reported to cause allergic hepatitis, including semisynthetic penicillins, ceftriaxone, erythromycin, nitrofurantoin, and sulfonamides. Many of these also induce antibodies directed against liver organelles (mitochondria, microsomes), smooth muscle, or nuclear components [46].

**3.** An immunologic mechanism is suspected for drug-induced allergic hepatitis because these reactions are not dose dependent, are accelerated on rechallenge, and are associated with eosinophilia in peripheral blood samples and on biopsy specimens. Antinuclear antibodies to single-stranded DNA also may be present [47].

**B. Hematologic reactions** include eosinophilia, thrombocytopenia, and hemolytic anemia. These have been noted with ampicillin, vancomycin, sulfonamides, and streptomycin antibiotics. Eosinophilia in the context of an ADR usually occurs with other commonly associated features of allergic drug reactions, such as dermatitis or hepatitis [7]. Eosinophils may be present in the urine of patients with methicillin-induced interstitial nephritis. Eosinophilia may be the only manifestation of drug hypersensitivity in some instances, such as that associated with intramuscular injections of gold thiomalate sodium.

**C. Other adverse reactions.** Less commonly, antibiotics, including β-lactams (especially methicillin), rifampin, and ciprofloxacin, can cause renal disease, with nephrosis or acute interstitial nephritis. Pulmonary infiltrates with peripheral eosinophilia have been associated with penicillin, sulfonamides, and nitrofurantoin.

## GUIDELINES FOR DIAGNOSIS AND MANAGEMENT OF ADRs

**I. General principles.** Published protocols are available for the diagnosis and management of a number of adverse reactions to drugs and biologic agents [7,13,48–53]. We have suggested a standardized approach to the management of patients with a previous adverse reaction who require treatment for the same indication (Fig. 24.1). A similar protocol is also available for patients who develop drug reactions while taking multiple drugs [13]. Table 24.2 lists antibiotics and concentrations useful in skin testing to detect the presence of drug-specific IgE.

**A.** Many patients with purported drug allergy have actually experienced type A reactions for which dose modification or drug substitution may be adequate intervention. Supervised administration of a small test dose for reassurance may be appropriate if a serious reaction after readministration appears unlikely and if therapeutic alternatives are unavailable. These challenges should be administered only in a setting where drug reactions can be treated promptly and adequately.

## ALLERGIC REACTIONS TO SPECIFIC ANTIBIOTICS

**I. Penicillin and other β-lactam antibiotics are responsible for most allergic drug reactions and drug-induced anaphylaxis.**

**A. Classified.** Allergic reactions to penicillin are classified according to the time of onset after initiation of therapy as immediate (within 1–45 minutes), accelerated (1–72 hours), or late/delayed (>72 hours and up to weeks afterward).

**1.** Immediate reactions result from the IgE-dependent mast cell and basophil release of histamine and other chemical mediators. These are the most dangerous antibiotic reactions and may be associated with urticaria, angioedema, laryngeal edema, bronchospasm, and anaphylaxis.

**2.** Accelerated reactions are IgE dependent but also are influenced by IgG. They share clinical features with immediate reactions but, in the absence of laryngeal edema, are generally not life threatening.

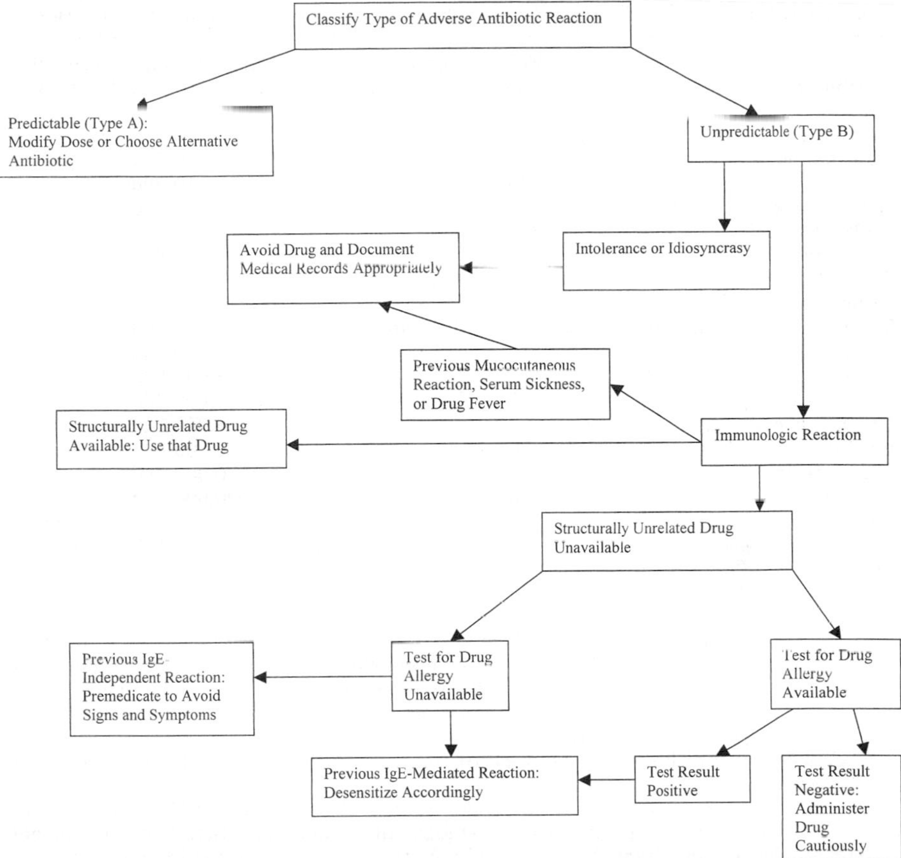


**FIG. 24.1** Systematic approach for evaluating the patient who reports a previous adverse antibiotic reaction and requires treatment for the same clinical indication. (Modified from deShazo RD, Kemp SF. Allergic reactions to drugs and biologic agents. *JAMA* 1997;278:1895–1906, with permission.)

3. Late/delayed reactions may account for 39% of all allergic reactions to penicillins and are mediated by T-lymphocytes. Morbilliform or maculopapular eruptions are the most common clinical features [38].

B. **Prevalence and incidence.** The estimated prevalence of penicillin allergy is 2%, but the reported incidence varies widely (1%–10%), depending on a number of factors, including the history of exposure, the route of administration, the duration of treatment, the elapsed time between the reaction and diagnostic testing or exposure, and the nature of the initial reaction [13,54].

1. **Anaphylactic reactions.** Because there is no system for tracking the incidence of ADRs accurately, the true incidence of antibiotic-induced anaphylactic reactions is unknown. In 1968, Idsoe et al. reported the international incidence of penicillin-induced anaphylaxis to be 0.015% to 0.04% (1.5–4/10,000) of treated patients [55].
2. In another study of 1,740 patients who received monthly prophylaxis with intramuscular penicillin G for an average of 3.4 years, allergic reactions occurred in 3.2%, with an anaphylaxis incidence of 1.23/10,000 injections. The risk of a

Table 24.2. Nonirritating Skin Test Concentrations of Selected Intravenous Antibiotics

| Antibiotic | Full-strength Concentration (mg/mL) | Nonirritating Concentration (dilution from full-strength) |
|---|---|---|
| Cefotaxime | 95 | 10-fold |
| Cefuroxime | 90 | 10-fold |
| Cefazolin | 330 | 10-fold |
| Ceftazidime | 250 | 10-fold |
| Ceftriaxone | 250 | 10-fold |
| Tobramycin | 40 | 10-fold |
| Ticarcillin | 200 | 10-fold |
| Clindamycin | 150 | 10-fold |
| Trimethoprim-sulfamethoxazole | 80 (sulfa component) | 100-fold |
| Gentamycin | 40 | 100-fold |
| Aztreonam | 50 | 1,000-fold |
| Levofloxacin | 25 | 1,000-fold |
| Erythromycin | 50 | 1,000-fold |
| Nafcillin | 250 | 10,000-fold |
| Vancomycin | 50 | 10,000-fold |
| Ciprofloxacin | 10 | 10,000,000-fold |

Reprinted from Solensky R, Mendelson LM. Systemic reactions to antibiotics. *Immunol Allergy Clin North Am* 2001;21:679–697, with permission.

fatality was 1/32,000 injections [56]. Similarly, two of 9,203 healthy military recruits developed anaphylaxis after prophylactic treatment with a single dose of intramuscular benzathine penicillin, for an incidence rate of 2.17/10,000 [57].

3. Anaphylactic reactions to penicillin occur most commonly in adults between the ages of 20 and 49 years [18].

C. **The clinical history is important** in identifying patients with a history of penicillin allergy.

1. The more remote the initial reaction from subsequent penicillin administration, the lower the risk of anaphylaxis following readministration. For example, only 20% of subjects with prior anaphylactic sensitivity to penicillin have persistent penicillin-specific IgE antibodies after 10 years of penicillin avoidance [54,58].
2. Selectively amoxicillin-allergic patients tend to lose sensitivity more quickly than those allergic to penicillin, suggesting at least two types of IgE response [59].
3. Because about one-third of penicillin-allergic patients have vague histories of penicillin allergy, it is prudent to assume penicillin allergy exists in a history-positive patient unless testing proves otherwise [60].

D. **Immunochemical etiology of penicillin allergy**

1. Ninety-five percent of penicillin is metabolized to the penicilloyl hapten, which is called the major determinant (see Fig. 24.2). The penicilloyl hapten is conjugated to polylysine (benzyl penicilloyl polylysine; [BPO-PLL or PPL]) as the commercially available skin testing Pre-Pen (Hollister-Stier, Spokane, WA).
2. The minor determinant mixtures (MDMs) comprise the remaining 5% of penicillin metabolites and include penicilloate, penicilloyl-amine, benzylpenicilloyl-*n*-propylamine, and penilloate. No commercial preparations of MDMs are available for diagnostic testing in the United States.
3. Immunochemical studies using human IgE antibodies have defined no predominance of a given penicillin determinant [61].
4. In addition, side chain–specific antibodies to amoxicillin, penicillin V, and antigenic determinants generated by penicillins demonstrate that additional epitopes exist [61,62].
5. Individuals experiencing anaphylaxis and most with serum sickness have circulating penicillin-specific IgE antibodies.

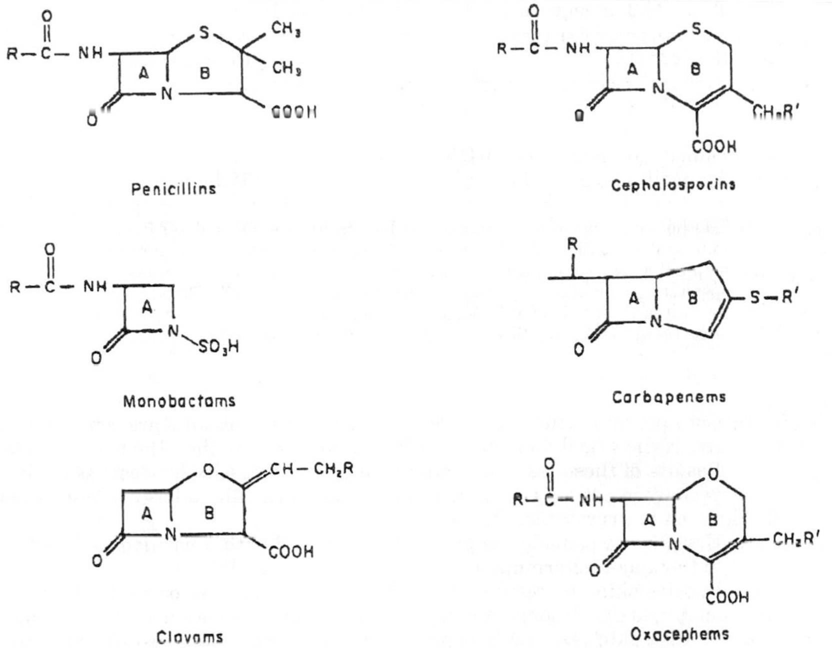

**FIG. 24.2** Structure and metabolism of $\beta$-lactam antibiotics. *R* represents the C-6 or C-7 side chain, *R′* is a second side chain, *A* is the $\beta$-lactam ring, and *B* is a fused ring. *All $\beta$-lactam antibiotics (penicillins, cephalosporins, monobactams, carbapenems, oxacephems, and clavams) possess a characteristic four-member $\beta$-lactam ring that, except for monobactams, is fused to a second five- or six-member ring. All except the clavams have a side chain attached to the $\beta$-lactam ring, and some cephalosporins, carbapenems, and oxacephems possess a side chain that is attached to the second ring. Aztreonam, clavulanic acid, imipenem/meropenem, and moxolactam are monobactams, clavams, carbapenems, and oxacephems, respectively. (Reprinted from Blanca M, Vega JM, Garcia J, et al. New aspects of allergic reactions to beta-lactams: cross-reactions and unique specificities. *Clin Exp Allergy* 1994;24:407–415, with permission.)

6. IgG and IgM antipenicillin antibodies are detected with penicillin-associated hemolytic anemia and serum sickness.

## E. Diagnostic testing for penicillin allergy

1. Skin test methods
   a. The probability that immediate or accelerated reactions will occur following readministration of penicillin in patients with histories suggestive of previous reactions can be determined by immediate hypersensitivity skin testing with a major determinant, MDMs (available in many research centers), and penicillin G. Table 24.3 lists reagents and concentrations used in skin testing for $\beta$-lactam allergy.
   b. Personnel skilled in the placement and interpretation of these tests should perform them in a setting where anaphylactic reactions can be treated promptly and correctly should they occur.
   c. Testing should be performed in the absence of antihistamines or medication with antihistamine properties. Percutaneous (prick) testing should always precede intracutaneous tests, and appropriate positive and negative controls should be used.

Table 24.3. Reagents Used in Penicillin Skin Testing

| Reagent | Concentration |
|---|---|
| Penicilloyl-polylysine (Pre-Pen) | $6 \times 10^{-5}$ *M* |
| Penicillin G | 10,000 units/mL |
| Penicilloate/penilloate (MDM)[a] | 0.01 *M* |
| Ampicillin/amoxicillin | 12.5 mg/mL |

[a]Method of preparation discussed in Macy E, Richter PK, Falkoff R, et al. Skin testing with penicilloate and penilloate prepared by an improved method: amoxicillin oral challenge in patients with negative skin test responses to penicillin reagents. *J Allergy Clin Immunol* 1997;100:586–591. Reprinted from Solensky R, Mendelson LM. Systemic reactions to antibiotics. *Immunol Allergy Clin North Am* 2001;21:679–697, with permission.

**d.** Both percutaneous and intracutaneous skin test results are considered positive if the wheal diameter is at least 3 mm greater than the negative control. Results of these tests may not preclude the necessity for desensitization, especially in patients with histories of severe penicillin allergy (see section **I.C**).

**2.** Skin test interpretation (Table 24.4)

**a.** Urticaria to penicillin is primarily associated with a positive skin test result to the major determinant.

**b.** Positive skin test results to the MDMs are strongly associated with a risk for anaphylaxis, although anaphylaxis may sometimes occur in the presence of a positive skin test result or positive radioallergosorbent test (RAST) result to the major determinant alone [63].

**c.** Delayed reactions to penicillins account for most allergic reactions. Although assessment of intradermal reactivity after 6 hours has been proposed as a method to diagnose these reactions (see section **I.A.3**), it has not been carefully evaluated.

**d.** The major factor limiting widespread use of penicillin skin testing in the United States has been the lack of commercial MDM preparations. Liquid solutions are unstable and generally are available only in research centers where they may be synthesized and lyophilized for storage [64].

**F. Utility of penicillin skin tests**

**1.** Routine penicillin skin testing can facilitate the safe use of penicillin without adverse reactions in 90% of individuals with a previous history of penicillin allergy [65].

**a.** Studies have reported the predictive value of a negative penicillin skin test result to be 97% to 99% for immediate hypersensitivity reactions [18,58,66].

**b.** To the contrary, the positive predictive value of skin testing to assess the risk for allergic reactions to penicillin is unclear because of the risk associated with penicillin challenge in a patient with a positive penicillin skin test result.

Table 24.4. Percutaneous and Intracutaneous Penicillin Skin Test Responses

| PPL | Penicillin-G | MDM | Allergic Reaction Expected |
|---|---|---|---|
| + | + | ± | Immediate |
| 0 | + | 0 | Immediate |
| 0 | 0 | + | Immediate |
| + | 0 | 0 | Accelerated |
| 0 | 0 | 0 | None; risk of adverse reaction <3% |

PPL, penicilloyl-polylysine (Pre-Pen); MDM, minor determinant mixture.

   **c.** Studies have reported allergic reaction rates ranging from 40% to 100% in history-positive patients with positive penicillin skin test results [49,67].
   **d.** Antibody to a minor determinant causes at least 7% of positive skin test results in penicillin-allergic patients [68].
   **e.** Penicillin-induced anaphylaxis has not been reported in subjects with negative skin test results when both major and minor determinant skin tests were performed [67]. Approximately 1% of history-positive, skin test–negative patients experience acute urticaria, and approximately 3% have other mild cutaneous reactions when penicillin is administered [69].
2. "Aged" penicillin is not useful in skin testing because spontaneous degradation of penicillin does not occur and amounts of minor determinant detectable by liquid chromatography or nuclear magnetic resonance are negligible [67]. Published practice parameters recommend skin testing with penicillin G diluted to 10,000 units/mL if MDM is unavailable, followed by an oral test using about 1/100 the desired therapeutic dose if the skin test results are negative [49]. The patient may safely receive the full dose after 60 minutes in most cases in which no drug reaction occurs [49].
3. Penicillin skin testing is a safe procedure. Combining data from five skin test trials, systemic reactions defined as urticaria beyond the skin test site or worse symptoms occurred in only 10 of 9,249 patients (0.11%) [18,66,70–72]. The prevalence of penicillin allergy is presumed to be about 10%, and approximately 10% of patients who have positive penicillin skin test results react only to MDM. This means that only about 1% (i.e., 10% of 10%) of penicillin-allergic patients will fail to be detected by skin testing that excludes MDM (i.e., using only penicillin 10,000 units and PPL) [69].

**G. Other information from penicillin skin tests**

1. A negative skin test outcome in the absence of a systemic reaction defines a dose of the test drug that can be tolerated. This permits selection of a drug dosage to be used for desensitization. The dose can then be increased incrementally based on the dose of the drug contained in the skin test. For example, duplicate 0.02-mL intradermal skin tests of a 1 mg/mL concentration of a test drug introduce approximately 40 $\mu$g into a patient [73].
2. Elective skin testing has been proposed as a method by which to correct erroneous labeling of patients as allergic to penicillin. Such testing may eliminate the use of more expensive or toxic drugs. A combination skin test and challenge procedure may be performed in an outpatient setting if the patient is well and has no immediate need for antibiotic therapy.
3. After negative skin tests, the first therapeutic dose can be administered in the office with a brief observation period, and followed by instructions to complete a subsequent 10-day therapeutic course of the medication [67].
4. Skin testing may be repeated several weeks later to exclude the possibility that the elective administration of penicillin has uncovered latent penicillin hypersensitivity (see section **I.H** below).

**H. Activation of latent hypersensitivity by penicillin skin testing**

1. Investigators have analyzed whether penicillin history–positive, skin test–negative patients who have tolerated a therapeutic course of penicillin may require skin testing prior to subsequent administration of a β-lactam antibiotic.
2. Reactivation of penicillin allergy in patients with previous penicillin allergy, termed resensitization, has an incidence ranging from approximately 1% to 14% in children [67,72] and 0% to 5% in adults following oral administration [67,74]. Less is known about the risk of penicillin resensitization following intravenous or intramuscular administration of the antibiotic.
3. Skin test conversion rates of 5% and 16% have been reported in adults following a single parenteral injection. To our knowledge, there are no published pediatric data on skin test conversion rates following penicillin treatment [67].
4. The sum of these data appear to support repeat skin testing to exclude resensitization in patients previously noted to be penicillin allergic and who receive a parenteral course of β-lactam antibiotic after negative penicillin skin tests.

**I. *In vitro* testing versus skin testing**

1. Most investigators consider skin tests for penicillin allergy to be more sensitive than RAST or ELISA [49,68].
2. RASTs with various determinants are of variable quality, and available data on penicillin RASTs are confusing. For instance, although *in vitro* determinations of specific IgE antibodies to the major determinant correspond to skin testing with the major determinant [75], Blanca et al. observed that some penicillin-allergic subjects with negative skin test results to the major determinant (BPO-PLL) and positive skin test results to the MDM had RAST positivity to the major determinant [76]. They also reported amoxicillin-allergic subjects with penicillin test–negative, selective IgE responses to amoxicillin who had negative skin test results to amoxicillin-PLL conjugates, positive skin test results to amoxicillin MDM, and positive RAST results to amoxicillin-PLL [75].
3. **These data suggest that the RAST, despite its limitations, may have a diagnostic role in patients for whom a high degree of clinical suspicion of allergy persists after negative β-lactam skin tests.** Further investigation on the role of RAST testing for β-lactam allergy is needed.

**J. Delayed (nonimmediate) allergic reactions to β-lactam antibiotics**

1. **Intracutaneous test versus patch testing or the LTT.** Several investigators have evaluated patch tests and the LTT in patients with nonimmediate reactions to β-lactams (i.e., those reactions that occur more than 1 hour after drug administration).
   a. The LTT reveals sensitization of T cells by an enhanced proliferative response of peripheral blood mononuclear cells to a specific drug. In one study, the specificity of the LTT was 92.8%, and its sensitivity (57.9%) exceeded that of skin testing (36.8%) for the nonimmediate group. However, results of the LTT in patients who received penicillin without allergic reactions were not included as controls. Skin testing sensitivity remained superior for immediate reactions, 77.4% versus 62% [77].
   b. A similar study reported a sensitivity of 78% and specificity of 85% for the LTT in patients with delayed reactions to β-lactams [78].
   c. Present data do not suggest the routine use of LTT in the evaluation of allergy to β-lactam antibiotics [49].

**K. Penicillin desensitization. Because skin tests are not always available and are not 100% reliable, we recommend desensitization of all patients with histories of life-threatening reactions to penicillin who require the drug, regardless of skin test results.**

1. Representative protocols of oral and intravenous penicillin desensitization are presented in Tables 24.5 and 24.6.
2. Oral penicillin desensitization is less likely than parenteral desensitization to induce anaphylaxis [14].
3. The underlying mechanism of desensitization is unclear. An attractive hypothesis is that IgE receptor aggregation may generate counterregulatory forces that actually extinguish activating signals rather than causing mast cell activation [79]. Thus, it is possible that slow rates of IgE receptor aggregation caused by the gradual increase in drug concentration, along with suppression of cellular activation signals, lead to antigen-specific desensitization and clinical tolerance.
4. Complications of oral β-lactam desensitization include mild pruritus and pruritic rashes in approximately 5% of patients during desensitization and approximately 25% during subsequent full-dose therapy.
5. Acute reactions during desensitization may require suppressive medication and adjustments in dosage and dose intervals. Approximately 5% of patients experience drug-induced serum sickness, hemolytic anemia, or nephritis late in the course of full-dose therapy, possibly as a result of increases in penicillin-specific IgG that occur during the desensitization process [80].
6. Premedication with antihistamines or corticosteroids is discouraged because they may mask early manifestations of systemic reactions, and there is no evidence

Table 24.5. Penicillin Oral Desensitization Protocol

| Step[a] | Penicillin (mg/mL) | Amount (mL) | Dose Given (mg) | Cumulative Dose (mg) |
|---|---|---|---|---|
| 1 | 0.5 | 0.1 | 0.05 | 0.05 |
| 2 | 0.5 | 0.2 | 0.1 | 0.15 |
| 3 | 0.5 | 0.4 | 0.2 | 0.35 |
| 4 | 0.5 | 0.8 | 0.4 | 0.75 |
| 5 | 0.5 | 1.6 | 0.8 | 1.55 |
| 6 | 0.5 | 3.2 | 1.6 | 3.15 |
| 7 | 0.5 | 6.4 | 3.2 | 6.35 |
| 8 | 5 | 1.2 | 6 | 12.35 |
| 9 | 5 | 2.4 | 12 | 24.35 |
| 10 | 5 | 5 | 25 | 49.35 |
| 11 | 50 | 1 | 50 | 100 |
| 12 | 50 | 2 | 100 | 200 |
| 13 | 50 | 4 | 200 | 400 |
| 14 | 50 | 8 | 400 | 800 |

The clinician should observe the patient for 30 minutes, then give full therapeutic dose by the desired route.

[a]Interval between doses is 15 minutes.

Adapted from Sullivan TJ. Drug allergy. In: Middleton E, Reed CE, Ellis EF, et al., eds. *Allergy: principles and practice,* 4th ed. St. Louis: CV Mosby, 1993:1726–1746; and Solensky R, Mendelson LM. Systemic reactions to antibiotics. *Immunol Allergy Clin North Am* 2001;21:679–697, with permission.

Table 24.6. Penicillin Intravenous Desensitization Protocol Using a Continuous Infusion Pump

| Step[a] | Penicillin (mg/mL) | Flow Rate (mL/h) | Dose Given (mg) | Cumulative Dose (mg) |
|---|---|---|---|---|
| 1 | 0.001 | 4 | 0.001 | 0.001 |
| 2 | 0.001 | 8 | 0.002 | 0.003 |
| 3 | 0.001 | 16 | 0.004 | 0.007 |
| 4 | 0.001 | 32 | 0.008 | 0.015 |
| 5 | 0.001 | 60 | 0.015 | 0.03 |
| 6 | 0.001 | 120 | 0.03 | 0.06 |
| 7 | 0.001 | 240 | 0.06 | 0.12 |
| 8 | 0.1 | 5 | 0.125 | 0.245 |
| 9 | 0.1 | 10 | 0.25 | 0.495 |
| 10 | 0.1 | 20 | 0.5 | 1 |
| 11 | 0.1 | 40 | 1 | 2 |
| 12 | 0.1 | 80 | 2 | 4 |
| 13 | 0.1 | 160 | 4 | 8 |
| 14 | 10 | 3 | 7.5 | 15 |
| 15 | 10 | 6 | 15 | 30 |
| 16 | 10 | 12 | 30 | 60 |
| 17 | 10 | 25 | 62.5 | 123 |
| 18 | 10 | 50 | 125 | 250 |
| 19 | 10 | 100 | 250 | 500 |
| 20 | 10 | 200 | 500 | 1,000 |

The clinician should observe the patient for 30 minutes, then give full therapeutic dose by the desired route.

[a]Interval between doses is 15 minutes.

Adapted from an oral presentation by Timothy Sullivan, MD, and from Solensky R, Mendelson LM. Systemic reactions to antibiotics. *Immunol Allergy Clin North Am* 2001;21:679–697, with permission.

that they prevent severe IgE-dependent reactions. Risk factors for complications during desensitization include poorly controlled chronic respiratory disease and concurrent treatment with β-adrenergic antagonists.

7. **Desensitization is transient and requires that ongoing drug exposure be maintained.** Otherwise, both skin test reactivity and clinical sensitivity may return within 48 hours after interruption of drug therapy. Long-term twice-daily oral penicillin therapy sustains desensitization between courses of parenteral therapy in individuals with cystic fibrosis or other conditions for which intermittent therapy with β-lactam antibiotics is required [14].

**L. Cross-reactivity of penicillin with other β-lactams**

1. Patients allergic to semisynthetic penicillins are often also allergic to penicillin because of the shared β-lactam ring. Thus, penicillin desensitization allows administration of other β-lactam antibiotics in most circumstances.
2. However, some patients may develop sensitivity to cephalosporins or semisynthetic penicillins without a concomitant allergy to penicillin. This unique sensitivity is presumably due to IgE antibodies specific for the side-chain antigenic determinants that distinguish these antibiotics from penicillin [81].
   - **a.** The side chains of cephalothin, cephaloridine, and cefamandole are similar to the penicillin side chain [82].
   - **b.** Cefadroxil has a side chain identical to amoxicillin, and cephalexin has the same side chain as ampicillin [83].
3. Penicillin skin testing may not identify patients with such unique sensitivities. Therefore, some investigators routinely use amoxicillin and ampicillin testing in all studies of penicillin-allergic patients for this reason. However, skin testing and desensitization with nonpenicillin β-lactams remain experimental since their haptenic determinants are unknown [83].
4. Rarely, selective immunologic reactions to clavulanic acid have also been reported [85]. This diagnosis should be considered when a patient has negative skin test results for both penicillin and amoxicillin after experiencing an immediate hypersensitivity drug reaction attributed to amoxicillin-clavulanic acid.
5. Clinical immunologic cross-reactivity is high between penicillin and the carbapenems (e.g., imipenem), less to cephalosporins, and least to monobactams (e.g., aztreonam).
   - **a.** Aztreonam cross-reacts minimally with most other β-lactam antibiotics, but its clinical spectrum is limited to the treatment of aerobic gram-negative bacilli.
   - **b.** Ceftazidime has the same side chain as aztreonam, but it is not known whether this structural similarity results in greater cross-reactivity between the two antibiotics [83].
6. Although, the data are contradictory, several studies suggest that patients with histories of penicillin allergy, regardless of skin test results, should be given other β-lactam antibiotics with caution, preferably under medical supervision by personnel prepared to treat anaphylaxis. For example:
   - **a.** Early cephalosporin antibiotic preparations contained trace amounts of penicillin, possibly leading early studies to overestimate the degree of cross-reactivity between cephalosporins and penicillin [86].
   - **b.** Current estimates of immunologic cross-reactivity between penicillin and cephalosporins range from 10% for first-generation cephalosporins to 1% to 3% for third-generation cephalosporins [87]. In one study, none of 120 history-positive patients with negative penicillin skin test results reacted to semisynthetic penicillinase-resistant agents, and about 2% of patients with positive penicillin skin test results had allergic reactions when treated with a cephalosporin [86]. Similarly, when 41 patients with penicillin allergy confirmed by skin test and/or provocation test were challenged with cefazolin, cefuroxime, and ceftriaxone, all agents without the penicillin side chain, and none reacted [84]. Eight (38%) of 21 subjects with selective response to amoxicillin had positive responses to cefadroxil, a cephalosporin with the same side chain as amoxicillin [88].
   - **c.** Conversely, 26 (87%) of 30 subjects with immediate allergic reactions to injectable cephalosporins displayed skin test and RAST reactivity to penicillin

Table 24.7. Intravenous Desensitization for Ceftazidime

| Step[a] | Ceftazidime (mg/L) | Flow Rate (mL/h) | Dose Given (mg) | Cumulative Dose (mg) |
|---|---|---|---|---|
| Day 1 | | | | |
| 1 | 100 | 1 | 0.025 | 0.025 |
| 2 | 100 | 2 | 0.05 | 0.075 |
| 3 | 100 | 3 | 0.1 | 0.175 |
| 4 | 100 | 6 | 0.2 | 0.375 |
| 5 | 100 | 12 | 0.4 | 0.775 |
| 6 | 100 | 25 | 0.83 | 1.63 |
| 7 | 100 | 50 | 1.66 | 3.3 |
| 8 | 100 | 100 | 2.5 | 5.8 |
| 9 | 1,000 | 25 | 6 | 11.8 |
| 10 | 1,000 | 50 | 12 | 23.8 |
| 11 | 1,000 | 100 | 25 | 48.8 |
| 12 | 1,000 | 200 | 50 | 98.8 |
| 13 | 1,000 | 400 | 100 | 198.8 |
| 14 | 1,000 | 600[b] | 307 | 505.8 |
| Day 2 | | | | |
| 1 | 2,000 | 1 | 0.5 | 0.5 |
| 2 | 2,000 | 2 | 1 | 1.5 |
| 3 | 2,000 | 3 | 2 | 3.5 |
| 4 | 2,000 | 6 | 4 | 7.5 |
| 5 | 2,000 | 12 | 8 | 15.5 |
| 6 | 2,000 | 25 | 16.5 | 32 |
| 7 | 2,000 | 50 | 32.3 | 64 |
| 8 | 2,000 | 100 | 50 | 114 |
| 9 | 2,000 | 200 | 100 | 214 |
| 10 | 2,000 | 400 | 200 | 414 |
| 11 | 2,000 | 600[b] | 586 | 1,000 |

[a]Interval between doses is 15 minutes.
[b]Until infusion has completed.
Adapted from Ghosal S, Taylor CJ. Intravenous desensitization to ceftazidime in cystic fibrosis patients. *J Antimicrob Chemother* 1997;39:556–557, with permission.

determinants and skin test positivity to cephalosporins. Fifteen (58%) reacted to the culprit cephalosporin alone [89].

**d.** These data must be interpreted with the recognition that skin tests with native cephalosporin have little predictive value [83].

**7.** Desensitization with cephalosporins remains experimental because their haptenic determinants are unknown. An intravenous desensitization protocol for ceftazidime is shown in Table 24.7 [90].

## II. Sulfonamides

**A.** Sulfonamide antibiotics possess *p*-aminobenzoic acid rings that are structurally similar to thiazide diuretics, furosemide, sulfonylurea oral hypoglycemic agents, chlorthalidone, and diazoxide. However, case reports of clinical cross-reactivity are rare [91].

**1.** Sulfonamides are metabolized primarily by hepatic *N*-acetylation and secondarily by cytochrome P-450–catalyzed *N*-oxidation.

**2.** Slow acetylators are more prone to generate metabolites with reactive oxygen species from sulfonamides. If glutathione reductase does not detoxify these metabolites, they also react efficiently with tissue proteins to produce hapten–carrier complexes [92].

**3.** The resulting clinical reactions are diverse. For instance, sulfamethoxazole alone may cause more than 20 types of reactions (Table 24.8) [93].

Table 24.8. Adverse Reactions to Sulfonamides

| | |
|---|---|
| Anaphylaxis | Hypersensitivity vasculitis |
| Aphthous stomatitis | Lichenoid eruption |
| Bullous eruption | Photodermatitis |
| Drug-associated lupus erythematosus | Pruritus |
| Erythema multiforme/Stevens-Johnson syndrome | Psoriasis |
| Erythema nodosum | Pustular eruption |
| Erythroderma | Serum sickness–like reaction |
| Exanthem | Sweet syndrome |
| Exfoliative dermatitis | Toxic epidermal necrolysis |
| Fixed drug eruption | Urticaria/angioedema |
| Generalized erythema | |

Modified from Gruchalla RS. Diagnosis of allergic reactions to sulfonamides. *Allergy* 1999;54(suppl 58): 28–32, with permission.

4. Rarely, immunologic reactivity to the TMP component of TMP-SMX causes clinical reactions. Three different epitopes have been identified on the TMP molecule: the entire TMP molecule, the 3,4-dimethoxybenzyl group, and the 2,4-diamino-5-(3,4-dimethoxybenzyl) pyrimidine group [94].
5. **Reactions in HIV-infected patients.** Adverse reactions to sulfonamides, dapsone, rifampin, and other drugs metabolized by hepatic *N*-acetylation occur 10 to 50 times more frequently in HIV-infected patients than in the general population [51,95].
   a. The most commonly observed reaction is a maculopapular rash that occurs in more than 3% of all sulfonamide recipients and in more than 50% of HIV-infected individuals. This reaction is more likely to occur in HIV-infected patients during high-dose induction therapy for *Pneumocystis carinii* pneumonia infection. Many patients, however, will tolerate a lower prophylactic dose of TMP-SMX after a short drug holiday. This suggests that the adverse reaction is due to a toxic metabolite and not true allergy.
   b. For unknown reasons, HIV-infected patients have decreased levels of glutathione reductase. More than 90% of HIV-infected patients treated with sulfonamides generate IgE or IgG antibodies to the $N_4$-sulfonamidoyl determinant; this may explain the frequently observed clinical features of both immunologic and toxic reactions.
6. **Approach to the patient who is sensitive to TMP-SMX**
   a. The combination of TMP and SMX is the preferred antibiotic regimen for both prophylaxis and treatment of *Pneumocystis carinii* infections in immunocompromised individuals. Because no reliable skin test or **in vitro** test is available, oral provocative dose challenge-desensitization protocols have been suggested, particularly where the nature of the previous reaction is uncertain. **Previous blistering reactions and aplastic anemia after administration of sulfa compounds are contraindications for these protocols.**
   b. A recommended test dose challenge and desensitization protocol begins with the administration of 1% of the full dose on day 1, 10% on day 2, 30% on day 3, and a full therapeutic dose on day 4 [48].
   c. More rapid oral or intravenous dosing may be attempted when the need for drug administration is urgent. TMP-SMX has been given intravenously at 20-minute intervals in doses of 0.8, 7.2, 40, 80, 400, and 680 mg of the SMX component [96]. An 8-hour protocol for TMP-SMX desensitization has been used successfully in seven of nine patients [97].
   d. A slower 10-day protocol may be used for less urgent circumstances or for any desensitization failures encountered while using the accelerated protocol (Table 24.9) [98].

Table 24.9. Ten-Day Challenge/Desensitization for Trimethoprim-Sulfamethoxazole (TMP-SMX)

| Day | Dose Administered | TMP-SMX Concentration (mg) |
|---|---|---|
| 1 | 1 mL of 1:20 vol/vol pediatric suspension | 0.4 mg/2 mg |
| 2 | 2 mL of 1:20 vol/vol pediatric suspension | 0.8 mg/4 mg |
| 3 | 4 mL of 1:20 vol/vol pediatric suspension | 1.6 mg/8 mg |
| 4 | 8 mL of 1:20 vol/vol pediatric suspension | 3.2 mg/16 mg |
| 5 | 1 mL of undiluted pediatric suspension | 8 mg/40 mg |
| 6 | 2 mL of undiluted pediatric suspension | 16 mg/80 mg |
| 7 | 4 mL of undiluted pediatric suspension | 32 mg/160 mg |
| 8 | 8 mL of undiluted pediatric suspension | 64 mg/320 mg |
| 9 | 1 single-strength tablet | 80 mg/400 mg |
| 10 | 1 double-strength tablet | 160 mg/800 mg |

Thereafter, TMP-SMX two double-strength tablets daily for isopsoriasis therapy or one tablet every Monday, Wednesday, and Friday for *Pneumocystis carinii* prophylaxis.
Modified from Absar N, Daneshvar H, Beall G. Desensitization to trimethoprim/sulfamethoxazole in HIV-infected patients. *J Allergy Clin Immunol* 1994;93:1001–1004, with permission.

**e.** Administration of corticosteroids and antihistamines may permit a patient to complete the recommended doses if febrile or a nonblistering cutaneous reaction develops during the desensitization process.

**f.** Desensitization is not risk free. Potential dangers include the development of Stevens-Johnson syndrome, exfoliative dermatitis, status asthmaticus, profound neutropenia, drug-induced hepatitis, or anaphylaxis [99,100].

**III. Vancomycin**

**A.** Vancomycin (Vancocin) may cause "red man syndrome," a dose-dependent reaction to vancomycin that is characterized by generalized erythema, pruritus, and a diffuse burning sensation. Vancomycin directly stimulates cutaneous mast cells to release histamine and other mediators. Decreasing the rate of the vancomycin infusion will reduce or prevent symptoms for most affected patients.

**B.** Desensitization protocols are available for the rare IgE-mediated, anaphylactic reactions [101–106].

**IV. Quinolones**

**A.** Approximately 50% of systemic reactions to ciprofloxacin are manifested after the first dose, and fatalities may occur [107].

1. A similar risk pertains to other quinolones, such as levofloxacin (package insert, Levaquin [levofloxacin] tablets/injection, Ortho-McNeil Pharmaceutical, Raritan, NJ; revised November 2000).
2. Ciprofloxacin, like vancomycin, directly degranulates mast cells to release histamine and other mediators.
3. Successful desensitization for IgE-dependent reactions to ciprofloxacin and levofloxacin has been reported [108–110].
4. The limited data available suggest that patients with allergic reactions to one quinolone are at high risk for reactions to other drugs of the same class.

## EDUCATION AND REPORTING OF ADRs

**I. Education is essential to risk reduction** in patients who have experienced ADRs. Patients with a history of life-threatening reactions should wear a medical warning bracelet or neck chain and carry epinephrine syringes for self-administration if they are at high risk for inadvertent exposure, as might occur in agriculture or industry. Since one study has reported that many subjects receive improper or no instructions on how to self-administer epinephrine, demonstration of proper technique with a placebo trainer is recommended.

**II. Surveillance.** The FDA maintains a surveillance system for ADRs. Physicians who observe an ADR should contact either the pharmaceutical manufacturer or the Office of Epidemiology and Biostatistics (HFN-700), Center for Drug Evaluation and Research, FDA, Parklawn Building, Rockville, MD 20857. The FDA MEDWatch may be contacted at 1-800-FDA-1088 (*www.fda.gov/medwatch/index.html*). The United States Pharmacopeia has also developed MedMARx, an anonymous, Internet-accessible, nationwide service for hospitals to report preventable adverse drug events and reactions [111].

## REFERENCES


1. Lazarou J, Pomeranz BH, Corey PN. Incidence of adverse drug reactions in hospitalized patients: a meta-analysis of prospective studies. *JAMA* 1998;279:1200–1205.
2. Chyka PA. How many deaths occur annually from adverse drug reactions in the United States? *Am J Med* 2000;109:122–130.
3. Ross SD. Drug-related adverse events: a reader's guide to assessing literature reviews and meta-analyses. *Arch Intern Med* 2001;161:1041–1046.
4. Classen DC, Pestotnik SL, Evans FS, et al. Computerized surveillance of adverse drug events in hospital patients. *JAMA* 1989;266:2847–2852.
5. Moore TJ, Psaty BM, Furberg CD. Time to act on drug safety. *JAMA* 1998;279:1571–1573.
6. Borda IT, Slone D, Jick H. Assessment of adverse reactions within a drug surveillance program. *JAMA* 1968;205:645–647.
7. DeSwarte RD, Patterson R. Drug allergy. In: Patterson R, Grammer LC, Greenberger PA, eds. *Allergic diseases. Diagnosis and management,* 5th ed. Philadelphia: Lippincott-Raven, 1997:317–412.
8. Lesar TS, Lomaestro BM, Pohl H. Medication-prescribing errors in a teaching hospital: a 9-year experience. *Arch Intern Med* 1997;157:1569–1576.
9. Coombs RRA, Gell PGH. Classification of allergic reactions responsible for clinical hypersensitivity and disease. In: Gell PGH, Coombs RRA, Lachmann PJ, eds. *Clinical aspects of immunology,* 3rd ed. Oxford: Blackwell Scientific, 1975:761–781.
10. Sell S. Immunopathology. In: Rich RR, Fleisher TA, Schwartz BD, et al., eds. *Clinical immunology: principles and practice.* St. Louis: CV Mosby, 1996:449–477.
11. Rawlins MD, Thompson W. Mechanisms of adverse drug reactions. In: Davies DM, ed. *Textbook of adverse drug reactions.* New York: Oxford University Press, 1991:18–45.
12. Parker CW, Kern M, Eisen HN. Polyfunctional dinitrophenol haptens as reagents for elicitation of immediate type allergic skin responses. *J Exp Med* 1962;115:789–801.
13. deShazo RD, Kemp SF. Allergic reactions to drugs and biological agents. *JAMA* 1997;278:1895–1906.
14. Stark BJ, Earl HS, Gross GN, et al. Acute and chronic desensitization of penicillin-allergic patients using oral penicillin. *J Allergy Clin Immunol* 1987;79:523–532.
15. Adkinson NF. Risk factors for drug allergy. *J Allergy Clin Immunol* 1984;74:567–572.
16. Attaway NJ, Jasin HM, Sullivan TJ. Familial drug allergy [Abstract]. *J Allergy Clin Immunol* 1991;87:227.
17. Kurtz KM, Beatty TL, Adkinson NF. Evidence for familial aggregation of immunologic drug reactions. *J Allergy Clin Immunol* 2000;105:184–185.
18. Gadde J, Spence M, Wheeler B, et al. Clinical experience with penicillin skin testing in a large inner-city STD clinic. *JAMA* 1993;270:2456–2463.
19. Sullivan TJ, Ong RC, Gilliam LK. Studies of the multiple drug allergy syndrome [Abstract]. *J Allergy Clin Immunol* 1989;83:270.
20. Kamada MM, Twarog F, Leung DYM. Multiple antibiotic sensitivity in a pediatric population. *Allergy Proc* 1991;12:347–350.
21. Khoury L, Warrington R. The multiple drug allergy syndrome: a matched-control retrospective study in patients allergic to penicillin. *J Allergy Clin Immunol* 1996:98:462–464.
22. Becker LC. Allergy in systemic lupus erythematosus. *Johns Hopkins Med J* 1973;133: 38–44.
23. Petri M, Allbritton J. Antibiotic allergy in systemic lupus erythematosus: a case-control study. *J Rheumatol* 1992;19:265–269.

24. Roujeau JC, Stern RS. Severe adverse cutaneous reactions to drugs. *N Engl J Med* 1994;331:1272–1285.
25. Kemp SF. Anaphylaxis: current concepts in pathophysiology, diagnosis, and management. *Immunol Allergy Clin North Am* 2001;21:611–634.
26. Rasmussen JE. Erythema multiforme: should anyone care about the standards of care? *Arch Dermatol* 1995;131:726–729.
27. Patterson R, Tripathi A. Stevens-Johnson syndrome: getting ready for the year 2000 and beyond. *Ann Allergy Asthma Immunol* 1999;83:339–340.
28. Patterson R, Miller M, Kaplan M, et al. The effectiveness of early therapy with corticosteroids in Stevens-Johnson syndrome: experience with 41 cases and a hypothesis regarding pathogenesis. *Ann Allergy Asthma Immunol* 1994;73:27–34.
29. Cheriyan S, Patterson R, Greenberger PA, et al. The outcome of Stevens-Johnson syndrome treated with corticosteroids. *Allergy Proc* 1995;16:151–155.
30. Tripathi A, Ditto AM, Grammer LC, et al. Corticosteroid therapy in an additional 13 cases of Stevens-Johnson syndrome: a total series of 67 cases. *Allergy Asthma Proc* 2000;21:101–105.
31. Roujeau JC, Kelly JP, Naldi L, et al. Medication use and the risk of Stevens-Johnson syndrome or toxic epidermal necrolysis. *N Engl J Med* 1995;333:1600–1607.
32. Viard I, Wehrti P, Bullani R, et al. Inhibition of toxic epidermal necrolysis by blockage of CD 95 with human intravenous immunoglobulin. *Science* 1998;282:490–493.
33. Hertl M, Bohlen H, Jugert F, et al. Predominance of epidermal $CD8^+$ T lymphocytes in bullous cutaneous reactions caused by β-lactam antibiotics. *J Invest Dermatol* 1993;101:794–799.
34. Barbaud AM, Béné MC, Schmutz JL, et al. Role of delayed cellular hypersensitivity and adhesion molecules in amoxicillin-induced morbilliform rashes. *Arch Dermatology* 1997;133:481–486.
35. Hertl M, Merck HF. Lymphocyte activation in cutaneous drug reactions. *J Invest Dermatol* 1995;105(suppl):95–98.
36. Romagnani S. Lymphokine production by human T cells in disease states. *Annu Rev Immunol* 1994;12:227–257.
37. Correia O, Delgado L, Ramos JP, et al. Cutaneous T-cell recruitment in toxic epidermal necrolysis: further evidence of $CD8^+$ lymphocyte involvement. *Arch Dermatol* 1993;129:626–628.
38. Terrados S, Blanca M, Garcia J. Nonimmediate reactions to betalactams: prevalence and role of the different penicillins. *Allergy* 1995;50:563–567.
39. Schnyder B, Pichler WJ. Skin and laboratory tests in amoxicillin- and penicillin-induced morbilliform skin eruption. *Clin Exp Allergy* 2000;30:590–595.
40. Romano A, Quaratino D, DiFonso M, et al. A diagnostic protocol for evaluating nonimmediate reactions to aminopenicillins. *J Allergy Clin Immunol* 1999;103:1186–1190.
41. Patriarca G, D'Ambrosio C, Schiavino D, et al. Clinical usefulness of patch and challenge tests in the diagnosis of cell-mediated allergy to betalactams. *Ann Allergy Asthma Immunol* 1999;83:257–266.
42. Podevin P, Broar M. Drug-induced "allergic hepatitis." *Clin Rev Allergy Immunol* 1995;13:223–244.
43. Lee WM. Drug-induced hepatotoxicity. *N Engl J Med* 1995;333:1118–1127.
44. Levine LR. Quantitative comparison of adverse reactions to cefaclor vs. amoxicillin in a surveillance study. *Pediatr Infect Dis J* 1985;4:358–361.
45. Parra FM, Igea JM, Martin JA, et al. Serum sickness-like syndrome associated with cefaclor therapy. *Allergy* 1992;47:439–440.
46. Kearns GL, Wheeler JG, Childress SH, et al. Serum sickness-like reactions to cefaclor: role of hepatic metabolism and individual susceptibility. *J Pediatr* 1994;125:805–811.
47. Mackowiak PA, LeMaistre CF. Drug fever: a critical appraisal of conventional concepts. *Ann Intern Med* 1987;106:728–733.
48. Patterson R, DeSwarte RD, Greenberger PA, et al. *Drug allergy and protocols for management of drug allergies,* 2nd ed. Providence, RI: OceanSide, 1995.
49. Joint Task Force on Practice Parameters, American Academy of Allergy, Asthma and Immunology, Joint Council of Allergy, Asthma and Immunology. Disease management of drug hypersensitivity: a practice parameter. *Ann Allergy Asthma Immunol* 1999;83:665–700.

50. Greenberger PA. Drug challenge and desensitization protocols. *Immunol Allergy Clin North Am* 1998;18:759–772.
51. Beall G, Sanwo M, Hussain H. Drug reactions and desensitization in AIDS. *Immunol Allergy Clin North Am* 1997;17:319–337.
52. Marshall GD Jr, Lieberman PL. Determining allergic versus nonallergic drug reactions. In: Kemp SF, Lockey RF, eds. *Diagnostic testing of allergic disease.* New York: Marcel Dekker, 2000:217–232.
53. Yates AB, deShazo RD. Drug allergies and hypersensitivity. In: Rich RR, Fleisher TA, Shearer WT, et al. *Clinical immunology: principles and practice,* 2nd ed. Philadelphia: Mosby-Year Book, 2001:54.1–54.15.
54. Salkind AR, Cuddy PG, Foxworth JW. Is this patient allergic to penicillin? An evidence-based analysis of the likelihood of penicillin allergy. *JAMA* 2001;285:2498–2505.
55. Idsoe O, Guthe T, Willcox RR, et al. Nature and extent of penicillin side-reactions, with particular reference to fatalities from anaphylactic shock. *Bull WHO* 1968;38:159–188.
56. Markowitz M, Lue HC. Allergic reactions in rheumatic fever patients on long-term benzathine penicillin G: the role of skin testing for penicillin allergy. *Pediatrics* 1996;97:981–983.
57. Napoli DC, Neeno TA. Anaphylaxis to benzathine penicillin G. *Pediatric Asthma Allergy Immunol* 2000;14:329–332.
58. Sullivan TJ, Wedner HJ, Schatz GS, et al. Skin testing to detect penicillin allergy. *J Allergy Clin Immunol* 1981;68:171–180.
59. Blanca M, Torres MJ, Garcia JJ, et al. Natural evolution of skin test sensitivity in patients allergic to beta-lactam antibiotics. *J Allergy Clin Immunol* 1999;103:918–924.
60. Solensky R, Earl HS, Gruchalla RS. Penicillin allergy: prevalence of vague history in skin test-positive patients. *Ann Allergy Asthma Immunol* 2000;85:195–199.
61. Baldo B, Pham NH. Detection and side-chain specificity of IgE antibodies to flucloxacillin in allergic subjects. *J Mol Recognition* 1995;8:1–7.
62. Blanca M, Vega JM, Garcia J, et al. New aspects of allergic reactions to betalactams: cross-reactions and unique specificities. *Clin Exp Allergy* 1994;24:407–415.
63. Torres MJ, Mayorga C, Pamies R, et al. Immunologic response to different determinants of benzylpenicillin, amoxicillin, and ampicillin. Comparison between urticaria and anaphylactic shock. *Allergy* 1999;54:936–943.
64. Macy E, Richter PK, Falkoff R, et al. Skin testing with penicilloate and penilloate prepared by an improved method: amoxicillin oral challenge in patients with negative skin test responses to penicillin reagents. *J Allergy Clin Immunol* 1997;100:586–591.
65. Lin RY. A perspective on penicillin allergy. *Arch Intern Med* 1992;152:930–937.
66. Sogn DD, Evans R III, Shepherd GM, et al. Results of NIAID collaborative clinical trial to test the predictive value of skin testing with major and minor penicillin derivatives in hospitalized adults. *Arch Intern Med* 1992;152:1025–1032.
67. Solensky R, Mendelson LM. Systemic reactions to antibiotics. *Immunol Allergy Clin North Am* 2001;21:679–697.
68. Mendelson LM. Adverse reactions to $\beta$-lactam antibiotics. *Immunol Allergy Clin North Am* 1998;18:745–757.
69. Weiss ME, Adkinson NF. Diagnostic testing for drug hypersensitivity. *Immunol Allergy Clin North Am* 1998;18:731–744.
70. Valyasevi MA, Van Dellen RG. Frequency of systemic reactions to penicillin skin tests. *Ann Allergy Asthma Immunol* 2000;85:363–365.
71. Macy E. Patterns of reactivity and adverse reactions associated with penicillin skin testing in 852 patients [Abstract]. *J Allergy Clin Immunol* 1999;103(suppl):64.
72. Pichichero ME, Pichichero DM. Diagnosis of penicillin, amoxicillin, and cephalosporin allergy: reliability of examination assessed by skin testing and oral challenge. *J Pediatr* 1998;132:137–143.
73. Sullivan TJ. Drug allergy. In: Middleton E, Reed CE, Ellis EF, et al., eds. *Allergy: principles and practice,* 4th ed. St. Louis, MO: Mosby-Year Book, 1993:1726–1746.
74. Solensky R, Earl HS, Gruchalla RS. Penicillin resensitization in patients with a history of penicillin allergy [Abstract]. *J Allergy Clin Immunol* 2000;105(suppl):272.
75. Blanca M, Torres MJ, Mayorga C, et al. *In vitro* methods for quantifying IgE antibodies to betalactams. *Allergy* 1999;54(suppl 58):8–12.

76. Blanca M, Vega JM, Garcia J, et al. Allergy to penicillin with good tolerance to other penicillins: study of the incidence in subjects allergic to betalactams. *Clin Exp Allergy* 1990;20:475–481.
77. Luque I, Leyva L, Torres MJ, et al. *In vitro* T-cell responses to $\beta$-lactam drugs in immediate and nonimmediate allergic reactions. *Allergy* 2001;56:611–618.
78. Nyfeler B, Pichler WJ. The lymphocyte transformation test for the diagnosis of drug allergy: sensitivity and specificity. *Clin Exp Allergy* 1997;27:175–181.
79. Sullivan TJ. Antigen-specific desensitization to prevent allergic reactions to drugs. *Ann Allergy* 1994;73:375–377.
80. Naclerio R, Mizrahi EA, Adkinson NF. Immunologic observations during desensitization and maintenance of clinical tolerance to penicillin. *J Allergy Clin Immunol* 1987;79:523–532.
81. Atkinson TP, Kaliner MA. Anaphylaxis. *Med Clin North Am* 1992;76:841–855.
82. Batchelor FR, Dewdney JM, Weston RD, et al. The immunogenicity of cephalosporin derivatives and their cross-reaction with penicillin. *Immunology* 1966;10:21–33.
83. Kelkar PS, Li JT-C. Cephalosporin allergy. *N Engl J Med* 2001;345:804–808.
84. Novalbos A, Sastre J, Cuesta J, et al. Lack of allergic cross-reactivity to cephalosporins among patients allergic to penicillins. *Clin Exp Allergy J* 2001;31:438–443.
85. Fernandez-Rivas M, Carral CP, Cuevas M, et al. Selective allergic reactions to clavulanic acid. *J Allergy Clin Immunol* 1995;95:748–750.
86. Saxon A, Beall GN, Rohr AS, et al. Immediate hypersensitivity reactions to beta-lactam antibiotics. *Ann Intern Med* 1987;107:204–215.
87. Anné S, Reisman RE. Risk of administering cephalosporin antibiotics to patients with histories of penicillin allergy. *Ann Allergy Asthma Immunol* 1995;74:167–170.
88. Miranda A, Blanca M, Vega JM, et al. Cross-reactivity between a penicillin and a cephalosporin with the same side chain. *J Allergy Clin Immunol* 1996;98:671–677.
89. Romano A, Mayorga C, Torres MJ, et al. Immediate allergic reactions to cephalosporins: cross-reactivity and selective responses. *J Allergy Clin Immunol* 2000;106:1177–1183.
90. Ghosal S, Taylor CJ. Intravenous desensitization to ceftazidime in cystic fibrosis patients. *J Antimicrob Chemother* 1997;39:556–557.
91. Shapiro LE, Knowles SR, Shear NH. Sulfonamide allergies—management in the nineties. *Allergy Clin Immunol Int* 1996;8:5–12.
92. Meekins CV, Sullivan TJ, Gruchalla RS. Immunochemical analysis of sulfonamide drug allergy: identification of sulfamethoxazole-substituted human serum proteins. *J Allergy Clin Immunol* 1994;94:1017–1024.
93. Gruchalla RS. Diagnosis of allergic reactions to sulfonamides. *Allergy* 1999;54(suppl 58):28–32.
94. Pham NH, Baldo BA, Manfredi M, et al. Fine structural specificity differences of trimethoprim allergenic determinants. *Clin Exp Allergy* 1996;26:1155–1160.
95. Coopman SA, Johnson RA, Platt R, et al. Cutaneous disease and drug reactions in HIV infection. *N Engl J Med* 1993;328:1670–1674.
96. Greenberger PA, Patterson R. Management of drug allergy in patients with acquired immunodeficiency syndrome. *J Allergy Clin Immunol* 1987;79:484–88.
97. Moreno JN, Poblete RB, Maggio C, et al. Rapid oral desensitization for sulfonamides in patients with the acquired immunodeficiency syndrome. *Ann Allergy Asthma Immunol* 1995;74:140–146.
98. Absar N, Daneshvar H, Beall G. Desensitization to trimethoprim/sulfamethoxazole in HIV-infected patients. *J Allergy Clin Immunol* 1994;93:1001–1004.
99. Greenberger PA. Desensitization and test-dosing for the drug-allergic patient. *Ann Allergy Asthma Immunol* 2000;85:250–251.
100. Sher MR, Suchar C, Lockey RF. Anaphylactic shock induced by oral desensitization to trimethoprim/sulfamethoxazole (TMP-SMX). *J Allergy Clin Immunol* 1986;77:133.
101. Anné S, Middleton E Jr, Reisman RE. Vancomycin anaphylaxis and successful desensitization. *Ann Allergy Asthma Immunol* 1994;73:402–404.
102. Chopra N, Oppenheimer J, Derimanov GS, et al. Vancomycin anaphylaxis and successful desensitization in a patient with end stage renal disease on hemodialysis by maintaining steady antibiotic levels. *Ann Allergy Asthma Immunol* 2000;84:633–635.
103. Lin RY. Desensitization in the management of vancomycin hypersensitivity. *Arch Intern Med* 1990;150:2197–2198.

104. Sorensen SJ, Wise SL, al-Tawfiq JA, et al. Successful vancomycin desensitization in a patient with end-stage renal disease and anaphylactic shock to vancomycin. *Ann Pharmacother* 1998;32:1020–1023.
105. Villavicencio AT, Hey LA, Patel D, et al. Acute cardiac and pulmonary arrest after infusion of vancomycin with subsequent desensitization. *J Allergy Clin Immunol* 1997;100:853–854.
106. Wong JT, Ripple RE, MacLean JA, et al. Vancomycin hypersensitivity: synergism with narcotics and "desensitization" by a rapid continuous intravenous protocol. *J Allergy Clin Immunol* 1994;94:189–194.
107. Landor M, Lashinsky A, Waxman J. Quinolone allergy? *Ann Allergy Asthma Immunology* 1996;77:273–276.
108. Gea-Banacloche JC, Metcalfe DD. Ciprofloxacin desensitization. *J Allergy Clin Immunol* 1996;97:1426–1427.
109. Lantner RR. Ciprofloxacin desensitization in a patient with cystic fibrosis. *J Allergy Clin Immunol* 1995;96:1001–1002.
110. Nelson MR, Loesevitz AW, Engler RJM. Emergent levofloxacin desensitization in acute myelogenous leukemia [Abstract]. *J Allergy Clin Immunol* 2001;107(suppl):5.
111. Cousins DD. Developing a uniform reporting system for preventable adverse drug events. *Clin Ther* 1998;20(suppl C):45–58.

# 25. MICROBIOLOGY LABORATORY TESTS

Paul S. Graman and Marilyn A. Menegus

## DIAGNOSTIC LABORATORY TESTS

### *Smear and Stain Techniques*

The most direct, rapid, and technically least restricted tests are the microscopic examination of stained and unstained smears of material from the site of infection. Direct microscopic evaluation can provide immediate data in such life-threatening illnesses as pneumonia and meningitis. Isolation of the potential etiologic agent may otherwise take hours to days (bacteria) or weeks (mycobacteria and fungi). Sometimes, as in malaria and other parasitic diseases, culture cannot be done [1].

**I. Gram stain**

**A.** Differential staining is based on cell wall lipid content and the cell wall's decreased permeability to organic solvents. Gram-positive organisms stain purple from the retained crystal violet–iodine complex, whereas gram-negative organisms do not retain this complex and stain red owing to a counterstain.

**B. Uses**

1. **Diagnostic aid.** Gram stains can help one make a clinical diagnosis by providing clues to the etiologic agent involved in an infection, which in turn will help one choose the appropriate antibiotic while awaiting culture results. (See Chapter 27A.)
2. **Adequacy of specimens** of culture material can be determined. When large numbers of epithelial cells (>10/low magnification field, ×10 objective) are present, it is likely that the sputum sample has been collected improperly and that cultures may contain colonizing species. Many laboratories will not culture these sputum samples.
3. **Purulence of a specimen.** Although many polymorphonuclear cells are more likely to be seen in infected, versus colonized, sputum specimens (see Chapter 11), their absence does not exclude an acute bacterial infection (e.g., in leukopenic patients).
4. **Quantitation of bacteria.** When one or more organisms per oil immersion field are seen on a Gram stain of a drop of fresh, unspun bodily fluid such as urine, the culture usually grows more than $10^5$ organisms per milliliter. This amount is required to cause disease.

**C. Technique of preparation**

1. The clinician should make a **thin smear** of the clinical specimen on a clean glass slide.
   - a. **Body fluids.** Cerebrospinal fluid (CSF), joint fluid, pleural fluid, and so forth can be applied directly to the slide or centrifuged (or cytocentrifuged) to concentrate the organisms. For CSF, greater sensitivity can be achieved by placing successive loops on the same spot, allowing the spot to dry between additions.
   - b. **Sputum.** The clinician should use purulent-appearing samples and spread the sample on the slide.
2. **The clinician should air-dry and gently heat-fix** the smear by passing the slide through a flame one or two times. *Making the slide too hot to touch causes artifacts*. Grossly bloody smears can be cleared by flooding with distilled water for 5 minutes after heat fixation.
   - a. **After cooling,** the slide may be flooded with **crystal or gentian violet** for 10 seconds and then rinsed.
   - b. **The clinician should flood the slide with Gram iodine** for 10 seconds and then rinse again. The duration of staining in the first two steps is not particularly critical.
   - c. **The clinician should decolorize** with 95% ethanol or an acetone-ethanol mixture (95% ethyl alcohol, 100 mL; acetone, 100 mL) and repeat the rinse. **Decolorization is the critical step.** Decolorization of the smear is complete when the blue stain is no longer visible and when the solvent is colorless as it runs from the slide.

Thick or purulent exudates resist decolorization. Attempts to clear all portions will result in excessive decolorization of the interpretable areas. Therefore, the clinician should decolorize only until the thin parts of the smear are colorless. Acetone-containing solvents act more rapidly than 95% ethanol. Decolorization should be performed for only 1 or 2 seconds.

d. **The clinician should counterstain** with safranin for 10 seconds, rinse, and air or blot dry.

D. **Factors affecting smear interpretation**

1. **Incomplete decolorization** results in excessive gram-positive staining, and gram-negative organisms could be read as gram positive. If the stain is inadequately decolorized, a new smear should be prepared. If the clinical sample is not available, the immersion oil should be removed with xylene and the decolorization and counterstaining steps repeated.
2. **Overdecolorization** can cause gram-positive organisms to appear gram-negative. Only gram-negative cells and bacteria are seen. The technique can be evaluated by parallel staining of a known gram-positive sample (e.g., oral secretions). A repeat smear should be made or the immersion oil should be removed with xylene and the entire staining process repeated if further specimens are unavailable.
3. **Precipitates of crystal violet are irregular in shape and more refractile but** may be misinterpreted as gram-positive cocci or fungi. They occur in the thick areas.
4. **Variations of morphologic features on Gram staining.** Gram-positive organisms may look gram negative or gram positive/gram negative (gram variable) when the organisms are old or exposed to antibiotics. Some organisms (e.g., *Acinetobacter* species and some *Bacillus* species) are naturally gram variable.
5. **Background interference.** The clinician should look carefully for small, pleomorphic, gram-negative organisms, such as *Haemophilus* species, which can easily be missed.
6. Almost any **gram-positive cocci** can appear in pairs or short chains, so a specific etiologic diagnosis is not possible. Staphylococci may appear as a single coccus.

II. **Acid-fast stains.** Organisms that stain well with carbol-fuchsin or auramine and resist decolorization with acid-alcohol are acid-fast bacilli (AFB). These include mycobacteria (which stain poorly or not at all with Gram stain) and *Nocardia* species. The initial diagnostic step for tuberculosis is to examine for AFB. Two types of acid-fast stains are available.

A. The basic fuchsin stain (**Kinyoun** or **Ziehl-Neelsen**) combined with light microscopy.

B. **Fluorochrome stains** offer the advantages of speed, greater sensitivity, and ease of observation because large areas can be examined. The most well established technique, Truant stain, uses auramine-rhodamine fluorescent dyes. Smears are examined under low power using a fluorescence microscope [2,3]. See Chapter 11 under Tuberculosis: Basic Concepts, including gastric and urine AFB smears.

C. **Application and interpretation**

1. The sensitivity of microscopy for the diagnosis of mycobacterial infection is relatively low, requiring approximately $5 \times 10^3$ bacilli per milliliter for detection. Therefore, all specimens examined by smear also should be cultured. **Whenever possible, sputum specimens should be concentrated.** Mycobacteria are recovered optimally from clinical specimens when methods that release them from cells (digestion) and reduce competing organisms (decontamination) are used. The N-acetyl-L-cysteine-sodium hydroxide method is used, and the N-acetyl-L-cysteine, a mucolytic agent, is added to digest tenacious sputum. Addition of sodium hydroxide is used for decontamination [2]. The sample can then be centrifuged and the sediment stained and cultured, with an improved yield of organisms compared with a direct stain of the patient's sputum.
2. Visible tubercle bacilli implies risk of transmission.
3. One cannot differentiate *Mycobacterium tuberculosis* from the atypical mycobacteria. However, in more than 90% of smear-positive cases, *M. tuberculosis* can be promptly identified in sputum concentrates by nucleic acid amplification (NAA)

assays. Culture followed by biochemical or probe assays takes days to weeks to complete.

4. *Nocardia* species are AFB but they retain acid-fast stains less tenaciously, so modified acid-fast stains with milder decolorization must be used to detect *Nocardia* reliably.

**III. Wet-mount preparations** of a variety of specimens can be examined microscopically for fungal, bacterial, parasitic, and other pathogens. A drop or small portion of specimen (feces, exudate, CSF, urine sediment, sputum, or scrapings) is mixed in a drop of physiologic saline on the surface of a glass slide. Coverslips prevent evaporation. A dim substage light with a ×10 or ×45 objective or dark field, depending on the organism sought, is used.

A. **Wet mounts with physiologic saline** are useful for trichomonads of the genital tract and intestinal parasites. They should be examined as soon as possible to avoid drying. Cold environments should be avoided because organisms become immobile. *Trichomonas vaginalis* appear as clear, actively motile forms, approximately the size of neutrophils in vaginal secretions, urethral discharges, or urine sediment. Cultures for *T. vaginalis* (not widely available), are more sensitive (20%–30%) than wet mounts [4]. (See Chapter 16 under Vulvovaginitis.)

B. **Potassium hydroxide** (KOH) is used primarily for identification of fungal forms.

1. **Specimens.** Cervical discharge, skin scrapings (taken with a no. 11 blade), sputum, and tissue scrapings can be examined using this technique.
2. **Method.** A drop of 10% to 20% KOH solution is mixed with the clinical specimen and allowed to stand for 10 to 15 minutes or the slide back can be gently heated. KOH lyses debris and background material, so fungal forms can be seen more easily.

C. **India ink preparations** are used to visualize the capsule of *Cryptococcus neoformans.*

1. **Technique.** Centrifuged cerebrospinal fluid or urine or exudates are mixed with a drop of India ink on a slide. A coverslip is applied and the specimen is examined when wet.
2. **Interpretation.** The mucoid capsule appears as a clear halo that surrounds the yeast cell. Mononuclear cells (especially lymphocytes) may be mistaken for *C. neoformans.* Budding forms must be seen to interpret as positive. **The latex test for polysaccharide antigen is now the preferred test because it is more sensitive** [5].

D. **Dark-field microscopy** is particularly useful in diagnosing primary syphilis. (See Chapter 16.)

**IV. Other useful staining methods.** A number of different stains are available.

A. **Giemsa and Wright stains** are available in every hematology laboratory.

1. **Malaria and babesiosis smears.** Thin smears of the patient's peripheral blood or a special malarial smear preparation (e.g., smear of platelet-depleted red blood cells [RBCs]) are suitable for screening for these intracellular parasites and eliminate many artifacts of thick smears. Platelets overlying RBCs can mimic intracellular parasites.
2. **Herpes simplex and varicella-zoster viral skin lesions** can be diagnosed by a Giemsa or Wright stain of a scraping of the periphery of the base of an unroofed vesicle. Herpetic lesions show the characteristic multinucleate giant cells and, rarely, intranuclear inclusions. Methylene blue (**Tzanck preparation**) and Papanicolaou smears are better suited to visualize nuclear detail.
3. *Pneumocystis carinii, Toxoplasma gondii, Histoplasma capsulatum,* yeast, and bacteria can be detected in **Giemsa stains of touch preparations of tissue.**

B. **Silver stains** (Gomori's methenamine silver, Warthin-Starry, and Dieterle) are difficult to perform properly and should be used only by skilled individuals. They are most useful for the detection of *Treponema pallidum,* fungi, *P. carinii, Legionella* species, rickettsiae, and *Bartonella henselae,* the organism associated with cat-scratch disease.

C. **Periodic acid-Schiff (PAS) and calcofluor white stains** are used to demonstrate fungi. PAS and Gomori methenamine silver stains often reveal fungi not well visualized by more conventional techniques (e.g., hematoxylin-eosin and Gram stain).

D. **Calcofluor** white is a nonspecific fluorochrome that binds to cellulose and chitin. The stain is useful for demonstrating fungi, *Pneumocystis,* and some parasites using a fluorescence microscope. Stained organisms fluoresce brightly against a dim background.

E. **Acridine orange,** a fluorochrome DNA stain, detects a variety of microorganisms (e.g., bacteria, fungi, and trichomonads) better than Gram stain for bacteria because organisms are seen under low power, and antibiotic-damaged organisms can still be detected [1].

F. **Methylene blue smears for fecal leukocytes** are discussed in Chapter 13.

G. **Fluorescent antibody and immunocytochemical stains** are discussed later in this chapter.

## *General Principles for Specimen Collection and Handling*

This topic has recently been reviewed in detail [6].

I. **The clinician should obtain specimens before initiating or changing antibiotic therapy.**

II. **Specimens should be collected in a manner that minimizes contamination by resident bacterial flora.**

   A. Many potential pathogens can be transient colonizers. Their isolation does not necessarily establish clinical significance. On the other hand, recovery of certain organisms such as *Neisseria gonorrhoeae* or *M. tuberculosis* is significant in any clinical specimen.

   B. Suprapubic bladder aspiration, transtracheal or percutaneous lung aspiration, and percutaneous aspiration of vesicles, bullae, or abscesses all avoid contamination.

III. **Specimens should be collected** in clean, sterile containers free of residual detergents or disinfectants. Antibacterial preservatives should be avoided (e.g., tissue aspirates). Lidocaine also has antibacterial activities that affect recovery of organisms from bronchoscopy samples. **Cotton swab collection generally is less satisfactory than syringe or catheter aspiration, which** provides sufficient material for both culture and Gram stain. Anaerobes are sensitive to atmospheric oxygen and desiccation, so special care is needed. Specimens aspirated into a syringe and air expelled can be transported or inoculated into a special oxygen-free system.

IV. **Transportation to the laboratory**

   A. **Rapid transport to the laboratory is preferable over transport media.** Except in acute settings, specimens should be collected when prompt inoculation and handling is possible. Aerobes such as *Streptococcus pneumoniae* and *Neisseria* species are fastidious and may not survive temperature extremes or drying. Long delays before inoculation can result in the growth of clinically insignificant bacterial contaminants in the specimen.

   B. **All specimens should be labeled** to avoid errors in later identification.

   C. **Clinicians should provide the laboratory with diagnostic questions** and note the source of specimen. The inoculation of highly selective media increases the probability of recovering certain organisms such as species of *Salmonella, Shigella, Campylobacter,* and *Yersinia.*

V. **Blood culture collection technique.** Strict attention to aseptic technique of skin preparation avoids contaminating blood cultures with resident skin flora (e.g., coagulase-negative staphylococci, diphtheroids, and *Propionibacterium acnes*) and decreases diagnostic confusion. Some organisms that are usually skin contaminants can be true blood-borne pathogens (e.g., catheter-related sepsis, prosthetic valve endocarditis).

   A. Technicians should wear gloves when drawing blood to reduce the risk of infection with blood-borne agents (e.g., hepatitis B, hepatitis C [HCV], and human immunodeficiency virus [HIV]).

   B. The equipment should be obtained and set up, including appropriate media, 2% tincture of iodine or povidone, alcohol swabs, tourniquet, syringe, and needles.

**C.** The caps should be removed from the culture bottles and the stopper swabbed twice with alcohol.

**D.** The venipuncture site (usually antecubital) should be selected. Starting at the puncture site, a circular area is scrubbed (radius approximately 2 inches) with povidone-iodine, using a circular motion with overlapping strokes and working toward the periphery. This is repeated once and allowed to dry. (With allergy to povidone-iodine, 70% isopropyl alcohol may be used for 1–2 minutes.)

**E.** For better visualization of the actual puncture site, povidone-iodine should be cleaned off the vein site with one or two alcohol swabs, using the same "clean-to-dirty" circular motion.

**F.** Venipuncture is carefully performed using the 10- to 20-mL syringe (for adults), taking care not to touch the needle or prepared skin site (a sterile glove may be used to palpate the site).

**G.** The needle is removed from the vein (not touching the needle to skin). For adults, **5 to 10 mL is transferred, using the maximum amount suggested by the manufacturer,** into each broth bottle, or the appropriate volume is transferred into the recommended blood culture tube.

**H.** The requisition is labeled with the **date** and **exact time of** the culture. **Blood drawn through intravascular catheters should be specifically identified.** This information is important in interpreting culture results.

## *Culture Techniques*

**I. Blood cultures** are indicated whenever there is suspected bacteremia or fungemia. In severely ill patients, blood cultures might be the only source demonstrating the causative agent.

**A. Blood culture methods.** Blood is placed into a broth medium or into an isolator tube in which the RBCs are lysed and the lysate is inoculated onto solid media [7].

**1. Broth culture bottles** are electronically monitored on a nearly continuous basis and the information gathered is analyzed using sophisticated computer algorithms to determine when growth has occurred. The majority of positive results are detected within 48 hours, but most laboratories monitor cultures for 5 days before discarding [7].

**a. Types of bacteremia.** Continuous bacteremia occurs in endocarditis and other intravascular infections. Intermittent bacteremia is the most common form and occurs in many different infections. Transient bacteremia is self-limited and often follows the manipulation of nonsterile mucosal surfaces or infected tissues [8–10].

**b. Volume of sample.** The ideal volume for broth culture is unknown. Because of the low density of most bacteremias, 10- to 20-mL samples (e.g., 5–10 mL per bottle, depending on the manufacturer's recommendation) for adults and 1- to 5-mL samples for children are recommended. A 1:5 to 1:10 dilution (or even higher [8–10]) of the blood appears to be best to reduce intrinsic serum antibacterial activity and to reduce the concentration of antimicrobials to subinhibitory levels.

**c. Timing and number of blood cultures.** Blood should be collected as soon as possible after the onset of fever or chills. **Two to three blood cultures, drawn at intervals of at least 20 minutes before antibiotics are initiated, are recommended both** because of the intermittent nature of most bacteremias and to establish continuous bacteremia [8–10]. (See discussions in Chapters 2 and 27A.)

**d. Media.** Many comparable broth media are available. Hypertonic media (usually prepared by the addition of 10% to 15% sucrose to a conventional broth media) appear to improve both the speed and overall recovery of certain organisms, especially organisms from patients being treated with antibiotics. In addition, resin devices and resin-containing media improve the recovery of organisms (staphylococci, in particular) from treated patients, but the usefulness is debated [7].

2. **Blood lysis tubes.** Two forms—one designed for centrifugation and concentration of organisms and the other, a smaller pediatric tube, from which the contents can be plated directly onto solid media—permit quantitation of organisms in blood. This may be useful to distinguish intravascular catheter-related sepsis from sepsis originating at another site (see Chapter 20). It also results in increased recovery and decreased detection time for certain microorganisms, among them dimorphic fungi, mycobacteria, and *Bartonella species* [7]. Major disadvantages include a high contamination rate, poor recovery of anaerobic organisms, and greater cost.

**B. Fastidious organisms.** Blood cultures for brucellosis, tularemia, leptospirosis, systemic fungal infections, *Bartonella henselae* (formerly *Rochalimaea henselae,* the organism believed to be responsible for cat-scratch disease [see Chapter 21]), and *Mycobacterium avium* require special media and incubation for optimal isolation. The Isolator lysis-centrifugation system (Wampole Laboratories, Cranbury, NJ) has detected *B. henselae* and *M. avium* complex. Laboratories should be alerted to these possibilities for specific recommendations regarding collection and processing of the specimens [7–10].

**II. Special methods for bacterial culture**

**A. Tissue specimens** can be cultured quantitatively or qualitatively. The former may be helpful for burns. Criteria based on the number of organisms per gram of tissue have been established for the diagnosis of burn wound sepsis. **Touch preparations** and subsequent staining for appropriate microorganisms may be helpful (e.g., rapid diagnosis of *P. carinii* pneumonia by staining of touch preparations of lung biopsy specimens).

**B. Foley catheter tips should not be submitted** because they are invariably contaminated.

**C. Intravenous catheters** are cultured qualitatively or semiquantitatively, depending on the laboratory. One technique involves rolling the catheter on **a blood** agar plate and reporting the total number of colonies of organisms grown. To interpret these results, blood cultures must be positive. Using this approach, 15 colonies or more correlate with bacteremia caused by catheter infection, whereas fewer represent extraneous contamination [11]. The optimal laboratory diagnostic method to define catheter-related sepsis has not been established. See related discussion in Chapter 20.

**D. Genital tract cultures** are more likely to yield *N. gonorrhoeae* if transported within 6 hours or if inoculated directly onto a selective medium. Special devices containing a layer of agar in a dish to which a $CO_2$-generating tablet (Jembec) is added are available.

**III. Anaerobic cultures.** Most anaerobic bacteria of clinical importance are oxygen tolerant. Nevertheless, special anaerobic containers often are recommended for specimen transport. Rapid processing is important to avoid overgrowth by facultative anaerobes [12,13].

**A. Whenever possible, specimens should be aspirated** and transported to the laboratory in the syringe used for collection or via an oxygen-free transport system.

**B. Swabs are less desirable** because of inadequate sample size, air exposure, and sample desiccation. If swabs must be used, they should be placed in an oxygen-free transport system.

**C. Sites for anaerobic culture.** Because many body sites are colonized by anaerobic organisms, only certain sites are appropriate for culture (Table 25.1).

**D. A Gram-stained smear should be performed on all specimens submitted for anaerobic culture.** Because anaerobic cultures take considerable time for processing and identification, the Gram stain can provide useful clues regarding the infecting organisms. **Anaerobes should be considered when organisms are seen on smear but do not grow on routine aerobic cultures.** The unique morphologic features of anaerobes is a clue to the experienced observer. Pale, unevenly stained, pleomorphic gram-negative rods with rounded ends and bipolar staining suggest *Bacteroides fragilis.* Broad gram-positive rods, generally without visible spores, suggest *Clostridium perfringens.* Other *Clostridium* species may be thin and gram variable, with or without spores.

Table 25.1. Sites of Culture for Anaerobic Specimens

| Appropriate Sites | Inappropriate Sites |
|---|---|
| Normally sterile bodily fluids, blood, bile; pleural, peritoneal, joint, and spinal fluid; surgical specimens from normally sterile sites | Specimens contaminated by indigenous anaerobic flora; sputum, throat swabs, fecal specimens, rectal and vaginal swabs |
| Abscess contents, deep-wound aspirates, surgical biopsy specimens | Superficial wound swabs, sites obviously contaminated by intestinal contents |
| Transtracheal or percutaneous lung aspirates | Sputum, bronchoscopy washings, nasopharyngeal or throat swabs |
| Suprapubic bladder aspirates | Voided or catheterized urine specimens |
| Culdocentesis fluid | Cervical or vaginal swabs |

**IV. Viral cultures.** Clinical differentiation of the specific infecting virus may be difficult, if not impossible (see Chapter 8). The etiology of a viral syndrome can often be established by viral culture, serologic tests, or both. Table 25.2 outlines the appropriate specimens. Rapid diagnostic tests are discussed later under Direct Detection of Microbial Antigens in Clinical Specimens.

**A. General guidelines**

1. **Specimens should be obtained from patients early in the course of illness,** when virus shedding is greatest, preferably within 3 days after the onset of symptoms.
2. Samples must be placed in viral transport media and transported promptly. Many specimens can be held at 4°C for up to 48 hours (even on wet ice) without decrease in virus recovery. For prolonged storage, specimens should be frozen at $-70$°C.
3. Samples collected on swabs (conjunctival, pharyngeal, nasopharyngeal, rectal) should be placed quickly in a liquid viral transport medium provided by the laboratory.
4. The type of specimen and clinical syndrome should be noted because different processing steps prior to attempted isolation are necessary for different types of samples.

**B. Specimen collection and transport guidelines**

1. **Blood.** Whole blood (anticoagulated with ethylenediaminetetraacetic acid [EDTA]) is used to obtain leukocytes for cytomegalovirus (CMV). Enteroviruses can be isolated from both serum and leukocytes. However, viremia usually is detected by molecular methods (e.g., HIV-1, hepatitis B and C viruses, CMV, Epstein-Barr virus, and enterovirus) [14,15].
2. **Nasal secretions.** A cotton swab on a fine wire is introduced through the anterior nares into the nasopharynx, or a cotton swab is inserted into each anterior naris and placed in a viral transport medium. **Nasal washings** (e.g., for respiratory syncytial virus [RSV]) are collected by instilling 4 to 5 mL of saline into each nostril while the patient extends his or her neck slightly and closes the posterior pharynx (by pushing against the *K* sound). The head is tilted forward, and a sample is collected in a clean container held beneath the nose.
3. **Pharynx.** A swabbing of the posterior pharynx should be accomplished by vigorously rubbing the swab over both tonsillar areas and the posterior pharyngeal wall.
4. **Vesicular fluid.** Without decontamination of overlying skin, lesion is aspirated with a small-gauge needle attached to a tuberculin syringe, or the vesicle is opened and fluids and cellular elements collected from the base onto a swab. If a crust is present, the crust should be lifted off; the fluid beneath the crust can then be swabbed.
5. **Cerebrospinal fluid.** The clinician should collect 1 to 3 mL into a sterile container.

Table 25.2. Viruses Associated with Specific Syndromes and Recommended Specimens for Viral Examination

| Syndrome | Common Agents | Less Common Agents | Source of Specimen for Viral Examination |
|---|---|---|---|
| Upper respiratory tract infection | Influenza A, B<br>Rhinovirus<br>Parainfluenza 1, 3<br>Respiratory syncytial virus<br>Adenovirus | Parainfluenza 2<br>Coxsackievirus A, B<br>Echovirus<br>Coronavirus | Nasal wash or aspirate<br>Nose or throat swab |
| Lower respiratory tract infection | | | |
| Child | Respiratory syncytial virus<br>Parainfluenza 3, 1, 2 | Adenovirus<br>Influenza B | Nasal wash or aspirate<br>Nose or throat swab |
| Adult | Influenza A, B | Adenovirus | Sputum |
| Pleurodynia | Coxsackievirus A, B | | Throat swab<br>Stool |
| Central nervous system infection | | | |
| Meningitis | Coxsackievirus A, B<br>Echovirus | HIV type 1<br>Lymphocytic choriomeningitis<br>Mumps | Cerebrospinal fluid<br>Throat swab<br>Stool |
| Encephalitis and encephalopathy | Herpes simplex virus type 1<br>HIV type 1<br>CMV | Arboviruses<br>Mumps | Cerebrospinal fluid<br>Blood, brain biopsy |
| Myocarditis and pericarditis | Coxsackievirus B | Coxsackievirus A<br>Influenza | Throat swab<br>Stool |
| Gastroenteritis | Rotavirus<br>Norwalk-like viruses | Adenovirus<br>Calicivirus<br>Astrovirus<br>Coronavirus | Stool |
| Hepatitis | Hepatitis A, B, C | | Blood |
| Urinary tract infection: acute hemorrhagic cystitis | Adenovirus 11<br>BK virus | | Urine |
| Parotitis | Mumps | | Throat swab |
| Exanthemas (nonspecific, with fever) | Coxsackievirus A9, A16<br>Echovirus 9, 16, 11 | Echovirus 1-6, 14, 18, 19<br>Coxsackievirus A (2, 4, 23)<br>Coxsackievirus B (1–5)<br>Adenovirus | Skin vesicle fluid<br>Throat swab<br>Stool |
| Herpangina | Coxsackievirus A (1–6, 8, 10, 16, 22) | Echovirus 9, 17<br>Coxsackievirus B | Skin vesicle fluid<br>Throat swab<br>Stool |
| Hand-foot-and-mouth disease | Coxsackievirus A<br>Enterovirus 71 | | Skin vesicle fluid<br>Throat swab<br>Stool |
| Nonspecific febrile illness | HIV type 1<br>CMV<br>EBV<br>Enteroviruses<br>Influenza A, B | Adenovirus | Urine (for CMV)<br>Nose and throat swab<br>Stool<br>Blood |

HIV, human immunodeficiency virus; CMV, cytomegalovirus; EBV, Epstein-Barr virus.
Adapted from Menegus MA, Douglas RG Jr. Viruses, Rickettsiae, Chlamydiae, and mycoplasmas. In Mandell GL, Douglas RG Jr, Bennett Jr, eds. *Principles and practice of infectious diseases*, 3rd ed. New York: Churchill Livingstone, 1990; with permission.

6. **Urine.** The patient provides 5 to 10 mL of a clean-catch, midstream urine into a sterile container, which is processed immediately or stored refrigerated. **Urine should never be frozen.**
7. **Feces.** A 2- to 5-g sample is placed into a clean specimen container without transport medium. A cotton tipped rectal swab (less satisfactory) is insert 5 cm into the rectum and gently rotated. In contrast to rectal cultures for the recovery of gonococci, some fecal material **should** be obtained when doing swabs for viral studies.

C. **Viruses use living cells to support their replication.** Cell cultures, rather than eggs or laboratory animals for virus isolation, are used. Specimens are inoculated and incubated at 33° to 36°C for 2 to 14 days. Periodically, the cultures are examined microscopically for evidence of viral growth. Most viruses are detected within 7 days [14,15].

V. **Mycobacterial cultures.** The major obstacle for recovering mycobacteria is the presence of large numbers of contaminating organisms. Prompt processing of individual fresh specimens is preferable to pooled samples, in which overgrowth of other microorganisms can occur.

A. **Appropriate specimens are obtained** (Table 25.3).

B. If delays are anticipated, specimens should be refrigerated at 4°C. **If gastric specimens cannot be processed promptly, they should be adjusted to pH 7** with sodium bicarbonate so that the gastric acidity will not affect the viability of the organisms.

C. Because mycobacteria may be present in low numbers, multiple large-volume specimens should be cultured when possible (sputum, fluid [CSF and pleural fluid in particular]).

D. Sterile, wide-mouth containers with fitted caps should be used. Mycobacteria sometimes adhere to wax-coated surfaces; therefore, **waxed containers should be avoided.**

E. During collection and handling, care should be taken to avoid the production of infectious aerosols. **Specimens should be labeled clearly to indicate a possible biologic hazard.**

F. *M. tuberculosis* usually grows on conventional solid media (e.g., Lowenstein-Jensen) in 2 to 4 weeks, but cultures routinely are observed for 6 to 10 weeks before being reported as negative. A radiometric system for mycobacteria has significantly shortened the time required for the recovery of *M. tuberculosis* as well as other *Mycobacterium* species [2,3].

G. Most laboratories differentiate between *M. tuberculosis* or mycobacteria other than tuberculosis (MOTT) using molecular methods or a few simple biochemical tests. This usually is accomplished within days to 1 or 2 weeks of isolation. Complete speciation of MOTT usually is done in some larger laboratories; whereas others send such isolates to reference laboratories for speciation [2,3,14]. See related discussion in Chapter 11.

H. **Nucleic acid probes.** In some laboratories, *M. tuberculosis* and *M. avium* are identified specifically through the use of commercially available nucleic acid probes [2,3]. See section **II** under Nucleic Acid Methods for the Characterization and Direct Detection of Microbial Pathogens in Clinical Specimens later in this chapter.

I. **Susceptibility tests.** Owing to the recent emergence of multidrug-resistant *M. tuberculosis,* the past practice of not performing susceptibility tests has changed. The **Centers for Disease Control and Prevention** (Atlanta) **now recommends that initial isolates from all patients be tested for susceptibility to first-line antituberculous drugs** [2,3] (see Antimicrobial Susceptibility Testing, under Laboratory Guidance in Therapy).

VI. **Chlamydiae.** Chlamydia trachomatis is an important cause of conjunctivitis, pneumonia in infancy, urethritis, cervicitis, and pelvic inflammatory disease. Chlamydiae, like viruses, are obligate intracellular parasites. Cultivation in living cells or by direct detection in clinical specimens using antigen, direct probe, or NAA assays assists in diagnosis [16,17].

A. **Diagnostic methods.** Specimens for culture (e.g., sputum, cervical scrapings, urethral discharge) are placed in special transport media and delivered promptly.

Table 25.3. Specimens for Culture of Mycobacteria

| Source | Recommended Number | Volume | Comments |
|---|---|---|---|
| Respiratory tract sputum | 3 | 5–10 mL | Saliva inappropriate |
| Bronchoscopy washing (e.g., bronchoalveolar lavage) | 1 | | See Chapter 9 |
| Gastric washing | 2–3 | 30–50 mL | Useful if respiratory secretions are not available; early morning specimens required before eating or activity; small volume of sterile water can be used in the tube placement (20–30 mL); requires rapid delivery (within 30–60 min) to microbiology laboratory to prevent inactivation of organism; stains may at times be helpful (saprophytes may cause false positive smears) (see Chapter 9) |
| Urine | 2–3 | Maximum volume of single specimen | Use first-voided midstream collections; avoid 24-h collection (too much bacterial overgrowth); stains may at times be helpful (saprophytes may cause false positive smears) (see Chapter 9) |
| Cerebrospinal fluid | | Maximum volume available | |
| Other: joint, pleural, and peritoneal fluid | | Maximum volume available | |
| Blood | 1–2 | 10 mL | Useful for the recovery of *Mycobacterium avium* from patients with AIDS (see Chapter 19) |

Chlamydia is demonstrated by staining with iodine, Giemsa, or fluorescent antibody 2 to 3 days after cell inoculation. NAA methods are now thought to be more sensitive than culture.

**B. Direct detection** of *C. trachomatis* in clinical specimens using antigen, direct nucleic acid probe, and NAA assays is now more widely available than cell culture.

1. Antigen assays are available in enzyme immunoassay (EIA) formats for laboratory use and in single test devices for office use. In addition, the elementary body of *C. trachomatis* can be detected in clinical specimens by direct immunofluorescence. In general, antigen assays are less sensitive than all other methods available for *Chlamydia* detection.

2. Direct probe assays are intermediate in sensitivity between antigen detection and NAA assays. The Gen-Probe Pace 2 is the most widely used. It offers the advantage of detecting both *N. gonorrhoeae* and *C. trachomatis* in the specimen.
3. A number of NAA assays are available, including the Roche PCR, Becton Dickinson strand displacement assay (SDA), Abbott ligase chain reaction (LCR), and Gen-Probe transcription-mediated amplification assay (TMA). The NAA assays are more sensitive than all other methods for *C. trachomatis* detection. However, problems with specificity have been reported [16]. NAA assays can be used to detect both *N. gonorrhoeae* and *C. trachomatis* in a single specimen as well as to detect the organisms in urine, which provides a convenient approach for screening patients for sexually transmitted diseases.

VII. **Mycoplasma.** Despite the clinical importance of *Mycoplasma pneumoniae* in respiratory infections, techniques to culture *M. pneumoniae* from clinical specimens are not widely available. This organism is slow growing, and positive culture results often are not available for 7 to 14 days. Therefore, serologic studies (cold-agglutinin titers or complement-fixing antibodies) are still most commonly used for diagnosis (see Chapter 11).

VIII. **Tests for bacterial exotoxins**

A. **Exotoxins** are the major virulence determinant for a number of organisms. Well-known exotoxin-induced disease processes include tetanus, diphtheria, toxic shock syndrome, botulism, cholera, and diarrhea caused by *Clostridium difficile* or enterotoxigenic *Escherichia coli*. Most tests for bacterial toxins are complex and technically difficult. **With the exception of *C. difficile*, tests for bacterial toxin generally are performed only in reference laboratories** and only under special circumstances.

B. *C. difficile* appears to cause up to 25% of antibiotic-associated diarrhea and plays an important role in the development of pseudomembranous colitis. A variety of assays are available, but tests based on demonstration of cytotoxic activity in cell culture that are sensitive and correlate with the presence of disease [18] are viewed as the gold standard.

## *Interpretation of Culture Results*

I. **Isolation of organisms.** Microorganisms in culture do not necessarily represent infection.

A. **Contamination** refers to the introduction of extraneous organisms into the culture during specimen collection or processing. They may originate from the skin of the patient, the clinician, or the technician, or from laboratory materials and the inanimate environment.

B. **Colonization** of a body site is the **presence of organisms,** including potential pathogens, that are **not causing infection** (no evidence of illness, tissue invasion, or inflammation). Colonizing bacteria inhabit the oropharynx, skin, colon, vagina, and wound surfaces.

C. **To determine the clinical significance of culture data, the clinician must interpret all culture results in the context of (a) the clinical condition of the patient, (b) the site cultured, (c) the method of specimen collection, and (d) the identity and quantity of organisms recovered.** See chapters on specific infections for further discussion; for example, wound infections in Chapter 4, and pneumonia in Chapter 11.

II. **Failure to culture or detect a suspected pathogen** can be caused by a number of factors; many are related to improper collection and transport.

A. **Incorrect diagnosis** can occur. Infection may not be present or may be caused by organisms that are not cultured routinely (e.g., viruses, rickettsiae, or mycoplasmas).

B. **Misinterpretations of Gram stain results** occur. Artifacts might be interpreted as organisms.

C. **Specimens** that do not represent material at the infection site may be examined.

D. **Improper technique or delayed transport of specimens** may cause overgrowth by indigenous flora or loss of anaerobes or fastidious organisms.

E. **Antimicrobial therapy** prior to specimen collection may inhibit the growth of organisms.

F. **Improper culture methods** may be used. Special isolation techniques are necessary for anaerobes, mycobacteria, viruses, and certain fungi and bacteria. The physician must communicate with the laboratory so that appropriate cultures can be performed.

III. **Preliminary identification of bacteria,** although not definitive, may assist the clinician in early diagnosis and choice of empiric antibiotic therapy. Clinical microbiology personnel can provide guidance in the interpretation of preliminary results. In addition to the Gram stain, results of several tests often are available before an organism is finally identified [19,20].

A. **Gram-positive cocci**

1. **Blood agar hemolysis.** Streptococci produce various patterns of hemolysis.
   a. **Beta hemolysis** is a clear, colorless zone surrounding colonies of group A (*S. pyogenes*), group B (*S. agalactiae*), and other less common streptococci.
   b. **Alpha hemolysis,** or partial hemolysis, refers to a greenish zone surrounding colonies of *S. pneumoniae* and many species of viridans streptococci.
   c. **Gamma hemolysis** actually denotes **nonhemolysis** and is observed typically with group D streptococci, including enterococcal and nonenterococcal species.
   d. Note that the **Lancefield serogrouping** of streptococci (groups A, B, C, D, etc.), based on antigenic differences in cell wall carbohydrates, is an independent classification system that **should not be confused with the hemolytic patterns.**
2. **Catalase test.** The Gram stain often distinguishes between streptococci (chains or pairs) and staphylococci (clusters). If uncertain, a simple catalase test can be helpful. Hydrogen peroxide bubbles on exposure to catalase-positive organisms. Streptococci are catalase negative, and **staphylococci are catalase positive.**
3. **Coagulase test.** Coagulase-positive staphylococci produce an enzyme that coagulates rabbit plasma. A coagulase **slide test** can be performed in minutes but is less sensitive than an overnight coagulase **tube test.** Negative results of a coagulase slide test should be confirmed with a coagulase tube test. ***S. aureus* is coagulase positive;** *S. epidermidis, S. saprophyticus,* and other staphylococcal species test negative. Many laboratories have adopted latex agglutination tests in place of the traditional coagulase test for differentiation between *S. aureus* and other staphylococcal species.
4. **Nomenclature of gram-positive cocci** is a frequent source of confusion.
   a. **Group A** $\beta$-hemolytic streptococci are *S. pyogenes.*
   b. **Group B** $\beta$-hemolytic streptococci are *S. agalactiae.*
   c. **Group D** streptococci include the following:
      (1) Enterococcal species. The majority of clinical isolates of enterococci will be *Enterococcus faecalis* (80%–90%) and *E. faecium* (5%–10%). Infrequently, *E. avium, E. raffinosus,* and *E. gallinarum* are found.
      (2) Nonenterococcal species (*S. bovis*). See Chapter 2, under Blood Cultures.
   d. **Viridans group streptococci,** often referred to as strep viridans, encompass not just one but many species, including the *S. milleri* group (*S. anginosus, S. constellatus, S. intermedius*), *S. mitis, S. mutans, S. salivarius,* and *S. sanguis* [21].

B. **Gram-negative bacilli**

1. **Lactose fermentation.** MacConkey agar plates promote selective growth of gram-negative bacilli. Colonies of **lactose fermenters** (*E. coli, Klebsiella, Enterobacter,* and *Citrobacter*) appear red on MacConkey plates within 24 hours. **Nonlactose fermenters** (*Proteus, Serratia, Salmonella, Shigella, Pseudomonas,* and others) appear colorless or white. **Caution:** Although certain species are typically lactose fermenters (e.g., *E. coli*), some strains are nonlactose fermenters.
2. **Oxidase test.** Oxidase reagent turns certain colonies purple. *Pseudomonas* species are oxidase positive and Enterobacteriaceae are oxidase-negative.

C. **Gram-positive bacilli** often are contaminants. At times, they may be true pathogens. These organisms can be spore forming or non–spore forming. The most commonly isolated non–spore-forming bacilli are diphtheroids—corynebacteria that normally inhabit the skin. However, when repeatedly isolated from normally sterile fluids or sites, they may be pathogenic (e.g., prosthetic device infection) [19]. When isolated from blood or CSF, it is important to distinguish corynebacteria from another non–spore-forming bacillus, *Listeria monocytogenes,* which is motile at room temperature and may cause meningitis in newborn infants, immunocompromised hosts [19], and the elderly. The clinical significance of gram-positive bacilli and *Bacillus* species is reviewed in detail elsewhere [22]. (**Note:** Anaerobic gram-positive bacilli may be clostridial species.)

## *Direct Detection of Microbial Antigens in Clinical Specimens*

Immunodiagnostic tests can detect microbial antigens in clinical specimens. The basis for all such tests is the reaction of an antibody with the target antigen in the clinical specimen.

**I. Antigen detection methods** have successfully been applied to the diagnosis of virtually all classes of microorganisms: bacteria, fungi, parasites, and viruses (Table 25.4) [4,5,23,24].

**II. There are advantages and disadvantages specific to each method.**

**A. Latex agglutination** tests generally are rapid (10–15 minutes) and can be performed by individuals with minimal training. However, in some cases, interpretation of the agglutination reactions may pose a problem for the unskilled reader.

**B. Immunofluorescent** (IF) **and immunocytochemical stains** (e.g., peroxidase, antiperoxidase) are especially useful for detecting and localizing virus-infected cells in infected organs and tissues. IF stains also are widely used to detect virus-infected cells in specimens from the respiratory tract, *C. trachomatis* elementary bodies in cervical and urethral discharge, and a variety of bacteria (e.g., *T. pallidum, Bordetella pertussis, Legionella* species) in clinical specimens.

**C. ELISAs (enzyme-linked immunosorbent assays)** have largely replaced their predecessors, the **radioimmunoassays,** as tools for antigen detection in clinical laboratories. Although some ELISAs remain complex and must be performed in the laboratory setting, a number of simple tests are now available in cassette or strip form that can be performed in the office with reasonable accuracy. Simple kits for group A $\beta$-hemolytic streptococci, rotavirus, RSV, and influenza viruses are commercially available and are as reliable as their more complex laboratory counterparts.

**III. Monoclonal and polyclonal antibodies** are used as both capture and detector antibodies in antigen detection tests. Although monoclonal antibodies are not suitable for all tests, they are preferred because they represent a consistent and reliable antibody source.

**IV.** The **sensitivity and specificity of antigen detection tests** varies depending both on the test and the target organism. **In general, they are not as sensitive or specific as culture,** but they often do produce results more rapidly and are a less expensive alternative than culture.

**V. Clinical applications**

**A.** The sensitivity of immunodetection tests in patients with **meningitis** on initial evaluation of CSF ranges from 82% to 95% for *H. influenzae,* from 40% to 80% for *N. meningitidis,* and from 70% to 80% for *S. pneumoniae.* Unfortunately, they are less sensitive in gram-negative cases. Few laboratories now offer such testing (see Chapter 6) [23].

**B.** The rapid diagnosis of infections with ***Legionella pneumophila*** is important because cultures may take as long as 3 to 5 days to become positive. Unfortunately, the sensitivity of IF is low (25%–50%), and although its specificity is high, the generally low prevalence of disease compromises the predictive value of positive results [23] (see Chapter 11). The ***Legionella*** **urinary antigen** test was discussed in Chapter 11, section **VI.F,** under Specific Considerations and Specific Therapy, and has been reviewed recently [25]. The test, a commercially available EIA kit (Binax, Portland, ME) detects *L. pneumophila* serogroup 1 antigen in the urine. In a recent report, it proved useful for the diagnosis of legionella pulmonary infection [23,25,26]. Although the urinary assay detects only *L. pneumophila* serogroup 1, this serogroup causes about 80% of cases of Legionnaires disease [25,26]. Because antigen may persist for days to weeks after initiation of antibiotic therapy, the assay results may be positive when other diagnostic test results are negative; the test results could also be positive from a prior and no longer active infection.

Table 25.4. Microorganisms Commonly Detected in Clinical Specimens by Nucleic Acid Amplification Methods for the Diagnosis of Laboratory Infectious Diseases

| Agent | Specimens | Uses | Comments |
|---|---|---|---|
| *Bordetella pertussis* | Nasopharyngeal | Diagnosis of pertussis | Significantly more sensitive than culture and FA |
| *Chlamydia trachomatis* | Genital tract specimens | Diagnosis | 10%–30% more sensitive than culture<br>Several FDA-cleared assays available |
| CMV | CSF, blood, ocular fluid, amniotic fluid | CNS infection, systemic infection, retinitis, congenital infection, preemptive therapy | Approximately twice as sensitive as culture for systemic infection<br>Quantitative assays used to distinguish between disease and asymptomatic infection |
| EBV | CSF, blood | AIDS-associated primary CNS lymphoma, PTLD | Quantitative measures used to monitor for PTLD post-transplantation |
| Enteroviruses (coxsackie, ECHO, and poliovirus) | CSF, blood | Encephalitis, meningitis | 30%–50% more sensitive than culture |
| Hepatitis B virus | | Monitor therapeutic efficacy | |
| Hepatitis C virus | Blood | Diagnose active infection and monitor therapeutic efficacy | FDA-cleared qualitative assay available |
| HIV (RNA/DNA) | Blood (EDTA or ACD tube) | RNA: prognosis and monitoring therapeutic efficacy<br>DNA: diagnosis of infected infants | Several FDA-cleared quantitative RNA assays in widespread use<br>No FDA-cleared tests for diagnosis |
| HSV | CSF, ocular fluid, blood | Encephalitis, meningitis, acute retinal necrosis | Method of choice for CNS disease and acute retinal necrosis |
| JC virus | CSF | Progressive multifocal leukoencephalopathy | No other detection methods available |
| *Mycobacterium tuberculosis* | Sputum | Diagnosis in conjunction with culture | Same day diagnosis in >90% of smear-positive specimens<br>Approximately 50% sensitive for smear-negative specimens<br>FDA cleared for smear-positive sputum specimens |
| *Neisseria gonorrhoeae* | Genital tract specimens | Diagnosis | Specificity problems in CAP surveys |
| Parvovirus B19 | Serum, amniotic fluid | Chronic infection in immunocompromised patients, aplastic crisis in patients with hemoglobinopathies, congenital infection | No culture methods available and serology insensitive in certain settings<br>NAA additive diagnostically |
| *Toxoplasma gondii* | CSF, amniotic fluid, ocular fluid, tissue, blood, BAL | Toxoplasma encephalitis, retinitis, systemic infection, congenital infection | Culture insensitive and generally unavailable |
| VZV | CSF, ocular fluid, dermal lesions | Encephalitis, myelitis, congenital infection | Significantly more sensitive than culture in all settings |

FA, fluorescent antibody; FDA, U.S. Food and Drug Administration; CMV, cytomegalovirus; CSF, cerebrospinal fluid; CNS, central nervous system; EBV, Epstein-Barr virus; AIDS, acquired immunodeficiency syndrome; PTLD, posttransplant lymphoproliferative disorder; HIV, human immunodeficiency virus; EDTA, ethylenediaminetetraacetic acid; ACD, citric acid; HSV, herpes simplex virus; CAP, community acquired pneumonia; NAA, nucleic acid amplification; BAL, bronchoalveolar lavage; VZV, varicella-zoster virus.

**C.** The U.S. Food and Drug Administration (FDA) recently cleared a simple immunoassay that detects **pneumococcal antigen** in urine to aid in the diagnosis of pneumonia and meningitis. The test is similar to the antigen assay for *Legionella,* and its sensitivity in blood culture–positive cases is approximately 90%. The test is potentially useful because conventional methods for the diagnosis of pneumococcal disease are notoriously imperfect [23].

**D.** More than 20 different commercial immunodiagnostic kits are available for the detection of **group A $\beta$-hemolytic streptococci** in pharyngeal specimens. When compared with culture, the sensitivity of such tests ranges from 60% to 90% or more, and the specificity generally is found to be in excess of 95%. Many clinicians recommend culture for all antigen-negative specimens because of the reports of low sensitivity [23] (see Chapter 8).

**E.** ***Helicobacter pylori*** antibody assays are widely used as a screen in the management of patients with gastritis, but they do not distinguish between active and past infection. Detecting *Helicobacter pylori* antigens or DNA in feces (the latter via polymerase chain reaction) as alternatives to the $^{14}C$ breath test and biopsy/urease test is now being explored [23].

**F.** Tests for **group B streptococcal antigen** are used to screen pregnant women to aid in the diagnosis of sepsis in the newborn. However, in 1997 the FDA issued a safety alert describing risks with such testing. The FDA warned of both false-positive and false-negative clinical test results. This warning prompted a substantial decline in their use [23].

**G.** The most sensitive and specific test for *C. difficile* infection is the detection of the cytotoxin B in cell culture. However, the test takes 1 to 3 days to complete and requires cell culture facilities. Several ELISAs that detect toxin A or B in stool are also available. These assays have a sensitivity of 71% to 94% and a specificity of 92% to 98%. Because of the rapidity of testing and ease of performance, ELISAs for toxins A and B are now widely used by laboratories for diagnosis of *C. difficile* infection [23].

**H.** **Influenza direct antigen tests** were briefly discussed in Chapter 10, section **V.B,** under Influenza. At least five assays in cassette format are available for the diagnosis of influenza, and two are Clinical Laboratory Improvement Act (CLIA) waived for office use [24]. Newer tests detect both influenza A and B. Nasopharyngeal washes or aspirates are preferred because they have more viral particles than do nasal or pharyngeal swabs. In patients in whom wash or aspirate techniques are contraindicated, swabs can be used. When positive, such rapid tests (which generally take less than 1 hour to perform) are very useful. The manufacturers generally report sensitivities of more than 80% and specificities of 95%. However, lower values have been reported in independent studies. Therefore, antigen-negative specimens should be cultured to provide greater sensitivity. By using a direct antigen test as an adjunct to culture isolation in nursing homes or the acute care setting, influenza often can be identified rapidly so that antiviral therapy and isolation measures can be initiated [24].

**I.** Immunodiagnostic tests (IF and ELISA) for **RSV** now are used widely. Most have very good performance characteristics, with sensitivities and specificities in excess of 90% and 95%, respectively. In large measure, the good performance of such tests is due to gold standard deficiencies (cell culture growth) against which they are measured [24].

**J.** The **CMV antigenemia assay** is used to measure CMV-infected leukocytes in blood. The assay is performed by first lysing RBCs and then depositing the leukocytes on a slide by cytocentrifugation. Leukocytes are stained with a CMV-specific monoclonal antibody. Results are expressed as the number of infected cells per total examined. The antigenemia assay is more sensitive than culture and slightly less sensitive than PCR [24].

**K.** Antigen detection assays for ***Giardia* and *Cryptosporidium parvum*** alone and in combination are available in various immunoassay formats. The sensitivity of such assays is equivalent to traditional ova and parasite examinations. Many laboratories now use immunoassays in lieu of traditional methods for detecting these parasites because the latter are more labor intensive and require greater technical skill [4].

**L.** The polysaccharide antigen of *C. neoformans* is readily detected in both the CSF and the serum in active infection. Properly controlled, the **sensitivity of the cryptococcal latex agglutination test approximates that of culture** [5] (see Chapters 6 and 18).

## *Nucleic Acid Methods for the Characterization and Direct Detection of Microbial Pathogens in Clinical Specimens*

In recent years, nucleic acid techniques have been used to address a variety of problems in clinical microbiology. **Although many methods remain research tools, a number are already in use in clinical laboratories.**

**I. Molecular epidemiology.** A variety of typing methods are used to determine if multiple organisms represent a single strain or unrelated strains. **Phenotypic typing schemes** use characteristics expressed by the organism, include biotyping, antimicrobial susceptibility testing, serotyping, phage typing, and multilocus enzyme electrophoresis. Strain relatedness also can be established with **genotypic methods** based on direct analysis of chromosomal and extrachromosomal DNA [27–29].

**A.** Genotyping services for outbreak investigation methods are now readily available through reference and public health laboratories but not routinely in clinical laboratories.

**II. Nucleic acid probe assays** are based on the combination of labeled, single-stranded DNA or RNA molecules (probes) with single-stranded target nucleic acid. Several techniques, including filter, liquid, Southern blot, Northern blot, and *in situ* hybridization, are in common use. Probes are generally short nucleotide sequences, unique to a given organism or species that serve as a molecular fingerprint for identification [28].

**A. Nucleic acid probes can be used to directly detect a wide variety of microorganisms in clinical specimens.** The sensitivity and specificity of nucleic acid probe assays and antigen detection assays are generally similar. The most successful commercial probe systems are those for the direct detection of *N. gonorrhoeae* and *C. trachomatis* (Gen-Probe) [28] (see Chapter 16) and papillomavirus (Digene).

**B.** Nucleic acid probe–based tests are also used to identify organisms grown *in vitro,* to detect virulence determinants (e.g., toxins), and to localize antibiotic resistance determinants.

**1.** *Mycobacterium* species probes for the rapid identification of mycobacteria are now widely used to identify acid-fast organisms grown on solid media or in liquid media. Probes are available for *M. tuberculosis, M. avium* complex (MAC), *M. kansasii,* and *M. gordonae. M. tuberculosis* frequently can be identified in less than 2 weeks from the time of specimen collection. Mixed infections (e.g., *M. tuberculosis* and MAC) can likewise be identified [28] (see Chapter 11).

**2.** Probes also have simplified the identification of the dimorphic fungi, *Histoplasma capsulatum, Blastomyces dermatitidis,* and *Coccidioides immitis.*

**C.** The VERSANT HCV RNA 3.0 assay is a sandwich nucleic acid hybridization assay for the direct quantitation of RNA in human serum and plasma.

**III. Nucleic acid amplification assays.** In the mid-1980's, **PCR** acid was introduced. The usefulness of PCR as a tool for detecting microorganisms was immediately obvious, and because commercialization of PCR was restricted by patent, alternative strategies for NAA and nucleic acid detection were developed. The FDA-cleared NAA products now available are described below. In addition, many laboratories offer "home brew" PCR assays for infectious diseases. Such assays are devised and validated by the laboratory performing the assay. Significant variation in laboratory performance in proficiency test panels has been observed in blinded, interlaboratory comparisons. When the results of NAA testing are used clinically, the limitations of NAA assays, particularly home brew assays, should always be considered.

**A.** Using the **PCR,** more than 1 billion copies of DNA can be made from a single target segment of DNA or RNA (**reverse transcriptase (rt) PCR**). The amplified product can then be detected by any one of a number of methods. The specific advantage of the PCR is its enormous sensitivity. However, the sensitivity of PCR is also its Achilles heel. Contamination resulting in false-positive results should always be considered.

1. The **Roche Amplicor PCR** is the most widely used NAA technology. FDA-cleared kits are available to qualitatively detect *C. trachomatis, N. gonorrhoeae, M. tuberculosis,* and HCV in clinical specimens.
2. **Amplicor monitor** assays are designed to quantify virus in plasma. Amplicor monitor assays are now widely used to evaluate therapeutic efficacy in patients infected with HIV and HCV.
3. Several fully automated versions of Amplicor assays, **COBAS Amplicor** assays, are available. Their performance is similar to their semiautomated counterparts.
4. **Real-time PCR** measures the product of the PCR reaction as it is formed. A number of larger clinical laboratories now use the **Light Cycler** instrument, a capillary PCR device, to perform both quantitative and qualitative PCR assays.

**B. The Gen-Probe transcription mediated amplification assay (TMA)** isothermal nucleic amplification process, like PCR, can be used to detect both DNA and RNA. The current FDA-cleared menu includes direct tests for *M. tuberculosis* and *C. trachomatis.*

**C.** The second-generation **thermophilic strand displacement amplification (tSDA)** assay was designed by Becton Dickinson. Originally limited to the detection of DNA, the assay has recently been modified and can now be used to detect both DNA and RNA. The tSDA tests, known as **Probe Tec assays,** presently cleared by the FDA include only direct tests for *N. gonorrhoeae* and *C. trachomatis*.

**D.** The **LCR** is the DNA amplification technology developed by Abbott Laboratories. Currently it is the only FDA-cleared LCR assay for the direct detection of *N. gonorrhoeae* and *C. trachomatis*.

**E. Nucleic acid sequence-based amplification (NASBA)** is used to amplify RNA targets and mRNA expression targets. NucliSens assays, NASBA-based amplification assays, formerly marketed by Organon Teknika, are now marketed by bioMerieux. The NucliSens HIV-1 QT assay was recently cleared by the FDA for viral load monitoring.

## SERODIAGNOSTIC AND IMMUNE STATUS TESTS

When attempts to recover an infectious agent are unsuccessful or impractical, or when culture techniques or facilities are not available, **serologic studies** frequently are used to provide a specific diagnosis. Unfortunately, serologic diagnoses often are retrospective, and therapeutic decisions must frequently be made before the serology results are available. Examples of infectious diseases that commonly are diagnosed by serologic methods are syphilis, rubella, *M. pneumoniae,* leptospirosis, toxoplasmosis, Lyme disease, and infectious mononucleosis.

**I. General principles. Interpretation** depends on determination of antibody titers in blood.

**A. Many different assay techniques exist** for demonstrating antibody titers in various infections. Whether antibody is measured by agglutination, complement fixation, neutralization, ELISA, or other techniques depends on the nature of the antigen, the availability of the assay and, most important, the ability of a given serologic technique to detect antibody. For certain infections such as rubella, the titers obtained with different antibody tests can be used to help assess the likelihood of recent infection.

**B. Clotted blood specimens** are acceptable for most serologic tests. Blood should be collected in tubes without anticoagulant and can be refrigerated for 2 or 3 days prior to testing. If longer delays are anticipated, the serum should be frozen at $-20°C$.

**II. Clinical applications are for** diagnosis of acute infection and immune status determination.

**A. Diagnosis of acute infection** usually is accomplished by comparing acute and convalescent sera pairs. Occasionally, a single acute-phase serum or a single convalescent-phase serum also can be used to diagnose acute infection.

1. **Paired sera.** Using acute and convalescent sera, a conversion from seronegative to seropositive or a fourfold or greater increase in antibody titer is considered indicative of recent infection. A single blood specimen containing antibody to a

specific antigen may indicate that the patient has had prior exposure to that antigen or to a cross-reacting one. **In most cases, single titers are difficult to interpret.**

a. **Acute-phase serum** should be obtained as early in the course of the illness as possible. In any patient hospitalized with an undiagnosed febrile illness, a 5-mL serum specimen should be frozen for potential use as an acute-phase serum in future serologic studies. It can be discarded if not needed. Blood should be collected aseptically and, to avoid lipemia, preferably during fasting.
b. **Convalescent-phase serum** should be collected at least 10 days, but preferably 2 to 4 weeks, after the onset of the illness. **For testing to be valid, both the acute and convalescent sera should be analyzed simultaneously.**

2. **A single acute-phase serum may be helpful diagnostically in some cases.** Immunoglobulin M (IgM) antibody typically develops early during primary infection, persists for several weeks, and then becomes undetectable. Therefore, commercial kits are now available for detecting IgM to hepatitis A virus and to rubella virus.
3. **Use of a single convalescent-phase serum.** For example, a presumptive diagnosis of *Legionella* is made on the basis of a single elevated indirect fluorescent antibody titer (1:256 or greater), because high titers persist only transiently after infection.

B. **Immune status testing** of an individual may be important in certain situations. For example, rubella vaccine is recommended for seronegative women of childbearing age as a means of preventing congenital rubella syndrome. Because of the complexity and variety of serologic tests now available, communication with the microbiology laboratory or infectious diseases unit prior to ordering a test is often essential to ensure that the maximum amount of useful information is obtained from the test. **Chapters on individual infectious diseases should be consulted for specific serologic testing.**

## LABORATORY GUIDANCE IN THERAPY

The two general types of laboratory tests used as aids in therapy are *in vitro* tests that assess the susceptibility of the infecting organism to various antimicrobial agents and the measurement of antimicrobial concentration or activity in serum or other bodily fluids [18,19,31,32].

### *Antimicrobial Susceptibility Testing*

I. **Disk diffusion test (Kirby-Bauer).** Worldwide, the most widely used method for testing the activity of antimicrobials against bacteria is the disk diffusion test (also called the **agar diffusion test**). Although dilution tests are believed to be more exact, the Kirby-Bauer disk diffusion test is the initial susceptibility test used in most laboratories. It has ease of performance, reproducibility, and proven value as a guide to antimicrobial therapy.

A. **Method.** Paper disks impregnated with a standardized quantity of antimicrobial agent are applied to the surface of an agar plate that has been inoculated with a suspension of the organism to be tested. The antimicrobial agent diffuses through the agar in a continuously decreasing gradient. After 16 to 20 hours of incubation, a concentric zone of growth inhibition around the paper disk is measured. In general, large zones are associated with susceptibility to the antibiotic, and small or absent zones with resistance. Standards for interpretation of the zone sizes have been based on susceptibility or resistance by broth or agar dilution tests. The disc diffusion test is applicable only to rapidly growing organisms such as the Enterobacteriaceae and *Staphylococcus* and *Pseudomonas* species. Its reproducibility depends on strictly standardized methods.

B. **Clinical application.** Disk diffusion susceptibility testing is indicated for clinically significant isolates that have unpredictable sensitivity patterns, such as the Enterobacteriaceae and *Staphylococcus* and *Pseudomonas* species. Susceptibility testing also is indicated for any isolate from normally sterile bodily fluids such as blood and CSF. Disk diffusion testing need not be performed routinely for organisms that are uniformly sensitive or resistant to a particular antibiotic; for example, group A streptococci and *N. meningitidis* are uniformly sensitive to penicillin G.

C. **Interpretation.** A three-category system of reporting results often is used.

1. **Susceptible (sensitive)** implies that an infection due to the tested strain should respond to an appropriate dose of the antibiotic recommended for that type of infection.
2. **Resistant** indicates that the strain is not completely inhibited by antimicrobial concentrations within the therapeutic range, and it strongly predicts antibiotic failure.
3. **Intermediate** indicates that a clinical response may occur if unusually high concentrations of relatively nontoxic antibiotics can be achieved at the site of the infection. **For most situations, however, a strain classified as intermediate should be considered resistant until proven otherwise.** If clinical circumstances favor the use of that particular antimicrobial, dilution susceptibility testing may be performed to determine the actual sensitivity or resistance of the organism to the drug. **Some laboratories will routinely report all intermediate zones of inhibition as resistant.**

D. **Limitations**

1. **For some organisms, the disk diffusion method is not applicable.**
   a. Organisms that are fastidious, slow growing, or have special growth requirements (e.g., anaerobes) cannot be tested. See section **IV.**
   b. Mycobacterial and fungal susceptibility testing requires specialized techniques that are usually available only in reference laboratories.
   c. Normal flora of nonsterile body sites are not routinely tested.
2. Special techniques may be required to detect penicillin-resistant *S. pneumoniae,* oxacillin-resistant (or methicillin-resistant) *S. aureus*, and aminoglycoside resistant or penicillin-resistant enterococci. See Chapter 27 and the E test in section **III.B.**
3. Disk diffusion testing may indicate *in vitro* susceptibility, despite lack of therapeutic efficacy in actual practice. Examples are *Salmonella typhi* susceptibility to aminoglycosides and enterococcus susceptibility to cephalosporins.
4. **Standards for interpreting zones of growth inhibition are based on achievable serum levels of antimicrobials. Disk diffusion testing, therefore, is not always applicable to urinary tract isolates, because the achievable levels of certain antibiotics in urine are much higher than in serum [33].** For example, an enterococcal isolate resistant to ampicillin by disk diffusion testing may nevertheless be successfully treated with ampicillin if the infection is limited to the urinary tract.
5. Certain antibiotics cannot be accurately tested (e.g., methenamine mandelate and the polymyxins).
6. Bactericidal activity cannot be tested because the disk diffusion method yields bacteriostatic data only.
7. **Simple matching of antibiotic to infecting organism susceptibility pattern is a superficial approach to therapy.** The disk diffusion test is only one aid to assessing potential response of the infection. Host defense mechanisms; site of infection; underlying illnesses; route, dose, and penetration of the antibiotic into the infected site; and duration of antibiotic therapy must always be considered (see Chapter 27A).

II. **Dilution susceptibility tests** are used to determine the **minimum inhibitory concentration** (MIC) and the **minimum bactericidal concentration** (MBC) of an antibiotic for an infecting organism. The **MIC is defined as the lowest concentration of drug that prevents visible growth of the test organism** under a standardized set of conditions (Fig. 25.1). The **MBC of the drug is the lowest concentration that results in 99.9% killing of** the initial inoculum under standardized conditions. The MIC and MBC are usually expressed in micrograms of antibiotic per milliliter. This testing can be done by a broth dilution or agar dilution method.

A. **Methods**

1. **Broth dilution tests.** Serial, twofold dilutions of an antimicrobial are incorporated into broth-containing tubes, which are then inoculated with a standard

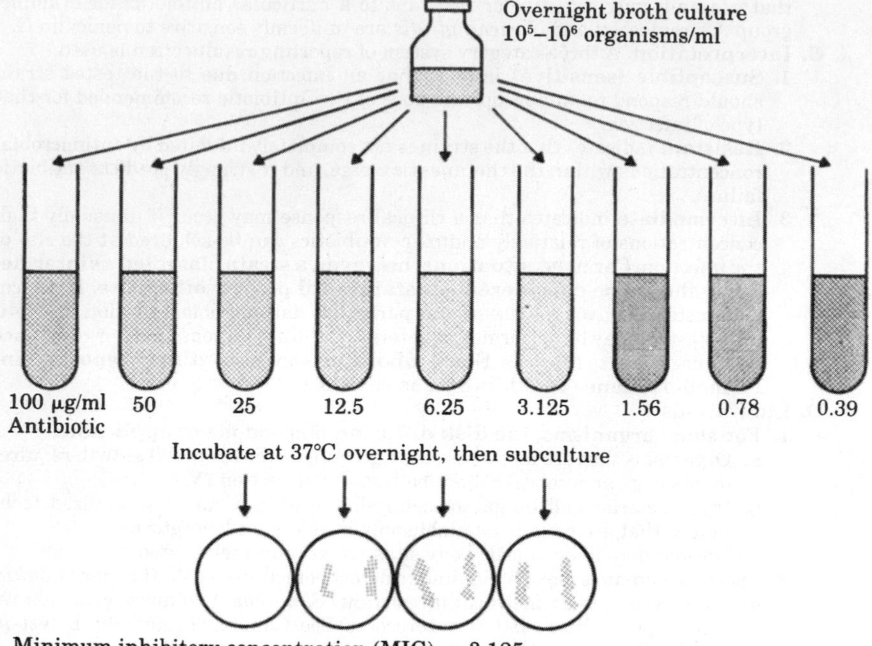


**FIG. 25.1** Dilution susceptibility testing for minimum inhibitory concentration and minimum bactericidal concentration determination.

number of organisms, usually $10^5$ to $10^6$ colony-forming units (CFU) per milliliter. After the culture has been incubated at 35°C for 16 to 20 hours, the tubes are inspected for visible growth. Rapid techniques are also available (see section **E.**) to determine the MIC. If the tubes with no visible growth are subcultured quantitatively to a drug-free medium, the MBC of the antimicrobial can be determined, as indicated in Figure 25.1. **Microdilution susceptibility** testing employs the same principles but uses wells on a microtiter tray rather than dilution tubes, permitting automation.

2. **The Agar dilution test** is similar to the broth technique except that the antibiotic dilutions are incorporated into a solid medium and the inoculum, usually $10^4$ CFU/mL, is applied as a spot to a small portion of the agar plate. The MIC is the lowest antibiotic concentration that prevents visible growth. The MBC cannot be determined.

**B. Clinical application.** Several commercially manufactured **semiautomated systems are now available that permit routine MIC determinations for all clinically significant bacterial isolates. If not routinely performed, dilution susceptibility testing (MIC and MBC determinations) should be considered in the following situations.**

1. Disk diffusion has yielded intermediate susceptibility to an antibiotic (e.g., an aminoglycoside) chosen to treat a serious infection.
2. Complicated or life-threatening infections exist owing to organisms with an unpredictable susceptibility pattern.
3. Serious infections are caused by organisms susceptible only to relatively toxic agents.
4. Determination of a bactericidal end point is desirable, as in endocarditis.

5. Disk diffusion results are unreliable, as with fastidious or slow-growing organisms.
6. An infection has failed to respond to an antibiotic, despite disk susceptibility.

C. **Interpretations.** The MIC of an organism may be useful in selecting an antibiotic that will be active against that organism at the site of the infection. Generally, if an antibiotic tissue level exceeds its MIC for the responsible organism, the infection should respond. A blood level that exceeds the MIC twofold to eightfold is a commonly accepted guideline. See time-dependent and concentration-dependent bactericidal activity in Chapter 27.

D. **Limitations**
1. Dilution tests for MIC and MBC often are more expensive and technically demanding.
2. Lack of interlaboratory standardization makes interpretation difficult.
3. The practitioner may experience difficulty in interpreting the MIC and MBC results. Assessment of susceptibility or resistance depends on a knowledge of the antibiotic levels achievable at the site of infection. For example, an MIC of piperacillin of 16 $\mu$g/mL to *Pseudomonas aeruginosa* may appear to be a high value, but a 3-g intravenous dose of piperacillin results in peak serum levels greater than 100 $\mu$g/mL. Conversely, an MIC of penicillin G of 0.5 $\mu$g/mL to viridans streptococci may appear to indicate susceptibility, but clinical experience has documented that endocarditis due to viridans streptococci with this MIC often fails penicillin therapy.

E. **Rapid versus conventional MIC methods.** In the past several years, a variety of instrument-assisted identification and susceptibility test methods have been developed that permit generation of test results in a period of 6 to 9 hours, as opposed to the 15- to 24-hour time frame required with traditional overnight methods [33a]. These newer "rapid" methods generally have been shown to provide test results nearly as accurate as those derived from traditional overnight tests, but the newer tests are more expensive [33a]. The clinical impact of this newer technology and whether it truly facilitates faster and more cost-effective patient care is undergoing clinical study. One study suggests the rapid tests have a positive impact on patient care [33a].

III. **Antimicrobial concentration gradient methods** combine features of disk diffusion and dilution susceptibility testing.

A. The **spiral gradient endpoint method** uses an agar plate containing a continuous gradient of antibiotic concentration from the center of the plate to the edge; the test organism is applied to the plate in a radial streak, and the MIC is determined by measuring the distance of growth from the edge of the plate.

B. **The E test** (AB Biodisk, Solna, Sweden) is based on the diffusion of a continuous concentration gradient of an antimicrobial from a plastic strip into an agar medium. In 1988 this technique was created to overcome several of the disadvantages of the disk diffusion and dilution techniques and also to retain the principle of the agar dilution method by producing an accurate, reproducible, quantitative MIC result [33b] (Fig. 25.2).

1. **Procedure**[33b]
   a. An inert thin plastic carrier strip with a predefined continuous concentration gradient of stabilized antibiotic on one side and a continuous MIC interpretive scale corresponding to a range of 15 $\log_2$ dilutions on the other side is used.
   b. After an agar plate is inoculated with a broth suspension of the test organism, four to six E strips can be placed on the plate, which is incubated.
2. **MIC result.** After incubation, an ellipse of inhibition is formed around the strip, and the MIC is read at the point where the ellipse intersects the strip edge (see Fig. 25.2). Studies evaluating E test performance compared with routine susceptibility testing methods have demonstrated excellent agreement [33b].
3. **Potential uses.** The role the E test will play in microbiology laboratories awaits further clinical study. However, it appears to be useful especially for *in vitro* susceptibility testing of organisms for which there is not a "routine" or "standardized" approach or **for fastidious organisms.** Examples include

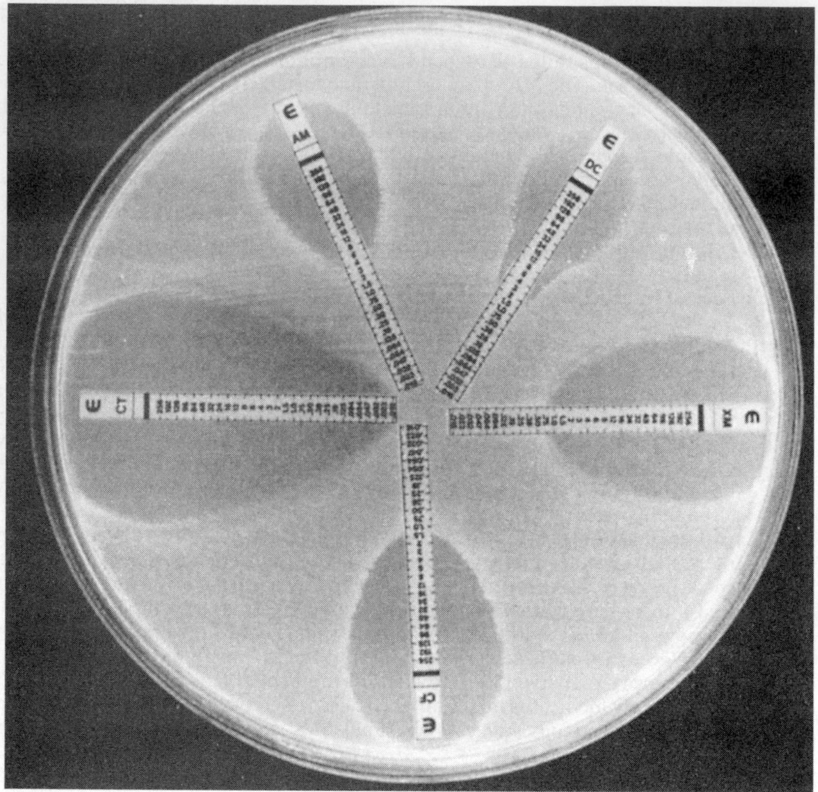


**FIG. 25.2** E tests with a $\beta$-lactamase–producing *Haemophilus influenzae* strain performed with HTM agar. Antibiotic abbreviations on the E-test strips and minimum inhibitory concentration interpretations (indexed to base 1) are as follows: *AM,* ampicillin, 8 $\mu$g/mL; *DC,* doxycycline, 4 $\mu$g/mL; *XM,* cefuroxime, 1 $\mu$g/mL; *CF,* cefaclor, 2 $\mu$g/mL; *CT,* cefotaxime, 0.015 $\mu$g/mL. (Reprinted from Jorgensen JH, et al. Quantitative antimicrobial susceptibility testing of *Haemophilus influenzae* and *Streptococcus pneumoniae* by using the E test. *J Clin Microbiol* 1991;29:109, with permission.)

*S. pneumoniae* [33c], *H. influenzae*, *Neisseria* species, anaerobes (see section **IV.B**), enterococci, methicillin-resistant *S. aureus*, and testing for the presence and susceptibility of extended-spectrum $\beta$-lactamase–producing organisms.

4. Its major drawback may be its relatively higher cost when compared with currently available susceptibility tests. However, in certain clinical situations **(e.g., in the isolation of *S. pneumoniae* from a normally sterile bodily fluid), this appears to be an easy and useful technique to determine whether the clinical isolate is susceptible, intermediately susceptible, or resistant to penicillin** (see Chapter 27C).

**IV. Susceptibility testing of anaerobic bacteria is not routinely available in most hospitals.** In recent years, however, anaerobic susceptibility patterns are known to be less predictable than once was believed [34]. For example, 10% or more of *B. fragilis* infections may be resistant to clindamycin in many institutions [35,36]. Hospitals may elect to monitor susceptibility patterns periodically to guide antibiotic use [18,36a].

**A. Susceptibility testing of specific anaerobic isolates can assist in the management of patients with selected infections** [34,37], as follows:

1. **Serious anaerobic infections** such as brain abscess, empyema, bone and

joint infections, or endocarditis, especially when the anaerobe is isolated in pure culture

2. **Anaerobic infections that persist or recur** despite presumed appropriate empiric antibiotic therapy directed at anaerobes

**B. Methods** of anaerobic susceptibility testing [18,19,21,34]

1. **Agar dilution** susceptibility tests are performed in reference laboratories but are time consuming and impractical for most clinical microbiology laboratories.
2. **Broth microdilution** tests are manageable for clinical laboratories. Microdilution trays are commercially available.
3. **Antimicrobial density gradient** methods (e.g., the E test) are applicable to anaerobes and are simple to perform (see section **II.B**). Although expensive, these simpler tests may play an increasing role in the hospital laboratory. The E test compared favorably with the reference agar dilution method in a recent study [37a].
4. **Determination of β-lactamase production.** Laboratories unable to perform susceptibility tests may assay gram-negative anaerobes for β-lactamase activity, which indicates resistance to penicillins and cephalosporins. A commercial disk test is available. However, a negative result must be interpreted with caution, because resistance to β-lactam antibiotics also may be mediated by mechanisms other than β-lactamase production.

**V. Susceptibility testing of antibiotic combinations** *in vitro* attempts to identify antibiotic combinations that are superior to single agents (see Chapter 27A, under Principles of Antibiotic Use). A combination of antibiotics is considered to be synergistic when the effect of the combination is greater than the sum of the independent effects of each agent and antagonistic when the combined effect of the two antibiotics is less than the effect of each single antibiotic [31,38].

Such testing has been advocated for certain situations such as *P. aeruginosa* sepsis in the immunocompromised patient [39,40]; but the techniques used to assess antibiotic synergy lack interlaboratory standardization and are cumbersome and often expensive.

## VI. Beta-lactamase test

**A. Principle and technique.** Resistance of *H. influenzae* and *N. gonorrhoeae* to the penicillin class of antibiotics may be due to plasmid-mediated β-lactamase enzymes. The development of rapid assays for β-lactamase permits an assessment of sensitivity before standard susceptibility testing results are available. Rapid acidometric, iodometric, and chromogenic cephalosporin methods are used to detect β-lactamase. Bacteria can be tested after overnight growth, and results usually are available within 30 minutes [19].

**B. Clinical application**

1. ***H. influenzae* infections** will not respond to ampicillin if the strain produces β-lactamase. Rapid testing for β-lactamase should be performed, and ampicillin should not be used if the test result is positive but can if the test result is negative. However, certain rare strains are negative by β-lactamase testing but are resistant to ampicillin by disk diffusion testing. Therefore, ideally, a negative β-lactamase test result (implying ampicillin sensitivity) should be confirmed by disk diffusion testing.
2. ***N. gonorrhoeae* strains.** Because of the high prevalence of β-lactamase–positive *N. gonorrhoeae* in the United States, treatment with a regimen (e.g., ceftriaxone) active against resistant strains of gonorrhea is required [41]. **Note:** Absence of β-lactamase does not guarantee susceptibility of *N. gonorrhoeae* to penicillin, because some strains may possess chromosomally mediated resistance to penicillin, which is independent of β-lactamase production (see Chapter 15).

**VII. Susceptibility testing of *M. tuberculosis*** is essential to the selection of appropriate antibiotic therapy, especially in the setting of increased prevalence of multidrug-resistant tuberculosis. Testing is performed on solid media or a radiometric method in liquid media (BACTEC system). In the proportion method (2–3 weeks after isolation), susceptibility is defined as growth on drug-containing medium that is less than 1% of growth on control medium. The radiometric BACTEC system measures and compares growth, by release of carbon 14, in a drug-containing vial compared with growth of the same organism in a control vial. Results may be available within 1 week after isolation of the organism. Isoniazid, rifampin, ethambutol, and streptomycin are tested in hospital laboratories; reference laboratories perform testing for pyrazinamide, cycloserine, ethionamide, and fluoroquinolones. Susceptibility testing of mycobacteria other than *M. tuberculosis* is less commonly performed, and correlations between *in vitro* drug susceptibility of these species and *in vivo* response to therapy are not well established [42,42a]. See Chapter 11, section **IV. A.**

**VIII. Fungal and viral susceptibility testing** is not routinely performed in clinical laboratories. Testing methods and interpretive criteria are not well standardized, and these tests are considered experimental. Infectious disease consultation is advised.

## *Monitoring Antimicrobial Therapy*

Two types of *in vitro* tests are used to monitor antimicrobial therapy: measurement of blood or bodily fluid inhibition of the responsible organism, and assay of antibiotic concentrations.

**I. The serum bactericidal test** determines the "killing power" **of patient serum** against the infecting organism. The result is expressed as the highest dilution of serum that kills **and is** shown schematically in Figure 25.3. **The serum inhibitory or bacteriostatic activity** is the highest dilution of serum that demonstrates a visible inhibitory effect. **The serum lethal or bactericidal activity** is similarly expressed as the highest dilution that produces a lethal effect, usually defined as a 99.9% or greater reduction of viable organisms in the initial inoculum. Bodily fluids such as CSF, urine, and synovial fluid also can be tested.

**A. Standards**

**1. Variables that influence interlaboratory standardization in the performance of these tests make it difficult to compare results between studies** [43,43a].

**2. Timing of sample.** Several investigators favor collection of the serum sample at peak, whereas others prefer trough levels. This remains controversial [43].

**B. Clinical application.** The test is the most reliable *in vitro* correlate of actual *in vivo* conditions because it accounts for other components of the antibacterial

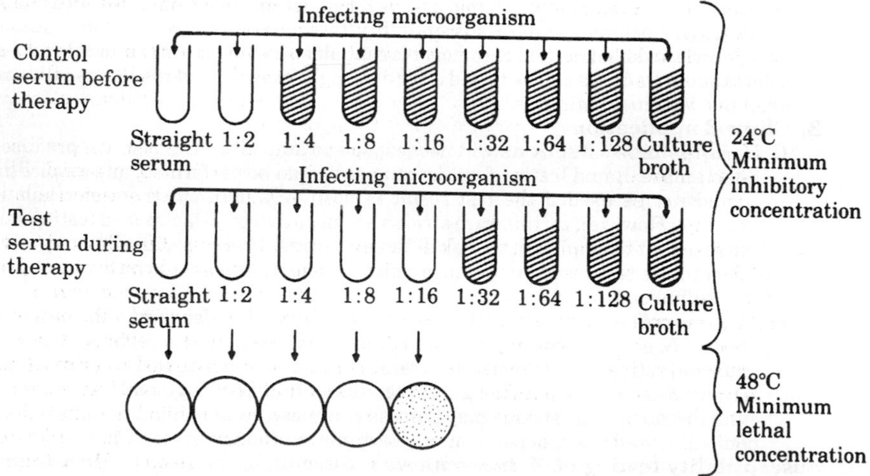


**FIG. 25.3** Dilution susceptibility testing for serum inhibitory and serum lethal activity. Serum minimum inhibitory concentration = 1:16; serum bactericidal concentration = 1:8. (Adapted from Sommers HM. Drug susceptibility testing in vitro—monitoring of antimicrobial therapy. In: Youmans GP, Paterson PY, Sommers HM, eds. *The biologic and clinical basis of infectious diseases,* 2nd ed. Philadelphia: WB Saunders, 1980, with permission.)

activity of serum in addition to the antibiotic (i.e., serum complement, opsonins, lysozymes). However, clinical applicability of the serum bactericidal titer remains to be proven rigorously [18,43,44]. **Infectious disease consultation is advised. A determination of serum bactericidal activity may prove useful in** guiding therapy, particularly in the following situations:

1. **Endocarditis.** However, the results are not necessarily predictive of survival or clinical cure, and the peak and trough bactericidal titers that best correlate with outcome are not yet clear [43,43a,45]. Although a peak titer of at least 1:8 is most frequently recommended, one study concluded that a peak titer of 1:64 or more and a trough titer of 1:32 or more were most predictive of cure; the test was a poor predictor of failure [46].
   - **a.** The organism is not highly sensitive to the antibiotics being used, and a synergistic combination of antibiotics might be more effective; less well established treatment regimens are used when the patient fails to improve on standard therapy; the serum bactericidal titer is high and drug toxicity is a significant risk; or the drug dose might be reduced without compromising antibacterial effect.
   - **b.** In acute and chronic **osteomyelitis,** serum bactericidal titers that exceed certain levels have been correlated with cure [47]. When changing to oral therapy of acute osteomyelitis in children, antibiotic doses are adjusted to achieve a bactericidal level of 1:8 or more [43a]. The usefulness in adults, remains uncertain.
   - **c.** In the **immunocompromised host,** maintaining an appropriate antibiotic level is correlated with successful outcome in bacteremia and soft-tissue infections [48].
   - **d.** For patients with acute pulmonary exacerbations of **cystic fibrosis,** peak serum bactericidal titers of 1:128 or greater against the patients' pulmonary pathogens have been correlated with favorable bacteriologic responses to therapy [49].

**II. Antimicrobial levels** may be obtained to assess the adequacy of the chosen dose and route of administration and to avoid toxicity [19].

**A. Methods**

1. **Correct timing of samples is necessary for accurate interpretation of the significance of antibiotic levels. Samples are collected without anticoagulant.**
   - **a. Peak blood levels** usually are obtained 1 hour after an intramuscular dose, 30 minutes after an intravenous infusion is over, or 1 to 2 hours after an oral dose. In renal failure, peak levels may be delayed 2 to 4 hours after an intramuscular or 1 hour after an intravenous dose.
   - **b. Trough blood levels** are obtained immediately before the next dose is due.
   - **c. Rapid processing is critical** (e.g., gentamicin is inactivated by penicillins).
   - **d.** The **requisition** should include the drug to be tested, other antibiotics, and timing of sample.
2. **Techniques for assay of antibiotic levels.** Bioassays (agar diffusion and broth dilution) have been largely supplanted by a variety of more accurate and reproducible methods (e.g., immunoassays and high-pressure liquid chromatography).
   - **a. Bioassays** use parallel dilution of both antibiotic standards and the patient's bodily fluid. This method cannot differentiate between the effects of two or more antibiotics in a bodily fluid. **Therefore, it is essential to submit information about combination antimicrobial therapy so that** the laboratory might be able to circumvent the problem by technical manipulations (e.g., add $\beta$-lactamase to inhibit penicillins, use multidrug-resistant indicator organisms, or remove antibiotics with cation-exchange resins). **Most bioassay systems are not as precise as other types of assays,** but the precision is adequate for clinical use.
   - **b. Immunologic assays** are presently the **most widely used.** and have gained widespread acceptance because they are rapid, accurate, specific, and easier to perform than bioassays. **Aminoglycoside** and **vancomycin** levels now are routinely available in many laboratories using the immunoassay method.

c. **High-pressure liquid chromatography** is a method for separating compounds; quantitation is subsequently achieved by analysis of the separated compounds. Liquid chromatographic procedures have been developed to measure almost all antibiotics in clinical specimens but are used most widely for chloramphenicol because no suitable immunoassay has been developed for this drug. Immunoassays generally are favored because they are simpler to perform.

B. **Clinical application.** Antibiotic levels may be considered in the following situations:

1. Pneumonia and bacteremia due to gram-negative organisms may respond more favorably to treatment when therapeutic plasma levels of aminoglycosides are achieved [50,51]. A high peak concentration of aminoglycoside relative to the MIC for the infecting organism has been correlated with improved clinical response to therapy [52]. For further discussion of the role of aminoglycoside levels, see Chapter 27I.
2. An antibiotic could have toxic side effects, particularly in the presence of altered hepatic or renal function (e.g., aminoglycosides; see Chapter 27I).
3. **An infection due to a sensitive organism may not respond to antibiotic** treatment and all other therapeutic approaches have been optimized.

C. **Interpretation.** It is anticipated that an infection will respond if a level of antibiotic greater than the MIC of the infecting organism can be achieved at the site of infection. However, factors other than an absolute serum level may be important (e.g., magnitude of level in comparison to MIC, duration of level above the MIC, and effect of serum protein binding). Other therapeutic modalities must always be optimized (e.g., draining abscesses, removing foreign bodies, and bolstering host defense mechanisms). See **time-dependent and concentration dependent bactericidal activity** in Chapter 27A).

## REFERENCES


1. Murray PR. Microscopy. In: Wentworth BB, ed. *Diagnostic procedures for bacterial infections.* Washington, DC: American Public Health Association, 1987:681–691.
2. Metchock BG, Nolte FS, Wallace RJ. Mycobacterium. In: Murray PR, et al., eds. *Manual of clinical microbiology,* 7th ed. Washington, DC: American Society for Microbiology, 1999:399–437.
3. Tenover FC, et al. The resurgence of tuberculosis: is your laboratory ready? *J Clin Microbiol* 1993;31:767–770.
4. Garcia LS. Diagnostic medical parisitology. In: Truant AL, ed. *Manual of commercial methods in clinical microbiology.* Washington, DC: American Society for Microbiology, 2002:274–305.
5. Wolk DM, Roberts GD. Commercial methods for identification and susceptibility testing of fungi. In: Truant AL, ed. *Manual of commercial methods in clinical microbiology.* Washington, DC: American Society for Microbiology, 2002:225–255.
6. Wilson MI. General principles of specimen collection and transport. *Clin Infect Dis* 1996;22:766.
7. Weinstein MP, Reller LB. Commercial blood culture systems and methods. In: Truant AL, ed. *Manual of commercial methods in clinical microbiology.* Washington, DC: American Society for Microbiology, 2002:12–21.
8. Reimer LG, Wilson ML, Weinstein MP. Update on detection of bacteremia and fungemia. *Clin Microbiol Rev* 1997;10:444–465.
9. Weinstein MP, et al. The clinical significance of positive blood cultures in the 1990s: a prospective comprehensive evaluation of the microbiology, epidemiology, and outcome of bacteremia and fungemia in adults. *Clin Infect Dis* 1997;24:584–602.
10. Smith-Elekes S, Weinstein MP. Blood cultures. *Infect Dis Clin North Am* 1993;9:221.
11. Mermel LA, et al. Guidelines for the management of intravascular catheter-related infections. *Infect Control Hosp Epidemiol* 2001;22:222–242.
12. Finegold SM, Jousimies-Somer HR, Wexler HM. Current perspectives in anaerobic infections. *Infect Dis Clin North Am* 1993;7:257–275.
13. Allen SD, Emery CL, Siders JA. Anaerobic bacteriology. In: Truant AL, ed. *Manual of*

*commercial methods in clinical microbiology.* Washington, DC: American Society for Microbiology, 2002:50–83.

14. Storch GA. Diagnostic virology. *Clin Infect Dis* 2000;31:739–751.
15. Menegus MA, Douglas RG Jr. Viruses, rickettsiae, chlamydiae, and mycoplasmas. In: Mandell GL, Douglas RG Jr, Bennett JE, eds. *Principles and practice of infectious diseases,* 3rd ed. New York: Churchill Livingstone, 1990.
16. Black CM. Current methods of laboratory diagnosis of *Chlamydia trachomatis* infections. *Clin Microbiol Rev* 1997;10:160–184.
17. Chernesky M, Morse S, Schachter J. Newly available and future laboratory tests for sexually transmitted diseases other than HIV. *Sexually Transmitted Dis* 1999;26(suppl): 8–11.
18. Mylonakis E, Ryan ET, Calderwood SB. *Clostridium difficile*–associated diarrhea: a review. *Arch Intern Med* 2001;161:525–533.
19. Woods GL, Washington JA. The clinician and the microbiology laboratory. In: Mandell GL, Bennett JE, Dolin R, eds. *Principles and practice of infectious diseases,* 4th ed. New York: Churchill Livingstone, 1995:169–199.
20. Murray P, et al., eds. *Manual of clinical microbiology,* 6th ed. Washington, DC: American Society for Microbiology, 1995.
21. Finegold SM, ed. Summary of current nomenclature, taxonomy, and classification of various microbial agents. *Clin Infect Dis* 1993;16:597–615.
22. Berkowitz FE. The gram-positive bacilli: a review of the microbiology, clinical aspects, and antimicrobial susceptibilities of a heterogeneous group of bacteria. *Pediatr Infect Dis J* 1994;13:1126.
23. Evangelista AT, Truant AL, Borbeau PP. Rapid methods and instruments for the identification of bacteria. In: Truant AL, ed. *Manual of commercial methods in clinical microbiology.* Washington, DC: American Society for Microbiology, 2002:22–49.
24. Menegus MA. Rapid systems and instruments for the identification of viruses. In: Truant AL, ed. *Manual of commercial methods in clinical microbiology.* Washington, DC: American Society for Microbiology, 2002:84–99.
25. Edelstein PH. Legionnaires' disease. *Clin Infect Dis* 1995;16:741.
26. Plouffe JF, et al. Reevaluation of the definition of Legionnaire's disease: use of the urinary antigen assay. *Clin Infect Dis* 1995;20:1286.
27. Struelens MJ, De Gheldre Y, Deplano A. Comparative and library epidemiological typing systems: outbreak investigations versus surveillance systems. *Infect Control Hosp Epidemiol* 1998;19:565–569.
28. Pfaller MA. Molecular epidemiology in the care of patients. *Arch Pathol Lab Med* 1999;123:1007–1010.
29. Tang Y, Persing DH. Molecular detection and identification of microorganisms. In: Murray PR, et al., eds. *Manual of clinical microbiology,* 7th ed. Washington, DC: American Society for Microbiology, 1999:215–244.
30. Jungkind D, Kessler HH. Molecular methods for diagnosis of infectious diseases. In: Truant AL, ed. *Manual of commercial methods in clinical microbiology.* Washington, DC: American Society for Microbiology, 2002:306–323.
31. Lorian V, ed. *Antibiotics in laboratory medicine,* 4th ed. Baltimore: Williams & Wilkins, 1996.
32. Rosenblatt JE. Laboratory tests used to guide antimicrobial therapy. *Mayo Clin Proc* 1991;66:942–948.
33. Stamey TA, et al. Serum versus urinary antimicrobial concentrations in cure of urinary tract infections. *N Engl J Med* 1974;291:1159–1163.

33a. Doern GV, et al. Clinical impact of rapid *in vitro* susceptibility testing and bacterial identification. *J Clin Microbiol* 1994;32:1757.

33b. Sanchez ML, Jones RN. E test, an antimicrobial susceptibility testing method with broad clinical and epidemiologic application. *Antimicrob News* 1992;8:1.

33c. Kiska DL, et al. Comparison of antimicrobial susceptibility methods for detection of penicillin-resistant *Streptococcus pneumoniae. J Clin Microbiol* 1995;33:229.

34. Finegold SM, Jousimies-Somer HR, Wexler HM. Current perspectives on anaerobic infections: diagnostic approaches. *Infect Dis Clin North Am* 1993;7:257–275.
35. Cuchural GJ, et al. Susceptibility of the *Bacteroides fragilis* group in the United States: analysis by site of isolation. *Antimicrob Agents Chemother* 1988;32:717.

36. Goldstein EJC, et al. Comparative susceptibility of the *Bacteroides fragilis* group species and other anaerobic bacteria to meropenem, imipenem, piperacillin, cefoxitin, ampicillin/sulbactam, clindamycin and metronidazole. *J Antimicrob Chemother* 1993;31:363–372.
36a. Wexler HM, Doern GV. Susceptibility testing of anaerobic bacteria. In: Murray PR, et al., eds. *Manual of clinical microbiology,* 6th ed. Washington, DC: American Society for Microbiology, 1995:1350–1355.
37. Finegold SM and the National Committee for Clinical Laboratory Standards. Susceptibility testing of anaerobic bacteria. *J Clin Microbiol* 1988;26:1253.
37a. Schieven BC, et al. Evaluation of susceptibility of anaerobic organisms by the E test and the reference agar dilution method. *Clin Infect Dis* 1995;20(suppl 2):5337.
38. Moellering RC. Antimicrobial synergism—an elusive concept. *J Infect Dis* 1979;140: 639.
39. Anderson ET, Young LS, Hewitt WL. Antimicrobial synergism in the therapy of gram-negative rod bacteremia. *Chemotherapy* 1978;24:45.
40. Kashuba AD, Bertino JS Jr, Nafziger AN. Dosing of aminoglycoside to rapidly attain pharmacokinetic goals and hasten therapeutic response by using individualized pharmacokinetic monitoring of patients with pneumonia caused by gram negative organisms. *Antimicrob Agents Chemother* 1998;42:1842–1844.
41. Centers for Disease Control and Prevention. Sexually transmitted disease treatment guidelines. *MMWR* 1993;42:1–102.
42. Witebsky FG, Conville PS. The laboratory diagnosis of mycobacterial diseases. *Infect Dis Clin North Am* 1993;7:359–376.
42a. Shinnick TM, Good RC. Diagnostic mycobacteriology laboratory practices. *Clin Infect Dis* 1995;21:291.
43. Wolfson JS, Swartz MN. Serum bactericidal activity as a monitor of antibiotic therapy. *N Engl J Med* 1985;312:968.
43a. Reller LB. The serum bactericidal test. *Rev Infect Dis* 1986;8:803.
44. Stratton CW. Bactericidal testing. *Infect Dis Clin North Am* 1993;7:445.
45. Coleman DL, Horwitz RI, Andriole VT. Association between serum inhibitory and bactericidal concentrations and therapeutic outcome in bacterial endocarditis. *Am J Med* 1982;73:260.
46. Weinstein MP, et al. Multicenter collaborative evaluation of a standardized serum bactericidal test as a prognostic indicator in infective endocarditis. *Am J Med* 1985; 78:262.
47. Weinstein MP, et al. Multicenter collaborative evaluation of a standardized serum bactericidal test as a predictor of therapeutic efficacy in acute and chronic osteomyelitis. *Am J Med* 1987;83:218.
48. Schentag JJ. Antimicrobial action and pharmacokinetics/pharmacodynamics: the use of AUIC to improve efficacy and avoid resistance. *J Chemother* 1999;11:426–439.
49. Cahen P, et al. Serum bactericidal test as a prognostic indicator in acute pulmonary exacerbations of cystic fibrosis. *Pediatrics* 1993;91:451–455.
50. Moore RD, Smith CR, Lietman PS. The association of aminoglycoside plasma levels with mortality in patients with gram-negative bacteremia. *J Infect Dis* 1984;149:443.
51. Kashuba AD, Nafziger AN, Drusano GL, et al. Optimizing aminoglycoside therapy for nosocomial pneumonia caused by gram negative bacteria. *Antimicrob Agents Chemother* 1999;43:623–629.
52. Moore RD, Leitman PS. Smith CR. Clinical response to aminoglycoside therapy: Importance of the ratio of peak concentration to minimal inhibitory concentration. *J Infect Dis* 1987;155:93–99.

# 26. INFECTIOUS DISEASE ASPECTS OF EMPLOYEE (OCCUPATIONAL) HEALTH: A BRIEF OVERVIEW

Keith A. Rosenbach, Sally H. Houston, John T. Sinnott, and JoAnn Palumbo Shea

## EMPLOYEE HEALTH AND SAFETY

Health-care workers (HCWs) are an important link in the control of infection. Many states already regulate minimal health and immunization requirements for employment in health-care facilities. A comprehensive employee health program should be developed using guidelines and regulations from the Centers for Disease Control and Prevention (CDC), Occupational Safety and Health Administration (OSHA), National Institute for Occupational Safety and Health, and state health departments. This discussion does not attempt to define such a comprehensive program, which has been addressed in other reports [1–5]. **Rather, the intent of this discussion is to alert** the student, house officer, practicing physician, and other **health-care providers about those employee health issues that overlap with infection control issues; that is, how to protect the HCW from acquiring or spreading infections in the hospital, clinic, or office setting.**

**I. Employee health program**

**A. Major objectives** of an employee health program should include the following:

1. To screen periodically to identify occupational health risks, implement preventive measures [1], and comply with respiratory agency minimal standards;
2. To provide management of occupationally related illness and communicable disease or blood-borne pathogen exposure among HCWs;
3. To monitor and investigate exposures and disease outbreaks among personnel;
4. To emphasize preventive health practices and health maintenance habits and promote individual responsibility for infection control.

**B. Baseline and periodic health assessment.** At the time of employment, it is useful to establish a baseline health and immunization history. If documentation of immunization is not possible, **serologic testing for rubella, rubeola, varicella-zoster virus,** and **hepatitis B virus** (HBV) is warranted [6]. A comprehensive medical history and physical examination is not necessary for infection-control purposes but may be required by state regulations, and it also serves as an important resource for determining preexisting medical problems. Many facilities have adopted "position-specific" screening that targets risks associated with specific tasks. Each worker's health status should be reassessed annually and immunizations updated [1].

**C. Tuberculosis control.** OSHA regulations include the following. A baseline intermediate purified protein derivative (PPD) tuberculin skin test is required for all new employees whose tuberculosis status is unknown or whose reaction is negative by history. Two-step testing eliminates potential false-positive PPD conversions as a result of the booster effect [7,8] (see Chapter 11 under Tuberculosis). A current chest roentgenogram to rule out active disease is recommended for individuals exhibiting a positive reaction to PPD, with assessment for active pulmonary disease and consideration of isoniazid prophylaxis (see Chapter 11). The need for repeat PPD testing should be dictated by exposure or the prevalence of tuberculosis in the hospital population or geographic area. State regulations may also affect this interval [1]. HCWs at increased risk for exposure to tuberculosis should be PPD tested every 3 to 6 months depending on hospital risk assessment data. Potential high-risk employees include emergency department personnel, respiratory therapists, microbiology laboratory workers, pathologists, specialists in pulmonary medicine, and nurses in some settings [8–10]. For further discussion, see Chapter 11 and related references [8,9].

**D. Immunization program.** Immunization of hospital staff helps reduce the risk of transmissible diseases [1,6,11,12] (see also Chapter 23).

1. **Rubella. All HCWs, regardless of age or gender, should be immune to rubella.** This is a vital strategy for preventing congenital rubella syndrome, and some states have made it mandatory. Many hospitals require immunity as a

condition of employment. **New employees** without documentation of immunization after his or her first birthday **should be screened for rubella antibody and offered immunization if seronegative** [11] (see Chapter 23).

2. **Hepatitis B immunization.** OSHA requires that all employees whose job activities place them at risk for blood exposure are **offered** the hepatitis B vaccine at the employer's expense. Although prescreening is not required unless specifically requested by the employee, it may be helpful and cost effective if risk factors for hepatitis B are present [13]. For the details of hepatitis B vaccination, see Chapters 14 and 23. Postvaccination testing for antibody to HBV surface antigen should be performed to document antibody response. This will assist in determining the need for further immunization or appropriate postexposure prophylaxis [14]. OSHA mandates that employers document vaccination history (including employee refusal of vaccine) and provide training in both the prevention of exposure to blood-borne pathogens and the correct use of personal protective equipment.
3. **Influenza.** Influenza can spread quickly through a health-care facility, particularly one with a residential environment. Therefore, aggressive efforts should be made to immunize staff, particularly those with direct patient contact, in November of each year [12] (see Chapter 10). Nosocomial transmission of influenza has been demonstrated and may have dramatic effects on patient outcome [6].
4. **Rubeola.** Measles may present a significant risk to both HCWs and their patients. Persons born before 1956 are, in general, considered immune to measles. Among HCWs born after 1956, up to 14% are susceptible to measles [15,16]. The Infectious Diseases Society of America recommends that hospitals require from all HCWs evidence of measles infection or receipt of two doses of live virus vaccine [17]. If this documentation is lacking, serologic testing should be done and live measles virus vaccine should be administered at employment and repeated 1 month later for all HCWs who are not immune. Live virus vaccines are contraindicated during pregnancy [17,18] (see Chapter 23).
5. **Tetanus-diphtheria.** It is important to update tetanus-diphtheria immunization at the time of employment (if need be) and every 10 years thereafter. See detailed discussion in Chapters 4 and 23.
6. **Mumps.** Susceptible adult HCWs, especially males, are candidates for vaccination [1] (see Chapter 23).
7. **Varicella.** Knowledge of the varicella-antibody status of employees who provide direct patient care has become more important as the immunosuppressed patient population increases. Consequently, most hospitals, particularly those with large pediatric or immunocompromised populations, have initiated varicella screening of all employees. Documentation of serology will prevent unnecessary work restrictions and disruption of patient services if exposure occurs [1,6].

   The live-attenuated varicella vaccine is discussed in detail in Chapter 23. Precise guidelines for the use of this vaccine in HCWs have not yet been published. Susceptible HCWs who have direct patient contact would appear to be potential candidates for this vaccine; this must be individualized until guidelines are available.
8. **Other immunizations.** Booster doses of poliomyelitis immunization are generally not indicated. Administration of oral poliovirus vaccine to an HCW is contraindicated because of the risk of transmitting the live virus. Some hospitals provide vaccine against pneumococcal pneumonia. Consideration should be given to offering hepatitis A vaccine to food handlers, hospital child-care workers, and selected research personnel (see Chapter 14).

E. **Screening for carriage of bacterial, viral, or parasitic pathogens.** Unless an HCW is or has been epidemiologically implicated in disease transmission or has symptoms of infection, routine screening for pathogens (e.g., HBV, human immunodeficiency virus [HIV], *Salmonella* species, vancomycin-resistant enterococci, group A *Streptococcus*, *Staphylococcus aureus,* including methicillin-resistant *S. aureus*) is not indicated (see section **II**). However, some state or local regulations may require screening of food handlers for enteric pathogens.

F. **Work restrictions for acute, chronic, or recurrent infections.** In certain situations, HCWs will need to be placed on work restrictions, complete or partial, depending on the infection and risk of transmission [1]. Table 26.1 summarizes these recommendations.

G. **Prophylaxis after exposure to various illnesses** has been reviewed elsewhere in this volume:

1. **Hepatitis A** (see Chapters 14 and 23).
2. **Hepatitis B** (see Chapters 14 and 23).
3. **Hepatitis C.** Results have been equivocal in studies attempting to assess the value of prophylaxis with immunoglobulins against parenterally transmitted non-A, non-B hepatitis. For persons with percutaneous exposure to blood from a patient with parenterally transmitted non-A, non-B hepatitis, it may be reasonable to administer immunoglobulin (0.06 mL/kg) as soon as possible after exposure [1]. A study indicated that treatment with interferon during the acute phase prevents the development of chronic HCV infection [19]. See related discussions in section **II.A.2** and Chapter 14.
4. **Meningococcal disease** (see Chapter 6).
5. **Rabies.** HCWs who have been bitten by a human with rabies or who have scratches, abrasions, open wounds, or mucous membranes contaminated with saliva or other potentially infective material from a human or animal with rabies should receive a full course of antirabies treatment [1] (see Chapter 4).

## II. Occupational issues related to blood-borne disease transmission

### A. Risk of transmission to HCWs

1. **HBV.** In the United States there are an estimated 1 to 1.25 million chronic carriers of HBV (hepatitis B surface antigen positive). These persons represent a continuous risk to uninfected persons. In the United States, between 200,000 and 300,000 new cases are reported annually. In part because of such figures, the CDC now recommends that all children in the United States receive hepatitis B vaccine [14] (see Chapters 14 and 23). Still, approximately 300 HCWs die annually of HBV or its complications [20]. Individuals in occupations that involve the performance of invasive procedures or frequent contact with blood are at increased risk of exposure. Surveys of personnel in high-risk occupations have shown high rates of seropositivity: between 5% and 30% or more for hospital-based physicians and laboratory personnel [11,12]. The risk for HBV infection after a single percutaneous exposure to blood contaminated with hepatitis B e antigen (HBeAg positive) is estimated to be 27% to 43%, with a 6% to 24% risk for subsequent development of clinical hepatitis [21]. **These data underscore the importance of hepatitis B immunization as a preventive measure** (see Chapter 23).
2. **Hepatitis C virus (HCV).** Third-generation immunoassays have improved the positive predictive value of the antibody test for HCV. However, the rate of HCV transmission and risk factors for transmission remain to be determined. OSHA guidelines regarding prevention of exposure to blood-borne pathogens were intended to prevent transmission of HCV and other yet to be identified blood-borne pathogens. Contraction of HCV infection has been documented to occur via needlestick transmission [21]. The risk of transmission appears to be less than 4%, compared with up to 67% for HBeAg-positive serum [22]. Approximately 50% of those infected with HCV will go on to develop chronic liver disease with increased risk for cirrhosis and hepatocellular carcinoma [23] (see related discussions in Chapter 14).
3. **HIV.** HCWs are at low risk for acquiring HIV from their patients. However, studies and individual case reports have documented several cases of occupational transmission [24]. Currently, the risk from a single percutaneous exposure to HIV-infected blood is estimated to be approximately 0.3% (see Chapter 18). Projections of individual lifetime risk have been proposed based on the seroprevalence of HIV in the geographic area and the frequency with which an individual sustains accidental injuries that represent a risk for blood-borne disease transmission [25]. As of June 2000, the CDC had reported approximately 56 cases of documented occupationally acquired HIV and an additional 138 possible occupationally acquired transmissions among HCWs [29]. Circumstances resulting in occupational **HIV transmission** have **involved blood or bloody fluids only,** and transmission has occurred primarily through hollow-bore needlestick injury [20]. **Prolonged**

Table 26.1. Work Restrictions for Hospital Workers Exposed to or Infected with Selected Infectious Diseases

| Disease or Problem | Relieve from Direct Patient Contact | Partial Work Restriction | Duration |
|---|---|---|---|
| Conjunctivitis, infectious | Yes | | Until discharge ceases |
| Cytomegalovirus infections | No | | |
| Diarrhea | | | |
| Acute stage (diarrhea with other symptoms) | Yes | | Until symptoms resolve and infection with *Salmonella* is ruled out |
| Convalescent stage *Salmonella* (nontyphoidal) | No | Personnel should not care for high-risk patients | Until stool is free of the infecting organism on two consecutive cultures not less than 24 h apart |
| Enteroviral infections | No | Personnel should not care for infants and newborns | Until symptoms resolve |
| Group A streptococcal disease | Yes | | Until 24 h after adequate treatment is started |
| Hepatitis, viral | | | |
| Hepatitis A | Yes | | Until 7 days after onset of jaundice |
| Hepatitis B | | | |
| Acute | Possibly | Personnel should use barrier precautions for procedures with mucous membranes on nonintact skin | Until antigenemia resolves |
| Chronic antigenemia | Possibly | HCWs who are HBeAg-positive may be restricted in certain situations | Until antigenemia resolves |
| Hepatitis C (parenterally transmitted non-A, non-B) | No | Personnel should use barrier precautions for procedures that involve trauma to tissues or contact with mucous membranes on nonintact skin | Period of infectivity has not been determined |
| Herpes simplex | | | |
| Genital | No | | |
| Hands (herpetic whitlow) | Yes | (Note: It is not known whether gloves prevent transmission) | Until lesions heal |
| Orofacial | No | Personnel should not care for high-risk patients | Until lesions heal |
| Human immunodeficiency virus | Possibly | HCWs may be restricted in certain situations | |

| | | | |
|---|---|---|---|
| Measles | | | |
| Active | Yes | | Until 7 days after the rash appears |
| Postexposure (susceptible personnel) | Yes | | From the 5th through the 21st day after exposure or 7 days after the rash appears |
| Mumps | | | |
| Active | Yes | | Until 9 days after onset of parotitis |
| Postexposure (susceptible personnel) | Yes | | From the 12th through the 26th day after exposure or until 9 days after onset of parotitis |
| Pertussis | | | |
| Active | Yes | | From the beginning of the catarrhal stage through the third week after onset of paroxysms or until 5 days after start of effective antimicrobial therapy |
| Postexposure (asymptomatic personnel) | No | | |
| Postexposure (symptomatic personnel) | Yes | | Same as active pertussis |
| Rubella | | | |
| Active | Yes | | Until 5 days after rash appears |
| Postexposure (susceptible personnel) | Yes | | From the 7th through the 21st day after exposure |
| Scabies | Yes | | Until treated |
| *Staphylococcus aureus* (skin lesions) | Yes | | Until lesions have resolved |
| Upper respiratory infections | No | Personnel with upper respiratory infections should not care for high-risk patients | Until acute symptoms resolve |
| Varicella (chickenpox) | | | |
| Active | Yes | | Until all lesions dry and crust |
| Postexposure (susceptible personnel) | Yes | | From the 10th through the 21st day after exposure and, if varicella occurs, until all lesions dry and crust |
| Zoster (shingles) | | | |
| Active | No, if lesions localized and covered | Appropriate barrier desirable | Until lesions dry and crust, personnel should not care for high-risk patients (regardless if lesions are covered) |
| Postexposure (personnel susceptible to chickenpox) | Yes | | From the 10th through the 21st day after exposure and, if varicella occurs, until all lesions dry and crust |

HBeAg, hepatitis B e antigen; HCWs, health-care workers.
From Polder JA, Tablan OC, Williams WW. Personnel health services. In: Bennett JV, Brachman PS eds. *Hospital infections,* 3rd ed. Boston: Little, Brown, 1992:36–37, with permission.

**contact** with HIV-positive blood on nonintact skin or mucous membranes also may have transmitted the virus [24]. Several instances of HIV transmission in laboratory settings have been documented [26]. This topic has been extensively reviewed elsewhere [27].

**B. Screening employees for HBV, HCV, or HIV.** Routine preemployment or periodic screening of employees for HBV, HCV, or HIV **has been discouraged** [28]. Such testing should be linked to the provision of employee health services (i.e., screening after hepatitis B vaccine administration or as part of postexposure management). **Screening should not be used, and is in fact prohibited in some states, to exclude or modify employment in health-care settings.**

**C. Postexposure management.** Employees who have sustained percutaneous or mucous membrane or nonintact skin exposures to blood or body fluids (i.e., serous fluids) that may contain a blood-borne virus should be evaluated, counseled, and offered appropriate medical follow-up. **When possible, individuals who are the source of such exposures should be screened for HBV, HCV, and HIV. Requirements for obtaining informed consent of the source patient vary from state to state.** In the past, recommendations for testing source patients for HCV were controversial [29]. Currently, most authorities would agree that testing of high-risk patients is reasonable. Testing for HIV in exposed employees should be accompanied by appropriate pretest and posttest counseling; informed consent must be obtained [26].

1. Chapters 14 and 23 provide guidelines for **HBV postexposure prophylaxis,** which takes into consideration the HBV status of both the source individual and the employee. The CDC recommendations (June 2001) for HBV postexposure prophylaxis include hepatitis B immune globulin and/or the HBV vaccination series, after the evaluation of the HBV surface antigen status of the source, as well as the vaccination history and titers in response to the vaccine of the exposed person [30]. Once again, it is important to emphasize the need to vaccinate all unexposed HCWs for HBV because of the high risk of transmission from a needlestick injury.
2. Gerberding and Henderson [31] recommend that an HCW exposed to HCV undergo testing for HCV antibody and liver function tests at the time of exposure. Follow-up testing should be repeated at 3 and 6 months, or sooner if the HCW becomes symptomatic [31]. Administration of serum immunoglobulin (ISG 0.06 mL/kg) to the HCW as soon as possible after parenteral exposure to a confirmed case of HCV has been suggested, but failures have been reported [29].
   - **a.** The CDC recommendations, June 2001, for HCV postexposure prophylaxis do not include intravenous immune globulin or antiviral agents [30]. Postexposure management involves determining the HCV status of the source and the exposed person. If the source is HCV antibody positive, then follow-up HCV testing is performed on the exposed HCW. Interestingly, one case has been reported in which an HCW did not seroconvert to HCV antibody positive after a needlestick injury involving a known HCV-infected source patient [32]. The HCW was documented by polymerase chain reaction (PCR) to have an acute HCV infection assay and has remained antibody negative at 1 year after exposure. Thus, clinical suspicion may be necessary in some cases, and liver function tests may also need to be followed.
   - **b.** For HCWs diagnosed in the acute phase of a HCV infection, treatment with interferon may be beneficial [19]. In one study, 44 subjects were diagnosed in the acute phase by documented seroconversion to HCV antibody positive, known or suspected exposure to HCV within the preceding 4 months, or marked elevation of serum alanine aminotransferase more than 350 U/L. All 44 subjects were HCV PCR positive and had elevated alanine aminotransferase levels. The study included subjects with different HCV genotypes. The patients resolved the HCV infection after 24 weeks of interferon alpha-2b monotherapy, preventing progression to chronic active disease. The regimen was 5 million units interferon alpha-2b subcutaneously injected daily for 4 weeks, followed by three times weekly for 20 weeks. At the end of 24 weeks, 42 of 43 (98%) subjects

had undetectable HCV RNA by the PCR-based assay. During the follow-up assays at 36 and 48 weeks, the serum from the 42 subjects remained free of detectable HCV RNA by the PCR-based assay. The level of detection is less than 600 copies/mL.

**e.** The important point is to treat early, before the more difficult to treat chronic infection is established. The success rate of 98% for treating HCV in the acute phase is quite remarkable, especially when compared with the success rate in chronic HCV infections treated with the most effective regimen to date. Chronic HCV infections treated for 48 weeks with pegylated-interferon plus ribavirin eliminated the virus in only 55% of cases [33,34].

**3.** HCWs who have been exposed to an HIV-positive source should be offered the following:

**a.** Baseline HIV antibody testing to determine the employee's serostatus at the time of exposure and periodically thereafter (e.g., 4 weeks, 3 and 6 months) to rule out seroconversion.

**b.** Pretest and posttest counseling is required in most states to manage postexposure anxiety and to provide risk-reduction education to prevent third-party transmission during the period when seroconversion may occur.

**c.** Any HCW exposed to a potential HIV-positive source should be offered postexposure prophylaxis with antiretroviral agents to reduce the risk of transmission, including the initial period of evaluating the HIV status of the potential source. The CDC recommends a basic regimen prescribed for 4 weeks: a two-drug regimen of nucleoside reverse transcriptase inhibitors for low-risk exposures and an expanded three-drug regimen, including two nucleoside reverse transcriptase inhibitors plus a protease inhibitor or nonnucleoside reverse transcriptase inhibitor for the higher risk exposures [30] (Tables 26.2 and 26.3). When the source patient is HIV positive and the virus is known to be resistant, based on genotype or phenotype results, or suspected to be resistant, the HCW should be given an expanded postexposure prophylaxis regimen of antiretroviral agents effective against these HIV subtypes.

Emphasis must be placed on decreasing the risk of exposure to blood-borne pathogens via proper barrier techniques and appropriate handling of sharps, as well as the implementation of needle safety devices [28]. For a more detailed discussion of this topic, see the report of Beekman and Henderson [27].

**D. Management of HCWs infected with HIV, HBV, or HCV.** This topic has been reviewed by a number of authors [21,35–37] and is also the subject of a thoughtful editorial by Gerberding [28].

**1. HIV-infected workers.** Every industry, including health care, has HIV-positive workers at all levels. A topic of some concern is whether infected HCWs pose a risk for HIV transmission to patients. Although a potential may exist in settings where invasive procedures are performed, as of March 1996 there was only one highly publicized reported case of suspected transmission [28,38–40]. Screening of more than 19,000 patients of HIV-infected HCWs has failed to reveal another case of HIV transmission from an infected HCW to patient [41]. Currently, the CDC recommends that individual institutions establish a task force with a mandate to define exposure-prone procedures and to evaluate the competency of HIV-infected and HBeAg-positive HCWs who perform such procedures [21,42,43]. According to a CDC analysis, the risk of death from HIV or HBV infection acquired during an invasive procedure performed by an infected surgeon is similar to that of acquiring HIV infection from a transfused unit of screened blood [28].

**2. HBV-infected workers.** Hepatitis B has uncommonly been transmitted from an HCW to a patient, despite the fact that the CDC estimates that approximately 1,900 U.S. surgeons are chronically infected with HBV [37]. An unusual outbreak of HBV was described recently in patients operated on by a surgeon who was positive for HBeAg [37]. Furthermore, HBV is known to have been transmitted during invasive procedures from 34 infected HCWs to at least 350 patients in the United States and elsewhere since the early 1970s [28].

It is suggested that HCWs who perform invasive procedures know their HBV status. However, if a worker is HBeAg positive or epidemiologically linked to

Table 26.2. Recommended HIV Postexposure Prophylaxis (PEP) for Percutaneous Injuries

| | Infection Status of Source | | | | |
|---|---|---|---|---|---|
| Exposure | HIV-Positive Class 1[a] | HIV-Positive Class 2[a] | Source of Unknown HIV Status[b] | Unknown Source[c] | HIV Negative |
| Less severe[d] | Basic 2-drug PEP | Expanded 3-drug PEP | Generally, no PEP warranted; however, consider basic 2-drug PEP[e] for source with HIV risk factors[f] | Generally, no PEP warranted; however, consider basic 2-drug PEP[e] in settings where exposure to HIV-infected persons is likely | No PEP warranted |
| More severe[g] | Expanded 3-drug PEP | Expanded 3-drug PEP | Same as above | Same as above | Same as above |

[a]HIV-positive, class 1: asymptomatic HIV infection or known low viral load (<1,500 RNA copies/mL). HIV-positive, class 2: symptomatic HIV infection, acquired immunodeficiency virus, acute seroconversion, or known high viral load. If drug resistance is a concern, obtain expert consultation. Initiation of PEP should not be delayed pending expert consultation, and because expert consultation alone cannot substitute for face-to-face counseling, resources should be available to provide immediate evaluation and follow-up care for all exposures.
[b]Source of unknown HIV status (e.g., deceased source person with no samples available for HIV testing).
[c]Unknown source (e.g., a needle from a sharps disposal container).
[d]Less severe (i.e., solid needle and superficial injuries).
[e]"Consider PEP" indicates that PEP is optional and should be based on an individualized decision between the exposed person and the treating clinician.
[f]If PEP is offered and taken and the source is later determined to be HIV negative, PEP should be discontinued.
[g]More severe (i.e., large-bore hollow needle, deep puncture, visible blood on device, or needle used in patient's artery or vein).
HIV, human immunodeficiency virus.
From Centers for Disease Control. Guidelines for the management of occupational exposures to HBV, HCV, and HIV and recommendations for postexposure prophylaxis. *MMWR Morb Mortal Wkly Rep* 2001;50(RR-11):1–54, with permission.

Table 26.3. Recommended HIV Postexposure Prophylaxis (PEP) for Mucous Membrane and Nonintact Skin[a] Exposures

| | Infection Status of Source | | | | |
|---|---|---|---|---|---|
| Exposure | HIV-Positive Class 1[b] | HIV-Positive Class 2[b] | Source of Unknown HIV Status[c] | Unknown Source[d] | HIV Negative |
| Small volume[e] | Basic 2-drug PEP | Basic 2-drug PEP | Generally, no PEP warranted; however, consider basic 2-drug PEP[c] for source with HIV risk factors[g] | Generally, no PEP warranted; however, consider basic 2-drug PEP[f] in settings where exposure to HIV-infected persons is likely | No PEP warranted |
| Large volume[h] | Basic 2-drug PEP | Expanded 3-drug PEP | Same as above | Same as above | Same as above |

[a]For skin exposures, follow-up is indicated only if there is evidence of compromised skin integrity (i.e., dermatitis, abrasion, or open wound).

[b]HIV-positive, class 1: asymptomatic HIV infection or known low viral load (<1,500 RNA copies/mL). HIV-positive, class 2: symptomatic HIV infection, acquired immunodeficiency, acute seroconversion, or known high viral load. If drug resistance is a concern, obtain expert consultation. Initiation of PEP should not be delayed pending expert consultation, and because expert consultation alone cannot substitute for face-to-face counseling, resources should be available to provide immediate evaluation and follow-up care for all exposures.

[c]Source of unknown HIV status (e.g., deceased source person with no samples available for HIV testing).

[d]Unknown source (e.g., a needle from a sharps disposal container).

[e]Small volume (i.e., a few drops).

[f]"Consider PEP" indicates that PEP is optional and should be based on an individualized decision between the exposed person and the treating clinician.

[g]If PEP is offered and taken and the source is later determined to be HIV negative, PEP should be discontinued.

[h]Large volume (i.e., major blood splash).

HIV, human immunodeficiency virus.

From Centers for Disease Control. Guidelines for the management of occupational exposures to HBV, HCV, and HIV and recommendations for postexposure prophylaxis. *MMWR Morb Mortal Wkly Rep* 2001;50(RR-11):1–54, with permission.

patient transmission, work practices should be reviewed, and if modifications cannot be reasonably accommodated, work restrictions should be imposed [11,21].

3. **HCV-infected workers.** Transmission of HCV occurs principally by the parenteral route (see related discussions in Chapter 14). A recent report identifies two patients who appeared to have contracted HCV from a cardiac surgeon infected with HCV [36]. Therefore, specific guidelines to reduce risk of transmission from infected HCWs to patients remain unclear. Proper handwashing, use of approved barriers, and appropriate surgical technique with regard to prevention of exposure to sharps should be emphasized [23].

III. **Education and training** of all HCWs is a vital component of the infection control and employee health program. All employees should receive initial job orientation and in-service education about disease transmission, their role and responsibility for disease prevention, the infection control aspects of employee health, and the use of employee health services [1]. Employees also should receive specific training on the use of barrier precautions and preventive practices as they relate to implementation of universal precautions. Such training has been mandated by OSHA.

IV. **OSHA regulations.** On December 6, 1991, OSHA published its standard, "Occupational Exposure to Bloodborne Pathogens" (*Federal Register* 29 CFR Part 1910.1030). By issuing this standard, OSHA indicated that HCWs face a significant health risk as a result of occupational exposure to blood-borne pathogens such as HBV and HIV.

A. **Purpose of the standard.** The purpose of this standard is to minimize or eliminate occupational risk to blood-borne diseases by the provision of engineering and work practice controls, personal protective equipment, training, vaccination, and postexposure evaluation and follow-up. This standard applies to employees in all health-care facilities, including hospitals, clinics, dentists' and physicians' offices, blood banks and plasma centers, long-term care homes, hospices, clinical laboratories, funeral homes, and institutions for the developmentally disabled.

B. **Components of the program**

1. **Exposure control plan.** This is a written plan that identifies employees with risk of occupational exposure. It contains a schedule and method for implementation of standard requirements and postexposure evaluation procedures. The plan should be reviewed and updated annually and should be made available to all employees at risk.
2. **Methods of compliance.** The standard requires employers to implement methods and training to comply with provisions for worker protection to minimize or eliminate exposures. Areas addressed include the following:
   a. Administration of policies and procedures;
   b. Engineering and work practice controls;
   c. Accessible personal protective equipment (PPE) to be used when indicated.
3. **Hepatitis B vaccination.** This standard requires that the hepatitis B vaccine is made available at no cost to all employees at risk of occupational exposure, within 10 days of initial job assignment, and after training on blood-borne pathogen exposure is completed. Employees declining vaccination must sign a declination form and may request vaccination at a later date.
4. **Postexposure evaluation and follow-up.** The employer must make a postexposure evaluation available immediately after the exposure incident. Requirements for HIV and HBV testing of the source individual and exposed employee, provision of postexposure prophylaxis, and counseling are included.
5. **Training program.** The OSHA standard requires that all employees at risk for occupational exposure attend a training program at the time of initial employment and annually thereafter. The components of the training program include an explanation of the epidemiology and transmission of blood-borne diseases, an explanation of methods to eliminate or minimize exposures (e.g., handwashing, use of personal protective equipment), and postexposure follow-up, in addition to labeling and record-keeping requirements.
6. **Record keeping.** Records of postexposure evaluations and hepatitis B vaccination must be kept for the length of employment plus 30 years.

## REFERENCES


1. Polder JA, Tablan OC, Williams WW. Personnel health services. In: Bennett JV, Brachman PS, eds. *Hospital infections,* 3rd ed. Boston: Little, Brown, 1992:31–62.
2. Sherertz RJ, Marosok RD, Streed SA. Infection control aspects of hospital employee health. In: Wenzel RP, ed. *Prevention and control of nosocomial infections.* Baltimore: Williams & Wilkins, 1993:295–332.
3. Rosenstock L, Cullen MR. *Textbook of clinical occupational and environmental medicine.* Philadelphia: WB Saunders, 1994.
4. Centers for Disease Control. *Guidelines for protecting the safety and health of health care workers.* Atlanta, GA: National Institute for Occupational Safety and Health (publication No. 88-119), 1988.
5. Mayhall CG, ed. *Hospital epidemiology and infection control.* Baltimore: Williams & Wilkins, 1996.
6. Williams WW, Pleblud SR, Reichelderfer PS, et al. Vaccines of importance in the hospital setting: problems and developments. *Infect Dis Clin North Am* 1989;3:701–719.
7. McGowan JE Jr. The booster effect—a problem for surveillance of tuberculosis in hospital employees. *Am J Infect Control* 1983;11:57.
8. Centers for Disease Control and Prevention. *Core curriculum on tuberculosis: what the clinician should know,* 4th ed. Atlanta:CDC, 2000. *www.cdc.gov/nchstp/tb/pubs/corecurr/* or CDC Voice and Fax Information System (1-888-232-3228).
9. Centers for Disease Control and Prevention. Essential components of a tuberculosis prevention and control program. *MMWR Morb Mortal Wkly Rep* 1995;44(RR-11):1–34.
10. Sepkowitz KA. AIDS, tuberculosis, and the health care worker. *Clin Infect Dis* 1995;20:232.
11. Williams WW. CDC guidelines for infection control in hospital personnel. *Infect Control* 1983;4[Suppl]:326–349.
12. Fedson DS. Immunization for health care workers and patients in hospitals. In: Wenzel RP, ed. *Prevention and control of nosocomial infections,* 2nd ed. Baltimore: Williams & Wilkins, 1993:214.
13. Centers for Disease Control. Protection against viral hepatitis. *MMWR Morb Mortal Wkly Rep* 1990;39:(RR-2):1–26.
14. Centers for Disease Control. Hepatitis B virus: a comprehensive strategy for eliminating transmission in the United States through universal childhood vaccination. Recommendations of ACIP. *MMWR Morb Mortal Wkly Rep* 1991;40(RR-13):1–25.
15. Kim M, Lapointe J, Liu F. Epidemiology of measles immunity in a population of health-care workers. *Infect Control Hosp Epidemiol* 1992;13:399–402.
16. Houck P, Scott-Johnson G, Krebs L. Measles immunity among community hospital employees. *Infect Control Hosp Epidemiol* 1991;12:663–668.
17. Krause PJ, Gross PA, Barrett TL, et al. Quality standard for assurance of measles immunity among health care workers. *Clin Infect Dis* 1994;18:431–436.
18. Centers for Disease Control. Measles prevention: recommendations of the Immunization Practices Advisory Committee (ACIP). *MMWR Morb Mortal Wkly Rep* 1989;38(S-9): 1–18.
19. Jaeckel E, Cornberg M, Wedemeyer H, et al. Treatment of acute hepatitis C with interferon alfa-2b. *N Engl J Med* 2001;345:1452–1457.
20. Fry DE. Occupational risks of infection in the surgical management of trauma patients. *Am J Surg* 1993;165[Suppl 2A]:26S–33S.
21. Doebbeling BN, Wenzel RP. Nosocomial viral hepatitis and infections transmitted by blood and blood products. In: Mandell GL, Bennett JE, Dolin R, eds. *Principles and practice of infectious diseases,* 4th ed. New York: Churchill Livingstone, 1995:2618.
22. Kiyosawa K, Sodeyama T, Tanaka E, et al. Hepatitis C in hospital employees with needlestick injuries. *Ann Intern Med* 1991;115:367–369.
23. Davis JM, Demling RH, Lewis FR, et al. The Surgical Infection Society's policy of human immunodeficiency virus and hepatitis B and C infection. *Arch Surg* 1992;127:218–221.
24. Centers for Disease Control. Update: acquired immune deficiency syndrome and HIV infection in health-care workers. *MMWR Morb Mortal Wkly Rep* 1989;37:229.

25. Centers for Disease Control. Guidelines for prevention and transmission of human immunodeficiency virus and hepatitis B virus to health care and public safety workers. *MMWR Morb Mortal Wkly Rep* 1989;38(S-6):1–37.
26. Centers for Disease Control. 1988 Agent summary statement for HIV and report on laboratory-acquired infection with HIV. *MMWR Morb Mortal Wkly Rep* 1988;37(S-4):1–17.
27. Beekman SE, Henderson DK. Nosocomial human immunodeficiency virus infection in health care workers. In: Mayhall CG, ed. *Hospital epidemiology and infection control.* Baltimore: Williams & Wilkins, 1996.
28. Gerberding JL. The infected health care provider. *N Engl J Med* 1996;334:594–595.
29. Lettau LA. The A, B, C, D, and E of viral hepatitis: spelling out the risks for healthcare workers. *Infect Control Hosp Epidemiol* 1992;13:77–81.
30. Centers for Disease Control and Prevention. Guidelines for the management of occupational exposures to HBV, HCV, and HIV and recommendations for postexposure prophylaxis. *MMWR Morb Mortal Wkly Rep* 2001;50(RR-11):1–54.
31. Gerberding JL, Henderson DK. Management of occupational exposures to bloodborne pathogens: hepatitis B virus, hepatitis C virus, and human immunodeficiency virus. *Clin Infect Dis* 1992;14:1179–1185.
32. Morand P, Dutertre N, Minazzi H, et al. Lack of seroconversion in a health care worker after polymerase chain reaction-documented acute hepatitis C resulting from a needlestick injury. *Clin Infect Dis* 2001;33:727–729.
33. Manns MP, McHutchison JG, Gordon SC, et al. Peginterferon alfa-2b in combination with ribavirin compared with interferon alfa-2b plus ribavirin for initial treatment of chronic hepatitis C: results of a randomized trial. *Lancet* 2001;358:958–965.
34. Fried MW, et al. Pegylated (40 kDa) interferon alfa-2a (PEGASYS) in combination with ribavirin: efficacy and safety results from a phase III, randomized, actively-controlled, multicenter study. *Gastroenterology* 2001;120[Suppl]:A-55.
35. Henderson DK. Human immunodeficiency virus in patients and providers. In: Wenzel RP, ed. *Prevention and control of nosocomial infections.* Baltimore: Williams & Wilkins, 1993:42–57.
36. Esteban JI, Gomez J, Martell M, et al. Transmission of hepatitis C virus by a cardiac surgeon. *N Engl J Med* 1996;334:555–560.
37. Harpaz R, Von Seidlein L, Averhoff FM, et al. Transmission of hepatitis B virus to multiple patients from a surgeon without evidence of inadequate infection control. *N Engl J Med* 1996;334:549–554.
38. Centers for Disease Control. Possible transmission of human immunodeficiency virus to a patient during an invasive dental procedure. *MMWR Morb Mortal Wkly Rep* 1990; 39:489–493.
39. Centers for Disease Control. Update: transmission of HIV infection during invasive dental procedures—Florida. *MMWR Morb Mortal Wkly Rep* 1991;40:21–27, 33.
40. Ciesielski C, Marianos D, Ou CY, et al. Transmission of human immunodeficiency virus in a dental practice. *Ann Intern Med* 1992;116:798–805.
41. Mishu B, Schaffner W. HIV-infected surgeons and dentists. Looking back and looking forward. *JAMA* 1993;269:1843–1844.
42. Centers for Disease Control. Recommendations for prevention of HIV transmission in health-care settings. *MMWR Morb Mortal Wkly Rep* 1987;36[Suppl 2S]:1S–19S.
43. Centers for Disease Control. Recommendations for preventing transmission of human immunodeficiency virus and hepatitis B virus to patients during exposure-prone procedures. *MMWR Morb Mortal Wkly Rep* 1991;40:1–9.

# 27. ANTIBIOTIC USE

Richard E. Reese and Robert F. Betts

## A. Principles of Antibiotic Use

**I. Introduction**

**A. Background.** The benefit to society of antibiotics is one of the most important advances in medicine of the twentieth century [1]. Empiric antibiotics for specific acute infectious processes improve clinical symptoms more quickly, and the eventual outcome is improved compared with delayed or inappropriate therapy. This has been especially true in the leukopenic patient with gram-negative bacteremia (see Chapters 2 and 20) but is also true in many other infections. As a consequence, clinicians initiate antibiotics for any clinical problem that might be a bacterial infection even when symptoms are mild and often even when symptoms are probably caused by a virus. **This "standard" approach has led to a striking overuse of antibiotics, which in turn has led to the evolution of bacteria (e.g., *Streptococcus pneumoniae* or *Staphylococcus aureus*) resistant to antibiotics that previously were effective.** This approach has placed antibiotics in jeopardy of no longer being effective for infections that used to be easily controlled.

**B. A different approach.** Clinicians need to consider new and different approaches to patients with symptoms suggestive of an infectious illness. This approach must provide effective management for those who are most ill and at the same time not use antibiotics when they are not indicated. **Two components of this approach are especially important.**

1. **First, of those who are seriously ill, the spectrum of the antibiotic regimen needs to include coverage of potentially resistant pathogens.** For example, in severe community-acquired pneumonia or bacterial meningitis, agents active against penicillin-resistant *S. pneumoniae* are needed (see Chapters 6 and 11). As a corollary to this, in community-acquired pneumonia it is useful to differentiate seriously ill patients from mildly ill patients (see Chapter 11).
2. **Second, antibiotic use must be minimized for situations where the patient will not benefit from an antibiotic.** A prime example is upper respiratory tract infections (see Chapter 8).
3. If we can do this successfully, we will benefit our patients and prolong the useful life of the new classes of antibiotics we have been forced to use. **If we are unsuccessful,** the pharmaceutical industry may not have sufficient time to provide new safe and effective agents with which to treat our patients.

**II. Ten important questions to ask before selecting an antibiotic.** The following 10 questions, summarized in Table 27A.1, help to provide a logical stepwise approach for antibiotic selection.

**A. Question 1.** Is an antibiotic indicated today, or even at all, on the basis of clinical findings?

1. **In the seriously ill,** empiric antibiotics are indicated after obtaining cultures. Examples are meningitis, acute endocarditis, or the neutropenic patient who suddenly develops a high fever.
2. **Although patients may be less ill than those mentioned above,** pneumonia and cellulitis are diseases for which antibiotics are indicated.
3. **The most common situation of antibiotic overuse is** in uncomplicated upper respiratory tract infection [2] or influenza, yet antibiotics are commonly prescribed in over 50% of these situations (see Chapter 8).
4. **For the individual who has had symptoms for 1 week or longer** and these symptoms are not rapidly accelerating, antibiotics **should not be started** until sufficient information and all possible cultures have been obtained to help guide future management. For the person with chronic symptoms, **antibiotics do not have to be started immediately** and, in fact, usually are not. Evaluate the situation and make sure all cultures have been obtained.

Table 27A.1. Important Questions to Answer Routinely Before Selecting an Antibiotic

1. Is an antibiotic **indicated?**
2. Have appropriate **specimens** been obtained, examined, and cultured?
3. **What organisms** are most likely?
4. If several antibiotics are available, **which is best?** (This question involves such factors as drugs of choice, pharmacokinetics, toxicology, cost, narrowness of spectrum, and bactericidal compared with bacteriostatic agents.)
5. Is an antibiotic **combination** appropriate?
6. What are the important **host factors?**
7. What is the best **route of administration?**
8. What is the appropriate **dose?**
9. Will initial therapy require **modification** after culture data are returned?
10. What is the optimal **duration** of treatment, **and** is development of **resistance** during prolonged therapy likely to occur?

**B. Question 2. Before antibiotics are initiated, have appropriate clinical specimens been obtained, examined, and cultured?**

1. **Gram stains** are one of the most useful tools available. Has wound drainage, sterile body fluids, sputum, or abscess fluid been sent to the laboratory for Gram stain (see Chapter 25). Often this helps identify whether the pathogens are gram-positive cocci or gram-negative bacilli. Further, it requires $10^5$ organisms in the specimen to be able to see them, and if there are many, there are $10^6$ to $10^7$ organisms present, the number that it requires to cause disease. Multiple morphotypes suggest anaerobic infection and, in the abdomen, perforation of a viscous.
2. **Site of infection cultures** (urine, sputum, wound drainage) must be obtained before starting antibiotics. **Of course, blood cultures** are almost always indicated. If the illness is low grade, three cultures can be spaced over 1 to 2 hours or even over 24 hours if subacute bacterial endocarditis is suspected. If it is an accelerating illness, three can be spaced over 20 to 30 minutes.

**C. Question 3. What organisms are likely?** Using clinical information and the always valuable Gram stain, an empiric regimen with good activity against the most likely pathogen(s) can be initiated. This is most important when the patient is only mildly or moderately ill and an organism may not be recovered from cultures. **For example,** if a patient presents with pneumonia and the Gram stain of the sputum shows many pleomorphic gram-negative coccobacillary organisms, therapy is aimed at *Haemophilus influenza* and not *S. pneumoniae*. Azithromycin does not need to be added to ceftriaxone.

1. **The organ system involved** (i.e., genitourinary, pulmonary, skin, or biliary) will strongly influence the decision about whether coverage will be directed against gram-positive, gram-negative, or anaerobic organisms. Acute cellulitis is usually due to gram-positive organisms and urinary tract infection (UTI), to gram-negative organisms. However, an elderly male with a UTI and gram-positive cocci on Gram stain must be treated for either enterococcus or *Staphylococcus.*
2. **Age** may provide clues. For example, in pneumonia, certain pathogens are common in different age groups (see Chapter 11). **In the elderly,** infections may present atypically with inadequate histories, blunted signs on examination, and lack of fever; yet **morbidity rates are higher** in the elderly with infections. Pneumonia is more apt to be associated with bacteremia and slow resolution. UTI is commonly associated with bacteremia. Intraabdominal infection is more commonly associated with perforation, bacteremia, or abscess formation than in younger patients. Therefore, **in the elderly, early empiric antibiotics, broad-spectrum antibiotics, careful dosing, and assessment of drug-drug interactions are especially important** [3–5].
3. **Hospital-acquired** infections are likely to be due to gram-negative bacilli resistant to many antibiotics, *S. aureus* resistant to methicillin (MRSA), or, in certain situations, enterococci resistant to vancomycin (see Chapters 20 and 27P). Severe

nosocomial infections may be due to *Pseudomonas* species, often necessitating initial use of an aminoglycoside.

4. **Severity of illness** dictates not only whether antibiotic therapy should be initiated but also, at times, whether multiple agents or very broad-spectrum agents should be used (see related discussion under section I.B.1).
5. **Prior culture data** often provide helpful clues. Do not forget to look at what was isolated last admission or in a posttreatment urine culture.

**D. Question 4. Which antibiotic among many should be chosen?**

1. Is there a **drug of choice** [6] (Table 27A.2)? If so, can this agent be used?
2. **Are there antibiotic allergies?** The penicillin-allergic patient must be presumed to be allergic to all the penicillin derivatives unless appropriate skin tests can be done to test specifically for cross-reactivity. It is important to **consider both trade and generic names of antibiotics** when evaluating a patient's allergic history (see the discussion of penicillin allergies in Chapter 24).
3. **Will the antibiotic penetrate** the infected area? This is especially important in meningitis, osteomyelitis, and prostatitis.
4. **What are the potential side effects?** Some agents may be contraindicated in certain settings. Examples include the following:
   a. **Tetracycline** use is limited to those over age 8 years who are not pregnant because of dental defects it produces.
   b. **Fluoroquinolones** may affect cartilage formation and therefore are not currently recommended for use in prepubertal children and pregnant women (see Chapter 27G).
5. **Bactericidal agents.** In minor infections of the healthy host, bacteriostatic agents are sufficient. However, in severe life-threatening infections (particularly bacteremia in leukopenic patients or patients with endocarditis or meningitis), bactericidal agents, which depend less on host factors, are necessary. Bactericidal agents include the penicillins, cephalosporins, aztreonam, imipenem, metronidazole for *Bacteroides*, aminoglycosides, vancomycin, and fluoroquinolones.
6. **Cost of antibiotics**
   a. **The cost of the antibiotic itself** is the easiest component to sort out (Appendix Table 1). **Generic preparations** should be ordered whenever possible [7], for example, generic oral trimethoprim-sulfamethoxazole (TMP-SMX). It is **essential for the clinician to recognize that the cost per day of the antibiotic itself is only one component of the cost of antibiotic administration in hospitalized patients.** Other factors are discussed later.
   b. **Frequency of administration** per day. The more frequently the antibiotic is given (every 4 hours vs. every 8 hours vs. every 24 hours), the more expensive it is to administer in terms of personnel time and materials used. Agents with longer half-lives may be more cost effective because they are given less often. In one study, the estimated average nonantibiotic cost associated with the mixing and administration of a single intravenous (i.v.) antibiotic dose was $3.35 [8].
   c. **Number of antibiotics.** Multiple antibiotics usually are more expensive than monotherapy. However, sometimes two antibiotics are less expensive than one (e.g., cefazolin plus metronidazole costs less than ampicillin-sulbactam for intraabdominal infection) (see Chapter 13).
   d. **Intravenous versus oral therapy.** The lower cost of equivalent oral agents coupled with ease of administration makes oral therapy very cost effective.
   e. **Monitoring of serum levels.** The potential for toxicity with certain agents (e.g., aminoglycosides) is real, and the toxicity, if it occurs, may prolong the patient's hospitalization, increase the level of care of the patient (e.g., dialysis), or may be associated with increased morbidity and even mortality. Monitoring of levels is expensive. This factor should always be considered.
   f. **Narrow versus broad spectrum of activity.** For empiric therapy in the seriously ill, antibiotics with a broad spectrum of activity are used initially. Once susceptibility data are known, it is preferable to use an agent with as narrow a spectrum as possible.

**E. Question 5. Is an antibiotic combination indicated?** In a few situations, this is appropriate.

Table 27A.2. Antibiotics of Choice for Common Pathogens

| Pathogen | Antibiotic of First Choice[a] | Alternative Agents[a] |
|---|---|---|
| Gram-positive cocci | | |
| *Staphylococcus aureus* or *S. epidermidis*[b] | | |
| Non-penicillinase producing | Penicillin | A first-generation cephalosporin preferred, vancomycin, imipenem, or clindamycin; a fluoroquinolone[c] |
| Penicillinase producing (methicillin sensitive) | Penicillinase-resistant penicillin (e.g., oxacillin or nafcillin) | A first-generation cephalosporin, vancomycin, clindamycin, imipenem, amoxicillin-clavulanic acid, ticarcillin-clavulanic acid, ampicillin-sulbactam, piperacillin-tazobactam; a fluoroquinolone[c] |
| Methicillin resistant | Vancomycin with or without gentamicin with or without rifampin | Linezolid, quinupristin-dalfopristin, TMP-SMX, minocycline; a fluoroquinolone[b] |
| Streptococci | | |
| Groups A, C, G | Penicillin | Clindamycin, a cephalosporin,[a] vancomycin, erythromycin; clarithromycin; azithromycin |
| Group B | Penicillin (or ampicillin) | A cephalosporin,[a] vancomycin, or erythromycin |
| Enterococcus[b] | | |
| Endocarditis or other serious infection | Penicillin (or ampicillin) with gentamicin | Vancomycin with gentamicin; linezolid, quinupristin/dalfopristin; (see Chapter 27 P) |
| Uncomplicated urinary tract infection | Ampicillin or amoxicillin | A fluoroquinolone, nitrofurantoin, fosfomycin |
| Viridans group[b] | Penicillin G (with or without gentamicin) | A cephalosporin,[a] vancomycin |
| *S. bovis* | Penicillin G | A cephalosporin,[a] vancomycin |
| *S. pneumoniae*[b] | See text (Chapters 6, 8, 11, 27C) | |

| | | |
|---|---|---|
| Gram-negative cocci | | |
| *Neisseria gonorrhoeae*[b] | Ceftriaxone or cefixime or ciprofloxacin or ofloxacin, or gatifloxacin see text (Chapter 16) | Cefotaxime, spectinomycin, cefoxitin (see Chapter 16) |
| *N. meningitidis* | Penicillin G | Third-generation cephalosporin, chloramphenicol |
| *Moraxella (Branhamella) catarrhalis* | Cefuroxime, a fluoroquinolone | TMP-SMX, amoxicillin-clavulanic acid; an erythromycin; clarithromycin, azithromycin, defuroxime, cefixime, third-generation cephalosporin, tetracycline |
| Gram-positive bacilli | | |
| *Clostridium perfringens* (and *Clostridium* species) | Penicillin G, clindamycin | Metronidazole, imipenem, meropenem, chloramphenicol |
| *Listeria monocytogenes* | Ampicillin with or without gentamicin | TMP-SMX |
| Gram-negative bacilli | | |
| *Acinetobacter* [b] | Imipenem or meropenem | Tobramycin, gentamicin, or amikacin, usually with ticarcillin or piperacillin (or similar agent); TMP-SMX; a ciprofloxacin |
| *Aeromonas hydrophila* | TMP-SMX | Gentamicin, tobramycin; imipenem; a fluoroquinolone |
| *Bacteroides*[b] | | |
| *Bacteroides* species (oropharyngeal) | Penicillin G or clindamycin | Cefoxitin, metronidazole, cefotetan, ampicillin, sulbactam, piperacillin-tazobactam, chloramphenicol |
| *B. fragilis* strains (gastrointestinal strains) | Metronidazole | Clindamycin; imipenem or meropenem; ampicillin-sulbactam; piperacillin-tazobactam; ticarcillin-clavulanic acid; cefoxitin,[d] cefotetan;[d] piperacillin;[d] chloramphenicol |

(*Continued*)

Table 27A.2. (*Continued*)

| Pathogen | Antibiotic of First Choice[a] | Alternative Agents[a] |
|---|---|---|
| *Campylobacter fetus*[b] | Imipenem or meropenem | Gentamicin |
| *Campylobacter jejuni*[b] | Erythromycin or azithromycin; | A fluoroquinolone a tetracycline, gentamicin |
| *Enterobacter* species[b] | Imipenem or meropenem | An aminoglycoside and piperacillin or ticarcillin or mezlocillin; a third-generation cephalosporin;[e] TMP-SMX; aztreonam; ciprofloxacin |
| *Escherichia coli*[b] | | |
| Uncomplicated urinary tract infection | TMP-SMX[b] or ciprofloxacin (see Chapters 15, 27G, 27L) | A cephalosporin or a fluoroquinolone |
| Recurrent or systemic infection | A third-generation cephalosporin[f] | Ampicillin with or without an aminoglycoside, TMP-SMX, oral fluoroquinolones useful in recurrent infections, ampicillin-sulbactam, ticarcillin-clavulanic acid, piperacillin-tazobactam, aztreonam |
| *Haemophilus influenzae* (coccobacillary)[b] | | |
| Life-threatening infections | Cefotaxime or ceftriaxone | Chloramphenicol; cefuroxime (for pneumonia but not meningitis), meropenem |
| Upper respiratory infections and bronchitis | TMP-SMX | Cefuroxime; cefuroxime-axetil; third-generation cephalosporin, amoxicillin-clavulanic acid, cefaclor, tetracycline; ampicillin or amoxicillin; clarithromycin; azithromycin; cefixime, a fluoroquinolone |
| *Klebsiella pneumoniae*[b] | A cephalosporin[f] | An aminoglycoside, imipenem or meropenem, TMP-SMX, ticarcillin-clavulanic acid, ampicillin-sulbactam piperacillin-tazobactam; aztreonam; a fluoroquinolone; amoxicillin-clavulanic acid |

| | | |
|---|---|---|
| *Legionella* species | Azithromycin or a fluoroquinolone with or without rifampin | Doxycycline ± rifampin; TMP-SMX, erythromycin |
| *Pasteurella multocida* | Penicillin G | Tetracycline, cefuroxime, cefuroxime-axetil; amoxicillin-clavulanic acid ampicillin-sulbactam, piperacillin-tazobactam |
| *Proteus* species, indole positive[b] | Cefotaxime, ceftizoxime ceftriaxone or cefepime[g] | An aminoglycoside; ticarcillin or piperacillin or mezlocillin; TMP-SMX; amoxicillin-clavulanic acid, ticarcillin-clavulanic acid, ampicillin-sulbactam, piperacillin-tazobactam; a fluoroquinolone; aztreonam; imipenem, meropenem |
| *Providencia stuartii*[b] | Cefotaxime, ceftizoxime, ceftriaxone or cefepime[g] | Imipenem or meropenem; an aminoglycoside often combined with ticarcillin or piperacillin or similar agent; ticarcillin-clavulanic acid; piperacillin-tazobactam; TMP-SMX; a fluoroquinolone; aztreonam |
| *Pseudomonas aeruginosa*[b] | | |
| Non-urinary tract infection | Gentamicin or tobramycin or amikacin (combined with ticarcillin, piperacillin, etc., for serious infections) | An aminoglycoside and ceftazidime; imipenem or meropenem, or aztreonam plus an aminoglycoside; cefepime plus an aminoglycoside; ciprofloxacin |
| Urinary tract infections | Ciprofloxacin | Carbenicillin; ticarcillin, piperacillin, or mezlocillin; ceftazidime; imipenem or meropenem; aztreonam, an aminoglycoside; cefepime |
| *Burkholderia (Pseudomonas) cepacia*[b] | TMP-SMX | Ceftazidime, chloramphenicol, imipenem |

(*Continued*)

Table 27A.2. (*Continued*)

| Pathogen | Antibiotic of First Choice[a] | Alternative Agents[a] |
|---|---|---|
| *Salmonella typhi*[b] | Ceftriaxone or a fluoroquinolone | TMP-SMX, chloramphenicol; ampicillin, amoxicillin |
| Other species | Cefotaxime or ceftriaxone or a fluoroquinolone | TMP-SMX, chloramphenicol; ampicillin or amoxicillin |
| *Serratia*[b] | Imipenem or meropenem | Gentamicin or amikacin; cefotaxime or ceftriaxone or cefepime; TMP-SMX; ticarcillin, piperacillin, or mezlocillin, which can be combined with an aminoglycoside; aztreonam; a fluoroquinolone |
| *Shigella*[b] | A fluoroquinolone | TMP-SMX; ceftriaxone; ampicillin, azithromycin |
| *Stenotrophomonas maltophilia*[h] | TMP-SMX | Minocycline, a fluoroquinolone |
| *Vibrio cholerae* (cholera) | A tetracycline | TMP-SMX; a fluoroquinolone |
| *Vibrio vulnificus* | A tetracycline | Cefotaxime |
| *Yersinia enterocolitica*[b] | TMP-SMX | A fluoroquinolone; an aminoglycoside; cefotaxime or ceftizoxime |
| *Yersinia pestis* (plague) | Streptomycin ± a tetracycline | Chloramphenicol; gentamicin, TMP-SMX |

*Note:* The fluoroquinolones should be used only in adults except pregnant women. See Chapter 27G.

[a]See later individual discussions of agents for details of agent use and contraindications of use. Choice presumes susceptibility studies indicate that the pathogen is susceptible to the agent.

[b]Resistance may be a problem; susceptibility tests should be performed. See Chapter 25.

[c]The experience with fluoroquinolone use in staphylococcal infections is relatively limited. Resistance during therapy may occur. See Chapter 27G.

[d]Up to 15–20% of strains may be resistant.

[e]*Enterobacter* species may develop resistance to the cephalosporins. See discussion in Chapter 27F.

[f]Specific choice will depend on susceptibility studies. Third-generation cephalosporins and cefepime may be exquisitely active against many gram-negative bacilli (e.g., *E. coli, Klebsiella* species). In some geographic areas, 20%–25% of community-acquired *E. coli* infections may be resistant to ampicillin (amoxicillin).

[g]In severely ill patients, this often is combined with an aminoglycoside while awaiting susceptibility data.

[h]Formerly called *Pseudomonas maltophilia.*

TMP-SMX, trimethoprim-sulfamethoxazole.

Modified from Medical Letter. The choice of antibacterial drugs. *Med Lett Drugs Ther* 2001;43:69; with permission.

1. **Synergism.** When one antibiotic greatly enhances the activity of another, with more than an additive effect, this interaction is called **synergy** (see Chapter 25). Examples include the following:
   a. **One antibiotic enhances the penetration of another.** It is believed that enterococci are impermeable to aminoglycosides. The synergistic interaction between **penicillin** (or ampicillin) **and aminoglycosides against enterococci** is due to penicillin altering the cell wall, allowing the aminoglycoside to penetrate the bacteria and thereby act effectively at the ribosomal level.
   b. **An extended-spectrum penicillin (e.g., piperacillin) and an aminoglycoside are often synergistic against *Pseudomonas aeruginosa* and Enterobacteriaceae.**
   c. **Serial inhibition of microbial growth.** Fixed combinations of TMP (80 mg) and SMX (400 g) block successive steps in the synthesis of folic acid (see Chapter 27L).
2. **In the febrile, bacteremic, leukopenic patient,** use of a synergistic combination is associated with improved outcome over a single agent [7].
3. **In infections in which multiple organisms are likely or proven** (e.g., intraabdominal or pelvic abscess), more than one antibiotic may be required for adequate treatment.
4. **Limiting or preventing the emergence of resistance.** This principle applies primarily to the treatment of tuberculosis. More than one agent is used in an attempt to prevent the replication of preexisting resistant mycobacteria. Whether or not two agents minimize the occurrence of resistance with gram-negative bacilli is unclear [9], but available data suggest they do not.
5. **$\beta$-Lactam–$\beta$-lactamase combinations** (e.g., ampicillin-sulbactam, Unasyn) are used so that the $\beta$-lactamase inhibitor protects the $\beta$-lactam antibiotic (see Chapter 27E).
6. **In the unique drug combination imipenem-cilastatin,** the enzyme inhibitor (cilastatin) prevents metabolic breakdown of imipenem by the kidney (see Chapter 27H).
7. **Disadvantages of multiple antibiotics**
   a. **An increased risk of drug allergies or toxicity** is present when more agents are used.
   b. **An increased risk of colonization with a resistant bacterial organism** may occur. If superinfection develops, such resistant organisms are more difficult to treat.
   c. **Antagonism** occurs when the combined effect of two drugs is less than the effect of either drug alone; one of the drugs appears to interfere with the action of the second. How often this occurs clinically is unknown [9]. A combination of tetracycline and penicillin for treatment of meningitis resulted in a higher mortality than when penicillin was used alone, presumably due to the inhibition of growth by tetracycline, which interferes with the bactericidal action of penicillin.
   d. **Higher costs.** Combination antibiotics often are more expensive than single agents.
   e. **False sense of security.** Although appealing at times, the use of multiple agents to treat all possible organisms often is not possible, practical, or necessary and may be associated with an increase in side effects.

**F. Question 6. Are there important host factors?** There may be special characteristics of the host that must be considered in choosing an antibiotic for use in individual patients.

1. **Special risks**
   a. A febrile person with an artificial heart valve should never receive antibiotics without first obtaining blood cultures.
   b. A person with lymphoma or a collagen vascular disease should be approached entirely differently from a person with the same type of infection who lacks these risk factors. Pneumonia in a lymphoma patient may be cryptococcal and not pneumococcal.
2. **Renal function.** Renal failure may affect not only the choice of antibiotic but also its dosages [10] (see discussions of individual agents). Consequently, **renal**

Table 27A.3. Major Pathways of Antibiotic Excretion

| Antibiotics Primarily Excreted by the Liver[a] | Antibiotics Primarily Excreted by the Kidneys |
|---|---|
| Cefoperazone | Aminoglycosides |
| Chloramphenicol | Aztreonam |
| Clindamycin | Cephalosporins (other than cefoperazone) |
| Doxycycline | Imipenem |
| Erythromycin | Fluoroquinolones[b] |
| Metronidazole | Penicillin and penicillin derivatives |
| Nafcillin | Trimethoprim |
| Rifampin | Tetracycline |
| Sulfamethoxazole | Vancomycin |

[a] In renal failure, dosages usually do not need modifications. See individual chapter discussions.
[b] The fluoroquinolones are excreted by the kidneys to a variable degree depending on the specific agent (see Chapter 27G).

**function should be monitored in patients treated with antibiotics that are potentially nephrotoxic** and primarily excreted by the kidney. **These are summarized in Table 27A.3.** Serum antibiotic levels, especially when aminoglycosides are used, should be monitored, as should serum creatinine, every 2 to 4 days.

a. **Dosages of antibiotics renally excreted are modified based on the creatinine clearance.**
b. **The serum creatinine may not accurately reflect the patient's renal function, especially in the elderly,** who may have decreased creatinine production. The **creatinine clearance is a better measure** of renal function. By modifying the equation of Cockcroft and Gault [11], it is possible to estimate the patient's creatinine clearance from the patient's age, gender, body weight (in kilograms), and serum creatinine as follows:
   (1) **Male estimated creatinine clearance =**
      (a) **Female estimated creatinine clearance = 85% of male value**
      (b) **Some prefer to use ideal body weight,** which can be calculated as
      Male = 50 kg + 2.3 kg per each inch over 5 feet (in height)
      Female = 45.5 kg + 2.3 kg per each inch over 5 feet
      (c) **In the obese patient,** we use ideal body weight to estimate the creatinine clearance.
   (2) **In patients with severe hepatic insufficiency,** this formula may overestimate the creatinine clearance (see section **F.3.d**).

3. **Liver function.** Our understanding of modifying dosages in hepatic insufficiency is not as sophisticated as it is for renal insufficiency [12]. However, **four issues deserve special emphasis** in patients with hepatic insufficiency.
   a. **Aminoglycoside use in patients with cirrhosis may be associated with an increased risk of nephrotoxicity,** as reviewed in Chapter 27I.
   b. **$\beta$-Lactam antibiotic use** in one study was **associated with an increased risk of leukopenia** when standard doses of $\beta$-lactam antibiotics were used in patients with underlying liver disease [13]. The probable mechanism is impaired hepatic metabolism of the $\beta$-lactam antibiotics, resulting in bone marrow suppression of white cell precursors from excessive antibiotic concentrations. In our experience, nafcillin at standard doses is more likely to cause nephrotoxicity in subjects with cirrhosis. A reduction in dosage of $\beta$-lactam antibiotic when used in patients with significant hepatic dysfunction was proposed [13].
   c. **Drugs primarily metabolized by the liver** (e.g., chloramphenicol, clindamycin) **need to have dose adjustments.** Other drugs to be used with caution or serum levels obtained include fluconazole, itraconazole, nitrofurantoin, and pyrazinamide [9] (Table 27A.3).

**d.** When selecting a dose for a drug cleared by renal mechanisms, creatinine clearance should be estimated (just as in the elderly) even when the serum creatinine is normal [14]. In patients with underlying liver disease, a low creatinine may overestimate the creatinine clearance (two- to threefold) as measured by the inulin clearance. This may be accounted for by underproduction of creatinine resulting from diminished muscle mass or by a decreased rate of hepatic production of creatine, the substrate for the production of creatinine in muscles [14]. **In practice, for those with an estimated creatinine clearance and severe hepatic disease, we assume their estimated creatinine clearance may be approximately 50% of the calculated estimate using the above formula.**

**4. In neutropenic patients,** bactericidal agents are preferred whenever possible.

**5. Genetic factors.** Patients with glucose-6-phosphate dehydrogenase deficiency may develop hemolysis from sulfonamides, nitrofurantoin, or chloramphenicol [9].

**6. Pregnancy and lactation.** Certain drugs may pose special problems (e.g., the tetracyclines, which may cause hepatotoxicity in the mother and dentition problems in the infant). Because of the physiologic changes that occur in the mother during pregnancy, serum antibiotic levels are lower during gestation. Therefore in critical infections, serum levels of antibiotics may need to be monitored and compensatory dosage adjustments may be necessary [15].

**a. Placental transfer of antibiotics.** Whenever possible, pregnant women should avoid all drugs because of the risk of fetal toxicity. This topic has been reviewed elsewhere [15,16] and is summarized as follows:

**(1) Antibiotics considered safe in pregnancy** include the penicillins (with the possible exception of ticarcillin) [9], the cephalosporins, erythromycin base, and probably aztreonam.

**(2) Antibiotics to be used with caution** include the aminoglycosides, vancomycin, clindamycin, imipenem/cilastatin, TMP, and nitrofurantoin.

**(3) Antibiotics contraindicated in pregnancy** include chloramphenicol, erythromycin estolate, tetracycline, fluoroquinolones, and TMP-SMX (Bactrim, Septra). Although controversial, we would try to avoid using metronidazole because of its carcinogenic potential (see Chapter 27Q). Sulfonamides should be avoided in the last trimester of pregnancy. Some experts suggest avoiding ticarcillin, because it has been shown to be teratogenic in rodents [9] (see Chapter 27E).

**b. Antibiotics in breast milk.** Data regarding adverse effects in nursing neonates from maternal antibiotics are limited. If possible, nursing mothers should avoid all drugs (see section **a.(1) to (3)** above).

**c. The U.S. Food and Drug Administration's use-in-pregnancy drug-rating system is shown in Table 27A.4.** These pregnancy categories are based on the degree to which available information has ruled out risk to the fetus balanced against the drug's potential benefits to the patient. This topic has been reviewed [15].

**7.** Prosthetic device infections may be difficult to eradicate (see Chapters 5 and 12).

**G. Question 7. What is the best route of administration?**

**1. Intravenous antibiotics are preferred in serious infections.** They provide high peaks with hopefully greater potential for diffusion into tissue rendered ischemic by the acute process. Many antibiotics have unpredictable oral absorption, but even in those that are very well absorbed (e.g., linezolid is 104% bioavailable), the very high peaks are not achieved (see individual chapter discussions).

**2. Continuous versus intermittent bolus i.v. infusion.** Whether intravenously administered antibiotics should be given by continuous infusion or by intermittent bolus remains controversial [9] and is undergoing evaluation and is reviewed elsewhere [17–19].

**a. Continuous** infusions may result in less vein irritation and phlebitis. Results from animal model studies suggested that concentrations of penicillins and cephalosporins in fibrin clots were related to peak serum levels achieved; therefore intermittent bolus therapy seemed appropriate for endocarditis and tissue infections [9]. Recent data from animal models suggest that the clinical

Table 27A.4. U.S. Food and Drug Administration (FDA) Use-in-Pregnancy Ratings

The FDA's use-in-pregnancy rating system weighs the degree to which available information has ruled out risk to the fetus against the drug's potential benefit to the patient. The ratings, and their interpretation, are as follows:

| Category | Interpretation |
|---|---|
| A | **Controlled studies show no risk.** Adequate well-controlled studies in pregnant women have failed to demonstrate a risk to the fetus in any trimester of pregnancy. |
| B | **No evidence of risk in humans.** Adequate well-controlled studies in pregnant women have not shown increased risk of fetal abnormalities despite adverse findings in animals, or, in the absence of adequate human studies, animal studies show no fetal risk. The chance of fetal harm is remote, but remains a possibility. |
| C | **Risk cannot be ruled out.** Adequate well-controlled human studies are lacking, and animal studies have shown a risk to the fetus or are lacking as well. There is a chance of fetal harm if the drug is administered during pregnancy, but the potential benefits may outweigh the potential risk. |
| D | **Positive evidence of risk.** Studies in humans, or investigational or post-marketing data, have demonstrated fetal risk. Nevertheless, potential benefits from the use of the drug may outweigh the potential risk. For example, the drug may be acceptable if needed in a life-threatening situation or serious disease for which safer drugs cannot be used or are ineffective. |
| X | **Contraindicated in pregnancy.** Studies in animals or humans, or investigational or post-marketing reports, have demonstrated positive evidence of fetal abnormalities or risk which clearly outweighs any posible benefit to the patient. |

*Physicians' desk reference* 56th ed. Montvale, NJ: Medical Economics, 2002:343, with permission.

effectiveness of $\beta$-lactam antibiotics is optimal when the concentration at the site of infection exceeds the minimum inhibitory concentration of the infecting organism for a prolonged time (50% of the 24-hour period) [9]. This is called time-dependent bactericidal activity. Drug levels just above those required to inhibit the organism are as effective as levels many fold above the inhibitory concentration. $\beta$-lactam antibiotics and vancomycin function by time-dependent killing [19]. Intermittent infusion remains the method used with $\beta$-lactam antibiotics.

**b. Intermittent infusions** may be preferred for antibiotics that exhibit **concentration-dependent bactericidal activity.** With these antibiotics the rate and extent of bactericidal action increase with increasing concentrations above the minimum bactericidal concentration (MBC) up to a point of maximum effect, usually 5 to 10 times the MBC [19]. The **aminoglycosides and fluoroquinolones** demonstrate concentration dependent killing [9,19]; the **higher the drug level, the greater the rate of bacterial clearance,** which slows as the drug level falls [19]. Large infrequently administered doses of concentration-dependent agents that achieve maximal concentrations at peak at the site of infection should produce optimal bactericidal effect. This is in large part the **basis for once-daily regimens of aminoglycoside** dosing, which is discussed in detail in Chapter 27I. However, clinical studies to prove this are still not available [9,19].

**3. Oral therapy** is effective for mild to moderately severe outpatient infections and for completion of therapy of focal infections initially treated with i.v. antibiotics. In special circumstances, oral therapy is used for relatively severe infections such as TMP-SMX in *Pneumocystis carinii* pneumonia and clindamycin in osteomyelitis (see individual sections).

4. **Home i.v. antibiotics** are used in selected settings for stable infections requiring prolonged or repeated courses of i.v. antibiotics (e.g., subacute endocarditis, prosthetic joint infections, recurrent pulmonary infection in patients with cystic fibrosis, or bronchiectasis). This topic is reviewed in detail elsewhere [20]. This is a cost-effective approach to therapy that many patients obviously prefer over hospitalization.

H. **Question 8. What is the appropriate dose?** To reduce the frequency of side effects, the potential of superinfection, and the cost of therapy, the lowest dose of an antibiotic that will be effective is used.
   1. **Dosage in neonates** (see Chapter 3).
   2. **Dosage in children and adults** (see discussions under individual agents).

I. **Question 9. What guides modification after culture data are available?** Once the results of cultures and antibiotic susceptibility data are available, the antibiotic regimen should be modified when possible. Some general guidelines follow:
   1. Conversion from a broad-spectrum to a narrow-spectrum agent should be carried out if susceptibility data show a decreased risk of colonization and possible superinfection with resistant organisms and/or selection of resistant flora.
   2. ***S. aureus*** **susceptible to nafcillin.** If vancomycin was initiated, and recovered *S. aureus* organisms are susceptible to nafcillin, this narrow-spectrum agent should be used both because it is more effective and its spectrum is more focused.
   3. **Gram-negative infections.** For the individual presumptively placed on an aminoglycoside, if the identified pathogen is susceptible to a narrow-spectrum agent (e.g., ampicillin or a cephalosporin), barring allergy, a change should be made [6].
   4. **No growth or normal flora only in initial cultures.** Other diagnostic possibilities should be considered. For example, if the patient with pneumonia receiving ceftriaxone is doing poorly, other infectious agents (mycoplasma, *Mycobacterium tuberculosis, Legionella* species) or even noninfectious possibilities (e.g., pulmonary infarct, pulmonary vasculitis) must be considered.
   5. **Evaluation of clinical response and culture results.** It is important for the clinician to assess the clinical response of the patient before making changes based on culture results. For example, colonization with new organisms is expected with antibiotic use. **New colonization must be differentiated from new infection.** If the patient is improving and an organism resistant to the antibiotic is isolated on follow-up sputum or wound cultures, it can usually be ignored (see Chapters 11 and 4).

J. **Question 10. What is the optimal duration of therapy?**
   1. **Duration.** The optimal duration of antibiotic therapy may be well established, such as a minimum of 6 weeks in osteomyelitis or relatively empiric 10 to 14 days for peritonitis. **Recommended duration** of therapy for common problems is shown in **Table 27A.5.** However, this must often be individualized. Because resistant organisms eventually colonize those who are treated for a prolonged period, it is important for the clinician to treat the patient for an adequate, but not an unnecessarily prolonged, period.
   2. **Development of resistance.** The growing problem of antibiotic resistance and its relationship to antibiotic use is discussed below under Antibiotic Resistance.
      a. **Broad versus narrow antibiotic therapy.** What has become increasingly clear is that **using a broader spectrum agent than necessary** (e.g., a third-generation cephalosporin rather than a first-generation cephalosporin) **will result in colonization of the individual with an organism resistant to the third- rather than the first-generation cephalosporin.** If superinfection ensues, patients infected with antibiotic-resistant organisms are more likely to require hospitalization, have a longer hospital stay, and have an increased risk of death [21].
      b. **Therefore it is particularly important for the clinician to use the new broad-spectrum agents carefully to help minimize the development of bacterial resistance** [21]. This usually involves some type of hospital-wide antibiotic control program and rational use of antibiotics. Cautious conservation is advocated in the use of new antimicrobial agents (see Antibiotic Resistance, below).

Table 27A.5. Duration of Antibiotic Therapy for Common Infections

| Diagnosis | Duration of Therapy (days) |
|---|---|
| Meningococcal meningitis | 7–10 |
| Pneumococcal meningitis | 10–14 |
| *Haemophilus influenzae* type b meningitis | 10–14 |
| Streptococcal group A pharyngitis | 10 |
| Otitis media | 7–10 |
| Bacterial sinusitis | 10–14 |
| Pneumococcal pneumonia | ? Optimal[a] |
| Gram-negative pneumonias (*Klebsiella, Enterobacter, Pseudomonas*) | ? 21[b] |
| *Mycoplasma* pneumonia | 14[c] |
| *Legionella* pneumonia | 21[c] |
| Endocarditis (nonprosthetic) | |
| Viridans streptococci | 28 |
| Staphylococcal | 28–42 |
| Peritonitis | 10–14 |
| Septic arthritis (nongonococcal) | 14–21[d] |
| Osteomyelitis (acute) | 28–42[e] |

[a]Most experts agree that therapy should be continued at least 3 days after the temperature returns to normal. Elderly patients may deserve 7 days of parenteral therapy.
[b]Difficult to eradicate; patients may require even longer courses.
[c]To prevent relapse, a full therapeutic course should be given.
[d]Four weeks of therapy may be indicated in patients with gram-negative infections, slowly responding infections (despite adequate drainage), or infections with virulent organisms such as *S. aureus*.
[e]In vertebral osteomyelitis, patients often are treated for 6 weeks.

## ANTIBIOTIC RESISTANCE

**Increasing bacterial resistance** has been emphasized in recent reviews [2,22–28] and in the lay media. **Although an extensive discussion of this topic is beyond the scope of this chapter, several issues deserve special emphasis.** For complete related discussion, see the Centers for Disease Control and Prevention website (*www.cdc.gov*).

**I. Background.** After the introduction of sulfonamides in the middle to late 1930's and penicillin in the early 1940's, pharmaceutical companies introduced a series of antibiotics to combat resistant bacteria. These agents included, in the late 1950's, the semisynthetic penicillins to treat penicillin-resistant *S. aureus* and, in the 1960's through the 1980's, cephalosporins and aminoglycosides for hospital-acquired organisms, especially gram-negative bacilli. Vancomycin (available in 1958) has been useful in treating increasing problems associated with MRSA. **The concept of an untreatable bacterial disease is foreign to most physicians in the developing world, but if recent bacterial-resistant trends continue, it may become a reality.**

**II. Current dilemma.** In the past decade, there has been a **worrisome rise in resistance,** often multidrug, to **bacteria,** not only in hospital-acquired bacteria but also in community-acquired bacteria and *M. tuberculosis* in the United States and worldwide.

**A. Nosocomial infections.** In the past decade, gram-positive bacteria have emerged as the most frequent causes of nosocomial infection [23,26].

1. **Coagulase-negative staphylococci** commonly cause prosthetic device- and catheter-related infections, and 60% to 90% of strains are methicillin resistant [23].
2. **MRSA** accounts for 5% to 40% of *S. aureus* infections, depending on the size and type of the hospital. MRSA is occurring in individuals with no hospital contact [28] (see Chapter 27D).
3. **Enterococci** are the third most common nosocomial pathogen after *S. aureus* and *Escherichia coli*. In 1993 vancomycin-resistant enterococci were reported in

up to 14% of intensive care unit enterococcal isolates, a 20-fold increase since 1987 [23] (see Chapter 27P).

4. **Multidrug-resistant** *P. aeruginosa* and *Stenotrophomonas maltophilia* have become common in patients with cystic fibrosis. These organisms, as well as multidrug-resistant *Acinetobacter* species, are present in intensive care units [23].
5. Outbreaks of extended-spectrum β-lactamases *Klebsiella* species have been reported [24], presumably related to selection pressure from widespread use of late-generation cephalosporins; they usually are susceptible to imipenem.

B. **Community-acquired infections**

1. The increasing and ominous problem of ***S. pneumoniae*** **resistant to penicillin [29]** and other antibiotics is discussed in detail in Chapters 6, 8 11, and 27C.
2. In recent years, *Neisseria gonorrhoeae* (see Chapter 16), *Salmonella*, and *Shigella* species (see Chapter 13) have shown increasing resistance. Ampicillin-resistant *H. influenzae* and *Branhamella catarrhalis* are discussed in Chapters 8 and 11.
3. **Multidrug-resistant** ***M. tuberculosis*** is a serious and increasing problem in the United States and worldwide. Case fatality rates in patients infected with these organisms of 40% to 60% occur even when immunity is normal, and 80% mortality occurs in the immunocompromised [23].

III. **Risk factors** for emergence of resistant bacteria **are partially understood** and reviewed in detail elsewhere [22–28]. Several points should be emphasized.

A. **Antibiotic use** selects out resistant bacteria.

B. **Often antibiotics are used inappropriately.** In the United States, antimicrobial agents are the second most commonly used class of drugs [30,31] (second to agents used for cardiovascular disorders). In hospitals, approximately 25% to 40% of patients receive an antibiotic, accounting for nearly 25% of total drug acquisition, whereas about 15% of office-based private practice prescriptions are for antibiotics [32]. Several **studies suggest that approximately 50% of antibiotic use in the United States is inappropriate** (i.e., not indicated, wrong drug, wrong dose or duration). Kunin [32] reviewed this problem and potential approaches to it in detail. Guidelines are often available to help hospitals improve their use of antibiotics.

C. **New antibiotics are often used excessively.** Resistance develops more rapidly than anticipated because of excess use. In a relatively short time, the agent has lost its effectiveness. Kunin [22] emphasized "the pattern of discovery, exuberant use, and predictable obsolescence has been repeated after the introduction of each new antimicrobial drug."

D. **Long-term use** of antibiotics may pose a greater risk for antimicrobial resistance than short-term use or prophylaxis.

E. **Use of antibiotics in animals.** Prolonged use either to prevent infection or to stimulate growth selects for resistant bacteria that then colonize humans through food [33–36]. Supplementing animal feed with antibiotics to enhance growth is estimated to constitute more than half the total antimicrobial use worldwide [35,36]. Subtherapeutic concentrations may help select out resistant *Campylobacter* and *Salmonella* species [33,34]. Glycopeptides in animal feed is linked to vancomycin-resistant enterococci in humans [35].

F. **Microbial characteristics** may facilitate the development of resistance [37].

1. The **propensity to exchange genetic material easily and/or the ability to mutate** and adapt to a changing environment are important properties of bacteria.
2. **Reservoirs** or "niches" may be important to allow the organisms to proliferate. Patients who harbor resistant organisms may be reservoirs and spreaders of resistant pathogens.
3. The **intrinsic resistance** of an organism may help facilitate resistance. Enterococci are intrinsically resistant to cephalosporins, and when cephalosporins are used excessively, these agents may facilitate increased colonization and eventual infection with enterococci.
4. The ability of an organism such as *Clostridium difficile* to survive on inanimate surfaces may allow it to spread and survive.

G. **Society and environmental aspects** [37]
1. **Day-care centers** allow "sharing" of many bacteria, with secondary spread to family members and other attendees.
2. **Crowding, homelessness, poor nutrition,** and **inadequate care** are conducive to the transmission of infectious diseases and therefore promote multidrug-resistant organisms such as *M. tuberculosis.*
3. **Poor sanitation and crowding** facilitate the spread of bacteria in developing countries.
4. **Behavioral aspects** of a society can affect the spread of bacteria, as in the sexual transmission of gonococci and disease associated with i.v. drug use.
5. **Erosion of the public health infrastructure in the United States** due to cost-containing policies has decreased public health activities such as supervised therapy for tuberculosis and surveillance of important infectious diseases [37]. For example, national surveillance of drug-resistant *M. tuberculosis* was discontinued in 1984 and was only reinstituted in 1993. Surveillance of food-borne disease is inadequate in most areas of the United States, and many outbreaks go undetected. Programs have recently been instituted to correct this.
6. **Changes in food production, processing, and distribution** may compromise food safety and increase food-borne illnesses.

H. **Other contributing factors** [37]
1. **International travel** exposes the traveler to resistant pathogens in both developing and developed countries and allows the traveler to spread infection from one country to another.
2. As **patients live longer and undergo more immunosuppression,** a larger population is at risk for infection, invasive procedures, and antibiotic therapy.
3. **Invasive procedures** (including central venous catheters) **and foreign bodies** as a consequence of these procedures expose patients to nosocomial infectious complications.
4. **Resistant bacteria are as virulent as susceptible bacteria.** Because of the disproportionately high incidence of multidrug-resistant bacteria in hospitals, the argument has been made that resistant pathogens are dangerous only to severely ill patients [23] and overall may be less virulent, especially to "normal hosts." This does not appear to be the case. Both methicillin-resistant and methicillin-susceptible *S. aureus* can produce toxins, and the frequency and spectrum of staphylococcal diseases caused by susceptible and resistant strains appear to be the same [23,28].

IV. **Urgency of situation with multidrug-resistant bacteria.** In a 1994 Rockefeller University Workshop on multidrug-resistant bacteria, the participants concluded that the epidemiologic data in the United States suggest the following:

> [We have already] reached the point that health agencies should be able to (and need to) take steps to avert a potential crisis. In particular, the acquisition of resistance to vancomycin, either by MRSA or resistant *S. pneumoniae,* would create highly invasive clones that could not be controlled by any currently available chemotherapeutic agent. Indeed, the transfer and expression of vancomycin resistance to staphylococci have already been demonstrated in the laboratory, and their emergence in clinical strains may only be a matter of time [23].

Recently, vancomycin (glycopeptide) resistant *S. aureus* strains have been described clinically (see Chapter 27P).

V. **Proposed solutions to the problem** [23–32,38]

A. **Awareness of the problem.** Special efforts should be made to bring the issue of antibiotic resistance to the attention of microbiologists, government health authorities, physicians [23], and especially lay public in an appropriate manner. Ideally, a national and multidisciplinary approach is needed. To this end, **in 1999 the *Public Health Action Plan to Combat Antimicrobial Resistance (Action Plan)* was developed** by an interagency task force co-chaired by the Centers for Disease Control and Prevention, the U.S. Food and Drug Administration, and the National Institutes of Health with input from a variety of agencies, including the Department of Agriculture, the Environmental Protection Agency, and the Department of Veterans Affairs. The *Action Plan* had input from many groups, including health agencies, health-care delivery organizations, universities, professional societies, pharmaceutical companies, agricultural producers, and consumer groups. The plan focuses on four areas: surveillance, prevention and control, research and product development (e.g., rapid viral diagnostic tests). **The Action Plan, first annual report, and many issues related to antibiotic resistance are available at *www.cdc.gov/drugresistance.*** Initially domestic issues will be addressed and then eventually, the international problem of antibiotic resistance.

**B. More prudent use of antibiotics in humans and animals is critical** in developing and developed countries [22–24,31,36,39]. These are **global issues,** not ones applicable only to the United States.
  1. Provider education, antibiotic control programs, shorter courses of antibiotics, and narrow-spectrum agents when feasible are all appropriate approaches. The unrealistic demand for and, at times, poor compliance with antibiotic regimens by patients must also be dealt with. Targeting obvious areas of abuse, such as antibiotic use in upper respiratory tract infection, is important (see Chapter 8).
  2. **Appropriate pharmaceutical advertising and promotion is essential** [40,41].
  3. Antimicrobial use in animals must be reviewed and improved [33–38]. For a comprehensive discussion of this topic, see a special 2002 symposium [36].

**C. Improved surveillance.** Funding for, and interest in, surveillance systems at the state and national level declined in the 1970's and 1980's in the United States [8,9,23,42]. This needs to be and is being rectified. In recent years there has been an improvement in tracking regional and national antibiotic-resistant organisms, but more needs to be done. Better global surveillance has also been suggested [23].

**D. Increase in funding for basic research** in mechanisms of resistance, vaccine development, and development of novel interventions is needed. By the early to mid-1990's the funding for research of bacterial disease was reduced substantially by the National Institutes of Health [23].

**E. New antibacterial agents** [23,38,39]. With initial success of antibiotics released in the late 1980's and early 1990's, many pharmaceutical companies reduced their antibacterial research efforts in the early to mid-1990's. As a result, it is expected that fewer antibiotics will be released in the immediate future. New research in this area is needed. It is hoped that development can be expedited, possibly even with a "fast track" for new antibiotics for multidrug-resistant bacteria.

**F. Prevention of transmission with infection control** practices, **improved sanitation** conditions in developing countries, and **improved care of the homeless and** those in crowded conditions also are needed. Rapid diagnostic tests and rapid treatment with effective antimicrobials also will help reduce transmission.

**G. Hospital administrations** are encouraged to support and pursue a multidisciplinary systems oriented approach to these problems, as emphasized in a 1996 report [43]. Each hospital should establish its own strategies to optimize the prophylactic, empiric, and therapeutic use of antimicrobials in the hospital and to detect, report, and prevent transmission of antimicrobial-resistant microorganisms [43].

**VI. Summary.** To deal with this increasing problem of multidrug-resistant bacteria and reverse this trend, we agree with Dr. Levy:

> The answer lies in efforts from all of us, physician, patient, microbiologist, manufacturer, public health and governmental policy officials. No one can sit back and expect someone else to solve the problem. In the past, we have relied on the pharmaceutical companies to develop new drugs to deal with resistance and they have largely succeeded. But, the ability to stay one step ahead of the bacteria has led to a complacency about the resistance problem. We can no longer maintain this attitude [39].

## END OF LIFE ISSUES

Use of antibiotics for patients nearing the end of life is a topic of paramount importance [44–47]. Because in most patients with fever the physician initiates antibiotics to be certain that his or her patient does not suffer the consequences of infection, it is a natural step to do the same for the terminally ill. However, one report from Wales in 1989 indicated that on the basis of a questionnaire of a hypothetical case of a terminally ill patient, only 16% of respondents (72/448) indicated they would use antibiotics if the terminally ill patient became febrile [47]. From observations made in the hospital, this does not seem to be the practice. Use of antibiotics in the terminally ill is not addressed in the literature. **We offer the following suggestions.**

**I. For patients designated "comfort care"**

**A.** Because other therapeutic agents are discontinued in comfort care patients, it is ethically reasonable to discontinue antibiotics unless their continued use is necessary for specific comfort (see section **B** below). This approach in a small way could provide not only the most rational care but also reduce resistance risks for the broader community.

**B. In special situations, directed antibiotic use with narrow-spectrum agents may be indicated for comfort.** Although therapy for a symptomatic UTI or cellulitis or pneumonia with a hacking cough may well be indicated, whether to treat or not must be individualized.

1. **UTI.** Usually UTI develops because of an indwelling catheter. If fever develops in this setting, it usually will resolve in 24 to 48 hours without therapy. If treatment is given, bacteria will be cleared and fever will disappear only to reappear with the next infection. Treatment may lead to greater discomfort.
2. **Cellulitis** with its rapidly advancing border is almost always due to a gram-positive organism and very often a penicillin susceptible $\beta$ streptococcus, often group B. Rarely does a gram-negative organism produce this picture. Occasionally MRSA contributes, however.
3. **Aspiration** can usually be managed with good pulmonary toilet. Antibiotics often lead to *Clostridium difficile* and great patient discomfort.

**II. For patients in whom broad-spectrum antibiotics are being considered,** simply because the infection has developed in the hospital the issue is more complex and raises ethical issues beyond the scope of this handbook. If the clinician would not consider surgical procedures, pacemakers, or resuscitation, why use antibiotics "just in case?" We offer a few considerations.

**A.** Often resistant organisms are simply colonizers, are not very invasive, and no therapy is indicated, even with fever.

**B.** With attention to nursing measures, especially to wounds, to catheters, and to measures to avoid aspiration, excellent comfort care can be provided with use of antibiotics.

**C.** In the intubated patient where extubation is not planned, most growth from the endotracheal tube represents colonization and does not require treatment even with fever. That will disappear, like in the bladder-catheterized patient, without treatment. If infection develops, it will often progress rapidly to death, for the ultimate good of the patient.

**D.** The inserted catheters and tracheostomies make eradication of the colonizing bacteria very difficult, and often treatment leads to resistance.

**E.** In these situations we have found that an open discussion with families allows development of a plan that will provide the most comfort to the patient, citing the above factors just discussed.

**F. An ethics consultation,** if available, can help the care-giving team deal with the ethical issues raised by the question of whether or not to treat when therapy may produce more discomfort than it prevents. Although the decision to withhold broad-spectrum antibiotics can be difficult, especially if the patient is young and competent, our ethics committee has believed it is ethically defensible (appropriate) when it is weighed against community needs.

## REFERENCES

1. Hager M. Antibiotics: the power of invention. *Newsweek* 1997;130:70. (See related discussion by Centers for Diseases Control and Prevention. Control of infectious diseases. *MMWR Morb Mortal Wkly Re* p 1999;48:621.)
2. Gonzales R, et al. Excessive antibiotic use for acute upper respiratory infections in the United States. *Clin Infect Dis* 2001;33:757.

3. Toshikawa TT. Unique aspects of infection in older adults. In: Toshikawa TT, Norman DC, eds. *Antimicrobial therapy in the elderly patient.* New York: Marcel Dekker, 1994:1–7.
4. Yohikawa TT, Norman DC. Treatment of infections in elderly patients. *Med Clin North Am* 1995;79;651.
5. Crossley KB, Peterson PK. Infections in the elderly. *Clin Infect Dis* 1996;22:209.
6. Medical Letter. The choice of antimicrobial drugs. *Med Lett Drugs Ther* 2001;43:39.
7. Medical Letter. Generic drugs. *Med Lett Drug Ther* 1999;41:47.
8. Foran RM, Brett JL, Wulf PH. Evaluating the cost impact of intravenous antibiotic dosing frequencies. *DICP Ann Pharmacother* 1991;25:546.
9. Moellering R Jr. Principles of anti-infective therapy. In: Mandell GL, Bennett JE, Dolin R, eds. *Principles and practice of infectious diseases,* 4th ed. New York: Churchill Livingstone, 1995:199–212.
10. Aronoff GR, et al. *Drug prescribing in renal failure: dosing guidelines for adults,* 4th ed. Philadelphia: American College of Physicians, 1999.
11. Cockcroft DW, Gault MH. Prediction of creatinine clearance from serum creatinine. *Nephron* 1976;16:31. (See also Levey A, et al. A more accurate method to estimate glomerular filtration rate from serum creatinine: a new prediction equation. *Ann Intern Med* 1999;130:461.)
12. Tschida SJ, et al. Anti-infective agents and hepatic disease. *Med Clin North Am* 1995;79:895.
13. Singh N, et al. β-Lactam antibiotic-induced leukopenia in severe hepatic dysfunction: risk factors and implications for dosing in patients with liver disease. *Am J Med* 1993;94:251.
14. Westphal JF, Jehl F, Vetter D. Pharmacological, toxicological, and microbiological considerations in the choice of initial antibiotic therapy for serious infections in patients with cirrhosis of the liver. *Clin Infect Dis* 1994;18:324.
15. Korzeniowski OM. Antibacterial agents in pregnancy. *Infect Dis Clin North Am* 1995;9:639.
16. Medical Letter. Safety of drugs in pregnancy. *Med Lett Drugs Ther* 1987;28:61.
17. Nightingale CH, Quintiliani R, Nicolau DP. Intelligent dosing of antimicrobials. *Curr Clin Top Infect Dis* 1994;14:252.
18. Nicolau DP, et al. Antibiotic kinetics and dynamics for the clinician. *Med Clin North Am* 1995;79:477.
19. Levinson ME. Pharmacodynamics of antimicrobial agents: bactericidal and post-antibiotic effects. *Infect Dis Clin North Am* 1995;9:483.
20. Tice AD, et al. Outpatient parenteral antibiotic therapy. *Infect Dis Clin North Am* 1998;12:827–1034.
21. Chow JW, et al. *Enterobacter* bacteremia: clinical features and emergence of antibiotic resistance during therapy. *Ann Intern Med* 1991;115:585.
22. Kunin CM. Resistance to antimicrobial drugs: a worldwide calamity. *Ann Intern Med* 1993;118:557.
23. Tomasz A. Multiple-antibiotic-resistant pathogenic bacteria: a report of the Rockefeller University Workshop. *N Engl J Med* 1994;330:1247.
24. Tenover FC, et al. Antimicrobial resistance. *Infect Dis Clin North Am* 1997;11:757.
25. Moellering RC Jr, et al. Bacterial resistance: laboratory explanations and clinical consequences. *Clin Infect Dis* 1998;27[Suppl 1]:S1.
26. Moellering RC Jr, et al., eds. The specter of glycopeptide resistance: current trends and future considerations. *Am J Med* 1998;104(5A):1S.
27. Bartlett JG, et al. Attempting to avoid antibiotic resistance: lessons for the primary care physician. *Am J Med* 1999;106(5A):1S–52S.
28. Kak V, Levine DP. Community-acquired methicillin-resistant *Staphylococcus aureus* infections: where do we go from here. *Clin Infect Dis* 1999;29:801.
29. Thornsberry C, Sahm DF, Kelley LJ, et al. Regional trends in antimicrobial resistance among clinical isolates of *Streptococcus pneumoniae, Haemophilus influenzae,* and *Moraxella catarrhalis* in the United States: results from the TRUST surveillance program, 1999–2000. *Clin Infect Dis* 2002;34:[Suppl 1]:S4–S16.
30. McCaig LF, Hughes JM. Trends in antimicrobial drug prescribing among office-based physicians in the United States. *JAMA* 1995;273:214.

31. Winker MA, et al. Emerging and reemerging global microbial threats: call for papers. *JAMA* 1995;273:241.
32. Kunin CM. Problems in antibiotic usage. In: Mandell GL, Douglas RG Jr, Bennett JE, eds. *Principles and practice of infectious diseases,* 3rd ed. New York: Churchill Livingstone, 1990:427.
33. Smith KE, et al. Quinolone-resistant *Campylobacter jejuni* infections in Minnesota 1992–1998. *N Engl J Med* 1999;240:1525.
34. Wegener HC. The consequences for food safety of the use of fluoroquinolones in food animals. *N Engl J Med* 1999;340:1581.
35. Wegener HC, et al. Use of antimicrobial growth promoters in food animals and *Enterococcus faecium* resistance to therapeutic antimicrobial drugs in Europe. *Emerg Infect Dis* 1999;5:329.
36. Barza M, Gorbach SL. The need to improve antimicrobial use in agriculture: ecological and human consequences. *Clin Infect Dis.* 2002;34[Suppl 3]:S71–S143.
37. Cohen ML. Epidemiology of drug resistance: implications for a post-antimicrobial era. *Science* 1992;257:1050.
38. Moellering RC Jr. Antibiotic resistance: lessons for the future. *Clin Infect Dis* 1998;27[Suppl 1]:S135.
39. Levy SB. Confronting multi-drug resistance: a role for each of us. *JAMA* 1993;269:1840.
40. Waud DR. Pharmaceutical promotions: a free lunch? *N Engl J Med* 1992;327:351.
41. Orlowski JP, et al. The efforts of pharmaceutical firm enticements on physician prescribing habits. *Chest* 1992;102:270.
42. Berkelmen RL, et al. Infectious disease surveillance: a crumbling foundation. *Science* 1994;264:368.
43. Goldmann D, et al. Consensus statement: strategies to prevent and control the emergence and spread of antimicrobial-resistant microorganisms in hospitals—a challenge to hospital leadership. *JAMA* 1996;275:234.
44. Carron AT, Lynn J, Keaney P. End-of-life care in medical textbooks. *Ann Intern Med* 1999;130:82.
45. Rabow MW, Brody RV. *Care at the end-of-life. Current medical diagnosis and treatment 1999,* 38th ed. New York: Lange Medical Books/McGraw-Hill, 1999.
46. Improving end-of-life care: a conference of nursing and medical publishers, Sorros Center, New York, March 12, 1999. Sponsored by the Robert Wood Johnson Foundation.
47. Marin PP, et al. Attitudes of hospital doctors in Wales to use of intravenous fluids and antibiotics in the terminally ill. *Postgrad Med J* 1989;65:650.

## B. Prophylactic Antibiotics

**I. Introduction.** Use of prophylactic antibiotics involves a risk-to-benefit assessment. Two types of situations exist for use of prophylaxis. The first is to prevent postoperative infection. For the second, long-term prophylaxis is used to prevent a specific type of infection such as $\beta$ streptococcus in the individual with prior rheumatic fever or pneumococcus in the splenectomized. In the tables to follow, a variety of options is summarized.

**II. Short-term use in surgical procedures**

**A. Incidence of infection.** Antimicrobial prophylaxis reduces the incidence of infection, particularly wound infection, after certain operations. However, this must be weighed against the risks of toxic and allergic reactions, emergence of resistant bacteria, drug interactions, superinfection, and cost. Studies from the literature conclude that antimicrobial prophylaxis should be used only for procedures with high infection rates, such as surgery (a) involving mucosal surfaces, so-called clean-contaminated; (b) involving implantation of prosthetic material; and (c) where the consequences of infection are especially serious.

**B. Definitions.** Clean surgery is any procedure where no mucosal surface is involved in the incision. Prosthetic material insertion includes any of the many situations in orthopedic surgery such as artificial joint or tendon, general surgery where meshes are used, or cardiac valve replacement. Clean-contaminated involves a mucosal surface such as oropharynx, bowel, vagina, or gallbladder, including endoscopic retrograde cholangiopancreatography [1]. Contaminated surgery includes gun shot abdominal wounds. See Table 27B.1 for surgical procedures where prophylaxis is believed to be important [2].

**C. Organisms involved.** The major pathogen in postoperative clean surgery is ***Staphylococcus aureus.*** Potential resistant organisms such as methicillin-resistant *S. aureus* (MRSA) should be considered in clean procedures when MRSA is prevalent in an institution. With foreign body insertion, coagulase-negative staphylococcal species is more common than *S. aureus*. Gram-negative bacteria and anaerobes cause wound infections after the surgery of colon, gram-negative bacteria and $\beta$ streptococcus after gynecologic surgery, and gram-negative bacteria alone after genitourinary surgery. For head and neck surgery, oral anaerobes and other normal oral flora predominate.

**D. Timing of antibiotic administration.** Antibiotics must be given so that good tissue levels are present at the time of the procedure and for the first 3 to 4 hours after the surgical incision. Reviews suggest that the optimal time to give an antibiotic is **30 to 60 minutes before the incision is made** [2–5]. For cesarean section it should be delayed until the umbilical cord is clamped. Stone et al. [6] showed that antibiotics given 24 hours before the procedure are no more effective than when given just before the procedure. Furthermore, if infection develops in the former, the organisms involved are more resistant than when it develops from the use of perioperative antibiotics [6].

**E. Duration**

1. In most instances, a single dose is sufficient. Some experts suggest continuing the antibiotics throughout the first 24 hours after surgery. For prosthetic device insertion, up to 48 hours is used.
2. If the procedure lasts several hours, redosing is suggested. For example, in colonic surgery cefotetan requires one dose every 6 to 8 hours. Therefore, it has become preferred over cefoxitin, in a long gastrointestinal procedure, because the latter must be given every 2 hours to maintain high intraoperative levels.

**F. Antibiotic choices (Table 27B.1)**

1. Cephalosporins are favored because of their spectrum and safety. Because cefazolin is more active against *S. aureus* than the newer cephalosporins, is less expensive, and does not suppress all bacteria, leaving a void for resistant organisms, this agent is preferred for most surgical procedures. Furthermore, cefazolin has a moderately long serum half-life. In colorectal surgery and appendectomy, cefotetan is preferred because of additional activity against bowel anaerobes (also see section **E** above).
2. Vancomycin is often used for antistaphylococcal activity if the patient is allergic to cephalosporins or MRSA is a major hospital pathogen and prosthetic devices are being inserted.
3. For colon surgery, metronidazole and gentamicin can be substituted for cefotetan.

**III. Nonsurgical short-term prophylaxis**

**A. Bacterial endocarditis prophylaxis. Valve risk and procedure risk guide use.** Adequate clinical trials on which to base endocarditis prophylaxis have not been done. Discussion on whether to reduce the use in this situation is ongoing. The 1997 guidelines published by the American Heart Association assist practitioners in their decision making [7].

1. **At-risk cardiac lesions (Table 27B.2)**
   a. Previous endocarditis, artificial valve, mitral regurgitation, aortic stenosis, or insufficiency and small ventricular septal defect are underlying lesions that require prophylaxis.
   b. **In mitral valve prolapse without regurgitation,** the risk of endocarditis is as low as that of the heart without valvular lesions so **prophylaxis is not indicated** [7,8].
2. **Dental and surgical procedures** at risk and recommended antibiotics are shown in Tables 27B.3 to 27B.6. In general, clean procedures do not require prophylaxis. Bacteria released are negligible. For procedures during which even low quantities (simple teeth cleaning) of bacteria are released, prophylaxis is administered to those with high risk lesions, but only high quantity release procedures

Table 27B.1. Recommended Antimicrobial Regimens

| Surgical Procedure | Recommended Regimen |
|---|---|
| Biliary tract surgery | |
| High risk<br>>60 yr<br>Obstructive jaundice<br>Acute cholecystitis<br>Cholangitis<br>Common duct stone<br>Previous biliary surgery<br>Nonfunctioning gall bladder | Cefazolin 1–2 g i.v. × 1 dose or gentamicin 1.7 mg/kg i.v. q8h × 1 or 2 doses[a] |
| Low risk | Not recommended |
| Gastrointestinal surgery | |
| Elective colorectal | **Oral GI prep;** Neomycin 1 g p.o. and erythromycin base 1 g p.o. given at 1 PM, 2 PM, 11 PM on day prior to surgery with or without cefoxitin 2 g i.v. q6h × 1 or 2 doses or cefotetan 2 g i.v. × 1 dose or metronidazole 500 mg i.v. and gentamicin 1.7 mg/kg i.v. q8h × 1 or 2 doses[a] (see text) |
| Nonelective colorectal | Cefoxitin or cefotetan or metronidazole and gentamicin[a] (at above doses) |
| Gastroduodenal procedures | |
| High risk: GI bleeding, obstruction, gastric ulcer or malignancy, decreased gastric acidity, obesity. | Cefazolin 1–2 g i.v. × 1 dose |
| Low risk | Not recommended |
| Appendectomy (perforated appendix will need full therapeutic regimen.) | Cefoxitin 2 g i.v. q6h × 1–3 dose(s) or cefotetan 2 g i.v. q12h × 1 or 2 doses or metronidazole 500 mg i.v. q8h and gentamicin 1.7 mg/kg i.v. q8h × 1–3 dose(s)[a] |
| Gynecological surgery | |
| Hysterectomy (abdominal or vaginal) | Cefazolin 1 g i.v. × 1 dose or doxycycline 200 IV × 1 dose[a] or clindamycin 900 mg i.v. × 1 dose[a] |
| Cesarean section | Cefazolin 1 g i.v. × 1 dose or metronidazole 500 mg i.v. × 1 dose[a] (after cord clamping) |
| High-risk patients (i.e., premature membrane rupture, active labor) | |
| Low risk | Not recommended |
| Therapeutic abortion | Cefazolin 1 g i.v. × 1 dose |
| First trimester with previous PID or midtrimester | |
| Head and neck surgery | |
| Incision through oral or pharyngeal mucosa | Clindamycin 600 mg i.v. and gentamicin 1.7 mg/kg i.v. × 1 dose or ampicillin-sulbactam |
| Uncontaminated | Not recommended |
| Neurosurgery | |
| CSF shunt | Not recommended |
| Craniotomy | Cefazolin 1 g i.v. × 1 dose or vancomycin[b] |

(continued)

Table 27B.1. (*Continued*)

| Surgical Procedure | Recommended Regimen |
|---|---|
| Orthopedics | |
| Closed reduction of a fracture | Not recommended |
| Open reduction of a fracture | Cefazolin 1–2 g i.v. × 1 dose |
| Prosthetic joint replacement | Cefazolin 1–2 g i.v. q6h or vancomycin i.v.; either, up to 24h |
| Amputation | Cefoxitin 2 g i.v. × 1 dose |
| Laminectomy and spinal fusion | |
| Hardware implantation | Cefazolin 1–2 g i.v. × 1 dose |
| No hardware implantation | Not recommended |
| Urologic surgery | |
| If the urine is sterile | Not recommended |
| If the urine is infected | Sterilize urine before surgery |
| Transrectal prostate biopsy | Ciprofloxacin 500 mg po or 400 mg i.v. up to 48h |
| Vascular and cardiothoracic surgery | |
| Pulmonary resection | Cefazolin 1 i.v. q8h or cefuroxime 750 mg i.v. q8h up to 48h |
| Prosthetic valve, CABG, pacemaker or defibrillator implant | Cefazolin 1–2g i.v. q8h or cefuroxime 1.5g i.v. q8h or vancomycin IV[b], doses given for up to 24–48h (see text) |
| Cardiac catheterization | Not recommended |
| Peripheral vascular surgery | Cefazolin 1–2 g i.v. × 1 dose |

[a]Alternative in cephalosporin-allergic patient. (Gentamicin dose assumes normal renal function. See Chapter 27I.)
[b]For hospitals in which MRSA commonly cause post-op wounds or in patients allergic to cephalosporins.
PID, pelvic inflammatory disease; CABG, coronary artery bypass grafts; CSF, cerebrospinal fluid; GI, gastrointestinal.
Modified from Reese RE, Betts RF, Gumustop B. Prophylactic antibiotics. *Handbook of Antibiotics,* 3rd ed. Philadelphia: Lippincott Williams & Wilkins, 2000; and from Medical Letter. Antimicrobial prophylaxis in surgery. *Med Lett Drugs Ther* 2001;43:92, with permission.

are grounds for prophylaxis in low risk valve lesions. Amoxicillin is used for oral procedures unless penicillin allergy is an issue, and then clindamycin is used. A wallet card is available from the American Heart Association.

3. **Unresolved issues.** Although studies concluding that antibiotic prophylaxis is effective are lacking [7,8], the practice is entrenched in the United States. Failure to use prophylaxis has led to malpractice claims [9]. Some studies challenged the value of antibiotic use before dental procedures in low risk patients. Durack [9] discussed this issue in a recent editorial.

B. **Influenza** chemoprophylaxis is discussed in detail in Chapter 10.

C. **Prophylaxis in those with total joint replacement** [10–15]. Evidence to show benefit from prophylaxis is lacking. Infection with the same oral flora that cause endocarditis occurs rarely and then proximal to the original surgery. Some reviews of the data suggest that antibiotics usually add little except expense. It has been recommended that **most patients** with indwelling prosthetic joints generally **do not require** antimicrobial **prophylaxis** when undergoing dental, gastrointestinal, or genitourinary procedures [3]. **However, for surgery in an infected area,** including periodontal disease and drainage of abscess; **procedures** with a **high inoculum of bacteria;** and **procedures lasting more than 45 minutes, prophylaxis may be advisable** [13–15].

D. **Bacterial meningitis.** With the disappearance of *Haemophilus influenza* type b only meningococcal disease requires prophylaxis. Only family members and intimate

Table 27B.2. Cardiac Conditions Associated with Endocarditis

| |
|---|
| Endocarditis prophylaxis recommended |
| High-risk category |
| Prosthetic cardiac valves, including bioprosthetic and homograft valves |
| Previous bacterial endocarditis |
| Complex cyanotic congenital heart disease (e.g., single ventricle states, transposition of the great arteries, tetralogy of Fallot) |
| Surgically constructed systemic pulmonary shunts or conduits |
| Moderate-risk category |
| Most other congenital cardiac malformations (other than above and below) |
| Acquired valvular dysfunction (e.g., rheumatic heart disease) |
| Hypertrophic cardiomyopathy |
| Mitral valve prolapse with valvar regurgitation and/or thickened leaflets |
| Endocarditis prophylaxis not recommended |
| Negligible-risk category (no greater risk than the general population) |
| Isolated secundum atrial septal defect |
| Surgical repair of atrial septal defect, ventricular septal defect, or patent ductus arteriosus (without residua beyond 6 mo) |
| Previous coronary artery bypass graft surgery |
| Mitral valve prolapse without valvular regurgitation |
| Physiologic, functional, or innocent heart murmurs |
| Previous Kawasaki disease without valvular dysfunction |
| Previous rheumatic fever without valvular dysfunction |
| Cardiac pacemakers (intravascular and epicardial) and implanted defibrillators |

From Dajani AS, et al. Prevention of bacterial endocarditis: recommendations by the American Heart Association. *JAMA* 1997;277:1794, with permission.

contacts, but not health-care workers unless they perform mouth to mouth resuscitation, should receive prophylaxis. A single 500-mg dose of ciprofloxacin is effective [16] (see Chapters 6 and 26).

E. **Traveler's diarrhea.** Prophylactic antibiotics are not advised for healthy travelers. Travelers to risk areas should bring antibiotics to be used if symptoms develop, as discussed in Chapters 13 and 22.

F. **Oral antibiotics in the leukopenic host.** Multiple studies indicate that prophylaxis given at the outset of chemotherapy does not reduce use of empiric parenteral antibiotics in neutropenic fever. However, ciprofloxacin reduces the incidence of gram-negative bacteremia, which seems to be of benefit [17]. The risks are that the frequency of ciprofloxacin resistance increases.

G. **Oral fluconazole in neutropenic subjects.** Daily fluconazole reduces the incidence of disseminated candidiasis but not the use of empiric parenteral antifungals. Although some studies show benefit, results in others are less convincing [18]. There is a hint that gram-negative bacteremia is increased in fluconazole recipients and observations of increased incidence of fluconazole resistant candidal infection [19].

H. **Endoscopic retrograde cholangiopancreatography.** Although antibiotics have often been given for this procedure, data now support their use in this setting [1].

IV. **Prophylaxis of medical conditions: long-term use to prevent a specific problem**

A. **Recurrent urinary tract infections** are discussed in Chapter 15.

B. **Rheumatic fever.** Prevention is discussed in detail elsewhere [20]. Either daily oral penicillin or monthly benzathine penicillin is effective. Most at risk maintain penicillin until age 35. Those who have contact with young children, such as school teachers, continue for that duration.

C. **Prevention of serious infections after splenectomy** [21–23]. Overwhelming infection due to encapsulated organisms such as *Streptococcus pneumoniae* and, rarely, *H. influenzae* or *Neisseria meningitidis* occur after splenectomy. How to prevent these

Table 27B.3. Dental Procedures and Endocarditis Prophylaxis

| |
|---|
| Endocarditis prophylaxis recommended[a] |
| Dental extractions |
| Periodontal procedures including surgery, scaling and root planing, probing, and recall maintenance |
| Dental implant placement and reimplantation of avulsed teeth |
| Endodontic (root canal) instrumentation or surgery only beyond the apex |
| Subgingival placement of antibiotic fibers or strips |
| Initial placement of orthodontic bands but not brackets |
| Intraligamentary local anesthetic injections |
| Prophylactic cleaning of teeth or implants where bleeding is anticipated |
| Endocarditis prophylaxis not recommended |
| Restorative dentistry[b] (operative and prosthodontic) with or without retraction cord[c] |
| Local anesthetic injections (nonintraligamentary) |
| Intracanal endodontic treatment; post placement and buildup |
| Placement of rubber dams |
| Postoperative suture removal |
| Placement of removable prosthodontic or orthodontic appliances |
| Taking of oral impressions |
| Fluoride treatments |
| Taking of oral radiographs |
| Orthodontic appliance adjustment |
| Shedding of primary teeth |

[a]Prophylaxis is recommended for patients with high- and moderate-risk cardiac conditions.
[b]This includes restoration of decayed teeth (filling cavities) and replacement of missing teeth.
[c]Clinical judgment may indicate antibiotic use in selected circumstances that may create significant bleeding.
From Dajani AS, et al. Prevention of bacterial endocarditis: recommendations by the American Heart Association. *JAMA* 1997;277:1794, with permission.

overwhelming infections, which can occur months or years after splenectomy, remains unclear and controversial. Children may be at particularly high risk, but overwhelming pneumococcal sepsis during which organisms are often seen in peripheral blood smears can also occur in adults. Recognition that adults and children are at increased risk of infection years after splenectomy has led to consideration of spleen-sparing surgical approaches after trauma.

1. **Identification warning.** Because these patients are at risk of fulminant sepsis, we encourage each patient to have some form of personal identification such as a medical alert necklace or bracelet, or note in his or her wallet or purse indicating that he or she has undergone splenectomy. The patient's family should be aware of this potential complication. The patient's medical record should clearly indicate this information.
2. **Vaccines.** If an elective splenectomy is performed, pneumococcal vaccine should be administered at least 2 weeks before the elective splenectomy [21]. Efficacy of **meningococcal vaccine** in this setting has not been established, but it seems to be a reasonable consideration and has been suggested [23]. A single-dose vial of the quadrivalent vaccine is available now in the United States.
3. **Prophylactic antibiotics.** Some experts recommend penicillin V, 125 mg twice daily in children and 250 mg twice daily in adults, for at least 2 to 4 years after splenectomy. Whether to use prophylactic penicillin routinely in adults who are not otherwise compromised is a controversial issue [21–23]. We do not routinely treat adults with prophylactic antibiotics but use penicillin in adults with Hodgkin disease who have undergone splenectomy, chemotherapy, or radiation.
4. **Early therapeutic antibiotics.** Patients can be given a supply of antibiotics for use if an acute illness develops [23]; they should also seek immediate medical

Table 27B.4. Other Procedures and Endocarditis Prophylaxis

| |
|---|
| Endocarditis prophylaxis recommended |
| Respiratory tract |
| Tonsillectomy and/or adenoidectomy |
| Surgical operations that involve respiratory mucosa |
| Bronchoscopy with a rigid bronchoscope |
| Gastrointestinal tract[a] |
| Sclerotherapy for esophageal varices |
| Esophageal stricture dilation |
| Endoscopic retrograde cholangiography with biliary obstruction |
| Biliary tract surgery |
| Surgical operations that involve intestinal mucosa |
| Genitourinary tract |
| Prostatic surgery |
| Cystoscopy |
| Urethral dilation |
| Endocarditis prophylaxis not recommended |
| Respiratory tract |
| Endotracheal intubation |
| Bronchoscopy with a flexible bronchoscope, with or without biopsy[b] |
| Tympanostomy tube insertion |
| Gastrointestinal tract |
| Transesophageal echocardiography[b] |
| Endoscopy with or without gastrointestinal biopsy |
| Genitourinary tract |
| Vaginal hysterectomy[b] |
| Vaginal delivery[b] |
| Cesarean section |
| In uninfected tissue |
| Urethral catheterization |
| Uterine dilatation and curettage |
| Therapeutic abortion |
| Sterilization procedures |
| Insertion or removal of intrauterine devices |
| Other |
| Cardiac catheterization, including balloon angioplasty |
| Implanted cardiac pacemakers, implanted defibrillators, and coronary stents |
| Incision or biopsy of surgically scrubbed skin |
| Circumcision |

[a]Prophylaxis is recommended for high-risk patients; optional for medium-risk patients.
[b]Prophylaxis is optional for high-risk patients.
From Dajani AS, et al. Prevention of bacterial endocarditis: recommendations by the American Heart Association. *JAMA* 1997;277:1794, with permission.

attention. Oral penicillin and amoxicillin have been used. When these patients present with nonspecific febrile illnesses, often flu-like, early antibiotic therapy is rational. Ideally, appropriate cultures should be obtained, but if facilities for culture analysis are not immediately available, starting antibiotics without cultures is reasonable [21]. In community-acquired bacteremia of unclear primary focus of infection, therapy aimed at the likely pathogens should be instituted early while awaiting cultures. Ceftriaxone plus vancomycin are indicated until susceptibility data are available (see Chapter 2).

**D. Prevention of recurrent cholangitis.** Selected patients with a compromised biliary system such as an endoprosthesis *in situ* or history of choledochojejunostomy, hepaticojejunostomy, or sphincteroplasty who are prone to develop recurrent bouts of cholangitis may benefit from chronic daily prophylactic antibiotics. The aim of

Table 27B.5. Prophylactic Regimens for Dental, Oral, Respiratory Tract, or Esophageal Procedures

| Situation | Agent | Regimen[a] |
|---|---|---|
| Standard general prophylaxis | Amoxicillin | Adults: 2 g; children: 50 mg/kg orally 1 h before procedure |
| Unable to take oral medications | Ampicillin | Adults: 2 g intramuscularly (i.m.) or intravencusly (i.v.); children: 50 mg/kg i.m. or i.v. within 30 min before procedure |
| Allergic to penicillin | Clindamycin | Adults: 600 mg; children: 20 mg/kg orally 1 h before procedure |
| | *or* | |
| | Cephalexin[b] or cefadroxil[b] | Adults: 2 g; children; 50 mg/kg orally 1 h before procedure |
| | *or* | |
| | Azithromycin or clarithromycin | Adults: 500 mg; children: 15 mg/kg orally 1 h before procedure |
| Allergic to penicillin and unable to take oral medications | Clindamycin | Adults: 600 mg; children: 20 mg/kg i.v. within 30 min before procedure |
| | *or* | |
| | Cefazolin[b] | Adults: 1 g; children: 25 mg/kg i.m. or i.v. within 30 min before procedure |

[a]Total children's dose should not exceed adult dose.

[b]Cephalosporins should not be used in individuals with immediate-type hypersensitivity reaction (urticaria, angioedema, or anaphylaxis) to penicillins.

From Dajani AS, et al. Prevention of bacterial endocarditis: recommendations by the American Heart Association. *JAMA* 1997;277:1794, with permission.

Table 27B.6. Prophylactic Regimens for Genitourinary Gastrointestinal (Excluding Esophageal) Procedures

| Situation | Agents[a] | Regimen[b] |
|---|---|---|
| High-risk patients | Ampicillin plus gentamicin | Adults: ampicillin 2 g intramuscularly (i.m.) or intravenously (i.v.) plus gentamicin 1.5 mg/kg (not to exceed 120 mg) within 30 min of starting the procedure; 6 h later, ampicillin 1 g i.m./i.v. or amoxicillin 1 g orally<br>Children: ampicillin 50 mg/kg i.m. or i.v. (not to exceed 2 g) plus gentamicin 1.5 mg/kg within 30 min of starting the procedure; 6 h later, ampicillin 25 mg/kg i.m./i.v. or amoxicillin 25 mg/kg orally |
| High-risk patients allergic to ampicillin/amoxicillin | Vancomycin plus gentamicin | Adults: vancomycin 1 g i.v. over 1–2 h plus gentamicin 1.5 mg/kg i.v./i.m. (not to exceed 120 mg); complete injection/infusion within 30 min of starting the procedure<br>Children: vancomycin 20 mg/kg IV over 1–2 h plus gentamicin 1.5 mg/kg i.v./i.m.; complete injection/infusion within 30 min of starting the procedure |
| Moderate-risk patients | Amoxicillin or ampicillin | Adults: amoxicillin 2 g orally 1 h before procedure, or ampicillin 2 g i.m./i.v. within 30 min of starting the procedure<br>Children: amoxicillin 50 mg/kg orally 1 h before procedure, or ampicillin 50 mg/kg i.m./i.v. within 30 min of starting the procedure |
| Moderate-risk patients allergic to ampicillin/amoxicillin | Vancomycin | Adults: vancomycin 1 g i.v. over 1–2 h; complete infusion within 30 min of starting the procedure<br>Children: vancomycin 20 mg/kg i.v. over 1–2 h; complete infusion within 30 min of starting the procedure |

[a]Total children's dose should not exceed adult dose.
[b]No second dose of vancomycin or gentamicin is recommended.
From Dajani AS, et al. Prevention of bacterial endocarditis: recommendations by the American Heart Association. *JAMA* 1997;277:1794, with permission.

suppressive antibiotic therapy is to prevent flare-ups of clinically overt cholangitis. Both trimethoprim-sulfamethoxazole and fluoroquinolones have been used. This topic has been reviewed elsewhere [24].

**E. Recurrent otitis media.** Pneumococcal prophylaxis is discussed in Chapter 8.

**F. Prophylaxis** in patients with acquired immunodeficiency syndrome to prevent opportunistic infections such as *Pneumocystis carinii* has recently been reviewed [25] and is discussed in Chapter 18.

**G. Spontaneous bacterial peritonitis** (see Chapter 13). For those with one proven episode, norfloxacin 400 mg daily taken orally has reduced the 1-year recurrence rate from 68% to 20% [26]. Despite this, ciprofloxacin is generally used. Trimethoprim-sulfamethoxazole has also been used in this setting [27]. This topic was reviewed [28].

## REFERENCES


1. Byl B, et al. Antibiotic prophylaxis for infectious complications after therapeutic endoscopic retrograde cholangiopancreatography: a randomized, double-blind, placebo-controlled study. *Clin Infect Dis* 1995;20:1236.
2. Polk HC Jr, Christmas AB. Prophylactic antibiotics in surgery and surgical wound infection. *Am Surg* 2000;66:105.
3. Medical Letter. Antimicrobial prophylaxis in surgery. *Med Lett Drugs Ther* 2001;43:92.
4. Dellinger EP, et al. Quality standard for antimicrobial prophylaxis in surgical procedures. *Clin Infect Dis* 1994;18:422.
5. Classen DC, et al. The timing of prophylactic administration of antibiotics and the risk of surgical wound infection. *N Engl J Med* 1992;326:281.
6. Stone HH, Haney BB, Kolb LD, et al. Prophylactic and preventive antibiotic therapy: timing, duration, and economics. *Ann Surg* 1979;189:691–699.
7. Dajani AS, et al. Prevention of bacterial endocarditis: recommendations by the American Heart Association. *JAMA* 1997;277:1794.
8. Medical Letter. Prevention of bacterial endocarditis. *Med Lett Drugs Ther* 2001;43:98.
9. Durack DT. Antibiotics for prevention of endocarditis during dentistry: time to scale back? *Ann Intern Med* 1998;129:829.
10. Haas DW, Kaiser AB. Antimicrobial prophylaxis of infections associated with foreign bodies. In: Bisno AL, Waldvogel FA, eds. *Infections associated with indwelling medical devices,* 2nd ed. Washington, DC: American Society for Microbiology, 1994.
11. Wahl MJ. Myths of dental-induced prosthetic device infections. *Clin Infect Dis* 1995;20:1420.
12. Steckelberg JM, Osmon DR. Prosthetic joint infections. In: Bisno AL, Waldvogel FA, eds. *Infections associated with prosthetic indwelling medical devices,* 2nd ed. Washington, DC: American Society for Microbiology, 1994:259–290.
13. American Dental Association, American Academy of Orthopedic Surgeons. Advisory statement: antibiotic prophylaxis for dental patients with total joint replacement. *J Am Dent Assoc* 1997;128:1004.
14. Waldman BJ, Mont MA, Hungerford DS. Total knee arthroplasty infections associated with dental procedures. *Clin Orthop Relat Res* 1997;343:164.
15. LaPorte DM, Waldman BJ, Mont MA. Infections associated with dental procedures in total hip arthroplasty. *J Bone Joint Surg [Br]* 1999;81:56.
16. Lieberman JM, Greenberg DP, Ward JI. Prevention of bacterial meningitis: vaccine and chemoprophylaxis. *Infect Dis Clin North Am* 1990;4:703.
17. Warren RE, Wimperis JZ, Bablin TP, et al. Prevention of infection by ciprofloxacin in neutropenia. *J Antimicrob Chemother* 1990;26[Suppl F]:109–123.
18. Rotstein C, Bow EJ, Laverdiere M, et al. Randomized placebo-controlled trail of fluconazole prophylaxis for neutropenic cancer patients: benefit based on purpose and intensity of cytotoxic therapy. The Canadian Study Group. *Clin Infect Dis* 1999;28:331–340.
19. Wingard JR, Merz WG, Rinaldi MG, et al. Increase in *Candida krusei* infection among patients with bone marrow transplantation and neutropenia treated prophylactically with fluconazole. *N Engl J Med* 1991;325:1274–1277.
20. Dajani A, et al. Treatment of acute streptococcal pharyngitis and prevention of rheumatic fever: a statement for health professionals. *Pediatrics* 1995;96:758.

21. Styrt B. Infection associated with asplenia: risks, mechanisms, and prevention. *Am J Med* 1990;88[Suppl 5N]:33N.
22. Reid MM. Splenectomy, sepsis, immunization, and guidelines. *Lancet* 1994;344:970–971.
23. Buchanan CR. Chemoprophylaxis in asplenic adolescents and young adults. *Pediatr Infect Dis J* 1993;12:892.
24. Van der Hazel SJ, et al. Role of antibiotics in treatment and prevention of acute and recurrent cholangitis. *Clin Infect Dis* 1994;19:279.
25. USPHS/IDSA Prevention of Opportunistic Infections Working Group. 1999 USPHS/IDSA guidelines for the prevention of opportunistic infections in persons infected with human immunodeficiency virus. *Ann Intern Med* 1999;131:873.
26. Gins P, et al. Norfloxacin prevents spontaneous bacterial peritonitis in cirrhosis: results of a double-blind, placebo-controlled trial. *Hepatology* 1990;12:716.
27. Singh N, et al. Trimethoprim-sulfamethoxazole for the prevention of spontaneous bacterial peritonitis in cirrhosis: a randomized trial. *Ann Intern Med* 1995;122:595.
28. Gins P, Navasa M. Antibiotic prophylaxis for spontaneous bacterial peritonitis: how and whom? *J Hepatol* 1998;29:490.

## C. Penicillin

The term **penicillin** is the generic term for a broad group of agents, including but not limited to penicillin G, penicillin V, oxacillin, nafcillin, ampicillin, ticarcillin, piperacillin, amoxicillin, and dicloxacillin. The major mechanism of action of penicillin is binding to proteins in the cell wall, called penicillin-binding protein. This binding promotes lysis of the bacteria. Thus penicillin is **bactericidal.** Penicillin has other mechanisms of action that are not fully understood.

Some penicillins are excreted primarily by the kidney by both glomerular filtration and tubular secretion; others are excreted via the liver. Penicillin is mainly eliminated via the kidney.

**I. Structure** [1]. The penicillin nucleus and breakdown products are shown in Figure 27C.1.

**A. Structural modifications.** Penicillins with differing antimicrobial activity can be synthesized from 6-aminopenicillanic acid by substitution of side chains. This results in compounds with a broader spectrum of activity, resistance to penicillinase, or stability in acid pH (important in oral preparations) and other different pharmacokinetic characteristics.

**B. Common nucleus.** An intact $\beta$-lactam ring (the penicillin nucleus of the molecule) is necessary for biologic activity. In addition, as a result of the common ring in the penicillins, the **potential for allergic cross-sensitivity** is high.

**C. Penicillinase is a $\beta$-lactamase enzyme that splits the $\beta$-lactam ring** (Fig. 27C.1, site 1). The resulting penicilloic acid is inactive against bacteria. The penicilloic acid and other breakdown molecules that result may mediate allergic reactions. The penicillins resistant to breakdown have less potential for allergic reactions. Penicillinase production is a principal mechanism of penicillin resistance in coagulase-positive *Staphylococcus aureus, Pseudomonas* species, and *Bacteroides fragilis* and one of the mechanisms of resistance in *Escherichia coli* and *Proteus* species. **When a penicillin is combined with a $\beta$-lactamase inhibitor (clavulanic acid,** sulbactam, or tazobactam), the penicillin escapes breakdown (see Chapter 27E).

**II. Penicillin G: spectrum of activity**

**A. Gram-positive aerobic cocci**

1. Penicillin is bactericidal against *S. pyogenes* (group A), *S. bovis,* and penicillin-susceptible *S. aureus* and against most *Streptococcus pneumoniae* and viridans streptococci. Against enterococci, penicillin G is bacteriostatic.
2. **Resistance of *S. pneumoniae* to penicillin is being seen with increased frequency** [2–6].This topic is discussed in Chapters 8, 11, and 25.

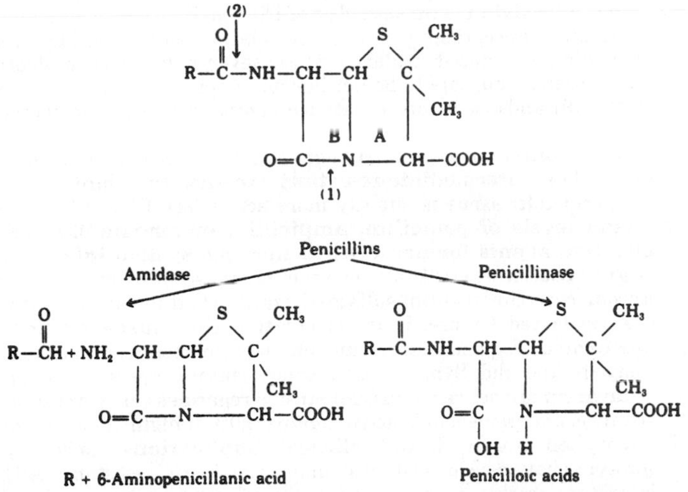

Penicillins

Amidase

Penicillinase

R + 6-Aminopenicillanic acid

Penicilloic acids

**FIG. 27C.1** Penicillin nucleus and breakdown products. [1] Site of $\beta$-lactamase activity. [2] Site of amidase activity. Amidase, an enzyme produced by microorganisms, cleaves penicillin at site 2.

**a. Laboratory definitions** [2–6]

**(1) Susceptible strains** have minimum inhibitory concentrations (MIC) (see Chapter 25) to penicillin of 0.1 $\mu$g/mL.

**(2) Intermediate resistance** is defined as strains with MIC of 0.12 to 1 $\mu$g/mL.

**(3) High resistance** is defined as MIC $\geq$2 $\mu$g/mL. These strains are resistant to other penicillins, including those that are $\beta$-lactamase inhibitors such as ampicillin/sulbactam, and are more likely to be resistant to other antibiotics as well. Strains resistant to three or more antibiotics are defined as multidrug resistant [7].

**(4) Laboratory testing.** The National Committee for Clinical Laboratory Standards recommends screening of pneumococcus isolated from blood or sterile fluid for penicillin resistance by disk diffusion, using a 1-$\mu$g oxacillin disk. For those organisms that are not susceptible by screening, MIC should be determined (see Chapter 25).

**b. Prevalence and frequency.** Penicillin resistance was uncommon in the United States through 1987, but the incidence has increased significantly [2–6]. Recent data from the United States suggested that 33% to 36% of *S. pneumoniae* are penicillin resistant, with most isolates intermediately resistant but identified more and more as highly resistant (see Chapter 11).

**c. Mechanisms and spread** [1–6]. Pneumococcal resistance to penicillin results from **alterations in the genetic structure** of the organism, **giving rise to changes in one** or **more of the penicillin binding proteins.** This reduces affinity of binding and, in turn, activity. This is a relative resistance that is partially overcome with higher concentrations of penicillin.

Selective pressure exerted by antibiotic use is a chief factor responsible for the initial development of resistance. Thereafter, most of the increase of resistance is due to the spread of resistant organisms from one individual to another. Those at highest risk to become colonized are the young, those attending a day-care center (especially a large center), or those residing in a nursing home. Resistant strains may be transported to geographically distant areas, where spread is influenced by these factors.

d. **Effect of resistance on severity of illness.** In experimental animal models using Swiss mice, there is a direct correlation between reduced resistance to penicillin and reduced virulence [8]. However, in humans, antibiotic-resistant pneumococcus appears to be neither more nor less virulent than susceptible strains [9], and disease presentation and progression is equal if proper therapy is not delayed.

e. **Susceptibility of penicillin-resistant *S. pneumoniae* to other antibiotics. For intermediate-resistant strains,** the third-generation cephalosporin ceftriaxone is slightly more active (see Chapter 27F). **Also high serum levels of penicillin, ampicillin, or amoxicillin are clinically effective agents for non-central nervous system infections** [5,10,11]. **Highly resistant strains** are very often resistant to erythromycin and clarithromycin, trimethoprim-sulfamethoxazole, and tetracycline. If these drugs are considered for use, **it is imperative that susceptibility testing is performed.** Expanded-spectrum fluoroquinolones (e.g., moxifloxacin), vancomycin, linezolid, Synercid, and experimental drugs such as daptomycin or oritavancin are active against all strains regardless of degree of penicillin resistance, and imipenem is active against 90% of highly resistant organisms.

f. **Serotypes involved and clinical implications.** Currently, only six serotypes have developed intermediate or high level resistance. All but type 6A is present in the 23-valent pneumococcal capsular polysaccharide vaccine. Therefore **the pneumococcal vaccine should be aggressively promoted** and **routinely administered.**

g. **Clinical implications of penicillin-resistance** includes the following:

   (1) **Pneumococcal meningitis.** Until susceptibilities have returned, gram-positive organisms seen on Gram stain should be considered as high level penicillin resistant and thus resistant to third-generation cephalosporins (cefotaxime and ceftriaxone). Therapy must include vancomycin and either cefotaxime or ceftriaxone for all individuals older than age 1 month [12] (see Chapter 6).

   (2) **Sepsis and pneumonia.** High-dose penicillin (150,000 to 200,000 units/kg/day) is effective therapy against strains resistant at the intermediate level [10]. For patients who are severely ill when high level penicillin resistance is a possibility, such as in a grandparent in contact with children who attend day care, a fluoroquinolones such as moxifloxacin or gatifloxacin or vancomycin should be used (see related discussions in Chapter 11).

   (3) **Otitis media.** Amoxicillin is recommended for initial therapy. The *2000 Red Book* emphasizes the following [12]. Based on concentrations in middle ear fluid and *in vitro* activity, no currently available $\beta$-lactam antibiotic, including the oral cephalosporins, has better activity than amoxicillin against penicillin-resistant *S. pneumoniae.* Cefuroxime axetil, cefpodoxime, and cefprozil are the only oral cephalosporins that have comparable, but not greater, activity than amoxicillin for highly resistant strains. Recently, doses of amoxicillin of 60 to 90 mg/kg/day have been suggested to achieve middle ear concentrations active against resistant strains [12,13] (see Chapter 8).

h. **Methods to control** the rising incidence of penicillin-resistant *S. pneumoniae* are being evaluated. These include more careful use of antibiotics in the community, shorter courses of antibiotics, and use of narrower spectrum antibiotics [14,15].

3. Resistance of group A streptococci to penicillin has not been observed.

B. **Gram-negative aerobes.** Penicillin remains the antibiotic of choice for *N. meningitidis* and *Pasteurella multocida* [16] but not for *N. gonorrhoeae.*

C. **Anaerobes.** Penicillin is very effective against anaerobic species [16], including *Clostridium, Fusobacterium,* and *Actinomyces israelii* (actinomycosis). Although penicillin is active against many *Bacteroides* species, particularly oropharyngeal strains, it is not active against some of the oral gram-negative anaerobes and

*B. fragilis*. If *B. fragilis* infections are suspected (e.g., intraabdominal or pelvic infections), another agent should be selected.

**D. Spirochetes.** Penicillin is the drug of choice for *Treponema pallidum* [16] infection (see Chapter 16) and is active against *Borrelia burgdorferi*.

**III. Parenteral preparations of penicillin G (benzyl penicillin).** There are three main forms of parenteral penicillin G. The pharmacokinetics differs markedly.

**A. Aqueous penicillin G** is available in potassium and sodium salt forms. Ordinarily, the potassium salt form is used. Aqueous penicillin is given intravenously and therefore produces **high blood levels.** Excretion is rapid, yielding undetectable penicillin blood levels 4 hours after a dose. Therefore for serious infections, the aqueous form should be given at least every 4 hours.

1. **High-dose therapy. In adults with normal renal function,** 3 to 4 million units every 4 hours is **used in serious infections,** such as meningitis due to susceptible organisms, in some forms of endocarditis due to mildly penicillin-resistant organisms, and in severe clostridia infections. A continuous infusion of 20 to 24 million units per day can be used [1].
2. **Intermediate doses** of aqueous penicillin (9 to 12 million units daily) are used in adults with aspiration pneumonia or lung abscess and in moderate to severe soft tissue infection due to group A streptococci. This dose of 9 to 12 million units/day is also used in conjunction with an aminoglycoside such as gentamicin to provide synergy against enterococci (those without high level resistance to gentamicin) and other resistant streptococci in endocarditis. This dose is active for pneumonia caused by intermediate-resistant *S. pneumoniae* (see Chapter 11).
3. **Low doses.** Procaine penicillin or oral penicillin is an option once the susceptibilities of the pneumococcus return. If the aqueous intravenous form of penicillin is used in known **penicillin-susceptible** pneumococcal pneumonia, the dose can be kept at 2.4 million units/day. High doses of penicillin may only increase the chances of superinfection (see prior discussion in section **II.A.2**).
4. **Pediatric dose.** For children, 25,000 to 300,000 units/kg/day is recommended, depending on the severity of the infection.

**B. Procaine penicillin G.** This repository form of penicillin has been developed to prolong the duration of penicillin in the blood. **Doses** usually are given **every 12 hours intramuscularly.** Peak levels (1–2 $\mu$g/mL) are reached in 2 to 4 hours, and detectable levels are present for 12 to 24 hours. This preparation should not be given intravenously because of the risk of procaine toxicity. To increase the peak serum levels, two separate intramuscular injections must be used. Very few clinical situations exist for its use, but procaine penicillin is used in some of the alternative regimens for syphilis (see Chapter 16).

**C. Benzathine penicillin G** (long acting) is an insoluble salt obtained by combining an ammonium base with penicillin G. **Very low blood levels** are achieved (approximately 0.10 to 0.15 units/mL), which persist for prolonged periods of time (i.e., 3–4 weeks). Injection-related pain limits its use. **Benzathine penicillin is used most commonly in the following conditions:**

1. **Syphilis** (primary, secondary, and latent), in which a prolonged blood level is necessary to kill the slowly dividing *Treponema* organisms. *T. pallidum* remains very sensitive to penicillin (MIC = 0.03 unit/mL) (see Chapter 16).
2. **Rheumatic fever prophylaxis.** A monthly injection will provide a serum level above that necessary to inhibit group A $\beta$-hemolytic streptococci [17].
3. **Streptococcal pharyngitis.** In the high-risk patient (e.g., prior rheumatic fever) or the poorly compliant patient, benzathine penicillin administration will ensure maintenance of adequate levels. Cure rates using penicillin for group A streptococcal pharyngitis are highest with a single dose of benzathine penicillin of 600,000 units in children less than 60 pounds and 1.2 million units in adults and children over 60 pounds [17].

**IV. Oral penicillin.** Oral penicillin G is partially inactivated by gastric acid. With a minor modification of the side chain, **penicillin V** (phenoxymethyl penicillin) is formed, and this oral congener **resists gastric acid breakdown** and therefore provides acceptable serum levels.

A. **Dosage.** The usual adult dosage is 250 mg (400,000 units) to 500 mg (800,000 units) every 6 hours. A 500-mg dose results in a peak level of 3 to 5 $\mu$g/mL. In children, the usual dosage is 25,000 to 100,000 units/kg/day (16 to 65 mg/kg/day) divided into doses every 6 hours.

B. **Uses.** Oral therapy is useful in pharyngitis, minor oral or dental infections, in minor soft tissue infections due to susceptible organisms, and for completion of courses of treatment after initial intravenous penicillin therapy. **Group A streptococci remain uniformly susceptible to all penicillins** and cephalosporins. The American Heart Association [17] and the American Academy of Pediatrics recommend a single dose of intramuscular benzathine penicillin or a 10-day course of oral **penicillin** V for group A streptococci. The suggested dose is 500 mg two or three times a day for those older than 12 years and 250 mg two or three times a day for children younger than 12 years.

C. **The spectrum of activity** of penicillin V is similar to that of penicillin G.

V. **Allergic and toxic reactions**

A. **Penicillin allergy and hypersensitivity reactions.** See Chapter 24 for a detailed discussion. However, several comments deserve emphasis.

1. **Allergic reactions to penicillin.** Adverse reactions to penicillin are estimated to occur in 1% to 10% of patients, with a fatal reaction occurring in 0.002% of patients (see Chapter 24).

   a. **Immediate reactions.** Hypotension or bronchospasm occur within the first 2 to 30 minutes. This is due to release of histamine and other vasoactive amines. The IgE-sensitized mast cells and basophils interact with penicillin or its breakdown products. Death can ensue.

   b. **Accelerated reactions occur in the first 1 to 72 hours** and except for laryngeal edema, which may cause asphyxia, are usually not life threatening. These reactions are also IgE mediated but not modified by IgG.

   c. **Serum sickness.** This can develop while on therapy or more often after completion of a course. Arthritis, skin rash, and nephritis are common features. IgE and IgG acting in conjunction mediate serum sickness reaction. Skin testing done at this time will be positive.

2. **Late reactions.** These are the **most frequent** type of reaction and **are not immunologically mediated.** They account for 80% to 90% of reactions and occur days after initiation of therapy.

   a. **Morbilliform rash.** No definite allergic mechanism has been demonstrated for this reaction. It is not IgE mediated. This rash cannot be predicted or diagnosed by skin tests.

   b. **Fever** may be the only manifestation of a penicillin reaction, and its occurrence does not preclude use of penicillin in the future. However, because fever may accompany vasculitis, patients with a drug fever history require careful observation on reexposure.

   c. **Eosinophilia** occurs with penicillin use. When the level exceeds 15% of the peripheral white blood cell count, patients may go on to more serious drug reactions (see Chapter 24).

   d. **Interstitial nephritis** may occur at high doses with any penicillin [18], at any age, and may be a hypersensitivity reaction. Fever, hematuria, proteinuria, morbilliform rash, peripheral eosinophilia, and renal failure (50% of cases) occur several days into therapy. Some patients have eosinophils in their urine sediments, which is a helpful diagnostic clue. Renal biopsy reveals an interstitial nephritis with eosinophilic aggregations.

      The offending agent should be discontinued. Whether cephalosporins can be used safely is uncertain, but we would be inclined not to use another $\beta$-lactam antibiotic.

   e. **Central nervous system toxicity.** High blood levels lead to excessively high spinal fluid levels of penicillin. This occurs with high doses in renal failure because penicillin diffuses into the spinal fluid and then competes with the other organic acids to be transported out (see section **VI.A.1**). **Myoclonic twitching** is an early clue. The patient may develop **seizures.**

3. **Cross-reactions (also see Chapter 24)**
   a. **Other penicillins.** Patients with a history of allergy to a penicillin should be presumed to be allergic to other penicillins unless skin tests prove otherwise.
   b. **Cephalosporins and imipenem.** In penicillin-allergic patients, studies suggest that risk of cross-allergy to a cephalosporin ranges from 5% to 15%. The more stable third-generation cephalosporins may cross-react as infrequently as 1% [1,19–21]. **When there is a history of immediate penicillin reaction, cephalosporins skin tests should be performed before their use. Patients allergic to penicillin may cross-react to imipenem.** In the patient with a history of delayed mild reaction to penicillin, cephalosporins or imipenem, in our experience, are used without difficulty [1,20,21].
   c. **Aztreonam.** Patients allergic to penicillin can receive aztreonam without risk.
4. **Documentation of allergic history.** Because the distinction between an immediate versus a delayed allergic reaction is crucial for determining future antibiotic administration, it is important to elicit this history carefully and to document it in the patient's record.

VI. **Special considerations**

A. **Dosage modification in renal failure**
1. **High dose regimens of aqueous penicillin.** In moderate to severe renal failure and in the elderly, **to avoid central nervous system toxicity, penicillin G doses must be reduced (Table 27C.1).**
2. When **moderate intravenous doses** (i.e., 9–12 million units/day) are to be used in patients with renal failure, we tend to reduce doses proportionately (Table 27C.1).
3. With **low dose intravenous** or oral penicillin regimens, standard doses are used.

B. **Hemodialysis** removes variable amounts of penicillin. For a high dose regimen, reduce the dose but supplement with 500,000 units after each 6-hour dialysis (Table 27C.1). For a moderate or low dose regimen, supplement with 500,000 units

Table 27C.1. Equivalent Doses of Aqueous Penicillin G for High-dose Therapy in Renal Failure[a]

| Endogenous Creatinine Clearance (mL/min) | Penicillin G Dose[b] and Dose Interval[c] (units) |
|---|---|
| 125 | 1.7–2.0 million q2h or 2.6–3.0 million q3h |
| 60 | 1.8–2.0 million q4h |
| 40 | 1.3–1.5 million q4h |
| 20 | 800,000–1 million q4h |
| 10 | 800,000–1 million q6h |
| 0 | 500,000–800,000 q6h or 700,000–1.1 million q8h |
| <10[d] | 500,000 q8h |

[a]**To achieve mean blood levels equivalent to 24 million units per day** in the adult with normal renal function, the above doses and dose intervals can be used in patients with renal failure. **A loading dose** of 750,000–1,200,000 units is suggested in patients with a creatinine clearance of less than 20 mL/min, and then the above doses and intervals can be followed. In patients with a creatinine clearance exceeding 20 mL/min, no loading dose is suggested.
[b]The lower dose is calculated to provide a mean serum level of 20 μg/mL for the "average patient." The higher dose is an overestimate.
[c]After hemodialysis, an additional 500,000 units should be given to replace expected losses for an average full 6-h dialysis.
[d]Because the extrarenal clearance of penicillin is impaired by liver disease, in patients with hepatic and renal failure (creatinine clearance < 10 mL/min), even lower doses of penicillin G are suggested.
Adapted from Bryan CS, Stone WJ, "Comparable massive" penicillin G therapy in renal failure. *Ann Intern Med* 1975;82:189.

every other dialysis. **Peritoneal dialysis** likewise removes a variable amount of penicillin. No supplementation is provided.

**C. Probenecid use.** Approximately 90% of penicillin is eliminated by tubular secretion and 10% by glomerular filtration. Probenecid blocks the renal tubular secretory transport, and this in turn results in higher (usually approximately twofold) and more prolonged blood levels of penicillin.

1. **Dosage.** Probenecid 500 mg orally four times a day. The major side effect is gastrointestinal, but rash frequency occurs.
2. **Uses.** Because probenecid increases side effect frequency, **we seldom use probenecid with oral therapy.** Amoxicillin may be preferred becuase this agent will provide higher serum levels.

## REFERENCES

1. Wright AJ. The penicillins. *Mayo Clin Proc* 1999;74:290.
2. Moellering RC, ed. The clinical significance of drug-resistant *Streptococcus pneumoniae* for the treatment of community-acquired pneumonia. *Clin Infect Dis* 2002;34[Suppl 1]: S1–S46.
3. Breiman RF, et al. Emergence of drug-resistant pneumococcal infections in the United States. *JAMA* 1994;271:1831.
4. Whitley CG, et al. Increasing prevalence of multidrug resistant *Streptococcus pneumoniae* in the United States. *N Engl J Med* 2000;343:1917.
5. Musher DM, Bartlett JG, Doern GV. A fresh look at the definition of susceptibility of *Streptococcus pneumoniae* to $\beta$-lactam antibiotics. *Arch Intern Med* 2001;161:2538–2544.
6. Center for Disease Control and Prevention. Assessment of susceptibility testing practices for *Streptococcus pneumoniae*—United States. *MMWR Morb Mortal Wkly Rep* 2002;51:392–394.
7. Clavo-Sanchez AJ, et al. Multivariate analysis of risk factors for infection due to penicillin-resistant and multidrug-resistant *Streptococcus pneumoniae:* a multicenter study. *Clin Infect Dis* 1997;24:1052.
8. Azoulay-Dupuis E, Rieux V, Muffat-Jolly M, et al. Relationship between capsular type, penicillin susceptibility, and virulence of human *Streptococcus pneumoniae* isolates in mice. *Antimicrob Agents Chemother* 2000;44:1575–1577.
9. Arditi M, Mason EO Jr, Tan TQ, et al. Three year multicenter surveillance of pneumococcal meningitis in children: clinical characteristics and outcome related to penicillin susceptibility and dexamethasone use. *Pediatrics* 1998;102:1087–1097.
10. Tomasz A. The pneumococcus at the gates. *N Engl J Med* 1995;333:514.
11. Appelbaum PC. Resistance among *Streptococcus pneumoniae*: implications for drug selection. *Clin Infect Dis* 2002;34:1613.
12. American Academy of Pediatrics. *2000 Red Book: report of the Committee on Infectious Diseases,* 24th ed. Elk Grove Village, IL: American Academy of Pediatrics, 2000:457.
13. Poole MD. Implications of drug-resistant *Streptococcus pneumoniae* for otitis media. *Pediatr Infect Dis J* 1998;17:953.
14. Jernigan DB, et al. Minimizing the impact of drug-resistant *Streptococcus pneumoniae* (DRSP): a strategy from the DRSP working group. *JAMA* 1996;275:206.
15. Center for Disease Control and Prevention. Methods of control of resistant pneumococcus. *MMWR Morb Mortal Wkly Rep* 1996;45:1.
16. The Medical Letter. The choice of antibacterial drugs. *Med Lett Drugs Ther* 2000;43: 69.
17. Dajani AS, et al. Treatment of streptococcal pharyngitis and prevention of rheumatic fever: a statement of health professionals on rheumatic fever, endocarditis, and Kawasaki disease of the Council on Cardiovascular Disease in the Young, the American Heart Association. *Pediatrics* 1995;96:758.
18. Murray KM, Keane WR.. Review of drug-induced acute interstitial nephritis. *Pharmacotherapy* 1992;12:462.
19. Donowitz GR. Third-generation cephalosporins. *Infect Dis Clin North Am* 1989;3:595.
20. Anne S, Reisman RE. Risk of administering cephalosporin antibiotics to patients with histories of penicillin allergy. *Ann Allerg Asthma Immunol* 1995;74:167.
21. Kelkar PS, Li JTC. Cephalosporin allergy. *N Engl J Med* 2001;345:804.

## D. Penicillinase-resistant Penicillins

Penicillinase-resistant penicillins are synthesized by modifying the side chain of the common penicillin nucleus. The substituted side chain inhibits penicillinase (a $\beta$-lactamase) by preventing opening of the $\beta$-lactam ring. **These bactericidal agents are used primarily to treat penicillinase-producing** *Staphylococcus aureus* [1,2].

I. **Available agents.** Two parenteral (nafcillin and oxacillin) and two oral (cloxacillin and dicloxacillin) agents are available. Methicillin, which is nephrotoxic, is no longer available.

II. **Spectrum of activity**

A. ***S. aureus*** **penicillin resistant**

1. **Methicillin-susceptible** *S. aureus* (MSSA)

a. ***In vitro*** The minimum inhibitory concentration (MIC) of MSSA to nafcillin or oxacillin ranges from 0.78 to 1.56 $\mu$g/mL.

b. **Clinical** Compared with the other agents that have activity (cefazolin, vancomycin), both nafcillin and oxacillin produce a higher cure rate [3,4]. In MSSA bacteremia, gentamicin is often used (1 mg/kg every 8 hours) in the first few days of therapy.

2. Methicillin-resistant *S. aureus* (MRSA) [5,6]. Although MRSA was previously considered only a nosocomial pathogen, recent data show that MRSA is becoming more common as a community-acquired pathogen [6]; see related discussion in Chapters 4 and 5.

a. Neither nafcillin nor oxacillin has any meaningful activity against MRSA, whose resistance is mediated by change in the penicillin binding proteins [6].

b. A small percent of MRSA are resistant because of a high concentration of $\beta$-lactamase. Increasing the dose of nafcillin or oxacillin can overcome this resistance.

B. **Other gram-positive aerobes.** Nafcillin and oxacillin are active against penicillin-susceptible *Streptococcus pneumoniae, S. pyogenes,* and *S. aureus,* but the MICs for these organisms are higher than for penicillin, making penicillin the preferred agent [1,4] **even for penicillin-susceptible *S. aureus*.** They are not useful in penicillin-resistant *S. pneumoniae* infections and are only minimally active against enterococci. **The penicillinase-resistant penicillins are drugs of first choice only for penicillinase-producing MSSA** [4].

C. **Gram-negative aerobes.** These agents are **not active against** the Enterobacteriaceae The penicillinase-resistant penicillins **are not recommended in the treatment of gonorrhea.** For patients with infections due to *Pasteurella multocida,* penicillin is the preferred agent [4]. In animal bite wounds with mixed flora, amoxicillin-clavulanate (or ampicillin-sulbactam) is suggested (see Chapter 4).

D. **Anaerobes.** The penicillinase-resistant penicillins are less active than penicillin against penicillin-susceptible anaerobes and, like penicillin, are not active against *Bacteroides fragilis*.

III. **Clinical activity parenteral preparations.** There are no adequate studies to determine which antistaphylococcal agent is more effective [1–4]. Overall, oxacillin and nafcillin are very similar and, except as noted later, are probably interchangeable. Methicillin was more commonly associated with interstitial nephritis, especially in adults; it is no longer available in the United States [2].

A. **Nafcillin**

1. **Dosage.** In adults, 6 g/day intravenously is recommended for moderate infections. For severe infections, 9 to 12 g/day intravenously has been suggested, but limiting the dose to 9 g/day seems to avoid excessive side effects. Because this antibiotic kills by concentration-dependent effects, the MIC simply needs to be exceeded and the 1.5-g dose is sufficient. In children, the usual dose is 100 to 200 mg/kg/day in divided doses every 4 to 6 hours. Because the half-life is short (40 minutes) and levels are undetectable at 2.5 to 3.0 hours, a 4-hour dose interval is preferred. Dosages for neonates are shown in Appendix Table 1. **Nafcillin should not be**

**used in infants with jaundice.** It is excreted primarily by hepatic mechanisms that may be deficient in these neonates or infants [1].

a. **In renal failure and dialysis, dosage modification is not necessary** [7]. **Nafcillin is an excellent choice in renal failure** when a semisynthetic penicillin is needed.

b. **Hepatic failure.** Dose reduction is required in hepatic failure. Even when renal function is normal, renal toxicity occurs if standard doses are used in the presence of significant hepatic dysfunction simply because high levels are exposed to the kidney.

2. **Central nervous system penetration.** Studies have shown adequate penetration of nafcillin into the spinal fluid, particularly when inflammation is present. Some authors suggest nafcillin is the **drug of choice in MSSA staphylococcal meningitis** [1,2].

3. **Side effects.** Penicillin-like allergic reactions may occur. Rarely, neutropenia has been observed. Interstitial nephritis appears to occur less frequently than with methicillin (see above). Phlebitis and/or pain often develops at the infusion site and is much more common with nafcillin than with oxacillin [1].

**B. Oxacillin**

1. **Dose** is similar to nafcillin and should be limited to 1.5 g every 4 hours in adults and older children.

a. **Renal failure.** Because oxacillin is excreted mainly by the liver and somewhat by the kidney, in renal failure doses do not have to be modified. **The exception is the individual with hepatic failure. Hemodialysis and peritoneal dialysis** do not remove oxacillin [7].

b. **Hepatic failure (see section A.1.b)**

2. **Side effects.** Oxacillin-related **hepatitis** in prolonged intravenous use has been described [8]. Therefore **weekly liver function tests are advisable for patients receiving prolonged therapy.** *Clostridium difficile* diarrhea may occur. Interstitial nephritis may occur with oxacillin use, but it is less frequent than after methicillin use (see section **A.3**). Neutropenia also occurs.

**IV. Oral preparations** (cloxacillin, dicloxacillin)

**A. Indications for use.** Oral penicillinase-resistant penicillins often are considered the oral drugs of choice for known or highly suspected penicillin-resistant mild staphylococcal infections. They are useful in treating soft tissue infections due to susceptible *S. aureus* or mixed *S. aureus* and *S. pyogenes* (group A streptococci). However, the first-generation oral cephalosporins have less frequent gastrointestinal side effects and are therefore often preferred over cloxacillin or dicloxacillin (see section **C**).

**B. Agents available.** These are better absorbed in the fasting state.

1. **Cloxacillin** is available in a solution (125 mg/5 mL) and in 250- and 500-mg capsules. Usual dosage in children is 50 to 100 mg/kg/day and in adults, 1 to 2 g/day divided into four equal doses.

2. **Dicloxacillin** is available as a suspension (62.5 mg/5 mL) and in 125- and 250-mg capsules. The usual dosage in children is 25 to 50 mg/kg/day; in adults, the usual dosage is 1 to 2 g/day divided into four equal doses. The higher dose range may be preferable for adequate antistaphylococcal activity.

**C. Side effects.** Mild **gastrointestinal symptoms** are common; often the standard oral dosages (e.g., 500 mg every 6 hours in adults) cannot be tolerated. Furthermore, the poor taste of the oral suspension may adversely affect compliance in children [9]. A first-generation oral cephalosporin is better tolerated and therefore often preferred. If severe or persistent diarrhea occurs, antibiotic-related diarrhea must be considered.

## REFERENCES

1. Reese RE, Betts RF. Penicillinase-resistant penicillin. In: Reese RE, Betts RF, Gumustop B, eds. *Handbook of antibiotics,* 3rd ed. Philadelphia: Lippincott Williams & Wilkins, 2000.
2. Wright AJ. The penicillins. *Mayo Clin Proc* 1999;74:290.

3. Fowler VG Jr, Sanders LL, Sexton DJ, et al. Outcome of *Staphylococcus aureus* bacteremia according to compliance with recommendations of infectious disease s specialists: experience with 244 patients. *Clin Infect Dis* 1998;27:478–486.
4. The Medical Letter. The choice of antibacterial drugs. *Med Lett Drug Ther* 1999;41:95.
5. Frainow HS, Abrutyn E. Pathogens resistant to antimicrobial agents: epidemiology, molecular mechanisms and clinical management. *Infect Dis Clin North Am* 1995;9:497.
6. Kak V, Levine DP. Community-acquired methicillin-resistant *Staphylococcus aureus* infections: where do we go from here? *Clin Infect Dis* 1999;29:801.
7. Aronoff GR, et al. *Drug prescribing in renal failure: dosing guidelines for adults,* 4th ed. Philadelphia: American College of Physicians, 1999. (Also see 3rd ed., 1994, for oxacillin dose reduction.)
8. Bruckstein AH, Attia AA. Oxacillin hepatitis. *Am J Med* 1978;64:519.
9. Ruff ME, et al. Antimicrobial drug suspensions: a blind comparison of taste of fourteen common pediatric drugs. *Pediatr Infect Dis J* 1991;10:30.

## E. Broad-spectrum Penicillins and β-Lactam–β-Lactamase Combinations

Several side-chain modifications of penicillin have been made to provide enhanced activity of the broad-spectrum penicillins (Table 27E.1).

I. **Aminopenicillins: ampicillin** and **amoxicillin** [1,2].
   A. **Spectrum of activity.** In addition to being active against penicillin-susceptible organisms, **ampicillin is** more active than penicillin against enterococci, *Listeria monocytogenes,* and β-lactamase–negative *Haemophilus influenzae.*
      1. **Drug of choice:** For *L. monocytogenes*, group B streptococci (*S. agalactiae*), *Proteus mirabilis,* and *Eikenella corrodens* [3].
      2. **Useful when proven active:** Many *Escherichia coli, Salmonella* species, and *Shigella* species are susceptible, so that ampicillin is a good choice once susceptibility studies are available [3]. About 50% of *E. coli* are susceptible but far fewer *Salmonella.*
      3. **Predictably inactive:** Ampicillin should not be used for penicillinase-producing *Staphylococcus aureus* or β-lactamase–positive *H. influenzae* or *Moraxella catarrhalis.*
      4. **Amoxicillin: Only** available for **oral** use. It is closely related to ampicillin in both chemical structure and antibacterial activity. Amoxicillin provides twice the serum level of oral ampicillin. Amoxicillin is given three times a day rather than the four times a day for ampicillin. Consequently, **amoxicillin has replaced oral ampicillin** [1,2], except that ampicillin is still preferred for susceptible *Shigella* species [3].
      5. **The combination of amoxicillin-clavulanate (Augmentin) is discussed separately** in section **III.B.**

Table 27E.1. Available β-lactamase Inhibitors and β-lactam Antibiotic Combinations

| Active Antibiotics | β-Lactamase Inhibitor | Trade Name | Comment |
|---|---|---|---|
| Amoxicillin | Clavulanate | Augmentin | Only as oral agent |
| Ticarcillin | Clavulanate | Timentin | Only parenteral |
| Ampicillin | Sulbactam | Unasyn | Only parenteral |
| Piperacillin | Tazobactam | Zosyn | Only parenteral; most active antibiotic *in vitro* |

**B.** Clinical usage

1. **Ampicillin intravenously** should be limited to those situations where susceptibilities are known. It is an excellent choice for susceptible enterococcal or group B streptococcal infections.
2. **Use is discouraged in combination therapy for the following:**
   a. **Pyelonephritis** with an aminoglycoside. Pyelonephritis due to enterococcus is uncommon, except in older men, and usually is relatively mild. For gram-negative organisms other single agents make more sense.
   b. **Intraabdominal infections.** Though used in combination with gentamicin and clindamycin for intraabdominal and gynecologic infections, use of three antibiotics increases the side effect potential and is inconvenient. The same coverage can be provided by piperacillin/tazobactam.
3. **Amoxicillin,** available as an **oral** agent **only,** is used for the following:
   a. **Acute otitis media,** as discussed in Chapter 8.
   b. **Acute sinusitis persisting for 10 days or longer** (see Chapter 8).
   c. **Exacerbation of chronic bronchitis,** as discussed in Chapter 8.
   d. **Susceptible** pathogens in nonbacteremic **urinary tract infection (UTI).**
   e. "Step-down" therapy after completion of intravenous ampicillin (see section **1**).
   f. Oral prophylactic antibiotic regimens to prevent endocarditis after dental manipulations (see section **B,** above, and Chapter 12).

**C. Dosage**

1. **Ampicillin**
   a. **Intravenous. In adults,** 6 to 12 g daily is given depending on the organism involved and the severity and site of the infection. In adults with moderately severe infections, 1 g should be given every 4 to 6 hours. The half-life is about 120 minutes. For more severe infections, 1.5 g every 4 hours may be necessary and, in *Listeria meningitis* in the adult, 2 g every 4 hours is used. **In children,** the usual dosage range is 100 to 200 mg/kg/day in divided doses every 6 hours. Neonatal doses are shown in the Appendix Table.
   b. **Oral.** The usual adult dose is 250 to 500 mg every 6 hours **on an empty stomach.** In children, 50 to 100 mg/kg/day in divided doses every 6 hours is suggested. Amoxicillin has replaced oral ampicillin.
   c. **Intramuscular.** Ampicillin can be given intramuscularly, but intravenous is preferred.
   d. **Renal failure.** Because ampicillin is excreted by the kidney, dosage is modified in patients with significant renal impairment, particularly when high dose regimens are used. If the creatinine clearance is 10 to 50 mL/min, the standard dose can be given every 6 to 12 hours. If the creatinine clearance is less than 10 mL/min, the standard dose can be given every 12 to 24 hours [4].
   e. **Dialysis.** Ampicillin is partially removed by hemodialysis. After dialysis, a supplemental dose is required. Peritoneal dialysis does not significantly lower ampicillin serum levels. For oral therapy, 250 mg every 12 hours has been used [4].
   f. **Pregnancy.** Ampicillin crosses the placenta and should be used conservatively in pregnancy.
   g. **Nursing mothers.** Ampicillin is excreted in human milk. The neonate could be sensitized by ampicillin in the mother's milk, so this agent should be used conservatively in nursing mothers.
2. **Amoxicillin**
   a. **Adults and children.** Since its introduction, the adult dose has been 250 to 500 mg every 8 hours, and the fasting state is not essential. More recently, **the suggested adult dose has been increased to 1.0 g every 8 hours**. In children, 20 to 40 mg/kg/day is given in divided doses every 8 hours. An oral suspension is available with 250 mg/5 mL and 125 mg/5 mL. **For otitis media in children, the high-dose regimen is discussed in Chapter 8.**
   b. **Renal failure.** If the creatinine clearance is 10 to 50 mL/min, the standard dose can be given every 12 hours. If the clearance is less than 10 mL/min, the standard dose can be given every 24 hours [4].

**c. Dialysis.** Dosage is as described for ampicillin; see the preceding discussion. In chronic ambulatory peritoneal dialysis patients, 250 mg every 12 hours has been suggested [4].

**d. Pregnancy.** The package insert notes that safety for use in pregnancy has not been established.

**e. Nursing mothers.** Amoxicillin is excreted in human milk (see section **1.g**, above).

**D. Adverse effects** of ampicillin (and amoxicillin)

**1.** These are similar to those described under penicillin discussed previously in this chapter.

**2. Rash.** Epstein-Barr virus infection (mononucleosis), acute lymphocytic leukemia, or cytomegalovirus infection increases the risk for an ampicillin (or amoxicillin) maculo papular rash to 60% to 100%. This does not appear to be mediated by IgE [5] and should not be interpreted as an allergic reaction. Morbilliform rashes, occurring unassociated with Epstein-Barr virus, are more common with ampicillin (amoxicillin) than with penicillin for unclear reasons [5].

**II. Extended-spectrum penicillins.** The carboxypenicillins include **carbenicillin (only oral available)** and **ticarcillin** and ureidopenicillins, **piperacillin.** They were introduced for more resistant gram-negative bacteria, including *Pseudomonas aeruginosa* [1,2].

**A. Spectrum of activity**

**1. Gram negative.** This group of antibiotics is active against many but not all Enterobacteriaceae, most *P. aeruginosa,* and other nosocomial gram-negative bacteria. Susceptibility testing is required. The extended-spectrum penicillins are synergistically active when used in conjunction with aminoglycosides. They are inactive against $\beta$-lactamase producing *Haemophilus* species, *N. gonorrhea*, and *Moraxella catarrhalis.*

**2. Gram positive.** Activity mimics that of ampicillin. The ureidopenicillins (not the carboxypenicillins) are active against ampicillin-susceptible enterococci at doses used for gram-negative bacilli. They are inactive against both *Staphylococcus aureus* and penicillin-resistant *Streptococcus pneumoniae.*

**B. Overview of uses**

**1.** For susceptible pathogens, prospective comparative studies have failed to demonstrate clinical superiority of one of these agents over another [1,2]. Except against *P. aeruginosa,* these agents are not **"drugs of choice"** [3].

**2.** For severe *P. aeruginosa* infection (e.g., pneumonia, sepsis), **monotherapy** with these agents is associated with the rapid emergence of resistance that requires any one of these to be combined with an aminoglycoside to decrease that likelihood of selecting resistant organisms. [1–3].

**3.** For hospital-acquired gram-negative organisms, including *P. aeruginosa,* one of these agents is combined with an aminoglycoside. Often the combination is synergistic (see discussions in Chapters 2 and 20).

**4.** These agents are active against anaerobes, including bowel anaerobes, but are considered "second-line" agents.

**5.** One of these agents combined with an aminoglycoside has historically been a useful combination for empiric therapy of the febrile neutropenic patient (see Chapter 20).

**C. Which agent?**

**1. Ticarcillin versus piperacillin.** Generally, the pharmacy and therapeutics committee of each hospital selects one of these agents for routine use.

**a. Piperacillin compared with ticarcillin** has lower sodium load per daily dose, is more active *in vitro,* and has less acquired platelet dysfunction, thereby reducing the likelihood for bleeding after surgery and/or in patients with renal failure [6]. However, the bactericidal mechanism may be more effective for ticarcillin.

**b. Because piperacillin** overall is about four times more active against ***P. aeruginosa*** than is ticarcillin [2], **piperacillin** is generally preferred because the situation in which they are most often used is when *P. aeruginosa* is the likely or the proven cause of the infection.

**D. Dosages**

1. **Adults**. Because of a relatively short half-life in normal renal function, the dose interval should be 4 hours, and a dose of 3 g is reasonable. Piperacillin, due to its nonlinear pharmacokinetics, may be dosed as 4 g every 6 hours. For UTI, 6 g/day can be used.
2. **Children.** In children 12 years of age or older, 200 to 300 mg/kg/day intravenously (not to exceed the adult daily dose) in divided doses every 4 (or sometimes 6) hours is suggested. Dosages for children younger than 12 years have not been established, and the safety of this agent in neonates is not known.
3. **Renal failure.** No dose reduction is necessary until the creatinine clearance is less than 50 mL/min. If the creatinine clearance is 10 to 50 mL/min, 3 to 4 g is given every 6 hours, and if less than 10 mL/min, 3 to 4 g is given every 8 hours [4].
   a. **Hemodialysis.** Because dialysis removes 30% to 50% of the serum levels, a dose of 2 g every 8 hours, with a supplemental 1-g dose after hemodialysis, is recommended. A 3- to 4-g dose every 8 hours with a dose after dialysis has been used with piperacillin [4].
   b. **With peritoneal dialysis** the doses for renal failure less than 10 mL/min can be used [4].
4. **For both hepatic and renal insufficiency occurring together,** 3.0 g per day is given, and ideally, levels monitored.
5. **Pregnancy.** This is a category B agent (see Chapter 16). Because there are no well-controlled studies in pregnant women, this drug should be used during pregnancy only if clearly needed.
6. **Nursing mothers.** These drugs are excreted in low concentrations in milk; therefore caution should be exercised when these agents are administered to nursing mothers.
7. **Cost** data are shown in Appendix Table 1.
8. **Side effects.** The side effects seen with penicillin may occur with these agents.
   a. Hypokalemia occurs less commonly with piperacillin than with carbenicillin [1,2].
   b. Platelet dysfunction is uncommon with piperacillin [1,2].

**III. β-Lactam–β-lactamase combinations:** an overview

**A. Background.** Because structural modification of the penicillin side chain has limitations, new strategies of extending the antibacterial spectrum of the penicillin family were explored. Because the primary mechanism of bacterial resistance to penicillins is through β-lactamase (enzyme) production, inactivation of these enzymes was the next logical step [1,2]. Therefore a β-lactamase inhibitor (e.g., clavulanate, sulbactam, or tazobactam) was combined with certain extended penicillins. These β-lactamase inhibitors bind **irreversibly to the β-lactamase** (plasmid mediated) and the bound β-lactamase cannot hydrolyze the penicillin [7]. Hence, the penicillin is free to interact with the penicillin binding proteins and exerts its antibacterial effect [2]. The benefit is provided only when the bacterial resistance is the result of β-lactamase production [1]. Worldwide, more than 90% of *S. aureus* and *B. fragilis* are β-lactamase producers [8].

**B. Spectrum of activity**

1. **Susceptible.** The inhibitors are effective against β-lactamases produced by *S. aureus, H. influenzae, M. catarrhalis, Bacteroides* species, many *Escherichia coli,* and Enterobacteriaceae.
2. **Resistant.** Some species of *Enterobacter, Citrobacter, Serratia, Morganella*, and *Pseudomonas*, among others, produce β-lactamases that are usually chromosomally encoded and are not inhibited by these β-lactamase inhibitors [2].
3. **Determinant of antimicrobial activity.** The *in vitro* activity of the active antibiotic is very important. For example, piperacillin/tazobactam activity against gram-negative organisms is greater than that of ticarcillin/clavulanate or ampicillin/sulbactam because of the relative greater activity of piperacillin [8]. If the mechanism of resistance is to the penicillin and not mediated by β-lactamase, these antibiotics are not effective. As such, methicillin-resistant

*S. aureus* (MRSA), high level penicillin-resistant pneumococcus, and vancomycin-resistant enterococci are resistant to the $\beta$-lactam–$\beta$-lactamase combination.

**C. Oral agents.** Amoxicillin-clavulanate (Augmentin) is the only oral combination agent available.

1. **Activity.** Separate susceptibility testing must be performed with the combination. Clavulanic acid inhibits the $\beta$-lactamase of *S. aureus, N. gonorrhoeae, H. ducreyi, M. catarrhalis,* and *H. influenzae* (10%–30% of these organisms are $\beta$-lactamase positive). In addition, clavulanic acid inhibits $\beta$-lactamase produced by many gram-negative bacilli, including *E. coli, Klebsiella,* and *Proteus* species. Therefore the combination of amoxicillin-clavulanate is active against amoxicillin-susceptible and many previously amoxicillin-resistant organisms. This includes 97% to 100% of oxacillin-susceptible *S. aureus,* most streptococci (including most enterococci), *N. gonorrhoeae, H. influenzae, E. coli,* and *Klebsiella* species. It is not active against the $\beta$-lactamase produced by *Enterobacter* species, *Pseudomonas* species, and *Serratia* species. High level penicillin-resistant *S. pneumoniae* are resistant to amoxicillin-clavulanate.
2. **Pharmacokinetics**
   a. Both components are **well absorbed.** Peak levels occur at 1 hour, independent of meals, antacids, or milk.
   b. The drugs penetrate peritoneal and pleural fluids well. **Very high urine levels** are achieved compared with modest serum levels. There is only fair penetration into pulmonary secretions; therefore higher doses are necessary in pulmonary infections.
3. **Clinical uses**
   a. **Human and animal bite wounds.** Because of the polymicrobial nature of these infections, **this agent is the drug of choice** in this setting (see detailed discussion in Chapter 4).
   b. **Alternate therapy in acute otitis media.** Amoxicillin remains the drug of choice in this setting, but for patients who fail amoxicillin or as initial therapy in areas with very high resistant rates of *H. influenzae,* Augmentin is very effective [9,10] (see related discussions in Chapter 8).
   c. **Acute bacterial sinusitis** can often be managed with amoxicillin, but amoxicillin-clavulanate is preferred in some situations (see Chapter 8).
   d. **UTI.** Although the fluoroquinolones and trimethoprim-sulfamethoxazole are commonly used in UTI, for susceptible pathogens amoxicillin-clavulanate provides another possible oral agent; it is not used for uncomplicated UTI caused by amoxicillin-susceptible organisms.
   e. **Pulmonary infections.** It is useful in exacerbation of chronic bronchitis and in mild community-acquired pneumonia in children and adults (see Chapters 8 and 11). (N.B. It is not active against *Mycoplasma pneumoniae, Chlamydia pneumoniae,* or *Legionella.*)
   f. **Other considerations** include mild diverticulitis (see Chapter 13) and wound infections due to susceptible pathogens.
4. **Dosages.** This agent **should be administered** at the start of a meal to decrease the incidence of gastrointestinal (GI) side effects. It is available in the United States only in an oral form.
   a. Oral **chewable tablets** are in doses of **250 mg amoxicillin and 62.5 mg clavulanate; 125 mg amoxicillin and 31.25 mg clavulanate** are for pediatric use.
   b. **Oral suspension** is available in doses of 125 mg amoxicillin and 31.25 mg clavulanate/5 mL, 250 mg amoxicillin and 62.5 mg clavulanate/5 mL, and 400 mg amoxicillin and 57 mg clavulanate/5 mL.
   c. **Adult-sized tablets:** 250 mg amoxicillin and 125 mg clavulanate given three times a day, 500 mg amoxicillin and 125 mg clavulanate given three times a day, and 875 mg amoxicillin and 125 mg clavulanate given every 12 hours.

      Note: Two of the 250-mg amoxicillin/125-mg clavulanate tablets should not be taken at one time, because the double dose of clavulanate is more likely to cause GI toxicity. To provide a 500-mg dose, give one 250-mg amoxicillin/125-mg clavulanate tablet with one 250-mg generic tablet of amoxicillin. **The**

**chewable tablets and adult tablets have different amoxicillin-to-clavulanate ratios, as noted above, and should not be interchanged.**

d. **For adults** the usual dose is one 250-mg tablet every 8 hours or one 500-mg tablet every 12 hours. For more severe infections and respiratory tract infections, one 875-mg tablet every 12 hours or one 500-mg tablet every 8 hours is advised. (**N.B.** The every 12 hour regimen is associated with fewer GI side effects.)

e. **Children. Suspension or tablets for children: For otitis media when there is amoxicillin failure,** higher doses of the amoxicillin component are advised, 80 to 90 mg/kg/day, using the new formulation to keep the dose of clavulanate at about 10 mg/kg/day [10]. Before the era of increasing penicillin resistance, regimens used 40 to 45 mg/kg/day of the amoxicillin component (see Chapter 8). For sinusitis, lower respiratory tract infections, and more severe infections, the amoxicillin component of 45 mg/kg/day divided every 12 hours or 40 mg/kg/day divided every 8 hours has been used. For less severe infection 25 mg/kg/day divided every 12 hours or 20 mg/kg/day divided every 8 hours has been suggested. **Children weighing 40 kg or more can follow adult dose regimens.** The adult-sized 250-mg tablet should not be used unless the child weighs more than 40 kg.

f. **Renal failure.** The package insert does not suggest dose modification if renal failure is modest (i.e., creatinine clearance of more than 30 mL/min). With a creatinine clearance of less than 30 mL/min, do not use the 875-mg tablet. With a creatinine clearance of 10 to 30 mL/min, use 250 or 500 mg every 12 hours, depending on the severity of the infection. With creatinine clearance of less than 10 mL/min, use 250 or 500 mg every 24 hours, depending on the severity of infection. **Hemodialysis patients** should receive 250 or 500 mg every 24 hours, depending on the severity of infection. Patients should receive an additional dose during and at the end of dialysis.

g. **Pregnancy.** This is a category B agent (see Chapter 16). Because there are no adequate and well-controlled studies in pregnant women, this agent should be used during pregnancy only if clearly needed. The combination has been safe in pregnant women with bacteruria or UTI.

h. **Nursing mothers.** Because amoxicillin is excreted in breast milk, the package insert suggests exercising caution if this agent is administered to a nursing woman.

5. **Side effects**

a. The usual side effects of penicillin can occur with amoxicillin-clavulanate.

b. **GI side effects**—nausea, vomiting, diarrhea, and abdominal cramps—occur in 10% or more of patients [10]. These are related in part to the dose of clavulanate (i.e., more symptoms at higher doses) and can be **minimized if the drug is taken at the start of a meal** [1,10]. **Also, the every 12 hour regimens** are associated with fewer side effects than the every 8 hour regimens (see section **C.4.c**).

6. **Cost.** This is a relatively **expensive** agent (see Appendix Table 1).

D. **Intravenous β-lactam and β-lactamase combinations**

1. **Ampicillin-sulbactam (Unasyn)** was approved in 1987.

a. ***In vitro* activity.** Sulbactam inhibits many bacterial β-lactamases, thereby extending the activity of ampicillin. The combination *in vitro* is active against β-lactamase–producing strains of *H. influenzae, M. catarrhalis, N. gonorrhoeae,* many anaerobes (including *B. fragilis*), *E. coli, Proteus* species, *Klebsiella* species, *Acinetobacter calcoaceticus, S. aureus,* and *S. epidermidis.*

(1) **Ampicillin-sulbactam is not active against MRSA, *P. aeruginosa* and certain Enterobacteriaceae strains *(Serratia, Enterobacter,* and *Citrobacter* species)** (see section **III.B.3**).

(2) ***E. coli*: Approximately 20% to 25% or more of *E. coli*** (including community-acquired) **are resistant** to this combination [10]. Most of these *E. coli* strains have minimal inhibitory concentrations that are very close to the breakpoint concentration for determining susceptibility ($\leq 8$ μg/mL). Although the clinical significance of this laboratory

observation is unknown, a study in an animal model of infection caused by an ampicillin-sulbactam–resistant isolates of *E. coli* found the agent to be ineffective [11]. Overall, not as many gram-negative bacilli are inhibited by ampicillin-sulbactam *in vitro* as by many cephalosporins or other intravenous $\beta$-lactam–$\beta$-lactamase combinations (Table 27E.2).

**b. Pharmacokinetics** of ampicillin are not altered by the coadministration of sulbactam. **Excretion**, of both components, is primarily in the urine. **Tissue levels** are achieved in extravascular fluids, bile, and peritoneal and cerebrospinal fluids.

**c. Clinical uses** [1–3]. This agent has been very useful, especially in the **mixed aerobic and anaerobic** infections, including mild to moderately severe community-acquired intraabdominal infection, aspiration pneumonia, community-acquired pneumonia (although it does not cover *Legionella* or *Mycoplasma*), UTI, pelvic infection, deep neck infection, and soft tissue infection, including diabetic foot infection.

**d. Dosage**

(1) **Adults.** The **usual dose** for mild to moderate infection is **1.5 g** (1 g ampicillin plus 0.5 g sulbactam) **every 6 hours** if renal function is normal. **In severe infection and/or most intraabdominal infections**, 3 g (2 g ampicillin and 1 g sulbactam) every 6 hours is used. **It is important to adjust doses in the elderly and those with renal dysfunction** to avoid excess serum levels and to provide cost-effective dosing (Table 27E.3).

(2) **Pediatrics.** The package insert notes that the safety and effectiveness of ampicillin-sulbactam has been established for pediatric patients 1 year of age and older for skin and soft tissue infections. The dose used in children is 300 mg/kg/day divided up every 6 hours.

(3) **In renal failure,** the elimination of ampicillin and sulbactam is similarly affected, and dose modification is necessary (Table 27E.3).

**e. Special considerations**

(1) **Pregnancy.** This is a category B agent (see Chapter 16). Because there are no adequate studies in pregnant women, this drug should be used during pregnancy only if clearly indicated.

(2) **Nursing mothers.** Low concentrations of this combination are excreted into breast milk. Therefore caution should be exercised when ampicillin-sulbactam is administered to a nursing woman.

(3) **Contraindicated in ampicillin-allergic patients.** Because this agent contains ampicillin, it is contraindicated in patients allergic to ampicillin or other penicillins (unless skin testing is performed). This seems obvious but is **a concern if physicians order antibiotics by a trade name (Unasyn) rather than its generic name.** This concern also applies to the combination of ticarcillin-clavulanate (Timentin) and piperacillin-tazobactam (Zosyn), discussed later.

**f. Side effects.** These are the same as those known to occur with ampicillin [2].

(1) **Ampicillin** skin **reactions. Rashes are common. Many are not allergic** (see Chapter 24).

(2) **Minor enzyme elevations** (serum aspartate aminotransferase and alanine aminotransferase) occur in approximately 6% of recipients.

(3) Ampicillin-sulbactam may have a marked **effect on oral flora,** leading to *Clostridium difficile* colitis.

**g. Cost** (see Appendix Table 1)

**h. Conclusion.** Although it is a very popular agent for polymicrobial infections, diabetic foot ulcer infections, mild to moderate community-acquired intraabdominal and pelvic infections, mixed aerobic/anaerobic soft tissue infections, selected cases of aspiration pneumonia, and severe UTI, there are drawbacks. The antibiotic is often selected in situations where *E. coli* is anticipated, yet 20% to 40% of *E. coli* are resistant, making this a less than optimal choice. Other agents with greater *E. coli* activity are more

Table 27E.2. Comparison of *In Vitro* Susceptibility Data

| Organism | Number Tested | Antimicrobial | Percent Susceptible |
|---|---|---|---|
| *Escherichia coli* | 10,942 | Piperacillin-tazobactam | 91.5 |
| | | Ticarcillin-clavulanate | 88.8 |
| | | Ampicillin-sulbactam | 65.4 |
| | | Cefoxitin | 96.1 |
| | | Cefotetan | 99.3 |
| | | Ceftriaxone | 99.2 |
| | | Imipenem | 99.7 |
| | | Aztreonam | 98.1 |
| | | Ciprofloxacin | 99.0 |
| *Klebsiella pneumoniae* | 4,405 | Piperacillin-tazobactam | 90.9 |
| | | Ticarcillin-clavulanate | 91.3 |
| | | Ampicillin-sulbactam | 75.2 |
| | | Cefoxitin | 90.3 |
| | | Cefotetan | 97.4 |
| | | Ceftriaxone | 95.2 |
| | | Imipenem | 99.6 |
| | | Aztreonam | 94.1 |
| | | Ciprofloxacin | 94.5 |
| *Proteus mirabilis* | 3,822 | Piperacillin-tazobactam | 96.2 |
| | | Ticarcillin-clavulanate | 95.0 |
| | | Ampicillin-sulbactam | 90.4 |
| | | Cefoxitin | 94.7 |
| | | Cefotetan | 97.7 |
| | | Ceftriaxone | 98.5 |
| | | Imipenem | 82.9 |
| | | Aztreonam | 91.7 |
| | | Ciprofloxacin | 96.6 |
| *Serratia marcescens* | 1,392 | Piperacillin-tazobactam | 86.9 |
| | | Ticarcillin-clavulanate | 84.3 |
| | | Ampicillin-sulbactam | 9.1 |
| | | Cefoxitin | 16.7 |
| | | Cefotetan | 94.3 |
| | | Ceftriaxone | 85.8 |
| | | Imipenem | 90.5 |
| | | Aztreonam | 86.0 |
| | | Ciprofloxacin | 86.0 |
| *Pseudomonas aeruginosa* | 2,941 | Piperacillin | 88.6 |
| | | Piperacillin-tazobactam | 91.5 |
| | | Ticarcillin-clavulanate | 86.3 |
| | | Ampicillin-sulbactam | 2.1 |
| | | Cefoxitin | 1.5 |
| | | Cefotetan | 3.2 |
| | | Ceftriaxone | 17.5 |
| | | Imipenem | 88.0 |
| | | Ciprofloxacin | 79.4 |
| *Staphylococcus aureus* | 4,454 | Piperacillin-tazobactam | 96.6 |
| | | Ticarcillin-clavulanate | 98.1 |
| | | Ampicillin-sulbactam | 98.0 |
| | | Cefoxitin | 98.1 |
| | | Ceftriaxone | 98.4 |
| | | Imipenem | 98.7 |
| | | Ciprofloxacin | 91.7 |

*(continued)*

Table 27E.2. *(Continued)*

| Organism | Number Tested | Antimicrobial | Percent Susceptible |
|---|---|---|---|
| *Streptococcus agalactiae (group B)* | 701 | Piperacillin-tazobactam | 98.2 |
| | | Ticarcillin-clavulanate | 97.0 |
| | | Ampicillin-sulbactam | 99.6 |
| | | Cefoxitin | 96.6 |
| | | Ceftriaxone | 97.0 |
| | | Imipenem | 99.4 |
| | | Ciprofloxacin | 92.9 |
| *Streptococcus faecalis* | 2,624 | Piperacillin-tazobactam | 94.7 |
| | | Ticarcillin-clavulanate | 23.2 |
| | | Ampicillin-sulbactam | 97.0 |
| | | Cefoxitin | 2.1 |
| | | Ceftriaxone | 7.0 |
| | | Imipenem | 95.5 |
| | | Ciprofloxacin | 62.5 |

Adapted from Murray PR, et al. and the In Vitro Susceptibility Surveillance Group. Multicenter evaluation of the in vitro activity of piperacillin-tazobactam compared with eleven selected $\beta$-lactam antibiotics and ciprofloxacin against more than 42,000 aerobic gram-positive and gram-negative bacteria. *Diagn Microbiol Infect Dis* 1994;19;111, with permission.

rational. We **would not use** ampicillin-sulbactam as monotherapy for patients with severe or life-threatening intraabdominal infection or mixed aerobic/anaerobic soft tissue infections but prefer a combination of antibiotics in this setting (e.g., a third-generation cephalosporin and metronidazole or piperacillin/tazobactam). **See section D for how this agent compares with similar** $\beta$-lactam/$\beta$-lactamase combinations; piperacillin-tazobactam may be preferred. In addition, we would not use this agent alone for severe nosocomial infections, because many hospital-acquired gram-negative bacteria, including *E. coli* and *Klebsiella* species, may be resistant; *Pseudomonas* species are also resistant. An aminoglycoside could be combined with it. It should not be used to treat methicillin-resistant staphylococcal infections. Ampicillin-sulbactam has not been studied extensively for treatment of infections in immunocompromised patients [12].

2. **Ticarcillin-clavulanate (Timentin)** [1,2,7]
   a. **Spectrum of activity** is very similar to that for ampicillin-sulbactam (see section **A.1**) except

Table 27E.3. Ampicillin-sulbactam Dosages in Patients with Renal Impairment

| Creatinine Clearance (mL/min) | Recommended Dosage |
|---|---|
| >50 | 1.5–3.0 g q6h |
| 30–50 | 1.5–3.0 g q6–8h |
| 15–29 | 1.5–3.0 g q12h |
| 5–14 | 1.5–3.0 g q24h |

In patients undergoing hemodialysis, preliminary data suggest the ampicillin will be partially removed (approximately 60%) but not the sulbactam. One could therefore give a supplemental dose of ampicillin after dialysis or time the daily dose of ampicillin-sulbactam so that it is given after dialysis.

(1) The concerns with *E. coli in vitro* susceptibilities are not as prominent with ticarcillin-clavulanate. Nevertheless, many hospital-acquired *E. coli* are resistant.
(2) Enterococci are less susceptible than to ampicillin-sulbactam or piperacillin-tazobactam.
(3) This agent is active against many strains of *P. aeruginosa* but is not as active as piperacillin-tazobactam (Table 27E.2).

b. **Clinical uses.** This combination is effective for a variety of polymicrobial infections with susceptible pathogens, including intraabdominal infection, pelvic infection, osteomyelitis, pneumonia, bacteremia, UTI, and skin and soft tissue infections.

c. **Pharmacokinetics.** The half-life of each agent is approximately 1 hour, necessitating a 4- to 6-hour dose interval. Ticarcillin is excreted primarily by the kidney, producing very high urine levels. Dosage adjustments in significant renal failure are required. The combination penetrates tissues well.

d. **Dosages**

(1) **Adults.** Ticarcillin-clavulanate is available in vials containing 3 g ticarcillin and 0.1 g clavulanic acid as the potassium salt. The usual dosage for systemic infections is one 3.1-g vial every 4 to 6 hours. For moderately severe gynecologic infections, a 3.1-g dose every 6 hours and for severe infection, 3.1 g every 4 hours. For patients weighing less than 60 kg, the recommended dose is 200 to 300 mg/kg/day (based on the ticarcillin content) divided every 4 to 6 hours. A vial containing 3 g ticarcillin and 0.2 g clavulanic acid is also available. This has been used in UTIs, with a dosage of 3.2 g given every 8 hours, per the package insert, when renal function is normal.
(2) **Children** ($\geq$3 months). In children weighing less than 60 kg, 50 mg/kg based on the ticarcillin component is administered as follows: For mild to moderate infections, a dose every 6 hours and for severe infections, dose every 4 hours. In children weighing more than 60 kg: For mild to moderate infections, 3.1 g every 6 hours and for severe infections, 3.1 g every 4 hours.
(3) **In renal failure,** in adults use a normal loading dose. Thereafter, for a creatinine clearance of 30 to 60 mL/min, 2 g every 4 hours; for a creatinine clearance of 10 to 30 mL/min, 2 g every 8 hours; and for creatinine clearance less than 10 mL/min, 2 g every 12 hours. If there is hepatic dysfunction as well, then the latter dose is given every 24 hours. For hemodialysis, give 2 g every 12 hours supplemented with 3.1 g after each dialysis, and for peritoneal dialysis give 3.1 g every 12 hours.

e. **Penicillin allergy precludes the use of this agent** unless skin testing is done.

f. **Pregnancy.** This is a category B agent. Because there are no adequate and well-controlled studies in pregnant women, the package insert suggests this agent should be used during pregnancy only if clearly indicated.

g. **Nursing mothers.** It is not known whether this agent is excreted in human breast milk, but it should not be used in nursing women unless necessary.

h. **Side effects** are similar to those for penicillin, ampicillin, and/or ticarcillin. See prior discussions. The potential for hypokalemia and for platelet abnormalities exists.

i. **Cost** (see Appendix Table 1)

j. **Conclusion.** The main indication for ticarcillin-clavulanate is for polymicrobial infections with susceptible aerobic and anaerobic infections. Because of its safety and activity against possible etiologic organisms, this is used frequently in obstetrics/gynecology services for pelvic and intraabdominal infections. **There are insufficient data** to use it as monotherapy for severe or life-threatening infections or for severe nosocomial infections, because many hospital-acquired gram-negative bacteria may be resistant. In febrile neutropenic cancer patients, ticarcillin-clavulanate has been evaluated primarily in combination with an aminoglycoside [12–15]. Other options are available in this setting (see Chapter 20). **See section D above for** a comparison of β-lactam–β-lactamase combinations. Piperacillin-tazobactam may be preferred.

3. **Piperacillin-tazobactam (Zosyn)** became available in the United States in 1993 [7,12,13].
   a. **Spectrum of activity.** Of the available β-lactam/β-lactamase antibiotics, piperacillin-tazobactam is the most active *in vitro*, in large part reflecting the enhanced *in vitro* activity of piperacillin over ampicillin and ticarcillin (see section **III.A.4**). This agent has an *in vitro* spectrum of activity comparable with that of imipenem-cilastatin and superior to that of ceftazidime, ticarcillin-clavulanate, and ampicillin-sulbactam [12] (Table 27E.2).
      (1) **Gram-positive aerobes.** This combination is active against *S. pyogenes, S. agalactiae, S. pneumoniae* (not highly penicillin-resistant strains), and methicillin-susceptible *S. aureus.* Although it is active against *Enterococcus faecalis,* it is not active against *E. faecium* and MRSA [12]. However, in an animal model, piperacillin/tazobactam is excreted into the bile in sufficiently high concentrations to prevent colonization after *E. faecium* oral challenge, whereas cefepime does not prevent colonization after this challenge [16].
      (2) **Enterobacteriaceae.** Most community-acquired Enterobacteriaceae (e.g., *E. coli, Klebsiella* species) are susceptible, but because of poor activity of piperacillin-tazobactam against many of the class 1 β-lactamases, *E. aerogenes, E. cloacae, Citrobacter* species, *Serratia* species, and *P. aeruginosa* may be resistant (Table 27E.2) (see section **III.B.3**).
      (3) **Other gram-negative bacteria.** Piperacillin-tazobactam has excellent activity against *H. influenzae, M. catarrhalis, Yersinia enterocolitica,* and *Plesiomonas shigelloides* but not *Salmonella* species or *Stenotrophomonas maltophilia.*
      (4) **Anaerobes.** Piperacillin-tazobactam has good activity against *B. fragilis* (but less than that of imipenem), *Bacteroides* species, and *Clostridium perfringens* [17]. Oral anaerobes are usually susceptible to penicillin and piperacillin. Although some reviewers conclude there are no significant differences between the activity against anaerobes of piperacillin-tazobactam and other β-lactamase inhibitor combination agents [12], other reviewers have concluded that piperacillin-tazobactam inhibits a broader spectrum of anaerobes than does ampicillin-sulbactam and ticarcillin-clavulanate [18].
   b. **Pharmacokinetics.** Preparations contain an 8:1 ratio of piperacillin to tazobactam; tazobactam does not interfere with the pharmacokinetics of piperacillin. Renal excretion accounts for 50% to 60% of the administered dose. Doses must be reduced in patients with a creatinine clearance of less than 40 mL/min [17]. As noted earlier, piperacillin is excreted into the biliary tract in sufficient concentration to inhibit *E. faecium*, reducing the likelihood of colonization of the GI track in the orally challenged animal [16].
   c. **Clinical use.** Piperacillin-tazobactam has been used in **polymicrobial infections.** Early clinical studies have been summarized [17–19]. The combination is approved for use in moderate to severe infections with susceptible pathogens and appears effective in the following situations:
      (1) **Intraabdominal infections** (especially appendicitis, including cases complicated by rupture or abscess). The combination appears as effective as imipenem or clindamycin plus gentamicin [2].
      (2) **Pelvic infections** in women.
      (3) **Mixed** aerobic **skin and soft tissue** infections, including diabetic foot infections.
      (4) **Community-acquired pneumonia.** This is not a usual agent; however, its activity against β-lactamase–producing *H. influenzae, Klebsiella pneumoniae, P. aeruginosa, Acinetobacter calcoaceticus,* and *Moraxella*

*catarrhalis* makes it a useful agent when Gram stain shows pure gram-negative organisms or when the patient has recently been hospitalized and returns for admission. However, this agent is not active against *Mycoplasma* or *Legionella* [17].

**(5) Nosocomial pneumonia.** When **Gram stain shows gram-negative organisms,** this agent, used in conjunction with an aminoglycoside pending susceptibilities, is an excellent choice [17]. Alternative therapy should be used if Gram stain shows gram-positive cocci in clusters.

**(6) Clinical investigation.** Piperacillin-tazobactam both with and without an aminoglycoside has been used for empiric therapy of the febrile leukopenic patient without a focal infection [14,15,17]. It is not listed as a drug of choice in this setting [15]. Currently a study comparing it with cefepime as monotherapy is underway. The potential for piperacillin/tazobactam to prevent colonization with vancomycin-resistant enterococci because of high biliary concentrations is a key point of evaluation in that study [16].

**d. Dosages**

**(1) Adults.** The **usual dose** is **3 g/0.375 g every 6 hours** if the creatinine clearance is higher than 40 mL/min. For empiric therapy nosocomial pneumonia, the package insert suggests a 3.375-g dose every 4 hours along with an aminoglycoside to ensure activity against *P. aeruginosa.* If *P. aeruginosa* is not isolated, then the aminoglycoside can be discontinued. If ***P. aeruginosa* is isolated, then piperacillin alone can be used with an aminoglycoside because** in documented pseudomonas infection, tazobactam does not enhance the activity of piperacillin against this pathogen [17]. **An alternate approach for high dose** therapy is to use a 4.5-g vial (piperacillin 4 g and tazobactam 0.5 g) every 6 hours, along with an aminoglycoside for empiric therapy of nosocomial infections and possible pseudomonas infection [18].

**(2) Children.** As of 2002, the package insert indicates the safety and efficacy in pediatric patients has not been established.

**(3) Renal failure. Dose reductions** are **shown in Table 27E.4.** For patients receiving **hemodialysis,** the maximum dose of piperacillin-tazobactam is 2 g/0.25 g every 8 hours. Because hemodialysis will remove 30% to 40% of the dose in a 4-hour dialysis, one additional dose of 0.75 g can be given after dialysis. **In chronic ambulatory peritoneal dialysis,** approximately 10% of the piperacillin dose is recovered [17]. Until further guidelines are available, in chronic ambulatory peritoneal dialysis patients select the dose as if the creatinine clearance is less than 10 mL/min (Table 27E.4).

**(4)** In **cirrhosis** or other hepatic disease, no dosage modifications are required [17].

**(5) Pregnancy.** This is a category B agent (see Chapter 16). There are no adequate and well-controlled studies with piperacillin-tazobactam in pregnant women. Therefore the drug should be used during pregnancy only if clearly indicated [12].

**(6) Nursing mothers.** Piperacillin is excreted in low concentrations in human breast milk; whether tazobactam is in human breast milk has not

Table 27E.4. Piperacillin-tazobactam Dosages in Renal Failure

| Creatinine Clearance (mL/min) | Recommended Dosage Regimen |
|---|---|
| >40 | 12 g/1.5 g/day in divided doses of 3.375 g q6h |
| 20–40 | 8 g/1.0 g/day in divided doses of 2.25 g q6h |
| <20 | 6 g/0.75 g/day in divided doses of 2.25 g q8h |

From *Physician's desk reference,* 56th ed. Montvale, NJ: Medical Economics, 2002:1893, with permission.

been studied. Therefore the package insert suggests that caution should be used if this agent is administered to a nursing woman.

e. **Side effects.** The toxicity of piperacillin-tazobactam is similar to that of other penicillins and $\beta$-lactam antibiotics [17–19]. The most common side effects include the following:
   (1) **GI** disorders, primarily diarrhea and nausea, occur in 4.6% of recipients.
   (2) Skin reactions occur in 2.2% of recipients. Fewer than 1% have a rash.
   (3) No significant hepatic or renal dysfunction has been noted in early reports.
   (4) Mild hypokalemia can occur, presumably due to the nonresorbable anions presented to the distal tubules, which cause an increase in the pH and a secondary loss of potassium ions.

4. **Ticarcillin-clavulanate versus ampicillin-sulbactam versus piperacillin-tazobactam.** The optimal agent for selected polymicrobial infections has not been clearly delineated in the medical literature. None of these $\beta$-lactam–$\beta$-lactamase combinations is listed as the antibiotic of first choice for any specific pathogen [3]. In a review [12], the authors concluded that "because of its broad spectrum of antibacterial activity, it [piperacillin-tazobactam] appears to be the best suited for treatment of mixed infections." In a 1996 summary of piperacillin-tazobactam, after an extensive review of the literature, the authors concluded, "The proven and theoretical advantages of piperacillin-tazobactam in comparison with those of ticarcillin-clavulanate appear to more than offset the modest difference in cost between the two compounds" [18].
   a. **When one of these drugs is indicated, we would offer the following considerations:**
      (1) For situations in which *E. coli* is a likely pathogen, because 20% to 25% are resistant to ampicillin-sulbactam, piperacillin-tazobactam is advised, although ticarcillin-clavulanate may be a reasonable alternative if one of these agents is to be used.
      (2) Because cefazolin is effective against most community-acquired *E. coli* strains, the more expensive $\beta$-lactam–$\beta$-lactamase inhibitor combinations should be used selectively. For community-acquired intraabdominal or pelvic infections, the most cost-effective cefazolin-metronidazole combination is reasonable (see Chapter 13).
      (3) **Piperacillin-tazobactam can be used selectively** in the following situations:
         (a) Severe (limb-threatening) diabetic foot ulcer infections, as discussed in Chapters 4 and 5.
         (b) Selected patients with severe head and neck infections.
         (c) As monotherapy in nosocomial pneumonia not acquired in an intensive care unit and where risk for *P. aeruginosa* infection is low and it is desirable to avoid an aminoglycoside.
         (d) Selected intensive care unit nosocomial pneumonia. While awaiting cultures, it is advisable to combine it with an aminoglycoside. Piperacillin and an aminoglycoside combination is more cost effective.
      (4) **Serious nosocomial infections.** None of these agents should be used as monotherapy for known or highly suspected severe *P. aeruginosa* infection.
      (5) **Versus imipenem.** For the situation in which monotherapy is indicated and there is a choice between one of these $\beta$-lactam–$\beta$-lactamase combinations and imipenem, most institutions reserve imipenem for those patients who may have or develop resistant pathogens.

E. **Drug resistance** to $\beta$-lactam–$\beta$-lactamase inhibitor compounds has been reviewed recently [7]. The extended spectrum $\beta$-lactamase–producing bacteria are resistant to these agents. The most common organisms carrying this resistance are *E. coli* and *Klebsiella* species. The frequency with which these are found depends on the total gram use of expanded spectrum cephalosporin antibiotics [7]. Carbapenem antibiotics (see Chapter 27H) are selected in infections caused by extended spectrum $\beta$-lactamase–producing bacteria instead of the combinations discussed in this chapter [6]. Piperacillin/tazobactam-resistant *P. aeruginosa* have also emerged. A predisposing risk factor appears to be the quantity of ciprofloxacin use. This factor needs to be considered when treating ventilator-associated pneumonia caused by *P. aeruginosa* [20].

## REFERENCES


1. Bush LM, Johnson CC. Ureidopenicillins and beta lactam/beta lactamase inhibitor combinations *Infect Dis Clin North Am* 2000;14:409–433.
2. Wright AJ. The penicillins. *Mayo Clin Proc* 1999;74:290.
3. The Medical Letter. The choice of antimicrobial drugs. *Med Lett Drugs Ther* 2001;43:69–78; 1999;41:95; 1998;40:33.
4. Aronoff GR, et al. *Drug prescribing in renal failure: dosage guidelines for adults,* 4th ed. Philadelphia: American College of Physicians, 1999.
5. Boguniewiez M, Leung YM. Hypersensitivity reactions to antibiotics commonly used in children. *Pediatr Infect Dis J* 1995;14:221.
6. Sattler FR, et al. Impaired hemostasis caused by beta-lactam antibiotics. *Am J Surg* 1988;155:30.
7. Lee NIS, et al. Beta lactam antibiotic and beta lactamase inhibitor combinations. *JAMA* 2001;285:386.
8. Moellering RC Jr. Importance of beta-lactamase inhibitors in overcoming bacterial resistance. *Infect Dis Clin Pract* 1995;4[Suppl 1]:S1.
9. Dagan R, Johnson CE, McLinn S, et al. Bacteriological and clinical efficacy of amoxicillin/clavulanate vs. azithromycin in acute otitis media. *Pediatr Infect Dis J* 2000;19:95.
10. Dowell SF, et al. Acute otitis media: management and surveillance in an era of pneumococcal resistance–a report from the drug-resistance *Streptococcus pneumoniae* Therapeutic Working Group. *Pediatr Infect Dis J* 1999;18:1.
11. Rice L, Carias L, Shlaes D. Efficacy of ampicillin-sulbactam versus that cefoxitin on treatment of *Escherichia coli* infections in a rat intra-abdominal model. *Antimicrob Agents Chemother* 1993;37:610.
12. Bush LM, Calmon J, Johnson CC. Newer penicillins and beta-lactamase inhibitors. *Infect Dis Clin North Am* 1995;9:653.
13. Giamarellou H, Antoniadou A. Anti-pseudomonal antibiotics. *Med Clin North Am* 2001;85:19.
14. Del Favero A, et al. A multi-center, double-blind placebo controlled trial comparing piperacillin/tazobactam with and without amikacin as empiric therapy for neutropenic patients. *Clin Infect Dis* 2001;33:1295.
15. Hughes WT, et al. 2002 Guidelines for the use of antimicrobial agents for neutropenic patients with cancer. *Clin Infect Dis* 2002;34:730.
16. Donskey CJ, Hanrahan JA, Hutton RA, et al. Effect of parenteral antibiotic administration on the establishment of colonization with vancomycin-resistant *Enterococcus faecium* in the mouse gastrointestinal tract. *J Infect Dis* 2000;181:1830–1833.
17. Bryson HM, Brogden RN. Piperacillin/tazobactam: a review of its antibacterial activity, pharmacokinetic properties, and therapeutic potential. *Drugs* 1994;47:506.
18. Sanders WE Jr, Sanders CC. Piperacillin-tazobactam: a critical review of evolving clinical literature. *Clin Infect Dis* 1996;22:107.
19. Moellering RC, et al. Piperacillin-tazobactam: a new dimension in antibiotic therapy. *Infect Dis Clin Pract* 1996;4[Suppl 1]:S1.
20. Trouilett JL, et al. *Pseudomonas aeruginosa* ventilator-associated pneumonia: comparison of episodes due to piperacillin-resistant versus piperacillin-susceptible organisms. *Clin Infect Dis* 2002;34.


## F. The Cephalosporins

The cephalosporins [1–3] are **bactericidal** agents that inhibit bacterial cell wall synthesis. They are widely used agents because they are safe, familiar to the clinician, and active against penicillinase-producing methicillin-susceptible *Staphylococcus aureus* (MSSA). They can be used for patients with delayed penicillin allergies. Unless special skin tests can be performed, **cephalosporins should be avoided in patients with a history of an**

**immediate severe reaction to a penicillin** (or cephalosporin), such as anaphylaxis or angioedema (see section **IV.A**).

**I. Introduction**

**A. Agents available.** The currently available cephalosporins are shown in Table 27F.1. **The goal of this chapter is to summarize and to emphasize a limited number of agents that are particularly useful** and have withstood the test of time.

1. **From a historical standpoint,** it is useful to note that the different "generations" of parenteral cephalosporins had a logical sequence of development by the pharmaceutical industry [1].

   a. **The first-generation** agents are active against MSSA, penicillin-susceptible *Streptococcus pneumoniae,* and other common gram-positive bacteria, such as streptococci groups A and B and viridans streptococci, and many community-acquired gram-negative bacteria. These agents remain active and useful against these pathogens.

   b. **Second-generation** agents, cefamandole and later cefuroxime, were developed, in part, because of their activity against ampicillin-susceptible and -resistant *Haemophilus influenzae* (and *Moraxella catarrhalis*). They maintained activity against *S. pneumoniae.* Cefoxitin was the first cephalosporin to have activity against bowel anaerobes, especially *Bacteroides fragilis;* it was also active against *Neisseria gonorrhoeae,* including penicillinase-producing strains. Although still useful, these agents enjoy less popularity than in the past, for reasons to be discussed.

   c. **Third-generation** agents can be divided into two subsets. One type, ceftazidime, was initially touted as having enhanced gram-negative activity, including activity against hospital-acquired pathogens such as *Pseudomonas aeruginosa.* This still holds. The other had excellent activity against community type bacteria but was not nearly as active against hospital-acquired organisms. Once-daily ceftriaxone has significant gram-positive activity and has found many clinical roles in those admitted from home but not for hospital-acquired gram-negative organisms.

   d. **Cefepime** has sometimes been called a **fourth-generation agent [3],** but it may be better summarized as a "hybrid" of cefotaxime (which has similar activity to ceftriaxone) and ceftazidime, two third-generation agents. In many

Table 27F.1. The Major Cephalosporins

| First Generation | Second Generation | Third Generation |
|---|---|---|
| Parenteral | Parenteral | Parenteral |
| Cephalothin (Keflin) | Cefamandole (Mandol) | Cefotaxime (Claforan) |
| Cefazolin (Ancef, Kefzol) | Cefoxitin (Mefoxin)[a] | Cefoperazone (Cefobid) |
| Cephapirin (Cefadyl) | Cefuroxime (Zinacef) | Ceftizoxime (Cefizox) |
| Cephradine (Velosef) | Cefotetan (Cefotan)[a] | Ceftriaxone (Rocephin) |
| | | Ceftazidime (Fortaz, Tazidime, or Tazicef) |
| | | Cefepime (Maxipime)[b] |
| Oral | Oral | Oral |
| Cephalexin (Keflex) | Cefuroxime axetil (Ceftin) | Cefixime (Suprax) |
| Cephradine (Velosef, Anspor) | Cefprozil (Cefzil) | Cefpodoxime (Vantin) |
| Cefadroxil (Duricef) | Loracarbef (Lorabid)[a] | Ceftibuten (Cedax) |
| | Cefaclor (Ceclor) | Cefdinir (Omnicef) |
| | | Cefditoren pivoxil (Spectracef) |

[a] A cephalosporin-like antibiotic.
[b] Some authors have referred to this agent as a fourth-generation cephalosporin; see text.

Table 27F.2. Pharmacokinetic Properties of Parenteral Cephalosporins (in Adults)

| | Half-Life (h) | Standard Dose (g) | Usual Dose Interval (h) | Half-Life (h) in End-Stage Renal Disease |
|---|---|---|---|---|
| Cephalothin | 0.6 | 1.0–2.0 | 4 | 10 |
| Cefoxitin | 0.9 | 1.0–2.0 | 4–6–8 | 10–22 |
| Cefotaxime | 1.0[a] | 1.0–2.0 | 6–8 | 3 |
| Cefuroxime | 1.0 | 0.75–1.5 | 6–8 | 15–20 |
| Cefazolin | 1.8 | 1.0 | 6–8 | 18–36 |
| Cefoperazone | 1.8 | 2.0 | 6–8 | 2 |
| Ceftizoxime | 1.8 | 2.0 | 8 | 25–35 |
| Ceftazidime | 1.8 | 1.0–2.0 | 8 | 16–25 |
| Cefepime | 2.0 | 1.0–2.0 | 12 | 14 |
| Cefotetan | 4.5 | 1.0–2.0 | 12 | 12–35 |
| Ceftriaxone | 7.0 | 1.0–2.0 | 24[b] | 12–15 |

[a]Cefotaxime has a half-life of 1 h in persons with normal renal function but is metabolized to a desacetyl derivative, which has a half-life of 1.6 h and possesses significant antimicrobial activity and may interact synergistically with the parent compound [1].
[b]For non–central nervous system infections; for meningitis doses are given q12h. See text.

centers, cefepime has replaced ceftazidime because it includes the latter's activity and extends it.

2. The cephalosporin "antibiotic market domination" of the late 1980's has been diminished somewhat by the advent of the newer quinolones released in the late 1980's and the newer macrolides (clarithromycin and azithromycin) released in the early 1990's.

**B. Side effects.** Cephalosporins are **well tolerated.** Their side effects are reviewed in section **IV** except for special considerations with an individual agent, which are discussed under that agent.

**C. Pharmacokinetics** data are summarized in Table 27F.2. Like the penicillins, the antimicrobial effects of the cephalosporins depend on maintaining concentrations of active drug above the minimum inhibitory concentration (MIC) of the infecting organism for 50% of the 24-hour period (**time-dependent killing;** see Chapter 25).

**D. Resistance issues**

1. **Mechanisms of action and bacterial resistance.** Penicillin binding proteins are targets of the cephalosporins that exert their antimicrobial effect by interfering with the synthesis of peptidoglycan, a major component of the bacterial cell wall [2]. The three most common mechanisms that mediate resistance are (a) production of enzymes, $\beta$-lactamases, to inactivate drugs before they reach the penicillin binding proteins; (b) alteration of the penicillin binding proteins; or (c) changes in the outer membrane that limit the ability of the drug to reach the target [2].

   a. **$\beta$-Lactamase production.** Some of the $\beta$-lactamases are plasmid mediated by plasmids that are transferred between bacteria. Some are inducible and are chromosomally mediated. These inducible enzymes develop in certain species (*Enterobacter* species, *Citrobacter* species, *P. aeruginosa*). Clinically, this phenomenon manifests as treatment failure and emergence of drug-resistant organisms despite initial susceptibility to the cephalosporin used [1,2].

   **"Extended-spectrum $\beta$-lactamases"** have recently been described, especially with nosocomial *Klebsiella pneumonia.* They confer high level resistance to all $\beta$-lactams. However, *in vitro* testing indicated resistance mainly to ceftazidime but suggested susceptibility to other cephalosporins when used in clinical situations tends to be resistant [2].

   b. **Alteration of penicillin binding proteins.** Gram-positive organisms such as *S. pneumoniae* or *S. aureus* represent excellent examples of this resistance development.

c. **Porin alterations and resistance.** *P. aeruginosa* very quickly changes its porins to exclude drugs like ceftazidime.

2. **Antibiotic pressure and resistance.** Because hospitalized patients are compromised, there is a tendency to initiate antibiotics such as ceftazidime or cefepime at the first sign of instability. As a result, organisms that are merely colonizers and not causing infection become resistant. Furthermore their excess use tends to select for vancomycin-resistant enterococci [4]. When true disease develops, they do not respond to the selected antibiotic.
3. **Intrinsic resistance.** Some organisms are always resistant to cephalosporins (e.g., all enterococci, *Listeria monocytogenes,* and the organisms of nonbacterial pneumonia [*Legionella, Mycoplasma,* and *Chlamydia* species]) [2].

## II. Rational approach to use of intravenous preparations

A. **First generation. Cefazolin (Ancef, Kefzol)** is the most commonly used agent. It can be given intravenously (i.v.) or intramuscularly every 6 to 8 hours rather than every 4 to 6 hours, which other first-generation agents require.

1. **This first-generation agent has activity against MSSA** and is active against most community acquired gram-negative organisms. Therefore it is useful in the following:
   a. **Routine surgical prophylaxis.**
   b. Known or suspected **MSSA,** but not methicillin-resistant *S. aureus* (MRSA) infections. There is some evidence that about 50% of *MSSA* that appear to be susceptible to cefazolin, produce a $\beta$-lactamase that has high activity against cefazolin. Although appearing susceptible by disk, when these organisms are present at concentrations above $10^6$/mL, the infection they are causing responds less well to cefazolin than it does to nafcillin.
   c. An alternative agent for penicillin-susceptible *S. pneumoniae, S. pyogenes,* viridans streptococci, and *S. agalactiae* (streptococci group B).
2. **Infection caused by community-acquired gram-negative organisms** (e.g., *E. coli, K. pneumoniae,* etc.), such as cholecystitis and in initial cases of community-acquired pyelonephritis.

   The combination of cefazolin (active against gram-negative organisms) and metronidazole (active against bowel anaerobes) is a very cost-effective regimen for community-acquired intraabdominal infections (see related discussion in Chapter13).
3. **Situations in which to avoid cefazolin.** Cefazolin does not penetrate the cerebrospinal fluid adequately and is not indicated in meningitis. **All cephalosporins are inactive against enterococci and therefore are not indicated in enterococcal endocarditis.** However, in most mixed aerobic and anaerobic intraabdominal infections, enterococci do not require specific antimicrobial treatment (see Chapter 13).
4. **Pregnancy and nursing.** All cephalosporins, both intravenous and oral, are category B agents and should be used in pregnancy only when clearly indicated. They are all excreted into the breast milk and could sensitize the newborn.
5. **Dosing** (Table 27F.3).
6. **Side effects** (see section **IV**)
7. **Cost** (see Appendix Table)

B. **Second-generation** cephalosporins

1. **Cefamandole (Mandol)** use has largely been replaced by cefuroxime or third-generation cephalosporins. From a **historical standpoint,** it is important to emphasize that **this agent was associated with a significant risk of hypoprothrombinemia** (more than 10% of recipients), **presumably related to the *N*-methylthiotetrazole (NMTT) side chain,** which interferes with prothrombin synthesis. Although controversial, **similar concerns persist in newer agents (e.g., cefotetan) that have this same side chain.**
2. **Cefuroxime (Zinacef, Kefurox)** was introduced in the middle to late 1980's and has replaced cefamandole. Because of its spectrum of activity (see section **a,** below), it is used for respiratory infections in some centers. In 1993, the American Thoracic Society [5] favored its use in empiric therapy of community-acquired pneumonia (CAP), especially in adults with comorbid illness. However, with the

Table 27F.3. Typical Dosages and Summary of Parenteral (i.v.) Cephalosporins

| Agent | Common Adult Single i.v. Dose[a] | Usual Dose Interval in Normal Renal Function[b] (h) | Typical Total Adult Daily Dose (g) | Pediatric Dose | Dose Interval (h) with Decreased Creatinine Clearance | | | | CSF Penetration | Potential for Bleeding Side Effects |
|---|---|---|---|---|---|---|---|---|---|---|
| | | | | | <50 | 30–49 | 10–29 | <10 | | |
| First generation | | | | | | | | | | |
| Cefazolin (Ancef, Kefzol) | 0.5–1 g | 8 | 1.5–3.0 | 25–100 mg/kg/d; divided into q6–8h equal doses | 8 | 12 | 24 | 24–48 | Poor | In renal failure |
| Second generation | | | | | | | | | | |
| Cefoxitin (Mefoxin) | 2 g | 6–8 | 6–8 | 80–160 mg/kg/d; divided into q4–6h doses | 6–8 | 8–12 | 12–24 | 24[c] | Poor | |
| Cefuroxime (Zinacef) | 750 mg–1.5 g | 8 | 2.25–4.5 | 75–100 mg/kg/d; divided into q8h | 8 | 8 | 12 | 24 | Modest | No |
| Cefotetan (Cefotan) | 1–2 g | 12 | 2–4 | Not advised | 12 | 12 | 24 | 48 | Poor | Yes |
| Third generation | | | | | | | | | | |
| Cefotaxime (Claforan) | 1–2 g | 8[d] | 3–6 | 50–180 mg/kg/d; divided into q6h[e] | 8[d] | 8–12 | 12 | 24 | Excellent | No |
| Ceftriaxone (Rocephin) | 1–2 g[f] | 24[f] | 1–2 | In meningitis, loading dose of 75 mg/kg and then 100 mg/kg/d (not to exceed 4 g/d) divided q12h. In other infections, 50–75 mg/kg/d (not to exceed 2 g) divided q12h or once-daily doses | 24[g] | 24[g] | 24[g] | See text | Excellent | No |

| | | | | | | | | | | |
|---|---|---|---|---|---|---|---|---|---|---|
| Ceftazidime (Fortaz, Tazidime, Tazicef) | 1–2 g | 8 | 3–6 | 90–150 mg/kg/d; divided q8h (to maximum 6 g/d) | 8 | 12–24[a] | 24–48[a] | 48–72[c] | Excellent | No |
| Expanded spectrum or fourth generation | | | | | | | | | | |
| Cefepime (Maxipime) | 1–2 g | 12[b] | 4 | 50 mg/kg/dose q12h[h] if over 2 months of age | Usual; see text | | | | Modest | |

[a]Doses suggested for moderately severe infections; higher dose in severe infection.
[b]Or in patients with creatinine clearance > 50 mL/min.
[c]Dose is also reduced 50%. See text.
[d]Dose interval for cefotaxime in children is usually q6h.
[e]Higher dose range of cefotaxime used in meningitis. Use adult dosages in children weighing > 50 kg. Neonatal dosages shown in Chapter 3.
[f]In meningitis, 2 g q12h is advised (see text). In less severe infections, 1 g daily may be used. See text.
[g]In CNS infections, a q12h regimen is preferred. See text.
[h]In neutropenic patients, a higher dose regimen is used: 2 g q8h in adults, and 50 mg/kg/dose q8h in children.

recent increased incidence of penicillin-resistant *S. pneumoniae* and the *in vitro* data suggesting cefuroxime is not an optimal agent for this pathogen, its role as of 2002 has undergone considerable reassessment (see Chapters 11 and 27C).

**a. *In vitro* activity**

(1) **Gram-positive organisms.** Cefuroxime is very active against group A and B streptococci and viridans streptococci but not enterococci. Generally, cefuroxime is less active against MSSA than cefazolin, but cefuroxime is still active, with an $MIC_{90}$ $\leq$1.6 $\mu$g/mL. **In a recent *in vitro* study of more than 1,500 respiratory isolates of *S. pneumoniae*, cefuroxime was active against 99.1% of penicillin-susceptible strains, 53% of penicillin intermediate susceptible strains, and none of the high level penicillin-resistant strains** [6] (see related discussions in Chapter 11).

(2) **Gram-negative organisms.** Cefuroxime is very active against ampicillin-susceptible or -resistant *H. influenzae* and *M. catarrhalis* as well as *Neisseria meningitidis, N. gonorrhoeae* (including penicillinase producers), and *Pasteurella multocida.* It is active against many community-acquired gram-negative bacteria (e.g., *E. coli, Klebsiella* species, etc) but is less active *in vitro* than the third-generation cephalosporins against gram-negative bacteria. Many hospital-acquired gram-negative organisms and most *Pseudomonas* species and *Providencia* species are resistant.

(3) **Anaerobes.** Cefuroxime is not as active as cefoxitin or cefotetan against bowel anaerobes. Practically speaking, we would not rely on cefuroxime for anaerobic activity.

(4) ***Borrelia burgdorferi*** (agent of Lyme disease) are susceptible.

**b. Pharmacokinetics** (Table 27F.2)

**c. Clinical uses.** Cefuroxime has commonly been used for CAP [7], postinfluenza pneumonia, orbital cellulitis, complicated sinusitis, and epiglottitis. However, it is now less favored in these clinical settings due to increasing antimicrobial resistance of the organisms causing these syndromes (see section **a,** above). Oral cefuroxime (cefuroxime axetil, Ceftin) is considered one of the drugs of choice for early Lyme disease (i.e., erythema chronicum migrans) [8].

**d. Doses** (Table 27F.3)

**e. Pregnancy and nursing mothers.** Category B.

**f. Cost** (See Appendix Table 1)

**g. Side effects** (see section **IV**)

**3. Cefoxitin (Mefoxin)** is a cephamycin antibiotic (cephalosporin-like) that has enhanced anaerobic activity.

**a. *In vitro* activity**

(1) **Gram-positive bacteria.** Cefoxitin is slightly less active than the first-generation agents.

(2) **Gram-negative bacteria.** Cefoxitin remains active against many community-acquired gram-negative bacteria but is not active against many hospital-acquired gram-negative bacteria (e.g., *Pseudomonas* species, *Enterobacter cloacae*). It is active against *N. gonorrhoeae,* including penicillinase producers.

(3) **Anaerobes.** Cefoxitin is active *in vitro* against 80% to 90% of strains of *B. fragilis* at clinically achievable concentrations, although in well-established anaerobic infections, cefoxitin may not be as effective *in vivo.* **Generally, cefoxitin is viewed as the cephalosporin with the best activity *in vitro* against oral and bowel anaerobes.**

**b. Pharmacokinetics** (Table 27F.2)

**c. Clinical uses**

(1) **Community-acquired mild to moderate intraabdominal infections.** Cefoxitin has been useful in the management of mixed gastrointestinal (GI) flora infections, especially before an abscess develops. Cefoxitin remains a useful agent in diverticulitis, very early appendix rupture, and early to mild bowel perforation before *B. fragilis* has become established in high titers. However, there are many antibiotic options for these infections,

including ampicillin-sulbactam, ticarcillin-clavulanate, and piperacillin-tazobactam (see Chapter 13). **Cefoxitin and the β-lactam–β-lactamase inhibitor combinations are expensive. Thus a combination of cefazolin and metronidazole** for mild to moderate community-acquired intraabdominal infections (see Chapter 13) and pelvic infections that do not involve *N. gonorrhoeae* is an alternative (see section **(2)**, below).

(2) **Pelvic infections.** Because cefoxitin is active against *N. gonorrhoeae,* many gram-negative bacilli, and most anaerobes, it has been clinically successful in a variety of pelvic infections, early pelvic abscesses, and pelvic inflammatory disease regimens [9] (see Chapter 16).

(3) **Mixed aerobic/anaerobic soft tissue infections** may respond well to cefoxitin. The best results may occur when the duration of illness, before initiation of antibiotics, is short. Cefoxitin has been used in mixed-flora foot infections in diabetic patients; it is not active against enterococci whose role in this setting is often unclear (see Chapter 4).

(4) **Note. Cefoxitin should not be relied on as monotherapy in** very ill patients with **bacteremia due to *B. fragilis,*** because cefoxitin may not be active against 5% to 15% of these isolates. **The same is true for hospital-acquired intraabdominal sepsis** that is often caused by resistant gram-negative bacteria.

d. **Dosing** (Table 27F.30)

e. **Pregnancy and nursing mothers** (see section **II.A.4**)

f. **Side effects** (see section **IV**)

g. **Cost** (see Appendix Table)

4. **Cefotetan (Cefotan)** has been promoted as a cost-effective **cefoxitin-like agent** with good anaerobic activity because cefotetan can be given every 12 hours rather than every 6 to 8 hours.

a. *In vitro* **activity**

(1) **Gram-positive organisms.** Cefotetan is two to four times less active than cefoxitin [10].

(2) **Gram-negative aerobes.** *In vitro,* cefotetan is more active than cefoxitin against enteric gram-negative bacilli but less active than the third-generation cephalosporins. It is active against gonococci but is inactive against many hospital-acquired gram-negative organisms, including many strains of *Enterobacter* species and most strains of *P. aeruginosa* and *Acinetobacter* species.

(3) **Anaerobes.** Cefotetan is considered comparable with cefoxitin *in vitro* against *B. fragilis* but is less active against other species within the *B. fragilis* group [1].

b. **Side effects. Interference with prothrombin synthesis.** Cefotetan contains the NMTT side chain, which may be related to an increased incidence of hypoprothrombinemia (see section **II.B.1**). The exact incidence of this with cefotetan is unclear. Of interest, the package insert warning for cefotetan (but not cefoxitin) indicates that cefotetan "may be associated with a fall in prothrombin activity and possible subsequent bleeding. Those at increased risk include patients with renal or hepatobiliary impairment or poor nutritional status, the elderly, and patients with cancer. Prothrombin times should be monitored and exogenous vitamin K administered as indicated" [10]. Barza [10] concluded that this needs to be considered when choosing between these agents.

c. Other side effects (see section **IV**)

d. **Clinical use** of cefotetan

(1) For young otherwise healthy women with pelvic infections, endometritis, pelvic inflammatory disease, or mild to moderate community-acquired intraabdominal infections, cefotetan is reasonable. A similar view was presented in a publication of clinical practice guidelines. The Committee on Antimicrobial Agents of the Canadian Infectious Disease Society suggested that cefotetan could be considered an alternative single agent for prophylaxis of infection in patients undergoing elective bowel surgery.

It may be used to treat patients with acute pelvic inflammatory disease and endometritis, but hypoprothrombinemia in debilitated patients is a concern [11].

(2) Cefotetan's useful role in **GI surgical prophylaxis** is reviewed in Chapter 27B.

(3) **For patients with underlying risk factors for hypoprothrombinemia (see section b), we do not recommend using cefotetan.**

e. **Dosing** (Table 27F.3). The safety and efficacy in children has not been established.

f. **Pregnancy and nursing mothers** (see section **II.A.4**)

g. **Cost** (see Appendix Table 1)

5. **Cefonicid** (Monocid). This agent is no longer available in the United States.

C. **Third-generation cephalosporins** are **useful in several settings,** as shown in Table 27F.4. These agents are drugs of choice for only a limited number of organisms (Table 27F.4).

1. ***In vitro* activity**

a. **Gram-positive aerobes** [12,13]

(1) ***S. pneumoniae.*** Cefotaxime, ceftizoxime, and ceftriaxone are very active against the highly and intermediate susceptible organisms but less so against penicillin-resistant ***S. pneumoniae.*** In one large *in vitro* report, ceftriaxone was found to be active against 92% of intermediate level but only 27% of high level penicillin-resistant strains [6,13].

(2) ***S. aureus.*** The first- and some second-generation cephalosporins are at least two- to fourfold more active than cefotaxime, ceftizoxime, and ceftriaxone against penicillin-susceptible *S. aureus* and against some, but not all, $\beta$-lactamase–producing strains. When considering cefotaxime, ceftizoxime, or ceftriaxone in suspected sepsis in which staphylococci cannot be excluded, any of these three cephalosporins would provide the necessary activity against staphylococci [12]. In patients with documented severe MSSA infections (e.g., endocarditis), an oxacillin or nafcillin or cefazolin is preferable.

(3) **Coagulase-negative staphylococci.** If the organisms are methicillin resistant, a cephalosporin is not recommended, even if the *in vitro* data suggest that a cephalosporin may be active. If methicillin susceptible, cephalosporins are potential agents, although vancomycin often is used.

(4) **Group A streptococci.** Some third-generation cephalosporins (cefotaxime, ceftizoxime, and ceftriaxone) are very active against these pathogens, with MICs less than 0.03 $\mu$g/mL, comparable with benzyl penicillin and, in fact, more active than cefazolin or cefoxitin.

(5) **Group B streptococci *(S. agalactiae)*** are also very susceptible to cefotaxime, ceftizoxime, and ceftriaxone, with an MIC comparable with penicillin G and lower than cefazolin. **Groups C and G streptococci** are also very susceptible to the aforementioned third-generation agents.

(6) **Most viridans streptococci and *Streptococcus bovis*** have lower MICs for these third-generation agents than the first- or second-generation cephalosporins. This has implications in alternate endocarditis therapeutic regimens (e.g., ceftriaxone once daily).

(7) **Inactive** *L. monocytogenes,* enterococci, MRSA, and, as mentioned above, most high level penicillin-resistant *S. pneumoniae* are resistant.

b. **Gram-negative aerobes** [12,14]

(1) ***H. influenzae*** (and other *Haemophilus* species) and ***N. gonorrhoeae*** are very susceptible to the third-generation cephalosporins, including strains that produce $\beta$-lactamases.

(2) ***N. meningitidis*** and ***M. catarrhalis*** likewise.

(3) **Community-acquired Enterobacteriaceae.** The excellent *in vitro* activity of the third-generation cephalosporins against gram-negative organisms is a major advantage of these agents over the first- and second-generation cephalosporins. Bacteria resistant to the older cephalosporins

Table 27F.4. Common Uses of Third-Generation Cephalosporins

| Setting | Agent Commonly Used | Comment |
|---|---|---|
| Gram-negative enteric meningitis (e.g., *E. coli, Klebsiella* species) | Cefotaxime,[a] Ceftriaxone, Ceftazidime | An unusual clinical problem. Seen in neonates, or post neurosurgery. |
| Bacterial meningitis | Cefotaxime,[a] ceftriaxone[b] | Excellent for *H. influenzae,*[b] *N. meningitidis,* and penicillin susceptible *S. pneumoniae.* For penicillin-resistant *S. pneumoniae* need vancomycin (see Chapters 6 and 27) and for *Listeria monocytogenes* need ampicillin or TMP-SMZ. |
| Febrile neutropenic patient without a focal source | Ceftazidime, cefepime[c] | Ceftazidime not active against gram (+) cocci. If there is a Hickman catheter infection, would need to add i.v. vancomycin until culture data are available. Cefepime not active against MRSA. Also see Chapter 2. |
| *S. viridans* endocarditis | Ceftriaxone | Once-a-day dose. |
| *P. aeruginosa* activity | Ceftazidime, cefepime | For synergy (e.g., in pneumonia) combined with an aminoglycoside. Ceftazidime has little gram-positive activity. Ceftriaxone not active against *P. aeruginosa.* |
| Broad-spectrum activity (see text) | Ceftriaxone (cefepime also an option) | Ceftazidime has little gram-positive activity. Ceftriaxone not active against *P. aeruginosa.* |
| Gram-negative pathogens (e.g., *E. coli, K. pneumoniae;* indole-positive *Proteus, P. vulgaris; Morganella morganii; Providence stuartii, Serratia* species | Ceftriaxone, cefotaxime, ceftazidime; cefepime | Active against most community-acquired gram negatives. Certain hospital-acquired gram negatives may be resistant. |
| *N. gonorrhoeae* infections | Ceftriaxone[b] | See Chapter 16. |
| *Pseudomonas pseudomallei* | Ceftazidime[b] | Rare problem. |
| *Haemophilus ducreyi* (chancroid) | Ceftriaxone[b] | Azithromycin is also an agent of choice |
| *Borrelia burgdorferi* (Lyme disease) | Ceftriaxone | See *Med Lett Drugs Ther* 2000;42:37 |

[a] For neonates, use cefotaxime, not ceftriaxone. See text.

[b] Agent considered a "drug of choice" [5].

[c] In patients at high risk for severe infection (including patients with a history of recent bone marrow transplantation, with hypotension at presentation, with underlying hematologic malignancy or with severe or prolonged neutropenia) the package insert notes monotherapy may not be appropriate. Insufficient data exist to support efficacy in such patients.

and, at times, even the aminoglycosides are often susceptible to the third-generation cephalosporins. ***E. coli*** is usually very susceptible to the third-generation agents. **Most *Klebsiella*** species and ***P. mirabilis*** remain susceptible.

(4) **Hospital-acquired gram-negative organisms.** Even hospital-acquired gram-negative organisms that are resistant to first- and second-generation agents and even occasionally to aminoglycosides are usually susceptible to specific third-generation drugs [14]. ***E. coli, Providencia, Citrobacter*** species, **and *P. vulgaris*** generally are inhibited by very low concentrations. Occasionally, nosocomial strains of ***Klebsiella*** species isolated in the United States are resistant (and these usually are susceptible to imipenem). ***Enterobacter*** species, especially ***E. cloacae,*** which are important nosocomial pathogens, **is a major weakness of the third-generation cephalosporins.** Approximately 10% to 30% of *E. cloacae* may initially be resistant to the third-generation cephalosporins, but even the isolates of *E. cloacae* with MICs of 1 μg/mL or less contain subpopulations of organisms that are easily selected for resistance to the third-generation cephalosporins (see section **I.D.2**). Presumably, the general use of cephalosporins, including the first- and second-generation cephalosporins, has caused the increase in isolation of this species over the last two decades. Also, ***C. freundii*** similarly develops resistance, although it has not become as prominent a nosocomial pathogen.

(5) **Susceptibility tests for hospital gram-negative organisms.** Because of the variability of *in vitro* susceptibility data, testing is needed for each third-generation cephalosporin that may be used. **For *P. aeruginosa,* cefepime, which has largely replaced ceftazidime and cefoperazone, can be considered a potential agent.** Because cefoperazone is less active (and has the NMTT side chain), we believe that **cefepime is the better third-generation cephalosporin for these situations [14].** Cefepime $MIC_{90}$ for ***P. aeruginosa*** is 8 μg/mL, signifying only modest activity. Some *Burkholderia cepacia* strains are inhibited by ceftazidime.

c. **Anaerobes.** The activity of the third-generation cephalosporins against anaerobes was summarized elsewhere [12], but a few points deserve emphasis. The anaerobic activity of cefotaxime, ceftizoxime, and ceftriaxone is suitable for respiratory pathogens (i.e., oral anaerobes). None of the third-generation agents is considered a drug of first choice for **bowel-related *B. fragilis*** [12], although cefotaxime has been very effective in clinical situations [15]. **Cefoxitin** and **cefotetan** are **more active** *in vitro* **against anaerobes than most but not all [11] third-generation agents.**

2. **Pharmacokinetics** is shown in Table 27F.2.
3. **Dosages** are shown in Table 27F.3, including doses in renal failure.
4. **Pregnancy and nursing mothers** (see section **II.A.4**)
5. **Clinical use: third-generation agents for community acquired infection**

a. **Ceftriaxone (Rocephin)** is a **widely used agent** both due to its broad spectrum of activity and its long half-life, allowing for every 24-hour dosing in non–central nervous system (CNS) infections (Table 27.F.2). It has been effective against serious infections and is the primary agent for CAP.

(1) **Dosing (Table 27F.3).** For non–CNS infections, **in adults** a single dose given once daily is preferred, usually 1 g every 24 hours. For CNS infections (e.g., meningitis, brain abscess), maximal doses are used, 2 g every 12 hours in adults. **In children,** with meningitis or severe infection, use every 12 hour regimen.

(2) **Renal failure.** Ceftriaxone has dual renal (60%) and hepatic (40%) excretion; in renal failure, hepatic excretion increases [2]. Dose adjustments are not necessary in renal failure [1,2]. If both hepatic and renal failure is present, half-life is prolonged. If serum levels are not available and ceftriaxone is clearly the agent of choice, 500 mg every 24 hours for non-CNS infections in adults [1] is used though serum monitoring is preferred.

For patients on hemodialysis, the package insert suggests serum levels be monitored.

(3) **Side effects** are **discussed in section IV. Rarely,** ceftriaxone may cause "sludge" to form in the gallbladder, especially in children, causing **"biliary pseudolithiasis."** Associated symptoms may include nausea, vomiting, and right upper quadrant abdominal pain [16].

b. **Cefotaxime (Claforan)** was the first third-generation cephalosporin introduced and is still the **preferred agent in neonates,** both because of greater experience and because it does not interfere with bilirubin metabolism in the neonate. Otherwise, ceftriaxone has for the most part replaced cefotaxime because of the single daily dose. The one exception is for bowel-perforated intraabdominal infections for which the parent drug cefotaxime plus its desacetyl breakdown product are very effective [15].

c. **Ceftizoxime (Cefizox)** must be given every 8 to 12 hours for severe infections and every 4 hours for life-threatening infections. **It has largely been replaced by ceftriaxone given once daily.**

6. **Clinical use: third-generation agents for hospital-acquired infection**

a. **Cefepime (Maxipime)** is an expanded-spectrum cephalosporin released in 1996 [13,14,17,18].

(1) ***In vitro* activity.** It has activity against gram-positive organisms comparable with cefotaxime and activity against gram-negative aerobic organisms comparable or superior to ceftazidime. Cefepime is less active against MSSA than cefazolin. Among the antibiotics with activity against *P. aeruginosa,*it has more frequent *in vitro* activity than ceftazidime [14]. One of the mechanisms by which it might impart resistance is by inhibiting adherence of the organism to epithelial cells [19]. However, some strains are susceptible to ceftazidime and not to cefepime [20]. It is not active against enterococci, MRSA, *B. fragilis,* or high level penicillin-resistant *S. pneumoniae* [13].

(2) **Pharmacokinetics** (Table 27F.2)

(3) **Approved indications** include therapy of susceptible pathogens in (a) uncomplicated and complicated urinary tract infection (UTI) [10], (b) uncomplicated skin infections, (c) moderate to severe pneumonia [13], and (d) empiric therapy for the febrile neutropenic patient [21–23]. (**N.B.** The package insert does not list meningitis as an indication for use.)

(4) **Dosages**

(a) **For adults** usually 1 to 2 g i.v. (or intramuscularly) every 12 hours, depending on the severity of infection. At 2 g every 12 hours, time above the MIC of *P. aeruginosa* for 60% to 70% of a 24-hour period [24]. In the febrile leukopenic patient, 2 g every 8 hours is advised [21–23].

(b) **For children** more than 2 months of age. If weight is less than 40 kg, 50 mg/kg/dose every 12 hours for most infections but every 8 hours in the febrile neutropenic patient. Maximum dose per day should not exceed adult doses. If weight is more than 40 kg, adult doses can be used.

(c) **Renal failure.** Normal doses are indicated for a creatinine clearance of more than 60 mL. **If the creatinine clearance is 30 to 60 mL/min and the interval selected is every 12 hours,** give the usual dose every 24 hours; for a creatinine clearance of 10 to 30 mL/min, give 50% of the usual dose every 24 hours; for a creatinine clearance of less than 10 mL/min, give 25% of the usual dose every 24 hours. **If the interval selected is every 8 hours** and the creatinine clearance is 30 to 60 mL/min, give the usual dose every 12 hours; for a clearance of 10 to 30 mL/min give the usual dose every 24 hours; and for a clearance of less than 10 mL/min, give 50% of the usual dose every 24 hours.

(5) **Side effects** (see section **IV**)

(6) **Cost** (see Appendix Table 1)

(7) **Summary.** Many institutions have replaced ceftazidime with cefepime. As with other broad-spectrum agents (e.g., imipenem, piperacillin-tazobactam), if these agents are used excessively, bacterial resistance will presumably develop. This is especially true in those associated with a foreign body. It has been suggested that emergence of resistance of *E. cloacae* and other gram-negative organisms with inducible β-lactamase potential will not be as common as it has been with ceftazidime [3].

b. **Ceftazidime (Fortaz, Tazidime, or Tazicef)** and cefepime are the most active cephalosporins against ***P. aeruginosa.*** **Ceftazidime has poor activity against gram-positive aerobes.** It has in many institutions been replaced with cefepime, but its niche involves therapy against known or potential ***P. aeruginosa*** infection, including the following:

(1) **Febrile neutropenic patients** without an obvious source of infection [22,25] (see Chapter 20).

(2) ***P. aeruginosa*** **meningitis.** In this rare problem, infectious disease consultation is advised.

(3) **In combination with an aminoglycoside for *P. aeruginosa* tissue or bloodstream infections in a patient with a delayed penicillin allergy.**

(4) **Nosocomial pneumonia** when a Gram stain or culture has ruled out *S. aureus.* In this setting resistance can develop on therapy (e.g., with hospital-acquired ***Enterobacter*** species).

(5) **Malignant external otitis**

(6) **Cystic fibrosis.** Early lower respiratory tract infections in cystic fibrosis patients.

D. **Cefoperazone (Cefobid)** is not quite as active as cefepime against *P. aeruginosa* and contains the NMTT side chain, which appears associated with hypoprothrombinemia (see section **II.B.1**) **We do not favor the use of this agent.**

III. **Oral cephalosporins** (Table 27F.5). Although **these are expensive agents** (see Appendix Table), they are commonly used. Adults will have less GI upset with cephalexin or cephradine than with oral antistaphylococcal agents (dicloxacillin). In children, taste and aftertaste are important in compliance. In one report, oral cephalosporin suspensions were more "acceptable" than other agents [26]. In general, these agents are rapidly and thoroughly absorbed [2].

**All these agents are category B in pregnancy and all are excreted in breast milk** (see section **II.A.4**). **The indications and uses** for these agents have been **summarized in** Tables 27F.4 and 27F.6 It is helpful to summarize these agents as first-, second-, and third-generation agents.

A. **First-generation oral agents** are useful for mild to moderately severe penicillin- and methicillin-susceptible *S. aureus* and group A streptococcal infections of the skin and soft tissue and susceptible UTI pathogens.

1. **Cephalexin (Keflex)** is well absorbed, but because of the relatively high MICs of the susceptible gram-negative organisms, **this agent is not useful in soft tissue infections due to gram-negative bacteria.** For UTI, even for uncomplicated UTI, a 7-day course, not 3-day course, is advised (see Chapter 15).

a. **Dosage. When treating significant *S. aureus* soft tissue infection in adults, a dose of 1,000 mg every 6 hours is used initially and the course completed with 500 mg every 6 hours [27].** This dose is required to provide adequate serum levels because cephalexin is excreted very rapidly,. The suggested adult dose for UTI is 250 to 500 mg every 6 hours. In children, 25 to 50 mg/kg/day is divided into four equal doses. In streptococcal pharyngitis, a twice daily regimen at the UTI dose can be used.

b. **In renal failure** with creatinine clearance less than 10 mL/min, the interval is prolonged to every 12 hours [24,29]; for dialysis patients, a single dose of 500 mg daily suffices and is an excellent regimen to complete treatment of a MSSA infection. When creatinine clearance is 10 to 50 mL/min, a dose is given every 8 to 12 hours, depending on disease severity and renal failure.

c. **Side effects** (see section **IV**)

Table 27F.5. Oral-Cephalosporins

| Agent | Indication | Comment |
|---|---|---|
| First generation<br>Cephalexin (Keflex), or<br>Cephradine (Anspor, Velosef) | Mild/minor soft-tissue infections due to methicillin-susceptible *S. aureus* and/or *S. pyogenes* (strep A). | Use an adequate dose since activity against *S. aureus* is modest and excretion is rapid. See text. |
| | Susceptible UTI. | Probably prudent to use 7-day course for uncomplicated UTI rather than 3-day course. |
| | Alternative in strep pharyngitis.[a] | |
| Second generation<br>Cefuroxime (Ceftin), or<br>Cefprozil (Cefzil), or<br>Loracarbef (Lorabid) | Alternative therapy in otitis media, sinusitis, bronchitis. See Chapter 8. | These are relatively expensive agents. See Appendix Table. |
| | Cefuroxime axetil (Ceftin) has been used in Lyme disease. | Cefaclor falling out of favor in children, for it may cause serum sickness. |
| | Alternate therapy in early selected cases of community-acquired pneumonia (CAP). See Chapter 11. | Oral cefuroxime has a poor taste vs "bubble-gum" flavored cefprozil, which is b.i.d. dosing. |
| Third generation<br>Cefixime (Suprax) | Alternate therapy for *H. influenzae* and *M. catarrhalis* therapy in otitis media | Less active against *S. pneumoniae* and not active for *S. aureus*. |
| | Susceptible UTI or mild soft-tissue infections due to susceptible pathogens. | Do *in vitro* susceptibility data to show activity. |
| | Alternate for uncomplicated GC therapy. | See Chapter 16. |
| | No unique niche. | |
| Cefpodoxime (Vantin) | No unique role. | See text. |
| Ceftibuten (Cedax) | No unique role. | |
| | Possible alternative in flares of bronchitis. | See text. |
| Cefdinir (Omnicef) | No unique role. | See text. |
| Cefditoren (Spectracef) | No unique role. | See text. |

[a] Although second- and third-generation cephalosporins have been used for strep pharyngitis, the first-generation agents are the most cost effective.
UTI, urinary tract infection; GC, gonococcal infection.

Table 27F.6. Common Clinical Uses of Oral Cephalosporins

| Setting | Particularly Useful Agents | Comments |
|---|---|---|
| Soft-tissue infections, cellulitis | First-generation agent preferred (e.g., cephalexin, cephradine) | When *S. aureus* and streptococci activity is desired. Agents provide poor gram-negative tissue levels. (Cefixime, ceftibuten, and cefditoren have poor *S. aureus* activity; good gram-negative activity.) |
| Otitis media | Cefprozil | Useful in delayed penicillin-allergic patients and when ampicillin-resistant *H. influenzae* are known or highly suspected. See Chapter 8. |
| | Cefixime, ceftibuten, and cefditoren | Have less activity against *S. pneumoniae,* so do not use for initial empiric therapy; are used for possible *H. influenzae* and *M. catarrhalis* infections. |
| Sinusitis | Cefuroxime axetil (adults)<br>Cefprozil (children or adults) | Especially if cannot use less expensive agents (i.e., TMP-SMZ, amoxicillin). See Chapter 8. |
| Bronchitis | Cefuroxime, cefprozil | Alternative agents for delayed penicillin-allergic patients or patients on rotating antibiotic regimens. See Chapter 8. Cefixime and ceftibuten are not as active against *S. pneumoniae.* |
| Streptococcal pharyngitis | First-generation agent | Most cost-effective alternative in the penicillin-allergic patient when a macrolide is not used. See Chapter 8. |
| Urinary tract infection | Cephalexin, cephradine<br>Cefaclor, cefuroxime<br>Cefixime | When susceptibility data support use. For uncomplicated UTI, a 7-day (not 3-day) course is preferred. See Chapter 15. |
| Community-acquired pneumonia, mild and typically when >55 y.o. | Cefuroxime | For completion of therapy when intravenous cefuroxime has been used (see text); selected cases for oral therapy. (See Chapter 11.) |

d. **Pregnancy and nursing mothers** (see section **II.A.4**)
e. **Cost** (see Appendix Table)

2. **Cephradine (Anspor, Velosef)** is considered equivalent to cephalexin and may be preferred if available locally at a lower cost than cephalexin.
a. **Dosages:** same as for cephalexin.
b. **In renal failure,** if the creatinine clearance is more than 50 mL/min, a normal dose is given every 6 hours. If the clearance is 10 to 50 mL/min, 50% of the usual dose is given at normal intervals. With a creatinine clearance of less than 10 mL/min, 25% of the usual dose is given at usual intervals. A dose is advised after dialysis. In chronic ambulatory peritoneal dialysis (CAPD), doses similar to those with a creatinine clearance of less than 10 mL/min can be used [28,29].
c. **Side effects** (see section **IV**)
d. **Cost** (see Appendix Table)
e. **Pregnancy and nursing mothers** (see section **II.A.4**)

3. **Cefadroxil (Duricef)** is a very expensive agent with no unique niches. **We do not advocate its use.**

B. **Second-generation oral cephalosporins** have enjoyed immense popularity primarily for upper respiratory (acute otitis media, sinusitis) and lower respiratory tract infections (acute exacerbations of chronic bronchitis, early CAP) (see Chapters 8 and 11). They are active against penicillin-susceptible *S. pneumoniae,* and **some of them are active against some intermediate penicillin-resistant *S. pneumoniae*** but not high level penicillin-resistant *S. pneumoniae.* They are also active against *M. catarrhalis* and *H. influenzae*—including $\beta$-lactamase–positive pathogens, streptococci group A—and have modest activity against MSSA. **All these agents are relatively expensive.** For streptococcal pharyngitis in the allergic patient, if a cephalosporin is indicated, a first-generation agent (e.g., cephalexin) is preferred (see Chapter 8).

1. **Cefuroxime axetil (Ceftin)** has an unpalatable taste, including the suspensions, and therefore an **alternate agent (e.g., cefprozil) seems prudent in children** in an attempt to improve compliance. It is active against $\beta$-lactamase–positive and–negative *M. catarrhalis, S. aureus,* group A and B streptococci, penicillin-susceptible *S. pneumoniae,* and some intermediate-level penicillin-resistant *S. pneumoniae* (see Chapters 8 and 11). In adults, oral cefuroxime has been used to complete therapy initiated with parenteral cefuroxime (see section **II.B.2**) and as an alternative agent for sinusitis or bronchitis, especially in an allergic patient (see Chapter 8).
a. **Dosage.** For children more than 13 years of age and adults, 250 to 500 mg twice daily, depending on the severity of infection. In early Lyme disease (erythema chronicum migrans) use 500 mg twice daily.
b. In **mild or moderate to even severe renal failure,** usual doses are given [28,29].
c. **Cost.** This is expensive (see Appendix Table). (Pregnancy and nursing, see section **II.A.4**).
d. **Side effects** (see section **IV**)
e. **Pregnancy and nursing mothers** (see section **II.A.4**)

2. **Cefprozil (Cefzil)** has similar *in vitro* activity as cefuroxime axetil. Because it is available in a bubble-gum–flavored suspension and can be **given twice daily,** it is commonly used in **otitis media** when there is amoxicillin allergy or when amoxicillin has failed. It also can be used in **sinusitis** and **acute exacerbations of chronic bronchitis.**
a. **Dosage.** Cefprozil is available as a 250- or 500-mg tablet as well as a liquid bubble-gum–flavor oral suspension of 125 mg/5 mL and 250 mg/5 mL. **In adults** with exacerbations of bronchitis, 500 mg twice daily is given. In sinusitis, a similar dose could be used. **In children** (6 months to 12 years) 15 mg/kg every 12 hours is suggested per package insert.
b. **Renal failure.** If the creatinine clearance is over 30 mL/min, use standard doses. For a creatinine clearance less than 30 mL/min, use 50% of the standard

dose at normal intervals. Because cefprozil is partially removed after dialysis, a dose should be given after completion of dialysis. In CAPD, use doses as if creatinine clearance was less than 10 mL/min [28,29].

c. **Cost** (see Appendix Table)

d. **Side effects** (see section **IV**)

e. **Pregnancy and nursing mothers** (see section **II.A.4**)

3. **Loracarbef (Lorabid)** has a cephalosporin-like structure. Its spectrum of activity is similar to cefuroxime axetil and cefprozil. Loracarbef has been used especially in acute otitis media, sinusitis, acute bronchitis, and selected cases of CAP similar to the indications for cefuroxime axetil and cefprozil. **It has no special niches and we seldom use it.**

a. **Dosing.** The ingestion of food will decrease and delay the peak serum concentration; **doses should be given 1 hour before or 2 hours after meals.** The suspension is more rapidly absorbed than the capsules, and the **suspension is recommended for otitis media.**

Loracarbef is available in 200-mg pulvules and a suspension (100 mg/5 mL and 200 mg/5 mL). **In adults** and children 13 years of age or more, for acute exacerbations of chronic bronchitis, CAP, sinusitis, and uncomplicated pyelonephritis, 400 mg every 12 hours has been suggested. **In children** (6 months to 12 years), for otitis the suspension preparation at 30 mg/kg/day in divided doses every 12 hours.

b. **In renal failure.** When creatinine clearance is 10 to 49 mL/min, a normal dose at twice the usual dose interval is given (i.e., every 24 hours). In patients with creatinine clearance of less than 10 mL/min who are not undergoing hemodialysis, the usual dose can be given every 3 to 5 days [24]. Patients undergoing hemodialysis should receive a supplemental dose after dialysis. For patients with CAPD, there are no data. Dose as if creatinine clearance is less than 10 mL/min [28,29].

c. **Side effects** (see section **IV**)

d. **Cost** (see Appendix Table 1)

e. **Pregnancy and nursing mothers** (see section **II.A.4**)

4. **Cefaclor (Ceclor)** produces serum sickness in children (see section **IV**), and 10% to 15% or more of ampicillin-resistant ***H. influenzae*** are resistant to cefaclor. Furthermore, its activity against ***S. pneumoniae*** is inferior. **Consequently, there is very little use for this agent** [1].

C. **Third-generation oral cephalosporins** are expensive and occasionally useful in the allergic patient and in the special circumstances discussed later. Because most microbiology laboratories can only perform susceptibility data on a limited number of agents, the susceptibility data of these agents often are not available. **We use these agents in a very limited fashion.**

1. **Cefixime (Suprax)** is more active than other oral cephalosporins against many gram-negative organisms (*E. coli, Klebsiella* species, *P. mirabilis,* and *S. marcescens*) but has no useful activity against *Pseudomonas* species, many strains of *Enterobacter* species, and *Acinetobacter* species. It is very active against *N. gonorrhoeae, H. influenzae,* and *M. catarrhalis,* including $\beta$-lactamase producers. However, **it is not active against *S. aureus*** and has decreased activity against *S. pneumoniae* when compared with other oral cephalosporins [1]. Cefixime is not active against anaerobes.

a. **Clinical use.** The exact role for this agent introduced in 1989 is still evolving. It can be considered especially in [1] **uncomplicated gonococcus infection** [9] (see Chapter 16) and ***H. influenzae or M. catarrhalis*** otitis media infections, **but** because cefixime is not as active against ***S. pneumoniae*** (a common pathogen in otitis), **cefixime is not a first-line agent for otitis;** it has been used when amoxicillin has failed (see Chapter 8) **In selected cases of UTI or gram-negative soft tissue infections,** when susceptibility data allow, cefixime may occasionally be useful, especially when allergies preclude using more conventional less expensive regimens. When it was first introduced, the general consensus was that it offered little. A recent study comparing cefixime to intravenous antibiotics in low risk febrile neutropenic patients with negative blood cultures, cefixime fared well [30]. Further studies are awaited.

  b. **Dosing.** The oral suspension is absorbed more rapidly and completely than the tablets and is preferred in the treatment of otitis media. Tablets are available in 200 and 400 mg, the oral suspension contains 100 mg/5 mL. **In adults and children older than 12 years of age,** 200 mg twice daily or 400 mg once daily is suggested. **In children** more than 6 months of age, 8 mg/kg/day of the suspension once daily or two divided doses are suggested.
  c. **Renal failure.** If the creatinine clearance is 10 to 50 mL/min, 75% of the standard dosage at the standard interval is given. Patients whose clearance is less than 10 mL/min or patients on CAPD may be given half the standard dose at the standard interval. Patients on hemodialysis can be given 300 mg after dialysis [28,29].
  d. **Side effects** (see section **IV**)
  e. **Pregnancy and nursing mothers** (see section **II.A.4**)
  f. **Cost** (see Appendix Table)

2. **Cefpodoxime (Vantin)** was approved in 1992. It is modestly active against MSSA, $MIC_{90} = 2.0\ \mu g/mL$, and against common respiratory pathogens, including penicillin-susceptible *S. pneumoniae; H. influenzae,* and $\beta$-lactamase–positive or–negative *M. catarrhalis,* and *Streptococcus* groups A and B. It is active against many Enterobacteriaceae but not against *Enterobacter, Serratia, Morganella,* or *Pseudomonas* species. It has been used in UTI, CAP, acute otitis, bronchitis, and single-dose therapy of uncomplicated gonorrhea.
   a. **Dosing.** Both 100- and 200-mg tablets and an oral suspension (50 mg/5 mL and 100 mg/5 mL) are available. **In adults** and children 13 years of age or more, 200 mg every 12 hours for moderately severe infection is used. **For children** (6 months to 12 years), the dose is 10 mg/kg/day divided every 12 hours (maximum 400 mg/day) for 10 days for otitis media. The oral suspension has a bad taste that can effect compliance in children.
   b. **In renal failure,** the dose interval can be changed [28,29]. If the creatinine clearance is 10 to 50 mL/min, a standard dose can be given every 16 hours; if the creatinine clearance is less than 10 mL/min, a standard dose can be given every 24 to 48 hours. In patients undergoing hemodialysis, 200 mg after dialysis only is suggested. For patients undergoing CAPD, dose as if the creatinine clearance is less than 10 mL/min [28,29].
   c. **Pregnancy and nursing mothers** (see section **II.A.4**)
   d. **Comment.** Shortly after its release, **the *Medical Letter*** reviewed this agent and concluded the following: "**Cefpodoxime is a broad-spectrum oral cephalosporin that offers no clear advantage over previously available drugs for the treatment of any infection**" [31]. In the woman with many antibiotic allergies, when susceptibility data allow, it may be useful in selected episodes of UTI.

3. **Ceftibuten (Cedax)** was approved in late 1995. The *in vitro* activity of this "third-generation" oral agent is similar to that of cefixime in that it has **enhanced activity against many Enterobacteriaceae, but many gram-positive organisms are resistant** (including *S. aureus, S. agalactiae,* and viridans streptococci). Ceftibuten has limited activity against *S. pneumoniae.* Specifically, strains of pneumococci that are intermediate or high level penicillin resistant are ceftibuten resistant. Anaerobes are not susceptible. Ceftibuten is not active against *Acinetobacter* species and *Pseudomonas* species. Susceptibility data are available [32].
   a. Although approved for pharyngitis and tonsillitis, less expensive agents are available. It should not be used for empiric therapy of otitis media because it is not active against many pneumococcal infections. Ceftibuten is a consideration for acute bacterial exacerbations of chronic bronchitis due to susceptible *H. influenzae* and *M. catarrhalis* especially.
   b. **Dosages.** Ceftibuten is available in 400-mg capsules and a suspension (90 mg/5 mL and 180 mg/5 mL). **Adults and children more than 12 years of age** are given 400 mg once daily. **Children more than 6 months of age**

should receive 9 mg/kg/day as a single dose up to a maximum of 400 mg/day. The **suspension must be administered 2 hours before or 1 hour after a meal.**

c. **Renal failure.** If creatinine clearance is between 10 to 50 mL/min, 50% of the usual dose is given every 24 hours; if the creatinine clearance is less than 10 mL/min, 25% of the usual dose is given every 24 hours [28,29]. In patients undergoing hemodialysis, a single 300-mg dose or 9 mg/kg (maximum of 300 mg) should be administered at the end of each hemodialysis session. There are no data for CAPD patients as of early 2000; use doses as if creatinine clearance is less than 10 mL/min [28,29].

d. **Pregnancy and nursing mothers** (see section **II.A.4**)

e. **Comment.** So far, this agent has no unique niches. Ceftibuten is another agent that could be used for acute exacerbations of chronic bronchitis, especially when a once-daily regimen is highly desirable or as an agent to rotate with other antibiotics in this setting. A recent review [3] and the *Medical Letter* [33] did not give this agent a very good report; in its review in 1996 the *Medical Letter* [33] concluded "ceftibuten is an expensive new oral cephalosporin that seems like a poor choice for the indications for which it is being marketed. In particular, recommending a drug for use in acute otitis media except when caused by pneumococcus makes no sense; pneumococcus are a frequent cause of otitis media and in clinical practice, the pathogen is usually not identified."

4. **Cefdinir (Omnicef)** was approved for use in mid-1998 and reviewed [2,34,35].

a. ***In vitro* activity** [34]. Cefdinir is similar to cefpodoxime in antibacterial activity. Cefdinir is active against MSSA; penicillin-susceptible *S. pneumoniae, H. influenzae, M. catarrhalis,* and *N. gonorrhoeae;* and many gram-negative bacteria but not against *Pseudomonas* species.

Cefdinir is not active against MRSA, atypical pathogens (*Legionella, Mycoplasma, Chlamydia*), enterococcus, and many anaerobes. It is not active against high level penicillin-resistant *S. pneumoniae,* and we view its activity against intermediately penicillin-resistant *S. pneumoniae* as inadequate. In one report, the $MIC_{90}$ of cefdinir against these strains was 3.1 $\mu$g/mL, with the average peak serum levels after a 600-mg dose of only 2.9 $\mu$g/mL [36].

b. **Pharmacokinetics.** Cefdinir is absorbed somewhat slowly from the GI tract with bioavailability of the capsules of only about 20% and 25% for the suspension. Food does not affect absorption. The drug is not metabolized and is excreted in the urine [36]. Because children find it to have a smell and taste they enjoy, compliance may be good.

c. **Approved uses** include therapy of susceptible pathogens in acute maxillary sinusitis, otitis media, acute exacerbations of chronic bronchitis, CAP, and skin infections and for pharyngitis in young children.

d. **Dosages** per package insert are as follows: **For adults,** 300 mg every 12 hours or 600 mg every 24 hours (the once-daily regimen is not advised in pneumonia or skin infections). **For children** (6 months to 12 years of age), 7 mg/kg every 12 hours or 14 mg/kg every 24 hours.

e. **Renal failure.** For patients **with creatinine clearance less than 30 mL/min** the package insert suggests the following: **In adults,** 300 mg once a day; **in children,** 7 mg/kg (up to 300 mg) given once a day. **In hemodialysis, which removes cefdinir,** the above reduced doses can be given every other day, with a dose after dialysis.

f. **Pregnancy and nursing mothers** (see section **II.A.4**)

g. **Side effects.** Like other oral cephalosporins, cefdinir is well tolerated. Diarrhea and vaginal candidiasis are the most common side effects [34].

h. **Cost.** This is an expensive agent: cost to the pharmacist for 10 days in an adult is $67 [34] for the 300 mg every 12 hour regimen (see Appendix Table).

i. **Summary.** In a review, the *Medical Letter* concluded the following: "cefdinir is an oral third-generation cephalosporin similar to cefpodoxime. **Older, better established drugs are preferred"** [34]. However, in a recent symposium, discussants concluded that the acceptability in children provides an alternative for a child who has failed penicillin for strep throat [35].

5. **Cefditoren** pivoxil (Spectracef) is a new oral third-generation cephalosporin approved by the U.S. Food and Drug Administration in late 2001. The drug has been used in Japan for 7 years [37].
   a. ***In vitro* activity.** This is similar to cefdinir and cefpodoxime.
   b. **Pharmacokinetics.** Cefditoren is well absorbed, with peak levels achieved in 1.5 to 3 hours. The drug's half-life (1.6 hours) permits dosing every 12 hours. It is excreted mainly by the kidneys. The inactive metabolite pivalate is eliminated by the kidneys in combination with carnitine as pivaloylcarnitine (see section **e.(2),** below).
   c. **Approved clinical uses in adults or children 12** or more years of age include therapy of acute exacerbation of chronic bronchitis, pharyngitis/tonsillitis, and uncomplicated skin and soft tissue infection.
   d. **Dosage.** 200-mg tablets should be taken with meals (absorption is increased with fatty meals). For pharyngitis and skin infections, 200 mg every 12 hours is advised; for exacerbation of acute bronchitis, 400 mg every 12 hours is advised.
   e. **Adverse effects.** For short-term use, this agent is generally well tolerated.
      (1) Common adverse side effects include diarrhea, nausea, and vaginal candidiasis.
      (2) Cefditoren decreases serum concentrations of carnitine, which is the substrate for carnitine acyltransferases involved in fatty acid metabolism and transport of long-chain fatty acids into mitochondria. In normal patients, the significance of this is unclear, and 7 to 10 days after stopping the drug, serum carnitine levels normalize. Patients with disorders of fatty acid metabolism associated with carnitine deficiency can develop progressive muscle weakness and rhabdomyolysis, but neither has been reported with cefditoren use [37].
      (3) **Cefditoren tablets** contain sodium caseinate, a milk protein. Therefore these **should not be given to patients with milk hypersensitivity** [37].
   f. **Drug interactions.** Absorption can be reduced when cefditoren is taken with antacids with magnesium or aluminum or $H_2$ receptor agonists such as ranitidine [37].
   g. **Cost.** As with other third-generation cephalosporins, a 10-day supply of cefditoren is expensive, although cefditoren is less expensive than cefdinir or cefpodoxime [37] (see Appendix Table).
   h. **Summary.** Cefditoren has no unique clinical niche. In early 2002 the *Medical Letter* concluded the following: "it offers no clinical advantage over cefdinir or cefpodoxime, but it costs less" [37]. Older cephalosporins (e.g., cephalexin for skin infections and cefuroxime for acute exacerbation of chronic bronchitis), the *Medical Letter* went on to conclude, "that have narrower spectrums of activity are as effective as cefditoren for the approved conditions. They are less likely to promote emergence of resistance. Penicillin remains the drug of choice for streptococcal pharyngitis or tonsillitis" [37].

IV. **Side effects of cephalosporins.** Both oral and intravenous formulations are very **well tolerated.**

A. **Primary allergic reactions.** There is approximately a **1% to 3% incidence** of primary allergic reactions to cephalosporins: urticarial and morbilliform rashes, fevers, eosinophilia, and serum sickness. Anaphylaxis is rare, occurring in less than 0.02% of recipients [2]. In individuals with a history of penicillin allergy, risk of an allergic reaction to cephalosporin is up to eight times higher than in those without that history. However, if the history-positive individual is tested and is negative, that excess risk disappears [38] (see Chapter 24). If skin tests are unavailable, the following approach is suggested:

1. **With a history of an immediate reaction to penicillin** (i.e., anaphylaxis, bronchospasm, hypotension, etc.), **cephalosporins should be avoided** [39].
2. **In the patient with a delayed mild reaction** (e.g., morbilliform rash) **to penicillins, cephalosporins are commonly used with caution.** The risk with the

third-generation cephalosporins in this setting is as low as 1%, similar to those without that history [40].

3. **Serum sickness has been observed more in recipients of cefaclor** [40] and with cefprozil [41,42]. Loracarbef may have a risk of serum sickness because its structure is similar to cefaclor.

**B. Nephrotoxicity** is infrequent with cephalosporin monotherapy [1,2]. Interstitial nephritis has occurred as a hypersensitivity response.

**C. Hematologic effects**

1. **Positive Coombs reactions** are relatively common (3%) while on high-dose parenteral therapy [2]. Although hemolytic anemia is quite uncommon, it occurs after cefotetan use [43,44].
2. **Granulocytopenia** and/or **thrombocytopenia** are rare complications. With severe underlying hepatic dysfunction, various $\beta$-lactam antibiotics, including the cephalosporins, have been associated with leukopenia; lower doses of $\beta$-lactam antibiotics should be used [45].
3. **Hypoprothrombinemia** associated with NMTT side chain is discussed in sections **II.B.1** and **II.B.4.** It has also been described with cefazolin use in patients with renal failure because of the side chain similar in structure to NMTT in cefazolin.

**D. Phlebitis** with intravenous use is reported in 1% to 2% and is related more to the known risks of intravenous catheters than to a particular thrombogenic potential of the cephalosporins [2].

**E. Ethanol intolerance.** Disulfiram-like reactions (flushing, tachycardia, nausea, vomiting, headache, hypotension) have been described with patients receiving **cefoperazone, cefotetan,** and cefazolin. The reaction may be related to the NMTT structure. Patients receiving these agents should be advised *not* to consume alcohol or alcohol-containing medications [1,2].

**F. *Clostridium difficile* diarrhea** may occur more often in recipients of second- and third-generation cephalosporins [46], including the oral third-generation agents.

## REFERENCES


1. Reese RE, Betts RF. Cephalosporins. In: Reese RE, Betts RF, Gumustop B, eds. *Handbook of antibiotics,* 3rd ed. Philadelphia: Lippincott Williams & Wilkins, 2000;365–400.
2. Marshall WF, Blair JE. The cephalosporins. *Mayo Clin Proc* 1999;74:187.
3. Asbel LE, Levison ME. Cephalosporins, carbapenems and monobactams. *Infect Dis Clin North Am* 2000;14:1435.
4. Fridkin SK, et al. The effect of vancomycin and third-generation cephalosporins on prevalence of vancomycin-resistant enterococci in 126 intensive care units. *Ann Intern Med* 2001;135:175.
5. Niederman MS, et al. Guidelines for the initial management of adults with community-acquired pneumonia: diagnosis, assessment of severity, and initial antimicrobial therapy. *Am Rev Respir Dis* 1993;148:1418.
6. Thornsberry C, et al. Surveillance of antimicrobial resistance in *Streptococcus pneumoniae, Haemophilus influenzae,* and *Moraxella catarrhalis* in the United States in the 1996–1997 respiratory season. *Diagn Microbiol Infect Dis* 1997;29:249.
7. Medical Letter. The choice of antibacterial drugs. *Med Lett Drugs Ther* 2001;43:69.
8. Medical Letter. Treatment of Lyme disease. *Med Lett Drugs Ther* 2000;42:37.
9. Center for Disease Control and Prevention. Sexually transmitted diseases guidelines 2002. *MMWR Morb Mortal Wkly Rep* 2002;51(RR-6):1.
10. Barza M. Cefotetan: summary of the symposium from an internists viewpoint. *Am J Surg* 1988;155:103.
11. Committee on Antimicrobial Agents, Canadian Infectious Disease Society. Cefotetan: a second-generation cephalosporin active against anaerobic bacteria. *Can Med Assoc J* 1994;151:537.
12. Neu H. Pathophysiologic basis for the use of third generation cephalosporins. *Am J Med* 1990;88[Suppl 4A]:3S.
13. Mathai D, Lewis MT, Kugler KC, et al. The SENTRY Participant Group North America. Antibacterial activity of 41 antimicrobials tested against over 2773 bacterial isolates from hospitalized patients with pneumonia. I. Results from The SENTRY Antimicrobial

Surveillance Program (North America, 1998). *Diagn Microbiol Infect Dis* 2001;39:105–116.

14. Mathai D, Jones RN, Pfaller MA. The SENTRY Participant Group North America. Epidemiology and frequency of resistance among pathogens causing urinary tract infections in 1,510 hospitalized patients: a report of the SENTRY Antimicrobial Surveillance Program North America. *Diagn Microbiol Infect Dis* 2001;40:129–136.
15. Feliciano DV, Gentry LO, Bitondo CG, et al. Single agent prophylaxis for penetrating abdominal trauma. Results and comments on emergence of enterococcus. *Am J Surg* 1986;152:674–681.
16. Lopez AJ, et al. Ceftriaxone-induced cholelithiasis. *Ann Intern Med* 1991;115:712.
17. Barradell LB, Bryson HM. Cefepime: a review of its antimicrobial activity, pharmacokinetic properties, and therapeutic uses. *Drugs* 1994;47:471.
18. Cunha BA, Gill MA. Cefepime. *Med Clin North Am* 1995;79:8–721.
19. Ferrara A, Dos Santos C, Lupi A. Effect of different antibacterial agents and surfactant-A (SP-A) on adherence of some respiratory pathogens to bronchial epithelial cells. *Int J Antimicrob Agents* 2001;17:401–405.
20. Aubert D, Poirel L, Chevalier J, et al. Oxacillinase-mediated resistance to cefepime and susceptibility to ceftazidime in *Pseudomonas aeruginosa. Antimicrob Agents Chemother* 2001;45:1615–1620.
21. Yamamura D, et al. Open randomized study of cefepime versus piperacillin-gentamicin for the treatment of febrile neutropenic cancer patients. *Antimicrob Agents Chemother* 1997;41:1704.
22. Hughes WT, et al. 1997 Guidelines for the use of antimicrobial agents in neutropenic patients with unexplained fever. *Clin Infect Dis* 1997;25:551.
23. Biron P, et al. Cefepime versus imipenem: cilastatin as empirical monotherapy in 400 febrile patients with short duration neutropenia. *J Antimicrob Chemother* 1998;42:511.
24. Ambrose PG, Owens RC Jr, Garvey MJ, et al. Pharmacodynamic considerations in the treatment of moderate to severe pseudomonal infections with cefepime. *J Antimicrob Chemother* 2002;49:445–453.
25. DePauw BE, et al. Ceftazidime compared with piperacillin and tobramycin for empiric treatment of fever in neutropenic patients with cancer: a multi-center randomized trial. *Ann Intern Med* 1994;120:834.
26. Ruff ME, et al. Antimicrobial drug suspensions: a blind comparison of taste of fourteen pediatric drugs. *Pediatr Infect Dis J* 1991;10:30.
27. Baxter R, Chapman J, Drew WI. Comparison of bactericidal activity of five antibiotics against *Staphylococcus aureus. J Infect Dis* 1990;161:23.
28. Aronoff GR, et al. *Drug prescribing in renal failure: dosage guidelines for adults,* 4th ed. Philadelphia: American College of Physicians, 1999.
29. Livornese LL, Slavin D, Benz RL, et al. Use of antibacterial agents in renal failure. *Infect Dis Clin North Am* 2000;14:371–390.
30. Shenep JL, et al. Oral cefixime is similar to continued intravenous antibiotics in the empirical treatment of febrile neutropenic children with cancer. *Clin Infect Dis* 2001;32:36.
31. Medical Letter. Cefpodoxime proxetil: a new oral cephalosporin. *Med Lett Drugs Ther* 1992;34:107.
32. Jones R. Ceftibuten: a review of antimicrobial activity, spectrum and other microbiologic features. *Pediatr Infect Dis J* 1995;14:S77.
33. Medical Letter. Ceftibuten: a new oral cephalosporin. *Med Lett Drugs Ther* 1996;38:23.
34. Medical Letter. Cefdinir: a new oral cephalosporin. *Med Lett Drugs Ther* 1998;40:85.
35. Klein JD, McCracken GH. Summary: role of new oral cephalosporin, cefdinir for therapy of infections in infants and children. *Pediatr Infect Dis* 2000;19[Suppl 1]:81.
36. Fukuoka T, et al. *In vitro* and *in vivo* activities of CS-834, a novel oral carbapenem. *Antimicrob Agents Chemother* 1997;41:2652.
37. Medical Letter. Cefditoren (Spectracef)—a new oral cephalosporin. *Med Lett Drugs Ther* 2002;44:5.
38. Keller PS, Li JTC. Cephalosporin allergy. *N Engl J Med* 2001;345:804.
39. Fekety FR. Safety of parenteral third-generation cephalosporins. *Am J Med* 1990;88[Suppl 4A]:38S.
40. Donowitz GR. Third generation cephalosporins. *Infect Dis Clin North Am* 1989;3:595.

41. Heckbert SR, et al. Serum sickness in children after antibiotic exposure: estimates of occurrence and morbidity in a health maintenance organization population. *Am J Epidemiol* 1990;132:336.
42. Lowery N, et al. Serum sickness-like reactions associated with cefprozil therapy. *J Pediatr* 1994;125:325.
43. Naylor CS, et al. Cefotetan induced hemolysis associated with antibiotic prophylaxis for Cesarean delivery. *Am J Obstet Gynecol* 2000;182:1427.
44. Moes GS, MacPherson BR. Cefotetan-induced hemolytic anemia: a case report and review of the literature. *Arch Pathol Lab Med* 2000; 124:1344–1346.
45. Singh N, et al. B-lactam antibiotic-induced leukopenia in severe hepatic dysfunction: risk factors and implications for dosing patients with liver disease. *Am J Med* 1993;94:251.
46. Nelson DE, et al. Epidemic *Clostridium difficile*-associated diarrhea: role of second- and third-generation cephalosporins. *Infect Control Hosp Epidemiol* 1994;15:88.

## G. Fluoroquinolones

Quinolone antibiotics have been available since the mid-1960's [1–5]. Thousands of different quinolone structures have been synthesized, but fewer than 10 U.S. Food and Drug Administration (FDA)-approved agents are clinically useful [2]. Quinolones can be categorized based on spectrum of antibacterial activity **as shown in Table 27G.1** [4]. The more recently introduced third- and fourth-generation fluoroquinolones are referred to as "expanded-spectrum" fluoroquinolones, in contrast to the earlier second-generation agents such as ciprofloxacin.

Because bacterial resistance to the first-generation quinolones (nalidixic acid, oxolinic acid, cinoxacin) developed rapidly and they are no longer used, they are not mentioned further. The second-generation agents (norfloxacin and ciprofloxacin, followed by ofloxacin) were released between 1986 and 1992. These agents have been very useful clinically for gram-negative or

Table 27G.1. Classification of Quinolones

| |
|---|
| First generation |
| Nalidixic acid[a] |
| Oxolinic acid[a] |
| Cinoxacin[a] |
| Second generation |
| Norfloxacin |
| Ciprofloxacin[b] |
| Ofloxacin |
| Enoxacin[a] |
| Lomefloxacin[a] |
| Third and fourth generation[c] |
| Levofloxacin[d] |
| Sparfloxacin |
| Gatifloxacin[e] |
| Grepafloxacin[f] |
| Trovafloxacin[f] |
| Moxifloxacin[e] |

[a]Withdrawn. See text.
[b]Most potent against *Pseudomonas*.
[c]More potent against *Pneumococcus* and/or anaerobes than were earlier compounds.
[d]Although classified by some as second-generation agent [2], becuase of its expanded spectrum against *S. pneumoniae*, including penicillin-resistant strains (see Chapter 11), it seems appropriate to view this as a third-generation agent.
[e]Most active *in vitro* against *S. pneumoniae*. See text.
[f]More potent against anaerobes but rarely indicated. See text.
Modified from Walker RC. The fluoroquinolones. *Mayo Clin Proc* 1999;74:1030.

mycobacterial infection, but they lack consistent activity against gram-positive cocci such as *Streptococcus pneumoniae* and anaerobes. The recently introduced expanded-spectrum third- and fourth-generation fluoroquinolones, which include sparfloxacin, levofloxacin, gatifloxacin, and moxifloxacin, were introduced after 1997 (Table 27G.1). The third- and fourth-generation quinolones have enhanced gram-positive activity, including penicillin-susceptible and penicillin-resistant *S. pneumoniae,* and modest anaerobic activity. They also have gram-negative activity, except for pseudomonas, and activity against the nonbacterial organisms that cause pneumonia, such as *Mycoplasma pneumoniae,* as well as against *Legionella pneumophila*. This spectrum, plus excellent bioavailability, good tissue penetration, long serum half-life, and safety, have made the fluoroquinolones very attractive agents. **The challenge for the health-care provider is to limit their use to clinical settings that call for their enhanced spectrum.** By doing so, the clinician **will reduce the rate of** resistance selection. These steps will lengthen the useful life of these agents.

In this chapter the terms "fluoroquinolones" and "quinolones" are used interchangeably.

**I. An overview of the fluoroquinolones**

**A. Structure**. Many structural modifications can be made to the basic synthetic nucleus to achieve specific goals such as enhanced gram-positive or anaerobic activity.

**B. Mechanism of action** is reviewed elsewhere [4]. Fluoroquinolones **inhibit DNA gyrase,** a bacterial enzyme essential for DNA replication, and thus inhibit DNA supercoiling. They promote gyrase-mediated double-stranded DNA breakage at specific sites.

**C. *In vitro* activity of the fluoroquinolones** is summarized in Table 27G.2 [4].

1. **Gram-positive bacteria.** Compared with the earlier quinolones, gatifloxacin, moxifloxacin, and to a lesser degree levofloxacin have enhanced activity against *S. pneumoniae,* including penicillin-susceptible and moderately and highly penicillin-resistant strains [6,7] (see Chapters 8, 11, and 27C). However, against penicillin-susceptible *S. pneumoniae,* penicillin is as active *in vitro* as are the quinolones. Some strains of *S. aureus* are susceptible to quinolones, but against methicillin-susceptible *S. aureus,* similarly nafcillin is as active as fluoroquinolones [7] (Table 27G.2) and methicillin-susceptible *S. aureus* is far less likely to develop resistance to nafcillin.
2. **Gram-negative bacteria.** All the fluoroquinolones are very active against gram-negative cocci and bacilli, which cause infections in community-residing individuals, including organisms like *Haemophilus influenzae, Moraxella catarrhalis,* and *Escherichia coli*. Recently, however, a study of sex workers in the Philippines demonstrated that *Neisseria gonorrhoeae* has developed high level resistance to ciprofloxacin; from 1994 through 1996 to 1997, resistance of gonococcal isolates increased from 9% to 49% [8]. This led to a significant number of clinical failures. Against *Pseudomonas aeruginosa* and other hospital gram-negative organisms, the activity of quinolones can be summarized as follows: ciprofloxacin > levofloxacin = gatifloxacin = moxifloxacin = ofloxacin. Sparfloxacin is not approved for pseudomonas.
3. **Anaerobes.** Gatifloxacin and moxifloxacin have some activity. Trovafloxacin is the most active *in vitro* [5] and has been approved for use in anaerobic infections; however, it is rarely used (see later discussion). The others have limited activity against anaerobes.
4. ***Chlamydia/Mycoplasma.*** The recently introduced fluoroquinolones are active against *Mycoplasma pneumoniae, Chlamydia pneumoniae,* and *C. trachomatis*. Ofloxacin is active against *C. trachomatis* (Table 27G.2).
5. ***Legionella pneumophila*.** Ciprofloxacin is quite active, as are the third- and fourth-generation fluoroquinolones. Ofloxacin, though active, is less so.
6. **$\beta$-Lactam-resistant organisms. All fluoroquinolones lack significant activity against** methicillin-resistant *S. aureus,* vancomycin-resistant enterococci, and multidrug-resistant nosocomial gram-negative organisms (e.g., *Stenotrophomonas maltophilia*).
7. **Miscellaneous. In foreign body infection,** there is laboratory evidence that quinolones are relatively more active against bacteria attached to foreign bodies than are the $\beta$-lactams. Furthermore, the quinolones adhere to such

Table 27G.2. Comparative *In Vitro* Minimum Inhibitory Concentrations ($MIC_{90}$) ($\mu$g/mL)

| Organism | Levofloxacin | Moxifloxacin | Gatifloxacin | Ciprofloxacin | Ofloxacin |
|---|---|---|---|---|---|
| *S. aureus* (MSSA) | 0.25 | 0.06 | 0.10–0.13 | 0.5–8 | 0.25–0.05 |
| *S. aureus* (MRSA) | 16 | 4 | 0.20–16 | 1–64 | 16–32 |
| *S. aureus* (CRSA) | 8 | 2 | 6.25 | CRSA | — |
| *S. epidermidis* | 0.5–1 | 0.13 | 0.20–0.25 | — | — |
| *E. faecalis* | 1–3.13 | 1 | 0.78–2 | 1–8 | 2–8 |
| *E. faccium* | 3.13–8 | 1–4 | 1.56–4 | >16 | >16 |
| *S. pneumoniae* | 1–3.13 | 0.12–0.25 | 0.5 | 1–4 | 1–4 |
| *S. pyogenes* | 1 | 0.25 | 0.39–0.5 | 0.5 | 2 |
| *E. cloacae* | 0.06 | 0.06 | 0.06–0.20 | 1–2 | 0.06–4 |
| *E. coli* | 0.03 | 0.008 | 0.016–0.1 | <0.015–0.5 | 0.05–0.12 |
| Ampicillin-resistant *E.coli* | 16 | 8 | 8 | — | — |
| *H. influenzae* | 0.06 | 0.06 | 0.013–0.016 | 0.02–0.06 | 0.03–0.06 |
| *K. pneumoniae* | 0.13 | 0.013 | 0.10–0.39 | 0.06–4 | 1–2 |
| Ceftazidime-resistant *K. pneumoniae* | 16 | 8 | 4 | — | — |
| *M. catarrhalis* | 0.03 | 0.03 | 0.013–0.6 | — | — |
| *N. gonorrhoeae* | 0.016 | 0.016 | 0.006–0.025 | 0.008 | 0.03 |
| *P. aeruginosa* | 2–8 | 1–4 | 3.13–32 | 0.25–>16 | 2–>16 |
| *Salmonella* species | 0.03 | 0.13 | 0.06–0.25 | 0.03 | 0.25 |
| *S. marcescens* | 8 | 8 | 1.56–12.5 | 0.12–2 | 0.5–4 |
| *B. fragilis* | 2 | 0.12 | 0.25–1 | 4–64 | 4–64 |
| *C. difficile* | 8 | — | 1–2 | — | — |
| *Peptostreptococcus* species | 3.13–>4 | 2 | 1 | 0.25–8 | 0.5–8 |
| *M. pneumoniae* | — | 0.06–0.12 | 0.05 | 1 | 1 |
| *L. pneumophila* | 0.032 | 0.015 | 0.016 | 0.015 | 0.015 |
| *C. trachomatis* | 0.25–0.5 | 0.03–0.125 | 0.063–0.125 | 2 | 1 |
| *C. pneumoniae* | 0.25–0.5 | 0.03–1 | 0.063–0.125 | — | — |
| *U. urealyticum* | — | — | 0.78 | 16 | 2 |

MSSA, methicillin-sensitive *S. aureus*; MRSA, methicillin-resistant *S. aureus*; CRSA, ciprofloxacin-resistant *S. aureus.*
Modified from O'Donnell JA, Gelone SP. Fluoroquinolones. *Infect Dis Clin North AM* 2000;14:489 for data on levofloxacin, moxifloxacin, and gatifloxacin; and from Garey KW, Amsden GW. Trovofloxacin: an overview. *Pharmacotherapy* 1999;19:21 for data on ciprofloxacin and ofloxacin.

foreign bodies as ureteral stents at concentrations that exceed the minimum inhibitory concentration of possible infecting organisms [9]. This has led to their use in artificial joint infection, sometimes combined with rifampin (see related discussions in Chapters 5 and 27R).

**D. Pharmacokinetics**

1. **Oral absorption.** Fluoroquinolones are **well absorbed** [1–4,10]. In obese subjects, weight-adjusted dosing yielded higher serum concentrations but similar tissue fluid concentrations compared with those occurring in nonobese subjects receiving standard doses [11]. **Certain drugs taken concomitantly will interfere with the absorption of quinolones.** If antacids, sucralfate, magnesium, aluminum, iron, zinc, calcium, or didanosine are taken together with an oral fluoroquinolone, absorption of the latter is reduced.
2. **Intravenous (i.v.) preparations** are available for ciprofloxacin, ofloxacin, trovafloxacin, levofloxacin, gatifloxacin, and moxifloxacin. **Oral regimens provide similar serum levels** as the more expensive i.v. formulations, and thus oral should be used preferentially [1,2]. The i.v. formulations are indicated for patients who cannot take anything by mouth or have active nausea and vomiting. If enteral nutrition is possible, patients can be on oral therapy [1,2].
3. **Tissue penetration.** Fluoroquinolones penetrate tissue well, including lung, bronchial mucosa, kidney, prostate, bone, and the genital tract.
4. **Renal excretion varies** [2]. All quinolones require dose reduction in the setting of both renal and hepatic dysfunction.
   a. **Levofloxacin and ofloxacin** depend entirely on renal excretion; dosage modification is required in renal failure.
   b. **Ciprofloxacin, sparfloxacin, and gatifloxacin:** moderate dosage adjustments are necessary in renal failure.
   c. **About 50% of moxifloxacin** is metabolized in the liver; dosage reduction is not necessary.
   d. **Trovafloxacin** is eliminated entirely by the hepatic route. No dosage change is necessary except in hepatic failure.
5. **Concentration-dependent killing.** Like gentamicin, fluoroquinolones have **"concentration-dependent killing"** and postantibiotic effect against gram-negative organisms [2,10] (see Chapter 25). If high peak serum concentration to minimum inhibitory concentration ratios are achieved, some experts believe the emergence of resistant bacteria may be reduced [12] (also see section **V.B**).
6. **Drug interactions** are discussed in section **F.4**.
7. **Topical** solutions are available for certain eye and ear infections (see Chapters 7 and 8 and section **II.B.12.f**).

**E. Adverse reactions.** Fluoroquinolones are well tolerated [1,2,13–15]. Although the clinical impression has been that side effects may be more common in the elderly (i.e., those older than 65 years of age), recently that opinion has been challenged [15]. **Side effects have recently been reviewed [13,14] and include the following:**

1. **Gastrointestinal symptoms,** primarily nausea but also anorexia, vomiting, and/or diarrhea, occur in about 5% or more. *C. difficile* diarrhea occurs but is uncommon, perhaps because of the quinolones minimal effect on anaerobic flora [13].
2. **Cutaneous reactions,** including nonspecific rashes and urticaria, occur in 1% to 2%. **Sparfloxacin** has **increased** rates of **phototoxicity** (see section **III.C.1**).
3. **Hepatotoxicity.** Liver function test abnormalities and hepatic toxicity are minimal in the commonly used quinolones. The exception is trovafloxacin [1,3,14], which has been associated with severe hepatotoxicity. During the 18 months after the release of this drug, several cases of severe liver toxicity, including acute liver failure and some deaths, were reported. In mid-1999, the FDA recommended that trovafloxacin should be used only for life-threatening or limb-threatening infections with initial i.v. therapy started in an inpatient setting; see related discussions under section **III.C.2.**
4. **Central nervous system symptoms** occur in 1% to 4% of patients, mainly the elderly. The most common symptoms are headaches (mild), slight dizziness, mild sleep disturbance, and alteration of mood with agitation, anxiety, or depression.

**Seizures** have rarely been reported and may occur in patients receiving other medications simultaneously, such as nonsteroidal antiinflammatory agents with any quinolone: theophylline with ciprofloxacin and moxifloxacin with metronidazole.

5. **QT prolongation with torsades de pointes** has been described with the use of some of the quinolones. This is an evolving area of interest, and up to date information is available from two excellent websites, *www.qtdrugs.org* and *www.Torsades.org,* which provide listings of drugs with this possible complication and current references for drugs that may prolong the QTc interval and/or may be associated with torsades. In recent discussions of this topic [16,16a], the authors conclude that moxifloxacin, levofloxacin, and gatifloxacin **should not be used in patients with risk factors predisposing them to prolonged QTc interval and therefore torsades.** Risk factors included female gender; presence of underlying cardiac disease, including congestive heart failure; advanced age; hypokalemia; hypomagnesemia; and use of concomitant drugs known to prolong the QTc, interval such as the class Ia (e.g., quinidine, procainamide) and III antiarrhythmics such as amiodarone or sotalol [17].

   See section III. under individual agents also.
6. **Tendon rupture** [10]. Postmarketing data suggest that quinolone use may be associated with tendon rupture, primarily the Achilles tendon (unilateral or bilateral) but also in the shoulder and hand. *In vitro* studies indicate that ciprofloxacin interferes with collagen synthesis. Tendon rupture is more common in men over age 50 and in those on steroids. **Therefore at the first sign of tendon pain or inflammation, quinolone should be discontinued** and exercise avoided until the tendonitis has subsided. This topic has recently been reviewed [18].
7. **Drug interactions** (see section **F.4**)

F. **Precautions in use** [19–24]

1. **Do not use in patients allergic to either the early analogues** (e.g., nalidixic acid, oxolinic acid, or cinoxacin) or other fluoroquinolones.
2. **Avoid systemic use in children.** Fluoroquinolones produce cartilage erosion in young animals. The clinical importance of this has not been demonstrated. Although topical preparations have been used in ear and eye infections (see section **II.B.12.f**), the *Red Book* [20], Centers for Disease Control and Prevention [25], and other experts [19,21] do not recommend systemic (oral or i.v.) fluoroquinolones for use in children with the following exceptions [1,2,19–21,26]:
   a. **Cystic fibrosis** patients, because the benefits are believed to outweigh the potential risks. Investigations of ciprofloxacin use in this setting have demonstrated no adverse effects [19].
   b. **In special circumstances** fluoroquinolones may be justified in children younger than 18 years when alternatives are not available [20,21]. For a detailed discussion see the *Red Book* [20]. For children over 45 kg, the Centers for Disease Control and Prevention policy is that adult quinolone regimens can be used and adult doses are advised [25].
   c. Topical agents have been used in eye and ear infections (see Chapter 7 and section **II.B.12.f**).
3. **Avoid in pregnancy and nursing mothers** because of the potential effect on developing cartilage (see section **2**). The fluoroquinolones are **category C** agents (see Chapter 27A).
4. **Drug interactions**
   a. **Antacids** containing magnesium or aluminum markedly diminish absorption. This effect is minimized if the antacid is taken 2 to 3 hours after the fluoroquinolone. **Other multivalent metal cations** impair absorption (see prior discussion in section **D**).
   b. **Theophylline levels** are **increased by ciprofloxacin.** See individual agents.
   c. **Caffeine.** Fluoroquinolones, especially **ciprofloxacin, can increase caffeine levels.** Avoid fluoroquinolones late in the evening with a heavy caffeine load.
   d. **Warfarin.** Whether a warfarin–fluoroquinolone interaction occurs remains

unanswered [22]. Close monitoring of prothrombin time while on warfarin and fluoroquinolones seems prudent.

e. **Cyclosporine.** Interaction of cyclosporine and fluoroquinolones is unclear. Monitoring of serum concentrations of cyclosporine and measures of renal function has been suggested [22].

G. **Cost.** In general, fluoroquinolones are expensive agents (see Appendix Table).

II. **Clinical indications**

A. **Drugs of choice.** Although the fluoroquinolones have an FDA-approved indication for many infections, they are drugs of choice **only for the following** [23]:

1. *Salmonella or Shigella* species
2. *Neisseria gonorrhoeae* (with ceftriaxone and cefixime)
3. *P. aeruginosa* urinary tract infections (UTIs)
4. *Legionella* species rifampin (azithromycin is also a drug of choice) N.B. For indications 1 to 3 above, many fluoroquinolones are effective, but ciprofloxacin has often been used for *Legionella* infections.

B. **Common empiric uses,** but not antibiotic of choice. They are used when the infecting organism is suspected to be resistant to the preferred agent or if the illness is severe (Table 27G.3). Certain issues need special emphasis.

1. **UTIs.** Most uncomplicated community-acquired UTI is due to pathogens susceptible to trimethoprim-sulfamethoxazole (TMP-SMX), so this is usually the preferred agent. However, as discussed in Chapter 27L, the incidence of TMP-SMX resistance for community-acquired *E. coli* is rising and is 15% to 20% in some regions of the United States. Hence, in some areas of the United States and for pyelonephritis or for UTI in diabetics, use ciprofloxacin until susceptibility data are available. Ciprofloxacin is preferred for anyone if *P. aeruginosa* is suspected. **See the related discussions in Chapters 15 and 27L.** The fluoroquinolones are very useful for complex UTI due to susceptible pathogens and many but not all nosocomial UTI.

Table 27G.3. An Overview of the Fluoroquinolones

| Setting | Suggested Agent[a] | Related Discussions |
|---|---|---|
| UTI | Ciprofloxacin | Chapter 15 |
| Prostatitis | Ciprofloxacin | Chapter 15 |
| Urethritis/PID | Ofloxacin | Chapter 16 |
| Intraabdominal infection | Ciprofloxacin + metronidazole, (or clindamycin) | Chapter 13 |
| Traveler's diarrhea | Ciprofloxacin | Chapter 13 |
| Bacterial diarrhea | Ciprofloxacin | Chapter 13 |
| Diabetic foot infections | Ciprofloxacin and anaerobic therapy in advanced infections | Chapter 4 |
| CAP | Moxifloxacin,[b,c] or gatifloxacin,[b,c] or levofloxacin[b,c] | Chapter 11 |
| Nosocomial pneumonia | Choice guided by susceptibility data. See text. | Chapter 11 |
| Selected cases of sinusitis, refractory otitis, acute exacerbations of COPD (see text) | Moxifloxacin,[b] or gatifloxacin,[b] or levofloxacin[b,c] | Chapter 8 |
| Septic arthritis, osteomyelitis[d] | Ciprofloxacin | Chapter 5 |

[a] Seems prudent to use the narrowest-spectrum fluoroquinolone that will do the job.
[b] Optimal agent is unclear. See text sec. III.B.3 and III.B.9.
[c] An advanced-generation fluoroquinolone, with activity against penicillin resistant *S. pneumoniae* is preferred. This agent is also active against common CAP pathogens and atypical pathogens.
[d] Primarily due to susceptible gram negatives. See Chapter 5.

2. **Prostatitis.** TMP, TMP-SMX, and the fluoroquinolones all penetrate the prostate well. Based on susceptibility data and/or side effect profile, fluoroquinolones are often used in this setting [24], although both TMP and TMP-SMX are more cost effective (see Chapter 15).
3. **Urethritis/cervicitis/pelvic inflammatory disease. Ofloxacin** is currently the preferred fluoroquinolone [25,26] and the agent with which there is the most experience (see Chapter 16).
4. **Intraabdominal infections.** Ciprofloxacin plus metronidazole (or clindamycin) provides good gram-negative and anaerobic activity, respectively. The many other antibiotic options one can use in this setting are discussed in Chapter 13.
5. **Traveler's diarrhea.** The fluoroquinolones (ciprofloxacin) are preferred (see Chapters 13 and 22).
6. **Diabetic foot infections** and therapeutic options are discussed in **Chapter 5.** There has been the greatest clinical experience with ciprofloxacin in this setting, and it remains the most active currently available fluoroquinolone against *P. aeruginosa.*
7. **Refractory sinusitis/otitis media.** When antibiotic therapy is indicated, amoxicillin remains the agent of choice for acute sinusitis and otitis media. When this agent fails or in the patient with multiple antibiotic allergies, moxifloxacin or gatifloxacin, with activity against penicillin-resistant *S. pneumoniae,* may be indicated (see Chapter 8).
8. **Acute exacerbation of chronic bronchitis** can usually be treated with less expensive and narrower spectrum antibiotics **(see Chapter 11).** Occasionally, in the allergic patient or with culture-proven resistant pathogens, a 5-day course of either moxifloxacin or gatifloxacin that are active against *S. pneumoniae* and *Haemophilus* species is reasonable.
9. **Community-acquired pneumonia (CAP)** is **discussed** in **Chapter 11.** The advanced-generation fluoroquinolones such as moxifloxacin or gatifloxacin and, to a lesser degree, levofloxacin are active against the common pathogens causing CAP, including penicillin-susceptible or -resistant *S. pneumoniae, H. influenzae, M. catarrhalis* and the atypical organisms, including *Mycoplasma* and *Chlamydia* species and *Legionella pneumophila* [6,7,27]. Consequently, these advanced quinolones have become very popular in the therapy of CAP. They are included as agents of possible choice in the therapeutic guidelines for CAP [28]. To avoid the rapid development of bacterial resistance, fluoroquinolones should be used judiciously in CAP [29]. See related discussion in section **V.B** and in Chapter 11.
   a. **Macrolides** remain agents of choice for CAP in those under 50 years of age.
   b. Advanced fluoroquinolones are useful in patients with known or highly likely penicillin-resistant *S. pneumoniae* pneumonia and/or if very ill with pneumonia and multilobar disease, requiring intensive care unit care while awaiting susceptibility data and other information (see Chapter11). These agents are indicated in other selected cases.
10. **Nosocomial pneumonia** usually occurs in ventilated patients, so-called ventilator-associated pneumonia.
    a. When fever develops in the patient on a ventilator, very frequently the cause is far from clear. It has recently been shown that in the patient who did not fulfill the criteria for definite pneumonia, ciprofloxacin, initiated at the onset of the fever, could be safely stopped after 3 days instead of continuing a full 7 to 10 days. When this was done, the patients had equal or better outcome [30] compared with those in whom the drug was continued for 7 to 10 days. **In those with clear-cut ventilator-associated pneumonia, initial empiric therapy** often involves combination therapy (e.g., antipseudomonal penicillin and an aminoglycoside) until culture data are available. An advanced fluoroquinolone (with or without) aztreonam may be useful in the allergic patient. See related discussions in Chapter 11.
    b. **For completion of therapy** an oral fluoroquinolone can often be used; the agent selected will depend on culture data, if available, or local susceptibility patterns and trends.

11. **Septic arthritis and osteomyelitis** due to susceptible pathogens, primarily gram-negative organisms, have been treated with fluoroquinolones, most commonly ciprofloxacin (see Chapter 5). More recently, ciprofloxacin with rifampin has been shown to be effective in staphylococcal infections of artificial hips. **The quinolone was chosen to be combined with rifampin** because of the quinolone's superior activity against gram-positive organisms attached to foreign material. However, when ciprofloxacin is used by itself, development of resistance, and clinical failure, is common [31]. See related discussions in section **I.C.7** and Chapters 5 and 27R.
12. **Miscellaneous**
    a. **Meningococcal carrier state.** Ciprofloxacin is a drug of choice (see Chapter 6).
    b. **Cat scratch disease,** due to *Bartonella henselae,* has been treated with ciprofloxacin [32], although azithromycin is listed as the drug of choice for this pathogen [23], with ciprofloxacin listed as an alternative agent.
    c. **Fever of unclear etiology in the leukopenic patient.** In an attempt to avoid hospitalization or minimize the hospital stay, oral antibiotics are being evaluated in these patients. Ciprofloxacin, which is very active against gram-negative organisms, combined with an agent for gram-positive organisms such as amoxicillin-clavulanate, has been studied [33–35]. For the hospitalized patient, ciprofloxacin plus piperacillin appears to be useful [36]. See related discussions in Chapter 20.
    d. **Mycobacterial infections** are sometimes treated with fluoroquinolones [32,37] (see Chapter 11). Infectious disease and/or pulmonary consultation is advised.
    e. **Patients with cystic fibrosis** and pulmonary colonization/infection with *Pseudomonas* have been treated with ciprofloxacin (see section **I.F.2**).
    f. **Selected ear infections in children have been treated with topical agents.** Ciprofloxacin HC otic suspension has been used for **otitis externa** (see Chapter 8) and ofloxacin otic solution has been approved for use in otitis externa, **chronic suppurative otitis media,** and the otorrhea of acute otitis media that occurs **in children with tympanostomy tubes** 1 year of age and older. The use of these topical agents has been reviewed in detail in a recently published symposium devoted to this topic [38].

III. **Brief comment on individual agents.** Although several agents are available, in the past decade of using these antibiotics, **certain common practices and special niches have often evolved** that have allowed the clinician to use selected agents effectively while eliminating other agents (Table 27G.3). In addition to the general comments made in section **I,** we emphasize the following:

A. **Second-generation agents**

1. **Norfloxacin (Noroxin),** available in 1986, provides good urinary and gastrointestinal levels but does not provide acceptable serum levels or nonrenal tissue levels. It is potentially a useful agent in uncomplicated UTI, traveler's diarrhea, and for spontaneous bacterial peritonitis prophylaxis in cirrhosis. It **has been replaced by ciprofloxacin,** even for the latter indications.
2. **Ciprofloxacin (Cipro)** was released in late 1987 and **remains a very useful agent.** It **remains more active against *P. aeruginosa* than any other fluoroquinolone.** However, it is not as active against penicillin-susceptible or -resistant pneumococci or against anaerobes, as are the third- and fourth-generation agents. Ciprofloxacin can raise theophylline and caffeine levels and causes central nervous system symptoms in the elderly but is otherwise well tolerated (see section **I.E**).
3. **Ofloxacin (Floxin)** was released in 1990. In the review in *Medical Letter* the contributors concluded that ofloxacin "appears to be equivalent to ciprofloxacin" for UTI, prostatitis, skin and soft tissue infections, lower respiratory tract infections, and "can be used for chlamydial infections" [39]. Ofloxacin is active against *C. trachomatis,* and there is considerable experience with its use for these infections. It has therefore achieved a special niche in the therapy of **nongonococcal urethritis, where it remains the quinolone of choice and is part of some**

**of the regimens for pelvic inflammatory disease** [25] (see Chapter 16). Ofloxacin **does not interfere with theophylline or caffeine** metabolism as may ciprofloxacin. It is not approved for osteomyelitis.

**B. Third- and fourth-generation agents: expanded spectrum.** There are three currently available agents in common use, levofloxacin, moxifloxacin, and gatifloxacin. The latter two were approved in late December 1999 for use in CAP, acute bacterial exacerbations of chronic bronchitis, and acute sinusitis [6,7,41–45]. Both agents are active against *Legionella* species and *M. pneumoniae* and both have less than optimal activity against some anaerobes. Neither drug affects the cytochrome P450 enzyme system [41]. Because of the potential **for prolongation of the QT interval** with both of these agents [41], while awaiting further clinical experience **we believe it is prudent to limit their use in patients who have other risk factors for QT prolongation. See related discussion under section I.E.5.**

1. **Levofloxacin (Levaquin)** became available in late 1997 [40]. This expanded-spectrum fluoroquinolone **has good activity against penicillin-resistant** *S. pneumoniae* (see Chapter 11) **and other CAP pathogens.** However, the minimum inhibitory concentration of *S. pneumoniae* is very close to the maximum achievable serum levels, and in some experts' opinions this fact may be contributing to the development of resistance in quinolones [3,12] (also see section **V.B**). It has been used in selected cases of CAP and selected cases of refractory sinusitis, otitis in adults, and acute exacerbations of chronic obstructive pulmonary disease (see Chapter 8). It is also used in some of the regimens for sexually transmitted diseases (e.g., nongonococcal urethritis, gonococcal (GC) urethritis, pelvic inflammatory disease regimens, etc.) [25]. The oral formulation is extremely well absorbed. **Oral and i.v. formulations are 99% bioequivalent.** One dose per day is needed; the dose interval is prolonged in renal failure.
2. **Moxifloxacin (Avelox)** has improved gram-positive activity over levofloxacin [40,41,45], including penicillin-resistant *S. pneumoniae,* but is less active against Enterobacteriaceae than ciprofloxacin and has little activity against *Pseudomonas* species. In addition to the indications listed in section **B** above, it is approved for use in uncomplicated skin and soft tissue infections due to susceptible *S. aureus* or *Streptococcus pyogenes.*
   a. **Dosage.** In adults, 400 mg orally is given once daily, without dose adjustment in renal failure. It does not interfere with theophylline or warfarin and has a low propensity for phototoxicity and central nervous system side effects.
   b. **Side effects** (see section **I.E**)
   c. **Cost** (see Appendix Table 1)
3. **Gatifloxacin (Tequin)** has similar *in vitro* activity [6,7,41,42] to moxifloxacin. In a recent report, gatifloxacin was about fourfold more active *in vitro* against *S. pneumoniae* than levofloxacin [42]. In addition to the respiratory tract infections listed under section **3** above, gatifloxacin is approved for used in uncomplicated and complicated UTI and for uncomplicated gonococcal infections (see Chapter 16).
   a. **Dosage.** Oral tablets and an i.v. preparation are available. The usual adult dose is 400 mg orally or intravenously every 24 hours with reduction if the creatinine clearance is less than 40 mL/min (Table 27G.4).
   b. **Cost** (see Appendix Table)
4. **Levofloxacin versus moxifloxacin versus gatifloxacin.** The optimal quinolone for use in CAP due to known or highly suspected penicillin-resistant *S. pneumoniae* is unclear as of mid-2002. There is more clinical experience with levofloxacin, but as discussed in earlier sections either gatifloxacin or moxifloxacin provides a greater therapeutic ratio that may be advantageous. The precise risk of QTc-related problems with any of these agents continues to undergo study and awaits further clinical experience. Clinically significant QTc prolongation appears to be rare and, when it occurs, may be more likely to take place in patients with more than one risk factor associated with QTc prolongation (see section **I.E.5**). Therefore, in patients with more than one risk factor for QTc prolongation, we would favor using an alternative class of antibiotic (see Chapter 11).

Table 27G.4. Dose Adjustments in Renal Failure

| | Creatinine Clearance (mL/min) | | | | |
|---|---|---|---|---|---|
| | >50 | 10–50 | <10 | Hemodialysis (HD) | CAPD |
| Ciprofloxacin | 100%[a] | 50–75%[a] | 50%[a] | 250 mg p.o. or 200 mg i.v. q12h | 250 mg p.o. q8h or 200 mg i.v. q8h |
| Ofloxacin | 100%[a] | 200–400 mg q24h | 200 mg q24h | 100–200 mg after HD | Same as for creatinine clearance <10 mL/min |
| Levofloxacin | 100%[a] | 250 mg q24–48h after usual 500-mg initial dose | 250 mg q48h after usual 500-mg initial dose | Same as for creatinine clearance <10 mL/min | |
| Gatifloxacin | 100% | [b] | [b] | [b] | [b] |
| Moxifloxacin | 100% | 100% | 100% | [c] | [c] |

[a]Refers to % of usual dose, when renal function is normal.
[b]For gatifloxacin, if the creatinine clearance is <40 mL/min, an initial dose of 400 mg can be given followed by subsequent doses (beginning day 2) of 200 mg q.d. A similar regimen is advised for patients on hemodialysis or undergoing CAPD.
[c]Dosages in hemodialysis and CAPD have not been studied yet per 2002 package insert.
Modified from Aronoff GR, et al, eds. *Drug prescribing in renal failure: dosing guidelines for adults,* 4th ed. Philadelphia: American College of Physicians, 1999; and *Physicians desk reference,* 56th ed. Montvale, N J: Medical Economics Co, 2002, with permission.

Because these are evolving issues, at this point we would advise discussing the optimal agent with an infectious disease subspecialist, especially if there are risk factors associated with QTc prolongation.

**C. Rarely used or recently withdrawn agents** include the following.

1. **Sparfloxacin (Zagam).** This agent was introduced in late 1997. A generic preparation is available but because this agent has been associated with significant problems with photosensitivity and QT prolongation with torsades, **we would use an alternate quinolone.**
2. **Trovofloxacin (Trovan)** was approved for use in early 1998. *In vitro,* this agent is active against pathogens causing CAP, many gram-negative bacilli, and anaerobes. It has good bioavailability, and both oral and i.v. formulations are available. **Because of the hepatotoxicity discussed previously (see section I.E.3) and the availability of other quinolones or other classes of antibiotics, we do not use this agent.** We would not suggest using trovafloxacin unless in a special circumstance and in consultation with an infectious disease specialist. Therefore this agent is not discussed further. Of interest, trovafloxacin is not listed as an important quinolone in the recent *Medical Letter* [23].
3. **Enoxacin** has been **withdrawn.**
4. **Lomefloxacin (Maxaquin)** was released in 1992, but patients on this agent had **moderate to severe phototoxic reactions.** This agent has been **withdrawn.**
5. **Grepafloxacin (Raxar)** was approved for use in late 1997. It was associated with prolongation of the QT interval, and in late 1999 it was voluntarily **withdrawn** from the market due to severe cardiovascular adverse reactions [14].

**IV. Dosages of fluoroquinolones**

**A. With normal renal function, see Table 27G.5.**

**B. In renal failure, see Table 27G.4.**

**V. Miscellaneous**

**A. Cost.** In general, the fluoroquinolones are **expensive** agents (see Appendix Table). Nevertheless, they may be cost-effective agents if they can shorten the hospital stay, or the oral form is used to avoid hospitalization for i.v. antibiotic administration, or early switch from the i.v. formulation to the oral form is carried out.

**B. Resistance to fluoroquinolones** [2,8,46–52]. With widespread use of the fluoroquinolones, selective pressure is exerted, particularly in intensive care and specialized care units in hospitals [2]. This has resulted in the emergence of quinolone-resistant bacteria [2]. Resistance develops by mechanisms of reduced drug penetration, altered regulation of active efflux mechanisms [2,3], and DNA gyrase mutations.

1. **Nosocomial pathogens**
   - a. **Methicillin-resistant *S. aureus*** is resistant to available fluoroquinolones or will become so with use in a patient.
   - b. ***P. aeruginosa.*** Resistance is common with infections involving a foreign body, such as a Foley catheter or a tracheostomy, or with prolonged use as occurs in cystic fibrosis respiratory infections. At this time approximately 15% to 30% of *P. aeruginosa* are resistant to all available fluoroquinolones.
   - c. ***Serratia marcescens,* other *Pseudomonas* species,** and ***Acinetobacter* species** often are resistant. *S. maltophilia* is resistant, even when laboratory tests report susceptibility. In a recent report [48], 56% of extended-spectrum $\beta$-lactamase–producing *E. coli* and *Klebsiella pneumoniae* isolates were resistant to the fluoroquinolones.
2. **Community-acquired** resistance of bacteria has been uncommon. Recently, pneumococci with decreased susceptibility to quinolones have been described [50], and treatment failures with levofloxacin have occurred [51,52]. Some experts believe that recent exposure to a fluoroquinolone should be a contraindication to the use of another fluoroquinolone for the empiric treatment of CAP [51,52]. Although fluoroquinolone-resistant *N. gonorrhoeae* have been isolated in the Far East, such strains fortunately have only been rarely isolated in the United States [8,49]. There is concern that resistance may increase due to use of fluoroquinolones in

Table 27G.5. Dosages in Normal Renal Function

| | | |
|---|---|---|
| Ciprofloxacin p.o.[a] | | |
| UTI | | |
| Acute, uncomplicated | 100 mg p.o. bid | × 3 days |
| Mild and moderate | 250 mg p.o. bid | 10–14 days |
| Severe, complicated, pyelonephritis | 500 mg p.o. bid | 14 days |
| Prostatitis | 500 mg p.o. bid | 2–4 weeks. See text |
| Intraabdominal infection[b] | 500 mg p.o. bid | 10–14 days |
| Traveler's diarrhea | 500 mg p.o. bid | 3 days |
| Bacterial diarrhea | 500 mg p.o. bid | 5–7 days[c] |
| Susceptible lower respiratory tract gram negatives (e.g., hospital-acquired pneumonia) | 500–750 mg p.o. bid | At least 14 days total treatment. See text. |
| Septic arthritis, osteomyelitis due to susceptible pathogens | 500–750 mg p.o. bid | See Chapter 5. |
| Ofloxacin (p.o./i.v.) | | |
| Acute, uncomplicated urethral and cervical gonorrhea | 400 mg, single dose | 1 day |
| Nongonococcal cervicitis/urethritis due to *C. trachomatis* | 300 mg bid | 7 days |
| Mixed infection of the urethra and cervix due to *C. trachomatis* and *N. gonorrhoeae* | 300 mg bid | 7 days |
| Acute pelvic inflammatory disease[d] | 400 mg bid | 14 days |
| Levofloxacin (p.o./i.v.) | | |
| CAP | 500 mg q24h | 10–14 days |
| Susceptible lower respiratory infections in hospitalized patients | 500 mg q24h | 10–14 days |
| Selected cases of sinusitis, bronchitis | 500 mg q24h | 5–7 days |
| Gatifloxacin (p.o./i.v.) | | |
| CAP | 400mg q24h | 7–14 days |
| Selected cases of | | |
| Sinusitis | 400mg q24h | 10 days |
| Bronchitis in COPD | 400mg q24h | 5–7 days |
| Moxifloxacin (p.o./i.v.) | | |
| CAP | 400mg q24h | 10 days |
| Selected cases of | | |
| Sinusitis | 400mg q24h | 10 days |
| Bronchitis In COPD | 400mg q24h | 5 days |

[a] Ciprofloxacin can be given i.v.: for mild to moderate UTI 200 mg i.v. q12h; for severe or complicated UTI 400 mg q12h. Doses given over 60 min. A 500-mg p.o. dose and a 400-mg i.v. dose provide similar serum levels.
[b] Needs to be combined with an anaerobic agent (e.g., metronidazole or clindamycin). See Chapter 13.
[c] Typhoid fever is treated with 10 days.
[d] Ofloxacin is combined with metronidazole. See details of therapy of PID in Chapter 16.

both human and animal food [47]; quinolone-resistant *Salmonella* species have been isolated [53,54].

## REFERENCES


1. Reese RE, Betts RF. Fluoroquinolones. In: Reese RE, Betts RF, Gumustop B, eds. *Handbook of antibiotics,* 3rd ed. Philadelphia: Lippincott Williams & Wilkins, 2000.
2. Walker RC. The fluoroquinolones. *Mayo Clin Proc* 1999;74:1030;544–563.
3. O'Donnell JA, Gelone SP. Fluoroquinolones. *Infect Dis Clin North Am* 2000;14:489.
4. Andriole VT. The quinolones: prospects. In: Andriole VT, ed. *The quinolones,* 2nd ed. San Diego: Academic Press, 1998;117–142.
5. Garey KW, Amsden GW. Trovofloxacin: an overview. *Pharmacotherapy* 1999;19:21.
6. Barman-Balfour JA, Wiseman LR. Moxifloxacin. *Drugs* 1999;57:363.
7. Perry CM, Balfour JA, Lamb HM. Gatifloxacin. *Drugs* 1999;58:683.
8. Aplasca De Los Reyes MR, Pato-Mesola V, Klausner JD, et al. A randomized trial of ciprofloxacin versus cefixime for treatment of gonorrhea after rapid emergence of gonococcal ciprofloxacin resistance in the Philippines. *Clin Infect Dis* 2001;32:1313.
9. Reid G, Habash M, Vachon D, et al. Oral fluoroquinolone therapy results in drug adsorption on ureteral stents and prevention of biofilm formation. *Int J Antimicrob Agents* 2001;17:317–319.
10. Lode H, Borner K, Koeppe P. Pharmacodynamics of fluoroquinolones. *Clin Infect Dis* 1999;27:33.
11. Hollenstein UM, Brunner M, Schmid R, et al. Soft tissue concentrations of ciprofloxacin in obese and lean subjects following weight adjusted dosing. *Int J Obesity Relat Metab Dis* 2001;25:354–358.
12. Craig WA. Does dose matter? *Clin Infect Dis* 2001;33[Suppl 3]:S233.
13. Lipsky BA, Baker C. Fluoroquinolone toxicity profiles: a review focusing on newer agents. *Clin Infect Dis* 1999;28:352.
14. Mandell LA, Ball P, Tillotson G. Antimicrobial safety and tolerability: differences and dilemmas. *Clin Infect Dis* 2001;32[Suppl 1]:S572.
15. Heyd A, Haverstock D. Retrospective analysis of the safety profile of oral and intravenous ciprofloxacin in a geriatric population. *Clin Therap* 2000;22:1239–1250.
16. Owens RC Jr, Ambrose PG. Torsades de pointes associated with fluoroquinolones. *Pharmacotherapy* 2002;22:663.

16a. Frothingham R. Rates of torsades de points associated with ciprofloxacin, ofloxacin, levofloxacin, gatifloxacin, and moxifloxacin. *Pharmacotherapy* 2001;21:468.

17. Bertino JB Jr, et al. Gatifloxacin-associated corrected QT interval prolongation, torsades de pointes and ventricular fibrillation in patients with known risk factors. *Clin Infect Dis* 2002;34:861.
18. Casparian JM, et al. Quinolones and tendon ruptures. *South Med J* 2000;93:488.
19. Schaad UB. Use of quinolone in pediatrics. In: Andriole VT, ed. *The quinolones,* 3rd ed. San Diego: Academic Press, 2000.
20. *Red Book 2000: Report of the Committee on Infectious Diseases,* 25th ed. Elk Grove, IL: American Academy of Pediatrics, 2000:645–646.
21. Schaad UB. Pediatric use of quinolones. *Pediatr Infect Dis J* 1999;18:469–470.
22. Radandt JM, Marchbanks CR, Dudley MN. Interactions of fluoroquinolones with other drugs: mechanisms, variability, clinical significance, and management. *Clin Infect Dis* 1992;14:272.
23. Medical Letter. The choice of antibacterial drugs. *Med Lett Drugs Ther* 2001;43:69.
24. Lipsky BA. Prostatitis and urinary tract infection in men: what's new, what's true? *Am J Med* 1999;106:327.
25. Centers for Disease Control and Prevention. Sexually transmitted disease treatment guidelines 2002. *MMWR Morb Mortal Wkly Rep* 2002;51:(RR-6):42–43.
26. Medical Letter. Drugs for sexually transmitted infections. *Med Lett Drugs Ther* 1999; 41:85
27. File TM, et al. A multicenter, randomized study comparing the efficacy and safety of intravenous and/or oral levofloxacin versus ceftriaxone and/or cefuroxime axetil in the treatment of adults with community-acquired pneumonia. *Antimicrob Agents Chemother* 1997;41:1965.

28. Mandell LA. Guidelines for community-acquired pneumonia: a tale of 2 countries. *Clin Infect Dis* 2000;31:422.
29. Williams JH Jr. Fluoroquinolones for respiratory infections: too valuable to overuse. *Chest* 2001;120:1771.
30. Singh N, Rogers P, Atwood CW, et al. Short course empiric antibiotic therapy for patients with pulmonary infiltrates in the intensive care unit. A proposed solution for indiscriminate antibiotic prescription. *Am J Respir Crit Care Med* 2000;162(2 Pt 1): 505–511.
31. Zimmerli W, Widmer AF, Blatter M, et al. Role of rifampin for treatment of orthopedic implant-related staphylococcal infections: a randomized controlled trial. Foreign Body Infection (FBI) Study Group. *JAMA* 1998;279:1575–1577.
32. Hooper DC. Expanding use of fluoroquinolones: opportunities and challenges. *Ann Intern Med* 1998;129:908.
33. Freifeld A, et al. A double-blind comparison of empirical oral and intravenous antibiotic therapy for low risk febrile patients with neutropenia during cancer chemotherapy. *N Engl J Med* 1999;341:305.
34. Kern WV, et al. for the International Antimicrobial Therapy Cooperative Group of the European Organization for Research and Treatment of Cancer. Oral versus intravenous empirical antimicrobial therapy for fever in patients with granulocytopenia who are receiving cancer chemotherapy. *N Engl J Med* 1999;341:312.
35. Talcott JA, Finberg RW. Fever and neutropenic: how to use a new strategy. *N Engl J Med* 1999;341:362.
36. Griggs JJ, Blair EA, Norton JR, et al. Ciprofloxacin plus piperacillin is an equally effective regimen for empiric therapy in febrile neutropenic patients compared with standard therapy. *Am J Hematol* 1998;58:293–297.
37. Alangaden GJ, Lerner SA. The clinical use of fluoroquinolones for the treatment of mycobacterial disease. *Clin Infect Dis* 1997;25:1213.
38. Klein JO, McCraken GH Jr. Summary and conclusions (on floxacin otic in children). *Pediatr Infect Dis J* 2001;20:123.
39. Medical Letter. Ofloxacin. *Med Lett Drugs Ther* 1991;33:71.
40. Medical Letter. Levofloxacin. *Med Lett Drugs Ther* 1997;39:41.
41. Medical Letter. Gatifloxacin and moxifloxacin: two new fluoroquinolones. *Med Lett Drugs Ther* 2000;42:15.
42. Perry CM, et al. Gatifloxacin: a review of its use in the management of bacterial infections. *Drugs* 2002;62:169.
43. Meyer RD, Goldstein EJC. Moxifloxacin: on a journey toward improving antimicrobial therapy. *Clin Infect Dis* 2001;32[Suppl 1]:S1–S72.
44. Felmingham D, Tesfaslasie Y, Robbins MJ. The *in vitro* activity of moxifloxacin against 817 isolates of *S. pneumoniae* collected from 27 centers throughout the U.K. and Ireland during the 1997–1998 cold season. *39th Interscience Conference on Antimicrobial Agents and Chemotherapy,* San Francisco, Abstract 379, September 1999.
45. Huczko E, et al. Susceptibility of bacterial isolates to gatifloxacin and ciprofloxacin from the clinical trials during the 1997–1998 period. *39th Interscience Conference on Antimicrobial Agents and Chemotherapy,* San Francisco, Abstract 351, September 1999.
46. Kohler T, Pechere JC. Bacterial resistance to quinolones: mechanisms and clinical implications. In: Andriole VT, ed. *The quinolones,* 2nd ed. San Diego: Academic Press, 1998;117–142.
47. Acar JF, Goldstein FW. Trends in bacterial resistance to fluoroquinolones. *Clin Infect Dis* 1997;24[Suppl 1]:S67.
48. Lautenbach E, Strom BL, Bilker WB, et al. Epidemiological investigation of fluoroquinolone resistance in infections due to extended-spectrum *B*-lactamase-producing *Escherichia coli* and *Klebsiella pneumoniae. Clin Infect Dis* 2001;33: 1288.
49. Centers for Disease Control and Prevention. Fluoroquinolone-resistant *Neisseria gonorrhoeae.* Hawaii, 1999. *MMWR Morb Mortal Wkly Rep* 2000;49:834.
50. Chen DK, et al. Decreased susceptibility of *Streptococcus pneumoniae* to fluoroquinolones in Canada. *N Engl J Med* 1999;341:233.
51. Davidson R, Cavalcanti R, Brunton JL, et al. Resistance to levofloxacin and failure of treatment of pneumococcal pneumonia. *N Engl J Med* 2002;346:747.

52. Weiss K, et al. A nosocomial outbreak of fluoroquinolone-resistant *Streptococcus pneumoniae. Clin Infect Dis* 2001;33:917.
53. Molbak K, Baggesen DL, Aarestrup FM, et al. An outbreak of multidrug-resistant, quinolone-resistant *Salmonella enterica* serotype typhimurium DT104. *N Engl J Med* 1999;341:1420.
54. Swartz MN. Human disease caused by foodborne pathogens of animal origin. *Clin Infect Dis* 2002;34[Suppl 3]:S111.

## H. Unique $\beta$-Lactam Antibiotics: Monobactams and Carbapenems (Aztreonam, Imipenem, Meropenem, and Ertapenem)

**I. Aztreonam (Azactam)** is the first clinically useful monobactam. It is active against most of the gram-negative aerobes without the nephrotoxicity of aminoglycosides [1].

**A. Mechanism of action.** Aztreonam binds to the penicillin binding proteins of **bacterial walls.**

**B.** *In vitro* **activity.** Aztreonam is **unique among the $\beta$-lactam antibiotics because it is active only against gram-negative aerobes.**

1. **Gram-negative aerobes**
   a. **Highly susceptible organisms** include $\beta$-lactamase and non–$\beta$-lactamase–producing strains of *Haemophilus influenzae* and *Neisseria gonorrhoeae,* as well as *N. meningitidis.*
   b. **Most Enterobacteriaceae** are inhibited by less than 1 $\mu$g/mL [1], except for resistant strains shown in section **d** below.
   c. ***Pseudomonas aeruginosa.*** Aztreonam inhibits 50% at 4 $\mu$g/mL and 90% at 16 to 32 $\mu$g/mL; concentrations required to inhibit usually are twofold greater than those for ceftazidime [2]. At least 12% of strains of *P. aeruginosa* are resistant [3,4]. The combination of aztreonam and piperacillin (or mezlocillin) is synergistic against some strains of *P. aeruginosa* and *Enterobacter* species but not as frequently as piperacillin plus an aminoglycoside [5,6].
   d. **Resistant strains** typically include *Citrobacter freundii, Enterobacter aerogenes,* some *E. cloacae, Legionella pneumophilia,* and *Acinetobacter* species. Cefoxitin antagonizes the activity of aztreonam against *Enterobacter* species. [1].
2. **Gram-positive aerobes:** little or no activity.
3. **Anaerobes:** little or no activity.

**C. Pharmacokinetics** [1,6].

1. **Absorption.** Aztreonam is poorly absorbed after oral administration but can be given intramuscularly (i.m.) or intravenously (i.v.).
2. **Excretion** is primarily by the **kidneys** and doses are reduced in renal failure.
3. **Penetration/distribution.** Aztreonam penetrates body fluids well but has limited penetration into the cerebrospinal fluid. After i.v. infusion of 0.5-, 1-, and 2-g doses, mean peak serum levels of more than 60, 160, and 250 $\mu$g/mL, respectively, are achieved [1]. Urinary concentrations are very high with urinary concentrations of more than 250 $\mu$g/mL and more than 700 $\mu$g/mL achieved 4 to 6 hours after a single i.v. 500-mg or 1-g dose, respectively, in patients with normal renal function [1].

**D. Clinical role. Because aztreonam is active against gram-negative aerobes only, combination therapy is necessary for mixed infections with gram-positive organisms and/or anaerobes.** Aztreonam has been successfully used in the following [1,6]:

1. **Urinary tract infection** as single agent for susceptible gram-negative organisms.
2. **Intraabdominal** (including peritonitis) and/or **pelvic** infections **in combination with antianaerobic agents** such as clindamycin or metronidazole [7].
3. **Bacteremia.** For empiric therapy, additional coverage is necessary. Once a gram-negative bacteria is isolated, this becomes an excellent choice.

Table 27H.1. Aztreonam Intravenous Dosage Guidelines (Normal Renal Function)

| Type of Infection | Dose[a] | Frequency (Hours) |
|---|---|---|
| **Adults[b]** | | |
| Urinary tract infections | 500 mg or 1 g | 8 or 12 |
| Moderately severe systemic infections | 1 g | 8 |
| Severe systemic or life-threatening infections | 2 g | 6 or 8[c] |
| **Pediatric patients[b]** | | |
| Mild-to-moderate infections | 30 mg/kg | 8 |
| Moderate-to-severe infections | 30 mg/kg | 6 or 8 |

[a]Higher doses are used in more severe infection.
[b]Maximum recommended dose is 8 g/day.
[c]In systemic or severe *P. aeruginosa* infections 2 g q6–8h is suggested.
[d]Maximum recommended dose is 120 mg/kg/day.
Modified from *Physicians' desk reference,* 56th ed. Montvale, NJ: Medical Economics Data, 2002, with permission.

4. **Gram-negative pneumonia** due to susceptible pathogens [8]. Because some nosocomially acquired *P. aeruginosa* may be resistant to aztreonam, an aminoglycoside is initially preferred until susceptibility data are available.
5. **Skin and soft tissue** infection after the gram-negative organism is identified.
6. **Bone and joint** infections due to susceptible pathogens have been treated with aztreonam i.v. Usually an oral fluoroquinolone is preferred in this setting.
7. **Febrile neutropenic patients** have been treated with aztreonam combined with an aminoglycoside. Vancomycin is added for patients when gram-positive infection is suspected (e.g., patients with central venous catheters or chemotherapy ports) (see Chapters 2 and 20).

E. **Dosing.** Aztreonam may be administered **i.v. or i.m.** The i.v. route is recommended for patients requiring more than 1 g per dose and in those patients with bacteremia, abscess, peritonitis, or other severe or life-threatening infections.
   1. **Adult and pediatric** (more than 9 months of age) **dosages are summarized in Table 27H.1.**
   2. **Renal failure** dose reduction is shown in Table 27H.2.
      a. **Doses for patients on hemodialysis** are similar to those whose clearance is <10 mL/min. Thereafter, one-eighth of the initial dose (or 500 mg) is given after each hemodialysis [9].

Table 27H.2. Dosing of Aztreonam in Renal Failure

| Estimated Creatinine Clearance | Adult Dose | Pediatric Dose |
|---|---|---|
| >30 mL/min | See Table 27H.1 | See Table 27H.1 |
| 10–30 mL/min | Initial dose as in Table 27H.1, then give half of the usual dose at the standard interval | Insufficient data[a] |
| <10 mL/min | Initial dose as in Table 27H.1, then one quarter the usual dose at the usual fixed interval | Insufficient data[a] |

[a]As per the 2002 package insert, there are insufficient data to support recommendations for dosing aztreonam in renally impaired pediatric patients.

b. **Chronic ambulatory peritoneal dialysis (CAPD).** Dosing guidelines followed for a clearance less than 10 mL/mm can be followed [9].

3. **Penicillin-allergic or cephalosporin-allergic patients.** For patients with immunologically mediated reactions to penicillins or cephalosporins there is little risk of cross-sensitivity. Repetitive courses of aztreonam may rarely provoke a hypersensitivity reaction [10].
4. **Pregnancy.** Aztreonam is a category B agent; it should be used during pregnancy only if clearly indicated.
5. **Nursing mothers.** Aztreonam is excreted in breast milk. The package insert suggests consideration should be given to temporary discontinuation of nursing and use of formula feedings while the mother receives aztreonam.

F. **Toxicity** [1,6]. Aztreonam is a safe agent with side effects similar to other $\beta$-lactams.

1. Serious **nephrotoxicity or ototoxicity has not been reported. Aztreonam is promoted for the treatment of gram-negative aerobic infections as safer than the aminoglycosides.**
2. **Adverse reactions** of rash, nausea, diarrhea, eosinophilia, and mild hepatic transaminase elevations have been seen as with other $\beta$-lactam antibiotics.

G. **Cost** (see Appendix Table 1). Although monotherapy costs compared with third-generation cephalosporins are competitive, aztreonam is much more expensive than gentamicin or tobramycin; thus combination therapy with aztreonam is more expensive.

H. **Summary. Guidelines for the optimal use of aztreonam continue to evolve** [1,6,11]. In moderate to severe nosocomial infections, aminoglycoside therapy for gram-negative organisms for the initial 48 to 72 hours while awaiting cultures is prudent unless an aminoglycoside is contraindicated. Once susceptibility data are back, if the organism is resistant to cephalosporins and quinolones but susceptible to aztreonam, aztreonam could be used. The development of resistance while on therapy is usually not a concern with aminoglycosides but with aztreonam is not fully delineated. If the approach just outlined is used, the risk of resistance may be minimized. There may be an increased incidence of *Clostridium difficile* diarrhea associated with the common use of advanced cephalosporins. Aztreonam appears to be associated less often with these problems and therefore may be an appealing alternative. Because aztreonam is active only against gram-negative bacilli, when it is used empirically for mixed infections, combination therapy will be necessary, thereby increasing costs. In some circumstances, an aminoglycoside may still be the preferred agent as, for example, in combination therapy against enterococcus and *Listeria monocytogenes* and in combination with anti-*Pseudomonas* penicillin in severe *P. aeruginosa* infections.

II. **Imipenem (Primaxin),** a carbapenem released in 1985, has a very broad spectrum of activity. It is combined with cilastatin, a potent enzyme inhibitor, which prevents the inactivation of imipenem in the kidney by inactivating enzymes in the brush border cells. This ensures good urinary concentrations. Cilastatin also appears to have a "nephroprotective" effect [1,6].

A. **Mechanism of action.** Imipenem binds with high affinity to penicillin-binding proteins, causing lysis of many gram-positive and gram-negative bacteria. Its ability to penetrate the cell membrane of multiple gram-negative bacilli and its resistance to $\beta$-lactamases produced by gram-positive and gram-negative bacilli help explain its broad spectrum [1].

B. *In vitro* **activity [12].** Some resistance has developed over time [1,13].

1. **Gram-positive aerobes**

a. **Very susceptible,** with a minimum inhibitory concentration $(MIC)_{90}$ typically of 0.1 $\mu$g/mL or less: penicillin-susceptible *Streptococcus pneumoniae,* group A and B streptococci, *Streptococcus bovis,* methicillin-susceptible *Staphylococcus aureus, S. saprophyticus,* intermediate penicillin-resistant *S. pneumoniae,* and many high level resistant strains [1,6] (see Chapters 11 and 27C).

b. **Moderately susceptible.** Amoxicillin-susceptible enterococci usually are susceptible, with the $MIC_{90}$ of susceptible *Enterococcus faecalis* approximately

1 to 3 μg/mL. Imipenem is bacteriostatic against susceptible enterococci. Imipenem-aminoglycoside combinations may be synergistic against *E. faecalis.* However, many strains of *E. faecium* are resistant to imipenem.

c. **Resistant.** Methicillin-resistant *S. aureus* (MRSA), coagulase-negative staphylococcus, *Corynebacterium JK,* and vancomycin-resistant enterococci (VRE) are resistant to imipenem.

2. **Gram-negative aerobic bacteria**

a. **Enterobacteriaceae.** In an early review of more than 8,000 isolates, three levels of imipenem activity were recognized [14]. An $MIC_{90}$ of 1.0 μg or less (very susceptible) was seen with *Escherichia coli, Klebsiella* species, *Salmonella, Shigella* species, *Citrobacter diversus, Hafniae alvei, and Yersinia enterocolitica. Enterobacter* species, *C. freundii,* and *Serratia* species have $MIC_{90}$ of approximately 1 to 2 μg/mL (susceptible). An $MIC_{90}$ of 2 to 4 μg/mL (less susceptible) is noted, especially with the *Proteus* species. Although some Enterobacteriaceae has developed resistance to imipenem, it remains more active than noncarbapenem β-lactam antibiotics [1,13].

b. *Pseudomonas.* The $MIC_{90}$ for *P. aeruginosa* is typically higher (e.g., 5 μg/mL in more than 1,600 strains in early testing) [14]. Although some strains have developed resistance to imipenem over time, in one 1996 report of more than 6,600 intensive care unit isolates, 87% of strains were susceptible to imipenem. Against these same strains, 89%, 93%, and 65% of strains were susceptible to amikacin, tobramycin, and gentamicin, respectively [13].

Similar MICs were noted for *P. fluorescens.* Imipenem may show synergism with tobramycin or other aminoglycosides against *P. aeruginosa* [1,6]. Risk factors for imipenem-resistant *Pseudomonas* have recently been reviewed [15].

c. *Burkholderia cepacia* and *Stenotrophomonas maltophilia* are **resistant. The latter produces a β-lactamase that easily hydrolyzes imipenem.** *Acinetobacter calcoaceticus* species are usually quite susceptible, but nosocomial infections due to resistant species can occur.

d. **Community-acquired pathogens.** The MICs for β-lactamase–positive and–negative *N. gonorrhoeae* are identical and similar to *N. meningitidis.* They have a $MIC_{90}$ of less than 0.20 μg/mL, and *H. influenzae* with a, $MIC_{90}$ of 0.6 μg/mL are very susceptible. Although imipenem is active *in vitro,* it is not considered appropriate treatment for *Legionella* pneumonia because of the intracellular location of the organism [1,6].

C. **Pharmacokinetics**

1. **Intravenous or i.m.** but not oral route is available. Lower serum levels are reached after i.m. doses. In adults of average size with normal renal function, 500- and 1,000-mg doses i.v. provide peak serum levels of 30 to 40 and 60 to 70 μg/mL, respectively [1].
2. **Excretion** is primarily by the kidneys, and doses must be reduced in renal failure. Little of the drug is found in the feces, so there is relatively little impact on bowel flora; *C. difficile* diarrhea has been reported (see section **F.3**).
3. **Penetration/distribution.** Imipenem-cilastatin penetrates body fluids well, with at least modest penetration of the inflamed meninges.

D. **Clinical role.** Imipenem-cilastatin is especially useful in infections caused by pathogens resistant to other agents or for infections that would otherwise require multiple antibiotics. It is particularly useful in complex nosocomial infections [1,5].

1. **See Table 27H.3** for a summary.
2. **Miscellaneous uses**

a. **Eye infections.** Its broad spectrum leads to its use for some eye infections [16] (see Chapter 7).

b. **Acute necrotizing pancreatitis.** Imipenem is detected in high concentrations in pancreatic tissue but not in the bile. It has been used to try to prevent or treat pancreatic infections, but other choices seem better for biliary sepsis [17] (see Chapter 13).

c. ***Nocardia.*** Alternate agent for *Nocardia* infections. It may be useful in selected infections due to high-level resistant *S. pneumoniae* (see Chapters 11 and 17).

Table 27H.3. Clinical Use of Imipenem (or Meropenem)

For **serious nosocomical infections** (e.g., bacteremia, pneumonia, complex UTI, severe perineal soft tissue infection, osteomyelitis), **especially** those **involving resistant organisms,** or polymicrobial infections (mixed anaerobes, aerobic, gram-positive and -negative, especially for diabetics)[a]

Used as an alternative to combination therapy for complex **nosocomial intraabdominal infections,** thus avoiding ototoxic and nephrotoxic effects of aminoglycosides[b]

For *Pseudomonas* infections caused by organisms resistant to other antipseudomonal $\beta$-lactam agents but, where possible, use in combination with an aminoglycoside.

Monotherapy in **febrile granulocytopenic patients** (see Chapter 20).

A **"drug of choice"** for severe nosocomial *Enterobacter* or *Serratia* or *Acinetobacter* spp., and *C. freundii* infections; also for *Campylobacter fetus* infections [8].

**When *not* to use imipenem (or meropenem)**

**Not** alone in treatment of serious *Pseudomonas* infections[c] especially pneumonia
**Not** for most community-acquired infections
**Not** for surgical prophylaxis
**Not** for methicillin-resistant staphylococcal infections or VRE
**Not** alone in therapy for serious enterococcal infections (*E. faecalis*)
**Not** in therapy for non–aeruginosa pseudomonal infections

[a]Editors' note: We "save for use" imipenem and meropenem for when cultures reveal or are likely to reveal resistant pathogens in someone usually already on antibiotics or who has recently received antibiotics. *C. freundii, Acinetobacter,* and *Enterobacter* species. may be resistant to other antibiotics.

[b]Editors' note: Not for mild to moderate community-acquired infections where less broad agents are effective (e.g., cefazolin combined with metronidazole, cefoxitin, cefotetan, ampicillin-sulbactam, ticarcillin-clavulanate). See Chapter 13. Particularly useful in hospital-acquired intraabdominal infections in which resistant organisms may be involved.

[c]Editors' note: For susceptible *P. aeruginosa* infections, an antipseudomonal penicillin and an aminoglycoside are preferred. (See Chapter 27I.)

Modified from Sobel JD. Imipenem and aztreonam. *Infect Dis Clin North Am* 1989;3:613, with permission.

d. **Prophylaxis.** Imipenem is not advised for prophylaxis because of the risks of promoting antimicrobial resistance. However, when a hospitalized patient who has had many courses of antibiotics requires surgery, it is reasonable to consider this possibility.

E. **Dosages.** For a given patient, the dose of imipenem **depends on** the **severity** of infection, **renal function, and weight of the patient** (with dose reductions if the patient weighs less than 70 kg). The dose of imipenem-cilastatin refers to the amount of the imipenem [1].

1. **A table for dosages for adults of less than 70 kg and different degree of renal dysfunction is** in the package insert and the *Physicians' desk reference,* which is readily available.
   a. **Serious infections in adults weighing 70 kg with normal creatinine clearance,** 500 mg every 6 hours are suggested [1,6]. For life-threatening infections, 1 g every 6 to 8 hours has been used.
   b. **Adults under 70 kg:** 25 mg/kg/day divided every 6 hours has been suggested [1].
   c. **Renal failure.** Fifty percent of the usual dose is given when creatinine clearance is between 10 to 50 mL/min and 25% of the usual dose when the creatinine clearance is less than 10 mL/min [9]. **Hemodialysis** removes 40% to 70% of the imipenem, so half a dose is given after dialysis. In patients undergoing **CAPD,** dosages are given as above in patients with a creatinine clearance of less than 10 mL/min [9].
2. **Children.** Intravenous imipenem has recently been approved. **For those older than 3 months,** the recommended dose is 15 to 25 mg/kg/dose i.v. every 6 hours

(to a maximum of 2 g daily). Higher doses have been used in children with pseudomonas infections and/or cystic fibrosis. See package insert for use in children less than 3 months. For neonates, see Chapter 3. For children less than 30 kg with impaired renal function there are no data.

3. **Central nervous system infections. Imipenem is not advised** because of the risk of seizures. See related discussions of meropenem in section **IV.**
4. **Pregnancy.** Imipenem is **category C.** The package insert indicates there are no adequate and well-controlled studies in pregnant women. Therefore this agent should be used during pregnancy only if the potential benefit justifies the potential risk to the mother and fetus.
5. **Nursing mothers.** It is not known whether imipenem is excreted in human milk. Because many drugs are excreted in human milk, caution should be exercised when this agent is administered to a nursing woman.

**F. Side effects and toxicity.** Overall, imipenem is well tolerated [1,6].

1. **Seizures** have occurred in less than 1% but occur more frequently in patients with closed head trauma, with a previous history of seizures, after neurosurgery, and if high doses and decreased renal function were present. **Dosage reduction in the elderly and in renal insufficiency is indicated.** If a seizure, tremor, or myoclonus occurs, need for imipenem should be reassessed and anticonvulsant therapy should be considered. **Imipenem use in patients with closed head injury or with meningitis is usually avoided; meropenem is preferred in these patients.** Whether seizures occur more often than with other antibiotics, when proper doses are used, is not established [1,6] (see section **5**).
2. **Allergic reactions** such as drug fever, pruritus, rash, and urticaria are uncommon. **Patients allergic to penicillin should be skin tested before imipenem use** [18]. In addition, imipenem should be avoided or administered under close monitoring to patients with a history of IgE-mediated hypersensitivity to other β-lactam antibiotics, although the exact incidence of cross over allergy is unknown [19,20].
3. **Gastrointestinal symptoms** occasionally occur. Decreasing the infusion rate or the dose decreases nausea and vomiting [1]. *C. difficile* diarrhea occurs.
4. **Nephrotoxicity and hepatotoxicity are rare.**
5. **Drug interactions.** Seizures have been reported in patients receiving **ganciclovir** and imipenem. These drugs should not be used concomitantly unless the benefit outweighs risks. **Probenecid** increases imipenem concentrations. Avoid concomitant use. **Imipenem may induce β-lactamases that inactivate** other β-lactams [1,6].

**G. Resistance** can develop especially against *P. aeruginosa* [15]. In severe infections due to this pathogen, monotherapy with imipenem should be avoided.

**H. Cost.** This is an expensive agent but may be competitive if it replaces multiple other agents (see Appendix Table 1).

**III. Ertapenem (Invanz)** is a new i.v. **carbapenem** agent released in early 2002 [21].

**A. Mechanism of action.** Like other β-lactam antibiotics, ertapenem inhibits bacterial cell wall synthesis. It is relatively resistant to hydrolysis by β-lactamases, including extended-spectrum β-lactamases.

**B. *In vitro* activity.** Ertapenem has a narrower spectrum of activity than imipenem or meropenem.

1. **Gram-positive aerobes.** Although active against many gram-positive aerobes, ertapenem is less active than imipenem. Although active against MSSA, group A streptococcus., penicillin-susceptible *S. pneumoniae,* and many strains of intermediately resistant pneumococci, it has **little activity against highly penicillin-resistant pneumococci, MRSA, or *Enterococcus faecium* or *faecalis* [21].**
2. **Gram-negative aerobes.** Ertapenem is more **active** than imipenem and similar to meropenem **against Enterobacteriaceae, but unlike imipenem and meropenem ertapenem has little or no activity against *P. aeruginosa* or *Acinetobacter*** species [21]. It is not active against *Stenotrophomonas maltophilia.*
3. **Anaerobes.** Ertapenem has good activity against most anaerobes, including *B. fragilis* [22]

4. **Miscellaneous. Ertapenem is not active against "atypical" respiratory pathogens** such as *Mycoplasma pneumoniae, Legionella* species, or *Chlamydia* species.

C. **Pharmacokinetics**

1. **Half-life.** Ertapenem has a **longer half-life than imipenem/meropenem:** 4 hours versus 1 hour. Therefore, **ertapenem has** been approved for a **once-daily dose** regimen [21].
2. **Metabolism/excretion.** Ertapenem is partly metabolized by hydrolysis and 80% is excreted by the kidney [21].

D. **Clinical role [21]**

1. **U.S. Food and Drug Administration approved uses.** Based on early clinical studies, ertapenem was approved for **once daily i.m./i.v.** therapy of complicated intraabdominal infections, urinary tract infection, skin and skin structure infections, acute pelvic infections, and community-acquired pneumonia.
2. As discussed in previous chapters on the above infections, there are already many commonly used regimens for each of these infections. The potential usefulness of this broad new agent must be weighed against the likelihood of selecting our resistance and greater expense, compared with other regimens. **See section H below for a summary of its potential role.**

E. **Dosing**

1. In adults, 1 g i.v. or i.m. is recommended [21].
2. **In renal failure,** the dose should be reduced by 50% in patients with a creatinine clearance less than 30 mL/min. For patients on chronic hemodialysis, the dose should be given 6 hours before dialysis; if given less than 6 hours before, an extra dose of 150 mg should be given after dialysis [21].
3. **In children,** the safety and efficacy of ertapenem have not been established and therefore should not be used in patients less than 18 years old.
4. **Pregnancy.** This is a category B drug and should be used only if clearly indicated during pregnancy.
5. **Nursing mothers.** Ertapenem is excreted in breast milk and should be given to nursing mothers only when clearly indicated.

F. **Toxicity.** In early reports, ertapenem has generally been well tolerated. Diarrhea, nausea, vomiting, increased serum aminotransferase levels, and local complications at the infusion site, including phlebitis, have occurred. Seizures have occurred in 0.5% of patients.

G. **Cost** (see Appendix Table). Ertapenem is less expensive than imipenem, meropenem, and piperacillin-tazobactam [21].

H. **Summary. The precise role of ertapenem awaits further clinical experience with this agent.**

1. **In their 2002 review, the *Medical Letter* concluded the following** [21]: "ertapenem is a broad-spectrum, once-daily, parenteral antibiotic that offers better anaerobic coverage than ceftriaxone and fewer doses per day than piperacillin/tazobactam (and related agents) and other drugs used to treat infections that may involve anaerobes. It might be a good choice for home treatment of some infections (since given once daily), but offers no advantage over ceftriaxone for treatment of community-acquired bacterial pneumonia. Unlike imipenem and meropenem, ertapenem is not active against *Pseudomonas* and *Acinetobacter,* and therefore **should not be used for empiric treatment of nosocomial infections."**
2. This new agent does not solve the clinician's problem of treating resistant pathogens. This agent is not active against many hospital-acquired gram-negative organisms (including *Pseudomonas, Acinetobacter* species), MRSA, high level penicillin-resistant pneumococci, and enterococci, including VRE. Also, ertapenem is not active against atypical respiratory pathogens.

IV. **Meropenem (Merrem)** is a new i.v. carbapenem, approved in 1996, which is **very similar to imipenem.** Meropenem has been reviewed elsewhere [1,6,23–28]. Meropenem is stable to human renal dehydropeptidase and therefore can be given without cilastatin.

**A. Susceptibilities.** ***In vitro,*** it is similar to **imipenem.** It is slightly more active against gram-negative organisms, whereas imipenem is slightly more active against gram-positive organisms (1,16,18). Whether these minor *in vitro* differences have clinical relevance is unknown, but no differences have been detected in the initial comparative trials [1].

1. **Gram-positive organisms.** Meropenem, like imipenem, is active *in vitro* against many penicillin-resistant *S. pneumoniae,* including many high level resistant forms. Meropenem is not active against MRSA, *E. faecium,* and VRE strains of enterococci.
2. **Gram-negative organisms** include *S. maltophilia* and some strains of *P. aeruginosa.*

**B. Pharmacokinetics.** The pharmacokinetics of meropenem is similar to those of imipenem [1,5]. Only an i.v. formulation is available. About 70% of each dose is recovered in the urine. Hemodialysis removes most of the drug. Its serum half-life is about 1 hour, so it is given every 8 hours. Meropenem reaches therapeutic concentrations in the cerebrospinal fluid in patients with meningitis [26].

**C. Clinical role.** Meropenem has been **approved for** i.v. therapy as follows [1,6,26]:

1. **Intraabdominal infections in adults and children** over 3 months of age. **Complex mixed aerobic and anaerobic and nosocomial infections** [27,29]. For mild to moderate community-acquired abdominal infections, other options are available. (Imipenem is chosen in adults unless possibly in a patient with recent seizures or there is renal failure, where dose modification is easier with meropenem.)
2. **Bacterial meningitis in children** more than 3 months of age, although meropenem has been used [29,30] and is approved for susceptible *H. influenzae, S. pneumoniae,* and *N. meningitidis* in children. A third-generation cephalosporin is preferred because of greater experience (see Chapter 6). For a case of known *S. pneumoniae* resistant to penicillin but susceptible to meropenem, **meropenem provides an alternative agent to vancomycin** (see Chapter 6), and meropenem is preferred over imipenem.
3. **Other.** Meropenem has been shown to be effective in a variety of clinical conditions, including pneumonia, febrile neutropenic patients, bacteremia, and complex urinary tract infection [1].

**D. Dosages**

1. **Adults.** The usual dose is 1 g i.v. every 8 hours. In the management of febrile neutropenic adult patients 1 g every 8 hours was as effective as 2 g every 8 hours of ceftazidime alone and/or ceftazidime and amikacin [1]. In bacterial meningitis, 2 g every 8 hours has been effective [1].
2. **In pediatrics,** for intraabdominal infections 20 mg/kg (maximum of 1 g) every 8 hours and for meningitis 40 mg/kg (maximum 2 g) every 8 hours. Patients more than 50 kg can be given adult doses.
   a. **Renal failure.** If the creatinine clearance is 26 to 50 mL/min, the regular dose is given every 12 hours. If the creatinine clearance is 10 to 25 mL/min, one-half of the usual dose is given every 12 hours. If the creatinine clearance is less than 10 mL/min, one-half of the usual dose is given every 24 hours. As of mid-2000, the package insert indicates no dose recommendations for pediatric patients with renal failure (i.e., no experience).
   b. **In dialysis.** As of mid-2000, there is inadequate information regarding the dose of meropenem in patients on hemodialysis and peritoneal dialysis, per the package insert.
3. **In hepatic disease,** the package insert indicates no dosage adjustments are needed (in adults).
4. **In pregnancy.** The package insert notes this is a **category B** agent and should be used during pregnancy only if clearly needed.
5. **In nursing mothers.** It is not known if this agent is excreted in human milk. Caution should be exercised when i.v. meropenem is administered to a nursing woman.

E. **Side effects. There are differences in the tolerability of imipenem and meropenem [1].**
   1. **Meropenem is unlikely to cause seizures** that have been reported with imipenem [26,31].
   2. Meropenem has been less likely to cause nausea and vomiting as well as inflammation at the i.v. site compared with imipenem [1].
   3. The frequency and severity of adverse events with meropenem does not seem to escalate at higher doses as with imipenem [1].
   4. Rashes, diarrhea, and reversible increases in aminotransferase enzymes have occurred as with other $\beta$-lactam antibiotics [1,6,26].

F. **Cost.** Meropenem is an **expensive** i.v. agent to use, even more so than imipenem [26] (see Appendix Table).

G. **Summary.** In their review, the *Medical Letter* concluded the following [26]: "meropenem is an expensive new parenteral antibiotic similar to imipenem, possibly with less potential for causing seizures. Meropenem, like imipenem, could be used for treatment of hospital-acquired infections that may be resistant to other antibiotics [27]. For treatment of intraabdominal infections or bacterial meningitis, meropenem generally offers no clear advantage over less costly older drugs."

   We would add that except for very selected cases of meningitis in which meropenem may be useful (infectious disease consultation is advised in these difficult cases), the indications for meropenem are the same as those for imipenem (see section **II.D**). In selected patients, the decreased side effects with meropenem may be important.

## REFERENCES


1. Hellinger WC, Brewer NS. Carbapenems and monobactams: imipenem, meropenem, and aztreonam. *Mayo Clin Proc* 1999;74:420.
2. Neu HC. Aztreonam activity, pharmacology, and clinical uses. *Am J Med* 1990;88[Suppl 3C]:2S.
3. Ennis DM, Cobbs CG. The newer cephalosporins, aztreonam, and imipenem. *Infect Dis Clin North Am* 1995;9:687.
4. Asbel LE, Levison ME. Cephalosporins, carbapenems, and monobactams. *Infect Dis Clin North Am* 2000;14:435.
5. Greenberg RN, Meade DW, Danko LS. Comparison of the synergistic activity of aztreonam or tobramycin plus piperacillin or mezlocillin. *J Antimicrob Chemother* 1993;32:342.
6. Reese RE, Betts RF. Unique $\beta$-lactam antibodies. In: Reese RE, Betts RF, Gumustop B, eds. *Handbook of antibiotics,* 3rd ed. Philadelphia: Lippincott Williams & Wilkins, 2000;401–414.
7. Holzhelmer RG, Dralle H. Antibiotic therapy in intra-abdominal-infection: a review of randomized clinical trails. *Eur J Med Res* 2001;6:277.
8. Boucher BA. Role of aztreonam in the treatment of nosocomial pneumonia in the critically ill surgical patient. *Am J Surg* 2000;179[2A Suppl]:45S.
9. Aronoff GR, et al, eds. *Drug prescribing in renal failure: dosing guidelines for adults,* 4th ed. Philadelphia: American College of Physicians, 1999.
10. Moss RB, et al. Evaluation of the immunologic cross-reactivity of aztreonam in patients with cystic fibrosis who are allergic to penicillin and/or cephalosporin antibiotics. *Rev Infect Dis* 1991;13[Suppl 7]:S598.
11. Medical Letter. The choice of antibacterial drugs. *Med Lett Drugs Ther* 2001;43:69.
12. Hellinger WC, Brewer NS. Imipenem. *Mayo Clin Proc* 1991;66:1074.
13. Itokazen GS, et al. Antimicrobial resistance rates among aerobic gram-negative bacilli recovered from patients in intensive care units: evaluation of a national post marketing surveillance program. *Clin Infect Dis* 1996;23:779.
14. Jones RN. Review of the *in vitro* spectrum of activity of imipenem. *Am J Med* 1985; 78:22.
15. Harris AD, et al. Risk factors for imipenem-resistant *Pseudomonas aeruginosa* among hospitalized patients. *Clin Infect Dis* 2002;34:340.
16. Axelrod JL, et al. Penetration of imipenem in human aqueous and vitreous humor. *Am J Ophthalmol* 1987;104:649.

17. Buchler MW, et al. Acute necrotizing pancreatitis: treatment strategy according to the status of infection. *Ann Surg* 2000;232:619.
18. Saxon A, et al. Immediate hypersensitivity reactions to beta-lactam antibiotics. *Ann Intern Med* 1987;127:204.
19. Sobel JD. Imipenem and aztreonam. *Infect Dis Clin North Am* 1989;3:613.
20. McConnell SA, et al. Incidence of imipenem hypersensitivity reactions in febrile neutropenic bone marrow transplant patients with a history of penicillin allergy. *Clin Infect Dis* 2000;31:1512.
21. Medical Letter. Ertapenem (Invanz)—a new parenteral carbapenem. *Med Lett Drugs Ther* 2002;44:25.
22. Goldstein EJC, et al. Comparative *in vitro* activities of ertapenem (MK 0826) against 1001 anaerobes isolated from human intra-abdominal infections. *Antimicrob Agents Chemother* 2000;44:2389.
23. Finch RG, et al. Meropenem: focus on clinical performance. *J Antimicrob Chemother* 1995;36[Suppl A]:1–223.
24. Wiseman LR, et al. Meropenem: a review of its antibacterial activity, pharmacokinetics and clinical efficacy. *Drugs* 1995;50:73–101.
25. Norrby SR. Carbapenems: efficacy and safety profiles-focus on meropenem. *Scand J Infect Dis* 1995;96[Suppl]:5–48.
26. Medical Letter. Meropenem: a new parenteral broad spectrum antibiotic. *Med Lett Drugs Ther* 1996;38:88.
27. Alvarez Lerma F. Serious Infection Study Group. Efficacy of meropenem as monotherapy in the treatment of ventilator-associated pneumonia. *J Chemother* 2001;13:70–81.
28. Norrby SR, Faulkner KL. Differentiating meropenem and imipenem/cilastatin. *Infect Dis Clin Pract* 1997;6:291.
29. Henry NK, et al. Antimicrobial agents for infants and children: guidelines for the in-patient and out-patient practice of pediatric infectious disease. *Mayo Clin Proc* 2000;75:86.
30. Odio CM, et al. Prospective, randomized, investigator-blinded study of the efficacy and safety of meropenem vs. cefotaxime therapy in bacterial meningitis in children, Meropenem Meningitis Study Group. *Pediatr Infect Dis J* 1999;18:581.
31. Norrby SR, Gildon KM. Safety profile of meropenem: a review of nearly 5,000 patients treated with meropenem. *Scand J Infect* 1999;31:3.

## I. Aminoglycosides

The role of aminoglycoside antibiotics in clinical medicine has decreased somewhat as third-generation cephalosporins, aztreonam, and fluoroquinolones have become available [1]. Nevertheless, because of the rare development of bacterial resistance, the low incidence of *Clostridium difficile* diarrhea, the low risk of allergic reactions, the better understanding of their toxicity, and cost considerations, the aminoglycosides remain very useful. **These agents are, in most instances, bactericidal.** However, the precise mechanism through which the aminoglycosides cause bacterial cell death remains unclear [2]. They penetrate the cell wall and membrane and bind irreversibly to the 30S bacterial ribosome. The most commonly used aminoglycosides are gentamicin, tobramycin, and amikacin, so these agents are emphasized here [1–3]. Netilmicin is no longer manufactured in the United States.

**I. Introduction: important principles of aminoglycoside use**

**A. When?** Aminoglycosides are active against almost all aerobic gram-negative rods.

**1. Community versus nosocomial infections.** Although aminoglycosides are active against community-acquired gram-negative bacteria, cephalosporins are preferred for empiric use. **In contrast, aminoglycosides are particularly useful in hospital-acquired infections,** especially for *Pseudomonas* species. A change to aztreonam after initial aminoglycoside treatment of a gram-negative bacteria when prolonged therapy is contemplated reduces toxicity. Ciprofloxacin is useful empirically when most gram-negative

Table 27I.1. Aminoglycoside Activity

| Typically Active Against | Not Usually Active Against |
|---|---|
| *Acinetobacter* species[a] | |
| *Citrobacter* species[a] | |
| *Enterobacter* species[a] | |
| *Escherichia coli*[b] | *Pseudomonas (Burkholderia) cepacia* |
| *Klebsiella* species[b] | |
| *Morganella morganii*[b] | *Stenotrophomonas maltophilia*[c] |
| *Proteus* species[b] | |
| *Providence* species[b] | |
| *Pseudomonas aeruginosa*[d] | |
| *P. fluorescens* | |
| *Serratia* species[b] | |
| *Yersinia enterocolitica* | |

[a]Although aminoglycosides may be active *in vitro,* imipenem or meropenem are viewed as "drugs of choice" [3].
[b]Although aminoglycosides are active *in vitro,* cephalosporins usually preferred [3].
[c]Formerly called *Pseudomonas maltophilia* or *Xanthomonas maltophilia.*
[d]Aminoglycosides, often in combination with piperacillin, are drugs of choice for severe infections. For UTIs, ciprofloxacin (a quinolone) preferred [3].

organisms occurring in that setting are susceptible or after the offending bacteria has been isolated and tested.

2. **Modifying initial therapy.** Regardless of the circumstances under which the aminoglycoside are initiated, if the isolated pathogen is susceptible to a narrow-spectrum agent, appropriate modifications should be made.

**B. Special problems with aminoglycoside use**

1. **Toxicity. The aminoglycosides have considerable intrinsic toxicity, both nephrotoxicity and eighth nerve.** Risk factors for toxicity include older age, treatment with aminoglycosides for more than 2 weeks, and the concurrent use of other ototoxic toxic or nephrotoxic agents. This risk of toxicity must be considered, especially with use for any extended time (>7 days) (see section **VI**). Aminoglycoside toxicity is rare before 7 days.
2. **Toxic-therapeutic ratio.** The margin between effective and toxic concentrations is narrow.
3. **Monitoring of serum levels.** Serum levels must be measured to ensure effective levels and minimize toxicity. This topic is discussed in detail in section **V.**

**II. *In vitro* activity (Note peak serum levels are 8 ug/ml for gentamicin and tobramycin and 25 ug/ml for amikacin)**

**A. Gram-negative aerobes (Table 27I.1)**

1. **Community-acquired** gram-negative organisms. All aminoglycosides are equally active in proportion to achievable serum levels.
2. **Hospital-acquired gram-negative organisms.** In general, tobramycin *in vitro* is two to four times more active than gentamicin against *Pseudomonas aeruginosa,* although the clinical implications of this are unclear. Against *Serratia* species, gentamicin has two to four times the bactericidal activity of tobramycin. For other nosocomial organisms, the aminoglycosides are equally active in proportion to achievable serum levels [1]. Against organisms resistant to one or more aminoglycosides, amikacin is the most frequently active, tobramycin is the next, and gentamicin is the least frequently active.

**B. Gram-positive aerobes.** The aminoglycosides have some activity against some organisms (e.g., staphylococci) but **alone are never the preferred agents** [3]. Gentamicin, together with ampicillin or penicillin, usually is **bactericidal against enterococci.** However, in recent years, at major medical centers, there has

Table 27I.2. Expected Peak and Trough Levels of Respective Aminoglycosides (in μg/mL) with Conventional or Individualized Dosing

| | Peak[a,b] | Trough[c] | Toxic[b] |
|---|---|---|---|
| Gentamicin | 6–10 | 1–2 | >10 |
| Tobramycin | 6–10 | 1–2 | >10 |
| Amikacin | 15–30 | 5–10 | >35 |

These ranges for peak and trough concentrations are used commonly, but their exact implications remain controversial, as reviewed by McCormack JP, Jewesson PJ. A critical reevaluation of the "therapeutic range" of aminoglycosides. *Clin Infect Dis* 1992;14:320.
[a]Drawn one-half hour after a half-hour i.v. infusion. See text. For pneumonia therapy, the higher levels of peaks are desirable.
[b]These peak toxic levels are with conventional dosage regimens. With once-a-day dosages, higher acceptable peak levels will routinely be achieved. See text.
[c]Level just before next dose.

been an increasing incidence of high level gentamicin-resistant enterococci. These enterococci are resistant to more than 2,000 μg/mL of gentamicin and therefore to the combination of gentamicin and penicillin. In one report, 26% of enterococci demonstrated high level gentamicin resistance [2]. The details of this problem and alternative therapeutic approaches are reviewed elsewhere [4].

C. **Anaerobes** are not susceptible.

D. ***Nocardia*** is susceptible to amikacin [3].

E. **Mycobacterium.** Most *Mycobacterium tuberculosis* are susceptible to streptomycin and amikacin; most *M. avium-intracellulare* isolates are susceptible to amikacin [3].

## III. Pharmacokinetics

A. **Gentamicin and tobramycin have similar pharmacokinetics;** therefore standard doses, peak levels achieved, and serum half-lives are essentially the same (Table 27I.2). Amikacin is a semisynthetic kanamycin derivative with pharmacokinetics nearly identical to those of kanamycin. The **intravenous route is preferred,** but the intramuscular route can be used if hypotension or thrombocytopenia is absent.

B. **Variation in pharmacokinetics.** There is striking variation in the volume of distribution and rate of excretion of aminoglycosides in individual patients with normal renal function [5]. **Thus it is important to monitor serum levels in all patients regardless of volume status or renal function** (see section **V**) to ensure adequate levels. Peak and trough level measures can be repeated every 3 to 4 days if the patient is stable. In a patient who has major changes in hydration status or renal function, levels have to be repeated more frequently (Table 27I.2).

1. **Peak levels** [1] are measured 30 minutes after completion of an intravenous infusion or 45 to 60 minutes after intramuscular injection. In renal failure, the peak sample is drawn 120 to 150 minutes after the intramuscular dose, because the drug continues to be absorbed and not excreted. **Peak** serum **level** is obtained to ensure that enough drug was administered for therapeutic efficacy. A peak level is obtained after the first or second maintenance dose or after dosage adjustments.
2. **Trough levels** are obtained just before the next dose. If trough levels are elevated, the dose needs to be reduced or the dose interval prolonged. In renal failure, the trough level should ideally be obtained after the same dose in which the peak was measured.

C. **Aminoglycoside excretion is entirely renal,** mandating dose reductions in renal failure.
D. **Tissue penetration.** Aminoglycosides achieve reasonable concentrations in bone, synovial fluid, and peritoneal fluid. Urinary concentrations are high and usually exceed serum concentration by 100 times in patients with normal renal function [2]. There is limited penetration into the central nervous system and probably intraabdominal abscesses [1]. Drug levels in bronchial secretions are poor [2].

IV. **Clinical use** [1,2]

A. **Aminoglycosides as drugs of choice** for specific pathogens [3]

1. **For *P. aeruginosa* infections other than urinary tract infection (UTI),** an aminoglycoside is combined with piperacillin or similar antibiotic except in delayed penicillin allergy where cefepime is often substituted. In ***P. aeruginosa* UTI,** ciprofloxacin is preferred [3].
2. **Gentamicin** is **used in combination** with another agent **to achieve synergy** with: (a) penicillin, ampicillin, or vancomycin against gentamicin-susceptible enterococci or viridans streptococci [1,2]; (b) ampicillin against *Listeria monocytogenes;* (c) an extended-spectrum penicillin (e.g., piperacillin) against *P. aeruginosa* and susceptible *Enterobacter* species (see section **1** above); (d) vancomycin and rifampin against *S. epidermidis* prosthetic valve infection; (e) ampicillin (or vancomycin) for endocarditis prophylaxis in high-risk patients before genitourinary or gastrointestinal procedures; (f) an antistaphylococcal penicillin for right-sided endocarditis caused by *S. aureus;* and (g) doxycycline for brucellosis [1–3].
3. **Amikacin** has been used in certain atypical mycobacterium infection. Amikacin (plus clarithromycin) is the drug of choice for *M. fortuitum* complex infections [3].
4. **Streptomycin (or gentamicin)** is an agent of choice for *Yersinia pestis* (plague); streptomycin remains a useful agent for *M. tuberculosis* therapy and for *M. kansasii* infections.

B. **Other situations.** Gentamicin is a primary agent. Tobramycin or amikacin are alternates [3].

1. **As empiric therapy in life-threatening community-acquired gram-negative** infections.
2. **Infections occurring in a hospital setting or in a patient who has recently been hospitalized;** an aminoglycoside is indicated while awaiting culture data.
   a. **In most community hospitals** where resistance to gentamicin is uncommon, we favor gentamicin because it is less expensive. An exception is the patient who has already received gentamicin and is possibly infected with a relatively resistant gram-negative bacterium. Until susceptibility data are available, tobramycin or amikacin are the preferred agents.
   b. **Amikacin versus gentamicin** [1]. **In large medical centers or specialized areas** (e.g., intensive care units, burn units) where the frequency of resistance to gentamicin, tobramycin, or netilmicin may be high, amikacin is preferred until susceptibility data are available. If gentamicin resistance is low (e.g., 1%–5%), gentamicin is the most rational cost-effective choice unless the patient has recently received gentamicin. In that instance amikacin should be used while awaiting culture results. Amikacin is the aminoglycoside of choice for the treatment of gentamicin-resistant gram-negative bacteria [2,6].
   c. **Note.** If a patient is potentially at high risk for aminoglycoside toxicity (e.g., in hepatic failure or is frail and elderly; see section **VI.A.4**), an alternate should be considered (e.g., aztreonam).
3. In the **leukopenic febrile patient** with no obvious focus of infection, an aminoglycoside and an extended-spectrum penicillin (e.g., piperacillin) have commonly been used (see Chapter 20).
4. **For susceptible pathogens in which a less toxic agent is unavailable,** aminoglycosides have been used effectively to treat susceptible gram-negative

organisms causing UTI, bone and joint infections, pneumonia, and sometimes gram-negative bacillary endocarditis.

5. **In nosocomial intraabdominal infections** (see Chapter 13). Resistant gram-negative organisms are present when peritonitis develops in a patient who has been in the hospital.
6. **For therapy for organisms that may develop resistance to monotherapy with a third-generation cephalosporin** such as *Enterobacter cloacae, Citrobacter freundii,* and *Acinetobacter* species. In this setting, an aminoglycoside is often combined with an extended-spectrum penicillin (e.g., piperacillin) for synergy. However, imipenem or meropenem is preferable for nosocomially acquired *Acinetobacter* species and some *Enterobacter* species [3].

C. **Aminoglycoside effectiveness** is not optimal in the following situations [1]:

1. **In lower respiratory tract infections,** the low pH of bronchial secretions may decrease the activity of aminoglycosides. One cannot **rely on aminoglycosides alone** in major lower respiratory tract infections such as *Pseudomonas* pneumonia.
2. **Sterilization of abscesses** with aminoglycosides may be difficult because of poor activity in the presence of the low pH, anaerobic conditions, and bivalent cations.
3. **Prostatitis.** Aminoglycosides do not achieve useful levels in prostate tissue.

V. **Aminoglycoside dosing.** Numerous dosage regimens have been proposed, but studies showing that one method is clearly superior are not available. **What is widely accepted is that in the very ill patient, giving a routine conventional dose (e.g., 1.5 mg/kg** every 8 hours) **to adults with normal renal function is not an acceptable dose regimen** because of the variability in levels achieved. Zaske et al. [5] emphasized this when they studied more than 200 surgical patients. In that carefully done study in patients with normal renal function, if this standard approach was used, 47% of the patients would be underdosed and 14% would be overdosed.

**Three acceptable approaches are** single daily dose regimens for short-use duration, individualized dosing with a pharmacokinetics model, and conventional dosing with serum levels used to adjust doses by someone skilled in the use of aminoglycoside.

A. **Single daily aminoglycoside dosing** has been evaluated in several settings [7–14].

1. **The underlying principles** of this approach include the following:
   a. **Concentration-dependent killing.** The rate of bactericidal killing by aminoglycosides increases as the antibiotic concentration is increased (see Chapter 25) and the increased killing persists for a prolonged period. In addition, data suggest that once daily dosing is less toxic than thrice daily dosing, although this could be the more effective level achieved initially [5].
   b. **Postantibiotics effect (PAE)** is persistent suppression of growth after short antibiotic exposure. Aminoglycosides demonstrate a PAE against aerobic gram-negative bacilli both *in vitro* and in animal models. The duration of the PAE correlates with the height of the peak. PAE remains after the serum level falls below the minimum inhibitory concentration. In the animal model with normal neutrophils, the presence of neutrophils doubled the duration of the *in vivo* PAE [7]. The importance of the PAE in humans has not been completely studied.
   c. Nephrotoxicity and probably ototoxicity are related to time-dependent drug accumulation. **Single daily dosing (SDD) seems less toxic** than multiple doses, perhaps because little or no tissue accumulation occurs during the several hours when serum levels are low before the next infusion [13] or perhaps because higher levels are guaranteed to occur initially [5].
2. **Clinical studies** have been summarized in detail elsewhere [7–14]. SDD appears to be comparable and in some cases superior in efficacy to traditional aminoglycoside dosing. However, in the studies of SDD, therapy has been for short duration plus a second effective agent has been part of the regimen and most study subjects have been under 55 years of age.

Table 27I.3. Exclusions for Using Single Daily Dosing

| |
|---|
| Moderate to severe renal insufficiency (creatinine clearance < 40 mL/min) |
| Serious burns (> 20% body surface area) |
| Ascites |
| Severe sepsis syndrome |
| Cystic fibrosis |
| Fluid overload postoperatively |
| Dialysis |
| Neonates/children |
| Pregnant patients |
| Documented invasive *P. aeruginosa* infection in neutropenic patients |
| Patients receiving other nephrotoxic agents (amphotericin B, cis-platinum, radiocontrast material, nonsteroidal anti-inflammatory drugs) |
| Endocarditis |
| Mycobacterial disease |
| Patients needing protracted courses, >7 days[a] |
| Patients with significant underlying hepatic disease[b] |

[a]For example, in *P. aeruginosa* pneumonia in which the patient may need 2–3 weeks of antibiotics.
[b]See text. We try to avoid aminoglycosides in these patients.
Modified from Gerberding JL. Aminoglycoside dosing: timing is of the essence. *Am J Med* 1998;105:256, with permission.

**3. Limitations of use of SDD (Table 27I.3)**

a. **In reduced creatinine clearance,** high-dose aminoglycoside treatment will produce sustained serum concentrations, drug accumulation, and increased potential for toxicity. Therefore these patients have been excluded from published trials [12].

b. **Situations of uncertain volume of drug distribution or clearance** [12], including ascites, sepsis syndrome, severe burns, cystic fibrosis, or recipients of large volumes of fluid infusion.

c. **Pregnant women, children, and neonates.** There are incomplete data for SDD [12].

d. **Endocarditis (e.g., enterococci).** Animal studies reveal SDD regimens are inferior [13].

e. **Prolonged SDD regimens.** Because there are limited data on the toxicity, we prefer individualized dosing in patients needing aminoglycosides for more than 7 days.

f. **Significant underlying hepatic disease (e.g., cirrhosis).** In general, **we try to avoid aminoglycosides here** because of the risk of nephrotoxicity. If they must be used, infectious disease consultation and individualized dosing are suggested.

**4. Dosing regimens for gentamicin and tobramycin.** Doses used have ranged from 5 to 7.5 mg/kg infused over 60 minutes [12]. For older subjects, the lower dose regimen of **5 mg/kg** is favored [6,7]. For the younger subject, the higher dose is reasonable.

a. **Ideal body weight (IBW) in kilograms [15]:** If the weight is more than 20% to 30% over IBW, an obese dosing weight is used.

(1) **To estimate IBW**

**Women** = 45 kg + 2.3 kg per inch of height over 5 feet
**Men** = 50 kg + 2.3 kg per inch of height over 5 feet
**For example,** for a male patient 5 ft 10 in. tall, an estimated IBW would be 50 + 2.3[10], or 50 + 23 = 73 kg

(2) **For weight more than 20% above IBW,** an obese dosing weight (ODW) is more reliable [15].

ODW = IBW + 40% (of excess weight; i.e., actual weight minus IBW)

Table 27I.4. Once-daily Aminoglycoside Maintenance Dosing Regimens for Gentamicin and Tobramycin

| Estimated Creatinine Clearance (mL/min) | Dose in mg/kg (Given q24h) Over 60 Min |
|---|---|
| >80 | 5 |
| 60–80 | 4 |
| 50–60 | 3.5 |
| 40–50 | 2.5 |
| <40 | Individualized pharmacokinetics advised |

Modified from Gilbert DN. Aminoglycosides. In: Root RK, et al., eds. *Clinical infectious diseases: a practical approach*. New York: Oxford University Press, 1999:273–284, with permission.

**For example,** an obese woman has a wound infection requiring gentamicin or tobramycin. Her actual weight is 100 kg; her ideal weight is 60 kg.

Obese dosing weight

= IBW + 20% (100 minus 60)
= 60 + 20% (40) = 60 + 8
= 68 kg, and this weight can be used in Table 27I.4.

b. **For estimating the creatinine clearance for doses**, a modification of the equation of Cockcroft and Gault is used (see Tables 27I.4 and 27I.5).

5. **Dosing in patients with renal dysfunction.** One convenient method is to determine the half-life and then give one-half the dose every half-life. However, data are not available to ensure the superiority of that method over extension of the interval [13] (see Tables 27I.4 and 27I.5).
   a. **Prolonging the dose interval.** See detailed guidelines for this approach [13].
   b. **Single daily dose with lowering the total daily aminoglycoside dose.** For patients with mild to moderate renal insufficiency, this approach is less cumbersome. Here, it is important to document that the 18-hour serum concentration is low (<2 μg/mL for gentamicin or tobramycin) or undetectable [12]. Gilbert [13] suggested that if the gentamicin or tobramycin serum level is more than 1 μg/mL at 18 hours, one should repeat serum creatinine and recalculate the estimated creatinine clearance and reassess the dose.

Table 27I.5. Once-daily Aminoglycoside Dosing Regimen for Amikacin

| Estimated Creatinine Clearance (mL/min) | Dose in mg/kg (Given q24h) Over 60 Min |
|---|---|
| >90 | 15 |
| 70–90 | 12 |
| 50–70 | 7.5 |
| 40–50 | 4.0 |
| <40 | Individualized pharmacokinetics advised |

Modified from Gilbert DN. Aminoglycosides. In: Root RK, et al., eds. *Clinical infectious diseases: a practical approach*. New York: Oxford University Press, 1999:273–284, with permission.

6. **Serum monitoring** in SDD continues to undergo evaluation.
   a. A **trough** level before the second or third dose is advised. Troughs should be less than 1 μg/mL; if not, extend the dose interval (see section **5.b**). **Troughs** can be repeated every 48 to 72 hours.
   b. **Peak** levels are not indicated, except in severe sepsis where clearance is very rapid.
7. **Summary.** Unless contraindicated (see Table 27I.3), "the available data are sufficient to establish this strategy (i.e., SDD or extended dosing) as a standard approach for most serious infections where aminoglycoside treatment is indicated" [9].

B. **Pharmacokinetics model (Table 27I.3 and see section V.A.4)**
1. Zaske and colleagues devised a formula for the pharmacokinetics of aminoglycosides in individual patients with either normal or impaired renal function [5,16]. **A loading dose** is given (see section **C.1** below). Subsequently, timed serum samples are used to determine the volume of distribution and the half-life of the aminoglycoside. Using a kinetic model, the appropriate dose needed to achieve a desired peak and trough is calculated. Acceptable peak and trough levels can be maintained by adjusting doses and dose intervals. (See Table 27I.2 **for desirable levels.**)
   a. Because of the **variations in the volume of drug distribution** and the patient's ability to excrete aminoglycosides, there is marked variation in levels achieved with conventional dosing (see section **C** below). The patient's age, renal function, state of hydration, presence or absence of fever, and degree of obesity affect serum levels. **Individualized dosing allows adjustment for each patient** by measuring serum levels and calculating the aminoglycoside's half-life.
   b. **Patients with shorter half-lives.** Higher and more frequent doses are required to maintain adequate aminoglycoside peaks and to avoid prolonged periods of subtherapeutic levels. The converse is true for those with longer half-lives [5].
   c. **Protracted therapy required.** The pharmacokinetic model is favored over SDD (Table 27I.3).

C. **Conventional dosing, careful level monitoring, and dose adjustment** [10,12]
1. **Loading dose,** independent of creatinine clearance, achieves therapeutic plasma levels rapidly. **IBW** in kilograms **is used for adult patients.** In the patient weighing 20% more than IBW, an obese weight is calculated as per section **V.A.4.** First, calculate the IBW/ODW for the patient. **For gentamicin and tobramycin,** use a loading dose of 2 mg/kg. **For amikacin,** a dose of 7.5 mg/kg is suggested.
   a. **Children.** A loading dose of 2 to 2.5 mg/kg is suggested for gentamicin and tobramycin. For amikacin, 5 to 7.5 mg/kg has been used (maximum of 500 mg).
   b. **Neonates** (see Chapter 3)
2. For **maintenance doses**
   a. **Adult, normal serum creatinine.** Gentamicin or tobramycin at 1.0 to 1.7 mg/kg/dose is given at an 8-hour interval in young to middle-aged patients and every 12 hours in older patients. The low dose is used for UTI and the higher dose is used for tissue or bloodstream infections. For amikacin 5 mg/kg is given every 8 hours up to middle age and every 12 hours in older patients.
   b. **Children.** Aminoglycosides are eliminated more rapidly, so the follow-up doses are the same as the loading dose (2 to 2.5 mg/kg/dose of gentamicin or tobramycin) given every 8 hours. The dose of amikacin is 5 to 7.5 mg/kg (maximum of 500 mg) given every 8 hours.
   c. **Renal failure. Two options exist and** the optimal approach is unclear. **The usual dose interval can be prolonged or doses can be given every half-life.** Serum monitoring after the first dose and at 48 hours is essential;

this dosing regimen is only an estimate. Further dosing can be adjusted as needed by someone experienced in aminoglycoside use to maintain appropriate peaks and troughs (Table 27I.2).

(1) **Prolonging the interval. For gentamicin and tobramycin:** Multiply the serum creatinine by 8 to estimate the interval. If the serum creatinine is 2.0, the maintenance dose can be given (serum creatinine of 2 × 8) every 16 hours (every 18 hours for convenience). **For amikacin:** Multiply the serum creatinine by 9, that is, creatinine is 2.0 and the interval is 18 hours.

(2) **Dosage every half-life.** This avoids very prolonged intervals of low serum trough levels, and half the dose can be given at the estimated half-life interval. For example, if the serum creatinine is 3.5, for gentamicin the estimated prolonged interval is 8 × 3.5 = 36 hours; 50% of the dose can be given every 18 hours (i.e., at half the extended interval). **In renal failure we prefer "individualized dosing" (see section B above).** Dosing based on **nomograms** alone is **not advised.**

**D. Overview of methods of dosing aminoglycosides.** Until further studies clarify this issue, a reasonable approach for those patients in whom it is not clear if they are infected with an aminoglycoside-requiring organism to dose aminoglycosides using a once daily regimen for empiric short courses (e.g., 3–5 days). If an aminoglycoside is genuinely required in the very ill patient and in certain complex patient settings where SDD is contraindicated (Table 27I.3), individualized dosing is preferable and may also be superior for courses longer than 7 days.

**E. Hemodialysis** reduces levels by approximately 50%. One-half of the dose is given after dialysis. Because the duration of dialysis and type of dialysis machine affect the amount of drug removed, **monitoring serum aminoglycoside levels is necessary.**

**F. Peritoneal dialysis.** One-third to one-half of a usual single dose is administered daily. Serum aminoglycoside levels are advised.

**G. Direct administration into infection sites.** Aminoglycosides have been administered into the site of infection to gain benefit of activity while at the same time avoiding their toxicity.

1. **Chronic ambulatory peritoneal dialysis.** Aminoglycosides in peritoneal dialysis fluid are used for chronic ambulatory peritoneal dialysis peritonitis but not for systemic infections. Because of the diffusion of an aminoglycoside across the peritoneum, serum levels of the aminoglycoside should be monitored. Infectious diseases consultation is recommended for these complicated patients [17].
2. **Aerosolized aminoglycosides** have been used in special settings: in cystic fibrosis patients with *P. aeruginosa* in their sputum [18–23], to prevent early colonization with *P. aeruginosa* in cystic fibrosis [21] and to treat selected cases of purulent *P. aeruginosa* tracheobronchitis without pneumonia in elderly patients [19], and as adjunctive therapy for persistent smear positive pulmonary tuberculosis [23]. Infectious disease consultation is advised.
3. **Artificial joint cement or gentamicin beads.** After removal of infected artificial joints, cement containing tobramycin has been used in anticipation of later artificial joint replacement. In addition, gentamicin-containing bead chains have been inserted into infected osteomyelitis cavities and have demonstrated a high success rate and virtually no toxicity [24].

**VI. Toxicity.** Hypersensitivity reactions are uncommon. Important side effects include the following [1,2,25]:

**A. Nephrotoxicity** occurs at the level of the proximal tubule, but how injury or death of proximal tubule cells results in a decrease in the glomerular filtration rate is uncertain. The overall incidence of aminoglycoside nephrotoxicity is about 5% to 10% [1,2]. **Serum creatinine levels** should be obtained every 2 to 4 days in patients receiving aminoglycosides.

1. **Definition.** Initial creatinine was normal: nephrotoxicity is either the elevation of creatinine to 1.5 or higher or an absolute increase of 0.4 mg/dL. Initial serum

creatinine is elevated but less than 3.0 mg/dL: nephrotoxicity is an increase of at least 0.5 mg/dL. Initial creatinine exceeded 3.0: a rise in serum creatinine of more than 1.0 mg/dL defines nephrotoxicity [25].

2. **Manifestations.** A rising blood urea nitrogen and creatinine, proteinuria, or oliguria or nonoliguric renal failure. Changes are **usually reversible with discontinuation.** Progression to dialysis is uncommon.
3. **Comparative toxicity.** No proof exists that gentamicin is more toxic than tobramycin [1,2].
4. **Risk factors** are [1,2,25] as follows:
   a. **Concomitant liver disease.** In particular, when prothrombin time is prolonged due to liver disease or in patients with known hepatorenal syndrome. Use other options if possible.
   b. **Concomitant drug use.** Vancomycin, amphotericin B, cyclosporine, furosemide, nonsteroidal antiinflammatory agents, and foscarnet appear to increase the frequency of nephrotoxicity.
   c. **Other risk factors.** Advanced age, previous courses of aminoglycosides (within 1 year), greater total dose of aminoglycoside, and prior renal disease may be associated with toxicity.
5. **Prevention** of nephrotoxicity is not fully understood. Considerations are as follows:
   a. **Use aminoglycosides only when indicated and for** the **shortest appropriate course.**
   b. **Management of fluid status:** Correct hypovolemia and/or congestive heart failure.
   c. **Avoid with underlying liver disease** (see section **4** above).
   d. **SDD regimens** for short courses of therapy.
   e. **Individualized dosing** for longer courses (>7 days) of therapy (see sections **V.A** and **V.B** ).
   f. **Monitoring of levels** is appropriate. However, even when levels are maintained at those that are recommended, toxicity may still occur [26].

B. **Ototoxicity is frequently irreversible** [1,2,25] and may appear during or after therapy. Repeated exposure engenders cumulative risk. Older patients are at greater risk for ototoxicity. A given patient may develop cochlear damage, vestibular damage, or, rarely, both.

1. **Cochlear (auditory) toxicity.** Audiometric studies show that 2% to 14% of recipients demonstrate hearing loss, but clinically detected hearing loss is uncommon. Patients particularly at risk to develop clinical signs are those who have received a high cumulative dose or a protracted course of aminoglycosides. **In general,** if renal function is normal, **routine audiograms are not recommended.** In a cooperative patient who needs protracted aminoglycoside therapy (e.g., more than 2 weeks), serial audiograms are reasonable. **Serum levels should be monitored carefully and adjusted. Protracted courses of aminoglycosides should be avoided whenever possible.**
2. **Vestibular dysfunction** manifested by nausea, vomiting, vertigo, dizziness, and unsteady gait with nystagmus is more difficult to evaluate in ill patients but presumably is related to the same predisposing factors that cause auditory toxicity. This appears to occur in 1% to 3% of patients and is usually irreversible.
3. **Interruption of therapy.** If a patient develops symptoms of hearing loss, tinnitus, vertigo, or nystagmus, the aminoglycoside should be discontinued and the situation reevaluated.

C. **Neuromuscular paralysis,** though rare, has occurred after intraperitoneal lavage (no longer used or recommended) or after rapid intravenous bolus therapy, particularly in the setting of myasthenia gravis or concurrent use of succinylcholine or curare. This is usually reversible.

VII. **Cost.** Gentamicin is less expensive than all other aminoglycosides and cephalosporins. A daily dose for SDD costs under $5 and monitoring costs are lower. Hospitals have estimated that SDD administration may reduce hospital costs of aminoglycoside administration 50% to 60% [2]. Amikacin is the most expensive aminoglycoside (see Appendix Table).

**VIII. Resistance**

**A. Gram-negative organisms.** With the exception of streptomycin, aminoglycoside resistance **evolves very slowly** [1,2], but use is eventually followed by the development of resistance. When gentamicin resistance of nosocomial gram-negative organisms exceeds 10%, it is reasonable to use amikacin, especially if resistant blood isolates have been detected.

**B. Mechanisms in gram-negative organisms. Diffusion mediated resistance.** Changes in porins of the cell wall restrict diffusion into the cell. This may be aminoglycoside specific. The minimum inhibitory concentration increases, but use with a $\beta$-lactam may still mediate synergy. **Inactivation of the aminoglycoside** inside the cell by six specific enzymes. All of these enzymes inactivate gentamicin; five of the six inactivates tobramycin, and one of the six inactivates amikacin.

**C. High level gentamicin-resistant enterococci** have increased significantly [2] (see section **II.B**).

1. **Clinical significance.** These enterococci are potentially very important nosocomial pathogens because of intrinsic cephalosporin resistance. Their epidemiology is very similar to that of methicillin-resistant *S. aureus* and of multidrug-resistant gram-negative bacilli. Therefore all enterococci isolated from normally sterile body fluids (e.g., blood) or serious wound infections should be tested **for high level aminoglycoside resistance,** as well as ampicillin and vancomycin susceptibility.
2. **Therapy.** Optimal therapy is unclear; **infectious disease consultation is advised.**

**IX. Other aminoglycosides are used less frequently and are discussed only briefly.**

**A. Streptomycin** was introduced in 1944 and was effective against many gram-negative bacteria and *M. tuberculosis.* Gram-negative resistance to streptomycin is now prevalent. Hospital pharmacies can order streptomycin by calling 1-800-254-4445 (Monday through Friday 8:30 A.M. to 5 P.M. EST).

1. **Current uses**
   a. **Tularemia.** Streptomycin (or gentamicin) is the drug of choice for susceptible strains of *Francisella tularensis* [3].
   b. **Antituberculous therapy.** Although its use has diminished, it is still used [3].
   c. **Uncommon diseases** in which streptomycin is a drug of choice or alternative drug [3] are brucellosis (with tetracycline), glanders *Pseudomonas (Burkholderia) mallei,* and plague due to *Yersinia pestis.* Streptomycin has been used for treatment of endocarditis due to those strains of enterococci exhibiting high level resistance to gentamicin but preserved susceptibility to streptomycin [2]. Streptomycin may be used as an alternate agent in rat-bite fever due to *Streptobacillus moniliformis* or *Spirillum minus* [3] or in granuloma inguinale.
2. **Dosage.** With normal renal function, for tularemia or plague, 500 to 1,000 mg intramuscularly every 12 hours can be used. In children, 20 to 30 mg/kg/day is given and divided into every 12 hour doses.
   a. **Renal failure.** Ototoxicity is the risk. Therefore, gentamicin with monitoring of levels is an acceptable alternative or the dose of streptomycin must be reduced. One approach [27] is to give a 1-g loading dose and then prolong the interval. If the creatinine clearance is 10 to 50 mL/min, use a dose interval of 24 to 72 hours. If the creatinine clearance is less than 10 mL/min, use a dose interval of 72 to 96 hours. Streptomycin is removed by hemodialysis and peritoneal dialysis. If streptomycin must be used in dialysis, monitoring of serum levels using the disk diffusion method is a possibility. Obtain infectious disease consultation.
   b. **Tuberculosis therapy** (see **Chapter 11)**
3. **Toxicity.** Avoid streptomycin in patients older than 55 years if an alternate agent is available.
   a. **Ototoxicity.** When given 2 g daily for more than 60 days, most patients develop vestibular toxicity. The incidence is reduced by half if the dosage

is reduced to 1 g daily. Deafness can occur. Risks include impaired renal function, old age, and prolonged therapy.

b. **Nephrotoxicity** is much less common with streptomycin than with the other aminoglycosides.

c. **Hypersensitivity** reactions include rash and drug fever.

B. **Paromomycin (Humatin).** Paromomycin sulfate is structurally related to streptomycin. It is too toxic for parenteral administration. It is available in an amorphous powder with a saline taste [28]. Because it is not absorbed from the intestinal tract, it can be used safely as alternative therapy for symptomatic infections due to *Entamoeba histolytica* [29] and has been used in patients with acquired immunodeficiency syndrome infected with the protozoa *Cryptosporidium parvum* [29].

1. **Pharmacokinetics.** Although paromomycin is poorly absorbed from the gastrointestinal tract, impaired gastrointestinal motility or ulcerations may facilitate absorption of the drug. Therefore paromomycin must be administered with caution to patients with ulcerative intestinal lesions. Accumulation may occur in patients with impaired renal function, making the drug contraindicated in this setting.
2. **Uses for parasitic infections.** Paromomycin is a drug of choice for a symptomatic carrier of *E. histolytica* and *Dientamoeba fragilis* infections. It is also an alternative agent for infections due to *Giardia lamblia* [29]. **Cryptosporidiosis in acquired immunodeficiency syndrome.** In a recent study, paromomycin was found to be no more effective than placebo [30]. Hence it is no longer indicated for therapy [29].
3. **Side effects** [18]. Anorexia, nausea, vomiting, epigastric burning, cramps, and diarrhea are the most frequent. Rash, eosinophilia, and headache and overgrowth of *Candida* may occur.

## REFERENCES

1. Reese RE, Betts RF. Aminoglycosides. In: Reese RE, Betts RF, Gumustop B. eds. *Handbook of antibiotics,* 3rd ed. Philadelphia: Lippincott Williams & Wilkins, 2000;415–434.
2. Edson RS, Terrelly CL. The aminoglycosides. *Mayo Clin Proc* 1999;74:519.
3. Medical Letter. The choice of antibacterial drugs. *Med Lett Drugs Ther* 2001;43:69–74.
4. Wells VD, et al. Infections due to beta-lactamase-producing, high-level gentamicin-resistant *Enterococcus faecalis*. *Ann Intern Med* 1992;116:285.
5. Zaske DE, Cipolle RJ, Strate RJ. Gentamicin dosage requirements: wide interpatient variations in 242 surgery patients with normal renal function, *Surgery* 1980;87:164.
6. Dubois V, Arpin C, Melon M, et al. Nosocomial outbreak due to a multi-resistant strain of *Pseudomonas aeruginosa P12*: efficacy of cefepime-amikacin therapy and analysis of beta-lactam resistance. *J Clin Microbiol* 2001;39:2072–2078.
7. Urban AW, Craig WA. Daily dosing of aminoglycosides. *Curr Clin Top Infect Dis* 1997;17:236.
8. Bailey TC, et al. A meta-analysis of extended-interval dosing versus multiple daily dosing of aminoglycosides. *Clin Infect Dis* 1997;24:786.
9. Gilbert DN. Editorial response: meta-analyses are no longer required for determining the efficacy of single daily dosing of aminoglycosides. *Clin Infect Dis* 1997;24:816.
10. Bertino JS Jr, Rotschafer JC. Editorial response: single daily dosing of aminoglycosides: a concept whose time has not come. *Clin Infect Dis* 1997;34:820.
11. Beringer PM, et al. Pharmacokinetics of tobramycin in adults with cystic fibrosis: implications for once-daily administration. *Antimicrob Agents Chemother* 2000;44:809.
12. Gerberding JL. Aminoglycoside dosing: timing is of the essence. *Am J Med* 1998;105:256.
13. Gilbert DN. Aminoglycosides. In: Root RK, et al, eds. *Clinical infectious diseases: a practical approach*. New York: Oxford University Press, 1999:273–284.
14. Miron D. Once daily dosing of gentamicin in infants and children. *Pediatr Infect Dis* 2001;20:1169.

15. Traynor AM, Nafziger AN, Bertino JS Jr. Aminoglycoside dosing weight correction factors for patients with various body sizes. *Antimicrob Agents Chemother* 1995;39: 545.
16. Cipolle RJ, et al. Systemically individualized tobramycin dosage regimens. *J Clin Pharmacol* 1980;20:570.
17. Keane WF, et al. Adult peritoneal dialysis-related peritonitis treatment recommendations: 2000 update. *Perit Dial Int* 2000;20:396.
18. Ramsey BW, et al. Efficacy of aerosolized tobramycin in patients with cystic fibrosis. *N Engl J Med* 1993;328:1740.
19. Barker AF, Couch L, Fiel SB, et al. Tobramycin solution for inhalation reduces sputum *Pseudomonas aeruginosa* density in bronchiectasis. *Am J Respir Crit Care Med* 2000; 162(2 Pt 1):481–485.
20. Prober CG, et al. Technical report: precautions regarding the use of aerosolized antibiotics. Committee on Infectious Diseases and Committee on Drugs. *Pediatrics* 2000;106:E89.
21. Ratjen F, Doring G, Nikolaizik WH. Effect of inhaled tobramycin on early colonization in patients with cystic fibrosis. *Lancet* 2001;358:983–984.
22. Moss RB. Long-term benefits of inhaled tobramycin in adolescent patients with cystic fibrosis. *Chest* 2002;121:55.
23. Sacks LV, et al. Adjunctive salvage therapy with inhaled aminoglycosides for patients with persistent smear-positive pulmonary tuberculosis. *Clin Infect Dis* 2001;32:44. (See Commentary found in *Clin Infect Dis* 2001;33:267.)
24. Klemm K. The use of antibiotic-containing bead chains in the treatment of chronic bone infection. *Clin Microbiol Infect* 2001;7:28–31.
25. Gilbert D. Aminoglycosides. In: Mandell GL, Bennett JE, Dolin R, eds. *Principles and practice of infectious diseases,* 5th ed. New York: Churchill Livingstone, 2000;307–329.
26. McCormack JP, Jewesson PJ. A critical reevaluation of the "therapeutic range" of aminoglycosides. *Clin Infect Dis* 1992:14:320–339.
27. Aronoff GR, et al., eds. *Drug prescribing in renal failure: dosing guidelines for adults,* 4th ed. Philadelphia: American College of Physicians, 1999.
28. McEvoy GK, et al. *Drug information.* American Society of Hospital Pharmacists. Bethesda, MD: American Hospital Formulary Service, 2002:50.
29. Medical Letter. Drugs for parasitic infections. *Med Lett Drugs Ther* 2002;44:1.
30. Hewitt RG, et al. Paromomycin: no more effective than placebo for treatment of cryptosporidiosis in patients with advanced human immunodeficiency virus infection. AIDS Clinical Trial Group. *Clin Infect Dis* 2000;31:1084.

## J. Clindamycin

Clindamycin, introduced in 1966, is an important antibiotic for intraabdominal or pelvic infections involving anaerobes [1,2]. In addition, it is a second-line alternative agent in penicillin-allergic patients for the treatment of susceptible gram-positive infections. Depending on the bacterial species, inoculum of bacteria, and concentration of antibiotic available, clindamycin is bactericidal for some organisms but generally is bacteriostatic. Clindamycin inhibits protein synthesis at the ribosomal level.

**I. Spectrum of activity**

**A. Gram-positive aerobes.** Clindamycin is active against group A streptococci, and in necrotizing fasciitis it is the drug of choice (see section **III.D** below). It is also active against most *Staphylococcus aureus* strains. **Of hospital isolates, at least 5% to 20% of strains of *S. aureus* are resistant to clindamycin** [1,3,4]. The emergence of clindamycin-resistant *S. aureus* has been noted in clindamycin-treated patients, especially when the organisms initially had erythromycin resistance at the onset of treatment. **Clindamycin-susceptible but erythromycin-resistant organisms should be considered resistant to clindamycin.** Some methicillin-resistant strains of *S. aureus* are susceptible to clindamycin, but this must be documented in the microbiology laboratory before treatment. Clindamycin is not active against enterococci. Although active against penicillin-susceptible *Streptococcus pneumoniae,* the susceptibility of penicillin-resistant *S. pneumoniae* strains is variable. In some areas, penicillin-resistant pneumococci remain clindamycin-sensitive, but in many areas penicillin-resistant pneumococci are clindamycin resistant. It is prudent that clinicians routinely review the susceptibility patterns of *S. pneumoniae* in their locale (see Chapters 11 and 27C).

**B. Anaerobes.** Clindamycin is active against gram-positive and gram-negative anaerobes, including most *Bacteroides fragilis* and *Clostridium perfringens* strains. In the past decade, susceptibility data have shown increasing resistance of *Bacteroides* species to clindamycin at many but not all institutions. For example, in a report from six hospitals in Chicago, rates of resistance within this one city varied from 0 to 20% [5]. Other data suggest that 6% to 11% or more of *B. fragilis* isolates are resistant to clindamycin [1–3,6]. Approximately 10% to 20% of clostridial species, other than *C. perfringens,* and 10% to 20% of peptococci strains are resistant [1,2].

**C. Gram-negative aerobes.** Clindamycin has **no useful activity** against gram-negative aerobes.

**D.** Clindamycin is not active against *Mycoplasma pneumoniae* but is against certain strains of *Toxoplasma gondii, Babesia microti, Pneumocystis carinii,* and some malarial species [1,2,4].

## II. Pharmacokinetics

**A. Oral and parenteral. Clindamycin is well absorbed from the gastrointestinal tract** (i.e., 90%), and food does not decrease its absorption. Therapeutic blood levels can be achieved by the oral, intramuscular, or intravenous route.

**B. Tissue penetration.** Clindamycin penetrates most body tissues well, including sputum, bile, bone, prostate, and pleural fluid, but not the cerebrospinal fluid. It crosses the placenta.

**C. Metabolism and excretion.** Clindamycin is metabolized primarily by the liver. **In severe hepatic insufficiency, the half-life of clindamycin is prolonged** to 8 to 12 hours; **therefore doses of clindamycin should be reduced** in severe liver or combined liver and renal failure [7].

Enterohepatic circulation of clindamycin and its metabolites can lead to a prolonged antimicrobial presence in stool, with changes in gut flora lasting up to 2 weeks after discontinuation of clindamycin. Some have suggested that perhaps this accounts for clindamycin causing *C. difficile* diarrhea [4].

## III. Indications for use

**Indications for use** [1,2,4]. Although, except for *Bacteroides* species, it is not generally considered the drug of choice for any other organism, it has become recognized as the drug of choice for certain clinical situations discussed below.

**A. Intraabdominal/pelvic infections.** *Bacteroides fragilis* plays an important role in these infections. Traditionally, clindamycin is listed as a drug of choice [8] for *Bacteroides* species, but many infectious disease experts have turned to metronidazole. It must be combined with an agent active against gram-negative organisms. In the animal model with well-established intraabdominal abscess due to *B. fragilis,* metronidazole is superior to clindamycin. In endocarditis or other intravascular infection due to *B. fragilis,* metronidazole, a bactericidal agent, is preferred.

**B. For mixed aerobic and anaerobic soft tissue infections** (e.g., perineum), clindamycin has an advantage over metronidazole in that clindamycin is also active against group A or B streptococci and *S. aureus* as well as anaerobes, whereas metronidazole is not. In polymicrobial infections in adults, it is combined with an anti–gram-negative agent (e.g., ciprofloxacin).

**C. Alternative drug in allergic patients.** For patients allergic to both penicillin and cephalosporins, clindamycin is an effective alternative for susceptible aerobic gram-positive cocci (e.g., *S. aureus, Streptococcus pyogenes*) causing skin and soft tissue infection. For *S. aureus* endocarditis or a staphylococcal bacteremia of unknown source, a bactericidal agent such as a vancomycin is required. Clindamycin is considered a second-line alternative agent for penicillin-susceptible *S. pneumoniae.* Testing using a clindamycin disk can identify high level macrolide resistant pneumococci [9].

D. **Necrotizing fasciitis. This disease is caused by invasive group A streptococcal that often leads to** streptococcal toxic shock syndrome, and bacteremia [10]. Clindamycin is more effective in the animal model and is thought more effective in the clinical situation, perhaps because of its activity against nongrowing organisms against which penicillin appears to be less active because the penicillin binding protein is not expressed [11,12]. Furthermore, clindamycin appears to interfere with toxin production [13] (see discussions in Chapters 2 and 4). Initial therapy for these infections combines penicillin with clindamycin until susceptibilities return. **The same thinking applies in severe cellulitis** of an extremity (see discussion in Chapter 4).

E. **Osteomyelitis.** Clindamycin penetrates bone very well, so it is a useful alternative for susceptible organisms in the allergic patient and has been used in carefully monitored oral programs. Some pediatric infectious disease experts use it as a first-line agent in childhood osteomyelitis due to susceptible pathogens.

F. **Lung abscess.** These infections are usually related to poor dental hygiene. For aspiration of oral anaerobes, penicillin has historically been the drug of choice, although clindamycin is also favored. Some experts favor clindamycin for those who are seriously ill with this problem, to ensure coverage for anaerobes that may be resistant to penicillin.

G. **Diabetic foot infections.** Clindamycin, combined with an agent with good activity against aerobic gram-negative rods (e.g., ciprofloxacin), is commonly used.

H. **Miscellaneous uses**
   1. **Alternative for endocarditis prophylaxis for oral/dental procedures** (see Chapters 12 and 27B).
   2. **Odontogenic infections.** A dental source that contains anaerobic streptococcus may lead to Ludwig's angina, maxillary sinusitis, and retropharyngeal and parapharyngeal abscesses with a major anaerobic component. Clindamycin is favored over penicillin or metronidazole.
   3. **Posttraumatic endophthalmitis** due to *Bacillus cereus*. Clindamycin has fairly good penetration into the eye.
   4. **Chronic sinusitis or chronic otitis.** Culture data have implicated anaerobic organisms.
   5. **Bacterial vaginosis** usually is treated with metronidazole, but topical clindamycin as clindamycin ovules once at bedtime for 3 days is an alternative [14].
   6. **Streptococcal group A pharyngitis, recurrent.** For susceptible $\beta$ streptococcus clindamycin is the most effective agent in recurrent disease or for penicillin allergic patients.
   7. **Acne vulgaris.** A 1% **topical** clindamycin **gel** and lotion has been used in this setting.
   8. **Other.** Clindamycin has been used in special settings, including central nervous system toxoplasmosis (in combination with pyrimethamine), *Pneumocystis carinii* pneumonia in acquired immunodeficiency syndrome (with primaquine, when standard therapy has failed), and babesiosis [15] and malaria regimens.

IV. **Route and dosage**

A. **Oral. In children,** the recommended oral dosage is 10 to 25 mg/kg/day divided into every 6 hour doses or for mild to moderately severe infections; 20 to 30 mg/kg/day in four divided doses has been used. In severe infections in children, such as osteomyelitis, 30 to 40 mg/kg/day (up to 50 kg of body weight) divided into every 6 hour doses has been used. **In adults,** 300 to 450 mg every 6 to 8 hours can be given, depending on the severity of the illness. However, some patients may have many gastrointestinal side effects at the 450-mg regimen.

B. **Parenteral**
   1. **In adults** 600 mg every 8 hours is usually recommended. For tubo-ovarian abscess and possibly in the therapy of morbidly obese patients, 900 mg intravenously every 8 hours is preferred.
   2. **In children** older than 1 month, 20 to 40 mg/kg/day is suggested, divided into every 6 to 8 hour doses.
   3. **In neonates,** doses are summarized in Appendix Table 1.

C. **Clindamycin 2% vaginal cream,** 5 g intravaginally once daily for 7 days [7] (see Chapter 16).

D. **In renal failure, no change in the dosage** is required. Clindamycin is **not removed by either peritoneal dialysis or hemodialysis [16].**

E. **In hepatic insufficiency,** the half-life is prolonged. **Doses should be reduced,** the dosage interval prolonged, or, if possible, an alternative agent should be used (see discussion in section **II.C**). Patients with moderate to severe liver disease should be given about half the usual dose, and further reductions may be necessary if the patient also has renal disease [2].

F. **Pregnancy.** This is a category B drug (see Chapter 27A). The package insert suggests that this drug should be used in pregnancy only if clearly indicated. Limited data have not revealed adverse effects on fetal development [4].

G. **Nursing mothers.** Clindamycin is detected in breast milk. Because of the potential for adverse reactions in neonates, the package insert suggests that the decision to discontinue the drug should be made, taking into account the importance of the drug to the mother.

H. **Potential for antagonism** exists with the macrolides and chloramphenicol, which also act at the ribosomal level and may competitively inhibit the action of each other. These drugs **should not be used in combination** with clindamycin.

I. **Cost.** Clindamycin is a relatively expensive agent (see Appendix Table).

V. **Side effects**

A. **Gastrointestinal.** Diarrhea is the most significant adverse reaction due to clindamycin [4].

1. **Antibiotic-associated diarrhea** occurs in up to 20% of patients receiving clindamycin, presumably because of alternations of anaerobic bowel flora [4].
2. ***C. difficile* diarrhea** can occur as a side effect of any antibiotic [17]. The incidence of clindamycin-induced *C. difficile* diarrhea in hospitalized patients varies considerably by institution [4]. The overall incidence is presumably less than 1%, unless there are nosocomial outbreaks within a given institution. When this occurs, restriction of clindamycin use has been beneficial [18]. It is much less common in outpatients receiving clindamycin.
3. Anorexia, nausea, vomiting, flatulence, bitter taste, and abdominal distention can occur [2]. **A metallic taste** in the mouth when clindamycin is given parenterally occurs infrequently.

B. **Allergic reactions,** eosinophilia, rashes, (with fever), and, rarely, anaphylaxis occur [1,2,4,19].

C. **Hepatotoxicity.** Minor reversible elevations of hepatocellular enzymes are frequent.

D. **Nephrotoxicity.** Clindamycin does not cause significant renal toxicity.

E. **Bone marrow suppression.** Neutropenia and thrombocytopenia have been reported.

## REFERENCES

1. Klein NC, Cunha BA. New uses of older antibiotics. *Med Clin North Am* 2001;85:125.
2. Kasten MJ. Clindamycin, metronidazole, and chloramphenicol. *Mayo Clin Proc* 1999;74:825.
3. Steigbigel NH. Macrolides and clindamycin. In: Mandell GL, Bennett JE, Dolin R, eds. *Principles and practice of infectious diseases,* 5th ed. New York: Churchill Livingstone, 2000:366–382.
4. Gold HS, Moellering RC Jr. Macrolides and clindamycin. In: Root RK, et al. *Clinical infectious diseases: a practical approach*. New York: Oxford University Press, 1999;291–297.
5. Hecht DW, Osmolski JR, O'Keefe JP. Variation in the susceptibility of *Bacteroides fragilis* group isolates from six Chicago hospitals. *Clin Infect Dis* 1993;16[Suppl 4]:S367.
6. Snydman DR, et al. Multicenter study of in vitro susceptibility of the *Bacteroides fragilis* group, 1995 to 1996, with comparison of resistant trends from 1990 to 1996. *Antimicrob Agents Chemother* 1999;43:2417.

7. Falagas ME, Gorbach SL. Clindamycin and metronidazole. *Med Clin North Am* 1995;79:845.
8. Medical Letter. The choice of antibacterial drugs. *Med Lett Drugs Ther* 2001;43:69.
9. Waites K, Johnson C, Gray B, et al. Use of clindamycin disks to detect macrolide resistance mediated by ermB and mefE in *Streptococcus pneumoniae* isolates from adults and children. *J Clin Microbiol* 2000;38:1731–1724.
10. Stevens DL. The flesh-eating bacterium: what's next? *J Infect Dis* 1999;179[Suppl 2]:S366.
11. Zimbelman J, et al. Improved outcome of clindamycin compared with beta-lactam antibiotic treatment for invasive *Streptococcus pyogenes* infection. *Pediatr Infect Dis J* 1999;18:1096.
12. Sharkawy A, et al. Severe group A streptococcal soft-tissue infections in Ontario: 1992–1996. *Clin Infect Dis* 2002;34:454.
13. Herbert S, Barry P, Novick RP. Sub-inhibitory clindamycin differentially inhibits transcription of exoprotein genes in *Staphylococcus aureus. Infect Immun* 2001;69:2996–3003.
14. Center for Diseases Control and Prevention. Sexually transmitted diseases: treatment guidelines 2002. *MMWR Morb Mortal Wkly Rep* 2002;51(RR-6):1–77.
15. Krause J. Babesiosis. *Med Clin North Am* 2002;86:361.
16. Aronoff GR, et al., eds. *Drug prescribing in renal failure: dosing guidelines for adults,* 4th ed. Philadelphia: American College of Physicians, 1999.
17. Bartlett JG. Antibiotic associated diarrhea. *N Engl J Med* 2002;346:334.
18. Climo MW, et al. Hospital-wide restriction on clindamycin: effect on the incidence of *Clostridium difficile*-associated diarrhea and cost. *Ann Intern Med* 1998;128:989.
19. Mazer N, Greenberger PA, Regaldo J. Clindamycin hypersensitivity appears to be rare. *Ann Allergy Asthma Immunol* 1999;82:443.


## K. Chloramphenicol

Chloramphenicol has been available since 1949. Because of the rare case of irreversible fatal aplastic anemia that is associated with its use, chloramphenicol should be used only when clearly indicated. In Third World countries, because it is readily available, inexpensive, and efficacious in many serious infections [1,2], it is widely used. In the United States, however, chloramphenicol is rarely used, and most young physicians are completely unfamiliar with the drug.

I. **Mechanism of action.** Chloramphenicol inhibits protein synthesis at the ribosomal level. Although active against *Staphylococcus aureus,* group B streptococci, and Enterobacteriaceae, chloramphenicol is bacteriostatic against these organisms. However, against meningeal pathogens, *Haemophilus influenzae,* penicillin-susceptible *Streptococcus pneumoniae,* and *Neisseria meningitidis,* chloramphenicol is bactericidal [3].

II. **Spectrum of activity** [1,2]. Chloramphenicol has a broad-spectrum antibiotic active against many gram-positive and gram-negative bacteria, rickettsiae, chlamydiae, and mycoplasma. However, **it is not listed as the drug of first choice for any common pathogen** [4].

   A. **Gram-positive bacteria.** Many gram-positive cocci, both aerobic and anaerobic, are susceptible to chloramphenicol, although the minimum inhibitory concentrations are relatively high. Alternate agents are preferred. Chloramphenicol is not considered a drug of choice against enterococci or staphylococci. Methicillin-resistant *S. aureus* usually is resistant to chloramphenicol. However, with the recent increase in vancomycin-resistant enterococci, which are resistant to most available antibiotics (see Chapter 27P), there is renewed interest in chloramphenicol, because it is active *in vitro* against many strains of vancomycin-resistant enterococci, probably because of its previous infrequent use [5].

   B. **Gram-negative bacteria.** *N. meningitidis* and almost all *H. influenzae* strains are susceptible. Chloramphenicol has variable activity against other gram-negative bacilli; therefore susceptibility studies are necessary. Salmonella species are often susceptible. *Pseudomonas* species are resistant.

C. **Anaerobes**. Chloramphenicol has **excellent activity against gram-positive and gram-negative anaerobes,** including *Bacteroides fragilis* [1,2].

D. **Miscellaneous.** Chloramphenicol is active against the rickettsiae that cause Rocky Mountain spotted fever, Q fever, and typhus, and it is active against *Ehrlichia chaffaenis* (4).

III. **Pharmacokinetics** [1,2]

A. **Absorption.** Chloramphenicol is rapidly absorbed orally, although variable absorption occurs in children. It penetrates body tissues well, including the spinal fluid and the unobstructed biliary tree. **Approximately 30% to 50% of serum levels appear in the cerebrospinal fluid** in both the inflamed and noninflamed meninges [1,2].

B. **Inactivation.** Chloramphenicol is metabolized and inactivated primarily in the **liver** by glucuronyl transferase.

C. **Excretion. In renal failure,** the plasma half-life of the biologically active free chloramphenicol is not prolonged. Consequently, chloramphenicol is given in normal doses in renal failure [6].

IV. **Toxicity**

A. **Dose-related bone marrow reversible suppression may occur in any patient** on chloramphenicol. Anemia, reticulocytopenia, and neutropenia can occur. Occasionally, only thrombocytopenia occurs. Bone marrow suppression is increased substantially in patients with ascites or jaundice [2]. This **suppression** is due to a direct pharmacologic effect of the antibiotic.

1. **Monitoring patients**

   a. **Serial blood counts. A complete blood cell count and platelet assessment every 2 or 3 days** is suggested. If suppression occurs, the dose should be reduced and drug reassessed. If the bone marrow suppression progresses, usually the drug is discontinued.

   b. **Serum levels.** Direct bone marrow toxicity is related to levels of free chloramphenicol. **Therapeutic levels are between 10 and 20 μg/mL. The risk of direct bone marrow suppression increases when unconjugated (free drug) levels exceed 25 μg/mL [1]. Serum should be monitored, especially in neonates and with prolonged use.**

2. **Recovery.** Complete recovery, **in this reversible form,** occurs approximately 2 weeks after stopping the chloramphenicol.

B. **Aplastic anemia** is rare, occurring only in 1 in 25,000 to 40,000 courses of chloramphenicol, **and usually is fatal.** The precise mechanism is unknown, but there is a genetic predisposition. The aplasia is not dose related and can become manifest weeks to months after use. Whether topical ophthalmic use of chloramphenicol can cause aplasia remains controversial [7].

C. **Gray baby syndrome.** Premature infants and newborns younger than 2 weeks have immature hepatic and renal function. Chloramphenicol accumulates in the blood of these infants, which can cause vasomotor collapse and death especially when higher doses of the drug are used. This is the so-called gray baby syndrome. **Therefore chloramphenicol should be avoided in the premature infant and in the first 2 weeks of life except in extreme life-threatening situations, in which decreased doses should be used and serum levels monitored.**

D. **Glucose-6-phosphate dehydrogenase deficiency.** Chloramphenicol may precipitate hemolysis in patients with a severe deficit of glucose-6-phosphate dehydrogenase [1].

V. **Clinical indications.** Chloramphenicol is not listed as the drug of first choice for any common pathogen [4]. **Because this agent is used so infrequently, before use, discuss with an infectious disease subspecialist.** The package insert clearly notes the pharmaceutical manufacturer's warning that chloramphenicol **"must not be used when less potentially dangerous agents will be effective." Because of the availability of less toxic antibiotics, chloramphenicol is** seldom used except in special settings or in the allergic patient.

A. **Potential important indications for chloramphenicol use include the following:**

1. **Alternative for life-threatening *H. influenzae* infections.** The third-generation cephalosporins are the drugs of choice in the empiric therapy of meningitis and acute epiglottitis in children [4]. If there is an allergic history that precludes the use of a cephalosporin, chloramphenicol is an acceptable alternative.
2. **Brain abscess.** Chloramphenicol may be used in selected cases.
3. **Alternative agent in severe anaerobic infection.**
4. **Alternative drug [4] in** *Salmonella typhi* infections, brucellosis, glanders (*P. pseudomallei*), plague, *Chlamydia psittaci* infections (psittacosis), tularemia, and intraocular infections due to susceptible pathogens.
5. **Rickettsial infections** Rocky Mountain spotted fever, endemic typhus (murine), scrub typhus, epidemic typhus (louse-borne), and Q fever. **Chloramphenicol may be the preferred agent when the patients require parenteral therapy, in young children, and in pregnancy** when a tetracycline cannot be used. Infectious disease consultation is advised.
6. **In susceptible** infections due to **vancomycin-resistant enterococci,** chloramphenicol may provide a possible alternative [5,8,9], although the availability of linezolid and quinupristin/dalfopristin have led away from the use of chloramphenicol.

**VI. Route and dosage**

**A. Neonatal doses.** Serum levels should be monitored in neonates. Infectious disease consultation is advised in this setting.

**B. Children and adults**

1. **Intravenous.** The usual dosage is 50 to 100 mg/kg/day in divided 6-hour doses, with a maximum dose of 1.5 g every 6 hours. Serial blood cell counts should be monitored (see section **IV.A.1**). Because children vary greatly in their ability to metabolize the drug, monitoring of levels is important [2].
   - a. **In renal failure, hemodialysis, or peritoneal dialysis,** no dosage adjustments are required [6].
   - b. **Hepatic failure.** If chloramphenicol must be used, serum levels should be monitored. In adults, an initial loading dose of 1 g followed by 500 mg every 6 hours sometimes is suggested; the course should be limited to 10 to 14 days [1].
2. **Oral chloramphenicol** is no longer available in the United States, although it is available in some countries (e.g., Mexico).
3. **Drug interactions.** Chloramphenicol can prolong the half-life of chlorpropamide, phenytoin, tolbutamide, and warfarin derivatives. The prothrombin time of patients receiving anticoagulation therapy must be closely monitored [2].

## REFERENCES


1. Klein NC, Cunha BA. New uses of older antibiotics. *Med Clin North Am* 2001;85:125.
2. Kasten MJ. Clindamycin, metronidazole, and chloramphenicol. *Mayo Clin Proc* 1999; 74:825.
3. Rahal JJ Jr, Simberkoff MS. Bactericidal and bacteriostatic action of chloramphenicol against meningeal pathogens. *Antimicrob Agents Chemother* 1979;16:13.
4. Medical Letter. The choice of antibacterial drugs. *Med Lett Drugs Ther* 2001;43:69.
5. Lautenbach E, et al. The role of chloramphenicol in the treatment of bloodstream infection due to vancomycin-resistant enterococcus. *Clin Infect Dis* 1999;27:1259.
6. Aronoff GR, et al. *Drug prescribing in renal failure: dosing guidelines for adults*, 4th ed. Philadelphia: American College of Physicians, 1999.
7. Walker S, et al. Lack of evidence for systemic toxicity following topical chloramphenicol use. *Eye* 1998;12:875.
8. Norris AH, et al. Chloramphenicol for the treatment of vancomycin-resistant enterococcal infections. *Clin Infect Dis* 1995;20:1137.
9. Perez MS, et al. Vancomycin-resistant *Enterococcus faecium* meningitis successfully treated with chloramphenicol. *Pediatr Infect Dis J* 1999;18:483.

## L. Sulfonamides and Trimethoprim-Sulfamethoxazole

I. **Sulfonamides.** Sulfonamides were the first effective systemic antibacterial drugs used in humans and were initially introduced in the late 1930's. The sulfonamides, which are primarily **bacteriostatic,** act by interfering with bacterial synthesis of folic acid [1].

A. **Pharmacokinetics.** Sulfonamides generally are used in the oral form. They are metabolized in the liver by acetylation and glucuronidation. Free drug and its metabolites are excreted by the kidney. Preparations less apt to become crystallized in urine have attained more widespread use. Sulfonamides compete for binding sites on plasma albumin. By so doing they may increase blood levels of unconjugated bilirubin (see section **I.E**).

B. **Spectrum of activity. Routine disk antibiotic susceptibility testing is unreliable.** Because testing is not used, susceptibilities of most organisms are unknown. Many community-acquired *Escherichia coli* are susceptible, particularly to levels achieved in the urine. The sulfonamides also are active against many strains of *Neisseria meningitidis, Chlamydia, Toxoplasma,* and some *Nocardia* species. **A sulfonamide alone is not the drug of first choice for any bacterial pathogen** [2]. Sulfonamides have *in vitro* activity against *Streptococcus pyogenes* and have been used to prevent recurrent rheumatic fever [3], but they are not advised for treatment of streptococcal pharyngitis.

C. **Current clinical uses**

1. **Situations in which sulfonamides are useful** include the following:
   a. ***Toxoplasma gondii*** infections (e.g., sulfadiazine with pyrimethamine).
   b. ***Nocardia asteroides*** infections respond well to sulfonamides. Trimethoprim-sulfamethoxazole (TMP-SMX) often is listed as the agent of choice [2].
2. **Miscellaneous indications** for sulfonamide use are the following:
   a. **Rheumatic fever prophylaxis [3].** Although sulfadiazine is effective as prophylaxis, it is ineffective in established streptococcal pharyngitis infections.
   b. ***Chlamydia trachomatis*** **pneumonia.** Alternate agent.
   c. **Otitis media prophylaxis.** Sulfonamides have been used in selected patients to prevent recurrences (see Chapter 8).
   d. ***E. coli.*** Because at least 25% to 35% of strains that cause cystitis are resistant to sulfonamides, sulfonamides are no longer the agents of choice for empiric therapy of initial uncomplicated urinary tract infection (UTI) (see section **II**) [1].

D. **Preparations available and dosage regimens** [1–4]. Sulfonamides are acetylated or glucuronated in the liver. These inactive metabolites and free drug are actively secreted into the urine [4]. Sulfonamide dosage is reduced for creatinine clearance of less than 50 mL/min; no dosage modification is necessary with hepatic impairment [4]. Sulfonamides penetrate pleural, peritoneal, synovial, and cerebrospinal fluid (CSF); they cross the placenta and are detectable in breast milk.

1. **Short-acting** preparations usually are given four (and sometimes six) times daily.
   a. **Sulfisoxazole** (e.g., Gantrisin, Azo Gantrisin) are no longer listed in the *Physicians' Desk Reference* and are not discussed here.
   b. **Pediazole.**This is a fixed combination of sulfisoxazole and erythromycin. Use of combinations when a single drug will do exposes the individual to excess toxicity.
   c. **Sulfadiazine** (e.g., Neotrizine) is less soluble in urine and therefore less suitable for use in UTI. It is less protein-bound than sulfisoxazole, which yields good blood and CSF levels. It is useful for **nocardial infection, toxoplasmosis, or for rheumatic fever prophylaxis** in the penicillin-allergic patient. Although it has a longer half-life than sulfisoxazole, sulfadiazine is given four times daily. The usual dose in adults is a 2-g loading dose with a maintenance dose of 1 g four times per day. For the treatment of toxoplasmosis or nocardiosis infectious disease consultation is advisable.

d. **Triple sulfa drug** (Trisem) usually is made up of sulfadiazine and two other sulfa preparations. Theoretically, each drug maintains its solubility in the urine to decrease the chances for crystalluria. In adults, the usual dose is 1 g four times daily.

2. **Intermediate-acting** sulfonamides are given two or three times daily. **Sulfamethoxazole** (e.g., Azo Gantanol) is given twice daily and has been used in UTI. Because it can cause crystalluria, it is important to ensure a high urine output. The dose in adults is 2 g followed by 1 g twice daily. In children older than 2 months, the initial dose is 50 mg/kg, then 25 to 30 mg/kg per dose is given twice daily. **Sulfamethoxazole combined with trimethoprim is available as cotrimoxazole (Bactrim, Septra) (see section II).**
3. **Long-acting sulfonamides** are **no longer recommended** because these preparations have the capacity to produce hypersensitivity reactions (e.g., Stevens-Johnson syndrome), which then become a prolonged problem. The exception is sulfadoxine, which is a component of Fansidar, which is still used in some antimalarial regimens (see section III).
4. **Topical sulfonamides** [5]. Mafenide acetate (Sulfamylon) is used on burns to help prevent bacterial colonization, particularly by pseudomonas. Its use has been limited by the side effect of metabolic acidosis. Silver sulfadiazine (Flamazine) has fewer side effects and is used extensively for burns. Outbreaks of silver-resistant infections may ultimately limit its usefulness [5]. Sulfonamides are used also in ophthalmic preparations and in vaginal suppositories and creams.
5. **Sulfasalazine** (Azulfidine) is used in the treatment of ulcerative colitis.

E. **Toxicity** [4,5]

1. **Pregnancy and neonates. Sulfonamides should not be used in the last trimester of pregnancy (especially the last month)** because they are transplacentally transmitted and compete for bilirubin-binding sites on plasma albumin, increasing the risk for kernicterus. Sulfonamides are **not recommended for therapy in neonatal infections or in nursing mothers** because the neonate's hepatic enzyme system may be immature.
2. **Hematology.** Sulfonamides should be **avoided in patients with glucose-6-phosphate dehydrogenase (G6PD) deficiency,** because hemolysis can be precipitated. However, one study showed that G6PD-deficient patients who received TMP-SMX did not have hemolytic reactions during therapy [6]. Anemia, leukopenia, or thrombocytopenia occurs with sulfonamide use, especially in those with folate deficiency.
3. **Hypersensitivity reactions** with rashes, vasculitis, erythema nodosum, erythema multiforme, and Stevens-Johnson syndrome can occur. These were particularly common with the long-acting compounds, which are no longer recommended.
4. **Gastrointestinal disturbances** with nausea, vomiting, and diarrhea occur in 3% to 5% of patients.
5. **Renal dysfunction** due to tubular deposition of sulfonamide is now rare.

F. **Important drug interactions.** Sulfonamides may displace drugs from albumin-binding sites, increasing the clinical effect of the displaced drug [5].

1. **Oral anticoagulants.** Sulfonamides compete for albumin-binding sites and, in effect, increase the activity of a given anticoagulant dose. Therefore **doses of oral anticoagulants** (e.g., warfarin sodium) **should be reduced** and serial prothrombin times monitored.
2. **Methotrexate.** Because sulfonamides displace methotrexate from its bound protein, **risk of methotrexate toxicity increases. Therefore sulfonamides** should be avoided.
3. **Oral hypoglycemic agents.** The hypoglycemic effect of sulfonylureas may be exaggerated by sulfonamides, although the precise mechanisms for this are unclear.
4. **Methenamine** compounds should not be given concomitantly with sulfonamides because there is an increased risk of insoluble urinary precipitate formation.

G. **Sulfonamide use in renal failure.** Because sulfonamides are excreted by way of the kidney, in renal failure **doses must be reduced or dose intervals prolonged** [7].

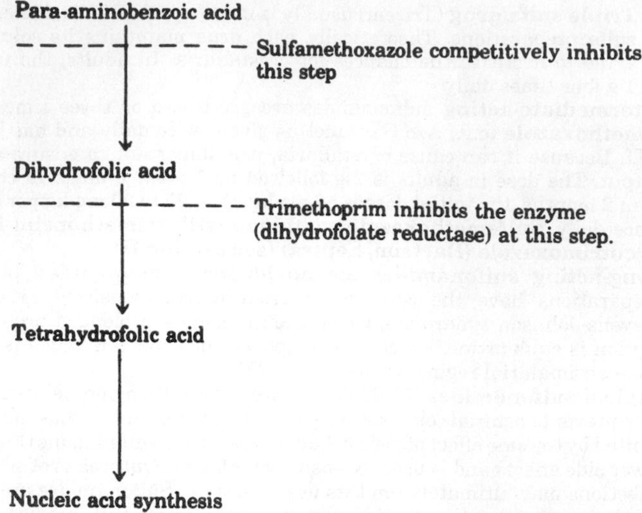


**FIG. 27L.1.** Mechanism of action of trimethoprim-sulfamethoxazole. Most bacteria cannot use exogenous folate but must make their own folate for nucleic acid synthesis. Trimethoprim-sulfamethoxazole can sequentially block the formation of tetrahydrofolic acid and thereby interfere with cell replication.

**II. TMP-SMX** [1,5,8,9], formerly called **cotrimoxazole,** is available commercially as **Bactrim or Septra as well as in generic** preparations. This unique preparation was specifically formulated to include a combination of agents that would inhibit activity in two sequential steps of bacterial metabolism. It became available in the United States in 1973. The combination has two theoretic advantages: It decreases the chances of bacterial resistance and the combination may act synergistically. The combination is available in oral and intravenous forms. The regular tablets contain 80 mg TMP and 400 mg SMX to provide an ideal blood ratio of 1:20 for optimal synergy. However, it is noteworthy that in different body fluids, the ratios of TMP to SMX are virtually never 1:20, so the value of the ideal ratio in the blood is uncertain. **Alone, each agent is bacteriostatic, but together they are bactericidal and synergistic *in vitro*.** Currently, sulfonamides are used most frequently in this combination [5].

**A. Mechanism of action.** TMP-SMX sequentially blocks two steps in the synthesis of folic acid by bacteria (Figure 27L.1).

**B. Pharmacokinetics** [1,4,5]. **Oral TMP-SMX is well absorbed.** Peak serum levels occur 1 to 4 hours after ingestion. The intravenous preparation provides excellent blood levels. Serum half-lives of TMP and SMX are 8 to 10 hours and 10 hours, respectively [4]. TMP-SMX is excreted primarily by the kidneys, so doses must be reduced in renal failure. **Because the pH of the urine dictates which component is excreted more rapidly in renal failure, this makes dosage selection difficult.** Excretion occurs over several hours, and this permits twice-daily dosing. Each drug is distributed widely and can be detected in most tissues of the body. This agent penetrates the CSF well (20%–40% of serum levels). Concentrations of TMP in prostatic fluid usually are at least three times those of the serum concentration [1].

**C. Spectrum of activity.** TMP by itself has a wide spectrum of activity against gram-positive and gram-negative bacteria (see Chapter 27M). SMX is less active alone, but it enhances the activity of TMP when combined with it.

1. **Gram-positive cocci.** TMP-SMX is active against most *Staphylococcus aureus, S. epidermidis,* penicillin-susceptible *S. pneumoniae* strains, and viridans streptococci. In a survey of penicillin-resistant strains of *S. pneumoniae* in Atlanta, Georgia, published in 1995, 75% of the isolates resistant to penicillin were resistant to TMP-SMX [10] (see related discussions in Chapter 11). This agent is active against many methicillin-resistant *S. aureus* species. Despite the apparent *in vitro* sensitivity of methicillin-resistant *S. aureus,* some reviews emphasize that clinical success with TMP-SMX therapy for methicillin-resistant *S. aureus* is extremely variable and unpredictable [8]. It is not useful clinically against enterococci.
2. **Gram-negative bacilli and cocci**
   a. **Enterobacteriaceae are usually susceptible,** although a higher percent of these and of ***Salmonella*** **and** ***Shigella*** species are now resistant than in the past.
   b. ***Haemophilus influenzae*** (ampicillin-susceptible and ampicillin-resistant) **and** ***Moraxella catarrhalis*** are usually susceptible. TMP-SMX has activity against *Pasteurella multocida* [11], although it is usually not listed as an alternative agent for this pathogen [2].
   c. ***Stenotrophomonas*** (formerly ***Xanthomonas maltophilia***) are susceptible. Even when they are labeled resistant, a slightly higher dose will be clinically effective. *Burkholderia cepacia* (formerly *P. cepacia*) are usually susceptible.
   d. ***Pseudomonas aeruginosa.*** TMP-SMX is **not active.**
3. **Anaerobes.** TMP-SMX is not particularly active against anaerobes, including *Bacteroides fragilis* [1,9].
4. **Miscellaneous** [1,2,9].
   a. TMP-SMX is active against *Listeria monocytogenes, Yersinia enterocolitica, Aeromonas* species, *Legionella micdadei,* and *Legionella pneumophila.*
   b. *Pneumocystis carinii* (a parasite) is susceptible but resistance has been noted [12], the meaning of which is uncertain.
   c. **Many** ***Nocardia*** species are susceptible.
   d. ***Treponema pallidum*** is resistant.
5. **Resistance to TMP-SMX** has recently been reviewed [8,13].
   a. **Bacterial resistance** to both TMP and SMX has developed, although there are significant geographic variations. Resistance to the sulfonamides is usually more common than is resistance to TMP. In developed and developing countries, levels of resistance to TMP-SMX for *S. pneumoniae* range from 10% to 50%. In the United States, for *H. influenzae* over 30% and for *M. catarrhalis* from 2% to 50% of strains are resistant to TMP-SMX. Many penicillin-resistant pneumococci are also resistant to TMP-SMX [13]. Because of increasing resistance, TMP-SMX is no longer the drug of choice for *Salmonella* species or *Shigella* species [2,13]. **At least 30% to 35% of nosocomial urinary pathogens are resistant to TMP-SMX** [8]. In recent reports of susceptibility studies in **community-acquired acute uncomplicated cystitis** in women aged 18 to 50 years, **the incidence of resistance of** ***E. coli*** **has risen to 16% to 20%** [14–16].This rise in resistance in community-acquired *E. coli* now has affected empiric antibiotic therapy for uncomplicated cystitis (see section **D.1.a** below and Chapter 15).
   b. ***P. carinii.*** TMP-SMX has been widely used to prevent infections in underlying human immunodeficiency virus (HIV) infection [17]. Selection pressure caused by prolonged use of TMP-SMX in this setting has been associated with an increase in the levels of resistance to TMP-SMX among clinically important bacterial species infecting HIV patients [13]. Furthermore, TMP-SMX resistant strains of *P. carinii* have been isolated but only from cases that were treated successfully [12]. Because resistance to TMP-SMX is in large part governed by resistance to TMP, this topic is discussed further in Chapter 27M.

D. **Indications for use [1,2,8,9]. TMP-SMX is the first-line drug [2] for the treatment of infections caused by** *Burkholderia cepacia, S. maltophilia, Nocardia* species, and *P. carinii* as well as *Y. enterocolitica* or *Aeromonas* species. TMP-SMX has been extensively used in the treatment of acute bronchitis and upper respiratory infections. Of concern, however, has been increasing TMP-SMX resistance amongst strains of *H. influenzae* and *S. pneumonia.* It is important for clinicians to know the susceptibility of these common respiratory pathogens to TMP-SMX in their local practice environment.

1. **UTIs. See related discussion in Chapter 15.**
   a. **Acute initial uncomplicated UTI.** Because many strains of community-acquired *E. coli* are resistant to sulfonamides alone and amoxicillin (ampicillin), for empiric therapy of community-acquired uncomplicated UTI, TMP-SMX is often preferred [2]. However, with community-acquired *E. coli* showing an increased frequency of resistance to TMP-SMX (see section **C.5.a** above) and up to 8% of strains of *S. saprophyticus* resistant to TMP-SMX [14], these factors must be considered in empiric therapy of cystitis [14–16], and especially pyelonephritis. Although we still commonly use empiric TMP-SMX in the healthy young female with an uncomplicated UTI, if the patient has underlying diabetes or repetitive infections or a possible early pyelonephritis, we would favor a quinolone.
   b. **Pyelonephritis.** Because TMP-SMX penetrates tissue well, it is a useful agent in this setting **for susceptible pathogens [14–16],** especially because it can be given both intravenously and orally. **If the Gram stain of unspun urine reveals gram-positive cocci, suggesting enterococci, TMP-SMX should not be used.**
   c. **Recurrent UTI in adult women.** In women prone to recurrent UTI, TMP-SMX has helped decrease the rate of recurrence, presumably in part by decreasing colonization at the periurethral area [1]. However, enterococcal colonization may result. An alternative regimen is a short course of self-administered antibiotic with a twice-daily dose of TMP-SMX for 3 days at the onset of symptoms.
   d. **Prostatitis recurrent UTI in men.** In the absence of other genitourinary pathology, men with recurrent UTI often have chronic **bacterial prostatitis.** [18,19]. Organisms in the prostate are extremely difficult to eradicate, because most antibiotics do not penetrate the prostate well. TMP-SMX penetrates the prostatic fluid and is very useful in these patients. Often trimethoprim by itself is used. The fluoroquinolones also are useful in this setting.
   e. **Postcoital antibiotic prophylaxis for recurrent UTI** with TMP-SMX has been shown to be a safe, effective, and inexpensive approach to management in carefully selected young women with recurrent UTI [20].
2. **Respiratory infections**
   a. ***P. carinii.* TMP-SMX is considered the drug of choice in children and adults,** with or without HIV, for the treatment and prevention of ***P. carinii* pneumonia** (PCP) [17,21,22]. A high incidence of adverse effects occurs in patients with acquired immunodeficiency syndrome (AIDS) who are treated with TMP-SMX, especially when maximal doses are used (see related discussion in section **G.2**). Usually the starting dose for PCP is 20 mg/kg/day TMP equivalent, which can be reduced to 10 mg/kg/day TMP over 48 to 72 hours. This reduced dose remains effective and a decrease in incidence of side effects occurs.
   b. **Acute exacerbations of chronic bronchitis.** Because TMP-SMX is active against penicillin-susceptible *S. pneumoniae, H. influenzae,* and *M. catarrhalis,* it is a useful agent in this setting [1,5] or as part of a rotating antibiotic regimen (see Chapter 8).
   c. **Pneumonia.** For susceptible gram-negative pathogens, intravenous TMP-SMX has been used for lower respiratory tract infections [5]. TMP-SMX is an alternative agent for *L. micdadei* and *L. pneumophila* infections when erythromycin or a fluoroquinolone cannot be used [2].
   d. **Acute otitis media.** TMP-SMX has been used as an alternative agent for acute otitis media, especially if ampicillin-resistant *H. influenzae* is a concern (see Chapter 8).
   e. **Sinusitis.** With the advent of penicillin (and TMP-SMX) resistant *S. pneumoniae,* TMP-SMX may be less effective for sinusitis therapy (see Chapter 8).

3. **Gastrointestinal infections. See Chapter 13 for additional discussion.**
   a. **Shigellosis.** TMP-SMX resistance has increased significantly. Thus, TMP-SMX should be used for bacterial enteritis caused by *Shigella* strains only if susceptibility is known [2].
   b. ***Salmonella.*** Although ceftriaxone or a quinolone are drugs of choice for *S. typhi* or other *Salmonella* species infections requiring treatment, TMP-SMX is an excellent alternative agent [2].
   c. **Traveler's diarrhea.** In the past, TMP-SMX was the most common agent used to treat traveler's diarrhea. Now the fluoroquinolones often are preferred in adults because TMP resistance has become common.
   d. **Spontaneous bacterial peritonitis.** Prevention in patients with underlying cirrhosis is discussed in Chapter 13.
   e. **Meningitis.** Gram-negative bacillary meningitis caused by organisms (e.g., *Enterobacter cloacae, Serratia marcescens*) only **moderately susceptible** or resistant to **third-generation cephalosporins** or (*P. cepacia, Acinetobacter* species) may be candidates for TMP-SMX treatment if the organisms are susceptible [1,5,9,23]. TMP-SMX is an alternate agent in meningitis due to *L. monocytogenes* [2] when ampicillin cannot be used.
4. **Neutropenic patients.** Although TMP-SMX has been used for **prevention of infection,** a recent panel of experts concluded that use of TMP-SMX should be avoided in this setting [9,24].
5. **Miscellaneous**
   a. **Endocarditis.** TMP-SMX has been used as an alternative agent for susceptible pathogens causing bacteremia or endocarditis [1,5]. Infectious disease consultation is advised.
   b. **Nosocomial infections.** Gram-negative nosocomial infections due to bacteria resistant to many antibiotics may be susceptible to TMP-SMX (e.g., *Enterobacter, Klebsiella,* and *Proteus* species), and patients will respond to this therapy. *Burkholderia cepacia* infections that have relapsed or failed other agents often have responded well to TMP-SMX. **Before using TMP-SMX for these types of infections, *in vitro* data should show susceptibility.**
   c. ***Nocardia.*** TMP-SMX is an important agent for these infections and sometimes is viewed as the agent of choice [2].
   d. ***Y. enterocolitica*** and ***Aeromonas*** species infections can be treated with TMP-SMX.
   e. **Brucellosis.** TMP-SMX is an alternative agent for brucellosis [2].
   f. **Renal transplantation recipients.** Prophylaxis with TMP-SMX significantly reduces the incidence of bacterial infection after renal transplantation (especially infection of the urinary tract and bloodstream), can provide protection against PCP, and is cost beneficial [25]. Patients appear to tolerate this regimen well in this setting [25].
   g. **Prevention of infection in patients with chronic granulomatous disease.** TMP-SMX prophylaxis is useful in the prevention of infectious complications [1,9].
   h. ***Mycobacterium marinum.*** TMP-SMX is an alternative agent [2].
   i. **Gastrointestinal infections** TMP-SMX is viewed as the drug of choice for *Cyclospora, Isospora,* and **coccidian parasites** in HIV-infected patients [16,26].

**E. Dosage forms available**

1. **Oral. Single strength** tablets contain 80 mg TMP and 400 mg SMX. **Double strength** tablets contain 160 mg of TMP and 800 mg SMX. There are unflavored and cherry-flavored **suspensions** containing 40 mg TMP and 200 mg SMX per 5 mL.
2. **Parenteral.** An intravenous form of TMP-SMX is supplied in 5-mL ampules that contain 80 mg TMP and 400 mg SMX. The intravenous preparation is recommended for the following: (a) **severe UTI** in patients who are vomiting or otherwise too ill to take an oral medication, (b) patients with severe **PCP,** (c) **severe *Shigella* infections,** and (d) certain serious multiresistant enteric gram-negative bacillary infections in which TMP-SMX is active *in vitro.* Infectious disease consultation is advisable in this setting. The intravenous form has also been

used in the treatment of pneumonia, bacteremia, meningitis, and other serious infections.

**For severe or complicated UTI,** due to known susceptible organisms, 8 to 10 mg/kg/day (based on the TMP component) is recommended. The dose is divided into an every 6 or 12 hour schedule until the patient improves enough to allow oral therapy (Table 27L.1).

**F. Preferred route.** Because TMP-SMX is well absorbed, **the oral route is usually preferred** unless the patient has nausea, is vomiting, is taking nothing by mouth, or is critically ill. If intravenous therapy is initially used, one can often switch to oral therapy when the patient improves. Adequate fluid intake should be encouraged to prevent sulfonamide crystalluria [1].

1. **See Table 27L.1.**
2. **In children,** TMP-SMX is **not recommended for infants less than 2 months** of age because of the risk of kernicterus. For otitis media and other infections 8 mg/kg TMP (and 40 mg/kg SMX) per 24 hours is given in two divided doses every 12 hours for 10 days (see Chapters 3 and 8) (Table 27 L.2). An identical dosage is given for 5 days for shigellosis.
3. **In pregnancy**
   - **a.** TMP-SMX is **not recommended at term** because sulfonamides cross the placenta and may cause kernicterus.
   - **b.** TMP-SMX is a **category C** drug (see Chapter 27A). It is generally not recommended for use in pregnancy unless the benefits justify the risks to the fetus [5] (see section **G.4** below).
4. **Nursing mothers.** Because sulfonamides are excreted in human breast milk and may cause kernicterus, avoid the **use** of TMP-SMX for nursing mothers (see section **G.4**).
5. **In renal failure, dosages** must be **modified.** The optimal approach is not well defined. The package insert suggests that standard doses can be used for a creatinine clearance of more than 30 mL/min. For a creatinine clearance of 15 to 30 mL/min, half the usual dose is suggested. For a creatinine clearance of less than 15 mL/min, use is not recommended.
   - **a.** In a recent review [9], the author suggested (a) usual doses for a creatinine clearance of more than 50 mL/min, (b) 50% of the standard dose be given every 12 hours or the standard dose of 18 to 24 hours if the creatinine clearance is 10 to 50 mL/min, and (c) a standard dose every 24 hours if the creatinine clearance is less than 10 mL/min. Because TMP-SMX is **removed by hemodialysis,** standard doses can be administered after dialysis, with perhaps a supplemental fractional dosing provided on nondialysis days [9]. Infectious disease input is advised. Adults on chronic ambulatory peritoneal dialysis should receive the equivalent of one double strength tablet every 48 hours [5].
6. In **significant hepatic failure,** TMP-SMX should be avoided.

**G. Toxicity and side effects.** Although skin rashes are common, this combination **usually is well tolerated,** even for prolonged periods. Reactions occur either to the TMP (see Chapter 27M) or, more commonly, to the sulfonamide component (see section **I.E**). Adverse reactions have been reviewed [1,4,9,27]. **In patients with AIDS, drug toxicity** (rash, fever, neutropenia, thrombocytopenia, and transaminase elevation) **occurs more frequently** [28] than in non-AIDS patients, but dose reduction and the use of corticosteroids, commonly used in PCP, may help reduce these reactions.

1. **Mild gastrointestinal symptoms,** including nausea, vomiting, diarrhea, cramps, and similar symptoms, occur in 3% to 3.5% of patients [21] and are the most frequent adverse effects [8].
2. **Skin rashes are relatively common,** occurring in 3% to 5% [1,9]. They are usually typical drug eruptions with a **diffuse maculopapular** rash **or mild toxic erythema.** Most rashes are benign and resolve with discontinuation of therapy. However, exfoliative dermatitis, Stevens-Johnson syndrome, or toxic epidermal necrolysis may occur. An increased frequency of rashes occurs in AIDS patients receiving TMP-SMX [28]. With a history of cutaneous sensitivity or other

Table 27L.1. Dosing of TMP-SMX

| Indication | Dosage[a]/Day (Normal Renal Function) | Duration and Comments |
|---|---|---|
| Uncomplicated cystitis in women | 1 DS bid | For 3 days |
| Conventional therapy in UTI, UTI in elderly | 1 DS bid | For 7–10 days |
| Pyelonephritis | i.v. or p.o., 1 DS bid p.o. | For at least 14 days. See text for i.v. doses. For children use dose as in acute otitis media. |
| Prophylaxis of recurrent UTI in women | ½ or 1 SS every other night or ½ SS tab nightly qhs | Typically for at least 6–12 mo; the urine should be sterilized first. See Chapter 15. |
| Prostatitis | 1 DS bid | For 3–4 weeks or more. See Chapter 15. |
| Acute exacerbations of COPD | 1 DS bid | Usually for 5–7 days. See Chapter 8. |
| Acute otitis media (AOM) | In children > 2 mo, TMP 8 mg/kg/day and SMX 40 mg/kg/day given in divided doses q12h See Table 27L.2 | 5 days to 10 days. See Chapter 8. |
| Sinusitis | 1 DS bid in adults. In children, see AOM doses | Usually for 10 days. See Chapter 8. |
| Pneumonia | i.v. initially (see text) | After improvement, switch to po, 1 DS bid in adults, duration must be individualized. See Chapter 11. |
| *Salmonella, Shigella* when susceptible | Dosages used for UTI | For 5 days |
| Traveler's diarrhea | 1 DS bid | For 3 days in adults. Many *E. coli* now resistant to TMP-SMX. See text and Chapter 22. Quinolones usually preferred unless contraindicated. |
| Susceptible, gram-negative meningitis[b] | 10 mg/kg/day (based on TMP component) i.v. divided q6h[b] | Probably for 2 weeks. Infectious disease consultation advised. |
| Bacteremias and nosocomial infections | i.v. 8–10 mg/kg/day (based on TMP component) divided q6 or q12h schedule. | Go to oral doses when patient improves. |
| Prevention of *Pneumocystis carinii* pneumonia (PCP) in immunocompromised e.g., AIDS[c] | 1 DS p.o. qd or 1 SS p.o. qd | While CD4 count is <200/$\mu$L or oropharyngeal candidiasis |
| Therapy of PCP | Initially, begin at 5 mg/kg of TMP component q6h for 3–5 days, then q8h for another 3–5 days, then 4 mg/kg of TMP q8h component until course completed. | Total course of 21 days. By tapering doses, side effects may be minimized. In very ill patients, i.v. therapy is initially used and converted to oral therapy as the patient improves. |

[a]DS, double-strength tablet; SS, single-strength tablet. The DS tablet of TMP-SMX is a large tablet; some patients may prefer two of the smaller SS tablets.
[b]See Levitz AE, Quintiliani R. Trimethoprim-sulfamethoxazole for bacterial meningitis. *Ann Intern Med* 1984;100:881.
[c]Guidelines for prevening opportunistic infections among HIV-infected persons—2002. *MMWR* 2002;51 (RR-8):4–5, with permission.
UTI, urinary tract infection; COPD, chronic obstructive pulmonary disease.

Table 27L.2. Pediatric Dosages of TMP-SMX for UTI, Otitis Media, Shigellosis, and the like[a] (Pediatric Suspension)

| Weight | | Dose (q12h) | |
|---|---|---|---|
| lbs. | Kg | Teaspoonfuls | Tablets |
| 22 | 10 | 1 tsp. (5 mL) | — |
| 44 | 20 | 2 tsp. (10 mL) | 1 tablet[b] |
| 66 | 30 | 3 tsp. (15 mL) | 1 ½ tablets |
| 88 | 40 | 4 tsp. (20 mL) | 2 tablets or 1 DS tablet |

[a]For children 2 months of age or older.
[b]Author's note: tablet = single strength.
DS, double strength; UTI, urinary tract infection.
*Physicians' desk reference,* 56th ed. Montvale, NJ: Medical Economics Data, 2002, with permission.

TMP-SMX intolerance, desensitization has been successful with oral desensitization protocols [9,29–31].

3. **Bone marrow and peripheral blood.** Megaloblastic bone marrow changes are uncommon except in those patients with preexisting depleted folate stores (e.g., alcoholics, the elderly, pregnant women, malnourished patients, and patients receiving phenytoin). Except for bone marrow transplant recipients in whom engraftment may be delayed, occasionally in pediatric patients, and in AIDS patients, severe hematologic reactions to TMP-SMX are rare [27]. Thrombocytopenia occurs as it does with sulfonamide use. Although neutropenia has been attributed to TMP-SMX, the precise relationship to drug therapy is difficult to determine, as neutropenia (a) is common in randomly sampled young children (control subjects); (b) is seen with viral illnesses for which the patient, especially children, may receive antibiotics; and (c) in reviews has been seen with similar frequency in patients receiving amoxicillin therapy [1]. Further studies are necessary to clarify this question. If neutropenia occurs in a patient receiving TMP-SMX, it is prudent to discontinue the TMP-SMX and use an alternative agent.

   **Use of folinic acid.** It has been suggested that concomitant administration of folinic acid may reverse the antifolate effects of TMP-SMX, especially in patients not infected with HIV, without interfering with its antimicrobial effect (see **Chapter 18**). In one report, adjunctive folinic acid with TMP-SMX for PCP **in AIDS patients was associated with an increased risk of therapeutic failure and death** [32]. Therefore empiric addition of folinic acid in this setting is not advised [32].

   Hemolysis may rarely be precipitated with TMP-SMX use in patients with G6PD deficiency (see section **I.E.2**). However, in one study, G6PD-deficient patients who received TMP-SMX did not have hemolytic reactions during therapy [6]. In patients with AIDS who receive TMP-SMX for PCP, dose reduction may help reduce bone marrow suppression.

4. **Pregnancy and lactation. Because of the teratogenic effect seen in animal studies, TMP-SMX is generally contraindicated in pregnant** [5] **or lactating women.** Furthermore, because the sulfonamide component displaces bilirubin from albumin-binding sites and may therefore increase the risk of kernicterus, **TMP-SMX is contraindicated in infants younger than 2 months and in pregnant women near term.**

5. **Drug-drug interactions.** The **sulfonamide-related interactions are reviewed in section I.F.** and include interactions with oral anticoagulants and oral hypoglycemic agents. We try to avoid using sulfonamides, including TMP-SMX, in patients receiving **warfarin.** If TMP-SMX is used, prothrombin times should be monitored. Often the dose of warfarin will need to be reduced. TMP-SMX may prolong the half-life of phenytoin.

**Methotrexate** concentrations can be increased, and toxicity may ensue as a result of displacement from plasma-binding sites [9]. A review of drug interactions has recently been published [33].

6. **Nephrotoxicity** does not appear to be a significant side effect [1]. Clinically insignificant elevations of creatinine can occur with TMP (see Chapter 27M).
7. **Hyperkalemia** may occur in patients with AIDS during treatment for PCP with TMP-SMX (see discussion in **Chapter 18**).
8. **Local thrombophlebitis** uncommonly occurs with intravenous administration.
9. **Acquisition of resistance** is discussed in Chapter 27M.

H. **Cost** (see Appendix Table)

III. **Fansidar** tablets are a combination of pyrimethamine (25 mg), a folate antagonist, and sulfadoxine (500 mg), a long-acting sulfonamide. This combination is still used in some antimalarial treatment regimens [21].

## REFERENCES


1. Reese RE, Betts RF. Sulfonamides and trimethoprim-sulfamethoxazole. In: Reese RE, Betts RF, Gumustop B, eds. *Handbook of antibiotics,* 3rd ed. Philadelphia: Lippincott, Williams & Wilkins, 2000;446–462.
2. Medical Letter. The choice of antibacterial drugs. *Med Lett Drugs Ther* 2000;43: 69.
3. Dajani A, et al. Treatment of acute streptococcal pharyngitis and prevention of rheumatic fever: a statement for health professionals. *Pediatrics* 1995;96:758.
4. Sanche SE, Ronald AR. Sulfonamides and trimethoprim. In: Root RK, et al., eds. *Clinical infectious diseases: a practical approach.* New York: Oxford University Press, 1999;313–317.
5. Zinner SH, Mayer KH. Sulfonamides and trimethoprim. In: Mandell GL, Bennett JE, Dolin R, eds. *Principles and practice of infectious diseases,* 5th ed. New York: Churchill Livingstone, 2000:394–404.
6. Markowitz N, Saravolatz LD. Use of trimethoprim-sulfamethoxazole in a glucose-6-phosphate dehydrogenase-deficient population. *Rev Infect Dis* 1987;9:S218.
7. Aronoff GR, et al. *Drug prescribing in renal failure: dosing guidelines for adults,* 4th ed. Philadelphia: American College of Physicians, 1999.
8. Lundstrom TS, Sobel JD. Vancomycin, trimethoprim-sulfamethoxazole, and rifampin. *Infect Dis Clin North Am* 1995;9:747.
9. Smilack JD. Trimethoprim-sulfamethoxazole. *Mayo Clin Proc* 1999;74:730.
10. Hofman J, et al. The prevalence of drug-resistant *Streptococcus pneumoniae* in Atlanta. *N Engl J Med* 1995;333:481.
11. Sands M, et al. Trimethoprim-sulfamethoxazole therapy of *Pasteurella multocida* infection. *J Infect Dis* 1989;160:354.
12. Navin TR, Beard CB, Huang L, et al. Effect of mutations in *Pneumocystis carinii* dihydropteroate synthase gene on outcome of *P. carinii* pneumonia in patients with HIV-1: a prospective study. *Lancet* 2001;358:545–549.
13. Huovinen P. Resistance to trimethoprim-sulfamethoxazole. *Clin Infect Dis* 2001;32: 1608.
14. Gupta K, Scholes D, Stamm WE. Increasing prevalence of antimicrobial resistance among uropathogens causing acute uncomplicated cystitis in women. *JAMA* 1999; 281:736.
15. Gupta K, Hooton TM, Stamm WE. Increasing antimicrobial resistance and the management of uncomplicated community-acquired urinary tract infection. *Ann Intern Med* 2001;135:41.
16. Brown PD, Freeman A, Foxman B. Prevalence and predictors of trimethoprim-sulfamethoxazole resistance among uropathogenic *Escherichia coli* isolates in Michigan. *Clin Infect Dis* 2002;34:1061.
17. Center for Disease Control and Prevention. Guidelines for preventing opportunistic infections among HIV-infected patients-2002. *MMWR Morb Mortal Wkly Rep* 2002; 51(RR-8):4.

18. Smith JW, et al. Recurrent urinary tract infections in men: characteristics and response to therapy. *Ann Intern Med* 1980;91:544.
19. Lipsky BA. Prostatitis and urinary tract infections: what's new; what's true? *Am J Med* 1999;106:327.
20. Stapleton A, et al. Postcoital antimicrobial prophylaxis for recurrent urinary tract infection: a randomized, double-blind, placebo-controlled trial. *JAMA* 1990;264:703.
21. Medical Letter. Drugs for parasitic infection. *Med Lett Drugs Ther* 1998;40:1.
22. Sepkowitz KA. *Pneumocystis carinii* pneumonia without acquired immunodeficiency syndrome: who should receive prophylaxis? *Mayo Clin Proc* 1996;71:102.
23. Levitz AE, Quintiliani, R. Trimethoprim-sulfamethoxazole for bacterial meningitis. *Ann Intern Med* 1984;100:881.
24. Hughes WT, et al. 1997 Guidelines for the use of antimicrobial agents in neutropenic patients with unexplained fever. *Clin Infect Dis* 1997;25:551.
25. Fox BC, et al. A prospective, randomized, double-blind study of trimethoprim-sulfamethoxazole for prophylaxis of infection in renal transplantation: clinical efficacy, absorption of trimethoprim-sulfamethoxazole, effects on microflora, and the cost-benefit of prophylaxis. *Am J Med* 1990;89:225.
26. Goodgame RW. Understanding intestinal spore forming protozoa: cryptosporidia, microsporidia, isospora, and cyclospora. *Ann Intern Med* 1996;124:429.
27. Gutman LT. The use of trimethoprim-sulfamethoxazole in children: a review of adverse reactions and indications. *Pediatr Infect Dis J* 1984;3:349.
28. Lee BL. Drug interactions and toxicities in patients with AIDS. In: Sande MA, Volberding PA, eds. *The medical management of AIDS,* 5th ed. Philadelphia: W.B. Saunders, 1997: 125–142.
29. Glucksteiny D, Ruskin J. Rapid oral desensitization to trimethoprim-sulfamethoxazole (TMP-SMX): use in prophylaxis for *Pneumocystis carinii* pneumonia in patients with AIDS who were previously intolerant to TMP-SMX. *Clin Infect Dis* 1995;20: 849.
30. Caumes E, et al. Efficacy and safety of desensitization with sulfamethoxazole and trimethoprim in 48 previously hypersensitive patients infected with human immunodeficiency virus. *Arch Dermatol* 1997;133:465.
31. Demoly P, et al. Six-hour trimethoprim-sulfamethoxazole-graded challenge in HIV infected patients. *J Allergy Clin Immun* 1998;102:1033.
32. Safrin S, Lee BL, Sande MA. Adjunctive folinic acid with trimethoprim-sulfamethoxazole for *Pneumocystis carinii* in AIDS patients is associated with an increased risk of therapeutic failure and death. *J Infect Dis* 1994;170:912.
33. Gregg CR. Drug interactions and anti-infective therapies. *Am J Med* 1999;106:227.

## M. Trimethoprim

Trimethoprim (TMP) not in combination with sulfamethoxazole (SMX) is available and is approved for use in uncomplicated urinary tract infections (UTIs) [1–3].

I. **Mechanism of action.** By inhibiting dihydrofolate reductase, TMP interferes with the production of tetrahydrofolic acid in bacterial cells (see Fig. 27L.1).

II. **Spectrum of activity.** TMP is bactericidal against many gram-positive aerobic cocci and many species of gram-negative bacteria, except *Pseudomonas aeruginosa* and other *Pseudomonas* species [3]. Enterococci usually are resistant. It is **active against community-acquired urinary tract pathogens** such as *Escherichia coli, Proteus mirabilis, Klebsiella pneumoniae,* and *Enterobacter* species Most anaerobes and *Chlamydia* species are resistant [2]. Its spectrum of activity is **very similar to that of the TMP-SMX combination.**

III. **Pharmacokinetics.** TMP is **well absorbed** from the gastrointestinal tract. It is excreted primarily unchanged in the urine. Urinary concentrations are considerably higher than in blood. Dosage must be altered in renal failure. **TMP penetrates prostatic** and vaginal secretions well [1,3]. It achieves high tissue levels in the kidney [3] and is excreted in breast milk. This drug increases the half-life of phenytoin.

## IV. Dosage

**A. Oral.** TMP is available in 100-mg doses. The effectiveness of TMP as a single agent in children younger than 12 years has not been established. The safety of TMP in infants younger than 2 months of age has not been demonstrated.

**B. In renal failure,** the interval is adjusted. For creatinine clearance of 10 to 50 mL/min, the usual dose is given every 18 hours, and for creatinine clearance less than 10 mL/min, the usual dose can be given every 24 hours [4].

**C. Pregnancy.** TMP is a **category C agent** (see Chapter 27A) and should be used during pregnancy only if the potential benefit justifies the potential risk to the fetus (see section **VI.B.6**).

**D. Nursing mothers.** TMP is excreted in human breast milk. Because TMP may interfere with folic acid metabolism, caution should be exercised for a nursing woman (see section **VI.B.6**).

## V. Current clinical uses

**A. Uncomplicated UTI.** Some experts prefer TMP alone to TMP-SMX because of equal spectrum and less common adverse effects [5]. A 3-day regimen is preferred over one dose. Adult dose is 100 mg every 12 hours or 200 mg every 24 hours for 3 or 10 days.

**B. Recurrent UTI** in women. TMP has been used in suppressive regimens of 100 mg at bedtime [1,2,5]. Urine should be sterilized before suppressive therapy is started (see Chapter 15).

**C. Prostatitis.** TMP, 100 mg every 12 hours or 200 mg every 24 hours is given for 4 to 12 weeks. It is effective for both acute and chronic prostatitis [1,2,5]. It is especially useful in the sulfa allergic. TMP-SMX and oral fluoroquinolones are alternative agents (see Chapter 15).

**D. Traveler's diarrhea.** TMP, 100 mg twice daily for 3 or, at most, 5 days has been effective [6]; quinolones are preferred (see Chapters 13, 22, and 27G, section **II.B.5.**).

**E. *Pneumocystis carinii*.** TMP cannot be substituted for TMP-SMX. A combination of **dapsone and TMP,** 200 mg every 8 hours **is effective for moderate *P. carinii*** in acquired immunodeficiency syndrome (AIDS) [7,8] (see Chapter 18).

## VI. Potential problems and adverse effects

**A. Resistance to TMP.** The topic of TMP and TMP-SMX has been reviewed [9–13] (see also **Chapter 27L, section II.C.5**). TMP resistance governs whether there is resistance to the combination. Resistance of *Escherichia coli* has been occurring with increasing frequency. For example, from 1978 to 1981, *E. coli* resistance to TMP rose modestly from 2% to 6% in Boston, from 8% to 30% in Paris, and to even higher rates (40%) in developing countries [9,11] (25%–68% in South America, Asia, and Africa [10]). In some developing countries, antibiotics are often available without prescription, and TMP is used as monotherapy. Resistance to *Salmonella typhi* is worldwide. Also, resistance of *Shigella* species, of methicillin-resistance *S. aureus,* and, recently, *S. pneumoniae* to TMP has become more common [3]. In two recent studies, it was shown that prior exposure to antibiotics, especially to TMP, predicted that organisms causing a current UTI would be resistant to TMP [12,13]. See related discussion in Chapters 15 and 27L.

**B. Adverse effects.** TMP is well tolerated in standard regimens.

1. **Skin rashes** have been noted in approximately 3% of patients, compared with 6% of patients receiving TMP-SMX [1] when conventional doses are used. In high dose regimens, TMP is associated with a higher incidence of rashes and other adverse drug effects [14].
2. **Anaphylaxis** has been described after TMP use [15,16]. **For a history of a delayed diffuse rash from TMP-SMX,** unless there was an immediate reaction associated, it is reasonable to use TMP alone as sulfonamides cause rashes more commonly.
3. **Hyperkalemia** [17–20] is seen commonly in patients with AIDS who are treated with high doses of TMP-SMX or TMP and dapsone and has occurred in hospitalized patients without AIDS who were treated with TMP-SMX. TMP is a sodium channel inhibitor and functions as a potassium-sparing diuretic agent.
4. **Bone marrow effects.** TMP is a weak human folic acid metabolic inhibitor, particularly in the elderly or alcoholic folate-deficient patient [1,5]. Megaloblastic

anemia, neutropenia, and thrombocytopenia have been described with prolonged use. The administration of 10 mg of folinic acid daily prevents this side effect, presumably without reducing the antibacterial activity of TMP, but folinic acid is expensive. However, adjunctive folinic acid with TMP-SMX for *P. carinii* pneumonia in AIDS patients was associated with an increased risk of therapeutic failure and death in one series [21]. Folinic acid must be used cautiously.

5. **Modest evaluations of serum creatinine** levels may occur in patients receiving TMP, but these are probably clinically insignificant [14]. **Abnormal liver function tests** can occur [22].
6. Teratogenicity of TMP in humans has not been clearly established. **It seems prudent to use an alternate agent in pregnancy and nursing women** [2].
7. **Drug interaction.** TMP may predispose to **phenytoin** toxicity by increasing free levels of phenytoin [5].

**C. Cost** (see Appendix Table)

## REFERENCES

1. Reese RE, Betts RF. Trimethoprim. In: Reese RE, Betts RF, Gumustop B, eds. *Handbook of antibiotics,* 3rd ed. Philadelphia: Lippincott, Williams & Wilkins 2000;463–467.
2. Zinner SH, Mayer KH. Sulfonamides and trimethoprim. In: Mandell GL, Bennett JE, Dolin R, eds. *Principles and practice of infectious diseases,* 5th ed. New York: Churchill Livingstone, 2000:394–404.
3. Lundstrom TS, Sobel JD. Vancomycin, trimethoprim-sulfamethoxazole, and rifampin. *Infect Dis Clin North Am* 1995;9:747.
4. Aronoff GR, et al. *Drug prescribing in renal failure: dosing guidelines for adults,* 4th ed. Philadelphia: American College of Physicians, 1999.
5. Sanche SE, Ronald AR. Sulfonamides and trimethoprim. In: Root RK, et al., eds. *Clinical infectious diseases: a practical approach*. New York: Oxford University Press, 1999:313–317.
6. Dupont HL, et al. Treatment of traveler's diarrhea with trimethoprim/sulfamethoxazole and with trimethoprim alone. *N Engl J Med* 1982;20:841.
7. Medina I, et al. Oral therapy for *Pneumocystis carinii* pneumonia in the acquired immunodeficiency syndrome: a controlled trial of trimethoprim-sulfamethoxazole versus trimethoprim-dapsone. *N Engl J Med* 1990;323:776.
8. Medical Letter. Drugs for parasitic infection. *Med Lett Drugs Ther* 2002;44:1.
9. Goldstein FW, et al. The changing pattern of trimethoprim resistance in Paris, with a review of worldwide experience. *Rev Infect Dis* 1986;8:725.
10. Houvinen P, et al. Trimethoprim and sulfonamide resistance. *Antimicrob Agents Chemother* 1995;39:279.
11. Houvinen P. Resistance to trimethoprim-sulfamethoxazole. *Clin Infect Dis* 2001;32:1608.
12. Steinke DT, Seaton RA, Phillips G, et al. Prior trimethoprim use and trimethoprim-resistant urinary tract infection: a nested case-control study with multivariant analysis for other risk factors. *J Antimicrob Chemother* 2001;47:781–787.
13. Howard AJ, Magee JT, Fitzgerald KA, et al. Factors associated with antibiotic resistance in coliforms organisms from community urinary tract infection in Wales. *J Antimicrob Chemother* 2001;47:305–313.
14. Naderer O, Nafziger AN, Bertino JS Jr. Effects of moderate-dose versus high-dose trimethoprim on serum creatinine and creatinine clearance and adverse reactions. *Antimicrob Agents Chemother* 1997;41:2466.
15. Alonso MD, et al. Hypersensitivity to trimethoprim. *Allergy* 1992;47:340.
16. Bijl AM, et al. Anaphylactic reactions associated with trimethoprim. *Clin Exp Allergy* 1998;28:510.
17. Choi MJ, et al. Brief report: trimethoprim-induced hyperkalemia in a patient with AIDS. *N Engl J Med* 1993;328:703.
18. Valazquez H, et al. Renal mechanism of trimethoprim-induced hyperkalemia. *Ann Intern Med* 1993;119:296.
19. Alappan R, et al. Hyperkalemia in hospitalized patients treated with trimethoprim-sulfamethoxazole. *Ann Intern Med* 1996;124:316.

20. Perazella MA. Trimethoprim-induced hyperkalemia: clinical data, mechanism, prevention, and management. *Drug Safety* 2000;22:227.
21. Safrin S, Lee BL, Sande MA. Adjunctive folinic acid with trimethoprim-sulfamethoxazole in *Pneumocystis carinii* in AIDS patients is associated with an increased risk of therapeutic failure and death. *J Infect Dis* 1994;170:912.
22. Lindgren A, Olsson R. Liver reactions from trimethoprim. *J Intern Med* 1994;236:281.


## N. Macrolides: Erythromycin, Clarithromycin, and Azithromycin*

Erythromycin and the semisynthetic derivatives of erythromycin, clarithromycin and azithromycin, have structural modifications to improve tissue penetration and broaden their spectrum of activity [1–4] and are available in the United States. The macrolides inhibit RNA-dependent protein synthesis by reversibly binding to the 50S ribosomal subunits of susceptible microorganisms. Although generally bacteriostatic, they may be bactericidal under certain conditions or against certain microorganisms [1,3]. Because the structure of the macrolides differs from that of $\beta$-lactams, macrolides are useful for patients who are allergic to $\beta$-lactams.

### ERYTHROMYCIN

**I. Spectrum of activity.** Erythromycin's spectrum includes many gram-positive bacteria, some gram-negative bacteria, mycoplasma, chlamydiae, treponema, and rickettsiae.

- **A. See Table 27N.1.**
- **B. Aerobic bacteria.** Certain points deserve emphasis.
  - **1. Gram-positive organisms**
    - **a.** Erythromycin is usually active against **group A streptococci** (GAS). In the United States, until recently less than 5% of GAS were resistant to erythromycin [5,6]. Resistance of GAS to erythromycin in some countries has been a problem (e.g., Finland). In 2002, a sudden outbreak was reported of a macrolide-resistant GAS in which 48% of throat isolates were resistant to erythromycin. Given these findings, an editorial encouraged research to document prevalence of macrolide resistance throughout the United States so that individual physicians know the likelihood of erythromycin-resistant GAS in their local area [7].
    - **b.** Penicillin-susceptible ***Streptococcus pneumoniae*** are susceptible to erythromycin, but many penicillin-resistant strains are also resistant *in vitro* to macrolides. The exact clinical significance of this remains debated [8] (see Chapters 8 and 11). Strains resistant to one macrolide are resistant to all macrolides [1].
    - **c.** Many other streptococci are susceptible (groups B, C, G, etc.), but **group D (enterococci) is resistant.**
    - **d. Methicillin-susceptible *Staphylococcus aureus*** are often susceptible to erythromycin, but resistance may emerge during therapy [9]. Interestingly, the *Medical Letter* does not list the macrolides as alternative agents for methicillin-susceptible *S. aureus* [10]. **Methicillin-resistant *S. aureus* (MRSA)** are resistant to macrolides.
    - **e. Erythromycin** is the drug of choice for *Corynebacterium diphtheriae* and **alternative agent** for ***Bacillus anthracis*** **(anthrax) [10].**
  - **2.** Gram-negative organisms
    - **a.** Erythromycin is an **agent of choice** for *Campylobacter jejuni, Bordetella pertussis* (whooping cough), bacillary angiomatosis caused by *Bartonella henselae,* and trench fever caused by *B. quintana.* [10].
    - **b.** Erythromycin is an **alternative agent** for ***Haemophilus ducreyi*** **(chancroid),** ***Eikenella corrodens,*** **and** ***Moraxella catarrhalis*** **[10].**

*Adapted from Reese ER, Betts RF. Macrolides: erythromycin, clarithromycin, and azithromycin. In: Reese RE, Betts RF, Gumustop B, eds. *Handbook of antibiotics,* 3rd ed. Philadelphia: Lippincott Williams and Wilkins, 2000:468–492.

Table 27N.1. *In Vitro* Activity of the Macrolides

| Organism | Mean $MIC_{90}$ (mg/L)[a] | | |
|---|---|---|---|
| | Erythromycin (≤0.5 mg/L)[b] | Clarithromycin (≤2 mg/L)[b] | Azithromycin (≤2 mg/L)[b] |
| Oral or respiratory | | | |
| *Moraxella catarrhalis* | 0.25 | 0.25 | 0.06 |
| Group A streptococci | 0.03 | <0.12 | 0.12 |
| *Streptococcus pneumoniae* (1994/1997) | | | |
| Penicillin sensitive | ≤0.25/0.12 | 32 | 4.0/0.5 |
| Intermediate resistance to penicillin | ≤0.25/8 | 16 | 2.0/16 |
| Penicillin resistant | ≤0.25/8 | >32 | 8/16 |
| *Haemophilus influenzae* | | | |
| β-Lactamase positive | 4–16 | 8–16[c] | 1–4[d] |
| β-Lactamase negative | 0.5–8 | 8–16 | 1–4[d] |
| *Bordetella pertussis* | 0.03 | 0.03 | 0.06 |
| *Neisseria meningitidis* | 0.5–4.0 | 1.0 | 0.12–2.0 |
| Atypical respiratory | | | |
| *Mycoplasma pneumoniae* | ≤0.01 | 0.0078–0.5 | ≤0.01 |
| *Legionella pneumophila* | 0.5 | 0.06 | 0.5 |
| *L. longbeachae* | 0.5 | 0.12 | 0.5 |
| *Chlamydia pneumoniae* | 0.5 | 0.25 | 0.25 |
| STD or GU | | | |
| *N. gonorrhoeae* (all) | 0.5–4.0 | 0.5–2.0 | 0.06–0.5 |
| *C. trachomatis* | ≤0.125 | ... | ≤0.125 |
| *H. ducreyi* | 0.03 | ... | 0.004 |
| *M. hominis* | ≥128 | 64 | 4–32 |
| *Ureaplasma urealyticum* | 1–4 | 0.2 | 0.5–4 |
| *Gardnerella vaginalis* | ≤0.03 | ... | ≤0.03 |
| *Mobiluncus species* | ≤0.03 | ... | 0.06 |
| Other gram positive | | | |
| *Staphylococcus aureus* | | | |
| MSSA | 1–8 | 0.5 | 1.0 |
| MRSA | >64 | ... | >128 |
| *S. epidermidis* | | | |
| MSSE | >8, >64 | >32 | >32, >128 |
| MRSE | >8, >64 | >32 | >32, >128 |
| *Streptococci* | | | |
| Group B | ≤0.12 | 0.06 | 0.12–0.1 |
| Group C, F, G | 0.5 | ... | 0.25 |
| *S. bovis* | 1.0–2.0 | 0.5 | 1.0–4.0 |
| *S. faecalis* / *S. faecium* | >8 | >32 | >32 |
| Viridans streptococci | 0.06–2.0 | 0.03 | 0.12–16 |
| Mycobacteria | | | |
| *Mycobacterium avium* complex | ≥64 | 4–16 | ≥32 |
| *M. chelonae* subsp. *chelonae* | 8.0 | 0.25 | 2.0 |
| *M. chelonae* subsp. *abscessus* | >8 | 0.5 | 8.0 |
| Miscellaneous | | | |
| *Borrelia burgdorferi* | 0.006–0.03 | 0.015–0.06 | 0.015–0.03 |
| *Helicobacter pylori* | 0.25 | 0.03 | 0.25 |

[a]Values for MIC cutoff for susceptibility. MIC of clarithromycin alone; 14-hydroxy metabolite of clarithromycin may contribute to antimicrobial activity. All MICs broth dilution, inoculum $10^{-4}$–$10^{-6}$; at least 10 strains from each source.
[b]Recommended susceptibility breakpoints.
[c]Recommended breakpoint ≤8 mg/L.
[d]Recommended breakpoint ≤4 mg/L.
GU, genitourinary; MIC, minimal inhibitory concentration; $MIC_{90}$, minimal concentration that will inhibit 90% of clinical isolates; MRSA, methicillin-resistant *Staphylococcus aureus;* MRSE, methicillin-resistant *Staphylococcus epidermidis;* MSSA, methicillin-sensitive *Staphylococcus aureus;* MSSE, methicillin-sensitive *Staphylococcus epidermidis;* STD, sexually transmitted disease; subsp, subspecies.
Modified from Alvarez-Elcoro S, Enzler MJ. The macrolides: erythromycin, clarithromycin, and azithromycin. *Mayo Clin Proc* 1999;74:613.

c. Most strains of *H. influenzae* [3] are resistant to erythromycin [1], and thus it is not viewed as an alternative agent for this pathogen, although clarithromycin and azithromycin are considered active against respiratory isolates of *H. influenzae* [10].

d. **Enterobacteriaceae** such as ***Escherichia coli and Klebsiella* species** are resistant.

C. Anaerobes. **Erythromycin has activity against some species of gram-negative anaerobes, but *Bacteroides fragilis* strains and *Fusobacterium* species usually are resistant [9].**

D. Nonbacterial pathogens

1. Mycoplasma. **Erythromycin is active against *Mycoplasma pneumoniae* and is a** drug of choice **for this pathogen as well as the drug of choice for *Ureaplasma urealyticum* [10].**
2. **Chlamydiae.** Erythromycin is active against *Chlamydia trachomatis* and *C. pneumoniae.*
3. **Spirochetes.** Erythromycin is active against *Borrelia burgdorferi,* the causative agent of Lyme disease. Azithromycin and clarithromycin are alternative agents for this pathogen [10]. It also is active against *Treponema pallidum* but seldom is used for this purpose.

II. Pharmacokinetics **[1–4,9,11]**

A. **Oral absorption.** Erythromycin is acid labile. In the stomach, it rapidly decomposes to two inactive metabolites, one of which may contribute to gastrointestinal (GI) side effects. As a result of this instability and depending on the salt form, the rate of absorption may be unpredictable (35% ± 25%) [11]. Preparations for oral use have been synthesized with a goal of diminishing destruction by gastric acid and promoting better absorption [9].

1. Food in the stomach may decrease absorption of some forms.
2. Average serum levels achieved by the available oral preparations are similar; therefore no single oral formulation of erythromycin offers a clear advantage in adults [9].
3. In children, erythromycin estolate has better bioavailability than the ethylsuccinate [9].
4. Four hours after an oral dose of 500 mg, peak serum concentrations are 1 to 2 $\mu$m/mL [1].

B. **Intravenous (i.v.).** Serum concentrations 1 hour after 500 mg to 1 g i.v. are approximately 10 to 15 $\mu$g/mL [1]. Erythromycin should not be administered intramuscularly. Intravenous preparations should be used to treat serious infections requiring erythromycin.

C. **Half-life and excretion.** The serum half-life of erythromycin is approximately 1 to 2 hours, and levels persist for approximately 6 hours [1,3]. Because erythromycin is excreted primarily in the bile, this fact must be considered in patients with liver disease. Dose reduction is not necessary in mild to moderate renal failure.

D. **Miscellaneous**

1. As a single agent, erythromycin provides **adequate middle-ear levels for penicillin-susceptible *S. pneumoniae* and *S. pyogenes,*** but these levels probably are not adequate to eradicate *H. influenzae* consistently [9].
2. **Erythromycin crosses the placenta,** but it is not known to be teratogenic. It is a category B agent (see Chapter 27A and section **IV.F.**). It also is excreted into breast milk [1].
3. **Synovial fluid.** Limited data from patients with septic arthritis suggest that erythromycin penetrates the synovial fluid poorly [9].
4. **Brain tissue and cerebrospinal fluid (CSF).** Because of limited preparation, we would not use erythromycin in central nervous system infections.

III. Indications for use

A. **Erythromycin** is considered **a drug of choice [10]** in the following infections:

1. ***Mycoplasma pneumoniae* pneumonia.** Tetracycline can also be used, but erythromycin is nearly 50 times more potent than tetracycline against *M. pneumoniae in vitro* [9].

2. ***Chlamydia trachomatis* pneumonia,** in newborns. Erythromycin is also used for *C. trachomatis* conjunctivitis or pelvic infections, especially during pregnancy [9].
3. **Miscellaneous.** Erythromycin is also used in whooping cough, for both therapy and prophylaxis; *Campylobacter jejuni* infections; *Corynebacterium diphtheriae* infections or carrier states; *B. henselae,* the agent of bacillary angiomatosis [10,13]; and *Ureaplasma urealyticum* infections (e.g., urethritis).

**B. Other indications**

1. **Community-acquired pneumonia (CAP).** Erythromycin, and especially azithromycin, have been commonly used in mild to moderate **CAP,** especially when it occurs in young to middle-aged adults. (See related discussions in Chapter 11 and under azithromycin later in this chapter.)
2. ***Legionella* infections.** Erythromycin was the first agent used. It has been replaced by azithromycin [10].
3. **Surgical prophylaxis, before elective GI procedures.** Oral erythromycin has been used with oral neomycin in (see Chapter 27B).
4. ***Lymphogranuloma venereum* and *C. trachomatis* [12].** It is used in both of these infections (see Chapter 16).

**C. Erythromycin is not recommended for the following:**

1. **Meningitis or endocarditis.**
2. **For dental/oral procedures for infective endocarditis prophylaxis** because of GI intolerance and unpredictable blood levels (see Chapter 27B).

**D. Erythromycin as an alternative in the penicillin-allergic** for the following conditions:

1. **Group A streptococcal (GAS) pharyngitis** (see Chapter 8 [7]).
2. ***Streptococcus pneumoniae* pneumonia (penicillin-susceptible strains) (see Chapter 11).**
3. **Minor staphylococcal skin infections.** Resistance to erythromycin may develop with its use over time, and erythromycin alone is not advised for deep-seated staphylococcal infections [9].
4. **Rheumatic fever prophylaxis [14].**
5. **Miscellaneous.** Erythromycin has been used in early syphilis.

**IV.** Preparations available and dosage

**A. Oral forms.** Several oral preparations are available: erythromycin base, stearate salt, ethylsuccinate ester, and the estolate form. Although the blood levels achieved vary somewhat, when the agents are used against very sensitive organisms, these minor differences are not clinically significant [1]. Also, no one formulation causes substantially less GI upset than others [1]. (The newer macrolides have less GI intolerance.)

1. **Children.** Erythromycin **estolate is more bioavailable than erythromycin ethylsuccinate** [15]. It rarely causes hepatitis, and it appears to be better absorbed, better tolerated, and more effective than ethylsuccinate [15]. Absorption is not affected by food [9].
2. **Adults.** Erythromycin estolate is no longer recommended because of the associated incidence **of cholestatic hepatitis [9].**

**B. Oral dosages**

1. **Adults.** The dose is 250 to 500 mg every 6 hours. Higher doses cause intolerable GI symptoms.
2. **Children.** The usual dose is 30 to 50 mg/kg/day divided into every 6 hour doses. In infants younger than 4 months, 20 to 40 mg/kg/day divided into doses every 6 hours has been suggested. Erythromycin estolate and erythromycin ethylsuccinate are the most widely used preparations, because they are both tasteless and available in suspensions.

**C. Parenteral forms** of erythromycin are available (e.g., erythromycin lactobionate 1–4 g/day, divided every 6 hour doses) for more serious infections requiring higher blood levels or for inability to take oral medications. Intravenous use may be associated **with thrombophlebitis.** This may be avoided by dilution in at least 250 mL of fluid [9] and infusion over 40 to 60 minutes into a large peripheral vein or through a central venous line. For children, 50 mg/kg/day is recommended, divided every

6 hours. Avoid intramuscular use. Intravenous azithromycin, which can be given once daily, is preferred for patients more than 16 years of age (see later discussion).

- **D. Topical.** Erythromycin gel or solution 1.5% or 2% applied twice daily for treatment of acne skin lesions. An ophthalmic ointment is used for bacterial conjunctivitis.
- **E. Renal failure.** In moderate renal failure, dose modification is not necessary [9,16]. With a creatinine clearance of 10 mL/min or less, **the drug may accumulate** and toxic side effects occur **[1] (e.g., transient hearing loss) [3].** Therefore in severe renal failure, 50% to 75% of dose can be given at standard intervals [16]. **Erythromycin is not removed by peritoneal dialysis or hemodialysis [16].**
- **F. Pregnancy. Erythromycin estolate should not be used in pregnancy** (see section **VI.A.3**). Other erythromycin agents are safe in pregnancy; they are category B agents (see section **II.D**).
- **G. Nursing. Erythromycin is excreted in breast milk;** caution should be exercised when erythromycin is administered to a nursing woman.
- **H. Hepatic insufficiency.** Erythromycin is metabolized primarily by the liver. It should be avoided in patients with severe liver disease. If absolutely needed, **dosages should be reduced and serum levels should be monitored.**
- **I. Cost** (see Appendix Table 1)

**V. Toxicity and side effects.** Erythromycin is considered one of the least toxic commonly used antibiotics [1,3,9], but drug-drug interactions may occur.

- **A. GI side effects.** With oral use, epigastric distress is common, **as is diarrhea, but** both can be diminished by taking the drug with meals. Symptoms often improve if the dose is reduced. GI symptoms can occur with oral and i.v. therapy [9]; a slow i.v. infusion (e.g., more than 60 minutes) may help to decrease the i.v. use associated nausea and vomiting, which may be seen more frequently in patients younger than 40 years [1].
  1. **Newer macrolides.** Because of these GI side effects, the newer macrolides are often preferred, and of these azithromycin appears to have the fewest GI side effects (see later).
  2. **Erythromycin in diabetic gastroparesis [17,18].** Although, the GI side effects are due to the GI motility-stimulating effect of the macrolides, erythromycin may have therapeutic value in this clinical entity.
  3. **Infantile hypertrophic pyloric stenosis.** Recent data suggest an association between systemic erythromycin use in infants (especially those <2 weeks of age) and subsequent infantile hypertrophic pyloric stenosis. Therefore, erythromycin should be used with prudence in early infancy [19].
- **B. Allergic reactions. Rash, fever, and eosinophilia are** uncommon, **generally mild,** and occur in approximately 0.5% to 2.0% of treated patients; rashes are usually maculopapular but sometimes urticarial. Fixed drug eruptions, contact dermatitis, and anaphylaxis occur rarely. The risk appears to be higher in patients allergic to other antibiotics [20].
- **C. Cholestatic hepatitis** is rare and, although associated with the estolate preparation in adults, usually after approximately 10 days of use [1] occurs with other erythromycins.
- **D. Deafness,** which occurs most frequently in elderly patients with renal failure receiving a high-dose [9], usually reverses several days after decreasing or discontinuing erythromycin.
- **E. *Clostridium difficile* diarrhea** occurs rarely with the use of erythromycin [9].
- **F. Drug interactions**
  1. **Erythromycin inhibits the metabolism** of numerous drugs presumably mediated by interfering with cytochrome P450 enzyme [1,3]. As a result, blood levels increase of theophylline, warfarin, carbamazepine, cyclosporine, triazolam, alfentanil, bromocriptine [3,9], and the "statins." Macrolide antibiotics inhibit CYP3A4 enzyme systems.
     - **a. Statins.** Erythromycin increases plasma concentrations of lovastatin, simvastatin, and atorvastatin. Because these interactions are sufficient to increase **the risk of myopathy and/or rhabdomyolysis,** the doses of these statins should be reduced by 50% during treatment with erythromycin or other macrolides [21]. Because pravastatin does not undergo CYP450 metabolism

and fluvastatin is metabolized by the CYP2C9 isoenzyme, statin-macrolide drug interactions do not occur with these statins, and no dosage modification is necessary when using macrolides with pravastatin or fluvastatin [21].

b. **Theophylline.** The dose should be reduced by 25% to 40% to compensate.

c. **Carbamazepine** doses may require a 50% reduction.

2. **Digoxin.** Erythromycin may improve digoxin absorption in some patients because it apparently inhibits one or more bacteria in the bowel that can break down some of the administered digoxin before it is absorbed [1].

3. **Prolonged QT interval.** Because erythromycin, especially i.v., may produce a long QT syndrome, erythromycin should probably be avoided in patients with a history of prolonged QT syndrome, especially drug induced [22]. Rarely, i.v. erythromycin has caused cardiac rhythm disturbances in premature infants [23].

4. **Cisapride (Propulsid).** Rare cases of serious cardiovascular adverse events—including torsade de pointes, other ventricular arrhythmias, and cardiac arrest—have occurred when these agents have been given concomitantly.

VI. **Resistance to macrolides.** This topic recently has been reviewed [24] and is beyond the scope of this chapter. However, a few clinical points deserve emphasis.

A. **Cross-resistance.** As previously stated, resistance to one macrolide implies cross-resistance to other macrolides [1,2,24].

B. **GAS** resistance to macrolides has occurred in the United States (see section **I.B.1** [6]).

C. **Penicillin-resistant *S. pneumoniae*.** In general, the higher the rate of penicillin resistance, the higher the rate of macrolide resistance. For example, only 4% of the penicillin-susceptible isolates were resistant to clarithromycin, but 34.8% and 60.1% of the penicillin intermediate and highly resistant strains, respectively, were macrolide resistant [2].

D. **Country to country comparisons.** Wide variations in the levels of resistance of certain pathogens to macrolides occur from country to country or within countries [24].

E. **Stable susceptibility.** Of interest, intracellular pathogens such as *Legionella, Chlamydia,* and *Mycoplasma* species are seldom resistant to macrolides [24].

## CLARITHROMYCIN (BIAXIN)

Clarithromycin differs chemically from erythromycin by having an O-methyl substitution at position 6 of the macrolide ring. Its spectrum of activity is similar to that of erythromycin, except for enhanced *H. influenzae* activity and activity against atypical mycobacterium. It has better pharmacokinetics, including once and twice daily doses [25–27].

I. ***In vitro* activity.** This is similar to erythromycin except as noted later (Table 27N.1).

A. Aerobes

1. **Gram-positive bacteria** resistant to erythromycin are resistant to clarithromycin (e.g., MRSA, high level penicillin-resistant and many intermediate level *S. pneumoniae*).

2. Gram-negative bacteria

a. ***H. influenzae.*** Clarithromycin is more active *in vitro* than erythromycin, in part due to the additive effect of its active metabolite, 14-OH clarithromycin, which *in vitro* decreases the minimum inhibitory concentration against these organisms [1,3]. The clinical significance of this is unclear [3].

b. ***M. catarrhalis*** strains are susceptible.

c. **Enterobacteriaceae.** Clarithromycin is not an active agent against these pathogens.

B. **Anaerobes.** Clarithromycin activity like erythromycin [27] is only modest.

C. **Miscellaneous**

1. ***M. pneumoniae.*** Similar to that of erythromycin.

2. ***H. pylori.*** Clarithromycin is also active.

3. ***Mycobacteria.*** Clarithromycin is active against ***M. avium* complex (MAC), *M. chelonei, M. chelonei abscessus,* and other atypical mycobacteria [1,3].** Clarithromycin is **a drug of choice** for MAC [28] and *H. pylori* and an alternative

for *S. pyogenes, M. catarrhalis, H. influenzae* (upper respiratory strains), and *B. burgdorferi* [10].

**4.** ***Ureaplasma urealyticum.*** Clarithromycin is active.

**II.** Pharmacokinetics

**A. Absorption.** Clarithromycin is acid stable and well absorbed orally with an absolute bioavailability of about 50% [1,6]. Its absorption is better and more reliable than erythromycin [1,2]. When taken with meals, bioavailability increases [26]. There is no i.v. preparation.

**B. Half-life.** The half-life of oral clarithromycin and its 14-OH metabolite is approximately 3 to 4 hours, which allows a twice daily dose schedule. An **extended release tablet** (Biaxin XL) is available, which allows a **once daily** schedule.

**C. Distribution.** Clarithromycin **penetrates tissue well,** including lung, kidney, liver, nasal mucosa, and tonsils [27], **but not into the CSF** of humans adequately. Clarithromycin and its OH metabolite penetrate middle-ear effusions adequately, with antibiotic concentrations exceeding the minimum inhibitory concentrations of the most susceptible otitis pathogens.

**D. Metabolism and elimination.** Clarithromycin is metabolized extensively in the liver by the hepatic cytochrome P450 enzyme system, and the excretion of clarithromycin and the 14-OH metabolite is by renal mechanisms [3] (see section **V.E**).

**III.** Indications for use **in adults**

**A.** Approved uses in adults

**1. Upper respiratory tract infections.** Clarithromycin has been used to treat (a) GAS pharyngitis, although penicillin is the agent of choice (see Chapter 8); (b) acute maxillary sinusitis (see Chapter 8); (c) acute exacerbation of chronic bronchitis (see Chapter 8); and (d) mild CAP, especially in the young to middle-aged adult (see Chapter 11).

**2. MAC.** Clarithromycin has been useful in the prevention and treatment of MAC infections in patients with acquired immunodeficiency syndrome (AIDS). This topic is reviewed in detail elsewhere [1,3,10,28–30].

**3.** ***H. pylori*** has been effectively treated with clarithromycin and omeprazole [1,3,10,31].

**4.** ***S. pyogenes*** **or** ***S. aureus*** susceptible uncomplicated skin and skin structure infections **[26].** More conventional therapy such as erythromycin, dicloxacillin, or oral first-generation cephalosporins may be more cost effective. In the penicillin-allergic patient or the patient who has GI side effects from erythromycin, clarithromycin provides a useful alternative but azithromycin may be even better tolerated.

**B.** Approved uses in children **[32–35]**

**1. Pharyngitis, tonsillitis, acute maxillary sinusitis, or mild CAP** (due to mycoplasma, susceptible *S. pneumoniae,* or *C. pneumoniae*).

**2. Skin and soft tissue infections,** when the susceptibilities are known.

**3. Otitis media.** Clinical trials in the treatment of otitis media have shown similar efficacy for clarithromycin, amoxicillin, amoxicillin-clavulanate, and cefaclor.

**C. Rapidly growing atypical mycobacterial infections, Lyme disease, or toxoplasmosis.** Investigation is ongoing [1,3,36]. Clarithromycin is listed as an agent for Lyme disease [10].

**IV. Dosages.** Administer with or without meals.

**A. Adult dosages.** A dose of 250 to 500 mg twice daily is used depending on the severity of infection. The Biaxin XL film tablets are available in 500 mg, and two tablets are given once daily with food for 14 days for acute maxillary sinusitis and for 7 days for acute exacerbation of chronic bronchitis.

**B. Pediatric dosage.** For children 6 months of age or older, 15 mg/kg/day divided every 12 hours for 10 days is recommended. Suspensions are available with 125 mg/5 mL and 250 mg/5 mL.

**C. Renal failure.** When the creatinine clearance is 10 to 50 mL/min, 75% of the usual dose is suggested. If creatinine clearance is less than 10 mL, use 50% to 75% of the usual dose [16]. **After hemodialysis,** some sources suggest a dose, although data are limited. **In chronic ambulatory peritoneal dialysis,** no dose adjustments are necessary [16].

D. **Hepatic failure.** No dose adjustments. There is an increase in renal clearance [9].
E. **Pregnancy.** Clarithromycin is a category C drug (i.e., used only if there is no alternative) (see Chapter 16). Clarithromycin has demonstrated adverse effects on pregnancy and embryo fetal development in animals. High doses of clarithromycin have caused cardiovascular anomalies in rats, cleft palates in mice, and fetal growth retardation in monkeys [37]. There are no adequate and well-controlled studies in pregnant women. Clarithromycin should be used in pregnancy only if the potential benefit justifies the potential risk to the fetus. **If pregnancy occurs while on this drug, the patient should be apprised of the risks.**
F. **Nursing mothers.** The package insert notes that it is not known whether clarithromycin is excreted in human breast milk, and caution should be exercised when administering clarithromycin to a nursing mother because clarithromycin is excreted in the milk of lactating animals and other drugs of this class are excreted in human milk.

V. **Toxicity and side effects.** Clarithromycin is relatively nontoxic [3,38].
A. **GI.** Occasionally, clarithromycin in standard doses causes nausea, diarrhea, abdominal pain, and metallic taste [3] but fewer GI side effects than erythromycin [39].
B. **Hepatic, renal, or hematologic.** No significant toxicity appears to occur [38] with clarithromycin. Minor hepatic enzyme elevations can occur. In fewer than 1% of recipients, leukopenia and prothrombin time prolongation have been noted.
C. **Headache** may occur in up to 2% of recipients [38].
D. **High-dose regimens.** For therapy of MAC in AIDS patients or of atypical mycobacterial infections in the elderly, more adverse reactions, (nausea, vomiting, metallic taste, abnormal liver function blood tests, and central nervous system side effects) may occur [3].
E. **Drug interactions [1,3].** As with erythromycin, drug interactions with clarithromycin are extremely important **[3].**
1. **Hepatic P450 system** Because clarithromycin inhibits **the hepatic P450 system,** it may result in increased levels of multiple medications metabolized by the liver **[3].**
a. **Carbamazepine.** Concomitant administration of clarithromycin and carbamazepine causes a major change in carbamazepine levels.
b. **Caffeine, nicotine, and midazolam,** as well as other potential interactions, including those discussed in section **V.F** under erythromycin, above [3].
2. **Antiretrovirals.** Clarithromycin lowers zidovudine levels. Similar interactions occur with other antiretroviral agents [3] (see Chapter 19).
F. **Cost.** Oral clarithromycin is a relatively expensive agent (see Appendix Table 1).

## AZITHROMYCIN (ZITHROMAX)

Azithromycin was approved in 1991 and developed to overcome the shortcomings of erythromycin such as GI intolerance, low bioavailability, and somewhat limited spectrum of activity [1,3]. It is an azalide antibiotic. Its nuclear structure differs from that of erythromycin in that the lactone ring contains a nitrogen atom. This molecular rearrangement has resulted in a compound with remarkable and **unique properties** [40], including high and sustained tissue antibiotic levels, which are much greater than the serum antibiotic levels. It has a prolonged tissue half-life, decreasing the doses per course of therapy and duration of therapy [1,3]. It also has an expanded *in vitro* spectrum of activity. Azithromycin inhibits protein synthesis, in a similar manner to erythromycin.

I. **Spectrum of activity.** The broad-spectrum *in vitro* activity of azithromycin is summarized in Table 27N.1. If erythromycin is active against pathogens, azithromycin is also, but azithromycin is also more active against some organisms (e.g., *H. influenzae*).
A. **Gram-positive aerobes.** Azithromycin is active against erythromycin-susceptible *S. aureus* (approximately 80% of strains), *S. pyogenes,* many *S. pneumoniae, S. agalactiae,* and coagulase-negative staphylococci, but overall erythromycin and clarithromycin are more active against these gram-positive cocci. Enterococci usually are resistant [26]. Strains of these organisms resistant to erythromycin will be resistant to azithromycin, including many intermediate and most high level

penicillin-resistant *S. pneumoniae* (see Chapters 11 and 27C). MRSA strains are resistant to erythromycin and azithromycin. In addition, azithromycin is two- to eightfold **less active than erythromycin against staphylococci and streptococci** [37].

**B. Gram-negative aerobes.** Most gram-negative bacteria are intrinsically resistant to the macrolides because of the inability of the macrolide to penetrate the outer cell membrane effectively. Azithromycin appears to be able to penetrate the outer membrane better than erythromycin and therefore has activity against some gram-negative organisms normally resistant to erythromycin [41].

1. ***H. influenzae, M. catarrhalis* and *Neisseria* species** Azithromycin is severalfold more active against *H. influenzae* than is erythromycin or clarithromycin. It is also more active than erythromycin against *M. catarrhalis* and *Neisseria* species.
2. **Enterobacteriaceae.** Azithromycin is not active against *E. coli, Klebsiella* species.
3. **Nonfermenters such as *Pseudomonas* species, [42].** It is not active.
4. ***H. pylori.*** Azithromycin is active against *H. pylori,* although not listed as an alternative agent for these infections [10].
5. **Gastroenteritis pathogens.** It is active against *Shigella* species and *C. jejuni* [10] **but not *Salmonella.***

**C. Anaerobes.** Azithromycin inhibits some anaerobes similar to erythromycin but is not useful against bowel anaerobes [10].

**D.** Miscellaneous

1. ***Legionella* species [3].** Azithromycin is the most active macrolide against *Legionella* species. (The fluoroquinolones and azithromycin are viewed as the agents of choice for *Legionella* infections [10].) See Chapter 11.
2. **Most *B. burgdorferi* strains** are inhibited by 0.015 $\mu$g/mL, suggesting azithromycin is more active *in vitro* than erythromycin or clarithromycin [26].
3. ***Mycoplasma pneumoniae*** is very susceptible at 0.25 $\mu$g/mL [26], as are *C. pneumoniae* [43].
4. **Sexually transmitted pathogens.** *C. trachomatis, U. urealyticum, N. gonorrhoeae,* and *T. pallidum* are susceptible to azithromycin [3].
5. **Atypical mycobacterium** are overall more susceptible to clarithromycin than azithromycin or erythromycin [3].
6. ***Babesia microti* [44].** Azithromycin is active against this agent.
7. ***Chlamydia* pneumonia and coronary arteries.** This is undergoing intense investigation [45].

**E. Resistance.** Resistance to erythromycin implies cross-resistance with azithromycin **[26,42].** See related discussion under Erythromycin, section **VI.**

**II. Pharmacokinetics.** For adults, **both an oral and i.v. formulation are available** (see section **IV**). For children less than 16 years of age, only the oral formulation is approved as of mid-2002.

Compared with other available antimicrobial agents, azithromycin has unique pharmacokinetic properties. It yields high and sustained tissue levels in excess of serum levels. This involves active movement from the serum into the intracellular sites. Therefore for tissue infections azithromycin can provide excellent antibiotic levels.

**A. Absorption.** Azithromycin is more stable than erythromycin at various pH ranges seen in the stomach, and approximately 37% of a single capsule dose is absorbed, compared with 25% absorption of erythromycin [46]. Although adsorption of the capsular formation of azithromycin was decreased in the presence of food, the new tablet formation is equally absorbed in the fasting or fed state [3].

**B. Tissue kinetics [27,46].** The unique pharmacokinetic profile of azithromycin reflects a rapid and extensive uptake from the circulation into intracellular compartments followed by slow release [3].

1. **Serum levels** are lower than those of erythromycin or clarithromycin **[1,3].**
2. **Tissue levels.** Azithromycin penetrates tissues rapidly and extensively to yield very high steady-state tissue concentrations that exceed serum levels by 10- to 100-fold **[1,3]** (e.g., lung [100-fold], sputum [30-fold], cervix [70-fold], and skin [35-fold]) [3].

3. **Intracellular accumulation.** Azithromycin is rapidly and highly concentrated in a number of cell types, including polymorphonuclear leukocytes, monocytes, alveolar macrophages, and fibroblasts [46].
   a. **Polymorphonuclear leukocyte function** is not affected by antibiotic uptake [46]. By migrating to sites of infection, these polymorphonuclear leukocytes may play a role in the transport of azithromycin to the actual site of infection. **Azithromycin is released spontaneously and slowly from phagocytes (and fibroblasts).**
   b. **Tissue concentrations** do not peak until 48 hours after administration and persist for several days afterward [41].
4. **Half-life.** The average tissue half-life is between 2 and 4 days.
5. **Tissue persistence.** With recommended dosages daily for 5 days, therapeutic concentrations of azithromycin persist at the tissue level for 5 days or more after the completion of therapy.
6. **Aqueous humor or CSF.** Very little or none of the drug is detectable in aqueous humor or CSF, although azithromycin is widely distributed in brain tissue [3].

C. Metabolism and excretion **[1,3]**
1. **Eliminated unchanged.** Most of the absorbed dose of azithromycin is eliminated unchanged principally in the feces [3]. **Urinary excretion** of the unchanged drug is **minor.**
2. **Liver disease.** No dosage modification is necessary for patients with class A or B cirrhosis [3].

**III. Indications for use**

A. Approved uses in adults
1. **CAP** due to *S. pneumoniae, Mycoplasma, H. influenzae,* and *C. pneumonia.* Mild to moderate CAP is commonly treated with oral regimens of azithromycin in young to middle-aged adults. For hospitalized patients, the i.v. formulation, approved for *S. pneumonia, M. pneumoniae, M. catarrhalis, S. aureus,* and *L. pneumophilia,* is used initially (see related discussions in Chapter 11). **N.B. For very ill hospitalized patients, because azithromycin often is not active against high level penicillin-resistant *S. pneumoniae* and many intermediate level resistant strains, monotherapy with azithromycin is not advised** (see Chapter 11).
2. **Acute exacerbation of chronic bronchitis** has successfully been treated with azithromycin, which is active against common pathogens, including most *S. pneumoniae, M. catarrhalis,* and *H. influenzae* (see related discussions in Chapter 8).
3. **Pharyngitis/tonsillitis due to GAS.** Azithromycin is an alternative to first-line therapy (i.e., penicillin) for the allergic [1,3]. Erythromycin-resistant strains of GAS will be resistant to azithromycin. (Of note, the package insert suggests susceptibility tests with azithromycin for GAS should be performed in this setting.) This topic is discussed in detail in Chapter 8. When compliance is a major concern, one dose daily for 5 days may be useful. Other alternative regimens are less expensive (see Chapter 27A, Tables 27A.2 and 27A.3).

   Data establishing the **efficacy of azithromycin in the prevention of subsequent rheumatic fever** are not available [3]. Overall, we believe that azithromycin will have a very limited role in this setting [1].
4. **Methicillin-susceptible *S. aureus,* GAS, or group B streptococci** uncomplicated skin and soft tissue infections. Similar efficacy is achieved with 5 days of azithromycin or 10 days of cephalexin [26].
5. **Sexually transmitted disease [12] (see Chapter 16)**
   a. **Urethritis and cervicitis** due to *C. trachomatis* can be treated with azithromycin. For *N. gonorrhoeae,* other agents are preferred.
   b. ***H. ducreyi*** (chancroid) genital ulcer disease has been treated with azithromycin.
   c. **Pelvic inflammatory disease** due to *N. gonorrhoeae, C. trachomatis,* and *M. hominis* have been treated initially with the i.v. formulation. (i.v. azithromycin 500 mg for 1 or 2 days followed by 250 mg orally daily to complete a 7-day course). If anaerobic microorganisms are suspected, an antianaerobic

agent (e.g., metronidazole) is added [3]. However, experience with this regimen compared with other Centers for Disease Control and Prevention regimens for pelvic inflammatory disease is summarized in Chapter 16 [12].

6. **Pharyngitis and tonsillitis (see discussion in section B.3 below).**
7. **Currently unapproved uses (as of early 2002).** Conventional uses of azithromycin include the following; the clinical studies supporting the use of azithromycin in these settings are reviewed elsewhere [3].
   a. **Sinusitis,** especially acute maxillary [26].
   b. **For MAC.** Azithromycin (1,200 mg once per week) is effective in preventing the first episode of MAC in AIDS patients at risk (i.e., CD4 count <50 $\mu$L). Because azithromycin does not have major drug interactions, it is preferred over clarithromycin [3,30]. For therapy **of established disseminated MAC in AIDS patients,** studies suggest that combination regimens including clarithromycin convert blood cultures to negative more quickly and more often than azithromycin-containing regimens [3].
   c. **Infective endocarditis prophylaxis.** Either clarithromycin or azithromycin is an alternative in patients allergic to penicillin and who require antibiotic prophylaxis before oral, dental, esophageal, or respiratory procedures [3] (see Chapter 12).
8. For investigational uses, see section **C.**

**B. Approved uses in children.** The oral suspension for pediatric use was approved by the U.S. Food and Drug Administration in 1995; it is approved for children more than 6 months of age. The i.v. preparation of azithromycin is approved, per the package insert, for children more than 16 years of age.

1. **Acute otitis media** caused by *S. pneumoniae, H. influenzae,* or *M. catarrhalis* (see Chapter 8).
2. **Mild CAP** due to *S. pneumoniae, M. pneumoniae, C. pneumoniae,* and *H. influenzae.*

   N.B. Even the package insert emphasizes that **azithromycin should not be used in moderate to severe pneumonia** or **in children with risk factors such as cystic fibrosis, nosocomial pneumonia, known or suspected bacteremia, immunodeficiency, or illness sufficiently severe to require hospitalization.**
3. **Pharyngitis/tonsillitis** due to GAS infection as an alternative when first-line therapy cannot be used (see related discussion section **III.A.4**).

**C. Investigational uses** have recently been reviewed [3,36].

1. **Lyme disease (*B. burgdorferi*)** in which azithromycin is listed as an alternative agent [10], although its precise role remains to be established [3].
2. ***Shigella* infections.** Azithromycin has been shown to be very active *in vitro* against *Shigella* species and is a potential alternative agent [10].
3. ***H. pylori.*** The role of azithromycin for the treatment of this pathogen remains to be determined; it is not approved [3] or recommended [10] even though clarithromycin is useful for *H. pylori* eradication (see section **III.A.3** under Clarithromycin).
4. ***Bartonella* infections (e.g., bacillary angiomatosis, cat scratch):** azithromycin is listed as an alternate agent [10].
5. **Secondary prevention antibiotic treatment trials for coronary artery disease (CAD).** There is considerable interest in the potential causative role of *C. pneumoniae* in CAD and the prevention of this with antibiotics. Because azithromycin is active against this pathogen and penetrates tissue well, there are two large CAD treatment trials underway to see if azithromycin can help reduce cardiac events in chronic CAD. Results are not expected until late 2003 [43].
6. **Miscellaneous areas of clinical investigation [3]** include the use of azithromycin in malaria prophylaxis, toxoplasmosis therapy, *Babesia microti* infection, and trachoma therapy.
7. **Babesiosis.** A recent report indicates a regimen of atovaquone and azithromycin is as effective as a regimen of clindamycin and quinine and is associated with fewer adverse reactions [44].

Table 27N.2. Dosages of Azithromycin

| | Setting | Dose/Route | Duration |
|---|---|---|---|
| **Adults** | CAP (community-acquired pneumonia) | i.v. 500 mg 1–3 days[a] then p.o. 250 mg qd | Usually 5 days total |
| | *Legionellosis* | i.v. 500 mg 1–7 days[b] | Usually 7 days |
| | Acute bronchitis | Z pack | 5 days total |
| | Pharyngitis | Z pack | 5 days total |
| | Uncomplicated skin infections | Z pack | 5 days total |
| | STDs | | |
| | Urethritis | 1 g p.o. | Once only. See text and Chapter 10. |
| | Cervicitis | 1 g p.o. | Once only. See text and Chapter 10. |
| | Chancroid | 1 g p.o. | Once only. See Chapter 10. |
| | PID | See text | |
| | Sinusitis | Z pack | |
| | MAC | | |
| | Prevention | 1,200 mg once weekly | While CD4 counts depressed (<50 cells/UL) |
| | Therapy | Infectious disease consult suggested | |
| | SBE prophylaxis | See Chapter 15 | |
| **Children** (over 6 mo) | Acute otitis media (AOM) | 10 mg/kg day 1 followed by 5 mg/kg on days 2–5 | 5 days |
| | Mild CAP | Same as AOM | 5 days |
| | Pharyngitis | 12 mg/kg day 1–5 (not to exceed 500 mg daily)[c] | 5 days |

[a]For mild, early CAP, a standard Z pack is often used. See text.
[b]Precise guidelines not available. For moderate to severe cases, i.v. and/or oral therapy for 7 days presumably provides 21 days of tissue levels and therefore a 7-day course seems prudent. For patients doing very well, i.v. may be converted to oral, 250–500 mg qd, to complete 7-day course.
[c]Failures at 10 mg/kg daily for 5 days have been reported. Therefore a higher dose is suggested. Penicillin is the preferred agent. See Chapter 8.
STDs, sexually transmitted diseases; MAC, *Mycobacterium arium* complex; SBE, subacute bacterial endocarditis.

**IV.** Dosages

**A.** See Table 27N.2

1. **Azithromycin** is available as a 250-mg tablet (or capsule) commonly distributed in a "Z pack" containing six tablets for a standard 5-day regimen in adults (two tablets [500 mg] day 1 and then one 250-mg tablet daily on days 2–5). Tablets can be taken with or without food. Capsules should not be taken with food.
2. **The flavored oral suspension** comes in 100 mg/5 mL and 200 mg/5 mL. The suspension should be given 1 hour before or 1 hour after meals.
3. **For MAC prophylaxis,** 600-mg tablets are available.
4. **Nongonococcal urethritis.** A 1-g oral suspension single dose packet is also available and should be taken in the fasting state.

5. **Intravenous azithromycin.** A dose of 500 mg i.v. once daily is infused over at least 60 minutes in patients 16 years of age and older [47].

B. **Pregnancy.** Azithromycin is a category B agent (i.e., used only if clearly needed) (see Chapter 27A). It does not produce abnormalities in pregnant animals.

C. **Nursing mothers.** The package insert indicates that it is not known whether azithromycin is excreted in human breast milk and that caution should be exercised when azithromycin is administered to a nursing woman. However, it should be presumed that azithromycin is in human breast milk because it is present in the milk of lactating animals and because other macrolides are excreted into human breast milk [26].

D. **Renal failure.** No dosage adjustments are necessary in renal failure, including situations in which patients are on hemodialysis or chronic ambulatory peritoneal dialysis [16].

E. **Erythromycin allergy.** In the rare patient who has a history of a severe allergic reaction to erythromycin, until further data are available azithromycin should be avoided.

F. **Drug interactions** have been reviewed in detail elsewhere [48]. Human clinical and pharmacokinetic studies have shown no major drug-drug interactions between azithromycin and numerous other agents, including carbamazepine, theophylline, midazolam, terfenadine, zidovudine, or cimetidine [3]. This is a distinct advantage of azithromycin over erythromycin and clarithromycin. **Coadministration of antacids does not affect absorption of azithromycin [3].**

G. **Limitation.** Because azithromycin typically produces low serum levels, we believe this precludes its use as a potential alternative agent in the allergic prone patient with endocarditis, although little data exist on this topic.

V. **Toxicity and side effects.** Initial studies in about 4,000 adults and 2,000 children indicate this is a very well-tolerated agent [27,49], and continued extensive clinical experience supports this.

A. **GI complaints** are far less common than erythromycin and less so than clarithromycin. Diarrhea, nausea, and mild abdominal discomfort can occur, more so with higher doses.

B. **Central nervous system.** Mild headache and dizziness can occur.

C. **Ototoxicity, severe liver toxicity, or nephrotoxicity** do not seem to occur with conventional dosing [49]. In high-dose regimens (e.g., for therapy of atypical mycobacterium), reversible dose-related hearing loss has been described [1].

D. **Rash** appears to be uncommon.

VI. **Cost** (see Appendix Table 1)

A. **Although a typical Z pack** (actual wholesale price) is about $37, this is often competitive and at times less expensive than other conventional regimens. Also, the convenience of once daily doses for only 5 days enhances compliance and satisfaction.

B. **Intravenous azithromycin,** 500 mg daily, costs about $24 per day. This is about as much as i.v. generic erythromycin drug acquisition costs per day (i.e., for four 500-mg doses), but it is more cost-effective to give i.v. azithromycin daily versus the every 6 hour regimen for erythromycin.

VII. **An overview of the macrolides**

A. **For i.v. use.** Because there is no i.v. clarithromycin and because i.v. azithromycin is more cost effective and lacks the drug interactions seen with erythromycin, **we favor i.v. azithromycin** when i.v. therapy is used in patients older than age 16.

B. **Oral macrolide therapy**

1. Generic oral erythromycin is still the most cost-effective regimen **and 250 mg four times a day for 10 days (average wholesale price) is about $7.25 versus the $37 (average wholesale price) of the azithromycin Z pack.** However, the GI side effects of erythromycin, four times a day dosing schedule often for 10 to 14 days, and drug interactions must be balanced with the ease and fewer side effects of azithromycin.
2. **Azithromycin is preferred** to maximize compliance and/or minimize GI side effects and/or minimize drug interactions. **Azithromycin can be used in pregnant women.**

3. **Clarithromycin** can be given twice daily but still requires conventional durations of therapy and has the potential of multiple drug interactions. It must be avoided in pregnancy, if possible. It is the macrolide of choice for *H. pylori* eradication regimens and for combination therapy of MAC bacteremia in AIDS patients **(see prior discussions).**

## REFERENCES


1. Reese RE, Betts RF. Erythromycin, azithromycin, and clarithromycin. In: Reese RE, Betts RF, Gumustop B, eds. *Handbook of antibiotics,* 3rd ed. Philadelphia: Lippincott, Williams & Wilkins, 2000;468–492.
2. Zuckermann JM. The newer macrolides: azithromycin and clarithromycin. *Infect Dis Clin North Am* 2000;14:449.
3. Alvarez-Elcoro S, Enzler MJ. The macrolides: erythromycin, clarithromycin, and azithromycin. *Mayo Clin Proc* 1999;74:613.
4. Gold HS, Moellering RC Jr. Macrolides and clindamycin. In: Root RK, et al., eds. *Clinical infectious diseases: a practical approach.* New York: Oxford University Press, 1999;291–297.
5. Bisno AL, et al. Diagnosis and management of group A streptococcal pharyngitis: a practice guideline. *Clin Infect Dis* 1997;25:574.
6. Kaplan EL, et al. Susceptibility of group A beta-hemolytic streptococci to thirteen antibiotics: examination of 301 strains isolated in the United States between 1994 and 1997. *Pediatr Infect Dis J* 1999;18:1069.
7. Huovine P. Macrolide-resistant group A streptococcus: now in the United States. *N Engl J Med* 2002;346:1243.
8. Amsden GW. Pneumococcal macrolide resistance: myth or reality. *J Antimicrob Chemother* 1999;44:1.
9. Steigbigel NH. Macrolides and clindamycin. In: Mandell GL, Bennett JE, Dolin R, eds. *Principles and practice of infectious diseases,* 5th ed. New York: Churchill Livingstone, 2000:366–382.
10. Medical Letter. The choice of antibacterial drugs. *Med Lett Drugs Ther* 2000;43:69.
11. Kanatani MS, Guglicimo BJ. The new macrolides: azithromycin and clarithromycin. *West J Med* 1994;160:31.
12. Sexually transmitted diseases treatment guidelines: 2002. *MMWR Morb Mortal Wkly Rep* 2002;51(RR-6):1–77.
13. Tappero JW, et al. The epidemiology of bacillary angiomatosis and bacillary peliosis. *JAMA* 1993;269:770.
14. Dajani A, et al. Treatment of acute streptococcal pharyngitis and prevention of rheumatic fever: a statement for health professionals. *Pediatrics* 1995;96:758.
15. Hoppe JE. the Erythromycin Study Group. Comparison of erythromycin estolate and erythromycin ethylsuccinate for treatment of pertussis. *Pediatr Infect Dis J* 1992;11: 189.
16. Aronoff GR, et al. *Drug prescribing in renal failure: dosing guidelines for adults,* 4th ed. Philadelphia: American College of Physicians, 1999.
17. Janssens J, et al. Improvement of gastric emptying in diabetic gastroparesis by erythromycin. *N Engl J Med* 1990;322:1028.
18. Chapman MJ, et al. Erythromycin improves gastric emptying in critically ill patients intolerant of nasogastric feeding. *Crit Care Med* 2000;28:2334.
19. Mahon BE, Rosenman MB, Kleinman MB. Maternal and infant use of erythromycin and other macrolide antibiotics as a risk factor for infantile hypertrophic pyloric stenosis. *J Pediatr* 2001;139:380–384.
20. Boguniewicz M, Leung DYM. Hypersensitivity reactions to antibiotics commonly used in children. *Pediatr Infect Dis J* 1995;14:221.
21. Chong P, et al. Clinically relevant differences between the statins: implications for therapeutic selection. *Am J Med* 2001;111:390.
22. Nattel S, et al. Erythromycin-induced long QT syndrome: concordance with quinidine and underlying cellular electrophysiologic mechanism. *Am J Med* 1990;89:235.

23. Farrar HC, et al. Cardiac toxicity associated with intravenous erythromycin lactobionate: two case reports and a review of the literature. *Pediatr Infect Dis J* 1993;12:688.
24. LeClerg R. Mechanisms of resistance to macrolides and lincosamides: nature of the resistance elements and there clinical implications. *Clin Infect Dis* 2002;34:482.
25. Neu HC. The development of macrolides: clarithromycin in perspective. *J Antimicrob Chemother* 1991;27[Suppl A]:1.
26. Eisenberg E, Barza M. Azithromycin and clarithromycin. *Curr Clin Top Infect Dis* 1994;14:52.
27. Piscitelli SC, Danziger LH, Rodvold KA. Clarithromycin and azithromycin: new macrolide antibiotics. *Clin Pharmacol Ther* 1992;11:137.
28. Chaisson RE, et al. Clarithromycin therapy for bacteremic *Mycobacterium avium* complex disease: a randomized, double-blind, dose-ranging study in patients with AIDS. *Ann Intern Med* 1994;121:905.
29. Benson CA, Elner JJ. *Mycobacterium avium complex* infection and AIDS. Advances in theory and practice. *Clin Infect Dis* 1993;17:7.
30. Guidelines for the prevention of opportunistic infections among HIV-infected—2002. *MMWR Morb Mortal Wkly Rep* 2002;51(RR-8):1.
31. Howden CW, Hunt RH. Guidelines for the management of *Helicobacter pylori* infection. *Am J Gastroenterol* 1998;93:2330.
32. Nelson JD, McCracken GH Jr, eds. Clinical perspectives on clarithromycin in pediatric infections. *Pediatr J Infect Dis* 1993;12[Suppl 3]:S98.
33. Aspin M, et al. Comparative study of the safety and efficacy of clarithromycin and amoxicillin-clavulanate in the treatment of acute otitis media in children. *J Pediatr* 1994;125:136.
34. Reed MD, Blumer JL. Azithromycin: a critical review of the first azalide antibiotic and its role in pediatric practice. *Pediatr Infect Dis J* 1997;16:1069.
35. Langtry HD, Balfour JA. Azithromycin: a review of its use in pediatric infectious diseases. *Drugs* 1998;56:273.
36. Tarlow MJ, et al. Future indications for macrolides. *Pediatr Infect Dis J* 1997;16:457.
37. Medical Letter. Clarithromycin and azithromycin. *Med Lett Drugs Ther* 1992;34:45.
38. Wood MJ. The tolerance and toxicity of clarithromycin. *J Hosp Infect* 1991;19[Suppl A]:39.
39. Anderson G, et al. A comparative safety and efficacy study of clarithromycin and erythromycin stearate in community-acquired pneumonia. *J Antimicrob Chemother* 1991;27[Suppl A]:117.
40. Moellering RC, Jr. Introduction: revolutionary changes in the macrolide and azalide antibiotics. *Am J Med* 1991;91[Suppl 3A]:1S.
41. Zuckerman JM, Kaye KM. The newer macrolides: azithromycin and clarithromycin. *Infect Dis Clin North Am* 1995;9:731. (See related review by Schlossberg D. Azithromycin and clarithromycin. *Med Clin North Am* 1995;79:803.)
42. Neu HC. Clinical microbiology of azithromycin. *Am J Med* 1991;91[Suppl 3A]:12S.
43. Grayston T. Secondary prevention antibiotic treatment trials for coronary artery disease. *Circulation* 2000;102:1742.
44. Krause PJ, et al. Atovaquone and azithromycin for treatment of babesiosis. *N Engl J Med* 2000;343:1454.
45. Parchure N, et al. Effect of azithromycin treatment on endothelial function in patients with coronary artery disease and evidence of *Chlamydia pneumoniae* infection. *Circulation* 2002;105:1298.
46. Schentag JJ, Ballow CH. Tissue directed pharmacokinetics. *Am J Med* 1991;91[Suppl 3A]:5S.
47. Garey KW, Amsden GW. Intravenous azithromycin. *Ann Pharmacother* 1999;33:218.
48. Amsden GW. Macrolides versus azalides: a drug interaction update. *Ann Pharmacother* 1995;29:906.
49. Hopkins S. Clinical toleration and safety of azithromycin. *Am J Med* 1991;91[Suppl 3A]:40S.

## O. Tetracyclines

Discovered more than 50 years ago, the tetracyclines remain one of the most widely prescribed antibiotic classes in the United States, especially by office-based physicians [1,2]. **Bacteriostatic** tetracyclines act by interfering with protein synthesis at the ribosomal level. The superior pharmacokinetic properties, enhanced compliance, lesser toxicity, and reasonable cost of doxycycline make it the tetracycline of choice (see section **II**).

**I. Spectrum of activity**

**A. Tetracyclines, especially doxycycline,** are active against a wide variety of pathogens [1–14] (Table 27O.1).

**1.** Community-acquired respiratory tract pathogens, including *Haemophilus influenzae, Moraxella catarrhalis*, and *Mycoplasma, Legionella,* and *Chlamydia*

Table 27O.1. Broad-spectrum Activity of Tetracyclines [13,14]

**Bacteria**
- *S. pneumoniae*[a] (penicillin-susceptible) (see text)
- *H. influenzae*[a] (ampicillin-susceptible and resistant)
- *M. catarrhalis*[a] (ampicillin-susceptible and resistant)
- *Brucella* species[b] (with rifampin)
- *Calymmatobacterium* granulomatis[a] (granuloma inguinale)
- *Vibrio cholera*[b] (cholera)
- *Vibrio vulnificus*[b]
- *Helicobacter pylori*[b]
- *Pasteurella multocida*[a]
- *Bartonella henselae*[a] (bacillary angiomatosis)
- *Yersinia pestis-plague* [14] (with streptomycin)
- *Francisella tularensis*[a]

**Ehrlichia**[b]
- *Ehrlichia chaffeenis*
- Agent of human granulocytic ehrlichiosis

**Chlamydiae**
- *C. psittaci* (psittacosis)[b]
- *C. trachomatis* (trachoma)[a] (urethritis, cervicitis)[b] (lymphogranuloma venereum)[b]
- *C. pneumoniae* (TWAR)[b]

**Spirochetes**
- *Borrelia burgdorferi*[b] (Lyme disease)[c]
- *Borrelia recurrentis*[b] (relapsing fever)
- *Treponema pallidum*[a] (syphilis)
- *Treponema pertenue*[a] (yaws)
- *Leptospire* species[a]

**Rickettsia**[b]
- Rocky Mountain spotted fever
- Endemic typhus (murine)
- Epidemic typhus (louse-borne)
- Scrub typhus
- Trench fever
- Q fever

**Mycoplasmas**
- *M. pneumoniae*[b]
- *Ureaplasma urealyticum*[a]

**Mycobacterium**
- *M. marinum* (minocycline)[b]
- *M. fortuitum* complex[a]

**Miscellaneous**
- *Nocardia*[c]
- *Actinomyces israeli*[a]
- Malaria[a]

[a] Alternative agent for (3).
[b] Drug of choice for (3).
[c] Including prevention regimens [13]. Also see Chapter 17.
[d] See reference 8.

Table 27O.2. Commonly Used Oral Tetracyclines in Adults

| Name | Usual Capsule Dose (mg) | Usual Interval Between Doses (h) | Usual Total Daily Dose (mg) (See Text) | Approximate Cost (Dollars) for 10 Days[a] |
|---|---|---|---|---|
| **Short acting** | | | | |
| Tetracycline hydrochloride[b] | 250–500 | 6 (without food)[c] | 1,000–2,000 | 2.50–5.00 |
| **Long acting** | | | | |
| Doxycycline hyclate[d] | 100 | 12–24 (with or without food) | 200 | $14.00 (generic form 100 mg bid) |
| Minocycline[e] | 100 | 12 (with or without food) | 200 | — |

[a] Approximate actual wholesale price in 2000.
[b] Trade names include Achromycin, Panmycin, Sumycin, Tetracyn.
[c] No food in preceding 2 h.
[d] Trade names include Vibramycin, Doroyx, Doxycin.
[e] Trade name is Minocin.

species [4] and penicillin-susceptible *Streptococcus pneumoniae* (see section **3** below).

2. Although any of the available agents (Table 27O.2) can often be used, against some organisms doxycycline and minocycline are the more potent [2].
   a. **Doxycycline** is more active against the following:
      (1) *S. pneumoniae* [4,5], including most intermediate penicillin-resistant strains. Strains resistant to tetracycline are often susceptible to doxycycline [5].
      (2) *M. fortuitum* and *M. chelonei* [2].
   b. **Minocycline** is more active against
      (1) *S. aureus,* including many strains of methicillin-resistant *S. aureus* and coagulase-negative staphylococci [2].
      (2) *M. marinum* [2].

B. Tetracyclines are not reliably active against *Neisseria gonorrhoeae* or *Bacteroides fragilis*. They are active against parasites such as *E. histolytica* and *Plasmodium falciparum* [6].

II. **Pharmacokinetics.** Oral tetracyclines are used for most infections except for treatment of pelvic inflammatory disease (PID) (see Chapter 16), where the intravenous route is often used.

A. **Gastrointestinal (GI) absorption.** These agents are incompletely absorbed from the GI tract. Absorption is impaired by milk, aluminum hydroxide, calcium, magnesium (e.g., in antacids), or iron preparations. The tetracyclines combine with the metallic ion calcium or magnesium, forming inactive chelates. Absorption is improved, even with the better adsorbed doxycycline, if the antibiotic is taken 1 hour before or 2 hours after meals [2].

B. **Blood levels.** Following the above, therapeutic blood levels are achieved. The twice daily dosing of doxycycline improves compliance (Table 27O.2).

1. **Short-acting agents. Tetracycline** is preferred over oxytetracycline and is cost effective.
2. **Long-acting agents** can be given once or twice daily.
   a. **Doxycycline** half-life (15–18 hours), permits dosing every 12 to 24 hours, improving compliance.
   b. **Minocycline** has a similar half-life.
   c. Both are dosed at 200 mg and then 100 mg once or twice daily.

C. **Distribution.** The tetracyclines diffuse reasonably well into sputum, urine, and peritoneal and pleural fluids. Levels in synovial fluid and sinuses approach serum concentrations. Because of its lipophilic properties, doxycycline yields higher concentrations in the brain and cerebrospinal fluid than other tetracyclines. This supports its use for oral therapy for Lyme disease [7].

D. **Excretion.** Tetracyclines are excreted via **the urine** except for doxycycline, which is excreted (90%) in the feces. **Hepatic failure** does not lead to elevated serum levels of the tetracyclines. However, these drugs have been noted to cause hepatotoxicity.

E. **Drug interactions** [2]

1. **Anticonvulsants** (e.g., carbamazepine, barbiturates, phenytoin) induce hepatic microsomal metabolism of tetracyclines, decreasing tetracycline serum concentrations.
2. **Cholestyramine and colestipol** can reduce GI absorption of tetracycline.
3. **Warfarin anticoagulation** may be potentiated by tetracyclines. Prothrombin time should be monitored.
4. **Oral contraceptive** efficacy may be decreased with concurrent use of tetracyclines.

III. **Indications for use.** Because of their broad-spectrum nature (Table 27O.1), these agents are useful in several settings [1,2,7,8] (Table 27O.3).

IV. **Contraindications to use** [1,2]

A. **Pregnancy and lactation.** Tetracyclines (including doxycycline) are **category D** agents (see Chapter 27A). Tetracycline may cause hepatotoxicity in pregnant women. Furthermore, it is transferred across the placenta and has caused **dental deformities and dental discoloration in children** whose mothers received tetracycline while pregnant. Tetracycline is excreted in breast milk. Therefore, the **tetracyclines should be avoided by pregnant or lactating women.**

B. **Children less than 8 years old.** Except in patients with Rocky Mountain spotted fever or ehrlichiosis, tetracycline should be given only when there is no alternative [1].

V. **Dosages.** The doxycycline twice daily dosing improves compliance. Doxycycline is usually preferred [1,2] unless minocycline is needed for its unique susceptibility profile (see section **I.A**).

A. **Route.** Generic tetracycline or doxycycline usually is given **orally** as capsules or tablets, but liquid forms are available. Oral preparations should be taken **while fasting.**

B. **Dosage regimens**

1. **Oral.** The common oral preparations available are shown in Table 27O.2.

a. **Tetracycline**

(1) **In adults,** 250 to 500 mg as the hydrochloride every 6 hours, or four times a day, can be used.

(2) **In children more than 8 years of age,** 20 to 40 mg/kg/day is divided into every 6 hour doses.

b. **Doxycycline**

(1) **In adults,** start with 200 mg initially or 100 mg every 12 hours and then 100 mg every 12 to 24 hours, depending on the severity of the infection. **Oral drug has the same bioavailability as does intravenous [8].**

(2) **In children older than 8 years of age** who weigh less than 45 kg, 4.4 mg/kg is given on the first day, divided into two doses given at 12-hour intervals, followed by 2.2 mg/kg/day as a single dose or divided into every 12 hour doses. Adult regimens can be used for children weighing more than 45 kg.

c. **Minocycline** is used **as an alternative therapy** for *Nocardia* or methicillin-resistant *S. aureus.* Infectious disease consultation is advised. If renal function is normal, 100 mg twice daily has been used in adults.

d. **In renal failure,** doxycycline is preferred. Neither **peritoneal dialysis** nor **hemodialysis** alters the half-life of doxycycline. Dosage changes are not needed in renal failure or post-dialysis [9].

2. **Parenteral** (**tetracycline hydrochloride** is no longer commercially available).

a. **Doxycycline** is used intravenously in selected patients in PID regimens, in Lyme disease, and occasionally in other settings. Because of pain associated

Table 27O.3. Major Clinical Conditions for Which Tetracyclines May be Used[a]

| |
|---|
| Respiratory infections |
| Community-acquired pneumonia in an outpatient setting |
| **Atypical pneumonia** (*Mycoplasma pneumoniae, Chlamydia pneumoniae,* psittacosis) |
| Acute exacerbation of chronic bronchitis |
| Legionellosis[b] |
| Genital infections |
| *Chlamydia trachomatis* **(nongonococcal urethritis, pelvic inflammatory disease,** epididymitis, prostatitis, **lymphogranuloma venereum)** |
| Granuloma inguinale[b] |
| Syphilis[b] |
| Systemic infections |
| **Rickettsiae (Rocky Mountain spotted fever, endemic and epidemic typhus, Q fever)** |
| **Brucellosis** in combination with rifampin (or streptomycin) |
| **Lyme borreliosis** |
| **Ehrlichiosis** |
| **Relapsing fever (*Borrelia recurrentis*)** |
| ***Vibrio* (cholera, *V. vulnificus,*** and ***V. parahaemolyticus*)** |
| Tularemia[b] |
| Bacillary angiomatosis (bartonellosis)[b] |
| Leptospirosis[b] |
| Other (local and systemic) infections |
| Methicillin-resistant *Staphylococcus aureus* and *S. epidermidis*[b] (minocycline) when vancomycin or other agents are not considered appropriate |
| *Pasteurella multocida*[b] |
| *Mycobacterium marinum*[b] |
| ***Helicobacter pylori*** (in combination with bismuth subsalicylate and metronidazole or clarithromycin) |
| *Yersinia pestis* (combined with streptomycin) |
| Other conditions |
| Acne vulgaris |
| Malaria [8] |
| Prophylaxis of mefloquine resistant *Plasmodium falciparum* malaria [8] |
| Therapy of certain forms of malaria |

[a] Tetracyclines are a drug of choice for the infections that are in **boldface.**
[b] Infections for which a tetracycline is an acceptable alternative to standard agents.
Modified from Smilack JD. The tetracyclines. *Mayo Clin Proc* 1999;74:727, with permission.

with intravenous infusion, doxycycline should be administered orally when possible even when the patient is hospitalized. For adults and for children older than 8 years weighing more than 45 kg, 200 mg day 1 is given in one or two divided infusions, followed by 200 mg every 24 hours or 100 mg every 12 hours. In children older than 8 years who weigh less than 45 kg, 4.4 mg/kg is given on day 1 in two divided doses at 12-hour intervals and then 2.2 mg/kg/day once daily subsequently. **In PID regimens,** oral doxycycline 100 mg twice daily is often used to complete a 14-day course [10]. However, its continued use is under question because of lower efficacy [11] (see Chapter 16). Nonetheless, data from a recent study indicate no difference in reproductive outcome between women randomized to inpatient or outpatient treatment [11].

**VI. Toxicity and side effects** [1,2]

**A. Teeth and bone.** Tetracycline can cause depression of bone growth, permanent gray-brown discoloration of the teeth, and enamel hypoplasia when given during tooth development. However, more than a single course seems to be required to produce this effect.

**B. Hypersensitivity** reactions such as anaphylaxis, urticaria, and rashes are uncommon. **Toxic photosensitivity reactions** consisting of a red rash on areas exposed to intense sunlight can occur with all tetracyclines. Patients receiving doxycycline, especially high doses, should avoid intense sun exposure or use sunscreens with a protection factor of 18 or above.

**C. GI effects** are usually minor. Epigastric distress and nausea can occur after oral administration, and these symptoms are somewhat dose related. Esophageal ulcerations can occur with doxycycline. To minimize this, give oral doses with adequate amounts of fluid.

**D. Accentuated prerenal azotemia.** Tetracyclines appear to aggravate preexisting renal failure by inhibiting protein synthesis.

**E. Benign intracranial hypertension.** This rare entity is seen in women on tetracycline.

**F. Hepatitis** occurs after high intravenous doses or in pregnant women as acute fatty necrosis.

**G. Skin pigmentation changes and blue-black oral pigmentation** changes can occur with prolonged minocycline use.

**H. Thrombophlebitis** can occur with intravenous use.

**I. Vestibular** side effects, including dizziness, ataxia, and vertigo, can occur with minocycline.

**J. Superinfections with** candida of the oral and anogenital region occurs.

## REFERENCES

1. Klein NC, Cunha BA. New uses of older antibiotics. *Med Clin North Am* 2001;85:125.
2. Smilack JD. The tetracyclines. *Mayo Clin Proc* 1999;74:727.
3. Medical Letter. The choice of antibacterial drugs. *Med Lett Drugs Ther* 2001;43:69.
4. Bartlett JG, et al. Community-acquired pneumonia in adults: guidelines for management. *Clin Infect Dis* 1998;26:811.
5. Shea K, et al. Doxycycline activity against *Streptococcus pneumoniae. Chest* 1995; 106:1775.
6. Taylor WR, Widaja H, Richie TL, et al. Chloroquine/doxycycline combination versus chloroquine alone and doxycycline alone for treatment of *Plasmodium falciparum* and *Plasmodium vivax* malaria in northeastern Irian Jaya, Indonesia. *Am J Trop Med Hyg* 2001;54:223–228.
7. Dotevall L, Hagberg L. Penetration of doxycycline into cerebrospinal fluid in patients treated for suspected Lyme neuroborreliosis. *Antimicrob Agents Chemother* 1989;33:1078.
8. Medical Letter. Drugs for parasitic infection. *Med Lett Drugs Ther* 2002;44:1.
9. Aronoff GR, et al. *Drug prescribing in renal failure: dosing guidelines for adults,* 4th ed. Philadelphia: American College of Physicians, 1999.
10. Center for Disease Control and Prevention. Sexually transmitted diseases treatment guidelines. *MMWR Morb Mortal Wkly Rep* 2002;51(RR-6):1–77.
11. Ross JD. Outpatient antibiotics for pelvic inflammatory disease: continued use of oral doxycycline and metronidazole is hard to justify. *BMJ* 2001;322:251–252.
12. Ness RB, et al. Effectiveness of in-patient and out-patient treatment strategies for women with pelvic inflammatory disease: results from the Pelvic Inflammatory Disease Evaluation and Clinical Health (PEACH) randomized trial. *Am J Obstet Gynecol* 2002;186:929.
13. Nadelman RB, et al. Prophylaxis with a single dose of doxycycline for the prevention of Lyme disease after an *Ixodes scapularis* tick bite. *N Engl J Med* 2001;345:79 (also see editorial).
14. Inglesby TV, et al. Plague as a biological weapon: medical and public health management. Working group on civilian biodefense. *JAMA* 2000;283:2281.

## P. Vancomycin, Quinupristin/Dalfopristin, and Linezolid

With the emergence of methicillin-resistant *Staphylococcus aureus* (MRSA) (see Chapters 4 and 12) and penicillin-resistant *S. pneumoniae* (see Chapter 11), vancomycin has become an extremely important agent [1–3]. Because of clinicians concern about the above organisms, vancomycin is used very frequently when the need may not really exist. This excessive use has contributed to the emergence of vancomycin-resistant *Enterococcus faecium*(VREF), vancomycin, (glycopeptide) intermediate *S. aureus* (**GISA**) and now even vancomycin completely resistant *S. aureus* (see section **II**). **Prudent use of vancomycin is essential to preserve the effectiveness of this important antibiotic.**

**I. Spectrum of activity.** Vancomycin is active **only** against **gram-positive bacteria,** particularly aerobes. There is no cross-resistance between vancomycin and penicillin [1].

**A. Gram-positive bacteria.** Except for enterococci and MRSA, vancomycin is bactericidal.

1. **Staphylococci.** Vancomycin is active against MRSA, coagulase-negative staphylococci (SSCN), and methicillin-susceptible *S. aureus* (MSSA), but not as active as nafcillin against the latter.
2. **Enterococci.** Vancomycin is **bacteriostatic against** Enterococcus faecalis, but in combination**with gentamicin it is bactericidal,** except for those that are high level gentamicin-resistant (see Chapter 27I). A common clinical dilemma is when to treat enterococcus. It is a pathogen with very low virulence. It occurs as part of mixed aerobicanaerobic flora in intraabdominal (see Chapter 13) and in pelvic (see Chapter 16) and surgical wound infections or in superficial cultures in diabetic foot infections (see Chapter 5). In these situations, **enterococci usually do not require specific treatment** (see Chapter 13).

   By contrast there are situations where enterococci need to be treated. *E. faecalis* occasionally is involved in osteomyelitis (see Chapter 5). It also causes urinary tract infection in older men. Bacteremias or endocarditis due to *E. faecalis* may follow gynecologic or genitourinary or gastrointestinal (GI) procedures or occur as a complication of a focal infection at these sites, but this is relatively uncommon [8] (see Chapter 12). *E. faecalis* , susceptible to vancomycin but not to ampicillin, infrequently causes nosocomial bacteremia.
3. **Streptococci.** Vancomycin is bactericidal against *Streptococcus pyogenes,* group C and G streptococci, viridans streptococci, and *S. pneumoniae,* including multidrug and high level penicillin-resistant strains [2] (see Chapter 11).
4. **Miscellaneous:** Vancomycin is active against *Corynebacterium JK* and *Clostridium difficile.*

**B. Gram-negative bacteria.** Vancomycin has no clinically useful activity [1].

**C. Anaerobes.** Although vancomycin has some activity against *Clostridium* species and anaerobic streptococci, it is not used as an agent for anaerobic infections [1].

**II. Vancomycin resistance.**

**A. Enterococcus. VREF** has emerged and is increasing in frequency in the intensive care unit (ICU), in the bone marrow transplant unit, and in hospital locations where patients with leukemia are treated. *E. faecium* is discussed further later in this chapter under quinupristin-dalfopristin (Q-D) and linezolid. It is resistant by virtue of containing one of the resistance determinants vanA, vanB, vanD, vanE, vanF, or vanG.

**B. *S. aureus***

1. **In 1997, *S. aureus* with intermediate levels of resistance to vancomycin—also referred to as GISA** because vancomycin is a glycopeptide antibiotic, with a minimum inhibitory concentration (MIC) of 6 μg/mL or more—was first isolated [4]. GISA are intermediately susceptible because the organism secretes an extracellular product, d-alanine-d-alanine, that binds vancomycin, not permitting it to reach the vancomycin-binding site. These organisms do not contain the resistance binding moieties found in VREF.

2. However, in a report published in early July 2002, a *S. aureus* that **had an MIC of 32 μg/mL** was isolated from a patient who had received vancomycin and other antibiotics. After treatment of an infection with a vancomycin-containing regimen, the *S. aureus* was repeatedly isolated, with **an MIC of more than 128 μg/mL** [5]. Unlike previous GISA, this *Staphylococcus* **contained the vanA resistance determinant.** Widespread use of vancomycin presumably contributes to the emergence of these resistant staphylococci.
3. **Patients** with documented GISA, and especially those strains with the vanA resistant determinant, **need to be isolated** to prevent nosocomial spread, and isolates should be reported through state and local health departments to the Centers for Disease Control and Prevention [6,7]. **Infectious disease consultation is advised for patients colonized or infected with GISA or with true vancomycin-resistant *S. aureus*.**

**III. Pharmacokinetics** [1,2]. Vancomycin demonstrates **time-dependent bactericidal activity** rather than concentration-dependent bactericidal activity [2] (see Chapter 25).

**A. Intravenous (i.v.) preparation.** Intramuscular vancomycin causes severe pain and is not advised.

1. **Therapeutic levels** are achieved in synovial, ascitic, pericardial, and pleural fluids after i.v. administration [1,2]. **Bile levels are low,** and ocular penetration is poor. Low bile levels help explain why vancomycin has little meaningful activity against *C. difficile* when given i.v. **Vancomycin penetrates inflamed meninges variably** [1,2]. Adequate cerebrospinal fluid (CSF) levels cannot be ensured [12].
2. **Peritoneal dialysis fluid.** Penetration is unpredictable. In dialysis-related peritonitis, the intraperitoneal route is recommended and convenient [13].
3. **Renal excretion.** Vancomycin is excreted primarily by glomerular filtration. **The dose must be reduced in renal failure. Vancomycin is not removed by dialysis** . The **half-life** of vancomycin in adults with normal renal function is 4 to 8 hours and in anuria, 7 to 12 days.
4. **Liver metabolism.** The liver also contributes to a lesser extent in the disposition of vancomycin. Dose adjustments may be needed with severe liver dysfunction [2].

**B. Oral preparation.** Vancomycin is **poorly absorbed** [1,2]. Very high stool concentrations are achieved after oral administration, making this agent active against *C. difficile* diarrhea and staphylococcal enterocolitis.

**IV. Indications for use.** Clinicians should be aware that vancomycin is less rapidly bactericidal and thus **less effective than β-lactam agents for β-lactam–susceptible staphylococci** (e.g., MSSA). Furthermore, because the use of vancomycin is a risk factor for colonization/infection with VREF and/or GISA [4–6], **prudent use of vancomycin is emphasized** [6,14]. **Guidelines for proper use of vancomycin should be a part of a hospital's quality improvement program** and should include the participation of the pharmacy and therapeutics committee, infection control, and infectious disease, medical, and surgical staffs.

**A. Vancomycin use is appropriate for the following infections** caused by β-lactam–resistant **gram-positive** bacteria. Those infections include the following [1–3]:

1. **MRSA. Vancomycin is treatment of choice** [15]. At times, gentamicin and/or rifampin are added for synergy [15] (see Chapters 4, 5, and 12). To achieve greatest success, some experts suggest troughs of no less than 15 μg/mL should be maintained.
2. **Bacterial meningitis in adults or in children older than 1 month, with gram-positive cocci suggestive of *S. pneumoniae*** [15,16] on Gram stain **or in those patients believed to be at risk for pneumococcal meningitis** (see Chapter 6). Vancomycin is added to cefotaxime or ceftriaxone, until susceptibility data are available, specifically to cover intermediate and high level **penicillin-resistant *S. pneumoniae*.** Because penetration of vancomycin in adult CSF may be compromised by steroid use, **some experts will also add rifampin** until susceptibility data are available [12,15,16] (see Chapter 6).

Outside the central nervous system, high-dose β-lactams or newer second-generation fluoroquinolones (e.g., gatifloxacin) are alternatives even for high-level resistant **penicillin-resistant *S. pneumoniae*** (Chapter 11).

3. **SSCN infections.** Surveys indicate that 35% to 65% of SSCN isolates are resistant to methicillin. Vancomycin, sometimes combined with gentamicin and/or rifampin, is the treatment of choice for these infections. Vancomycin combined with rifampin is effective in prosthetic device infections and CSF shunt infections. It also is effective against SSCN nosocomial infections in intensive care nurseries [1].
4. **Selected febrile neutropenic patients.** Whether to use vancomycin empirically in this setting is an area of **clinical debate** (see section **D.3** below and Chapter 20). Generally agreed on situations for use **for 72 hours pending cultures are as follows:** an epidemiologic situation of **β-lactam–resistant viridans streptococci,** when the treated subject has known colonization with MRSA, when more than one blood culture has yielded gram-positive bacteria (see section **D.2** below) but susceptibility data are pending, or if the situation is life-threatening [17,18].
5. **Central catheter infections.** When catheter exit site has clear-cut surrounding cellulitis, empiric vancomycin is used while awaiting culture results (see [17] and Chapter 2).
6. ***Corynebacterium* infections** such as endocarditis of prosthetic valves or CSF shunt infections, especially if penicillin resistant such as the JK bacillus.
7. **Miscellaneous**
   a. MRSA **hemodialysis shunt infections.**
   b. Chronic ambulatory peritoneal dialysis is often complicated by SSCN **peritonitis** [12] (see Chapter 13).
   c. For the rare **staphylococcal enterocolitis,** oral vancomycin is indicated.

B. **Vancomycin is used in patients with a history of anaphylaxis or severe reactions to β-lactam antimicrobials** for the following:
   1. **Serious *S. aureus* (coagulase-positive) infections.**
   2. **Endocarditis** due to enterococci or to viridans streptococci or other susceptible streptococci, (e.g., *S. bovis*). Because vancomycin is bacteriostatic against enterococci, vancomycin plus an aminoglycoside is required (see Chapter 12).
   3. ***S. aureus* or other gram-positive bacterial central nervous system infections.** The penetration of vancomycin into the CSF is variable. Infectious disease consultation is advisable to help adjust doses and/or monitor CSF drug levels.

C. **Prophylaxis**
   1. **Endocarditis.** The American Heart Association recommends vancomycin for patients at risk who are amoxicillin-allergic and are undergoing GI or genitourinary manipulations, in patients with an artificial heart valve, or in other high-risk patients undergoing dental procedures (see Chapters 12 and 27B).
   2. **Implantation of prosthetic devices.** A single dose administered immediately preoperatively with a repeat dose if the procedure lasts more than 6 hours is sufficient to reduce attack rate of **MRSA or SSCN** (see detailed discussion in Chapter 5).

D. **Vancomycin use is discouraged for the following situations** [11,14,19,20]:
   1. **Routine surgical prophylaxis** (see Chapter 27B).
   2. **SSCN single positive blood culture out of several** drawn in the same time frame. This is almost always either a contaminant or clinically unimportant bacteremia.
   3. **Culture-negative neutropenic fever.** There is a higher rate of rash and abnormal liver function tests and no obvious benefit if vancomycin is continued when there is no microbiological reason for its use [21–23]. Most of those who do develop positive blood cultures requiring therapy aimed at gram-positive organisms, which is a small minority of the febrile group, do as well if vancomycin is started after the blood culture data become available as when it is used empirically.

4. **Systemic or i.v. catheter "lock" prophylaxis** to prevent infection or colonization of indwelling central or peripheral intravascular catheters or vascular grafts.
5. **Selective decontamination of the digestive tract.**
6. **Eradication of MRSA colonization.**
7. **Treatment of *C. difficile* diarrhea.** Although oral vancomycin is often selected either when there is relapse of *C. difficile* diarrhea after metronidazole therapy or when *C. difficile* diarrhea is severe and potentially life-threatening, there is no proof that it is superior to metronidazole for these purposes. Because of the concern for selecting VREF and because i.v. vancomycin does not achieve levels in the bowel, vancomycin is not the primary treatment of *C. difficile* diarrhea (see Chapter 13). Oral metronidazole remains the drug of choice in this setting (see Chapter 27Q).
8. **Prophylaxis** for very low birth weight infants.
9. **Prophylaxis** for patients on continuous ambulatory peritoneal dialysis.
10. **Treatment (chosen for dosing convenience)** of $\beta$-lactam–sensitive gram-positive infections in patients who have renal failure.
11. **Vancomycin solution** for topical application or irrigation.

**V. Continued inappropriate use of vancomycin has contributed to the emergence of VREF, GISA, and the recent vancomycin completely resistant *S. aureus*** (see section **II.B.2**).

A. Despite published Centers for Disease Control and Prevention guidelines (see section **IV**), several investigators have reported that **30% to 80% of vancomycin used in hospitals is inappropriate** [24–26].

B. **Vancomycin is often part of empiric antibiotic regimens, especially in hospitalized patients,** because of concern for MRSA and SSCN line-associated bacteremia [26].

1. Vancomycin use could be controlled better by infection control measures to reduce MRSA rates and central-line infections [26], thereby reducing the need to use vancomycin so frequently.
2. **Infection control practices** , include the following [26]:
   a. **Better handwashing** and more use of the "user-friendly" soapless/waterless soaps.
   b. **New technology** (e.g., new i.v. catheters bonded with antiinfectives) are undergoing clinical evaluation.

**VI. Dosage**

A. **Intravenous** [1,2]

1. **Adults**
   a. **One gram every 12 hours.** A convenient and cost-effective dosage regimen in subjects with **normal renal function is** 1 g every 12 hours (over 2 hours to avoid red man syndrome; see section **VIII.A** ).
   b. **Mayo Medical Center vancomycin dosing nomogram (Table 27P.1).** Conventional dosing mentioned in section **1** above does not take into account variability in patient"s weight and renal function. **In obese** patients, ideal body weight can be used to determine the creatinine clearance, but actual total body weight is used in dose calculations [2] (see section **C.2** below).
   c. **Combined vancomycin and aminoglycoside.** Some authorities recommend either a reduced dose of 500 mg every 8 hours or, preferably, pharmacokinetic monitoring.
   d. **Prophylaxis in cardiac surgery.** Some authors favor a single 15-mg/kg preoperative dose (see Chapter 12).
2. **Children and neonates.** There is less experience with the use of vancomycin in children. For infants and children with non-central nervous system infections, 10-mg/kg doses i.v. over 60 minutes every 6 hours (40 mg/kg/day) often are suggested. In central nervous system infections, 15 mg/kg doses i.v. over 60 minutes every 6 hours are suggested to attain peak serum concentrations between 30 and 40 $\mu$g/mL [12]. **In neonates,** close monitoring of vancomycin serum levels is important to ensure therapeutic efficacy without toxicity (see Chapter 3 for dose regimens in neonates).

Table 27P.1. Mayo Medical Center i.v. Vancomycin Dosing Nomogram[a,b]

| Creatinine Clearance | Dosing Interval |
|---|---|
| >80 | Every 12 h |
| 65–80 | Every 12 to 18 h |
| 50–64 | Every 24 h |
| 35–49 | Every 24 to 36 h[c] |
| 21–34 | Every 48 h[c] |

[a]Use a dose of 15 mg/kg (actual body weight). The dosing interval is based on renal function. It can be estimated by using the estimated creatinine clearance. See Chapter 27A, and the table above.
[b]If the estimated renal function is near the border of two dosing intervals, it may be reasonable to begin with the more aggressive interval; the dose can then be modified if necessary according to serum levels.
[c]Patients with serious infection in whom the initial dosing interval is >24 h should have serum level monitoring performed before steady state to ensure that the levels are not subtherapeutic. It may be advisable to measure a random level about 24 h after the first dose. This level can be interpreted with respect to the seriousness of the infection to determine whether the dosage regimen needs to be modified.
Modified from Wilhelm MP, Estes L. Vancomycin. *Mayo Clin Proc* 1999;74:928.

**B. Oral.** An oral preparation is available but its appropriate use is extremely limited.

1. **For *C. difficile* diarrhea** in adults [1], 125 mg every 6 hours for 10 to 14 days is as effective a regimen as 500 mg orally four times a day. In children, the dose is 40 mg/kg/day in four divided doses (see Chapter 13). Metronidazole is the preferred drug, as discussed in Chapters 13 and 27Q.
2. **For staphylococcal enterocolitis,** 500 mg every 6 hours in adults has been suggested. It is unclear whether this entity really exists.

**C. Doses in renal failure. In renal failure, maintenance doses must be reduced.**

1. **The Mayo Clinic Center vancomycin dosing nomogram** can be used (Table 27P.1). However, nomograms may not work well in anuric patients or patients with rapidly changing renal function; serum drug level monitoring is useful in these patients (see section **VII**).
2. Figure 27P.1 shows a very useful nomogram designed to achieve peak and trough concentrations of 30 and 7.5 μg/mL, respectively. After an **initial loading dose of 25 mg/kg** (infused at 500 mg/h), the vancomycin **maintenance** dose remains constant at **19 mg/kg** (infused at 500 mg/h), but the dosage interval depends on the creatinine clearance. **Doses are based on actual total weight,** not ideal patient weight. (See Chapter 27A for instructions on estimation of **creatinine clearance based on ideal body weight.**)
3. **Individualized dosing.** Ideally, vancomycin dosage can be "individualized" based on serum concentrations, using pharmacokinetic consultation. Initial vancomycin dosage is calculated on a per body weight basis with the use of the nomogram (see section **2** above). Adjustments are made to attain peak serum levels of 30 to 40 μg/mL and trough levels of 5 to 10 μg/mL. For treatment of **MRSA, troughs of 15 μg/mL** have been recommended by some experts.
4. **Hemodialysis** or **peritoneal dialysis does not remove significant amounts of vancomycin.** Individualized dosing is preferred in this setting, with a loading dose of 25 mg/kg infused at 500 mg/h and maintenance dose of 19 mg/kg every 5 to 7 days. If on day 5 the level is less than 10 μg/mL (<16μg/mL for MRSA) a maintenance dose is given. If on day 5 the level is more than 10 μg/mL (more than 18 μg/mL for MRSA), the maintenance dose can be given usually on day 7. When treating MRSA, it seems prudent to keep the trough 15 or possibly even as high as 20 μg/mL.

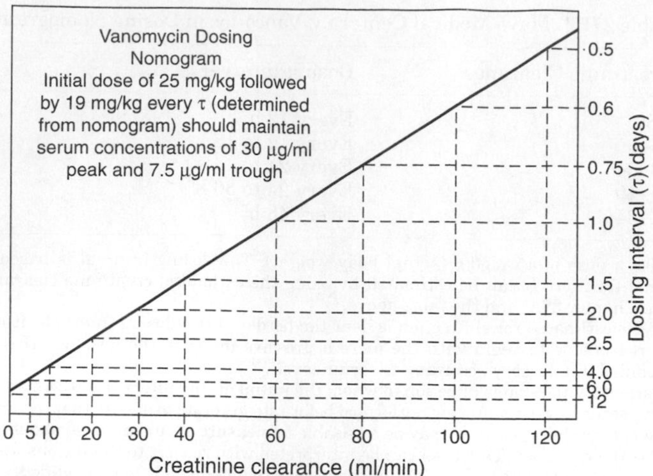


**FIG.27P.1.** Nomogram for vancomycin dosage in patients with renal failure. (From Matzke GR, et al. Pharmacokinetics of vancomycin in patients with varying degrees of renal function. *Antimicrob Agents Chemother* 1984;25:433, with permission.)

**D. Intraperitoneal administration.** Vancomycin dosage is discussed elsewhere [13].

**E. Vancomycin administration into the CSF.** Because of the somewhat variable vancomycin CSF penetration, for inadequately responding meningitis, intrathecal injection is a consideration. This has been reviewed [12]. **Infectious disease consultation is advised.**

**VII. Monitoring serum vancomycin.** The theoretical optimal serum level range for vancomycin is **peaks of 20 to 40 $\mu$g/mL and troughs of 5 to 10 $\mu$g/mL** [2], but some experts, as noted, suggest troughs of **15 $\mu$g/mL if treating MRSA.**

**A. Vancomycin pharmacokinetics** is sufficiently predictable that adequate serum drug concentrations can be obtained by empiric dosing methods (e.g., see section **III**). These take into account the patient's age, weight, and renal function. This is especially true when renal function is normal. Therefore, **routine serum monitoring is not advised** [27,28]. In a thoughtful editorial comment on vancomycin serum level monitoring, Moellering [28] suggested a limited number of clinical settings in which following serum or body fluid levels of vancomycin may be prudent:

1. **Vancomycin/aminoglycoside combination** administration.
2. **Anephric patients** undergoing hemodialysis with systemic infection and receiving infrequent doses of vancomycin.
3. **Patients receiving higher than usual doses of vancomycin** such as treatment of high level penicillin-resistant *S. pneumoniae* meningitis.
4. **Patients with rapidly changing renal function.**
5. **In addition, we would monitor levels early in therapy of those with MRSA** infection as noted above in an attempt to ensure a trough of about 15 $\mu$g/mL.

   **Note:** Vancomycin serum monitoring is indicated, especially initially to be certain that you have achieved adequate serum concentrations.

**B.** In a review [2], the authors emphasize that **if monitoring is done, only trough levels** are needed. Maintaining adequate trough levels may correlate with a better outcome. Furthermore, if nephrotoxicity is, in fact, related to trough levels, nephrotoxicity can be avoided.

**VIII. Toxicity** [1–3]

A. **Red man syndrome.** If vancomycin is infused too rapidly, it may cause flushing of the face, neck, or torso; pruritus; or hypotension [29]. This is a **nonimmunologically mediated** histamine release precipitated by the hyperosmolarity associated with the rapid infusion of vancomycin. Rapid bolus infusions also can cause pain and muscle spasms of the chest and back.

1. **Infusion rate. To avoid these reactions, infuse vancomycin slowly, at 500 mg/h.**
2. **Clinical implications.** Because red man syndrome is **not immunologically mediated,** it does not preclude continued use. **Bronchospasm and angioedema are not part of red man syndrome and suggest a true allergic reaction to vancomycin.**

B. **Rashes** other than red man syndrome occur in approximately 5% of patients. Stevens-Johnson syndrome may occur rarely. **Anaphylaxis** has been described with vancomycin use.

C. **Nephrotoxicity** is very uncommon. Currently available purified parenteral preparations are very well tolerated. Only when **another drug with nephrotoxic potential** such as an aminoglycoside **is used simultaneously** is there significant risk of these toxicities. If there is renal failure or vancomycin is used with an aminoglycoside, monitoring levels of both antibiotics will decrease the risk of toxicity.

D. **Ototoxicity** is a potential side effect, is relatively **uncommon,** and **occurs with very high serum levels** (>80 μg/mL) or in combination with aminoglycosides or other ototoxic drugs. Serum level monitoring as in section **VII.B** above will avoid this [1].

E. **Phlebitis** at the site of infusion **can be minimized if the vancomycin is diluted in 100 to 200 mL dextrose and water or saline and infused slowly** at a rate not exceeding 15 mg/min.

F. **Fever and chills** after i.v. administration are uncommon but occur occasionally.

G. **Neutropenia** can occur, especially with prolonged use, and agranulocytosis has been described [30]. **Blood counts weekly are indicated with prolonged vancomycin therapy.**

**IX. Cost. Oral** vancomycin is **expensive** (see Appendix Table).

## TEICOPLANIN

**Teicoplanin** (Targocid) is an antibiotic chemically similar to vancomycin but with important differences responsible for the unique physical and chemical properties of the complex. Although widely used in Europe for the treatment of gram-positive infections, teicoplanin was an investigational agent in the United States until late 1995, and at that point **clinical investigations were suspended.** As of mid-2002, we are not aware of "compassionate-use" availability of this agent in the United States. This agent is discussed elsewhere [3].

## QUINUPRISTIN/DALFOPRISTIN (SYNERCID) [31]

**I. Introduction.** Quinupristin/dalfopristin (Synercid) **is a combination of two antibiotics and is the first agent from a new class of antibiotics called streptogramins. In September 1999, it was** given accelerated approval by the U.S. Food and Drug Administration for bloodstream infections due to VREF **[31–33]. This was based on a demonstrated effect on a surrogate end point that is likely to predict clinical benefit, the ability to clear VREF from the bloodstream.**

**II. The problem. Vancomycin-resistant enterococci, usually *E. faecium* (VREF).** It is important to be aware of the new problem posed by this organism.

A. **Incidence.** VREF are being isolated more frequently [10,11,34,35], especially in larger hospitals. From January 1989 through March 1993, nosocomial VREF increased 20-fold. During this time, ICU isolates increased from 0.4% to 13.9% [36]. Now about 50% of enterococci isolates from ICUs are VREF [9]. Initially, **all strains of VREF were identical to one another,** carrying the vanA resistance determinant. This indicates that **resistance was not induced in the treated patient but instead** that the VREF was **transmitted from one** antibiotic-treated individual **to another.**

**B. Clinical problems**

1. **Colonization is more common** with VREF**than infection.** Because VREF colonizes the GI tract, **cultures of either stool or rectal swabs are the best way to identify carriers,** with stool cultures being superior.
   a. **Infection control.** Because "person to person" and "fomites to person" spread is critical in maintaining a reservoir, **infection control practices must be followed diligently.** Acquisition of infection occurs from thermometers and from personnel and is closely related to proximity to colonized and, even more so, infected patients (see Chapter 20). **Handwashing and change of gloves between every patient are mandatory.** Gowns probably add an additional measure of protection, but studies are inconclusive.
   b. **Investigational observations.** Preliminary data suggest that if VREF is given orally to animals or human volunteers, simultaneous administration of piperacillin reduces the potential to colonize because of the high biliary levels piperacillin produces. The levels are sufficient to inhibit the organism and prevent establishment of colonization. By contrast, cephalosporins do not prevent colonization in this model. However, once colonization is established, antibiotics with antianaerobic activity lead to higher fecal titers of VREF and hence to its potential to spread or cause disease. **Prudent use of all antibiotics, including vancomycin, may help decrease the incidence of VREF.** This has led some to speculate that the use of piperacillin-tazobactam, when treatment of gram-negative bacteria is needed, in the ICU may reduce VREF colonization; this will require careful study.
2. **Infection. Patients infected with VREF often are very debilitated and have had prolonged hospitalizations.** They have **often received multiple antibiotics,** including vancomycin [1–3,34–36]. Individuals with VREF bacteremia have a higher death rate than those with susceptible enterococcal bacteremia [34,35]. **Two specific groups at risk to develop VREF infection are patients who have undergone liver transplants and patients with hematologic malignancy.** Colonization (see section **B.1** above) precedes infection. **In liver transplant patients,** once enterococci colonize the gut they migrate and find an ecological niche in the biliary tract. A major complication of liver transplant is hepatic artery thrombosis. Because the peribiliary duct anatomic areas of the liver are served only by the hepatic artery and not simultaneously by the portal system, this leads to necrosis of those areas. Abscess forms due to the necrosis. If that individual has previously been colonized with VREF, it replicates to high titer when antibiotics active against gut flora suppress competing bacteria. **In the patient with leukemia,** when antibiotics are administered for neutropenic fever, other flora are suppressed and VREF emerges, enters the bloodstream through the gut compromised by mucositis, and then disseminates.

**III. Use of Q-D for VREF and other gram-positive infections**

**A. Mechanism of action.** The two antibiotics work synergistically by interfering with protein synthesis: Dalfopristin inhibits the early phase, whereas quinupristin interferes with the late phase of protein synthesis. Resistance is associated with resistance to both components. However, if the staphylococcus is resistant to macrolide-lincosamide-streptogramin B, Q-D is less efficacious than if the organism is susceptible to macrolide-lincosamide-streptogramin B [37]. Clindamycin susceptibility appears to identify organisms susceptible to macrolide-lincosamide-streptogramin B [38].

**B. *In vitro* activity.** Q-D is not active against gram-negative organisms.

1. Q-D is **bacteriostatic against VREF and may be bactericidal against MSSA and group A streptococcus (GAS), but it is not active against *E. faecalis.***
2. Q-D also is active against *Streptococcus pneumoniae,* regardless of penicillin susceptibility; MRSA; *S. agalactiae; Corynebacterium jeikeium; S. epidermidis;* and group C $\beta$ hemolytic streptococcus.
3. *Ureaplasma urealyticum, Mycoplasma pneumoniae,* and *Mycoplasma hominis* are susceptible *in vitro* [39].
4. *Borrelia* and *Leptospira* species are susceptible *in vitro* [40].

C. **Pharmacokinetics.** Synercid consists of 30% quinupristin and 70% dalfopristin, each of which is converted into several active major metabolites.

1. **Elimination half-lives** of quinupristin and dalfopristin are less than 1 hour.
2. **Biliary excretion,** and hence fecal excretion, constitutes the major elimination of both parent drugs and their metabolites.
3. **Renal failure.** Doses do not require modification in renal failure.
4. **Cytochrome P450 3A. Q-D is a major inhibitor of the activity of cytochrome P450 3A4 isoenzyme and can interfere with the metabolism of other drugs** (see section **V.G**).

IV. **Indications for use** [32,41–43]

A. **VREF infection.** Q-D is approved for **serious or life-threatening infections associated with VREF.** Because of the difficulty in eradicating these infections, **infectious disease consultation is advised.**

B. Skin and skin structure infections caused by MSSA or GAS. Although approved for this use, other very active agents are available for these infections (see Chapter 4), and we do not suggest using Q-D in this setting unless there is VREF bacteremia associated with MSSA or GAS wound infection. Infectious disease consultation is advised.

C. MRSA. Although U.S. Food and Drug Administration approval has not been issued, success is reported using Q-D when vancomycin has failed. It may find a role also in GISA and vancomycin-resistant *S. aureus.*

V. **Dosages and administration.** Only an i.v. preparation is available.

A. **Dose ranges.** The dose is diluted in at least 250 mL D5W and infused over 60 minutes.

1. **VREF.** An i.v. dose, infused over 1 hour, of 7.5 mg/kg every 8 hours is recommended with duration dependent on clinical response.
2. **For complex skin and skin structure infections,** 7.5 mg/kg every 12 hours i.v. for 7 days is suggested.

B. **Pediatric use.** The safety and efficacy in those under 16 has not been established.

C. **Pregnancy.** Q-D is a **category B** agent (see Chapter 27A). It should be used during pregnancy only if clearly needed.

D. **Nursing.** Q-D is excreted in milk in animals; it is not known if it is excreted in human breast milk. Caution should be exercised administering Synercid to nursing women.

E. **In renal failure** no dosage adjustment is required, including patients undergoing dialysis.

F. **In hepatic failure,** no special dose changes are recommended at this time, but only preliminary data are available.

G. **Drug interactions**

1. **Cytochrome P450 3A4. Q-D** significantly **inhibits cytochrome P450 3A4 metabolism** of **cyclosporin A, midazolam, nifedipine,** and **terfenadine.** Therefore concomitant administration of these or other drugs metabolized by the cytochrome P450 enzyme system may result in increased plasma concentrations of these drugs. **Monitoring levels** of cyclosporin is indicated.
2. **QTc prolongation potential.** Q-D itself does not seem to increase the QTc interval. However, **medications metabolized by cytochrome P450 3A4 that prolong the QTc interval should be avoided when using Q-D.** For up-to-date drug information on drugs that may affect the QTc interval, see *www.qt.org,* and for drugs associated with drug interactions causing torsades, see *www.torsades.org*
3. **Other serum drug level increases. Examples of drugs whose concentrations may be raised by** concomitant use of **Q-D** have been summarized in the package insert and **include** the following: antihistamines (astemizole, terfenadine); anti-human immunodeficiency virus (non-nucleaside reverse transcriptase inhibitors [NNRTI] and protease inhibitors; e.g., delavirdine, nevirapine, indinavir, ritonavir); antineoplastic agents: vinca alkaloids (e.g., vinblastine), docetaxel, and paclitaxel; benzodiazepams (midazolam, diazepam); calcium channel blockers; HMG-CoA reductase inhibitor; cholesterol-lowering agents (statins);

cisapride; cyclosporine; tacrolimus; methylprednisolone; carbamazepine; quinidine; disopyramide; and lidocaine.

VI. **Side effects**
   A. **Arthralgia** and/or **myalgias** are common. These are the number one reason that the drug is discontinued. Reducing the dose helps [44].
   B. **Intravenous site inflammation, pain, edema, and local reactions** are common and if severe may be reduced by increasing the infusion volume to 500 or 750 mL of D5W.
   C. **Hyperbilirubinemia** is relatively common.
   D. **GI side effects** (nausea, vomiting, diarrhea) occur in a small percent (<5%).

## LINEZOLID (ZYVOX): A NEW PROTEIN SYNTHESIS INHIBITOR ANTIBIOTIC

Linezolid belongs to a **new class of antibiotics, the oxazolidinones.** It was approved in early 2000. It interferes with bacterial protein synthesis by binding at the 50S ribosomal area but at a site different from that to which erythromycin binds [32,45–48].

I. **Spectrum of activity [31] and related issues**
   A. **Gram-positive bacteria.** It is active against all *S. aureus,* including MRSA; VREF; *S. faecalis;* and penicillin-resistant or -susceptible *S. pneumoniae* [49].
      1. **It is bacteriostatic** for most gram-positive bacteria, although it may be bactericidal against pneumococcus.
      2. **Serum inhibitory levels** for these organisms range from 0.5 to 2.0 μg/mL.
   B. **Gram-negative aerobes.** Linezolid is not active against gram-negative aerobes.
   C. **Miscellaneous.** *In vitro,* it is also active against *Legionella pneumophila, M. pneumoniae,* and *C. pneumoniae.*
   D. **Resistance.** VREF resistance develops in liver transplant patients who are continuously on this drug [50]. Resistant organisms are transmitted person to person [51]. MRSA resistance to linezolid has been described. [52].

II. **Pharmacokinetics**
   A. **Oral drug is 100% bioavailable.** Intravenous or oral administration yields the same serum levels. The oral and i.v. doses are 600 mg yielding serum levels approximating 20 μg/mL.
   B. **Dose interval** is every 12 hours.
   C. **Hepatic or renal failure.** There is **no dose modification** for hepatic or renal failure.
   D. **Bone levels** are about 50% of serum levels [53]. **CSF penetration** is poor, but penetration into **skin and soft tissue** is excellent.

III. **Clinical results.** These studies have been carried out in multicenter trials. **Usually studies were designed as initial i.v. followed by oral therapy.**
   A. ***S. aureus***—soft tissue infection or pneumonia
      1. **MSSA. Oxacillin/dicloxacillin versus linezolid:** Cure rates were similar [54].
      2. **MRSA soft tissue, pulmonary, and urinary tract infection.** Vancomycin versus linezolid were compared. Linezolid was as effective as vancomycin against MRSA with similar clinical cure rates and similar microbiologic eradication [55]. In a nosocomial pneumonia study in which several but not all isolates were MRSA, linezolid plus aztreonam was as effective as vancomycin plus aztreonam [56].
   B. ***S. pneumoniae.*** Trials have compared i.v. with oral linezolid versus ceftriaxone followed by oral cefixime.
      1. **Nonbacteremic pneumonia.** Linezolid was equally effective to ceftriaxone. In a pediatric trial, linezolid was quite successful.
      2. **Bacteremic pneumonia.** Linezolid was more effective than ceftriaxone ($p < 0.01$). Most cases were caused by penicillin-susceptible *S. pneumoniae.*
   C. **Enterococcus. In trials against VREF,** linezolid was effective in treating urinary tract infection, soft tissue infection, extravascular body fluid infection such as ascites, and source unknown bacteremia. Linezolid has been effective in cases where Q-D has failed [57]. Case reports of efficacy in VREF endocarditis are reported [58]. Linezolid is also active against *E. faecalis.*

**IV. Side effects and toxicity**

**A. GI.** GI side effects that did not result in drug cessation were more common than in vancomycin-treated subjects. Both diarrhea and nausea and/or dyspepsia were manifest. An occasional patient cannot continue oral linezolid because of severe nausea, but most tolerate the drug to the end of the treatment course [55].

**B. Rash** has not been prominent with linezolid and in one study occurred less frequently than occurred with vancomycin [56].

**C. Hematologic** [59–61]. Thrombocytopenia has been observed in those treated for more than 3 weeks but is reversible on drug cessation in those where it has occurred. The frequency is low. Mild neutropenia was observed in one study of treatment of pneumonia in children but did not lead to cessation of drug. Mild reversible neutropenia and thrombocytopenia are certainly not totally unexpected in a drug whose action interferes with protein synthesis. Reversible red blood cell aplasia has been described.

**D. Monoamine oxidase inhibition [62].** Because of its biochemical structure there was concern that linezolid could pose a risk with certain dietary products. However, this has not been borne out with clinical experience or with studies in normal volunteers.

**E. Drug interactions [63].** When linezolid is administered in conjunction with pseudoephedrine or phenylpropanolamine, a minimal increase in both blood pressure and serum levels of the coadministered drugs was observed but no serious adverse events developed. When administered in conjunction with dextromethorphan, a serotonin uptake inhibitor, there was only minimal change in the clearance of a metabolic breakdown product of dextromethorphan. There was no change in the pharmacokinetics of linezolid. **There is no anticipated interaction between CYP 450 drug-drug interactions.**

**V. Indications for Use [31,55,59–61,64].** Because of the **high expense** of linezolid and the need to **use it only when clearly indicated** so that resistance will be minimized, **infectious disease consultation is advised before prescribing** this agent. This is a very expensive agent (see Appendix Table).

**A. MRSA soft tissue infection** is a primary indication for its use. Compared with vancomycin it is similarly effective, and linezolid offers the advantage of switch to oral therapy with the potential for shorter hospital stay and reduced risk of line-related infection [55]. Although resistance has been reported [52], if appropriated debridement is carried out accompanying the antibiotic this risk is probably small. MRSA resistant to vancomycin has also been observed [4,5], so special attention to management of the MRSA infections, regardless of what antibiotic is chosen, is very important.

**B. VREF infection.** Considerable experience and success has been reported [31].

**C. Probable or known severe pneumococcal pneumonia** in a $\beta$-lactam highly allergic individual [60].

**D. MRSA osteomyelitis.** Data are limited. Tissue levels in bone and hematoma are promising [53]. In a large series of patients treated under emergency use protocol, linezolid treatment resulted in cure of osteomyelitis due to either MSSA or MRSA [64]. Although linezolid is effective against MSSA, there are other available drugs with which to treat that infection.

## AN INVESTIGATIONAL DRUG FOR GRAM-POSITIVE INFECTIONS: DAPTOMYCIN (CIDECIN)

**I. Mechanism of action [64].** Daptomycin is a novel lipopeptide antibiotic derived from the fermentation of *Streptomyces roseosporus.* It belongs to a new class of antibiotics. Daptomycin appears to kill bacteria by a mode of attack at more than one site that is rapid and distinct from resistance mechanisms against usual organisms. It may inhibit peptidoglycan biosynthesis, it disrupts cell membrane permeability, it reduces synthesis of lipoteichoic acids, and it may even disrupt trans-membrane electrochemical gradient.

**II. Resistance potential.** *In vitro* evaluation indicates that it has an extremely low resistance potential ($<10^{-10}$) for *S. aureus* when challenged at eight times the MIC value.

III. **Spectrum of activity** [65]

A. **Gram-positive aerobes.** Daptomycin is active against all gram-positive cocci, including MSSA; MRSA; enterococcus, including VREF; *S. pneumoniae;* and SSCN species. MIC for *S. aureus is* 1 μg/mL and for enterococci is 2 μg/mL.

B. **Gram-negative bacteria.** It has no activity against gram-negative bacteria.

IV. **Pharmacokinetics**

A. **Bactericidal activity.** Vancomycin exhibits time-dependent bactericidal activity. By contrast, daptomycin demonstrates **concentration-dependent bactericidal activity** (see Chapter 25). Its rate of bactericidal activity is faster than vancomycin.

B. **Serum levels.** At a dose of 4 mg/kg/dose $C_{max}$ is approximately 54.6 μg/mL.

C. **Excretion.** The major route of excretion is of unmetabolized drug via the kidney. There are very limited data on dose reduction in renal failure.

V. **Side effects and toxicity**

A. **Muscle enzyme changes.** In a small proportion of treated individuals, creatine phosphate kinase levels become elevated after 2 weeks of therapy. Usually the individual is asymptomatic and creatine phosphate kinase levels return to normal on drug cessation.

B. **Other side effects.** Preliminary data suggest no renal, hepatic, or bone marrow toxicity, but the number of individuals receiving the drug is limited.

VI. **Clinical experience**

A. **Skin and soft tissue.** Efficacy appears similar to conventional agents.

B. **Bacteremia.** Daptomycin sterilized blood cultures in all (of a small number) of treated individuals and its use was associated with a high cure rate.

VII. **Summary.** This is an interesting new antibiotic that is currently undergoing phase III clinical trials for *S. aureus* and *E. faecium* bacteremia.

## REFERENCES


1. Reese RE, Betts RF. Vancomycin. In: Reese RE, Betts RF, Gumustop B, eds. *Handbook of antibiotics,* 3rd ed. Philadelphia: Lippincott Williams & Wilkins, 2000:503–526.
2. Wilhelm MP, Estes L. Vancomycin. *Mayo Clin Proc* 1999;74:928.
3. Sulaiman AS, Rakita RM, Murray BE. Glycopeptides. In: Root RK, et al., eds. *Clinical infectious diseases: a practical approach.* New York: Oxford University Press, 1999.
4. Hiramatsu K, Hanaki H, Ino T, et al. Methicillin-resistant *Staphylococcus aureus* clinical strain with reduced vancomycin susceptibility. *J Antimicrob Chemother* 1997;40:135–136.
5. Centers for Disease Control and Prevention. *Staphylococcus aureus* resistant to vancomycin—United States, 2002. *MMWR Morb Mortal Wkly Rep* 2002;51:565–567.
6. Centers for Disease Control and Prevention. Interim guidelines for prevention and control of staphylococcal infections associated with reduced susceptibility to vancomycin. *MMWR Morb Mortal Wkly Rep* 1997;46:626–628, 635.
7. Waldvogel FA. New resistance in *Staphylococcus aureus. N Engl J Med* 1999;340:556.
8. Besnier JM, Leport C, Bure A, et al. Vancomycin-aminoglycoside combinations in therapy of endocarditis caused by enterococcus species and *Streptococcus bovis. Eur J Clin Microbiol Infect Dis* 1990;9:130–133.
9. Moellering RC Jr. Vancomycin-resistant enterococci. *Clin Infect Dis* 1998;36:1196.
10. French GL. Enterococci and vancomycin-resistance. *Clin Infect Dis* 1998;27[Suppl 1]:S75.
11. Murray BE. Vancomycin resistant enterococci infections. *N Engl J Med* 2000;342:710.
12. Ahmed A. A critical evaluation of vancomycin for treatment of bacterial meningitis. *Pediatr Infect Dis J* 1997;16:895.
13. Keane WF, et al. Adult peritoneal-dialysis related peritonitis treatment recommendations: 2000 update. *Perit Dial Int* 2000;20:396.
14. Centers for Disease Control and Prevention. Preventing the spread of vancomycin resistance: report from the Hospital Infection Control Practice Advisory Committee. *MMWR Morb Mortal Wkly Rep* 1995;44(RR-12):1.
15. Medical Letter. The choice of antibacterial drugs. *Med Lett Drugs Ther* 2001;43:69.

16. Peter G, et al. *Red Book 2000: Report of the Committee on Infectious Diseases,* 25th ed. Elk Grove, IL: American Academy of Pediatrics, 2000:420.
17. Hughes WT, et al. 1997 Guidelines for use of antimicrobial agents in neutropenic patients with unexplained fever. *Clin Infect Dis* 1997;25:551 (updated 2002;34:730).
18. Feld R. Vancomycin as part of initial empirical antibiotic therapy for febrile neutropenic patients with cancer: pros and cons. *Clin Infect Dis* 1999;29:503.
19. Murray BE. What can we do about vancomycin-resistant enterococci? *Clin Infect Dis* 1995;20:1134.
20. Fisher MC. Control of methicillin-resistant *Staphylococcus aureus* and vancomycin-resistant enterococcus in hospitalized children. *Pediatr Infect Dis J* 1998;17:823.
21. European Organization for Research and Treatment of Cancer (EORTC) International Antimicrobial Therapy Cooperative Group and National Cancer Institute of Canada Clinical Trials Group. Vancomycin added to empirical combination antibiotic therapy for fever in granulocytopenic cancer patients. *J Infect Dis* 1991;163:951–958.
22. Ramphal R, Bolger M, Oblon DJ, et al. Vancomycin is not an essential component of the initial treatment regimen for febrile neutropenic patients receiving ceftazidime: a randomized prospective study. *Antimicrob Agents Chemother* 1992;36:1062–1067.
23. Dompeling EC, Donnelly JP, Dereinski SC, et al. Early identification of neutropenic patients at risk for Gram positive bacteremia and the impact of empirical administration of vancomycin. *Eur J Cancer* 1996;32A:1332–1339.
24. Fridkin SK, et al. Determinants of vancomycin use in adults intensive care units in 41 United States hospitals. *Clin Infect Dis* 1999;28:1119.
25. Jarvis WR. Epidemiology, appropriateness, and cost of vancomycin use. *Clin Infect Dis* 1998;26:1200.
26. Wenzel RPWong MT. Editorial response: managing antibiotic use-impact of infection control. *Clin Infect Dis* 1999;28:1126.
27. Cantu TG, Yamanaka-Yuen NA, Leitman PS. Serum vancomycin concentrations: reappraisal of their clinical value. *Clin Infect Dis* 1994;18:533.
28. Moellering RC Jr. Monitoring serum vancomycin levels: climbing the mountain because it is there? *Clin Infect Dis* 1994;18:544.
29. Wallace MR, Mascola JR, Oldfield EC III. Red man syndrome: incidence, etiology, and prophylaxis. *J Infect Dis* 1991;164:1180.
30. Adrouny A, et al. Agranulocytosis related to vancomycin therapy. *Am J Med* 1986;81: 1059.
31. Hamilton DC, Ludlam H. New anti-Gram-positive agents. *Curr Opin Crit Care* 2001;7:232–237.
32. Moellering RC Jr. A novel antimicrobial agent joins battle against resistant bacteria. *Ann Intern Med* 1999;130:155.
33. Dowzicky M, et al. Evaluation of *in vitro* activity of quinupristin/dalfopristin and comparator antimicrobial agents against worldwide clinical trial and other laboratory isolates. *Am J Med* 1998;104[Suppl 5A]:34S.
34. Lucas GM, et al. Vancomycin-resistant and vancomycin-susceptible enterococcal bacteremia: comparison of clinical features and outcomes. *Clin Infect Dis* 1998;26:1127.
35. Vergis EN, Hayden MK, Chow JW, et al. Determinants of vancomycin resistance and mortality rates in enterococcal bacteremia: a prospective multicenter study. *Ann Intern Med* 2001;135:484–492.
36. Centers for Disease Control. Nosocomial enterococci resistant to vancomycin: United States, 1989–1993. *MMWR Morb Mortal Wkly Rep* 1993;30:597.
37. Vouillamoz J, Entenza JM, Feger C, et al. Quinupristin/dalfopristin combined with beta-lactams for treatment of experimental endocarditis due to *Staphylococcus aureus* constitutively resistant to macrolides-lincosamide-streptogramin B antibiotics. *Antimicrob Agents Chemother* 2000;44:1789–1795.
38. Fuchs PC, Barry AL, Brown SD. Bactericidal activity of quinupristin-dalfopristin against *Staphylococcus aureus:* clindamycin susceptibility as a surrogate indicator. *Antimicrob Agents Chemother* 2000;44:2880–2882.
39. Kenney GE, Cartwright FD. Susceptibilities of *Mycoplasma pneumoniae, Mycoplasma hominis and Ureaplasma urealyticum* to GAR-936, dalfopristin, dirithromycin, evernimicin, gatifloxacin, linezolid, moxifloxacin, quinupristin-dalfopristin, and telithromycin

compared to their susceptibilities to reference macrolides, tetracyclines and quinolones. *Antimicrob Agents Chemother* 2001;45:2604–2608.
40. Murgia R, Cinco M. Sensitivity of Borrelia and Leptospira to quinupristin-dalfopristin (Synercid) *in vitro. N Microbiol* 2001;24:193–196.
41. Moellering RC Jr, et al. The efficacy and safety of quinupristin/dalfopristin for the treatment of infections caused by vancomycin-resistant *Enterococcus faecium*. Synercid-Emergency Use Study Group. *J Antimicrob Chemother* 1999;44:251.
42. Nichols RL, et al. Treatment of hospitalized patients with complicated gram-positive skin and soft tissue structure infections: two randomized, multicenter studies of quinupristin/dalfopristin versus cefazolin, oxacillin, or vancomycin. Synercid Skin and Skin Structure Infection Group. *J Antimicrob Chemother* 1999;44:263.
43. Medical Letter. Quinupristin/dalfopristin. *Med Lett Drugs Ther* 1999;41:109.
44. Olsen KM, Rebuck JA, Rupp ME. Arthralgias and myalgias related to quinupristin-dalfopristin administration. *Clin Infect Dis* 2001;32:e83–e86.
45. Chien JW, Kucia ML, Salata RA. Use of linezolid, an oxazolidinone, in the treatment of multidrug-resistant gram-positive bacterial infection. *Clin Infect Dis* 2000;30: 146.
46. Pharmacia and UpJohn Clinical Protocol (M/1260/0025), 1998.
47. Rybak MJ, et al. Comparative *in vitro* activities and post-antibiotic effects of the oxazolidinone compounds eperezolid and linezolid versus vancomycin against *Staphylococcus aureus,* coagulase-negative staphylococci, *Enterococcus faecalis,* and *Enterococcus faecium. Antimicrob Agents Chemother* 1998;42:721.
48. Patel R, et al. In vitro activity of linezolid against vancomycin-resistant enterococci, methicillin-resistant Staphylococcus aureus and penicillin-resistant Streptococcus pneumoniae. *Diagn Microbiol Infect Dis* 1999;34:119.
49. Noskin GA, et al. Successful treatment of persistent vancomycin-resistant *Enterococcus faecium* bacteria with linezolid and gentamicin. *Clin Infect Dis* 1999;28:689.
50. Gonzales RD, Schreckenberger PC, Graham MB, et al. Infections due to vancomycin resistant *Enterococcus faecium* resistant to linezolid. *Lancet* 2001;357:1179.
51. Herrero IA, Issa NC, Patel R. Nosocomial spread of linezolid-resistant, vancomycin resistant *Enterococcus faecium. N Engl J Med* 2002;346:867–868.
52. Tsiodras S, Gold HS, Sakoulas G, et al. Linezolid resistance in an isolate of *Staphylococcus aureus. Lancet* 2001;358:207–208.
53. Lovering AM, Zhang J, Bannister GC, et al. Penetration of linezolid into bone, fat, muscle, and hematoma of patients undergoing routine hip replacement. *J Antimicrob Chemother* 2002;50:73–77.
54. Stevens DL, Smith LG, Bruss JB, et al. Randomized comparison of linezolid ((PNU-100766) versus oxacillin/dicloxacillin for treatment of complicated skin and soft tissue infections. *Antimicobial Agents Chemother* 2000;44:3408–3413.
55. Stevens DL, Herr D, Lampris H, et al. Linezolid versus vancomycin for the treatment of methicillin-resistant *Staphylococcus aureus* infections. *Clin Infect Dis* 2002;34:1481–1490
56. Rubinstein E, Cammarata SK, Oliphant TH, et al. Linezolid (PNU-100766) versus vancomycin in the treatment of hospitalized patients with nosocomial pneumonia: a randomized double-blind multi-center study. *Clin Infect Dis* 2001;32:402–412.
57. McNeil SA, Clark NM, Chandrasekar PH, et al. Successful treatment of vancomycin-resistant *Enterococcus faecium* bacteremia with linezolid after failure with Synercid (quinupristin-dalfopristin). *Clin Infect Dis* 2000;30:403–404.
58. Babcock HM, Ritchie DJ, Christiansen E, et al. Successful treatment of vancomycin-resistant Enterococcus endocarditis with oral linezolid. *Clin Infect Dis* 2001;32:1373–1375.
59. Fung HB, Kirschenbaum HL, Ojofeitimi BO. Linezolid: an oxazolidinone antimicrobial agent [Review]. *Clin Therap* 2001;23:356–391.
60. Kaplan SL, Patterson L, Edwards KM, et al. Linezolid for the treatment of community acquired pneumonia in hospitalized children. Linezolid Pediatric Pneumonia Study Group. *Pediatr Infect Dis J* 2001;20:488–494.
61. Perry CM, Jarvis B. Linezolid: a review of its use in the management of serious gram-positive infections. *Drugs* 2001;61:525–551.
62. Antal EJ, Hendershot PE, Batts DH, et al. Linezolid, a novel oxazolidinone antibiotic:

assessment of monoamine oxidase inhibition using pressor response to oral tyramine. *J Clin Pharmacol* 2001;41:552–562.

63. Hendershot PE, Antal EJ, Welshman IR, et al. Linezolid: pharmacokinetic and pharmacodynamic evaluation of co-administration with pseudoephedrine HCl, phenylpropanolamine HCL and dextromethorphan HBr. *J Clin Pharmacol* 2001;41:563–572.
64. Birmingham MC, Rayner C, Meagher AK, et al. Linezolid in the treatment of multidrug-resistant gram-positive infections: results of compassionate use experience. *Clin Infect Dis* (in press).
65. Tally FP, Zeckel M, Wasilewski MM, et al. Daptomycin: a novel agent for Gram-positive infections. *Exp Opin Invest Drugs* 1999;8:1223–1238.

## Q. Metronidazole

Metronidazole, introduced in 1959, has become an extremely important agent for the treatment of anaerobic infections [1–4]. It inhibits DNA synthesis, regardless of the growth phase of the organism, and is rapidly bactericidal.

**I. Spectrum [2–4]**

**A. Anaerobic activity**

1. **Gram-negative anaerobes.** Metronidazole is bactericidal against *Bacteroides fragilis,* other *Bacteroides* species, and *Fusobacterium* species [1,2].
2. **Gram-positive anaerobes.** Against some gram-positive anaerobes, including *Clostridium perfringens* and *C. difficile,* metronidazole is very active. The activity against anaerobic gram-positive cocci is much more variable, with resistance in up to 50% of tested isolates [2]. Strains of *Actinomyces* and *Propionibacterium* (e.g., *P. acnes*) are resistant [2].

**B. Aerobic activity.** *Gardnerella (Haemophilus) vaginalis* and *Helicobacter pylori* are susceptible to metronidazole. However, unlike clindamycin, metronidazole is not active against gram-positive aerobic bacteria such as *Staphylococcus aureus* and $\beta$ streptococcus group A.

**C. Parasites.** Metronidazole is very active against *Entamoeba histolytica, Giardia lamblia,* and *Trichomonas vaginalis.*

**II. Resistance.** Susceptible bacteria rarely develop resistance. During a 10-year period at the Mayo Clinic, no increase in resistance occurred among *Bacteroides* or *Fusobacterium* species [2].

**III. Pharmacokinetics** [1–4]

**A. Oral absorption.** Metronidazole is **very well absorbed. Serum levels are similar after equivalent oral and intravenous doses** [1,2]. Metronidazole can be taken with food.

**B. Tissue penetration.** Metronidazole has **excellent penetration** into almost all sites and provides therapeutic levels in bone, unobstructed biliary tract, cerebrospinal fluid, brain abscess contents, empyema fluid, hepatic abscesses, middle ear, pelvic tissue, and vaginal secretions.

**C. Metabolism and excretion.** Metronidazole is metabolized primarily in the liver and excreted in the kidney. Dose reductions are advised in severe renal failure [5].

**D. Placenta and breast milk.** Metronidazole readily crosses the placenta and penetrates breast milk.

**IV. Clinical uses**

**A. Drug of choice.** Metronidazole is indicated for *C. difficile, Bacteroides* species, susceptible *H. pylori,* and *G. vaginalis* [6]. In addition, it is the drug of choice for *Entamoeba histolytica, Giardia lamblia,* and other less common parasites [7] (Table 27Q.1).

**B. Anaerobic infections.** Metronidazole alone or in combination is indicated for the following:

1. **Mixed aerobic/anaerobic soft tissue or intraabdominal and pelvic infections:** with antiaerobic antibiotics. (See related discussions in Chapters 13 and 16.)

Table 27Q.1. Metronidazole Dosage Regimens

| Indication | Route of Administration | Adult Dosage[a] |
|---|---|---|
| Susceptible anaerobic infections | i.v. | Loading dose of 15 mg/kg, then 7.5 mg/kg q6h. For the average adult (70 kg) a 1-g load followed by 500 mg q6h. |
| | p.o. | 1–2 g/day in 2–4 doses q6–12h. For the average-sized adult, 500 mg q6–8h is often used. |
| *C. difficile* diarrhea | p.o. | 500 mg tid or 250 mg qid for 10 days [7a] |
| | i.v. (see text) | 500 mg q6–8h |
| *Trichomonas* vaginitis | p.o. | 2 g in a single dose or 500 mg bid × 7 days |
| Bacterial vaginosis (nonspecific vaginitis, *Gardnerella vaginalis* vaginosis) | p.o. | 500 mg bid for 7 days |
| | Topical | See footnote[b] |
| Giardiasis | p.o. | 250 mg tid for 5 days[c] |
| Amebiasis (intestinal or extraintestinal) | i.v. or p.o. | 500–750 mg tid for 10 days[d] |

[a]Dosages must be modified if creatinine clearance <10 mL/min or if there is significant hepatic dysfunction. See text.
[b]A 0.75% vaginal gel formulation of metronidazole (MetroGel-Vaginal) is available in a 70-g tub-and packaged with a 5-g vaginal applicator. The dose is 5 g intravaginally bid for 5 days. For use of metronidazole in pregnancy see reference 10 and Chapter 16.
[c]In children, giardiasis has been treated with 5 mg/kg/dose tid for 5 days.
[d]In amebiasis therapy, after 10 days of metronidazole, iodoquinol, 650 mg tid for 20 days, is recommended in adults. The pediatric dose of metronidazole is 35–50 mg/kg/day divided into three doses for 10 days; iodoquinol, 30–40 mg/kg/day (max. 2 g) in three divided doses, given (after completion of metronidazole) for 20 days.
Modified from Mathisen GE, Finegold SM. Metronidazole and other nitroimidazoles. In: Gorbach SL, Bartlett JG, Blacklow NR, eds. *Infectious diseases.* Philadelphia: WB Saunders, 1992:262; and Medical Letter. Drugs for parasite diseases. *Med Lett Drugs Ther* 2002;44:1 (April 2002), with permission.

2. ***B. fragilis* bacteremia with endocarditis or other vascular infections.** Metronidazole is bactericidal against *B. fragilis.* It is active against the 5% to 15% of isolates of *B. fragilis* that are resistant to clindamycin. Metronidazole costs less than clindamycin and is associated with less *C. difficile* diarrhea than clindamycin. **It is the agent of choice.**
3. **Brain abscess.** Metronidazole penetrates brain abscesses and is bactericidal. It is used with anti–gram-positive antibiotics.
4. **Antibiotic-associated diarrhea due to *C. difficile.*** Metronidazole is the drug of choice. [1,2,6,8] (see Chapter 13). Oral therapy is more effective and less expensive than intravenous therapy, but intravenous therapy may be effective in patients who cannot receive oral therapy.
5. **Tetanus.** Some data suggest metronidazole, not penicillin, may be the preferred agent [6,9].
6. **Anaerobic pleuropulmonary infections.** Failures have occurred, perhaps because these infections are polymicrobial [2] and because microaerophilic streptococci are resistant [1,4].

C. **Other infectious agents**

1. **Trichomoniasis** and **bacterial vaginosis [10]** (see Chapter 16) and **Giardiasis** (see Chapter 13).
2. **Amebiasis** [7].
3. ***H. pylori* in peptic ulcer disease** [1–4,6].
4. **Miscellaneous.** Metronidazole is adjunctive to debridement in severe **gingivitis and**

a. **Bacterial overgrowth conditions** such as Crohn disease and the perineal disease associated with **Crohn disease** [1,2].

b. **Periodontitis,** including those with human immunodeficiency virus infection [2].

5. **Topical metronidazole gel** is an effective and safe therapeutic agent for **rosacea.** A 0.75% vaginal gel formulation is available for treatment of bacterial vaginosis (see Chapter 16).

V. **Use in pregnancy.** Metronidazole has been shown to have **carcinogenic potential. It is** carcinogenic in mice and rats. The precise risk for humans is unclear and remains controversial. Metronidazole has not been shown to be teratogenic. However, many experts agree metronidazole use in the second and third trimesters of pregnancy should be restricted to those patients in whom alternative treatment has been inadequate. The use of metronidazole in the first trimester should be carefully evaluated because metronidazole crosses the placenta barrier and its effects on human fetal organogenesis are not known. The **pros and cons of using metronidazole in pregnancy,** especially the first trimester, have **recently** been **reviewed** [11]. In his commentary, the reviewer emphasizes that the "preponderance of published human experience does not support a teratogenic effect in any trimester" [11]. He believes that pending further data, metronidazole should be avoided in the first trimester except for serious or life-threatening infections. After organogenesis is complete, metronidazole could be considered for significant infections when other equally effective options are not available or are contraindicated [11]. In a recent report, investigators found no increase in late incidence of cancer after short-term metronidazole use in more than 5,000 women followed for a median of more than 12.5 years [12]. **Because metronidazole is excreted into breast milk, nursing should be discontinued during and for 2 days after therapy**[1].

VI. **Preparations and doses.** Seriously ill patients should receive metronidazole intravenously. Because blood levels are comparable after intravenous and oral drug, oral is indicated when clinically reasonable [1,2].

A. **Adult dosage regimens** (Table 27Q.1). The intravenous dose is infused over 60 minutes. Because of the relatively long half-life of metronidazole, oral doses can be given every 6, 8, or 12 hours, although higher doses, given at one time, may be associated with more gastrointestinal side effects.

B. **Renal failure.** No dose modification is needed, except with creatinine clearance of less than 10 mL/min, where a 50% reduction in the usual dose is suggested [5] to prevent the accumulation of toxic metabolites. **A** dose after hemodialysis, but not peritoneal dialysis, is recommended because of drug removal. Furthermore, some sources suggest a 50% dose reduction for patients undergoing chronic ambulatory peritoneal dialysis [5].

C. **In significant hepatic impairment, doses** should be **reduced** by at least 50% [1,2].

D. **Pediatrics.** The safety and efficacy of metronidazole in pediatric patients has not been established except in the treatment of amebiasis. [7].

VII. **Adverse effects.** In general, metronidazole is well tolerated [1,2].

A. **Alcohol intolerance.** Because of a disulfiram-like effect (i.e., nausea, vomiting, headaches), alcoholic beverages should not be consumed while taking metronidazole [13].

B. **Peripheral neuropathy,** manifested as numbness and tingling of the extremities, may occur in those on long-term therapy. This is usually reversible if the drug is stopped [2]. **Seizures,** encephalopathy, or cerebellar dysfunction are rare. Some advise caution with a history of central nervous system disorders. If neurologic symptoms develop on therapy and there is no other obvious cause, metronidazole should be stopped [2].

C. **Anticoagulation interference.** Metronidazole can potentiate the effect of warfarin.

D. **Miscellaneous. Mild gastrointestinal symptoms** of nausea, abdominal discomfort, and diarrhea can occur. Patients complain of a **metallic unpleasant taste** while on oral therapy. Metronidazole may be a cause of **acute pancreatitis.**

VIII. **Cost.** Generic oral formulations are inexpensive (see Appendix Table 1).

## REFERENCES


1. Klein NC, Cunha BC. New uses of older antibiotics. *Med Clin of North Am* 2001;85:125.
2. Kasten JJ. Clindamycin, metronidazole, and chloramphenicol. *Mayo Clin Proc* 1999; 74:825.
3. Finegold SM. Metronidazole. In: Mandell GL, Bennett JE, Dolin R, eds. *Principles and practice of infectious diseases,* 5th ed. New York: Churchill Livingstone, 2000:361–366.
4. Dow G, Ronald AR. Miscellaneous and antibacterial drugs. In: Root RK, et al., eds. *Clinical infectious diseases: a practical approach.* New York: Oxford University Press, 1999;319–325.
5. Aronoff GR, et al., eds. *Drug prescribing in renal failure: dosing guidelines for adults,* 4th ed. Philadelphia: American College of Physicians, 1999.
6. Medical Letter. The choice of antibacterial drugs. *Med Lett Drugs Ther* 2001;43:69.
7. Medical Letter. Drugs for parasitic infections. *Med Lett Drugs Ther* 2002;44:1.
8. Bartlett JG. Antibiotic associated diarrhea. *N Engl J Med* 2002;346:334.
9. Ahmadsyah I, Salim A. Treatment of tetanus: an open study to compare the efficacy of procaine penicillin and metronidazole. *Br Med J* 1985;291:648.
10. Centers for Disease Control and Prevention. Sexually transmitted disease treatment guidelines 2002. *MMWR Morb Mortal Wkly Rep* 2002;51(RR-6):42–43.
11. Coustan DR. Use of metronidazole in pregnancy. *Pediatr Infect Dis J* 1999;18:79. (See also *N Engl J Med* 2000;342:534.)
12. Falagas ME, et al. Late incidence of cancer after metronidazole use: a matched metronidazole user/non-user study. *Clin Infect Dis* 1998;26:384.
13. Williams CS, Woodcock KR. Do ethanol and metronidazole interact to produce a disulfiram-like infection? *Ann Pharmacother* 2000;34:255.


## R. Rifampin, Rifapentine, and Rifabutin

### RIFAMPIN (RIFADIN) [1–4]

Rifampin, discovered in 1965, inhibits DNA-dependent RNA polymerase by binding to the subunit of the enzyme, thus interfering with protein synthesis [1]. Rifampin is bactericidal. Resistant strains of bacteria have altered RNA polymerase that is not inhibited by rifampin [1].

I. **Spectrum of activity.** Rifampin is a **broad-spectrum** agent active against bacteria, mycobacteria, and chlamydiae [1,2]
   A. **Bacteria.** The *in vitro* activity of rifampin as a single agent is summarized in Table 27R.1.
   B. **Mycobacteria.** Most strains of *Mycobacterium tuberculosis* are susceptible to rifampin, but **resistant strains have been isolated** with greater frequency in recent years [3,4]. The susceptibility of other mycobacteria is variable: *M. kansasii* and *M. marinum* are susceptible, whereas *M. fortuitum* and *M. chelonei* are resistant [1]. (See related discussions in Chapter 11.)
   C. **Chlamydiae.** Many species of *Chlamydia,* particularly *C. trachomatis,* are susceptible.

II. **Resistance. Monotherapy.** Rapid emergence of resistant bacteria occurs with monotherapy [1]. Except for short-term **prophylaxis,** rifampin should not be used alone [1].

III. **Pharmacokinetics and preparations.** Rifampin is red-orange in color in the crystalline state. The **oral** form is well absorbed from the gastrointestinal (GI) tract in the fasting state. In late 1989, an **intravenous preparation** of rifampin became available for use when the oral route is not an option; this preparation should not be given intramuscularly [1,2].

*Adapted from Reese RE, Betts RF. Rifampin, rifapentine, and rifabutin. In: Reese RE, Betts RF, Gumustop B, eds. *Handbook of antibiotics,* 3rd ed. Philadelphia: Lippincott Williams and Wilkins, 2000: 527–541.

Table 27R.1. *In Vitro* Activity of Rifampin

| Organism | $MIC_{90}$ ($\mu$g/mL)[a] |
|---|---|
| **Gram positive** | |
| *Staphylococcus aureus*[b] | 0.015 |
| *S. epidermidis*[b] | 0.015 |
| *Streptococcus pyogenes* | 0.12 |
| *S. pneumoniae (penicillin susceptible)* | 4.0 |
| *Viridans streptococci* | 0.12 |
| *Enterococcus faecalis* | 16.0 |
| *J K diphtheroids* | 0.05 |
| *Listeria monocytogenes* | 0.25 |
| *Clostridium difficile* | ≤0.2 |
| *C. perfringens* | ≤0.1 |
| *Peptococcus, Peptostreptococcus species* | 1.6 |
| *Proprionibacterium acnes* | ≤0.1 |
| **Gram negative** | |
| *Neisseria gonorrhoeae* | 0.5 |
| *N. meningitidis* | 0.12 |
| *Moraxella (Branhamella) catarrhalis* | 0.03 |
| *Haemophilus influenzae* | 0.5 |
| *H. ducreyi* | 0.03 |
| *Legionella pneumophila* | 0.03 |
| *Brucella species* | 1.25 |
| *Escherichia coli* | 16.0 |
| *Klebsiella pneumoniae* | 32.0 |
| *Enterobacter species* | 64.0 |
| *Pseudomonas aeruginosa* | 64.0 |
| *Bacteroides fragilis* | 0.8 |
| *B. melaninogenicus* | 0.2 |

Source: Modified from Craig WA. Rifampin and related drugs. In: Gorbach SL, Bartlett JG, Blacklow NR, eds. *Infectious diseases.* Philadelphia: WB Saunders, 1992:265–266.
[a]$MIC_{90}$ = concentration below which 90% of tested organisms are inhibited.
[b]In most cases, the MIC for methicillin-resistant strains is similar to those for methicillin-susceptible strains (1).

A. **Distribution.** Body fluids and tissue levels are similar to those observed in serum. Therapeutic concentrations are obtained in serum, urine, saliva, bone, pleura, pancreatic juice, and cerebrospinal fluid [1,2].

B. **Metabolism.** Rifampin is cleared from the circulation primarily by hepatic metabolism and biliary excretion. Its half-life is 2 to 5 hours and is prolonged in hepatic disease, perhaps more so with jaundice. **In renal failure,** only modest dose adjustments are advised (see section **VI.B**).

C. **Peak serum concentrations** after an oral dose of 600 mg or 10 mg/kg are variable but usually are in the range of 7 to 15 $\mu$g/mL [1].

IV. **Clinical use.** Rifampin has U.S. Food and Drug Administration approval only for treatment of patients with tuberculosis and carriers of *N. meningitidis* [4].

A. **Tuberculosis.** Rifampin is an important agent in the treatment of *M. tuberculosis* and for some of the atypical mycobacteria [5–7]. Rifampin or rifampin plus pyrazinamide are options for chemoprophylaxis of tuberculosis. One hesitates to use this in contacts of human immunodeficiency virus (HIV)-infected subjects because of the high risk of the index case having infection with multidug resistant *M. tuberculosis* [6–9]. Because of the risk of drug-drug interactions of rifampin in HIV-infected patients on antiretroviral therapy, rifabutin is preferred for these patients (see section **V.D.2** and Chapter 11).

**B. Bacterial meningitis contacts.** Rifampin has been used successfully in eradicating the carrier state of close **contacts of meningococcal or *Haemophilus influenzae* meningitis.** This is one of the rare uses of rifampin as monotherapy, but the use is legitimate because it is used for a very short time. See the rationale and specific recommendations in Chapter 6.

**C. Investigational studies.** When rifampin is used alone for specific infections, resistance rapidly develops. Thus there has been increased interest in the **use of rifampin with other antibiotics to avoid this** and yet take advantage of its excellent *in vitro* activity [10–12].

1. **Methicillin-resistant *Staphylococcus aureus* (MRSA)**
   - a. **MRSA nasal carriage.** Rifampin in combination with a second agent (e.g., trimethoprim-sulfamethoxazole) has been used to try to eradicate nasal carriage of MRSA [13]. Topical nasal mupirocin has also been used to eradicate MRSA nasal carriers [14]. See the related discussion in Chapter 27D.
   - b. **MRSA infections.** Vancomycin is the therapy of choice [5] (see Chapter 27P). There are no data to support the routine addition of rifampin to vancomycin, but if there is an inadequate response to vancomycin alone, then the addition of rifampin, gentamicin, or both should be considered [5]. In his review, Farr [12] emphasized that rifampin resistance has been reported during therapy for MRSA infections with rifampin plus vancomycin, and the addition of gentamicin to the regimen may help prevent the development of rifampin resistance.
2. **Endocarditis.** Rifampin has been studied particularly in **endocarditis** due to *S. aureus* and *S. epidermidis*[12]. For *S. aureus,* there are conflicting *in vitro* data, because antagonism may be seen with combination therapy [15,16]. Infectious disease consultation is advised. Bactericidal levels should be compared before and after adding rifampin. **In the animal model of endocarditis** caused by MRSA, the combination of vancomycin with rifampin was significantly more effective than vancomycin alone [15]. In the same model with *S. epidermidis,* the addition of gentamicin or rifampin to vancomycin was beneficial, even though *in vitro* synergistic studies may not predict a beneficial effect [15]. See related discussions in Chapter 12.
3. ***Legionella* infections.** In severe pneumonia caused by *Legionella pneumophila* or other *Legionella* species, rifampin has often been combined with a macrolide, usually azithromycin, or a fluoroquinolone [5,10]. See related discussion in Chapter 11.
4. **Cerebrospinal fluid shunt infections.** In combination with vancomycin, rifampin has been used to treat staphylococcal coagulase-negative infections [17]. See discussion in Chapter 6.
5. **Chronic osteomyelitis** due to *S. aureus* has been treated with a combination of nafcillin and rifampin [1,2]. This complex and difficult problem is discussed elsewhere [12]. In these difficult cases, infectious disease consultation is advised (see Chapter 5).
6. ***Brucella* infections.** Prolonged therapy with doxycycline plus rifampin has a clinical response similar to that of tetracycline plus streptomycin [1,5,10].
7. **Orthopedic implant infections.** Patients with prosthetic device infections have been treated with rifampin-containing antibiotic combinations [18–20]. In a 1998 report, patients with stable implants and short duration of staphylococcal infection (<21 days) were treated with initial debridement and intravenous antibiotics. If patients could then tolerate long-term therapy with 3 to 6 months therapy of rifampin-ciprofloxacin, cure of the infection without device removal was commonly achieved [20–22]. Only patients with quinolone-susceptible staphylococci should be candidates for this form of therapy [22]. See related discussions in Chapter 5.
8. **Penicillin-resistant *S. pneumoniae* meningitis** merits therapy with vancomycin. Some experts have suggested that rifampin may be added [5]. If cefotaxime or ceftriaxone is used, rifampin in combination may improve results [23] (see Chapters 6, 11, 27C, and 27P).

9. **Miscellaneous uses** include combination therapy with penicillin for eradication of group A streptococcal carrier states and combination regimens for severe cat scratch disease [11].

V. **Adverse reactions.** Adverse reactions of rifampin often are classified into four types [2]:

A. **Immunosuppression.** In animal and *in vitro* studies, rifampin has been shown to suppress the secretion of migration inhibition factor by lymphocytes, the response of lymphocytes to stimulation by nonspecific mitogen, and the production of antibody by cultured lymph node cells. The precise implications of these studies for humans are unclear [12]. In addition, patients tuberculin skin test reactivity may be diminished by rifampin therapy.

B. **Immunologic reactions**

1. **Allergic or hypersensitivity reactions** such as drug fever, skin rashes, and eosinophilia are uncommon.
2. **A flu-like syndrome** with fever, malaise, and headache can occur, particularly with irregular administration. It is very infrequent with daily or twice weekly tuberculosis regimens. Renal failure, thrombocytopenia, hemolysis, and the hepatorenal syndrome can occur in this flu-like syndrome [12]. Interstitial nephritis is a rare complication. Most patients improve with supportive care and withdrawal of the agent. Presumably, the risk of these reactions can be reduced if the doses are given on a regular schedule.
3. **Red-orange coloring of the urine, saliva, feces, sweat, and tears.** The most common side effect observed with rifampin is a harmless orange-red discoloration of the urine (see section **III**). Permanent staining of soft contact lenses can occur during rifampin therapy [1]. Patients should be forewarned of this to prevent unnecessary anxiety.
4. **Hepatotoxicity** has been seen in patients with overdose, prior hepatic disease, and concurrent use of hepatotoxic agents (e.g., halothane anesthesia). For patients with mild liver function test abnormalities, rifampin must be used with caution. Liver function tests ideally should be monitored carefully if the drug is used. For nonmycobacterial infections, if there is no underlying hepatic dysfunction, serial liver function tests are not routinely recommended.
   a. **Isoniazid and rifampin.** There is some concern about whether this combination increases hepatotoxicity. In one review, Craig [1] emphasized that although elevated liver enzyme values are observed in approximately 5% to 10% of recipients of rifampin, "hepatitis occurs in only 0.15% to 0.43%. The incidence of hepatitis rises to 2.5% with multiple drug regimens for tuberculosis. However, most studies suggest that rifampin does not enhance hepatotoxicity of isoniazid" [1].
   b. **Rifampin and pyrazinamide.** The new guidelines for use in treatment of latent tuberculosis infection (+PPD) were published in 2000 [8] (see Chapter 11).
      (1) In these 2000 recommendations, for contacts of patients with isoniazid-resistant rifampin-susceptible tuberculosis, rifampin and pyrazinamide given daily for 2 months was one option [8].
      (2) Unexpected severe hepatotoxicity developed in some recipients. This option is no longer advised for HIV-negative patients [24]. In addition, for those patients who are still candidates for the rifampin-pyrazinamide combination therapy, careful monitoring was advised [24] (see Chapter 11).
5. **Renal injury** is uncommon [12].
6. **Exudative conjunctivitis,** which is reversible with drug cessation, has been reported.

C. **Drug interactions.** Rifampin induces increased hepatic excretion of a number of drugs by stimulating an increase in activity of hepatic microsomal cytochrome P450-related enzymatic reactions and other compounds metabolized by the liver [1,2,12]. The interactions of rifampin have been reviewed in detail [25–28]. The **drugs that may interact with rifampin are summarized from these reports in Tables 27R.2 through 27R.6,** respectively.

Table 27R.2. Previously Described Rifampin Drug Interactions,[a] Part I

| Drug | Comments |
|---|---|
| Anticoagulants, oral[b] | Increase anticoagulant dose based on monitoring of prothrombin time |
| β-Blockers | May need to increase propranolol or metoprolol dose |
| Chloramphenicol | Monitor serum chloramphenicol concentrations; increase dose if needed |
| Contraceptives, oral[b] | Use other forms of birth control; document patient counseling in chart |
| Cyclosporine[b] | Monitor serum cyclosporine concentrations; increased dose will likely be needed |
| Digitoxin[b] | Monitor serum digitoxin concentrations; monitor for arrhythmia control and signs and symptoms of heart failure; increase dose if needed |
| Digoxin | Monitor serum digoxin concentrations; monitor for arrhythmia control and signs and symptoms of heart failure; clinically significant interaction most likely in patients with decreased renal function |
| Glucocorticoids[b] | Increase glucocorticoid dose twofold to threefold with concomitant rifampin therapy |
| Ketoconazole[b] | Avoid this combination if possible; monitor serum ketoconazole concentrations; increase dose if needed; space rifampin and ketoconazole doses by 12 h |
| Methadone[b] | Increase methadone dose with concurrent rifampin therapy; control withdrawal symptoms |
| Phenytoin[b] | Monitor serum phenytoin concentrations; increase phenytoin dose if needed |
| Quinidine[b] | Monitor serum quinidine concentrations; monitor for arrhythmia control; increase dose if needed |
| Sulfonylureas | Increase sulfonylurea dose based on blood glucose control; monitor blood glucose with discontinuation of rifampin therapy |
| Theophylline[b] | Monitor serum theophylline concentrations; increased dose will likely be needed |
| Verapamil[b] | Use alternative agent to verapamil if possible, because even very large increase in oral verapamil may not be sufficient; monitor serum verapamil concentrations; monitor patient for clinical response |

[a]Carefully adjust doses when rifampin is discontinued; enzyme induction effect is gradually reduced over 1–2 weeks. For details see Borcherding SM, Baciewicz AM, Self TH. Update on rifampin drug interactions, II. *Arch Intern Med* 1992;152:711.
[b]Major clinical significance is well established.
From Borcherding SM, Baciewicz AM, Self TH. Update on rifampin drug interactions. *Arch Intern Med* 1992;152:711, with permission.

1. **Antiretroviral therapy.** Of the available rifamycins, rifampin is the most potent CYP450 inducer, followed by rifapentine and then rifabutin, which has substantially less activity as an inducer [28,29]. Although this topic is reviewed in detail elsewhere, a few points deserve special emphasis. Also see related discussions in Chapter 19.
   a. **Protease inhibitors** and **nonnucleside reverse transcriptase inhibitors.** Drug-drug interactions occur with rifamycins, principally because of the induction or inhibition of the cytochrome CYP450 enzyme system. For example, if a protease inhibitor is administered with rifampin, blood

Table 27R.3. Rifampin Drug Interactions,[a] Part II

| Drug | Comments |
|---|---|
| Antacids | May need to space rifampin and aluminum hydroxide doses apart by several hours; more study needed |
| Haloperidol | Monitor serum haloperidol concentrations; alter dosing regimen if needed; limited initial study indicates serum concentrations and half-life are reduced by about 50% |
| Tocainide | Monitor arrhythmia control; increase dose if needed; 1 trial in healthy subjects found nearly 30% decrease in tocainide serum half-life |
| Disopyramide | Monitor arrhythmia control; increase dose if needed; initial study indicates decrease in disopyramide serum half-life of about 50% |
| Propafenone | Monitor plasma propafenone concentrations; monitor arrhythmia control; increase dose if needed |
| Ciprofloxacin | No interaction noted in humans to date; more study needed |
| Dapsone | Decrease serum concentrations; studies needed in patients with *Pneumocystis carinii* pneumonia |
| Fluconazole | May need to increase fluconazole dose; monitor signs and symptoms of infection; one trial in healthy subjects found 22% decrease in fluconazole serum half-life |
| Nifedipine | Monitor clinical response; may need to increase dose; controlled study needed |
| Diltiazem[b] | Consider alternative agent to diltiazem if possible, because even very large increase in oral diltiazem may not be sufficient; may monitor serum diltiazem concentrations (see Table 27R.2 regarding similar interaction with verapamil); monitor clinical response |
| Diazepam | Monitor clinical response; may need to increase diazepam dose; 300% increase in diazepam oral clearance has been reported |

[a]Agents available in the United States; for each interaction, carefully adjust doses when rifampin is discontinued; enzyme induction effect is reduced gradually over 1–2 weeks.
[b]More study needed in patients; probably of major clinical significance.
From Borcherding SM, Baciewicz AM, Self TH. Update on rifampin drug interactions. *Arch Intern Med* 1992;152:711, with permission.

concentrations of the protease inhibitor decrease markedly and most of the antiviral activity decreases as well [29] (see Chapter 19). **Rifabutin is a less potent inducer with less of an effect** on the drug levels of antiretrovirals (Table 27R.5).

b. **Rifabutin is preferred.** Because rifampin markedly lowers the blood levels of these antiretrovirals, which results in suboptimal antiretroviral therapy, rifampin is always contraindicated [29] (see Chapter 19).

c. **Rifapentine** is not recommended as a substitute for rifampin because its safety and effectiveness have not been established for the treatment of patients with HIV-related tuberculosis [29].

2. **Oral contraceptives.** As shown in Table 27R.2, **rifampin impairs the effectiveness of oral contraceptives;** this topic has recently been reviewed [30].

D. **Thrombophlebitis** can occur with the parenteral form [11].

VI. **Dosages and precautions**

A. **Dosages.** Capsules are available in 150- and 300-mg sizes. The oral regimen is preferred and is given 1 hour before or 2 hours after meals. For special needs, a liquid suspension can be made according to the package insert. The same dose per day is given orally or intravenously.

Table 27R.4. Rifampin Drug Interaction,[a] Part III

| Type of Drug | Comments |
|---|---|
| Clarithromycin | Monitor signs and symptoms of infection; more study needed. |
| Delavirdine | Avoid concomitant use if possible. |
| Doxycycline | Monitor clinical response and serum doxycycline concentrations; increased dosage may be needed. |
| Itraconazole | Monitor clinical response; increased dosage will likely be needed. |
| Midazolam | Monitor for decreased efficacy; increase dosage as necessary. |
| Nifedipine | Alternative class of agents should be considered; monitor clinical response; dosage increase may be needed.[b] |
| Nortriptyline | Monitor clinical response and serum nortriptyline concentrations. |
| Pefloxacin | Moderate rifampin induction effect; pending further research, no dosage adjustment recommended. |
| Protease inhibitors | Most significant decreases in serum concentrations seen with saquinavir mesylate, indinavir sulfate, and nelfinavir mesylate; ritonavir appears to have less reduction in serum concentrations; adjust dosage as necessary. |
| Tacrolimus | Monitor serum tacrolimus concentrations and clinical respones; increased dosage may be needed. |
| Triazolam | Monitor for decreased efficacy; incrrease dosage as necessary. |
| Zidovudine | Monitor clinical response; increased dosage may be necessary. |

[a]Carefully adjust dosage when rifampin use is discontinued. Enzyme induction effect is gradually reduced during a 1- to 2-week period or longer. Based on small numbers of reports; further studies are needed for most of these agents.
[b]See also verapamil (Table 27R.2) and diltiazem (Table 27R.3).
From Stayhorn VA, Baciewicz AM, Self TH. Update on rifampin drug interactions, III. *Arch Intern Med* 1997;157:2453, with permission.

1. **Tuberculosis:** A single daily dose of 10 mg/kg up to 600 mg for adults and 10 to 20 mg/kg, not to exceed 600 mg/day, for children is used. The same doses are used in the intermittent regimen [2]. See detailed discussion in Chapter 11.
2. **In meningococcal meningitis and *H. influenzae* meningitis contacts,** dose regimens are discussed in Chapter 16.
3. **Doses for other regimens**
   a. ***S. epidermidis* prosthetic valve endocarditis.** Vancomycin given in combination with rifampin (300 mg every 8 hours) and gentamicin (1.0–1.3 mg/kg every 8 hours) is advocated in adults [31]. All three drugs are given for 2 weeks, and vancomycin and rifampin are continued for an additional 4 weeks (see Chapter 12).
   b. **Prosthetic device infections.** Rifampin 450 mg every 12 hours [16] and 300 mg every 8 to 12 hours have been used (see Chapter 5). Another antibiotic such as ciprofloxacin or vancomycin is always used.

B. **Renal failure.** Dose modifications are suggested [32]. For a creatinine clearance of 10 to 50 mL/min, 50% to 100% of the usual dose is suggested. For a creatinine clearance of less than 10 mL/min or for the patient on chronic ambulatory peritoneal dialysis, 50% of the usual dose is suggested [32].

Table 27R.5. Parcentage by Which Rifampin and Rifabutin Lower the AUC of PIs and NNRTIs

| | Indinavir | Nelfinavir Mesylate | Saquinavir Mesylate | Amprenvir | Ritonavir | Ritonavir and Lopinavir | Efavirenz | Nevirapine | Delavirdine Mesylate |
|---|---|---|---|---|---|---|---|---|---|
| Rifampin | 89 | 32 | 84 | 82 | 35 | 75 | 25 | 34 | 96 |
| Rifabutin | 32 | 32 | 40 | 15 | 0 | 0 | 0 | 16 | 30 |

AUC, area under the concentration–time curve; PI, protease inhibitor; NNRTI, non-nucleoside reverse transcriptase inhibitor.

Table 27R.6 Updated Rifampin Drug Interactions,[a] Part IV

| Type of Drug | Comments |
|---|---|
| **Controlled drug interaction studies** | |
| Selective serotonin receptor ($5\text{-}HT_3$) antagonist | Monitor clinical response, increase dose if needed; use another agent if needed |
| Buspirone hydrochloride | Monitor clinical response; increased dose will likely be needed or use another agent if possible |
| 3-Hydroxy-3-methylglutaryl coenzyme A reductase inhibitors | Monitor lipid panel; increased dose will likely be needed for simvastatin; further research needed for other agents in this class |
| Metronidazole | Monitor for decreased clinical response; increase dose if needed or use another agent if possible |
| Opiates (morphine or codeine) | Monitor pain control and clinical response; increased dose may be needed in extensive metabolizers; use another agent if possible; may be associated with ethnic variability |
| Propafenone hydrochloride | Monitor clinical response; increased dose may be needed or use another agent if possible |
| Tamoxifen citrate or toremifene citrate | Monitor clinical response; increased dose likely needed |
| Zolpidem tartrate | Monitor clinical response; increased dose may be needed or use another agent if possible |
| **Potential interactions based on case reports**[b] | |
| Clozapine | Monitor clinical response; increase dose if needed or use another agent if possible |
| Levothyroxine sodium | Monitor thyrotropin level; increase dose likely needed |
| Sertraline hydrochloride | Monitor clinical response; increase dose if needed |

[a]Carefully adjust dosage when rifampin use is initiated and discontinued. The enzyme induction is gradually reduced during a 1- to 2-week period or longer when rifampin therapy is discontinued. Based on the small number of reports, further studies are needed for most of these agents.
[b]Controlled study is needed to establish the importance and extent of the interaction.

C. **Pregnancy.** Rifampin is a **category C** agent (see Chapter 27A). Rifampin crosses the placenta readily and is teratogenic in animals. There are no adequate and well-controlled studies in pregnant women in terms of the effects on the fetus. The package insert emphasizes that rifampin should be used during pregnancy only if the potential benefits justify the potential risks to the fetus [4]. Rifampin has been used to treat severe cases of tuberculosis in pregnant women [1]. Rifampin is not recommended for pregnant women who are contacts of infected patients with *H. influenzae* meningitis. Pregnant women in close contact with an index case of *N. meningitidis* can be treated with ceftriaxone (see the related discussion in Chapter 6).

D. **Nursing mothers.** Because of the potential for tumorigenicity of rifampin shown in animal studies, a decision should be made whether to discontinue nursing or to discontinue the drug, taking into account the importance of the drug to the mother [4].

E. **Liver disease.** The use of rifampin in patients with liver disease is not recommended except in case of necessity; in such patients, the drug's half-life usually is doubled [1].

F. **Drug interactions** (see section **V.C** and Table 27R.6)

## RIFAPENTINE (PRIFTIN)

Rifapentine (Priftin) **is a long-acting analogue of rifampin** that became available in late 1998 for oral use, with at least one other drug, in the treatment of pulmonary tuberculosis. It inhibits DNA-dependent RNA polymerase [33].

I. **Activity.** Rifapentine is active against *M. tuberculosis,* but strains resistant to rifampin are also resistant to rifapentine. Rifapentine is also active against *M. avium* and *Toxoplasma gondii* [33].

II. **Pharmacokinetics.** Rifapentine is well absorbed, especially when taken with food. It is excreted mostly in the feces (70%). It is metabolized to a desacetyl form that is microbiologically active, contributing 40% of the drug's overall activity [33].

III. **Clinical trials.** Only limited data are available so far about the clinical efficacy of this agent in pulmonary tuberculosis regimens [33]. Further clinical studies are needed before the precise role of this agent is clarified. See related discussions in Chapter 11.

IV. **Dosage.** Tablets of 150 mg are available. The recommended dosage of rifapentine in adults is 600 mg twice weekly (with at least 72 hours between doses) for the first 2 months of therapy and then 600 mg once a week, always in combination with other antituberculosis drugs [33].

V. **Adverse effects.** Like other rifamycins, rifapentine causes red-orange discoloration of body fluids and stains contact lenses. In clinical trials with isoniazid, rates of adverse reactions were similar to those with rifampin and rifapentine. The only adverse effect that occurred more often with rifapentine than with rifampin was hyperuricemia when the drug was given twice weekly [33] (see related discussions under Rifampin, above).

VI. **Drug interactions** (see related discussion in section **V.C** under Rifampin). In terms of other drugs, until further experience is available, it seems prudent to assume rifapentine may have the same drug interactions as rifampin (see above discussion under Rifampin).

VII. **Conclusion.** In its February 1999 review of this agent, the ***Medical Letter* concluded:** "rifapentine has the advantage over rifampin of requiring only twice-weekly doses for initial therapy of tuberculosis and once-weekly doses during the continuous phase of treatment. **It is not clear that rifapentine in the dosages currently recommended is as effective as rifampin. Until more data become available, rifampin is preferred" [33].** We concur with this conclusion (see related discussions in Chapter 11).

## RIFABUTIN (ANSAMYCIN)

**Rifabutin (Mycobutin)** [34–43] is a semisynthetic ansamycin approved in 1992 for the prevention of disseminated *Mycobacterium avium* complex (MAC) in patients with advanced HIV infection [39]. It also is used in regimens to treat disseminated MAC [5]. Because of the concerns with drug-drug interactions in HIV-infected patients on antiretroviral drugs, rifabutin is preferred over rifampin in therapy of tuberculosis [29] (see section **V.B.2** under Rifampin). Rifabutin is active against most strains of MAC isolated from HIV-positive and HIV-negative people. The minimal inhibitory concentration $(MIC)_{†90}$ of MAC is typically approximately 2 μg/mL [1]. Rifabutin is also active against all rifampin-sensitive *M. tuberculosis* strains and about one-third of rifampin-resistant strains [12].

I. **Pharmacokinetics.** The drug is taken up by all tissues and is especially concentrated in the lungs, where levels may be 10 times higher than in the serum [12]. Rifabutin has excellent solubility in lipids, which results in good intracellular penetration; cerebrospinal fluid concentrations are about 50% of those in the serum [42].
   A. **Bioavailability.** Rifabutin is absorbed rapidly, and absolute bioavailability is in the range of approximately 20% [1].
   B. **Metabolism** is similar to that for rifampin. The elimination half-life is long (45 hours), and as a result of a very large volume of distribution, average plasma concentrations remain relatively low after repeated standard doses [34]. Animal models suggest rifabutin has less of an effect on hepatic microsomal enzyme activity than rifampin [28,29] (see section **V.B** under Rifampin).

II. **Clinical studies**
   A. **Therapy of *M. tuberculosis* in HIV-infected patients on antiretroviral drugs.** (See related discussion in section **IV.A** and **V.C** under Rifampin.) In these patients, rifabutin is preferred [28,29].
   B. **MAC. [39,42]** Rifabutin is used as an **alternative regimen to prevent MAC** in patients with HIV infection. This topic has been reviewed elsewhere [39], but

prophylaxis should be considered for HIV-infected adults and adolescents who have $CD4^+$ lymphocyte counts of less than 50/$mm^3$. **Clarithromycin or azithromycin are the preferred prophylactic agents** with rifabutin as an alternate. Because the combination of clarithromycin and rifabutin is no more effective than clarithromycin alone and is associated with a higher rate of adverse effects than either agent alone, this combination should not be used [39]. Disseminated MAC should be ruled out before starting prophylaxis (i.e., with a negative blood culture for mycobacterium). Because treatment with rifabutin could result in the development of resistance to rifampin in persons who have active tuberculosis, tuberculosis should be excluded before rifabutin is used for prophylaxis [39].

**C. MAC therapy.** Rifabutin has also been used **in therapeutic regimens** for disseminated MAC in patients with acquired immunodeficiency syndrome [5,36,38]. Infectious disease consultation is advised.

**III. Dosages.** A 150-mg capsule is available.

**A. MAC prophylaxis.** When patients with advanced HIV cannot tolerate clarithromycin or azithromycin, 300 mg administered orally once daily is recommended [39]. If there is a propensity to nausea, vomiting, or other GI upset, 150 mg twice daily is given with meals.

**B. Treatment of disseminated MAC** with rifabutin 300 to 450 mg orally daily has been suggested, along with clarithromycin or azithromycin and/or ethambutol and/or ciprofloxacin [5,40,42]. Because of the potential side effects at higher doses (see section **IV**), 300 mg/day of rifabutin may be a rational compromise [41]. Infectious disease consultation is suggested. For *M. tuberculosis,* see regimens in Chapter 11.

**C. Pediatric use.** The safety and effectiveness of rifabutin for prophylaxis of MAC in children have not been established, per the package insert. However, preliminary recommendations suggest consideration of rifabutin for children infected with HIV and depressed $CD4^+$ cell counts who cannot tolerate clarithromycin or azithromycin [39,42]. Candidates for prophylaxis include the following $CD4^+$ thresholds (cells/$\mu$L): children 6 years of age or more, less than 50; children aged 2 to 6 years, less than 75; children aged 1 to 2 years, less than 500; and children below 12 months of age, less than 750 [39]. A liquid formulation of rifabutin is under development. The drug can be mixed with foods such as applesauce for administration to children [42]. A dosage of 5 mg/kg of rifabutin has been used per package insert.

**D. Pregnancy.** Rifabutin is viewed as a **category B** agent (see Chapter 27A). The package insert suggests that rifabutin should be used in pregnant women only if the potential benefit justifies the potential risk to the fetus. Chemoprophylaxis for MAC should be administered to pregnant women and other adults and adolescents [39]. However, because of general concern about administering drugs during the first trimester of pregnancy, some providers may choose to withhold prophylaxis during the first trimester. **Azithromycin is the agent of choice for prevention of MAC in pregnancy** (see Chapter 27N). Experience with rifabutin in this setting is limited [39].

**E. Nursing mothers.** It is not known whether rifabutin is excreted in human breast milk. The package insert suggests that a decision should be made about whether to continue nursing or discontinue rifabutin, taking into account the importance of the drug to the mother. (See Chapter 27N regarding the association between macrolide use in infants and hypertrophic pyloric stenosis.)

**F. In renal failure** no dosage modifications are necessary. Neither hemodialysis nor chronic ambulatory peritoneal dialysis requires dosage adjustment [32].

**G. In hepatic dysfunction,** the package insert does not currently advise any dosage modifications.

**IV. Side effects.** Rifabutin is generally well tolerated at the prophylaxis dose of 300 mg/day. Rash, GI intolerance, and neutropenia are seen in 2% to 4% of recipients [4]. In therapeutic regimens for MAC and at higher doses (e.g., 600 mg/day or more), adverse effects can be seen in most patients, especially leukopenia, GI intolerance, diffuse polyarthralgia syndrome (19%), and **anterior uveitis** (6%) [41,43]. Use of rifabutin may cause an orange-brown discoloration of urine, feces, saliva, tears, and soft contact lenses [42].

Rifabutin is metabolized in the liver and induces activity of the hepatic cytochrome P450 enzyme group, which may lead to pharmacokinetic interaction with other drugs administered concurrently [42]. The extent to which this occurs, compared with rifampin, is discussed in section **V.D** under Rifampin. Concurrent administration of fluconazole or clarithromycin can increase serum concentrations of rifabutin by 60% to 100% and potentially increase toxicity (e.g., increase the risk of uveitis) [43].

**V. Investigational uses.** Rifabutin is undergoing clinical investigation for the treatment of Crohn disease [44]. It is also being used in multiple drug regimens designed to treat difficult to eradicate *H. pylori* infections [45].

## REFERENCES


1. Craig WA. Rifampin and related drugs. In: Gorbach SL, Bartlett JG, Blacklow NR, eds. *Infectious diseases.* Philadelphia: WB Saunders, 1992:265–271.
2. Reese RE, Betts RF. Rifampin and rifabutin. In: Reese RE, Betts RF, Gumustop B, eds. *Handbook of antibiotics,* 3rd ed. Philadelphia: Lippincott Williams & Wilkins, 2000;527–541.
3. Freiden TR, et al. The emergence of drug-resistant tuberculosis in New York City. *N Engl J Med* 1993;328:522.
4. *Physicians' desk reference,* 56th ed. Montvale, NJ: Medical Economics Data, 2000:765–772, 2838–2840.
5. Medical Letter. The choice of antibacterial drugs. *Med Lett Drugs Ther* 2001;43:69.
6. American Thoracic Society and Centers for Disease Control. Treatment of tuberculosis and tuberculosis infection in adults and children. *Am J Resp Crit Care Med* 1994;149:1359.
7. Horsburgh CR Jr, Feldman S, Ridzon R. Practice guidelines for the treatment of tuberculosis. *Clin Infect Dis* 2000;31:633.
8. American Thoracic Society and Centers for Disease Control and Prevention. Targeted tuberculosis testing and treatment of latent tuberculosis infection. *Am J Resp Crit Care Med* 2000;161[Suppl]:S221–S247.
9. Van Scoy RE, Wilkowske CJ. Antimycobacterial therapy. *Mayo Clin Proc* 1999; 74:1038.
10. Morris AB, et al. Use of rifampin in nonstaphylococcal, nonmycobacterial disease. *Antimicrob Agents Chemother* 1993;37:1.
11. Loeffler AM. Uses of rifampin for infections other than tuberculosis. *Pediatr Infect Dis J* 1999;18:631.
12. Farr BM. Rifamycins. In: Mandell GL, Bennett JE, Dolin R, eds. *Principles and practice of infectious diseases,* 5th ed. New York: Churchill Livingstone, 2000: 348–361.
13. Mulligan ME, et al. Methicillin-resistant *Staphylococcus aureus*: a consensus review of the microbiology, pathogenesis, and epidemiology with implications for prevention and management. *Am J Med* 1993;94:313.
14. Wenzel RP, et al. Methicillin-resistant *Staphylococcus aureus* outbreak: a consensus panel's definition and management guidelines. *Am J Infect Control* 1998;26: 102.
15. Fantin B, Carbon C. *In vivo* antibiotic synergism: contribution of animal models. *Antimicrob Agents Chemother* 1992;36:907.
16. Kaatz GW, et al. Ciprofloxacin and rifampin, alone and in combination, for therapy of experimental *Staphylococcus aureus* endocarditis. *Antimicrob Agents Chemother* 1989;33:1184.
17. Bisno AL, Sternau L. Infections of central nervous system shunts. In: Bisno AL, Waldvogel FA, eds. *Infections associated with indwelling devices.* Washington, DC: ASM Press, 1994;91–109.
18. Widner AF, et al. Antimicrobial treatment of orthopedic implant-related infections with rifampin combinations. *Clin Infect Dis* 1992;14:1251.
19. Drancourt M, et al. Oral rifampin plus ofloxacin for treatment of staphylococcal-infected orthopedic implants. *Antimicrob Agents Chemother* 1993;37:1214.
20. Zimmerli W, et al. Role of rifampin for treatment of orthopedic implant-related staphylococcal infections: a randomized controlled trial. *JAMA* 1998;279:1537.

21. Konig DP, et al. Treatment of staphylococcal implant infection with rifampin-ciprofloxacin in stable implants. *Arch Orthop Trauma Surg* 2001;121:297.
22. Zavasky DM, Sande MA. Reconsideration of rifampin: a unique drug for a unique infection. *JAMA* 1998;279:1575.
23. Bradley JS, Scheld WM. The challenge of penicillin-resistant *Streptococcus pneumoniae* meningitis: current antibiotic therapy in the 1990s. *Clin Infect Dis* 1997;24[Suppl]:S213.
24. Centers for Disease Control and Prevention. Update: fatal and severe liver injuries associated with rifampin and pyrazinamide for latent tuberculosis infection and revisions in the American Thoracic Society/CDC recommendations—United States, 2001. *MMWR Morb Mortal Wkly Rep* 2001;50:733.
25. Baciewicz AM, et al. Update on rifampin drug interactions. *Arch Intern Med* 1987;147: 565.
26. Borcherding SM, Baciewicz AM, Self TH. Update on rifampin drug interactions. II. *Arch Intern Med* 1992;152:711.
27. Stayhorn VA, Baciewicz AM, Self TH. Update on rifampin drug interactions. III. *Arch Intern Med* 1997;157:2453.
28. Finch CK, et al. Rifampin and rifabutin drug interactions. *Arch Intern Med* 2002;162: 985.
29. Centers for Disease Control and Prevention. Prevention and treatment of tuberculosis among patients infected with the human immunodeficiency virus: principles of therapy and revised recommendations. *MMWR Morb Mortal Wkly Rep* 1998;47(RR-20):11–15.
30. Dickinson DD, et al. Drug interactions between oral contraceptives and antibiotics. *Obstet Gynecol* 2001;98:853.
31. Wilson W, et al. Antibiotic treatment of adults with infective endocarditis due to streptococci, enterococci, staphylococci, and HACEK microorganisms. *JAMA* 1995;274: 1706.
32. Aronoff GR, et al. *Drug prescribing in renal failure: dosing guidelines for adults,* 4th ed. Philadelphia: American College of Physicians, 1999.
33. Medical Letter. Rifapentine: a long-acting rifamycin for tuberculosis. *Med Lett Drugs Ther* 1999;41:21.
34. Skinner MH, Blaschke TF. Clinical pharmacokinetics of rifabutin. *Clin Pharmacokinet* 1995;28:115.
35. Brogden RN, Fitton A. Rifabutin: a review of its antimicrobial activity, pharmacokinetic properties and therapeutic efficacy. *Drugs* 1994;47:983.
36. Medical Letter. Rifabutin. *Med Lett Drugs Ther* 1993;35:36.
37. Gordin FM, et al. Rifabutin: the research continues. *Clin Infect Dis* 1996;22[Suppl]:S1–S61.
38. Sullam PM, et al. Efficacy of rifabutin in the treatment of disseminated infection due to *Mycobacterium avium* complex. *Clin Infect Dis* 1994;19:84.
39. USPHS/IDSA guidelines for the prevention of opportunistic infections among HIV-infected persons–2002. *MMWR Morb Mortal Wkly Rep* 2002;51(RR-8):8–11.
40. Medical Letter. Drugs for AIDS and associated infections. *Med Lett Drugs Ther* 1995;37:87, and 1997;39:14–16.
41. Griffith DE, et al. Adverse events associated with high-dose rifabutin in macrolide-containing regimens for the treatment of *Mycobacterium avium* complex lung disease. *Clin Infect Dis* 1995;21:594.
42. McFenson LM. Rifabutin. *Pediatr Clin Infect Dis J* 1998;17:71.
43. Khan MA, et al. Rifabutin-induced uveitis with inflammatory vitreous infiltrate. *Eye* 2000;14:344.
44. Gui GP, et al. Two-year outcomes analysis of Crohn's disease treated with rifabutin and macrolide antibiotics. *J Antimicrob Chemother* 1997;39:393.
45. Bock H, et al. Rifabutin-based triple therapy after failure of *Helicobacter pylori* eradication treatment: preliminary experience. *J Clin Gastroenterol* 2000;31:222.

## S. Spectinomycin

Spectinomycin (Trobicin) was approved in 1971. The structure of spectinomycin is similar, but not identical, to aminoglycosides and inhibits ribosomal protein synthesis. It is bactericidal against gonococci. **Spectinomycin is used only as an alternative agent for *Neisseria gonorrhoeae*** [1–4].

I. **Indications.** Alternative regimens for gonococcal infections (see Chapter 16).

A. **Uncomplicated urethral, endocervical, or rectal infections.** When the drugs of choice (cephalosporin or quinolone) cannot be used, spectinomycin is an alternative [1–4]. It is active against penicillin-resistant strains of gonococci. In published trials, cure rates of 98.2% of uncomplicated urogenital and anorectal injections have been achieved with spectinomycin [2].

B. **Treatment of gonococcal infections in pregnancy.** Pregnant women who cannot tolerate cephalosporins can be treated with spectinomycin [2].

C. **Disseminated gonococcal infections.** Patients who are allergic to $\beta$-lactams and quinolones (or for whom quinolones are contraindicated) can be treated with spectinomycin [2].

II. **Contraindications and limitations to use** [1–4]

A. **Pharyngeal gonococcal infection.** Spectinomycin **is ineffective** against this infection, probably because the drug is not secreted in saliva in adequate concentrations.

B. **Incubating syphilis. Spectinomycin will not abort incubating syphilis** and may actually prolong the incubation period. Thus **syphilis serology** at the time of treatment and again in 2 to 3 months to rule out this associated diagnosis is indicated.

C. **Nonspecific urethritis** (nongonococcal urethritis). At least 50% of cases that are not susceptible to spectinomycin are due to *Clostridium trachomatis*.

III. **Actual or potential resistance.** Spectinomycin does not produce sustained high bactericidal levels in blood. Resistant strains have occurred in the United States and elsewhere [4]. Prior data suggest that extensive use of spectinomycin in initial gonococcal therapy might lead to the emergence of spectinomycin-resistant gonorrhea [5]. Careful use of spectinomycin has also been emphasized in a report by Boslego et al. [6]. After only 3 years of using spectinomycin as the primary treatment for uncomplicated gonococcal urethritis in U.S. military men in the Republic of Korea, more than 8% of recipients were treatment failures [6] (see Chapter 16).

IV. **Route and dosage.** Spectinomycin **intramuscularly** is well absorbed. In uncomplicated anogenital gonococcal infection, 2 g spectinomycin is given as a single dose in men or women and in children, 40 mgkg (maximum 2 g) [2]. As an alternative agent in disseminated gonococcal infection, 2 g intramuscularly every 12 hours can be used [2]; optimal duration is not well defined, but a 7-day course seems prudent [2].

**In renal failure,** no dose adjustment is required. Neither hemodialysis nor chronic ambulatory peritoneal dialysis removes spectinomycin [7]. It is relatively expensive (see Appendix Table).

V. **Toxicity** appears very limited, perhaps because the total dose is low. There are no known serious adverse reactions.

VI. **Conclusions.** Spectinomycin has a **limited but useful role in gonococcal infections.** The best use of this agent is in the treatment of gonorrhea in persons who cannot tolerate or be treated with cephalosporins or quinolones [2].

### REFERENCES

1. Medical Letter. The choice of antibacterial drugs. *Med Lett Drugs Ther* 1999;41:95.
2. Centers for Disease Control and Prevention. 1998 Sexually transmitted disease treatment guidelines. *MMWR Morb Mortal Wkly Rep* 2002;51(RR-6):37–39.
3. Gilbert DN. Aminoglycosides. In: Mandell GL, Bennett JE, Dolin R, eds. *Principles and practice of infectious diseases*, 5th ed. New York: Churchill Livingstone, 2000.

4. Reese RE, Betts RF. Spectinomycin. In: Reese RE, Betts RF, eds. *A practical approach to infectious diseases,* 4th ed. Boston: Little, Brown, 1996:1346–1347.
5. Karney WW, et al. Spectinomycin versus tetracycline for the treatment of gonorrhea. *N Engl J Med* 1987;296:889.
6. Boslego JW, et al. Effect of spectinomycin use on the prevalence of spectinomycin-resistant and the penicillinase-producing *Neisseria gonorrhoeae*. *N Engl J Med* 1987;317: 272.
7. Aronoff GR, et al. *Drug prescribing in renal failure,* 4th ed. Philadelphia: American College of Physicians, 1999.

## T. Urinary Antiseptics

**Urinary antiseptics** are agents that concentrate in the urine but do not produce therapeutic levels in the serum. Therefore these agents are useful only in the **prevention or therapy of lower urinary tract infection** (UTI) but are not indicated for pyelonephritis or associated systemic infection [1–3]. This unique feature has **advantages, including** reduced suppression of normal flora compared with other antimicrobials used for UTI, decreased rates of resistance, low rates of yeast overgrowth, and minimization of teratogenic risk and fetal toxicity [3].

**I. Nitrofurantoin** inhibits various enzymes within bacteria, and nitrofurantoin intermediates also damage DNA directly, leading to DNA strand breakage [2,3].

**A. Spectrum of activity.** Nitrofurantoin is active against most *Escherichia coli, Enterobacter* and *Klebsiella* species. *Pseudomonas* species are resistant, as are most *Proteus* species. Nitrofurantoin also is active against gram-positive bacteria that sometimes produce a UTI, such as enterococci or coagulase-negative staphylococci [1–3]. Of note, some isolates of vancomycin-resistant enterococci remain susceptible to nitrofurantoin, and this agent may be useful in the treatment of selected patients with lower UTI caused by this difficult to treat organism. Infectious diseases consultation is recommended for these patients.

**B. Pharmacokinetics.** Nitrofurantoin is well absorbed from the gastrointestinal (GI) tract, but it **does not reach therapeutic concentrations in tissue, only in urine.** Bioavailability increases when taken with food. Therapeutic **urinary concentrations** of the drug are present for up to 6 hours. Tubular reabsorption provides levels in renal medullary tissue. The liver is the principal site of metabolic inactivation [2,3].

**The drug is contraindicated in renal failure** (i.e., creatinine clearance of less than 50 mLmin) [4] because adequate urinary antibiotic levels may not be achieved and serum levels increase in renal failure, presumably increasing the toxicity of this agent. In alkaline urine, the antibacterial effect of nitrofurantoin is decreased; therefore the urine should not be alkalinized [2].

**C. Resistance.** Nitrofurantoin's *in vitro* activity has remained stable despite four decades of use. This has been explained in part by its broad mechanisms of action, high oral bioavailability, and low concentrations at mucosal surfaces [3].

**D. Preparations.** All are equally active, and sections **1** and **2** below have similar pharmacokinetics.

1. **Furadantin** is the **microcrystalline** form and has been available since 1953.
2. **Macrodantin** is the macrocrystalline form. It appears to be associated with a **lower incidence of GI side effects** [2]. This is the preferred agent.
3. **Nitrofurantoin monohydrate** (75 mg) macrocrystals (25 mg) (Macrobid) is a slow-release formulation, in a capsule, equivalent to 100 mg nitrofurantoin.
4. An intravenous preparation of nitrofurantoin is no longer available.

**E. Uses.** Nitrofurantoin is used in the treatment of susceptible uncomplicated (lower) UTI or the prophylaxis of recurrent UTI [1–3,5]. Cure rates for lower UTI range from 70% to 95%. Nitrofurantoin **should not be used for symptomatic upper UTI or complex UTI** in which therapeutic levels of antibiotic may not be attained at the site of infection [1–3].

1. **Therapy** for 3 to 7 days at 100 mg twice daily taken with meals in adults with normal renal function is suggested [3]. **In children** older than 1 month of age, 5 to 7 mg/kg/day is given in divided doses four times a day, commonly for 7 days. **Therapy in pregnancy** is discussed in section **5**. In lower UTI due to **susceptible enterococci,** nitrofurantoin may provide an alternative **agent** for the ampicillin-allergic patient [5].
2. **UTI prophylaxis.** Macrodantin has been given daily at bedtime or after coitus as a single 50- or 100-mg dose to women with recurrent uncomplicated UTI (see Chapter 15). In children older than 1 month of age, 1 to 2 mg/kg/day in one daily dose has been used. Prolonged use requires periodic clinical assessment for pulmonary and neurologic toxicity as well as complete blood count and transaminase determinations [3] (see section **F**).
3. **If creatinine clearance** is less than 50 mL/min, **the drug is contraindicated** [4] (see section **B**).
4. **In hepatic failure,** the drug should be avoided because of its association with hepatotoxicity.
5. **In pregnancy,** caution should be used; this is a **category B agent** (see Chapter 27A). This topic has been reviewed elsewhere [3,6]. Nitrofurantoin is considered a safe and effective agent when ampicillin (amoxicillin) cannot be used because of allergies or resistance. However, a single 200-mg dose of nitrofurantoin for asymptomatic bacteriuria has been associated with a failure rate of 27%, similar to other single dose failure rates. Symptomatic bacteriuria (acute cystitis) or relapse after single dose has been treated with nitrofurantoin 100 mg two to four times a day for 3 to 7 days [3,6]; more experience is available with 7 days [6]. Follow-up urine cultures are important. Suppressive therapy may be indicated if a repeat course of therapy does not sterilize the urine [6]. Nitrofurantoin is safe in pregnancy postcoital or nightly at a dose of 50 mg [3].

F. **Toxicity**. The side effects of nitrofurantoin have been well documented and reviewed in detail elsewhere [7]. **GI irritation** is the **most common** side effect, with anorexia, nausea, and vomiting. This may be decreased by using the macrocrystalline preparation (Macrodantin) and may be dose related [1,3]. Serious adverse reactions have occurred at approximately 28 per million treatment courses [3,7]. **Because major adverse events are more common in the elderly,** with reduced renal function of aging, we agree with the recommendation that **nitrofurantoin is rarely warranted in people 60 years of age or more** [3]. The **frequency** of these **serious adverse reactions** in more than 120 million treatment courses is shown in Table 27T.1; some reactions are fatal.

Table 27T.1. Nitrofurantion and Serious Adverse Events

| Adverse Event | Patients Worldwide | Incidence[a] (Reactions/Million Treatment Courses) |
|---|---|---|
| Acute pulmonary | 1,138 | 9.4 |
| Subacute pulmonary | 22 | 0.2 |
| Chronic pulmonary | 281 | 2.3 |
| Miscellaneous pulmonary | 283 | 2.3 |
| Hepatic | 312 | 2.6 |
| Neurologic | 847 | 7.0 |
| Hematologic | 500 | 4.1 |
| Total | 3,383 | 27.8 |

[a]Based on 121.43 million courses of therapy.
From Darcy P. Nitrofurantoin. *Drug Intell Clin Pharmac* 1985;19:540–547; and Dow G, Ronald AR. Miscellaneous drugs. In: Root RK, et al., eds. *Clinical infectious disease: a practical approach.* New York: Oxford University Press, 1999, with permission.

1. **Pulmonary reactions are the most common severe problem** [1–3,7,8].
   a. **Acute pneumonitis** with fever, cough, and eosinophilia may occur after a few hours or days of therapy. On chest roentgenography, pulmonary alveolar-interstitial infiltrates or pleural fluid is seen. This pneumonitis probably is hypersensitivity phenomenon and is rapidly reversible by discontinuing treatment. Acute reactions do not generally progress to chronic reactions [1–3]. Corticosteroids may be used in patients with severe reactions [3].
   b. **Subacute** presentations are less likely to have fever and eosinophilia and are slower to resolve. **Chronic** pulmonary reactions with interstitial infiltrates are rare and occur when the drug has been prescribed for more than 6 months [3]. This latter syndrome has an **insidious onset** (malaise, cough, dyspnea on exertion). Fever and eosinophilia are seen less frequently. This reaction presumably represents a cumulative toxic drug effect. In some cases, improvement occurs with discontinuation [1–3]. A beneficial effect of corticosteroid therapy has not been convincingly demonstrated in patients with chronic nitrofurantoin pulmonary reactions [2]. Histopathology reveals chronic pneumonitis and fibrosis [3].
2. **Polyneuropathies** (ascending sensorimotor) with demyelination and degeneration of sensory and motor nerves may occur, more often in patients with renal failure or on chronic therapy [1–3]. The mechanisms are unclear, but it is believed to be related to a direct toxic effect of the drug. Sensory symptoms usually begin within 6 weeks of starting therapy followed by motor neuropathy; total recovery occurs in one-third of cases, with partial recovery in one-half [3]. **The drug should be stopped if early signs of a neuritis, such as paresthesias, develop.**
3. **Hepatic reactions** are rare and of two types [1–3].
   a. **Acute cholestatic hepatitis** with fever, rash, eosinophilia, and jaundice. This appears to be immunologically mediated and resolves with discontinuation of nitrofurantoin [1–3].
   b. **Chronic active hepatitis** has an insidious onset after prolonged therapy (more than 6 months). Recovery is seen in most patients if the nitrofurantoin is discontinued.
   c. **Monthly liver function tests** for patients on chronic nitrofurantoin are suggested by some [9].
4. **Bone marrow depression** or megaloblastic anemia may occur. **In patients with glucose-6-phosphate dehydrogenase deficiency, acute hemolysis may be precipitated.** However, based on one report, clinically important hemolytic reactions appear to be rare [10].
5. **Maculopapular rashes, urticaria, and angioneurotic edema** occur in 1% to 5% of recipients [3]; these resolve rapidly with discontinuation of therapy.
6. **In children,** there has been concern that the side effects of nitrofurantoin may outweigh the benefits. However, it has been concluded that **serious adverse reactions in children are rare** and that most patients recovered from their reactions once the drug was discontinued. Therefore **nitrofurantoin remains potentially useful** in pediatric patients [11,12].

G. **Contraindications to use** [3]
   1. **Renal insufficiency** (see section **I.B**)
   2. **Children less than 1 month** of age (nitrofurantoin can cause hemolysis)
   3. **Pregnant woman near delivery** (to avoid transplacental transfer at the time of birth)

II. **Methenamine** [2,3] is not an active antibacterial agent but has been used as a urinary antiseptic since 1895 [3]. It has the advantage of economy, tolerability, minimal effect on GI flora, and absence of bacterial resistance [3]. With the emergence of bacterial resistance, this is a **potentially useful UTI suppressive agent.**

A. **Mechanism of action.** Under acid pH, methenamine is hydrolyzed to form formaldehyde and ammonia. **Formaldehyde is the active agent** that yields protein denaturation. It is bacteriostatic at low and bactericidal at higher levels [3]. Formaldehyde formation depends on several factors:

1. **Acid environment.** For hydrolysis to occur, an acid pH is required. Ideally, the **urine pH must be 6.0 or less [2].** In many patients, in the absence of diuresis, the pH of the urine is low enough to liberate free formaldehyde. Fluid restriction may also help (see section **D**).
2. **Kinetics.** At least 2 to 3 hours are necessary to generate adequate concentrations of formaldehyde. Therefore **in a patient with a chronic indwelling bladder catheter, it is not surprising that it is ineffective** [13]. However, this agent may be helpful for patients with prostatic hypertrophy where retention provides adequate contact time. The same is true for preventing UTI in patients with neurogenic bladders who are in a program of intermittent catheterization and bladder retraining [14].
3. **High dosage.** Adequate doses of methenamine are needed to provide sufficient formaldehyde.

**B. Spectrum of activity.** If sufficient formaldehyde is generated, **all bacteria are susceptible, and** bacteria do not become resistant.

**C. Pharmacokinetics.** Methenamine is well absorbed from the GI tract and is excreted into the urine. Under ideal urine pH, only 2% to 20% is converted into free formaldehyde. Because ammonia is also generated, **the agent is contraindicated in hepatic insufficiency** [2].

**D. Preparations available.** Therapeutically available agents combine methenamine with acids to help acidify the urine. These include methenamine mandelate (Mandelamine) and methenamine hippurate (Hiprex or Urex). However, in the usual recommended doses, these organic acids generally are inadequate to acidify the urine [2]. Methenamine alone has been given with large doses of ascorbic acid (2–6 g daily) to achieve the desired result.

**Fluid restriction** has been suggested as a more useful method **to acidify urine.** This acts to reduce voiding frequency, acidify the urine, and allow more formaldehyde generation. **Patients should be asked to reduce voiding frequency and restrict fluids to 1,200 to 1,500 mL/day so that the urine specific gravity is maintained at a level of 1.015 or greater** [3].

**E. Uses.** Methenamine and ascorbic acid (or methenamine hippurate [15]) are used primarily in **chronic suppressive therapy** for patients without an indwelling catheter. They are **not indicated for acute UTI.** This regimen may be particularly useful in partial obstruction. **It is important to sterilize the urine initially with another agent** [16]. In UTI due to *Proteus* species it may be impossible to achieve adequate pH levels because of the high urinary pH generated.

**F. Dosage**

1. In **adults,** 1 g of methenamine mandelate or methenamine hippurate orally two to four times a day. Fluid restriction is useful to provide adequate acidification (see section **D**). Ascorbic acid (e.g., 1 g orally four times a day) may be given in an attempt to acidify the urine adequately and keep the pH less than or equal to 6.0. Ideally, urine pH should be monitored daily or every other day. Higher doses of ascorbic acid may be necessary when reduction of the pH to 6 is not achieved with 4 to 6 g daily.
2. **For children between 6 and 12 years of age**, the dose is 500 mg to 1 g twice daily. A suspension (methenamine mandelate 500 mg/5 mL) is available for younger children; for children less than 6 years of age, the usual dose is 250 mg per 30 pounds of body weight orally four times a day [2].
3. **In renal failure,** limited guidelines are available. Methenamine alone is nontoxic and urinary methenamine is readily converted to formaldehyde in the azotemic state [3]. Methenamine-acid combinations are not advised if the creatinine clearance is less than 50 mL/min [4]. They may exacerbate acidosis or precipitate in renal tubules.
4. **In patients with gout or hyperuricemia, these agents should be avoided.** Acidification of the urine and the use of acid salts may promote uric acid crystals and calculi formation.
5. **Methenamine and sulfonamides contraindicated.** The latter may precipitate when formaldehyde is released (see Chapter 27L).

6. **In hepatic insufficiency, methenamine should not be used** because of the ammonia produced [2], which may induce or exacerbate hepatic encephalopathy.
7. **In pregnancy,** the safety of methenamine and its salts has not been established [3].

G. **Toxicity.** Methenamine generally is well tolerated, especially in children [3]. Minor GI side effects, such as gastric discomfort, nausea, and vomiting, occur, especially at high doses. With prolonged high doses, some patients note urinary frequency, dysuria, and hematuria, perhaps due to formaldehyde irritating the mucosal lining of the genitourinary tract. The dysuria often diminishes with continued use as the mucosa becomes less sensitive.

III. **Fosfomycin tromethamine (Monurol)** was approved in the United States in 1997 **for single dose oral treatment of uncomplicated susceptible** *Escherichia coli* and *Enteroccocus faecalis* **UTI in women.** The drug interferes with the formation of bacterial cell wall [17].

A. **Spectrum of activity.** Fosfomycin is moderately active *in vitro* against *E. coli* and many other gram-negative bacteria, as well as some strains of *S. saprophyticus* and most enterococci [17,18] that cause community-acquired uncomplicated UTI. In addition, vancomycin-resistant enterococci are susceptible to fosfomycin [19,20]. *Pseudomonas* species are usually, but not always, resistant [17].

B. **Pharmacokinetics.** Oral fosfomycin is rapidly absorbed and is excreted unchanged in the urine, reaching bactericidal concentrations that persist for 24 to 48 hours or longer [3,17,21].

C. **Clinical trials.** There are three randomized trials in women with uncomplicated UTI comparing a single 3-g dose of fosfomycin with nitrofurantoin (50 mg four times a day for 7 days) or norfloxacin (400 mg twice daily for 5 days) or cephalexin (500 mg four times a day for 5 days). Eradication rates with fosfomycin were similar to those with norfloxacin and nitrofurantoin and superior to those with cephalexin [17]. Additional data in more than 1,000 patients found that a single dose of fosfomycin was less effective than 7 days of ciprofloxacin or 10 days of trimethoprim-sulfamethoxazole [17].

D. **Dosage. A single oral dose of 3 g is used** for uncomplicated UTI in women over age 17. The $25 cost to the pharmacist [17] is more expensive than 3 days of standard therapy (see Chapter 15). The dose that has been used in *Pseudomonas* infection is 1 sachet every other day for 3 days.

1. **Pediatric use.** Safety and efficacy in children under 12 years of age have not been established.
2. **In renal failure,** no special recommendations are available in the 2002 package insert [4].
3. **Pregnancy.** This is a **category B** agent (see Chapter 27A). There are no adequate and well-controlled studies in pregnant women per the package insert.
4. **Nursing.** The package insert indicates it is not known whether fosfomycin is excreted into human breast milk; a decision should be made about whether to discontinue nursing or not after administering the drug, taking into account the importance of the drug to the mother.

E. **Adverse effects.** Fosfomycin is generally well tolerated, with diarrhea the most common side effect (9%). Vaginitis can occur [17].

F. **Overview.** In their 1997 review, the *Medical Letter* concluded: "A single dose of fosfomycin is **moderately effective** for treatment of uncomplicated UTI in women and should improve compliance; but it is **expensive.** How the new drug compares with a three-day course of TMP-SMX, an effective regimen that costs much less, has not been established" [17]. Fosfomycin may play a useful role in some settings where compliance is a major issue. Fosfomycin is an alternative for uncomplicated UTI in women due to susceptible enterococci [5].

An interesting recent report revealed that many vancomycin-resistant enterococci are susceptible *in vitro* to fosfomycin [18]. Because the drug is safe, because it would not induce dangerous resistance, and because there are not many options for this, it is certainly reasonable to attempt therapy with this agent for that problem (see Appendix Table).

**IV. Cranberry juice** may be useful in the prophylaxis of UTI [3], and its **benefit** has been demonstrated in **elderly women** in whom prophylaxis with 300 mL of cranberry juice cocktail per day significantly reduced bacteriuria and pyuria compared with those receiving placebo [22]. Its mechanism of action has been attributed to the inhibition of bacterial adherence [3]. However, recent Cochrane Database reviews emphasized that further properly designed studies are indicated before concluding that cranberry juice is efficacious. [23,24] (see related discussion in **Chapter 15**).

## REFERENCES


1. Reese RE, Betts RF. Urinary antiseptics. In: Reese RE, Betts RF, Gumustop B, eds. *Handbook of antibiotics,* 3rd ed. Philadelphia: Lippincott, Williams and Wilkins 2000;564–573.
2. Hooper DC. Urinary tract agents: nitrofurantoin and methenamine. In: Mandell GL, Bennett JE, Dolin R, eds. *Principles and practice of infectious diseases,* 5th ed. New York: Churchill Livingstone, 2000:423–428.
3. Dow G, Ronald AR. Miscellaneous antibacterial drugs. In: Root RK, et al., eds. *Clinical infectious diseases: a practical approach*. New York: Oxford University Press, 1999:319.
4. Aronoff GR, et al., eds. *Drug prescribing in renal failure,* 4th ed. Philadelphia: American College of Physicians, 1999.
5. Medical Letter. The choice of antibacterial drugs. *Med Lett Drugs Ther* 2000;43:69.
6. Patterson TF, Andriole VT. Detection, significance, and therapy of bacteriuria in pregnancy: update in the managed health care era. *Infect Dis Clin North Am* 1997;11:593.
7. Darcy P. Nitrofurantoin. *Drug Intell Clin Pharm* 1985;19:540.
8. Jick SS, et al. Hospitalizations for pulmonary reactions following nitrofurantoin use. *Chest* 1989;96:512.
9. Sharp JR, et al. Chronic active hepatitis and severe hepatic necrosis associated with nitrofurantoin. *Ann Intern Med* 1980;92:14.
10. Gait JE. Hemolytic reactions to nitrofurantoin in patients with glucose-6-phosphate dehydrogenase deficiency: theory and practice. *DICP* 1990;24:1210.
11. Coraggio MJ, Gross TP, Rocelli JD. Nitrofurantoin toxicity in children. *Pediatr Infect Dis J* 1989;8:163.
12. Guay DR. An update on the role of nitrofurantoin in the management of urinary tract infections. *Drugs* 2001;61:353.
13. Vainrub B, Musher DM. Lack of effect of methenamine in suppression of or prophylaxis against chronic urinary tract infection. *Antimicrob Agents Chemother* 1977;12:625.
14. Kevorkian CG, Merritt JL, Ilstrup DM. Methenamine mandelate with acidification: an effective urinary antiseptic in patients with neurogenic bladders. *Mayo Clin Proc* 1984;59:523.
15. Cronberg S, et al. Prevention of recurrent acute cystitis by methenamine hippurate: double-blind cross-over long-term study. *Br Med J* 1987;294:1507.
16. Freeman RB, et al. Long-term therapy for chronic bacteriuria in men: U.S. Public Health Service cooperative study. *Ann Intern Med* 1975;83:133.
17. Medical Letter. Fosfomycin for urinary tract infections. *Med Lett Drugs Ther* 1997;39:66.
18. Patel SS, Balfour JA, Bryson HM. Fosfomycin tromethamine: a review of its antibacterial activity, pharmacokinetic properties, and therapeutic efficacy as a single-dose oral treatment for acute uncomplicated lower urinary tract infections. *Drugs* 1997;53:637.
19. Perri MB, Herschberber E, Ionescu M, et al. *In vitro* susceptibility of vancomycin-resistant enterococci (VRE) to fosfomycin. *Diagn Microbial Infec Dis* 2002;42:269.
20. Murry B. Vancomycin-resistant enterococcal infections. *N Engl J Med* 2000;342:710.
21. Stein GE. Single-dose treatment of acute cystitis with fosfomycin tromethamine. *Ann Pharmacother* 1998;32:215.
22. Avorn J, et al. Reduction of bacteriuria and pyuria after ingestion of cranberry juice. *JAMA* 1994;271:751.
23. Jepson RG, et al. Cranberries for preventing urinary tract infections. *Cochrane Data Base Syst Rev* 2001;(3):CD001321.
24. Jepson RG, et al. Cranberries for treating urinary tract infections. *Cochrane Data Base Syst Rev* 2000;(3):CD001322.

## APPENDIX

Appendix 1: Cost of Common Oral Regimens

| Drug | Daily Dosage | Cost Per Day (AWP) | Cost for 10 Days (AWP) | FUL Cost Per Day | FUL Cost for 10 Days |
|---|---|---|---|---|---|
| Penicillin V potassium | 250 mg q.i.d. | | | | |
| Allscripts (generic) | | $0.26 | $2.60 | | |
| Veetids | | $0.29 | $2.85 | | |
| Dicloxacillin | 250 mg q.i.d. | | | | |
| Teva (generic) | | $1.68 | $16.81 | | |
| Cloxacillin | 250 mg q.i.d. | | | | |
| PD-RX Pharm (generic) | | $1.57 | $15.67 | | |
| Amoxicillin | 250 mg t.i.d. | | | $0.19 | $1.91 |
| Teva (generic) | | $0.75 | $7.50 | | |
| Trimox | | $0.75 | $7.47 | | |
| Ampicillin | 250 mg q.i.d. | | | $0.34 | $3.40 |
| Teva (generic) | | $0.48 | $4.77 | | |
| Principen | | $0.47 | $4.69 | | |
| Augmentin | t.i.d. | | | | |
| 250 mg tablets | | $8.43 | $84.34 | | |
| 250 mg chewables | | $7.61 | $76.06 | | |
| 500 mg tablets | | $12.41 | $124.10 | | |
| 125 mg chewables | | $3.99 | $39.88 | | |
| 125 mg suspension | | $3.99 | $39.88 | | |
| 875 mg tablets | 875 mg b.i.d. | $11.04 | $110.44 | | |
| Carbenicillin (Geocillin) | 382 mg q.i.d. | $8.87 | $88.70 | | |
| | 2 × 382 tab q.i.d. | $17.74 | $177.41 | | |
| Cephalexin | 250 mg q.i.d. | | | $0.60 | $6.00 |
| Teva (generic) | | $2.56 | $25.56 | | |
| Keflex | | $6.59 | $65.88 | | |
| Teva (generic) | 500 mg q.i.d. | $5.04 | $50.38 | | |
| Keflex | | $12.95 | $129.48 | | |
| Cefadroxil | 1 g b.i.d. | | | $12.32 | $123.16 |
| Ivax (generic) | | $13.12 | $131.18 | | |
| Duricef | | $14.19 | $141.92 | | |
| Cefaclor (Ceclor) | 250 mg t.i.d. | | | $1.98 | $19.80 |
| Mylan (generic) | | $5.97 | $59.69 | | |
| | 500 mg t.i.d. | | | $3.87 | $38.70 |
| Mylan (generic) | | $11.69 | $116.85 | | |
| Loracarbef (Lorabid) | 200 mg b.i.d. | $9.06 | $90.63 | | |
| Cefprozil (Cefzil) | 250 mg b.i.d. | $7.51 | $75.13 | | |
| Cefuroxime axetil (Ceftin) | 125 mg b.i.d. | $4.30 | $43.02 | | |
| | 250 mg b.i.d. | $8.82 | $88.20 | | |
| | 500 mg b.i.d. | $16.07 | $160.73 | | |
| Ceflxime (Suprax) | 400 mg q24 | $8.01 | $80.08 | | |
| Ceftibuten (Cedax) | 400 mg daily | $8.14 | $81.35 | | |
| Cefpodoxime Proxetil (Vantin) | 200 mg b.i.d. | $8.71 | $87.10 | | |
| Cefdinir (Omnicef) | 300 mg b.i.d. | $8.56 | $85.63 | | |
| Clindamycin | 300 mg t.i.d. | | | $5.51 | $55.08 |
| Allscripts (generic) | | $7.15 | $71.47 | | |
| Cleocin | | $12.72 | $127.16 | | |

*(continued)*

Appendix 1: *(continued)*

| Drug | Daily Dosage | Cost Per Day (AWP) | Cost for 10 Days (AWP) | FUL Cost Per Day | FUL Cost for 10 Days |
|---|---|---|---|---|---|
| Erythromycin (base) | 250 mg q.i.d. | | | | |
| Abbott Pharm (generic) | | $0.59 | $5.92 | | |
| Ery-Tab | | $1.01 | $10.07 | | |
| Allscript (delayed release) | | $1.08 | $10.80 | $0.76 | $7.56 |
| Erythromycin stearate | 250 mg q.i.d. | | | | |
| Consolidated Midland (generic) | | $0.53 | $5.30 | | |
| Erythrocin | | $0.58 | $5.84 | | |
| Dirithromycin (Dynabac) | 500 mg daily | $7.74 | $77.36 | | |
| Azithromycin (Zithromax) | 1 g once only | | $22.30 | | |
| | 500 mg day 1 then 250 mg days 2–5 (Z-pak) | | $43.09 | | |
| Clarithromycin (Biaxin) | 250 mg b.i.d | $8.41 | $84.09 | | |
| | 500 mg b.i.d | $8.41 | $84.09 | | |
| Extended release | 1g daily | $9.18 | $91.75 | | |
| Doxycycline | 100 mg b.i.d | | | $0.23 | $2.34 |
| URL (generic) | | $2.32 | $23.20 | | |
| Vibra-Tabs | | $8.70 | $86.99 | | |
| Minocycline | 100 mg b.i.d | | | $1.58 | $15.75 |
| Watson (generic) | | $4.92 | $49.20 | | |
| Minocin | | $3.72 | $37.22 | | |
| Vancomycin (Vancocin) | 125 mg q.i.d | $25.73 | $257.28 | | |
| Trimethoprim | 100 mg b.i.d | | | | |
| Watson (generic) | | $1.37 | $13.68 | | |
| Proloprim | | $2.22 | $22.25 | | |
| TMP/SMX | 1 double strength b.i.d | | | | |
| Bactrim | | $3.23 | $32.30 | | |
| Schein (generic) | | $2.18 | $21.80 | | |
| Metronidazole | 500 mg q.i.d | | | $0.54 | $5.38 |
| Watson (generic) | | $2.86 | $28.62 | | |
| Flagyl | | $13.85 | $138.55 | | |
| Linezolid (Zyvox) | 600 mg b.i.d | $112.63 | $1,126.25 | | |
| Ciprofloxacin (Cipro) | 250 mg b.i.d | $8.46 | $84.61 | | |
| | 500 mg b.i.d | $9.90 | $99.04 | | |
| | 750 mg b.i.d | $10.23 | $102.34 | | |
| Ofloxacin (Floxin) | 200 mg b.i.d | $8.68 | $86.76 | | |
| | 300 mg b.i.d | $10.32 | $103.25 | | |
| | 400 mg b.i.d | $10.89 | $108.89 | | |
| Levofloxacin (Levaquin) | 250 mg daily | $7.60 | $75.99 | | |
| | 500 mg daily | $8.93 | $89.29 | | |
| | 750 mg daily | $10.82 | $108.20 | | |
| Gatifloxacin (Tequin) | 200 mg daily | $8.22 | $82.21 | | |
| | 400 mg daily | $8.22 | $82.21 | | |
| Moxifloxacin (Avelox) | 400 mg daily | $9.42 | $94.23 | | |

AWP, average wholesale price to pharmacist from *Red Book,* 2002; FUL, federal upper limit prices for Medicaid reimbursement, *Red Book,* 2002; q.i.d., 4 times daily; t.i.d., 3 times daily; b.i.d., 2 times daily. Retail and patient prices will be different based on local mark-up and bidding practices.

Appendix 2: Cost of Common Parenteral Regimens

| Drug | Daily Dosage | Cost Per Day (AWP) | Cost Per 10 Days (AWP) |
|---|---|---|---|
| Penicillin G | | | |
| Watson (generic) | 5 million units | $3.44 | $34.44 |
| Pfizerpen | 5 million units | $3.44 | $34.44 |
| Pfizerpen | 20 million units | $10.09 | $100.90 |
| Nafcillin | | | |
| Geneva (generic) | 1 g q4 | $16.73 | $167.28 |
| | 2 g q4 | $28.13 | $281.28 |
| Oxacillin | | | |
| Geneva (generic) | 1 g q4 | $17.25 | $172.50 |
| | 2 g q4 | $32.63 | $326.28 |
| Ampicillin | | | |
| Geneva (generic) | 2 g q4 | $15.38 | $153.78 |
| | 2 g q6 | $10.25 | $102.52 |
| Ampicillin Sulbactam | 1.5 g q6 | $34.52 | $345.24 |
| (Unasyn) | 3 g q6 | $63.40 | $634.00 |
| Ticarcillin (Ticar) | 3 g q6 | $53.72 | $537.24 |
| Ticarcillin Clavulanate | 3 g q6 | $61.48 | $614.80 |
| (Timentin) | | | |
| Piperacillin (Pipracil) | 3 g q6 | $90.87 | $908.72 |
| | 4 g q6 | $121.15 | $1,211.52 |
| Piperacillin Tazobactam | 3.375 g q6 | $66.12 | $661.16 |
| (Zosyn) | 4.5 g q8 | $83.34 | $833.40 |
| Imipenem (Primaxin) | 500 mg q6 | $128.21 | $1,282.10 |
| Meropenem (Merrem) | 1 g q8 | $157.32 | $1,573.20 |
| Ertapenem (Invanz) | 1 g q24 | $47.69 | $476.69 |
| Aztreonam (Azactam) | 1 g q8 | $56.67 | $566.70 |
| | 2 g q8 | $113.07 | $1,130.70 |
| Cefazolin | 1 g q8 | | |
| Allscripts (generic) | | $5.94 | $59.40 |
| Ancef | | $13.00 | $130.03 |
| Cefotetan (Cefotan) | 1 g q12 | $25.27 | $252.72 |
| | 2 g q12 | $49.58 | $495.84 |
| Cefoxitin | | | |
| Lederle (generic) | 2 g q6 | $90.00 | $900.00 |
| | 2 g q8 | $67.50 | $675.00 |
| Mefoxin | 2 g q6 | $95.49 | $954.93 |
| | 2 g q8 | $71.62 | $716.20 |
| Cefuroxime | 1.5 g q8 | | |
| Geneva (generic) | | $40.38 | $403.80 |
| Zinacef | | $41.82 | $418.17 |
| Cefotaxime | | | |
| APP (generic) | 1 g q8 | $33.00 | $330.00 |
| | 2 g q8 | $66.00 | $660.00 |
| | 2 g q6 | $88.00 | $880.00 |
| Claforan | 1 g q8 | $38.44 | $384.40 |
| | 2 g q8 | $71.18 | $711.79 |
| | 2 g q6 | $94.90 | $949.05 |
| Ceftizoxime (Cefizox) | 1 g q8 | $34.17 | $341.70 |
| | 2 g q8 | $63.42 | $634.20 |

(continued)

Appendix 2: (*continued*)

| | | | |
|---|---|---|---|
| Ceftriaxone (Rocephin) | 1 g q24 | $49.07 | $490.67 |
| | 2 g q12 | $195.00 | $1,950.04 |
| Cefoperazone (Cefobid) | 2 g q12 | $71.98 | $719.78 |
| Ceftazidime (Fortaz) | 2 g q8 | $85.00 | $850.50 |
| | 2 g q12 | $56.91 | $569.06 |
| Cefepime (Maxipime) | 2 g q8 | $94.89 | $948.90 |
| | 2 g q12 | $63.26 | $632.60 |
| Ciprofloxacin (Cipro) | 400 mg q12 | $60.02 | $600.24 |
| Levofloxacin (Levaquin) | 500 mg q24 | $41.39 | $413.90 |
| | 750 mg q24 | $54.92 | $549.20 |
| Gatifloxacin (Tequin) | 400 mg q24 | $38.20 | $382.00 |
| Moxifloxacin (Avelox) | 400 mg q24 | $525.00 | $5,250.00 |
| Gentamicin | 360 mg (1.5 mg/kg q8 for 80 kg patient) | | |
| APP (generic) | | $5.69 | $56.88 |
| Garamycin | | $27.25 | $272.47 |
| Tobramycin | 360 mg (1.5 mg/kg q8 for 80 kg patient) | | |
| Abbott (generic) | | $28.00 | $280.00 |
| Nebcin | | $32.78 | $327.80 |
| Amikacin | 1,200 mg (7.5 mg/kg q12 for 80 kg patient) | | |
| Abbott (generic) | | $52.08 | $520.80 |
| Amikin | | $82.24 | $822.24 |
| Clindamycin | | | |
| Abbott (generic) | 600 mg q6 | $17.24 | $172.43 |
| | 600 mg q8 | $12.93 | $129.32 |
| | 900 mg q8 | $25.47 | $254.72 |
| Cleocin | 600 mg q6 | $41.75 | $417.53 |
| | 600 mg q8 | $31.31 | $313.15 |
| | 900 mg q8 | $38.26 | $382.56 |
| Erythromycin (Erythrocin) | 500 mg q6 | $14.77 | $147.72 |
| Azithromycin (Zithromax) | 500 mg q24 | $25.98 | |
| Doxycycline | 100 mg q12 | | |
| Allscripts (generic) | | $29.50 | $295.00 |
| Minocycline (Minocin) | 100 mg q12 | $88.86 | $888.60 |
| Vancomycin | 1 g q12 | | |
| Lilly (generic) | | $31.20 | $312.01 |
| Vancocin | | $69.12 | $691.20 |
| TMP/SMX | | | |
| Elkins-Sinn (generic) | 1,400 mg TMP (5 mg TMP/kg q6 for 70 kg patient) | $56.18 | $561.75 |
| | 700 mg TMP (5 mg TMP/kg q12 for 70 kg patient) | $28.09 | $280.88 |
| Septra | 1,400 mg TMP | $91.09 | $910.88 |
| | 700 mg TMP | $45.54 | $455.44 |
| Metronidazole | 500 mg q6 | | |
| Baxter (generic) | | $61.36 | $613.60 |
| Flagyl | | $49.48 | $494.83 |
| Linezolid (Zyvox) | 600 mg q12 | $152.38 | $1,523.80 |
| Quinupristin/Dalfopristin (Synercid) | 525 mg q8 (7.5 mg/kg for 70 kg patient) | $338.40 | $3,384.05 |
| | 525 mg q12 | $225.60 | $2,256.03 |

AWP, average wholesale price to pharmacist from Redbook, 2002.
Patient prices will be different based on local mark-up and bidding practices.

# SUBJECT INDEX

Note: Page numbers followed by *f* indicate figures; those followed by *t* indicate tables.

## H

## J

## K



## L

## Q

## T